Quick Table of Contents

Essentials of Pathophysiology
CONCEPTS OF ALTERED HEALTH STATES

Edition 4

(Physiology), FAHA

s, College of Nursing

Wisconsin–Milwaukee

Milwaukee, Wisconsin

Consultant

N J. GASPARD, PhD

ate Professor Emeritus

Wisconsin–Milwaukee

College of Nursing

Milwaukee, Wisconsin

. Wolters Kluwer

Philadelphia · Baltimore · New York · London
Buenos Aires · Hong Kong · Sydney · Tokyo

Publisher: Lisa McAllister
Executive Editor: Sherry Dickinson
Associate Product Development Editor: Dawn Lagrosa
Developmental Editor: Laura Bonazzoli
Editorial Assistant: Dan Reilly
Design Coordinator: Joan Wendt
Art Direction, Illustration: Jennifer Clements
Illustrator, 4th Edition: Wendy Beth Jackelow, MFA, CMI
Production Project Manager: Marian A. Bellus
Manufacturing Coordinator: Karin Duffield
Production Service: SPi Global

4th edition

This book is dedicated to

All the Students who use the book, for it is for them that the book was written.

CAROL MATTSON PORTH

Contributors

Jacqueline M. Akert, RNC, MSN, WHNP-BC
Nurse Practitioner, Women's Health
Aurora Health Care
Waukesha, Wisconsin
(Chapters 40, 41 with Patricia McCowen Mehring)

Aoy Tomita-Mitchell, PhD
Associate Professor
Department of Surgery
Medical College of Wisconsin
Children's Research Institute
Milwaukee, Wisconsin
(Chapters 5, 6)

Diane Book, MD
Associate Professor, Neurology
Co-Director Stroke & Neurovascular Program
Froedtert Hospital & Medical College of Wisconsin
Milwaukee, Wisconsin
(Chapter 37)

Freddy W. Cao, MD, PhD
Clinical Associate Professor
College of Nursing
University of Wisconsin–Milwaukee
Milwaukee, Wisconsin
(Chapters 18, 34)

Paula Cox-North, PhD, ARNP
Hepatitis & Liver Clinic
Harborview Medical Center
Clinical Assistant Professor
University of Washington School of Nursing
Seattle, Washington
(Chapters 29, 30)

Herodotos Ellinas, MD, FAAP, FACP
Assistant Professor, Department of Anesthesiology
Med–Anesthesia and PGY-1 Program Director
Medical College of Wisconsin
Milwaukee, Wisconsin
(Chapters 11, 12, 13)

Jason R. Faulhaber, MD
Division of Infectious Diseases, Carilion Clinic
Assistant Program Director, Fellowship in Infectious Diseases, Carilion Clinic
Assistant Professor, Virginia Tech, Carilion School of Medicine
Adjunct Professor, Department of Biomedical Sciences, Jefferson College of Health Sciences
Roanoke, Virginia
(Chapters 15, 16)

Anne M. Fink, RN, PhD
Postdoctoral Research Associate
University of Illinois–Chicago
College of Nursing
Chicago, Illinois
(Chapters 19, 20 with Karen M. Vuckovic)

Susan A. Fontana, PhD, APRN-BC
Associate Professor and Family Nurse Practitioner
University of Wisconsin–Milwaukee
College of Nursing
Milwaukee, Wisconsin
(Chapter 38)

Kathleen E. Gunta, MSN, RN, OCNS-C
Clinical Nurse Specialist
Aurora St. Luke's Medical Center
Milwaukee, Wisconsin
(Chapter 43)

Nathan A. Ledeboer, PhD, D(ABMM)
Associate Professor of Pathology
Medical College of Wisconsin
Milwaukee, Wisconsin
(Chapter 14)

Kim Litwack, PhD, RN, FAAN, APNP
Associate Dean for Academic Affairs
Family Nurse Practitioner
Advanced Pain Management
University of Wisconsin–Milwaukee
Milwaukee, Wisconsin
(Chapter 35)

Glenn Matfin, MSc (Oxon), MB, ChB, FACE, FACP, FRCP
Medical Director
International Diabetes Center
Clinical Professor of Medicine
University of Minnesota
Minneapolis, Minnesota
(Chapters 10, 31, 32, 33, 39)

Patricia McCowen Mehring, RNC, MSN, WHNP
Nurse Practitioner
Women's Health
Milwaukee, Wisconsin
(Chapter 40, 41 with Jacqueline M. Akert)

Carrie J. Merkle, PhD, RN, FAAN
Associate Professor
College of Nursing
The University of Arizona
Tucson, Arizona
(Chapters 1, 2, 3, 4, 7)

Kathleen Mussatto, PhD, RN
Nurse Scientist, Herma Heart Center
Children's Hospital of Wisconsin
Assistant Clinical Professor of Surgery
Medical College of Wisconsin
Milwaukee, Wisconsin
(Chapter 19, Heart Disease in Infants and Children)

Debra Bancroft Rizzo, RN, MSN, FNP-BC
Nurse Practitioner
Division of Rheumatology
University of Michigan
Ann Arbor, Michigan
(Chapter 44)

Jonathan Shoopman, MD
Assistant Professor of Anesthesiology and Critical Care
Medical College of Wisconsin
Milwaukee, Wisconsin
(Chapters 22, 23)

Gladys Simandl, RN, PhD
Professor
Columbia College of Nursing
Milwaukee, Wisconsin
(Chapters 45, 46)

Karen M. Vuckovic, RN, PhD, ACNS-BC
Assistant Clinical Professor
University of Illinois–Chicago
College of Nursing
Chicago, Illinois
(Chapters 19, 20 with Anne M. Fink)

Jill M. Winters, RN, PhD, FAHA
President and Dean
Columbia College of Nursing
Milwaukee, Wisconsin
(Chapter 9)

Reviewers

Louise Boudreault, PhD
Professor of Practical Nursing
Algonquin College
Ottawa, Ontario

Freddy W. Cao, MD, PhD
Clinical Associate Professor
College of Nursing
University of Wisconsin–Milwaukee
Milwaukee, Wisconsin

Lori Hendrickx, MSN, EdD
Professor of Nursing
South Dakota State University
Brookings, South Dakota

Lisa Hight, EdD
Associate Professor of Biology
Baptist College of Health Sciences
Memphis, Tennessee

Mini Jose, PhD, RN
Assistant Professor
University of Texas Medical Branch
School of Nursing
Galveston, Texas

Michelle McDonald, MS
Assistant Professor of Biology
Baptist College of Health Sciences
Memphis, Tennessee

Sandra McLeskey, PhD, RN
Professor
University of Maryland School of
    Nursing
Baltimore, Maryland

Cheryl Neudauer, PhD
Biology Faculty
Center for Teaching and Learning
    Co-Leader
Minneapolis Community and Technical
    College
Minneapolis, Minnesota

Paige Wimberley, MSN, PhD(c)
Assistant Professor of Nursing
Arkansas State University
Jonesboro, Arkansas

As the 21st century unfolds, more information is available to more people at a faster pace than ever before. This ever-evolving ability to communicate has produced phenomenal advances in the ability to understand and treat disease. Yet despite these advances, we are also reminded that illness and disease continue to occur and impact the physiologic, social, psychological, and economic well-being of individuals, their families, the community, and the world.

As a nurse–physiologist, my major emphasis with this edition, as in previous editions, is to relate normal body functioning to the physiologic changes that participate in disease production and occur as a result of disease, as well as the body's remarkable ability to compensate for these changes. The beauty of physiology is that it integrates all of the aspects of human genetics, molecular and cellular biology, and organ anatomy and physiology into a functional whole that can be used to explain both the physical and psychological aspects of altered health. Indeed, it has been my philosophy to share the beauty of the human body and to emphasize that in disease, as in health, there is more "going right" in the body than is "going wrong."

With the creation of this text, I focused on presenting information that is fundamental to understanding the physiologic processes of altered health states; information that necessary to support an understanding pathophysiology. One of the strengths of *Essentials of Pathophysiology* is that it is a book to grow with. Although intended as a course textbook for students, it is also designed to serve as a reference book that students can take with them and use in their practice once the course is finished.

Updated to reflect state-of-the-art science, content remains organized in a manner that is logical, understandable, and draws readers into the wonders of the human body. Concepts build on one another, with concepts from physiology, biochemistry, physics, and other sciences reviewed as deemed appropriate. A conceptual model that integrates the developmental and preventative aspects of health has been used. Selection of content was based on common health problems, including the special needs of children, pregnant women, and elderly persons. The fourth edition expands the art program, increasing the number of photographs depicting clinical manifestations of selected disorders while also providing more than 500 full-color illustrations, many created specifically to supplement and expand the concepts presented.

Newly created Summary Concepts follow each section and provide a review of material that focuses on integrating and linking concepts rather than fostering rote memorization. Once again, the "Understanding" feature depicts physiologic processes and phenomena, breaking them down into an easy-to-follow sequence for easier learning. "Clinical Features" are illustrations that depict the clinical features of persons with selected diseases. As with other types of illustrations in this edition, they are designed to help the reader develop a visual memory—in this case, the memory of the entire spectrum of clinical manifestations that are associated with a disease state.

Review exercises appear at the end of each chapter and assist the reader in using the conceptual approach to solving problems related to chapter content. The glossary defines the specialized terms of pathophysiology. Tables of normal laboratory values provide a handy reference of conventional and SI units, as well as conversion units.

As with previous editions, every effort has been taken to make the text as accurate and up to date as possible. This was accomplished through an extensive review of the literature and through the use of critiques provided by students, faculty, and content specialists. This book is an extension of my career and, as such, of my philosophy. It is my hope that readers will learn to appreciate the marvelous potential of the body, incorporating it into their own philosophy and ultimately sharing it with their clients.

Carol Mattson Porth

A Comprehensive Package for Teaching and Learning

To further facilitate teaching and learning, a carefully designed ancillary package has been developed to assist faculty and students.

Instructor Resources

Tools to assist you with teaching your course are available upon adoption of this text at http://thePoint.lww.com/PorthEssentials4e.

- A thoroughly revised and augmented **Test Generator** contains more than 1,100 NCLEX-style questions mapped to chapter learning objectives.
- An extensive collection of materials is provided for each book chapter:
  - **Pre-Lecture Quizzes** (and answers) allow you to check students' reading.
  - **PowerPoint Presentations** provide an easy way to integrate the textbook with your students' classroom experience; multiple-choice questions are included to promote class participation.
  - **Guided Lecture Notes** offer corresponding PowerPoint slide numbers to simplify preparation for lecture.
  - **Discussion Topics** (and suggested answers) can be used in the classroom or in online discussion boards to facilitate interaction with your students.

- **Assignments** (and suggested answers) include group, written, clinical, and Web assignments to engage students in varied activities and assess their learning.
- **Case Studies** with related questions (and suggested answers) give students an opportunity to apply their knowledge to a client case similar to one they might encounter in practice.
- A **QSEN Competency Map** identifies content and special features in the book related to competencies identified by the QSEN Institute.
- An **Image Bank** lets you use the photographs and illustrations from this textbook in your course materials.
- **Strategies for Effective Teaching** provide general tips for instructors related to preparing course materials and meeting student needs.
- Access to all **Student Resources** is provided so that you can understand the student experience and use these resources in your course as well.

Student Resources

An exciting set of free learning resources is available to help students review and apply vital concepts of pathophysiology. For the fourth edition, multimedia engines have been optimized so that students can access many of these resources on mobile devices. Students can activate the codes printed in the front of their textbooks at http://thePoint.lww.com/activate to access these resources:

- **Student Review Questions** for each chapter, totaling more than 900 questions, help students review important concepts and practice for certification examinations.
- Interactive learning resources appeal to a variety of learning styles. Icons in the text direct readers to relevant resources:
    - **Concepts in Action Animations** bring physiologic and pathophysiologic concepts to life.
    - Interactive **Clinical Simulation Case Studies** present case scenarios and offer interactive exercises and questions to help students apply what they have learned.
- A **Spanish–English Audio Glossary** provides helpful terms and phrases for communicating with patients who speak Spanish.
- **Journal articles** offer access to current articles relevant to each chapter and available in Lippincott Williams & Wilkins journals to familiarize students with health care literature.

Study Guide

A comprehensive study aid for reviewing key concepts, *Study Guide for Porth's Essentials of Pathophysiology,* **4th edition,** has been thoroughly revised and presents a variety of exercises, including case studies and practice NCLEX-style questions, to reinforce textbook content and enhance learning.

Adaptive Learning | Powered by PrepU

Updated to accompany the 4th edition, Lippincott Adaptive Learning | Powered by PrepU helps every student learn more, while giving instructors the data they need to monitor each student's progress, strengths, and weaknesses. The adaptive learning system allows instructors to assign quizzes or students to take quizzes on their own—quizzes that adapt to each student's individual mastery level. Visit at http://thePoint.lww.com/PrepU to learn more.

A Comprehensive, Digital, Integrated Course Solution

Lippincott CoursePoint is the only integrated digital course solution for health care education, combining the power of digital course content, interactive resources, and Adaptive Learning | Powered by PrepU. Pulling these resources together into one solution, the integrated product offers a seamless experience for learning, studying, applying, and remediating.

Lippincott CoursePoint provides a personalized learning experience that is structured in the way students study. It drives students to immediate remediation in their text; digital course content and interactive course resources like case studies, videos, and journal articles are also immediately available in the same digitally integrated course solution to help expand on concepts and bring them to life. After students complete an adaptive, formative assessment on the reading, the results identify students' specific weaknesses and, at the moment it's identified they don't understand the material, they can immediately remediate to that content. Instructors also have a powerful and measurable way to assess their students' understanding and to help engage them in the course content. Knowing where students are struggling allows instructors to adapt class time as appropriate.

Lippincott CoursePoint can bring Adaptive Learning | Powered by PrepU and digital resources together on the same platform to provide all of the aids that students need to study more effectively, score higher on exams, and prepare for clinical practice. The SmartSense links feature included throughout CoursePoint integrates all of the content, offering immediate remediation and additional learning resources at the click of a mouse. With Lippincott CoursePoint, instructors can collaborate with students at any time, identify common misunderstandings, evaluate student comprehension, and differentiate instruction as needed. This unique offering creates an unparalleled learning experience for students because they can learn and retain course material in an adaptive, personalized way.

Contact your Wolters Kluwer Health sales representative or visit http://thePoint.lww.com/coursepoint-porthessentials4e for more information about Lippincott CoursePoint solution.

It is with pleasure that we introduce these resources— the textbook, ancillary resources, and additional supplements and learning tools—to you. One of our primary goals in creating these resources has been to help students learn how to provide quality care to patients and families across health care settings. We hope that we have succeeded in that goal, and we welcome feedback from our readers.

To the Reader

This book was written with the intent of making the subject of pathophysiology an exciting exploration that relates normal body functioning to the physiologic changes that occur as a result of disease, as well as the body's remarkable ability to compensate for these changes. Indeed, it is these changes that represent many of the signs and symptoms of disease.

Using a book such as this can be simplified by taking time out to find what is in the book and how to locate information when it is needed. The *Table of Contents* provides an overall view of the organization and content of the book. The *Index* can be viewed as a roadmap for locating content. Using the Index, readers can quickly locate related content in different chapters of the book or answer questions that come up in other courses.

Organization

The book is organized into units and chapters. The *units* identify broad areas of content, such as alterations in the circulatory system. Many of the units have *introductory chapters* that contain information about the normal structure and function of the body systems discussed in the unit. These chapters, which are intended as a review of content from previous courses as well as an update on recent scientific advances in genetic and molecular biology, provide the foundation for understanding the pathophysiology content presented in the subsequent chapters. The *disorder chapters* focus on specific areas of pathophysiology content, such as heart failure and circulatory shock. The *chapter outline* that appears at the beginning of each chapter provides an overall view of the chapter content and organization. *Icons* identify specific content related to infants and children , pregnant women , and older adults .

Reading and Learning Aids

In an ever-expanding world of information, you will not be able to read, let alone remember, everything that is in this (or any other) book. With this in mind, we have developed a number of special features that will help you focus on and master the essential content for your current as well as future needs.

It is essential for any professional to use and understand the vocabulary of his or her profession. Throughout the text, you will encounter terms in *italics*. This is a signal that a word and the ideas associated with

it are important to learn. To help, the *Glossary* contains concise definitions of frequently encountered terms. If you are unsure of the meaning of a term you encounter in your reading, check the Glossary in the back of the book before proceeding.

Summary Concepts

Summary concepts at the end of each section provide a review and a reinforcement of the main content that has been covered. One of the ways to approach learning is to focus on the major ideas or concepts rather than trying to memorize significant amounts of information. As you have probably already discovered, it is impossible to memorize everything that is in a particular section or chapter of the book. Not only does your brain have a difficult time trying to figure out where to store all the different bits of information, your brain doesn't know how to retrieve the information when you need it. Most important of all, memorized lists of content can seldom, if ever, be applied directly to an actual clinical situation. Summary concepts guide you in identifying the major ideas or concepts that form the foundation for truly understanding the major areas of content. When you understand the concepts in these sections, you will have a framework for remembering and using the facts given in the text.

SUMMARY CONCEPTS

■ Chromosomal disorders result from a change in chromosome structure or number. They reflect events that occur at the time of meiosis, such as defective movement of an entire chromosome or breakage of a chromosome with loss, gain, or translocation of genetic material.

■ A change in chromosome number is called *aneuploidy*. *Monosomy* involves the presence of only one member of a chromosome pair as is seen in Turner syndrome, in which there is monosomy of the X chromosome in females. *Polysomy* refers to the presence of more than two chromosomes in a set, as occurs in Klinefelter syndrome, which involves polysomy of the X chromosome in males. Trisomy 21 (i.e., Down syndrome) is the most common disorder of the autosomal chromosomes, and occurs in both sexes.

Tables, Charts, and Boxes

Tables, charts, and *boxes* are designed to present complex information in a format that makes it more meaningful and easier to remember. Tables have two or more columns, and are often used for the purpose of comparing or contrasting information. Charts have one column and are used to summarize information. Boxes highlight key information.

TABLE 6-2	Some Disorders of Organ Systems Associated with Mitochondrial DNA Mutations
Disorder	Manifestations
Chronic progressive external ophthalmoplegia	Progressive weakness of the extraocular muscles
Deafness	Progressive sensorineural deafness, often associated with aminoglycoside antibiotics
Kearns-Sayre syndrome	Progressive weakness of the extraocular muscles of early onset with heart block, retinal pigmentation
Leber hereditary optic neuropathy	Painless, subacute, bilateral visual loss, with central blind spots (scotomas) and abnormal color vision
Leigh disease	Proximal muscle weakness, sensory neuropathy, developmental delay, ataxia, seizures, dementia, and visual impairment due to retinal pigment degeneration
MELAS	Mitochondrial Encephalomyopathy (cerebral structural changes), Lactic Acidosis, and Strokelike syndrome, seizures, and other clinical and laboratory abnormalities; may manifest only as diabetes mellitus
MERRF	Myoclonic Epilepsy, Ragged Red Fibers in muscle; ataxia; sensorineural deafness
Myoclonic epilepsy with ragged red fibers	Myoclonic seizures, cerebellar ataxia, mitochondrial myopathy (muscle weakness, fatigue)

CHART 6-1 Teratogenic Agents*

Radiation
Drugs and Chemical Substances
  Alcohol
  Anticoagulants
  Warfarin
  Anticonvulsants
  Cancer drugs
  Aminopterin
  Methotrexate
  6-Mercaptopurine
  Isotretinoin (Accutane)
  Propylthiouracil
  Tetracycline
  Thalidomide

Infectious Agents
Viruses
  Cytomegalovirus
  Herpes simplex virus
  Measles (rubella)
  Mumps
  Varicella-zoster virus (chickenpox)
Nonviral factors
  Syphilis
  Toxoplasmosis

*Not inclusive.

BOX 8-1 Measurement Units

Laboratory measurements of electrolytes in body fluids are expressed as a concentration or amount of solute in a given volume of fluid, such as milligrams per deciliter (mg/dL), milliequivalents per liter (mEq/L), or millimoles per liter (mmol/L).

The use of *milligrams (mg) per deciliter* expresses the weight of the solute in one tenth of a liter (dL). The concentration of electrolytes such as calcium, phosphate, and magnesium is often expressed in mg/dL.

The *milliequivalent* is used to express the charge equivalency for a given weight of an electrolyte: 1 mEq of sodium has the same number of charges as 1 mEq of chloride, regardless of molecular weight. The number of milliequivalents of an electrolyte in a liter of solution can be derived from the following equation:

$$mEq = \frac{mg/100 \ mL \times 10 \times valence}{atomic \ weight}$$

The Système Internationale (SI) units express electrolyte concentration in *millimoles per liter* (mmol/L). A millimole is one thousandth of a mole, or the molecular weight of a substance expressed in milligrams. The number of millimoles of an electrolyte in a liter of solution can be calculated using the following equation:

$$mmol/L = \frac{mEq/L}{valence}$$

Illustrations and Photographs

The full-color *illustrations* will help you to build your own mental image of the content that is being presented. Each drawing has been developed to fully support and build upon the ideas in the text. Some illustrations are used to help you picture the complex interactions of the multiple phenomena that are involved in the development of a particular disease; others can help you visualize normal function or understand the mechanisms whereby the disease processes exert their effects. In addition, *photographs* depicting clinical manifestations and detailing pathologic processes provide a realistic view of selected disorders and pathologic processes.

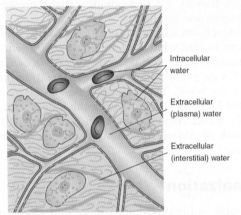

FIGURE 8-1. Distribution of body water. The extracellular space includes the vascular compartment and the interstitial spaces.

Intracellular water

Extracellular (plasma) water

Extracellular (interstitial) water

Clinical Features

This edition retains the illustrations that depict the *clinical features* of persons with selected diseases. This feature is designed to help you visualize the entire spectrum of clinical manifestations that are associated with these disease states.

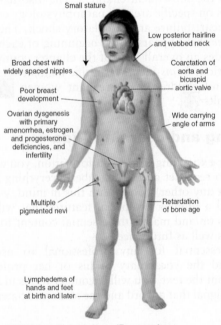

Small stature

Low posterior hairline and webbed neck

Coarctation of aorta and bicuspid aortic valve

Wide carrying angle of arms

Retardation of bone age

Broad chest with widely spaced nipples

Poor breast development

Ovarian dysgenesis with primary amenorrhea, estrogen and progesterone deficiencies, and infertility

Multiple pigmented nevi

Lymphedema of hands and feet at birth and later

FIGURE 6-11. Clinical features of Turner syndrome.

Understanding Physiologic Processes

Included in a number of chapters is an *Understanding* feature that focuses on the physiologic processes and phenomena that form the basis for understanding disorders presented in the text. This feature breaks a process or phenomenon down to its component parts and presents them in a sequential manner, providing an insight into the many opportunities for disease processes to disrupt the sequence.

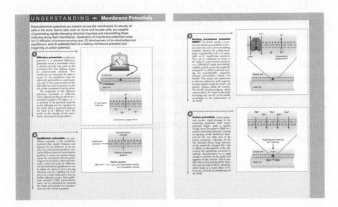

Material for Review

An important feature has been built into the text to help you verify your understanding of the material presented. After you have finished reading and studying the chapter, work on answering the *Review Exercises* at the end of the chapter. They are designed to help you integrate, conceptualize, and apply material from the text. If you are unable to answer a question, reread the relevant section in the chapter.

REVIEW EXERCISES

1. A 23-year-old woman with sickle cell disease and her husband want to have a child, but worry that the child will be born with the disease.

   A. What is the mother's genotype in terms of the sickle cell gene? Is she heterozygous or homozygous?

   B. If the husband is found not to have the sickle cell gene, what is the probability of their child having the disease or being a carrier of the sickle cell trait?

2. A couple has a child who was born with a congenital heart disease.

   A. Would you consider the defect to be the result of a single-gene or a polygenic trait?

   B. Would these parents be at greater risk of having another child with a heart defect, or would they be at equal risk of having a child with a defect in another organ system, such as cleft palate?

3. A couple has been informed that their newborn child has the features of Down syndrome. It was suggested that genetic studies be performed.

   A. The child is found to have trisomy 21. Use Figure 6-8 to describe the events that occur during meiosis to explain the origin of the third chromosome.

   B. If the child had been found to have the robertsonian chromosome, how would you explain the origin of the abnormal chromosome?

4. A 26-year-old woman is planning to become pregnant.

   A. What information would you give her regarding the effects of medications and drugs on the fetus? What stage of fetal development is associated with the greatest risk?

   B. What is the rationale for ensuring that she has an adequate intake of folic acid before conception?

   C. She and her husband have an indoor cat. What precautions should she use in caring for the cat?

Appendix

The *Lab Values* tables in the appendix provide rapid access to normal values for many laboratory tests in conventional and SI units, as well as a description of the prefixes, symbols, and factors (e.g., micro, μ, 10^{-6}) used for describing these values. Knowledge of normal values can help you put abnormal values in context.

We hope that this guide has given you a clear picture of how to use this book. Good luck and enjoy the journey!

Acknowledgments

As in past editions, many persons participated in the creation of this work. The contributing authors deserve a special mention. Dr. Gaspard, in particular, deserves thanks. Her wide breadth of knowledge and skillful assistance were invaluable in preparing the text and developing the illustrations for the book. Another person who deserves recognition is Georgianne Heymann, who assisted in editing the manuscript. As with previous editions, she provided not only excellent editorial assistance but also encouragement and support when the tasks associated with manuscript preparation became most frustrating. I would also like to acknowledge Jody Erickson, RN, BSN, DNP, FNP, BC for her assistance with selected work in the text.

Special thanks also to those at Wolters Kluwer Health who participated in the development of this edition:

Sherry Dickinson, executive editor; Dawn Lagrosa, associate product development editor; Joan Wendt, design coordinator; and Marian Bellus, production project manager. Thanks also to Wendy Beth Jackelow, MFA, CMI, for her talent and expertise in creating and modifying the illustrations.

The students in the classes I have taught over the years also deserve a special salute, for they are the inspiration upon which this book was founded. They provided the questions, suggestions, and contact with the "real world" of patient care that directed the organization and selection of content for the book.

Last, but certainly not least, I would like to acknowledge my family and friends for their unlimited patience, understanding, and encouragement throughout the entire process.

Contents

Introduction to Pathophysiology

Pathophysiology, which is the focus of this book, may be defined as the physiology of altered health. The term combines the words *pathology* and *physiology*. Pathology (from the Greek *pathos*, meaning "disease") deals with the study of the structural and functional changes in cells, tissues, and organs of the body that cause or are caused by disease. Physiology deals with the functions of the human body. Thus, pathophysiology deals not only with the cellular and organ changes that occur with disease, but also with the effects that these changes have on total body function. In addition, pathophysiology focuses on the mechanisms of the underlying disease process and provides the background for preventive as well as therapeutic health care measures and practices.

Disease

Disease may be defined as an interruption, cessation, or disorder of a body system or organ structure that is characterized usually by a recognized etiologic agent or agents, an identifiable group of signs and symptoms, or consistent anatomic alterations.[1] The aspects of the disease process include etiology, pathogenesis, morphologic changes, and clinical manifestations.

Etiology

The causes of disease are known as *etiologic factors*.[2] Among the recognized etiologic agents are biologic agents (e.g., bacteria, viruses), physical forces (e.g., trauma, burns, radiation), chemical agents (e.g., poisons, alcohol), and nutritional excesses or deficits. At the molecular level, it is important to distinguish between abnormal molecules and molecules that cause disease.[3] This is true of diseases such as cystic fibrosis, sickle cell anemia, and familial hypercholesterolemia, in which the genetic abnormality of a single amino acid, transporter molecule, or receptor protein produces widespread effects on health.

Most disease-causing agents are nonspecific, and many different agents can cause disease of a single organ. A single agent or traumatic event can, however, lead to disease of a number of organs or systems. Although a disease-causing agent can affect more than a single organ and a number of disease-causing agents can affect the same organ, most disease states do not have a single cause. Instead, the majority of diseases are multifactorial in origin. This is particularly true of diseases such as cancer, heart disease, and diabetes. The multiple factors that predispose to a particular disease often are referred to as *risk factors*.[4]

One way to view the factors that cause disease is to group them into categories according to whether they were present at birth or acquired later in life. *Congenital conditions* are defects that are present at birth, although they may not be evident until later in life. Congenital conditions may be caused by genetic influences, environmental factors (e.g., viral infections in the mother, maternal drug use, irradiation, or intrauterine crowding), or a combination of genetic and environmental factors. *Acquired defects* are those that are caused by events that occur after birth. These include injury, exposure to infectious agents, inadequate nutrition, lack of oxygen, inappropriate immune responses, and neoplasia. Many diseases are thought to be the result of a genetic predisposition and an environmental event or events that serve as a trigger to initiate disease development.

Pathogenesis

Pathogenesis is the sequence of cellular and tissue events that take place from the time of initial contact with an etiologic agent until the ultimate expression of a disease.[2] Etiology describes what sets the disease process in motion, while pathogenesis describes how the disease process evolves. Although the two terms often are used interchangeably, their meanings are quite different. For example, atherosclerosis often is cited as the cause or etiology of coronary heart disease. In reality, the progression from fatty streak to the occlusive vessel lesion seen in persons with coronary heart disease represents the pathogenesis of the disorder. The true etiology of atherosclerosis remains largely uncertain.

Morphology

Morphology refers to the fundamental structure or form of cells or tissues. *Morphologic changes* are concerned with both the gross anatomic and microscopic changes that are characteristic of a disease.[2] *Histology* deals with the study of the cells and extracellular matrix of body tissues. The most common method used in the study of tissues is the preparation of histologic sections—thin, translucent sections of human tissues and organs—that can be examined with the aid of a microscope. Histologic sections play an important role in the diagnosis of many types of cancer. A *lesion* represents a pathologic or traumatic discontinuity of a body organ or tissue. Descriptions of lesion size and characteristics often can be obtained through the use of radiographs, ultrasonography, and other imaging methods. Lesions also may be sampled by biopsy and the tissue samples subjected to histologic study.

Clinical Manifestations

Diseases can manifest in a number of ways. Sometimes the condition produces manifestations, such as fever, that make it evident that the person is sick. In other cases, the condition is silent at the onset and is detected during examination for other purposes or after the disease is far advanced.

Signs and *symptoms* are terms used to describe the structural and functional changes that accompany a disease.[3] A *symptom* is a subjective complaint that is noted by the person with a disorder, whereas a *sign* is a manifestation that is noted by an observer. Pain, difficulty in breathing, and dizziness are symptoms of a disease. An elevated temperature, a swollen extremity, and changes in pupil size are objective signs that can be observed by someone other than the person with the disease. Signs and symptoms may be related to the primary disorder or they may represent the body's attempt to compensate for the altered function caused by the pathologic condition. Many pathologic states are not observed directly—one cannot see a sick heart or a failing kidney. Instead, what can be observed is the body's attempt to compensate for changes in function brought about by the disease, such as the tachycardia that accompanies blood loss or the increased respiratory rate that occurs with pneumonia.

A *syndrome* is a compilation of signs and symptoms (e.g., chronic fatigue syndrome) that are characteristic of a specific disease state. *Complications* are possible adverse extensions of a disease or outcomes from treatment. *Sequelae* are lesions or impairments that follow or are caused by a disease.

Diagnosis

A *diagnosis* is the designation as to the nature or cause of a health problem (e.g., bacterial pneumonia or hemorrhagic stroke). The diagnostic process usually requires a careful history and physical examination. The history is used to obtain a person's account of his or her symptoms and their progression, and the factors that contribute to a diagnosis. The physical examination is done to observe for signs of altered body structure or function.

The development of a diagnosis involves weighing competing possibilities and selecting the most likely one from among the conditions that might be responsible for the person's clinical presentation.[4] The clinical probability of a given disease in a person of a given age, gender, race, lifestyle, and locality often is influential in arriving at a presumptive diagnosis. Laboratory tests, radiologic studies, computed tomography (CT) scans, and other tests often are used to confirm a diagnosis.

An important factor when interpreting diagnostic test results is the determination of whether they are normal or abnormal. Is a blood count above normal, within the normal range, or below normal? What is termed a *normal* value for a laboratory test is established statistically from test results obtained from a selected sample of people. The normal values refer to the 95% distribution (mean plus or minus two standard deviations [mean ± 2 SD]) of test results for the reference population.[4-6] Thus, the normal levels for serum sodium (136 to 145 mEq/L) represent the mean serum level for the reference population ± 2 SD. The normal values for some laboratory tests are adjusted for sex or age. For example, the normal hemoglobin range for women is 12.0 to 16.0 g/dL, and for men, 14.0 to 17.4 g/dL.[7] Serum creatinine levels often are adjusted for age in the elderly, and normal values for serum phosphate differ between adults and children.

The quality of data on which a diagnosis is based may be judged for their validity, reliability, sensitivity, specificity, and predictive value.[4,7,8] *Validity* refers to the extent to which a measurement tool measures what it is intended to measure. This often is assessed by comparing a measurement method with the best possible method of measure that is available. For example, the validity of blood pressure measurements obtained by a sphygmomanometer might be compared with those obtained by intra-arterial measurements. *Reliability* refers to the extent to which an observation, if repeated, gives the same result. A poorly calibrated blood pressure machine may give inconsistent measurements of blood pressure, particularly of pressures in either the high or low range. Reliability also depends on the persons making the measurements. For example, blood pressure measurements may vary from one observer to another because of the technique used (e.g., different observers may deflate the cuff at a different rate, thus obtaining different values), the way the numbers on the manometer are read, or differences in hearing acuity.

In the field of clinical laboratory measurements, *standardization* is aimed at increasing the trueness and reliability of measured values. Standardization relies on the use of written standards, reference measurement procedures, and reference materials.[9] In the United States, the Food and Drug Administration (FDA) regulates in vitro diagnostic devices, including clinical laboratory instruments, test kits, and reagents. Manufacturers who propose to market new diagnostic devices must submit information on their instrument, test kit, or reagent to the FDA, as required by existing statutes and regulations. The FDA reviews this information to decide whether the product may be marketed in the United States.

Measures of sensitivity and specificity are concerned with determining how likely or how well the test or observation will identify people with or without the disease.[4] *Sensitivity* refers to the proportion of people with a disease who are positive for that disease on a given test or observation (called a *true-positive* result). If the result of a very sensitive test is negative, it tells us the person does not have the disease and the disease has been excluded or "ruled out." *Specificity* refers to the proportion of people without the disease who are negative on a given test or observation (called a *true-negative* result). Specificity can be calculated only from among people who do not have the disease. A test that is 95% specific correctly identifies 95 of 100 normal people. The other 5% are *false-positive* results. A false-positive test result can be unduly stressful for the person being tested, whereas a *false-negative* test result can delay diagnosis and jeopardize the outcome of treatment.

Predictive value is the extent to which an observation or test result is able to predict the presence of a given disease or condition.[4,10] A *positive predictive value* refers to the proportion of true-positive results that occurs in a given population. In a group of women found to have "suspect breast nodules" in a cancer screening program, the proportion later determined to have breast cancer would constitute the positive predictive value. A *negative predictive value* refers to the true-negative observations in a population. In a screening test for breast cancer, the negative predictive value represents the proportion of women without suspect nodules who do not have breast cancer. Although predictive values rely in part on sensitivity and specificity, they depend more heavily on the prevalence of the condition in the population. Despite unchanging sensitivity and specificity, the positive predictive value of an observation rises with prevalence, whereas the negative predictive value falls.

Clinical Course

The clinical course describes the evolution of a disease. A disease can have an acute, subacute, or chronic course. An *acute disorder* is one that is relatively severe, but self-limiting. *Chronic disease* implies a continuous, long-term process. A chronic disease can run a continuous course or can present with exacerbations (aggravation of symptoms and severity of the disease) and remissions (a period during which there is a decrease in severity and symptoms). *Subacute disease* is intermediate or between acute and chronic: it is not as severe as an acute disease and not as prolonged as a chronic disease.

The spectrum of disease severity for infectious diseases, such as hepatitis B, can range from preclinical to persistent chronic infection. During the *preclinical stage*, the disease is not clinically evident but is destined to progress to clinical disease. As with hepatitis B, it is possible to transmit a virus during the preclinical stage. *Subclinical disease* is not clinically apparent and is not destined to become clinically apparent. It is diagnosed with antibody or culture tests. Most cases of tuberculosis are not clinically apparent, and evidence of their presence is established by skin tests. *Clinical disease* is manifested by signs and symptoms. A persistent chronic infectious disease persists for years—sometimes for life. *Carrier status* refers to an individual who harbors an organism but is not infected, as evidenced by antibody response or clinical manifestations. This person still can infect others. Carrier status may be of limited duration or it may be chronic, lasting for months or years.

Perspectives and Patterns of Disease

The health of individuals is closely linked to the health of the community and to the population it encompasses. The ability to traverse continents in a matter of hours has opened the world to issues of populations at a global level. Diseases that once were confined to limited areas of the world now pose a threat to populations throughout the world.

As we move through the 21st century, we are continually reminded that the health care system and the services it delivers are targeted to particular populations. Managed care systems are focused on a population-based approach to planning, delivering, providing, and evaluating health care. The focus of health care also has begun to emerge as a partnership in which individuals are asked to assume greater responsibility for their own health.

Epidemiology and Patterns of Disease

Epidemiology is the study of disease occurrence in human populations.[4] It was initially developed to explain the spread of infectious diseases during epidemics and has emerged as a science to study risk factors for multifactorial diseases, such as heart disease and cancer. Epidemiology looks for patterns, such as age, race, dietary habits, lifestyle, or geographic location, of persons affected with a particular disorder. In contrast to biomedical researchers, who seek to elucidate the mechanisms of disease production, epidemiologists are more concerned with whether something happens than how it happens. For example, the epidemiologist is more concerned with whether smoking itself is related to cardiovascular disease and whether the risk of heart disease decreases when smoking ceases. The biomedical researcher, however, is more concerned about the causative agent in cigarette smoke and the pathway by which it contributes to heart disease.

Much of our knowledge about disease comes from epidemiologic studies. Epidemiologic methods are used to determine how a disease is spread, how to control it, how to prevent it, and how to eliminate it. Epidemiologic methods also are used to study the natural history of disease, to evaluate new preventative and treatment strategies, to explore the impact of different patterns of health care delivery, and to predict future health care needs. As such, epidemiologic studies serve as a basis for clinical decision making, allocation of health care dollars, and development of policies related to public health issues.

Measures of disease frequency are an important aspect of epidemiology. They establish a means for predicting what diseases are present in a population and provide an indication of the rate at which they are increasing or decreasing. A *disease case* can be either an existing case or the number of new episodes of a particular illness that are diagnosed within a given period. *Incidence* reflects the number of new cases arising in a population at risk during a specified time. The population at risk is considered to be persons who are without the disease but are at risk for developing it. It is determined by dividing the number of new cases of a disease by the population at risk for development of the disease during the same period (e.g., new cases per 1000 or 100,000 persons in the population who are at risk). The cumulative incidence estimates the risk of developing the disease during that period of time. *Prevalence* is a measure of existing disease in a population at a given point in time (e.g., number of existing cases divided by the current population).[9] The prevalence is not an estimate of risk of developing a disease because it is a function of both new cases and how long the cases remain in the population. Incidence and prevalence are always reported as rates (e.g., cases per 100 or cases per 100,000).

Morbidity and mortality statistics provide information about the functional effects (morbidity) and death-producing (mortality) characteristics of a disease. These statistics are useful in terms of anticipating health care needs, planning of public education programs, directing health research efforts, and allocating health care dollars.

Mortality statistics provide information about the causes of death in a given population. In most countries, people are legally required to record certain facts such as age, sex, and cause of death on a death certificate.

Internationally agreed-upon classification procedures (the International Classification of Diseases [ICD] by the World Health Organization) are used for coding the cause of death, and these data are expressed as death rates.[11] Crude mortality rates (i.e., number of deaths in a given period) do not account for age, sex, race, socioeconomic status, and other factors. For this reason, mortality often is expressed as death rates for a specific population, such as the infant mortality rate. Mortality also can be described in terms of the leading causes of death according to age, sex, race, and ethnicity.

Morbidity describes the effects an illness has on a person's life. Many diseases, such as arthritis, have low death rates but a significant impact on quality of life. Morbidity is concerned not only with the occurrence or incidence of a disease but also the persistence and long-term consequences of the disease.

Determination of Risk Factors

Conditions suspected of contributing to the development of a disease are called *risk factors*. They may be inherent to the person (high blood pressure or overweight) or external (smoking or drinking alcohol). There are different types of studies used to determine risk factors, including cross-sectional studies, case–control studies, and cohort studies. *Cross-sectional studies* use the simultaneous collection of information necessary for classification of exposure and outcome status. They can be used to compare the prevalence of a disease in those with the factor (or exposure) with the prevalence of a disease in those who are unexposed to the factor, such as the prevalence of coronary heart disease in smokers and nonsmokers. *Case–control studies* are designed to compare persons known to have the outcome of interest (*cases*) with those known not to have the outcome of interest (*controls*).[4] Information on exposures or characteristics of interest is then collected from persons in both groups. For example, the characteristics of maternal alcohol consumption in infants born with a fetal alcohol spectrum disorder (cases) can be compared with those in infants born without one of these disorders (controls).

A *cohort* is a group of persons who were born at approximately the same time or share some characteristics of interest.[4] Persons enrolled in a cohort study (also called a *longitudinal study*) are followed over a period of time to observe a specific health outcome. A cohort may consist of a single group of persons chosen because they have or have not been exposed to suspected risk factors; two groups specifically selected because one has been exposed and the other has not; or a single exposed group in which the results are compared with the general population.

One of the best-known examples of a cohort study is the Framingham Study, which was carried out in Framingham, Massachusetts.[12] Framingham was selected because of the size of its population, the relative ease with which the people could be contacted, and the stability of the population in terms of moving into and out of the area. This longitudinal study, which began in 1950, was set up by the U.S. Public Health Service to study the characteristics of people who would later develop coronary heart disease. The study consisted of 5000 persons, aged 30 to 59 years, selected at random and followed for an initial period of 20 years, during which time it was predicted that 1500 of them would develop coronary heart disease. The advantage of such a study is that it can explore a number of risk factors at the same time and determine the relative importance of each. Another advantage is that the risk factors can later be related to other diseases, such as stroke.

A second well-known cohort study is the Nurses' Health Study, which was developed by Harvard University and Brigham and Women's Hospital. The study began in 1976 with a cohort of 121,700 female nurses, 30 to 55 years of age, living in the United States.[13] Initially designed to explore the relationship between oral contraceptives and breast cancer, nurses in the study have provided answers to detailed questions about their menstrual cycle, smoking habits, diet, weight and waist measurements, activity patterns, health problems, and medication use. They have given urine and blood samples, and even provided researchers with their toenail clippings. In selecting the cohort, it was reasoned that nurses would be well-organized, accurate, and observant in their responses, and that physiologically they would be no different from other groups of women. It also was anticipated that their childbearing, eating, and smoking patterns would be similar to those of other working women.

Natural History

The *natural history* of a disease refers to the progression and projected outcome of the disease without medical intervention.[4] By studying the patterns of a disease over time in populations, epidemiologists can better understand its natural history. Knowledge of the natural history can be used to determine disease outcome, establish priorities for health care services, determine the effects of screening and early detection programs on disease outcome, and compare the results of new treatments with the expected outcome without treatment.

There are some diseases for which there are no effective treatment methods available, or for which the current treatment measures are only effective in certain people. In this case, the natural history of the disease can be used as a predictor of outcome. For example, the natural history of hepatitis C indicates that 80% of people who become infected with the virus fail to clear the virus and progress to chronic infection.[14] Information about the natural history of a disease and the availability of effective treatment methods provides directions for preventive measures. In the case of hepatitis C, careful screening of blood donations and education of intravenous drug abusers can be used to prevent transfer of the virus. At the same time, scientists are striving to develop a vaccine that will prevent infection in persons exposed to the virus. The development of vaccines to prevent the spread of infectious diseases such as polio and hepatitis B undoubtedly has been motivated by knowledge about the natural history of these diseases and the lack of effective intervention measures. With other diseases, such as breast cancer, early detection through use of clinical breast examination and mammography increases the chances for a cure.

Prognosis refers to the probable outcome and prospect of recovery from a disease. It can be designated as chances for full recovery, possibility of complications, or anticipated survival time. Prognosis often is presented in relation to treatment options—that is, the expected outcomes or chances for survival with or without a certain type of treatment. The prognosis associated with a given type of treatment usually is presented along with the risk associated with the treatment.

Levels of Prevention

Leading a healthy life contributes to the prevention of disease. There are three fundamental types of prevention: primary prevention, secondary prevention, and tertiary prevention.[4,15] It is important to note that all three levels are aimed at prevention. *Primary prevention* is directed at keeping disease from occurring by removing all risk factors. Examples of primary prevention include the administration of folic acid to pregnant women and women who may become pregnant to prevent fetal neural tube defects, giving immunizations to children to prevent communicable disease, and counseling people to adopt healthy lifestyles as a means of preventing heart disease. Primary prevention is often accomplished outside the health care system at the community level. Some primary prevention measures are mandated by law (e.g., wearing seat belts in automobiles and helmet use on motorcycles). Other primary prevention activities (e.g., use of earplugs or dust masks) occur in specific occupations. *Secondary prevention* detects disease early when it is still asymptomatic and treatment measures can affect a cure or stop the disease from progressing. The use of a Papanicolaou (Pap) smear for early detection of cervical cancer is an example of secondary prevention. Screening also includes history taking (asking if a person smokes), physical examination (blood pressure measurement), laboratory tests (cholesterol level determination), and other procedures (colonoscopy) that can be applied to asymptomatic people. Most secondary prevention is done in clinical settings. All types of health care professionals (e.g., physicians, nurses, dentists, audiologists, optometrists) participate in secondary prevention. *Tertiary prevention* is directed at clinical interventions that prevent further deterioration or reduce the complications of a disease once it has been diagnosed.

REFERENCES

1. *Stedman's Medical Dictionary.* 28th ed. Philadelphia, PA: Lippincott Williams & Wilkins; 2006:855.
2. Kumar V, Abbas AK, Fausto N, et al. *Robbins and Cotran Pathologic Basis of Disease.* 8th ed. Philadelphia, PA: Saunders Elsevier; 2012:4,5.
3. Waldenstrom J. Sick molecules and our concepts of illness. *J Intern Med.* 1989;225:221–227.
4. Fletcher RH, Fletcher SW, Fletcher G. *Clinical Epidemiology: The Essentials.* 5th ed. Philadelphia, PA: Wolters Kluwer Health/Lippincott Williams & Wilkins; 2014:1–16, 17–29, 31–49, 50–59, 93–104, 108–130.
5. Brigden ML, Heathcote JC. Problems with interpreting laboratory tests. *Postgrad Med.* 2000;107(7):145–162.
6. Mayer D. *Essentials of Evidence-Based Medicine.* New York, NY: Cambridge University Press; 2004.
7. Fischbach F, Dunning MB. *A Manual of Laboratory and Diagnostic Tests.* 8th ed. Philadelphia, PA: Wolters Kluwer Health/Lippincott Williams & Wilkins; 2009;74:964.
8. Dawson B, Trapp RG, Trapp R. *Basic and Clinical Biostatistics.* New York, NY: Lange Medical Books/ McGraw-Hill; 2004.
9. Michaud GY. The role of standards in the development and implementation of clinical laboratory tests: A domestic and global perspective. *Cancer Biomark.* 2005;1:209–216.
10. Montori VM, Wyer P, Newman TB, et al. Tips for learning of evidence-based medicine: 5. The effect of spectrum of disease on performance of diagnostic tests. *Can Med Assoc J.* 2005;173:385–390.
11. World Health Organization. About WHO: Definition of health; disease eradication/elimination goals. 2007. Available at: http://www.who.int/about/definition/en/. Accessed September 2, 2013.
12. Framingham Heart Study. Framingham Heart Study: Design, rationale, objectives, and research milestones. 2011. Available at: http://www.framinghamheartstudy.org. Accessed September 2, 2013.
13. Channing Laboratory. Nurses' Health Study. 2011. Available at: http://www.channing.harvard.edu/nhs/. Accessed September 2, 2013.
14. Liang J, Reherman B, Seeff LB, et al. Pathogenesis, natural history, treatment, and prevention of hepatitis C. *Ann Intern Med.* 2000;132:296–305.
15. Neis MA, McEwan M. *Community Health Nursing.* 5th ed. St. Louis, MO: Mosby; 2011:1–90.

Cell Structure and Function

The cell is the smallest functional unit of life. Cells are the smallest unit capable of self-reproduction and are vehicles for transmitting genetic information that defines the organism. Cells with similar specialized functions are often organized into larger functional aggregates called *tissues*. These tissues in turn combine to form the various body structures and organs. Although the cells of different tissues and organs vary in structure and function, they are remarkably similar in their ability to exchange materials with their immediate environment, obtain energy from organic nutrients, synthesize complex molecules, and replicate themselves. Because most diseases begin at the cellular level, an understanding of cell function is crucial to understanding the disease process. Some diseases affect the cells of a single organ, others affect the cells of a particular tissue type, and still others affect the cells of the entire organism.

This chapter discusses the structural and functional components of the cell, basic cellular mechanisms, and tissue types.

Functional Components of the Cell

Although diverse in their organization, all eukaryotic cells (cells with a true nucleus) have in common structures that perform unique functions. Under a light microscope, three primary components of the eukaryotic cell become evident: the plasma membrane, the nucleus, and the cytoplasm, while numerous structures are visible by higher magnification electron microscopy (Fig. 1-1).

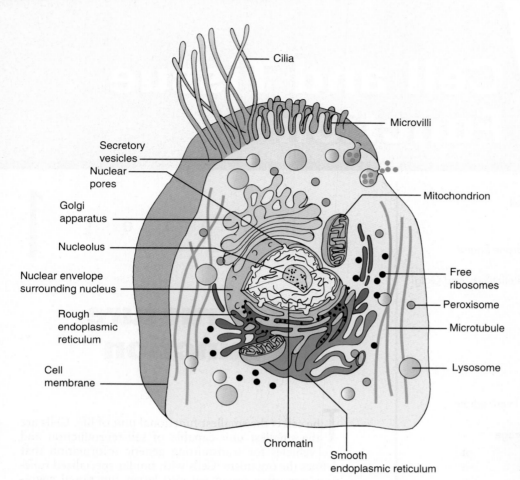

FIGURE 1-1. Composite cell designed to show in one cell all of the various components of the nucleus and cytoplasm.

Two distinct regions exist in the cell: the *cytoplasm*, which lies outside the nucleus, and the *nucleoplasm*, which lies inside the nucleus. The cytoplasm contains membrane-enclosed organelles ("little organs") and inclusions in an aqueous gel called the *cytoplasmic matrix*. The matrix consists of a variety of solutes including inorganic ions (Na^+, K^+, Ca^+) and organic molecules such as intermediate metabolites, carbohydrates, lipids, proteins, and RNA. The nucleus is the largest organelle within the cell and its nucleoplasm contains the genome along with the enzymes necessary for deoxyribonucleic acid (DNA) and ribonucleic acid (RNA) transcription.

The Cell Membrane

In many respects, the cell membrane (also called the plasma membrane) is one of the most important parts of the cell. It acts as a semipermeable structure that separates the intracellular and extracellular environments. It controls the transport of materials from the extracellular fluids to the interior of the cell, holds and binds receptors for hormones and other biologically active substances, participates in the generation and conduction of electrical currents in nerve and muscle cells, and aids in the regulation of cell growth and proliferation.

The cell membrane is a dynamic and fluid structure consisting of an organized arrangement of lipids, carbohydrates, and proteins (Fig. 1-2). A main structural component of the membrane is its lipid bilayer that consists primarily of phospholipids, cholesterol, and glycoproteins. This lipid bilayer provides the basic fluid structure of the membrane and serves as a relatively impermeable barrier to all but lipid-soluble substances. The most abundant lipids are phospholipids, each with a hydrophilic (water-soluble) head and a hydrophobic (water-insoluble) tail. Phospholipid molecules along with the glycolipids are aligned such that their hydrophilic heads face outward on each side of the membrane and their hydrophobic tails project toward the middle of the membrane. The presence of cholesterol makes the membrane regionally less deformable and less permeable to small water soluble molecules.

Although the lipid bilayer provides the basic structure of the cell membrane, proteins carry out most of the specific functions. The *integral proteins* span the entire lipid bilayer and are part of the membrane. Because most of the integral proteins pass directly through the membrane, they are also referred to as *transmembrane proteins*. Other proteins, called the *peripheral proteins*, are bound to one or the other side of the membrane and do not pass into the lipid bilayer.

The manner in which proteins are associated with the cell membrane often determines their function. Thus, peripheral proteins are associated with functions involving the inner or outer side of the membrane where they

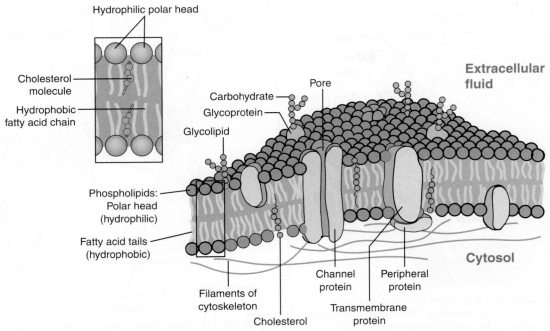

FIGURE 1-2. Structure of the plasma (cell) membrane showing the hydrophilic (polar) heads and the hydrophobic (fatty acid) tails (*inset*), and the position of the integral and peripheral proteins in relation to the interior and exterior of the cell.

are found. Several peripheral proteins serve as receptors or are involved in intracellular signaling systems. By contrast, only the transmembrane proteins can function on both sides of the membrane or transport molecules across it. Many integral transmembrane proteins form the ion channels found on the cell surface. These channel proteins have a complex morphology and are selective with respect to the substances they transmit.

A fuzzy-looking layer, called the *cell coat* or *glycocalyx*, surrounds the cell surface. It consists of long, complex carbohydrate chains attached to protein molecules that penetrate the outside portion of the membrane (i.e., glycoproteins); outward-facing membrane lipids (i.e., glycolipids); and carbohydrate-binding proteins called lectins. The cell coat participates in cell-to-cell recognition due to antigens that label cells as self or nonself and are important in tissue transplantation. The cell coat of a red blood cell contains the ABO blood group antigens.

The Nucleus

The nucleus of a nondividing cell appears as a rounded or elongated structure situated near the center of the cell (see Fig. 1-1). It is enclosed in a nuclear envelope and contains chromatin, the genetic material of the nucleus, and a distinct region called the *nucleolus*. All eukaryotic cells have at least one nucleus (prokaryotic cells, such as bacteria, lack a nucleus and nuclear membrane).

The nucleus is regarded as the control center for the cell. It contains the DNA that is essential to the cell because its genes encode the information necessary for the synthesis of proteins that the cell must produce to stay alive. The genes also represent the individual units of inheritance that transmit information from one generation to another. The nucleus also is the site for the synthesis of the three types of RNA that move to the cytoplasm and carry out the actual synthesis of proteins. Messenger RNA (mRNA) copies and carries the DNA instructions for protein synthesis to the cytoplasm; ribosomal RNA (rRNA) is the site of protein synthesis; and transfer RNA (tRNA) transports amino acids to the site of protein synthesis for incorporation into the protein being synthesized (see Chapter 5).

The complex structure of DNA and DNA-associated proteins dispersed in the nuclear matrix is called *chromatin*. Depending on its transcriptional activity, chromatin may be condensed as an inactive form of chromatin called *heterochromatin* or extended as a more active form called *euchromatin*. Because heterochromatic regions of the nucleus stain more intensely than regions consisting of euchromatin, nuclear staining can be a guide to cell activity. The nucleus also contains the darkly stained round body called the *nucleolus* that is the site of rRNA synthesis and initial ribosomal assembly. Cells that are actively synthesizing proteins can be recognized because their nucleoli are large and prominent and the nucleus as a whole is euchromatic or slightly stained.

Surrounding the nucleus is the *nuclear envelope* formed by an inner and outer nuclear membrane containing a *perinuclear* space between them (Fig. 1-3). The inner nuclear membrane is supported by a rigid network of protein filaments called *nuclear lamina* that bind to chromosomes and secure their position in the nucleus. The outer nuclear membrane resembles and is continuous with the membrane of the endoplasmic reticulum.

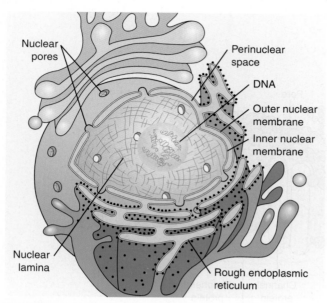

FIGURE 1-3. Schematic drawing of the inner and outer membranes of the nuclear envelope. The double-membrane envelope is penetrated by pores in which nuclear pore complexes are positioned and continuous with the rough endoplasmic reticulum. The nuclear lamina on the surface of the inner membrane binds to DNA and holds the chromosomes in place. DNA, deoxyribonucleic acid.

At the site where the inner and outer membranes fuse, the nuclear envelope is penetrated by pores containing *nuclear pore complexes*. Structures of the nuclear pore complexes act as barriers and enable selective transportation of RNA, ribosomes, and lipids and proteins with signaling functions between the nucleus and cytoplasm to coordinate events such as gene transcription and metabolic activities.

The Cytoplasm and Its Membrane-Bound Organelles

The cytoplasm surrounds the nucleus, and it is in the cytoplasm that the work of the cell takes place. Embedded in the cytoplasm are various membrane-enclosed organelles (e.g., endoplasmic reticulum [ER], Golgi apparatus, mitochondria, and lysosomes) and complexes without membranes (e.g., ribosomes and proteasomes) that have important functions in cells.

Ribosomes, Endoplasmic Reticulum, and Golgi Apparatus

The endoplasmic reticulum (with its associated ribosomes) and Golgi apparatus represent the primary sites of protein synthesis in the cell (Fig. 1-4). Following protein synthesis in the ribosomes, the endoplasmic reticulum and Golgi apparatus use transport vesicles to move newly synthesized proteins, membrane components, and soluble molecules from one organelle to another.

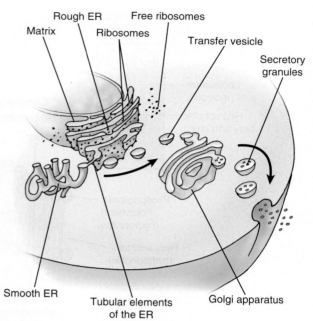

FIGURE 1-4. Three-dimensional view of the rough and the smooth endoplasmic reticula (ER) and the Golgi apparatus. The ER functions as a tubular communication system through which substances can be transported from one part of the cell to another and as the site of protein (rough ER), carbohydrate, and lipid (smooth ER) synthesis. Most of the proteins synthesized by the rough ER are sealed into transfer vesicles and transported to the Golgi apparatus, where they are modified and packaged into secretory granules.

Ribosomes. The ribosomes are small particles of nucleoproteins (rRNA and proteins) that are held together by a strand of mRNA. Poly Ribosomes exist as isolated clusters of free ribosomes within the cytoplasm or attached to the membrane of the ER (see Fig. 1-4). Free ribosomes are involved in the synthesis of proteins that remain in the cell as cytoplasmic structural or functional elements, whereas those attached to the ER translate mRNAs that code for proteins to be bound in membranes or destined for secretion.

Endoplasmic Reticulum. The endoplasmic reticulum is an extensive dynamic system of interconnected membranous tubes and sac-like cisternae (see Figs. 1-3 and 1-4). Within the lumen of the ER is a matrix that connects the space between the two membranes of the nuclear envelope to the cell periphery. The ER functions as a tubular communication system for transporting various substances from one part of the cell to another. A large surface area and multiple enzyme systems attached to the ER membranes also provide the machinery for many cellular metabolic functions.

Two forms of ER exist in cells: rough and smooth. *Rough ER* is studded with ribosomes attached to specific binding sites on the membrane. These ribosomes, with their accompanying strand of mRNA, synthesize proteins destined to be incorporated into cell membranes, used in the generation of lysosomal enzymes, or exported from the cell. The *smooth ER* is free of ribosomes and is continuous with the rough ER. It does not participate in protein synthesis; instead, its enzymes are involved in the synthesis of lipid and steroid hormone molecules, regulation of intracellular calcium, and metabolism and detoxification of certain hormones and drugs. The sarcoplasmic reticulum of skeletal and cardiac muscle cells is a form of smooth ER. Calcium ions needed for muscle contraction are stored and released from cisternae of the sarcoplasmic reticulum. The smooth ER of the liver is involved in glycogen storage and metabolism of lipid-soluble drugs.

Golgi Apparatus.

The Golgi apparatus, sometimes called the *Golgi complex*, consists of stacks of thin, flattened vesicles or sacs (see Fig. 1-4). These Golgi bodies are found near the nucleus and function in association with the ER. Substances produced in the ER are transported to the Golgi complex in small, membrane-bound transport vesicles. Many cells synthesize proteins that are larger than the active product. The Golgi complex modifies these substances and packages them into secretory granules or vesicles. Insulin, for example, is synthesized as a large, inactive proinsulin molecule that is cleaved to produce a smaller, active insulin molecule within the Golgi complex of the beta cells of the pancreas. In addition to producing secretory granules, the Golgi complex is thought to produce large carbohydrate molecules that are added to proteins produced by the rough ER to form glycoproteins.

Lysosomes

The lysosomes, which can be viewed as digestive organelles in the cell, are small, membrane-bound sacs filled with hydrolytic enzymes. These enzymes can break down excess and worn-out cell parts as well as foreign substances that are taken into the cell. All of the lysosomal enzymes are acid hydrolases, which means that they require an acid environment. The lysosomes provide this environment by maintaining a pH of approximately 5.0 in their interior. The pH of the cytosol and other cellular components is approximately 7.2. Like all other cellular organelles, lysosomes not only contain a unique collection of enzymes, but also have a unique surrounding membrane that prevents the release of its digestive enzymes into the cytosol.

Lysosomes are formed from digestive vesicles called *endosomes*. These vesicles fuse to form multivesicular bodies called *early endosomes* (Fig. 1-5). The early endosomes mature into *late endosomes* as they recycle lipids, proteins, and other membrane components back to the plasma membrane in vesicles called *recycling vesicles*. Lysosomal enzymes are synthesized in the rough ER and then transported to the Golgi apparatus, where they are biochemically modified and packaged for transport to the endosomes. The late endosomes mature into lysosomes as they progressively accumulate newly synthesized acid hydrolases from the Golgi apparatus and attain digestive abilities.

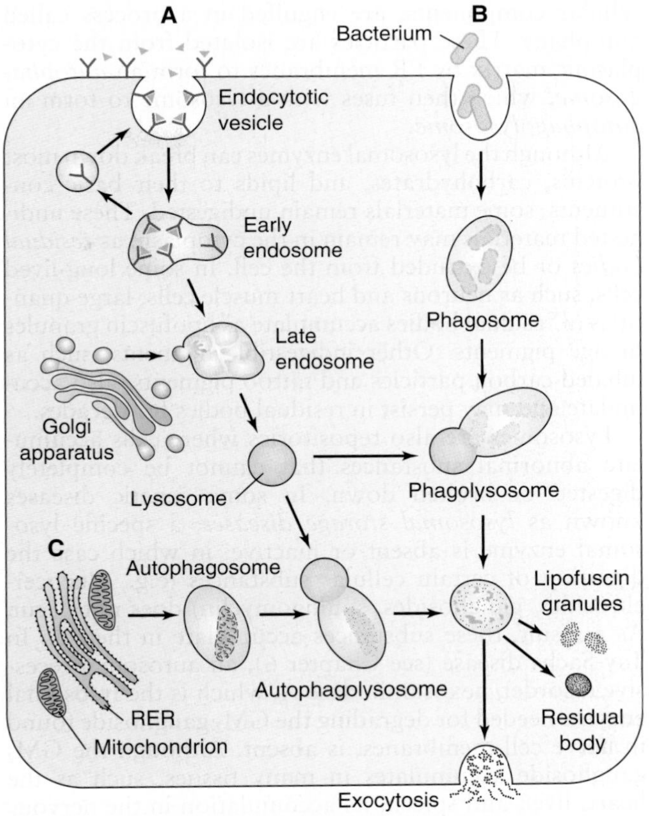

FIGURE 1-5. Pathways for digestion of materials by lysosomes. **(A)** Receptor-mediated endocytosis with formation of lysosome from early and late endosomes. Vesicle contents are sorted in the early endosome with receptors and lipids being sent back to the membrane. Transport vesicles carry lysosomal enzymes to the late endosomes, converting them into lysosomes that digest proteins and other components acquired from the endocytotic vesicles. **(B)** Phagocytosis involving the delivery of large extracellular particles such as bacteria and cellular debris to the lysosomes via phagosomes. **(C)** Autophagy is the process in which worn-out mitochondria and other cell parts are surrounded by a membrane derived from the rough endoplasmic reticulum (RER). The resulting autophagosome then fuses with a lysosome to form an authophagolysosome. Undigested material may be extruded from the cell or remain in the cytoplasm as lipofuscin granules or membrane-bound residual bodies.

Depending on the nature of the substance, different pathways are used for lysosomal degradation of unwanted materials (see Fig. 1-5). Small extracellular particles such as extracellular proteins and plasma membrane proteins form endocytotic vesicles after being internalized by pinocytosis or receptor-mediated endocytosis. These vesicles are converted into early and late endosomes, after which they mature into lysosomes. Large extracellular particles such as bacteria, cell debris, and other foreign particles are engulfed in a process called *phagocytosis*. A *phagosome*, formed as the material is internalized within the cell, fuses with a lysosome to form a *phagolysosome*. Intracellular particles, such as entire organelles, cytoplasmic proteins, and other cellular components, are engulfed in a process called autophagy. These particles are isolated from the cytoplasmic matrix by ER membranes to form an *autophagosome*, which then fuses with a lysosome to form an *autophagolysosome*.

Although the lysosomal enzymes can break down most proteins, carbohydrates, and lipids to their basic constituents, some materials remain undigested. These undigested materials may remain in the cytoplasm as *residual bodies* or be extruded from the cell. In some long-lived cells, such as neurons and heart muscle cells, large quantities of residual bodies accumulate as lipofuscin granules or age pigments. Other indigestible pigments, such as inhaled carbon particles and tattoo pigments, also accumulate and may persist in residual bodies for decades.

Lysosomes are also repositories where cells accumulate abnormal substances that cannot be completely digested or broken down. In some genetic diseases known as *lysosomal storage diseases*, a specific lysosomal enzyme is absent or inactive, in which case the digestion of certain cellular substances (e.g., glucocerebrosides, gangliosides, sphingomyelin) does not occur. As a result, these substances accumulate in the cell. In Tay-Sachs disease (see Chapter 6), an autosomal recessive disorder, hexosaminidase A, which is the lysosomal enzyme needed for degrading the GM_2 ganglioside found in nerve cell membranes, is absent. Although the GM_2 ganglioside accumulates in many tissues, such as the heart, liver, and spleen, its accumulation in the nervous system and retina of the eye causes the most damage.

Peroxisomes

Spherical membrane-bound organelles called *peroxisomes* contain enzymes that are used in oxidative reactions. Reactions occurring in peroxisomes use oxygen to produce peroxides and convert hydrogen peroxide to water. Unless degraded, these highly unstable reactive oxygen species and free radicals (see Chapter 2) would damage other cellular molecules and structures. Peroxisomes also contain the enzymes needed for breaking down very–long-chain fatty acids, which are ineffectively degraded by mitochondrial enzymes. In liver cells, peroxisomal enzymes are involved in the formation of the bile acids.

Proteasomes

Proteasomes are cytoplasmic protein complexes that are not bound by membranes. Proteasomes are responsible for proteolysis of malformed and misfolded proteins and have roles in many cellular responses and events. The process of cytosolic proteolysis is carefully controlled by the cell and requires that the protein be targeted for degradation. This process involves *ubiquitination*, a process whereby several small ubiquitin molecules (a small 76-amino-acid polypeptide chain) are attached to an amino acid residue of the targeted protein. Once a protein is so tagged, it is degraded by proteasomes. After the targeted protein has been degraded, the resultant amino acids join the intracellular pool of free amino acids and the ubiquitin molecules are released and recycled.

Mitochondria

The mitochondria are literally the "power plants" of the cell because they contain the enzymes needed for capturing most of the energy in foodstuffs and converting it into cellular energy. This multistep process requires oxygen and is often referred to as *aerobic metabolism*. Much of this energy is stored in the high-energy phosphate bonds of adenosine triphosphate (ATP) that serves to power various cell activities. Mitochondria are found close to the site of energy consumption in the cell (e.g., near the myofibrils in muscle cells). The number of mitochondria in a given cell type is largely determined by the type of activity the cell performs and how much energy is needed to undertake the activity. For example, a dramatic increase in mitochondria occurs in skeletal muscle repeatedly stimulated to contract.

The mitochondria are composed of two membranes: an outer membrane that encloses the periphery of the mitochondrion and an inner membrane that forms shelflike projections, called *cristae* (Fig. 1-6). The narrow space between the outer and inner membranes is called the *intermembrane space*, whereas the large space enclosed by the inner membrane is termed the *matrix space*. The outer mitochondrial membrane contains a large number of transmembrane porins, through which inorganic ions and metabolites may pass. The inner membrane contains the respiratory chain enzymes and transport proteins needed for the synthesis of ATP.

Mitochondria contain their own DNA and ribosomes and are self-replicating. The DNA is found in the mitochondrial matrix and is distinct from the chromosomal DNA found in the nucleus. Mitochondrial DNA, known as the "other human genome," is a double-stranded, circular molecule that encodes the rRNA and tRNA required for intramitochondrial synthesis of the proteins needed for the energy-generating function of the mitochondria. Although mitochondrial DNA directs the synthesis of 13 of the proteins required for mitochondrial function, the DNA of the nucleus encodes the structural

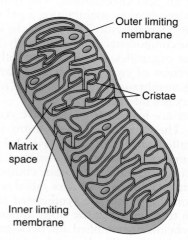

FIGURE 1-6. Mitochondrion. The inner membrane forms transverse folds called cristae, where the enzymes needed for the final step in adenosine triphosphate (ATP) production (i.e., oxidative phosphorylation) are located.

proteins of the mitochondria and other proteins needed to carry out cellular respiration.

Mitochondrial DNA is inherited matrilineally (i.e., from the mother) and provides a basis for familial lineage studies. Mutations have been found in each of the mitochondrial genes, and an understanding of the role of mitochondrial DNA in certain diseases and of mechanisms to maintain the integrity of the mitochondrial genome is beginning to emerge. Most tissues in the body depend to some extent on oxidative metabolism and can therefore be affected by mitochondrial DNA mutations.

Mitochondria also function as key regulators of apoptosis or programmed cell death (discussed in Chapter 2). The initiation of the mitochondrial pathway for apoptosis results from an increase in mitochondrial membrane permeability and the subsequent release of proapoptotic molecules into the cytoplasm. One of these proapoptotic molecules, cytochrome c, is well known for its role in cellular respiration. In the cytosol, cytochrome c binds to a protein called the *apoptosis protease activating factor-1* protein, initiating the molecular events involved in the apoptosis cascade. Other apoptotic proteins also enter the cytoplasm, where they bind to and neutralize the various apoptotic inhibitors, whose normal function consists of blocking the apoptotic cascade. Both the formation of reactive oxygen species (e.g., peroxide) and the activation of the p53 tumor-suppressor gene by DNA damage or other means initiate apoptotic signaling through the mitochondria. Dysregulated apoptosis (too little or too much) has been implicated in a wide range of diseases, including cancer, in which there is an inappropriately low rate of apoptosis, and neurodegenerative diseases, in which there is an increased or excessive rate of apoptosis.

The Cytoskeleton

In addition to its organelles, the cytoplasm contains a network of microtubules, microfilaments, and intermediate filaments (Fig. 1-7). Because they control cell shape and movement, these structures are a major component of the structural elements called the *cytoskeleton*.

Microtubules

Microtubules are slender and rigid tubular structures composed of globular proteins called *tubulin*. Each microtubule consists of parallel protofilaments, each composed of α- and β-tubulin dimers. Microtubules function in many ways, including the development and maintenance of cell form; participation in intracellular transport mechanisms, including axoplasmic transport in neurons; and formation of the basic structure for several complex cytoplasmic organelles, including the cilia, flagella, and centrioles. *Cilia* and *flagella* are microtubule-filled cellular extensions extending from the cell membrane that are capable of sweeping movements. Cilia are found on the apical (luminal) surfaces of many epithelial linings, including the nasal sinuses and passages of the upper respiratory system.

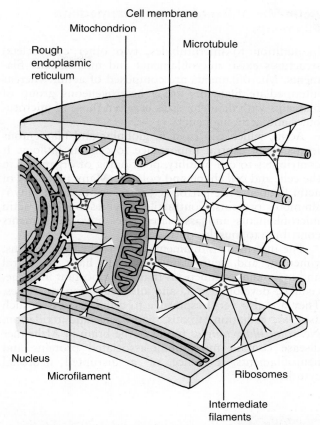

FIGURE 1-7. Three-dimensional view of the network of microtubules, microfilaments, and intermediate filaments that supports the organelles within the cell cytoplasm.

Removal of mucus from the respiratory passages is highly dependent on the proper functioning of the cilia. Flagella form the tail-like structures that provide motility for sperm. Centrioles are small, barrel-shaped bodies oriented at right angles to each other. In dividing cells, the two cylindrical centrioles form the mitotic spindle that aids in the separation and movement of the chromosomes during cell division.

Abnormalities of the microtubules occur in a number of pathologic states. These abnormalities may be manifested by an abnormal appearance and function, aberrant movements of intracellular organelles, and defective cell locomotion. Defective organization of the microtubules can cause sterility by inhibiting sperm motility, as well as defective motility of cilia in the epithelial lining of the respiratory tract, resulting in chronic respiratory tract infections. Proper functioning of the microtubules is also essential for various stages of leukocyte migration. Drugs that bind to tubulin molecules and prevent their assembly of microtubules (*colchicine*) are useful in the treatment of gout, in which symptoms are due to movement of leukocytes toward urate crystals in the tissues. Since microtubules form the mitotic spindle, which is essential for cell proliferation, drugs that bind microtubules (e.g., vinca alkaloids) are useful in the treatment of cancer.

Actin Microfilaments and Intermediate Filaments

In addition to microtubules, two other cytoskeletal structures exist: microfilaments and intermediate filaments. Microfilaments are composed of actin, whereas intermediate filaments are a heterogeneous group of filaments with diameter sizes between those of microtubules and actin filaments.

Actin, which can exist in globular and filamentous forms, is of central importance to cellular biology. It contributes to cell motility, positioning of organelles in the cell, and cell shape and polarity. Many functions of actin filaments are performed in association with myosin motor proteins. Contractile activities involving actin microfilaments and associated thick myosin filaments contribute to muscle contraction.

The intermediate filaments include the cytokeratins, vimentin, and neurofilaments. They have structural and maintenance functions that are important in tissue, cellular, developmental, and differentiation processes. They are also very responsive to cellular stresses, such as heat, radiation, toxins, pathogens and oxidation. *Neurofibrillary tangles* found in the brain in Alzheimer disease contain microtubule-associated proteins and neurofilaments, evidence of a disrupted neuronal cytoskeleton.

SUMMARY CONCEPTS

- Cells are the smallest functional unit of the body. They are autonomous units that contain structures that are strikingly similar to those needed to maintain total body function.

- The cell membrane is a protein-studded lipid bilayer that surrounds the cell and separates it from its surrounding external environment. It contains receptors for hormones and other biologically active substances, participates in the electrical events that occur in nerve and muscle cells, and aids in the regulation of cell growth and proliferation. The cell surface is surrounded by a fuzzy-looking layer called the *cell coat* or *glycocalyx*. The cell coat participates in cell-to-cell recognition and adhesion, and it contains tissue transplant antigens.

- The nucleus is the control center for the cell. It contains deoxyribonucleic acid (DNA), which provides the information necessary for the synthesis of the various proteins that the cell must produce to stay alive and to transmit information from one generation to another.

- The cytoplasm contains the cell's organelles. *Ribosomes* serve as sites for protein synthesis

in the cell. The *endoplasmic reticulum* (ER) functions as a tubular communication system through which substances can be transported from one part of the cell to another and as the site of protein (rough ER), carbohydrate, and lipid (smooth ER) synthesis. The *Golgi apparatus* modifies materials synthesized in the ER and packages them into secretory granules for transport within the cell or export from the cell. *Lysosomes*, which can be viewed as the digestive system of the cell, contain hydrolytic enzymes that digest worn-out cell parts and foreign materials. The mitochondria serve as power plants for the cell because they transform food energy into ATP, which is used to power cell activities. They contain their own extrachromosomal DNA, which is used in the synthesis of certain proteins required for mitochondrial function.

- In addition to its organelles, the cytoplasm also contains a network of microtubules, actin microfilaments, and intermediate filaments called the *cytoskeleton*. Microtubules are slender, stiff tubular structures that influence cell shape, provide a means of moving organelles through the cytoplasm, and form cilia, flagella, and centrioles. Actin microfilaments are dynamic, thin, threadlike cytoplasmic structures that are important in cell movement and organelle positioning. Many types of intermediate filaments function in supporting and maintaining the shape of cells and participate in numerous cellular processes.

Cell Metabolism and Energy Storage

Energy metabolism refers to the chemical processes involved in converting carbohydrates, fats, and proteins from the foods we eat into the energy needed for cell functions. Cells use oxygen to transform the breakdown products of the foods we eat into the energy needed for muscle contraction; the transport of ions and other molecules across cell membranes; and the synthesis of enzymes, hormones, and other macromolecules.

The special "unit of currency" for transferring energy in living cells is ATP. Adenosine triphosphate molecules consist of adenosine, a nitrogenous base; ribose, a five-carbon sugar; and three phosphate groups (Fig. 1-8). The last two phosphate groups are attached to the remainder of the molecule by two high-energy bonds. Each bond releases a large amount of energy when hydrolyzed. Adenosine triphosphate is hydrolyzed to form adenosine

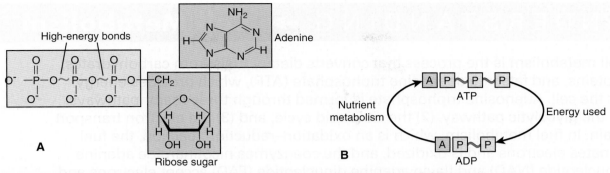

FIGURE 1-8. Adenosine triphosphate (ATP) is the major source of cellular energy. **(A)** Each molecule of ATP contains two high-energy bonds, each containing about 12 kcal of potential energy. **(B)** The high-energy ATP bonds are in constant flux. They are generated by substrate (glucose, amino acid, and fat) metabolism and are consumed as the energy is expended. ADP, adenosine diphosphate.

diphosphate (ADP) with the loss of one high-energy bond and to adenosine monophosphate (AMP) with the loss of two such bonds. The energy liberated from the hydrolysis of ATP is used to drive reactions that require free energy, such as muscle contraction and active transport mechanisms. Energy from foodstuffs is used to convert ADP back to ATP. Hence ATP is often called the *energy currency* of the cell; energy can be "saved" or "spent" using ATP as an exchange currency.

Two types of energy production are present in the cell: the *anaerobic* (i.e., without oxygen) glycolytic pathway, occurring in the cytoplasm, and the *aerobic* (i.e., with oxygen) pathway, occurring in the mitochondria. The glycolytic pathway serves as the prelude to the aerobic pathway.

Anaerobic Metabolism

Glycolysis is the anaerobic process by which energy is liberated from glucose. It is an important source of energy for cells that lack mitochondria. The process also provides a temporary source of energy for cells that are deprived of an adequate supply of oxygen. Glycolysis involves a sequence of reactions that convert glucose to pyruvic acid, with the concomitant production of ATP from ADP. The net gain of energy from the glycolytic metabolism of one molecule of glucose is two ATP molecules. Although relatively inefficient as to energy yield, the glycolytic pathway is important during periods of decreased oxygen delivery, such as occurs in skeletal muscle during the first few minutes of exercise.

Glycolysis requires the presence of nicotinamide adenine dinucleotide (NAD$^+$), a hydrogen carrier. The end products of glycolysis are pyruvate and NADH (the reduced form of NAD$^+$) plus H$^+$. When oxygen is present, pyruvic acid moves into the aerobic mitochondrial pathway, and NAD$^+$ is regenerated as NADH delivers its electron and proton (H$^+$) to the oxidative electron transport system. Under anaerobic conditions, such as cardiac arrest or circulatory shock, pyruvic acid is converted to lactic acid, which diffuses out of the cells into the extracellular fluid. Conversion of pyruvate to lactic

acid is reversible, and once the oxygen supply has been restored, lactic acid is converted back to pyruvic acid and used directly for energy or to synthesize glucose.

Aerobic Metabolism

Aerobic metabolism, which supplies 90% of the body's energy needs, occurs in the cell's mitochondria and requires oxygen. It is here that the hydrogen and carbon molecules from dietary fats, proteins, and carbohydrates are broken down and combined with molecular oxygen to form carbon dioxide and water as energy is released. Unlike lactic acid, which is an end product of anaerobic metabolism, carbon dioxide and water are relatively harmless and easily eliminated from the body. In a 24-hour period, oxidative metabolism produces 150 to 300 mL of water.

The citric acid cycle, sometimes called the *tricarboxylic acid* (TCA) or *Krebs* cycle, provides the final common pathway for the metabolism of nutrients. In the citric acid cycle, which takes place in the matrix of the mitochondria, an activated two-carbon molecule of acetyl-coenzyme A (acetyl-CoA) condenses with a four-carbon molecule of oxaloacetic acid and moves through a series of enzyme-mediated steps. This process produces hydrogen atoms and carbon dioxide. As hydrogen is generated, it combines with NAD$^+$ or flavin adenine dinucleotide (FAD) for transfer to the electron transport system. Besides pyruvate from the glycolysis of glucose, products of amino acid and fatty acid degradation enter the citric acid cycle and contribute to the generation of ATP.

Oxidation of electrons from the hydrogen atoms generated during glycolysis and the citric acid cycle takes place in the electron transport system located on the inner mitochondrial membrane. The electrons are used to reduce elemental oxygen, which combines with hydrogen to form water. During this sequence of oxidative reactions, large amounts of energy are released and used to convert ADP to ATP. Because the formation of ATP involves the addition of a high-energy phosphate bond to ADP, the process is called *oxidative phosphorylation*.

(text continues on page 12)

UNDERSTANDING → Cell Metabolism

Cell metabolism is the process that converts dietary fuels from carbohydrates, proteins, and fats into adenosine triphosphate (ATP), which provides energy for the cell. Adenosine triphosphate is formed through three major pathways: (1) the glycolytic pathway, (2) the citric acid cycle, and (3) the electron transport chain. In fuel metabolism, which is an oxidation–reduction reaction, the fuel donates electrons and is oxidized, and the coenzymes nicotinamide adenine dinucleotide (NAD) and flavin adenine dinucleotide (FAD) accept electrons and are reduced.

1

Glycolytic Pathway. Glycolysis, which occurs in the cytoplasm of the cell, involves the splitting of the six-carbon glucose molecule into two three-carbon molecules of pyruvic acid. Because the reaction that splits glucose requires two molecules of ATP, there is a net gain of only two molecules of ATP from each molecule of glucose that is metabolized. The process is anaerobic and does not require oxygen (O_2) or produce carbon dioxide (CO_2). When O_2 is present, pyruvic acid moves into the mitochondria, where it enters the aerobic citric acid cycle. Under anaerobic conditions, pyruvate is converted to lactic acid, allowing glycolysis to continue as a means of supplying cells with ATP when O_2 is lacking.

2

Citric Acid Cycle. Under aerobic conditions, both of the pyruvic acid molecules formed by the glycolytic pathway enter the mitochondria, where each combines with acetyl-coenzyme to form acetyl-coenzyme A (acetyl-CoA). The formation of acetyl-CoA begins the reactions that occur in the citric acid cycle. Some reactions release CO_2 and some transfer electrons from the hydrogen atom to NADH or FADH. In addition to pyruvic acid from the glycolysis of glucose, fatty acid and amino acid breakdown products can also enter the citric acid cycle. Fatty acids, which are the major source of fuel in the body, are oxidized by a process called β-*oxidation* to acetyl-CoA for entry into the citric acid cycle.

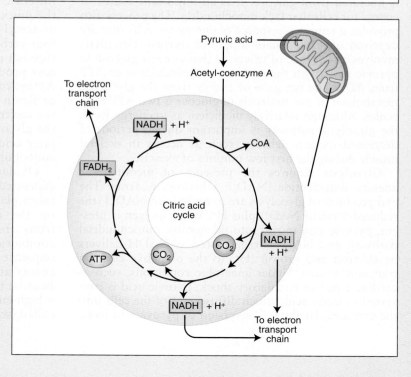

3 **Electron Transport Chain.** At the completion of the citric acid cycle, each glucose molecule has yielded only four new molecules of ATP (two from glycolysis and two from the citric acid cycle). In fact, the principal function of these earlier stages is to make the electrons (e^-) from glucose and other food substrates available for oxidation. Oxidation of the electrons carried by NADH and $FADH_2$ is accomplished through a series of enzymatically catalyzed reactions in the mitochondrial electron transport chain. During these reactions, protons (H^+) combine with O_2 to form water (H_2O), and large amounts of energy are released and used to add a high-energy phosphate bond to adenosine diphosphate (ADP), converting it to ATP. There is a net yield of 36 molecules of ATP from 1 molecule of glucose (2 from glycolysis, 2 from the citric acid cycle, and 32 from the electron transport chain). In general, the net amount of ATP formed from each gram of protein that is metabolized is less than for glucose, whereas that obtained from fat is greater (e.g., each 16-carbon fatty acid molecule yields about 129 molecules of ATP).

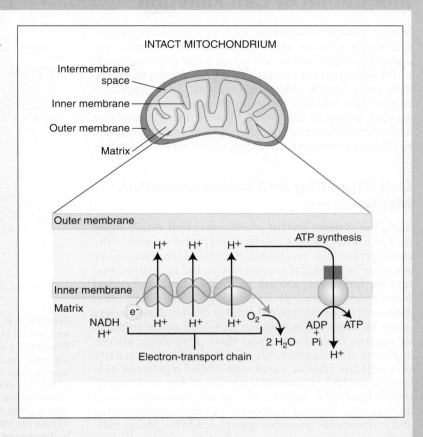

INTACT MITOCHONDRIUM

Intermembrane space
Inner membrane
Outer membrane
Matrix

Outer membrane

Inner membrane
Matrix

H^+ H^+ H^+

ATP synthesis

e^-

NADH
H^+ H^+ H^+ H^+ O_2 ADP + Pi   ATP

2 H_2O H^+

Electron-transport chain

SUMMARY CONCEPTS

- Metabolism is the process whereby the carbohydrates, fats, and proteins from the foods we eat are broken down and subsequently converted into the energy needed for cell function. Energy is stored in the high-energy phosphate bonds of adenosine triphosphate (ATP), which serves as the energy currency for the cell.

- Two sites of energy conversion are present in cells: the *anaerobic glycolytic pathway* in

the cytoplasm and the *aerobic pathways* in the mitochondria. The most efficient of these pathways is the aerobic citric acid cycle and electron transport chain in the mitochondria. This pathway, which requires oxygen, produces carbon dioxide and water as end products and results in the release of large amounts of energy that is used to convert adenosine diphosphate (ADP) to ATP. The glycolytic pathway in the cytoplasm involves the breakdown of glucose to form ATP. This pathway can function without oxygen by producing lactic acid.

(text continued from page 9)

Integration of Cell Function

Within a complex organism, such as a human being, different organs, tissues, and individual cell types develop specialized functions and needs. Yet each cell must contribute to the integrated life process as the body grows, differentiates, and adapts to changing conditions. Such integration requires that cells have the ability to communicate with one another, transport substances between their intracellular and extracellular environments, and generate and respond to changes in the electrical charge of membrane potentials.

Cell Signaling and Communication Mechanisms

Signaling systems consist of receptors that reside either on the cell membrane (surface receptors) or within the cells (intracellular receptors). Receptors are activated by a variety of chemical messengers including neurotransmitters, hormones, growth factors, and other chemical messengers, as well as signaling proteins called *cytokines* and *lipids*. Some lipid-soluble chemical messengers move through the membrane and bind to cytoplasmic or nuclear receptors to exert their physiologic effects. Signaling systems often rely on the intermediary activity of a separate class of membrane-bound regulatory proteins to convert extracellular signals, or first messengers, into intracellular signals, or second messengers, such as a unique form of adenosine monophosphate called *cyclic adenosine monophosphate* (cAMP). Many molecules involved in signal transduction within cells are enzymes and other proteins. Some of the enzymes are protein kinases that catalyze the phosphorylation of proteins, thereby changing their activity and function.

Cell Surface Receptors

Each cell type in the body contains numerous receptor proteins, which as a set may characterize the cell type, that enable it to respond to a complementary set of ligands (i.e., molecules with a high affinity for a receptor) or signaling molecules in a specific, preprogrammed way. These receptors, which span the cell membrane, relay information to a series of intracellular intermediates that eventually pass the signal to its final destination. There are three major classes of cell surface receptor proteins: G protein–linked receptors, enzyme-linked receptors, and ion channel–linked receptors.

G Protein–Linked Receptors.
G protein–linked receptors mediate cellular responses for numerous types of first messengers through regulatory proteins called *G proteins* that bind to guanine nucleotides such as guanine diphosphate (GDP) and guanine triphosphate (GTP). With more than 1000 members, G protein–linked receptors are the largest family of cell surface receptors.

Although there are differences among the G protein–linked receptors, all share a number of features. They all have a ligand-binding extracellular receptor component,

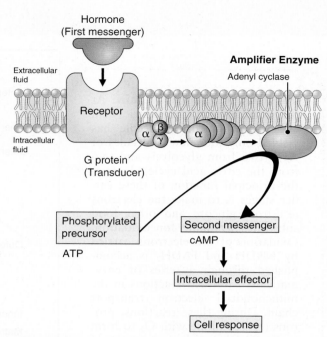

FIGURE 1-9. Activation of a G-protein-linked receptor and production of cyclic adenosine monophosphate (cAMP). Binding of a hormone (the first messenger) causes the activated receptor to interact with the inactive, guanine diphosphate (GDP)-bound G protein. This results in activation of the G protein and dissociation of the G protein α, β, and γ subunits. The activated α subunit of the G protein can then interact with and activate the membrane protein adenyl cyclase to catalyze the conversion of adenosine triphosphate (ATP) to the second messenger cAMP. The second messenger then activates an internal effector, which leads to the cell response.

which recognizes a specific ligand or first messenger. Upon ligand-binding, they all undergo conformational changes that activate the G protein found on the cytoplasmic side of the cell membrane (Fig. 1-9). All G proteins incorporate the *guanosine triphosphatase (GTPase) cycle*, which functions as a molecular switch that exists in two states: an activated (on) state and an inactivated (off) state. Receptor activation causes the α subunit to dissociate from the receptor and the β and γ subunits and transmit the signal from the first messenger to a membrane-bound intermediate called an *effector*. Often, the effector is an enzyme that converts an inactive precursor molecule into a second messenger, which diffuses into the cytoplasm and carries the signal beyond the cell membrane. One common effector is the enzyme *adenylyl cyclase*, which converts the precursor ATP to the second messenger cAMP, transferring the two phosphate groups to other proteins. This transfer changes the conformation and function of these proteins. Such changes eventually produce the cell response initiated by the first messenger, whether it is a secretion, muscle contraction or relaxation, or change in metabolism. Sometimes it is the opening of membrane channels involved in calcium or potassium influx.

Enzyme-Linked Receptors.
Like G protein–linked receptors, enzyme-linked receptors are transmembrane

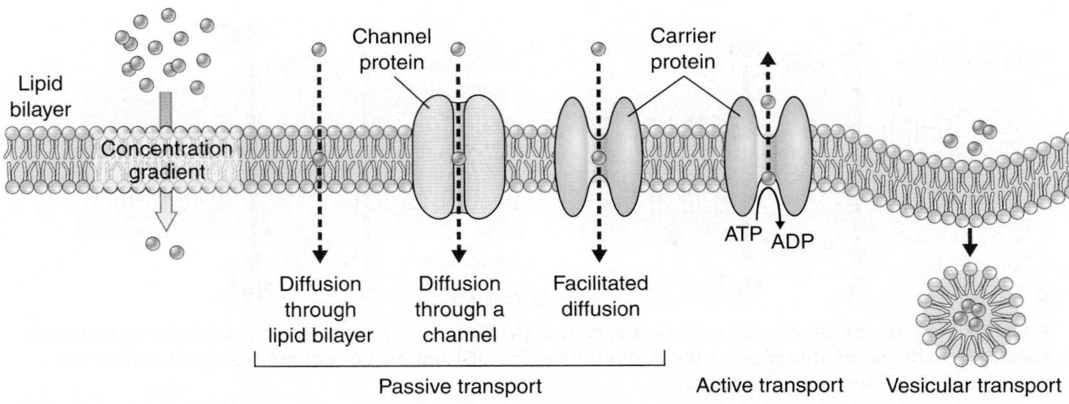

FIGURE 1-10. Mechanisms of membrane transport. Passive transport represents the net movement from a region of higher to lower concentration and active transport (energy requiring) from a region of lower to higher concentration. Vesicular transport involves the formation of membrane-enclosed vesicles or sacs that serve as transport vehicles from extracellular materials that are being moved into the cell (endocytosis) or intracellular materials that are being moved out of the cell (exocytosis). ADP, adenosine diphosphate; ATP, adenosine triphosphate.

proteins with their ligand-binding site on the outer surface of the cell membrane. Instead of having a cytosolic domain that associates with a G protein, their cytosolic domain either has intrinsic enzyme activity or associates directly with an enzyme. There are several classes of enzyme-linked receptors, including one widely used in hormonal control of cell function. The binding of the hormone to a special transmembrane receptor results in activation of the enzyme adenylyl cyclase at the intracellular portion of the receptor. This enzyme then catalyzes the formation of the second messenger cAMP, which has multiple effects on cell function. Insulin, for example, acts by binding to an enzyme-linked receptor (see Chapter 33).

Ion Channel–Linked Receptors. Ion channel–linked receptors are involved in the rapid synaptic signaling between electrically excitable cells. Many neurotransmitters mediate this type of signaling by transiently opening or closing ion channels formed by integral proteins in the cell membrane (to be discussed). This type of signaling is involved in the transmission of impulses in nerve and muscle cells.

Intracellular Receptors

Some messengers, such as thyroid hormone and steroid hormones, do not bind to membrane receptors but move directly across the lipid bilayer of the cell membrane and are transported to the cell nucleus, where they influence DNA activity (see Chapter 31). Many of these hormones bind to a receptor within the cytoplasm, and the receptor–hormone complex enters the nucleus. There it binds to DNA, initiating processes that increase the production of proteins that alter cell function.

Membrane Transport Mechanisms

The lipid layer of the cell membrane serves as a barrier against the movement of water and water-soluble substances between the intracellular and extracellular fluids, while allowing a few lipid-soluble (e.g., alcohols with lower numbers of hydrocarbons, oxygen, nitrogen) and uncharged molecules (glycerol, water) to cross the cell membrane by simple diffusion. The cell membrane also contains large numbers of protein molecules, many of which insert completely through the membrane (Fig. 1-10). Most ions and small molecules rely on these proteins for transport.

Different membrane proteins function in different ways. For example, *channel proteins* form water-lined passageways through the membrane and allow free movement of water as well as selected ions or molecules. *Membrane transport proteins* bind molecules or ions and undergo a series of conformational changes to transfer the bound solute across the membrane. Some transport proteins, called *uniporters*, simply mediate the movement of a single solute from one side of the membrane to the other, whereas others function as coupled transporters in which the transfer of one solute depends on the transfer of a second solute (Fig. 1-11). This coupled transport involves either the simultaneous transport in the same direction, performed by transporters called *symporters*, or the transport of a second solute in the opposite direction, by transporters called *antiporters*.

All channels and many transporters allow solutes to cross the membrane only passively by *passive transport* or *facilitated diffusion*. Cells also require transport proteins that actively pump certain solutes across the membrane against an electrochemical gradient, in a process called *active transport*. Active transport is directional and requires an energy source such as ATP. The cell membrane can also engulf substances, forming a membrane-bound vesicle; this vesicle is brought into the cell by *endocytosis*. The process by which cellular vesicles fuse to the cell membrane releasing contents outside of the cell is called *exocytosis*.

Many integral transmembrane proteins form the ion channels found on the cell surface. These channel proteins have a complex morphology and are selective with respect to the substances that can transverse the channel.

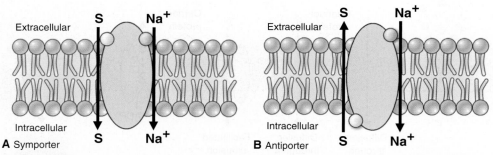

FIGURE 1-11. Secondary active transport systems. **(A)** Symport or cotransport carries the transported solute (S) in the same direction as the sodium (Na⁺) ion. **(B)** Antiport or countertransport carries the solute and Na⁺ in the opposite direction.

A host of genetic disorders known as *channelopathies* involve mutations in channel proteins. For example, in cystic fibrosis (see Chapter 23), the primary defect resides in an abnormal chloride channel, which results in increased sodium and water reabsorption that causes respiratory tract secretions to thicken and occlude the airways.

Diffusion

Diffusion refers to the passive process by which molecules and other particles in a solution become widely dispersed and reach a uniform concentration because of energy created by their spontaneous kinetic movements. In the process of reaching a uniform concentration, these molecules and particles move "downhill" from an area of higher to an area of lower concentration. If the molecules or particles carry a net charge, both the concentration gradient and the electrical potential difference across the membrane influence transport.

Lipid-soluble molecules, such as oxygen, carbon dioxide, alcohol, and fatty acids, become dissolved in the lipid matrix of the cell membrane and diffuse through the membrane in the same manner that diffusion occurs in water. Other substances diffuse through minute pores of the cell membrane.

Simple Diffusion. Simple diffusion means that the kinetic movement of molecules or ions occurs through a membrane opening or through intermolecular spaces without any interaction with a carrier protein. The rate of diffusion depends on how many particles are available for diffusion, the kinetic movement of the particles, and the number and size of the openings in the membrane through which the molecules or ions can move.

Facilitated Diffusion. Like simple diffusion, facilitated diffusion occurs down a concentration gradient; thus, it does not require input of metabolic energy. Unlike simple diffusion, however, facilitated diffusion requires a transport protein. Some substances, such as glucose, cannot pass unassisted through the cell membrane because they are not lipid soluble or they are too large to pass through the membrane's pores. These substances combine with special transport proteins at the membrane's

outer surface, are carried across the membrane attached to the transporter, and then are released. In facilitated diffusion, a substance can move only from an area of higher concentration to one of lower concentration. The rate at which a substance moves across the membrane by facilitated diffusion depends on the difference in concentration between the two sides of the membrane. Also important are the availability of transport proteins and the rapidity with which they can bind and release the substance being transported. It is thought that insulin, which facilitates the movement of glucose into cells, acts by increasing the availability of glucose transporters in the cell membrane.

Ion Channels and Gates. Ion channels (leak channels) are integral proteins that span the width of the membrane and are normally composed of several polypeptides or protein subunits that form a gating system (Fig. 1-12). Specific stimuli cause the protein subunits to undergo conformational changes to form an open channel or gate through which the ions can move. In this way, ions do not need to cross the lipid-soluble portion of the membrane but can remain in the aqueous solution that fills the ion channel. Many of the ion channels are highly selective for transport of one or more specific ions or molecules. This selectivity results from the characteristics of the channel itself, such as its diameter, its shape, and the nature of electrical charges and chemical bonds along its inside surface.

The cell membrane contains two basic groups of ion channels: leakage channels and gated channels. Leakage channels are open even in the unstimulated state, whereas gated channels open and close in response to specific stimuli. Three main types of gated channels are present in the cell membrane: *voltage-gated channels*, which have electrically operated channels that open when the membrane potential changes beyond a certain point; *ligand-gated channels*, which are chemically operated and respond to specific receptor-bound ligands, such as the neurotransmitter acetylcholine; and *mechanically gated channels*, which open or close in response to such mechanical stimulations as vibrations, tissue stretching, or pressure.

Movement of Water Across the Cell Membrane. Water molecules move through adjacent phospholipid

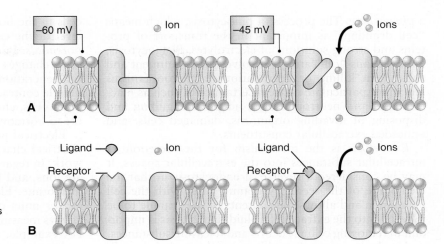

FIGURE 1-12. Gated ion channels that open in response to specific stimuli. **(A)** Voltage-gated channels are controlled by a change in the membrane potential. **(B)** Ligand-gated channels are controlled by binding of a ligand to a receptor.

molecules in the cell membrane by osmosis without actually dissolving in the region occupied by the fatty acid side of the chains. Osmosis is regulated by the concentration of nondiffusible particles on either side of the membrane, with water moving from the side with the lower concentration of particles to the side with the higher concentration. The cell membranes of most cells also contain transmembrane proteins, called *aquaporins*, that function as water channels. Aquaporins are especially abundant in cells that must transport water at particularly high rates, such as certain cells of the kidney.

Active Transport

The process of diffusion describes particle movement from an area of higher concentration to one of lower concentration, resulting in an equal distribution of permeable substances across the cell membrane. Sometimes, however, different concentrations of a substance are needed in the intracellular and extracellular fluids. For example, to function, a cell requires a higher intracellular concentration of potassium ions than is present in the extracellular fluid, while maintaining a much lower concentration of sodium ions than the extracellular fluid. In these situations, energy is required to pump the ions "uphill" or against their concentration gradient. When cells use energy to move ions against an electrical or chemical gradient, the process is called *active transport*. Two types of active transport systems exist: primary active transport and secondary active transport.

Primary Active Transport. Among the substances that are transported by primary active transport are sodium, potassium, calcium, and hydrogen ions. The active transport system studied in the greatest detail is the sodium/potassium (Na^+/K^+)-adenosine triphosphatase (ATPase) membrane pump. The Na^+/K^+–ATPase membrane pump moves sodium from inside the cell to the extracellular region, where its concentration is approximately 14 times greater than inside; the pump also returns potassium to the inside, where its concentration is approximately 35 times greater than it is outside the cell. If it were not for the activity of the Na^+/K^+–ATPase

membrane pump, the osmotically active sodium particles would accumulate in the cell, causing cellular swelling because of an accompanying influx of water.

Secondary Active Transport. Secondary active transport mechanisms harness the energy derived from the primary active transport of one substance, usually sodium, for the cotransport of a second substance. For example, when sodium ions are actively transported out of a cell by primary active transport, a large concentration gradient develops (i.e., high concentration on the outside and low on the inside). This concentration gradient represents a large storehouse of energy because sodium ions are always attempting to diffuse into the cell. Similar to facilitated diffusion, secondary transport uses membrane transport proteins. These proteins have two binding sites: one for sodium and the other for the substance undergoing secondary transport. Secondary active transport systems are classified into two groups: cotransport, or symport systems, in which sodium and the solute are transported in the same direction, and countertransport, or antiport systems, in which sodium and the solute are transported in the opposite directions. An example of cotransport occurs in the intestine, where the absorption of glucose and amino acids is coupled with sodium transport.

Vesicular Transport

Vesicular transport is a mechanism in which materials are transported in membrane-bound vesicles. There are two types of vesicular transport: *endocytosis*, in which materials are moved into a cell in a vesicle formed from the cell membrane, and *exocytosis*, in which materials are moved out of a cell by fusion of a vesicle with the cell membrane.

Endocytosis is the process by which cells engulf materials from their surroundings. In the process, the material is progressively enclosed in small portions of the cell membrane, which first invaginates (folds inward) and then pinches off to become an endocytotic vesicle. If the vesicle is small (>150 nm in diameter), the process is called *pinocytosis*, and the vesicle is called a *pinocytotic vesicle*; if the vesicle is large (>250 nm in diameter), the process is called *phagocytosis*, and the vesicle is called a *phagosome*. The process of pinocytosis, which means "cell drinking," is important in the transport of proteins and strong solutions of electrolytes. Phagocytosis, which means "cell eating," involves the engulfment and subsequent killing or degradation of microorganisms and other particulate matter. Certain cells, such as macrophages and neutrophils, are adept at engulfing and disposing of invading organisms, damaged cells, and unneeded extracellular constituents.

Exocytosis is the mechanism for the secretion of intracellular substances into the extracellular spaces. It may be considered a reverse of endocytosis in that the membrane of the secretory granule fuses with the cell membrane and allows the contents of the granule to be released into the extracellular fluid. Exocytosis is important in removing cellular debris and releasing substances, such as hormones and cytokines, synthesized in the cell.

Receptor-mediated endocytosis involves the binding of substances to a receptor on the cell surface. Many of these receptor proteins are concentrated in *clathrin-coated pits*, which are specific areas of the cell where the membrane is lined on its cytoplasmic side by a peripheral protein called *clathrin*. The interaction between the proteins in the receptor–ligand complex causes the membrane to invaginate. The edges of the membrane around the clathrin-coated pit then fuse, and a portion of the membrane pinches off as an endocytic vesicle. Almost immediately after it is formed, the vesicle loses its clathrin coat and becomes fused with an early endosome in a manner similar to that involved in non–receptor-mediated endocytosis. The uptake of cholesterol transported in the blood as low-density lipoprotein (LDL) relies on receptor-mediated removal associated with clathrin-coated pits. This pathway for cholesterol removal is disrupted in persons who inherit defective genes for encoding LDL receptors (see Chapter 18).

In addition to clathrin-coated pits and vesicles, there are a number of other mechanisms by which cells can form endocytotic vesicles. One of these pathways involves the formation of small invaginations or "little cavities" in the cell membrane, called *caveolae*, that extend inward, indenting the cell membrane and the cytoplasm. These cavities may pinch off and form free vesicles within the cytoplasm. Caveolae are considered to be sites for uptake of material into the cell, for expulsion of material from the cell, and for addition or removal of cell membrane components. In smooth muscle, caveolae project into the cytoplasm and, analogous to the T tubules in striated muscle, play an important role in regulating intracellular calcium concentration and smooth muscle tone. In addition to transport, caveolae are involved in a number of other functions such as signal transduction and may be involved in the pathogenesis of a number of diseases, including muscular dystrophy.

Generation of Membrane Potentials

Living organisms have electrical properties in which current flow involves the movement of ions in water. Electrical potentials exist across the membranes of most cells in the body. Because these potentials occur at the level of the cell membrane, they are called *membrane potentials*. In excitable tissues, such as nerve or muscle cells, changes in the membrane potential are necessary for generation and conduction of nerve impulses and muscle contraction. In other types of cells, such as glandular cells, changes in the membrane potential contribute to hormone secretion and other functions.

Electrical potentials describe the ability of separated electrical charges of opposite polarity (+ and –) to do work. In regard to cells, the oppositely charged particles are ions, and the barrier that separates them is the cell membrane. Electrical potentials are measured in volts (V) or units of electromotive force (EMF). Voltage is always measured with respect to two points in a system. For example, the voltage in a car battery (6 or 12 V) is the potential difference between the two battery terminals. In a cell it is the potential difference between the inside and outside of the cell membrane. Because the total amount of charge that can be separated by a biologic membrane is small, the potential differences are small and are therefore measured in millivolts (mV), or 1/1000 of a volt.

There are two main factors that alter membrane potentials: the difference in the concentration of ions on the inside and outside of the membrane and the permeability of the membrane to these ions. Extracellular and intracellular fluids are electrolyte solutions containing approximately 150 to 160 mmol/L of positively charged ions and an equal concentration of negatively charged ions. The diffusion of these current-carrying ions is responsible for generating and conducting membrane potentials. A *diffusion potential* describes the voltage generated by ions that diffuse across the cell membrane.

An *equilibrium potential* is one in which there is no net movement of a particular ion across a membrane because the diffusion potential and electrical forces generated by the movement of the ion are exactly balanced. The magnitude of the equilibrium potential, also known as the *Nernst potential*, is determined by the ratio of the concentration of a specific ion on the two sides of the membrane. The greater the ratio, the greater the tendency for the ion to diffuse in one direction, and therefore the greater the electrical forces required to prevent further diffusion. The Nernst equation (described in the figure on Understanding Membrane Potentials) can be used to calculate the equilibrium potential for any univalent ion at a given concentration difference, assuming that membrane is permeable to the ion. When using the equation, it is generally assumed that the electrical potential of the extracellular fluid outside the membrane remains at zero and the potential being calculated is the electrical potential inside the membrane. It is also assumed that the sign of the potential is negative (–) if a positively charged ion diffuses from the inside to the outside of the membrane and positive (+) if a positively charged ion diffuses from the outside to the inside of the membrane.

The *resting membrane potential* represents the period of time when excitable cells, such as nerve fibers, are not transmitting signals. Because resting cell membranes are more permeable to potassium than sodium, the resting membrane reflects the diffusion of potassium ions. The Na$^+$/K$^+$-ATPase membrane pump, which removes three Na$^+$ from inside the cell while returning two K$^+$ to the inside, assists in maintaining the resting membrane potential. During an action potential, the cell membrane becomes more permeable to sodium, causing its polarity to change so that it is positive on the inside and negative on the outside (discussed in Chapter 34).

SUMMARY CONCEPTS

■ Cells communicate with each other by chemical messenger systems. Chemical messengers bind to receptors on or near the cell surface. There are three classes of cell surface receptor proteins: G protein-linked, enzyme-linked, and channel-linked. *G protein–linked receptors* rely on a class of molecules called G proteins that function as an on–off switch to convert external signals (first messengers) into internal signals (second messengers). *Enzyme-linked receptors* have intrinsic enzyme activity or rely on enzymes that are closely associated with the receptor they activate. One type of enzyme-linked receptor is widely used in hormonal control of cell function and involves the activation of the enzyme adenylyl cyclase, which catalyzes the formation of cAMP, a second messenger that has multiple effects inside the cell. Activation of *ion channel–linked receptors* (e.g., by neurotransmitters) may trigger signaling to transiently open or close ion channels formed by integral proteins in the cell.

■ Substances that enter or leave the cell must cross the cell membrane. *Diffusion* is a process by which substances such as ions move from areas of greater concentration to areas of lesser concentration until reaching a uniform distribution. *Facilitated diffusion* is a passive process, in which molecules that cannot normally pass through the cell's membranes do so with the assistance of a carrier molecule. *Active transport* requires the cell to expend energy in moving ions against a concentration gradient. The Na$^+$/K$^+$-ATPase membrane pump is the best-known type of active transport. *Vesicular transport* is a mechanism in which a cell encloses extracellular material in a membrane-bound vesicle. There are two types of vesicular transport: *endocytosis*, in which materials are brought into the cell by invagination of the cell membrane to form a vesicle, and *exocytosis*, in which materials are exported from the cell by fusion of a vesicle with the cell membrane.

■ Electrical potentials, which are measured in volts, describe the ability of separated electrical charges of opposite polarity (+ and −) to do work. In regard to cells, the oppositely charged particles are ions, and the barrier that separates them is the cell membrane. There are two main factors that alter membrane potentials and excitability: the difference in concentration of ions on the inside and outside of the membrane and the permeability of the membrane to these ions. An *equilibrium potential* is one in which there is no net movement of a particular ion across a membrane because the *diffusion* and *electrical forces* generated by the movement of the ions are exactly balanced. The resting membrane potential (− outside and + inside) is essentially a potassium equilibrium potential that results from the selective permeability of the membrane to the potassium ion and the large difference in potassium concentration that exists between the inside and the outside of the membrane. During an action potential, the cell membrane becomes highly permeable to sodium, causing it to depolarize and reverse its polarity (− inside and + outside).

Tissues

In the preceding sections, we discussed the individual cell, its metabolic processes, and mechanisms of signaling and communication. Although cells have similarities, their structures and functions vary according to the specific needs of the body. For example, muscle cells are specialized to perform different functions from skin cells or nerve cells. Groups of cells that are closely associated in structure and have common or similar functions are called *tissues*. Four categories of tissue exist: (1) epithelial, (2) connective, (3) muscle, and (4) nervous. These tissues do not exist in isolated units but in association with each other and in variable proportions, forming different structures and organs of the body. This section of the chapter provides a brief overview of the cells in each of the four tissue types, the structures that hold these cells together, and the extracellular matrix in which they live.

Embryonic Origin of Tissue Types

After conception, the fertilized ovum undergoes a series of divisions, ultimately forming different cell types that comprise the various tissues of the body. The formation of different, more specialized types of cells and

(*text continues on page 20*)

UNDERSTANDING ➡ Membrane Potentials

Electrochemical potentials are present across the membranes of virtually all cells in the body. Some cells, such as nerve and muscle cells, are capable of generating rapidly changing electrical impulses and transmitting these impulses along their membranes. Generation of membrane potentials relies on (1) diffusion of current-carrying ions, (2) development of an electrochemical equilibrium, and (3) establishment of a resting membrane potential and triggering an action potential.

1 **Diffusion potentials.** A diffusion potential is a potential difference generated across a membrane when a current-carrying ion, such as the potassium (K^+) ion, diffuses down its concentration gradient. Two conditions are necessary for this to occur: (1) the membrane must be selectively permeable to a particular ion, and (2) the concentration of the diffusible ion must be greater on one side of the membrane than the other.

The magnitude of the diffusion potential, measured in millivolts (mV), depends on the size of the concentration gradient. The sign (+ or −) or polarity of the potential depends on the diffusing ion. It is negative on the inside when a positively charged ion such as K^+ diffuses from the inside to the outside of the membrane, carrying its charge with it.

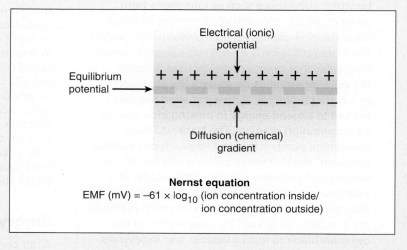

Concentration gradient for K^+

2 **Equilibrium potentials.** An equilibrium potential is the membrane potential that exactly balances and opposes the net diffusion of an ion down its concentration gradient. As a cation diffuses down its concentration gradient, it carries its positive charge across the membrane, thereby generating an electrical force that will eventually retard and stop its diffusion. An electrochemical equilibrium is one in which the *chemical forces* driving diffusion and the *repelling electrical forces* are exactly balanced so that no further diffusion occurs. The equilibrium potential (EMF, electromotive force) can be calculated by inserting the inside and outside ion concentrations into the Nernst Equation.

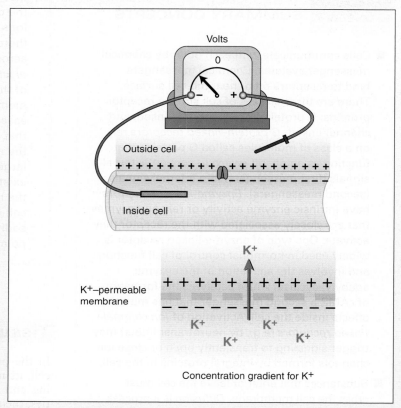

Nernst equation

EMF (mV) = −61 × $\log_{10}$ (ion concentration inside/ ion concentration outside)

③ Resting membrane potential (RMP). The RMP, which is necessary for electrical excitability, is present when the cell is not transmitting impulses. Because the resting membrane is permeable to K^+, it is essentially an K^+ equilibrium potential. This can be explained in terms of the large K^+ concentration gradient (e.g., 140 mEq/L inside and 4 mEq/L outside), which causes the positively charged K^+ to diffuse outward, leaving the nondiffusible, negatively charged intracellular anions (A^-) behind. This causes the membrane to become polarized, with negative charges aligned along the inside and positive charges along the outside. The Na^+/K^+ membrane pump, which removes three Na^+ from inside while returning only two K^+ to the inside, contributes to the maintenance of the RMP.

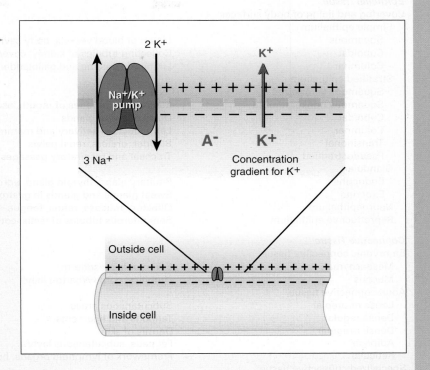

④ Action potentials. Action potentials involve rapid changes in the membrane potential. Each action potential begins with a sudden change from the negative RMP to a positive threshold potential, causing an opening of the membrane channels for Na^+ (or other ions of the action potential). Opening of the Na^+ channels allows large amounts of the positively charged Na^+ ions to diffuse to the interior of the cell, causing the membrane potential to undergo depolarization or a rapid change to positive on the inside and negative on the outside. This is rapidly followed by closing of Na^+ channels and opening of the K^+ channels, which leads to a rapid efflux of K^+ from the cell and reestablishment of the RMP.

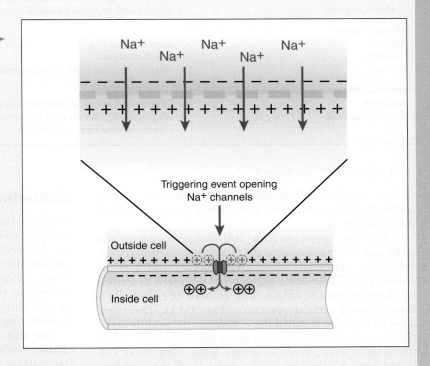

TABLE 1-1	Classification of Tissue Types
Tissue Type	**Location**
Epithelial Tissue	
Covering and lining of body surfaces	
Simple epithelium	
Squamous	Lining of blood vessels, body cavities, alveoli of lungs
Cuboidal	Collecting tubules of kidney; covering of ovaries
Columnar	Lining of intestine and gallbladder
Stratified epithelium	
Squamous keratinized	Skin
Squamous nonkeratinized	Mucous membranes of mouth, esophagus, and vagina
Cuboidal	Ducts of sweat glands
Columnar	Large ducts of salivary and mammary glands; also found in conjunctiva
Transitional	Bladder, ureters, renal pelvis
Pseudostratified	Tracheal and respiratory passages
Glandular	
Endocrine	Pituitary gland, thyroid gland, adrenal and other glands
Exocrine	Sweat glands and glands in gastrointestinal tract
Neuroepithelium	Olfactory mucosa, retina, tongue
Reproductive epithelium	Seminiferous tubules of testis; cortical portion of ovary
Connective Tissue	
Embryonic connective tissue	
Mesenchymal	Embryonic mesoderm
Mucous	Umbilical cord (Wharton jelly)
Adult connective tissue	
Loose or areolar	Subcutaneous areas
Dense regular	Tendons and ligaments
Dense irregular	Dermis of skin
Adipose	Fat pads, subcutaneous layers
Reticular	Framework of lymphoid organs, bone marrow, liver
Specialized connective tissue	
Bone	Long bones, flat bones
Cartilage	Tracheal rings, external ear, articular surfaces
Hematopoietic	Blood cells, myeloid tissue (bone marrow)
Muscle Tissue	
Skeletal	Skeletal muscles
Cardiac	Heart muscles
Smooth	Gastrointestinal tract, blood vessels, bronchi, bladder, and others
Nervous Tissue	
Neurons	Central and peripheral neurons and nerve fibers
Supporting cells	Glial and ependymal cells in central nervous system; Schwann and satellite cells in peripheral nervous system

(*text continued from page 17*)

tissues is called *cell differentiation*, a process that is controlled by mechanisms that switch genes on and off (see Chapter 4).

All of the approximately 200 different cells of the body can be classified into the four basic or primary tissue types: epithelial, connective, muscle, and nervous (Table 1-1). These basic tissue types are often described by their embryonic origin. The embryo is essentially a three-layered tubular structure (Fig. 1-13). The outer layer of the tube is called the *ectoderm*; the middle layer, the *mesoderm*; and the inner layer, the *endoderm*. All of the mature tissue types originate from these three cellular layers. Epithelium has its origin in all three embryonic layers, connective tissue and muscle develop mainly from the mesoderm, and nervous tissue develops from the ectoderm.

Epithelial Tissue

Epithelial tissue forms sheets that cover the body's outer surface, line the internal surfaces, and form glandular tissue. Underneath all types of epithelial tissue is a fibrous extracellular layer, called the *basement membrane*, which serves to attach the epithelial cells to adjacent connective tissue and may serve other functions, such as providing a barrier against cancer cell invasion and contributing to the filtration function of the glomerulus.

The cells that make up epithelium have three general characteristics: (1) they have three distinct surfaces: a free surface or apical surface, a lateral surface, and a basal surface; (2) they are closely apposed and joined by cell-to-cell adhesion molecules, which form specialized cell junctions; and (3) their basal surface is attached

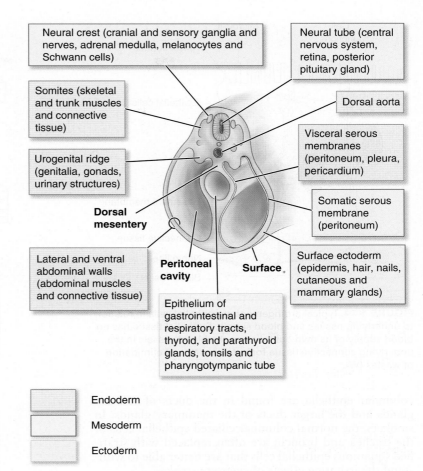

Neural crest (cranial and sensory ganglia and nerves, adrenal medulla, melanocytes and Schwann cells)

Neural tube (central nervous system, retina, posterior pituitary gland)

Somites (skeletal and trunk muscles and connective tissue)

Dorsal aorta

Visceral serous membranes (peritoneum, pleura, pericardium)

Urogenital ridge (genitalia, gonads, urinary structures)

Dorsal mesentery

Somatic serous membrane (peritoneum)

Lateral and ventral abdominal walls (abdominal muscles and connective tissue)

Peritoneal cavity

Surface

Surface ectoderm (epidermis, hair, nails, cutaneous and mammary glands)

Epithelium of gastrointestinal and respiratory tracts, thyroid, and parathyroid glands, tonsils and pharyngotympanic tube

Endoderm

Mesoderm

Ectoderm

FIGURE 1-13. Cross-section of human embryo illustrating the development of the somatic and visceral structures.

to the underlying basement membrane (Fig. 1-14). The characteristics and geometric arrangement of the cells in the epithelium contribute to their function. In an epithelium formed from a single layer of epithelial cells, the free or apical surface is directed toward the exterior surface or lumen of an enclosed cavity or tube, the lateral surface communicates with adjacent cells and is characterized by specialized attachment areas, and the basal surface rests on the basement membrane anchoring the cell to the surrounding connective tissue.

Epithelial tissues are classified according to the shape of the cells and the number of layers that are present: simple, stratified, and pseudostratified. Glandular epithelial tissue is formed by cells specialized to produce a fluid secretion. The terms *squamous* (thin and flat), *cuboidal* (cube shaped), and *columnar* (resembling a column) refer to the cells' shape (Fig. 1-15).

Simple Epithelium

Simple epithelium contains a single layer of cells, all of which rest on the basement membrane. Simple squamous epithelium is adapted for filtration; it is found lining the blood vessels, lymph nodes, and alveoli of the lungs. The single layer of squamous epithelium lining the heart and blood vessels is known as the *endothelium*. A similar type of layer, called the *mesothelium*, forms the serous

membranes that line the pleural, pericardial, and peritoneal cavities and covers the organs of these cavities. A *simple cuboidal epithelium* is found on the surface of the ovary and in the thyroid. *Simple columnar epithelium* lines the intestine. One form of a simple columnar epithelium has hair-like projections called *cilia*, often with specialized mucus-secreting cells called *goblet cells*. This form of simple columnar epithelium lines the airways of the respiratory tract.

Stratified and Pseudostratified Epithelium

Stratified epithelium contains more than one layer of cells, with only the deepest layer resting on the basement membrane. It is designed to protect the body surface. *Stratified squamous keratinized epithelium* makes up the epidermis of the skin. *Keratin* is a tough, fibrous protein that polymerizes to form intermediate filaments that are abundant in the outer cells of skin. A stratified squamous keratinized epithelium is made up of many layers. The layers closest to the underlying tissues are cuboidal or columnar. The cells become more irregular and thinner as they move closer to the surface. Surface cells become totally filled with keratin and die, are sloughed off, and then replaced by the deeper cells. A stratified squamous nonkeratinized epithelium is found on moist surfaces such as the mouth and tongue. Stratified cuboidal and

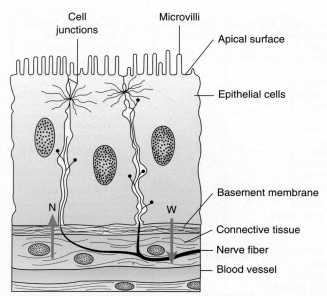

FIGURE 1-14. Typical arrangement of epithelial cells in relation to underlying tissues and blood supply. Epithelial tissue has no blood supply of its own but relies on the blood vessels in the underlying connective tissue for nutrition (N) and elimination of wastes (W).

columnar epithelia are found in the ducts of salivary glands and the larger ducts of the mammary glands. In smokers, the normal columnar ciliated epithelial cells of the trachea and bronchi are often replaced with stratified squamous epithelial cells that are better able to withstand the irritating effects of cigarette smoke.

Pseudostratified epithelium is a type of epithelium in which all of the cells are in contact with the underlying intercellular matrix, but some do not extend to the surface. A pseudostratified ciliated columnar epithelium with goblet cells forms the lining of most of the upper respiratory tract. All of the tall cells reaching the surface of this type of epithelium are either ciliated cells or mucus-producing goblet cells. The basal cells that do not reach the surface serve as stem cells for ciliated and goblet cells.

Transitional epithelium is a stratified epithelium characterized by cells that can change shape and become thinner when the tissue is stretched. Such tissue can be stretched without pulling the superficial cells apart. Transitional epithelium is well adapted for the lining of organs that are constantly changing their volume, such as the urinary bladder.

Glandular Epithelium

Glandular epithelial tissue is formed by cells specialized to produce a fluid secretion. This process is usually accompanied by the intracellular synthesis of macromolecules. The chemical nature of these macromolecules is variable. The macromolecules typically are stored in the cells in small membrane-bound vesicles called *secretory granules*. For example, glandular epithelia can synthesize, store, and secrete proteins (e.g., insulin), lipids (e.g., adrenocortical hormones), secretions of the sebaceous

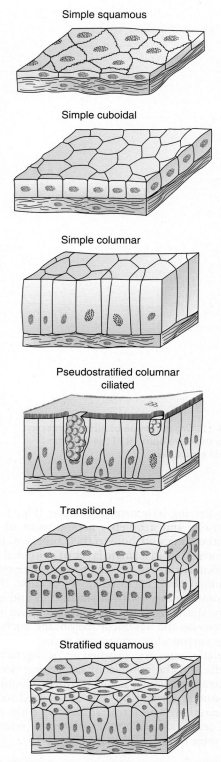

FIGURE 1-15. Representation of the various epithelial tissue types.

glands), and complexes of carbohydrates and proteins (e.g., saliva). Less common are secretions that require minimal synthetic activity, such as those produced by the sweat glands.

All glandular cells arise from surface epithelia by means of cell proliferation and invasion of the underlying connective tissue. Epithelial glands can be divided into two groups: exocrine and endocrine glands. Exocrine glands, such as the sweat glands and lactating mammary glands, retain their connection with the surface epithelium from which they originated. This connection takes the form of epithelium-lined tubular ducts through which the secretions pass to reach the surface. Endocrine glands are epithelial structures that have had their connection with the surface obliterated during development. These glands are ductless and produce secretions (i.e., hormones) that move directly into the bloodstream.

Epithelial Cell Renewal

Cells making up the epithelial tissues generally exhibit a high rate of turnover, which is related to their location and function. The rate of cell turnover is characteristic of specific epithelium. For example, the epithelial cells of the small intestine are renewed every 4 to 6 days by regenerative cells in the lower portion of the intestinal glands (crypts). Similarly, the cells of the stratified squamous epithelium of the skin are constantly being renewed at the basal layer by cell division.

Connective Tissue

Connective or supportive tissue is the most abundant tissue in the body. As its name suggests, it connects and binds or supports the various tissues. Connective tissue is unique in that its cells produce the extracellular matrix that supports and holds tissues together. The proximity of the extracellular matrix to blood vessels allows it to function as an exchange medium through which nutrients and metabolic wastes pass.

The functions of the various connective tissues are reflected by the types of cells and fibers present in the tissue and the characteristics of the extracellular matrix (Fig. 1-16). The capsules that surround organs of the body are composed of connective tissue. Bone, adipose tissue, and cartilage are specialized types of connective tissue that function to support the soft tissues of the body and store fat. One type of cell, the fibroblast, is responsible for synthesis of collagen, elastic, reticular fibers, and ground substance of the extracellular matrix. Other cells, such as lymphocytes, plasma cells, macrophages, and eosinophils, are associated with body defense systems.

Adult connective tissue can be divided into two types: connective tissue proper, which is the focus of the discussion in this chapter, and specialized connective tissue (cartilage, bone, and blood cells), which is discussed in other chapters. There are four recognized types of connective tissue proper: loose (areolar), adipose, reticular, and dense connective tissue.

Loose Connective Tissue

Loose connective tissue, also known as areolar tissue, is soft and pliable. It fills spaces between muscle sheaths, forms a layer that encases blood and lymphatic vessels, and provides support for epithelial tissues and the means

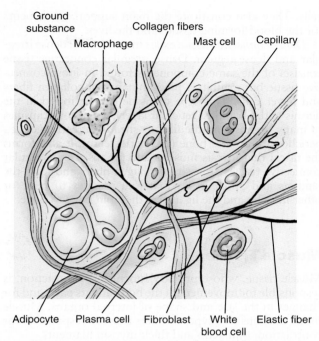

FIGURE 1-16. Diagrammatic representation of cells that may be seen in loose connective tissue. The cells lie in an intercellular matrix that is bathed in tissue fluid that originates in the capillaries.

by which these tissues are nourished. Loose connective tissue is characterized by an abundance of ground substance and tissue fluid housing the fixed connective tissue cells: fibroblasts, mast cells, adipose or fat cells, macrophages, and leukocytes. Fibroblasts are the most abundant of these cells. They produce all three fiber types—collagen, elastic, and reticular fibers—found in loose connective tissue, and synthesize the ground substance that fills the intercellular tissue spaces.

Adipose Tissue

Adipose tissue is a special form of connective tissue in which adipocytes predominate. Adipocytes do not generate an extracellular matrix but maintain a large intracellular space. These cells store large quantities of triglycerides and are the largest repository of energy in the body. Adipose tissue helps fill spaces between tissues and to keep organs in place. The subcutaneous fat helps to shape the body. Because fat is a poor conductor of heat, adipose tissue serves as thermal insulation for the body. Adipose tissue exists in two forms: unilocular and multilocular. Unilocular (white) adipose tissue is composed of cells in which the fat is contained in a single, large droplet in the cytoplasm. Multilocular (brown) adipose tissue is composed of cells that contain multiple droplets of fat and numerous mitochondria.

Reticular and Dense Connective Tissue

Reticular and dense connective tissue is characterized by a network of fibers interspersed with macrophages and fibroblasts that synthesize collagen fibers. *Reticular fibers* provide the framework for capillaries, nerves, and muscle cells. They also constitute the main supporting elements for the blood-forming tissues and the liver.

Dense connective tissue exists in two forms: dense irregular and dense regular. Dense irregular connective tissue consists of the same components found in loose connective tissue but exhibits a predominance of collagen fibers and fewer cells. This type of tissue can be found in the dermis of the skin (i.e., reticular layer), the fibrous capsules of many organs, and the fibrous sheaths of cartilage (i.e., perichondrium) and bone (i.e., periosteum). It also forms the fascia that invests muscles and organs. Dense regular connective tissues are rich in collagen fibers and form the tendons and aponeuroses that join muscles to bone or other muscles and the ligaments that join bone to bone.

Muscle Tissue

Muscle tissue, whose primary function is contraction, is responsible for movement of the body and its parts and for changes in the size and shape of internal organs. Muscle tissue contains two types of fibers that are responsible for contraction: thin actin and thick myosin filaments.

There are three types of muscle tissues: skeletal, cardiac, and smooth. *Skeletal* and *cardiac muscles* are striated muscles, in which the actin and myosin filaments are arranged in large parallel arrays in bundles, giving the muscle fibers a striped or striated appearance when observed with a microscope. *Smooth muscle* lacks striations and is found in the iris of the eye; the walls of blood vessels; hollow organs, such as the stomach and urinary bladder; and hollow tubes, such as the ureters and common bile duct that connect internal organs.

Although the three types of muscle tissues differ significantly in structure, contractile properties, and control mechanisms, they have many similarities. In the following section, the structural properties of skeletal muscle are presented as the prototype of striated muscle tissue. Smooth muscle and the ways in which it differs from skeletal muscle are also discussed. Cardiac muscle is described in Chapter 17.

Skeletal Muscle

Skeletal muscle is the most abundant tissue in the body, accounting for 40% to 45% of the total body weight. Most skeletal muscles are attached to bones, and their contractions are responsible for movements of the skeleton.

Skeletal Muscle Structure. Skeletal muscle fibers are packaged into skeletal muscles that attach to and cover the body skeleton. Each skeletal muscle is a discrete organ made up of hundreds or thousands of muscle fibers. Although muscle fibers predominate, substantial amounts of connective tissue, blood vessels, and nerve fibers are present. In an intact muscle, several different layers of connective tissue hold the individual muscle fibers together. Skeletal muscles such as the biceps brachii are surrounded by a dense irregular connective tissue covering called the *epimysium* (Fig. 1-17A). Each muscle is subdivided into smaller bundles called *fascicles*, which are surrounded by a connective tissue covering called the *perimysium*. The number of fascicles and their size vary among muscles. Fascicles consist of many elongated structures called *muscle fibers*, each of which is surrounded by connective tissue called the *endomysium*.

Skeletal muscles are syncytial or multinucleated structures, meaning there are no true cell boundaries within a skeletal muscle fiber. The cytoplasm or sarcoplasm of the muscle fiber is contained within the sarcolemma, which

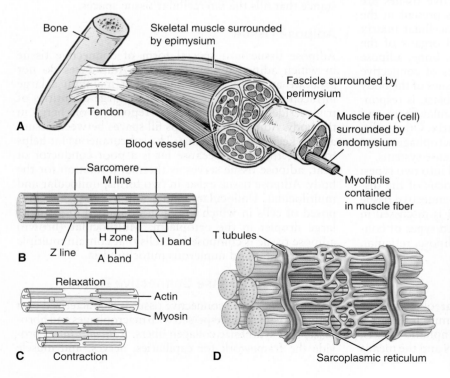

FIGURE 1-17. **(A)** Connective tissue components of a skeletal muscle. **(B)** Striations of the myofibril showing the overlap of contractile proteins and the A and I bands, the H zone, and the Z and M lines. **(C)** The relaxed and contracted states of the myofibril showing the position of actin filaments (*blue*) between the myosin filaments (*pink*) in the relaxed muscle (*top*) and pulling of the Z membranes toward each other (*bottom*) as the muscle contracts. **(D)** The sarcoplasmic reticulum with T tubules.

represents the cell membrane. Embedded throughout the sarcoplasm are the contractile elements actin and myosin, which are arranged in parallel bundles (i.e., *myofibrils*). Each myofibril consists of regularly repeating units called *sarcomeres* along its length.

Sarcomeres, which are the structural and functional units of striated muscle, extend from one Z line to another Z line (Fig. 1-17B). The central portion of the sarcomere contains the dark band (A band) consisting mainly of myosin filaments, with some overlap with actin filaments. Straddling the Z line, the lighter I band contains only actin filaments; therefore, it takes two sarcomeres to complete an I band. An H zone is found in the middle of the A band and represents the region where only myosin filaments are found. In the center of the H zone is a thin, dark band, the M band or M line, produced by linkages between the myosin filaments. Z lines consist of short elements that interconnect and provide the thin actin filaments from two adjoining sarcomeres with an anchoring point. Muscle contraction involves the actin filaments sliding inward among the myosin filaments (Fig. 1-17C). In the relaxed state, the ends of the actin filaments extend from two successive Z lines, barely overlapping one another. In the contracted state, these actin filaments have been pulled inward among the myosin filaments so their ends overlap one another.

The *sarcoplasmic reticulum*, which is comparable to the smooth ER, is composed of longitudinal tubules that run parallel to the muscle fiber and surround each myofibril (Fig. 1-17D). This network ends in enlarged, saclike regions called the *lateral sacs* or *terminal cisternae*. These sacs store calcium that is released during muscle contraction. A second system of tubules consists of the *transverse* or *T tubules*, which are extensions of the cell membrane and run perpendicular to the muscle fiber. The hollow portion or lumen of the T tubule is continuous with the extracellular fluid compartment. Action potentials, which are rapidly conducted over the surface of the muscle fiber, are in turn propagated by the T tubules into the sarcoplasmic reticulum. As the action potential moves through the lateral sacs, the sacs release calcium, initiating muscle contraction. The membrane of the sarcoplasmic reticulum also has an active transport mechanism for pumping calcium ions back into the reticulum. This prevents interactions between calcium ions and the actin and myosin myofilaments after cessation of a muscle contraction.

Skeletal Muscle Contraction. Muscle contraction involves the sliding of the thick myosin and thin actin filaments over each other to produce shortening of the muscle fiber, while the actual length of the individual thick and thin filaments remains unchanged. The thick myosin filaments consist of a thin tail, which provides the structural backbone for the filament, and a globular head that forms cross-bridges with the thin actin filaments (Fig. 1-18A). Myosin molecules are bundled together side by side in the thick filaments such that one half have their heads toward one end of the filament and their tails toward the other end, and the other half are arranged in the opposite manner. Each globular myosin head contains a site able to bind to a complementary site on the actin molecule. Besides the binding site for actin, each myosin head has a separate active site that catalyzes the breakdown of ATP to provide the energy needed to activate the myosin head so it can form a cross-bridge with actin. After contraction, myosin also

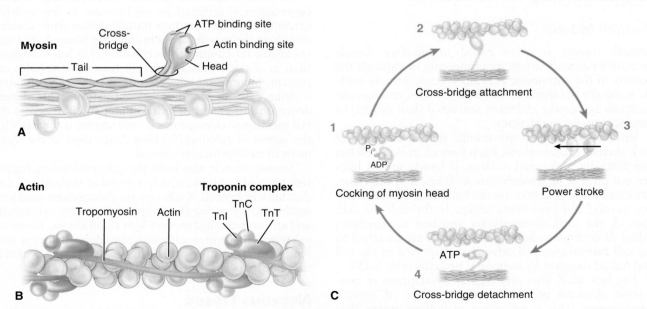

FIGURE 1-18. Molecular structure of the thicker myosin filament (**A**) and the thinner actin filament (**B**) of striated muscle. The thin filament is a double-stranded helix of actin molecules with tropomyosin and troponin molecules lying along the grooves of the actin strands. (**C**) Sequence of events involved in sliding of adjacent actin and myosin filaments: (1) cocking of the myosin head, which occurs as adenosine triphosphate (ATP) is split to adenosine diphosphate (ADP); (2) cross-bridge attachment; (3) power stroke during which the myosin head bends as it moves the actin forward; and (4) cross-bridge detachment, which occurs as a new ATP attaches to the myosin head.

binds ATP, thus breaking the linkage between actin and myosin.

The thin filaments are composed mainly of actin, a globular protein lined up in two rows that coil around each other to form a long helical strand (Fig. 1-18B). Associated with each actin filament are two regulatory proteins, tropomyosin and troponin. *Tropomyosin*, which lies in grooves of the actin strand, provides the site for attachment of the globular heads of the myosin filament. In the noncontracted state, *troponin* covers the tropomyosin-binding sites and prevents formation of cross-bridges between the actin and myosin. During an action potential, calcium ions released from the sarcoplasmic reticulum diffuse to the adjacent myofibrils, where they bind to troponin. The binding of calcium to troponin uncovers the tropomyosin-binding sites such that the myosin heads can attach and form cross-bridges.

Muscle contraction begins with activation of the cross-bridges from the myosin filaments and uncovering of the tropomyosin-binding sites on the actin filament (Fig. 1-18C). When activated by ATP, the heads of the myosin filaments swivel in a fixed arc, much like the oars of a boat, as they become attached to the actin filament. During contraction, each myosin head undergoes its own cycle of movement, forming a bridge attachment and releasing it, then moving to another site where the same sequence of movement occurs. This pulls the thin and thick filaments past each other. Energy from ATP is used to break the actin and myosin cross-bridges, stopping the muscle contraction. After the linkage between actin and myosin, the concentration of calcium around the myofibrils decreases as calcium is actively transported into the sarcoplasmic reticulum by a membrane pump that uses energy derived from ATP.

Smooth Muscle

Smooth muscle is often called *involuntary muscle* because its activity arises spontaneously or through the activity of the autonomic nervous system. Smooth muscle is usually arranged in sheets or bundles and its contractions are slower and more sustained than skeletal or cardiac muscle contractions.

Smooth muscle cells are spindle shaped and smaller than skeletal muscle fibers. Each smooth muscle cell has one centrally positioned nucleus. Z bands and M lines are not present in smooth muscle fibers, and the cross-striations are absent because the bundles of filaments are not parallel but criss-cross obliquely through the cell. Instead, the actin filaments are attached to structures called *dense bodies*. Some dense bodies are attached to the cell membrane, and others are dispersed in the cell and linked together by structural proteins (Fig. 1-19).

The lack of Z lines and regular overlapping of contractile elements provide a greater range of tension development. This is important in hollow organs that undergo changes in volume, with consequent changes in the length of the smooth muscle fibers in their walls. Even with the distention of a hollow organ, the smooth muscle fiber retains some ability to develop tension, whereas such distention would stretch skeletal muscle beyond the area where the thick and thin filaments overlap.

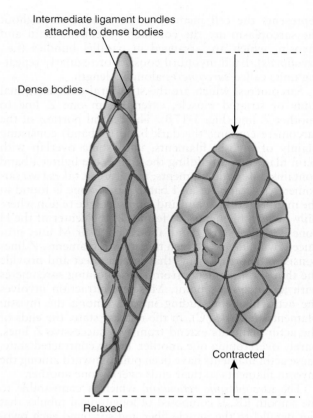

FIGURE 1-19. Structure of smooth muscle showing the dense bodies. In smooth muscle, the force of contraction is transmitted to the cell membrane by bundles of intermediate fibers.

As with cardiac and skeletal muscle, smooth muscle contraction is initiated by an increase in intracellular calcium. However, smooth muscle differs from skeletal muscle in the way its cross-bridges are formed. The sarcoplasmic reticulum of smooth muscle is less developed than in skeletal muscle, and no transverse tubules are present. Smooth muscle relies on the entrance of extracellular calcium for muscle contraction. This dependence on movement of extracellular calcium across the cell membrane during muscle contraction is the basis for the action of calcium-blocking drugs used in the treatment of cardiovascular disease.

Smooth muscle also lacks the calcium-binding regulatory protein troponin, which is found in skeletal and cardiac muscle. Instead, it relies on another calcium-regulated mechanism involving the cytoplasmic protein calmodulin and an enzyme called myosin light chain kinase. Increased calcium ions form a calcium–calmodulin complex that binds to and activates myosin light chain kinase, which in turn phosphorylates myosin to initiate contraction.

Nervous Tissue

Nervous tissue is distributed throughout the body as an integrated communication system. Nerve cells, which develop from the embryonic ectoderm, are highly differentiated and have long been considered incapable of regeneration in postnatal life. However, it is now known that parts of the brain, such as the hippocampus, contain areas where neurogenesis occurs from neural stem cells/ progenitor cells throughout life. Embryonic development of the nervous system and the structure and functions of the nervous system are discussed more fully in Chapter 34.

Structurally, nervous tissue consists of two cell types: nerve cells or neurons and supporting cells or neuroglia. Most nerve cells consist of three parts: the soma or cell body, dendrites, and the axon. The cytoplasm-filled dendrites, which are multiple elongated processes, receive and carry stimuli from the environment, sensory epithelial cells, and other neurons to the cell. The axon, which is a single cytoplasm-filled process, is specialized for generating and conducting nerve impulses away from the cell body to other nerve cells, muscle cells, and glandular cells.

Neurons can be classified as afferent and efferent neurons according to their function. Afferent or sensory neurons carry information toward the central nervous system; they are involved in the reception of sensory information from the external environment and from within the body. Efferent or motor neurons carry information away from the central nervous system (CNS); they are needed for control of muscle fibers and endocrine and exocrine glands.

Communication between neurons and effector organs, such as muscle cells, occurs at specialized structures called *synapses*. At the synapse, chemical messengers (i.e., neurotransmitters) alter the membrane potential to conduct impulses from one nerve to another or from a neuron to an effector cell. In addition, electrical synapses exist in which nerve cells are linked through gap junctions that permit the passage of ions from one cell to another.

Neuroglia (*glia* means "glue") are the cells that support neurons, form myelin, and have trophic and phagocytic functions. Four types of neuroglia are found in the CNS: astrocytes, oligodendrocytes, microglia, and ependymal cells. Astrocytes are the most abundant of the neuroglia. They have many long processes that surround blood vessels in the CNS. They provide structural support for the neurons, and their extensions form a sealed barrier that protects the CNS. In last decade, investigations have established important roles for astrocytes in the response of the brain to injury, calcium ion-based excitation, CNS metabolism, neural stem cell source, blood–brain barrier maintenance, and numerous diseases and pathological conditions. The oligodendrocytes provide myelination of neuronal processes in the CNS. The microglia are phagocytic cells that represent the mononuclear phagocytic system in the nervous system. Ependymal cells line the cavities of the brain and spinal cord and are in contact with the cerebrospinal fluid. In the peripheral nervous system, supporting cells consist of the Schwann and satellite cells. The Schwann cells provide myelination of the axons and dendrites, and the satellite cells enclose and protect the dorsal root ganglia and autonomic ganglion cells.

Extracellular Tissue Components

The discussion thus far has focused on the cellular components of the different tissue types. Within tissues, cells are held together by cell junctions, and adhesion molecules form intercellular contacts.

Cell Junctions

The junctions between tissue cells are important in governing the shape of the body, transmitting mechanical stresses from one cell to another, and creating pathways for communication. Cell junctions occur at many points in cell-to-cell contact, but they are particularly plentiful and important in epithelial tissue. These specialized junctions enable cells to form barriers to the movement of water, solutes, and cells from one body compartment to the next. Three basic types of intercellular junctions are observed: tight junctions, adhering junctions, and gap junctions (Fig. 1-20).

Tight or *occluding junctions* (i.e., zonula occludens), which are found in epithelial tissue, seal the surface membranes of adjacent cells together. This type of intercellular junction prevents fluids and materials such as macromolecules present in the intestinal contents from entering the intercellular space.

Adhering junctions represent sites of strong adhesion between cells. The primary role of adhering junctions may be that of preventing cell separation. Adhering junctions are not restricted to epithelial tissue; they provide adherence between adjacent cardiac muscle cells as well. Adhering junctions are found as continuous, beltlike adhesive junctions (i.e., zonula adherens) or scattered, spotlike adhesive junctions, called *desmosomes* (i.e., macula adherens). A special feature of the adhesion belt junction is that it provides an anchoring site to the cell membrane for actin filaments. In epithelial desmosomes, bundles of keratin intermediate filaments (i.e., tonofilaments) are anchored to the junction on the cytoplasmic area of the cell membrane. A primary disease of desmosomes is pemphigus, which is caused by antibody binding to the desmosome proteins and the resulting separation of neighboring cells. Affected persons have skin and mucous membrane blistering. *Hemidesmosomes*, which resemble a half desmosome, are another type of junction. They are found at the base of epithelial cells and help attach the epithelial cell to the underlying connective tissue.

Gap or *nexus junctions* involve the close adherence of adjoining cell membranes with the formation of channels that connect the cytoplasm of the two cells. Because they are low-resistance channels, gap junctions are important in cell-to-cell conduction of electrical signals (e.g., between cells in sheets of smooth muscle or between adjacent cardiac muscle cells, where they function as electrical synapses). Gap junctions also enable ions and small molecules to pass directly from one cell to another.

Extracellular Matrix

Tissues are not made up solely of cells. A large part of their volume is made up of an extracellular matrix. This matrix is composed of a variety of proteins and polysaccharides (i.e., polymers made up of many sugar monomers). These proteins and polysaccharides are secreted locally and are organized into a supporting meshwork in close association with the cells that produced them. The amount and composition of the matrix vary with the different tissues and their function. In bone, for example, the matrix is more plentiful than the cells that surround it; in the brain, the cells are much more abundant and the matrix is only a minor constituent.

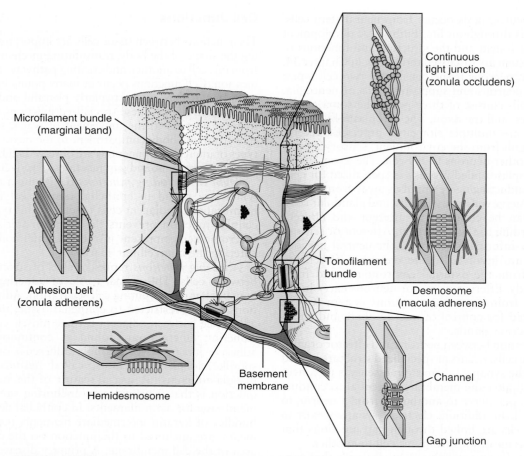

Continuous tight junction (zonula occludens)

Microfilament bundle (marginal band)

Tonofilament bundle

Adhesion belt (zonula adherens)

Desmosome (macula adherens)

Hemidesmosome

Basement membrane

Channel

Gap junction

FIGURE 1-20. Three types of intercellular junctions found in epithelial tissue: the continuous tight junction (zonula occludens); the adhering junction, which includes the adhesion belt (zonula adherens), desmosomes (macula adherens), and hemidesmosomes; and the gap junction.

Two main classes of extracellular macromolecules make up the extracellular matrix. The first is an amorphous gel-like material called *ground substance*. Ground substance is composed of polysaccharide chains of proteins called *glycosaminoglycans* (GAGs), which are usually found linked to protein as proteoglycans. The second type consists of the fibrous proteins (i.e., collagen and elastin) and the fibrous adhesive proteins (i.e., fibronectin and laminin) that are found in the basement membrane. Members of each of these two classes of extracellular macromolecules come in a variety of shapes and sizes.

Ground Substance. The proteoglycan and GAG molecules form a highly hydrated, gel-like substance, or tissue gel, in which the fibrous proteins are embedded. The polysaccharide gel resists compressive forces; the collagen fibers strengthen and help organize the matrix; the rubberlike elastin adds resilience; and the adhesive proteins help cells attach to the appropriate part of the matrix. Polysaccharides in the tissue gel are highly hydrophilic, and they form gels even at low concentrations. They also produce a negative charge that attracts cations such as sodium, which are osmotically active, causing large amounts of water to be sucked into the matrix. This creates a swelling pressure, or turgor, that enables the matrix to withstand extensive compressive forces. For example,

the cartilage matrix that lines the knee joint can support pressures of hundreds of atmospheres by this mechanism.

Fibrous Proteins. Three types of fibers are found in the extracellular space: collagen, elastin, and reticular fibers. *Collagen* is the most common protein in the body. It is a tough, nonliving, white fiber that serves as the structural framework for skin, ligaments, tendons, and many other structures. *Elastin* acts like a rubber band; it can be stretched and then returns to its original form. Elastin fibers are abundant in structures subjected to frequent stretching, such as the aorta and some ligaments. *Reticular fibers* are extremely thin fibers that create a flexible network in organs subjected to changes in form or volume, such as the spleen, liver, uterus, or intestinal muscle layer.

Cell Adhesion Molecules

Important classes of extracellular macromolecules are the cell adhesion molecules (CAMs). Cell adhesion molecules can be cell-to-cell or cell-to-matrix adhesion molecules. There are four major classes of CAMs: cadherins, selectins, integrins, and the immunoglobulin (Ig) superfamily of proteins. These proteins are located on the cell surface where they function as receptors, or they can be stored in the cytoplasm. As receptors, CAMs can bind to similar or different molecules in other cells, providing for interaction between the same cell types or different cell types.

Cadherins. Cadherins are the major CAMs responsible for calcium-dependent cell-to-cell adhesion junctions. The word *cadherin* is derived from the term "calcium-dependent adhesion protein." There are over 90 members of the cadherin superfamily. The first three cadherins that were discovered were named according to the main tissues in which they were found: the E-cadherins, which are present in many types of epithelial cells; the N-cadherins, which are present in nerve and muscle cells; and the P-cadherins, which are found on cells in the placenta and epidermis. All are found in various other tissues; N-cadherin, for example, is expressed in fibroblasts, and E-cadherin is expressed in parts of the brain.

Most cadherins function as transmembrane adhesive proteins that indirectly link the actin cytoskeletons of cells they join together, an arrangement that occurs in adhering junctions. Cadherins also form desmosomes that interact with intermediate filaments of the cytoskeleton, rather than the actin filaments. Cell-to-cell interactions mediated by cadherins play a major role in regulating cell motility, proliferation, and differentiation.

Selectins. Selectins are cell surface carbohydrate-binding proteins (lectins) that mediate a variety of transient, cell-to-cell adhesion interactions in the bloodstream. They are found on activated endothelial cells of blood vessels, on leukocytes, and on platelets. Selectins, together with integrins and immunoglobulins, participate in leukocyte movement through the endothelial lining of blood vessels during inflammation.

Integrins. Integrins usually assist in attaching epithelial cells to the underlying basement membrane. Extracellularly, they are attached to fibronectin and laminin, the two major components of the basement membrane. Like the cadherins, their intracellular portion is linked to actin. One group of integrins is associated with hemidesmosomes, whereas others are associated with the surface of white blood cells, macrophages, and platelets. Integrins usually have a weak affinity for their ligands unless they are associated with cellular focal contacts and hemidesmosomes. This allows some movement between cells except where a firm attachment is required to attach epithelial cells to the underlying connective tissue.

Certain integrins play an important role in allowing white blood cells to pass through the vessel wall, a process called *transmigration*. Persons affected with leukocyte adhesion deficiency are unable to synthesize appropriate integrin molecules. As a result, they experience repeated bacterial infections because their white blood cells are not able to transmigrate through vessel walls.

Immunoglobulin Superfamily. The Ig superfamily consists of a group of one or more immunoglobulin-like adhesion proteins that are similar structurally to those of antibody molecules. They have many functions outside the immune system that are unrelated to immune defenses. The best-studied example of Ig superfamily proteins are the neural cell adhesion molecules (N-CAMs), which are expressed in a variety of cells, including most nerve cells. During early development, N-CAMs play an important role in connecting the neurons of the developing nervous system.

SUMMARY CONCEPTS

- Body cells are organized into four basic tissue types: epithelial, connective, muscle, and nervous. The epithelium covers and lines the body surfaces and forms the functional components of glandular structures. Epithelial tissue is classified into three types according to the shape of the cells and the number of layers that are present: simple, stratified, and pseudostratified.

- Connective tissue supports and connects body structures; it forms the bones and cartilage, the joint structures, the dermis of the skin, the sheaths of blood vessels and nerves, adipose tissue, lymphatic tissues, and blood. Fibroblasts are the most abundant connective tissue cells. They are responsible for the synthesis of collagen, elastic, and reticular fibers and the gel-like ground substance that fills the intercellular spaces.

- Muscle tissue is a specialized tissue designed for contractility. Three types of muscle tissue exist: skeletal, cardiac, and smooth. Actin and myosin filaments interact to produce muscle shortening, a process activated by the presence of calcium. In skeletal muscle, calcium is released from the sarcoplasmic reticulum in response to an action potential. Smooth muscle is often called *involuntary muscle* because it contracts spontaneously or through the activity of the autonomic nervous system. It differs from skeletal muscle in that its sarcoplasmic reticulum is less defined and it depends on the entry of extracellular calcium ions for muscle contraction.

- Nervous tissue is designed for communication purposes and includes the neurons, the supporting neural structures, and the ependymal cells that line the ventricles of the brain and the spinal canal.

- Within tissues, cells are held together by cell junctions, which are especially plentiful in epithelial tissues. There are three basic types of cell junctions: tight junctions, adhering or adhesive-type junctions, and gap junctions. The ability of cells to adhere together (cell to cell) or to components of the extracellular matrix (cell to matrix) is mediated by cell adhesion molecules (cadherins, selectins, integrins, and the immunoglobulin superfamily of proteins).

REVIEW EXERCISES

1. Persons who drink sufficient amounts of alcohol display rapid changes in central nervous system function, including both motor and behavioral changes, and the odor of alcohol can be detected on their breath.

   A. Use the concepts related to the lipid bilayer structure of the cell membrane to explain these observations.

2. Tattoos consist of pigments that have been injected into the skin.

   A. Explain what happens to the dye once it has been injected and why it does not eventually wash away.

3. Insulin is synthesized in the beta cells of the pancreas as a prohormone and then secreted as an active hormone.

   A. Using your knowledge of the function of DNA, the RNAs, the endoplasmic reticulum, and the Golgi complex, propose a pathway for the synthesis of insulin.

4. Mitochondrial disorders, whether due to mutations in mitochondrial or nuclear genes, often produce muscle weakness, sometimes with severe involvement of the muscles that move the eyes, other neurologic symptoms, lactic acidosis, and cardiomyopathy.

   A. Mitochondrial disorders that are responsible for these manifestations are often classified as mitochondrial encephalomyopathies. Propose an explanation for the propensity to develop encephalopathies and myopathies with mitochondrial disorders rather than disorders of other body systems such as the kidney or digestive tract.

   B. Relate the function of the mitochondria in terms of oxidative metabolism to the development of lactic acidosis.

5. The absorption of glucose from the intestine involves a cotransport mechanism in which the active primary transport of sodium is used to provide for the secondary transport of glucose.

   A. Hypothesize how this information might be used to design an oral rehydration solution for someone who is suffering from diarrhea.

BIBLIOGRAPHY

Alberts B, Johnson A, Lewis J, et al. *Molecular Biology of the Cell.* 5th ed. New York and London: Garland Publishing; 2008.

Alexeyev M, Shokolenko I, Wilson G, et al. The maintenance of mitochondrial DNA integrity-critical analysis and update. *Cold Spring Harb Perspect Biol.* 2013;5:a012641.

Doherty GJ, McMahon HT. Mechanisms and endocytosis. *Annu Rev Biochem.* 2009;78:857–902.

Dominguez R, Holmes KC. Actin structure and function. *Annu Rev Biophys.* 2011;40:169–186.

Ferdinandusse S, Denis S, Faust PL, et al. Bile acids: the role of peroxisomes. *J Lipid Res.* 2009;50:2139–2147.

Finley D. Recognition and processing of ubiquitin-protein conjugates by the proteosome. *Annu Rev Biochem.* 2009;78:477–513.

MacAskill AF, Kittler JT. Control of mitochondrial transport and localization in neurons. *Trends Cell Biol.* 2009;20: 102–112.

Mizuno Y, Isotani E, Huang J, et al. Myosin light chain kinase and calcium sensitization in smooth muscle in vivo. *Am J Physiol Cell Physiol.* 2008;295:C358–C336.

Parton RG, del Pozo MA. Caveolae as plasma membrane sensors, protectors and organizers. *Nat Rev Mol Cell Biol.* 2013;14:98–112.

Ross MH, Pawlina W. *Histology: Text and Atlas.* 6th ed. Philadelphia, PA: Wolters Kluwer Health/Lippincott Williams & Wilkins; 2011.

Rudrabhatia P, Jaffe H, Pant HC. Direct evidence of phosphorylated neuronal intermediate filament proteins in neurofibrillary tangles (NFTs): phosphoproteomics of Alzheimer's NFTs. *FASEB J.* 2011;25:3896–3905.

Sofroniew MV, Vinters HV. Astrocytes: biology and pathology. *Acta Neuropathol.* 2010;119:7–35.

Strambio-De-Castillia C, Niepel M, Rout MP. The nuclear pore complex: bridging nuclear transport and gene regulation. *Nat Rev Mol Cell Biol.* 2010;11:490–501.

Su X, Ohi R, Pellman D. Move in for the kill: motile microtubule regulators. *Trends Cell Biol.* 2012;22:567–575.

Tirone F, Fariola-Vecchioli S, Micheli L, et al. Genetic control of adult neurogenesis: interplay of differentiation, proliferation and survival modulates new neurons function, and memory circuits. *Front Cell Neurosci.* 2013;7:59.

Toivola DM, Strnad P, Habtezion A, et al. Intermediate filaments take the heat. *Trends Cell Biol.* 2010;20:79–91.

Verkman AS. Aquaporins in clinical medicine. *Annu Rev Med.* 2012;63:303–316.

Voshol PJ, Rensen PC, van Dijk KW, et al. Effect of plasma triglyceride metabolism on lipid storage in adipose tissue: studies using genetically engineered mouse models. *Biochimica Biophys Acta.* 2009;1791:479–485.

Walde S, Kehlenbach RH. The part and the whole: functions of nucleoporins in nucleocytoplasmic transport. *Trends Cell Biol.* 2010;20:461–469.

Wanders RJA, Waterham HR. Biochemistry of peroxisomes revisited. *Annu Rev Biochem.* 2006;75:295–332.

Porth Essentials Resources

Explore these additional resources to enhance learning for this chapter:

- NCLEX-Style Questions and Other Resources on the**Point**, http://thePoint.lww.com/PorthEssentials4e
- Study Guide for Essentials of Pathophysiology
- Concepts in Action Animations
- Adaptive Learning | Powered by PrepU, http://thepoint.lww.com/prepu

C h a p t e r 2

Cellular Responses to Stress, Injury, and Aging

In their simplest form, all diseases exert their effects on the smallest living unit of the body—the cell. When confronted with stresses that endanger its normal structure and function, the cell undergoes adaptive changes that permit survival and maintenance of function. It is only when the stress is overwhelming or adaptation is ineffective that injury, maladaptive changes, and cell death occur. Biologic aging produces its own changes in cell structure and function.

Cellular Responses to Persistent Stress

Cells adapt to changes in the internal environment just as the total organism adapts to changes in the external environment. Cells may adapt by undergoing changes in size, number, and type. These changes, occurring singly or in combination, may lead to atrophy, hypertrophy, hyperplasia, metaplasia, and dysplasia (Fig. 2-1). Cellular stresses also include intracellular accumulations and storage of products in abnormal amounts.[1,2]

Adaptations of Growth and Differentiation

Numerous molecular mechanisms mediate cellular adaptation, including factors in the cellular microenvironment and the cells themselves. These mechanisms largely depend on extracellular signals and cues, which in turn activate intracellular signaling mechanisms transmitted by chemical messengers that alter gene expression. Once the primary stimulus for adaptation is removed, the cause of changing gene expression patterns is removed and the cell may revert back to its previous state. Whether adaptive cellular changes are normal or abnormal depends in part on whether the response was mediated by an appropriate stimulus. Normal adaptive responses occur in response to need and an appropriate

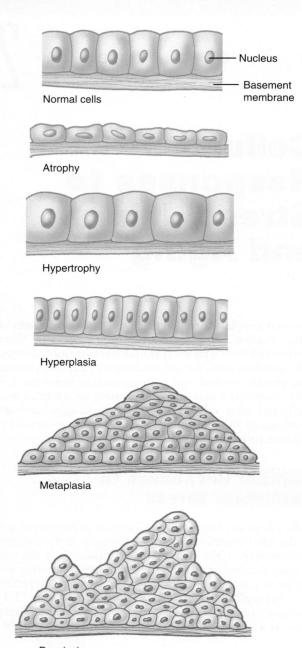

Normal cells

Nucleus

Basement membrane

Atrophy

Hypertrophy

Hyperplasia

Metaplasia

Dysplasia

FIGURE 2-1. Adaptive cell and tissue responses involving a change in cell size (hypertrophy and atrophy), number (hyperplasia), cell type (metaplasia), or size, shape, and organization (dysplasia). (From Anatomical Chart Company. *Atlas of Pathophysiology.* Springhouse, PA: Springhouse; 2002:4.)

stimulus. After the need has been removed, the adaptive response ceases.

Atrophy

When confronted with a decrease in work demands or adverse environmental conditions, most cells are able to revert to a smaller size and a lower and more efficient level of functioning that is compatible with survival.[1,2] This decrease in cell size is called *atrophy*. Cells that are atrophied reduce oxygen consumption and other cellular functions by decreasing the number and size of their organelles and other structures. There are fewer mitochondria, myofilaments, and endoplasmic reticulum structures. When a sufficient number of cells are involved, the entire tissue atrophies.

Cell size, particularly in muscle tissue, is related to workload. As the workload of a cell declines, oxygen consumption and protein synthesis decrease. Furthermore, proper muscle mass is maintained by sufficient levels of insulin/insulin-like growth factor-1 (IGF-1). When insulin/IGF-1 levels are low or catabolic signals are present, muscle atrophy occurs by a variety of mechanisms. One such mechanism is increased proteolysis by the ubiquitin-proteasome system, in which intracellular proteins destined for destruction are covalently bonded to a small protein called *ubiquitin* and then degraded by small cytoplasmic organelles called *proteasomes* (see Chapter 1). Other mechanisms, such as reduced synthetic (anabolic) processes and apoptosis (programmed cell death), are also involved (to be discussed).[3]

The general causes of atrophy can be grouped into five categories: (1) disuse, (2) denervation, (3) loss of endocrine stimulation, (4) inadequate nutrition, and (5) ischemia or decreased blood flow. Disuse atrophy occurs when there is a reduction in skeletal muscle use. An extreme example of disuse atrophy is seen in the muscles of extremities that have been encased in casts. Because atrophy is adaptive and reversible, muscle size is restored after the cast is removed and muscle use is resumed. Denervation atrophy is a form of disuse atrophy that occurs in the muscles of paralyzed limbs. Lack of endocrine stimulation produces a form of disuse atrophy. In women, the loss of estrogen stimulation during menopause results in atrophic changes in the reproductive organs. With malnutrition and decreased blood flow, cells decrease their size and energy requirements as a means of survival.

Hypertrophy

Hypertrophy represents an increase in cell size, and with it an increase in the amount of functioning tissue mass. It results from an increased workload imposed on an organ or body part and is commonly seen in cardiac and skeletal muscle tissue, which cannot adapt to an increase in workload through mitotic division and formation of more cells. Hypertrophy involves an increase in the functional components of the cell that allows it to achieve equilibrium between demand and functional capacity. For example, as muscle cells hypertrophy, additional actin and myosin filaments, cell enzymes, and adenosine triphosphate (ATP) are synthesized.

Hypertrophy may occur as the result of normal physiologic or abnormal pathologic conditions. The increase in muscle mass associated with exercise is an example of physiologic hypertrophy. Pathologic hypertrophy occurs as the result of disease conditions and may be adaptive or compensatory. Examples of adaptive hypertrophy are the thickening of the urinary bladder from long-continued obstruction of urinary outflow and myocardial hypertrophy from valvular heart disease or hypertension. Compensatory hypertrophy is the enlargement of a remaining organ or tissue after a portion has been surgically removed or rendered inactive. For instance, if one kidney is removed, the remaining kidney enlarges to compensate for the loss.

The initiating signals for hypertrophy appear to be complex and related to ATP depletion, mechanical forces such as stretching of the muscle fibers, activation of cell degradation products, and hormonal factors. In the case of the heart, initiating signals can be divided into two broad categories: (1) biomechanical and stretch-sensitive mechanisms and (2) neurohumoral mechanisms associated with the release of hormones, growth factors, cytokines, and chemokines.[4] Internal stretch-sensitive receptors for the biochemical signals and an array of membrane-bound receptors for the specific neurohumoral ligands, such as IGF-1 and epidermal growth factor (EGF), activate specific signal transduction pathways. These pathways control myocardial growth by altering gene expression to increase protein synthesis and reduce protein degradation, thereby causing hypertrophic enlargement of the heart. A limit is eventually reached beyond which further enlargement of the tissue mass is no longer able to compensate for the increased work demands. The limiting factors for continued hypertrophy might be related to limitations in blood flow. In hypertension, for example, the increased workload required to pump blood against an elevated arterial pressure results in a progressive increase in left ventricular muscle mass and need for coronary blood flow (Fig. 2-2).

There continues to be interest in the signaling pathways that control the arrangement of contractile elements in myocardial hypertrophy. Research suggests that certain signal molecules can alter gene expression controlling the size and assembly of the contractile proteins in hypertrophied myocardial cells. For example, the hypertrophied myocardial cells of well-trained athletes have proportional increases in width and length. This is in contrast to the hypertrophy that develops in dilated cardiomyopathy, in which the hypertrophied cells have a relatively greater increase in length than width. In pressure overload, as occurs with hypertension, the hypertrophied cells have greater width than length.[5] It is anticipated that further elucidation of the signal pathways that determine the adaptive and nonadaptive features of cardiac hypertrophy will lead to new targets for treatment.

Hyperplasia

Hyperplasia refers to an increase in the number of cells in an organ or tissue. It occurs in tissues with cells that are capable of mitotic division, such as the epidermis, intestinal epithelium, and glandular tissue.[1,2] Certain cells, such as neurons, rarely divide and therefore have little (if any) capacity for hyperplastic growth. There is evidence that hyperplasia involves activation of genes controlling cell proliferation and the presence of intracellular messengers that control cell replication and growth. As with other normal adaptive cellular responses, hyperplasia is a controlled process that occurs in response to an appropriate stimulus and ceases after the stimulus has been removed.

The stimuli that induce hyperplasia may be physiologic or nonphysiologic. There are two common types of physiologic hyperplasia: hormonal and compensatory. Breast and uterine enlargement during pregnancy are examples of a physiologic hyperplasia that results from estrogen stimulation. The regeneration of the liver that occurs after partial hepatectomy (i.e., partial removal of the liver) is an example of compensatory hyperplasia. Hyperplasia is also an important response of connective tissue in wound healing, during which proliferating fibroblasts and blood vessels contribute to wound repair. Although hypertrophy and hyperplasia are two distinct processes, they may occur together and are often triggered by the same mechanism.[1] For example, the pregnant uterus undergoes both hypertrophy and hyperplasia as a result of estrogen stimulation.

Most forms of nonphysiologic hyperplasia are due to excessive hormonal stimulation or the effects of growth factors on target tissues.[2] Excessive estrogen production can cause endometrial hyperplasia and abnormal menstrual bleeding (see Chapter 40). Benign prostatic hyperplasia, which is a common disorder of men older than 50 years of age, is thought to be related to the action of androgens (see Chapter 39). Skin warts are an example of hyperplasia caused by growth factors produced by certain viruses, such as the papillomaviruses.

Metaplasia

Metaplasia represents a reversible change in which one adult cell type (epithelial or mesenchymal) is replaced by another adult cell type.[1,2] These changes are thought

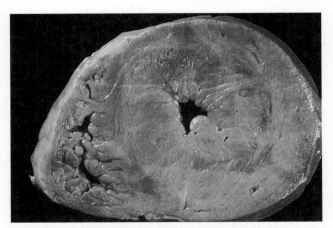

FIGURE 2-2. Myocardial hypertrophy. Cross-section of the heart in a patient with long-standing hypertension. (From Strayer DS, Rubin E. Cell adaptation, cell injury and cell death. In: Rubin R, Strayer DS, eds. *Rubin's Pathology: Clinicopathologic Foundations of Medicine.* 6th ed. Philadelphia, PA: Wolters Kluwer Health | Lippincott Williams & Wilkins; 2012:4.)

to involve the reprogramming of undifferentiated stem cells that are present in the tissue undergoing the metaplastic changes.

Metaplasia usually occurs in response to chronic irritation and inflammation and allows for substitution of cells that are better able to survive under circumstances in which a more fragile cell type might succumb. However, the conversion of cell type never oversteps the boundaries of the primary tissue type (e.g., one type of epithelial cell may be converted to another type of epithelial cell, but not to a connective tissue cell). An example of metaplasia is the adaptive substitution of stratified squamous epithelial cells for the ciliated columnar epithelial cells in the trachea and large airways of a habitual cigarette smoker. Although the squamous epithelium is better able to survive in these situations, the protective function that the ciliated epithelium provides for the respiratory tract is lost. Also, continued exposure to the influences that cause metaplasia may predispose to cancerous transformation of the metaplastic epithelium.

Dysplasia

Dysplasia is characterized by deranged cell growth of a specific tissue that results in cells that vary in size, shape, and organization. Minor degrees of dysplasia are associated with chronic irritation or inflammation.[1] The pattern is most frequently encountered in areas of metaplastic squamous epithelium of the respiratory tract and uterine cervix. Although dysplasia is abnormal, it is adaptive in that it is potentially reversible after the irritating cause has been removed. Dysplasia is strongly implicated as a precursor of cancer. In cancers of the respiratory tract and the uterine cervix, dysplastic changes have been found adjacent to the foci of cancerous transformation. Through the use of the Papanicolaou (Pap) test, it has been documented that cancer of the uterine cervix develops in a series of incremental epithelial changes ranging from severe dysplasia to invasive cancer (discussed in Chapter 40). However, dysplasia is an adaptive process and as such does not necessarily lead to cancer. In many cases, the dysplastic cells revert to their former structure and function.

Intracellular Accumulations

Intracellular accumulations represent the buildup of substances that cells cannot immediately use or eliminate. The substances may accumulate in the cytoplasm (frequently in the lysosomes) or in the nucleus. In some cases the accumulation may be an abnormal substance that the cell has produced, and in other cases the cell may be storing exogenous materials or products of pathologic processes occurring elsewhere in the body. These substances can be grouped into three categories: (1) normal body substances, such as lipids, proteins, carbohydrates, melanin, and bilirubin, that are present in abnormally large amounts; (2) abnormal endogenous

products, such as those resulting from inborn errors of metabolism; and (3) exogenous products, such as environmental agents and pigments that cannot be broken down by the cell.[2] These substances may accumulate transiently or permanently, and they may be harmless or, in some cases, toxic.

Under some conditions cells may accumulate abnormal amounts of various substances, some of which may be harmless while others may be associated with varying degrees of injury. Frequently, normal substances accumulate because they are synthesized at a rate that exceeds their metabolism or removal. An example of this type of process is a condition called fatty liver, which is due to intracellular accumulation of triglycerides. Liver cells normally contain some fat, which is either oxidized and used for energy or converted to triglycerides. This fat is derived from free fatty acids released from adipose tissue. Abnormal accumulation occurs when the delivery of free fatty acids to the liver is increased, as in starvation and diabetes mellitus, or when the intrahepatic metabolism of lipids is disturbed, as in alcoholism.

Intracellular accumulation can result from genetic disorders that disrupt the enzymatic degradation of selected substances or their transport to other sites. A normal enzyme may be replaced with an abnormal one, resulting in the formation of a substance that cannot be used or eliminated from the cell, or an enzyme may be missing, so that an intermediate product accumulates in the cell. For example, there are at least 10 genetic disorders that affect glycogen metabolism, most of which lead to the accumulation of intracellular glycogen stores. In the most common form of this disorder, von Gierke disease, large amounts of glycogen accumulate in the liver and kidneys because of a deficiency of the enzyme glucose-6-phosphatase. Without this enzyme, glycogen cannot be broken down to form glucose. The disorder leads not only to an accumulation of glycogen but also to a reduction in blood glucose levels. In Tay-Sachs disease, another genetic disorder, abnormal lipids accumulate in the brain and other tissues, causing motor and mental deterioration beginning at approximately 6 months of age, followed by death at 2 to 3 years of age (see Chapter 6).

Pigments are colored substances that may accumulate in cells. They can be endogenous (i.e., arising from within the body) or exogenous (i.e., arising from outside the body). Icterus, also called *jaundice*, is characterized by a yellow discoloration of tissue due to the retention of bilirubin, an endogenous bile pigment. This condition may occur because of increased bilirubin production from red blood cell destruction, obstruction of bile passage into the intestine, or diseases that affect the liver's ability to remove bilirubin from the blood. Lipofuscin is a yellow-brown pigment that results from the accumulation of the indigestible residues produced during normal turnover of cell structures (Fig. 2-3). The accumulation of lipofuscin increases with age and is sometimes referred to as the *wear-and-tear pigment*. It is more common in heart, nerve, and liver cells than other

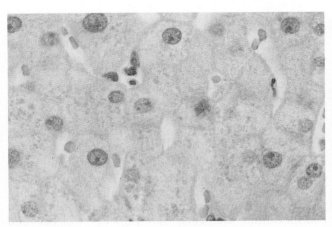

FIGURE 2-3. Accumulation of intracellular lipofuscin. A photomicrograph of the liver of an 80-year-old man shows golden cytoplasmic granules, which represent lysosomal storage of lipofuscin. (From Strayer DS, Rubin E. Cell adaptation, cell injury and cell death. In: Rubin R, Strayer DS, eds. *Rubin's Pathology: Clinicopathologic Foundations of Medicine.* 6th ed. Philadelphia, PA: Wolters Kluwer Health | Lippincott Williams & Wilkins; 2012:21.)

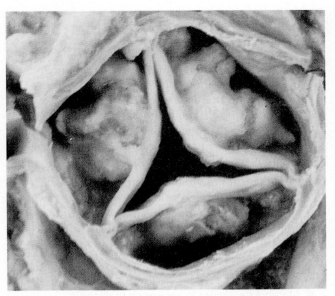

FIGURE 2-4. Calcific aortic stenosis. Large deposits of calcium salts are evident in the cusps and free margins of the thickened aortic valve as viewed from above. (From Strayer DS, Rubin E. Cell adaptation, cell injury and cell death. In: Rubin R, Strayer DS, eds. *Rubin's Pathology: Clinicopathologic Foundations of Medicine.* 6th ed. Philadelphia, PA: Wolters Kluwer Health | Lippincott Williams & Wilkins; 2012:13.)

tissues and is seen more often in conditions associated with atrophy of an organ.

One of the most common exogenous pigments is carbon in the form of coal dust. In coal miners or persons exposed to heavily polluted environments, the accumulation of carbon dust blackens the lung tissue and may cause serious lung disease. The formation of a blue lead line along the margins of the gum is one of the diagnostic features of lead poisoning. Tattoos are the result of insoluble pigments introduced into the skin, where they are engulfed by macrophages and persist for a lifetime.

The significance of intracellular accumulations depends on the cause and severity of the condition. Many accumulations, such as lipofuscin and mild fatty changes, have no effect on cell function. Some conditions, such as the hyperbilirubinemia that causes jaundice, are reversible. Other disorders, such as glycogen storage diseases, produce accumulations that result in organ dysfunction and other alterations in physiologic function.

Pathologic Calcifications

Pathologic calcification involves the abnormal tissue deposition of calcium salts, together with smaller amounts of iron, magnesium, and other minerals. It is known as *dystrophic calcification* when it occurs in dead or dying tissue and as *metastatic calcification* when it occurs in normal tissue.[1,2]

Dystrophic Calcification

Dystrophic calcification represents the macroscopic deposition of calcium salts in injured tissue. It is often visible to the naked eye as deposits that range from

gritty sand-like grains to firm, hard, rock-like material. The pathogenesis of dystrophic calcification involves the intracellular or extracellular formation of crystalline calcium phosphate. The components of the calcium deposits are derived from the bodies of dead or dying cells as well as from the circulation and interstitial fluid.

Dystrophic calcification is commonly seen in atheromatous lesions of advanced atherosclerosis, areas of injury in the aorta and large blood vessels, and damaged heart valves. While the presence of calcification may only indicate the presence of previous cell injury, as in healed tuberculosis lesions, it is also a frequent cause of organ dysfunction. For example, calcification of the aortic valve is a frequent cause of aortic stenosis in the elderly (Fig. 2-4).

Metastatic Calcification

In contrast to dystrophic calcification, which occurs in injured tissues, metastatic calcification occurs in normal tissues as the result of increased serum calcium levels (hypercalcemia). Almost any condition that increases the serum calcium level can lead to calcification in inappropriate sites such as the lung, renal tubules, and blood vessels. The major causes of hypercalcemia are hyperparathyroidism, either primary or secondary to phosphate retention in renal failure; increased release of calcium from bone as in immobilization, Paget disease, or cancer with metastatic bone lesions; and vitamin D intoxication.

SUMMARY CONCEPTS

■ Cells adapt to changes in their environment and in their work demands by changing their size, number, and characteristics. These adaptive changes are consistent with the needs of the cell and occur in response to an appropriate stimulus. The changes are usually reversed after the stimulus has been withdrawn.

■ When confronted with a decrease in work demands or adverse environmental conditions, cells *atrophy,* or reduce in size. When confronted with an increase in work demands they undergo *hypertrophy,* an increase in size. An increase in the number of cells in an organ or tissue is called *hyperplasia.*

■ *Metaplasia* occurs in response to chronic irritation and represents the substitution of cells of a type that are better able to survive under circumstances in which a more fragile cell type might succumb. *Dysplasia* is characterized by deranged cell growth of a specific tissue that results in cells that vary in size, shape, and appearance. It is often a precursor of cancer.

■ Under some circumstances, cells may accumulate abnormal amounts of various substances. If the accumulation reflects a correctable systemic disorder, such as the hyperbilirubinemia that causes jaundice, the accumulation is reversible. If the disorder cannot be corrected, as often occurs in many inborn errors of metabolism, the cells become overloaded, causing cell injury and death.

■ Pathologic calcification involves the abnormal tissue deposition of calcium salts. *Dystrophic calcification* occurs in dead or dying tissue, whereas *metastatic calcification* occurs in normal tissues as the result of elevated serum calcium levels.

Cell Injury, Death, and Senescence

Cells can be injured in many ways. The extent to which any injurious agent can cause reversible or irreversible cell injury and death depends in large measure on the intensity and duration of the injury and the type of cell that is involved, as well as variables such as blood supply, nutritional status, and regenerative capacity. Cell injury and death are ongoing processes, and in the healthy state, they are balanced by cell renewal.

Causes of Cell Injury

Cell damage can occur in many ways. For purposes of discussion, the ways by which cells are injured have been grouped into five categories: (1) injury from physical agents, (2) radiation injury, (3) chemical injury, (4) injury from biologic agents, and (5) injury from nutritional imbalances.

Injury from Physical Agents

Physical agents responsible for cell and tissue injury include mechanical forces, extremes of temperature, and electrical forces. They are common causes of injuries due to environmental exposure, occupational and transportation accidents, and physical violence and assault.

Mechanical Forces. Injury or trauma due to mechanical forces occurs as the result of body impact with another object. The body or the mass can be in motion or, as sometimes happens, both can be in motion at the time of impact. These types of injuries split and tear tissue, fracture bones, injure blood vessels, and disrupt blood flow.

Extremes of Temperature. Extremes of heat and cold cause damage to the cell, its organelles, and its enzyme systems. Exposure to low-intensity heat (43°C to 46°C), such as occurs with partial-thickness burns and severe heat stroke, causes cell injury by inducing vascular injury, accelerating cell metabolism, inactivating temperature-sensitive enzymes, and disrupting the cell membrane. With more intense heat, coagulation of blood and tissue proteins occurs. Exposure to cold increases blood viscosity and induces vasoconstriction by direct action on blood vessels and through reflex activity of the sympathetic nervous system. The resultant decrease in blood flow may lead to hypoxic tissue injury, depending on the degree and duration of cold exposure. Injury from freezing probably results from a combination of ice crystal formation and vasoconstriction. The decreased blood flow leads to capillary stasis and arteriolar and capillary thrombosis. Edema results from increased capillary permeability.

Electrical Forces. Injuries due to electrical forces can affect the body through extensive tissue injury and disruption of neural and cardiac impulses. The effect of electricity on the body is mainly determined by its voltage, the type of current (i.e., direct or alternating), its amperage, the resistance of the intervening tissue, the pathway of the current, and the duration of exposure.[6]

Lightning and high-voltage wires that carry several thousand volts produce the most severe damage.[2] Alternating current (AC) is usually more dangerous than direct current (DC) because it causes violent muscle contractions, preventing the person from releasing the electrical source and sometimes resulting in fractures and dislocations. In electrical injuries, the body acts as a conductor of the electrical current. The current enters the body from an electrical source, such as an exposed wire, and passes through the body and exits to another conductor, such as the moisture on the ground or a piece of metal the person is holding. The pathway that a current takes is critical because the electrical energy disrupts impulses in excitable tissues. Current flow through the brain may interrupt impulses from respiratory centers in the brain stem, and current flow through the chest may cause fatal cardiac arrhythmias.

The resistance to the flow of current in electrical circuits transforms electrical energy into heat. This is why the elements in electrical heating devices are made of highly resistive metals. Much of the tissue damage produced by electrical injuries is caused by heat production in tissues that have the highest electrical resistance.[2,7] Resistance to electrical current varies from the greatest to the least in bone, fat, tendons, skin, muscles, blood, and nerves. The most severe tissue injury usually occurs at the skin sites where the current enters and leaves the body (Fig. 2-5). After electricity has penetrated the skin, it rapidly passes through the body along the lines of least resistance—through body fluids and nerves. Degeneration of vessel walls may occur, and thrombi may form as current flows along the blood vessels. This can cause extensive muscle and deep tissue injury. Thick, dry skin is more resistant to the flow of electricity than thin, wet skin. It is generally believed that the greater the skin resistance, the greater is the amount of local skin burn; and the less the resistance, the greater are the deep and systemic effects.

Radiation Injury

Electromagnetic radiation comprises a wide spectrum of wave-propagated energy, ranging from ionizing gamma rays to radiofrequency waves. A photon is a particle

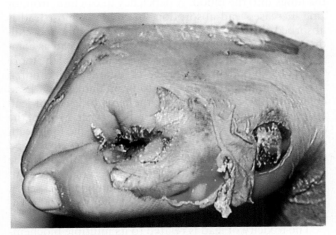

FIGURE 2-5. Electrical burn of the skin. The victim was electrocuted after attempting to stop a fall from a ladder by grasping a high-voltage line. (From Strayer DS, Rubin E. Environmental and nutritional pathology. In: Rubin R, Strayer DS, eds. *Rubin's Pathology: Clinicopathologic Foundations of Medicine.* 6th ed. Philadelphia, PA: Wolters Kluwer Health | Lippincott Williams & Wilkins; 2012:313.)

of radiation energy. Radiation energy with frequencies above the ultraviolet (UV) range is called *ionizing radiation* because the photons have enough energy to knock electrons off atoms and molecules. *Nonionizing radiation* refers to radiation energy at frequencies below those of visible light. *Ultraviolet radiation* represents the portion of the spectrum of electromagnetic radiation just above the visible range.

Ionizing Radiation. Ionizing radiation affects cells by causing ionization of molecules and atoms in the cell, by directly hitting the target molecules in the cell, or by producing free radicals (highly reactive chemical species) that destabilize molecules in critical cell components.[2,7] It can immediately kill cells, interrupt cell replication, or cause a variety of genetic mutations, which may or may not be lethal. Most radiation injury is caused by localized irradiation that is used in the treatment of cancer (see Chapter 7). Except for unusual circumstances such as the use of high-dose irradiation that precedes bone marrow transplantation, exposure to whole-body irradiation is rare.

The injurious effects of ionizing radiation vary with the dose, dose rate (a single large dose can cause greater injury than divided or fractionated doses), and the differential sensitivity of the exposed tissue to radiation injury. Because of the effect on deoxyribonucleic acid (DNA) synthesis and interference with mitosis, rapidly dividing cells of the bone marrow and intestine are much more vulnerable to radiation injury than tissues such as bone and skeletal muscle. Over time, occupational and accidental exposure to ionizing radiation can result in increased risk for the development of various types of cancers, including skin cancers, leukemia, osteogenic sarcomas, and lung cancer.

Many of the clinical manifestations of radiation injury result from acute cell injury, dose-dependent changes in the blood vessels that supply the irradiated tissues, and fibrotic tissue replacement. The cell's initial response to radiation injury involves swelling, disruption of the mitochondria and other organelles, alterations in the cell membrane, and marked changes in the nucleus. The endothelial cells in blood vessels are particularly sensitive to irradiation. During the immediate post-irradiation period, only vessel dilatation is apparent (e.g., the initial erythema of the skin after radiation therapy). Later or with higher levels of radiation, destructive changes occur in small blood vessels such as the capillaries and venules. Acute reversible necrosis is represented by such disorders as radiation cystitis, dermatitis, and diarrhea from enteritis. More persistent damage can be attributed to acute necrosis of tissue cells that are not capable of regeneration, or because of chronic ischemia. Chronic effects of radiation damage are characterized by fibrosis and scarring of tissues and organs in the irradiated area (e.g., interstitial fibrosis of the heart and lungs after irradiation of the chest). Because the radiation delivered in radiation therapy inevitably travels through the skin, radiation dermatitis is common. There may be necrosis of the skin, impaired wound healing, and chronic radiation dermatitis.

Ultraviolet Radiation. Ultraviolet radiation contains increasingly energetic rays that are powerful enough to disrupt intracellular bonds, cause sunburn, and increase the risk of skin cancers (see Chapter 46). The degree of risk depends on the type of UV rays, the intensity of exposure, and the amount of protective melanin pigment in the skin. Skin damage induced by UV radiation is thought to be caused by reactive oxygen species and by damage to melanin-producing processes in the skin. Ultraviolet radiation also damages DNA, resulting in the formation of pyrimidine dimers (i.e., the insertion of two identical pyrimidine bases into replicating DNA instead of one). Other forms of DNA damage include the production of single-stranded breaks and formation of DNA–protein cross-links. Normally, errors that occur during DNA replication are repaired by enzymes that remove the faulty section of DNA and repair the damage. The importance of DNA repair in protecting against UV radiation injury is evidenced by the vulnerability of persons who lack the enzymes needed to repair UV-induced DNA damage. In a genetic disorder called *xeroderma pigmentosum*, an enzyme needed to repair sunlight-induced DNA damage is lacking. This autosomal recessive disorder is characterized by extreme photosensitivity and a 2000-fold increased risk of skin cancer in sun-exposed skin.[2]

Nonionizing Radiation. Nonionizing radiation includes infrared light, ultrasound, microwaves, and laser energy.[1] Unlike ionizing radiation, which can directly break chemical bonds, nonionizing radiation exerts its effects by causing vibration and rotation of atoms and molecules. All of this vibrational and rotational energy is eventually converted to thermal energy. Low-frequency nonionizing radiation is used widely in radar, television, industrial operations (e.g., heating, welding, melting of metals, processing of wood and plastic), household appliances (e.g., microwave ovens), and medical applications (e.g., diathermy). Isolated cases of skin burns and thermal injury to deeper tissues have occurred in industrial settings and from improperly used household microwave ovens. Injury from these sources is mainly thermal and, because of the deep penetration of infrared or microwave rays, tends to involve dermal and subcutaneous tissue injury.

Chemical Injury

Chemicals capable of damaging cells are everywhere around us. Pollutants in the air, water, and soil, such as carbon monoxide, pesticides, and trace metals including lead, are capable of tissue injury, as are certain chemicals in foods.

Chemical agents can injure the cell membrane and other cell structures, block enzymatic pathways, coagulate cell proteins, and disrupt the osmotic and ionic balance of the cell. Corrosive substances such as strong acids and bases destroy cells as the substances come into contact with the body. Other chemicals may injure cells in the process of metabolism or elimination. For example, carbon tetrachloride (CCl_4), a chemical used in manufacturing, causes little damage until it is metabolized by liver enzymes to a highly reactive free radical that is extremely toxic to liver cells.

Drugs. Many drugs—alcohol, prescription drugs, over-the-counter drugs, and street drugs—are capable of directly or indirectly damaging tissues. Ethyl alcohol can harm the gastric mucosa, liver (see Chapter 30), developing fetus (see Chapter 6), and other organs. Antineoplastic (anticancer) and immunosuppressant drugs can directly injure cells. Other drugs produce metabolic end products that are toxic to cells. Acetaminophen, a commonly used over-the-counter analgesic drug, is detoxified in the liver, where small amounts of the drug are converted to a highly toxic metabolite. This metabolite is detoxified by a metabolic pathway that uses a substance (i.e., glutathione) normally present in the liver. When large amounts of the drug are ingested, this pathway becomes overwhelmed and toxic metabolites accumulate, causing massive liver necrosis.

Lead Toxicity. Lead is a particularly toxic metal. Small amounts accumulate to reach toxic levels. There are innumerable sources of lead in the environment, including flaking paint, lead-contaminated dust and soil, pottery glazes, traditional remedies, cosmetics, and wild game contaminated by lead shot. Adults often encounter lead through occupational exposure. Lead and other metal smelters, miners, welders, storage battery workers, and pottery makers are particularly at risk.[2,7] Children are exposed to lead through ingestion of peeling lead paint, by breathing dust from lead paint (e.g., during remodeling), playing in contaminated soil, or playing with toys or items made or decorated with lead.[8,9] Factors that increase the risk of lead toxicity include preschool age, low socioeconomic status, and living in housing built before 1960.[9]

Lead is absorbed through the gastrointestinal tract or the lungs into the blood. A deficiency in calcium, iron, or zinc increases lead absorption. In children, most lead is absorbed through the lungs. Although infants and children may have the same or a lower intake of lead as compared to adults, their absorption is greater. Also, the more permeable blood–brain barrier of infants and children makes them highly susceptible to brain damage.[2,7,9] Lead crosses the placenta, exposing the fetus to levels of lead that are comparable with those of the mother. Most of the absorbed lead (80% to 85%) is stored in bone (and teeth of young children), 5% to 10% remains in the blood, and the remainder accumulates in soft tissues.[2] Although the half-life of lead is hours to days, bone serves as a repository from which blood levels are maintained. In a sense, bone protects other tissues, but the slow turnover maintains blood levels for months to years.

The toxicity of lead is related to its multiple biochemical effects.[2,7] It has the ability to inactivate enzymes, compete with calcium for incorporation into bone, and interfere with nerve transmission and brain development. The major targets of lead toxicity are the red blood cells, the gastrointestinal tract, the kidneys, and the nervous system. Anemia is a cardinal sign of lead toxicity.

Lead competes with the enzymes required for hemoglobin synthesis and with the membrane-associated enzymes that prevent hemolysis of red blood cells. The life span of the red cell is decreased. The gastrointestinal tract is the main source of symptoms in the adult. This is characterized by "lead colic," a severe and poorly localized form of acute abdominal pain. A lead line formed by precipitated lead sulfite may appear along the gingival margins. The lead line is seldom seen in children. The kidneys are the major route for excretion of lead. Lead can cause diffuse kidney damage, eventually leading to renal failure. Even without overt signs of kidney damage, lead toxicity leads to hypertension.

In the nervous system, lead toxicity is characterized by demyelination of cerebral and cerebellar white matter and death of brain cells. When this occurs in early childhood, it can affect neurobehavioral development and result in lower IQ levels and poorer classroom performance.[9] Demyelination of peripheral nerves may occur in adults. The most serious manifestation of lead poisoning is acute encephalopathy. It is manifested by persistent vomiting, ataxia, seizures, papilledema, impaired consciousness, and coma. Acute encephalopathy may manifest suddenly, or it may be preceded by other signs of lead toxicity such as behavioral changes or abdominal complaints.

The threshold level at which lead causes subclinical and clinical disturbances has been redefined a number of times over the past 50 years. At one time, a blood level of 25 µg/dL was considered safe. Recent research suggests that even levels below 10 µg/dL are associated with declines in children's IQ at 3 to 5 years of age.[10,11]

Approximately 99% of children are identified by screening procedures, which are recommended for high-risk populations based on the likelihood of lead exposure. A screening value greater than 10 µg/dL requires repeat testing for a diagnosis and to determine the need for treatment. Treatment involves removal of the lead source and, in cases of severe toxicity, administration of a chelating agent. A public health team should evaluate the source of lead because meticulous removal is needed.

Mercury Toxicity. Mercury has been used for industrial and medical purposes for hundreds of years. Mercury is toxic, and the hazards of mercury-associated occupational and accidental exposures are well known. In recent times, the primary concern of the general public about the potential hazards of mercury has focused on exposure from eating certain fish, amalgams used in dentistry, and vaccines.[12] Mercury is present in four primary forms: mercury vapor, inorganic divalent mercury, methyl mercury, and ethyl mercury.[12] Depending on the form of mercury exposure, toxicity involving the central nervous system and kidney can occur.

In the case of dental fillings, the concern involves mercury vapor being released into the mouth. However, the amount of mercury vapor released from fillings is very small. There is no clear evidence supporting health risk from this type of exposure, and removal of amalgams may temporarily increase blood levels of mercury.[12] The main source of methyl mercury exposure is from consumption of long-lived fish, such as tuna and swordfish. Fish concentrate mercury from sediment in the water. Because the developing brain is more susceptible to mercury-induced damage, it is recommended that young children and pregnant and nursing women avoid consumption of fish known to contain high mercury content. Thimerosal is an ethyl mercury–containing preservative that helps prevent microbial growth in vaccines. Concern about potential adverse effects have led to the creation of single-dose vials that eliminate the need for thimerosal.[12] In the United States and Canada, most vaccines are either free of thimerosal or contain only trace amounts.

Injury from Biologic Agents

Biologic agents differ from other injurious agents in that they are able to replicate and can continue to produce their injurious effects (see Chapter 14). These agents range from submicroscopic viruses to the larger parasites. Biologic agents injure cells by diverse mechanisms. Viruses enter the cell and incorporate its genetic material into their cellular DNA, which then enables synthesis of new viruses. Certain bacteria produce exotoxins that may interfere with cellular protein synthesis. Other bacteria, such as the gram-negative bacilli, release endotoxins that cause cell injury and increased capillary permeability.

Injury from Nutritional Imbalances

Nutritional excesses and nutritional deficiencies predispose cells to injury. Obesity and diets high in saturated fats are thought to predispose persons to atherosclerosis. The body requires more than 60 organic and inorganic substances in amounts ranging from micrograms to grams. These nutrients include minerals, vitamins, certain fatty acids, and specific amino acids. Dietary deficiencies can occur because of a selective deficiency of a single nutrient. Iron-deficiency anemia, scurvy, beriberi, and pellagra are examples of injury caused by a lack of specific vitamins or minerals. The protein and calorie deficiencies that occur with starvation cause widespread tissue damage.

Mechanisms of Cell Injury

The mechanisms by which injurious agents cause cell injury and death are complex. Some agents, such as heat, produce direct cell injury; other factors, such as genetic derangements, produce their effects indirectly through metabolic disturbances and altered immune responses. There seem to be at least three major mechanisms whereby most injurious agents exert their effects: free radical formation, hypoxia and ATP depletion, and disruption of intracellular calcium homeostasis (Fig. 2-6).

Free Radical Injury

Cell injury in many circumstances involves the production of reactive chemical species known as free radicals.[1,2,13–15] These circumstances include ischemia-reperfusion injury,

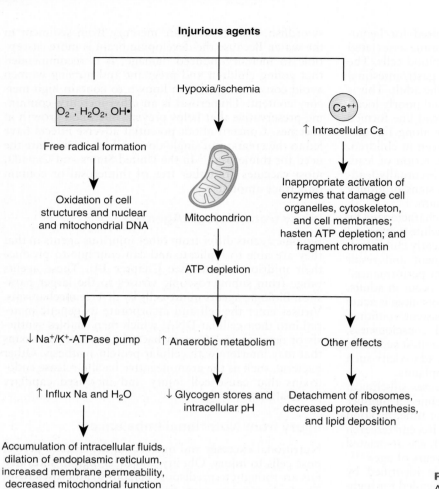

Injurious agents

O_2^-, H_2O_2, OH•

Hypoxia/ischemia

Ca^{++}

Free radical formation

↑ Intracellular Ca

Oxidation of cell structures and nuclear and mitochondrial DNA

Mitochondrion

Inappropriate activation of enzymes that damage cell organelles, cytoskeleton, and cell membranes; hasten ATP depletion; and fragment chromatin

ATP depletion

↓ Na^+/K^+-ATPase pump

↑ Anaerobic metabolism

Other effects

↑ Influx Na and H_2O

↓ Glycogen stores and intracellular pH

Detachment of ribosomes, decreased protein synthesis, and lipid deposition

Accumulation of intracellular fluids, dilation of endoplasmic reticulum, increased membrane permeability, decreased mitochondrial function

FIGURE 2-6. Mechanisms of cell injury. ATP, adenosine triphosphate.

chemical and radiation injury, toxicity from oxygen and other gases, cellular aging, responses to microbial infections, and tissue injury caused by inflammation.

Free radicals are highly reactive chemical species with an unpaired electron in the outer orbit (valence shell) of the molecule. In the literature, the unpaired electron is denoted by a dot, for example, NO•. The unpaired electron causes free radicals to be unstable and highly reactive, so that they react nonspecifically with molecules in the vicinity. Moreover, free radicals can establish chain reactions consisting of many events that generate new free radicals. In cells and tissues, free radicals react with proteins, lipids, and carbohydrates, thereby damaging cell membranes, inactivating enzymes, and damaging nucleic acids that make up DNA.

Many free radicals that are harmful in human physiology are derived from oxygen. These *reactive oxygen species* (ROS) include free radicals, such as superoxide anion (O_2^-) and hydroxyl radical (OH•), as well as reactive oxygen-containing species that are not free radicals, such as hydrogen peroxide (H_2O_2). Reactive oxygen species are normal products of mitochondrial respiration and energy metabolism, and are typically removed by cellular antioxidative systems. Exogenous causes, including ionizing and UV radiation, can also cause ROS production in the body. *Oxidative stress* is a condition

that occurs when the generation of ROS exceeds the ability of the body to neutralize and eliminate ROS. Oxidative stress can lead to oxidation of cell components, activation of signal transduction pathways, DNA damage, and changes in gene expression. In addition to focusing on nuclear DNA as a target of oxidative injury, current studies are focusing on mitochondrial DNA as a target of oxidation and subsequent cause of mitochondrial dysfunction.[16]

Although ROS and oxidative stress are clearly associated with cell and tissue damage, recent evidence suggests that ROS are not always acting in a random and damaging manner. Current studies find that ROS are also important signaling molecules that are used in healthy cells to regulate normal functions such as vascular smooth muscle tone and vascular endothelial growth factor (VEGF) signaling, and even function as a preconditioning factor to protect cells from injury.[17]

Antioxidants are natural and synthetic molecules that inhibit the reactions of ROS with biologic structures or that prevent the uncontrolled formation of ROS. Antioxidants include enzymatic and nonenzymatic compounds. Enzymes known to function as antioxidants include superoxide dismutase (SOD), catalase, glutathione peroxidase, and thioreductase. Superoxide dismutase forms hydrogen peroxide from superoxide. Catalase, present in peroxisomes, catalyzes the reaction that forms water from hydrogen peroxide. Nonenzymatic antioxidants include carotenes (e.g., vitamin A), tocopherols (e.g., vitamin E), ascorbate (vitamin C), glutathione, and flavonoids, as well as micronutrients such as selenium and zinc.[18] Nonenzymatic antioxidants often directly react with oxidants to "disarm" them. For example, vitamin C directly scavenges superoxide and hydroxyl radicals.[19]

Oxidative damage has been implicated in many diseases. Mutations in the gene for SOD are associated with amyotrophic lateral sclerosis (ALS; so-called *Lou Gehrig disease*).[20] Oxidative stress is thought to have an important role in the development of cancer.[21] Reestablishment of blood flow following loss of perfusion, as occurs during heart attack and stroke, is associated with oxidative injury to vital organs. The endothelial dysfunction that contributes to the development, progression, and prognosis of cardiovascular diseases is thought to be caused in part by oxidative stress.[22] In addition, oxidative stress has been associated with age-related functional declines.[23]

Hypoxic Cell Injury

Hypoxia deprives the cell of oxygen and interrupts oxidative metabolism and the generation of ATP. The actual time necessary to produce irreversible cell damage depends on the degree of oxygen deprivation and the metabolic needs of the cell. Some cells, such as those in the heart, brain, and kidney, require large amounts of oxygen to provide the energy to perform their functions. Brain cells, for example, begin to undergo permanent damage after 4 to 6 minutes of oxygen deprivation. A thin margin of time exists between reversible and irreversible cell damage. A classic study found that the epithelial cells of the proximal tubule of the kidney in the rat could survive 20 but not 30 minutes of ischemia.[24] Recent work has identified a group of proteins called *hypoxia-inducible factors* (HIFs). During hypoxic conditions, HIFs cause the expression of genes that stimulate red blood cell formation, manufacture glycolytic enzymes that produce ATP in the absence of oxygen, and increase angiogenesis[25] (i.e., the formation of new blood vessels).

Hypoxia can result from an inadequate amount of oxygen in the air, respiratory disease, ischemia (i.e., decreased blood flow due to vasoconstriction or vascular obstruction), anemia, edema, or inability of the cells to use oxygen. Ischemia is characterized by impaired oxygen delivery and impaired removal of metabolic end products such as lactic acid. In contrast to pure hypoxia, which depends on the oxygen content of the blood and affects all cells in the body, ischemia commonly depends on blood flow through limited numbers of blood vessels and produces local tissue injury. In some cases of edema, the distance for diffusion of oxygen may become a limiting factor in the delivery of oxygen. In hypermetabolic states, the cells may require more oxygen than can be supplied by normal respiratory function and oxygen transport. Hypoxia also serves as the ultimate cause of cell death in other injuries. For example, physical factors such as a cold temperature can cause severe constriction and impair blood flow.

Hypoxia causes a power failure in the cell, with widespread effects on the cell's structural and functional components. As oxygen tension in the cell falls, oxidative metabolism ceases, and the cell reverts to anaerobic metabolism, using its limited glycogen stores in an attempt to maintain vital cell functions. Cellular pH falls as lactic acid accumulates in the cell. This reduction in pH can have adverse effects on intracellular structures and biochemical reactions. Low pH can alter cell membranes and cause chromatin clumping and cell volume changes.

An important effect of reduced ATP is acute cell swelling caused by failure of the energy-dependent sodium/potassium (Na^+/K^+)-adenosine triphosphatase (ATPase) membrane pump, which extrudes sodium from and returns potassium to the cell. With impaired function of this pump, intracellular potassium levels decrease, and sodium and water accumulate in the cell. The movement of water and ions into the cell is associated with dilation of the endoplasmic reticulum, increased membrane permeability, and decreased mitochondrial function.[2] To a point, the cellular changes due to hypoxia are reversible if oxygenation is restored. However, if the oxygen supply is not restored there is continued loss of enzymes, proteins, and ribonucleic acid through the hyperpermeable cell membrane. Injury to the lysosomal membranes results in the leakage of destructive lysosomal enzymes into the cytoplasm and enzymatic digestion of cell components. Leakage of intracellular enzymes through the permeable cell membrane into the extracellular fluid provides an important clinical indicator of cell injury and death. These enzymes enter the blood and can be measured by laboratory tests.

Impaired Calcium Homeostasis

Calcium functions as an important second messenger and cytosolic signal for many cell responses. Various calcium-binding proteins, such as troponin and calmodulin, act as transducers for cytosolic calcium signaling. Calcium/calmodulin–dependent kinases indirectly mediate the effects of calcium on responses such as smooth muscle contraction and glycogen breakdown. Normally, intracellular calcium ion levels are kept extremely low compared with extracellular levels. These low intracellular levels are maintained by energy-dependent membrane-associated calcium/magnesium (Ca^{++}/Mg^{++})-ATPase exchange systems[2] and sequestration of calcium ions within organelles such as the mitochondria and smooth endoplasmic reticulum. Ischemia and certain toxins lead to an increase in cytosolic calcium because of the increased influx across the cell membrane and the release of calcium from intracellular stores. The increased calcium level may inappropriately activate a number of enzymes with potentially damaging effects. These enzymes include phospholipases that can damage the cell membrane, proteases that damage the cytoskeleton and membrane proteins, ATPases that break down ATP and hasten its depletion, and endonucleases that fragment chromatin. Although it is known that injured cells accumulate calcium, it is unknown whether this is the ultimate cause of irreversible cell injury.

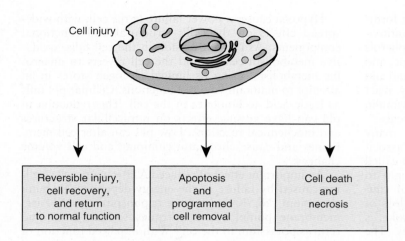

Cell injury

| Reversible injury, cell recovery, and return to normal function | Apoptosis and programmed cell removal | Cell death and necrosis |

FIGURE 2-7. Outcomes of cell injury: reversible cell injury, apoptosis and programmed cell removal, cell death, and necrosis.

Reversible Cell Injury and Cell Death

The mechanisms of cell injury can produce sublethal and reversible cellular damage or lead to irreversible injury with cell destruction or death (Fig. 2-7). Cell destruction and removal usually involve one of two mechanisms: apoptosis, which is designed to remove injured or worn-out cells, or cell death or necrosis, which occurs in irreversibly damaged cells.

Reversible Cell Injury

Reversible cell injury, although impairing cell function, does not result in cell death. Two patterns of reversible cell injury can be observed under the microscope: cellular swelling and fatty change. Cellular swelling occurs with impairment of the energy-dependent Na$^+$/K$^+$-ATPase membrane pump, usually as the result of hypoxic cell injury.

Fatty changes are linked to intracellular accumulation of fat. When fatty changes occur, small vacuoles of fat disperse throughout the cytoplasm. The process is usually more ominous than cellular swelling, and although it is reversible, it usually indicates severe injury. These fatty changes may occur because normal cells are presented with an increased fat load or because injured cells are unable to metabolize the fat properly. In obese persons, fatty infiltrates often occur within and between the cells of the liver and heart because of an increased fat load. Pathways for fat metabolism may be impaired during cell injury, and fat may accumulate in the cell as production exceeds use and export. The liver, where most fats are synthesized and metabolized, is particularly susceptible to fatty change, but fatty changes may also occur in the kidney, the heart, and other organs.

Programmed Cell Death

In most normal nontumor cells, the number of cells in tissues is regulated by balancing cell proliferation and cell death. Cell death occurs by necrosis or a form of programmed cell death called *apoptosis*.

Apoptosis, from the Greek *apo* for "apart" and *ptosis* for "fallen," means "fallen apart." Apoptosis is a highly selective process that eliminates injured and aged cells, thereby controlling tissue regeneration.[26] Cells undergoing apoptosis have characteristic morphologic features, as well as biochemical changes. As shown in Figure 2-8, shrinking and condensation of the nucleus and cytoplasm occur. The chromatin aggregates at the nuclear envelope, and DNA fragmentation occurs. Then, the cell becomes fragmented into multiple apoptotic bodies in a manner that maintains the integrity of the plasma membrane and does not initiate inflammation. Changes in the plasma membrane induce phagocytosis of the apoptotic bodies by macrophages and other cells, thereby completing the degradation process.

Apoptosis is thought to be responsible for several normal physiologic processes, including the programmed destruction of cells during embryonic development, hormone-dependent involution of tissues, death of immune cells, cell death by cytotoxic T cells, and cell death in proliferating cell populations. During embryogenesis, in the development of a number of organs such as the heart, which begins as a pulsating tube and is gradually modified to become a four-chambered pump, apoptotic cell death allows for the next stage of organ development.

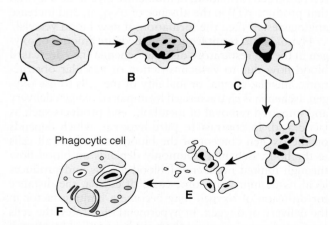

FIGURE 2-8. Apoptotic cell removal. **(A)** Shrinking of the cell structures. **(B, C)** Condensation and fragmentation of the nuclear chromatin. **(D, E)** Separation of nuclear fragments and cytoplasmic organelles into apoptotic bodies. **(F)** Engulfment of apoptotic fragments by phagocytic cell.

It also separates the webbed fingers and toes of the developing embryo. Apoptotic cell death occurs in the hormone-dependent involution of endometrial cells during the menstrual cycle and in the regression of breast tissue after weaning from breast-feeding. The control of immune cell numbers and destruction of autoreactive T cells in the thymus have been credited to apoptosis. Cytotoxic T cells and natural killer cells are thought to destroy target cells by inducing apoptotic cell death.

Apoptosis is linked to many pathologic processes and diseases. For example, interference with apoptosis is known to be a mechanism that contributes to carcinogenesis.[27] Apoptosis is also known to be involved in the cell death associated with viral infections, such as hepatitis B and C.[27,28] Apoptosis may also be implicated in neurodegenerative disorders such as ALS, Alzheimer disease, and Parkinson disease. However, the exact mechanisms involved in these diseases remains under investigation.

Two basic pathways for apoptosis have been described (Fig. 2-9). These are the extrinsic pathway, which is death receptor dependent, and the intrinsic pathway, which is death receptor independent. The execution phase of both pathways is carried out by proteolytic enzymes called *caspases* (cysteine proteases that cleave aspartate residues), which are present in the cell as *procaspases* and are activated by cleavage of an inhibitory portion of their polypeptide chain.[2,29]

The *extrinsic pathway* involves extracellular signaling proteins that bind to cell surface molecules called *death receptors* and trigger apoptosis. The prototype death receptors are tumor necrosis factor (TNF) receptor and the Fas ligand receptor.[29] Fas ligand may be expressed on the surface of certain cells, such as cytotoxic T cells, or appear in a soluble form. When Fas ligand binds to its receptor, proteins congregate at the cytoplasmic end of the Fas receptor to form a death-initiating complex. The complex then converts procaspase-8 to caspase-8. Caspase-8, in turn, activates a cascade of caspases that execute the process of apoptosis. The end result includes activation of endonucleases that cause fragmentation of DNA and cell death. In addition to TNF and Fas ligand, primary signaling molecules known to activate the extrinsic pathway include TNF-related apoptosis-inducing ligand (TRAIL); the cytokine interleukin-1 (IL-1); and lipopolysaccharide (LPS), the endotoxin found in the outer cell membrane of gram-negative bacteria.

The *intrinsic pathway*, or *mitochondrion-induced pathway*, of apoptosis is activated by conditions such as DNA damage, ROS, hypoxia, decreased ATP levels, cellular senescence, and activation of the p53 protein by DNA damage. The intrinsic pathway is tightly regulated to ensure that cells kill themselves only when appropriate. A major class of intracellular regulators of apoptosis is the Bcl-2 family of proteins. Some of these proteins insert into the mitochondrial membrane opening channels through which proteins escape into the cytoplasm.[29] A crucial protein released from the mitochondria is cytochrome c, a component of the mitochondrial electron transport chain (see Chapter 1). When released into the cytoplasm, cytochrome c binds to a procaspase-activating protein that activates caspases,

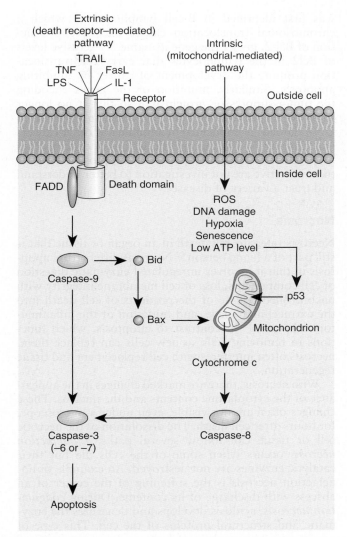

FIGURE 2-9. Pathways for apoptosis. The *extrinsic pathway* is activated by signals such as TNF-related apoptosis-inducing ligand (TRAIL) and Fas ligand (FasL) that, upon binding to the Fas receptor, form a death-inducing complex by joining the Fas-associated death domain (FADD) to the death domain of the Fas receptor. The *intrinsic pathway* is activated by signals, such as reactive oxygen species (ROS) and DNA damage, which induce the release of cytochrome c from mitochondria into the cytoplasm. Both pathways activate caspases to execute apoptosis, with activation of the pro-apoptotic proteins Bid and Bax by caspase-8 serving to bridge the two systems. ATP, adenosine triphosphate; DNA, deoxyribonucleic acid; IL-1, interleukin-1; LPS, lipopolysaccharide; TNF, tumor necrosis factor.

including caspase-3. Caspase-3 activation is a common step to both the extrinsic and intrinsic pathways. Activation of caspase-8 in the extrinsic pathway can also lead to activation of pro-apoptotic proteins, such as Bid and Bax, thereby bridging the two pathways for apoptosis.[2,29] While some members of the Bcl-2 family are pro-apoptotic, others are anti-apoptotic and inhibit apoptosis by binding to pro-apoptotic proteins, either on the mitochondrial membranes or in the cytoplasm.

Inhibitors of apoptosis are thought to contribute to cancer and autoimmune diseases.[29–31] The Bcl-2 gene was first identified in B-cell lymphoma, in which a chromosomal translocation causes excessive production of Bcl-2, giving the gene its name.[29] Excessive levels of Bcl2 in the lymphocytes that carry the translocation promote the development of cancer by inhibiting apoptosis. Similarly, mutation of the genes encoding the tumor-suppressor protein p53 so that it no longer suppresses apoptosis or cell cycle arrest in response to DNA damage is implicated in a number of other cancers (see Chapter 7). The therapeutic actions of certain drugs may induce or facilitate apoptosis. Apoptosis continues to be an active area of investigation to better understand and treat a variety of diseases.

Necrosis

Necrosis refers to cell death in an organ or tissue that is still part of a living person.[32] Necrosis differs from apoptosis in that it involves unregulated enzymatic digestion of cell components, loss of cell membrane integrity with uncontrolled release of the products of cell death into the extracellular space, and initiation of the inflammatory response.[32] In contrast to apoptosis, which functions in removing cells so new cells can replace them, necrosis often interferes with cell replacement and tissue regeneration.

With necrosis, there are marked changes in the appearance of the cytoplasmic contents and the nucleus. These changes often are not visible, even under a microscope, for hours after cell death. The dissolution of the necrotic cell or tissue can follow several paths. *Liquefaction necrosis* occurs when some of the cells die but their catalytic enzymes are not destroyed. An example of liquefaction necrosis is the softening of the center of an abscess with discharge of its contents. During *coagulation necrosis*, acidosis develops and denatures the enzymatic and structural proteins of the cell. This type of necrosis is characteristic of hypoxic injury and is seen in infarcted areas. *Infarction* (i.e., tissue death) occurs when an artery supplying an organ or part of the body becomes occluded and no other source of blood supply exists. As a rule, the shape of the infarction is conical and corresponds to the distribution of the artery and its branches. An artery may be occluded by an embolus, a thrombus, disease of the arterial wall, or pressure from outside the vessel.

Caseous necrosis is a distinctive form of coagulation necrosis in which the dead cells persist indefinitely as soft, cheese-like debris.[1] It is most commonly found in the center of tuberculosis granulomas, or tubercles, and is thought to result from immune mechanisms (see Chapter 22).

The term *gangrene* is applied when a considerable mass of tissue undergoes necrosis. Gangrene may be classified as dry or moist. In dry gangrene, the part becomes dry and shrinks, the skin wrinkles, and its color changes to dark brown or black. The spread of dry gangrene is slow, and its symptoms are not as marked as those of wet gangrene. The irritation caused by the dead tissue produces a line of inflammatory reaction (i.e., line of

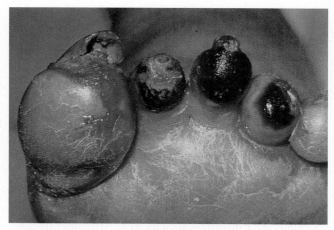

FIGURE 2-10. Gangrenous toes. (Biomedical Communications Group, Southern Illinois University School of Medicine, Springfield, IL.)

demarcation) between the dead tissue of the gangrenous area and the healthy tissue (Fig. 2-10). Dry gangrene usually results from interference with arterial blood supply to a part without interference with venous return and is a form of coagulation necrosis.

In moist or wet gangrene, the area is cold, swollen, and pulseless. The skin is moist, black, and under tension. Blebs form on the surface, liquefaction occurs, and a foul odor is caused by bacterial action. There is no line of demarcation between the normal and diseased tissues, and the spread of tissue damage is rapid. Systemic symptoms are usually severe, and death may occur unless the condition can be arrested. Moist or wet gangrene primarily results from interference with venous return from the part. Bacterial invasion plays an important role in the development of wet gangrene and is responsible for many of its prominent symptoms. Dry gangrene is confined almost exclusively to the extremities, but moist gangrene may affect the internal organs or the extremities. If bacteria invade the necrotic tissue, dry gangrene may be converted to wet gangrene.

Gas gangrene is a special type of gangrene that results from infection of devitalized tissues by one of several *Clostridium* bacteria, most commonly *Clostridium perfringens*. These anaerobic and spore-forming organisms are widespread in nature, particularly in soil; gas gangrene is prone to occur in trauma and compound fractures in which dirt and debris are embedded. Some species have been isolated in the stomach, gallbladder, intestine, vagina, and skin of healthy persons. The bacteria produce toxins that dissolve cell membranes, causing death of muscle cells, massive spreading edema, hemolysis of red blood cells, hemolytic anemia, hemoglobinuria, and renal failure.[33] Characteristic of this disorder are the bubbles of hydrogen sulfide gas that form in the muscle. Gas gangrene is a serious and potentially fatal disease. Antibiotics are used to treat the infection and surgical methods are used to remove the infected tissue. Amputation may be required to prevent spreading infection involving a limb. Hyperbaric oxygen therapy has been used, but clinical data supporting its efficacy has not been rigorously assessed.

Cellular Aging

Aging is a complex natural process in which there are physiologic and structural alterations in almost all organ systems.[1,2,34-38] Even in the absence of disease, beginning in the fourth decade of life, there is a progressive decline in muscle strength, cardiac reserve, vital capacity, nerve conduction time, and glomerular filtration rate. Although the biologic basis of aging is poorly understood, there is general consensus that its elucidation should be sought at the cellular level. Many cell functions decline with age. Oxidative phosphorylation by the mitochondria is reduced, as is synthesis of nucleic acids and transcription factors, cell receptors, and cell proteins.

A number of theories have been proposed to explain the cause of aging. The main theories are based on scientific observations at the molecular, cellular, organ, and system levels. In general, these theories can be divided into either programmed or error theories. The *programmed theories* propose that the changes that occur with aging are genetically programmed, whereas the *damage* or *error theories* maintain that the changes result from an accumulation of random events or environmental agents or influences that are associated with DNA damage.[35-39] Evidence suggests that the process of aging and longevity is multifaceted, with both genetic and environmental factors playing a role. In animal studies, genetics accounted for less than 35% of the effects of aging, whereas environmental influences accounted for over 65%.[36] In humans, long life appears to have a stronger genetic basis, which explains why centenarians and near centenarians tend to cluster in families.[40]

Replicative Senescence

Replicative senescence implies that cells have a limited capacity for replication. At the cellular level, Hayflick and Moorhead observed more than 40 years ago that cultured human fibroblasts have a limited ability to replicate (approximately 50 population doublings) and then die.[41] Before achieving this maximum, they slow their rate of division and manifest identifiable and predictable morphologic changes characteristic of senescent cells.

One explanation of replicative senescence is related to the length of the outermost regions of each chromosome, called *telomeres,* that contain short repeat sequences of DNA bases.[1,2,35] During mitosis, the molecular machinery that replicates DNA cannot copy the extreme ends of the chromosome. Thus, with each cell division, a small segment of telomeric DNA is lost. Over time, it is theorized that as the telomeres become progressively shorter, the DNA at the ends of the chromosomes cannot be protected, resulting in inhibition of cell replication. The lengths of the telomeres are normally maintained by an enzyme called *telomerase,* which is present in low levels in stem cells, but is usually absent in most adult cells. Therefore, as cells age, their telomeres become shorter and they lose their ability to replicate and replace damaged or senescent cells. Moreover, oxidative stress induces single-stranded damage to telomeric DNA, and this defect cannot be repaired in telomeres. In theory, such mechanisms could also provide a safeguard against uncontrolled cell proliferation of abnormal cells. It has been shown that telomerase is reactivated and telomeres are not shortened in immortal cancer cells, suggesting that telomere elongation may be important in tumor formation.

Genetic Influences

There is ongoing interest in genes that determine longevity. Longevity genes have been found in fruit flies and roundworms, organisms that have attracted considerable attention from scientists because of their short life span and their well-characterized genomes. One example is the mutation of the *Indy* (I'm Not Dead Yet) gene in the fruit fly, which can double the length of its life.[35] Scientists have also found genetic clues to the aging process in the tiny roundworm, *Caenorhabditis elegans*. By altering one of its *daf-2* genes, which codes for a protein that is similar to insulin and insulin growth factor (IGF)-1 receptors found in humans, researchers can substantially extend the longevity of these worms.[1,35] Pathways related to the *daf-2* gene, for example, may be responsible for relationships between caloric restriction and prolonged life span in rodents and other animals. Whether human counterparts of genes found in these laboratory organisms exist and whether they have similar effects remain an ongoing area of inquiry.

However, many genes that are associated with human life span are not intrinsically "longevity genes," per se. For example, because mutations in the tumor-suppressor genes BRAC1 and BRAC2 increase mortality associated with breast and ovarian cancer, they are rare among long-lived women.[40] Conversely, genes that reduce the risk of atherosclerosis may be more common in long-lived individuals. Genetic studies of biologic aging have also explored the involvement of variants of genes encoding apolipoproteins (proteins that bind lipids for transport in the circulatory system), in particular, the APOE gene encoding the synthesis of apolipoprotein E. The presence of the variant apoE4 is associated with an increased incidence of cardiovascular and neurodegenerative diseases, thereby shortening life span.[37,41]

Accumulation of Environmental and Genetic Damage

In addition to the importance of timing and a genetic clock, cellular life span may be determined by a balance between cellular damage resulting from metabolic events occurring within the cell and molecular responses that repair the damage. The damage eventually accumulates to a level sufficient to result in the physiologic decline associated with aging. The most prominent example of the damage theory is the somatic mutation theory of aging, which states that the longevity and function of cells in various tissues of the body are determined by the double-stranded DNA molecule and its specific repair enzymes. Deoxyribonucleic acid undergoes continuous change in response to both exogenous agents and intrinsic processes. It has been suggested that aging results from conditions that produce mutations in DNA or deficits in DNA repair mechanisms.

The oxidative free radical explanation of aging is an error theory in which aging is thought to result partially from oxidative stress and the effects of free radical damage. The major by-products of oxidative metabolism include superoxides that react with DNA, ribonucleic acid, proteins, and lipids, leading to cellular damage and aging. Blood glucose is another suspect in cellular deterioration. In a process called *nonenzymatic glycation*, glucose molecules attach to proteins, setting in motion a chain of chemical reactions that ends with proteins binding together or cross-linking, thus altering their structure and function. Investigators hypothesize that glycation and oxidation are interdependent, since free radicals and cross-links seem to accelerate the formation of one another. Cross-links, also known as *advanced glycation end products (AGEs),* tend to stiffen tissues and cause some of the deterioration associated with aging.[2,35] For example, AGEs may help trap low-density cholesterol in arterial walls and thus contribute to atherosclerosis. They also have been linked to cataract formation, reduced kidney function, and neurologic disorders such as Alzheimer disease.

Syndromes of Premature Aging

The syndromes of premature aging, or *progeria*, represent a range of phenotypes seen in usual aging, but with much earlier ages of onset and more rapid rates of progression.[1] Hutchinson-Gilford progeria syndrome is a rare fatal genetic disorder characterized by accelerated aging in children.[42] The disorder is caused by a mutation in the *LMNA* gene, which codes for a precursor of lamin A—a scaffolding protein that lines the nucleus. The mutant gene leads to abnormal nuclear structure and altered gene regulation and DNA replication. Although they are born looking healthy, children with the disorder begin to display many characteristics of accelerated aging at around 18 to 24 months of age. Progeria signs include growth failure, loss of body fat and hair, aged-looking skin, cataracts, and coronary artery disease and stroke (Fig. 2-11). Death occurs at an early age of atherosclerotic heart disease (average age 13 years).

Other progeroid syndromes include Werner syndrome, also known as adult progeria, which does not have an onset until the late teens, with a life span into the 40s and 50s.[1] The gene responsible for the disorder has been localized to chromosome 8 and appears to code for an enzyme involved in unwinding DNA, a process that is necessary for DNA repair and replication.

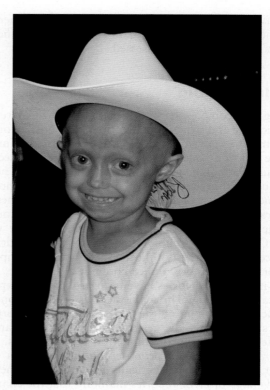

FIGURE 2-11. A 5-year-girl with progeria. (From National Human Genome Research Institute, National Institutes of Health.)

SUMMARY CONCEPTS

- Cell injury can be caused by a number of agents, including physical agents, chemicals, biologic agents, and nutritional factors.

- Among the physical agents that generate cell injury are mechanical forces that produce tissue trauma, extremes of temperature, and electrical forces. Ionizing radiation can directly break chemical bonds, whereas nonionizing radiation exerts its harmful effects by causing vibration and rotation of atoms and molecules. Chemical agents can block enzymatic pathways, cause coagulation of tissues, or disrupt the osmotic or ionic balance of the cell. Biologic agents differ from other injurious agents in that they are able to replicate and continue to produce injury. Among the nutritional factors that contribute to cell injury are excesses and deficiencies of total energy, as well as individual nutrients.

- Injurious agents exert their effects largely through generation of reactive oxygen species (ROS) and free radicals, promotion of cell hypoxia, or impaired regulation of intracellular calcium levels. Free radicals are an important cause of cell injury in hypoxia and after exposure to radiation and certain chemical agents. Lack of oxygen, which underlies the pathogenesis of cell injury in hypoxia and ischemic, can result from inadequate oxygen in the air, cardiopulmonary disease, cardiorespiratory disease, anemia, or the inability of the cells to use oxygen. Increased intracellular calcium activates a number of enzymes with potentially damaging effects.

■ Injurious agents may produce sublethal and reversible cellular damage or may lead to irreversible cell injury and death. Cell death can involve two mechanisms: apoptosis or necrosis. *Apoptosis* involves controlled cell destruction and is the means by which the body removes and replaces cells that have been produced in excess, developed improperly, have genetic damage, or are worn out. *Necrosis* refers to cell death that is characterized by cell swelling, rupture of the cell membrane, and inflammation.

■ A number of body functions decline with age, including muscle strength, cardiac reserve, vital capacity, nerve conduction time, and glomerular filtration rate. At the cellular level, oxidative phosphorylation by the mitochondria is reduced, as is the synthesis of nucleic acids and transcription factors, cell receptors, and structural and enzymatic proteins.

REVIEW EXERCISES

1. A 30-year-old man sustained a fracture of his leg 2 months ago. The leg has been encased in a cast and he has just had the cast removed. He is amazed at the degree to which the muscles in his leg have shrunk.

   A. Explain.

2. A 45-year-old woman has been receiving radiation therapy for breast cancer.

   A. Explain the effects of ionizing radiation in eradicating the tumor cells.
   B. Why is the radiation treatment given in small divided, or fractionated, doses rather than as a single large dose?
   C. Partway through the treatment schedule, the woman notices that her skin over the irradiated area has become reddened and irritated. What is the reason for this?

3. People who have had a heart attack may experience additional damage once blood flow has been restored, a phenomenon referred to as *reperfusion injury*.

   A. What is the proposed mechanism underlying reperfusion injury?
   B. What factors might influence this mechanism?

4. Every day blood cells in our body become senescent and die without producing signs of inflammation, yet massive injury or destruction of tissue, such as occurs with a heart attack, produces significant signs of inflammation.

   A. Explain.

REFERENCES

1. Strayer DS, Rubin E. Cell adaptation, cell injury, and cell death. In: Rubin R, Strayer CS, eds. *Rubin's Pathology: Clinicopathologic Foundations of Medicine.* 6th ed. Philadelphia, PA: Wolters Kluwer Health/Lippincott Williams & Wilkins; 2012:1–46.
2. Kumar V, Abbas AK, Fauusto N, et al. *Robbins Basic Pathology.* 8th ed. Philadelphia, PA: Saunders Elsevier; 2010:3–42.
3. Heszele MFC, Price SR. Insulin-like growth factor 1: the yin and yang of muscle atrophy. *Endocrinology.* 2004;145:4803–4805.
4. Heineke J, Molkentin JD. Regulation of cardiac hypertrophy by intracellular signalling pathways. *Nat Rev Mol Cell Biol.* 2006;7:589–600.
5. Hunter JJ, Chien KR. Signaling pathways in cardiac hypertrophy and failure. *N Engl J Med.* 1999;341:1276–1283.
6. Anastassios C, Koumbourlis MD. Electrical injuries. *Crit Care Med.* 2002;30(suppl):S424–S430.
7. Strayer DS, Rubin E. Environmental and nutritional pathology. In: Rubin R, Strayer CS, eds. *Rubin's Pathology: Clinicopathologic Foundations of Medicine.* 6th ed. Philadelphia, PA: Lippincott Williams & Wilkins; 2012:293–328.
8. Centers for Disease Control and Prevention. *Preventing Lead Poisoning in Young Children: A Statement by the Centers for Disease Control and Prevention.* Atlanta, GA: U.S. Department of Health and Human Services, Public Health Service; 2005.
9. Warniment C, Tsang K, Galazka SK. Lead poisoning in children. *Am Fam Physician.* 2010;81(6):751–760.
10. Chandran L, Cataldo R. Lead poisoning: basics and new substances. *Pediatr Rev.* 2010;31(10):399–405.
11. Canfield RL, Henderson CR Jr, Cory-Slechta DA, et al. Intellectual impairment in children with blood lead concentrations below 10 μg per deciliter. *N Engl J Med.* 2003;348:1517–1526.
12. Clarkson TW, Magos L, Myers GJ. The toxicity of mercury—Current exposures and clinical manifestations. *N Engl J Med.* 2003;349:1731–1737.
13. McCord JM. The evolution of free radicals and oxidative stress. *Am J Med.* 2000;108:652–659.
14. Poljsak B. Strategies for reducing or preventing the generation of oxidative stress. *Oxid Med Cell Longev.* 2011(H):1–15.
15. Chuyanyu CL, Jackson RM. Reactive species mechanisms of cellular hypoxia-reoxygenation injury. *Am J Physiol Cell Physiol.* 2002;282:C227–C241.
16. Lagouge M, Larsson NG. The role of mitochondrial DNA mutations and free radicals in disease and ageing. *J Intern Med.* 2013;273:529–543.
17. Finkel T. Oxidant signals and oxidative stress. *Curr Opin Cell Biol.* 2003;15:247–254.

18. Brenneistein P, Steinbrenner H, Seis H. Selenium, oxidative stress, and health aspects. *Mol Aspects Med.* 2005;26:256–267.

19. Comhair SA, Erzuum SC. The regulation and role of extracellular glutathione peroxidase. *Antioxid Redox Signal.* 2005;7:72–79.

20. Johnson F, Giulivi C. Superoxide dismutases and their impact upon human health. *Mol Aspects Med.* 2005;26:340–352.

21. Klaunig JE, Kamendulis LM. The role of oxidative stress in carcinogenesis. *Annu Rev Pharmacol Toxicol.* 2004;44:239–267.

22. Fenster BE, Tsao PS, Rockson SG. Endothelial dysfunction: clinical strategies for treating oxidant stress. *Am Heart J.* 2003;146:218–226.

23. Martin I, Grotewiel MS. Oxidative damage and age-related functional declines. *Mech Ageing Dev.* 2006;127:411–423.

24. Vogt MT, Farber E. On the molecular pathology of ischemic renal cell death: reversible and irreversible cellular and mitochondrial metabolic alterations. *Am J Pathol.* 1968;53:1–26.

25. Marx J. How cells endure low oxygen. *Science.* 2004;303:1454–1456.

26. Favaloro B, Allocati N, Di Ilio C, et al. Role of apoptosis in disease. *Aging.* 2012;4(5):330–345.

27. Vermeulen K, Van Bockstaele DR, Berneman ZN. Apoptosis: mechanisms and relevance in cancer. *Ann Hematol.* 2005;84:627–639.

28. Cruise MW, Lukens JR, Nguyen AP, et al. Fas ligand is responsible for CXCR3 chemokine induction in CD4+ T cell-dependent liver damage. *J Immunol.* 2006;176:6235–6244.

29. Alberts B, Johnson A, Lewis L, et al. *Molecular Biology of the Cell.* 5th ed. New York, NY: Garland Press; 2008:1115–1129.

30. Malhi H, Gores GJ, Lemasters JJ. Apoptosis and necrosis in the liver: a tale of two deaths? *Hepatology.* 2006;43(2 suppl 1):S31–S44.

31. Dorner T, Lipsky PE. Signalling pathways in B cells: implications for autoimmunity. *Curr Top Microbiol Immunol.* 2006;305:213–240.

32. Proskuryakov SY, Konoplyannikov AG, Gabai VL. Necrosis: a specific form of programmed cell death. *Exp Cell Res.* 2003;283:1–16.

33. Kasper DL, Madoff LC. Gas gangrene and other clostridial infections. In: Kasper DL, Braunwald E, Fauci A, et al., eds. *Harrison's Principles of Internal Medicine.* 16th ed. New York, NY: McGraw-Hill; 2005:845–849.

34. Weinert BT, Timiras PS. Invited review: theories of aging. *J Appl Physiol.* 2003;95:1706–1716.

35. National Institute of Aging. *Biology of Aging: Research Today for a Healthier Tomorrow.* 2011. Available at: http://www.nia.nih.gov/sites/default/files/biology_of_aging.pdf/. Accessed August 27, 2013.

36. Hayflick L. Biological aging is no longer an unsolved problem. *Ann N Y Acad Sci.* 2007;1100:1–13.

37. Martin GM. The biology of aging: 1985–2010 and beyond. *FASEB J.* 2011;25:3756–3762.

38. Kim S. Molecular biology of aging. *Arch Surg.* 2003;138:1051–1054.

39. Fredarko NS. The biology of aging and frailty. *Clin Geriatr Med.* 2011;27(1):27–37.

40. Browner WS, Kahn AJ, Ziv E, et al. The genetics of human longevity. *Am J Med.* 2004;117:851–860.

41. Vijg J, Suh Y. Genetics of longevity and aging. *Annu Rev Med.* 2005;56:193–212.

42. Warner HH. Research on Hutchinson-Gilford progeria syndrome. *J Gerantol.* 2008;63A(3):775–786.

Porth Essentials Resources

Explore these additional resources to enhance learning for this chapter:

- NCLEX-Style Questions and Other Resources on the**Point**, http://thePoint.lww.com/PorthEssentials4e
- Study Guide for Essentials of Pathophysiology
- Adaptive Learning | Powered by PrepU, http://thepoint.lww.com/prepu

Chapter **3**

Inflammation, the Inflammatory Response, and Fever

Inflammation is a complex nonspecific response to tissue injury intended to minimize the effects of injury or infection, remove the damaged tissue, generate new tissue, and facilitate healing. As part of the innate immune system, inflammation dilutes, destroys, and gets rid of damaged or necrotic tissues and foreign agents, such as microbes. Although first described over 2000 years ago, the inflammatory response has been the subject of intense research during the past several decades. As a result, it is now recognized as playing a key role in both the contributing factors and consequences of numerous diseases and altered health states including, but not limited to, atherosclerosis, obesity and diabetes, many types of cancers, stroke, bronchial asthma, rheumatoid arthritis, and certain dementias, including Alzheimer disease.

The discussion in this chapter is divided into four sections: (1) the general features of inflammation, (2) acute inflammation, (3) chronic inflammation, and (4) systemic manifestations of inflammation, including fever. The innate and adaptive immune responses that are closely intertwined with the inflammatory response are discussed in Chapter 15.

General Features of Inflammation

Inflammation is the reaction of vascularized tissues to cell injury or death. It is characterized by the production and release of inflammatory mediators and the movement of fluid and leukocytes from the vasculature into the extravascular tissues.[1-4] Inflammatory conditions are commonly named by adding the suffix *-itis* to the affected organ or system. For example, *appendicitis* refers to inflammation of the appendix, *pericarditis* to inflammation of the pericardium, and *neuritis* to inflammation of the nerve.

Inflammation can be acute or chronic.[1,2] *Acute inflammation* is triggered by noxious stimuli, such as infection or tissue injury, is rapid in onset (typically minutes), and is of relatively short duration, lasting from a few minutes to several days. It is characterized by the exudation of fluid and plasma proteins and emigration of leukocytes. *Chronic inflammation* is of a longer duration, lasting for days to years, and is often associated with the proliferation of blood vessels (angiogenesis), tissue necrosis, and fibrosis (scarring). Acute and chronic inflammation may coexist, with episodes of acute inflammation being superimposed on chronic inflammation.

Cells of Inflammation

Many cells and tissue components are involved in the inflammatory process, including the endothelial cells that line blood vessels and form capillaries, circulating platelets and leukocytes, cells in the connective tissue (mast cells, fibroblasts, tissue macrophages), and components of the extracellular matrix (Fig. 3-1).[1–3] The principal leukocytes in acute inflammation are neutrophils, whereas macrophages, lymphocytes, eosinophils, and mast cells predominate in chronic infection.

Endothelial Cells

Endothelial cells, which make up the single-cell-thick linings of blood vessels, help to separate the intravascular and extravascular spaces.[1,2,5] They normally have a nonthrombogenic surface and produce agents that maintain vessel patency, as well as vasodilators and vasoconstrictors that regulate blood flow. Endothelial cells are also key players in the inflammatory response. As such, they provide a selective permeability barrier to exogenous (microbial) and endogenous inflammatory stimuli; regulate leukocyte extravasation by expression of adhesion molecules and receptor activation; contribute to the regulation and modulation of immune responses through synthesis and release of inflammatory mediators; and regulate immune cell proliferation through secretion of hematopoietic colony-stimulating factors (CSFs). Endothelial cells also participate in the repair process that accompanies inflammation through the production of growth factors that stimulate angiogenesis and extracellular matrix synthesis.

Platelets

Platelets or thrombocytes are small, membrane-bound disks circulating in the blood that play an active role in normal hemostasis (see Chapter 12). Activated platelets also release a number of potent inflammatory mediators, thereby increasing vascular permeability and altering the chemotactic, adhesive, and proteolytic properties of the endothelial cells.[6,7] When a platelet undergoes activation, over 300 proteins are released. While the functions of only a relatively small proportion of these proteins have been fully elucidated, it appears that many help mediate inflammation.[6] The association between the platelet and inflammatory diseases is highlighted by the number of inflammatory disease processes (e.g., atherosclerosis, migraine headaches, systemic lupus erythematosus) shown to be associated with platelet activation.[6]

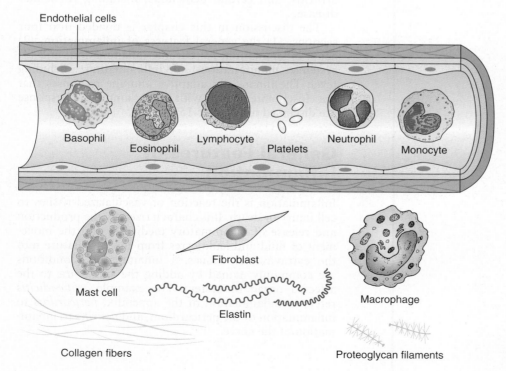

Endothelial cells

Basophil

Eosinophil

Lymphocyte

Platelets

Neutrophil

Monocyte

Mast cell

Fibroblast

Elastin

Collagen fibers

Macrophage

Proteoglycan filaments

FIGURE 3-1. Cells involved in the inflammatory process.

Leukocytes

Leukocytes or white blood cells are the major cellular components of the inflammatory response. They include the granulocytes (neutrophils, eosinophils, and basophils), which contain specific cytoplasmic granules and a multilobed nucleus, and the agranulocytes (monocytes/macrophages and lymphocytes), which lack cytoplasmic granules and have a single nucleus.

Neutrophils. Neutrophils are the most numerous leukocytes in the circulating blood, accounting for 60% to 70% of all white blood cells. These leukocytes have nuclei that are divided into three to five lobes; therefore, they often are referred to as *polymorphonuclear neutrophils (PMNs)*. Because of their ability to form pseudopods used in ameboid movement, neutrophils are highly mobile, and are the first cells to appear at the site of acute inflammation, usually arriving within 90 minutes of injury (Fig. 3-2A). Neutrophils are scavenger cells capable of engulfing bacteria and other cellular debris through phagocytosis. Their cytoplasmic granules, which resist staining and remain a neutral color, contain enzymes and other antibacterial substances that are used in destroying and degrading engulfed microbes and dead tissue.[3,8,9] Neutrophils also have oxygen-dependent metabolic pathways that generate toxic reactive oxygen (e.g., hydrogen peroxide) and nitrogen (e.g., nitric oxide) species that aid in the destruction of engulfed pathogens. Neutrophils have a short life span. They die by apoptosis and disappear within 24 to 48 hours after entering the site of inflammation.

Eosinophils. Eosinophils account for 2% to 3% of circulating leukocytes and are recruited to tissues in a similar way as the neutrophils. Their appearance at the site of inflammation occurs 2 to 3 hours after the neutrophils. This is, in part, because of their slower mobility and comparatively slower reaction to chemotactic stimuli.

The granules of eosinophils, which stain pink with the acid dye eosin, contain a protein that is highly toxic to large parasitic worms that cannot be phagocytized. Eosinophils also play an important role in allergic reactions by controlling the release of specific chemical mediators. They interact with basophils and are prominent in allergic reactions such as hay fever and bronchial asthma. Eosinophils have a longer life span than neutrophils and therefore are present in chronic inflammation.

Basophils and Mast Cells. Basophils are granulocytes with granules that stain blue with a basic dye. Although they account for less than 1% of the circulating leukocytes, they are important participants in inflammatory reactions and are most prominent in allergic reactions mediated by immunoglobulin E (IgE). Binding of IgE triggers release of histamine and vasoactive agents from the basophil granules.

Mast cells derive from the same hematopoietic stem cells as basophils but do not develop until they leave the circulation and lodge in tissue sites. They are particularly prevalent along mucosal surfaces of the lung, gastrointestinal tract, and dermis of the skin.[2,10] This distribution places them in a sentinel position between environmental antigens and the host for a variety of acute and chronic inflammatory conditions.[2] Activation of mast cells

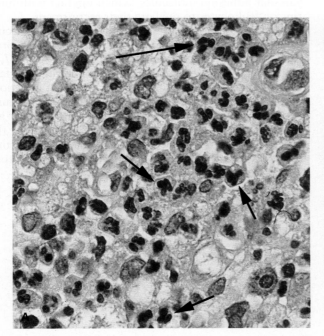
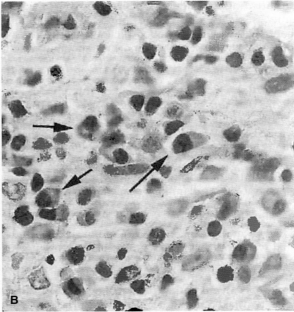

FIGURE 3-2. Inflammatory cells of acute and chronic inflammation. **(A)** Acute inflammation with densely packed polymorphonuclear neutrophils with multilobed nucleus (*arrows*). **(B)** Chronic inflammation with lymphocytes, plasma cells (*arrows*), and a few macrophages. (From Murphy HS. Inflammation. In: Rubin R, Strayer DS, eds. *Rubin's Pathology: Clinicopathologic Foundations of Medicine.* 5th ed. Philadelphia, PA: Wolters Kluwer Health/Lippincott Williams & Wilkins; 2008:39.)

results in release of the preformed contents of their granules (e.g., histamine, proteases, cytokines such as tumor necrosis factor-α [TNF-α] and interleukin-16 [IL-16], growth factors such as vascular endothelial growth factor [VEGF]) and synthesis of lipid mediators derived from cell membrane precursors (arachidonic acid metabolites, such as prostaglandins, and platelet-activating factor). Finally, the release of mast cell contents stimulates cytokine and chemokine synthesis by other inflammatory cells such as monocytes and macrophages.

Monocyte/Macrophages. *Monocytes* constitute 3% to 8% of the white blood cell count. They have a single kidney-shaped nucleus and are the largest of the circulating leukocytes. The half-life of circulating monocytes is about a day, after which they begin to migrate to the site of injury and mature into larger macrophages, which have a longer half-life and greater phagocytic ability than do blood monocytes. Circulating monocytes have been linked to a number of inflammatory disorders, particularly atherosclerosis, in which they are transformed into macrophages that accumulate in atherosclerotic plaques and turn into lipid-laden foam cells (see Chapter 18).

Monocyte/macrophages produce potent vasoactive mediators including prostaglandins and leukotrienes, platelet-activating factor (PAF), inflammatory cytokines, and growth factors that promote regeneration of tissues.[8,9] As their name implies, macrophages are capable of phagocytosis and are active in bacterial killing. They engulf larger and greater quantities of foreign material than the neutrophils, and their circulating life span is three to four times longer than that of any granulocyte. These longer-lived phagocytes help to destroy the causative agent, aid in the signaling processes of immunity, serve to resolve the inflammatory process, and contribute to initiation of the healing processes. Macrophages are especially important in maintaining chronic inflammation.

Lymphocytes and Plasma Cells. Lymphocytes are the smallest of the leukocytes and have a thin rim of cytoplasm surrounded by a deeply staining nucleus (Fig. 3-2B). They participate in immune-mediated inflammation caused by infectious agents as well as non–immune-mediated inflammation associated with cell injury and death. Both T and B lymphocytes (T and B cells) migrate into inflammatory sites using some of the same adhesion molecules and chemokines that recruit neutrophils and other leukocytes (discussed in Chapter 15). Lymphocytes and macrophages communicate in a bidirectional way, and these interactions play an important role in chronic inflammation. Macrophages display antigen to T cells, express membrane molecules called costimulators (meaning that their response requires the action of two signaling molecules), and produce cytokines that stimulate T-cell responses.[2] Activated T cells, in turn, produce cytokines that activate macrophages, increasing antigen presentation and further cytokine production. (Cytokines and other inflammatory mediators are discussed later in this chapter.) The result is a perpetuating cycle of cellular responses that fuel and sustain chronic inflammation.

Plasma cells develop from B lymphocytes that have become activated after encountering an antigen and receiving T cell help. In the inflammatory site, they produce antibodies directed against persistent antigens and altered tissue components. In some intense, chronic inflammatory reactions, plasma cells and other lymphocytes may accumulate to form geminal centers that resemble lymph nodes.[2] This pattern of lymphocyte accumulation, with formation of germinal centers, is often seen in the inflamed synovium of persons with long-standing rheumatoid arthritis.

Cell Adhesion Molecules

Several families of cell adhesion molecules, including selectins, integrins, and the immunoglobulin superfamily, are involved in leukocyte recruitment and trafficking (see Chapter 1).[8,11,12] The *selectins* are a family of three closely related proteins (E-selectin, L-selectin, P-selectin) that differ in their cellular distribution but all function in adhesion of leukocytes or platelets to endothelial cells. The *integrins* consist of different types of structurally similar transmembrane receptor proteins that function as heterodimers to promote cell-to-cell and cell–to–extracellular matrix interactions. The name *integrin* derives from the hypothesis that they *integrate* the signals of extracellular ligands with cytoskeleton-dependent motility, shape change, and phagocytic responses of immune cells. *Cell adhesion molecules* of the immunoglobulin superfamily include intercellular adhesion and vascular adhesion molecules, which interact with integrins on leukocytes to mediate their recruitment.

The importance of the leukocyte adhesion molecules is demonstrated in persons with an inherited disorder called *leukocyte adhesion deficiency (LAD) type I*, in which deficiency of a member of the integrin superfamily leads to severe leukocytosis and recurrent infections. A similar deficiency is seen in individuals with impaired expression of a member of the selectin superfamily and has been labeled *LAD type 2*.[8] There is also evidence that excessive expression of cell adhesion molecules or their receptors contributes to the pathogenesis of some chronic inflammatory diseases such as rheumatoid arthritis.

SUMMARY CONCEPTS

■ Inflammation is the body's response to injury and is characterized by the elaboration of chemical mediators and movement of fluid and leukocytes from the vascular compartment into the extravascular tissue space.

■ There are two types of inflammation: *acute inflammation,* which is of short duration and characterized by the exudation of fluid and plasma proteins, and *chronic inflammation*, which is associated with angiogenesis, tissue necrosis, and fibrosis (scarring).

■ Many cells and tissue components contribute to the inflammatory response, including the endothelial cells that form capillaries and line blood vessels, circulating platelets and white blood cells, cells in connective tissue, and components of the extracellular matrix.

Acute Inflammation

Acute inflammation is the early or almost immediate reaction of local tissues and their blood vessels to injury. It typically occurs before the adaptive immune response becomes established (see Chapter 15) and is aimed primarily at removing the injurious agent and limiting the extent of tissue damage. Acute inflammation can be triggered by a variety of stimuli, including infections, immune reactions, blunt and penetrating trauma, physical or chemical agents (e.g., burns, frostbite, irradiation, caustic chemicals), and tissue necrosis from any cause.

The classic description of inflammation has been handed down through the ages. In the first century AD, the Roman physician Aulus Celsus described the local reaction of injury in terms that are now known as the *cardinal signs* of inflammation.[1] These signs are *rubor* (redness), *tumor* (swelling), *calor* (heat), and *dolor* (pain). In the second century AD, the Greek physician Galen added a fifth cardinal sign, *functio laesa* (loss of function). In addition to the cardinal signs that appear at the site of injury, systemic manifestations (e.g., fever) may occur as chemical mediators (e.g., cytokines) produced at the site of inflammation lead to increased levels in the plasma. The constellation of systemic manifestations and increases in serum proteins that may occur during acute inflammation is known as the *acute-phase response*.

Stages of Acute Inflammation

Acute inflammation has two stages: vascular and cellular. The vascular stage is characterized by increased blood flow (vasodilation) and structural changes (increased vascular permeability) that allow plasma proteins to leave the circulation. The cellular stage involves the emigration of leukocytes (mainly neutrophils) from the microcirculation and their accumulation at the site of injury or infection.

Vascular Stage

The vascular changes that occur with inflammation involve the arterioles, capillaries, and venules of the microcirculation. These changes begin almost immediately after injury and are characterized by vasodilation and changes in blood flow followed by increased vascular permeability and leakage of protein-rich fluid into the extravascular tissue space.[1,2]

Vasodilation, which is one of the earliest manifestations of inflammation, follows a transient constriction of the arterioles, lasting a few seconds. Dilation begins in the arterioles and opens capillary beds in the area. As a result, the area becomes congested, causing the redness (erythema) and warmth associated with acute inflammation. Vasodilation is induced by the action of several mediators, most notably histamine and nitric oxide.

Vasodilation is quickly followed by increased permeability of the microvasculature, with the outpouring of a protein-rich fluid (exudate) into the extravascular spaces. The loss of fluid results in an increased concentration of blood constituents (red blood cells, leukocytes, platelets, and clotting factors), stagnation of flow, and clotting of blood at the site of injury. This aids in limiting the spread of infectious microorganisms. The loss of plasma proteins reduces the intracapillary osmotic pressure and increases the osmotic pressure of the interstitial fluid, increasing fluid movement from the vascular compartment into the tissue space and producing the swelling, pain, and impaired function that are the cardinal signs of acute inflammation. The exudation of fluid into the tissue spaces also serves to dilute the offending agent.

The increased permeability characteristic of acute inflammation results from formation of endothelial gaps in the venules of the microcirculation. Binding of the chemical mediators to endothelial receptors causes contraction of endothelial cells and separation of intercellular junctions. This is the most common mechanism of vascular leakage and is elicited by histamine, bradykinin, leukotrienes, and many other classes of chemical mediators.

Depending on the severity of injury, the vascular changes that occur with inflammation follow one of three patterns of responses.[2] The first pattern is an *immediate transient response*, which occurs with minor injury. It develops rapidly after injury and is usually reversible and of short duration (15 to 30 minutes). The second pattern is an *immediate sustained response*, which occurs with more serious types of injury and continues for several days. It affects all levels of the microcirculation (arterioles, capillaries, and venules) and is usually due to direct damage of the endothelium by injurious stimuli, such as burns or the products of bacterial infections.[2] Neutrophils that adhere to the endothelium may also injure endothelial cells. The third pattern is a *delayed response*, in which the increased permeability begins after a delay of 2 to 12 hours, lasts for several hours or even days, and involves venules as well as capillaries.[2] A delayed response often accompanies injuries due to radiation, such as sunburn.

Cellular Stage

The cellular stage of acute inflammation is marked by changes in the endothelial cells lining the vasculature and movement of phagocytic leukocytes into the area of

(*text continues on page 56*)

U N D E R S T A N D I N G ➡ Acute Inflammation

Acute inflammation is the immediate and early response to an injurious agent. The response, which serves to control and eliminate altered cells, microorganisms, and antigens, occurs in two phases: (1) the vascular phase, which leads to an increase in blood flow and changes in the small blood vessels of the microcirculation; and (2) the cellular phase, which leads to the migration of leukocytes from the circulation and their activation to eliminate the injurious agent. The primary function of the inflammatory response is to limit the injurious effect of the pathologic agent and remove the injured tissue components, thereby allowing tissue repair to take place.

1

Vascular Phase. The vascular phase of acute inflammation is characterized by changes in the small blood vessels at the site of injury. It begins with momentary vasoconstriction followed rapidly by vasodilation. Vasodilation involves the arterioles and venules with a resultant increase in capillary blood flow causing heat and redness, which are two of the cardinal signs of inflammation. This is accompanied by an increase in vascular permeability with outpouring of protein-rich fluid (exudate) into the extravascular spaces. The loss of proteins reduces the capillary osmotic pressure and increases the interstitial osmotic pressure. This, coupled with an increase in capillary pressure, causes a marked outflow of fluid and its accumulation in the tissue spaces, producing the swelling, pain, and impaired function that represent the other cardinal signs of acute inflammation. As fluid moves out of the vessels, stagnation of flow and clotting of blood occur. This aids in localizing the spread of infectious microorganisms.

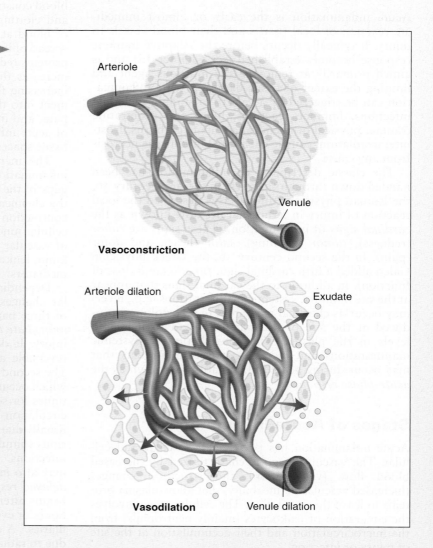

Arteriole

Venule

Vasoconstriction

Arteriole dilation

Exudate

Vasodilation

Venule dilation

2

Cellular Phase: Leukocyte Margination, Adhesion, and Transmigration. The cellular phase of acute inflammation involves the delivery of leukocytes, mainly neutrophils, to the site of injury so they can perform their normal functions of host defense. The delivery and activation of leukocytes can be divided into the following steps: adhesion and margination, transmigration, and chemotaxis. The recruitment of leukocytes to the precapillary venules, where they exit the circulation, is facilitated by the slowing of blood flow and margination along the vessel surface. Leukocyte adhesion and transmigration from the vascular space into the extravascular tissue is facilitated by complementary adhesion molecules (e.g., selectins, integrins) on the leukocyte and endothelial surfaces. After extravasation, leukocytes migrate in the tissues toward the site of injury by chemotaxis, or locomotion oriented along a chemical gradient.

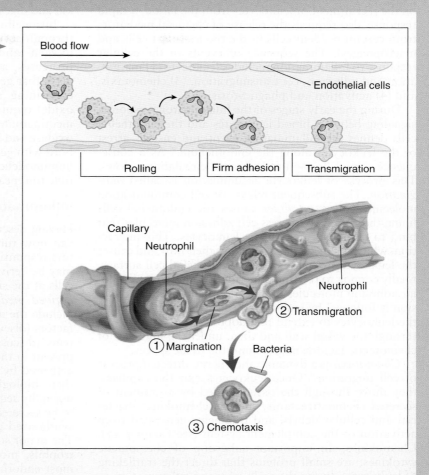

3

Leukocyte Activation and Phagocytosis. Once at the sight of injury, the products generated by tissue injury trigger a number of leukocyte responses, including phagocytosis and cell killing. Opsonization of microbes (1) by complement factor C3b and antibody facilitates recognition by neutrophil C3b and the antibody Fc receptor. Receptor activation (2) triggers intracellular signaling and actin assembly in the neutrophil, leading to formation of pseudopods that enclose the microbe within a phagosome. The phagosome (3) then fuses with an intracellular lysosome to form a phagolysosome into which lysosomal enzymes and oxygen radicals (4) are released to kill and degrade the microbe.

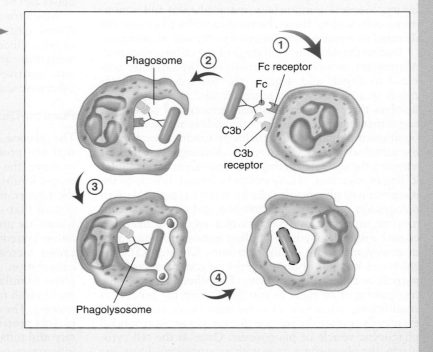

(*text continued from page 53*)

injury or infection. Although attention has been focused on the recruitment of leukocytes from the blood, a rapid response also requires the release of chemical mediators from certain resident cells in the tissues (mast cells and macrophages). The sequence of events in the cellular response to inflammation includes leukocyte (1) margination and adhesion, (2) transmigration, (3) chemotaxis, and (4) activation and phagocytosis.[1–3]

During the early stages of the inflammatory response, signaling between blood leukocytes and the endothelial cells defines the inflammatory event and ensures arrest of the leukocytes along the endothelium.[9] As a consequence, blood flow—and leukocyte circulation—slows. This process of leukocyte accumulation is called *margination*. The subsequent release of cell communication molecules called *cytokines* causes the endothelial cells lining the vessels to express cell adhesion molecules that bind to carbohydrates on the leukocytes. This interaction, which is called *tethering,* slows their flow and causes the leukocytes to roll along the endothelial cell surface, finally coming to rest and adhering strongly to intercellular adhesion molecules on the endothelium.[1,2] The adhesion is followed by endothelial cell separation, allowing the leukocytes to extend pseudopodia and *transmigrate* through the vessel wall and then, under the influence of chemotactic factors, migrate into the tissue spaces.

Chemotaxis is a dynamic and energy-directed process of cell migration.[1] Once leukocytes exit the capillary, they move through the tissue guided by a gradient of secreted chemoattractants, such as chemokines, bacterial and cellular debris, and fragments generated from activation of the complement system (see Chapter 15). Chemokines, an important subgroup of chemotactic cytokines, are small proteins that direct the trafficking of leukocytes during the early stages of inflammation or injury.[13] Several immune (e.g., macrophages) and nonimmune cells secrete these chemoattractants to ensure the directed movement of leukocytes to the site of infection.

During the next and final stage of the cellular response, neutrophils, monocytes, and tissue macrophages are activated to engulf and degrade the bacteria and cellular debris in a process called *phagocytosis*.[1,2,14] Phagocytosis involves three distinct steps: recognition and adherence, engulfment, and intracellular killing. It is initiated by recognition and binding of particles by specific receptors on the surface of phagocytic cells. This binding is essential for trapping the agent, triggering engulfment, and intracellular killing of microbes. Microbes can be bound directly to the membrane of phagocytic cells by several types of pattern recognition receptors (e.g., toll-like and mannose receptors) or indirectly by receptors that recognize microbes coated with carbohydrate-binding lectins, antibody, and/or complement (see innate immunity, Chapter 15). The enhanced binding of an antigen to a coated microbe or particle is called *opsonization*. Engulfment follows the recognition of an agent as foreign. During the process of engulfment, extensions of cytoplasm move around and eventually enclose the particle in a membrane-surrounded phagocytic vesicle or *phagosome*. Once in the cell cytoplasm, the phagosome fuses with a cytoplasmic lysosome containing antibacterial molecules and enzymes that can kill and digest the microbe (see Chapter 1).

Intracellular killing of pathogens is accomplished through several mechanisms, including toxic reactive oxygen- and nitrogen-containing species, lysozymes, proteases, and defensins. The metabolic burst pathways that generate toxic reactive oxygen- and nitrogen-containing species (e.g., hydrogen peroxide, nitric oxide) require oxygen and metabolic enzymes such as nicotinamide adenine dinucleotide phosphate (NADPH) oxidase and nitric oxide synthetase. Individuals who are born with genetic defects in some of these enzymes have immunodeficiency conditions that make them susceptible to repeated bacterial infection.

Inflammatory Mediators

Having described the events of acute inflammation, we can now turn to a discussion of the chemical mediators responsible for the events. Inflammatory mediators may be derived from the plasma or produced locally by cells at the site of inflammation (Fig. 3-3). The *plasma-derived mediators*, which are synthesized in the liver, include the acute-phase proteins, coagulation (clotting) factors (discussed in Chapter 12), and complement proteins (discussed in Chapter 15). These mediators are present in the plasma in a precursor form that must be activated by a series of proteolytic processes to acquire their biologic properties. *Cell-derived mediators* are normally sequestered in intracellular granules that need to be secreted (e.g., histamine from mast cells) or newly synthesized (e.g., cytokines) in response to a stimulus. The major sources of these mediators are platelets, neutrophils, monocyte/macrophages, and mast cells, but most endothelial cells, smooth muscle cells, and fibroblasts can be induced to produce some of the mediators.

Mediators can act on one or a few target cells, have diverse targets, or have differing effects on different types of cells. Once activated and released from the cell, most mediators are short-lived. They may be transformed into inactive metabolites, inactivated by enzymes, or otherwise scavenged or degraded.

Plasma-Derived Mediators

The plasma is the source of inflammatory mediators that are products of three major protein cascades or systems: the kallikrein–kininogen system, which generates kinins; the coagulation system, which includes the important fibrin end product; and the complement system that includes the various complement proteins. Kinins are products of the liver and factors in the coagulation system (see Chapter 12). One kinin, bradykinin, causes increased capillary permeability and pain. The coagulation system also contributes to the vascular phase of inflammation mainly through formation of the fibrin mesh formed during the final steps of the clotting process. The complement system consists of a cascade of plasma proteins that play important roles in both immunity and inflammation. These proteins contribute to the inflammatory response by (1) causing vasodilation and

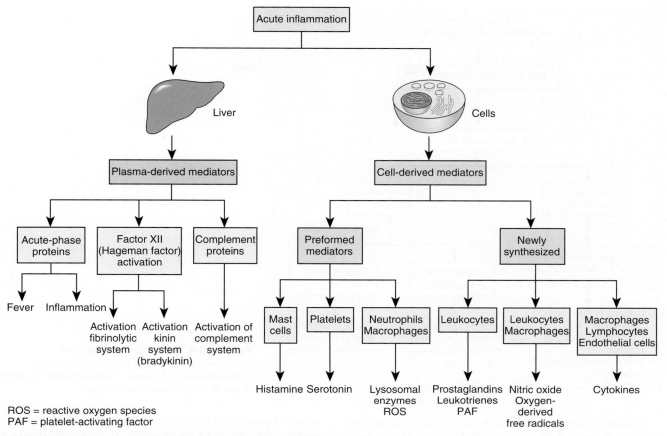

FIGURE 3-3. Plasma- and cell-derived mediators of acute inflammation.

increasing vascular permeability; (2) promoting leukocyte activation, adhesion, and chemotaxis; and (3) augmenting phagocytosis (see Chapter 15).

Cell-Derived Mediators

The cell-derived mediators are released from cells that are present at sites of inflammation. Tissue macrophages, mast cells, endothelial cells, as well as leukocytes that are recruited to the site from the blood are all capable of releasing the different mediators of inflammation, as are platelets, which are cellular fragments (see Fig. 3-3).

Histamine and Serotonin. Histamine and serotonin are classified as *vasoactive amines*, meaning they are derived from amino acids (histamine from histidine and serotonin from tryptamine) and act by producing changes in blood vessel tone. Both histamine and serotonin are stored as preformed molecules in mast cells and other cells and are among the first mediators to be released in acute inflammatory reactions.

Preformed histamine is widely distributed in tissues, the highest concentrations being found in mast cells adjacent to blood vessels.[1,2] It is also found in circulating platelets and basophils and is released in response to a variety of stimuli, including trauma and immune reactions involving binding of IgE to basophils and mast cells. Histamine produces dilation of arterioles

and increases the permeability of venules. It acts at the level of the microcirculation by binding to histamine$_1$ (H$_1$) receptors on endothelial cells and is considered the principal mediator of the immediate transient phase of increased vascular permeability in the acute inflammatory response. Antihistamine drugs (H$_1$ receptor antagonists), which bind to the H$_1$ receptors, act to competitively antagonize many of the effects of the immediate inflammatory response. Serotonin (5-hydroxytryptamine) is also a preformed vasoactive mediator, with effects similar to histamine. It is found primarily within platelet granules and is released during platelet aggregation.

Arachidonic Acid Metabolites. Arachidonic acid is a 20-carbon unsaturated fatty acid found in the phospholipids of cell membranes. Release of arachidonic acid by phospholipases initiates a series of complex reactions that lead to the production of the *eicosanoid* family of inflammatory mediators (prostaglandins, leukotrienes, and related metabolites).[15] Eicosanoid synthesis follows one of two pathways: the cyclooxygenase pathway, which culminates in the synthesis of prostaglandins; and the lipoxygenase pathway, which culminates in the synthesis of the leukotrienes (Fig. 3-4). The corticosteroid drugs block the inflammatory effects of both pathways by inhibiting phosphodiesterase activity and thus preventing the release of arachidonic acid.[16]

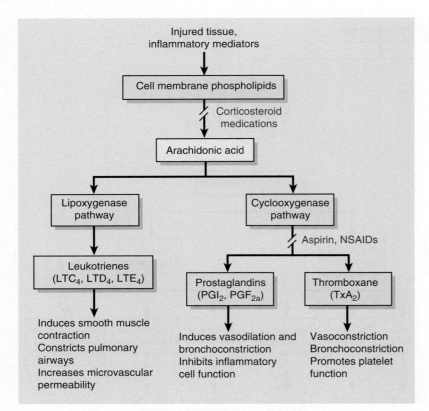

FIGURE 3-4. The cyclooxygenase and lipoxygenase pathways and sites where the corticosteroid and nonsteroidal anti-inflammatory drugs (NSAIDs) exert their action.

Several prostaglandins are synthesized from arachidonic acid through the cyclooxygenase metabolic pathway.[15] The prostaglandins (e.g., PGD_2, PGE_2, $PGF_{2\alpha}$, and PGI_2) induce inflammation and potentiate the effects of histamine and other inflammatory mediators. The prostaglandin thromboxane A_2 promotes platelet aggregation and vasoconstriction. Aspirin and the nonsteroidal anti-inflammatory drugs (NSAIDs) reduce inflammation by inactivating the first enzyme in the cyclooxygenase pathway for prostaglandin synthesis.

Like the prostaglandins, the leukotrienes are formed from arachidonic acid, but through the lipoxygenase pathway. Histamine and leukotrienes have similar functions; however, histamine is produced rapidly and transiently while the more potent leukotrienes are being synthesized. The leukotrienes also have been reported to affect the permeability of the postcapillary venules, the adhesion properties of endothelial cells, and the extravasation and chemotaxis of neutrophils, eosinophils, and monocytes. Leukotriene (LT) C_4, LTD_4, and LTE_4, collectively known as the *slow-reacting substance of anaphylaxis* (SRS-A), cause slow and sustained constriction of the bronchioles and are important inflammatory mediators in bronchial asthma and anaphylaxis.

Omega-3 Polyunsaturated Fatty Acids. There has been recent interest in dietary modification of the inflammatory response through the use of *omega-3 polyunsaturated fatty acids*. These include *eicosapentaenoic acid* and *docosahexaenoic acid*, which are present in oily fish and fish oil,[17,18] but can be derived in limited quantities from α-*linolenic acid*. The α-*linolenic acid*, which is present in flax seed, canola oil, green leafy vegetables, walnuts, and soybeans, is an essential omega-3 fatty acid that cannot be produced in the body and must be obtained through the diet. The omega-3 polyunsaturated fatty acids, which are considered antithrombotic and anti-inflammatory, are structurally different from the prothrombotic and proinflammatory omega-6 polyunsaturated fatty acids, which are present in most seeds, vegetable oils, and meats. Typically, the cell membranes of inflammatory cells contain high proportions of omega-6 arachidonic acid, which is the source of prostaglandin and leukotriene inflammatory mediators. Eating oily fish and other foods that are high in omega-3 fatty acids results in partial replacement of omega-6 arachidonic acid in inflammatory cell membranes by eicosapentaenoic acid, a change that leads to decreased production of arachidonic acid–derived inflammatory mediators. This response alone is a potentially beneficial effect of omega-3 fatty acids. However, omega-3 fatty acids may have a number of other anti-inflammatory effects that occur downstream of altered eicosanoid production or might be independent of this function.

Platelet-Activating Factor. Originally named for its ability to cause platelet aggregation and granulation, PAF is another phospholipid-derived mediator with a broad spectrum of inflammatory effects. Platelet-activating factor is generated from the membrane phospholipids of virtually all activated inflammatory cells and affects a variety of cell types. In addition to activating platelets, PAF stimulates neutrophils, monocytes/macrophages, endothelial cells, and vascular smooth muscle. Platelet activating factor-induced platelet aggregation and degranulation at the site of injury enhances serotonin release, thereby causing changes in vascular permeability. It also enhances leukocyte adhesion, chemotaxis, and leukocyte degranulation and stimulates the synthesis of other inflammatory mediators, especially the prostaglandins.

Cytokines and Chemokines. Cytokines are low-molecular-weight proteins that are important cellular messengers. They modulate the function of cells by paracrine and autocrine mechanisms to cause responses in neighboring cells and the cells that produced the cytokine, respectively. They are produced by many cell types, including activated macrophages and lymphocytes, endothelial cells, epithelial cells, and fibroblasts.[1,2,18] Although well known for their role in adaptive immune responses, these proteins also play important roles in both acute and chronic inflammation.

Tumor necrosis factor-α (TNF-α) and interleukin-1 (IL-1) are two of the major cytokines that mediate inflammation. The major cellular source of TNF-α and IL-1 is activated macrophages (Fig. 3-5). Interleukin-1 is also produced by many other cell types, including neutrophils, endothelial cells, and epithelial cells (e.g.,

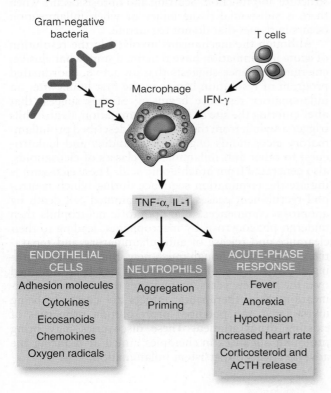

FIGURE 3-5. Central role of interleukin (IL)-1 and tumor necrosis factor (TNF)-α in inflammation. Lipopolysaccharide (LPS) and interferon (IFN)-γ activate macrophages to release inflammatory cytokines, principally IL-1 and TNF-α, responsible for directing both local and systemic inflammatory responses. ACTH, adrenocorticotrophic hormone. (From Murphy HS. Inflammation. In: Rubin R, Strayer DS, eds. *Rubin's Pathology: Clinicopathologic Foundations of Medicine.* 6th ed. Philadelphia, PA: Wolters Kluwer Health/Lippincott Williams & Wilkins; 2012:60.)

keratinocytes). The secretion of TNF-α and IL-1 can be stimulated by bacterial toxins, immune cells, injury, and a variety of inflammatory stimuli. TNF-α and IL-1 induce endothelial cells to express adhesion molecules and release other cytokines, chemokines, and reactive oxygen species. Tumor necrosis factor-α induces priming and aggregation of neutrophils, leading to augmented responses of these cells to other mediators. Interleukin-1 and TNF-α are also mediators of the acute-phase responses associated with infection or injury. Features of these systemic responses include fever, hypotension and increased heart rate, anorexia, release of neutrophils into the circulation, and increased levels of corticosteroid hormones.

Chemotactic cytokines, or *chemokines*, are a family of small proteins that act primarily as chemoattractants that both recruit and direct the migration of inflammatory and immune cells[20] (see Chapter 15). Chemokines generate a chemotactic gradient by binding to proteoglycans on the surface of endothelial cells or in the extracellular matrix.[20] As a result, high concentrations of chemokines persist at sites of tissue injury or infection. Two classes of chemokines have been identified: inflammatory chemokines and homing chemokines. Inflammatory chemokines are produced in response to bacterial toxins and inflammatory cytokines (i.e., IL-1, TNF-α). These chemokines recruit leukocytes during an inflammatory response. Homing chemokines are constantly produced, with the genes that control their production being up-regulated during inflammatory reactions.

Nitric Oxide. Nitric oxide (NO), which is produced by a variety of cells, plays multiple roles in inflammation, including relaxation of vascular smooth muscle; antagonism of platelet adhesion, aggregation, and degranulation; and as regulator of leukocyte recruitment.[2] Blocking of NO production under normal conditions promotes leukocyte rolling and adhesion to postcapillary venules and delivery of exogenous NO reduces leukocyte recruitment. Thus, production of NO appears to be an endogenous compensatory mechanism that reduces the cellular phase of inflammation. Impaired production of NO by vascular endothelial cells is implicated in the inflammatory changes that occur with atherosclerosis (see Chapter 18). Nitric oxide and its derivatives also have antimicrobial actions, and thus NO is also a host mediator against infection.

Reactive Oxygen Species. Reactive oxygen species may be released extracellularly from leukocytes after exposure to microbes, cytokines, and immune complexes, or in the phagocytic process that occurs during the cellular phase of the inflammatory process. The superoxide radical, hydrogen peroxide, and hydroxyl radical (discussed in Chapter 2) are the major species produced within the cell. These species can combine with NO to form other reactive nitrogen intermediates. Extracellular release of low levels of these potent mediators can increase the expression of cytokines and endothelial adhesion molecules, amplifying the cascade that elicits the inflammatory process,[2] and increase cell proliferation. However, at higher levels these mediators can produce endothelial cell damage, with a resultant increase in vascular permeability; inactivate antiproteases, such as α_1-antitrypsin, which protect against lung damage in smokers; and produce injury to other cell types, including red blood cells.[2] Thus, the influence of ROS in any inflammatory process depends on a balance between the generation and inactivation of these metabolites.

Local Manifestations

The local manifestations of acute inflammation, which are determined by severity of the reaction, its specific cause, and the site of involvement, can range from mild swelling and redness to abscess formation or ulceration. As part of the normal defense reaction, inflammation can also injure adjacent tissues.[2] In some infections, such as tuberculosis and certain viral infections, the host response can cause more damage than the microbe itself. As a normal attempt to clear damaged and dead tissues (e.g., after a myocardial infarction), the inflammatory response may prolong and exacerbate the injurious consequences of the infarction.

Characteristically, the acute inflammatory response involves the production of exudates. These exudates vary in terms of fluid type, plasma protein content, and presence or absence of cells. They can be serous, hemorrhagic, fibrinous, membranous, or purulent. Often the exudate is composed of a combination of these types. *Serous exudates* are watery fluids low in protein content that result from plasma entering the inflammatory site. *Hemorrhagic exudates* occur when there is severe tissue injury that causes damage to blood vessels or when there is significant leakage of red cells from the capillaries. *Fibrinous exudates* contain large amounts of fibrinogen and form a thick and sticky meshwork, much like the fibers of a blood clot. *Membranous* or *pseudomembranous exudates* develop on mucous membrane surfaces and are composed of necrotic cells enmeshed in a fibropurulent exudate.

A *purulent* or *suppurative exudate* contains pus, which is composed of degraded white blood cells, proteins, and tissue debris. The term *pyogenic* refers to "pus forming." Certain pyogenic microorganisms, such as *Staphylococcus*, are more likely to induce localized suppurative inflammation than others. An *abscess* is a localized area of inflammation containing a purulent exudate. Abscesses typically have a central necrotic core containing purulent exudates surrounded by a layer of neutrophils.[2] Fibroblasts may eventually enter the area and wall off the abscess. Because antimicrobial agents cannot penetrate the abscess wall, surgical incision and drainage may be required as a cure.

An *ulceration* refers to a site of inflammation where an epithelial surface (e.g., skin or gastrointestinal epithelium) has become necrotic and eroded, often with associated subepithelial inflammation. Ulceration may occur as the result of traumatic injury to the epithelial surface (e.g., peptic ulcer) or because of vascular compromise

(e.g., foot ulcers associated with diabetes). In chronic lesions where there is repeated insult, the area surrounding the ulcer develops fibroblastic proliferation, scarring, and accumulation of chronic inflammatory cells.[2]

Resolution

Although the manifestations of acute inflammation are largely determined by the nature and intensity of injury, the tissue affected, and the person's ability to mount a response, the outcome generally results in one of three processes: resolution, progression to chronic inflammation, or substantial scarring and fibrosis.[2] Resolution involves the replacement of any irreversibly injured cells and return of tissues to their normal structure and function.[21,22] It is seen with short-lived and minimal injuries and involves neutralization or degradation of inflammatory mediators, normalization of vascular permeability, and cessation of leukocyte infiltration. Progression to chronic inflammation may follow acute inflammation if the offending agent is not removed. Depending on the extent of injury, as well as the ability of the affected tissues to regenerate, chronic inflammation may be followed by restoration of normal structure and function. Scarring and fibrosis occurs when there is substantial tissue injury or when inflammation occurs in tissues that do not regenerate.

Although the mechanisms involved in the resolution of acute inflammation have remained somewhat elusive, emerging evidence suggests that an active, coordinated program of resolution begins in the first hours after an inflammatory response begins.[2,21] Studies suggest that after entering the site of acute inflammation, neutrophils trigger a switch from the previously described proinflammatory eicosanoids (e.g., prostaglandins and leukotrienes) to other anti-inflammatory classes of eicosanoids, also generated from arachidonic acid. These eicosanoids initiate the termination sequence during which neutrophil recruitment ceases and programmed cell death by apoptosis commences. The apoptotic neutrophils then undergo phagocytosis by macrophages, leading to their clearance and release of anti-inflammatory and reparative cytokines. Although much new information regarding the resolution of inflammation has been obtained over the past few years, many issues require further clarification. New therapeutic targets are currently being investigated and potential proresolution properties of existing drugs studied. These discoveries may bring profound advances in therapies aimed at reducing the adverse effects of persistent inflammation.

SUMMARY CONCEPTS

■ The classic signs of an acute inflammatory response are redness, swelling, local heat, pain, and loss of function. These manifestations can be attributed to the immediate vascular changes that occur (vasodilation and increased capillary permeability), the influx of inflammatory cells such as neutrophils, and, in some cases, the widespread effects of inflammatory mediators, which produce fever and other systemic signs and symptoms.

■ Chemical mediators are integral to initiation, amplification, and termination of inflammatory processes. The plasma is the source of mediators derived from three major protein cascades that are activated during inflammation. These protein cascades include the kallikrein-kininogen system, the coagulation system, and the complement system. Cell-derived mediators, including histamine, bradykinin, the arachididonic metabolites, platelet activating factor (PAF), and many others are released from cells at the site of inflammation.

■ Acute inflammation may involve the production of exudates containing serous fluid (serous exudate), red blood cells (hemorrhagic exudate), fibrinogen (fibrinous exudate), or tissue debris and white blood cell breakdown products (purulent exudate).

■ The outcome of acute inflammation generally results in one of three processes: resolution, progression to chronic inflammation, or substantial scarring and fibrosis.

Chronic Inflammation

In contrast to acute inflammation, which is usually self-limited and of short duration, chronic inflammation is self-perpetuating and may last for weeks, months, or even years.[1,2,23] It may develop as a result of a recurrent or progressive acute inflammatory process or from low-grade, smoldering responses that fail to evoke an acute response. Instead of the vascular permeability changes, edema, and predominantly neutrophilic infiltration seen in acute inflammation, chronic inflammation is characterized by infiltration with mononuclear cells (macrophages, lymphocytes, and plasma cells) and attempted connective tissue repair involving angiogenesis and fibrosis. Although it may follow acute inflammation, chronic inflammation often begins insidiously as a low-grade, smoldering, and asymptomatic process. This type of process is the cause of tissue damage in some of the most common disabling diseases such as atherosclerosis, chronic lung disease, rheumatoid arthritis, and inflammatory bowel disease.

There is also evidence that recurrent and persistent inflammation induces, promotes, and/or influences susceptibility to cancer by causing deoxyribonucleic acid (DNA) damage, inciting tissue reparative proliferation, and/or creating an environment that is enriched with cytokines and growth factors that favor tumor development and growth (see Chapter 7).[23] Among the cancers associated with chronic infection and inflammation are cervical cancer (human papillomavirus [HPV]), cancer of the liver (hepatitis B and C), cancer of the stomach (*Helicobacter pylori*), and cancer of the gallbladder (chronic cholecystitis and cholelithiasis).

Causes of Chronic Inflammation

Agents that evoke chronic inflammation typically are low-grade, persistent infections or irritants that are unable to penetrate deeply or spread rapidly.[1,2] Among the causes of chronic inflammation are foreign agents such as talc, silica, asbestos, and surgical suture materials. Many viruses provoke chronic inflammatory responses, as do certain bacteria, such as the tubercle bacillus and the actinomyces, as well as fungi, and larger parasites of moderate to low virulence. The presence of injured tissue such as that surrounding a healing fracture also may incite chronic inflammation. Diseases that cause excessive and inappropriate activation of the immune system are increasingly being recognized as causes of chronic inflammation. Under certain conditions, immune reactions may develop against the person's own tissues, leading to autoimmune disease.

Obesity is a newly suspected cause of chronic inflammation.[24-26] During the last decade, white adipose tissue was recognized to be an active endocrine organ and a source of a number of proinflammatory mediators. Many of the mediators appear to play an important role in the pathogenesis of obesity-related diseases including accelerated atherosclerosis and diabetes mellitus. The link between obesity and inflammation dates back to the discovery that adipose tissue was a source of the proinflammatory cytokine TNF-α, and that adipose tissue TNF-α concentrations are correlated with insulin resistance both in persons with and without type 2 diabetes mellitus. It was later found that obesity is related not only to increased number and size of adipocytes, but also to infiltration of adipose tissue by macrophages that possess the ability to produce TNF-α, nitric oxide, and other inflammatory mediators. The mechanisms mediating the proinflammatory state associated with obesity are still unclear, but recent studies suggest that circulating free fatty acids may play a role.

Granulomatous Inflammation

A granulomatous lesion is a distinctive form of chronic inflammation.[1,2] A granuloma typically is a small, 1- to 2-mm lesion in which there is a massing of macrophages surrounded by lymphocytes. The macrophages are modified and, because they resemble epithelial cells, sometimes are called epithelioid cells. Like other macrophages, these epithelioid cells are derived originally from blood monocytes. Granulomatous inflammation is associated with foreign bodies such as splinters, sutures, silica, and asbestos and with microorganisms that cause tuberculosis, syphilis, sarcoidosis, deep fungal

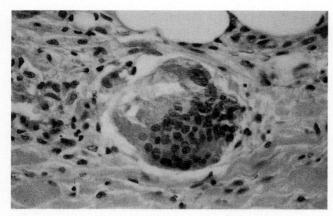

FIGURE 3-6. Foreign body giant cell. The numerous nuclei are randomly arranged in the cytoplasm. (From Rubin E, Farber LL. *Rubin's Pathology: Clinicopathologic Foundations of Medicine.* 3rd ed. Philadelphia, PA: Lippincott Williams & Wilkins; 1999:40.)

infections, and brucellosis. These types of agents have one thing in common: they are poorly degraded and usually are not easily controlled by other inflammatory mechanisms. The epithelioid cells in granulomatous inflammation may clump in a mass or coalesce, forming a multinucleated giant cell (often referred to as a foreign body giant cell) that attempts to surround the foreign agent (Fig. 3-6). A dense membrane of connective tissue eventually encapsulates the lesion and isolates it.

SUMMARY CONCEPTS

■ Chronic inflammation involves infiltration with macrophages, lymphocytes, and fibroblasts, leading to persistent inflammation, fibroblast proliferation, and scar formation.

■ Among the conditions associated with chronic inflammation and inappropriate activation of the immune system are low-grade inflammation associated with atherosclerosis and type 2 diabetes mellitus; autoimmune disorders; and susceptibility to cancer due to deoxyribonucleic acid damage, increased tissue proliferation, and creation of an environment rich in cytokines and growth factors that favor tumor cell development and growth.

■ A granulomatous lesion is a distinctive form of chronic inflammation characterized by aggregates of epithelioid macrophages that "wall off" the causal agent. Granulomatous inflammation is associated with foreign bodies such as splinters, sutures, silica, and asbestos and with microorganisms that cause tuberculosis, syphilis, sarcoidosis, deep fungal infections, and brucellosis.

Systemic Manifestations of Inflammation

Under optimal conditions, the inflammatory response remains confined to a localized area. In some cases, however, local injury can result in prominent systemic manifestations as inflammatory mediators are released into the circulation. The most prominent systemic manifestations of inflammation include the acute-phase response, alterations in white blood cell count (leukocytosis or leukopenia), and fever. Localized acute and chronic inflammation may extend to the lymphatic system and lead to a reaction in the lymph nodes that drain the affected area. Painful palpable lymph nodes are more commonly associated with inflammatory processes, whereas nonpainful nodes are more characteristic of neoplasms.

Acute-Phase Response

Along with the cellular responses that occur during the inflammatory response, a constellation of systemic effects called the *acute-phase response* occurs.[1,2] The acute-phase response, which usually begins within hours or days of the onset of inflammation or infection, includes changes in the concentrations of plasma proteins, skeletal muscle catabolism, negative nitrogen balance, elevated erythrocyte sedimentation rate, and increased numbers of leukocytes. Other manifestations of the acute-phase response include fever, increased heart rate, anorexia, somnolence, and malaise.

Acute-Phase Proteins

During the acute-phase response, the liver dramatically increases the synthesis of acute-phase proteins such as fibrinogen, C-reactive protein (CRP), and serum amyloid A protein (SAA) that serve several different defense functions.[1,2] The synthesis of these proteins is stimulated by cytokines, especially TNF-α, IL-1 (for SAA), and IL-6 (for fibrinogen and CRP).

C-reactive protein was named because it precipitated with the C fraction (C polypeptide) of pneumococci. The function of CRP is thought to be protective, in that it binds to the surface of invading microorganisms and targets them for destruction by complement and phagocytosis. Although everyone maintains a low level of CRP, this level rises when there is an acute inflammatory response.[27] Recent interest has focused on the use of high-sensitivity CRP (hsCRP) serum measurements as a marker for increased risk of myocardial infarction in persons with coronary heart disease.[28,29] It is believed that inflammation involving atherosclerotic plaques in coronary arteries may predispose to thrombosis and myocardial infarction (see Chapter 18).

During the acute-phase response, SAA protein replaces apolipoprotein A, a component of high-density lipoprotein (HDL) particles (see Chapter 18). This presumably increases the transfer of HDLs from liver cells to macrophages, which can then utilize these particles for energy. The rise in fibrinogen causes red blood cells to form stacks (rouleaux) that settle or sediment more rapidly than individual erythrocytes. This is the basis for the accelerated erythrocyte sedimentation rate (ESR) that occurs in disease conditions characterized by the systemic inflammatory response.

White Blood Cell Response

Leukocytosis, or the increase in white blood cells, is a frequent sign of an inflammatory response, especially those caused by bacterial infection. In acute inflammatory conditions, the white blood cell count commonly increases from a normal value of 4000 to 10,000 cells/μL to 15,000 to 20,000 cells/μL. After being released from the bone marrow, circulating neutrophils have a life span of only about 10 hours and therefore must be constantly replaced if their numbers are to be adequate. With excessive demand for phagocytes, immature forms of neutrophils (bands) are released from the bone marrow. The phrase "a shift to the left" in a white blood cell differential count refers to the increase in immature neutrophils seen in severe infections.

Bacterial infections produce a relatively selective increase in neutrophils (neutrophilia), while parasitic and allergic responses induce eosinophilia. Viral infections tend to produce a decrease in neutrophils (neutropenia) and an increase in lymphocytes (lymphocytosis).[3] A decrease in white blood cells (leukopenia) may also occur in persons with overwhelming infections or impaired ability to produce white blood cells.

Systemic Inflammatory Response

In severe bacterial infections (sepsis), the large quantities of microorganisms in the blood result in an uncontrolled inflammatory response with the production and release of enormous quantities of inflammatory cytokines (most notably IL-1 and TNF-α) and development of what is referred to as the *systemic inflammatory response syndrome* (see Chapter 20).[30] A decrease in total white blood cells (leukopenia) may occur in persons with overwhelming infections or impaired ability to produce white blood cells.

Fever

Fever (pyrexia) is an elevation in body temperature caused by an upward displacement of the set point of the thermoregulatory center in the hypothalamus.[31–33] It is one of the most prominent manifestations of the acute-phase response.[1,2]

Body Temperature Regulation

The temperature in the deep tissues of the body (core temperature) is normally maintained within a range of 36.0°C to 37.5°C (97.0°F to 99.5°F).[31,32] Within this range, there are individual differences and diurnal variations; internal core temperatures reach their highest point in late afternoon and evening and their lowest point in the early morning hours (Fig. 3-7). Virtually all biochemical processes in the body are affected by

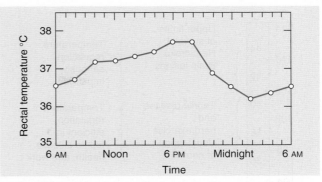

FIGURE 3-7. Normal diurnal variations in body temperature.

changes in temperature. Metabolic processes speed up or slow down depending on whether body temperature is rising or falling.

Body temperature, which reflects the difference between heat production and heat loss, is regulated by the *thermoregulatory center* in the hypothalamus. Body heat is generated in the tissues of the body, transferred to the skin surface by the blood, and then released into the environment surrounding the body. The thermoregulatory center regulates the temperature of the deep body tissues, or "core" of the body, rather than the surface temperature. It does so by integrating input from cold and warmth receptors located throughout the body and participating in negative feedback mechanisms.

The *thermostatic set point* of the thermoregulatory center is the level at which body temperature is regulated so that core temperature is maintained within the normal range. When body temperature begins to rise above this set point, heat-dissipating behaviors are initiated, and when the temperature falls below the set point, heat production is increased. A core temperature greater than 41°C (105.8°F) or less than 34°C (93.2°F) usually indicates that the body's thermoregulatory ability is impaired (Fig. 3-8). Body responses that produce, conserve, and dissipate heat are described in Table 3-1. Spinal cord injuries that transect the cord at T6 or above can seriously impair temperature regulation because the hypothalamus no longer can control skin blood flow or sweating.

In addition to physiologic thermoregulatory mechanisms, humans engage in voluntary behaviors to help regulate body temperature. These behaviors include the selection of proper clothing and regulation of environmental temperature through heating systems and air conditioning. Body positions that hold the extremities close to the body (e.g., huddling) prevent heat loss and are commonly assumed in cold weather.

Mechanisms of Heat Production. Metabolism is the body's main source of heat production. The sympathetic neurotransmitters epinephrine and norepinephrine, which are released when an increase in body temperature is needed, act at the cellular level to shift body metabolism to heat production rather than energy generation. This may be one of the reasons fever tends to produce feelings of weakness and fatigue. Thyroid hormone

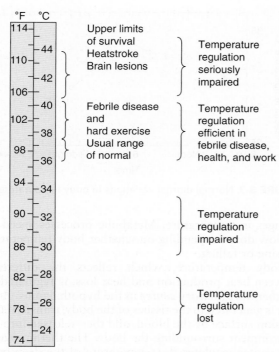

FIGURE 3-8. Body temperatures under different conditions. (From Dubois EF. *Fever and the Regulation of Body Temperature.* Springfield, IL: Charles C. Thomas; 1948.)

increases cellular metabolism, but this response usually requires several weeks to reach maximal effectiveness.

Fine involuntary actions such as shivering and chattering of the teeth can produce a threefold to fivefold increase in body temperature. *Shivering* is initiated by impulses from the hypothalamus. The first muscle change that occurs with shivering is a general increase in muscle tone, followed by an oscillating rhythmic tremor involving the spinal-level reflex that controls muscle tone. Because no external work is performed, all of the energy liberated by the metabolic processes from shivering is in the form of heat. Contraction of the *pilomotor muscles* of the skin, which raises the skin hair and produces goose bumps, reduces the surface area available for heat loss.

Physical exertion also increases body temperature. With strenuous exercise, more than three fourths of the increased metabolism resulting from muscle activity appears as heat within the body, and the remainder appears as external work.

Mechanisms of Heat Loss. Most of the body's heat is produced by the deeper core tissues (i.e., muscles and viscera) and then transferred in the blood to the body surface, where it is released into the environment.

There are numerous *arteriovenous (AV) shunts* under the skin surface that allow blood to move directly from the arterial to the venous system.[31] These AV shunts are much like the radiators in a heating system. When the shunts are open, body heat is freely dissipated to the skin and surrounding environment; when the shunts are closed, heat is retained in the body. The blood flow in the AV shunts is controlled almost exclusively by the sympathetic nervous system in response to changes in core temperature and environmental temperature. The transfer of heat to the body's surface is influenced by blood volume. In hot weather, the body compensates by increasing blood volume as a means of dissipating heat. Exposure to cold produces a cold diuresis and a reduction in blood volume as a means of controlling the transfer of heat to the body's surface.

Heat is lost from the body through radiation and conduction from the skin surface; through evaporation

TABLE 3-1	Heat Gain and Heat Loss Responses Used in Regulation of Body Temperature		
Heat Gain		**Heat Loss**	
Body Response	**Mechanism of Action**	**Body Response**	**Mechanism of Action**
Vasoconstriction of the superficial blood vessels	Confines blood flow to the inner core of the body, with the skin and subcutaneous tissues acting as insulation to prevent loss of core heat	Dilatation of the superficial blood vessels	Delivers blood containing core heat to the periphery where it is dissipated through radiation, conduction, and convection
Contraction of the pilomotor muscles that surround the hairs on the skin	Reduces heat loss from the skin	Sweating	Increases heat loss through evaporation
Assumption of the huddle position with the extremities held close to the body	Reduces the surface area for heat loss		
Shivering	Increases heat production by the muscles		
Increased production of epinephrine	Increases the heat production associated with metabolism		
Increased production of thyroid hormone	Is a long-term mechanism that increases metabolism and heat production		

of sweat and insensible perspiration; through exhalation of air that has been warmed and humidified; and through heat lost in urine and feces. Of these mechanisms, only heat losses that occur at the skin surface are directly under hypothalamic control.

Radiation involves the transfer of heat through the air or a vacuum. Heat loss through radiation varies with the temperature of the environment. Environmental temperature must be less than that of the body for heat loss to occur. About 60% of body heat loss typically occurs through radiation.[31] *Conduction* involves the direct transfer of heat from one molecule to another. Blood carries, or conducts, heat from the inner core of the body to the skin surface. Normally, only a small amount of body heat is lost through conduction to a cooler surface. Cooling blankets and mattresses that are used for reducing fever rely on conduction of heat from skin to the cooler surface of the mattress or blanket. Heat can also be conducted in the opposite direction—from the external environment to the body surface. For instance, body temperature may rise slightly after a hot bath.

Convection refers to heat transfer through the circulation of air currents. Normally, a layer of warm air tends to remain near the body's surface; convection causes continual removal of the warm layer and replacement with air from the surrounding environment. The wind-chill factor that often is included in the weather report combines the effect of convection caused by wind with the still-air temperature.

Evaporation involves the use of body heat to convert water on the skin to water vapor. Water that diffuses through the skin independent of sweating is called *insensible perspiration.* Insensible perspiration losses are greatest in a dry environment. Sweating occurs through the sweat glands and is controlled by the sympathetic nervous system, using acetylcholine as a neurotransmitter. This means that anticholinergic drugs, such as atropine, can interfere with heat loss by interrupting sweating.

Evaporative heat losses involve both insensible perspiration and sweating, with 0.58 calorie being lost for each gram of water that is evaporated.[31] As long as body temperature is greater than the atmospheric temperature, heat is lost through radiation. However, when the temperature of the surrounding environment becomes greater than skin temperature, evaporation is the only way the body can rid itself of heat. Any condition that prevents evaporative heat losses causes the body temperature to rise.

The Febrile Response

Fever, or pyrexia, describes an elevation in body temperature that is caused by a cytokine-induced upward displacement of the set point of the hypothalamic thermoregulatory center. It is resolved when the factor that caused the increase in the set point is removed. Fevers that are regulated by the hypothalamus usually do not rise above 41°C (105°F), suggesting a built-in thermostatic regulatory mechanism. Temperatures above that level are usually the result of superimposed activity, such as convulsions, hypermetabolic states, or direct impairment of the temperature control center.

Causes of Fever. Fever can be caused by a number of microorganisms and substances that are collectively called pyrogens.[33–35] Many proteins, including lipopolysaccharide toxins released from bacterial cell membranes, can raise the set point of the hypothalamic thermostat. Noninfectious disorders, such as myocardial infarction and pulmonary emboli, also produce fever. In these conditions, the injured or abnormal cells incite the production of fever-producing pyrogens. Some malignant cells, such as those of leukemia and Hodgkin disease, also secrete pyrogens.

Some pyrogens act directly and immediately on the hypothalamic thermoregulatory center to increase its set point. Other pyrogens, often referred to as *exogenous pyrogens,* act indirectly and may require several hours to produce their effect.[31] Exogenous pyrogens induce host cells, such as blood leukocytes and tissue macrophages, to produce fever-producing mediators called *endogenous pyrogens* (e.g., IL-1). For example, the breakdown products of phagocytosed bacteria that are present in the blood lead to the release of endogenous pyrogens. The endogenous pyrogens are thought to increase the set point of the hypothalamic thermoregulatory center through the action of prostaglandin E_2 (PGE_2) (Fig. 3-9).[31] In response to the sudden increase in set point, the hypothalamus initiates heat production behaviors (shivering and vasoconstriction) that increase the core body temperature to the new set point, and fever is established.

A fever that has its origin in the central nervous system is sometimes referred to as a *neurogenic fever.*[36] It usually is the result of damage to the hypothalamus caused by central nervous system trauma, intracerebral bleeding, or an increase in intracranial pressure. Neurogenic fevers are characterized by a high temperature that is resistant to antipyretic therapy and is not associated with sweating.

Purpose of Fever. The purpose of fever is not completely understood. However, from a purely practical standpoint, fever signals the presence of an infection and may legitimize the need for medical treatment. In ancient times, fever was thought to "cook" the poisons that caused the illness. With the availability of antipyretic drugs in the late 19th century, the belief that fever was useful began to wane, probably because most antipyretic drugs also had analgesic effects.

Fever Patterns. The patterns of temperature change in persons with fever vary and may provide information about the nature of the causative agent.[37] These patterns can be described as intermittent, remittent, sustained, or relapsing (Fig. 3-10). An intermittent fever is one in which temperature returns to normal at least once every 24 hours. Intermittent fevers are commonly associated with conditions such as gram-negative/-positive sepsis, abscesses, and acute bacterial endocarditis. In a remittent fever, the temperature does not return to normal and varies a few degrees in either direction.

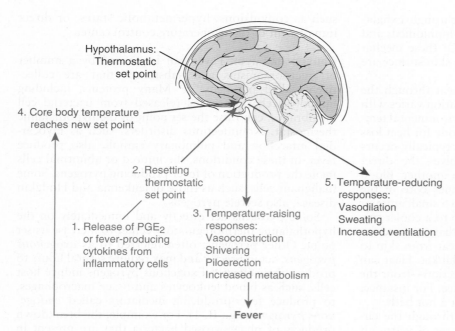

4. Core body temperature reaches new set point

2. Resetting thermostatic set point

1. Release of PGE$_2$ or fever-producing cytokines from inflammatory cells

3. Temperature-raising responses:
Vasoconstriction
Shivering
Piloerection
Increased metabolism

5. Temperature-reducing responses:
Vasodilation
Sweating
Increased ventilation

Hypothalamus: Thermostatic set point

Fever

FIGURE 3-9. Mechanisms of fever. (*1*) Release of prostaglandin E$_2$ (PGE$_2$) or fever-producing cytokines from inflammatory cells, (*2*) resetting of the thermoregulatory set point in the hypothalamus to a higher level (prodrome), (*3*) generation of hypothalamic-mediated responses that raise body temperature (chill), (*4*) development of fever with elevation of body to new thermostatic set point, and (*5*) production of temperature-lowering responses (flush and defervescence) and return of body temperature to a lower level.

In a sustained or continuous fever, the temperature remains above normal with minimal variations (usually less than 0.55°C or 1°F). Sustained fevers are seen in persons with drug-induced fever in which a drug inadvertently leads to a hypermetabolic fever-inducing state.[38] A recurrent or relapsing fever is one in which there is one or more episodes of fever, each as long as several days, with one or more days of normal temperature between episodes. Relapsing fevers may be caused by a variety of infectious diseases, including tuberculosis, fungal infections, Lyme disease, and malaria.

Critical to the analysis of a fever pattern is the relation of heart rate to the level of temperature elevation. Most persons respond to an increase in temperature with an appropriate increase in heart rate. The observation that a rise in temperature is not accompanied by the anticipated change in heart rate can provide useful information about the cause of the fever. For example, a heart rate that is slower than would be anticipated can occur with Legionnaires' disease and drug fever, and a heart rate that is more rapid than anticipated can be symptomatic of hyperthyroidism.

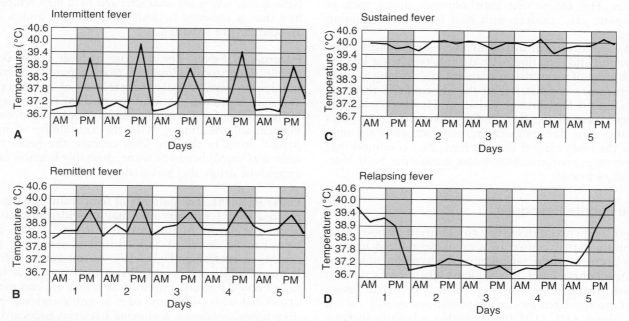

FIGURE 3-10. Schematic representation of fever patterns: **(A)** intermittent, **(B)** remittent, **(C)** sustained, and **(D)** recurrent or relapsing.

Manifestations of Fever

The physiologic behaviors that occur during the development of fever can be divided into four successive stages: a prodrome; a chill, during which the temperature rises; a flush; and defervescence (see Fig. 3-9). During the *first* or *prodromal* period, there are nonspecific complaints, such as mild headache and fatigue, general malaise, and fleeting aches and pains. During the *second stage* or *chill,* there is the uncomfortable sensation of being cold and the onset of generalized shaking, although the temperature is rising. Vasoconstriction and piloerection usually precede the onset of shivering. At this point the skin is pale and covered with goose flesh. There is an urge to put on more clothing or covering and to curl up in a position that conserves body heat. When the shivering has caused the body temperature to reach the new set point of the temperature control center, the shivering ceases, and a sensation of warmth develops. At this point, the *third stage* or *flush* begins, during which cutaneous vasodilatation occurs and the skin becomes warm and reddened. The *fourth,* or *defervescence,* stage of the febrile response is marked by the initiation of sweating. Not all persons proceed through all four stages of fever development. Sweating may be absent, and fever may develop gradually, with no indication of a chill or shivering.

Common manifestations of fever are anorexia, myalgia, arthralgia, and fatigue. These discomforts are worse when the temperature rises rapidly or exceeds 39.5°C (103.1°F). Respiration is increased, and the heart rate usually is elevated. Dehydration occurs because of sweating and the increased vapor losses caused by the rapid respiratory rate. The occurrence of chills commonly coincides with the introduction of pyrogen into the circulation. This is one of the reasons that blood cultures to identify the organism causing the fever are usually drawn during the first signs of a chill.

Many of the manifestations of fever are related to the increases in the metabolic rate, increased need for oxygen, and use of body proteins as an energy source. During fever, the body switches from using glucose (an excellent medium for bacterial growth) to metabolism based on protein and fat breakdown. With prolonged fever, there is increased breakdown of endogenous fat stores. If fat breakdown is rapid, metabolic acidosis may result (see Chapter 8).

Headache is a common accompaniment of fever and is thought to result from the vasodilatation of cerebral vessels occurring with fever. Delirium is possible when the temperature exceeds 40°C (104°F). In the elderly, confusion and delirium may follow moderate elevations in temperature. Because of the increasingly poor oxygen uptake by the aging lung, pulmonary function may prove to be a limiting factor in the hypermetabolism that accompanies fever in older persons. Confusion, incoordination, and agitation commonly reflect cerebral hypoxemia. Febrile seizures can occur in some children.[39] They usually occur with rapidly rising temperatures and/or at a threshold temperature that differs with each child.

Herpetic lesions, or fever blisters, develop in some persons during fever. They are caused by a separate infection by the type 1 herpes simplex virus that established latency in the regional ganglia and is reactivated by a rise in body temperature.

Management of Fever

Fever usually is a manifestation of a disease state, and as such, determining the cause of a fever is an important aspect of its treatment. Sometimes it is difficult to establish the cause. A prolonged fever for which the cause is difficult to ascertain is often referred to as *fever of unknown origin* (FUO). Fever of unknown origin is defined as a temperature of 38.3°C (101°F) or higher that is present for 3 weeks or longer.[40,41] Among the causes of FUO are malignancies (i.e., lymphomas, metastases to the liver or central nervous system); infections such as human immunodeficiency virus or tuberculosis, or abscessed infections; and drug fever. Malignancies, particularly non-Hodgkin lymphoma, are important causes of FUO in the elderly. Cirrhosis of the liver is another cause of FUO.

The methods of fever treatment focus on modifications of the external environment intended to increase heat transfer from the internal to the external environment, support of the hypermetabolic state that accompanies fever, protection of vulnerable body organs and systems, and treatment of the infection or condition causing the fever. Because fever is a disease symptom, its manifestation suggests the need for treatment of the primary cause.

Modification of the environment ensures that the environmental temperature facilitates heat transfer away from the body. Sponge baths with cool water or an alcohol solution can be used to increase evaporative heat losses. More profound cooling can be accomplished through the use of a cooling blanket or mattress, which facilitates the conduction of heat from the body into the coolant solution that circulates through the mattress. Care must be taken so that cooling methods do not produce vasoconstriction and shivering that decrease heat loss and increase heat production.

Adequate fluids and sufficient amounts of simple carbohydrates are needed to support the hypermetabolic state and prevent the tissue breakdown that is characteristic of fever. Additional fluids are needed for sweating and to balance the insensible water losses from the lungs that accompany an increase in respiratory rate. Fluids also are needed to maintain an adequate vascular volume for heat transport to the skin surface.

Antipyretic drugs, such as aspirin, ibuprofen, and acetaminophen, often are used to alleviate the discomforts of fever and protect vulnerable organs, such as the brain, from extreme elevations in body temperature. These drugs act by resetting the hypothalamic temperature control center to a lower level, presumably by blocking the activity of cyclooxygenase, an enzyme that is required for the conversion of arachidonic acid to prostaglandin E_2.

Fever in Children

Fever occurs frequently in infants and young children (i.e., ages 1 day to 3 years) and is a common reason for visits to the clinic or emergency department.[42,43] The differential diagnosis of fever is broad and includes both infectious and noninfectious causes, with the majority of febrile children having an underlying infection. The most common causes are minor or more serious infections of the respiratory system, gastrointestinal tract, urinary tract, or central nervous system. The epidemiology of serious bacterial disease has changed dramatically with the introduction of the *Haemophilus influenzae* and *Streptococcus pneumoniae* vaccines in developed countries. *H. influenzae* type b has been nearly eliminated and the incidence of pneumococcal disease has declined substantially. Febrile children who are younger than 1 year of age and females between 1 and 2 years of age should be considered at risk for a urinary tract infection (see Chapter 24).

While most children have identifiable causes for their fevers, many have fevers without localizing signs or symptoms. These fevers, which are usually of rapid onset and present for less than a week, are commonly referred to as *fever without source*. The American College of Emergency Physicians has developed clinical guidelines for use in the treatment of previously healthy infants and children ages 1 day to 3 years with fever without a source. The guidelines define fever in this age group as a rectal temperature of at least 38°C (100.4°F). The reliability of other methods of temperature measurements (e.g., axillary, ear) is lower and must be considered when making decisions about the seriousness of the fever.[43]

The approach to the young child who has fever without a source varies depending on the age of the child (neonate [0 to 28 days], young infant [1 to 3 months], and older infants and toddlers [3 to 36 months]).[44] All have decreased immunologic function and are more commonly infected with virulent organisms. Neonates are at particularly high risk for serious bacterial infections that can cause bacteremia or meningitis. Also, neonates and young infants demonstrate limited signs of infection, often making it difficult to distinguish between serious bacterial infections that require immediate medical attention and other causes of an elevated temperature.

Fever without source in children younger than age 3 months requires careful history and physical examination.[42] The temperature-lowering response to antipyretic medications does not change the likelihood of a child having a serious bacterial infection and should not be used as an indicator of infection severity.[45] Neonates with signs of toxicity (and high risk) including lethargy, poor feeding, hypoventilation, poor tissue oxygenation, and cyanosis usually require hospitalization and treatment with antibiotics. Diagnostic tests such as white blood cell count, blood and urine cultures, chest radiographs, and lumbar puncture usually are done to determine the cause of fever. Infants with fever who are considered to be at low risk for bacterial infections often are managed on an outpatient basis provided the parents or caregivers are deemed reliable. Older children with fever without source also may be treated on an outpatient basis.

Fever in the Elderly

In the elderly, even slight elevations in temperature may indicate serious infection, most often caused by bacteria, or disease. This is because the elderly often have a lower baseline temperature (36.4°C [97.6°F] in one study) than younger persons, and although their temperature increases during an infection, it may fail to reach a level that is equated with significant fever.[45,46] Therefore, it has been recommended that the definition of fever in the elderly be expanded to include an elevation of temperature of at least 1.1°C (2°F) above baseline values.

The absence of fever may delay diagnosis and initiation of antimicrobial treatment. Unexplained changes in functional capacity, worsening of mental status, weakness and fatigue, and weight loss are signs of infection in the elderly and should be viewed as possible signs of infection and sepsis when fever is absent. A thorough history and physical examination are critically important.[47] The probable mechanisms for the blunted fever response include a disturbance in sensing of temperature by the thermoregulatory center in the hypothalamus, alterations in release of endogenous pyrogens, and the failure to elicit responses such as vasoconstriction of skin vessels, increased heat production, and shivering that increase body temperature during a febrile response.

Another factor that may delay recognition of fever in the elderly is the method of temperature measurement. Oral temperature remains the most commonly used method, but research suggests that rectal and tympanic membrane methods are more effective in detecting fever in the elderly.[47] This is because conditions such as mouth breathing, tongue tremors, and agitation often make it difficult to obtain accurate oral temperatures in the elderly.

SUMMARY CONCEPTS

■ The systemic manifestations of inflammation include the effects of the acute-phase response, such as fever and lethargy; increased erythrocyte sedimentation rate (ESR), levels of C-reactive protein (CRP), other acute-phase proteins, and white blood cells; and enlargement of the lymph nodes that drain the affected area. In severe bacterial infections (sepsis), large quantities of microorganisms in the blood result in the production and release of enormous quantities of inflammatory cytokines and development of what is referred to as the *systemic inflammatory response syndrome.*

■ Fever, an elevation in body temperature, is one of the most prominent manifestations of the acute-phase response, especially if inflammation is caused by infection. It is produced in response to pyrogens that act by prompting the release of prostaglandin E$_2$ or fever-producing cytokines, which in turn resets the hypothalamic thermoregulatory center.

■ The reactions that occur during fever consist of four stages: a *prodromal period* with nonspecific complaints, such as mild headache and fatigue; a *chill,* during which the temperature rises; a *flush,* during which the skin becomes warm and flushed; and a *defervescence stage,* which is marked by the initiation of sweating.

■ The approach to fever in children varies depending on the age of the child. Infants and young children have decreased immunologic function and are more commonly infected with virulent organisms.

■ The elderly tend to have a lower baseline temperature, so that serious infections may go unrecognized because of the perceived lack of a significant fever.

REVIEW EXERCISES

1. A 15-year-old boy presents with abdominal pain, a temperature of 38°C (100.5°F), and an elevated white blood cell count of 13,000/μL, with an increase in neutrophils. A tentative diagnosis of appendicitis is made.

   A. Explain the significance of pain as it relates to the inflammatory response.
   B. What is the cause of the fever and elevated white blood cell count?
   C. What would be the preferred treatment for this boy?

2. Aspirin and other nonsteroidal anti-inflammatory drugs are often used to control the manifestations of chronic inflammatory disorders such as arthritis.

   A. Explain their mechanism of action in terms of controlling the inflammatory response.

3. Persons with long-standing ulcerative colitis, an inflammatory bowel disease, have a higher risk of colorectal cancer than the general population.

   A. Hypothesize on cancer-producing mechanisms of this chronic inflammatory disease.

4. A 3-year-old child is seen in a pediatric clinic with a temperature of 39°C (103°F). Her skin is warm and flushed, her pulse is 120 beats per minute, and her respirations are shallow and rapid at 32 breaths per minute. Her mother states that she has complained of a sore throat and has refused to drink or take medications to bring her fever down.

   A. Explain the physiologic mechanisms of fever generation.
   B. Are the warm and flushed skin, rapid heart rate, and respirations consistent with this level of fever?
   C. After receiving an appropriate dose of acetaminophen, the child begins to sweat, and the temperature drops to 37.2°C. Explain the physiologic mechanisms responsible for the drop in temperature.

REFERENCES

1. Murphy HS. Inflammation. In: Rubin E, Strayer D, eds. *Rubin's Pathology: Clinicopathologic Foundations of Medicine.* 5th ed. Philadelphia, PA: Wolters Kluwer Health/ Lippincott Williams & Wilkins; 2012:47–82.
2. Kumar V, Abbas AK, Fausto N, et al. *Robbins and Cotran Basic Pathology.* 8th ed. Philadelphia, PA: Saunders Elsevier; 2010:43–77.
3. Schmid-Schonbein GW. Analysis of inflammation. *Annu Rev Biomed Eng.* 2006;8:93–131.
4. Medzhitov R. Origin and physiological roles of inflammation. *Nature.* 2008;454(24):428–435.
5. Szekanecz Z, Koch AE. Vascular endothelium and immune responses: implications for inflammation and angiogenesis. *Rheum Dis Clin North Am.* 2004;30:97–114.
6. Steinhubl SR. Platelets as mediators of inflammation. *Hematol Oncol Clin North Am.* 2007;21:115–121.
7. Gawaz M, Langer H, May AE. Platelets in inflammation and atherogenesis. *J Clin Invest.* 2005;115(12):3378–3384.
8. Ricciotti E, Fitzgerald GA. Prostaglandins and inflammation. *Arterioscler Thromb Vasc Biol.* 2011;31(5):986–1000.
9. Ormenetti A, Gattorno M. Principles of inflammation for the pediatrician. *Pediatr Clin North Am.* 2012;59:225–243.
10. Bachelet I, Levi-Schaffer F, Mekori YA. Mast cells: not only in allergy. *Immunol Allergy Clin North Am.* 2006;26:407–425.
11. Frenette PS, Wagner DD. Adhesion molecules—parts I and II. *N Engl J Med.* 1996;334(23):1526–1529.
12. Bochner BS. Adhesion molecules as therapeutic targets. *Immunol Allergy Clin North Am.* 2004;24:615–630.
13. Stein DM, Nombela-Arrieta C. Chemokine control of lymphocyte trafficking: a general review. *Immunology.* 2005;116:1–12.
14. Underhill DM, Ozinsky A. Phagocytosis of microbes. *Annu Rev Immunol.* 2002;20:825–852.
15. Simmons DL, Botting RM, Hla T. Cyclooxygenase isoenzymes: the biology of prostaglandin synthesis and inhibition. *Pharmacol Rev.* 2004;56(3):387–437.
16. Barnes PJ. How corticosteroids control inflammation: Quintiles Prize Lecture 2005. *Br J Pharmacol.* 2006;14B:245–254.
17. Covington MB. Omega-3 fatty acids. *Am Fam Physician.* 2004;70(1):133–140.

18. Harper CR, Jacobson TA. Usefulness of omega-3 fatty acids and prevention of coronary heart disease. *Am J Cardiol.* 2005;96:1521–1529.

19. Gosain A, Gamelli RL. A primer on cytokines. *J Burn Care Rehabil.* 2005;26:7–12.

20. Charo I, Ransohoff RM. The many roles of chemokines and chemokine receptors in inflammation. *N Engl J Med.* 2006;354(6):610–621.

21. Serhan CN, Savill J. Resolution of inflammation: the beginning programs the end. *Nat Immunol.* 2005;6(12):1191–1197.

22. Serhan CN, Brain SD, Buckley CD, et al. Resolution of inflammation: state of the art, definitions and terms. *FASEB J.* 2007;21:325–332.

23. Schottenfeld D, Beebe-Dimmer J. Chronic inflammation: a common and important factor in the pathogenesis of neoplasia. *CA Cancer J Clin.* 2006;56:69–83.

24. Nathan C. Epidemic inflammation: pondering obesity. *Mol Med.* 2008;7(8):485–492.

25. Tateya S, Kim F, Tamori Y. Recent advances in obesity-related inflammation and insulin resistance. *Front Endocrinol (Lausanne).* 2013;4:93.

26. Greenberg AS, Obin MS. Obesity and the role of adipose tissue in inflammation and metabolism. *Am J Clin Nutr.* 2006;83(suppl):461S–465S.

27. Ridker PM. C-reactive protein, inflammation, and cardiovascular disease. *Curr Issues Cardiol.* 2005;32(3):384–386.

28. Ridker PM. High-sensitivity C-reactive protein: potential adjunct for global risk assessment in primary prevention of cardiovascular disease. *Circulation.* 2001;103:1813–1818.

29. Pearson TA, Mensah GA, Alexander RW, et al. Markers of inflammation and cardiovascular disease: application to clinical and public health practice: a statement for healthcare professionals from the Centers for Disease Control and Prevention and the American Heart Association. *Circulation.* 2003;107:499–511.

30. Hotchiss RS, Karl IE. The pathophysiology and treatment of sepsis. *N Engl J Med.* 2003;348(2):138–150.

31. Hall JE. *Guyton and Hall Textbook of Medical Physiology.* 12th ed. Philadelphia, PA: Saunders Elsevier; 2011:867–877.

32. Wilzmann FA. The regulation of body temperature. In: Rhoades RA, Bell DR. *Medical Physiology.* 2nd ed. Philadelphia, PA: Wolters Kluwer Health/Lippincott Williams & Wilkins; 2013:550–574.

33. Roth J, Rummel C, Barth SW, et al. Molecular aspects of fever and hyperthermia. *Neurol Clin.* 2006;24:421–439.

34. Blatteis CM. Endotoxic fever: new concepts of its regulation suggest new approaches to its management. *Pharmacol Ther.* 2006;111:194–223.

35. Blatteis CM, Li S, Li Z, et al. Cytokines, PGE_2, and endotoxic fever: a re-assessment. *Prostaglandins Other Lipid Mediat.* 2005;76:1–18.

36. Thompson HJ, Pinto-Martin J, Bullock MR. Neurogenic fever after traumatic brain 2011 injury: an epidemiological study. *J Neurol Neurosurg Psychiatry.* 2003;74:614–619.

37. Ogoina D. Fever, fever patterns and 2011 diseases called "fever"—A review. *J Infect Public Health* 2011;4(3):108–124.

38. Patel R, Gallagher JC. Drug fever. *Pharmacotherapy.* 2010;30(1):57–69.

39. Graves RC, Oehler K, Tingle LE. Febrile seizures: risks, evaluation, and prognosis. *Am Fam Physician.* 2012;85(2):149–153.

40. Cunha BA. Fever of unknown origin: clinical overview of and classic and current concepts. *Infect Dis Clin North Am.* 2007;21:867–915.

41. Horowitz HW. Fever of unknown origin or fever of too many origins. *N Engl J Med.* 2013;368(3):197–199.

42. Hamilton JL, John SP. Evaluation of fever in infants and young children. *Am Fam Physician.* 2013;87(4):254–260.

43. Ishimine P. Fever without source in children 0 to 36 months of age. *Pediatr Clin North Am.* 2006;53:167–194.

44. ACEP Clinical Policy Committee and Clinical Policies Subcommittee on Pediatric Care. Clinical policy for children less than 3 years presenting to the emergency department with fever. *Ann Emerg Med.* 2003;42(4):530–545.

45. Woolery WA, Franco FR. Fever of unknown origin: keys to determining the etiology in older patients. *Geriatrics.* 2004;59(10):41–45.

46. Norman DC, Wong MG, Yoshikawa TT. Fever of unknown origin in older persons. *Infect Dis Clin North Am.* 2007;21:937–945.

47. Outzen M. Management of fever in older adults. *J Gerontol Nurs.* 2009;35(5):17–23.

Porth Essentials Resources

Explore these additional resources to enhance learning for this chapter:

- NCLEX-Style Questions and Other Resources on thePoint, http://thePoint.lww.com/PorthEssentials4e
- Study Guide for Essentials of Pathophysiology
- Concepts in Action Animations
- Adaptive Learning | Powered by PrepU, http://thepoint.lww.com/prepu

Chapter 4

Cell Proliferation and Tissue Regeneration and Repair

Tissue repair, which overlaps the inflammatory process that was discussed in Chapter 3, refers to the restoration of tissue structure and function after an injury. Tissue repair can take the form of regeneration, in which injured cells are replaced with cells of the same type, sometimes leaving no residual trace of previous injury; or it can take the form of replacement by connective (fibrous) tissue, which leads to scar formation or fibrosis in organs such as the liver or lung. For many types of common injuries, both regeneration and connective tissue replacement contribute to tissue repair. This chapter is divided into two parts. The first part discusses cell proliferation and regeneration, the cell cycle, the role of stem cells, growth factors, and the extracellular matrix in tissue renewal. The second focuses on connective tissue repair, cutaneous wound healing, factors that affect wound healing, and the effect of aging on wound healing.

Cell Proliferation and Tissue Regeneration

Tissue repair involves the proliferation of various cells, and close interactions between cells and the extracellular matrix (ECM). Body organs and tissues are composed of two types of tissues: parenchymal and stromal. The parenchymal tissues consist of the functioning cells of an organ or body part: whereas, the stromal tissues contain the supporting connective tissues, blood vessels, fibroblasts, nerve fibers, and extracellular matrix.

Cell Proliferation Versus Differentiation

Cell proliferation refers to the process of increasing cell numbers by mitotic division. *Cell differentiation* is the process whereby a cell becomes more specialized in

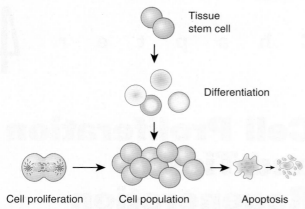

FIGURE 4-1. In normal tissues, the size of the cell population is determined by a balance of cell proliferation, death by apoptosis, and emergence of newly differentiated cells from stem cells.

terms of structure and function.[1,2] Stem cells are undifferentiated cells that have the capacity to generate multiple cell types (to be discussed). In normal tissue the size of the cell population is determined by a balance of cell proliferation, death by apoptosis (see Chapter 2), and emergence of newly differentiated cells from stem cells[2] (Fig. 4-1). Several cell types proliferate during tissue repair including remnants of injured parenchymal tissue cells, vascular endothelial cells, and fibroblasts. The proliferation of these cell types is driven by proteins called *growth factors*. The production of growth factors and the ability of these cells to respond and expand in sufficient numbers are important determinants of the repair process.

All of the different cell types in the body originate from a single cell—the fertilized ovum. As the embryonic cells increase in number, they differentiate, facilitating the development of all the different cells and organs of the body. The process of differentiation is regulated by a combination of internal processes involving the expression of specific genes and external stimuli provided by neighboring cells, the ECM, and a variety of growth factors. The process occurs in orderly steps, with each progressive step being exchanged for a loss of ability to develop different cell characteristics. As a cell becomes more highly specialized, the stimuli that are able to induce mitosis become more limited. Neurons, which are highly specialized cells, lose their ability to proliferate once development of the nervous system is complete. In other, less-specialized tissues, such as the skin and mucosal lining of the gastrointestinal tract, a high degree of cell renewal continues throughout life. Even in these continuously renewing cell populations, the more specialized cells are unable to divide. Many of these cell populations rely on *progenitor* or *parent cells* of the same lineage. Progenitor cells are sufficiently differentiated so that their daughter cells are limited to the same cell line, but they have not reached the point of differentiation that precludes the potential for active proliferation. Some cell populations have self-renewing multipotent stem cells, such as the epithelial stem

cells, that can differentiate into the different cell types throughout life.

The Cell Cycle

In order to understand cell proliferation, whether physiologic (as in tissue regeneration and repair) or pathologic (as in cancer), it is important to learn about the cell cycle, an orderly sequence of events in which a cell duplicates its genetic contents and divides. During the cell cycle, the duplicated chromosomes are appropriately aligned for distribution between two genetically identical daughter cells.

The cell cycle is divided into four distinct phases referred to as G_1, S, G_2, and M. Gap 1 (G_1) is the postmitotic phase during which deoxyribonucleic acid (DNA) synthesis ceases while ribonucleic acid (RNA) and protein synthesis and cell growth take place (see Understanding the Cell Cycle).[1–4] During the S *phase*, DNA synthesis occurs, giving rise to two separate sets of chromosomes, one for each daughter cell. G_2 is the premitotic phase and is similar to G_1 in that DNA synthesis ceases while RNA and protein synthesis continue. Collectively, G_1, S, and G_2 are referred to as *interphase*. The M *phase* is the phase of nuclear division and cytokinesis. Continually dividing cells, such as the stratified squamous epithelium of the skin, continue to cycle from one mitotic division to the next. When environmental conditions are adverse, such as nutrient or growth factor unavailability, or cells become terminally differentiated (i.e., highly specialized), cells may exit the cell cycle, becoming mitotically quiescent and reside in a special resting state known as G_0. Cells in G_0 may reenter the cell cycle in response to extracellular nutrients, growth factors, hormones, and other signals such as blood loss or tissue injury that trigger cell renewal. Highly specialized and terminally differentiated cells, such as neurons, may permanently stay in G_0.

Within the cell cycle are checkpoints where pauses or arrests can be made if the specific events in the phases of the cell cycle have not been completed. There are also opportunities for ensuring the accuracy of DNA replication. These DNA damage checkpoints allow for any defects to be edited and repaired, thereby ensuring that each daughter cell receives a full complement of genetic information, identical to that of the parent cell.[1–3]

The *cyclins* are a family of proteins that control the entry and progression of cells through the cell cycle.[1–4] Cyclins bind to (thereby activating) proteins called *cyclin-dependent kinases* (CDKs). Kinases are enzymes that phosphorylate proteins. The CDKs phosphorylate specific target proteins and are expressed continuously during the cell cycle but in an inactive form, whereas the cyclins are synthesized during specific phases of the cell cycle and then degraded once their task is completed. Different arrangements of cyclins and CDKs are associated with each stage of the cell cycle. For example, cyclin B and CDK1 control the transition from G_2 to M. As the cell moves into G_2, cyclin B is synthesized and binds to CDK1. The cyclin B–CDK1 complex then directs the events leading to mitosis, including DNA replication and assembly of the mitotic spindle. Although each phase of the cell cycle is monitored carefully, the transition from G_2 to M is believed to be one of the most important checkpoints in the cell cycle. In addition to the synthesis and degradation of the cyclins, the cyclin–CDK complexes are regulated by the binding of CDK inhibitors. The CDK inhibitors are particularly important in regulating cell cycle checkpoints during which mistakes in DNA replication are repaired. The finding that the cell cycle can be reactivated by removing CDK inhibitors in quiescent and nonproliferating cells has potential implications for tissue repair and cell replacement therapy.[4]

Proliferative Capacity of Tissues

The capacity for regeneration varies with the tissue and cell type. Body tissues are divided into three types depending on the ability of their cells to undergo regeneration: (1) continuously dividing, (2) stable, and (3) permanent tissues.[1,2]

Continuously dividing or *labile* tissues are those in which the cells continue to divide and replicate throughout life, replacing cells that are continually being destroyed. They include the surface epithelial cells of the skin, oral cavity, vagina, and cervix; the columnar epithelium of the gastrointestinal tract, uterus, and fallopian tubes; the transitional epithelium of the urinary tract; and bone marrow cells. These tissues can readily regenerate after injury as long as a pool of stem cells is preserved. Bleeding, for example, stimulates the rapid proliferation of replacement cells by the blood-forming progenitor cells of the bone marrow.

Stable tissues contain cells that normally stop dividing when growth ceases. Cells in these tissues remain quiescent in the G_0 stage of the cell cycle. However, these cells are capable of undergoing regeneration when confronted with an appropriate stimulus; thus, they are capable of reconstituting the tissue of origin. Stable cells constitute the parenchyma of solid organs such as the liver and kidney. They also include smooth muscle cells, vascular endothelial cells, and fibroblasts, the proliferation of which is particularly important to wound healing.

The cells in *permanent* tissues do not proliferate. The cells in these tissues are considered to be terminally differentiated and do not undergo mitotic division in postnatal life. The permanent cells include nerve cells, skeletal muscle cells, and cardiac muscle cells. These cells do not normally regenerate; once destroyed, they are replaced with fibrous scar tissue that lacks the functional characteristics of the destroyed tissue.

Stem Cells

Another type of tissue cell, called a *stem cell*, remains incompletely differentiated throughout life.[1,2,5] In most continuously dividing tissues, the mature cells are terminally differentiated and short lived. As mature cells die the tissue is replenished by the differentiation of cells

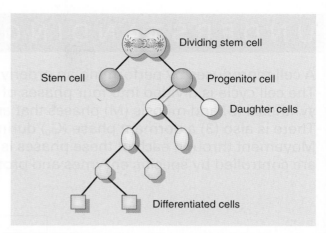

FIGURE 4-2. Mechanisms of stem cell–mediated cell replacement. Division of a stem cell with an unlimited potential for proliferation results in one daughter cell, which retains the characteristics of a stem cell, and a second daughter cell that differentiates into a progenitor or parent cell, with limited potential for differentiation and proliferation. As the daughter cells of the progenitor cell proliferate they become more differentiated, until they reach the stage where they are fully differentiated.

generated from stem cells. Stem cells are reserve cells that remain quiescent until there is a need for cell replenishment, in which case they divide, producing other stem cells and cells that can carry out the functions of the differentiated cell. When a stem cell divides, one daughter cell retains the stem cell characteristics, and the other daughter cell becomes a progenitor cell that undergoes a process that leads to terminal differentiation (Fig. 4-2).

Stem cells are characterized by three important properties: self-renewal, asymmetric replication, and differential potential.[1,2] *Self-renewal* means that the stem cells can undergo numerous mitotic divisions while maintaining an undifferentiated state. *Asymmetric replication* means that after each cell division, some progeny of the stem cell enter a differentiation pathway, while others remain undifferentiated, retaining their self-renewal capacity. The progeny of each progenitor cell follows a more restricted genetic program, with the differentiating cells undergoing multiple mitotic divisions in the process of becoming a more mature cell type, and with each generation of cells becoming more specialized. In this way, a single stem cell can give rise to the many cells needed for normal tissue repair or blood cell production.

The term *potency* is used to define the differentiation potential of stem cells. *Totipotent stem cells* are those produced by a fertilized ovum. The first few cells produced after fertilization are totipotent and can differentiate into embryonic and extraembryonic cells. Totipotent stem cells give rise to *pluripotent stem cells* that can differentiate into the three germ layers of the embryo. *Multipotent stem cells* are cells such as hematopoietic stem cells that give rise to a family of cells, including the red blood cells and all the various types of leukocytes. Finally, *unipotent stem cells* produce only one cell type but retain the property of self-renewal.

(*text continues on page 76*)

UNDERSTANDING ➜ The Cell Cycle

A cell reproduces by performing an orderly sequence of events called the *cell cycle.* The cell cycle is divided into four phases of unequal duration that include the (1) synthesis (S) and mitosis (M) phases that are separated by (2) two gaps (G₁ and G₂). There is also (3) a dormant phase (G₀) during which the cell may leave the cell cycle. Movement through each of these phases is mediated at (4) specific checkpoints that are controlled by specific enzymes and proteins called *cyclins.*

1

Synthesis and Mitosis. Synthesis (S) and mitosis (M) represent the two major phases of the cell cycle. The S phase, which takes about 10 to 12 hours, is the period of DNA synthesis and replication of the chromosomes. The M phase, which usually takes less than an hour, involves formation of the mitotic spindle and cell division with formation of two daughter cells.

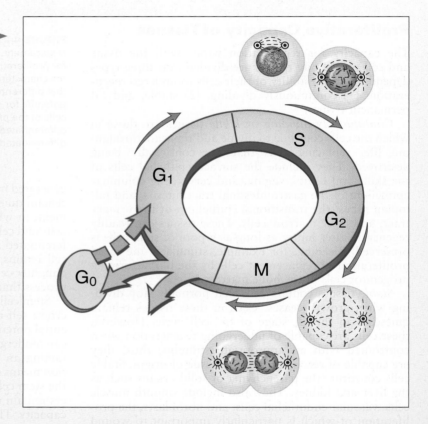

2

Gaps 1 and 2. Because most cells require time to grow and double their mass of proteins and organelles, extra gaps (G) are inserted into the cell cycle. G₁ is the stage during which the cell is starting to prepare for DNA replication and mitosis through protein synthesis and an increase in organelle and cytoskeletal elements. G₂ is the premitotic phase. During this phase, enzymes and other proteins needed for cell division are synthesized and moved to their proper sites.

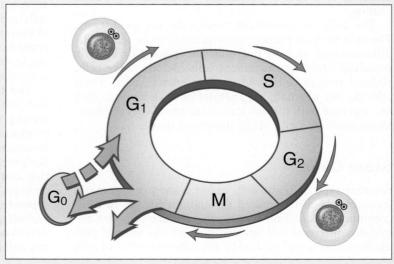

3

Gap 0. G_0 is the stage after mitosis during which a cell may leave the cell cycle and either remain in a state of inactivity or reenter the cell cycle at another time. Labile cells, such as blood cells and those that line the gastrointestinal tract, do not enter G_0 but continue cycling. Stable cells, such as hepatocytes, enter G_0 after mitosis but can reenter the cell cycle when stimulated by the loss of other cells. Permanent cells, such as neurons that become terminally differentiated after mitosis, leave the cell cycle and are no longer capable of cell renewal.

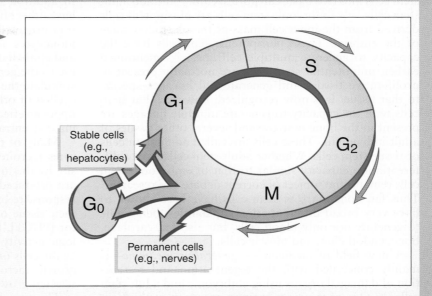

4

Checkpoints and Cyclins. In most cells there are several checkpoints in the cell cycle, at which time the cycle can be arrested if previous events have not been completed. For example, the G_1/S checkpoint monitors whether the DNA in the chromosomes is damaged by radiation or chemicals, and the G_2/M checkpoint prevents entry into mitosis if DNA replication is not complete.

The cyclins are a family of proteins that control entry and progression of cells through the cell cycle. They function by activating proteins called cyclin-dependent kinases (CDKs). Different combinations of cyclins and CDKs are associated with each stage of the cell cycle. In addition to the synthesis and degradation of the cyclins, the cyclin–CDK complexes are regulated by the binding of CDK inhibitors. The CDK inhibitors are particularly important in regulating cell cycle checkpoints during which mistakes in DNA replication are repaired.

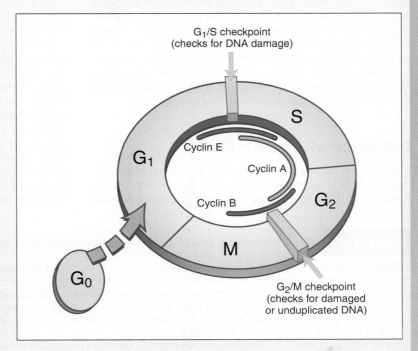

(*text continued from page 73*)

In recent years, it has become useful to categorize stem cells into two basic categories: embryonic and adult stem cells.[1,2,5,6] Embryonic stem cells are pluripotent cells derived from the inner cell mass of the blastocyst stage of the embryo. These pluripotent stem cells have the capacity to generate multiple cell lines. As mentioned earlier, unipotential stem cells are normally present in proliferative tissues and generate cell lineages specific to that tissue. It is now recognized, however, that stem cells with the capacity to generate multiple lineages are present in the bone marrow and several other tissues of adult individuals. These cells are called adult stem cells or tissue stem cells. Whether adult stem cells have a differentiation capacity similar to that of embryonic stem cells remains the subject of current debate and research.[2] Thus far, bone marrow stem cells have been shown to have very broad differentiation capabilities, being able to generate not only blood cells, but also fat, cartilage, bone, endothelial, and muscle cells.

A new field of medicine—*regenerative medicine*—is mainly concerned with the regeneration and restoration of damaged organs using embryonic and adult stem cells.[2,6,7] One of the most exciting prospects in this area is a type of stem cell therapy known as therapeutic cloning. Other potential therapeutic strategies that use stem cells involve the transplantation of stem cells into areas of injury, mobilization of stem cells from the bone marrow into injured tissues, and use of stem cell culture systems to produce large amounts of differentiated stem cells for transplantation into injured tissue.

Influence of Growth Factors

Cell proliferation can be triggered by chemical mediators including growth factors, hormones, and cytokines.[1,2,8–11] The term *growth factor* is generally applied to small proteins that increase cell size and cell division.[2] In addition to cell proliferation, most growth factors have other effects. They assist in regulating the inflammatory process; serve as chemoattractants for neutrophils, monocytes (macrophages), fibroblasts, keratinocytes, and epithelial cells; stimulate angiogenesis; and contribute to the generation of the ECM. Some growth factors stimulate the proliferation of some cells and inhibit the cycling of other cells. In fact, a growth factor can have opposite effects on the same cell depending on its changing concentration during the healing process.

Many of the growth factors are produced by leukocytes recruited to the site of injury or activated at the site by the inflammatory process. Other growth factors are produced by parenchymal cells or stromal cells in response to injury or loss. Growth factors are named for their tissue of origin (e.g., platelet-derived growth factor [PDGF], fibroblast growth factor [FGF]), their biologic activity (e.g., transforming growth factor [TGF]), or the cells on which they act (e.g., vascular endothelial growth factor [VEGF]). The sources and functions of selected growth factors are described in Table 4-1.

The signaling pathways for the growth factors are similar to those of other cellular receptors that recognize extracellular ligands. The binding of a growth factor to its receptor triggers a series of events by which extracellular signals are transmitted into the cell, leading to the stimulation or inhibition of gene expression. These genes typically have several functions—they relieve blocks on cell cycle progression (thus promoting cell proliferation), prevent apoptosis, and enhance synthesis of cellular proteins in preparation for mitosis. Signaling may occur in the cell producing the growth factor (autocrine signaling), in cells in the immediate vicinity of the cell releasing the growth factor (paracrine signaling), or in distant target cells through growth factors that are released into the bloodstream (endocrine signaling).

TABLE 4-1	Growth Factors Involved in Tissue Regeneration and Wound Healing

Growth Factor	Source	Function
Epidermal growth factor (EGF)	Activated macrophages, keratinocytes, and many other cells	Mitogenic for keratinocytes and fibroblasts; simulates keratinocyte migration and granulation tissue formation
Transforming growth factor-α (TGF-α)	Activated macrophages, T lymphocytes, keratinocytes, and many other cells	Similar to EGF; stimulates replication of hepatocytes and many epithelial cells
Transforming growth factor-β (TGF-β)	Platelets, macrophages, T lymphocytes, keratinocytes, smooth muscle cells, fibroblasts	Chemotactic for neutrophils, macrophages, fibroblasts, and smooth muscle cells; stimulates angiogenesis and production of fibrous tissue; inhibits proteinase production and keratinocyte proliferation
Vascular endothelial cell growth factor (VEGF)	Mesenchymal cells	Increases vascular permeability; mitogenic for endothelial cells of blood vessels
Platelet-derived growth factor (PDGF)	Platelets, macrophages, endothelial cells, keratinocytes, smooth muscle cells	Chemotactic for neutrophils, macrophages, fibroblasts, and smooth muscle cells; stimulates production of proteinases, fibronectin, and hyaluronic acid; stimulates angiogenesis and wound remodeling
Fibroblast growth factor (FGF)	Macrophages, mast cells, T lymphocytes, endothelial cells, fibroblasts, and many other tissues	Chemotactic for fibroblasts; mitogenic for fibroblasts and keratinocytes; stimulates angiogenesis, wound contraction, and matrix deposition
Keratinocyte growth factor (KGF)	Fibroblasts	Stimulates keratinocyte migration, proliferation, and differentiation

There is continued interest in developing growth factors as a means of increasing cell proliferation and enhancing wound healing as well as developing strategies to block growth factor signaling pathways that could be used to inhibit malignant cell proliferation in cancer.

Extracellular Matrix and Cell–Matrix Interactions

The understanding of tissue regeneration and repair has expanded over the past several decades to encompass the complex environment of the ECM. There are two basic forms of ECM: (1) the *basement membrane,* which surrounds epithelial, endothelial, and smooth muscle cells; and (2) the *interstitial matrix,* which is present in the spaces between cells in connective tissue and between the epithelium and supporting cells of blood vessels.

The ECM is secreted locally and assembles into a network of spaces surrounding tissue cells (see Chapter 1). There are three basic components of the ECM: fibrous structural proteins (e.g., collagen and elastin fibers), water-hydrated gels (e.g., proteoglycans and hyaluronic acid) that permit resilience and lubrication, and adhesive glycoproteins (e.g., fibronectin, laminin) that connect the matrix elements to one another and to cells[1-3,9] (Fig. 4-3). Integrins are a family of transmembrane glycoproteins that are the main cellular receptors for ECM components such as fibronectin and laminin. They bind to many ECM components, initiating signaling cascades that affect cell proliferation and differentiation. Fibroblasts, which reside in close proximity to collagen fibers, are responsible for the synthesis of collagen, elastic, and reticular fibers, and complex carbohydrates in the ground substance.

The ECM provides turgor to soft tissue and rigidity to bone; it supplies the substratum for cell adhesion; it is involved in the regulation of growth, movement, and differentiation of the cells surrounding it; and it provides for the storage and presentation of regulatory molecules that control the repair process. The ECM also provides the scaffolding for tissue renewal. Although the cells in many tissues are capable of regeneration, injury does not always result in restoration of normal structure unless the ECM is intact. The integrity of the underlying basement membrane, in particular, is critical to the regeneration of tissue. When the basement membrane is disrupted, cells proliferate in a haphazard way, resulting in disorganized and nonfunctional tissues.

Critical to the process of wound healing are transitions in the composition of the ECM. In the transitional process, the ECM components are degraded by proteases (enzymes) that are secreted locally by a variety of cells (fibroblasts, macrophages, neutrophils, synovial cells, and epithelial cells). Some of the proteases, such as the collagenases, are highly specific, cleaving particular proteins at a small number of sites.[10,11] This allows for the structural integrity of the ECM to be retained while healing occurs. Because of their potential to produce havoc in tissues, the actions of the proteases are tightly controlled. They are typically produced in an inactive form that must first be activated by certain chemicals likely to be present at the site of injury, and they are rapidly inactivated by tissue inhibitors. Recent research has focused on the unregulated action of the proteases in disorders such as cartilage matrix breakdown in arthritis and neuroinflammation in multiple sclerosis.[11]

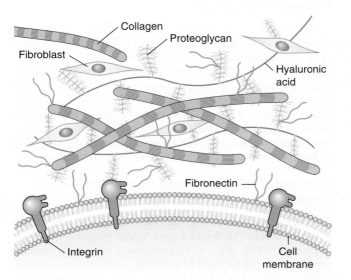

FIGURE 4-3. Components of the extracellular matrix and supporting connective tissue components involved in tissue repair.

SUMMARY CONCEPTS

- The process of tissue growth and repair involves proliferation of functioning parenchymal cells of an organ or body part and its supporting connective tissues and extracellular matrix.

- *Cell proliferation* refers to the process of increasing cell numbers by mitotic division. *Cell differentiation* is the process whereby a cell becomes more specialized in terms of structure and function. The periodic biochemical and structural events occurring during cell proliferation are called the *cell cycle*.

- Body cells are divided into types according to their ability to regenerate. *Labile cells,* such as the epithelial cells of the skin and gastrointestinal tract, are those that continue to regenerate throughout life. *Stable cells,* such as those in the liver, are those that normally do not divide but are capable of regeneration when confronted with an appropriate stimulus. *Permanent* or *fixed cells* are

(continued)

Healing by Connective Tissue Repair

The primary objective of the healing process is to fill the gap created by tissue destruction and to restore the structural continuity of the injured part. Tissue regeneration refers to the restoration of injured tissue to its normal structure and function by proliferation of adjacent surviving cells. As discussed earlier in the chapter, cell renewal occurs continuously in labile tissues such as gastrointestinal epithelium and skin. Regeneration can also occur in parenchymal organs with stable cell populations but, with the exception of the liver, is usually a limited process. It should be pointed out that extensive regeneration can occur only if the residual tissue is structurally and functionally intact. If the tissue is damaged by infection or inflammation, regeneration is incomplete and accomplished by replacement with scar tissue.

When regeneration cannot occur, healing by replacement with a connective (fibrous) tissue occurs, a process that terminates in *scar formation*. The term *fibrosis* is often used to describe the extensive deposition of collagen that occurs in organs that are incapable of regeneration.[2] When this occurs, fibrous tissue grows into the area of damage, converting it to a mass of fibrous tissue, a process called *organization*.[1,2] It can also occur in serous cavities (pleura, peritoneum) when excessive exudate accumulates and cannot be cleared. In the pericardium, fibroblasts secrete and organize collagen within fibrous strands, thereby binding the visceral and parietal pericardia together[1] (Fig. 4-4). Fibrous strands sometimes become organized within the peritoneal cavity following abdominal surgery or peritonitis. These strands of collagen, called *adhesions*, can trap loops of bowel and cause obstruction.[1]

Phases of Repair

Repair by connective tissue deposition can be divided into three phases: (1) hemostasis, angiogenesis, and ingrowth of granulation tissue; (2) emigration of fibroblasts and

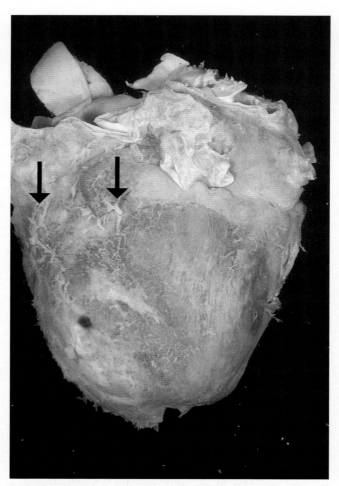

FIGURE 4-4. Organized strands of collagen (*arrows*) in constrictive pericarditis. (From Sephal GC, Davidson JM. Repair, regeneration, and fibrosis. In: Rubin R, Strayer DS, eds. *Rubin's Pathology: Clinicopathologic Foundations of Medicine.* 6th ed. Philadelphia, PA: Wolters Kluwer Health | Lippincott Williams & Wilkins; 2012:94.)

deposition of extracellular matrix; and (3) maturation and reorganization of the fibrous tissue (remodeling).[1,2,10–16] It usually begins within 24 hours of injury and is evidenced by the migration of fibroblasts and the induction of fibroblast and endothelial cell proliferation.[2] By 3 to 5 days, a special type of tissue called *granulation tissue* is apparent.[2] The granulation tissue then progressively accumulates connective tissue, eventually resulting in the formation of a scar, which is then remodeled.

Angiogenesis and Ingrowth of Granulation Tissue

Granulation tissue is a glistening red, moist connective tissue that fills the injured area while necrotic debris is removed[1,2] (Fig. 4-5). It is composed of newly formed capillaries, proliferating fibroblasts, and residual inflammatory cells. The development of granulation tissue involves the growth of new capillaries (angiogenesis). Angiogenesis is a tightly regulated process that includes migration of endothelial cells to the site of tissue injury,

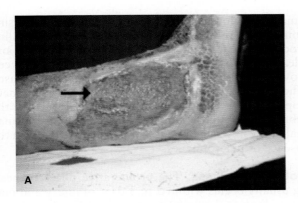

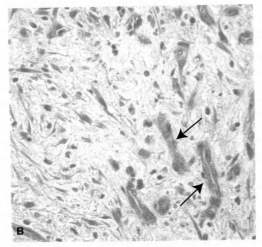

FIGURE 4-5. Granulation tissue. **(A)** A foot covered by granulation tissue. **(B)** A photomicrograph of granulation tissue shows the thin-walled vessels (*arrows*) embedded in a loose connective tissue matrix containing mesenchymal cells and occasional inflammatory cells. (From Sephal GC, Davidson JM. Repair, regeneration, and fibrosis. In: Rubin R, Strayer DS, eds. *Rubin's Pathology: Clinicopathologic Foundations of Medicine.* 6th ed. Philadelphia, PA: Wolters Kluwer Health | Lippincott Williams & Wilkins; 2012:94.)

formation of capillary buds, and proliferation of endothelial cells, followed by fusion and remodeling of the endothelial cells into capillary tubes. Several growth factors induce angiogenesis, but the most important are VEGF and basic FGF-2. In angiogenesis, VEGF stimulates both proliferation and motility of endothelial cells, thus initiating the process of capillary sprouting. FGF-2 participates in angiogenesis mainly by stimulating the proliferation of endothelial cells. During angiogenesis, new blood vessels are leaky because of incompletely formed interendothelial cell junctions and because VEGF increases vascular permeability. This leakiness explains the edematous appearance of granulation tissue and accounts in part for the swelling that may persist in healing wounds long after the acute inflammation has subsided.

Emigration of Fibroblasts and Deposition of Extracellular Matrix

Scar formation builds on the granulation tissue framework of new vessels and loose ECM. The process occurs in two phases: emigration and proliferation of fibroblasts into the site of injury, and deposition of extracellular matrix by these cells. The recruitment and proliferation of fibroblasts is mediated by a number of growth factors including FGF-2 and TGF-β. These growth factors are released from endothelial cells and from inflammatory cells that are present at the site of injury.

As healing progresses, the number of proliferating fibroblasts and formation of new vessels decrease and there is increased synthesis and deposition of collagen. Collagen synthesis is important to the development of strength in the healing wound site. Ultimately, the granulation tissue scaffolding evolves into a scar composed of largely inactive spindle-shaped fibroblasts, dense collagen fibers, fragments of elastic tissue, and other ECM components. As the scar matures, vascular degeneration eventually transforms the highly vascular granulation tissue into a pale, largely avascular scar.

Maturation and Remodeling of the Fibrous Tissue

The transition from granulation to scar tissue involves shifts in the modification and remodeling of the ECM. The outcome of the repair process is, in part, a balance between previously discussed ECM synthesis and degradation. The rate of collagen synthesis diminishes until it reaches equilibrium with collagen degradation. The degradation of collagen and other ECM proteins is achieved through a family of metalloproteinases, which require zinc for their activity. The metalloproteinases are produced by a variety of cell types (fibroblasts, macrophages, synovial cells, and some epithelial cells), and their synthesis and secretion are regulated by growth factors, cytokines, and other agents.[10,11] Their synthesis may be suppressed pharmacologically by corticosteroids. Metalloproteinases are typically released as inactive precursors that require activation by enzymes, such as proteases, that are present at sites of injury.

Cutaneous Wound Healing

Thus far, this chapter has focused on general aspects of tissue repair and wound healing. The following section specifically addresses healing of skin wounds (cutaneous wound healing). This is a process that involves both epithelial cell regeneration and connective tissue scar formation, and thus is illustrative of general principles that apply to all tissues.

Healing by Primary and Secondary Intention

Depending on the extent of tissue loss, wound closure and healing occur by primary or secondary intention (Fig. 4-6). A sutured surgical incision is an example of healing by primary intention. Larger wounds (e.g., burns and large surface wounds) that have a greater loss of tissue and contamination heal by secondary intention. Healing by secondary intention is slower than healing by primary intention and results in the formation of larger

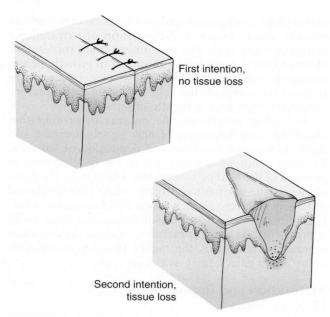

First intention, no tissue loss

Second intention, tissue loss

FIGURE 4-6. Healing by primary and secondary intention.

amounts of scar tissue. A wound that might otherwise have healed by primary intention may become infected and heal by secondary intention.

Phases of Healing

Cutaneous wound healing is commonly divided into three phases: (1) the inflammatory phase, (2) the proliferative phase, and (3) the remodeling phase.[1,2,17–19] The duration of the phases is fairly predictable in wounds healing by primary intention. In wounds healing by secondary intention, the process depends on the extent of injury and the healing environment.

Inflammatory Phase. The inflammatory phase of wound healing begins at the time of injury and is a critical period because it prepares the wound environment for healing.[18] It includes hemostasis (see Chapter 12) and the vascular and cellular phases of inflammation. Hemostatic processes are activated immediately at the time of injury. There is constriction of injured blood vessels and initiation of blood clotting by way of platelet activation and aggregation and deposition of fibrin. After a brief period of constriction, these same vessels dilate and capillaries increase their permeability, allowing plasma and blood components to leak into the injured area. In small surface wounds, the clot loses fluid and becomes a hard, desiccated scab that protects the area.

The cellular phase of inflammation follows and is evidenced by the migration of phagocytic white blood cells that digest and remove invading organisms, fibrin, extracellular debris, and other foreign matter. The neutrophils arrive within minutes and are usually gone by day 3 or 4. They ingest bacteria and cellular debris. Within 24 to 48 hours, macrophages, which are larger phagocytic cells, enter the wound area and

remain for an extended period. These cells, arising from blood monocytes, are essential to the healing process. Their functions include phagocytosis and release of growth factors that stimulate epithelial cell growth, angiogenesis, and attraction of fibroblasts. When a large wound occurs in deeper tissues, neutrophils and macrophages are required to remove the debris and facilitate closure. Although a wound may heal in the absence of neutrophils, it cannot heal in the absence of macrophages.

Proliferative Phase. The proliferative phase of healing usually begins within 2 to 3 days of injury and may last as long as 3 weeks in wounds healing by primary intention. The primary processes during this time focus on the building of new tissue to fill the wound space. The key cell during this phase is the *fibroblast*. The fibroblast is a connective tissue cell that synthesizes and secretes collagen and other intercellular elements needed for wound healing. Fibroblasts also produce numerous growth factors that induce angiogenesis and endothelial cell proliferation and migration.

As early as 24 to 48 hours after injury, fibroblasts and vascular endothelial cells begin proliferating to form the granulation tissue that serves as the foundation for scar tissue development. This tissue is fragile and bleeds easily because of the numerous, newly developed capillary buds. Wounds that heal by secondary intention have more necrotic debris and exudate that must be removed, and they involve larger amounts of granulation tissue. The newly formed blood vessels are leaky and allow plasma proteins and white blood cells to leak into the tissues.

The final component of the proliferative phase is epithelialization, which is the migration, proliferation, and differentiation of the epithelial cells at the wound edges to form a new surface layer that is similar to that destroyed by the injury. In wounds that heal by primary intention, these epithelial cells proliferate and seal the wound within 24 to 48 hours. Because epithelial cell migration requires a moist vascular wound surface and is impeded by a dry or necrotic wound surface, epithelialization is delayed in open wounds until a bed of granulation tissue has formed. When a scab has formed on the wound, the epithelial cells migrate between it and the underlying viable tissue; when a significant portion of the wound has been covered with epithelial tissue, the scab lifts off.

At times, excessive granulation tissue, sometimes referred to as *proud flesh,* may form and extend above the edges of the wound, preventing reepithelialization from taking place. Surgical removal or chemical cauterization of the defect allows healing to proceed.

As the proliferative phase progresses, there is continued accumulation of collagen and proliferation of fibroblasts. Collagen synthesis reaches a peak within 5 to 7 days and continues for several weeks, depending on wound size. By the second week, the white blood cells have largely left the area, the edema has diminished, and the wound begins to blanch as the small blood vessels become thrombosed and degenerate.

Remodeling Phase. The third phase of wound healing, the remodeling process, begins approximately 3 weeks after injury and can continue for 6 months or longer, depending on the extent of the wound. As the term implies, there is continued remodeling of scar tissue by simultaneous synthesis of collagen by fibroblasts and lysis by collagenase enzymes. As a result of these two processes, the architecture of the scar becomes reoriented to increase the tensile strength of the wound.

Most wounds do not regain the full tensile strength of unwounded skin after healing is completed. Carefully sutured wounds immediately after surgery have approximately 70% of the strength of unwounded skin, largely because of the placement of the sutures. This allows persons to move about freely after surgery without fear of wound separation. When the sutures are removed, usually at the end of the 1st week, wound strength is approximately 10%. It increases rapidly over the next 4 weeks and then slows, reaching a plateau of approximately 70% to 80% of the tensile strength of unwounded skin at the end of 3 months.[2] An injury that heals by secondary intention undergoes wound contraction during the proliferative and remodeling phases. As a result, the scar that forms is considerably smaller than the original wound. Cosmetically, this may be desirable because it reduces the size of the visible defect. However, contraction of scar tissue over joints and other body structures tends to limit movement and cause deformities. As a result of loss of elasticity, scar tissue that is stretched fails to return to its original length.

An abnormality in healing by scar tissue repair is *keloid* formation.[20] Keloids are benign tumor-like masses caused by excess production of scar tissue (Fig. 4-7). They tend to develop in genetically predisposed individuals and are more common in African Americans and other dark skinned people.[1,2,19] The majority of keloids lead to considerable cosmetic defects, but can grow to sufficient size to become symptomatic by causing deformity or limiting joint mobility. Thus far the majority of keloid research has focused on growth factors and signaling pathways, but unfortunately, reliable preventative or treatment measures have yet to be established.

Factors That Affect Wound Healing

Although many local and systemic factors impair healing, science has found only a few ways to promote wound repair. Among the causes of impaired wound healing are malnutrition; impaired blood flow and oxygen delivery; impaired inflammatory and immune responses; infection, wound separation, and foreign bodies; and age effects.[21]

Nutritional Status

Successful wound healing depends in part on adequate stores of proteins, carbohydrates, fats, vitamins, and minerals. It is well recognized that malnutrition slows the healing process, causing wounds to heal inadequately or incompletely.[22,23] Protein deficiencies prolong the inflammatory phase of healing and impair fibroblast proliferation, collagen and protein matrix synthesis, angiogenesis, and wound remodeling. Carbohydrates are needed as an energy source for white blood cells. Carbohydrates also have a protein-sparing effect and help to prevent the use of amino acids for fuel when they are needed for the healing process. Fats are essential constituents of cell membranes and are needed for the synthesis of new cells.

Although most vitamins are essential cofactors for the daily functions of the body, vitamins play an essential role in the healing process. Vitamin C is needed for collagen synthesis. In vitamin C deficiency, improper sequencing of amino acids occurs, proper linking of amino acids does not take place, the by-products of collagen synthesis are not removed from the cell, new wounds do not heal properly, and old wounds may pull apart. Administration of vitamin C rapidly restores the healing process to normal. Vitamin A functions in stimulating and supporting epithelialization, capillary formation, and collagen synthesis. Vitamin A also has been shown to counteract the anti-inflammatory effects of corticosteroid drugs and can be used to reverse these effects in persons who are on chronic steroid therapy. The B vitamins are important cofactors in enzymatic reactions that contribute to the wound-healing process. All are water soluble and must be replaced daily, with the exception of vitamin B_{12}, which is stored in the liver and must be replaced daily. Vitamin K plays an indirect role in wound healing by preventing bleeding disorders that contribute to hematoma formation and subsequent infection.

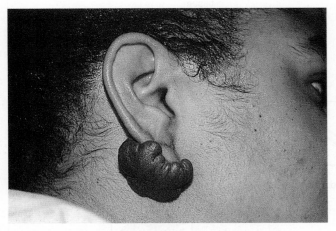

FIGURE 4-7. Keloid. A light-skinned black woman with keloid that developed after ear piercing. (From Sephal GC, Davidson JM. Repair, regeneration, and fibrosis. In: Rubin R, Strayer DS, eds. *Rubin's Pathology: Clinicopathologic Foundations of Medicine.* 6th ed. Philadelphia, PA: Wolters Kluwer Health | Lippincott Williams & Wilkins; 2012:113.)

(*text continues on page 83*)

UNDERSTANDING → Wound Healing

Wound healing involves the restoration of the integrity of injured tissue. The healing of skin wounds, which are commonly used to illustrate the general principles of wound healing, is generally divided into three phases: (1) the inflammatory phase, (2) the proliferative phase, and (3) the wound contraction and remodeling phase. Each of these phases is mediated through cytokines and growth factors.

1

Inflammatory Phase. The inflammatory phase begins at the time of injury with the formation of a blood clot and the migration of phagocytic white blood cells into the wound site. The first cells to arrive, the neutrophils, ingest and remove bacteria and cellular debris. After 24 hours, the neutrophils are joined by macrophages, which continue to ingest cellular debris and play an essential role in the production of growth factors for the proliferative phase.

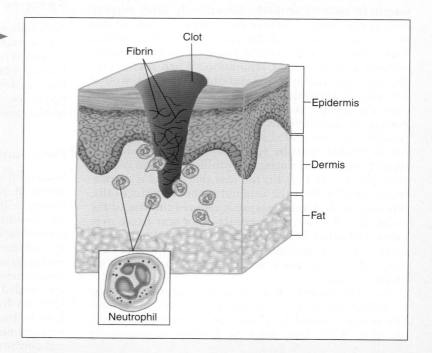

2

Proliferative Phase. The primary processes during this phase focus on the building of new tissue to fill the wound space. The key cell during this phase is the *fibroblast*, a connective tissue cell that synthesizes and secretes the collagen, proteoglycans, and glycoproteins needed for wound healing. Fibroblasts also produce a family of growth factors that induce angiogenesis (growth of new blood vessels) and endothelial cell proliferation and migration. The final component of the proliferative phase is epithelialization, during which epithelial cells at the wound edges proliferate to form a new surface layer that is similar to that which was destroyed by the injury.

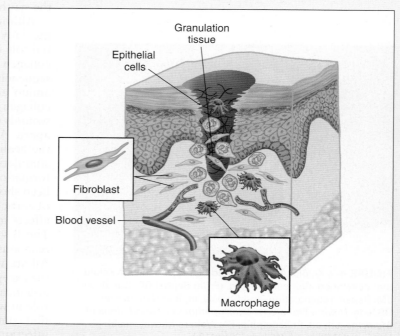

3

Wound Contraction and Remodeling Phase. This phase begins approximately 3 weeks after injury with the development of the fibrous scar, and can continue for 6 months or longer, depending on the extent of the wound. During this phase, there is a decrease in vascularity and continued remodeling of scar tissue by simultaneous synthesis of collagen by fibroblasts and lysis by collagenase enzymes. As a result of these two processes, the architecture of the scar becomes reoriented to increase its tensile strength, and the scar shrinks so it is less visible.

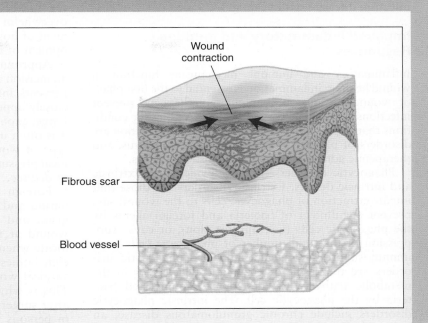

(text continued from page 81)

The role of minerals in wound healing is less clearly defined. The major minerals, including sodium, potassium, calcium, and phosphorus, as well as trace minerals such as copper and zinc, must be present for normal cell function. Zinc is a cofactor in a variety of enzyme systems responsible for cell proliferation. In animal studies, zinc has been found to aid in reepithelialization.

Blood Flow and Oxygen Delivery

Impaired healing due to poor blood flow and hypoxia may occur as a result of wound conditions (e.g., swelling) or preexisting health problems.[24,25] Arterial disease and venous pathology are well-documented causes of impaired wound healing. In situations of trauma, a decrease in blood volume may cause a reduction in blood flow to injured tissues.

For healing to occur, wounds must have adequate blood flow to supply the necessary nutrients and to remove the resulting waste, local toxins, bacteria, and other debris. Molecular oxygen is required for collagen synthesis and killing of bacteria by phagocytic white blood cells. It has been shown that even a temporary lack of oxygen can result in the formation of less-stable collagen.[24] Wounds in ischemic tissue become infected more frequently than wounds in well-vascularized tissue. Neutrophils and macrophages require oxygen for destruction of microorganisms that have invaded the area. Although these cells can accomplish phagocytosis in a relatively anoxic environment, they cannot digest bacteria. Oxygen also contributes to signaling systems that support wound healing. Recent research suggests that almost all cells in the wound environment are fitted with specialized enzymes to convert oxygen to reactive oxygen species (ROS).[24] These ROS function as cellular messengers that support wound healing, stimulating cytokine action, angiogenesis, cell motility, and extracellular matrix formation.

The availability of respired oxygen to wound tissues depends on vascular supply, vasomotor tone, the partial pressure of oxygen (PO_2) in arterial blood, and the diffusion distance for oxygen (see Chapter 21). The central area of a wound has the lower oxygen level, with dermal wounds ranging from a PO_2 of 0 to 10 mm Hg centrally to 60 mm Hg in the periphery, while the PO_2 of arterial blood is approximately 100 mm Hg.[24] Transcutaneous oxygen sensors are available for use in measuring wound oxygenation. From a therapeutic standpoint oxygen can be given systemically or administered locally using a topical device. Although topical oxygen therapy is not likely to diffuse into the deeper tissues, it does have the advantage of oxygenating superficial areas of the wound not supported by intact vasculature. Hyperbaric oxygen therapy delivers 100% oxygen at two to three times the normal atmospheric pressure at sea level.[26] The goal of hyperbaric oxygen therapy is to increase oxygen delivery to tissues by increasing the partial pressure of oxygen dissolved in the plasma. Hyperbaric oxygen is currently reserved for the treatment of problem wounds in which hypoxia and infection interfere with healing.

Impaired Inflammatory and Immune Responses

Inflammatory and immune mechanisms function in wound healing. Inflammation is essential to the first phase of wound healing, and immune mechanisms prevent infections that impair wound healing. Among the conditions that impair inflammation and immune function are disorders of phagocytic function, diabetes mellitus, and therapeutic administration of corticosteroid drugs.

Phagocytic disorders may be divided into extrinsic and intrinsic defects. Extrinsic disorders are those that impair attraction of phagocytic cells to the wound site, prevent engulfment of bacteria and foreign agents by the phagocytic cells (i.e., opsonization), or cause suppression of the total number of phagocytic cells (e.g., immunosuppressive agents). Intrinsic phagocytic disorders are the result of enzymatic deficiencies in the metabolic pathway for destroying the ingested bacteria by the phagocytic cell. The intrinsic phagocytic disorders include chronic granulomatous disease, an X-linked inherited disease in which there is a deficiency of myeloperoxidase and nicotinamide adenine dinucleotide peroxidase (NADPH)–dependent oxidase enzyme. Deficiencies of these compounds prevent generation of hydrogen superoxide and hydrogen peroxide needed for killing bacteria.

Wound healing is a problem in persons with diabetes mellitus, particularly those who have poorly controlled blood glucose levels.[27] Studies have shown delayed wound healing, poor collagen formation, and poor tensile strength in diabetic animals. Of particular importance is the effect of hyperglycemia on phagocytic function. Neutrophils, for example, have diminished chemotactic and phagocytic function, including engulfment and intracellular killing of bacteria, when exposed to altered glucose levels. Small blood vessel disease is also common among persons with diabetes, impairing the delivery of inflammatory cells, oxygen, and nutrients to the wound site.

The therapeutic administration of corticosteroid drugs decreases the inflammatory process and may delay the healing process. These hormones decrease capillary permeability during the early stages of inflammation, impair the phagocytic property of the leukocytes, and inhibit fibroblast proliferation and function.

Infection, Wound Separation, and Foreign Bodies

Wound contamination, wound separation, and foreign bodies delay wound healing. Infection impairs all dimensions of wound healing.[28] It prolongs the inflammatory phase, impairs the formation of granulation tissue, and inhibits proliferation of fibroblasts and deposition of collagen fibers. All wounds are contaminated at the time of injury. Although body defenses can handle the invasion of microorganisms at the time of wounding, badly contaminated wounds can overwhelm host defenses. Trauma and existing impairment of host defenses also can contribute to the development of wound infections.

Approximation of the wound edges (i.e., suturing of an incision type of wound) greatly enhances healing and prevents infection. Epithelialization of a wound with closely approximated edges occurs within 1 to 2 days. Large, gaping wounds tend to heal more slowly because it is often impossible to effect wound closure with this type of wound. Mechanical factors such as increased local pressure or torsion can cause wounds to pull apart, or *dehisce*.

Foreign bodies tend to invite bacterial contamination and delay healing. Fragments of wood, steel, glass, and other compounds may have entered the wound at the site of injury and can be difficult to locate when the wound is treated. Sutures are also foreign bodies, and although needed for the closure of surgical wounds, they are an impediment to healing. This is why sutures are removed as soon as possible after surgery. Wound infections are of special concern in persons with implantation of foreign bodies such as orthopedic devices (e.g., pins, stabilization devices), cardiac pacemakers, and shunt catheters. These infections are difficult to treat and may require removal of the device.

 ## Wound Healing in the Elderly

A number of structural and functional changes have been reported to occur in aging skin, including a decrease in dermal thickness, a decline in collagen content, and a loss of elasticity.[29,30] The observed changes in skin that occur with aging are complicated by the effects of sun exposure. Since the effects of sun exposure are cumulative, older persons show more changes in skin structure.

Wound healing is thought to be progressively impaired with aging. The elderly have alterations in wound-healing phases including hemostasis and inflammation, cell proliferation, and resolution.[30] Keratinocytes, fibroblasts, and vascular endothelial cells display a reduced rate of proliferation. There is also a reported decrease in angiogenesis and collagen synthesis, impaired wound contraction, and slower reepithelialization of open wounds. Although wound healing may be delayed, most wounds heal, even in the debilitated elderly patient undergoing major surgical procedures.

The elderly are more vulnerable to chronic wounds, chiefly pressure, diabetic, and ischemic ulcers, than younger persons, and these wounds heal more slowly. However, these wounds are more likely due to other disorders such as immobility, diabetes mellitus, or vascular disease, rather than aging.

SUMMARY CONCEPTS

- Tissue repair involves regeneration with the same cell type, or when regeneration cannot restore the injured tissue, by replacement with fibrous (scar) tissue.

- Cutaneous wound healing occurs by primary and secondary intention and is commonly divided into three phases: inflammatory, proliferative, and remodeling. In wounds healing by primary intention, such as occurs in a sutured surgical incision, the duration of the healing phases is fairly predictable and the edges of the wound are closely approximated. Larger wounds that have a greater loss of tissue heal by secondary intention, a process that is more unpredictable and results in formation of larger amounts of scar tissue.

- Wound healing can be impaired or complicated by factors such as malnutrition, poor blood flow, diminished inflammatory and immune responses, infection, wound separation, and the presence of foreign bodies.

REVIEW EXERCISES

1. Following a heart attack, the area of heart muscle that has undergone necrosis because of a lack of blood supply heals by replacement with scar tissue.

   A. Compare the functioning of the heart muscle that has been replaced by scar tissue with that of the normal surrounding heart muscle.

2. A 35-year-old man comes in with a large abscess on his leg. He tells you he injured his leg while doing repair work on his house and he thinks there might be a wood sliver in the infected area.

   A. Explain the events that lead to formation of an abscess.
   B. He is told that incision and drainage of the lesion will be needed so healing can take place. Explain.
   C. He is reluctant to have the procedure done and asks whether an antibiotic would work as well. Explain why antibiotics alone are usually not effective in eliminating the microorganisms contained in an abscess.

REFERENCES

1. Sephel GC, Davidson JM. Repair, regeneration, and fibrosis. In: Rubin R, Strayer DS, eds. *Rubin's Pathology: Clinicopathologic Foundations of Medicine*. 6th ed. Philadelphia, PA: Wolters Kluwer Health/Lippincott Williams & Wilkins; 2012:83–113.
2. Kumar V, Abbas AK, Fausto N, et al. *Robbins and Cotran Pathologic Basis of Disease*. 8th ed. Philadelphia, PA: Saunders Elsevier; 2010:79–110.
3. Alberts B, Johnson A, Lewis J, et al. *Molecular Biology of the Cell*. 5th ed. New York, NY: Garland Science; 2008:1053–1114, 1178–1195.
4. Pajalunga D, Maxxola A, Franchitto A, et al. The logic of cell cycle exit and reentry. *Cell Mol Life Sci*. 2008;65:8–15.
5. Vats A, Bielby RC, Tolley NS, et al. Stem cells. *Lancet*. 2005;366:592–602.
6. Körbling M, Estrov Z. Adult stem cells for tissue repair—A new therapeutic strategy. *N Engl J Med*. 2003;349:570–582.
7. Metcalfe AD, Ferguson MWJ. Skin stem cells and progenitor cells: using regeneration as a tissue-engineering strategy. *Cell Mol Life Sci*. 2008;65:24–32.
8. Werner S, Grose R. Regulation of wound healing by growth factors and cytokines. *Physiol Rev*. 2003;83:835–870.
9. Daley WP, Peters SB, Larsen M. Extracellular matrix dynamics in development and regenerative medicine. *J Cell Sci*. 2008;21(3):255–264.
10. Goldberg SR, Dieglmann RR. Wound healing primer. *Surg Clin North Am*. 2011;90:1113–1140.
11. Teller P, White TK. The physiology of wound healing: injury through maturation. *Surg Clin North Am*. 2009;89:598–610.
12. Whitney JD. Overview: acute and chronic wounds. *Nurs Clin North Am*. 2005;40:191–205.
13. Wei L, Dasgeb B, Phillips T, et al. Wound-healing perspectives. *Dermatol Clin*. 2005;23:181–192.
14. Strecker-McGraw MK, Jones TR, Baer DG. Soft tissue wounds and principles of healing. *Emerg Med Clin North Am*. 2007;25:1–22.
15. Li B, Wang JH. Fibroblasts and myofibroblasts in wound healing: force generation and measurement. *J Tissue Viability*. 2011;20(4):108–120.
16. Adamson R. Role of macrophages in normal wound healing: an overview. *J Wound Care*. 2009;18(8):349–351.
17. Bielefeld KA, Amini-Nik S, Alman BA. Cutaneous wound healing: recruiting developmental pathways for regeneration. *Cell Mol Life Sci*. 2013;70:2059–2061.
18. Koh TJ, Dipietro LA. Inflammation and wound healing: the role of the macrophage. *Expert Rev Mol Med*. 2013;13(e23):1–14.
19. Monaco JL, Lawrence WT. Acute wound healing: an overview. *Clin Plast Surg*. 2003;30:1–12.
20. Butler PD, Longaker MT, Yang GP. Current progress in keloid research and treatment. *J Am Coll Surg*. 2008;206(6):731–741.
21. Burns JL, Mancoll JS, Phillips LG. Impairments of wound healing. *Clin Plast Surg*. 2003;30:47–56.
22. Wild T, Raharnia A, Kellner M, et al. Basics in nutrition and wound healing. *Nutrition*. 2010;28(5):562–566.
23. Mechanick JI. Practical aspects of nutrition support for wound-healing patients. *Am J Surg*. 2004;188(Suppl):52S–56S.
24. Gordillo GM, Sen CK. Revisiting the essential role of oxygen in wound healing. *Am J Surg*. 2003;186:259–263.
25. Tandara AA, Mustoe TA. Oxygen and wound healing—More than a nutrient. *World J Surg*. 2004;28:294–300.

26. Zamboni WA, Browder LK, Martinez J. Hyperbaric oxygen and wound healing. *Clin Plast Surg*. 2003;30:67–75.

27. Greenhalgh DG. Wound healing and diabetes mellitus. *Clin Plast Surg*. 2003;30:37–45.

28. Hunt TK, Hopf HW. Wound healing and wound infection. *Surg Clin North Am*. 1977;77:587–605.

29. Sgonc R, Gruber J. Age-related aspects of cutaneous wound healing: a mini-review. *Gerontology*. 2013;59:159–164.

30. Gosain A, Dipietro LA. Aging and wound healing. *World J Surg*. 2004;28:321–326.

Porth Essentials Resources

Explore these additional resources to enhance learning for this chapter:

- NCLEX-Style Questions and Other Resources on **thePoint**, http://thePoint.lww.com/PorthEssentials4e
- Study Guide for Essentials of Pathophysiology
- Concepts in Action Animations
- Adaptive Learning | Powered by PrepU, http://thepoint.lww.com/prepu

C h a p t e r **5**

Genetic Control of Cell Function and Inheritance

Our hereditary information is stored in the chemical structure of *deoxyribonucleic acid* (DNA), an extremely stable macromolecule. Deoxyribonucleic acid contains within its structure the basic information needed to direct the function of our cells, influence our appearance, and how we respond to our environment, and serve as the unit of inheritance that is passed on from generation to generation. Our DNA can also influence disease susceptibility and how we react to drugs.

A gene is a locatable segment or segments of DNA sequence that encodes a set of functional products, typically proteins. Genetics is the study of genes. An understanding of the role that genetics plays in the pathogenesis of disease has expanded greatly over the past century. It is now apparent that many diseases, including cancer, diabetes, and cardiovascular diseases, have a genetic component. At the same time, genetic advances have led to new methods for early detection and more effective treatment. Advances in immunogenetics have made compatible blood transfusion and organ transplants a reality, and recombinant DNA technology has provided the methods for producing human insulin, growth hormone, and clotting factors. Perhaps the most extensive use of gene technology involved the Human Genome Project, begun in 1990 and completed in 2003. The goal of this international effort was to sequence the human genome and map all of its genes.

This chapter includes discussions of genetic control of cell function, chromosomes, patterns of inheritance, and gene technology.

Genetic Control of Cell Function

The genetic instructions for protein synthesis are encoded in the DNA contained in the cell nucleus. Because of its stable structure, the genetic information carried in DNA can survive the many stages of cell division involved in the day-to-day process of cell renewal and tissue growth. Its stable structure also allows the information to survive the many processes of reduction division involved in gamete (i.e., ovum and sperm) formation, the fertilization process, and the mitotic cell divisions involved in the formation of a new organism from the single-celled fertilized ovum called the *zygote*.

Although genes have gotten a lot of attention, it is the proteins that the genes encode that make up the majority of cellular structures and contribute to their function. Proteins are responsible for the functional diversity of cells, they perform most biologic functions, and it is at their level that many regulatory processes take place, many disease processes occur, and most drug targets are found. The term *proteome* is a relatively new term, created to define the complete set of proteins encoded by a genome. *Proteomics,* the study of the proteome, uses highly sophisticated technologic methods to examine the molecular and biochemical events in a cell.

DNA Structure and Function

The DNA molecule that stores the genetic information in the nucleus is a long, double-stranded, helical structure. Deoxyribonucleic acid is composed of *nucleotides*, which consist of phosphoric acid, a five-carbon sugar called *deoxyribose*, and one of four nitrogenous bases. These nitrogenous bases carry the genetic information and are divided into two groups: the *pyrimidine bases*, thymine (T) and cytosine (C), which have one nitrogen ring; and the *purine bases*, adenine (A) and guanine (G), which have two. The backbone of DNA consists of alternating groups of sugar and phosphoric acid, with the paired bases projecting inward from the sides of the sugar molecule.

Double Helix and Base Pairing

The native structure of DNA, as elucidated by James Watson and Frances Crick in 1953, is that of a spiral staircase, with the paired bases representing the steps (Fig. 5-1). A precise complementary pairing of purine and pyrimidine bases occurs in the double-stranded DNA molecule in which A is paired with T and G is paired with C. Each nucleotide in a pair is on one strand of the DNA molecule, with the bases on opposite DNA strands bound together by hydrogen bonds that are extremely stable under normal conditions. The double-stranded structure of DNA molecules allows them to replicate precisely by separation of the two strands, followed by synthesis of two new complementary strands. Similarly, the base complementary pairing allows for efficient and correct repair of damaged DNA molecules.

Several hundred to almost 1 million base pairs can represent a gene, the size being proportional to the protein product it encodes. Of the two DNA strands, only one is used in transcribing the information for the cell's protein-building machinery. The genetic information of one strand is meaningful and is used as a template for transcription; the complementary code of the other strand does not make sense and is ignored. Both strands, however, are involved in DNA duplication. Before cell division, the two strands of the helix separate and a complementary molecule is duplicated

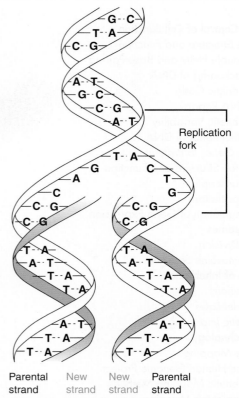

Replication fork

Parental strand | New strand | New strand | Parental strand

FIGURE 5-1. A replicating DNA helix. The parental strands separate at the replication fork. Each parental strand serves as a template for the synthesis of a new strand. The backbone of DNA consists of a sugar–phosphate backbone with paired pyrimidine bases (thymine [T] and cytosine [C] with their one nitrogen ring) and purine bases (adenine [A] and guanine [G] with their two nitrogen rings) projecting inward. (From Smith C, Marks AD, Lieberman M. *Marks' Basic Medical Biochemistry.* 2nd ed. Philadelphia, PA: Lippincott Williams & Wilkins; 2005:222.)

next to each original strand. Two strands become four strands. During mitotic cell division, the newly duplicated double-stranded molecules are separated and placed in each daughter cell by the mechanics of mitosis. As a result, each of the daughter cells again contains the meaningful strand and the complementary strand joined together as a double helix. In 1958, Meselson and Stahl characterized this replication of DNA as *semiconservative* replication, as opposed to *conservative* replication, in which the parental strands reassociate when the two strands are brought together (Fig. 5-2).

Although scientific discussion regarding the structure and functioning of a gene goes into explicit detail, it does not really address the question of what a gene is. Many scientists are now in agreement that the proteins encoded by DNA know no boundaries. This means that nucleotides from one part of the genome can combine with nucleotides from other regions at extreme distances on the DNA molecule. It is also proposed that the functions of some genes are controlled by regulatory regions, also at a distance. Moreover, researchers now recognize that many thousands of genes in the human genome do not code for protein assembly, but rather for segments of ribonucleic

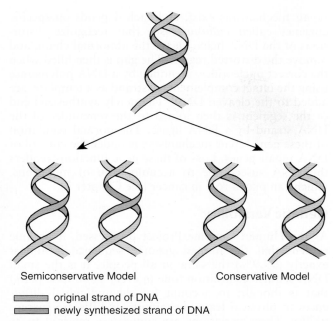

Semiconservative Model   Conservative Model

▭ original strand of DNA
▭ newly synthesized strand of DNA

FIGURE 5-2. Semiconservative versus conservative models of DNA replication as proposed by Meselson and Stahl in 1958. In semiconservative DNA replication, the two original strands of DNA unwind and a complementary strand is formed along each original strand.

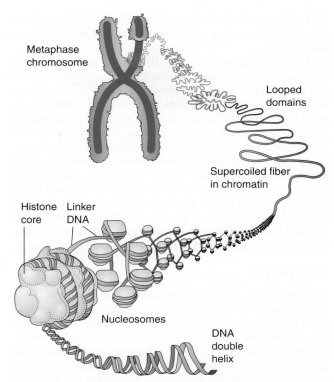

FIGURE 5-3. Increasing orders of DNA compaction in chromatin and mitotic chromosomes. (From Cormack DH. *Essential Histology*. Philadelphia, PA: J.B. Lippincott; 1993.)

acid (RNA). These and other current findings have put to rest the old hypothesis of "one gene–one protein."

Packaging of DNA

The genome is distributed in chromosomes, discrete bundles made up of one continuous, linear DNA helix. Each human somatic cell (cells other than the gametes) has 23 pairs of different chromosomes, with one chromosome of each pair derived from the individual's mother and the other from the father. One of the chromosome pairs consists of the sex chromosomes. Genes are arranged linearly along each chromosome. When unraveled, the DNA in the longest chromosome is more than 7 cm in length. If the DNA of all 46 chromosomes were placed end to end, the total DNA would span a distance of about 2 m (more than 6 feet).

Because of their enormous length, the DNA double helices are tightly coiled in a complex called *chromatin*, which consists of proteins called *histones* along with other less well-characterized proteins that appear to be critical for ensuring normal chromosome behavior and appropriate gene expression. The histones play a critical role in proper packaging of chromatin. They form a core around which a segment of DNA double helix winds, like thread around a spool (Fig. 5-3). About 140 base pairs of DNA are associated with each histone core, making about two turns around the core. After a short "spacer" segment of DNA, the next core DNA complex forms, and so on, giving chromatin the appearance of beads on a string. Each complex of DNA with a histone core is called a *nucleosome,* which is the basic structural

unit of chromatin. Each chromosome contains several hundred to over a million nucleosomes.

Although solving the structural problem of how to fit a huge amount of DNA into the nucleus, the chromatin fiber, when complexed with histones and packaged into various levels of compaction, makes the DNA inaccessible during the processes of replication and gene expression. To accommodate these processes, chromatin must be induced to change its structure, a process called *chromatin remodeling*. Several chemical interactions are now known to affect this process. One of these involves the acetylation of a histone amino acid group that is linked to opening of the chromatin fiber and gene activation. Another important chemical modification involves the methylation of histone amino acids, which is correlated with gene inactivation.

Genetic Code

Four bases—guanine, adenine, cytosine, and thymine—make up the alphabet of the genetic code. A sequence of three of these bases forms the fundamental triplet code for one of the 20 amino acids used in protein synthesis in humans. This triplet code is called a *codon*. The molecular link between the DNA code of genes and the amino acid sequence of proteins is RNA, a macromolecule similar in structure to DNA, except that uracil (U) replaces thymine (T) as one of the four bases. An example is the nucleotide sequence GCU (guanine, cytosine, and uracil), which is an RNA codon for the amino acid alanine (Table 5-1). *Start* and *stop codons,* which signal the beginning or end of a protein molecule, are also present.

Although there are only 20 amino acids, plus the start and stop codons, mathematically, the four bases can be arranged in 64 different combinations. As shown in Table 5-1, several triplets code for the same amino acid; therefore, the genetic code is said to be *redundant.* For example, there are four codons for the amino acid valine. Codons that specify the same amino acid are *synonymous.* Synonymous codons usually have the same first two bases but differ in the third base. Because the genetic code is a universal language used by most living cells, the codons for an amino acid are the same whether that amino acid is found in a bacterium, plant, or human being. Also notice that AUG is the codon for the start signal as well as the codon for the amino acid methionine.

DNA Repair

Accidental errors in the replication of DNA do arise. These errors are called *mutations.* Mutations can result from the substitution of one base pair for another, the loss or addition of one or more base pairs, or rearrangements of base pairs. Many of these mutations occur spontaneously through normal endogenous processes, whereas others occur because of exogenous or environmental agents such as chemical and radiation. Mutations may arise in somatic cells or in germ cells. Only those DNA changes that occur in germ cells can be inherited.

Considering the millions of base pairs that must be duplicated in each cell division, it is not surprising that random changes in replication occur. Most of these defects are corrected by DNA repair mechanisms. Several

repair mechanisms exist, and each depends on specific enzymes called *endonucleases* that recognize distortions of the DNA helix, cleave the abnormal chain, and remove the distorted region. The gap is then filled when the correct nucleotides, identified by a DNA polymerase using the intact complementary strand as a template, are added to the cleaved DNA. The newly synthesized end of the segment is then joined to the remainder of the DNA strand by a DNA ligase. The normal regulation of these gene repair mechanisms is under the control of DNA repair genes. Loss of these gene functions renders the DNA susceptible to accumulation of mutations, which can play a role in cancer (see Chapter 7).

Genetic Variability

As the Human Genome Project progressed, it became evident that the human genome sequence is almost exactly (99.9%) the same in all people. It is the small DNA sequence variation (one in every 1000 base pairs) that is thought to account for the individual differences in physical traits, behaviors, and disease susceptibility. These variations are sometimes referred to as *single nucleotide polymorphisms* (from the existence of more than one morphologic form in a population), or SNPs. An international effort has been organized to develop a genome-wide map of these variations as haplotypes (a combination of SNPs at adjacent locations which are inherited together) with the intent of providing a link between genetic variations and common complex diseases such as cancer, heart disease, diabetes, and some forms of mental disease (the International HapMap Project is discussed in the section under gene technology).

TABLE 5-1	Triplet Codes for Amino Acids				
Amino Acid	**RNA Codons**				
Alanine	GCU	GCC	GCA	GCG	
Arginine	CGU	CGC	CGA	CGG	AGA	AGG
Asparagine	AAU	AAC			
Aspartic acid	GAU	GAC			
Cysteine	UGU	UGC			
Glutamic acid	GAA	GAG			
Glutamine	CAA	CAG			
Glycine	GGU	GGC	GGA	GGG	
Histidine	CAU	CAC			
Isoleucine	AUU	AUC	AUA		
Leucine	CUU	CUC	CUA	CUG	UUA	UUG
Lysine	AAA	AAG			
Methionine	AUG				
Phenylalanine	UUU	UUC			
Proline	CCU	CCC	CCA	CCG	
Serine	UCU	UCC	UCA	UCG	AGC	AGU
Threonine	ACU	ACC	ACA	ACG	
Tryptophan	UGG				
Tyrosine	UAU	UAC			
Valine	GUU	GUC	GUA	GUG	
Start (CI)	AUG				
Stop (CT)	UAA	UAG	UGA		

Mitochondrial DNA

In addition to nuclear DNA, part of the DNA of a cell resides in the mitochondria. Mitochondrial DNA (mtDNA) is inherited from the mother (i.e., matrilineal inheritance). It is a double-stranded closed circle containing 37 genes, 24 of which are needed for mtDNA translation and 13 of which are needed for oxidative metabolism. Replication of mtDNA depends on enzymes encoded by nuclear DNA. Thus, the protein-synthesizing apparatus and molecular components for oxidative metabolism are jointly derived from nuclear and mitochondrial genes. Genetic disorders of mtDNA, although rare, commonly affect tissues such as those of the neuromuscular system that have a high requirement for oxidative metabolism (see Chapter 6).

From Genes to Proteins

Although DNA determines the type of biochemical product that is needed by the cell and directs its synthesis, it is RNA, through the process of transcription and translation, which is responsible for the actual assembly of the products.

RNA Structure and Function

RNA, like DNA, is a large molecule made up of a long string of nucleotides. However, it differs from DNA in three aspects of its structure. First, RNA is a single-stranded rather than a double-stranded molecule. Second, the sugar in each nucleotide of RNA is ribose instead of deoxyribose. Third, the pyrimidine base thymine in DNA is replaced by uracil in RNA.

Cells contain three types of RNA: messenger RNA (mRNA), ribosomal RNA (rRNA), and transfer RNA (tRNA). All three types of RNA are synthesized in the nucleus by RNA polymerase enzymes and then moved into the cytoplasm, where protein synthesis takes place. See Understanding DNA-Directed Protein Synthesis.

Messenger RNA. Messenger RNA is the template for protein synthesis. It is a long molecule containing several hundred to several thousand nucleotides. Each group of three nucleotides forms a codon that is exactly complementary to a nucleotide triplet of the DNA molecule. Messenger RNA is formed by a process called *transcription*. In this process, the weak hydrogen bonds of DNA are broken so that free RNA nucleotides can pair with their exposed DNA counterparts on the meaningful strand of the DNA molecule (see Fig. 5-1). As with the base pairing of the DNA strands, complementary RNA bases pair with the DNA bases.

Ribosomal RNA. The ribosome is the physical structure in the cytoplasm where protein synthesis takes place. Ribosomal RNA forms 60% of the ribosome, with the remainder of the ribosome composed of the structural proteins and enzymes needed for protein synthesis. Unlike the two other types of RNA, rRNA is produced in a specialized nuclear structure called the *nucleolus*.

The formed rRNA combines with ribosomal proteins in the nucleus to produce the ribosome, which is then transported into the cytoplasm. On reaching the cytoplasm, most ribosomes become attached to the endoplasmic reticulum and begin the task of protein synthesis.

Transfer RNA. *Transfer RNA* is a clover-shaped molecule containing only 80 nucleotides, making it the smallest RNA molecule. Its function is to deliver the activated form of an amino acid to the protein that is being synthesized in the ribosomes. At least 20 different types of tRNA are known, each of which recognizes and binds to only one type of amino acid. Each tRNA molecule has two recognition sites: the first is complementary for the mRNA codon, the second for the amino acid itself. Each type of tRNA carries its own specific amino acid to the ribosomes, where protein synthesis is taking place; there it recognizes the appropriate codon on the mRNA and delivers the amino acid to the newly forming protein molecule.

Transcription

Transcription occurs in the cell nucleus and involves the synthesis of RNA from a DNA template (Fig. 5-4B). Genes are transcribed by enzymes called *RNA polymerases* that generate a single-stranded RNA identical in sequence (with the exception of U in place of T) to one of the strands of DNA. It is initiated by the assembly of a transcription complex composed of RNA polymerase and other associated factors. This complex binds to the double-stranded DNA at a specific site called the *promoter region*. Within the promoter region is the so-called "TATA box" that contains the crucial thymine-adenine-thymine-adenine sequence that RNA polymerase recognizes and binds to, starting the replication process (Fig. 5-4A). The RNA polymerase continues to copy the meaningful DNA strand as it travels along the length of the gene, stopping only when it reaches a termination site with a stop codon. On reaching the stop signal, the RNA polymerase leaves the gene and releases the RNA strand. The RNA strand then is processed.

Processing involves the addition of certain nucleic acids at the ends of the RNA strand and cutting and splicing of certain internal sequences. Splicing often involves the removal of stretches of RNA (Fig. 5-5). Because of the splicing process, the final mRNA sequence is different from the original DNA template. The retained protein-coding regions of the mRNA sequences are called *exons* and the regions between exons are called *introns*. The functions of the introns are unknown. They are thought to be involved in the activation or deactivation of genes during various stages of development.

Splicing permits a cell to produce a variety of mRNA molecules from a single gene. By varying the splicing segments of the initial mRNA, different mRNA molecules are formed. For example, in a muscle cell, the original tropomyosin mRNA is spliced in as many as 10 different ways, yielding distinctly different protein products. This permits different proteins to be expressed from a single gene and reduces the amount of DNA contained in the genome.

(text continues on page 93)

UNDERSTANDING ➤ DNA-Directed Protein

Deoxyribonucleic acid (DNA) directs the synthesis of the many thousands of proteins that are contained in the different cells of the body. Although some of the proteins are structural proteins, the majority are enzymes that catalyze the different chemical reactions in the cell. Because DNA is located in the cell's nucleus and protein synthesis takes place in the cytoplasm, a second type of nucleic acid—ribonucleic acid (RNA)—participates in the actual assembly of the proteins. There are three types of RNA: messenger RNA (mRNA), ribosomal RNA (rRNA), and transfer RNA (tRNA) that participate in (1) the transcription of the DNA instructions for protein synthesis and (2) the translation of those instructions into the assembly of the polypeptides that make up the various proteins.

1

Transcription. Transcription involves copying the genetic code containing the instructions for protein synthesis from DNA to a complementary strand of mRNA. Once mRNA has been processed, it diffuses through the nuclear pores into the cytoplasm, where it controls protein synthesis.

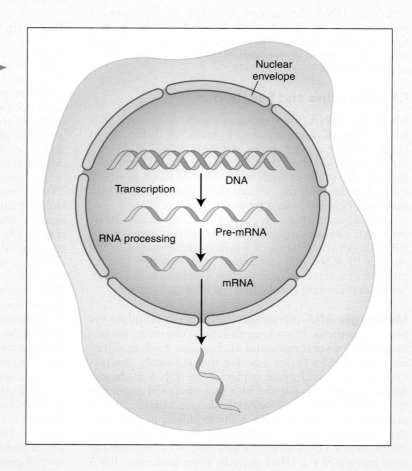

Nuclear envelope

Transcription

DNA

RNA processing

Pre-mRNA

mRNA

Synthesis

2 **Translation.** The process of translation involves taking the instructions transcribed from DNA to mRNA and transferring them to the rRNA of ribosomes located in the cytoplasm. It is the recognition of the mRNA codon by the tRNA anticodon that ensures the proper sequence of amino acids in a synthesized protein. In order to be functional, the newly synthesized protein must be folded into its functional form, modified further, and then routed to its final position in the cell.

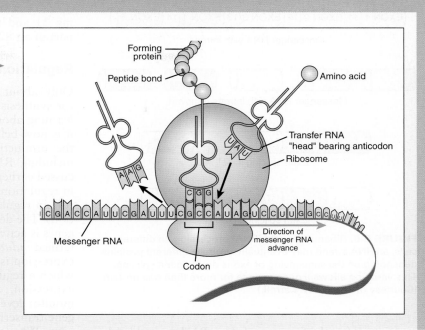

(text continued from page 91)

Translation

Proteins are made from a standard set of amino acids, which are joined end to end to form the long polypeptide chains of protein molecules. Each polypeptide chain may have as few as 100 to more than 300 amino acids in it. The process of protein synthesis is called *translation* because the genetic code is translated into the language of this polypeptide assembly.

Translation requires the coordinated actions of all three forms of RNA. It begins when mRNA contacts and passes through the ribosome, where it bonds to rRNA. As the RNA complex passes through the ribosome, tRNA translates its codons into complementary *anticodons*, which determine which amino acids it then delivers to the rRNA of ribosomes for attachment to the growing polypeptide chain. The long mRNA strand usually travels through and directs protein synthesis in more than one ribosome

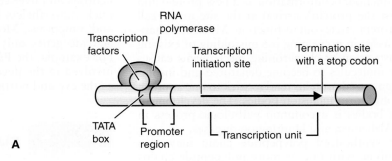

FIGURE 5-4. Transcription of messenger RNA (mRNA) from DNA double helix. **(A)** Transcription of mRNA involves attachment of RNA polymerase along with transcription factors to a specific nucleotide sequence, the TATA (thymine-adenosine-thymine-adenosine) region on the promoter region of the DNA. Transcription moves along the transcription unit and terminates at the stop codon. **(B)** Transcription creates a complementary copy mRNA from one of the DNA strands in the double helix. DNA, deoxyribonucleic acid; RNA, ribonucleic acid.

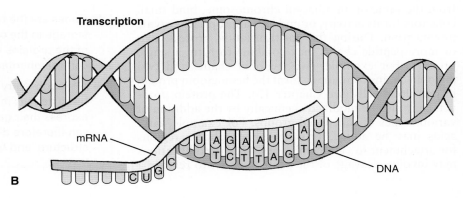

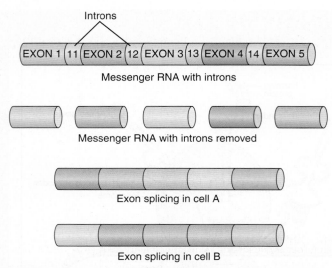

Introns

| EXON 1 | 11 | EXON 2 | 12 | EXON 3 | 13 | EXON 4 | 14 | EXON 5 |

Messenger RNA with introns

Messenger RNA with introns removed

Exon splicing in cell A

Exon splicing in cell B

FIGURE 5-5. Ribonucleic acid (RNA) processing. In different cells, an RNA strand may eventually produce different proteins depending on the sequencing of exons during gene splicing. This variation allows a gene to code for more than one protein. (Courtesy of Edward W. Carroll.)

at a time. After the first part of the mRNA is read by the first ribosome, it moves onto a second and a third. As a result, ribosomes that are actively involved in protein synthesis are often found in clusters called *polyribosomes*.

The process of translation is not over when the genetic code has been used to create the sequence of amino acids that constitute a protein. To be useful to a cell, this new polypeptide chain must be folded up into its unique three-dimensional conformation. The folding of many proteins is made more efficient by special classes of proteins called *molecular chaperones*. Typically, the function of a chaperone is to assist a newly synthesized polypeptide chain to attain a functional conformation as a new protein and then to assist the protein's arrival at the site in the cell where the protein carries out its function. Molecular chaperones also assist in preventing the misfolding of existing proteins. Disruption of chaperoning mechanisms causes intracellular molecules to become denatured and insoluble. These denatured proteins tend to stick to one another, precipitate, and form inclusion bodies. The development of inclusion bodies is a common pathologic process in Parkinson, Alzheimer, and Huntington diseases.

A newly synthesized polypeptide chain may also need to combine with one or more polypeptide chains from the same or an adjacent chromosome, bind small cofactors for its activity, or undergo appropriate enzyme modification. During the posttranslation process, two or more peptide chains may combine to form a single product. For example, two α-globin chains and two β-globin chains combine to form the hemoglobin protein in red blood cells (see Chapter 13). The protein products may also be modified chemically by the addition of various types of functional groups. For example, fatty acids may be added, providing hydrophobic regions for attachment to cell membranes. Other modifications may involve cleavage of the protein, either to remove a

specific amino acid sequence or to split the molecule into smaller chains. As an example, the two chains that make up the circulating active insulin molecule, one containing 21 and the other 30 amino acids, were originally part of an 82-amino-acid proinsulin molecule.

Regulation of Gene Expression

Only about 2% of the genome encodes instructions for synthesis of proteins. Although researchers are still learning about the functions of the other 98% of DNA, it is now believed to consist of sequences that code for the production of certain types of regulatory RNA, including RNA involved in the splicing process discussed earlier. Some of the remaining genes are involved in regulation of other genes; whereas others may play a role in regulating various nuclear or cytoplasmic functions. The degree to which a gene or particular group of genes is active is called *gene expression*. A phenomenon termed *induction* is an important process by which gene expression is increased. *Gene repression* is a process by which a regulatory gene acts to reduce or prevent gene expression. Activator and repressor sites commonly monitor levels of the synthesized product and regulate gene transcription through a negative feedback mechanism. Whenever product levels decrease, gene transcription is increased, and when product levels increase, gene transcription is repressed.

Although control of gene expression can occur in multiple steps, many regulatory events occur at the transcription level. As noted earlier, the initiation and regulation of transcription require the collaboration of a battery of proteins collectively termed *transcription factors*. After binding to their own specific DNA region, transcription factors can function to increase or decrease transcriptional activity of the genes. The role of transcription factors in gene expression explains why neurons and liver cells that have the same DNA in their nuclei nevertheless have completely different structures and functions. Moreover, some transcription factors activate genes only at specific stages of development. For example, the PAX family of transcription factors is involved in the development of such embryonic tissues as the eye and portions of the nervous system.

SUMMARY CONCEPTS

■ Genes are the fundamental unit of information storage in the cell. They code for the assembly of the proteins made by the cell and therefore control inheritance and day-to-day cell function.

■ Although every cell in the body contains the same basic genetic information, cells from our body express their genetic information differently, and can therefore differ vastly in their appearance, structure, and function.

- Genetic information is stored in a stable macromolecule called *deoxyribonucleic acid* (*DNA*). Genes transmit information contained in the DNA molecule as a triplet code consisting of an arrangement of the nitrogenous bases of the four nucleotides (i.e., adenine, guanine, thymine [or uracil in RNA], and cytosine).

- Gene mutations represent accidental errors in duplication, rearrangement, or deletion of parts of the genetic code. Fortunately, most mutations are corrected by DNA repair mechanisms in the cell.

- The production of proteins requires both DNA and a second type of macromolecule called *ribonucleic acid* (*RNA*). The process is accomplished by (1) the transcription of the DNA code onto *messenger RNA*, (2) the synthesis of proteins by ribosomal RNA, and (3) the translation of messenger RNA code by transfer RNA, which delivers the amino acids needed for protein synthesis to ribosomal RNA of ribosomes located in the cytoplasm.

- The degree to which a gene or particular group of genes is active is called *gene expression*. Gene expression involves a set of complex interrelationships among different levels of control including RNA transcription and posttranslational processing.

- Posttranslational processing involves the proper folding of the newly synthesized polypeptide chain into its unique three-dimensional conformation. Posttranslational processing may also involve the combination of polypeptide chains from the same or an adjacent chromosome, the binding of small cofactors, or enzyme modification.

Chromosomes

Most genetic information of a cell is organized, stored, and retrieved in discrete bundles of DNA called *chromosomes*. Although the chromosomes are visible only in dividing cells, they retain their integrity between cell divisions. The chromosomes are arranged in pairs: one member of the pair is inherited from the mother, the other from the father. The maternal and paternal chromosomes of a pair are called *homologous chromosomes* (homologs). Humans have 23 pairs of chromosomes (46 total). Of the 23 pairs, 22 are called *autosomes*. These have the same appearance in all individuals, males and females, and each has been given a numeric designation for classification purposes (Fig. 5-6). The sex chromosomes, which make up the 23rd pair of chromosomes, determine the sex of a person. All males have an X and Y chromosome (i.e., an X chromosome from the mother and a Y chromosome from the father); all females have two X chromosomes (i.e., one from each parent). The much smaller Y chromosome contains the *male-specific region* (MSY) that determines sex. This region comprises more than 90% of the length of the Y chromosome.

Only one X chromosome in the female is active in controlling the expression of genetic traits; however, both X chromosomes are activated during gametogenesis. In the female, the active X chromosome is invisible, but the inactive X chromosome can be visualized with appropriate nuclear staining. This inactive chromatin mass is called a *Barr body*. The genetic sex of a child can be determined by microscopic study of cell or tissue samples for the presence of a Barr body. For example, the cells of a normal female have one Barr body and therefore a total of two X chromosomes. A normal male has no Barr bodies. Males with Klinefelter syndrome (one Y, an inactive X, and an active X chromosome) exhibit one Barr body.

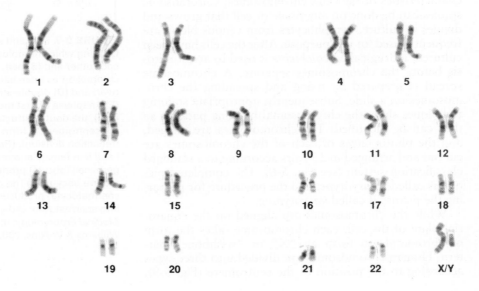

FIGURE 5-6. Karyotype of a normal male (xy). (From National Cancer Institute Visuals. No. AV-9700-4394.)

Cell Division

Cells reproduce by duplicating their chromosomes and dividing in two. There are two types of cell division: mitosis and meiosis. *Mitosis* is the cell cycle process in which nongerm cells are replicated. It provides a way for the body to replace cells that have a limited life span, such as skin and blood cells; increase tissue mass during periods of growth; and repair tissue, such as in wound healing.

Meiosis is limited to replicating germ cells and takes place only once in a cell line. It results in the formation of gametes or reproductive cells (i.e., ovum and sperm), each of which has only a single set of 23 chromosomes. Meiosis is typically divided into two distinct phases: meiosis I and meiosis II (Fig. 5-7). During meiosis I, homologous chromosomes pair up, forming a double-structured chromosome containing four chromatids (four strands) and therefore called a tetrad (two chromatids per chromosome). They are also sometimes called *bivalents.* The X and Y chromosomes are not homologs and do not form bivalents. While in meiosis I, an interchange of chromatid segments can occur (Fig. 5-8). This process, called *crossing over,* allows for new combinations of genes, increasing genetic variability.

After cell division I, each of the two daughter cells contains one member of each homologous pair of chromosomes and a sex chromosome (23 double-stranded chromosomes). No DNA synthesis occurs before meiotic division II. During cell division II, the 23 double-stranded chromosomes (two chromatids) of each of the two daughter cells from meiosis I divide at their centromeres (central regions where the chromatids meet). Each subsequent daughter cell receives 23 single-stranded chromatids. Thus, a total of four daughter cells are formed by a meiotic division of one cell.

Chromosome Structure

Cytogenetics is the study of the structure and numeric characteristics of the cell's chromosomes. Chromosome studies can be done on any tissue or cell that grows and divides in culture. Lymphocytes from venous blood are frequently used for this purpose. After the cells have been cultured, a drug called *colchicine* is used to arrest mitosis before the chromosomes separate. A chromosome spread is prepared by fixing and spreading the chromosomes on a slide. Subsequently, appropriate staining techniques show the chromosomal banding patterns so they can be identified. The chromosomes are imaged, and the photoimages of each of the chromosomes are cut out and arranged in 23 pairs according to a standard classification system (see Fig. 5-6). The completed picture is called a *karyotype,* and the procedure for preparing the picture is called *karyotyping.*

While the chromosomes are aligned on the equatorial plate of the cell, each chromosome takes the form of chromatids to form an "X" or "wishbone" pattern. Human chromosomes are divided into three types according to the position of the centromere (Fig. 5-9).

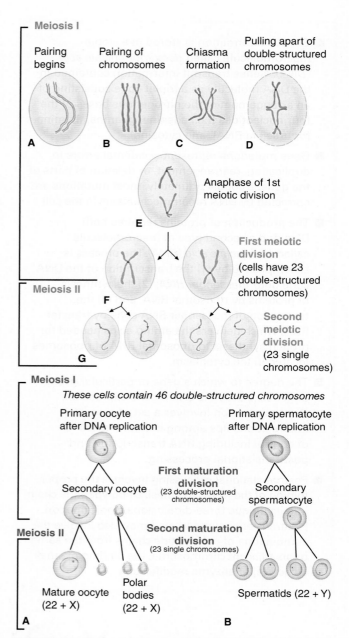

FIGURE 5-7. First and second meiotic divisions. (*Top*) Meiosis I, during which homologous chromosomes **(A)** approach each other and **(B)** pair; **(C)** intimately paired homologous chromosomes interchange chromatid fragments (crossing over) and **(D)** double-structured chromosomes pull apart. **(E)** Anaphase of first meiotic division. During meiosis II **(E, F)**, the double-structured chromosomes pull apart at the centromere to form four single-stranded chromosomes (reduction division). (*Bottom*) Events occurring during meiosis I and II in female and male gametes. **(A)** The primitive female germ cell (oocyte) produces only one mature gamete, the mature oocyte. **(B)** The primitive male germ cell (primary spermatocyte) produces four spermatids, all of which develop into spermatozoa. (Adapted from Sadler RW. *Langman's Medical Embryology*, 9th ed. Philadelphia, PA: Lippincott Williams & Wilkins; 2003.)

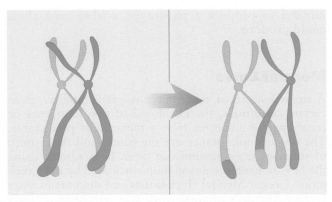

FIGURE 5-8. Crossing over of DNA at the time of meiosis.

If the centromere is in the center and the arms are of approximately the same length, the chromosome is said to be *metacentric*; if it is not centered and the arms are of clearly different lengths, it is *submetacentric*; and if it is near one end, it is *acrocentric*. The short arm of the chromosome is designated as "p" for "petite," and the long arm is designated as "q" for no other reason than it is the next letter of the alphabet. The arms of the chromosome are indicated by the chromosome number followed by the p or q designation (e.g., 15p). Chromosomes 13, 14, 15, 21, and 22 have small masses of chromatin called *satellites* attached to their short arms by narrow stalks.

The banding patterns of a chromosome are used in describing the geographic position of a gene on a chromosome, which can be useful, for example, in communicating the location of genes involved in genetic diseases. Each arm of a chromosome is divided into regions, which are numbered from the centromere outward (e.g., 1, 2). The regions are further divided into bands, which are also numbered (Fig. 5-10). These

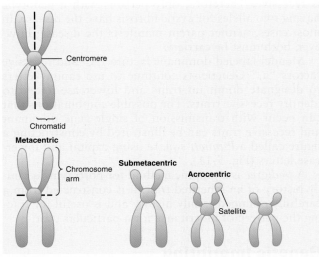

FIGURE 5-9. Three basic shapes and the component parts of human metaphase chromosomes. The relative size of the satellite on the acrocentric is exaggerated for visibility. (Adapted from Cormack DH. *Essential Histology.* Philadelphia, PA: J.B. Lippincott; 1993.)

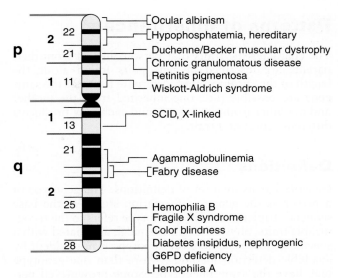

FIGURE 5-10. Localization of inherited diseases as represented on the banded karyotype of the X chromosome. Notice the nomenclature of arms (P, Q), regions (1, 2), and bands (e.g., 22 [region 2, band 2]). G6PD, glucose-6-phosphate dehydrogenase deficiency; SCID, severe combined immunodeficiency disease. (Modified from Peiper S, Strayer DS. In: Rubin R, Strayer DS, eds. *Rubin's Pathology: Clinicopathologic Foundations of Medicine.* 6th ed. Philadelphia, PA: Wolters Kluwer Health | Lippincott Williams & Wilkins; 2012:251.)

numbers are combined to designate the position of a gene; for example, Xp22 refers to band 2, region 2 of the short arm (p) of the X chromosome.

SUMMARY CONCEPTS

- The genetic information in a cell is organized, stored, and retrieved as small structures called *chromosomes.* There are 46 chromosomes arranged in 23 pairs, 22 of which are alike for males and females, and 1 pair of sex chromosomes, with XX pairing in females and XY pairing in males.

- Cell division involves the duplication of the chromosomes. Duplication of chromosomes in somatic cell lines involves mitosis, in which each daughter cell receives 23 pairs of chromosomes. Meiosis is limited to replicating germ cells (ovum and sperm) and results in formation of a single set of 23 chromosomes.

- A karyotype is an image of a person's chromosomes. It is prepared by special laboratory techniques in which body cells are cultured, fixed, and then stained to display identifiable banding patterns. A photomicrograph is then made. Often the individual chromosomes are cut out and regrouped according to chromosome number.

Patterns of Inheritance

The characteristic traits that persons inherit from their parents are inscribed in gene pairs found along the length of the chromosomes. Alternate forms of the same gene are possible (i.e., one inherited from the mother and the other from the father), and each may produce a different aspect of a trait.

Definitions

Genetics has its own set of definitions. The genotype of a person is the genetic information stored in the base sequence triplet code. The phenotype refers to the recognizable traits, physical or biochemical, associated with a specific genotype. Often, the genotype is not evident by available detection methods. More than one genotype may have the same phenotype. Some brown-eyed persons carry one copy of the gene that codes for blue eyes, and other brown-eyed persons do not. Phenotypically, these two types of brown-eyed persons are the same, but genotypically they are different.

With regard to a genetic disorder, not all persons with a mutant gene are affected to the same extent. *Expressivity* refers to the manner in which the gene is expressed in the phenotype, which can range from mild to severe. *Penetrance* represents the ability of a gene to express its function. Seventy-five percent penetrance means 75% of persons of a particular genotype present with a recognizable phenotype. Syndactyly (webbed fingers or toes) and blue sclera are genetic mutations that often do not exhibit 100% penetrance.

The position of a gene on a chromosome is called its *locus*. Because each chromosome is paired, each gene is paired, and the two copies of a gene at the same locus are called *alleles*. When only one pair of alleles is involved in the transmission of information, the term *single-gene trait* is used. For example, the inheritance of freckles is governed by the alleles (the two copies) of a single gene. Single-gene traits follow the mendelian laws of inheritance (to be discussed).

Polygenic inheritance involves multiple genes at different loci, with each gene exerting a small additive effect in determining a trait. Most human traits are determined by multiple pairs of genes, many with alternate codes, accounting for some dissimilar forms that occur with certain genetic disorders. Polygenic traits are predictable, but with less reliability than single-gene traits. *Multifactorial* inheritance is similar to polygenic inheritance in that multiple genes at different loci affect the outcome; however, environmental effects on the genes also affect the outcome.

Many other gene–gene interactions are known. These include *epistasis*, in which a gene in one locus masks the phenotypic effects of a gene at a different locus; *multiple alleles*, in which more than one allele affects the same trait (e.g., ABO blood types); *complementary genes*, in which each gene is mutually dependent on the other; and *collaborative genes*, in which two different genes influencing the same trait interact to produce a phenotype neither gene alone could produce.

Mendel Laws

A main feature of inheritance is predictability: given certain conditions, the likelihood of the occurrence or recurrence of a specific trait is remarkably predictable. The units of inheritance are the genes, and the pattern of single-gene expression can often be predicted using the laws of genetic transmission elucidated by the Czech monk Gregor Mendel. Techniques and discoveries since Gregor Mendel's original work was published in 1865 have led to some modification of his original laws.

During maturation, the primordial germ cells (i.e., sperm and ovum) of both parents undergo meiosis, or reduction division, in which the number of chromosomes is divided in half (from 46 to 23). At this time, the two alleles from a gene locus separate so that each germ cell receives only one allele from each pair. The alleles from the different gene loci segregate independently and recombine randomly in the zygote. Offspring in whom the two alleles of a given pair are the same are called *homozygotes*. For example, a plant may have two alleles for wrinkled peas. *Heterozygotes* have different alleles at a gene locus. For example, a plant may have one allele for wrinkled peas and one allele for round peas. In the latter case, what would the peas look like? Mendel discovered that the allele for round peas was *dominant*; that is, the trait it encodes is expressed in either a homozygous or a heterozygous pairing. The trait for wrinkled peas is *recessive*. It is expressed only in a homozygous pairing. All offspring with a dominant allele manifest that trait. In human genetics, a *carrier* is a person who is heterozygous for a recessive trait and does not manifest the trait. For example, the gene for the genetic disorder cystic fibrosis is recessive. Therefore, only persons with a genotype having two alleles for cystic fibrosis have the disease. In most cases, neither parent manifests the disease; however, both must be carriers.

Mendel labeled dominant factors "A" and recessive factors "a." Geneticists continue to use capital letters to designate dominant traits and lowercase letters to identify recessive traits. The possible combinations that can occur with transmission of single-gene dominant and recessive traits can be illustrated by constructing a figure called a *Punnett square* using capital and lowercase letters (Fig. 5-11).

A *pedigree* is a graphic method for portraying a family history of an inherited trait. It is constructed from a carefully obtained family history and is useful for tracing the pattern of inheritance for a particular trait.

Genetic Imprinting

According to Mendel the phenotype of an individual is established by whether a given allele is inherited from the mother or father. Recently, however, it has become increasingly apparent that this is not always true. For

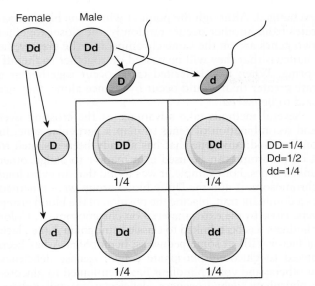

FIGURE 5-11. The Punnett square showing all possible combinations for transmission of a single gene trait (dimpled cheeks). The example shown is when both parents are heterozygous (dD) for the trait. The alleles carried by the mother are on the left and those carried by the father are on the top. The D allele is dominant and the d allele is recessive. The DD and Dd offspring have dimples and the dd offspring does not.

some human genes one of the alleles is transcriptional inactive (no RNA produced), depending on the parent from whom the allele is inherited. For example, an allele from the mother would be active and that from the father would be inactive. This process of gene silencing was given the name *genomic imprinting* by Helen Crouse in 1960. It is now more commonly known as *genetic imprinting*. In humans, it is estimated that approximately 100 genes exhibit genetic imprinting. Evidence suggests that a genetic conflict occurs in the developing embryo: the male genome attempts to establish larger offspring, whereas the female genome favors smaller offspring to conserve her energy for the current and subsequent pregnancies.

It was the pathologic analysis of ovarian teratomas (tumors made up of various cell types derived from an undifferentiated germ cell) and hydatidiform moles (gestational tumors) that yielded the first evidence of genetic imprinting. All ovarian teratomas were found to have a 46,XX karyotype. The results of detailed chromosomal polymorphism analysis confirmed that these tumors developed without the paternally derived genome. Conversely, analysis of hydatidiform moles suggested that they were tumors of paternal origin.

A related chromosomal disorder is *uniparental disomy*. This occurs when two chromosomes of the same number are inherited from one parent. Normally, this is not a problem except in cases where a chromosome has been imprinted by a parent. If an allele is inactivated by imprinting, the offspring will have only one working copy of the chromosome, resulting in possible problems.

SUMMARY CONCEPTS

- The transmission of information from one generation to the next is vested in genetic material transferred from each parent at the time of conception.

- Inheritance represents the likelihood of the occurrence or recurrence of a specific genetic trait.

- The *genotype* is the total sum of the genetic information that is stored in the genetic code of a person, whereas the *phenotype* represents the recognizable traits, physical and biochemical, associated with the genotype.

- *Expressivity* refers to the expression of a gene in the phenotype, and *penetrance* is the ability of a gene to express its function. The point on the DNA molecule that controls the inheritance of a particular trait is called a *gene locus*.

- Alleles are the alternate forms of a gene (one from each parent), and the locus is the position that they occupy on the chromosome. The alleles at a gene locus may carry recessive or dominant traits.

- Mendelian, or single-gene, patterns of inheritance include autosomal dominant and recessive traits that are transmitted from parents to their offspring in a predictable manner. *A recessive trait* is one expressed only when two copies (homozygous) of the recessive allele are present. *Dominant traits* are expressed with either homozygous or heterozygous pairing of the alleles.

- Polygenic inheritance, which involves multiple genes, and multifactorial inheritance, which involves multiple genes as well as environmental factors, are less predictable.

- A *pedigree* is a graphic method for portraying a family history of an inherited trait.

Gene Technology

The past several decades have seen phenomenal advances in the field of genetics. These advances have included the assembly of physical and genetic maps through the Human Genome Project; the establishment of the International HapMap Project (http://hapmap. ncbi.nlm.nih.gov) to map the haplotypes of the many adjacent single-nucleotide polymorphisms in the human genome; the establishment of the 1000 Genomes Project (http://www.1000genomes.org), and the development of methods for applying the technology of these projects to the diagnosis and treatment of disease.

Gene Mapping

Genetic mapping is the assignment of genes to specific chromosomes or parts of the chromosome. Another type of mapping strategy, the haplotype map, focuses on identifying the slight variations in the human genome that influence an individual's susceptibility to disease and responses to environmental factors such as microbes, toxins, and drugs.

There are two types of gene maps: genetic maps and physical maps. Genetic maps are like highway maps. They use linkage studies (e.g., dosage, hybridization) to estimate the distances between chromosomal landmarks (i.e., gene markers). Physical maps are similar to a surveyor's map. They make use of cytogenetic and molecular techniques to determine the actual physical locations of genes on chromosomes. Genetic mapping has been refined over the decades. The earliest mapping efforts localized genes on the X chromosome. The initial assignment of a gene to a particular chromosome was made in 1911 for the color blindness gene inherited from the mother (i.e., following the X-linked pattern of inheritance).

The Human Genome Project

The Human Genome Project, initiated in 1990, sought to sequence and identify all the genes in the human genome. The international project was charged with developing genetic and physical maps that allowed the precise location of genes. Some of what was revealed was quite unexpected, including the fact that humans have a mere approximately 21,000 genes, rather than the initially estimated 100,000, and that any two individuals share 99.9% of their DNA sequence, indicating that the remarkable diversity among individuals is vested in about 0.1% of our DNA.

To date, the locations of approximately 21,000 genes have been mapped to a specific chromosome, and most of them to a specific region on the chromosome. However, genetic mapping is continuing so rapidly that these numbers are constantly being updated. An excellent source of articles regarding specific chromosome sequencing in humans is the National Center for Biotechnology Information (NCBI) (www.ncbi.nlm.nih.gov/index.html). Another source is the Genome Data Base, a central database for mapped genes and an international repository for most mapping information.

Genetic Mapping Methods

Many methods have been used for developing genetic maps. The most important ones are family linkage studies, gene dosage methods, and hybridization studies. Often, the specific assignment of a gene is made using information from several mapping techniques.

Linkage Studies. Linkage studies assume that genes occur in a linear array along the chromosomes. During meiosis, the paired chromosomes of the diploid germ cell exchange genetic material because of the crossing-over phenomenon (see Fig. 5-8). This exchange usually involves more than one gene; large blocks of genes (representing large portions of the chromosome) are usually exchanged. Although the point at which one block separates from another occurs randomly, the closer together two genes are on the same chromosome, the greater the chance is that they will be passed on together to the offspring. When two inherited traits occur together at a rate greater than would occur by chance alone, they are said to be *linked*.

Several methods take advantage of the crossing over and recombination of genes to map a particular gene. In one method, any gene that has already been assigned to a chromosome can be used as a marker to assign other linked genes. For example, it was found that an extra long chromosome 1 and the Duffy blood group were inherited as a dominant trait, placing the position of the blood group gene close to the extra material on chromosome 1. Color blindness has been linked to classic hemophilia A (i.e., lack of factor VIII) in some pedigrees; hemophilia A has been linked to glucose-6-phosphate dehydrogenase deficiency in others; and color blindness has been linked to glucose-6-phosphate dehydrogenase deficiency in still others. Because the gene for color blindness is found on the X chromosome, all three genes must be found in a small section of the X chromosome. Linkage analysis can be used clinically to identify affected persons in a family with a known genetic defect. Males, because they have one X and one Y chromosome, are said to be *hemizygous* for sex-linked traits. Females can be homozygous (normal or mutant) or heterozygous for sex-linked traits. Heterozygous females are known as *carriers* for X-linked defects.

One autosomal recessive disorder that has been successfully diagnosed prenatally by linkage studies using amniocentesis is congenital adrenal hyperplasia (due to 21-hydroxylase deficiency), which is linked to an immune response gene (human leukocyte antigen [HLA] type). Postnatal linkage studies have been used in diagnosing hemochromatosis, which is closely linked to another HLA type. Persons with this disorder are unable to metabolize iron, and it accumulates in the liver and other organs. It cannot be diagnosed by conventional means until irreversible damage has been done. Given a family history of the disorder, HLA typing can determine if the gene is present, and if it is present, dietary restriction of iron intake may be used to prevent organ damage.

Gene Dosage Studies. Dosage studies involve measuring enzyme activity. Autosomal genes are normally arranged in pairs, and normally both are expressed. If both alleles are present and are expressed, the activity of the enzyme should be 100%. If one member of the gene pair is missing, only 50% of the enzyme activity is present, reflecting the activity of the remaining normal allele.

Hybridization Studies. A recent biologic discovery revealed that two somatic cells from different species, when grown together in the same culture, occasionally fuse to form a new hybrid cell. Two types of hybridization methods are used in genomic studies: somatic cell hybridization and in situ hybridization.

Somatic cell hybridization involves the fusion of human somatic cells with those of a different species (typically, the mouse) to yield a cell containing the chromosomes of both species. Because these hybrid cells are unstable, they begin to lose chromosomes of both species during subsequent cell divisions. This makes it possible to obtain cells with different partial combinations of human chromosomes. The enzymes of these cells are then studied with the understanding that for an enzyme to be produced, a certain chromosome must be present and, therefore, the coding for the enzyme must be located on that chromosome.

In situ hybridization involves the use of specific sequences of DNA or RNA to locate genes that do not express themselves in cell culture. Deoxyribonucleic acid and RNA can be chemically tagged with radioactive or fluorescent markers. These chemically tagged DNA or RNA sequences are used as probes to detect gene location. The probe is added to a chromosome spread after the DNA strands have been separated. If the probe matches the complementary DNA of a chromosome segment, it hybridizes and remains at the precise location (therefore the term *in situ*) on a chromosome. Radioactive or fluorescent markers are used to find the location of the probe.

Haplotype Mapping

As work on the Human Genome Project progressed, many researchers reasoned that identifying the common patterns of DNA sequence variations in the human genome would be possible. An international project, known as the *International HapMap Project,* was organized with the intent of developing a haplotype map of these variations. One of the findings of the Human Genome Project was that the genome sequence was 99.9% identical for all people. It is anticipated that the 0.1% variation may greatly affect an individual's response to drugs, toxins, and predisposition to various diseases. Sites in the DNA sequence where individuals differ at a single DNA base are called *single-nucleotide polymorphisms* (SNPs, pronounced "snips"). A haplotype consists of the many closely linked SNPs on a single chromosome that generally are passed as a block from one generation to another in a particular population. One of the motivating factors behind the HapMap project was the realization that the identification of a few SNPs was enough to uniquely identify the haplotypes in a block. The specific SNPs that identify the haplotypes are called *tag SNPs*. A HapMap is a map of these haplotype blocks and their tag SNPs. This approach should prove useful in reducing the number of SNPs required to examine an entire genome and make genome scanning methods much more efficient in finding regions with genes that contribute to disease development.

Recent improvements in sequencing technology ("Next-Gen" sequencing platforms) have dramatically reduced the cost of sequencing. The goal of the 1000 Genomes Project is to sequence the genomes of a large number of people and provide a comprehensive high resolution resource for human genetic variation (www.1000genomes.org). It is anticipated that the HapMap Project and the 1000 Genomes Project will provide a useful tool for disease diagnosis and management. Much attention has focused on the use of SNPs to decide whether a genetic variant is associated with a higher risk of disease susceptibility in one population versus another. Pharmacogenetics addresses the variability of drug response due to inherited characteristics in individuals. With the availability of SNPs, it may soon be possible to identify persons who can be expected to respond favorably to a drug and those who can be expected to experience adverse reactions. This would result in safer, more effective, and more cost-efficient use of medications.

Recombinant DNA Technology

The term *recombinant DNA* refers to a combination of DNA molecules that are not found together in nature. Recombinant DNA technology makes it possible to identify the DNA sequence in a gene and produce the protein product encoded by a gene. The specific nucleotide sequence of a DNA fragment can often be identified by analyzing the amino acid sequence and mRNA codon of its protein product. Short sequences of base pairs can be synthesized, radioactively labeled, and subsequently used to identify their complementary sequence. In this way, identifying normal and abnormal gene structures is possible.

Gene Isolation and Cloning

The gene isolation and cloning methods used in recombinant DNA technology rely on the fact that the genes of all organisms, from bacteria through mammals, are based on a similar molecular organization. Gene cloning requires cutting a DNA molecule apart, modifying and reassembling its fragments, and producing copies of the modified DNA, its mRNA, and its gene product. The DNA molecule is cut apart using a bacterial enzyme, called a *restriction enzyme,* that binds to DNA wherever a particular short sequence of base pairs is found and cleaves the molecule at a specific nucleotide site. In this way, a long DNA molecule can be broken down into smaller, discrete fragments, one of which presumably contains the gene of interest. Many restriction enzymes are commercially available that cut DNA at different recognition sites.

The restrictive fragments of DNA can often be replicated through insertion into a unicellular organism, such as a bacterium (Fig. 5-12). To do this a *plasmid,* which is a cloning vector such as a bacterial virus or a small DNA circle that is found in most bacteria, is used. Viral and plasmid vectors replicate autonomously in the host bacterial cell. During gene cloning, a bacterial vector and the DNA fragment are mixed and joined by a special enzyme called a *DNA ligase.* The recombinant vectors formed are then introduced into a suitable culture of bacteria, and the bacteria are allowed to replicate and express the recombinant vector gene. Sometimes, mRNA taken from a tissue that expresses a high level of the gene is used to produce a complementary DNA molecule that can be used in the cloning process. Because the fragments of the entire DNA molecule are used in the cloning process, additional steps are taken to identify and separate the clone that contains the gene of interest.

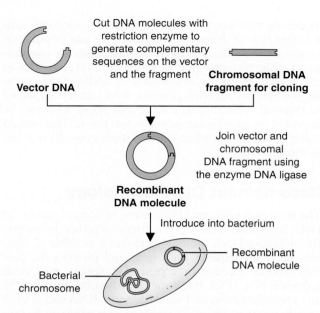

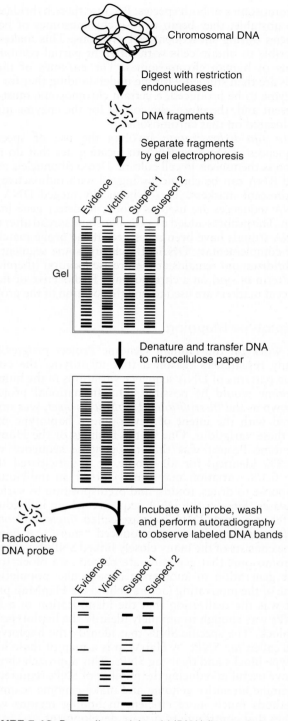

FIGURE 5-12. Recombinant DNA technology. By fragmenting DNA of any origin and inserting it in the DNA of rapidly reproducing foreign cells, billions of copies of a single gene can be produced in a short time. The DNA to be cloned is inserted into a plasmid (a small, self-replicating circular molecule of DNA) that is separate from chromosomal DNA. When the recombinant plasmid is introduced into bacteria, the newly inserted segment will be replicated along with the rest of the plasmid. DNA, deoxyribonucleic acid. (From Office of Biological and Environmental Research of the U.S. Department of Energy Office of Science. http://science.energy.gov/ber/)

Pharmaceutical Applications

Recombinant DNA technology has also made it possible to produce proteins that have therapeutic properties. One of the first products to be produced was human insulin. Recombinant DNA corresponding to the A chain of human insulin was isolated and inserted into plasmids that were in turn used to transform *Escherichia coli*. The bacteria then synthesized the insulin chain. A similar method was used to obtain the B chains. The A and B chains were then mixed and allowed to fold and form disulfide bonds, producing active insulin molecules. Human growth hormone has also been produced in *E. coli*. More complex proteins are produced in mammalian cell culture using recombinant DNA techniques. These include erythropoietin, which is used to stimulate red blood cell production; factor VIII, which is used to treat hemophilia; and tissue plasminogen activator (tPA), which is frequently administered after a heart attack to dissolve the thrombi that are obstructing coronary blood flow.

DNA Fingerprinting

The technique of DNA fingerprinting is based in part on those techniques used in recombinant DNA technology and on those originally used in medical genetics to detect slight variations in the genomes of different individuals. Using restriction enzymes, DNA is cleaved at specific regions (Fig. 5-13). The DNA fragments are separated

FIGURE 5-13. Deoxyribonucleic acid (DNA) fingerprinting. Restrictive enzymes are used to break chromosomal DNA into fragments, which are then separated by gel electrophoresis, denatured, and transferred to nitrocellulose paper; DNA bands are labeled with a radioactive probe and observed using autoradiography. (Modified from Smith C, Marks AD, Lieberman M. *Marks' Basic Medical Biochemistry.* 2nd ed. Philadelphia, PA: Lippincott Williams & Wilkins; 2005:309.)

according to size by electrophoresis. The single-stranded DNA is then transferred to nitrocellulose paper, baked to attach the DNA to the paper, and treated with a series of radioactive probes. After the radioactive probes have been allowed to bond with the denatured DNA, radiography is used to reveal the labeled DNA fragments.

When used in forensic pathology, this procedure is applied to specimens from the suspect and the forensic specimen. Banding patterns are then analyzed to see if they match. With conventional methods of analysis of blood and serum enzymes, a 1 in 100 to 1000 chance exists that the two specimens match because of chance. With DNA fingerprinting, these odds are 1 in 100,000 to 1 million.

When necessary, the polymerase chain reaction (PCR) can be used to amplify specific segments of DNA (see Chapter 14). It is particularly suited for amplifying regions of DNA for clinical and forensic testing procedures because only a small sample of DNA is required as the starting material. Regions of DNA can be amplified from a single hair or drop of blood or saliva.

Gene Therapy

Although quite different from inserting genetic material into a unicellular organism such as bacteria, techniques are available for inserting genes into the genome of intact multicellular plants and animals. The adenoviruses are promising delivery vehicles for these genes. These viruses are ideal vehicles because their DNA does not become integrated into the host genome; however, repeated inoculations are often needed because the body's immune system usually targets cells expressing adenovirus proteins. Sterically stable liposomes also show promise as DNA delivery mechanisms. This type of therapy is one of the more promising methods for the treatment of genetic disorders such as cystic fibrosis, certain cancers, and a number of infectious diseases.

Two main approaches are used in gene therapy: transferred genes can replace defective genes or they can selectively inhibit deleterious genes. Cloned DNA sequences are usually the compounds used in gene therapy. However, the introduction of the cloned gene into the multicellular organism can influence only the few cells that get the gene. An answer to this problem would be the insertion of the gene into a sperm or ovum; after fertilization, the gene would be replicated in all of the differentiating cell types. Even so, techniques for cell insertion are limited. Not only are moral and ethical issues involved, but these techniques cannot direct the inserted DNA to attach to a particular chromosome or supplant an existing gene by knocking it out of its place.

To date, gene therapy has been used successfully to treat children with severe combined immunodeficiency disease (see Chapter 16) and in a suicide gene transfer to facilitate treatment of graft-versus-host disease after donor lymphocyte infusion.

RNA Interference Technology

One method of gene therapy focuses on the previously described replacement of missing or defective genes. However, several genetic disorders are not due to missing genes, but to faulty gene activity. With this in mind, some scientists are approaching the problem by using *RNA interference* (RNAi) to stop genes from making unwanted disease proteins. RNA interference is a naturally occurring process in which small pieces of double-stranded RNA (small interfering RNA [siRNA]) suppress gene expression. Scientists believe that RNAi may have originated as a defense against viral infections and potentially harmful genomic invaders. In viral infections, RNAi would serve to control the infection by preventing the synthesis of viral proteins.

With the continued refinement of techniques to silence genes, RNAi has already had a major impact on molecular biology. For example, it has given scientists the ability to practice reverse genomics, in which a gene's function can be inferred through silencing its expression. Increasingly, pharmacologic companies are using RNAi to identify disease-related drug targets. There also is considerable interest in harnessing RNAi for therapeutic purposes, including the treatment of human immunodeficiency virus (HIV) infection and hepatitis C. Before this can occur, however, the therapeutic methods must be shown to be safe and effective, and obstacles to delivering RNAi into targeted cells must be overcome. It is difficult for RNA to cross the cell membrane, and it is quickly broken down by enzymes in the blood.

SUMMARY CONCEPTS

- The genome is the gene complement of an organism. Genomic mapping is a method used to assign genes to particular chromosomes or parts of a chromosome. The most important methods used are family linkage studies, gene dosage methods, and hybridization studies. *Linkage studies* assign a chromosome location to genes based on their close association with other genes of known location. *Dosage studies* involve measuring enzyme activity to determine if both members of a gene pair are present and functioning normally. *Hybridization studies* involve the fusion of human somatic cells with those of a different species to study gene location on chromosomes.

- Recombinant DNA studies involve the extraction of specific types of mRNA used in the synthesis of complementary DNA strands. The complementary DNA strands, labeled with a radioisotope, bind with the genes for which they are complementary and are used as gene probes.

- Genetic engineering has provided the methods for manipulating nucleic acids and recombining genes (recombinant DNA) into hybrid molecules that can be inserted into unicellular organisms

(continued)

SUMMARY CONCEPTS (continued)

and reproduced many times over. As a result, proteins that formerly were available only in small amounts (e.g., human insulin) can now be made in large quantities once their respective genes have been isolated. Deoxyribonucleic acid fingerprinting, which relies on recombinant DNA technologies and those of genetic mapping, is often used in forensic investigations.

■ A newer strategy for management of genetic disorders focuses on gene silencing by using ribonucleic acid interference (RNAi) technology to stop genes from making unwanted disease proteins.

REVIEW EXERCISES

1. The Human Genome Project has revealed that humans have only approximately 21,000 genes. Only about 2% of the genome encodes instructions for protein synthesis, whereas 50% consist of repeat sequences that do not code proteins.

    A. Use this information to explain how this small number of protein-encoding genes is able to produce the vast array of proteins needed for organ and structural development in the embryo, as well as those needed for normal function of the body in postnatal life.

2. A child about to undergo surgery is typed for possible blood transfusions. His parents are told that he is type O positive. Both his mother and father are type A positive.

    A. How would you go about explaining this variation in blood type to the parents?

3. The posttranslational folding of proteins is essential to their proper functioning and degradation.

    A. Hypothesize on how age-related changes in the folding of proteins in the central nervous system could contribute to the development of the neurofibrillary tangles that are characteristic of Alzheimer disease.

4. More than 100,000 people die of adverse drug reactions each year; another 2.2 million experience serious reactions; whereas others fail to respond at all to the therapeutic actions of drugs.

    A. Explain how the use of information about *single-nucleotide polymorphisms* might be used to map individual variations in drug responses.

5. Human insulin, prepared by recombinant DNA technology, is now available for the treatment of diabetes mellitus.

    A. Explain the techniques used for the production of a human hormone using this technology.

6. Cystic fibrosis is a disorder of the cell membrane chloride channel that causes the exocrine glands of the body to produce abnormally thick mucus resulting in the development of chronic obstructive lung disease, pancreatitis, and infertility in men.

    A. Explain how a single mutant gene can produce such devastating effects.
    B. The disease is transmitted as a single-gene recessive trait. Describe the inheritance of the disorder using Figure 5-11.

7. Adult polycystic kidney disease is transmitted as an autosomal dominant trait.

    A. Explain the parent-to-child transmission of this disorder.
    B. Although the disease is transmitted as an autosomal dominant trait, some people who inherit the gene may develop symptoms early in life, others may develop them later in life, and still others may never develop significant symptoms of the disease. Explain.

BIBLIOGRAPHY

Alberts B, Johnson A, Lewis J, et al. *Molecular Biology of the Cell.* 5th ed. New York, NY: Garland Science; 2008:195–499.

Bartolomei MS, Ferguson-Smith AC. Mammalian genomic imprinting. *Cold Spring Harb Perspect Biol.* 2011;3:w002592.

Cheng J, Kapranov P, Drenkow J, et al. Transcriptional maps of 10 human chromosomes at 5-nucleotide resolution. *Science.* 2005;308:1149–1154.

Fischer A, Cavazzana-Calvo M. Wither gene therapy? *The Scientist.* 2006;20(2):36–40.

Gibbs R. Deeper into the genome. *Nature.* 2005;437:1233–1234.

Gibson G, Muse SV. *A Primer of Genome Science.* Sunderland, MA: Sinauer Associates, Inc.; 2004.

Jegalian K, Lahn BT. Why the Y is so weird. *Sci Am* Feb. 2001:56–61.

Jorde LB, Carey JC, Bamshad MJ. *Medical Genetics.* 4rd ed. Phildelphia, PA: Mosby Elsevier; 2010.

Klug WS, Cummings MR. *Essentials of Genetics.* 5th ed. Upper Saddle River, NJ: Pearson Prentice Hall; 2005.

Lieberman M, Marks AD. *Marks' Basic Medical Biochemistry: A Clinical Approach.* 4th ed. Philadelphia, PA: Wolters Kluwer Health | Lippincott Williams & Wilkins; 2012:193–309.

McElheny VK. The human genome project. *The Scientist.* 2006;20(2):42–48.

Moore KL, Persaud TVN, Torchia MG. *The Developing Human: Clinically Orientated Embryology.* 9th ed. Philadelphia, PA: Elsevier Saunders; 2013.

Myers S, Bottolo L, Freeman C, et al. A fine-scale map of recombination rates and hotspots across the human genome. *Science.* 2005;310:321–324.

National Human Genome Project Research Institute. *An Overview of the Human Genome Project*. November 8, 2012. Available at: http://www.genome.gov/12011238/. Accessed October 10, 2013.

Nussbaum RL, McInnes RR, Willard HF. *Thompson & Thompson Genetics in Medicine*. 7th ed. Philadelphia, PA: Saunders Elsevier; 2007.

Phimister EG. Genomic cartography—presenting the HapMap. *N Engl J Med*. 2005;353(17):1766–1768.

Sadler RW. *Langman's Medical Embryology*. 9th ed. Philadelphia, PA: Lippincott Williams & Wilkins; 2003:3–30.

Shankar P, Manjunath N, Lieberman J. The prospect of silencing disease using RNA interference. *JAMA*. 2005;293(11):1367–1373.

Stevenson M. Therapeutic potential of RNA interference. *N Engl J Med*. 2004;351(17):1772–1777.

The International Hapmap 3 Consortium. Integrating common and rare genetic variations in diverse human populations. *Nature*. 2010;4672(2):82–88.

Villard J. Transcription regulation and human disease. *Swiss Med Wkly*. 2004;124:571–579.

Porth Essentials Resources

Explore these additional resources to enhance learning for this chapter:

- NCLEX-Style Questions and Other Resources on thePoint, http://thePoint.lww.com/PorthEssentials4e
- Study Guide for Essentials of Pathophysiology
- Concepts in Action Animations
- Adaptive Learning | Powered by PrepU, http://thepoint.lww.com/prepu

C h a p t e r **6**

Genetic and Congenital Disorders

Congenital disorders are abnormalities of a body structure, function, or metabolism that are present at birth. They affect about a quarter of a million babies in the United States each year and are the leading cause of infant death.[1,2] Congenital disorders may be caused by defective genes (single-gene or multifactorial inheritance), chromosomal aberrations, or environmental factors that are active during embryonic or fetal development (e.g., maternal exposure to infection or toxic chemicals during pregnancy). Although all congenital disorders are by definition present at birth, genetic disorders may make their appearance later in life.

The scientific understanding of congenital disorders has advanced significantly over the past three decades, largely as a result of the Human Genome Project. In fact, the molecular basis for many single-gene disorders is now known or will likely be known within the next few years. Such research has led to new and exciting insights not only in genetics, but also in the basic pathophysiology of disease.

This chapter provides an overview of genetic and other congenital disorders. It concludes with a brief survey of prenatal screening and diagnostic methods.

Disorders Involving Single or Multiple Genes

A genetic disorder can be described as a discrete event that affects gene expression in a group of cells during development. Most genetic disorders are caused by changes in the deoxyribonucleic acid (DNA) sequence that alter the synthesis of a single-gene product. However, some genetic disorders are caused by chromosomal rearrangements that result in deletion or duplication of a group of closely linked genes, or by an abnormal number of chromosomes resulting from mistakes that occur during meiosis or mitosis.[1–3] Chromosomal disorders are discussed separately.

As explained in Chapter 5, the genes on each person's two chromosomes are arranged in pairs and in strict order, with each gene occupying a specific location or *locus*. One member of each pair is derived from the person's father and the other from the person's mother. The term *allele* refers to different forms or DNA sequences that a gene may have in a population. If the members of a gene pair are identical (i.e., code the exact same gene product), the person is *homozygous*, and if the two members are different, the person is *heterozygous*. The genetic composition of a person is called a *genotype*, whereas the *phenotype* is the observable expression of a genotype in terms of morphologic, biochemical, or molecular traits. If the trait is expressed in the heterozygote (i.e., only one member of the gene pair codes for the trait), it is said to be *dominant;* if it is expressed only in the homozygote (i.e., both members of the gene pair code for the trait), it is *recessive.* Although gene expression usually follows a dominant or recessive pattern, it is possible for both alleles of a gene pair to be fully expressed in the heterozygote, a condition called *codominance.* Many genes have only one normal version, which geneticists call the *wild-type* allele. Other genes have more than one normal allele (alternate forms) at the same locus. This is called *polymorphism.* Blood group inheritance (e.g., AO, BO, AB) is an example of codominance and polymorphism.

A *gene mutation* is a biochemical event that results in a change in the DNA sequence of a gene. Mutations can involve the substitution of a single-nucleotide base (point mutation) or insertion or deletion of one or two base pairs. Those that affect the germ cells (ovum or spermatozoa) are transmitted to the progeny and may give rise to inherited diseases. Mutations in somatic (body) cells are not transmitted to the progeny but are important in the causation of cancers and some congenital disorders.

Single-Gene Disorders

Single-gene disorders are caused by a single defective or mutant gene. The defective gene may be present on an autosome or the X chromosome and may affect only one member of an autosomal gene pair (matched with a normal gene) or both members of the pair. Single-gene defects follow the mendelian pattern of inheritance (see Chapter 5) and are often called *mendelian disorders.*

A single mutant gene may be expressed in many different parts of the body. Marfan syndrome is a defect in connective tissue that has widespread effects involving skeletal, ocular, and cardiovascular structures. In other single-gene disorders, the same defect can be caused by mutations at several different loci. Childhood deafness can result from 16 different types of autosomal recessive mutations.

Virtually all single-gene disorders lead to formation of an abnormal protein or decreased production of a gene product. The disorder can result in a defective enzyme or decreased amounts of an enzyme, defects in receptor proteins and their function, alterations in nonenzyme proteins, or mutations resulting in unusual reactions to drugs. Table 6-1 lists some of the common single-gene disorders and their manifestations.

TABLE 6-1	**Some Disorders of Mendelian or Single-Gene Inheritance and Their Significance**
Disorder	**Significance**
Autosomal Dominant	
Achondroplasia	Short-limb dwarfism
Adult polycystic kidney disease	Chronic kidney disease
Huntington chorea	Neurodegenerative disorder
Familial hypercholesterolemia	Premature atherosclerosis
Marfan syndrome	Connective tissue disorder with abnormalities in the skeletal, ocular, and cardiovascular systems
Neurofibromatosis (NF)	Neurogenic tumors: fibromatous skin tumors, pigmented skin lesions, and ocular nodules in NF-1; bilateral acoustic neuromas in NF-2
Osteogenesis imperfecta	Brittle bone disease due to defects in collagen synthesis
Spherocytosis	Disorder of red blood cells
von Willebrand disease	Bleeding disorder
Autosomal Recessive	
Cystic fibrosis	Disorder of membrane transport of chloride ions in exocrine glands causing lung and pancreatic disease
Glycogen storage diseases	Excess accumulation of glycogen in the liver and hypoglycemia (von Gierke disease); glycogen accumulation in striated muscle in myopathic forms
Oculocutaneous albinism	Hypopigmentation of skin, hair, and eyes as a result of inability to synthesize melanin
Phenylketonuria (PKU)	Lack of phenylalanine hydroxylase with hyperphenylalaninemia and impaired brain development
Sickle cell disease	Red blood cell defect
Tay-Sachs disease	Deficiency of hexosaminidase A; severe mental and physical deterioration beginning in infancy
X-Linked Recessive	
Bruton-type hypogammaglobulinemia	Immunodeficiency
Hemophilia A	Bleeding disorder
Duchenne dystrophy	Muscular dystrophy
Fragile X syndrome	Mental retardation

Autosomal Dominant Disorders

In autosomal dominant disorders, a single mutant allele from an affected parent is transmitted to an off-spring regardless of sex. The affected parent has a 50% chance of transmitting the disorder to each offspring[1-4] (Fig. 6-1). The unaffected relatives of the parent or unaffected siblings of the offspring do not transmit the disorder. In many conditions, the age of onset is delayed, and the signs and symptoms of the disorder do not appear until later in life, as in Huntington disease (see Chapter 37).

In some cases, the person with an autosomal dominant disorder does not have an affected parent. Such persons owe their disorder to new mutations involving either the ovum or sperm from which they were derived. Their siblings are neither affected nor at increased risk of developing the disease. Whether the mutation is passed on to the next generation depends on the affected person's reproductive capacity. Many new autosomal dominant mutations are accompanied by reduced reproductive capacity; therefore, the defect is not perpetuated in future generations. If an autosomal defect is accompanied by a total inability to reproduce, essentially all new cases of the disorder will be due to new mutations. If the defect does not affect reproductive capacity, it is more likely to be inherited.

Although there is a 50% chance of inheriting a dominant genetic disorder from an affected parent, there can be wide variation in gene penetration and expression. When a person inherits a dominant mutant gene but fails to express it, the trait is described as having *reduced penetrance*. Penetrance is expressed in mathematical terms: a 50% penetrance indicates that a person who inherits the defective gene has a 50% chance of expressing the disorder. The person who has a mutant gene but does not express it is an important exception to the rule that unaffected persons do not transmit an autosomal dominant trait. These persons can transmit the gene to their descendants and so produce a skipped generation. Autosomal dominant disorders also can display *variable expressivity*, meaning that they can be expressed differently among individuals. Polydactyly or supernumerary digits, for example, may be expressed in either the fingers or the toes.

The gene products of autosomal dominant disorders usually are regulatory proteins involved in rate-limiting components of complex metabolic pathways or key components of structural proteins such as collagen.[2,3] Two disorders of autosomal inheritance, Marfan syndrome and neurofibromatosis (NF), are discussed here.

Marfan Syndrome. Marfan syndrome is an autosomal dominant disorder with an estimated prevalence of 1 per 20,000.[3] Approximately 75% of cases are of familial origin, with the rest arising from new mutations in the germ cells of parents. The pathogenesis of Marfan syndrome is related to mutations in a gene on chromosome 15 that codes for *fibrillin*, a major component of microfibrils found in the extracellular matrix.[3-5] Microfibrils serve as scaffolding for deposition of elastin and are considered integral components of elastic fibers. These fibers are essential for maintaining the tissue architecture of various body structures, most notably tendons and other elastin tissue–rich structures, such as heart valves and blood vessels.

Marfan syndrome affects several organ systems, including the ocular system (eyes), the cardiovascular system (heart and blood vessels), and the skeletal system (bones and joints).[3-6] There is a wide range of variation in the expression of the disorder. Persons may have abnormalities of one or all three systems. The skeletal deformities, which are the most obvious features of the disorder, include a long, thin body with exceptionally long extremities and long, tapering fingers, sometimes called *arachnodactyly* or *spider fingers*; hyperextensible joints; and a variety of spinal deformities, including kyphosis and scoliosis (Fig. 6-2). Chest deformities, pectus excavatum (i.e., deeply depressed sternum), or pectus carinatum (pigeon chest) deformity often is present and may require surgery. The most common eye disorder is bilateral dislocation of the lens due to weakness of the suspensory ligaments. Myopia and predisposition to retinal detachment also are common, the result of increased optic globe length due to altered connective tissue support of ocular structures. The most life-threatening aspects of the disorder, however, are the cardiovascular defects, which include mitral valve prolapse, progressive dilation of the aortic valve ring, and weakness of the aorta and other arteries. Dissection and rupture of the aorta may lead to premature death. In women, the risk of aortic dissection is increased in pregnancy.

Treatment plans for Marfan syndrome include echocardiograms and electrocardiograms to assess the status of the cardiovascular system, periodic eye examinations, and evaluation of the skeletal system, especially in children and adolescents. Low to moderate activity levels are usually well tolerated. Strenuous activities such as contact sports, weight training, high-impact aerobics, and scuba diving should usually be avoided. Surgical treatment may become necessary in cases of progressive aortic dilation or acute aortic dissection.

Neurofibromatosis. Neurofibromatosis is a condition involving neurogenic tumors that arise from Schwann cells and other elements of the peripheral nervous system.[2,3,7-12]

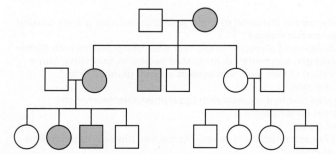

FIGURE 6-1. Simple pedigree for inheritance of an autosomal dominant trait. The *blue-colored square* (male) or *circle* (female) represents an affected persons with a mutant gene. An affected parent with an autosomal dominant trait has a 50% chance of passing the mutant gene on to each child regardless of sex.

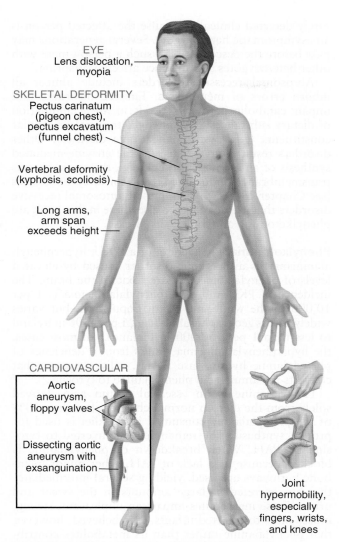

EYE
Lens dislocation, myopia

SKELETAL DEFORMITY
Pectus carinatum (pigeon chest), pectus excavatum (funnel chest)

Vertebral deformity (kyphosis, scoliosis)

Long arms, arm span exceeds height

CARDIOVASCULAR
Aortic aneurysm, floppy valves

Dissecting aortic aneurysm with exsanguination

Joint hypermobility, especially fingers, wrists, and knees

FIGURE 6-2. Clinical features of Marfan syndrome.

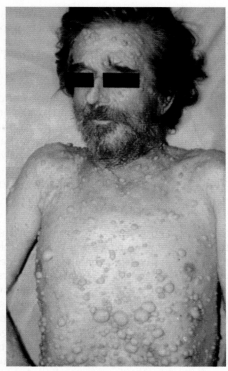

FIGURE 6-3. Neurofibromatosis, type I. Multiple cutaneous neurofibromas are noted on the face and trunk. (From Peiper S, Rubin DS. In: Rubin R, Strayer DS, eds. *Rubin's Pathology: Clinicopathologic Foundations of Medicine.* 6th ed. Philadelphia, PA: Wolters Kluwer Health/Lippincott Williams & Wilkins; 2012:238.)

There are at least two genetically and clinically distinct forms of the disorder: type 1 NF (NF-1), also known as *von Recklinghausen disease*, and type 2 bilateral acoustic NF (NF-2). Both of these disorders result from a genetic defect in a tumor-suppressor gene that regulates cell differentiation and growth. The gene for NF-1 has been mapped to chromosome 17 and the gene for NF-2 to chromosome 22.[3]

Type 1 NF is a relatively common disorder, with a frequency of 1 in 3500.[3] Approximately 50% of cases have a family history of autosomal dominant transmission, and the remaining 50% appear to represent a new mutation. The disorder is characterized by multiple neural tumors (neurofibromas) dispersed anywhere on the body; numerous pigmented skin lesions, some of which are café au lait spots; and pigmented nodules (Lisch nodules) of the iris.[7–11] The cutaneous neurofibromas, which vary in number from a few to many hundreds, manifest as soft, pedunculated lesions that project from the skin. They are the most common type of lesion, often are not apparent until puberty, and are present in greatest density over

the trunk (Fig. 6-3). The subcutaneous lesions grow just below the skin; they are firm and round, and may be painful. Plexiform neurofibromas involve the larger peripheral nerves. They tend to form large tumors that cause severe disfigurement of the face, overgrowth of an extremity, or skeletal deformities such as scoliosis. Pigmented nodules of the iris (Lisch nodules), which are specific to NF-1, usually are present after 6 years of age. They do not present any clinical problem but are useful in establishing a diagnosis.

A second major component of NF-1 is the presence of large (usually ≥15 mm in diameter), flat cutaneous pigmentations, known as *café au lait spots*. They are usually a uniform light brown in whites and darker brown in persons of color, with sharply demarcated edges. Although small single lesions may be found in normal children, larger lesions or six or more spots larger than 1.5 cm in diameter suggest NF-1. The skin pigmentations become more evident with age as the melanosomes in the epidermal cells accumulate melanin.

Children with NF-1 are also susceptible to neurologic complications. There is an increased incidence of learning disabilities, attention deficit disorders, and abnormalities of speech. Complex partial and generalized tonic-clonic seizures are a frequent complication. Neurofibromatosis-1 is also associated with increased incidence of other neurogenic tumors, including meningiomas, optic gliomas, and pheochromocytomas.[2]

Neurofibromatosis-2, which is characterized by tumors of the acoustic nerve and multiple meningiomas, is much less common than NF-1.[10-12] The disorder is often asymptomatic through the first 15 years of life. The most frequent symptoms are headaches, hearing loss, and tinnitus (i.e., ringing in the ears). There may be associated intracranial and spinal meningiomas. The condition is often made worse by pregnancy, and oral contraceptives may increase the growth and symptoms of tumors. Persons with the disorder should be warned that severe disorientation may occur during diving or swimming underwater, and drowning may result. Surgery may be indicated for debulking or removal of the tumors.

Autosomal Recessive Disorders

Autosomal recessive disorders are manifested only when both members of the gene pair are affected. In this case, both parents may be unaffected but are carriers of the defective gene. Autosomal recessive disorders affect both sexes. The occurrence risks in each pregnancy are one in four for an affected child, two in four for a carrier child, and one in four for a normal (noncarrier, unaffected) homozygous child[1-4] (Fig. 6-4). *Consanguineous mating* (mating of two related individuals), or inbreeding, increases the chance that two people who mate will be carriers of an autosomal recessive disorder.

With autosomal recessive disorders, the age of onset is frequently early in life; the symptomatology tends to be more uniform than with autosomal dominant disorders; and the disorders are characteristically caused by loss-of-function mutations, many of which impair or eliminate the function of an enzyme. In the case of a heterozygous carrier, the presence of a mutant gene usually does not produce symptoms because equal amounts of normal and defective enzymes are synthesized. This "margin of safety" ensures that cells with half their usual amount of enzyme function normally. By contrast, the inactivation of both alleles in a homozygote results in complete loss of enzyme activity. Although new mutations for recessive disorders do occur, they are

rarely detected clinically because the affected person is an asymptomatic heterozygote. Several generations may pass before the descendants of such a person mate with other heterozygotes and produce affected offspring.[3]

Autosomal recessive disorders include almost all inborn errors of metabolism. Enzyme disorders that impair catabolic pathways result in an accumulation of dietary substances (e.g., phenylketonuria) or cellular constituents (e.g., lysosomal storage diseases). Other disorders result from a defect in the enzyme-mediated synthesis of an essential protein (e.g., the cystic fibrosis transmembrane conductance regulator in cystic fibrosis [see Chapter 23]). Two examples of autosomal recessive disorders that are not covered elsewhere in this book are phenylketonuria and Tay-Sachs disease.

Phenylketonuria. Phenylketonuria (PKU, hyperphenylalaninemia) is a metabolic disorder caused by elevated levels of phenylalanine that are toxic to the brain. The incidence of PKU and hyperphenylalaninemia is 1 per 10,000 in the white and Asian population, but varies widely across geographic areas (e.g., 1 per 4500 in Ireland to less than 1 per 100,000 in Finland).[2] In most cases, the hyperphenylalaninemia results from a deficiency of phenylalanine hydroxylase (PAH), a liver enzyme that converts the amino acid phenylalanine to tyrosine.[1-3,13,14]

Phenylalanine is an essential amino acid derived solely from the diet. In normal children, less than 50% of the phenylalanine consumed in the diet is used for protein synthesis. The remainder is converted to tyrosine by PAH. When breakdown of phenylalanine is blocked because of a lack of PAH, other minor metabolic pathways are used, yielding several intermediates that are excreted in large amounts in the sweat and urine. These metabolites impart an unpleasant, strong, musty odor to affected infants. It is believed, however, that phenylalanine rather than its metabolites contributes to the brain damage in PKU. The lack of tyrosine, a precursor of melanin, is responsible for the light color of the hair and skin.

At the molecular level, approximately 400 mutant alleles for the PAH gene have been identified, some of which produce only mild deficiency while others produce severe deficiency.[3] The severity of hyperphenylalaninemia depends on the degree of PAH deficiency and can be classified as *classic PKU*, *mild PKU*, or *mild hyperphenylalaninemia* based on blood concentrations of phenylalanine.[13,14] Infants and children with classic and mild PKU require dietary protein restrictions to prevent intellectual impairment, microcephaly, and other signs of impaired neurologic development. Affected infants are normal at birth but within a few weeks begin to develop a rising phenylalanine level and signs of impaired brain development. Seizures, other neurologic abnormalities, decreased pigmentation of the hair and skin, and eczema often accompany the mental retardation in untreated infants.

Because the symptoms of untreated PKU develop gradually and would often go undetected until irreversible intellectual impairment had occurred, newborns are routinely screened for abnormal levels of serum phenylalanine.[13-15]

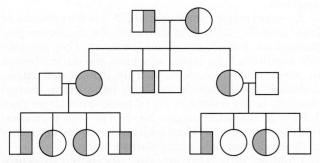

FIGURE 6-4. Simple pedigree for inheritance of an autosomal recessive trait. The half *blue-colored square* (male) and *circle* (female) represent a mutant gene. When both parents are carriers of a mutant gene, there is a 25% chance of having an affected child (*full blue-colored circle or square*), a 50% chance of a carrier child, and a 25% chance of an unaffected or noncarrier child, regardless of sex. All children (100%) of an affected parent are carriers.

Infants with hyperphenylalaninemia are treated with a special diet that restricts phenylalanine intake. The results of dietary therapy of children with PKU have been impressive. The diet can prevent intellectual impairment as well as other neurodegenerative effects of untreated PKU. However, dietary treatment must be started early in neonatal life to prevent brain damage. Infants with elevated phenylalanine levels should begin treatment by 7 to 10 days of age, indicating the need for early diagnosis. The duration of the dietary restriction remains controversial. Women with PKU who wish to have children require careful attention to their diet, both before conception and during pregnancy, as a means of controlling their phenylalanine levels.

Tay-Sachs Disease.

Tay-Sachs disease is a variant of a class of lysosomal storage diseases, known as the gangliosidoses, in which there is failure of lysosomes to break down the GM_2 ganglioside of cell membranes. Tay-Sachs disease is inherited as an autosomal recessive trait and is predominantly a disorder of Eastern European (Ashkenazi) Jews, in whom a carrier rate of 1 in 30 has been reported.[1-3]

The GM_2 ganglioside accumulates in the lysosomes of all organs in Tay-Sachs disease, but is most prominent in the brain neurons and retina. Microscopic examination reveals neurons ballooned with cytoplasmic vacuoles, each of which constitutes a markedly distended lysosome filled with gangliosides. In time, there is progressive destruction of neurons within the brain substance, including the cerebellum, basal ganglia, brain stem, spinal cord, and autonomic nervous system. Involvement of the retina is detected by ophthalmoscopy as a cherry-red spot on the macula.

Infants with Tay-Sachs disease appear normal at birth but begin to manifest progressive weakness, muscle flaccidity, and decreased attentiveness at approximately 6 to 10 months of age. This is followed by rapid deterioration of motor and mental function, often with development of generalized seizures. Retinal involvement leads to visual impairment and eventual blindness. The disease is invariably fatal, and death usually occurs before 4 to 5 years of age. Although there is no cure for the disease, analysis of the blood serum for the lysosomal enzyme hexosaminidase A, which is deficient in Tay-Sachs disease, allows for accurate identification of genetic carriers for the disease.

X-Linked Disorders

Sex-linked disorders are almost always associated with the X, female, chromosome, and the inheritance pattern is predominantly recessive.[1-4] Because of the presence of a normal paired X gene, female heterozygotes rarely experience the effects of a defective gene, whereas all males who receive the gene are typically affected. The common pattern of inheritance is one in which an unaffected mother carries one normal and one mutant allele on the X chromosome. This means that she has a 50% chance of transmitting the defective gene to her sons, and her daughters have a 50% chance of being carriers

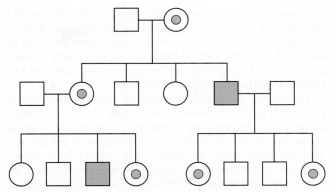

FIGURE 6-5. Simple pedigree for inheritance of an X-linked recessive trait. X-linked recessive traits are expressed phenotypically in the male offspring. A *small blue-colored circle* represents the X chromosome with the defective gene in the female and the *larger blue-colored square* represents the affected male. The affected male passes the mutant gene to all of his daughters, who become carriers of the trait and have a 50% chance of passing the gene to their sons and daughters, who in turn have a 50% chance of being carriers of the gene.

of the mutant gene (Fig. 6-5). When the affected son procreates, he transmits the defective gene to all of his daughters, who become carriers of the mutant gene. Because the genes of the Y chromosome are unaffected, the affected male does not transmit the defect to any of his sons, and they will not be carriers or transmit the disorder to their children. X-linked recessive disorders include glucose-6-phosphate dehydrogenase deficiency (see Chapter 13), hemophilia A (see Chapter 12), and X-linked agammaglobulinemia (see Chapter 16).

Single-Gene Disorders with Atypical Patterns of Inheritance

Several genetic disorders do not follow the mendelian pattern of inheritance. These include diseases caused by genomic imprinting, triplet repeat mutations, and mutations in mitochondrial genes.[3]

Genomic Imprinting

According to the mendelian pattern of inheritance, a mutant allele of an autosomal gene is equally likely to be transmitted from a parent to an offspring of either sex; similarly, a female is equally likely to transmit a mutated X-linked gene to either sex.[2] Originally, little attention was paid to whether the sex of the parent had any effect on expression of the genes each parent transmits. It is now known that in some genetic disorders, such as Prader-Willi and Angelman syndromes, the expression of the disease phenotype depends on whether the mutant allele was inherited from the father or the mother, a phenomenon known as *genomic imprinting*. Both syndromes exhibit intellectual disability as a common feature, and both involve the same deletion in chromosome 15. However, when the deletion is inherited from the mother, the infant presents with Angelman ("happy puppet") syndrome, which exhibits mental retardation along with paroxysms of laughter, ataxia, and seizures. In contrast, when the same deletion is inherited from the father, Prader-Willi syndrome results, and the child manifests intellectual impairment, uncontrolled appetite, obesity, and diabetes.

Figure 6-6 is a pedigree showing another inheritance pattern typical of genetic imprinting. In the example shown, gene expression is entirely "turned off" during spermatogenesis, so that any offspring who inherit the affected allele from the father will merely be carriers. Expression is "turned on" during oogenesis, however, so those who inherit the allele from the mother will express the disorder.

Triplet Repeat Mutations: Fragile X Syndrome

Fragile X syndrome is the prototype of disorders in which the mutation is characterized by a long repeating sequence of three nucleotides.[1-3] Thus far, about 40 diseases associated with neurodegenerative changes, including Huntington disease and myotonic dystrophy, have been classified as triplet repeat mutations, in which the expansion of specific sets of three nucleotides within a gene disrupts its function.

Fragile X syndrome, an abnormality in the X chromosome, is the common cause of inherited intellectual disability.[2,16-19] It is second only to Down syndrome as an identifiable cause of intellectual impairment. Because the syndrome is an X-linked disorder, it is more prevalent in males (1 in 4000) than females (1 in 8000).[19]

In addition to intellectual disability, the fragile X syndrome is characterized by distinctive features including a large face, a large mandible, and large, everted ears. Hyperextensible joints, a high-arched palate, and mitral

valve prolapse, which are observed in some cases, mimic a connective tissue disorder. Some physical abnormalities may be subtle or absent. The most distinctive feature, which is present in 90% of prepubertal boys, is macroorchidism, or large testes. Because girls have two X chromosomes, they are more likely to have relatively normal cognitive development, or they may show a learning disability in a particular area, such as mathematics. Women with the disorder may also experience premature ovarian failure or begin menopause earlier than women who are not affected by fragile X syndrome.

The term *fragile X* stems from the cytogenic observation of a constriction or fragile site on the long arm of the X chromosome. The fragile X syndrome results from a mutation in the *FMR1* (fragile X mental retardation 1) gene that has been mapped to this fragile site.[2,3] The protein product of the FMR1 gene, the *fragile X mental retardation protein* (FMRP), is a widely expressed ribonucleic acid (RNA)-binding protein. The protein travels from the cytoplasm to the nucleus, where it binds specific messenger RNAs (mRNAs) and then transports them from the nucleus to the synaptic ends of axons and dendrites, where the FMRP–mRNA complexes perform critical roles in regulating the translation of mRNA.[3]

The inheritance of the FMR1 gene follows the pattern of X-linked traits, with the father passing the gene on to all his daughters but not his sons. However, unlike other X-linked recessive disorders, approximately 20% of males who have been shown to carry the fragile X mutation are clinically and cytogenetically normal. These "carrier males" can transmit the disease to their grandsons through their phenotypically normal daughters. Another peculiarity is the presence of mental retardation in approximately 50% of carrier females. Both of these peculiarities have been related to the dynamic

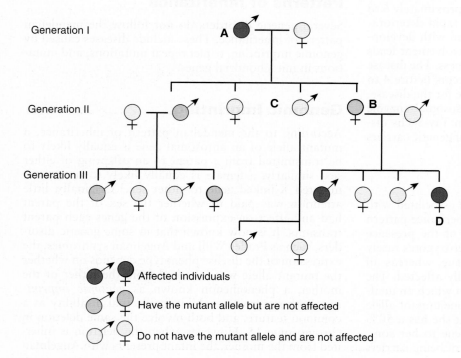

Generation I

Generation II

Generation III

Affected individuals

Have the mutant allele but are not affected

Do not have the mutant allele and are not affected

FIGURE 6-6. Pedigree of genetic imprinting. In generation I, male **(A)** has inherited a mutant allele from his affected mother (not shown); the gene is "turned off" during spermatogenesis, and therefore none of his offspring (generation II) will express the mutant allele, regardless of whether they are carriers. However, the gene will be "turned on" again during oogenesis in any of his daughters **(B)** who inherit the allele. All offspring (generation III) who inherit the mutant allele will be affected. All offspring of normal children **(C)** will produce normal offspring. Children of female **(D)** will all express the mutation if they inherit the allele.

nature of the mutation, which is sometimes maintained as a "premutation" (e.g., in carrier males) and sometimes advances to a full mutation (e.g., in affected males and carrier females who are nonetheless affected).

Mitochondrial Gene Disorders

The mitochondria contain their own DNA, which is distinct from the DNA contained in the cell nucleus. An understanding of the role of mitochondrial DNA (mtDNA) has evolved since 1988, when the first mutation of mtDNA was discovered.[20–22] Since that time, more than 100 different disease-related rearrangements and point mutations have been identified. In contrast to the mendelian pattern of inheritance of nuclear DNA, disorders of mtDNA have a maternal form of inheritance. This reflects the fact that sperm mitochondria are generally eliminated from the embryo so that disorders of the mtDNA are almost always inherited entirely from the mother.[1]

Mitochondrial DNA, which is packaged in a double-stranded circular chromosome located inside the mitochondria, is often referred to as the "other human genome."[20–22] It contains 37 genes: two ribosomal RNA (rRNA) genes; 22 transfer RNA (tRNA) genes; and 13 structural genes encoding subunits of the mitochondrial respiratory chain enzymes, which participate in oxidative phosphorylation and generation of adenosine triphosphate (ATP; see Chapter 1). Another 74 polypeptides that participate in oxidative phosphorylation are encoded by the nuclear genes. Although a rare disorder in nuclear encoded mitochondrial proteins has been described, most inherited defects in mitochondrial function result from mutations in the mitochondrial genome itself.

Mitochondrial DNA mutations generally affect tissues and organs that are highly dependent on oxidative phosphorylation to meet their high needs for metabolic energy. Thus, mitochondrial diseases frequently affect the brain and neuromuscular system and produce encephalomyopathies, retinal degeneration, loss of extraocular muscle function, lactic acidosis, and deafness.[21–23] The mitochondrial myopathies are often associated with the so-called *ragged red fibers*, a histologic phenotype resulting from degeneration of muscle fibers and massive accumulation of abnormal mitochondria. The range of mitochondrial diseases is broad, however, and may include liver dysfunction, bone marrow failure, pancreatic islet cell dysfunction, and diabetes, as well as other disorders. Table 6-2 describes representative examples of disorders due to mutations in mtDNA.

Multifactorial Inheritance Disorders

Multifactorial inheritance disorders are caused by multiple genes and, in many cases, environmental factors.[1–4] The exact number of genes contributing to multifactorial traits is not known, and these traits do not follow the same clear-cut pattern of inheritance as single-gene disorders. Multifactorial inheritance has been described as a threshold phenomenon in which the factors contributing to the trait can be compared with water filling a glass.[24] Using this analogy, it could be said that expression of the disorder occurs when the glass overflows. Disorders of multifactorial inheritance can be expressed during fetal life and be present at birth, or they may be expressed later in life. Congenital disorders that are thought to arise through multifactorial inheritance include cleft lip or palate, clubfoot, congenital dislocation of the hip, congenital heart disease, and urinary tract malformation. Environmental factors are thought to play a greater role in disorders of multifactorial inheritance that develop in adult life, such as coronary artery disease, diabetes mellitus, hypertension, cancer, and common psychiatric disorders such as bipolar disorder and schizophrenia.

Although multifactorial traits cannot be predicted with the same degree of accuracy as mendelian single-gene

TABLE 6-2	Some Disorders of Organ Systems Associated with Mitochondrial DNA Mutations
Disorder	**Manifestations**
Chronic progressive external ophthalmoplegia	Progressive weakness of the extraocular muscles
Deafness	Progressive sensorineural deafness, often associated with aminoglycoside antibiotics
Kearns-Sayre syndrome	Progressive weakness of the extraocular muscles of early onset with heart block, retinal pigmentation
Leber hereditary optic neuropathy	Painless, subacute, bilateral visual loss, with central blind spots (scotomas) and abnormal color vision
Leigh disease	Proximal muscle weakness, sensory neuropathy, developmental delay, ataxia, seizures, dementia, and visual impairment due to retinal pigment degeneration
MELAS	*M*itochondrial *E*ncephalomyopathy (cerebral structural changes), *L*actic *A*cidosis, and *S*trokelike syndrome, seizures, and other clinical and laboratory abnormalities; may manifest only as diabetes mellitus
MERRF	*M*yoclonic *E*pilepsy, *R*agged *R*ed *F*ibers in muscle; ataxia; sensorineural deafness
Myoclonic epilepsy with ragged red fibers	Myoclonic seizures, cerebellar ataxia, mitochondrial myopathy (muscle weakness, fatigue)

mutations, characteristic patterns exist. First, multifactorial congenital malformations tend to involve a single organ or tissue derived from the same embryonic developmental field. Second, the risk of recurrence in future pregnancies is for the same or a similar defect. This means that parents of a child with a cleft palate defect have an increased risk of having another child with a cleft palate, but not with spina bifida. Third, the increased risk (compared with the general population) among first-degree relatives of the affected person is 2% to 7%, and among second-degree relatives, it is approximately one-half that amount.[4] The risk increases with increasing incidence of the defect among relatives. This means that the risk is greatly increased when a second child with the defect is born to a couple. The risk also increases with severity of the disorder and when the defect occurs in the sex not usually affected by the disorder.

Cleft Lip and Cleft Palate

Cleft lip with or without cleft palate is one of the most common birth defects.[25–28] It is also one of the more conspicuous, resulting in an abnormal facial appearance and defective speech. The incidence varies among ethnic groups, ranging from 2 per 1000 live births among Native Americans and Asians, 1 per 1000 among people of European ancestry, to 1 per 2500 among Africans.[27] Cleft lip with or without cleft palate is more frequent among boys, whereas isolated cleft palate is twice as common among girls.

Developmentally, the defect has its origin at about the 35th day of gestation when the frontal prominences of the craniofacial structures fuse with the maxillary process to form the upper lip.[2] This process is under the control of many genes, and disturbances in gene expression (hereditary or environmental) at this time may result in cleft lip with or without cleft palate (Fig. 6-7). The defect may also be caused by teratogens (e.g., rubella, anticonvulsant drugs) and is often encountered in children with chromosomal abnormalities.

Cleft lip and palate defects may vary from a small notch in the vermilion border of the upper lip to complete separation involving the palate and extending into the floor of the nose. The clefts may be unilateral or bilateral and may involve the alveolar ridge. The condition may be accompanied by deformed, supernumerary, or absent teeth. Isolated cleft palate occurs in the midline and may involve only the uvula or may extend into or through the soft and hard palates.

Children with cleft lip or palate commonly have problems with feeding and speech. The immediate problem in an infant with cleft palate is feeding. Nursing at the breast or nipple depends on suction developed by pressing the nipple against the hard palate with the tongue. Although infants with cleft lip usually have no problems with feeding, those with cleft palate usually require specially constructed, soft artificial nipples with large openings and a squeezable bottle. A specially constructed plastic obturator that fits over the palate defect may be used to facilitate sucking for some infants.[25] Cleft lip and palate can also cause speech defects. The muscles of the soft palate and the lateral and posterior walls of the nasopharynx constitute a valve that separates the nasopharynx from the oropharynx during swallowing and in the production of certain vocal sounds such as *p, b, d, t, h,* and *y,* or the sibilants *s, sh,* and *ch.*

A child with cleft lip or palate may require years of special treatment by health care professionals, including a plastic surgeon, pediatric dentist, orthodontist, speech therapist, and nurse specialist.[25] Surgical closure of the lip is usually performed by 3 months of age, with closure of the palate usually done before 1 year of age. Depending on the extent of the defect, additional surgery may be required as the child grows. Displacement of the maxillary arches and malposition of the teeth usually require orthodontic correction.

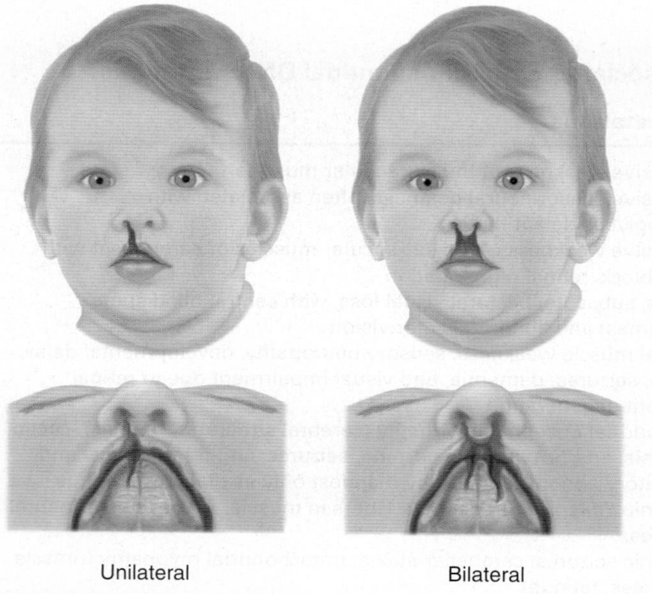

Unilateral   Bilateral

FIGURE 6-7. Cleft lip and cleft palate.

SUMMARY CONCEPTS

■ Genetic disorders can be caused by single gene (mendelian) or multiple gene (polygenic) inheritance. In single gene disorders the defective gene may be present on an autosome or on the X chromosome and they may be expressed as a dominant or recessive trait. In *autosomal dominant disorders,* a single mutant allele from an affected parent is transmitted to an offspring regardless of sex. The affected parent has a 50% chance of transmitting the disorder to each offspring. *Autosomal recessive disorders* are manifested only when both members of the gene pair are affected. Usually, both parents are unaffected but are carriers of the defective gene. Their chances of having an affected child are one in four.

- Sex-linked disorders, which are associated with the X chromosome, are those in which an unaffected mother carries one normal and one mutant allele on the X chromosome. She has a 50% chance of transmitting the defective gene to her sons, who are affected, and her daughters, who are carriers. Because of a normal paired gene, female heterozygotes rarely experience the effects of a defective gene.

- Several genetic disorders do not follow the mendelian pattern of inheritance. These include diseases caused by genomic imprinting, triplet repeat mutations, and mutations in mitochondrial genes. The fragile X syndrome is an inherited form of mental retardation that results from a repeating sequence of three (CGG) nucleotides on a fragile site on the long arm of the X chromosome. Disorders of mitochondrial DNA, which are inherited from the mother, interfere with production of cellular energy. The nervous system, and heart and skeletal muscles, which have a high need for cellular energy, tend to be the most seriously affected.

- Multifactorial inheritance disorders are caused by multiple genes and, in many cases, environmental factors. Although they cannot be predicted with the same accuracy as single-gene disorders, they tend to involve a single organ or tissue derived from the same embryonic developmental field. Cleft lip and cleft palate are common examples.

Chromosomal Disorders

Chromosomal disorders form a major category of genetic disease, accounting for a large proportion of reproductive wastage (early gestational abortions), congenital malformations, and intellectual disability. Specific chromosomal abnormalities can be linked to more than 60 identifiable syndromes that are present in 0.7% of all live births, 2% of all pregnancies in women older than 35 years of age, and 50% of all first-term abortions.[2]

During cell division (i.e., mitosis) in nongerm cells, the chromosomes replicate so that each cell receives a full diploid number. In germ cells, a different form of division (i.e., meiosis) takes place (see Chapter 5). During meiosis, the double sets of 22 autosomes and the two sex chromosomes (normal diploid number) are reduced to single sets (haploid number) in each gamete. At the time of conception, the haploid number in the ovum and that in the sperm join and restore the diploid number of chromosomes.

Occasionally, mitotic errors during cleavage of the fertilized ovum or in somatic cells give rise to two or more cell lines characterized by distinctive karyotypes, a condition referred to as *mosaicism*. Sometimes mosaicism consists of an abnormal karyotype and a normal one, in which case the physical deformities caused by the abnormal cell line usually are less severe.

Chromosomal abnormalities are commonly identified according to the shorthand description of the karyotype. In this system, the total number of chromosomes is given first, followed by the sex chromosome complement, and then the description of any abnormality. For example, a male with trisomy 21 is designated 47,XY,+21.

Structural Chromosomal Abnormalities

Aberrations in chromosome structure occur when there is a break in one or more of the chromosomes followed by rearrangement or deletion of the chromosome parts.[1-4] Among the factors believed to cause chromosome breakage are exposure to radiation sources, such as x-rays; influence of certain chemicals; extreme changes in the cellular environment; and viral infections. Several patterns of chromosome breakage and rearrangement can occur (Fig. 6-8). There can be a *deletion* of the broken portion of the chromosome. One of the most common deletion disorders is 22q11.2 deletion syndrome (to be discussed). When one chromosome is involved, the broken parts may be inverted. *Isochromosome formation* occurs when the centromere, or central portion, of the chromosome separates horizontally instead of vertically. *Ring formation* results from a break involving both ends of a chromosome, deletion of the outermost fragments, and joining of the remaining centric portion of the chromatids to form a ring. *Translocation* occurs when there are simultaneous breaks in two chromosomes from different pairs, with exchange of chromosome parts. With a balanced reciprocal translocation, no genetic information is lost; therefore, persons with translocations usually are normal. However, these persons are translocation carriers and may have normal and abnormal children.

A special form of translocation called a *centric fusion* or *Robertsonian translocation* involves two chromosomes in which the centromere is near the end, most commonly chromosomes 13 and 14 or 14 and 21. Typically, the break occurs near the centromere, affecting the short arm in one chromosome and the long arm in the other. Transfer of the chromosome fragments leads to one unusually long and one extremely short fragment. The short fragment is usually lost during subsequent divisions. In this case, the person has only 45 chromosomes, but the amount of genetic material that is lost is so small that it often goes unnoticed. The chief clinical importance of this type of translocation is that carriers of a robertsonian translocation involving chromosome 21 are at risk for producing a child with Down syndrome (to be discussed).

The manifestations of aberrations in chromosome structure depend to a great extent on the amount of genetic material that is lost. Many cells sustaining

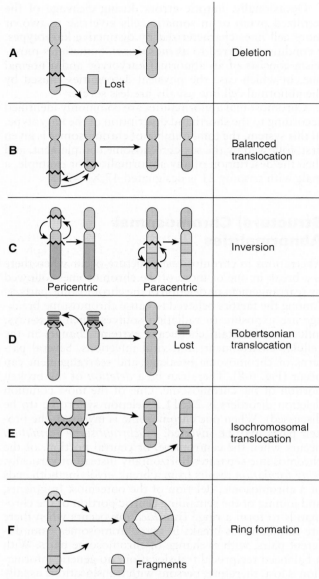

A Deletion
Lost

B Balanced translocation

C Inversion
Pericentric — Paracentric

D Robertsonian translocation
Lost

E Isochromosomal translocation

F Ring formation
Fragments

FIGURE 6-8. Structural abnormalities in the human chromosome. **(A)** Deletion of part of a chromosome leads to loss of genetic material and shortening of the chromosome. **(B)** A reciprocal translocation involves two nonhomologous chromosomes, with exchange of the acentric segment. **(C)** Inversion requires two breaks in a single chromosome, with inversion to the opposite side of the centromere (pericentric) or with the fragment inverting but remaining on the same arm (paracentric). **(D)** In robertsonian translocation, two nonhomologous acrocentric chromosomes break near their centromeres, after which the long arms fuse to form one large metacentric chromosome. **(E)** Isochromosomes arise from faulty centromere division, which leads to duplication of the long arm and deletion of the short arm, or the reverse. **(F)** A ring chromosome with breaks in both telomeric portions of a chromosome, deletion of acentric fragments, and fusion of the remaining centric portion. (Adapted from Peiper S, Strayer DS. In: Rubin R, Strayer DS, eds. *Rubin's Pathology: Clinicopathologic Foundations of Medicine.* 6th ed. Philadelphia, PA: Wolters Kluwer Health/Lippincott Williams & Wilkins; 2012:223.)

unrestored breaks are eliminated within the next few mitoses because of deficiencies that may in themselves be fatal. This is beneficial because it prevents the damaged cells from becoming a permanent part of the organism or, if it occurs in the gametes, from giving rise to grossly defective, nonviable zygotes. Some altered chromosomes, such as those that occur with translocations, are passed on to the next generation.

22q11.2 Deletion Syndrome

The 22q11.2 deletion syndrome (22q11.2 DS) is a particularly common inheritable deletion syndrome.[1] This autosomal dominant disease is caused by the deletion of a small piece of chromosome 22 and is characterized by a wide range of clinical phenotypes. While overall phenotypic penetrance for 22q11.2 DS is very high among deleted individuals, there are often marked phenotypic differences (variable expressivity) between related individuals with identical 22q11.2 microdeletions.[2,4,7] Clinical findings are diverse and include psychosocial abnormalities, cognitive abnormalities, developmental delay, psychiatric illnesses, palatal abnormalities, parathyroid insufficiency, growth retardation, immune defects, congenital heart defects, renal anomalies, and abnormal craniofacial findings.[1,2,4] Due to its highly variable phenotype, 22q11.2 DS has also been known by a variety of other names, including DiGeorge syndrome, velo-cardio-facial syndrome, conotruncal anomaly face syndrome, Shprintzen syndrome, and others. The most widely used approach to diagnose a patient with suspected 22q11.2 DS relies on the fluorescent *in situ* hybridization (FISH) cytogenetic test using a probe localized to the *TUPLE1* gene. More recently, clinical cytogenetic reference labs employ microarrays that carry millions of probes to detect smaller microdeletions. The early diagnosis of 22q11.2 DS is critically important to effectively treat this disorder.

Numeric Disorders Involving Autosomes

A change in chromosome number is referred to as *aneuploidy*. Among the causes of aneuploidy is a failure of the chromosomes to separate during oogenesis or spermatogenesis. This can occur in either the autosomes or the sex chromosomes and is called *nondisjunction* (Fig. 6-9). Nondisjunction gives rise to germ cells that have an even number of chromosomes (22 or 24). The products of conception formed from this even number of chromosomes have an uneven number of chromosomes, 45 or 47. *Monosomy* refers to the presence of only one member of a chromosome pair. The defects associated with monosomy of the autosomes are severe and usually cause abortion. Monosomy of the X chromosome (45,X), or Turner syndrome, causes less severe defects. *Polysomy*, or the presence of more than two chromosomes to a set, occurs when a germ cell containing more than 23 chromosomes is involved in conception. A variety of trisomies involving autosomal chromosomes 13, 18, 21, and 22 have been described.[2,3] With the exception of trisomy 21, most of these disorders are quite uncommon.

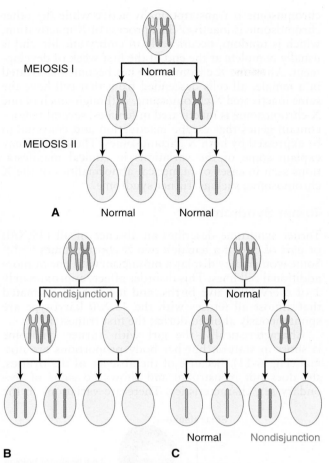

FIGURE 6-9. Nondisjunction as a cause of disorders of chromosomal numbers. **(A)** Normal distribution of chromosomes during meiosis I and II. **(B)** If nondisjunction occurs at meiosis I, the gametes contain either a pair of chromosomes or a lack of chromosomes. **(C)** If nondisjunction occurs at meiosis II, the affected gametes contain two copies of one parental chromosome or a lack of chromosomes.

Down Syndrome

First described in 1866 by John Langon Down, trisomy 21, or Down syndrome, causes a combination of birth defects including some degree of intellectual disability characteristic facial features, and other health problems.[1] According to the National Down Syndrome Association, it is the most common chromosomal disorder, occurring approximately once in every 691 births.[29]

Approximately 95% of cases of Down syndrome are caused by nondisjunction or an error in cell division during meiosis, resulting in a trisomy of chromosome 21. A rare form of Down syndrome can occur in the offspring of persons in whom there has been a Robertsonian translocation (see Fig. 6-7) in which the long arm of another chromosome (most often 14 or 22) is added to the normal long arm of chromosome 21; therefore, the person with this type of Down syndrome has 46 chromosomes, but essentially has a trisomy of 21.[2,3]

The risk of having a child with Down syndrome increases with maternal age. It begins to rise sharply at about age 30, reaching 1 in 25 births at 45 years of age.[2] The reason for the correlation between maternal age and nondisjunction is unknown, but is thought to reflect some aspect of aging of the oocyte. Although men continue to produce sperm throughout their reproductive life, women are born with all the oocytes they ever will have. These oocytes may change as a result of the aging process. With increasing age, there is a greater chance of a woman having been exposed to damaging environmental agents such as drugs, chemicals, and radiation. Unlike trisomy 21, Down syndrome due to a translocation shows no relation to maternal age.

The physical features of a child with Down syndrome are distinctive, and therefore the condition usually is apparent at birth.[1–4,29–32] These features include growth delay and a small and rather square head. There is a flatter facial profile, small nose, and somewhat depressed nasal bridge; small folds on the inner corners of the eyes (epicanthal folds) and upward slanting of the eyes; small, low-set, and malformed ears; a fat pad at the back of the neck; an open mouth; and a larger, protruding tongue (Fig. 6-10). The child's hands usually are short and stubby, with fingers that curl inward, and there usually is only a single palmar (i.e., simian) crease. There is excessive space between the large and second toe. Hypotonia and joint laxity also are present in infants and young children. There often are

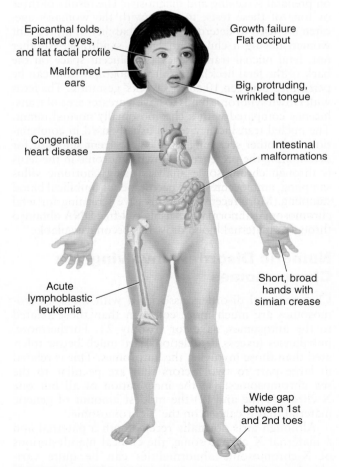

FIGURE 6-10. Clinical features of a child with Down syndrome.

accompanying congenital heart defects and an increased risk of gastrointestinal malformations. Approximately 1% of persons with trisomy 21 Down syndrome have mosaicism (i.e., cell populations with the normal chromosome number and cell populations with trisomy 21); these persons may be less severely affected. Of particular concern is the much greater risk of development of acute leukemia among children with Down syndrome—10 to 20 times greater than that of other children.[3] With increased life expectancy due to improved health care, it has also been found that there is an increased risk of Alzheimer disease among older persons with Down syndrome.

In the past few years, unprecedented breakthroughs have been made in the treatment of Down syndrome. These include the development of interventional and educational strategies to help affected individuals achieve their employment and independence goals based on their full potential. Several studies to determine safe and effective drugs to improve cognitive ability have been initiated (Down Syndrome Research and Treatment Foundation http://lumindfoundation.org/).

Several prenatal screening tests can help determine the risk of having a child with Down syndrome.[33] The most commonly used are blood tests that measure maternal serum levels of α-fetoprotein, human chorionic gonadotropin (hCG), unconjugated estriol, inhibin A, and pregnancy-associated plasma protein A (PAPP-A, see section on prenatal screening and diagnosis). The results of three or four of these tests, together with the woman's age, often are used to determine the probability of a pregnant woman having a child with Down syndrome. Another test, fetal nuchal translucency (sonolucent space on the back of the fetal neck), uses ultrasonography and can be performed between 10 and 13 weeks' gestation. The fetus with Down syndrome tends to have a greater area of translucency compared with a chromosomally normal infant. The nuchal translucency test is usually used in combination with other screening tests. The current standard for determining the presence of Down syndrome in the fetus is through chromosome analysis using chorionic villus sampling, amniocentesis, or percutaneous umbilical blood sampling. More recently, non-invasive screening for fetal chromosomal abnormalities using cell-free DNA obtained through a maternal blood draw has become available.

Numeric Disorders Involving Sex Chromosomes

Chromosomal disorders associated with the sex chromosomes are much more common than those related to the autosomes, save for trisomy 21. Furthermore, imbalances (excess or deletions) are much better tolerated than those involving the autosomes. This is related in large part to two factors that are peculiar to the sex chromosomes: (1) the inactivation of all but one X chromosome and (2) the modest amount of genetic material that is carried on the Y chromosome.

Although girls normally receive both a paternal and a maternal X chromosome, the clinical manifestations of X-chromosome abnormalities can be quite variable because in somatic cells of females only one X chromosome is transcriptionally active while the other chromosome is inactive.[1] The process of X inactivation, which is random, occurs early in embryonic life and is usually complete at the end of the first week of development. After one X chromosome has become inactivated in a female, all cells descended from that cell have the same inactivated X chromosome. Although much of one X chromosome is inactivated in females, several regions contain genes that escape inactivation and continue to be expressed by both X chromosomes. These genes may explain some of the variations in clinical manifestations seen in cases of numerical abnormalities of the X chromosome, such as Turner syndrome.

Turner Syndrome

Turner syndrome describes an absence of all (45,X/0) or part of one of a female's two X chromosomes.[2,3,34–42] Some women may display a mosaicism with one or more additional cell lines. This disorder affects approximately 1 of every 5000 live births, and it has been estimated that almost all fetuses with the 45,X/0 karyotype are spontaneously aborted during the first trimester.[2]

Characteristically, the girl with Turner syndrome is short in stature, but her body proportions are normal (Fig. 6-11). Because of the absence of the ovaries, she does not menstruate and shows no signs of secondary sex characteristics. There are variations in the

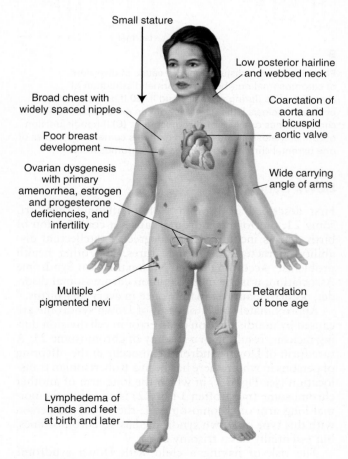

Small stature

Low posterior hairline and webbed neck

Broad chest with widely spaced nipples

Coarctation of aorta and bicuspid aortic valve

Poor breast development

Ovarian dysgenesis with primary amenorrhea, estrogen and progesterone deficiencies, and infertility

Wide carrying angle of arms

Multiple pigmented nevi

Retardation of bone age

Lymphedema of hands and feet at birth and later

FIGURE 6-11. Clinical features of Turner syndrome.

syndrome, with abnormalities ranging from essentially none to webbing of the neck with redundant skin folds, nonpitting lymphedema of the hands and feet, and congenital heart defects, particularly coarctation of the aorta and bicuspid aortic valve. There also may be abnormalities in kidney development (i.e., abnormal location, abnormal vascular supply, or double collecting system). There may be other abnormalities, such as changes in nail growth, high-arched palate, short fourth metacarpal, and strabismus. Although most women with Turner syndrome have normal intelligence, they may have problems with visuospatial organization (e.g., difficulty in driving, nonverbal problem-solving tasks such as mathematics, and psychomotor skills) and may have attention deficit disorder.

The diagnosis of Turner syndrome often is delayed until late childhood or early adolescence in girls who do not present with the classic features of the syndrome. Early diagnosis is an important aspect of treatment for Turner syndrome. It allows for counseling about the phenotypic characteristics of the disorder; screening for cardiac, renal, thyroid, and other abnormalities; and provision of emotional support for the girl and her family. Because of the potential for delay in diagnosis, it has been recommended that girls with unexplained short stature (height below the fifth percentile), webbed neck, peripheral lymphedema, coarctation of the aorta, or delayed puberty have chromosome studies done.[40]

The management of Turner syndrome begins during childhood and requires ongoing assessment and treatment. Growth hormone therapy is now standard treatment and can result in a gain of 6 to 10 cm in final height. Estrogen therapy, which is instituted around the normal age of puberty, is used to promote development and maintenance of secondary sexual characteristics.[34–36]

There are also health concerns for adult women with Turner syndrome.[34–42] Until recently, females with Turner syndrome received intensive medical care during childhood but were discharged from specialty clinics after induction of puberty and attainment of final height. It is now known that women with Turner disease have increased morbidity due to cardiovascular disease and gastrointestinal, renal, and endocrine disorders. Adults with Turner syndrome continue to have reduced bone mass, and this has been associated with increased risk of fractures.

Klinefelter Syndrome

Klinefelter syndrome is a condition of testicular dysgenesis accompanied by the presence of one or more extra X chromosomes in excess of the normal male XY complement.[2,43–47] Most males with Klinefelter syndrome have one extra X chromosome (47,XXY). In rare cases, there may be more than one extra X chromosome (48,XXXY). The presence of the extra X chromosome in the 47,XXY male results from nondisjunction during meiotic division in one of the parents.

Klinefelter syndrome is characterized by enlarged breasts, sparse facial and body hair, small testes, and the inability to produce sperm (Fig. 6-12).[45–47] Regardless

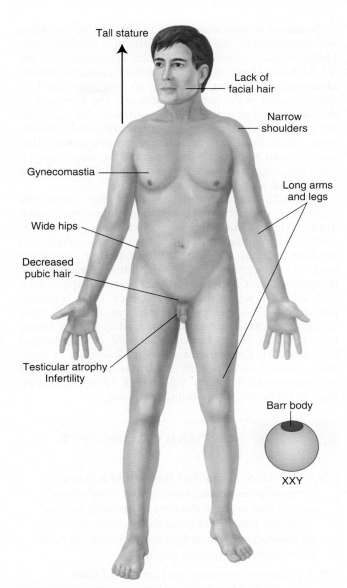

FIGURE 6-12. Clinical features of Klinefelter syndrome.

of the number of X chromosomes present, the male phenotype is retained. The condition often goes undetected at birth. The infant usually has normal male genitalia, with a small penis and small, firm testicles. At puberty, the intrinsically abnormal testes do not respond to stimulation from the gonadotropins and undergo degeneration. Low testosterone levels lead to tall stature with abnormal body proportions in which the lower part of the body is longer than the upper part. Later in life, the body build may become heavy, with a female distribution of subcutaneous fat and variable degrees of breast enlargement. There may be deficient secondary male sex characteristics, such as a voice that remains feminine in pitch and sparse beard and pubic hair. While the intellect usually is normal, most 47,XXY males have some degree of language impairment. They often learn to talk later than do other children and often have trouble with learning to read and write.

Based on studies conducted in the 1970s, including one sponsored by the National Institutes of Health and Human Development, it has been estimated that the 47,XXY syndrome is one of the most common genetic abnormalities known, occurring as frequently as 1 in 500 to 1000 male births.[32] Although the presence of the extra chromosome is fairly common, the signs and symptoms of Klinefelter syndrome are relatively uncommon. Many men live their lives without being aware that they have an additional chromosome. For this reason, it has been suggested that the term *Klinefelter syndrome* be replaced with *47,XXY male.*

Adequate management of Klinefelter syndrome requires a comprehensive neurodevelopmental evaluation. Men with Klinefelter syndrome have congenital hypogonadism, which results in inability to produce normal amounts of testosterone accompanied by an increase in hypothalamic gonadotrophic hormones (see Chapter 39). Androgen therapy is usually initiated when there is evidence of a testosterone deficit. This may begin as early as 12 to 14 years of age.[34] Because gynecomastia predisposes to breast cancer, breast self-examination should be encouraged for men with Klinefelter syndrome. Infertility is common in men with Klinefelter syndrome due to a decrease in sperm count. If sperm are present, cryopreservation may be useful for future family planning.

SUMMARY CONCEPTS

■ Chromosomal disorders result from a change in chromosome structure or number. They reflect events that occur at the time of meiosis, such as defective movement of an entire chromosome or breakage of a chromosome with loss, gain, or translocation of genetic material.

■ A change in chromosome number is called *aneuploidy. Monosomy* involves the presence of only one member of a chromosome pair as is seen in Turner syndrome, in which there is monosomy of the X chromosome in females. *Polysomy* refers to the presence of more than two chromosomes in a set, as occurs in Klinefelter syndrome, which involves polysomy of the X chromosome in males. Trisomy 21 (i.e., Down syndrome) is the most common disorder of the autosomal chromosomes, and occurs in both sexes.

Disorders Due to Environmental Influences

The developing embryo is subject to many nongenetic influences. After conception, development is influenced by the environmental factors that the embryo shares with the mother. The physiologic status of the mother—her hormone balance, her general state of health, her nutritional status, and the drugs she takes—undoubtedly influences fetal development. For example, diabetes mellitus is associated with increased risk of congenital anomalies. Smoking is associated with lower than normal neonatal weight. Alcohol consumption can cause fetal abnormalities. Some agents cause early abortion. Measles and other infectious agents cause congenital malformations. Other agents, such as radiation, can cause chromosomal and genetic defects and produce developmental disorders. Chart 6-1 lists some common agents.

Period of Vulnerability

The embryo's development is most easily disturbed during the period when differentiation and development of the organs are taking place. This time interval, which is often referred to as the period of *organogenesis*, extends from day 15 to day 60 after conception. Environmental influences during the first 2 weeks after fertilization may interfere with implantation and result in abortion or early resorption of the products of conception. Each organ has a critical period during which it is highly susceptible to environmental derangements[2,3,48] (Fig. 6-13). Often, the effect is expressed at the biochemical level just before the organ begins to develop. The same agent may affect different organ systems that are developing at the same time.

Teratogenic Agents

A teratogenic agent is an environmental agent that produces abnormalities during embryonic or fetal development. Maternal disease or altered metabolic state also can affect the environment of the embryo or fetus. Theoretically, environmental agents can cause birth defects in three ways: by direct exposure of the pregnant woman and the embryo or fetus to the agent; through exposure of the soon-to-be-pregnant woman with an agent that has a slow clearance rate such that a teratogenic dose is retained during early pregnancy; or as a result of mutagenic effects of an environmental agent that occur before pregnancy, causing permanent damage to a woman's (or a man's) reproductive cells. The developing embryo is subject to many nongenetic influences. After conception, development is influenced by the environmental factors that the embryo shares with the mother.

Radiation

Radiation is teratogenic and mutagenic, and there is the possibility of effecting inheritable changes in genetic materials. Heavy doses of ionizing radiation have been shown to cause microcephaly, skeletal malformations, and intellectual disability. There is no evidence that diagnostic levels of radiation cause congenital abnormalities. Because the question of safety remains, however, many agencies require that the day of a woman's last menstrual

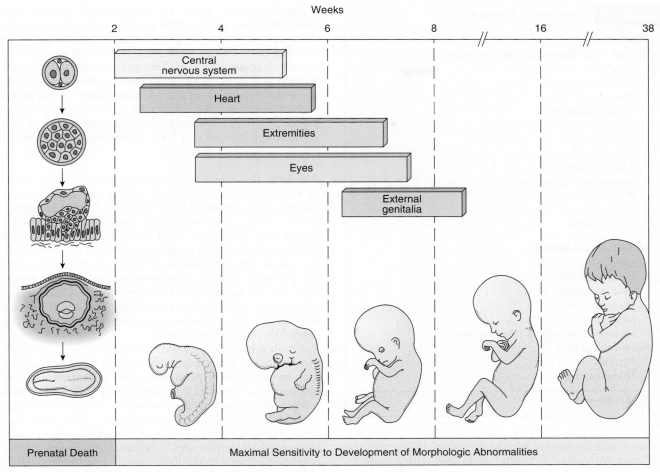

FIGURE 6-13. Sensitivity of specific organs to teratogenic agents at critical periods in embryogenesis. Exposure of adverse influences in the preimplantation and early postimplantation stages of development (*far left*) leads to prenatal death. Periods of maximal sensitivity to teratogens (*horizontal bars*) vary for different organ systems, but overall are limited to the first 8 weeks of pregnancy. (From Peiper S, Strayer DS. In: Rubin R, Strayer DS, eds. *Rubin's Pathology: Clinicopathologic Foundations of Medicine*. 6th ed. Philadelphia, PA: Wolters Kluwer Health/Lippincott Williams & Wilkins; 2012:216.)

period be noted on all radiologic requisitions. Other institutions may require a pregnancy test before any extensive diagnostic x-ray studies are performed. Administration of therapeutic doses of radioactive iodine (^{131}I) during the 13th week of gestation, the time when the fetal thyroid is beginning to concentrate iodine, has been shown to interfere with thyroid development.

Environmental Chemicals and Drugs

Environmental chemicals and drugs can cross the placenta and cause damage to the developing embryo and fetus. Some of the best-documented environmental teratogens are the organic mercurials, which cause neurologic deficits and blindness. Sources of exposure to mercury include contaminated food (fish) and water.[49] The precise mechanism by which chemicals and drugs exert their teratogenic effects is largely unknown. They may produce cytotoxic (cell-killing), antimetabolic, or

growth-inhibiting properties. Often their effects depend on the time of exposure (in terms of embryonic and fetal development) and extent of exposure (dosage).[48]

Medications and Illicit Drugs. Drugs top the list of chemical teratogens, probably because they are regularly used at elevated doses. Many drugs can cross the placenta and expose the fetus to both pharmacologic and teratogenic effects. Factors that affect placental drug transfer and drug effects on the fetus include the rate at which the drug crosses the placenta, the duration of exposure, and the stage of placental and fetal development at the time of exposure.[50] Lipid-soluble drugs tend to cross the placenta more readily and enter the fetal circulation. The molecular weight of a drug also influences the rate of transfer and the amount of drug transferred across the placenta. Drugs with a molecular weight of less than 500 can cross the placenta easily, depending on lipid solubility and degree of ionization;

CHART 6-1 **Teratogenic Agents***

Radiation

Drugs and Chemical Substances
   Alcohol
   Anticoagulants
   Warfarin
   Anticonvulsants
   Cancer drugs
   Aminopterin
   Methotrexate
   6-Mercaptopurine
   Isotretinoin (Accutane)
   Propylthiouracil
   Tetracycline
   Thalidomide

Infectious Agents
Viruses
   Cytomegalovirus
   Herpes simplex virus
   Measles (rubella)
   Mumps
   Varicella-zoster virus (chickenpox)
Nonviral factors
   Syphilis
   Toxoplasmosis

*Not inclusive.

those with a molecular weight of 500 to 1000 cross the placenta with more difficulty; and those with a molecular weight of more than 1000 cross very poorly.

A number of drugs are suspected of being teratogens, but only a few have been identified with certainty. Perhaps the best known of these drugs is thalidomide, which has been shown to give rise to a full range of malformations, including phocomelia (i.e., short, flipperlike appendages) of all four extremities.[2] Other drugs known to cause fetal abnormalities are the antimetabolites that are used in the treatment of cancer, the anticoagulant drug warfarin, several of the anticonvulsant drugs, ethyl alcohol, and cocaine. More recently, vitamin A and its derivatives (the retinoids) have been targeted for concern because of their teratogenic potential. Concern over the teratogenic effects of vitamin A derivatives became evident with the introduction of the acne drug isotretinoin (Accutane). Fetal abnormalities such as cleft palate, heart defects, retinal and optic nerve abnormalities, and central nervous system malformations were observed in women ingesting therapeutic doses of the drug during the first trimester of pregnancy.[51]

In 1979, the U.S. Food and Drug Administration established a system for classifying drugs according to probable risks to the fetus. This system classifies all drugs approved after 1983 into five pregnancy risk categories: A, B, C, D, and X. Drugs in category A are the least dangerous, and categories B, C, and D are increasingly more dangerous. Those in category X are contraindicated during pregnancy because of proven teratogenicity.[50]

Because many drugs are suspected of causing fetal abnormalities, and even those that were once thought to be safe are now being viewed critically, it is recommended that women in their childbearing years avoid unnecessary use of drugs. This pertains to nonpregnant women as well as pregnant women because many developmental defects occur early in pregnancy. As happened with thalidomide, the damage to the embryo may occur before pregnancy is suspected or confirmed. A drug that is often abused and can have deleterious effects on the fetus is alcohol.

Alcohol. The term fetal alcohol syndrome (FAS) refers to a constellation of physical, behavioral, and cognitive abnormalities resulting from maternal alcohol consumption.[52-56] It has been estimated that out of the 4 million babies born each year, 4000 to 6000 will be born with FAS.[2] Alcohol, which is lipid soluble and has a molecular weight between 600 and 1000, passes freely across the placental barrier; concentrations of alcohol in the fetus are at least as high as in the mother. Unlike other teratogens, alcohol exerts harmful effects that are not restricted to the sensitive period of early gestation but extend throughout pregnancy.

Alcohol has widely variable effects on fetal development, ranging from minor abnormalities to FAS. There may be prenatal or postnatal growth retardation; central nervous system (CNS) involvement, including neurologic abnormalities, developmental delays, behavioral dysfunction, intellectual impairment, and skull and brain malformation; and the characteristic set of facial features that include small palpebral fissures (i.e., eye openings), a thin vermillion (upper lip), and an elongated, flattened midface and philtrum (i.e., the groove in the middle of the upper lip) (Fig. 6-14). The facial features of FAS may not be as apparent in the newborn but become more prominent as the infant develops. As the children grow into adulthood, the facial features become more subtle, making diagnosis of FAS in older

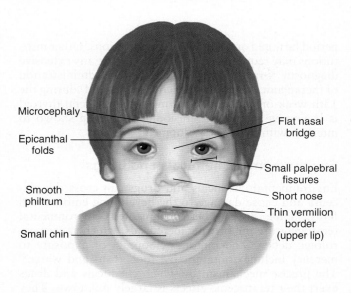

FIGURE 6-14. Clinical features of fetal alcohol syndrome.

individuals more difficult. Each of these defects can vary in severity, probably reflecting the timing of alcohol consumption in terms of the period of fetal development, amount of alcohol consumed, and hereditary and environmental influences.

In 2004, the National Task Force on Fetal Alcohol Syndrome and Fetal Alcohol Effects published guidelines for the referral and diagnosis of FAS.[52] The criteria for FAS diagnosis require the documented presence of three of the following findings: (1) three facial abnormalities (smooth philtrum, thin vermillion, and small palpebral fissures), (2) growth deficits (prenatal or postnatal height or weight, or both, below the 10th percentile), and (3) CNS abnormalities (e.g., head circumference below 10th percentile, global cognitive or intellectual deficits, motor functioning delays, problems with attention or hyperactivity).

The amount of alcohol that can be safely consumed during pregnancy is unknown. Even small amounts of alcohol consumed during critical periods of fetal development may be teratogenic. For example, if alcohol is consumed during the period of organogenesis, a variety of skeletal and organ defects may result. When alcohol is consumed later in gestation, when the brain is undergoing rapid development, there may be behavioral and cognitive disorders in the absence of physical abnormalities. Chronic alcohol consumption throughout pregnancy may result in a variety of effects, ranging from physical abnormalities to growth retardation and compromised CNS functioning. Evidence suggests that short-lived high concentrations of alcohol such as those that occur with binge drinking may be particularly significant, with abnormalities being unique to the period of exposure. Because of the possible effect on the fetus, it is recommended that women abstain from alcohol during pregnancy.

Infectious Agents

Many microorganisms cross the placenta and enter the fetal circulation, often producing multiple malformations. The acronym *TORCH* stands for *t*oxoplasmosis, *o*ther, *r*ubella (i.e., German measles), *c*ytomegalovirus, and *her*pes, which are the agents most frequently implicated in fetal anomalies.[2] Other infections include varicella-zoster virus infection, listeriosis, leptospirosis, Epstein-Barr virus infection, and syphilis. Human immunodeficiency virus (HIV) and human parvovirus (B19) have been suggested as additions to the list. The TORCH screening test examines the infant's serum for the presence of antibodies to these agents. These infections tend to cause similar clinical manifestations, including microcephaly, hydrocephalus, defects of the eye, and hearing problems.

Toxoplasmosis is a protozoal infection caused by *Toxoplasma gondii*. The infection can be contracted by eating raw or inadequately cooked meat or food that has come in contact with infected meat.[57] The domestic cat can carry the organism, excreting the protozoa in its feces. It has been suggested that pregnant women should avoid contact with excrement from the family cat. Although the introduction of the rubella vaccine has

virtually eliminated congenital rubella syndrome in most developed countries, it remains endemic in many developing countries, where it is the major preventable cause of hearing impairment, blindness, and adverse neurodevelopmental outcome. The epidemiology of cytomegalovirus infection is largely unknown. Some infants are severely affected at birth, and others, although having evidence of the infection, have no symptoms. In some symptom-free infants, brain damage becomes evident over a span of several years. There also is evidence that some infants contract the infection during the first year of life, and in some of them the infection leads to retardation a year or two later. Herpes simplex virus type 2 infection is considered to be a genital infection and usually is transmitted through sexual contact. The infant acquires this infection in utero or in passage through the birth canal.

Nutrient Deficiencies

Although most birth defects are related to exposure to a teratogenic agent, deficiencies of nutrients and vitamins also may be a factor. Folic acid deficiency has been implicated in the development of neural tube defects (e.g., anencephaly, spina bifida, encephalocele). Studies have shown a reduction in neural tube defects when folic acid was taken before conception and continued during the first trimester of pregnancy.[58,59] The Public Health Service recommends that all women of childbearing age should receive 400 micrograms (µg) of folic acid daily. These recommendations are particularly important for women who have previously had an affected pregnancy, for couples with a close relative with the disorder, and for women with diabetes mellitus and those taking anticonvulsant drugs who are at increased risk for having infants with birth defects.

Since 1998, all enriched cereal grain products in the United States have been fortified with folic acid. To achieve an adequate intake of folic acid, pregnant women should couple a diet that contains folate-rich foods (e.g., orange juice; dark, leafy green vegetables; and legumes) with sources of synthetic folic acid, such as fortified food products.[58]

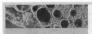 **SUMMARY CONCEPTS**

■ Teratogenic agents such as radiation, chemicals and drugs, and infectious organisms produce abnormalities in the developing embryo.

■ The stage of development of the embryo determines the susceptibility to teratogens. The period during which the embryo is most susceptible to teratogenic agents is the time during which rapid differentiation and development of body organs and tissues are taking place, usually from days 15 to 60 postconception.

(continued)

SUMMARY CONCEPTS *(continued)*

■ A number of environmental agents can be damaging to the unborn child, including radiation, environmental pollutants such as mercury, medications and illicit drugs, alcohol, and infectious agents. Because many of these agents have the potential for causing fetal abnormalities, often at an early stage of pregnancy, it is recommended that women of childbearing age avoid all unnecessary use of drugs and abstain from alcohol.

■ The acronym TORCH stands for *t*oxoplasmosis, *o*ther, *r*ubella, *c*ytomegalovirus, and *h*erpes, which are the infectious agents most frequently implicated in fetal anomalies.

■ It also has been shown that maternal folic acid deficiency can contribute to neural tube defects, and iodine deficiency can cause congenital hypothyroidism and impaired neurological development (cretinism).

Prenatal Screening and Diagnosis

The purpose of prenatal screening and diagnosis is not just to detect fetal abnormalities. Rather, it has the following objectives: to provide parents with information needed to make an informed choice about having a child with an abnormality; to provide reassurance and reduce anxiety among high-risk groups; and to allow parents at risk for having a child with a specific defect, who might otherwise forgo having a child, to begin a pregnancy with the assurance that knowledge about the presence or absence of the disorder in the fetus can be confirmed by testing.[1] Prenatal screening cannot be used to rule out all possible fetal abnormalities. It is limited to determining whether the fetus has (or probably has) designated conditions indicated by late maternal age, family history, or well-defined risk factors.

Screening and Diagnostic Methods

Among the methods used for prenatal screening and diagnosis are ultrasonography, maternal serum (blood) screening tests, amniocentesis, chorionic villus sampling, and percutaneous umbilical fetal blood sampling[1,33,60] (Fig. 6-15). Amniocentesis, chorionic villus sampling, percutaneous umbilical cord blood sampling, and fetal biopsy are invasive procedures that carry a small risk for the fetus.

Ultrasonography

Ultrasonography is a non-invasive diagnostic method that uses reflections of high-frequency sound waves to visualize soft tissue structures. Since its introduction

in 1958, it has been used during pregnancy to determine the number of fetuses, fetal size and position, the amount of amniotic fluid, and placental location. It also is possible to assess fetal movement, breathing movements, and heart pattern. There is also good evidence that early ultrasonography (i.e., before 14 weeks) accurately determines gestational age.

Improved resolution and real-time units have enhanced the ability of ultrasound scanners to detect congenital anomalies. With this more sophisticated equipment, it is possible to obtain information such as measurements of hourly urine output in a high-risk fetus. Ultrasonography makes possible the in-utero diagnosis of hydrocephalus, spina bifida, facial defects, congenital heart defects, congenital diaphragmatic hernias, disorders of the gastrointestinal tract, and skeletal anomalies. Cardiovascular abnormalities are the most commonly missed malformation. A four-chamber view of the fetal heart improves the detection of cardiac malformations. Intrauterine diagnosis of congenital abnormalities permits planning of surgical correction shortly after birth, preterm delivery for early correction, selection of cesarean section to reduce fetal injury, and, in some cases, intrauterine therapy. When a congenital abnormality is suspected, a diagnosis made using ultrasonography usually can be obtained by weeks 16 to 18 of gestation.

Maternal Serum Markers

Maternal blood testing began in the early 1980s with the test for α-fetoprotein (AFP). Since that time, many serum factors have been studied as screening tests for fetal anomalies. Current maternal testing uses three distinct tests (AFP, human chorionic gonadotropin [hCG], and unconjugated estriol) to screen for trisomy syndromes in low-risk women while incorporating the detection of neural tube defects.[61] The combined use of the three maternal serum markers between 15 and 22 weeks of pregnancy has been shown to detect as many as 60% of Down syndrome pregnancies.[1] The use of ultrasound to verify fetal age can reduce the number of false-positive tests with this screening method.

α-Fetoprotein is a major fetal plasma protein and has a structure similar to the albumin that is found in postnatal life. AFP is made initially by the yolk sac, gastrointestinal tract, and liver. Fetal plasma levels peak at approximately 10 to 13 weeks' gestation and then decline progressively until term, while maternal levels peak in the third trimester.[47] Maternal and amniotic fluid levels of AFP are elevated in pregnancies where the fetus has a neural tube defect (i.e., anencephaly and open spina bifida) or certain other malformations such as an anterior abdominal wall defect in which the fetal integument is not intact. Screening of maternal blood samples usually is done between weeks 16 and 18 of gestation.[1,61] Although neural tube defects have been associated with elevated levels of AFP, decreased levels have been associated with Down syndrome.

A complex glycoprotein, hCG is produced exclusively by the outer layer of the trophoblast shortly after

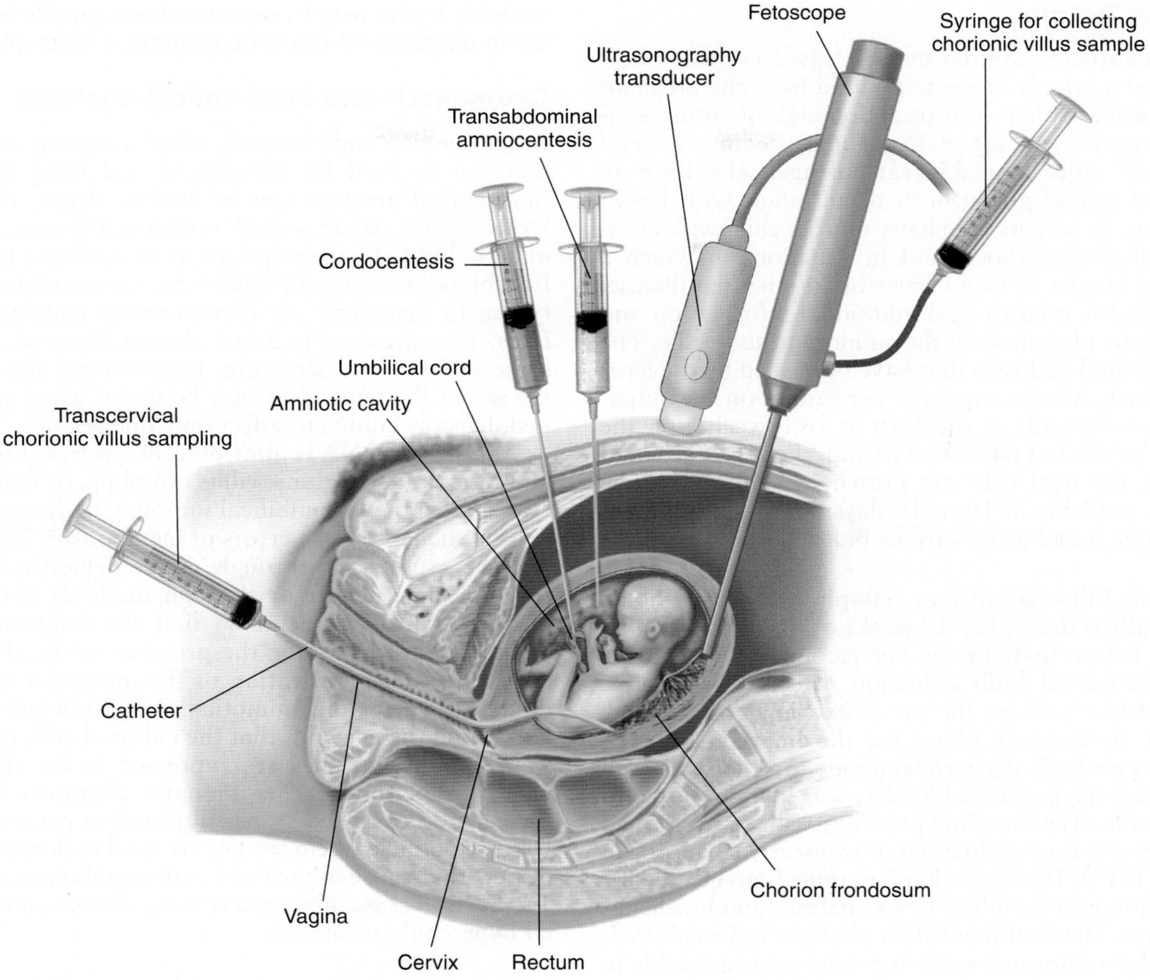

FIGURE 6-15. Methods of prenatal screening.

implantation in the uterine wall. It increases rapidly in the first 8 weeks of gestation, declines steadily until 20 weeks, and then plateaus. The single maternal serum marker that yields the highest detection rate for Down syndrome is an elevated level of hCG.

Unconjugated estriol is produced by the placenta from precursors provided by the fetal adrenal glands and liver. It increases steadily throughout pregnancy to a higher level than that normally produced by the liver. Unconjugated estriol levels are decreased in Down syndrome and trisomy 18.

Other maternal serum markers include pregnancy-associated plasma protein A (PAPP-A) and inhibin A.[62] PAPP-A, which is secreted by the placenta, has been shown to play an important role in promoting cell differentiation and proliferation in various body systems. In complicated pregnancies, the PAPP-A concentration increases with gestational age until term. Decreased PAPP-A levels in the first trimester (between 10 to 13 weeks) have been shown to be associated with Down syndrome. When used along with maternal age, free β-hCG, and ultrasound measurement of nuchal translucency, serum PAPP-A levels can reportedly detect

85% to 95% of affected pregnancies with a false-positive rate of approximately 5%.[62] Inhibin A, which is secreted by the corpus luteum and fetoplacental unit, is also a maternal serum marker for fetal Down syndrome.[63]

Non-Invasive Prenatal Testing (NIPT)

Circulating cell free DNA (cf-DNA) fragments are short fragments of DNA found in the blood. During pregnancy, there are cf-DNA fragments from both the mother and fetus in maternal circulation. It is possible to analyze cf-DNA from the maternal blood to detect common fetal trisomies such as Down syndrome as early as 10 weeks. Non-invasive prenatal testing using cf-DNA offers tremendous potential as a screening tool due to its increased accuracy over maternal serum markers and the nuchal translucency tests.[64] The recent and rapid adoption of non-invasive prenatal screening in high-risk pregnancies in the United States suggests that NIPT may change the standard of care for genetic screening (ACOG 2013).[11]

Invasive Testing

Amniocentesis. Amniocentesis involves the withdrawal of a sample of amniotic fluid from the pregnant uterus using either a transabdominal or transcervical approach[65] (see Fig. 6-15). The procedure is useful in women older than 35 years of age, who have an increased risk of giving birth to an infant with Down syndrome; in parents who have another child with chromosomal abnormalities; and in situations in which a parent is known to be a carrier of an inherited disease. Ultrasound is used to gain additional information and to guide the placement of the amniocentesis needle. The amniotic fluid and cells that have been shed by the fetus are studied. Amniocentesis is performed on an outpatient basis typically at the 15th to 16th week after the first day of the last menstrual period.[1] For chromosomal analysis, the fetal cells are grown in culture and the result is available in 10 to 14 days. The amniotic fluid also can be tested using various biochemical tests.

Chorionic Villus Sampling. Sampling of the chorionic villi usually is done after 10 weeks of gestation.[65] Doing the test before that time is not recommended because of the danger of limb reduction defects in the fetus. The chorionic villi are the site of exchange of nutrients between the maternal blood and the embryo—the chorionic sac encloses the early amniotic sac and fetus, and the villi are the primitive blood vessels that develop into the placenta. The sampling procedure can be performed using either a transabdominal or transcervical approach (see Fig. 6-15). The tissue that is obtained can be used for fetal chromosome studies, DNA analysis, and biochemical studies. The fetal tissue does not have to be cultured, and fetal chromosome analysis can be made available in 24 hours. Deoxyribonucleic acid analysis and biochemical tests can be completed within 1 to 2 weeks.

Percutaneous Umbilical Cord Blood Sampling. Percutaneous umbilical cord blood sampling involves the transcutaneous insertion of a needle through the uterine wall and into the umbilical artery. It is performed under ultrasound guidance and can be done any time after 16 weeks of gestation. It is used for prenatal diagnosis of hemoglobinopathies, coagulation disorders, metabolic and cytogenetic disorders, and immunodeficiencies. Fetal infections such as rubella and toxoplasmosis can be detected through measurement of immunoglobulin M antibodies or direct blood cultures. Results from cytogenetic studies usually are available within 48 to 72 hours. Because the procedure carries a greater risk of pregnancy loss than amniocentesis, it usually is reserved for situations in which rapid cytogenetic analysis is needed or in which diagnostic information cannot be obtained by other methods.

Fetal Biopsy. Fetal biopsy is done with a fetoscope under ultrasound guidance. It is used to detect certain genetic skin defects that cannot be diagnosed with DNA analysis. It also may be done to obtain muscle tissue for use in diagnosis of Duchenne muscular dystrophy.

Cytogenetic and Biochemical Analyses

Amniocentesis and chorionic villus sampling yield cells that can be used for cytogenetic and DNA analyses. Biochemical analyses can be used to detect abnormal levels of AFP and abnormal biochemical products in the maternal blood and in specimens of amniotic fluid and fetal blood. Cytogenetic studies are used for fetal karyotyping to determine the chromosomal makeup of the fetus. They are done to detect abnormalities of chromosome number and structure. Karyotyping also reveals the sex of the fetus. This may be useful when an inherited defect is known to affect only one sex.

Analysis of DNA is done on cells extracted from the amniotic fluid, chorionic villus sampling, or fetal blood from percutaneous umbilical sampling to detect genetic defects such as inborn errors of metabolism. The defect may be established through direct demonstration of the molecular defect or through methods that break the DNA into fragments so that the fragments may be studied to determine the presence of an abnormal gene. Direct demonstration of the molecular defect is done by growing the amniotic fluid cells in culture and measuring the enzymes that the cultured cells produce. Many of the enzymes are expressed in the chorionic villi; this permits earlier prenatal diagnosis because the cells do not need to be subjected to prior culture. Deoxyribonucleic acid studies are used to detect genetic defects that cause inborn errors of metabolism, such as Tay-Sachs disease, glycogen storage diseases, and familial hypercholesterolemia.

SUMMARY CONCEPTS

■ Prenatal diagnosis includes the use of ultrasonography, maternal blood screening, amniocentesis, chorionic villus sampling, and percutaneous umbilical fetal blood sampling.

■ Ultrasonography is used for determination of fetal size and position and for the presence of structural anomalies.

■ Maternal blood screening, which measures α-fetoprotein (AFP), unconjugated estriol, and chorionic gonadotropin (hCG), is used to assess for neural tube defects (AFP) and Down syndrome (AFP, unconjugated estriol, and hCG).

■ Amniocentesis, chorionic villus sampling, and percutaneous umbilical blood sampling are used to obtain specimens for cytogenetic and biochemical studies.

REVIEW EXERCISES

1. A 23-year-old woman with sickle cell disease and her husband want to have a child, but worry that the child will be born with the disease.

A. What is the mother's genotype in terms of the sickle cell gene? Is she heterozygous or homozygous?

B. If the husband is found not to have the sickle cell gene, what is the probability of their child having the disease or being a carrier of the sickle cell trait?

2. A couple has a child who was born with a congenital heart disease.

A. Would you consider the defect to be the result of a single-gene or a polygenic trait?

B. Would these parents be at greater risk of having another child with a heart defect, or would they be at equal risk of having a child with a defect in another organ system, such as cleft palate?

3. A couple has been informed that their newborn child has the features of Down syndrome. It was suggested that genetic studies be performed.

A. The child is found to have trisomy 21. Use Figure 6-8 to describe the events that occur during meiosis to explain the origin of the third chromosome.

B. If the child had been found to have the robertsonian chromosome, how would you explain the origin of the abnormal chromosome?

4. A 26-year-old woman is planning to become pregnant.

A. What information would you give her regarding the effects of medications and drugs on the fetus? What stage of fetal development is associated with the greatest risk?

B. What is the rationale for ensuring that she has an adequate intake of folic acid before conception?

C. She and her husband have an indoor cat. What precautions should she use in caring for the cat?

REFERENCES

1. Nassbaum RL, McInnes RR, Willard HF, et al. *Thompson & Thompson Genetics in Medicine.* 7th ed. Philadelphia, PA: Saunders Elsevier; 2007:33–94, 157–179, 359–389.

2. Pieper S, Rubin E, Strayer DS. Developmental and genetic diseases. In: Rubin R, Strayer DS, eds. *Rubin's Pathology: Clinicopathologic Foundations of Medicine.* 6th ed. Philadelphia, PA: Wolters Kluwer Health/Lippincott Williams & Wilkins; 2012:213–266.

3. Kumar V, Abbas AK, Fausto N, et al. *Robbins and Cotran Pathologic Basis of Medicine.* 8th ed. Philadelphia, PA: Saunders Elsevier; 2010:135–182.

4. Jorde LB, Carey JC, Barmshad MJ, et al. *Medical Genetics.* 3rd ed. St. Louis, MO: Mosby; 2006:57–101, 107–135, 248–278.

5. Gonzales EA. Marfan syndrome. *J Am Acad Nurse Pract.* 2009;21(12):663–670.

6. Dean JCS. Management of Marfan syndrome. *Heart* 2002;88:97–103.

7. Theos A, Korf BR. Pathophysiology of neurofibromatosis type I. *Ann Intern Med.* 2006;144(11):842–849.

8. Jouhilahi EM, Peltonen S, Heape AM, et al. The pathoetiology of neurofibromatosis 1. *Am J Pathol.* 2011;178(5):1932–1939.

9. Pasmant E, Vidaud M, Vidaud D, et al. Neurofibromatosis type 1: from genotype to phenotype. *J Med Genet.* 2012;49:483–489.

10. Yohay K. Neurofibromatosis type 1 and 2. *Neurologist.* 2006;12(2):86–93.

11. Ferner RE. Neurofibromatosis 1 and neurofibromatosis 2: a twenty first century perspective. *Lancet Neurol.* 2007;6:340–350.

12. Hoa M, Slattery WH. Neurofibromatosis 2. *Otolaryngol Clin North Am.* 2012;45(2):316–332.

13. Rezvani I, Melvin J. Phenylalanine. In: Kliegman Stamtpm BF, St. Gemille JW, et al, eds. *Nelson Textbook of Pediatrics*, 19th ed. Philadelphia, PA: Elsevier Saunders; 2011:418–421.

14. Blau N, van Spronsen FJ, Levy HI. Phenylketonuria. *Lancet.* 2010;376:1417–1427.

15. U.S. Preventative Services Task Force. *Screening for Phenylketonuria.* 2008. Available at: http://www.uspreventiveservicestaskforce.org/uspstf/uspsspku.htm. Accessed October 11, 2013.

16. Wang T, Bray SM, Warren ST. New perspectives on the biology of fragile X syndrome. *Curr Opin Genet Dev.* 2012;22(3):256–263.

17. Lubs HA, Stevenson RE, Schwartz CE. Fragile X and X-linked intellectual disability: four decades of discovery. *Am J Hum Genet.* 2012;90:S79–S90.

18. Hagerman RJ, Berry-Kravis E, Kaufmann WE, et al. Advances in treatment of fragile X syndrome. *Pediatrics.* 2009;123(1):378–390.

19. Healy A, Rush R, Ocain T. Fragile X syndrome: an update on developing treatment modalities. *ACS Chem Neurosci.* 2011;2:402–410.

20. Johns DR. Mitochondrial DNA and disease. *N Engl J Med.* 1995;333:638–644.

21. Dimauro S, Davidzon G. Mitochondrial DNA and disease. *Ann Med.* 2005;37:222–232.

22. Falk MJ, Sondheimer N. Mitochondrial genetic diseases. *Curr Opin Pediatr.* 2010;22(6):711–716.

23. McFarland R, Taylor R, Turnbull DM. A neurological perspective of mitochondrial disease. *Lancet Neurol.* 2010;9:829–840.

24. Riccardi VM. *The Genetic Approach to Human Disease.* New York, NY: Oxford University Press; 1977:92.

25. Tinanoff N. Cleft lip and palate. In: Behrman RE, Kliegman RM, Jensen HB, eds. *Nelson Textbook of Pediatrics.* 18th ed. Philadelphia, PA: Saunders Elsevier; 2011:1252–1253.

26. Mulliken JB. The changing faces of children with cleft lip and palate. *N Engl J Med.* 2004;351(8):745–747.

27. Marazita ML. The evolution of human genetic studies of cleft lip and cleft palate. *Annu Rev Genomics Hum Genet.* 2012;13:263–283.

28. Dixon MJ, Marazita ML, Beaty TH, et al. Cleft lip and palate: synthesizing genetic and environmental influences. *Nat Rev Genet.* 2011;12(3):167–178.

29. National Down Syndrome Society. *Down Syndrome Fact Sheet.* 2013. Available at: http://www.ndss.org/PageFiles/1474/NDSS%20Down%20Syndrome%20Fact%20Sheet%20English.ppt%20%5bCompatibility%20Mode%5d.pdf. Accessed October 10, 2013.

30. Roizen NJ, Patterson D. Down syndrome. *Lancet.* 2003;361: 1281–1289.

31. Weijerman ME, de Winter JP. The care of children with Down syndrome. *Eur J Pediatr.* 2010;169:1445–1452.

32. Wiseman FK, Afford KA, Tylbulewica VLJ, et al. Down syndrome—recent progress and future prospects. *Hum Mol Genet.* 2009;18:E75–E83.

33. Rappaport VJ. Prenatal diagnosis and genetic screening—integration into prenatal care. *Obstet Gynecol Clin North Am.* 2008;35:435–458.

34. Sybert VP, McCauley E. Turner's syndrome. *N Engl J Med.* 2004;351:1227–1238.

35. Morgan T. Turner syndrome: diagnosis and management. *Am Fam Physician.* 2007;76:405–410.

36. Gravholt CH. Epidemiological, endocrine and metabolic features in Turner syndrome. *Eur J Endocrinol.* 2004;151:657–687.

37. Elsheikh M, Dunger DB, Conway GS, et al. Turner syndrome in adulthood. *Endocr Rev.* 2002;21:120–140.

38. Frías JL, Davenport ML, American Academy of Pediatrics Committee on Genetics, Section on Endocrinology. Health supervision of children with Turner syndrome. *Pediatrics.* 2005;111:692–702.

39. Chacko E, Regelmann MO, Costin G. Updates on Turner and Noonan syndromes. *Endocrinol Metab Clin North Am.* 2012;41:713–734.

40. Gonxalez L, Witchel SF. The patient with Turner syndrome: puberty and medical management concerns. *Fertil Steril.* 2012;98(4):780–786.

41. Davenport ML. Approach to patient with Turner syndrome. *J Clin Endocrinol Metab.* 2010;95(4):1487–1495.

42. Pinsker JE. Turner syndrome: updating the paradigm of clinical care. *J Clin Endocrinol Metab.* 2012;97(6):E994–E1003.

43. National Institutes of Health. *Understanding Klinefelter Syndrome.* 2013. Available at: http://ghr.nlm.nih.gov/condition/klinefelter-syndrome. Accessed October 11, 2013.

44. Lanfranco F, Kamischke A, Zitzmann M, et al. Klinefelter syndrome. *Lancet.* 2004;364:273–283.

45. Wattendorf DJ, Muenke M. Klinefelter syndrome. *Am Fam Physician.* 2005;72(11):2259–2262.

46. Wikström A, Dunkel L. Klinefelter syndrome. *Best Pract Res Clin Endocrinol Metab.* 2011;25(2):239–250.

47. Groth KA, Skakkebaek A, Høst C, et al. Klinefelter syndrome—a clinical update. *J Clin Endocrinol Metab.* 2013;98(1):20–30.

48. Brent RL. Environmental causes of congenital malformations: the pediatrician's role in dealing with these complex clinical problems caused by a multiplicity of environmental and genetic factors. *Pediatrics.* 2004;113:957–968.

49. Steurerwald U, Weibe P, Jorgensen PJ, et al. Maternal seafood diet, methylmercury exposure, and neonatal neurologic function. *J Pediatr.* 2000;136:599–605.

50. Katzung BG, Masters SB, Trevor AJ. *Basic & Clinical Pharmacology.* 12th ed. New York, NY: McGraw-Hill Medical; 2013:1039–1043.

51. Ross SA, McCaffery PJ, Drager UC, et al. Retinoids in embryonal development. *Physiol Rev.* 2000;80:1021–1055.

52. Bertrand J, Floyd RL, Weber MK, et al.; for the National Task Force on Fetal Alcohol and Fetal Alcohol Effects. *Fetal Alcohol Syndromes: Guidelines for Referral and Diagnosis.* Atlanta, GA: Centers for Disease Control and Prevention; 2004.

53. Sokol RJ, Delaney-Black V, Nordstrom B. Fetal alcohol syndrome. *JAMA.* 2003;290(22):2996–2999.

54. Wattendorf DJ, Muenke M. Fetal alcohol spectrum disorders. *Am Fam Physician.* 2005;72(2):279–285.

55. Riley EP, McGee CL. Fetal alcohol spectrum disorders: an overview with emphasis on changes in brain and behavior. *Exp Biol Med.* 2005;230(6):357–365.

56. Riley EP, Infante MA, Warren KR. Fetal alcohol spectrum disorders: an overview. *Neuropsychol Rev.* 2011;21(3):75–80.

57. Centers for Disease Control and Prevention. Recommendations for use of folic acid to reduce the number of cases of spina bifida and other neural tube defects. *MMWR Morb Mortal Wkly Rep.* 1992;41:1–8.

58. Bailey LB. New standard for dietary folate intake in pregnant women. *Am J Clin Nutr.* 2000;71(Suppl):1304S–1307S.

59. Jones J, Lopez A, Wilson M. Congenital toxoplasmosis. *Am Fam Physician.* 2003;67:2131–2138.

60. Kirkham C, Harris S, Grzybowski S. Evidence-based prenatal care: part I. General prenatal care and counseling issues. *Am Fam Physician.* 2005;71(7):1307–1316.

61. Graves JC, Miller KE. Maternal serum triple analyte screening in pregnancy. *Am Fam Physician.* 2002;65(5):915–920.

62. Qin Q-P, Christiansen M, Pettersson K. Point of care time-resolved immunofluorometric assay of human pregnancy-associated plasma protein A: use in first-trimester screening for Down syndrome. *Clin Chem.* 2002;48(3):473–483.

63. Lambert-Messerlian GM, Canick JA. Clinical application of inhibin A measurement: prenatal serum screening for Down syndrome. *Semin Reprod Med.* 2004;22(3):235–242.

64. Ashoor G, Syngelaki A, Poon LCY, et al. Fetal fraction in maternal plasma cell-free DNA at 11–13 weeks' gestation: relation to maternal and fetal characteristics. *Ultrasound Obstet Gynecol.* 2013;41:26–32.

65. Wilson RD. Amniocentesis and chorionic villus sampling. *Curr Opin Obstet Gynecol.* 2000;12:81–86.

Porth Essentials Resources

Explore these additional resources to enhance learning for this chapter:

- NCLEX-Style Questions and Other Resources on **the**Point, http://thePoint.lww.com/PorthEssentials4e
- Study Guide for Essentials of Pathophysiology
- Adaptive Learning | Powered by PrepU, http://thepoint.lww.com/prepu

C h a p t e r ⁷

Neoplasia

Cancer is a major health problem in the United States and many other parts of the world. It is estimated that 1.66 million Americans were newly diagnosed with cancer in 2013 and 580,350 died of the disease.[1] Cancer affects all age groups, and is the second leading cause of death among children ages 1 to 14 years.[1] As age-adjusted cancer mortality rates increase and heart disease mortality decreases, it is predicted that cancer will soon become the leading cause of death. The good news, however, is that the survival rates have improved to the extent that almost 64% of people who develop cancer each year will be alive 5 years later.

Cancer is not a single disease. It can originate in almost any organ, with skin cancers being the most common site in persons in the United States. Excluding skin cancers, the prostate is the most common site in men and the breast is the most common site in women (Fig. 7-1). The ability of cancer to be cured varies considerably and depends on the type of cancer and the extent of the disease at the time of diagnosis. Cancers such as acute lymphoblastic leukemia, Hodgkin disease, testicular cancer, and osteosarcoma, which only a few decades ago had poor prognoses, are cured in many cases today. However, lung cancer, which is the leading cause of death in men and women in the United States,[1] remains resistant to therapy.

This chapter is divided into five sections: characteristics of benign and malignant neoplasms, etiology of cancer, clinical manifestations, diagnosis and treatment, and childhood cancers and late effects on cancer survivors. Hematologic malignancies (lymphomas and leukemias) are presented in Chapter 11.

Characteristics of Benign and Malignant Neoplasms

Cancer is a disorder of altered cell differentiation and growth. The resulting process is called *neoplasia,* and the new growth is called a *neoplasm.* Unlike the processes of hypertrophy and hyperplasia that are discussed in Chapter 2, the cell changes that occur with neoplasia tend to be relatively uncoordinated and autonomous, lacking normal regulatory controls over cell growth and division.

Normal renewal and repair involves two components: cell proliferation and differentiation (see Chapter 4). *Proliferation,* or the process of cell division, is an inherent

Estimated New Cases

Prostate (28%)	Breast (29%)
Lung and bronchus (14%)	Lung and bronchus (14%)
Colon and rectum (9%)	Colon and rectum (9%)
Urinary bladder (6%)	Uterine corpus (6%)
Melanoma of the skin (5%)	Thyroid (6%)
Kidney and renal pelvis (5%)	Non-Hodgkin lymphoma (4%)
Non-Hodgkin lymphoma (4%)	Melanoma of the skin (4%)
Leukemia (3%)	Ovary (3%)
Oral cavity and pharynx (3%)	Kidney and renal pelvis (3%)
Pancreas (3%)	Pancreas (3%)

Estimated Deaths

Lung and bronchus (28%)	Lung and bronchus (26%)
Prostate (10%)	Breast (14%)
Colon and rectum (9%)	Colon and rectum (9%)
Pancreas (6%)	Pancreas (7%)
Liver and intrahepatic bile duct (5%)	Ovary (5%)
Leukemia (4%)	Leukemia (4%)
Esophagus (4%)	Non-Hodgkin lymphoma (3%)
Urinary bladder (4%)	Uterine corpus (3%)
Non-Hodgkin lymphoma (3%)	Brain and other nervous system (2%)
Kidney and renal pelvis (3%)	Liver and intrahepatic bile duct (2%)

*Excludes basal and squamous cell skin cancers and in situ carcinomas except urinary bladder.
Note: Estimates are rounded to the nearest 10.

FIGURE 7-1. Ten leading cancer types for the estimated new cancer cases and deaths in the United States by sex and site, 2013. (Adapted from Siegel R, Naishadham D, Jemel A. Cancer statistics, 2013. *CA Cancer J Clin.* 2013;63[1]:11–30.)

adaptive mechanism for cell replacement when old cells die or additional cells are needed. Fundamental to the origin of all neoplasms are the genetic changes that allow excessive and uncontrolled proliferation that is unregulated by normal growth-regulating stimuli to occur.

Differentiation is the process of specialization whereby new cells acquire the structural, microscopic, and functional characteristics of the cells they replace. Neoplasms are commonly classified as benign or malignant. *Benign neoplasms* are composed of well-differentiated cells that resemble the normal counterpart both in terms of structure and function but have lost the ability to control cell proliferation. *Malignant neoplasms* are less differentiated and have lost the ability to control both cell differentiation and proliferation. In general, the better the differentiation of a neoplasm, the slower its rate of growth and the more completely it retains the functional capabilities found in its normal counterparts. For example, benign neoplasms and even well-differentiated cancers of endocrine glands frequently elaborate the hormones characteristic of their origin.

Apoptosis, which is discussed in Chapter 2, is a form of programmed cell death that eliminates senescent cells, deoxyribonucleic acid (DNA), and damaged or unwanted cells. In adult tissues, the size of a population of cells is determined by the rates of cell proliferation and death by apoptosis. In malignant neoplasms, the accumulation of neoplastic cells may result not only from excessive and uncontrolled proliferation, but also from evasion of apoptosis.

All tumors—benign and malignant—are composed of two types of tissue: (1) *parenchymal* or specific functional cells of an organ or tissue, and (2) connective tissue that forms the supporting tissue framework or stroma.[2,3] The *parenchymal* tissue, which is made up of the transformed or neoplastic cells of a tumor, determines its behavior and is the component for which the tumor is named. The supporting nonneoplastic stromal tissue component is made up of connective tissue, extracellular matrix, and blood vessels. It is essential to the growth of the tumor since it carries the blood supply and provides support for the parenchymal tumor cells.

Terminology

Cancers are commonly referred to as *tumors* or *neoplasms*. Although defined in the medical literature as a swelling that can be caused by a number of conditions, including inflammation and trauma, the term *tumor* is increasingly being used to describe a neoplasm. *Oncology*, from the Greek term *onkos*, for a "swelling," refers to the study or science of neoplasms. *Clinical oncology* deals with neoplastic disorders in the clinical setting, primarily in terms of diagnosis and treatment.

Benign tumors usually are named by adding the suffix *-oma* to the parenchymal tissue type from which the growth originated.[2] Thus, a benign epithelial neoplasm of glandular tissue is called an *adenoma*, and a benign tumor arising in fibrous tissue is called a *fibroma*. The term *carcinoma* is used to designate a malignant tumor of epithelial tissue origin. In the case of malignancies that originate from glandlike structures, the term *adenocarcinoma* is used, and for those that originate from squamous cells, the term *squamous cell carcinoma* is used. Malignant tumors of mesenchymal origin are called *sarcomas*. A cancer of fibrous tissue is a *fibrosarcoma* and a malignant tumor composed of chondrocytes is a *chondrosarcoma*.

Papillomas are benign microscopic or macroscopic fingerlike projections that grow on any surface. A *polyp* is a growth that projects from a mucosal surface, such as the intestine. Although the term usually implies a benign neoplasm, some malignant tumors also appear as polyps. Adenomatous polyps are considered precursors to adenocarcinomas of the colon. Table 7-1 lists the names and tissue types of selected benign and malignant tumors.

Biology of Benign and Malignant Tumors

The differences between benign and malignant tumors are determined by (1) the characteristics of the tumor cells, (2) the rate of growth, (3) local invasion, and (4) the ability to metastasize. The characteristics of benign and malignant neoplasms are summarized in Table 7-2.

TABLE 7-1	Names of Selected Benign and Malignant Tumors According to Tissue Types		
Tissue Type	**Benign Tumors**	**Malignant Tumors**	
Epithelial			
Surface	Papilloma	Squamous cell carcinoma	
Glandular	Adenoma	Adenocarcinoma	
Connective			
Fibrous	Fibroma	Fibrosarcoma	
Adipose	Lipoma	Liposarcoma	
Cartilage	Chondroma	Chondrosarcoma	
Bone	Osteoma	Osteosarcoma	
Blood vessels	Hemangioma	Hemangiosarcoma	
Lymph vessels	Lymphangioma	Lymphangiosarcoma	
Lymph tissue		Lymphosarcoma	
Muscle			
Smooth	Leiomyoma	Leiomyosarcoma	
Striated	Rhabdomyoma	Rhabdomyosarcoma	
Neural Tissue			
Nerve cell	Neuroma	Neuroblastoma	
Glial tissue	Glioma	Glioblastoma, astrocytoma, medulloblastoma, oligodendroglioma	
Nerve sheaths	Neurilemmoma	Neurilemmal sarcoma	
Meninges	Meningioma	Meningeal sarcoma	
Hematologic			
Granulocytic		Myelocytic leukemia	
Erythrocytic		Erythrocytic leukemia	
Plasma cells		Multiple myeloma	
Lymphocytic		Lymphocytic leukemia or lymphoma	
Monocytic		Monocytic leukemia	
Endothelial Tissue			
Blood vessels	Hemangioma	Hemangiosarcoma	
Lymph vessels	Lymphangioma	Lymphangiosarcoma	

Benign Neoplasms

Benign tumors are composed of well-differentiated cells that resemble the cells of the tissues of origin and are generally characterized by a slow, progressive rate of growth that may come to a standstill or regress.[2,3] For unknown reasons, benign tumors have lost the ability to suppress the genetic program for cell proliferation but have retained the program for normal cell differentiation.

They grow by expansion and remain localized to their site of origin and do not have the capacity to infiltrate, invade, or metastasize to distant sites. Because they expand slowly, they develop a surrounding rim of compressed connective tissue called a *fibrous capsule*.[3] The capsule is responsible for a sharp line of demarcation between the benign tumor and the adjacent tissues, a factor that facilitates surgical removal.

TABLE 7-2	Characteristics of Benign and Malignant Neoplasms	
Characteristics	**Benign**	**Malignant**
Cell characteristics	Well-differentiated cells that resemble cells in the tissue of origin	Cells are undifferentiated, with anaplasia and atypical structure that often bears little resemblance to cells in the tissue of origin
Rate of growth	Usually progressive and slow; may come to a standstill or regress	Variable and depends on level of differentiation; the more undifferentiated the cells, the more rapid the rate of growth
Mode of growth	Grows by expansion without invading the surrounding tissues; usually encapsulated	Grows by invasion, sending out processes that infiltrate the surrounding tissues
Metastasis	Does not spread by metastasis	Gains access to blood and lymph channels to metastasize to other areas of the body

Malignant Neoplasms

In contrast to benign tumors, malignant neoplasms tend to grow rapidly, invade and infiltrate nearby tissue, and spread to other parts of the body. They lack a well-defined capsule and their margins are not clearly separated from the normal surrounding tissue.[2,3] Because of their rapid rate of growth, malignant tumors may compress blood vessels and outgrow their blood supply, causing ischemia and tissue injury. Some malignancies secrete hormones and/or cytokines, liberate enzymes and toxins, and/or induce an inflammatory response that injures normal tissue as well as the tumor itself.

There are two categories of malignant neoplasms—solid tumors and hematologic cancers. Solid tumors initially are confined to a specific tissue or organ. As the growth of the primary solid tumor progresses, cells detach from the original tumor mass, invade the surrounding tissue, and enter the blood and lymph system to spread to distant sites, a process termed *metastasis*. Hematologic cancers involve cells normally found within the blood and lymph, thereby making them disseminated diseases from the beginning.

Cancer in situ is a localized preinvasive lesion. For example, in ductal carcinoma in situ of the breast, the malignant cells have not crossed the basement membrane. Depending on its location, an in situ lesion usually can be removed surgically or treated so that the chances of recurrence are small. For example, cancer in situ of the cervix is essentially 100% curable.

Tumor Cell Characteristics

Whether a tumor is benign or malignant is determined by an examination of its cells. Typically, such an examination includes macroscopic (naked eye) inspection to determine the presence or absence of a tumor capsule and invasion of the surrounding tissue, supplemented by microscopic examination of histologic sections of the tumor. Additional information may be obtained from electron microscopy, immunochemistry techniques, chromosomal studies, and DNA analysis. The growth and behavior of tumor cells may be studied using culture techniques.

Differentiation and Anaplasia. Differentiation refers to the extent to which the parenchymal (specific organ versus supportive tissue) cells of a tumor resemble their normal forbearers morphologically and functionally.[2,3] Malignant neoplasms that are composed of poorly differentiated or undifferentiated cells are described as being *anaplastic, anaplasia* literally means to "form backward" to an earlier dedifferentiated state. On histologic examination, benign tumors are composed of cells that resemble the tissue from which they have arisen. By contrast, the cells of malignant tumors are characterized by wide changes of parenchymal cell differentiation from well differentiated to completely undifferentiated.

Undifferentiated cancer cells are marked by a number of morphologic changes. Both the cells and nuclei display variations in size and shape, a condition referred to as *pleomorphism*.[2,3] Their nuclei are variable in size and bizarre in shape, their chromatin is coarse and clumped, and their nucleoli are often considerably larger than normal (Fig. 7-2A). Characteristically, the nuclei contain an abundance of DNA and are extremely dark staining. The cells of undifferentiated tumors usually display a large number of mitoses, reflecting a higher rate of proliferation. They also display atypical, bizarre mitotic figures, sometimes producing tripolar, tetrapolar, or multipolar spindles (Fig. 7-2B). Highly anaplastic cancer cells, whatever their tissue of origin, begin to resemble undifferentiated or embryonic cells more than they do their tissue of origin.

Some cancers display only slight anaplasia and others marked anaplasia. The cytologic/histologic grading of tumors is based on the degree of differentiation and the number of proliferating cells. The closer the tumor cells resemble comparable normal tissue cells, both morphologically (structurally) and functionally, the lower the

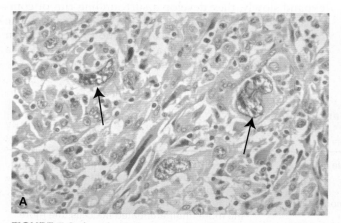
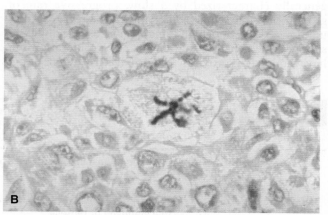

FIGURE 7-2. Anaplastic features of malignant tumors. **(A)** The cells of this anaplastic carcinoma are highly pleomorphic (i.e., they vary in size and shape). The nuclei are hyperchromatic and are large relative to the cytoplasm. Multinucleated tumor giant cells are present (*arrows*). **(B)** A malignant cell in metaphase exhibits an abnormal mitotic figure. (From Strayer DS, Rubin E. Neoplasia. In: Rubin R, Strayer DS, eds. *Rubin's Pathology: Clinicopathologic Foundations of Medicine.* 6th ed. Philadelphia, PA: Wolters Kluwer Health | Lippincott Williams & Wilkins; 2012:162.)

grade. Accordingly, on a scale ranging from grade I to IV, grade I neoplasms are well differentiated and grade IV are poorly differentiated and display marked anaplasia.[2]

Genetic Instability and Chromosomal Abnormalities.

Most cancer cells exhibit a characteristic called *genetic instability* that is often considered to be a hallmark of cancer.[3,4] The concept came about after the realization that uncorrected mutations in normal cells are rare due to many cellular mechanisms to prevent them. To account for the high frequency of mutations in cancer cells, it is thought that cancer cells have a genotype that is highly divergent from the genotype of normally transformed cells. Characteristics of genetic instability are alterations in growth regulatory genes and genes involved in cell cycle progression and arrest.

Genomic instability most commonly results in gross chromosomal abnormalities. Benign tumors usually have a normal number of chromosomes. By contrast, malignant cells often display a feature called *aneuploid*, in which they have an abnormal number of chromosomes.[2–4] The chromosomes may be structurally abnormal due to insertions, deletions, amplifications, or translocations of parts of their arms (see Chapter 6). They may also display microsatellite instability, which involves short repetitive sequences of DNA, and point mutations.

Growth Properties.

The characteristics of altered proliferation and differentiation are associated with a number of growth and behavioral changes that distinguish cancer cells from their normal counterparts. These include growth factor independence, lack of cell density–dependent inhibition, impaired cohesiveness and adhesion, loss of anchorage dependence, faulty cell-to-cell communication, and an indefinite cell life span or immortality.

Cell growth in test tubes or culture dishes is referred to as *in vitro cell culture* because the first containers used for these cultures were made of glass (*vitrium*, meaning "glass" in Latin). It is assumed that the in vivo (in the body) growth of tumor cells mimics that of in vitro studies. Most normal cells require a complex growth medium and survive for only a limited time in vitro. In the case of cancer cells, the addition of serum, which is rich in growth factors, is unnecessary for the cancers to proliferate. Some cancer cells produce their own growth factors and secrete them into the culture medium, while others have abnormal receptors or signaling proteins that may inappropriately activate growth-signaling pathways within the cells. Breast cancer cells that do not express estrogen receptors are an example. These cancer cells grow even in the absence of estrogen, which is the normal growth stimulus for breast duct epithelial cells.

Normal cells that are grown in culture tend to display a feature called *cell density–dependent inhibition,* in which they stop dividing after the cell population reaches a particular density.[5] This is sometimes referred to as *contact inhibition* since cells often stop growing when they come into contact with each other. In wound healing, for example, contact inhibition causes fibrous tissue growth to cease at the point where the edges of a wound come together. Malignant cells show no such contact inhibition

and grow rampantly without regard for adjacent tissue. There is also a reduced tendency of cancer cells to stick together (i.e., loss of *cohesiveness* and *adhesiveness*) owing, in part, to a loss of cell surface adhesion molecules. This permits shedding of the tumor's surface cells; these cells appear in the surrounding body fluids or secretions and often can be detected using cytologic examination.

Cancer cells also display a feature called *anchorage independence.*[5,6] Studies in culture show that normal cells, with the exception of hematopoietic cells, will not grow and proliferate unless they are attached to a solid surface such as the extracellular matrix. For some cell types, including epithelial tissue cells, even survival depends on such attachments. If normal epithelial cells become detached, they often undergo a type of apoptosis known as *anoikis* due to not having a "home." In contrast to normal cells, cancer cells often survive in microenvironments different from those of the normal cells. They frequently remain viable and multiply without normal attachments to other cells and the extracellular matrix. Another characteristic of cancer cells is faulty *cell-to-cell communication*, a feature that may contribute to the growth and survival of cancer cells. Impaired cell-to-cell communication may interfere with formation of intercellular connections and responsiveness to membrane-derived signals. For example, changes in gap junction proteins, which enable cytoplasmic continuity and communication between cells, have been described in some types of cancer.[7]

Cancer cells also differ from normal cells by being *immortal*; that is, they have an unlimited life span. If normal noncancerous cells are harvested from the body and grown under culture conditions, most cells divide a limited number of times, usually about 50 population doublings, then achieve senescence and fail to divide further. In contrast, cancer cells may divide an infinite number of times, and hence achieve immortality. Telomeres are short, repetitive nucleotide sequences at the outermost extremities of chromosome arms (see Chapter 2). Most cancer cells maintain high levels of telomerase, an enzyme that prevents telomere shortening, which keeps telomeres from aging and attaining a critically short length that is associated with cellular replicative senescence.

Functional Features.

Because of their lack of differentiation, cancer cells tend to function on a more primitive level than normal cells, retaining only those functions that are essential for their survival and proliferation. They may also acquire some new features and become quite different from normal cells. For example, many transformed cancer cells revert to earlier stages of gene expression and produce antigens that are immunologically distinct from the antigens that are expressed by cells of the well-differentiated tissue from which the cancer originated. Some cancers may elaborate fetal antigens that are not produced by comparable cells in the adult. Tumor antigens may be clinically useful as markers to indicate the presence, recurrence, or progressive growth of a cancer. Response to treatment can also be evaluated based on an increase or decrease in tumor antigens.

Cancers may also engage in the abnormal production of substances that affect body function. For example, cancer cells may produce procoagulant materials that affect the clotting mechanisms, or tumors of nonendocrine origin may assume the ability to engage in hormone synthesis. These conditions are often referred to as *paraneoplastic syndromes* (to be discussed).

Tumor Growth

The rate of growth in normal and cancerous tissue depends on three factors: (1) the number of cells that are actively dividing or moving through the cell cycle, (2) the duration of the cell cycle, and (3) the number of cells that are being lost relative to the number of new cells being produced. One of the reasons cancerous tumors often seem to grow so rapidly relates to the size of the cell pool that is actively engaged in cycling. It has been shown that the cell cycle time of cancerous tissue cells is not necessarily shorter than that of normal cells. Rather, cancer cells do not die on schedule and growth factors prevent cells from exiting the cell cycle and entering the G_0 or noncycling phase (see Chapter 4, Understanding the Cell Cycle). Thus, a greater percentage of cancer cells are actively engaged in cycling as compared to cells in normal tissue.

The ratio of dividing cells to resting cells in a tissue mass is called the *growth fraction*. The *doubling time* is the length of time it takes for the total mass of cells in a tumor to double. As the growth fraction increases, the doubling time decreases. When normal tissues reach their adult size, an equilibrium between cell birth and cell death is reached. Cancer cells, however, continue to divide until limitations in blood supply and nutrients inhibit their growth. When this occurs, the doubling time for cancer cells decreases. If tumor growth is plotted against time on a semilogarithmic scale, the initial growth rate is exponential and then tends to decrease or flatten out over time. This characterization of tumor growth is called the *Gompertzian model*.[5]

By conventional radiographic methods, a tumor usually is undetectable until it has doubled 30 times and contains more than 1 billion (10^9) cells. At this point, it is approximately 1 cm in size (Fig. 7-3). Methods to identify tumors at smaller sizes are under investigation; in some cases the application of ultrasound and magnetic resonance imaging (MRI) enable detection of tumors less than 1 cm. After 35 doublings, the mass contains more than 1 trillion (10^{12}) cells, which is a sufficient number to kill the host.

Invasion

The word *cancer* is derived from the Latin word meaning *crablike* because cancers grow and spread by sending crablike projections into the surrounding tissues. Unlike benign tumors, which grow by expansion and usually are surrounded by a capsule, cancer spreads by direct invasion into surrounding tissues, seeding of cancer cells in body cavities, and metastatic spread.

Most cancers synthesize and secrete enzymes that break down proteins and contribute to the infiltration, invasion, and penetration of the surrounding tissues. The lack of a sharp line of demarcation separating them from the surrounding tissue makes the complete surgical removal of malignant tumors more difficult than removal of benign tumors. Often it is necessary for the surgeon to excise portions of seemingly normal tissue bordering the tumor for the pathologist to establish that cancer-free margins are present around the excised tumor and to ensure that the remaining tissue is cancer free.

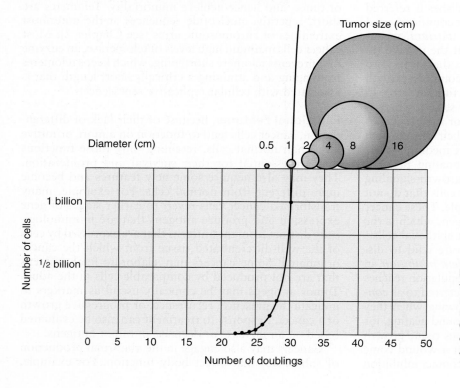

FIGURE 7-3. Growth curve of a hypothetical tumor on arithmetic coordinates. Notice the number of doubling times before the tumor reaches an appreciable size. (Adapted from Collins VP, Loeffler RK, Tivey H. Observations of growth rates of human tumors. *Am J Roentgenol Radium Ther Nucl Med.* 1956;76(5):988–1000.)

The *seeding* of cancer cells into body cavities occurs when a tumor erodes and sheds cells into these spaces.[2,3] Most often, the peritoneal cavity is involved, but other spaces such as the pleural cavity, pericardial cavity, and joint spaces may be involved. Seeding into the peritoneal cavity is particularly common with ovarian cancers. Similar to tissue culture, tumors in these sites grow in masses and often produce fluid (e.g., ascites, pleural effusion).[2] The seeding of cancers is often a concern during the surgical removal of cancers, where it is possible to inadvertently introduce free cancer cells into a body cavity such as the peritoneal cavity.[8]

Metastatic Spread

The term *metastasis* is used to describe the development of a secondary tumor in a location distant from the primary tumor.[2,3] Metastatic tumors frequently retain many of the microscopic characteristics of the primary tumor from which they were derived. Because of this, it usually is possible to determine the site of the primary tumor from the cellular characteristics of the metastatic tumor. Some tumors tend to metastasize early in their developmental course, while others do not metastasize until later. Occasionally, a metastatic tumor will be found far advanced before the primary tumor becomes clinically detectable.

Malignant tumors disseminate by one of two pathways: lymph channels (lymphatic spread) or blood vessels (hematogenous spread).[2] Lymphatic spread is more typical of carcinomas, whereas hematogenous spread is favored by sarcomas.

Lymphatic Spread. In many types of cancer, the first evidence of disseminated disease is the presence of tumor cells in the lymph nodes that drain the tumor area.[9] When metastasis occurs by way of the lymphatic channels, the tumor cells lodge first in the initial lymph node that receives drainage from the tumor site. Once in this lymph node, the cells may die because of the lack of a proper environment, remain dormant for unknown reasons, or grow into a discernible mass (Fig. 7-4). If they survive and grow, the cancer cells may spread from more distant lymph nodes to the thoracic duct, and then gain access to the blood vasculature. Furthermore, cancer cells may gain access to the blood vasculature from the initial node and more distant lymph nodes by way of tumor-associated blood vessels that may infiltrate the tumor mass.

The term *sentinel node* is used to describe the initial lymph node to which the primary tumor drains.[10] Because the initial metastasis in breast cancer is almost always lymphatic, lymphatic spread and, therefore, extent of disease may be determined through lymphatic mapping and sentinel lymph node biopsy. This is done by injecting a radioactive tracer and blue dye into the tumor to determine the first lymph node in the route of lymph drainage from the cancer. Once the sentinel lymph node is identified, it is examined to determine the presence or absence of cancer cells. The procedure is also used to map the spread of melanoma and other

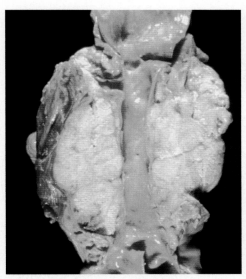

FIGURE 7-4. Metastatic carcinoma in periaortic lymph nodes. Aorta has been opened and nodes bisected. (From Strayer DS, Rubin E. Neoplasia. In: Rubin R, Strayer DS, eds. *Rubin's Pathology: Clinicopathologic Foundations of Medicine*. 6th ed. Philadelphia, PA: Wolters Kluwer Health | Lippincott Williams & Wilkins; 2012:167.)

cancers that have their initial metastatic spread through the lymphatic system.

Hematogenous Spread. With hematogenous spread, cancer cells commonly invade capillaries and venules, whereas thicker-walled arterioles and arteries are relatively resistant. With venous invasion, blood-borne neoplastic cells follow the venous flow draining the site of the neoplasm, often stopping in the first capillary bed they encounter. Since venous blood from the gastrointestinal tract, pancreas, and spleen is routed through the portal vein to the liver, and all vena caval blood flows to the lungs, the liver and lungs are the most frequent metastatic sites for hematogenous spread.[2,3]

Although the site of hematologic spread usually is related to vascular drainage of the primary tumor, some tumors metastasize to distant and unrelated sites. For example, prostatic cancer preferably spreads to bone, bronchogenic cancer to the adrenals and brain, and neuroblastomas to the liver and bones. The selective nature of hematologic spread indicates that metastasis is a finely orchestrated and multistep process, in which only a small, select clone of cancer cells has the right combination of gene products to perform all of the steps needed for establishment of a secondary tumor (Fig. 7-5). To metastasize, a cancer cell must be able to break loose from the primary tumor, invade the surrounding extracellular matrix, gain access to a blood vessel, survive its passage in the bloodstream, emerge from the bloodstream at a favorable location, invade the surrounding tissue, and begin to grow and establish a blood supply.

Considerable evidence suggests that cancer cells capable of metastasis secrete enzymes that break down the surrounding extracellular matrix, allowing them to

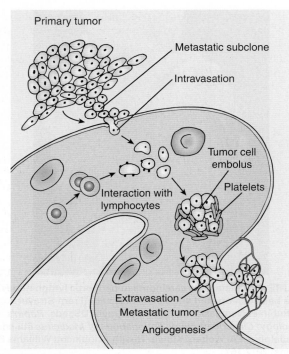

Primary tumor
Metastatic subclone
Intravasation
Tumor cell embolus
Interaction with lymphocytes
Platelets
Extravasation
Metastatic tumor
Angiogenesis

FIGURE 7-5. The pathogenesis of metastasis. (Adapted from Kumar V, Abbas AK, Fausto N, eds. *Robbins and Cotran Pathologic Basis of Disease*. 7th ed. Philadelphia, PA: Elsevier Saunders; 2005:311.)

move through the degraded matrix and gain access to a blood vessel. Once in the circulation, the tumor cells are vulnerable to destruction by host immune cells. Some tumor cells gain protection from the antitumor host cells by aggregating and adhering to circulating blood components, particularly platelets, to form tumor emboli. Exit of the tumor cells from the circulation involves adhesion to the vascular endothelium followed by movement through the capillary wall into the site of secondary tumor formation by mechanisms similar to those involved in invasion.

Once in the distant site, the process of metastatic tumor development depends on the establishment of blood vessels and specific growth factors that promote proliferation of the tumor cells. Tumor cells as well as other cells in the microenvironment secrete factors that enable the development of new blood vessels within the tumor, a process termed *angiogenesis* (to be discussed).[11–13] The presence of stimulatory or inhibitory growth factors correlates with the site-specific pattern of metastasis. For example, a potent growth-stimulating factor has been isolated from lung tissue, and stromal cells in bone have been shown to produce a factor that stimulates growth of prostatic cancer cells.

Recent evidence indicates that chemoattractant cytokines called *chemokines* that regulate the trafficking of leukocytes (white blood cells) and other cell types under a variety of inflammatory and noninflammatory conditions may play a critical role in cancer invasion and metastasis.[14,15] Tumor cells have been shown to express functional chemokine receptors, which can sustain cancer

cell proliferation, angiogenesis, and survival and promote organ-specific localization of metastasis. Insights into the presence and role of chemokines in cancer spread and metastasis provide directions for development of future diagnostic and treatment methods. The implications include methods to diminish metastasis by blocking the action of selected chemokines and/or their receptors.

SUMMARY CONCEPTS

- The term *neoplasm* refers to an abnormal mass of tissue in which the uncontrolled proliferation of cells exceeds and is uncoordinated with that of the normal tissues. Differentiation refers to the extent to which neoplastic cells resemble their normal counterparts.

- Neoplasms are commonly classified as being either benign or malignant. *Benign neoplasms* are well-differentiated tumors that resemble their tissues of origin, but have lost the ability to control cell proliferation. They grow by expansion, are enclosed in a fibrous capsule, and do not cause death unless their location is such that it interrupts vital body functions. *Malignant neoplasms* are less–well-differentiated tumors that have lost the ability to control both cell proliferation and differentiation. They grow in a disorganized and uncontrolled manner, invade surrounding tissues, have cells that break loose and travel to distant sites to form metastases, and inevitably cause suffering and death unless their growth can be controlled through treatment.

- *Anaplasia* is the loss of cell differentiation in cancerous tissue. Undifferentiated cancer cells are marked by a number of morphologic changes, referred to as *pleomorphism*. The characteristics of altered proliferation and differentiation are associated with a number of other changes including genetic instability, growth factor independence, loss of cell density–dependent inhibition, loss of cohesiveness, and anchorage dependence, faulty cell-to-cell communication, an indefinite cell life span (immortality), and expression of fetal antigens not produced by their normal adult counterparts, and abnormal production of hormones and substances that affect body function.

- The rate of growth of cancerous tissue depends on the ratio of dividing to resting cells (growth fraction) and the time it takes for the total mass of cells in the tumor to double (doubling time). A tumor is usually undetectable until it has doubled 30 times and contains more than a billion cells.

■ The spread of cancer occurs through three pathways: direct invasion and extension, seeding of cancer cells in body cavities, and metastatic spread through lymphatic or vascular pathways. Only a proportionately small clone of cancer cells is capable of metastasis. To metastasize, a cancer cell must be able to break loose from the primary tumor, invade the surrounding extracellular matrix, gain access to a blood vessel, survive its passage in the bloodstream, emerge from the bloodstream at a favorable location, and invade the surrounding tissue. Once in the distant tissue site, the metastatic process depends on the establishment of blood vessels and specific growth factors that promote proliferation of the tumor cells.

Etiology of Cancer

The cause or causes of cancer can be viewed from two perspectives: (1) the genetic and molecular mechanisms that characterize the transformation of normal cells into cancer cells and (2) the external and more contextual factors such as age, heredity, and environmental agents that contribute to its development and progression. Together, both mechanisms contribute to a multidimensional web of causation by which cancers develop and progress over time.

Genetic and Molecular Basis of Cancer

The pathogenesis of most cancers is thought to originate from genetic damage or mutation with resultant changes that transform a normally functioning cell into a cancer cell. Epigenetic factors that involve silencing of a gene or genes may also be involved. In recent years, the role of cancer stem cells in the pathogenesis of cancer has been identified. Finally, the cellular microenvironment that involves the extracellular matrix and a complex milieu of cytokines, growth factors, and other cell types is also recognized as an important contributor to cancer development and its growth and progression.

Cancer-Associated Genes

Most cancer-associated genes can be classified into two broad categories based on whether gene overactivity or underactivity increases the risk for cancer. The category associated with gene overactivity involves *proto-oncogenes*, which are normal genes that become cancer-causing genes if mutated.[2,3] Proto-oncogenes encode for normal cell proteins such as growth factors, growth factor receptors, transcription factors that promote cell growth, cell cycle proteins (cyclins or cyclin-dependent proteins), and inhibitors of apoptosis. The category of cancer-associated underactivity genes includes the *tumor-suppressor genes*, which, by being less active, create an environment in which cancer is promoted.

Genetic Events Leading to Oncogene Formation or Activation. There are a number of genetic events that can cause or activate oncogenes.[16] A common event is a point mutation in which there is a single nucleotide base change due to an insertion, deletion, or substitution. An example of an oncogene caused by point mutations is the ras oncogene, which has been found in many cancers.[2] Members of the ras proto-oncogene family are important signal-relaying proteins that transmit growth signals to the cell nucleus. Hence, activation of the ras oncogene can increase cell proliferation.

Chromosomal translocations have traditionally been associated with cancers such as Burkitt lymphoma and chronic myeloid leukemia. In Burkitt lymphoma the c-myc gene, which encodes a growth signal protein, is translocated from its normal position on chromosome 8 to chromosome 14, placing it at the site of an immunoglobulin gene.[2] The outcome of the translocation in chronic myeloid leukemia is the appearance of the so-called *Philadelphia chromosome* involving chromosomes 9 and 22 and the formation of an abnormal fusion protein that promotes cell proliferation[3] (see Chapter 11, Fig. 11-6). Recent advances in biotechnology and genomics are enabling the identification and increased understanding of how gene translocations, even within the same chromosome, contribute to the development of cancer.

Another genetic event that is common in cancer is gene amplification. Multiple copies of certain genes may cause overexpression with higher than normal levels of proteins that increase cell proliferation. For example, the human epidermal growth factor receptor-2 (HER-2/neu) gene is amplified in up to 30% of breast cancers and indicates a tumor that is aggressive with a poor prognosis.[17] One of the agents used in treatment of HER-2/neu overexpressing breast cancers is trastuzumab (Herceptin), a monoclonal antibody that selectively binds to HER-2, thereby inhibiting the proliferation of tumor cells that overexpress HER-2.

Genetic Events Leading to Loss of Tumor-Suppressor Gene Function. Normal cells have regulatory genetic mechanisms that protect them against activated or newly acquired oncogenes. These genes are called tumor-suppressor genes. When this type of gene is inactivated, a genetic signal that normally inhibits cell proliferation is removed, thereby causing unregulated growth to begin.[2,3] Mutations in tumor-suppressor genes are generally recessive, in that cells tend to behave normally until there is homologous deletion, inactivation, or silencing of both the maternal and paternal genes.

Two of the best-known tumor-suppressor genes are the p53 and retinoblastoma (RB) genes. The p53 gene, named after the molecular weight of the protein it encodes, is the most common target for genetic alteration in human cancers. Mutations in the p53 gene can occur in virtually every type of cancer including lung, breast, and colon cancer—the three leading causes of cancer death.[2] Sometimes called the "*guardian of the genome*," the p53 gene acts as a molecular police officer that prevents the propagation of genetically damaged cells.[2] Located on the short arm of chromosome 17, the p53 gene normally senses DNA damage and assists in DNA repair by causing arrest of the cell cycle in G_1 and inducing DNA repair or initiating apoptosis in a cell that cannot be repaired.[2,3] With homologous loss of p53 gene activity, DNA damage goes unrepaired and mutations occur in dividing cells leading to malignant transformations. The p53 gene also appears to initiate apoptosis in radiation- and chemotherapy-damaged tumor cells. Thus, tumors that retain normal p53 function are more likely to respond to such therapy than tumors that carry a defective p53 gene.[2]

The RB gene was isolated in studies involving a malignant tumor of the eye known as *retinoblastoma*. The tumor occurs in a hereditary and sporadic form and becomes evident in early life. Approximately 60% of cases are sporadic, and the remaining 40% are hereditary, inherited as an autosomal dominant trait.[2] Known as the "two hit" hypothesis of carcinogenesis, both normal alleles of the RB gene must be inactivated for the development of retinoblastoma (Fig. 7-6).[2,3] In hereditary cases, one genetic change ("first hit") is inherited from an affected parent and is therefore present in all somatic cells of the body, whereas the second mutation ("second hit") occurs in one of the retinal cells (which already carries the first mutation). In sporadic (noninherited) cases, both mutations ("hits") occur within a single somatic cell, whose progeny then form the cancer.

The RB gene represents a model for other genes that act similarly. In persons carrying an inherited mutation, such as a mutated RB allele, all somatic cells are perfectly normal, except for the risk of developing cancer. That person is said to be *heterozygous* or carrying one mutated gene at the gene locus. Cancer develops when a person becomes homozygous with two defective genes for the mutant allele, a condition referred to as *loss of heterozygosity*.[2] For example, loss of heterozygosity is known to occur in hereditary cancers, in which a mutated gene is inherited from a parent and other conditions (e.g., radiation exposure) are present that cause mutation of the companion gene, making an individual more susceptible to cancer.

Epigenetic Mechanisms

In addition to mechanisms that involve DNA and chromosomal structural changes, there are molecular and cellular mechanisms termed "epigenetic" mechanisms that involve changes in the patterns of gene expression without a change in the DNA.[18] Epigenetic mechanisms may "silence" genes, such as tumor-suppressor genes, so that even if the gene is present, it is not expressed and a cancer-suppressing protein is not made. One such mechanism of epigenetic silencing is by methylation of the promoter region of the gene, a change that prevents transcription and causes gene inactivity. Genes silenced

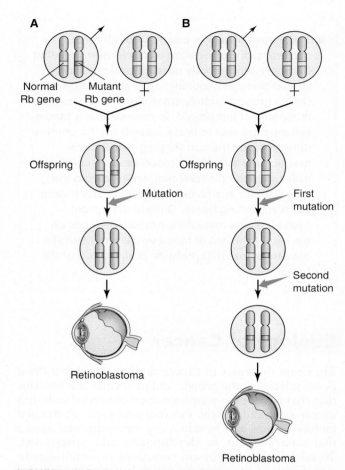

FIGURE 7-6. Pathogenesis of retinoblastoma. Two mutations of the mutant retinoblastoma (Rb) gene lead to development of neoplastic proliferation of retinal cells. **(A)** In the familial form all offspring become carriers of the mutant Rb gene. A second mutation affects the other Rb gene locus after birth. **(B)** In the sporadic form, both mutations occur after birth.

by hypermethylation can be inherited, and epigenetic silencing of genes can be considered a "first hit" in the "two hit" hypothesis described earlier.[19]

MicroRNAs (miRNA) are small, noncoding, single-stranded ribonucleic acids (RNAs), about 22 nucleotides in length, which function at the post-transcriptional level as negative regulators of gene expression.[2,3,20] miRNAs pair with messenger RNA (mRNA) containing a nucleotide sequence that complements the sequence of the microRNA, and through the action of the RNA-induced silencing, mediate post-transcriptional gene silencing. miRNAs have been shown to undergo changes in expression in cancer cells, and frequent amplifications and deletions of miRNA loci have been identified in a number of human cancers, including those of the lung, breast, colon, pancreas, and hematopoietic systems.[3] They can participate in neoplastic transformation by increasing the expression of oncogenes or reducing the expression of tumor suppressor genes. For example, down-regulation or deletion of certain miRNAs in some leukemias and lymphomas results in increased expression of BCL2, an anti-apoptotic protein that protects tumor cells from apoptosis.

Molecular and Cellular Pathways

Numerous molecular and cellular mechanisms with a myriad of associated pathways and genes are known or suspected to facilitate the development of cancer. These mechanisms include defects in DNA repair mechanisms, disorders in growth factor signaling pathways, evasion of apoptosis, development of sustained angiogenesis, and evasion of metastasis.

Mechanisms and genes that regulate repair of damaged DNA have been implicated in the process of oncogenesis (Fig. 7-7). The DNA repair genes affect cell proliferation and survival indirectly through their ability to repair nonlethal damage in other genes including proto-oncogenes, tumor-suppressor genes, and the genes that control apoptosis.[2,3] These genes have been implicated as the principal targets of genetic damage occurring during the development of a cancer cell. Such genetic damage may be caused by the action of chemicals, radiation, or viruses, or it may be inherited in the germ line. Significantly, it appears that the acquisition of a single-gene mutation is not sufficient to transform normal cells into cancer cells.

Instead, cancerous transformation appears to require the activation of many independently mutated genes.

A relatively common pathway by which cancer cells gain autonomous growth is by mutations in genes that control signaling pathways between growth factor receptors on the cell membrane and their targets in the cell nucleus.[2] Under normal conditions, cell proliferation involves the binding of a growth factor to its receptor on the cell membrane, activation of the growth factor receptor on the inner surface of the cell membrane, transfer of the signal across the cytosol to the nucleus via signal-transducing proteins that function as second messengers, induction and activation of regulatory factors that initiate DNA transcription, and entry of the cell into the cell cycle (Fig. 7-8). Many of the proteins involved in the signaling pathways that control the action of growth factors in cancer cells exert their effects through enzymes called *kinases* that phosphorylate proteins. In some types of cancer such as chronic myeloid leukemia, mutation in a proto-oncogene controlling tyrosine kinase activity occurs, causing unregulated cell growth and proliferation.

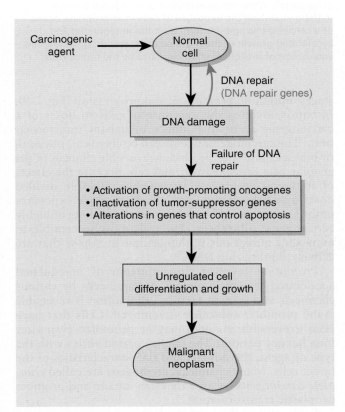

FIGURE 7-7. Flow chart depicting the stages in the development of a malignant neoplasm resulting from exposure to an oncogenic agent that produces DNA damage. When DNA repair genes are present (*red arrow*), the DNA is repaired and gene mutation does not occur.

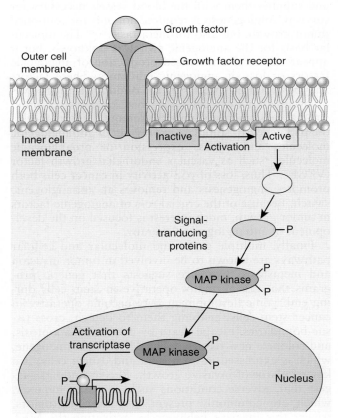

FIGURE 7-8. Pathway for genes regulating cell growth and replication. Stimulation of a normal cell by a growth factor results in activation of the growth factor receptor and signaling proteins that transmit the growth-promoting signal to the nucleus, where it modulates gene transcription and progression through the cell cycle. Many of these signaling proteins exert their effects through enzymes called *kinases* that phosphorylate (P) proteins. MAP, mitogen-activating protein.

The accumulation of cancer cells may result not only from the activation of growth-promoting oncogenes or inactivation of tumor-suppressor genes, but also from genes that regulate cell death through apoptosis or programmed cell death.[2,3,21,22] Faulty apoptotic mechanisms have an important role in cancer. The failure of cancer cells to undergo apoptosis in a normal manner may be due to a number of problems. There may be altered cell survival signaling, down-regulation of death receptors, stabilization of the mitochondria, or inactivation of proapoptotic proteins. Alterations in apoptotic and antiapoptotic pathways have been found in many cancers. One example is the high levels of the antiapoptotic protein BCL2 that occur secondary to a chromosomal translocation in certain B-cell lymphomas. The mitochondrial membrane is a key regulator of the balance between cell death and survival. Proteins in the BCL2 family reside in the inner mitochondrial membrane and are either proapoptotic or antiapoptotic. Since apoptosis is considered a normal cellular response to DNA damage, loss of normal apoptotic pathways may contribute to cancer by enabling DNA-damaged cells to survive.

Even with all the genetic abnormalities described earlier, tumors cannot enlarge unless angiogenesis occurs and supplies them with the blood vessels necessary for survival. Angiogenesis is required not only for continued tumor growth, but also for metastasis.[2,3,23] The molecular basis for the angiogenic switch is unknown, but it appears to involve increased production of angiogenic factors or loss of angiogenic inhibitors. These factors may be produced directly by the tumor cells themselves or by inflammatory cells (e.g., macrophages) or other stromal cells associated with the tumors. In normal cells, the p53 gene can stimulate expression of antiangiogenic molecules and repress expression of proangiogenic molecules, such as vascular endothelial growth factor (VEGF).[2] Thus, loss of p53 activity in cancer cells both promotes angiogenesis and removes an antiangiogenic switch. Because of the crucial role of angiogenic factors in tumor growth, much interest is focused on the development of antiangiogenesis therapy.

Finally, multiple genes and molecular and cellular pathways are known to be involved in tumor invasion and metastasis. Evidence suggests that genetic programs that are normally operative in stem cells during embryonic development may become operative in cancer stem cells, enabling them to detach, cross tissue boundaries, escape death by anoikis or apoptosis, and colonize new tissues.[24] The *MET* proto-oncogene, which is expressed in both stem and cancer cells, is a key regulator of invasive growth. Recent findings suggest that adverse conditions such as tissue hypoxia, which are commonly present in cancerous tumors, trigger this invasive behavior by activating the MET tyrosine kinase receptor.

Tumor Cell Transformation

The process by which carcinogenic agents cause normal cells to become cancer cells is hypothesized to be a multistep mechanism that can be divided into three

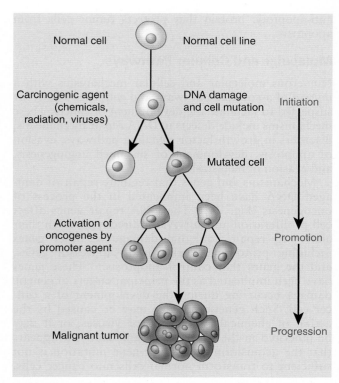

FIGURE 7-9. The processes of initiation, promotion, and progression in the clonal evolution of malignant tumors. Initiation involves the exposure of cells to appropriate doses of a carcinogenic agent; promotion, the unregulated and accelerated growth of the mutated cells; and progression, the acquisition of malignant characteristics by the tumor cells.

stages: initiation, promotion, and progression (Fig. 7-9). *Initiation* involves the exposure of cells to doses of a carcinogenic agent that induce malignant transformation.[2] The carcinogenic agents can be chemical, physical, or biologic, and they produce irreversible changes in the genome of a previously normal cell. Because the effects of initiating agents are irreversible, multiple divided doses may achieve the same effects as single exposures of the same comparable dose or small amounts of highly carcinogenic substances. The cells most susceptible to mutagenic alterations in the genome are those that are actively synthesizing DNA.

Promotion involves the induction of unregulated accelerated growth in already initiated cells by various chemicals and growth factors.[2] Promotion is reversible if the promoter substance is removed. Cells that have been irreversibly initiated may be promoted even after long latency periods. The latency period varies with the type of agent, the dosage, and the characteristics of the target cells. Many chemical carcinogens are called *complete carcinogens* because they can initiate and promote neoplastic transformation.

Progression is the process whereby tumor cells acquire malignant phenotypic changes. These changes may promote the cell's ability to proliferate autonomously, invade, or metastasize. They may also destabilize its karyotype.

Host and Environmental Factors

Because cancer is not a single disease, it is reasonable to assume that it does not have a single cause. More likely, cancers develop because of interactions among host and environmental factors. Among the host factors that have been linked to cancer are heredity, hormonal factors, obesity, and immunologic mechanisms. Environmental factors include chemical carcinogens, radiation, and microorganisms.

Heredity

The genetic predisposition for development of cancer has been documented for a number of cancerous and precancerous lesions that follow mendelian inheritance patterns. Two tumor suppressor genes, called *BRCA1* (breast carcinoma 1) and *BRCA2* (breast carcinoma 2), have been implicated in a genetic susceptibility to breast cancer.[2,3] These genes have also been associated with an increased risk of ovarian, prostate, pancreatic, colon, and other cancers.

Several cancers exhibit an autosomal dominant inheritance pattern that greatly increases the risk of developing a tumor. The inherited mutation is usually a point mutation occurring in a single allele of a tumor-suppressor gene. Persons who inherit the mutant gene are born with one normal and one mutant copy of the gene. In order for cancer to develop, the normal allele must be inactivated, usually through a somatic mutation. As previously discussed, retinoblastoma is an example of a cancer that follows an autosomal dominant inheritance pattern. Approximately 40% of retinoblastomas are inherited, and carriers of the mutant RB suppressor gene have a 10,000-fold increased risk of developing retinoblastoma, usually with bilateral involvement.[2] Familial adenomatous polyposis of the colon also follows an autosomal dominant inheritance pattern. In people who inherit this gene, hundreds of adenomatous polyps may develop, some of which inevitably become malignant.

Hormones

Hormones have received considerable research attention with respect to cancer of the breast, ovary, and endometrium in women and of the prostate and testis in men. Although the link between hormones and the development of cancer is unclear, it has been suggested that it may reside with the ability of hormones to drive the cell division of a malignant phenotype.[2] Because of the evidence that endogenous hormones affect the risk of these cancers, concern exists regarding the effects on cancer risk if the same or closely related hormones are administered for therapeutic purposes.

Obesity

There has been recent interest in obesity as a risk factor for certain types of cancer, including breast, endometrial, and prostate cancer.[25] The process relating obesity to cancer development is multifactorial and involves a network of metabolic and immunologic mechanisms.

Obesity has been associated with insulin resistance and increased production of pancreatic insulin, both of which can have a carcinogenic effect. Insulin enhances insulin-like growth factor-1 (IGF-1) synthesis and its bioavailability. Both insulin and IGF-1 are anabolic molecules that can promote tumor development by stimulating cell proliferation and inhibiting apoptosis. Obesity has also been associated with increased levels of sex hormones (androgens and estrogens), which act to stimulate cell proliferation, inhibit apoptosis, and therefore increase the chance of malignant cell transformation, particularly of endometrial and breast tissue, and possibly of other organs (e.g., prostate and colon cancer). And lastly, obesity has been related to a condition of chronic inflammation characterized by abnormal production of inflammatory cytokines that can contribute to the development of malignancies.

Immunologic Mechanisms

There is substantial evidence for the participation of the immune system in resistance against the progression and spread of cancer.[2,3,26] The central concept, known as the *immune surveillance hypothesis,* which was first proposed by Paul Ehrlich in 1909, postulates that the immune system plays a central role in protection against the development of tumors.[27] In addition to cancer–host interactions as a mechanism of cancer development, immunologic mechanisms provide a means for the detection, classification, and prognostic evaluation of cancers and a potential method of treatment. *Immunotherapy* (discussed later in this chapter) is a cancer treatment modality designed to heighten the patient's general immune responses so as to increase tumor destruction.

The *immune surveillance hypothesis* suggests that the development of cancer might be associated with impairment or decline in the surveillance capacity of the immune system. For example, increases in cancer incidence have been observed in people with immunodeficiency diseases and in those with organ transplants who are receiving immunosuppressant drugs. The incidence of cancer also is increased in the elderly, in whom there is a known decrease in immune activity. The association of Kaposi sarcoma with acquired immunodeficiency syndrome (AIDS) further emphasizes the role of the immune system in preventing malignant cell proliferation (discussed in Chapter 16).

It has been shown that most tumor cells have molecular configurations that can be specifically recognized by immune cells or antibodies. These configurations are therefore called *tumor antigens.* Some tumor antigens are found only on tumor cells, whereas others are found on both tumor cells and normal cells; however, quantitative and qualitative differences in the tumor antigens permit the immune system to distinguish tumor from normal cells.[2]

Virtually all of the components of the immune system have the potential for eradicating cancer cells, including T and B lymphocytes, natural killer (NK) cells, and macrophages (see Chapter 15). The T-cell response, which is responsible for direct killing of tumor cells and for activation of other components of the immune system, is one of the most important host responses for controlling the growth of tumor cells. The finding of tumor-reactive antibodies in the serum of people with cancer supports the role of the B lymphocyte as a member of the immune surveillance team. Antibodies cause destruction of cancer cells through complement-mediated mechanisms or through antibody-dependent cellular cytotoxicity, in which the antibody binds the cancer cell to another effector cell, such as the NK cell, that does the actual killing of the cancer cell. NK cells do not require antigen recognition and can lyse a wide variety of target cells.

Chemical Carcinogens

A carcinogen is an agent capable of causing cancer. The role of environmental agents in causation of cancer was first noted in 1775 by Sir Percivall Pott, a English physician who related the high incidence of scrotal cancer in chimneysweeps to their exposure to coal soot.[2,3] Coal tar has since been found to contain potent polycyclic aromatic hydrocarbons. Since then, many chemicals have been suspected of being carcinogens. Some have been found to cause cancers in animals, and others are known to cause cancers in humans (Chart 7-1).

Chemical carcinogens can be divided into two groups: (1) direct-reacting agents, which do not require

activation in the body to become carcinogenic, and (2) indirect-reacting agents, called *procarcinogens* or *initiators,* which become active only after metabolic conversion.[2,3] Direct- and indirect-acting initiators form highly reactive species (such as free radicals) that bind with residues on DNA, RNA, or cellular proteins. They then prompt cell mutation or disrupt protein synthesis in a way that alters cell replication and interferes with cell regulatory controls. The carcinogenicity of some chemicals is augmented by agents called *promoters* that, by themselves, have little or no cancer-causing ability. It is believed that promoters, in the presence of these carcinogens, exert their effect by altering gene expression, increasing DNA synthesis, enhancing gene amplification (i.e., number of gene copies that are made), and altering intercellular communication.

Exposure to many carcinogens, such as those contained in cigarette smoke, is associated with a lifestyle risk for development of cancer. Cigarette smoke contains both procarcinogens and promoters. It is directly associated with lung and laryngeal cancer and has been linked with cancers of the mouth, nasal cavities, pharynx, esophagus, pancreas, liver, kidney, uterus, cervix, and bladder and myeloid leukemias. Not only is the smoker at risk, but others passively exposed to cigarette smoke are at risk. Chewing tobacco increases the risk of cancers of the oral cavity and esophagus.

Occupational exposure to industrial chemicals is another significant risk factor for cancer. These include polycyclic aromatic hydrocarbons, which are metabolized in the liver.[5] For example, long-term exposure to vinyl chloride, the simple two-carbon molecule that is widely used in the plastics industry, increases the risk for hepatic angiosarcoma.[3]

There is also strong evidence that certain elements in the diet contain chemicals that contribute to cancer risk. Most known dietary carcinogens occur either naturally in plants (e.g., aflatoxins) or are produced during food preparation.[2] The polycyclic aromatic hydrocarbons are of particular interest because they are produced during several types of food preparation, including frying foods in animal fat that has been reused multiple times; grilling or charcoal-broiling meats; and smoking meats and fish. Nitrosamines, which are powerful carcinogens, are formed in foods that are smoked, salted, cured, or pickled using nitrites or nitrates as preservatives. Formation of these nitrosamines may be inhibited by the presence of antioxidants such as vitamin C found in fruits and vegetables. Cancer of the colon has been associated with high dietary intake of fat and red meat and a low intake of dietary fiber.[28] A high-fat diet is thought to be carcinogenic because it increases the flow of primary bile acids that are converted to secondary bile acids in the presence of anaerobic bacteria in the colon, producing carcinogens or promoters.

Heavy or regular alcohol consumption is associated with a variety of cancers. The first and most toxic metabolite of ethanol is acetaldehyde, a known carcinogen that interferes with DNA synthesis and repair and that causes point mutations in some cells.[28,29] The carcinogenic effect of cigarette smoke can be enhanced

---

CHART 7-1 **Major Chemical Carcinogens**[2,3]

Direct-Acting Alkylating Agents
- Anticancer drugs (e.g., cyclophosphamide, cisplatin, busulfan)

Polycyclic and Heterocyclic Aromatic Hydrocarbons
- Tobacco combustion (cigarette smoke)
- Animal fat in broiled and smoked meats
- Benzo(a)pyrene
- Vinyl chloride

Aromatic Amines and Azo Dyes
- β-Naphthylamine
- Aniline dyes

Naturally Occurring Carcinogens
- Aflatoxin B1
- Griseofulvin
- Betel nuts

Nitrosamines and Amides
- Formed in gastrointestinal tract from nitro-stable amines and nitrates used in preserving processed meats and other foods

Miscellaneous Agents
- Asbestos
- Chromium, nickel, and other metals when volatilized and inhaled in industrial settings
- Insecticides, fungicides
- Polychlorinated biphenyls

by concomitant consumption of alcohol; persons who smoke and drink considerable amounts of alcohol are at increased risk for development of cancer of the oral cavity, larynx and esophagus.

The effects of carcinogenic agents usually are dose dependent—the larger the dose or the longer the duration of exposure, the greater the risk that cancer will develop. Some chemical carcinogens may act in concert with other carcinogenic influences, such as viruses or radiation, to induce neoplasia. There usually is a time delay ranging from 5 to 30 years from the time of chemical carcinogen exposure to the development of overt cancer. This is unfortunate because many people may have been exposed to the agent and its carcinogenic effects before the association was recognized.

Radiation

The effects of *ionizing radiation* in carcinogenesis have been well documented in atomic bomb survivors, in patients diagnostically exposed, and in industrial workers, scientists, and physicians who were exposed during employment. Malignant epitheliomas of the skin and leukemia were significantly elevated in these populations. Between 1950 and 1970, the death rate from leukemia alone in the most heavily exposed population groups of the atomic bomb survivors in Hiroshima and Nagasaki was 147 per 100,000 persons, 30 times the expected rate.[30]

The type of cancer that developed depended on the dose of radiation, the sex of the person, and the age at which exposure occurred. The length of time between exposure and the onset of cancer is related to the age of the individual. For example, children exposed to ionizing radiation in utero have an increased risk for developing leukemias and childhood tumors, particularly 2 to 3 years after birth. Therapeutic irradiation to the head and neck can give rise to thyroid cancer years later. The carcinogenic effect of ionizing radiation is related to its mutagenic effects in terms of causing chromosomal breakage, translocations, and, less frequently, point mutations.[2]

The association between sunlight and the development of skin cancer (see Chapter 46) has been reported for more than 100 years. *Ultraviolet radiation* emits relatively low-energy rays that do not deeply penetrate the skin. The evidence supporting the role of ultraviolet radiation in the cause of skin cancer includes skin cancer that develops primarily on the areas of skin more frequently exposed to sunlight (e.g., the head and neck, arms, hands, and legs), a higher incidence in light-complexioned individuals who lack the ultraviolet-filtering skin pigment melanin, and the fact that the intensity of ultraviolet exposure is directly related to the incidence of skin cancer, as evidenced by higher rates occurring in Australia and the American Southwest. There also are studies that suggest that intense, episodic exposure to sunlight, particularly during childhood, is more important in the development of melanoma than prolonged low-intensity exposure. As with other carcinogens, the effects of ultraviolet

radiation usually are additive, and there usually is a long delay between the time of exposure and the time that cancer can be detected.

Viral and Microbial Agents

An oncogenic virus is one that can induce cancer. Many DNA and RNA viruses have proved to be oncogenic in animals. However, only four DNA viruses have been implicated in human cancers: the human papilloma virus (HPV), Epstein-Barr virus (EBV), hepatitis B virus (HBV), and human herpesvirus 8 (HHV-8).[2,4,31] HHV-8, which causes Kaposi sarcoma in persons with AIDS, is discussed in Chapter 16. There is also an association between infection with the bacterium *Helicobacter pylori* and gastric adenocarcinoma and gastric lymphomas[2,3] (discussed in Chapter 29).

There are over 70 genetically different types of HPV.[2] Some types (i.e., types 1, 2, 4, 7) have been shown to cause benign squamous papillomas (i.e., warts). By contrast, high-risk HPVs (e.g., types 16 and 18) are implicated in the pathogenesis of squamous cell carcinoma of the cervix and anogenital region.[2,3] Thus, cervical cancer can be viewed as a sexually transmitted disease, caused by transmission of HPV. In addition, at least 20% of oropharyngeal cancers are associated with high-risk HPVs.[2] A vaccine to protect against HPV types 6, 11, 16, and 18 is now available[32] (see Chapter 40).

Epstein-Barr virus is a member of the herpesvirus family. It has been implicated in the pathogenesis of several human cancers, including Burkitt lymphoma, a tumor of B lymphocytes. In persons with normal immune function, the EBV-driven B-cell proliferation is readily controlled and the person becomes asymptomatic or experiences a self-limited episode of infectious mononucleosis (see Chapter 11). However, in regions of the world where Burkitt lymphoma is endemic, such as parts of East Africa, concurrent malaria or other infections cause impaired immune function, allowing sustained B-lymphocyte proliferation. Epstein-Barr virus is also associated with B-cell lymphomas in immunosuppressed individuals, such as those with AIDS or with drug-suppressed immune systems (e.g., individuals with transplanted organs).

There is strong epidemiologic evidence linking chronic HBV and hepatitis C virus (HCV) infection with hepatocellular carcinoma (discussed in Chapter 30). It has been estimated that 70% to 85% of hepatocellular cancers worldwide are due to infection with HBV or HCV.[2] The precise mechanism by which these viruses induce hepatocellular cancer has not been fully determined. It seems probable that the oncogenic effects are multifactorial, with immunologically mediated chronic inflammation leading to persistent liver damage, regeneration, and genomic damage. The regeneration process is mediated by a vast array of growth factors, cytokines, chemokines, and bioactive substances produced by immune cells that promote cell survival, tissue remodeling, and angiogenesis.

Although a number of retroviruses (RNA viruses) cause cancer in animals, human T-cell leukemia virus-1

(HTLV-1) is the only known retrovirus to cause cancer in humans. Human T-cell leukemia virus-1 is associated with a form of T-cell leukemia that is endemic in certain parts of Japan and some areas of the Caribbean and Africa, and is found sporadically elsewhere, including the United States and Europe.[2] Similar to the AIDS virus, HTLV-1 is attracted to the CD4+ T cells, and this subset of T cells is therefore the major target for malignant transformation. The virus requires transmission of infected T cells by way of sexual intercourse, infected blood, or breast milk.

SUMMARY CONCEPTS

■ The etiology of cancer is highly complex, encompassing both molecular and cellular origins, and external and contextual factors such as heredity and environmental agents that influence its inception and growth. It is likely that multiple factors interact at the molecular and cellular level to transform normal cells into cancer cells.

■ The *molecular pathogenesis* of cancer is thought to have its origin in genetic damage or a mutation that changes the cell's physiology and transforms it into a cancer cell. The types of genes involved in cancer are numerous, but two main groups are the *proto-oncogenes,* which control cell growth and replication, and *tumor-suppressor genes,* which are growth-inhibiting regulatory genes.

■ Genetic and molecular mechanisms that increase susceptibility to cancer and/or facilitate cancer include defects in DNA repair mechanisms, defects in growth factor signaling pathways, evasion of apoptosis, development of sustained angiogenesis, invasion, and metastasis. Genetic and epigenetic damage may be the result of interactions between multiple risk factors or repeated exposure to a single carcinogenic (cancer-producing) agent.

■ Among the external and contextual risk factors that have been linked to cancer are heredity, hormonal factors, obesity, immunologic mechanisms, and environmental agents such as chemicals, radiation, and cancer-causing viruses and microbes.

Clinical Manifestations

There probably is not a single body function left unaffected by the presence of cancer. Even the presenting signs and symptoms may be localized or widespread.

Local and Regional Manifestations

Because tumor cells replace normally functioning parenchymal cells, the initial manifestations of cancer usually reflect the function of the primary site of involvement. For example, lung cancer initially produces impairment of respiratory function; as the tumor grows and metastasizes, other body structures become affected.

Cancer has no regard for normal anatomic boundaries; as it grows, it invades and compresses adjacent structures. Abdominal cancer, for example, may compress the viscera and cause bowel obstruction. Growing tumors may also compress and erode blood vessels, causing ulceration and necrosis along with frank bleeding and sometimes hemorrhage.

The development of effusions (i.e., fluid) in the pleural, pericardial, or peritoneal spaces may be the presenting sign of some tumors. Direct involvement of the serous surface seems to be the most significant inciting factor, although many other mechanisms such as obstruction of lymphatic flow may play a role. Most persons with pleural effusions are symptomatic at presentation with chest pain, shortness of breath, and cough. More than any other malignant neoplasms, ovarian cancers are associated with the accumulation of fluid in the peritoneal cavity. Complaints of abdominal discomfort, swelling and a feeling of heaviness, and increase in abdominal girth, which reflect the presence of peritoneal effusions or ascites, are the most common presenting symptoms in ovarian cancer, occurring in up to 65% of women with the disease.[33]

Systemic Manifestations

Cancer also produces systemic manifestations such as anemia, anorexia and cachexia, and fatigue and sleep disorders. Many of these manifestations are compounded by the side effects of methods used to treat the disease. In its late stages, cancer often causes pain (see Chapter 35). Pain is probably one of the most dreaded aspects of cancer, and pain management is one of the major treatment concerns for persons with incurable cancers. Although research has produced amazing insights into the causes and cures for cancer, only recently have efforts focused on the associated side effects of the disease.

Anemia

Anemia is common in persons with various types of cancers. It may be related to blood loss, iron deficiency, hemolysis, impaired red cell production, or treatment effects.[34–36] For example, drugs used in treatment of cancer are cytotoxic and can decrease red blood cell production. Also, there are many mechanisms through which erythrocyte production can be impaired in persons with malignancies including nutritional deficiencies, bone marrow failure, a blunted erythropoietin response to hypoxia, and an iron deficiency. Inflammatory cytokines generated in response to tumors decrease erythropoietin synthesis, resulting in a decrease in erythrocyte production. Iron deficiency may be due, in part, to a dysregulation of iron metabolism, leading to a functional iron deficiency.[37]

Cancer-related anemia is associated with reduced treatment effectiveness, increased mortality, increased transfusion requirements, and reduced performance and quality of life. Hypoxia, a characteristic feature of advanced solid tumors, has been recognized as a critical factor in promoting tumor resistance to radiotherapy and some chemotherapeutic agents.

Cancer-related anemia is often treated with iron supplementation and recombinant human erythropoietin (rHuEPO, epoetin alfa).[37] Since iron deficiency may result in failure to respond to erythropoietin, it has been suggested that iron parameters be measured before initiation of erythropoietin therapy. When treatment with supplemental iron is indicated, it has been suggested that it be given intravenously, since oral iron has been shown to be largely ineffective in persons with cancer.[37]

Anorexia and Cachexia

Many cancers are associated with weight loss and wasting of body fat and muscle tissue, accompanied by profound weakness, anorexia, and anemia. This wasting syndrome is often referred to as the *cancer anorexia–cachexia syndrome*.[38–40] It is a common manifestation of most solid tumors with the exception of breast cancer. The condition is more common in children and elderly persons and becomes more pronounced as the disease progresses. Persons with cancer cachexia also respond less well to chemotherapy and are more prone to toxic side effects.

The cause of the cancer anorexia–cachexia syndrome is probably multifactorial, resulting from a persistent inflammatory response in conjunction with production of specific cytokines and catabolic factors by the tumor. Although anorexia, reduced food intake, and abnormalities of taste are common in people with cancer and often are accentuated by treatment methods, the extent of weight loss and protein wasting cannot be explained in terms of diminished food intake alone. There also is a disparity between the size of the tumor and the severity of cachexia, which supports the existence of other mediators in the development of cachexia. It has been demonstrated that tumor necrosis factor (TNF)-α and other cytokines including interleukin-1 (IL-1) and IL-6 can produce the wasting syndrome in experimental animals.[3] High serum levels of these cytokines have been observed in persons with cancer, and their levels appear to correlate with progress of the tumor. Tumor necrosis factor-α, secreted primarily by macrophages in response to tumor cell growth or gram-negative bacterial infections, was the first identified cytokine associated with cachexia and wasting. It causes anorexia by suppressing satiety centers in the hypothalamus and increasing the synthesis of lipoprotein lipase, an enzyme that facilitates the release of fatty acids from lipoproteins so that they can be used by tissues. IL-1 and IL-6 share many of the features of TNF-α in terms of the ability to initiate cachexia.

Fatigue and Sleep Disorders

Fatigue and sleep disturbances are two of the side effects most frequently experienced by persons with cancer.[41–45] Cancer-related fatigue is characterized by feelings of tiredness, weakness, and lack of energy and is distinct from the normal tiredness experienced by healthy individuals in that it is not relieved by rest or sleep. It occurs both as a consequence of the cancer itself and as a side effect of cancer treatment. Cancer-related fatigue may be an early symptom of malignant disease and has been reported by as many as 40% of patients at the time of diagnosis.[42] Furthermore, the symptom often remains for months or even years after treatment.

The cause of cancer-related fatigue is largely unknown but is probably multifactorial and involves the dysregulation of several interrelated physiologic, biochemical, and psychological systems. The basic mechanisms of fatigue have been broadly categorized into two components: peripheral and central. Peripheral fatigue, which has its origin in the neuromuscular junction and muscles, results from the inability of the peripheral neuromuscular apparatus to perform a task in response to central stimulation. Mechanisms implicated in peripheral fatigue include a lack of adenosine triphosphate (ATP) and the buildup of metabolic by-products such as lactic acid. Central fatigue arises in the central nervous system (CNS) and is often described as the difficulty in initiating or maintaining voluntary activities. One hypothesis proposed to explain cancer-related fatigue is that cancer and cancer treatments result in dysregulation of brain serotonin (5-HT) levels or function. There is also evidence that proinflammatory cytokines, such as TNF-α, can influence 5-HT metabolism.

Paraneoplastic Syndromes

In addition to signs and symptoms at the sites of primary and metastatic disease, cancer can produce manifestations in sites that are not directly affected by the disease. Such manifestations are collectively referred to as *paraneoplastic syndromes*.[46,47] Some of these manifestations are caused by the elaboration of hormones by cancer cells, and others result from the production of circulating factors that produce hematopoietic, neurologic, and dermatologic syndromes (Table 7-3). These syndromes are most commonly associated with lung, breast, and hematologic malignancies.[2]

A variety of peptide hormones are produced by both benign and malignant tumors. Although not normally expressed, the biochemical pathways for the synthesis and release of peptide hormones are present in most cells.[47] The three most common endocrine syndromes associated with cancer are the syndrome of inappropriate antidiuretic hormone (ADH) secretion (see Chapter 8), Cushing syndrome due to ectopic adrenocorticotropic hormone (ACTH) production (see Chapter 32), and hypercalcemia (see Chapter 8). Hypercalcemia also can be caused by osteolytic processes induced by cancer such as multiple myeloma or bony metastases from other cancers.

Some paraneoplastic syndromes are associated with the production of circulating mediators that produce

TABLE 7-3	**Common Paraneoplastic Syndromes**	
Type of Syndrome	**Associated Tumor Type**	**Proposed Mechanism**
Endocrinologic		
Syndrome of inappropriate ADH	Small cell lung cancer, others	Production and release of ADH by tumor
Cushing syndrome	Small cell lung cancer, bronchial carcinoid cancers	Production and release of ACTH by tumor
Hypercalcemia	Squamous cell cancers of the lung, head, neck, ovary	Production and release of polypeptide factor with close relationship to PTH
Hematologic		
Venous thrombosis	Pancreatic, lung, other cancers	Production of procoagulation factors
Nonbacterial thrombolytic endocarditis	Advanced cancers	
Neurologic		
Eaton-Lambert syndrome	Small cell lung cancer	Autoimmune production of antibodies to motor end-plate structures
Myasthenia gravis	Thymoma	
Dermatologic		
Acanthosis nigricans	Gastric carcinoma	Possibly caused by production of growth factors (epidermal) by tumor cells

ACTH, adrenocorticotropic hormone; ADH, antidiuretic hormone; PTH, parathyroid hormone.

hematologic complications.[47] For example, a variety of cancers may produce procoagulation factors that contribute to an increased risk for venous thrombosis and nonbacterial thrombotic endocarditis. Sometimes, unexplained thrombotic events are the first indication of an undiagnosed malignancy. The precise relationship between coagulation disorders and cancer is still unknown. Several malignancies, such as mucin-producing adenocarcinomas, release thromboplastin and other substances that activate the clotting system.

The symptomatic paraneoplastic neurologic disorders are relatively rare with the exception of the Lambert-Eaton myasthenic syndrome, which affects about 3% of persons with small cell lung cancer, and myasthenia gravis, which affects about 15% of people with thymoma.[48,49] The *Lambert-Eaton syndrome*, or reverse myasthenia gravis, is seen almost exclusively in small cell lung cancer. It produces muscle weakness in the limbs rather than the initial mouth and eye muscle weakness seen in myasthenia gravis. The origin of paraneoplastic neurologic disorders is thought to be immune mediated. The altered immune response is initiated by the production of onconeural antigens (e.g., antigens normally expressed in the nervous system) by the cancer cells. The immune system, in turn, recognizes the onconeural antigens as foreign and mounts an immune response. In many cases, the immune attack controls the growth of the cancer.

The paraneoplastic syndromes may be the earliest indication that a person has cancer, and should be regarded as such. They may also represent significant clinical problems, may be potentially lethal in persons with cancer, and may mimic metastatic disease and confound treatment. Diagnostic methods focus on both identifying the cause of the disorder and locating the malignancy responsible. Techniques for precise identification of minute amounts of polypeptides may allow for early diagnosis of curable malignancies in asymptomatic individuals. The treatment of paraneoplastic syndromes involves concurrent treatment of the underlying cancer and suppression of the mediator causing the syndrome.

SUMMARY CONCEPTS

- There probably is no single body function left unaffected by the presence of cancer. Because tumor cells replace normally functioning parenchymal tissue, the initial manifestations of cancer usually reflect the primary site of involvement.

- Cancer compresses blood vessels, obstructs lymph flow, disrupts tissue integrity, invades serous cavities, and compresses visceral organs. It may result in development of effusions (i.e., fluid) in the pleural, pericardial, or peritoneal spaces.

- Systemic manifestations of cancer include anorexia and cachexia; fatigue and sleep disorders; and anemia.

- Cancer may also produce paraneoplastic syndromes that arise from the ability of neoplasms to elaborate hormones and other chemical mediators to produce endocrine, hematopoietic, neurologic, and dermatologic syndromes. Many of these manifestations are compounded by the side effects of methods used to treat the disease.

Screening, Diagnosis, and Treatment

Advances in the screening, diagnosis, and treatment of cancer have boosted 5-year survival rates to nearly 64%. When treatment cannot cure the disease, it may be used to slow its progression or provide palliative care.

Screening

Screening represents a secondary prevention measure for the early recognition of cancer in an otherwise asymptomatic population.[50,51] Screening can be achieved through observation (e.g., skin, mouth, external genitalia), palpation (e.g., breast, thyroid, rectum and anus, prostate, lymph nodes), and laboratory tests and procedures (e.g., Papanicolaou [Pap] smear, colonoscopy, mammography). It requires a test that will specifically detect early cancers or premalignancies, is cost effective, and results in improved therapeutic outcomes. For most cancers, stage at presentation is related to curability, with the highest rates reported when the tumor is small and there is no evidence of metastasis. For some tumors, however, metastasis tends to occur early, even from a small primary tumor. Unfortunately, no reliable screening methods are currently available for many cancers.

Cancers for which current screening or early detection has led to improvement in outcomes include cancers of the breast (breast self-examination and mammography, discussed in Chapter 40), cervix (Pap smear, Chapter 40), colon and rectum (rectal examination, fecal occult blood test, and flexible sigmoidoscopy and colonoscopy, Chapter 29), prostate (prostate-specific antigen testing and transrectal ultrasonography, Chapter 39), and malignant melanoma (self-examination, Chapter 46). While not as clearly defined, it is recommended that screening for other types of cancers such as cancers of the thyroid, testicles, ovaries, lymph nodes, and oral cavity be done at the time of periodic health examinations.

Diagnostic Methods

The methods used in the diagnosis and staging of cancer are determined largely by the location and type of cancer suspected. They include blood tests for tumor markers, cytologic studies, tissue biopsy, and gene profiling techniques as well as medical imaging, which is discussed with specific cancers later in this text.

Tumor Markers

Tumor markers are antigens expressed on the surface of tumor cells or substances released from normal cells in response to the presence of tumor.[2] Some substances, such as hormones and enzymes, that are normally produced by the involved tissue become overexpressed as a result of cancer. Tumor markers are used for screening, establishing prognosis, monitoring treatment, and detecting recurrent disease. Table 7-4 identifies some of the more commonly used tumor markers and summarizes their source and the cancers associated with them.

TABLE 7-4	**Tumor Markers**	
Marker	**Source**	**Associated Cancers**
Oncofetal Antigens		
α-Fetoprotein (AFP)	Fetal yolk sac and gastrointestinal structures early in fetal life	Primary liver cancers; germ cell cancer of the testis
Carcinoembryonic antigen (CEA)	Embryonic tissues in gut, pancreas, and liver	Colorectal cancer and cancers of the pancreas, lung, and stomach
Hormones		
Human chorionic gonadotropin (hCG)	Hormone normally produced by placenta	Gestational trophoblastic tumors; germ cell cancer of testis
Calcitonin	Hormone produced by thyroid parafollicular cells	Thyroid cancer
Catecholamines (epinephrine, norepinephrine) and metabolites	Hormones produced by chromaffin cells of the adrenal gland	Pheochromocytoma and related tumors
Specific Proteins		
Monoclonal immunoglobulin	Abnormal immunoglobulin produced by neoplastic cells	Multiple myeloma
Prostate-specific antigen (PSA)	Produced by the epithelial cells lining the acini and ducts of the prostate	Prostate cancer
Mucins and Other Glycoproteins		
CA-125	Produced by müllerian cells of ovary	Ovarian cancer
CA-19-9	Produced by alimentary tract epithelium	Cancer of the pancreas, and colon
Cluster of Differentiation		
CD antigens	Present on leukocytes	Used to determine the type and level of differentiation of leukocytes involved in different types of leukemia and lymphoma

The serum markers that have proven most useful in clinical practice are the human chorionic gonadotropin (hCG), prostate-specific antigen (PSA), CA-125, α-fetoprotein (AFP), CD blood cell antigens, and carcinoembryonic antigen (CEA). The hCG is a hormone normally produced by the placenta. It is used as a marker for diagnosing, prescribing treatment, and following the disease course in persons with high-risk gestational trophoblastic tumors. Prostate-specific antigen (PSA) is used as a marker in prostate cancer, and CA-125 is used as a marker in ovarian cancer. Markers for leukemia and lymphomas are grouped by so-called *clusters of differentiation* (CD) antigens (see Chapter 15). The CD antigens help to distinguish among T and B lymphocytes, monocytes, granulocytes, and natural killer cells and immature variants of these cells.[2,3]

Some cancers express fetal antigens that are normally present only during embryonal development and induced to reappear as a result of neoplasia.[2] The two that have proved most useful as tumor markers are alpha fetoprotein (AFP) and CEA. α-fetoprotein is synthesized by the fetal liver, yolk sac, and gastrointestinal tract and is the major serum protein in the fetus. Elevated levels are encountered in people with primary liver cancers and have also been observed in some testicular, ovarian, pancreatic, and stomach cancers. Carcinoembryonic antigen normally is produced by embryonic tissue in the gut, pancreas, and liver and is elaborated by a number of different cancers, including colorectal carcinomas, pancreatic cancers, and gastric and breast tumors. As with most other tumor markers, elevated levels of AFP and CEA are found in other, noncancerous conditions, and elevated levels of both depend on tumor size so that neither is useful as an early test for cancer.

As diagnostic tools, tumor markers have limitations. Nearly all markers can be elevated in benign conditions, and most are not elevated in the early stages of malignancy. Furthermore, they are not in themselves specific enough to permit a diagnosis of a malignancy, but once a malignancy has been diagnosed and shown to be associated with elevated levels of a tumor marker, the marker can be used to assess progress of the disease. Extremely elevated levels of a tumor marker can indicate a poor prognosis or the need for more aggressive treatment. Perhaps the greatest value of tumor markers is in monitoring therapy in people with widespread cancer. The level of most cancer markers tends to decrease with successful treatment and increase with recurrence or spread of the tumor.

Cytologic, Histologic, and Gene-Profiling Methods

Cytologic and histologic studies are laboratory methods used to examine tissues and cells. Several sampling approaches are available including cytologic smears, tissue biopsies, and needle aspiration.[2]

Papanicolaou Smear. The Pap smear is a cytologic method that consists of a microscopic examination of a properly prepared slide by a cytotechnologist or pathologist for the purpose of detecting the presence of abnormal cells. The usefulness of the Pap smear relies on the fact that cancer cells lack the cohesive properties and intercellular junctions that are characteristic of normal tissue; without these characteristics, cancer cells tend to exfoliate and become mixed with secretions surrounding the tumor growth. Although the Pap smear is widely used as a screening test for cervical cancer, it can be performed on other body secretions, including nipple drainage, pleural or peritoneal fluid, and gastric washings.

Tissue Biopsy. Tissue biopsy involves the removal of a tissue specimen for microscopic study. It is of critical importance in designing the treatment plan should cancer cells be found. Biopsies are obtained in a number of ways, including needle biopsy; endoscopic methods, such as bronchoscopy or cystoscopy, which involve the passage of an endoscope through an orifice and into the involved structure; and laparoscopic methods.

Fine needle aspiration involves withdrawing cells and attendant fluid with a small-bore needle. The method is most widely used for assessment of readily palpable lesions in sites such as the thyroid, breast, and lymph nodes. Modern imaging techniques have also enabled the method to be extended to deeper structures such as the pelvic lymph nodes and pancreas.

In some instances, a surgical incision is made from which biopsy specimens are obtained. Excisional biopsies are those in which the entire tumor is removed. The tumors usually are small, solid, palpable masses. If the tumor is too large to be completely removed, a wedge of tissue from the mass can be excised for examination. A quick frozen section may be done and examined by a pathologist to determine the nature of a mass lesion or evaluate the margins of an excised tumor to ascertain that the entire neoplasm has been removed.[3]

Immunohistochemistry. Immunohistochemistry involves the use of monoclonal antibodies to facilitate the identification of cell products or surface markers.[3] For example, certain anaplastic carcinomas, malignant lymphomas, melanomas, and sarcomas look very similar under the microscope, but must be accurately identified because their treatment and prognosis are quite different.

Immunohistochemistry can also be used to determine the site of origin of metastatic tumors. Many cancer patients present with metastasis. In cases in which the origin of the metastasis is obscure, immunochemical detection of tissue-specific or organ-specific antigens can often help to identify the tumor source. Immunochemistry can also be used to detect molecules that have prognostic or therapeutic significance. For example, detection of estrogen receptors on breast cancer cells is of prognostic and therapeutic significance because these tumors respond to antiestrogen therapy.

Microarray Technology. Microarray technology has the advantage of analyzing a large number of molecular changes in cancer cells to determine overall patterns of behavior that would not be available by conventional means. The technique uses "gene chips" that can perform miniature assays to detect and quantify the expression of large numbers of genes at the same time.[2] DNA arrays are now commercially available to assist in making clinical decisions regarding breast cancer treatment. In addition to identifying tumor types, microarrays have been used for predicting prognosis and response to therapy, examining tumor changes after therapy, and classifying hereditary tumors.[2]

Staging and Grading of Tumors

The two basic methods for classifying cancers are grading according to the histologic or cellular characteristics of the tumor and staging according to the clinical spread of the disease. Both methods are used to determine the course of the disease and aid in selecting an appropriate treatment or management plan.

Grading of tumors involves the microscopic examination of cancer cells to determine their level of differentiation and the number of mitoses. The closer the tumor cells resemble comparable normal tissue cells, both morphologically and functionally, the lower the grade. Accordingly, on a scale ranging from grade I to IV, grade I neoplasms are well differentiated and grade IV are poorly differentiated and display marked anaplasia.[2,3]

The *clinical staging* of cancers uses methods to determine the extent and spread of the disease. It is useful in determining the choice of treatment for individual patients, estimating prognosis, and comparing the results of different treatment regimens. The significant criteria used for staging that vary with different organs include the size of the primary tumor, its extent of local growth (whether within or outside the organ), lymph node involvement, and presence of distant metastasis.[2,3] This assessment is based on clinical and radiographic examination (CT and MRI) and, in some cases, surgical exploration. Two methods of staging are currently in use: the TNM system (T for primary tumor, N for regional lymph node involvement, and M for metastasis), which was developed by the Union for International Cancer Control, and the American Joint Committee (AJC) system.[2] In the TNM system, T1, T2, T3, and T4 describe *tumor* size, N0, N1, N2, and N3, lymph *node* involvement; and M0 or M1, the absence or presence of *metastasis*. In the AJC system, cancers are divided into stages 0 to IV incorporating the size of the primary lesions and the presence of nodal spread and distant metastasis.

Cancer Treatment

The goals of cancer treatment methods fall into three categories: curative, control, and palliative. The most common modalities are surgery, radiation, chemotherapy, hormonal therapy, and biotherapy. The treatment of cancer involves the use of a carefully planned program that combines the benefits of multiple treatment modalities and the expertise of an interdisciplinary team of specialists including medical, surgical, and radiation oncologists; clinical nurse specialists; nurse practitioners; pharmacists; and a variety of ancillary personnel.

Surgery

Surgery is used for diagnosis, staging of cancer, tumor removal, and palliation (i.e., relief of symptoms) when a cure cannot be achieved.[52] The type of surgery to be used is determined by the extent of the disease, the location and structures involved, the tumor growth rate and invasiveness, the surgical risk to the patient, and the quality of life the patient will experience after the surgery. If the tumor is small and has well-defined margins, the entire tumor often can be removed. If, however, the tumor is large or involves vital tissues, surgical removal may be difficult if not impossible.

Radiation Therapy

Radiation can be used as the primary method of treatment, as preoperative or postoperative treatment, with chemotherapy, or along with chemotherapy and surgery.[53–57] It can also be used as a palliative treatment to reduce symptoms in persons with advanced cancers. It is effective in reducing the pain associated with bone metastasis and, in some cases, improves mobility. Radiation also is used to treat several oncologic emergencies, such as spinal cord compression, bronchial obstruction, and hemorrhage.

Radiation therapy exerts its effects through ionizing radiation, which affects cells by direct ionization of molecules or, more commonly, by indirect ionization. Indirect ionization produced by x-rays or gamma rays causes cellular damage when these rays are absorbed into tissue and give up their energy by producing fast-moving electrons. These electrons interact with free or loosely bonded electrons of the absorber cells and subsequently produce free radicals that interact with critical cell components (see Chapter 2). It can immediately kill cells, delay or halt cell cycle progression, or, at dose levels commonly used in radiation therapy, cause damage to the cell nucleus, resulting in cell death after replication. Cell damage can be sublethal, in which case a single break in the strand can repair itself before the next radiation insult. Double-stranded breaks in DNA are generally believed to be the primary damage that leads to cell death. Cells with unrepaired DNA damage may continue to function until they undergo cell mitosis, at which time the genetic damage causes cell death.

The therapeutic effects of radiation therapy derive from the fact that the rapidly proliferating and poorly differentiated cells of a cancerous tumor are more likely to be injured by radiation therapy than are the more slowly proliferating cells of normal tissue. To some extent, however, radiation is injurious to all rapidly proliferating cells, including those of the bone marrow and the mucosal lining of the gastrointestinal tract. This results in many of the common adverse effects of radiation therapy, including infection, bleeding, and anemia due to loss of blood cells, and nausea and vomiting due to loss of gastrointestinal tract cells. In addition to its lethal effects, radiation also produces sublethal injury. Recovery from sublethal doses of radiation occurs in the interval between the first dose of radiation and subsequent doses. This is why large total doses of radiation can be tolerated when they are divided into multiple smaller, fractionated doses. Normal tissue is usually able to recover from radiation damage more readily than is cancerous tissue.

Therapeutic radiation can be delivered in one of three ways: external beam or teletherapy, with beams generated by a linear accelerator or cobalt-60 machine at a distance and aimed at the patient's tumor; brachytherapy, in which a sealed radioactive source is placed close to or directly in the tumor site; and systemic therapy, in which radioisotopes with a short half-life are given by mouth or injected into the tumor site.

Chemotherapy

Cancer chemotherapy has evolved as one of the major systemic treatment modalities.[58,59] Unlike surgery and radiation, cancer chemotherapy is a systemic treatment that enables drugs to reach the site of the tumor as well as distant sites. Chemotherapeutic drugs may be used as the primary form of treatment, or they may be used as part of a multimodal treatment plan. Chemotherapy is the primary treatment for most hematologic and some solid tumors, including choriocarcinoma, testicular cancer, acute and chronic leukemia, Burkitt lymphoma, Hodgkin disease, and multiple myeloma.

Most cancer drugs are more toxic to rapidly proliferating cells than to those incapable of replication or in phase G_0 of the cell cycle. Because of their mechanism of action, they are more effective against tumors with a high growth fraction. By the time many cancers reach a size that is clinically detectable, the growth fraction has decreased considerably. In this case, reduction in tumor size through the use of surgical debulking procedures or radiation therapy often causes tumor cells residing in G_0 to reenter the cell cycle. Thus, surgery or radiation therapy may be used to increase the effectiveness of chemotherapy, or chemotherapy may be given to patients with no overt evidence of residual disease after local treatment (e.g., surgical resection of a primary breast cancer).

For most chemotherapy drugs, the relationship between tumor cell survival and drug dose is exponential, with the number of cells surviving being proportional to drug dose, and the number of cells at risk for exposure being proportional to the destructive action of the drug. Exponential killing implies that a proportion or percentage of tumor cells is killed, rather than an absolute number (Fig. 7-10). This proportion is a constant percentage of the total number of cells. For this reason, multiple courses of treatment are needed if the tumor is to be eradicated.

A major problem in cancer chemotherapy is the development of cellular resistance. Acquired resistance develops in a number of drug-sensitive tumor types.[59] Experimentally, drug resistance can be highly specific to a single agent and is usually based on genetic changes in a given tumor cell type. In other instances, a multidrug-resistant phenomenon affecting anticancer drugs with differing structures occurs. This type of resistance often involves the increased expression of transmembrane transporter genes involved in drug efflux.

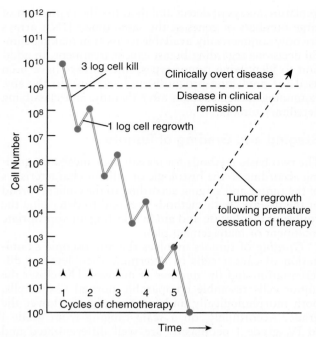

FIGURE 7-10. Relationship between tumor cell survival and administration of chemotherapy. The exponential relationship between drug dose and tumor cell survival dictates that a constant proportion, not number, of tumor cells is killed with each treatment cycle. In this example, each cycle of drug administration results in a 99.9% (3 log) cell kill, and 1 log of cell growth occurs between cycles. The *broken line* indicates what would occur if the last cycle of therapy were omitted: despite complete clinical remission of disease, the tumor ultimately would recur. (Reprinted by the permission from Raymond E. Lenhard Jr., et al. *The American Cancer Society's Clinical Oncology*. Atlanta, GA: American Cancer Society; 2001: 181. © American Cancer Society.)

Cancer chemotherapy drugs may be classified as either cell cycle specific or cell cycle nonspecific (see Understanding—The Cell Cycle, Chapter 4).[58] Drugs are *cell cycle specific* if they exert their action during a specific phase of the cell cycle. For example, methotrexate, an antimetabolite, acts by interfering with DNA synthesis and thereby interrupts the S phase of the cell cycle. *Cell cycle–nonspecific* drugs exert their effects throughout all phases of the cell cycle. The alkylating agents, which are cell cycle nonspecific, act by disrupting DNA when cells are in the resting state as well as when they are dividing. The site of action of chemotherapeutic drugs varies. Chemotherapy drugs that have similar structures and effects on cell function usually are grouped together, and these drugs usually have similar side effect profiles. Because chemotherapy drugs differ in their mechanisms of action, cell cycle–specific and cell cycle–nonspecific agents are often combined to treat cancer.

Combination chemotherapy has been found to be more effective than treatment with a single drug. With this method, several drugs with different mechanisms of action, metabolic pathways, times of onset of action and recovery, side effects, and onset of side effects are used. Drugs used in combinations are individually effective against the tumor and synergistic with each other. The maximum possible drug doses usually are used to ensure the maximum cell kill within the range of toxicity tolerated by the host for each drug. Routes of administration and dosage schedules are carefully designed to ensure optimal delivery of the active forms of the drugs to the tumor during the sensitive phase of the cell cycle.

Chemotherapy Side Effects. Unfortunately, chemotherapeutic drugs affect both cancer cells and the rapidly proliferating cells of normal tissue, producing undesirable side effects. Some side effects appear immediately or after a few days (acute), some within a few weeks (intermediate), and others months to years after chemotherapy administration (long term).

Most chemotherapeutic drugs suppress bone marrow function and formation of blood cells, leading to anemia, neutropenia, and thrombocytopenia. With neutropenia, there is risk for developing serious infections, whereas thrombocytopenia increases the risk for bleeding. The availability of hematopoietic growth factors (e.g., granulocyte colony-stimulating factor [G-CSF]); erythropoietin, which stimulates red blood production; and IL-11, which stimulates platelet production) has shortened the period of myelosuppression, thereby reducing the need for hospitalizations due to infection and decreasing the need for blood products.

Anorexia, nausea, and vomiting are common problems associated with cancer chemotherapy.[58] The severity of the vomiting is related to the emetic potential of the particular drug. These symptoms can occur within minutes or hours of drug administration and are thought to be due to stimulation of the chemoreceptor trigger zone in the medulla that stimulates vomiting (see Chapter 28). The chemoreceptor trigger zone responds to the level of chemicals circulating in the blood. The acute symptoms usually subside within 24 to 48 hours and often can be relieved by antiemetic drugs. The pharmacologic approaches to prevent chemotherapy-induced nausea and vomiting have greatly improved over several decades. The development of serotonin ($5-HT_3$) receptor antagonists has facilitated the use of highly emetic chemotherapy drugs by more effectively reducing the nausea and vomiting induced by these drugs.

Alopecia or hair loss results from impaired proliferation of the hair follicles and is a side effect of a number of cancer drugs; it usually is temporary, and the hair tends to regrow when treatment is stopped. The rapidly proliferating structures of the reproductive system are particularly sensitive to the action of cancer drugs. Women may experience changes in menstrual flow or have amenorrhea. Men may have a decreased sperm count (i.e., oligospermia) or absence of sperm (i.e., azoospermia). Many chemotherapeutic agents also may have teratogenic or mutagenic effects leading to fetal abnormalities.[58]

Chemotherapy drugs are toxic to all cells. Because they are potentially mutagenic, carcinogenic, and teratogenic, special care is required when handling or administering the drugs. Drugs, drug containers, and administration equipment require special disposal as hazardous waste.[60]

Hormone and Antihormone Therapy

Hormonal therapy consists of administration of drugs designed to deprive the cancer cells of the hormonal signals that otherwise would stimulate them to divide. It is used for cancers that are responsive to or dependent on hormones for growth and have specific hormone receptors.[61] Among the tumors that are known to be responsive to hormonal manipulation are those of the breast, prostate, and endometrium. Other cancers, such as Kaposi sarcoma and renal, liver, ovarian, and pancreatic cancer, are also responsive to hormonal manipulation, but to a lesser degree.

The therapeutic options for altering the hormonal environment in the woman with breast cancer or the man with prostate cancer include surgical and pharmacologic measures. Surgery involves the removal of the organ responsible for the hormone production that is stimulating the target tissue (e.g., ovaries in women or testes in men). Pharmacologic methods focus largely on reducing circulating hormone levels or changing the hormone receptors so that they no longer respond to the hormone. Pharmacologic suppression of circulating hormone levels can be effected through pituitary desensitization, as with the administration of androgens, or through the administration of *gonadotropin-releasing hormone* (GnRH) analogs that act at the level of the hypothalamus to inhibit gonadotropin production and release. Another class of drugs, the *aromatase inhibitors*, is used to treat breast cancer; these drugs act by interrupting the biochemical processes that convert the adrenal androgen androstenedione to estrone.[62]

Hormone receptor function can be altered by the administration of pharmacologic doses of exogenous hormones that act by producing a decrease in hormone receptors or by antihormone drugs (antiestrogens and antiandrogens) that bind to hormone receptors, making them inaccessible to hormone stimulation. Initially, patients often respond favorably to hormonal treatments, but eventually the cancer becomes resistant to hormonal manipulation, and other approaches must be sought to control the disease.

Biotherapy

Biotherapy involves the use of immunotherapy and biologic response modifiers as a means of changing a person's immune response and modifying tumor cell biology. It involves the use of monoclonal antibodies, cytokines, and adjuvants.[63]

Monoclonal Antibodies. Recent advances in the ability to manipulate the genes of immunoglobulins have resulted in the development of a wide array of monoclonal antibodies directed against tumor-specific antigens as well as signaling molecules.[64] These include *chimeric* human-murine (mouse) antibodies with human constant region and murine-variable regions (see Chapter 15, Figure 15-10), *humanized* antibodies in which the murine regions that bind antigen have been grafted into human immunoglobulin (Ig) G molecules, and *entirely human* antibodies derived from transgenic mice expressing immunoglobulin genes.[65] Some monoclonal antibodies are directed to block major pathways central to tumor cell survival and proliferation, whereas others are modified to deliver toxins, radioisotopes, cytokines, or other cancer drugs.

Currently approved monoclonal antibodies include rituximab (Rituxan), a chimeric IgG monoclonal antibody that targets the CD20 antigen on B cells and is used in the treatment of nonHodgkin lymphoma; bevacozumab (Avastin), a humanized IgG monoclonal antibody that targets vascular endothelial growth factor (VEGF) to inhibit blood vessel growth (angiogenesis) and is approved for treatment of colorectal, lung, renal, and breast cancer; and cetuximab (Erbitux), a chimeric monoclonal antibody that targets the epidermal growth factor receptor (EGFR) to inhibit tumor cell growth and is approved for treatment of colorectal cancer and squamous cell cancer of the head and neck.[64,65]

Cytokines. The biologic response modifiers include cytokines such as the interferons and interleukins. The *interferons* appear to inhibit viral replication and also may be involved in inhibiting tumor protein synthesis, prolonging the cell cycle, and increasing the percentage of cells in the G_0 phase. Interferons stimulate NK cells and T-lymphocyte killer cells. There are three major types of interferons, alpha (α), beta (β), and gamma (γ), with members of each group differing in terms of their cell surface receptors.[63] Interferon-γ has been approved for the treatment of hairy cell leukemia, AIDS-related Kaposi sarcoma, and chronic myelogenous leukemia, and as adjuvant therapy for patients at high risk for recurrent melanoma. Interferon-α has been used to treat some solid tumors (e.g., renal cell carcinoma, colorectal cancer, carcinoid tumors, ovarian cancer) and hematologic neoplasms (e.g., B-cell and T-cell lymphomas, cutaneous T-cell lymphoma, and multiple myeloma).[62] Research now is focusing on combining interferons with other forms of cancer therapy and establishing optimal doses and treatment protocols.

The *interleukins* (ILs) are cytokines that provide communication between cells by binding to receptor sites on the cell surface membranes of the target cells. Of the 18 known interleukins (see Chapter 15), IL-2 has been the most widely studied. A recombinant human IL-2 (rIL-2, aldesleukin) has been approved by the U.S. Food and Drug Administration (FDA) and is currently being used for the treatment of metastatic renal cell carcinoma and metastatic melanoma.[63]

Adjuvants. Adjuvants are substances such as Bacillus Calmette-Guérin (BCG) that nonspecifically stimulate or indirectly augment the immune system.[63] Instillations of BCG, an attenuated strain of the bacterium that causes bovine tuberculosis, are used to treat noninvasive bladder cancer after surgical ablation. It is assumed that BCG acts locally to stimulate an immune response, thereby decreasing the relapse rate.

Targeted Therapy

Researchers have been working diligently to produce drugs that selectively attack malignant cells while leaving normal cells unharmed.[66,67] The characteristics and capabilities of cancer cells have been used to establish a framework for the development of such targeted therapies, including those that disrupt molecular signaling pathways, inhibit angiogenesis, and harness the body's immune system. The first targeted therapies were the monoclonal antibodies. Researchers are now working to design drugs that can disrupt molecular signaling pathways, such as those that use the protein tyrosine kinases. The protein tyrosine kinases are intrinsic components of the signaling pathways for growth factors involved in the proliferation of lymphocytes and other cell types. Imatinib mesylate is a protein tyrosine kinase inhibitor indicated in the treatment of chronic myeloid leukemia (see Chapter 11). Angiogenesis is also being explored as a target for targeted cancer therapy.[66] One of the newerr antiangiogenic agents, bevacizumab, targets and blocks VEGF, which is released by many cancers to stimulate proliferation of new blood vessels.

SUMMARY CONCEPTS

- The methods used in the detection and diagnosis of cancer vary with the type of cancer and its location. Because many cancers are curable if diagnosed early, health care practices designed to promote early detection, such as screening, are important.

- Diagnostic methods include laboratory tests for the presence of tumor markers, cytologic and histologic studies using cells or tissue specimens, and gene profiling methods, in addition to medical imaging.

- There are two basic methods of classifying tumors: grading according to the histologic or tissue characteristics, and clinical staging according to spread of the disease. The Tumor, Node, Metastasis (TNM) system for clinical staging of cancer uses tumor size, lymph node involvement, and presence of metastasis.

- Treatment of cancer can include surgery, radiation, or chemotherapy. Other therapies include hormonal, immunologic, and biologic therapies, as well as molecularly targeted agents that disrupt molecular signaling pathways, inhibit angiogenesis, and harness the body's immune system. Treatment plans that use more than one type of therapy are providing cures for a number of cancers that a few decades ago had a poor prognosis, and are increasing the life expectancy in other types of cancer.

Childhood Cancers and Late Effects on Cancer Survivors

Despite progressively improved 5-year survival rates, from 56% in 1974 to 75% in 2000, cancer remains the leading cause of disease-related deaths among children between 1 to 14 years in the United States.[68] Leukemia (discussed in Chapter 11) accounts for one-third of cases of cancer in children ages 1 to 14 years.[1] Cancer of the brain and other parts of the nervous system are the second most common, followed by tissue sarcoma, neuroblastoma, renal cancer (Wilms tumor, discussed in Chapter 26), and non-Hodgkin and Hodgkin lymphoma (discussed in Chapter 11).[1]

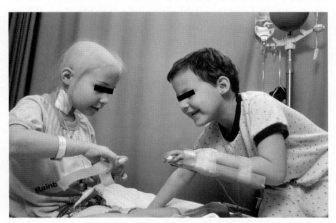

Two young girls with acute lymphocytic leukemia are receiving chemotherapy (From National Cancer Institute Visuals. No. AV-8503-3437.)

Incidence and Types of Childhood Cancers

The spectrum of cancers that affect children differs markedly from those that affect adults. Although most adult cancers are of epithelial cell origin (e.g., lung cancer, breast cancer, colorectal cancers), childhood cancers usually involve the hematopoietic system (leukemia), brain and other parts of the nervous system, soft tissues, kidneys (Wilms tumor), and bone.[1,68]

The incidence of childhood cancers is greatest during the first years of life, decreases during middle childhood, and then increases during puberty and adolescence.[68] During the first 2 years of life, embryonal tumors such as neuroblastoma, retinoblastoma, and Wilms tumor are among the most common types of tumors. Acute lymphocytic leukemia has a peak incidence in children 2 to 5 years of age. As children age, especially after they pass puberty, bone malignancies, lymphoma, gonadal germ cell tumors (testicular and ovarian carcinomas), and various carcinomas such as thyroid cancer and malignant melanoma increase in incidence.

A number of the tumors of infancy and early childhood are embryonal in origin, meaning that they exhibit features of organogenesis similar to that of embryonic

development. Because of this characteristic, these tumors are frequently designated with the suffix "-*blastoma*" (e.g., nephroblastoma [Wilms tumor], retinoblastoma, neuroblastoma).[2] Wilms tumor (discussed in Chapter 25) and neuroblastoma are particularly illustrative of this type of childhood tumor.

Biology of Childhood Cancers

As with adult cancers, there probably is no one cause of childhood cancer. Although a number of genetic conditions are associated with childhood cancer, such conditions are relatively rare, suggesting an interaction between genetic susceptibility and environmental exposures. The most notable heritable conditions that impart susceptibility to childhood cancer include Down syndrome (20- to 30-fold increased risk of acute lymphoblastic leukemia),[1] neurofibromatosis (NF) type 1 (neurofibromas, optic gliomas, brain tumors), NF type 2 (acoustic neuroma, meningiomas), xeroderma pigmentosum (skin cancer), ataxia-telangiectasia (lymphoma, leukemia), and the Beckman-Wiedemann syndrome (Wilms tumor).[2,69]

While constituting only a small percentage of childhood cancers, the biology of a number of these tumors illustrates several important biologic aspects of neoplasms, such as the two-hit theory of recessive tumor-suppressor genes (e.g., RB gene mutation in retinoblastoma); defects in DNA repair; and the histologic similarities between embryonic organogenesis and oncogenesis. Syndromes associated with defects in DNA repair include xeroderma pigmentosa, in which there is increased risk of skin cancers due to defects in repair of DNA damaged by ultraviolet light. The development of childhood cancers has also been linked to genetic imprinting, which is characterized by selective inactivation of one of the two alleles of a certain gene (discussed in Chapter 5).[69] The inactivation is determined by whether the gene is inherited from the mother or father. For example, normally the maternal allele for the insulin-like growth factor-2 (IGF-2) gene is inactivated (imprinted). The Beckwith-Wiedemann syndrome is an overgrowth syndrome characterized by organomegaly, macroglossia (enlargement of the tongue), hemihypertrophy (muscular or osseous hypertrophy of one side of the body or face), renal abnormalities, and enlarged adrenal cells.[2] The syndrome, which reflects changes in the imprinting of IGF-2 genes located on chromosome 11, is also associated with increased risk of Wilms tumor, hepatoblastoma, rhabdomyosarcoma, and adrenal cortical carcinoma.

Diagnosis and Treatment

Because many childhood cancers are curable, early detection is imperative. In addition, there are several types of cancers for which less therapy is indicated than for more advanced disease. Therefore, early detection often minimizes the amount and duration of treatment required for cure.

Unfortunately, there are no early warning signs or screening tests for cancer in children.[70,71] Prolonged fever, persistent lymphadenopathy, unexplained weight loss, growing masses (especially in association with weight loss), and abnormalities of central nervous system function should be viewed as warning signs of cancer in children. Because these signs and symptoms of cancer are often similar to those of common childhood diseases, they are frequently attributed to other causes.

Diagnosis of childhood cancers involves many of the same methods that are used in adults. Histologic examination is usually an essential part of the diagnostic procedure. Accurate disease staging is especially beneficial in childhood cancers, in which the potential benefits of treatment must be carefully weighed against potential long-term treatment effects.

The treatment of childhood cancers is complex and continuously evolving. It usually involves appropriate multidisciplinary and multimodal therapy, as well as the evaluation for recurrent disease and late effects of the disease and therapies used in its treatment. The treatment program should include specialized teams of health care providers.[72]

Several modalities are frequently used in the treatment of childhood cancer, with chemotherapy being the most widely used, followed in order of use by surgery, radiotherapy, and biologic agent therapy. Chemotherapy is more widely used in treatment of children with cancer than in adults because children better tolerate the acute adverse effects, and in general, pediatric tumors are more responsive to chemotherapy than adult cancers.

Radiation therapy is generally used sparingly in children because they are more vulnerable to the late adverse effects. As with care of adults, adequate pain management is critical.

Survivors of Childhood Cancers

With improvement in treatment methods, the number of children who survive childhood cancer is continuing to increase.[73–76] As a result of cancer treatment, almost 80% of children and adolescents with a diagnosis of cancer become long-term survivors.[72] Unfortunately, radiation and chemotherapy may produce late sequelae, such as impaired growth, neurologic dysfunction, hormonal dysfunction, cardiomyopathy, pulmonary fibrosis, and risk for second malignancies (Table 7-5). There is a special risk of second cancers in children with the retinoblastoma gene. Thus, one of the growing challenges is providing appropriate health care to survivors of childhood and adolescent cancers.

Children reaching adulthood after cancer therapy may have reduced physical stature because of the therapy they received, particularly radiation, which retards the growth of normal tissues along with cancer tissue. The younger the age and the higher the radiation dose, the greater the deviation from normal growth.

There is concern about the effect that CNS radiation has on cognition and hormones that are controlled by the hypothalamic-pituitary axis. Children younger than 6 years of age at the time of radiation and those receiving

TABLE 7-5	Long-term Effects of Childhood Cancer Treatment	
System	**Cancer Treatment**	**Risk**
Cardiac	Radiation, chemotherapy (anthracyclines)	Cardiomyopathy, conduction abnormalities, valve damage, pericarditis, left ventricular dysfunction
Pulmonary	Radiation, chemotherapy (carmustine, lomustine, bleomycin)	Reduction in lung volume with exercise intolerance, restrictive lung disease
Renal/urological	Radiation, chemotherapy (platinums, ifbsfamide and cyclophosphamide, cyclosporine A), nephrectomy	Kidney hypertrophy or atrophy, renal insufficiency or failure, hydronephrosis
Endocrine	Radiation, chemotherapy (alkylating agents)	Pituitary, thyroid, and adrenal dysfunction; growth failure; ovarian and testicular failure; delayed secondary sex characteristics; obesity; infertility
Central nervous system	Radiation, intrathecal (injected into subarachnoid or subdural space) chemotherapy	Learning disabilities
Musculoskeletal and bone	Radiation, chemotherapy (alkylating agents, topoisomerase II inhibitors), amputation	Disordered limb growth, disorders of ambulation and limb use
Hematologic and lymphatic systems	Radiation, chemotherapy (anthracyclines, alkylating agents, vinca alkyloids, antimetabolites), and corticosteroid medications	Leukemia Lymphoma
Second malignancy	Radiation, chemotherapy (alkylating agents, epipodophylotoxins)	Solid tumors, leukemia, lymphoma, brain tumors

Information from: Schmidt D, Anderson L, Bingen K, et al. Late effects in adult survivors of childhood cancer: Considerations for the general practitioner. *WMJ.* 2010;109(2):98–107; and Henderson TO, Friedman DL, Meadows AT. Childhood cancer survivors: Transition to adult-focused risk-based care. *Pediatrics.* 2010;126:127–136.

the highest radiation doses are most likely to have subsequent cognitive difficulties.[73-75] Growth hormone deficiency in adults is associated with increased prevalence of dyslipidemia, insulin resistance, and cardiovascular mortality.[77] Moderate doses of cranial radiation therapy (CRT) are also associated with obesity, particularly in female patients. For many years, whole-brain radiation or cranial radiation was the primary method of preventing CNS relapse in children with acute lymphocytic leukemia. Because of cognitive dysfunction associated with CRT, other methods of CNS prophylaxis are now being used.

Delayed sexual maturation in both boys and girls can result from chemotherapy with alkylating agents or from irradiation of the gonads. Cranial irradiation may result in premature menarche in girls, with subsequent early closure of the epiphyses and a reduction in final growth achieved. Data related to fertility and health of the offspring of childhood cancer survivors is just becoming available.

Vital organs such as the heart and lungs may be affected by cancer treatment. Children who received anthracyclines (i.e., doxorubicin or daunorubicin) may be at risk for developing cardiomyopathy and congestive heart failure. Pulmonary irradiation may cause lung dysfunction and restrictive lung disease. Drugs such as bleomycin, methotrexate, and busulfan also can cause lung disease.

SUMMARY CONCEPTS

- Although most adult cancers are of epithelial cell origin, most childhood cancers involve the hematopoietic system, nervous system, or connective tissue.

- Heritable forms of cancer tend to have an earlier age of onset, a higher frequency of multifocal lesions in a single organ, and bilateral involvement of paired organs or multiple primary tumors.

- The early diagnosis of childhood cancers often is overlooked because the signs and symptoms mimic those of other childhood diseases.

- With improvement in treatment methods, the number of children who survive childhood cancer is continuing to increase. As these children approach adulthood, there is continued concern that the life-saving therapy they received during childhood may produce late effects, such as impaired growth, cognitive dysfunction, hormonal dysfunction, cardiomyopathy, pulmonary fibrosis, and risk for second malignancies.

REVIEW EXERCISES

1. A 30-year-old woman has experienced heavy menstrual bleeding and is told she has a uterine tumor called a *leiomyoma*. She is worried she has cancer.

   A. What is the difference between a leiomyoma and leiomyosarcoma?

   B. How would you go about explaining the difference to her?

2. Among the characteristics of cancer cells are the lack of cell differentiation, impaired cell–cell adhesion, and loss of anchorage dependence.

   A. Explain how each of these characteristics contributes to the usefulness of the Pap smear as a screening test for cervical cancer.

3. A 12-year-old boy is seen in the pediatric cancer clinic with osteosarcoma. His medical history reveals that his father had been successfully treated for retinoblastoma as an infant.

   A. Relate the genetics of the retinoblastoma (RB) gene and "two hit" hypothesis to the development of osteosarcoma in this boy.

4. A 48-year-old man presents at his health care clinic with complaints of leg weakness. He is a heavy smoker and has had a productive cough for years. Subsequent diagnostic tests reveal he has a small cell lung cancer with brain metastasis. His proposed plan of treatment includes chemotherapy and radiation therapy.

   A. What is the probable cause of the leg weakness and is it related to the lung cancer?

   B. Relate this man's smoking history to the development of lung cancer.

   C. Explain the mechanism of cancer metastasis.

   D. Explain the mechanisms whereby chemotherapy and irradiation are able to destroy cancer cells while having less or no effect on normal cells.

5. A 17-year-old girl is seen by a guidance counselor at her high school because of problems in keeping up with assignments in her math and science courses. She tells the counselor that she had leukemia when she was 2 years old and was given radiation treatment to her brain. She confides that she has always had more trouble with learning than her classmates and thinks it might be due to the radiation. She also relates that she is shorter than her classmates and this has been bothering her.

   A. Explain the relationship between cranial radiation therapy and decreased cognitive function and short stature.

   B. What other neuroendocrine problems might this girl have as a result of the radiation treatment?

REFERENCES

1. Siegel R, Naishadham D, Jemal A. Cancer statistics, 2013. *CA Cancer J Clin.* 2013;63:71–81.
2. Striker TP, Kumanr V. Neoplasia. In: Kumar V, Abbas A, Fausto N, et al. *Robbins and Cotran Pathologic Basis of Disease.* 8th ed. Philadelphia, PA: Saunders Elsevier; 2010:259–330.
3. Strayer DS, Rubin E, et al. Neoplasia. In: Rubin R, Strayer DS, eds. *Rubin's Pathology: Clinicopathologic Foundations of Medicine.* 6th ed. Philadelphia, PA: Wolters Kluwer Health | Lippincott Williams & Wilkins; 2012:157–212.
4. Janssen A, Medema RH. Genetic instability: tipping the balance. *Oncogene.* 2013;32:4459–4470.
5. Alberts B, Johnson A, Lewis J, et al. *The Cell.* 5th ed. New York, NY: Garland Science; 2008:1133–1139, 1175–1176, 1230–1240.
6. Wang L. Molecular signaling regulating anchorage-independence growth in cancer cells. *Mt Sinai J Med.* 2004;71(6):361–367.
7. Carruba G, Webber MM, Quader STA, et al. Regulation of cell-to-cell communication in non-tumorigenic and malignant human prostate epithelial cells. *Prostate.* 2002;50:73–82.
8. Marutsuka T, Shimada S, Shiomori K, et al. Mechanisms of peritoneal metastasis after operation for non-serosa-invasive gastric carcinoma: an ultrarapid detection system for intra peritoneal free cancer cells and a prophylactic strategy for peritoneal metastasis. *Clin Cancer Res.* 2003;9:678–685.
9. Tobler NE, Detmar M. Tumor and lymph node lymphangiogenesis—Impact on cancer metastasis. *J Leukoc Biol.* 2006;8:691–696.
10. Chen SL, Iddings DM, Scheri R, et al. Lymphatic mapping and sentinel node analysis: current concepts and applications. *CA Cancer J Clin.* 2006;56:292–307.
11. Minn AJ, Massaguè J. Molecular biology of cancer: invasion and metastasis. In: DeVita VT Jr., Lawrence TS, Rosenberg SA, eds. *Cancer: Principles and Practice of Oncology.* 9th ed. Philadelphia, PA: Wolters Kluwer Health | Lippincott Williams & Wilkins; 2011:113–126.
12. Kerbel RS. Angiogenesis. *N Engl J Med.* 2008;358:2039–2049.
13. Harlozinska A. Progress in molecular mechanisms of tumor metastasis and angiogenesis. *Anticancer Res.* 2005;25:3327–3334.
14. Ruffini PA, Morandi P, Altundag K, et al. Manipulating the chemokine-chemokine receptor network to treat cancer. *Cancer.* 2007;109(12):2392–2404.
15. Kakinuma T, Twang ST. Chemokines, chemokine receptors, and cancer metastasis. *J Leukoc Biol.* 2006;79:639–651.
16. Crocce CM. Oncogenes and cancer. *N Engl J Med.* 2008;358(5):502–511.
17. Zhou BP, Hung MC. Dysregulation of cellular signaling by HER2/neu in breast cancer. *Semin Oncol.* 2003;30(5 Suppl 16):38–48.
18. Esteller M. Epigenetics in cancer. *N Engl J Med.* 2008;358(11):1148–1159.
19. Baylin SB. DNA methylation and gene silencing in cancer. *Nat Clin Pract Oncol.* 2005;2:S4–S11.
20. Iorio MV, Croce CM. microRNA involvement in human cancer. *Carcinogenesis.* 2012;33(6):1126–1133.
21. Schulze-Bergkamen H, Krammer PH. Apoptosis in cancer—Implications for therapy. *Semin Oncol.* 2004;31:90–119.
22. Mooi WJ, Peeper DS. Oncogene-induced cell senescence—Halting the road to cancer. *N Engl J Med.* 2006;355(10):1037–1046.
23. Kerbel RS. Tumor angiogenesis. *N Engl J Med.* 2008;358(19):2039.
24. Boccaccio C, Comoglio PM. Invasive growth: a *MET*-driven genetic programme for cancer and stem cells. *Nat Rev Cancer.* 2006;6:637–645.

25. Ceschi M, Gutzwiller F, Mody H, et al. Epidemiology and pathophysiology of obesity as a cause of cancer. *Swiss Med Wkly.* 2007;137:50–56.
26. Finn OJ. Cancer immunology. *N Engl J Med.* 2008;358(25):2704–2715.
27. Burnett FM. Immunologic aspects of malignant disease. *Lancet* 1967;1:1171.
28. Michels KB, Willett WC. Etiology of cancer: dietary factors. In: DeVita VT Jr, Lawrence TS, Rosenberg SA, eds. *Cancer: Principles and Practice of Oncology.* 9th ed. Philadelphia, PA: Wolters Kluwer Health | Lippincott Williams & Wilkins; 2011:217–226.
29. Seitz HK, Stickel F. Molecular mechanisms of alcohol-mediated carcinogenesis. *Nat Rev Cancer.* 2007;7:599–612.
30. Jablon S, Kato H. Studies of the mortality of A-bomb survivors: 5. Radiation dose and mortality, 1950–1970. *Radiat Res.* 1972;50:649–698.
31. Liao JB. Viruses and human cancer. *Yale J Biol Med.* 2006;79:115–122.
32. Centers for Disease Control and Prevention. *HPV vaccine information for young women—Fact sheet.* [Online]. Available at: http://www.cdc.gov/std/hpv/STDFact-HPV-vaccine-young-women.htm. Accessed September 26, 2013.
33. Cornett PA, Dea TO. Cancer. In: Papadakis MA, McPhee SJ, eds. *Current Medical Diagnosis and Treatment.* 52th ed. New York, NY: McGraw-Hill; 2013:1593–1663.
34. Knight K, Wade S, Balducci L. Prevalence and outcomes of anemia in cancer: a systematic review of the literature. *Am J Med.* 2004;116(7A):11S–26S.
35. Hurter B, Bush NJ. Cancer-related anemia: Clinical review and management update. *Clin J Oncol Nurs.* 2007;11(3):349–359.
36. Dicato M, Plawny L, Diederich M. Anemia in cancer. *Ann Oncol.* 2011;27(7):viii,167–172.
37. Pedrazzoli P, Rosti G, Secondino S, et al. Iron supplementation and erythropoiesis-stimulatory agents in the treatment of cancer anemia. *Cancer.* 2009;115:1169–1175.
38. Gordon JN, Green SR, Goggin PM. Cancer cachexia. *Q J Med.* 2005;98:779–788.
39. Tisdale MJ. Molecular pathways leading to cancer cachexia. *Physiology (Bethesda).* 2005;20:340–348.
40. Bennani-Baita N, Davis MP. Cytokines and cancer anorexia cachexia syndrome. *Am J Hosp Palliat Care.* 2008;25(5):407–441.
41. Wu H, Davis JE, Natavio T. Fatigue and disrupted sleep-wake patterns in patients with cancer: A shared mechanism. *Clin J Oncol Nurs.* 2012;16(2):E56–E68.
42. Ryan JL, Carroll JK, Ryan EP, et al. Mechanisms of cancer-related fatigue. *Oncologist.* 2007;12(Suppl 1):S1–S22.
43. Wang XS. Pathophysiology of cancer-related fatigue. *Clin J Oncol Nurs.* 2008;12(5 Suppl 1):11–20.
44. Hofman M, Ryan JL, Comar D, et al. Cancer-related fatigue: the scale of the problem. *Oncologist.* 2007;12(Suppl 1):4–10.
45. Barsevick AM, Newhall T, Brown S. Management of cancer-related fatigue. *Clin J Oncol Nurs.* 2008;12(5 Suppl 1):21–25.
46. Pelosof LC, Gerber DE. Paraneoplastic syndromes: an approach to diagnosis and treatment. *Mayo Clin Proc.* 2012;85(9):838–854.
47. Boyiadzis M, Lieberman FS, Geskin LJ, et al. Paraneoplastic syndromes. In: DeVita VT Jr, Lawrence TS, Rosenberg SA, eds. *Cancer: Principles and Practice of Oncology.* 9th ed. Philadelphia, PA: Wolters Kluwer Health | Lippincott Williams & Wilkins; 2011:2220–2238.
48. Dalmau J, Rosenfeld M. Paraneoplastic neurologic syndromes. In: Abeloff MD, Armitage JO, Niolerhuber JE, et al. *Clinical Oncology.* 4th ed. London, UK: Elsevier/Churchill Livingston; 2008:767–779.
49. Darnell RB, Posner JB. Paraneoplastic syndromes involving the nervous system. *N Engl J Med.* 2003;349(16):1543–1554.

50. Miser WF. Cancer screening in the primary care setting. *Prim Care* 2007;34:137–167.
51. Smith RA, Brooks D, Cokkinides V, et al. Cancer screening in the United States, 2013: a review of current American Cancer Society guidelines, current issues in cancer screening and lung cancer screening. *CA Cancer J Clin.* 2013;63(2):88–105.
52. Rosenberg SA. Cancer management: surgical oncology: general issues. In: DeVita VT Jr, Lawrence TS, Rosenberg SA, eds. *Cancer: Principles and Practice of Oncology.* 9th ed. Philadelphia, PA: Wolters Kluwer Health | Lippincott Williams & Wilkins; 2011:268–276.
53. Jeremic B. Radiation therapy. *Hematol Oncol Clin North Am* 2004;18:1–12.
54. Morgan MA, Ten Haken RK, Lawrence TS. Radiation oncology. In: DeVita VT Jr, Lawrence TS, Rosenberg SA, eds. *Cancer: Principles and Practice of Oncology.* 9th ed. Philadelphia, PA: Wolters Kluwer Health | Lippincott Williams & Wilkins; 2011:289–311.
55. Willers H, Held KD. Introduction to clinical radiation biology. *Hematol Oncol Clin North Am.* 2006;20:1–24.
56. Hogle WP. The state of the art in radiation therapy. *Semin Oncol Nurs.* 2006;22(4):212–220.
57. Ikushima H. Radiation therapy: state of the art and the future. *J Med Invest* 2010;97:1–11.
58. Chu E, Sartorelli AC. Cancer chemotherapy. In: Katzung BG, eds. *Basic and Clinical Pharmacology.* 10th ed. New York, NY. McGraw-Hill; 2012:949–975.
59. DeVita VT Jr, Lawrence TS, Rosenberg SA, eds. *Cancer: Principles and Practice of Oncology.* 9th ed. Philadelphia, PA: Wolters Kluwer Health/Lippincott Williams & Wilkins; 2011:360–498.
60. Neuss MN, Polocich M, McNiff K, et al. 2013 updated American Society of Clinical Oncology/Oncology Nursing Society chemotherapy administration safety standards including standards for safe administration and management of oral chemotherapy. *Oncol Nurs Forum.* 2013;40(3):325–233.
61. Hawkins R. Hormone therapy in cancer. *Oncol Nurs Updates.* 2002;9(3):1–16.
62. Altundag K, Ibrahim NK. Aromatase inhibitors in breast cancer: an overview. *Oncologist.* 2006;11:553–562.
63. Kuroki M, Miyamoto S, Morisaki T, et al. Biological response modifiers in cancer biotherapy. *Anticancer Res.* 2012;32:2229–2233.
64. Kirkwood JM, Butterfield LH, Tarhini A, et al. Immunotherapy in cancer 2012. *CA Cancer J Clin.* 2012;62(5):309–335.
65. Robinson MK, Borghaei H, Adams GP, et al. Monoclonal antibodies. In: DeVita VT Jr, Lawrence TS, Rosenberg SA, eds. *Cancer: Principles and Practice of Oncology.* 9th ed. Philadelphia, PA: Wolters Kluwer Health/Lippincott Williams & Wilkins; 2011:499–507.
66. Sharkey RM, Goldenberg DM. Targeted therapy of cancer: new prospects for antibodies and immunoconjugates. *CA Cancer J Clin.* 2006;56:226–243.
67. Goetsch CM. Genetic tumor profiling and genetically targeted cancer therapy. *Semin Oncol Nurs.* 2011;27(3):34–44.
68. Asselin BL. Epidemiology of childhood and adolescent cancer. In: Kliegman RM, Stanton BF, St. Geme JW, et al., eds. *Nelson Textbook of Pediatrics.* 19th ed. Philadelphia, PA: W.B. Saunders; 2011:1725–1727.
69. Smith LL. Molecular and cellular biology of cancer. In: Kliegman RM, Stanton BF, St. Geme JW, et al., eds. *Nelson Textbook of Pediatrics.* 19th ed. Philadelphia, PA: W.B. Saunders; 2011:1727–1728.
70. Richey K. Principles of diagnosis. In: Kliegman RM, Stanton BF, St. Geme JW, et al., eds. *Nelson Textbook of Pediatrics.* 19th ed. Philadelphia, PA: W.B. Saunders; 2011:1729–1731.
71. Fragkandrea J, Nixon JA, Panagopoulou P. Signs and symptoms of childhood cancer: a guide to early recognition. *Am Fam Physician.* 2013;88(3):185–192.
72. Bleyer A, Rtchey AK. Principles of treatment. In: Kliegman RM, Stanton BF, St. Geme JW, et al., eds. *Nelson Textbook of Pediatrics.* 19th ed. Philadelphia, PA: W.B. Saunders; 2011:1732–1741.
73. Armstrong GT, Stoval M, Robison LL. Long-term effects of radiation exposure among adult survivors of childhood cancer: results from the childhood cancer survivors study. *Radiat Res.* 2010;17:840–850.
74. Schmidt D, Anderson LA, Bingen K. Late effects in adult survivors of childhood cancer: Considerations for the general practitioner. *Wis Med J.* 2010;100(2):98–107.
75. Henderson TTO. Childhood cancer survivors: transition in adult-focused risk-based care. *Pediatrics.* 2010;126:127–136.
76. Oeffinger KC, Mertens AC, Sklar CA, et al. Chronic health conditions in adult survivors of childhood cancer. *N Engl J Med.* 2006;355:1572–1582.
77. Cohen LE. Endocrine late effects of cancer treatment. *Endocrinol Metab Clin North Am.* 2005;34:769–789.

Porth Essentials Resources

Explore these additional resources to enhance learning for this chapter:

- NCLEX-Style Questions and Other Resources on the**Point**, http://thePoint.lww.com/PorthEssentials4e
- Study Guide for Essentials of Pathophysiology
- Concepts in Action Animations
- Adaptive Learning | Powered by PrepU, http://thepoint.lww.com/prepu

(continued on page 160)

C h a p t e r 8

Disorders of Fluid, Electrolyte, and Acid–Base Balance

Fluids and electrolytes are present in body cells, in the tissue spaces between the cells, and in the blood that fills the vascular compartment. Body fluids transport gases, nutrients, and wastes; help generate the electrical activity needed to power body functions; take part in the transforming of food into energy; and otherwise maintain the overall function of the body. Although fluid volume and composition remain relatively constant in the presence of a wide range of changes in intake and output, conditions such as environmental stresses and disease can impair intake, increase losses, and otherwise interfere with mechanisms that regulate their volume, composition, and distribution.

This chapter is divided into five sections: composition and compartmental distribution of body fluids; disorders of sodium and water balance; disorders of potassium balance; disorders of calcium, phosphorus, and magnesium balance; and disorders of acid–base balance.

Composition and Compartmental Distribution of Body Fluids

Body fluids are distributed between the intracellular and extracellular fluid compartments.[1-3] The *intracellular fluid (ICF) compartment*, which consists of the fluid contained within all of the trillions of cells in the body, contains about two thirds of the body water in healthy adults. The remaining one third is in the *extracellular fluid (ECF) compartment*, which contains all the fluids outside the cells, including those in the interstitial or tissue spaces and the plasma in the blood vessels (Fig. 8-1).

The composition of the ECF and ICF are strikingly different. The ECF contains large amounts of sodium and chloride, moderate amounts of bicarbonate, but only small quantities of potassium, magnesium, calcium, and phosphate. In contrast, the ICF contains almost no calcium; small amounts of sodium, chloride, bicarbonate, and phosphate; moderate amounts of magnesium; and large amounts of potassium (Table 8-1). Although blood levels usually are representative of the total body levels of an electrolyte, this is not always the case, particularly with potassium, which is approximately 28 times more concentrated inside the cell than outside.

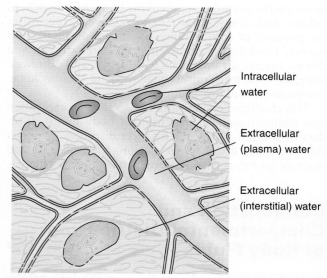

FIGURE 8-1. Distribution of body water. The extracellular space includes the vascular compartment and the interstitial spaces.

Intracellular water

Extracellular (plasma) water

Extracellular (interstitial) water

Movement of Body Fluids and Electrolytes Between Compartments

The lipid bilayer and transport proteins serve as the primary barriers to the movement of substances across the cell membrane that separates the ECF and ICF compartments (see Chapter 1, Fig. 1-11). Lipid-soluble substances (e.g., oxygen [O_2] and carbon dioxide [CO_2]), which dissolve in the lipid layer of the cell membrane, pass directly through the membrane. Many ions (e.g., sodium [Na^+] and potassium [K^+]) rely on transport proteins located in the cell membrane for movement across the membrane, accounting for the compartmental difference in their concentrations. Water crosses the cell membrane by osmosis using special transmembrane protein channels called aquaporins.

Dissociation of Electrolytes

Electrolytes are substances that dissociate in solution to form charged particles, or *ions*. For example, the sodium chloride (NaCl) molecule dissociates to form a positively charged Na^+ and a negatively charged Cl^- ion. Particles that do not dissociate into ions such as glucose and urea are called *nonelectrolytes*. Positively charged ions are called *cations* because they are attracted to the cathode of a wet electric cell, and negatively charged ions are called *anions* because they are attracted to the anode. The ions found in body fluids carry one charge (i.e., monovalent ion) or two charges (i.e., divalent ion). Because of their attraction forces, positively charged cations are always accompanied by negatively charged anions. Thus, both the ICF and ECF contain equal amounts of anions and cations. Cations and anions may be exchanged for one another, providing they carry the same charge. For example, a positively charged hydrogen ion (H^+) may be exchanged for a positively charged K^+, and a negatively charged bicarbonate ion (HCO_3^-) may be exchanged for a negatively charged chloride ion (Cl^-).

The concentration of electrolytes in the ICF and ECF can be expressed in several ways; for example, milligrams per deciliter (mg/dL), milliequivalents per liter (mEq/L), or millimoles per liter (mmol/L) (Box 8-1).

TABLE 8-1	Concentrations of Extracellular and Intracellular Electrolytes in Adults				
	Extracellular Concentration*			**Intracellular Concentration***	
Electrolyte	*Conventional Units*	*SI Units*		*Conventional Units*	*SI Units*
Sodium	135–145 mEq/L	135–145 mmol/L		10–15 mEq/L	10–15 mmol/L
Potassium	3.5–5.0 mEq/L	3.5–5.0 mmol/L		140–150 mEq/L	140–150 mmol/L
Chloride	98–106 mEq/L	98–106 mmol/L		3–4 mEq/L	3–4 mmol/L
Bicarbonate	24–31 mEq/L	24–31 mmol/L		7–10 mEq/L	7–10 mmol/L
Calcium	8.5–10.5 mg/dL	2.1–2.6 mmol/L		<1 mg/dL	<0.25 mmol/L
Phosphorus	2.5–4.5 mg/dL	0.8–1.45 mmol/L		4 mEq/kg[†]	75 mmol/L
Magnesium	1.3–2.1 mg/dL	0.65–1.1 mmol/L		variable[†]	variable[†]

*Values may vary among laboratories, depending on the method of analysis used.

[†]Values vary among various tissues and with nutritional status.

Osmosis and Tonicity

Despite the remarkable difference in the concentration of individual molecules in the ICF and ECF, the total concentration gradient is the same in both compartments because of the osmotic movement of water. *Osmosis* refers to the movement of water across a semipermeable membrane (i.e., one that is permeable to water but impermeable to most solutes).[1,3] As with solute particles, water diffuses down its concentration gradient, moving from the side of the membrane with a greater concentration of water and lesser concentration of solute particles to the side with a lesser concentration of water and greater concentration of solute particles (Fig. 8-2). As water moves across the semipermeable membrane, it generates a pressure called the *osmotic pressure*. The magnitude of the osmotic pressure represents the hydrostatic pressure (measured in millimeters of mercury [mm Hg]) needed to oppose the movement of water across the membrane.

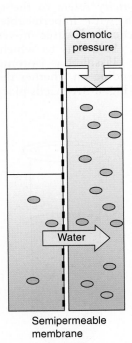

FIGURE 8-2. Movement of water across a semipermeable membrane. Water moves from the side that has fewer nondiffusible particles to the side that has more. The osmotic pressure is equal to the hydrostatic pressure needed to oppose water movement across the membrane.

The osmotic activity that nondiffusible particles exert in pulling water from one side of the semipermeable membrane to the other is measured by a unit called an *osmole*. In the clinical setting, osmotic activity usually is expressed in milliosmoles (one thousandth of an osmole) per liter. Each nondiffusible particle, large or small, is equally effective in its ability to pull water through a semipermeable membrane. Thus, it is the *number*, rather than the *size*, of the nondiffusible particles that determines the osmotic activity of a solution.

The osmotic activity of a solution may be expressed in terms of either its osmolarity or osmolality. *Osmolarity* refers to the osmolar concentration in 1 L of solution (mOsm/L H_2O) and *osmolality* to the osmolar concentration in 1 kg of water (mOsm/kg H_2O).[2] Osmolarity is often used when referring to fluids outside the body and osmolality for describing fluids inside the body. Because 1 L of water weighs 1 kg, the terms *osmolarity* and *osmolality* are often used interchangeably.

Serum osmolality, which is largely determined by Na^+ and its attendant anions (Cl^- and HCO_3^-), normally ranges between 275 and 295 mOsm/kg H_2O. Blood urea nitrogen (BUN) and glucose, which also are osmotically active, usually account for less than 5% of the total osmotic pressure in the ECF compartment. However, this can change, such as when blood glucose levels are elevated in persons with diabetes mellitus or when BUN levels change rapidly in persons with chronic kidney disease.

The term *tonicity* refers to the tension or effect that a solution with impermeable solutes exerts on cell size because of water movement across the cell membrane.[3] Solutions to which body cells are exposed can be classified as isotonic, hypotonic, or hypertonic depending on whether they cause cells to swell or shrink (Fig. 8-3A). Cells placed in an *isotonic solution*, which has the same effective osmolality as the ICF, neither shrink nor swell. An example of an isotonic solution is 0.9% sodium chloride. When cells are placed in a *hypotonic solution*, which has a lower osmolality than the ICF, they swell as water moves into the cell (Fig. 8-3B). When they are placed in a *hypertonic solution*, which has a greater osmolality than the ICF, they shrink as water is pulled out of the cell (Fig. 8-3C).

Compartmental Distribution of Body Fluids

Body water, which constitutes about 60% of body weight in the adult, is distributed between the ICF and ECF compartments.[1–4] The fluid in the ICF compartment constitutes approximately 40% of body weight, and that in the ECF approximately 20% of body weight.

The fluid in the ECF compartment is further divided into two major subdivisions: the *plasma compartment*, which constitutes approximately 5% of body weight, and the *interstitial compartment*, which constitutes approximately 14% of body weight (Fig. 8-4). The fluid in the interstitial compartment acts as a transport vehicle for gases, nutrients, wastes, and other materials that move between the vascular compartment and body cells. The interstitial fluid compartment also provides a reservoir from which vascular volume can be maintained during periods of hemorrhage or loss of vascular volume. An interstitial gel, which is a sponge-like material supported by collagen fibers, fills the tissue spaces and aids in even distribution of interstitial fluid. Normally, most of the fluid in the interstitium is in gel form.[2] The interstitial gel, which has a firmer consistency than water, opposes the outflow of water from the capillaries, preventing the accumulation of free water in the interstitial spaces.

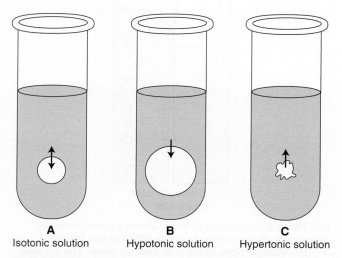

FIGURE 8-3. Tonicity: Red cells undergo no change in size in isotonic solutions (**A**). They increase in size in hypotonic solutions (**B**) and decrease in size in hypertonic solutions (**C**).

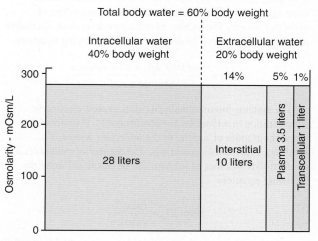

FIGURE 8-4. Approximate size of body compartments in a 70-kg adult.

A third, usually minor, subdivision of the ECF compartment is the *transcellular compartment*. It includes the cerebrospinal fluid and fluid contained in the various body spaces, such as the peritoneal, pleural, and pericardial cavities, and joint spaces. Normally, only about 1% of ECF is in the transcellular space. This amount can increase considerably in conditions such as ascites, in which large amounts of fluid are sequestered in the peritoneal cavity. When the transcellular fluid compartment becomes considerably enlarged, it is referred to as a *third space*, because this fluid is not readily available for exchange with the rest of the ECF.

Capillary/Interstitial Fluid Exchange

The transfer of water between the vascular and interstitial compartments occurs at the capillary level. There are four main forces that control the movement of water between the capillary and interstitial spaces: (1) the *capillary filtration pressure*, which *pushes* water out of the capillary into the interstitial spaces; (2) the *capillary colloidal osmotic pressure*, which *pulls* water back into the capillary; (3) the *interstitial* or *tissue hydrostatic pressure*, which *opposes* the movement of water out of the capillary; and (4) the *interstitial colloidal osmotic pressure*, which *pulls* water out of the capillary into the interstitial spaces.[1-3] Normally, the combination of these four forces is such that only a small excess of fluid remains in the interstitial compartment. This excess fluid is removed from the interstitium by the lymphatic system and returned to the systemic circulation.

Capillary filtration refers to the movement of water through capillary pores because of hydrostatic pressure, rather than an osmotic force. The capillary filtration pressure (about 30 to 40 mm Hg at the arterial end, 10 to 15 mm Hg at the venous end, and 25 mm Hg in the middle) is the pressure pushing water out of the capillary into the interstitial spaces.[2] It reflects the arterial and venous pressures, the precapillary (arterioles) and postcapillary (venules) resistances, and the force of gravity.[2] A rise in arterial or venous pressure increases capillary pressures throughout the body, whereas the force of gravity increases the capillary pressure in the dependent or lower parts of the body. In a person who is standing absolutely still, the weight of blood in the vascular column causes an increase of 1 mm Hg pressure for every 13.6 mm of distance from the heart.[2] Since this pressure results from the weight of water, it is called *hydrostatic pressure*. In the adult who is standing absolutely still, the pressure in the veins of the feet can reach 90 mm Hg.

The *capillary colloidal osmotic or oncotic pressure* (about 28 mm Hg) is the osmotic pressure generated by the plasma proteins that are too large to pass through the pores of the capillary wall.[2] The term *colloidal osmotic pressure* differentiates this type of osmotic pressure from the osmotic pressure that develops at the cell membrane from the presence of electrolytes and nonelectrolytes.

Because plasma proteins do not normally penetrate the capillary pores and because their concentration is greater in the plasma than in the interstitial fluids, it is capillary colloidal osmotic pressure that pulls fluids back into the capillary.

The interstitial fluid pressure (about −3 mm Hg) and interstitial colloidal osmotic pressure (about 8 mm Hg) contribute to movement of water into and out of the interstitial spaces.[2] The *interstitial hydrostatic fluid pressure*, which is normally negative, contributes to the outward movement of water into the interstitial spaces. The *interstitial colloidal osmotic pressure*, which reflects the small amount of plasma proteins that normally escape into the interstitial spaces from the capillary, also pulls water out of the capillary into the tissue spaces.

The lymphatic system represents an accessory route whereby fluid from the interstitial spaces can return to the circulation. More importantly, the lymphatic system provides a means for removing plasma proteins and osmotically active particulate matter from the tissue spaces, neither of which can be reabsorbed into the capillaries.

Edema

Edema can be defined as palpable swelling produced by an increase in interstitial fluid volume. The physiologic mechanisms that contribute to edema formation include factors that: (1) increase the capillary filtration pressure, (2) decrease the capillary colloidal osmotic pressure, (3) increase capillary permeability, or (4) produce obstruction to lymph flow. The causes of edema are summarized in Chart 8-1.

CHART 8-1   Common Causes of Edema

Increased Capillary Pressure

Increased vascular volume (e.g., heart failure, kidney disease)
Venous obstruction (e.g., thrombophlebitis)
Liver disease with portal vein obstruction
Acute pulmonary edema

Decreased Colloidal Osmotic Pressure

Increased loss of plasma proteins (e.g., protein-losing kidney diseases, extensive burns)
Decreased production of plasma proteins (liver disease, malnutrition)

Increased Capillary Permeability

Inflammation
Allergic reactions (e.g., hives, angioneurotic edema)
Malignancy (e.g., ascites, pleural effusion)
Tissue injury and burns

Obstruction of Lymphatic Flow

Malignant obstruction of lymphatic structures
Surgical removal of lymph nodes

(*text continues on page 165*)

UNDERSTANDING → Capillary Fluid

Movement of fluid between the vascular compartment and the interstitial fluid compartment surrounding the body cells occurs at the capillary level. The direction and amount of fluid that flows across the capillary wall are determined by: (1) the hydrostatic pressure of the two compartments, (2) the colloidal osmotic pressures of the two compartments, and (3) the removal of excess fluid and osmotically active particles from the interstitial spaces by the lymphatic system.

1

Hydrostatic Pressure. The hydrostatic pressure is the pushing force exerted by a fluid. Inside the capillaries, the hydrostatic pressure is the same as the capillary filtration pressure, about 30 mm Hg at the arterial end and 10 mm Hg at the venous end. The interstitial fluid pressure is the force of fluid in the interstitial spaces pushing against the outside of the capillary wall. Evidence suggests that the interstitial pressure is slightly negative (−3 mm Hg), contributing to the outward movement of fluid from the capillary.

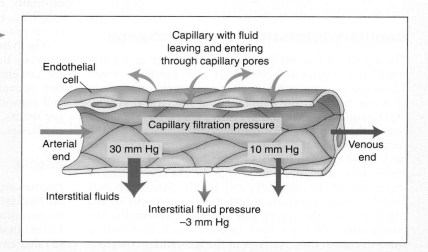

2

Colloidal Osmotic Pressure. The colloidal osmotic pressure is the pulling force created by the presence of evenly dispersed particles, such as the plasma proteins, that cannot pass through the pores of the capillary membrane. The capillary colloidal osmotic pressure is normally about 28 mm Hg throughout the length of the capillary bed. The interstitial colloidal osmotic pressure (about 8 mm Hg) represents the pulling pressure exerted by the small amounts of plasma proteins that leak through the pores of the capillary wall into the interstitial spaces. The capillary colloidal osmotic pressure, which is greater than both the hydrostatic pressure at the venous end of the capillary and the interstitial colloidal osmotic pressure, is largely responsible for the movement of fluid back into the capillary.

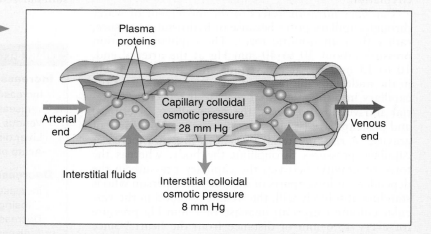

Exchange

3

Lymph Drainage. The lymphatic system represents an accessory system by which fluid can be returned to the circulatory system. Normally the forces moving fluid out of the capillary into the interstitium are greater than those returning fluid to the capillary. Any excess fluids and osmotically active plasma proteins that may have leaked into the interstitium are picked up by vessels of the lymphatic system and returned to the circulation. Without the function of the lymphatic system, excessive amounts of fluid would accumulate in the interstitial spaces.

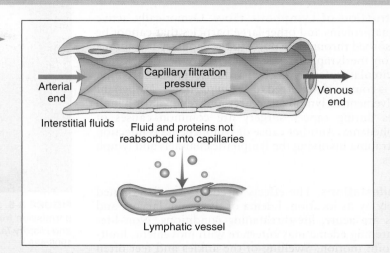

(text continued from page 163)

Increased Capillary Filtration Pressure. Edema due to increased capillary filtration pressure is usually the result of increased vascular volume. It is commonly seen in conditions such as congestive heart failure that produce fluid retention and venous congestion (see Chapter 20). Edema does not usually become evident until the interstitial volume has been increased by 2.5 to 3 L.[4] *Dependent edema* describes an accumulation of fluid in the lower parts of the body. Because of the effects of gravity, edema that results from increased capillary pressure commonly causes dependent edema. For example, edema of the ankles and feet becomes more pronounced during prolonged periods of standing. Lower extremity edema due to an increase in venous pressure is a common complication of venous insufficiency resulting from thrombophlebitis (development of a blood clot in one of the deep leg veins).

Decreased Capillary Colloidal Osmotic Pressure. Plasma proteins exert the osmotic force needed to pull fluid back into the capillary from the tissue spaces. The plasma proteins constitute a mixture of albumin, globulins, and fibrinogen. Albumin, the smallest of the plasma proteins, has a molecular weight of 69,000; globulins have molecular weights of approximately 140,000; and fibrinogen has a molecular weight of 400,000.[2] Because of its lower molecular weight, 1 g of albumin has approximately twice as many osmotically active molecules as 1 g of globulin and almost six times as many as 1 g of fibrinogen. Also, the concentration of albumin (approximately 4.5 g/dL) is greater than that of the globulins (2.5 g/dL) and fibrinogen (0.3 mg/dL).[2]

Therefore, albumin has the greatest effect on the colloidal osmotic pressure.

Edema caused by decreased capillary colloidal osmotic pressure usually is the result of inadequate production or excessive loss of plasma proteins, mainly albumin. The plasma proteins are synthesized in the liver. In persons with severe liver failure, the impaired synthesis of albumin results in a decrease in colloidal osmotic pressure. In starvation and malnutrition, edema develops because there is a lack of amino acids for plasma protein synthesis. The most common site of plasma protein loss is the kidney. In kidney diseases such as nephrotic syndrome, the glomerular capillaries become permeable to the plasma proteins, particularly albumin (see Chapter 25). When this occurs, large amounts of albumin are filtered out of the blood and lost in the urine. An excessive loss of plasma proteins also occurs when large areas of skin are injured or destroyed, such as occurs during the early stages of a burn.[5]

Because the plasma proteins are evenly distributed throughout the body and are not affected by the force of gravity, edema that is caused by a decrease in capillary colloidal osmotic pressure tends to produce generalized edema involving the face as well the legs and feet.

Increased Capillary Permeability. When the capillary pores become enlarged or the integrity of the capillary wall is damaged, capillary permeability is increased. When this occurs, plasma proteins and other osmotically active particles leak into the interstitial spaces, pulling fluid out of the capillary into the interstitium. Among the conditions that increase capillary permeability are burn injury, inflammation, and immune responses.

Obstruction of Lymphatic Flow. Osmotically active plasma proteins and other large particles that cannot be reabsorbed through the pores in the capillary membrane rely on the lymphatic system for movement back into the circulatory system. Edema due to impaired lymph flow is commonly referred to as *lymphedema*. Malignant involvement of lymph structures and removal of lymph nodes during cancer surgery are common causes of lymphedema. Another cause of lymphedema is infection and trauma involving the lymphatic channels and lymph nodes.

Manifestations. The effects of edema are determined largely by its location. Edema of the brain, larynx, and lungs are acute, life-threatening conditions. Non–life-threatening edema may interfere with movement, limiting joint motion. Swelling of the ankles and feet often is insidious in onset and may or may not be associated with disease. At the tissue level, edema increases the distance for diffusion of oxygen, nutrients, and wastes. Thus, edematous tissues usually are more susceptible to injury and development of ischemic tissue damage, including pressure ulcers. Edema can also compress blood vessels. For example, the skin of a severely swollen finger can act as a tourniquet, shutting off the blood flow. Edema can also be disfiguring, causing psychological effects and disturbances in self-concept, as well as making it difficult to obtain proper-fitting clothing and shoes.

Pitting edema occurs when the accumulation of interstitial fluid exceeds the absorptive capacity of the tissue gel. In this form of edema, the tissue water becomes mobile and can be translocated with pressure exerted by a finger. *Nonpitting edema* in which the swollen area becomes firm and discolored, occurs when plasma proteins have accumulated in the tissue spaces and coagulated. It is most commonly seen in areas of localized infection or trauma.

Assessment and Treatment. Methods for assessing edema include daily weight (1 L of water weighs 2.2 pounds), visual assessment, measurement of the affected part, and application of finger pressure to assess for pitting edema. Daily weight measurements taken at the same time each day with the same amount of clothing provide a useful index of water gain due to edema. Visual inspection and measurement of the circumference of an extremity can also be used to assess the degree of swelling. This is particularly useful when swelling is due to thrombophlebitis. Finger pressure can be used to assess the degree of pitting edema. If an indentation remains after the finger has been removed, pitting edema is identified. It is evaluated on a scale of +1 (minimal) to +4 (severe) (Fig. 8-5).

Distinguishing lymphedema from other forms of edema can be challenging, especially early in its course. *Papillomatosis,* a characteristic honeycomb appearance

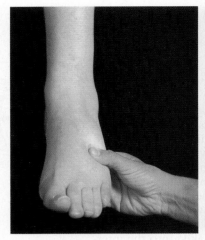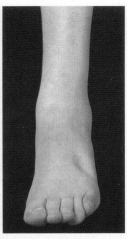

FIGURE 8-5. 3+ pitting edema of the left foot. (Used with permission from Bates B. *Bates' Guide to Physical Examination and History Taking.* 6th ed. Philadelphia, PA: J.B. Lippincott; 1995:438.)

of the skin due to dilated lymph vessels that are enveloped in fibrotic tissue, distinguishes lymphedema from other forms of edema. Computed tomography (CT) or magnetic resonance imaging (MRI) may be used to confirm the diagnosis.[6]

Treatment of edema usually is directed toward maintaining life when the swelling involves vital structures, correcting or controlling the cause, and preventing tissue injury. Edema of the lower extremities may respond to simple measures such as elevating the feet. Diuretic therapy commonly is used to treat edema associated with an increase in ECF volume. Serum albumin levels can be measured, and albumin administered intravenously to raise the plasma colloidal osmotic pressure when edema is caused by hypoalbuminemia.

Elastic support stockings and sleeves increase interstitial fluid pressure and resistance to outward movement of fluid from the capillary into the tissue spaces. These support devices typically are prescribed for patients with conditions such as venous or lymphatic obstruction and are most efficient if applied before the tissue spaces have filled with fluid—for example, in the morning before the effects of gravity have caused fluid to move into the ankles. Moderate to severe lymphedema is usually treated with light-pressure massage designed to increase lymph flow by encouraging opening and closing of lymph vessel valves; compression garments or pneumatic compression pumps; range-of-motion exercises; and scrupulous skin care to prevent infection.[6]

Third-Space Accumulation

Third spacing represents the loss or movement and trapping of ECF in a transcompartmental space. The serous cavities are part of the transcompartmental compartment (i.e., third space) located in strategic body areas where there is continual movement of body structures—the pericardial sac, the peritoneal cavity, and the pleural cavity. The serous cavities, which are closely linked with lymphatic drainage systems, use the same mechanisms for interstitial fluid exchange as other areas of the body. The milking action of the moving structures, such as the lungs, continually forces fluid and plasma proteins back into lymphatic channels, helping to keep these cavities empty. Thus any obstruction of lymph flow causes fluid to accumulate in the serous cavities. Although the accumulation of third-space fluids produces a gain in body weight, it does not contribute to the body's fluid reserve or function.

The prefix *hydro-* may be used to indicate the presence of excessive fluid in one of the serous cavitis, with *hydrothorax* referring to fluid in the pleural cavity. An accumulation of fluid in the peritoneal cavity as *ascites* and the transudation of fluid into the serous cavities is referred to as *effusion*. Effusion can contain blood, plasma proteins, inflammatory cells (i.e., pus), and extracellular fluid.

SUMMARY CONCEPTS

■ Body fluids, which contain water and electrolytes, are distributed between the intracellular fluid (ICF) and extracellular fluid (ECF) compartments of the body, with two thirds being contained in the ICF and one third in the ECF.

■ The cell membrane serves as a selective barrier to the movement of substances between the ICF and ECF. Lipid-soluble substances (e.g., oxygen [O_2] and carbon dioxide [CO_2]), which dissolve in the lipid layer of the cell membrane, pass directly through the membrane. Electrolytes, such as sodium [Na^+] and potassium [K^+], rely on transport proteins located in the cell membrane for movement across the membrane, accounting for the compartmental difference in their concentrations.

■ Water moves across a semipermeable membrane by *osmosis* moving from the side with the greater concentration of water and lesser concentration of solute particles to the side having the lesser water concentration and greater solute concentration. *Osmolarity* refers to the osmotic activity that nondiffusible particles exert in pulling water from one side of a semipermeable membrane to the other and *tonicity* to the tension or effect that the osmotic pressure of a solution with nondiffusible solutes exerts on cell size because of water movement. Cells remain the same size when placed in an *isotonic solution* with the same osmolarity as the ICF; swell when placed in a hypotonic solution that has an osmolality less than the

ICF; and shrink when placed in a hypertonic solution that has an osmolality greater than the ICF.

■ Edema represents the accumulation of fluid volume in the interstitial spaces of the ECF resulting from: (1) an increase in capillary filtration pressure, (2) a decrease capillary colloidal osmotic pressure, (3) an increase in capillary permeability, or (4) obstructed lymphatic flow. The effect that edema exerts on body function is determined by its location, with edema of the brain, larynx, or lungs representing an acute life-threatening situation.

■ Third spacing represents the loss or trapping of ECF in the transcellular space, such as in the pericardial sac, the peritoneal cavity, or the pleural cavity.

Water and Sodium Balance

The distribution of body fluids between the ICF and ECF compartments relies on the concentration of ECF water and sodium. Water provides approximately 90% to 93% of the volume of body fluids and sodium salts approximately 90% to 95% of ECF solutes. Normally, equivalent changes in sodium and water are such that the volume and osmolality of ECF are maintained within a normal range. Positive water balance (intake greater than output) results in a decrease in body fluid osmolality and ECF sodium concentration due to diluting effects of the excess water.[7] Likewise, a negative water balance (intake less than output) results in an increase in body fluid osmolality and ECF sodium concentration.

Regulation of Water Balance

Total body water (TBW) accounts for a large percentage of body weight. In young men, TBW accounts for approximates 60% of body weight and decreases to approximately 52% in elderly men. Because women usually have less lean muscle mass than men, TBW accounts for only about 50% of body weight in young women and decreases to approximately 46% in elderly women.[1,3] Obesity decreases TBW, with levels sometimes as low as 30% to 40% of body weight in adults (Fig. 8-6).

Infants normally have more TBW than older children or adults. Total body water constitutes approximately 75% to 80% of body weight in full-term infants and an even greater percentage in premature infants. In addition to having a greater percentage of body water than adults, infants have more than half of their TBW in their ECF compartment, as compared

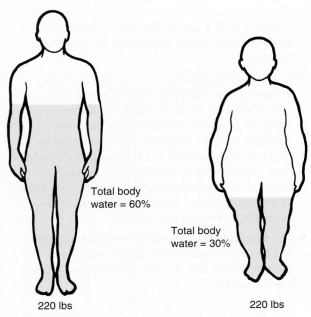

FIGURE 8-6. Body composition of a lean and an obese individual. (Adapted with permission from Statland H. *Fluids and Electrolytes in Practice.* 3rd ed. Philadelphia, PA: J.B. Lippincott; 1963.)

Total body
water = 60%

Total body
water = 30%

220 lbs   220 lbs

TABLE 8-2	Sources of Body Water Gains and Losses in the Adult		
Gains	**(approximate)**	**Losses**	**(approximate)**
Oral intake		Urine	1500 mL
As water	1000 mL	Insensible losses	
In food	1300 mL	Lungs	300 mL
Water of	200 mL	Skin	500 mL
oxidation		Feces	200 mL
Total	2500 mL	Total	2500 mL

to adults who have only about a third in their ECF compartment.[1,3] The greater ECF water content of an infant can be explained in terms of a higher metabolic rate, larger surface area in relation to its body mass, and inability to concentrate urine because of immature kidney structures. Because ECF is more readily lost from the body, infants are more vulnerable to fluid deficit than are older children and adults. As an infant grows older, TBW decreases, and by the second year of life, the percentages and distribution of body water approach those of an adult.

The main source of water gain is through oral intake and metabolic processes. Oral intake, including that obtained from liquids and solid foods, is absorbed from the gastrointestinal tract. The amount of water gained from metabolic processes is much less than from oral intake, varying from 150 to 300 mL/day, depending on the metabolic rate.

Normally, the largest loss of water occurs through the kidneys, with lesser amounts being lost through the skin, lungs, and gastrointestinal tract. Even when oral or parenteral fluids are withheld, the kidneys continue to produce urine as a means of ridding the body of metabolic wastes. The urine output that is required to eliminate these wastes is called the *obligatory urine output.* Water losses that occur through evaporative losses from skin and to moisten the air in the respiratory system are referred to as *insensible water losses* because they occur without a person's awareness. The amount of water lost from the skin through sweating varies depending on physical activity and environmental temperature. The sources of body water gains and losses are summarized in Table 8-2.

Regulation of Sodium Balance

Sodium is the most plentiful electrolyte in the ECF compartment, with a concentration ranging from 135 to 145 mEq/L (135 to 145 mmol/L).[3] Sodium does not readily cross the cell membrane; as a result, only a small amount (10 to 15 mEq/L [10 to 15 mmol/L]) is located in the ICF compartment.[1] As the major cation in the ECF compartment, Na+ and its attendant Cl− and HCO_3^- anions account for approximately 90% to 95% of the osmotic activity in the ECF. Thus, serum osmolality usually varies with changes in serum sodium concentration.

Sodium normally enters the body through the gastrointestinal tract, being derived from dietary sources. Although body needs for sodium usually can be met by as little as 500 mg/day, dietary intake frequently exceeds that amount.[3] As package labels indicate, many commercially prepared foods and soft drinks contain considerable amounts of sodium.

Most sodium losses occur through the kidney. The kidneys are extremely efficient in regulating sodium output. When sodium intake is limited or conservation of sodium is needed, the kidneys are able to reabsorb almost all the Na+ that has been filtered in the glomerulus, resulting in essentially sodium-free urine.

Usually, less than 10% of sodium intake is lost through the gastrointestinal tract and skin. Sodium losses increase with conditions such as vomiting, diarrhea, and gastrointestinal suction, all of which can remove sodium from the stomach or small intestine. Sodium leaves the skin by way of the sweat glands, which secrete a hypotonic solution containing both sodium and chloride. Although sodium losses due to sweating are usually negligible, they can increase greatly during heavy exercise and periods of exposure to a hot environment.[2]

Mechanisms of Water and Sodium Regulation

There are two major physiologic mechanisms for regulating body levels of water: thirst, which is primarily a regulator of water intake, and the antidiuretic hormone (ADH), which controls the output of water by the kidney. Thirst and ADH function in the maintenance of the *effective circulating volume*, which can be described as that portion of the ECF that fills the vascular compartment and is "effectively" perfusing the tissues.[1,2] The effective circulating volume is monitored by sensors that are located both in the vascular system and the kidney.

While thirst and ADH are the main regulators of water intake and output, the sympathetic nervous system and the renin-angiotensin-aldosterone system function in the regulation of sodium balance by the kidneys (see Chapter 18). The *sympathetic nervous system* responds to changes in arterial pressure and blood volume by adjusting the glomerular filtration rate and the rate at which sodium is filtered from the blood. Sympathetic activity also regulates renal reabsorption of sodium and renin release. The *renin-angiotensin-aldosterone system* exerts its action through angiotensin II and aldosterone. Angiotensin II acts directly on the renal tubules to increase sodium reabsorption. It also acts to constrict renal blood vessels, thereby decreasing the glomerular filtration rate and slowing renal blood flow so that less sodium is filtered and more is reabsorbed. Angiotensin II is also a powerful regulator of *aldosterone*, a hormone secreted by the adrenal cortex. Aldosterone acts to increase sodium reabsorption by the kidneys, while increasing potassium elimination.

Thirst and Disorders of Thirst

Like appetite and eating, thirst and drinking are two separate entities.[1,2,8,9] Thirst is the conscious sensation of the need to obtain and drink fluids high in water content. Drinking water or other fluids often occurs as the result of habit or for reasons other than those related to thirst. Most people drink without being thirsty, and water is consumed before it is needed. As a result, thirst is basically an emergency response. It usually occurs only when the need for water has not been anticipated.

Thirst is controlled by the thirst center in the hypothalamus. There are two stimuli for true thirst based on water need: (1) cellular dehydration caused by an increase in ECF osmolality, and (2) a decrease in the effective circulating volume, which may or may not be associated with a decrease in serum osmolality. Sensory neurons, called *osmoreceptors*, which are located in or near the thirst center in the hypothalamus, respond to changes in ECF osmolality by swelling or shrinking (Fig. 8-7). Thirst normally develops when there is as little as a 1% to 2% change in serum osmolality.[9] Stretch receptors in the vascular system that monitor the effective circulating volume also aid in the regulation of thirst. Thus, thirst is one of the earliest symptoms of hemorrhage and is often present before other signs of blood loss appear.

A third stimulus, the production of angiotensin II by the renin-angiotensin mechanism in the kidney, functions in the production of nonosmotic thirst. Angiotensin II increases in response to low blood volume and low blood pressure. This system is considered a backup

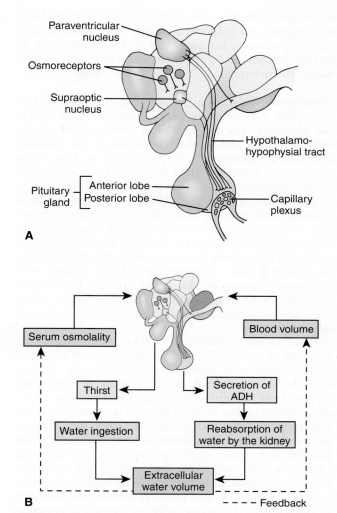

FIGURE 8-7. (A) Sagittal section through the pituitary and anterior hypothalamus. Antidiuretic hormone (ADH) is formed primarily in the supraoptic nucleus and to a lesser extent in the paraventricular nucleus of the hypothalamus. It is then transported down the hypothalamohypophysial tract and stored in secretory granules in the posterior pituitary, where it can be released into the blood. **(B)** Pathways for regulation of extracellular water volume by thirst and antidiuretic hormone. ADH, antidiuretic hormone.

system for thirst should other systems fail. Because it is a backup system, it probably does not contribute to the regulation of normal thirst. However, elevated levels of angiotensin II may lead to thirst in conditions such as congestive heart failure and chronic kidney disease, in which a decrease in renal blood flow leads to increased renin levels.

Hypodipsia. Hypodipsia represents a decrease in the ability to sense thirst. Water deficit is commonly associated with lesions in the area of the hypothalamus (e.g., head trauma, meningiomas, occult hydrocephalus, subarachnoid hemorrhage). There is also evidence that thirst is decreased and water intake reduced in elderly persons, despite higher serum sodium and osmolality levels.[10] The inability to perceive and respond to thirst is compounded in elderly persons who have had a stroke and may be further influenced by confusion, sensory deficits, and motor disturbances.

Polydipsia. Polydipsia, or excessive thirst, is normal when it accompanies conditions of water deficit, but abnormal when it results in excess water intake. Increased thirst and drinking behavior can be classified into two categories: (1) inappropriate or false thirst that occurs despite normal levels of body water and serum osmolality, and (2) compulsive water drinking. *Inappropriate* or *excessive thirst* may persist despite adequate hydration. It is a common complaint in persons with congestive heart failure and chronic kidney disease. Although the cause of thirst in these people is unclear, it may result from increased angiotensin II levels. Thirst is also a common complaint in those with dry mouth caused by decreased salivary function or treatment with drugs with an anticholinergic action (e.g., antihistamines, atropine) that lead to decreased salivary flow.

Psychogenic polydipsia involves compulsive water drinking and is usually seen in persons with psychiatric disorders, most commonly schizophrenia. Persons with the disorder drink large amounts of water and excrete large amounts of urine. The cause of excessive water drinking in these persons is uncertain. It has been suggested that it may share the same pathology as the psychosis because persons with the disorder often increase their water drinking during periods of exacerbation of their psychotic symptoms.[11] The condition may be compounded by antipsychotic medications that increase ADH levels and interfere with water excretion by the kidneys. Cigarette smoking, which is common among persons with psychiatric disorders, also stimulates ADH secretion. Excessive water ingestion coupled with impaired water excretion (or rapid ingestion at a rate that exceeds renal excretion) in persons with psychogenic polydipsia can lead to water intoxication (see section on hyponatremia). Treatment usually consists of water restriction and behavioral measures aimed at decreasing water consumption. Measurements of body weight can be used to provide an estimate of water consumption.[12]

Antidiuretic Hormone and Disorders of Antidiuretic Hormone

The antidiuretic hormone, also known as *vasopressin*, controls the reabsorption of water by the kidneys.[1,2,7] Antidiuretic hormone is a small peptide, nine amino acids in length, that is synthesized by cells in the supraoptic and paraventricular nuclei of the hypothalamus and then transported along a neural pathway (i.e., hypothalamic-hypophysial tract) to the posterior pituitary gland, where it is stored. When the supraoptic and paraventricular nuclei in the hypothalamus are stimulated by increased serum osmolality or other factors, nerve impulses travel down the hypothalamic-hypophyseal tract to the posterior pituitary gland, causing the stored ADH to be released into the circulation (see Fig. 8-7).

As with thirst, ADH levels are controlled by ECF volume and osmolality. Osmoreceptors in the hypothalamus sense changes in ECF osmolality and stimulate the production and release of ADH (see Fig. 8-7). A small increase in serum osmolality of 1% is sufficient to cause ADH release.[7] Stretch receptors that are sensitive to changes in blood pressure and the effective circulating volume also contribute to the regulation of ADH release (i.e., nonosmotic ADH secretion). A blood volume decrease of 5% to 10% produces a maximal increase in ADH levels.[7] As with many other homeostatic mechanisms, acute conditions produce greater changes in ADH levels than do chronic conditions.

Antidiuretic hormone exerts its effects through vasopressin receptors located in the collecting tubules of the kidney. In the presence of ADH, highly permeable water channels called *aquaporins* are inserted into the tubular membrane. The increased water permeability allows water from the urine filtrate to be reabsorbed into the blood, making the urine more concentrated (see understanding urine concentration, Chapter 24).

The abnormal synthesis and release of ADH occurs in a number of stress situations including severe pain, nausea, trauma, surgery, certain anesthetic agents, and some narcotics (e.g., morphine and meperidine). Among other drugs that affect ADH are nicotine, which stimulates its release, and alcohol, which inhibits it. Two important conditions that alter ADH levels are diabetes insipidus and the syndrome of inappropriate secretion of ADH.

Diabetes Insipidus. Diabetes insipidus (DI) is caused by a deficiency of ADH or a decreased renal response to ADH.[13] Persons with DI are unable to concentrate their urine during periods of water restriction and they excrete large volumes of urine, usually 3 to 20 L/day, depending on the degree of ADH deficiency or renal insensitivity to ADH. This large urine output is accompanied by excessive thirst. As long as the thirst mechanism is normal and fluid is readily available, there is little or no alteration in the fluid levels of persons with DI. The danger arises when the condition develops in someone who is unable to communicate the need for water or is unable to secure the needed water. In such cases, inadequate fluid intake rapidly leads to increased serum osmolality and hypertonic dehydration.

There are two types of DI: neurogenic or central DI, which occurs because of a defect in the synthesis or release of ADH, and nephrogenic DI, which occurs because the kidneys do not respond to ADH.[13–16] Most cases of *neurogenic DI* are caused by inflammatory, autoimmune, or vascular diseases that affect the hypothalamic-neurohypophyseal system, with less than 10% attributed to heritary forms of the disorder. In neurogenic DI, loss of 80% of ADH-secretory neurons is necessary before polyuria becomes evident.[14] Most persons with neurogenic DI have an incomplete form of the disorder and retain some ability to concentrate their urine. Temporary neurogenic DI may follow traumatic head injury[16] or surgery near the hypothalamic hypophyseal tract. *Nephrogenic DI* is characterized by impairment of urine-concentrating ability and free-water conservation. Congenital nephrogenic DI, which is present at birth, is caused by defective expression of the renal vasopressin receptors or vasopressin insensitive water channels.[16] Acquired forms of the disorder may occur with pyelonephritis, lithium toxicity,[17] and electrolyte disorders, such as potassium depletion or chronic hypercalcemia, that interfere with the actions of ADH on the collecting tubules of the kidney.

The manifestations of DI include complaints of intense thirst, a craving for ice water, and polyuria or excessive urination. The volume of ingested fluids may range from 2 to 20 L daily with corresponding large urine volumes. Partial DI usually presents with less-intense thirst and should be suspected in persons with enuresis or bed-wetting. DI may present with hypernatremia and dehydration, especially in persons without free access to water, or with damage to the hypothalamic thirst center and altered thirst sensation.

The management of central or neurogenic DI depends on the cause and severity of the disorder. Many persons with incomplete neurogenic DI maintain near-normal water balance when permitted to ingest water in response to thirst. Pharmacologic preparations of ADH (e.g., nasal and oral forms of desmopressin acetate [DDAVP]) are available for persons who cannot be managed by conservative measures. Both neurogenic and nephrogenic forms of DI respond partially to the thiazide diuretics (e.g., hydrochlorothiazide). These diuretics are thought to act by increasing sodium excretion by the kidneys, leading to ECF volume contraction, a decrease in the glomerular filtration, and an increase in sodium and water reabsorption.

Syndrome of Inappropriate Antidiuretic Hormone.
The syndrome of inappropriate ADH (SIADH) results from a failure of the negative feedback system that regulates the release and inhibition of ADH.[18–20] In persons with this syndrome, ADH secretion continues even when serum osmolality is decreased, causing marked water retention and dilutional hyponatremia.

The SIADH can occur as an acute transient condition or as a chronic condition. Stimuli such as surgery, pain, stress, and temperature changes are capable of stimulating ADH through the CNS. Drugs induce SIADH in different ways; some drugs are thought to increase hypothalamic production and release of ADH, and others are believed to act directly on the renal tubules to enhance the action of ADH. More chronic forms of SIADH may result from lung tumors, chest lesions, and CNS disorders. Tumors, particularly bronchogenic carcinomas and cancers of the lymphoid tissue, prostate, and pancreas, are known to produce and release ADH independent of normal hypothalamic control mechanisms (described in Chapter 7). Other intrathoracic

conditions, such as advanced tuberculosis, severe pneumonia, and positive-pressure breathing, can also cause SIADH. The suggested mechanism for SIADH in positive-pressure ventilation is activation of baroreceptors that respond to marked changes in intrathoracic pressure. Disease and injury to the CNS can cause direct pressure on or direct involvement of the hypothalamic–posterior pituitary structures. Examples include brain tumors, hydrocephalus, head injury, meningitis, and encephalitis. Human immunodeficiency virus (HIV) infection is an established cause of SIADH (e.g., related to associated infections, tumors, drugs).

The manifestations of SIADH are those of dilutional hyponatremia (to be discussed). Urine output decreases despite adequate or increased fluid intake. Urine osmolality is high and serum osmolality low. Hematocrit, serum sodium, and BUN levels are decreased because of the dilutional effects of an expanded blood volume. The severity of symptoms is usually related to the extent of sodium depletion and water intoxication.

The treatment of SIADH depends on its severity.[20] In mild cases, treatment consists of fluid restriction. If fluid restriction is not sufficient, diuretics such as mannitol and furosemide (Lasix) may be given to promote diuresis and free-water clearance. Lithium and the antibiotic demeclocycline inhibit the action of ADH on the renal collecting ducts and sometimes are used in treating the disorder. In cases of severe water intoxication, a hypertonic (e.g., 3%) sodium chloride solution may be administered intravenously.

Disorders of Water and Sodium Balance

Disorders of water and sodium can be divided into two main categories: (1) isotonic contraction or expansion of the ECF volume brought about by proportionate changes in sodium and water, and (2) hypotonic dilution or hypertonic concentration of the ECF brought about by disproportionate changes in sodium and water (Fig. 8-8).

Isotonic disorders usually are confined to the ECF compartment, producing a contraction (fluid volume deficit) or expansion (fluid volume excess) of the interstitial and vascular fluids. Disorders of sodium concentration produce a change in the osmolality of the ECF with movement of water from the ECF compartment into the ICF compartment (hyponatremia) or from the ICF compartment into the ECF fluid compartment (hypernatremia).

Isotonic Fluid Volume Deficit

Fluid volume deficit is characterized by a decrease in the ECF, including the circulating blood volume. Isotonic fluid volume deficit, which results when water and electrolytes are lost in isotonic proportions, is almost always caused by a loss of body fluids and is often accompanied by a decrease in fluid intake. This form of volume loss may follow a variety of disorders, including the loss of

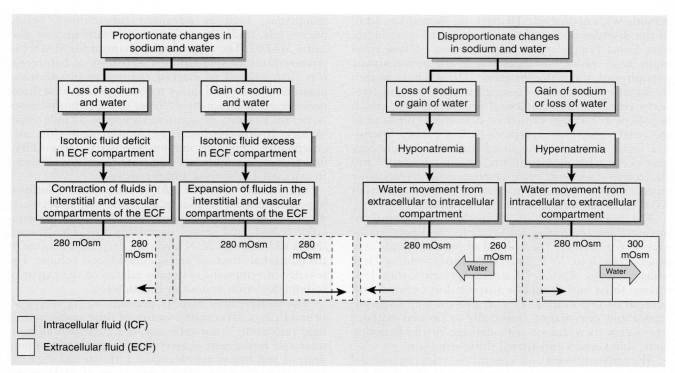

FIGURE 8-8. Effect of isotonic fluid excess and deficit and of hyponatremia and hypernatremia on movement of water between the extracellular fluid (ECF) and intracellular fluid (ICF) compartment.

gastrointestinal fluids such as occurs with severe vomiting, diarrhea, or gastrointestinal suction; excessive urinary losses, such as occurs with osmotic diuresis or injudicious use of diuretic therapy; excessive sweating due to fever and exercise; or endocrine disorders, such as adrenal insufficiency, in which reduced levels of aldosterone cause excessive sodium loss in the urine (see Chapter 32). Third-space losses cause sequestering of ECF in the serous cavities or extracellular spaces of injured tissue.

Isotonic fluid volume deficit is manifested by a decrease in ECF volume, as evidenced by a decrease in body weight. A mild ECF deficit exists when weight loss equals 2% of body weight. A moderate deficit equates to a 5% loss in weight and a severe deficit to an 8% or greater loss in weight (Table 8-3).[3] Because the ECF is trapped in the transcellular compartment of persons with third-space losses, their body weight may not decrease.

Thirst is a common symptom of fluid deficit, although it is not always present in early stages of isotonic fluid deficit. Urine output decreases and urine osmolality and specific gravity increase as ADH levels rise because of a decrease in vascular volume. Although there is an isotonic loss of fluid from the vascular compartment, blood components such as red blood cells and BUN become more concentrated.

The fluid content of body tissues decreases as fluid is removed from the interstitial spaces. The eyes assume a sunken appearance and feel softer than normal as the fluid content in the anterior chamber of the eye decreases. Fluids add resiliency to the skin and underlying tissues that is referred to as *tissue turgor.* Tissue turgor is assessed by pinching a fold of skin between the thumb and forefinger (Fig. 8-9). The skin should immediately return to its original configuration when the fingers are released. A loss of 3% to 5% of body water in children causes the resiliency of the skin to be lost, and the tissue remains elevated for several seconds.[3] Decreased tissue turgor is less predictive of fluid deficit in older persons (>65 years) because of the loss of tissue elasticity. In infants, fluid deficit may be evidenced by depression of the anterior fontanel due to a decrease in cerebrospinal fluid.

Arterial and venous volumes decline during periods of fluid deficit, as does filling of the capillary circulation, which can be assessed by applying pressure to a fingernail for 5 seconds and then releasing the pressure and observing the time (normally 1 to 2 seconds) that it takes for the color to return to normal (capillary refill time).[3] As the volume in the arterial system declines, the blood pressure decreases, the heart rate increases, and the pulse becomes weak and thready. Postural hypotension (a drop in blood pressure on standing) is an early sign of fluid deficit. On the venous side of the circulation, the veins become less prominent. When volume depletion becomes severe, signs of hypovolemic shock and vascular collapse appear (see Chapter 20).

Treatment of fluid volume deficit consists of fluid replacement and measures to correct the underlying cause. Usually, isotonic electrolyte solutions are used for fluid replacement. Acute hypovolemia and hypovolemic shock can cause renal damage; therefore, prompt

TABLE 8-3	Manifestations of Isotonic Fluid Volume Deficit and Excess

Fluid Volume Deficit	Fluid Volume Excess
Acute Weight Loss (% body weight)	***Acute Weight Gain (% body weight)***
Mild fluid volume deficit: 2%	Mild fluid volume excess: 2%
Moderate fluid volume deficit: 5%	Moderate fluid volume excess: 5%
Severe fluid volume deficit: >8%	Severe fluid volume excess: >8%
Signs of Compensatory Mechanisms	
Increased thirst	
Increased ADH: oliguria and high urine specific gravity	
Decreased Interstitial Fluid Volume	***Increased Interstitial Fluid Volume***
Decreased skin and tissue turgor	Edema
Dry mucous membranes	
Sunken and soft eyeballs	
Depressed fontanel in infants	
Decreased Vascular Volume	***Increased Vascular Volume***
Postural hypotension	Full and bounding pulse
Weak, rapid pulse	Venous distention
Decreased vein filling	Pulmonary edema (severe fluid excess)
Hypotension and shock (severe deficit)	Shortness of breath
	Crackles
	Dyspnea
	Cough

ADH, antidiuretic hormone.

assessment of the degree of fluid deficit and adequate measures to resolve the deficit and treat the underlying cause are essential.

Isotonic Fluid Volume Excess

Isotonic fluid volume excess, which represents an isotonic expansion of the ECF compartment with increases in both interstitial and vascular volumes, usually results from an increase in total body sodium that is accompanied by a proportionate increase in body water. Although it can occur as the result of excessive sodium intake, it is most commonly caused by a decrease in sodium and water elimination by the kidney. Among the causes of decreased sodium and water elimination are disorders of renal function, heart failure, liver failure,

and corticosteroid hormone excess. A condition called *circulatory overload* results from an increase in blood volume; it can occur during infusion of intravenous fluids or transfusion of blood if the amount or rate of administration is excessive.

Heart failure produces a decrease in the effective circulating volume and renal blood flow and a compensatory increase in sodium and water retention (see Chapter 20). Persons with severe congestive heart failure maintain a precarious balance between sodium and water intake and output. Even small increases in sodium intake can precipitate a state of fluid volume excess and a worsening of heart failure. Liver failure (e.g., cirrhosis of the liver) impairs aldosterone metabolism and decreases effective circulating volume and renal perfusion, leading to increased salt and water retention.

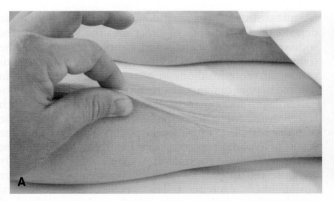 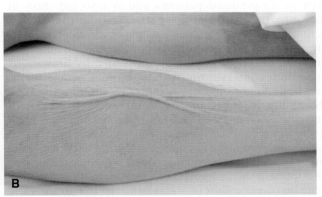

FIGURE 8-9. Decreased tissue turgor in a 61-year-old male with severe volume depletion. Skin was pinched over anterior leg **(A)** and continued to be tented after 10 minutes **(B)**. (From de Vries Feyers C. Decreased tissue turgor. Images in medicine. *N Engl J Med.* Jan 27, 2011;364:e6. Copyright © 2011. Massachusetts Medical Society.)

The corticosteroid hormones also increase sodium reabsorption by the kidneys; therefore, persons being treated with these medications and those with Cushing syndrome or disease often have problems with sodium retention (see Chapter 32).

Isotonic fluid volume excess is manifested by an increase in interstitial and vascular fluids, and is characterized by weight gain over a short period of time. Mild fluid volume excess represents a 2% gain in weight; moderate fluid volume excess, a 5% gain in weight; and severe fluid volume excess, a gain of 8% or more in weight (see Table 8-3).[3] The presence of edema is characteristic of isotonic fluid excess. When the fluid excess accumulates gradually, as often happens in debilitating diseases and starvation, edema may mask the loss of tissue mass. As vascular volume increases, central venous pressure increases, leading to distended neck veins, slow-emptying peripheral veins, a full and bounding pulse, and an increase in central venous pressure. There is often a dilutional decrease in hematocrit and BUN levels due to expansion of the plasma volume. When excess fluid accumulates in the lungs (i.e., pulmonary edema), there are complaints of shortness of breath and difficult breathing, respiratory crackles, and a productive cough. Ascites and pleural effusion may occur with severe fluid volume excess.

The treatment of fluid volume excess focuses on providing a more favorable balance between sodium and water intake and output. A sodium-restricted diet is often prescribed as a means of decreasing extracellular sodium and water levels. Diuretic therapy is commonly used to increase sodium elimination. When there is a need for intravenous fluid administration or transfusion of blood components, the procedure requires careful monitoring to prevent circulatory overload.

Hyponatremia

Hyponatremia is usually defined as a serum sodium concentration of less than 135 mEq/L (135 mmol/L).[3] It is one of the most common electrolyte disorders seen in hospitalized patients and is also common in the outpatient population, particularly in the elderly. A number of age-related events make the elderly population more vulnerable to hyponatremia, including a decrease in renal function accompanied by limitations in sodium conservation. Although older people maintain body fluid homeostasis under most circumstances, the ability to withstand environmental, drug-related, and disease-associated stresses often becomes progressively limited.

Hyponatremia can present as a hypovolemic, euvolemic, or hypervolemic state. Hyponatremia can also present as a *hypertonic hyponatremia* resulting from an osmotic shift of water from the ICF to the ECF, such as occurs with hyperglycemia. In this situation, the sodium in the ECF becomes diluted as water moves out of body cells in response to the osmotic effects of the elevated blood glucose level.[21,22]

Hypovolemic hypotonic hyponatremia is the most common type of hyponatremia. It occurs when water is used to replace the loss of iso-osmotic body fluids. Among the causes of hypovolemic hyponatremia is excessive sweating in hot weather, particularly during heavy exercise, which leads to loss of salt and water. Hyponatremia develops when water, rather than electrolyte-containing liquids, is used to replace fluids lost in sweating. Iso-osmotic fluid loss, such as occurs in vomiting or diarrhea, does not usually lower serum sodium levels unless these losses are replaced with disproportionate amounts of orally ingested or parenterally administered water. Gastrointestinal fluid loss and ingestion of excessively diluted formula are common causes of acute hyponatremia in infants and children. Hypovolemic hypotonic hyponatremia is also a common complication of adrenal insufficiency, in which a lack of aldosterone increases renal losses of sodium and a cortisol deficiency leads to increased release of ADH with water retention.

Euvolemic or *normovolemic hypotonic hyponatremia* represents retention of water with dilution of sodium while maintaining the effective circulatory volume within a normal range. It is usually the result of SIADH. The risk of normovolemic hyponatremia is increased during the postoperative period. During this time ADH levels are often high, producing an increase in water reabsorption by the kidney. The hyponatremia becomes exaggerated when electrolyte-free fluids (e.g., 5% glucose in water) are used for intravenous fluid replacement.

Hypervolemic hypotonic hyponatremia occurs in edematous states such as decompensated heart failure, advanced liver disease, and renal disease. Although the total body sodium is increased in heart failure, the baroreceptors often sense the effective circulatory volume as inadequate, resulting in fluid retention. Abuse of methylenedioxymethylamine (MDMA), also know as "ecstasy," can lead to severe neurologic symptoms, including seizures, brain edema, and herniation due to severe hyponatremia. MDMA and its metabolites have been shown to produce enhanced release of ADH from the hypothalamus.[3,22]

Manifestations. The manifestations of hyponatremia depend on the rapidity of onset and the severity of the sodium dilution. The signs and symptoms may be acute (refers to onset within 48 hours), as in severe water intoxication, or more insidious in onset and less severe, as in chronic hyponatremia. Because of water movement, hyponatremia produces an increase in intracellular water, which is responsible for many of the clinical manifestations of the disorder Muscle cramps, weakness, and fatigue reflect the effects of hyponatremia on skeletal muscle function and are often early signs of hyponatremia. These effects commonly are observed in persons with hyponatremia that occurs during heavy exercise in hot weather. Gastrointestinal manifestations such as nausea and vomiting, abdominal cramps, and diarrhea may also occur (Table 8-4).

The cells of the brain and nervous system are the most seriously affected by increases in intracellular water.[22-25]

TABLE 8-4	**Manifestations of Hyponatremia and Hypernatremia**
Hyponatremia	**Hypernatremia**
Laboratory Values Serum sodium <135 mEq/L (135 mmol/L) Decreased serum osmolality Dilutional decrease in blood components, including hematocrit, blood urea nitrogen (BUN)	*Laboratory Values* Serum sodium >145 mEq/L (145 mmol/L) Increased serum osmolality Increased concentrations of blood components, including hematocrit, BUN *Compensatory Mechanisms* Increased thirst Increased ADH with oliguria and high urine specific gravity *Decreased Intracellular Fluid* Dry skin and mucous membranes Decreased tissue turgor Decreased salivation and lacrimation Elevated body temperature

Hypo-osmolality and Movement of Water into Muscle and Neural Tissue
   Muscle cramps and weakness
   Depressed deep tendon reflexes
   Headache
   Disorientation
   Lethargy
   Seizures and coma (severe hyponatremia)
Gastrointestinal Tract
   Anorexia, nausea, vomiting
   Abdominal cramps, diarrhea
	Hyperosmolality and Movement of Water out of Neural Tissue
	Headache
	Disorientation and agitation
	Decreased reflexes
	Seizures and coma (severe hypernatremia)

ADH, antidiuretic hormone.

Symptoms include apathy, lethargy, and headache, which can progress to disorientation, confusion, gross motor weakness, and depression of deep tendon reflexes. Seizures and coma occur when serum sodium levels reach extremely low levels.[22] These severe effects, which are caused by cerebral edema, may be irreversible.

Treatment. The treatment of hyponatremia is determined by the underlying cause, severity, and timing of onset.[21–23] When hyponatremia is caused by water intoxication, limiting water intake or discontinuing medications that contribute to SIADH may be sufficient. The administration of a saline solution orally or intravenously may be needed when hyponatremia is caused by sodium deficiency. Symptomatic hyponatremia (i.e., neurologic manifestations) may be treated with hypertonic saline solution and a loop diuretic, such as furosemide, to increase water elimination. This combination allows for correction of serum sodium levels while ridding the body of excess water. The vasopressin receptor antagonists (vaptans) may be used in the treatment of euvolemic hyponatremia.[22,23]

The treatment of severe hyponatremia varies depending on the timing of the onset of the disorder. Cells, particularly those in the brain, tend to defend against changes in cell volume caused by changes in ECF osmolality by increasing or decreasing their concentration of organic osmotically active molecules (called *osmolytes*) that can't cross the cell membrane.[22,25] In the case of prolonged water intoxication (greater than 48 hours), brain cells reduce their concentration of osmolytes as a means of preventing an increase in cell volume.[22] It takes several days for brain cells to restore the osmolytes lost during hyponatremia. Thus, treatment measures that produce rapid changes in serum osmolality may cause a dramatic decrease in brain cell volume. One of the reported effects of rapid treatment of hyponatremia, called the *osmotic demyelination syndrome*, is characterized by destruction of the myelin sheath of the axons passing through the brain stem.[22,23,25] This syndrome can cause serious neurologic injury and sometimes death. In persons with acute-onset hyponatremia (i.e., onset within 48 hours), in whom cerebral adaptation has not had time to occur, rapid correction is less likely to result in osmotic demyelination.

Hypernatremia

Hypernatremia is characterized by a serum sodium level above 145 mEq/L (145 mmol/L) and a serum osmolality greater than 295 mOsm/kg H_2O.[3] Because sodium and its attendant anion is functionally an impermeable solute, hypernatremia increases ECF tonicity, causing movement of water out of the ICF, resulting in cellular dehydration.[3,26–28]

As with hyponatremia, hypernatremia can present as an *euvolemic state*, in which water from the ICF is pulled into the ECF preventing a change in volume; as a *hypovolemic state,* in which water loss is greater than sodium loss; or as a *hypervolemic state* if there is an addition of a hypertonic solution containing both sodium and water.[3,26–28]

All forms of hypernatremia represent a hypertonic state with an increase in intracellular osmolality that causes activation of the thirst mechanism and an increased ability of the kidneys to conserve water by producing concentrated urine. Thirst is highly effective in preventing hypernatremia. Therefore, hypernatremia is more likely to occur in infants and in persons who do not experience or cannot express their thirst or obtain water to drink.[28] Hypodipsia is particularly prevalent among the elderly. A defect in thirst or inability to obtain or drink water can interfere with water intake. An increase in the intracellular osmolality normally leads to an increase in ADH levels with increased reabsorption of water by the kidneys. Hypernatremia develops when there is impaired ability of the kidneys to conserve water by producing concentrated urine, most commonly due to acute or chronic renal failure.

Net water loss can occur through the urine, gastrointestinal tract, lungs, or skin. It can result from increased losses from the respiratory tract during fever or strenuous exercise, or from the gastrointestinal tract due to watery diarrhea or when highly osmotic tube feedings are given with inadequate amounts of water. With pure water loss, both the ICF and ECF compartments lose an equal percentage of their volume. Because ICF contains a greater percentage of water than the ECF, more actual water volume is lost from the ICF than the ECF compartment. The therapeutic administration of excess amounts of sodium-containing solutions may also cause hypernatremia.

Manifestations. The clinical manifestations of hypernatremia caused by water loss are largely those of ECF loss and cellular dehydration (see Table 8-4). The severity of signs and symptoms is greatest when the increase in serum sodium is large and occurs rapidly. Body weight is decreased in proportion to the amount of water that has been lost. Because blood plasma is roughly 90% to 93% water, the concentrations of blood cells and other blood components increase as ECF water decreases.

Thirst is an early symptom of water deficit, occurring when water losses are equal to 0.5% of body water. Urine output is decreased and urine osmolality increased because of renal water-conserving mechanisms. Body temperature frequently is elevated, and the skin becomes warm and flushed. Hypernatremia produces an increase in serum osmolality and results in water being pulled out of body cells.[3] As a result, the skin and mucous membranes become dry, and salivation and lacrimation are decreased. The mouth becomes dry and sticky, and the tongue becomes rough and fissured. Swallowing is difficult. The subcutaneous tissues assume a firm, rubbery texture. Most significantly, movement of water out of the CNS causes decreased reflexes, agitation, headache,

and restlessness. Coma and seizures may develop as hypernatremia progresses.

Treatment. Treatment of hypernatremia includes measures to treat the underlying cause of the disorder and fluid replacement therapy to treat the accompanying dehydration. Replacement fluids can be given orally or intravenously. Oral glucose–electrolyte replacement solutions are widely available in grocery stores and pharmacies for use in the treatment of acute hypernatremia due to diarrhea and other dehydrating disorders in infants and young children (see Chapter 29).[29] Oral replacement therapy is less expensive than intravenous therapy and has a lower complication rate. Intravenous therapy may be required for children and adults with severe dehydration.

One of the serious aspects of sustained hypernatremia is dehydration of brain and nerve cells. The treatment of sustained hypernatremia requires controlled gradual correction of sodium and water levels to avoid serious neurologic complications.[26–28] As with severe hyponatremia, brain cells protect against changes in cell volume by changing their concentration of organic osmolytes, increasing their concentration in hypernatremia to prevent water from being pulled into the ECF. If hypernatremia is corrected too rapidly—before the osmolytes have had a chance to dissipate—the plasma may become relatively hypotonic in relation to brain cell osmolality. When this occurs, water moves into the brain cells, causing cerebral edema and potentially severe neurologic impairment.

SUMMARY CONCEPTS

- The volume and distribution of body fluids between the intracellular fluid (ICF) and extracellular fluid (ECF) compartments depend on the concentration of water, which provides approximately 90% to 93% of its fluid volume, and sodium salts, which provide approximately 90% to 95% of the ECF solutes.

- The main determinant of water and sodium balance is the *effective circulating blood volume,* which is monitored by stretch receptors in the vascular system that exert their effects through thirst, which controls water intake, and the antidiuretic hormone (ADH), which controls urine concentration. The sympathetic nervous system and the renin-angiotensin-aldosterone system contribute to fluid balance through the regulation of sodium balance.

- Isotonic fluid disorders result from contraction or expansion of ECF volume brought about by proportionate changes in sodium and water. *Isotonic fluid volume deficit* (hypovolemia), which is characterized by a decrease in ECF volume, causes thirst, signs of decreased vascular volume, and a decrease in urine output along with an increase in urine specific gravity. *Isotonic fluid volume excess* (hypervolemia), which is characterized by an increase in ECF volume, is manifested by signs of increased vascular volume and edema.

■ Hyponatremia (sodium deficit) and hypernatremia (sodium excess) are brought about by disproportionate losses or gains in ECF sodium concentration, which cause water to move in or out of body cells. Because of water movement, hyponatremia produces an increase in ICF water causing cells to swell;, whereas hypernatremia produces an ICF water deficit and cellular dehydration.

Potassium Balance

Potassium (K^+) is the second most abundant cation in the body, with 98% located in the intracellular compartment, primarily in skeletal muscle.[30–32] Of the remaining 2% that is in the extracellular compartment, only about 0.4% is measurable in the plasma. This tiny amount is maintained at a fairly narrow serum concentration of 3.5 to 5.0 mEq/L (3.5 to 5.0 mmol/L).

Regulation of Potassium Balance

Potassium balance is normally regulated by dietary intake, urine output, and transcompartmental shifts between the ICF and ECF compartments. The kidneys are the main source of potassium loss. Approximately 80% to 90% of potassium loss occurs in the urine, with the remainder being lost in the stools from the gastrointestinal tract and in sweat from the skin.[30–34]

Potassium is filtered in the glomerulus, reabsorbed along with sodium and water in the proximal tubule and with sodium and chloride in the thick ascending loop of Henle, and then secreted into the late distal and collecting tubules for elimination in the urine. In contrast to other electrolytes, the regulation of potassium elimination by the kidney is mainly controlled by its secretion from the blood into the tubular filtrate rather than through its reabsorption from the tubular filtrate into the blood (see Chapter 24).

Aldosterone plays an essential role in regulating potassium elimination in the distal tubule of the kidney. In the presence of aldosterone, Na^+ is transported back into the blood and K^+ is secreted in the tubular filtrate for elimination in the urine. There is also a potassium/

hydrogen exchange mechanism in the collecting tubules of the kidney. When serum potassium levels increase, K^+ is secreted into the urine and H^+ is reabsorbed, leading to a decrease in pH and metabolic acidosis; when potassium levels are low, K^+ is reabsorbed and H^+ is secreted in the urine, leading to an increase in pH and metabolic alkalosis.

Among the factors that influence the ECF/ICF shift in potassium are serum osmolality, acid–base balance, insulin, and increased sympathetic nervous system activity (Fig. 8-10). An acute increase in *serum osmolality* causes water to move out of the cell; this in turn prompts an increase in K^+ concentration that causes it to move out into the ECF. *Acid–base disorders* rely on an ECF to ICF cation shift for buffering of the H^+ ion. In metabolic acidosis, for example, H^+ moves into body cells for buffering, causing K^+ to leave and move into the ECF. Both insulin and epinephrine (a β-adrenergic sympathetic neurontransmitter) increase cellular uptake of K^+ by increasing the activity of the Na^+/K^+-adenosine triphosphatase (ATPase) membrane pump.[4,30–33] Normally, it takes 6 to 8 hours for the kidneys to eliminate half of potassium that has been ingested in the diet.[4] After a meal, insulin release not only serves to regulate blood glucose levels, but also serves to control serum potassium levels by temporarily shifting the excess into cells until it can be eliminated by the kidneys.

Exercise can also produce compartmental shifts in potassium. Repeated muscle contraction causes potassium to be released into the ECF. Although the increase usually is small with modest exercise, it can be considerable during exhaustive exercise. Even the repeated clenching and unclenching of the fist during a blood draw can cause potassium to move out of cells causing an artificial elevation in serum potassium levels.

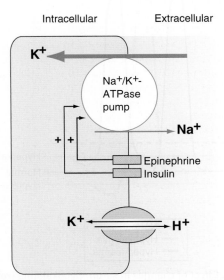

FIGURE 8-10. Mechanisms regulating transcellular shifts in potassium.

Disorders of Potassium Balance

As the major intracellular cation, potassium is critical to many body functions, including maintenance of the osmotic integrity of cells, acid–base balance, and the intricate chemical reactions that transform carbohydrates into energy and convert amino acids to proteins. Potassium also plays a critical role in conducting nerve impulses and controlling the excitability of skeletal, cardiac, and smooth muscle. It does this by regulating the resting membrane potential, the opening of sodium channels that control the flow of current during the action potential, and the rate of repolarization.[30,33] Changes in nerve and muscle excitability are particularly important in the heart, where alterations in serum potassium levels can produce serious cardiac arrhythmias and conduction defects. Changes in serum potassium levels also affect the electrical activity of skeletal muscles and the smooth muscle in the blood vessels and gastrointestinal tract.

The *resting membrane potential* is determined by the ratio of ECF to ICF potassium concentration (see Chapter 1, "Understanding Membrane Potentials"). A *decrease* in the ECF potassium concentration (hypokalemia) causes the resting membrane potential to become more negative, moving it further from the threshold for excitation (Fig. 8-11). Thus, it takes a greater stimulus to reach the threshold potential and open the sodium channels that are responsible for the action potential. An *increase* in serum potassium (hyperkalemia) has the opposite effect; it causes the resting membrane potential to become more positive, moving it closer to the threshold. With severe hyperkalemia, the resting membrane potential approaches the threshold potential, causing sustained subthreshold depolarization with a resultant inactivation of

the sodium channels and net decrease in excitability.[3] The *rate of repolarization* (return of the membrane potential toward its resting potential so it can undergo another action potential) also varies with serum potassium levels. It is more rapid in hyperkalemia and delayed in hypokalemia.

Hypokalemia

Hypokalemia refers to a decrease in serum potassium levels below 3.5 mEq/L (3.5 mmol/L). The causes of potassium deficit can be grouped into three categories: inadequate intake; excessive gastrointestinal, renal, and skin losses; and a shift between the ICF and ECF compartments.[3,30-33]

Inadequate dietary intake is a frequent cause of hypokalemia. Insufficient dietary intake may result from the inability to obtain or ingest food or from a diet that is low in potassium-containing foods. Potassium intake is often inadequate in persons on fad diets and those who have eating disorders. Elderly persons are particularly likely to have potassium deficits.

Excessive renal losses of potassium occur with diuretic therapy, metabolic alkalosis, magnesium depletion, trauma and stress, and an increase in aldosterone levels. Diuretic therapy, with the exception of potassium-sparing diuretics, is the most common cause of hypokalemia. Both thiazide and loop diuretics increase the loss of potassium in the urine. Magnesium depletion, which often coexists with potassium depletion due to diuretic therapy, produces additional urinary losses. Renal losses of potassium are accentuated by aldosterone. Primary aldosteronism, caused by either a tumor or hyperplasia of the cells of the adrenal cortex that secrete aldosterone, can produce severe losses by increasing potassium secretion in the distal renal tubule (see Chapter 32).

Although potassium losses from the skin and the gastrointestinal tract usually are minimal, these losses can become excessive under certain conditions. For example, burns increase surface losses of potassium. Intestinal secretions contain relatively large amounts of potassium (e.g., 85 to 90 mEq/L), thus diarrhea can produce large losses of potassium.[3]

Hypokalemia can also be caused by *intracellular shifting* of potassium from the ECF compartment (see Fig. 8-10). A wide variety of β_2-adrenergic agonist drugs (e.g., decongestants and bronchodilators) produce an intracellular shift in potassium, causing a transient decrease in serum potassium levels.[37] Insulin also increases the movement of potassium into the cell. Because insulin increases the movement of glucose and potassium into cells, potassium deficit often develops during treatment of diabetic ketoacidosis.

Manifestations. The manifestations of hypokalemia include alterations in neuromuscular, gastrointestinal, renal, and cardiovascular function[3,30-33] (Table 8-5). These manifestations reflect the effects of hypokalemia on the electrical activity of excitable tissues such as those of the neuromuscular systems as well as the body's

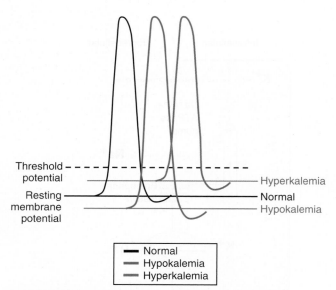

FIGURE 8-11. Effect of changes in serum hypokalemia (*red*) and hyperkalemia (*blue*) on the resting membrane potential in relation to the threshold potential.

TABLE 8-5	Manifestations of Hypokalemia and Hyperkalemia
Hypokalemia	**Hyperkalemia**

Hypokalemia	Hyperkalemia
Laboratory Values	**Laboratory Values**
Serum potassium <3.5 mEq/L (3.5 mmol/L)	Serum potassium >5.5 mEq/L (5.5 mmol/L)
Thirst and Urine	
Increased thirst	
Inability to concentrate urine with polyuria and urine with low specific gravity	
Effects of Changes in Membrane Potentials on Neural and Muscle Function	**Effects of Changes in Membrane Potentials on Neural and Muscle Function**
Gastrointestinal	**Gastrointestinal**
Anorexia, nausea, vomiting	Nausea, vomiting
Constipation, abdominal distention	Intestinal cramps
Paralytic ileus (severe hypokalemia)	Diarrhea
Neuromuscular	**Neuromuscular**
Muscle weakness, flabbiness, fatigue	Muscle weakness
Muscle cramps and tenderness	
Paresthesias	Paresthesias
Paralysis (severe hypokalemia)	Paralysis (severe hyperkalemia)
Central Nervous System	
Confusion, depression	
Cardiovascular	**Cardiovascular**
Postural hypotension	Electrocardiogram changes
Electrocardiogram changes	Risk of cardiac arrest with severe hyperkalemia
Cardiac arrhythmias	
Predisposition to digitalis toxicity	
Acid–Base Balance	
Metabolic alkalosis	

attempt to regulate ECF potassium levels within a more normal range. The signs and symptoms of hypokalemia seldom develop until serum potassium levels have fallen to less than 3.0 mEq/L (3.0 mmol/L).[3] They are typically gradual in onset, and therefore the disorder may go undetected for some time.

The renal mechanisms that serve to conserve potassium during hypokalemia interfere with the kidney's ability to concentrate urine. Urine output and plasma osmolality are increased, urine specific gravity is decreased, and complaints of polyuria, nocturia, and thirst are common. Metabolic alkalosis and renal chloride wasting are signs of severe hypokalemia.

There are numerous signs and symptoms associated with gastrointestinal function, including anorexia, nausea, and vomiting. Atony of the gastrointestinal smooth muscle can cause constipation, abdominal distention, and, in severe hypokalemia, paralytic ileus. When gastrointestinal symptoms occur gradually and are not severe, they often impair potassium intake and exaggerate the condition.

Complaints of weakness, fatigue, and muscle cramps, particularly during exercise, are common in moderate hypokalemia (serum potassium 2.5 to 3.0 mEq/L [2.5 to 3.0 mmol/L]). Muscle paralysis with life-threatening respiratory insufficiency can occur with severe hypokalemia. Leg muscles, particularly the quadriceps, are most prominently affected. Some people complain of muscle tenderness and paresthesias rather than weakness. In chronic potassium deficiency, muscle atrophy may contribute to muscle weakness.

The most serious effects of hypokalemia are on the heart.[3,31–33] Hypokalemia produces a decrease in the resting membrane potential, causing prolongation of the PR interval (see Chapter 17). It also prolongs the rate of ventricular repolarization and lengthens the relative refractory period, causing depression of the ST segment, flattening of the T wave, and appearance of a prominent U wave. Although these ECG changes usually are not serious, they may predispose to reentry ventricular arrhythmias. Hypokalemia also increases the risk of digitalis toxicity in persons being treated with the drug, and there is an increased risk of ventricular arrhythmias, particularly in persons with underlying heart disease. The dangers associated with digitalis toxicity are compounded in persons who are receiving diuretics that increase urinary losses of potassium.

In a rare genetic condition, called *hypokalemic familial periodic paralysis*, episodes of hypokalemia cause attacks of flaccid paralysis that last 6 to 48 hours if untreated.[30] The paralysis may be precipitated by situations that cause severe hypokalemia by producing an intracellular shift in potassium, such as ingestion of a high-carbohydrate meal or administration of insulin, epinephrine, or glucocorticoid drugs. The paralysis often can be reversed by potassium replacement therapy.

Treatment. When possible, hypokalemia caused by a potassium deficit is treated by increasing the intake of foods high in potassium content—meats, dried fruits, fruit juices (particularly orange juice), and bananas. Oral potassium supplements are prescribed for persons whose intake of potassium is insufficient in relation to losses. This is particularly useful in persons who are receiving diuretic therapy and those who are taking digitalis.

Potassium may be given intravenously when the oral route is not tolerated or when rapid replacement is needed. Magnesium deficiency may impair potassium correction; in such cases, magnesium replacement is indicated.[30] The rapid infusion of a concentrated potassium solution can cause death from cardiac arrest. Health personnel who assume responsibility for administering intravenous solutions that contain potassium should be fully aware of all the precautions pertaining to their dilution and flow rate.

Hyperkalemia

Hyperkalemia refers to an increase in serum levels of potassium in excess of 5.5 mEq/L (5.5 mmol/L).[3,30,31,34] It seldom occurs in healthy persons because the body is extremely effective in preventing excess potassium accumulation in the extracellular fluid.

There are three main causes of hyperkalemia: (1) decreased renal elimination, (2) a shift in potassium from the ICF to ECF compartment, and (3) excessively rapid rate of administration. The most common cause of serum potassium excess is *decreased renal function.* Chronic hyperkalemia is almost always associated with chronic kidney disease. Some kidney disorders, such as sickle cell nephropathy, lead nephropathy, and systemic lupus nephritis, can selectively impair tubular secretion of potassium without causing kidney failure.

A mineralocorticoid (aldosterone) deficiency, which increases tubular reabsorption of potassium in the distal renal tubule, is another cause of hyperkalemia. It can result from adrenal insufficiency, depression of aldosterone release due to a decrease in renin or angiotensin II, or impaired ability of the kidneys to respond to aldosterone. Potassium-sparing diuretics can produce hyperkalemia by means of the latter mechanism. Because of their ability to decrease aldosterone levels, the angiotensin-converting enzyme inhibitors and angiotensin II receptor blockers can also produce an increase in serum potassium levels.

A shift in potassium from the ICF into the ECF also can lead to elevated serum potassium levels. Acidosis tends to increase serum potassium levels by causing potassium to move from the ICF to the ECF. Tissue injury also causes release of intracellular potassium into the ECF compartment. For example, burns and crushing injuries cause cell death and release of potassium into the extracellular fluids. The same injuries often diminish renal function, which contributes to the development of hyperkalemia. Transient hyperkalemia may occur during exhaustive exercise or seizures, when muscle cells are permeable to potassium.

Potassium excess can also result from excessive oral ingestion or intravenous administration of potassium. Normally it is difficult to increase potassium intake to the point of causing hyperkalemia when renal function is adequate and the aldosterone Na+/K+ exchange system is functioning. An exception to this rule is the intravenous route of administration. In some cases, severe and fatal incidents of hyperkalemia have occurred when intravenous potassium solutions were infused too rapidly. Because the kidneys control potassium elimination, the administration of intravenous solutions that contain potassium should not be initiated until urine output has been assessed and renal function has been deemed to be adequate.

Manifestations. The signs and symptoms of potassium excess are closely related to a decrease in neuromuscular excitability (see Table 8-5). The neuromuscular manifestations of potassium excess usually are absent until the serum concentration exceeds 6 mEq/L (6 mmol/L).[30] The first symptom associated with hyperkalemia typically is paresthesia (a feeling of numbness and tingling). There may be complaints of generalized muscle weakness or dyspnea secondary to respiratory muscle weakness.

The most serious effect of hyperkalemia is on the heart. Hyperkalemia decreases membrane excitability, producing a delay in atrial and ventricular depolarization, and it increases the rate of ventricular repolarization.[3,4] As the serum potassium concentration rises, there is a characteristic sequence of changes in the ECG that are due to the effects of hyperkalemia on atrial and ventricular depolarization (represented by the P wave and QRS complex) and repolarization (represented by the T wave and QRS complex).[3] The earliest ECG changes are peaked and narrowed T waves and a shortened QT interval, which reflect abnormally rapid repolarization (Fig. 8-12). The alteration in T-wave configuration typically becomes prominent when the serum potassium concentration exceeds 6 mEq/L (6 mmol/L). If serum potassium levels continue to rise, delayed depolarization of the atria and ventricles produces further changes in the ECG. There is a prolongation of the PR interval; widening of the QRS complex with no change in its configuration; and decreased amplitude, widening, and eventual disappearance of the P wave. The heart rate may be slow. Ventricular fibrillation and cardiac arrest are terminal events. Detrimental effects of hyperkalemia on the heart are most pronounced when the serum potassium level rises rapidly.

Treatment. The treatment of potassium excess varies with the degree of increase in serum potassium and whether there are ECG and neuromuscular manifestations. On an emergent basis, calcium antagonizes the potassium-induced decrease in membrane excitability, restoring excitability toward normal.[30,31] The protective effect of calcium administration is usually short lived (15 to 30 minutes) and must be accompanied by other therapies to decrease the ECF potassium concentration. The redistribution of potassium from the ECF into the

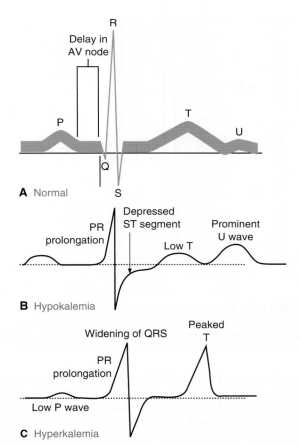

FIGURE 8-12. Comparison of the **(A)** normal electrocardiogram with electrocardiographic changes that occur with **(B)** hypokalemia and **(C)** hyperkalemia.

ICF compartment can be accomplished by the administration of sodium bicarbonate, β-agonists (e.g., nebulized albuterol), or insulin to rapidly decrease the ECF concentration.[30]

Less-emergent measures focus on decreasing or curtailing potassium intake or absorption, increasing renal excretion, and increasing cellular uptake. Decreased intake can be achieved by restricting dietary sources of potassium. The major ingredient in most salt substitutes is potassium chloride, and such substitutes should not be given to persons with kidney problems. Increasing potassium output often is more difficult. Persons with kidney failure may require hemodialysis or peritoneal dialysis to reduce serum potassium levels.

SUMMARY CONCEPTS

- Potassium is the second most abundant cation in the body, with 98% being located in the intracellular fluid (ICF) compartment. The high ICF concentration is required for many cell functions, including maintenance of the osmotic integrity of cells and acid–base balance, intricate chemical reactions that transform carbohydrates into energy, changing glucose into glycogen, and converting amino acids to proteins. Potassium also plays a critical role in conducting nerve impulses and controlling the excitability of skeletal, cardiac, and smooth muscles.

- Potassium is ingested in the diet and eliminated in the urine, with ICF and extracellular (ECF) levels being regulated by compartmental shifts between the ICF and ECF, and mechanisms that adjust renal excretion with dietary ingestion of potassium.

- Hypokalemia, or potassium deficit, can result from inadequate intake, excessive losses, or redistribution from the ECF to the ICF compartments. It is manifested by alterations in kidney, skeletal muscle, gastrointestinal, and cardiac function, reflecting the crucial role of potassium in cell metabolism and neuromuscular function.

- Hyperkalemia, or potassium excess, can result from decreased elimination of potassium by the kidney, a transcellular shift in potassium from the ICF into the ECF compartment, or excessively rapid intravenous administration of potassium. It is manifested by alterations in neuromuscular and cardiac function, the most serious being the development of serious and even fatal cardiac arrhythmias.

Calcium, Phosphorus, and Magnesium Balance

Calcium, phosphorus, and magnesium are the major divalent cations in the body. Most of these cations are deposited in bone, with only a small amount in the ECF. Homeostatic mechanisms that regulate serum calcium and phosphorus levels involve three organs—the intestine, kidney, and bone, principally through the complex interaction of parathyroid hormone and vitamin D [35–37] (Fig. 8-13).

The main function of *parathyroid hormone* (PTH) is to maintain ECF calcium concentrations.[35,37] It does this by stimulating the release of calcium and phosphorus from bone into the ECF; increasing renal reabsorption of calcium and excretion of phosphorus; and enhancing the gastrointestinal absorption of calcium and phosphorus through its effects on vitamin D synthesis. *Vitamin D*, which functions as a hormone, is synthesized by the skin and converted to its active form, *calcitriol*, in the kidney. The active form of vitamin D has several effects on the intestines, kidneys, and bone that increase serum levels of calcium and phosphorus and contribute to their

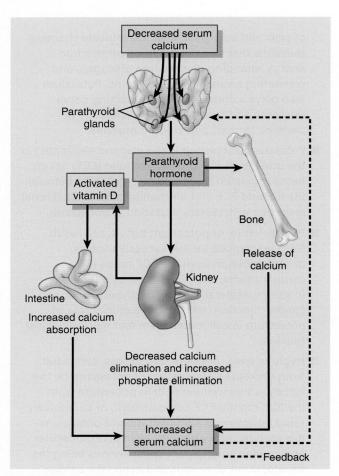

FIGURE 8-13. Regulation of serum calcium concentration by parathyroid hormone.

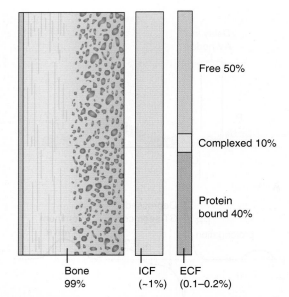

FIGURE 8-14. Distribution of body calcium between the bone and the intracellular fluid (ICF) and extracellular fluid (ECF) compartments. The percentages of free, complexed, and protein-bound calcium in extracellular fluids are indicated.

feedback regulation.[35,37] It stimulates the absorption of calcium, and to a lesser extent phosphorus, from the intestine; it increases calcium and phosphorus reabsorption by the renal tubules; and it inhibits PTH synthesis by the parathyroid glands. The role of PTH and vitamin D on the skeleton is discussed further in Chapters 42 and 43.

Disorders of Calcium Balance

Calcium is the major divalent cation in the body. Approximately 99% of body calcium is found in bone, where it provides strength and stability for the skeletal system and serves as an exchangeable source to maintain ECF calcium levels.[36,37] Most of the remaining calcium (approximately 1%) is located in the ICF, and only 0.1% to 0.2% (approximately 8.5 to 10.5 mg/dL [21 to 26 mmol/L]) of the remaining calcium is present in the ECF.

Extracellular calcium exists in three forms: (1) protein bound, (2) complexed, and (3) ionized (Fig. 8-14). Approximately 40% of serum calcium is bound to plasma proteins, mainly albumin. Another 10% is complexed (i.e., chelated) with substances such as citrate, phosphorus, and sulfate.[36] The remaining 50% of serum calcium is present in the ionized form. Only the ionized form of calcium (Ca^{++}) is free to leave the vascular compartment and participate in cellular functions. Since most of the protein-bound calcium combines with albumin, total serum calcium is significantly altered by serum albumin levels. As a general rule, a decrease in serum albumin of 1.0 g/dL below normal will decrease total serum Ca^{++} by 0.8 mg/dL.[3] Ionized Ca^{++} levels are inversely affected by the pH of the blood. For example, when the arterial pH increases in alkalosis, more calcium becomes bound to protein.[3] Although the total serum calcium remains unchanged, the ionized portion decreases.

Ionized Ca^{++} serves a number of functions. It participates in many enzyme reactions; exerts an important effect on membrane potentials and neuronal excitability; is necessary for contraction in skeletal, cardiac, and smooth muscle; participates in the release of hormones, neurotransmitters, and other chemical messengers; influences cardiac contractility and automaticity by way of slow calcium channels; and is essential for blood coagulation (see Chapter 12).

Regulation of Calcium Balance

Calcium enters the body through the gastrointestinal tract, is absorbed from the intestine under the influence of vitamin D, excreted by the kidney, and stored in bone. Approximately 35% of dietary calcium is absorbed from the duodenum and upper jejunum; the remainder is eliminated in the stool.[2]

Calcium is stored in bone and excreted by the kidney. The ionized form of Ca^{++} is filtered from the plasma into the glomerulus and then selectively reabsorbed back into the blood. The distal convoluted tubule is an important regulatory site for controlling the amount of Ca^{++} that enters the urine. Parathyroid hormone and possibly vitamin D stimulate Ca^{++} reabsorption in this segment of the nephron. Thiazide diuretics, which exert their effects in the distal convoluted tubule, enhance Ca^{++} reabsorption. Another factor that influences Ca^{++} reabsorption by the kidney is the serum concentration of phosphorus. An increase in serum phosphorus stimulates PTH, which increases Ca^{++} reabsorption by the renal tubules, thereby reducing Ca^{++} excretion. The opposite occurs with reduction in serum phosphorus levels.

Hypocalcemia

Hypocalcemia represents a total serum calcium level of less than 8.5 mg/dL (2.1 mmol/L) and an ionized Ca^{++} level of less than 4.6 mg/dL (1.2 mmol/L).[38] A pseudo-hypocalcemia is caused by hypoalbuminemia. It results in a decrease in protein-bound rather than ionized Ca^{++} and usually is asymptomatic.[35] Before a diagnosis of hypocalcemia can be made, the total calcium should be corrected for low albumin levels.

The most common causes of hypocalcemia are abnormal losses of calcium by the kidney, impaired ability to mobilize calcium from bone due to hypoparathyroidism, and increased protein binding or chelation such that greater proportions of calcium are in the nonionized form.[3,35] An important cause of hypocalcemia is renal failure, in which decreased production of activated vitamin D and hyperphosphatemia both play a role (see Chapter 26). Because of the inverse relation between calcium and phosphate, in renal failure serum Ca^{++} levels fall as phosphate levels rise.

The ability to mobilize calcium from bone depends on PTH levels. Decreased levels of PTH may result from primary or secondary forms of hypoparathyroidism. Suppression of PTH release may also occur with elevated levels of vitamin D. Magnesium deficiency inhibits PTH release and impairs the action of PTH on bone resorption. This form of hypocalcemia is difficult to treat with calcium supplementation alone and requires correction of the magnesium deficiency. Hypocalcemia is also a common problem in acute pancreatitis in which fat necrosis and precipitation of calcium soaps produce a decrease in serum calcium.

Since only the ionized Ca^{++} is able to leave the capillary and participate in body functions, conditions that alter the ratio of protein-bound to ionized calcium can also produce signs of hypocalcemia. This can occur in situations where an increase in pH, such as occurs with alkalosis, produces a decrease in Ca^{++}. For example, hyperventilation sufficient to cause respiratory alkalosis can produce a decrease in Ca^{++} sufficient to cause tetany. Free fatty acids also increase protein binding, causing a reduction in Ca^{++}. Elevations in free fatty acids sufficient to alter calcium binding may occur during stressful situations that cause elevations of epinephrine, glucagon, growth hormone, and adrenocorticotropic hormone levels.

Hypocalcemia has also been associated with many drugs, including those that inhibit bone resorption (e.g., biphosphonates), cause vitamin D deficiency or resistance (e.g., antiepileptics), increase urinary losses of calcium (loop diuretics), or decrease calcium absorption through reduced gastric acid production (proton-pump inhibitors, histamine 2-blockers).[38,39] Citrate, which is used as an anticoagulant in blood transfusion, can also produce a decrease in Ca^{++} if transfused too rapidly. Hypocalcemia is seen more commonly during the transfusion of plasma and platelets, which have high citrate concentrations.[3]

Manifestations. Hypocalcemia can manifest as an acute or chronic condition. Most persons with mild hypocalcemia are asymptomatic, whereas large or abrupt changes in ionized calcium lead to increased neuromuscular excitability and cardiovascular effects (Table 8-6).[3,35,36,38]

Ionized calcium stabilizes neuromuscular excitability, thereby making nerve cells less sensitive to stimuli. Nerves exposed to low ionized calcium levels show decreased thresholds for excitation, repetitive responses to a single stimulus, and, in extreme cases, continuous activity. The severity of the manifestations depends on the underlying cause, rapidity of onset, accompanying electrolyte disorders, and extracellular pH. Increased neuromuscular excitability can manifest as paresthesias (i.e., tingling around the mouth and in the hands and feet), tetany (i.e., muscle spasms of the muscles of the face, hands, and feet), and, in severe hypocalcemia, laryngeal spasm and seizures.[35,38] Chvostek and Trousseau tests can be used to assess for increased neuromuscular excitability (Fig. 8-15).[3,38] *Chvostek sign* is elicited by tapping the face just below the temple at the point where the facial nerve emerges. Tapping the face over the facial nerve causes spasm of the lip, nose, or face when the test result is positive. An inflated blood pressure cuff is used to test for *Trousseau sign*. The cuff is inflated 10 mm Hg above systolic blood pressure for 3 minutes. Contraction of the fingers and hands (i.e., carpopedal spasm) indicates the presence of tetany.

Cardiovascular effects of acute hypocalcemia include hypotension, cardiac insufficiency, cardiac arrhythmias (particularly heart block and ventricular fibrillation), and failure to respond to drugs such as digitalis, norepinephrine, and dopamine that act through calcium-mediated mechanisms.[3]

Treatment. Acute hypocalcemia is an emergency situation, requiring prompt treatment. An intravenous infusion containing calcium (e.g., calcium gluconate, calcium chloride) is used when tetany or acute symptoms are present or anticipated because of a decrease in the serum calcium level.[35,38]

Chronic hypocalcemia is treated with oral intake of calcium. Oral calcium supplements of carbonate, gluconate, or lactate salts may be used.[35] Long-term treatment may require the use of vitamin D preparations, especially in persons with hypoparathyroidism and chronic

TABLE 8-6	Manifestations of Hypocalcemia and Hypercalcemia	

Hypocalcemia	Hypercalcemia
Laboratory	*Laboratory*
Serum calcium <8.5 mg/dL (2.1 mmol/L)	Serum calcium >10.5 mg/dL (2.6 mmol/L)
	Inability to Concentrate Urine and Exposure of Kidney to Increased Concentration of Calcium
	Polyuria
	Increased thirst
	Signs of acute renal insufficiency
	Signs of kidney stones
Neural and Muscle Effects (Increased Excitability)	*Neural and Muscle Effects (Decreased Excitability)*
Paresthesias, especially numbness and tingling	Muscle weakness
Skeletal muscle cramps	Ataxia, loss of muscle tone
Abdominal muscle spasms and cramps	Lethargy
Hyperactive reflexes	Personality and behavioral changes
Carpopedal spasm	Stupor and coma (severe hypercalcemia)
Positive Chvostek and Trousseau tests	
Tetany	
Laryngeal spasm (severe hypocalcemia)	
Cardiovascular Effects	*Cardiovascular Effects*
Hypotension	Hypertension
Signs of cardiac insufficiency	Shortening of the QT interval
Decreased response to drugs that act by calcium-mediated mechanisms	Atrioventricular block
Prolongation of the QT interval predisposes to ventricular arrhythmias	
Skeletal Effects (Chronic Deficiency)	*Gastrointestinal Effects*
Osteomalacia	Anorexia
Bone pain	Nausea, vomiting
	Constipation

kidney disease. The active form of vitamin D is administered when the liver or kidney mechanisms needed for hormone activation are impaired. Synthetic PTH (1–34) can be administered by subcutaneous injection as replacement therapy in hypoparathyroidism.

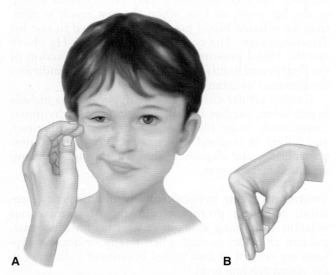

FIGURE 8-15. (A) The Chvostek sign: A contraction of the facial muscles elicited in response to a light tap over the facial nerve in front of ear. **(B)** The Trousseau sign: Carpopedal spasm induced by inflating a blood pressure cuff above systolic blood pressure. (Adapted from Bullock BA, Henze RJ. *Focus on Pathophysiology*. Philadelphia, PA: Lippincott Williams & Wilkins; 2000.)

Hypercalcemia

Hypercalcemia represents a total serum calcium concentration greater than 10.5 mg/dL (2.6 mmol/L).[40] Falsely elevated levels of calcium can result from prolonged drawing of blood with an excessively tight tourniquet. Increased serum albumin levels may also elevate the total serum calcium but not affect the ionized calcium.

Hypercalcemia occurs when calcium movement into the circulation overwhelms calcium regulatory hormones or the ability of the kidney to remove excess calcium ions. The two most common causes of hypercalcemia are increased bone resorption due to hyperparathyroidism and neoplasms.[40] Hypercalcemia is a common complication of malignancy, occurring in approximately 20% to 30% of persons with advanced disease.[40,41] A number of malignant tumors, including carcinoma of the lung, have been associated with hypercalcemia. Some tumors destroy the bone, while others produce humoral agents that stimulate bone resorption or inhibit bone formation.

Less common causes of hypercalcemia include prolonged immobilization, increased intestinal absorption of calcium, excessive doses of vitamin D, or the effects of drugs such as lithium and thiazide diuretics.[41] Prolonged immobilization and lack of weight bearing cause demineralization of bone and release of calcium into the bloodstream. Intestinal absorption of calcium can be increased by excessive doses of vitamin D or as the result of a condition called the *milk-alkali syndrome*.

The *milk-alkali* syndrome is caused by the ingestion of calcium (often in the form of milk) and absorbable antacids, particularly calcium carbonate.[42] The condition is characterized by hypercalcemia, hyperphosphatemia, alkalosis, and progressive renal failure. Because of the availability of nonabsorbable antacids, the condition is seen less frequently than in the past, but it may occur in women who are overzealous in taking calcium preparations for osteoporosis prevention. Discontinuation of the antacid repairs the alkalosis and increases calcium elimination.

A variety of drugs elevate calcium levels.[36] The use of lithium to treat bipolar disorders has been shown to cause hyperparathyroidism and hypercalcemia in some people. The thiazide diuretics increase calcium reabsorption in the distal convoluted tubule of the kidney. Although the thiazide diuretics seldom cause hypercalcemia, they can unmask hypercalcemia from other causes such as underlying bone disease and conditions that increase bone resorption.

Manifestations. The signs and symptoms of calcium excess reflect a decrease in neural excitability, alterations in cardiac and smooth muscle function, and exposure of the kidneys to high concentrations of calcium [3,35,40] (see Table 8-6). There may be a dulling of consciousness, stupor, weakness, and muscle flaccidity. Behavioral changes may range from subtle alterations in personality to acute psychoses. The heart responds to elevated levels of calcium with increased contractility and ventricular arrhythmias. Digitalis accentuates these responses. Gastrointestinal symptoms include constipation, anorexia, nausea, and vomiting, reflecting a decrease in smooth muscle activity. Bone pain can occur with hyperparathyroidism or malignancy. Excess PTH can lead to bone reabsorption with development of bone cysts or osteoporosis.

High calcium concentrations in the urine filtrate impair the ability of the kidneys to concentrate urine by interfering with the action of ADH (an example of nephrogenic DI). This causes salt and water diuresis and an increased sensation of thirst. Hypercalciuria also predisposes to the development of renal calculi. Pancreatitis is another potential complication of hypercalcemia and is probably related to stones in the pancreatic ducts.

Hypercalcemic crisis describes an acute life-threatening increase in the serum calcium level.[43] Hyperparathyroidism and malignant disease are the major causes of hypercalcemic crisis. Manifestations reflect those of severe hypercalcemia including polyuria, excessive thirst, dehydration, excessive muscle weakness, cardiac arrhythmias, disturbed mental state, and altered levels of consciousness.

Treatment. Treatment of calcium excess usually is directed toward rehydration and use of measures to increase urinary excretion of calcium and inhibit release of calcium from bone.[40] Fluid replacement is needed in situations of volume depletion. The excretion of sodium is accompanied by calcium excretion. Diuretics and sodium chloride can be administered to increase urinary elimination of calcium after the ECF volume has been restored. Loop diuretics commonly are used rather than thiazide diuretics, which increase calcium reabsorption.

The initial lowering of calcium levels is followed by measures to inhibit bone reabsorption. Drugs that are used to inhibit calcium mobilization include bisphosphonates, calcitonin, and corticosteroids.[3,40] The bisphosphonates, which act mainly by inhibiting osteoclastic activity, provide a significant reduction in calcium levels with relatively few side effects. Calcitonin inhibits osteoclastic activity, thereby decreasing bone resorption. The corticosteroids inhibit the conversion of vitamin D to its active form and are used to treat hypercalcemia due to vitamin D toxicity and hematologic malignancies.

Disorders of Phosphorus Balance

Phosphorus is mainly located in bone (about 85%) and in the ICF (about 14%).[3] Only about 1% is in the ECF compartment, and of that, only a minute proportion is in the plasma. In the adult, the normal serum phosphorus level ranges from 2.5 to 4.5 mg/dL (0.8 to 1.45 mmol/L).[3] Levels in children are greater, probably because of increased levels of growth hormone and decreased levels of gonadal hormones.

Regulation of Phosphorus Balance

Phosphorus is ingested in the diet and eliminated in the urine. It is derived from many dietary sources, including milk and meats. About 50% to 65% of ingested phosphorus is absorbed in the intestine, primarily in the jejunum.[35] Absorption is diminished by concurrent ingestion of substances that bind phosphorus, including calcium, magnesium, and aluminum. Renal elimination of phosphate is then regulated by an overflow mechanism in which the amount of phosphate lost in the urine is directly related to phosphate concentrations in the blood.

Phosphorus exists in two forms within the body—inorganic and organic. The inorganic form (phosphate [$H_2PO_4^-$ or HPO_4^{2-}]) is the principal circulating form of phosphorus and is the form that is routinely measured (and reported as phosphorus) for laboratory purposes.[3,36] Most of the intracellular phosphorus is in the organic form (e.g., nucleic acids, phospholipids, adenosine triphosphate [ATP]).

Phosphorus is essential to many bodily functions.[35] It plays a major role in bone formation; is essential to a number of metabolic processes, including the formation of ATP and the enzymes needed for glucose, fat, and protein metabolism; is a necessary component of several vital parts of the cell, being incorporated into the nucleic acids of DNA and RNA and the phospholipids of the cell membrane; and serves as an acid–base buffer in the ECF and in the kidney. Delivery of oxygen by the red blood cell depends on organic phosphorus in ATP and 2,3-diphosphoglycerate (2,3-DPG). Phosphorus is also needed for normal function of white blood cells and platelets.

Hypophosphatemia

Hypophosphatemia is commonly defined by a serum phosphorus level of less than 2.5 mg/dL (0.81 mmol/L) in adults; and is considered severe at a concentration of less than 1.0 mg/dL (0.32 mmol/L).[3,44] Hypophosphatemia may occur despite normal body phosphorus stores as a result of movement from the ECF into the ICF compartment. Serious depletion of phosphorus may exist with low, normal, or high plasma concentrations.

The most common causes of hypophosphatemia are depletion of phosphorus because of insufficient intestinal absorption, transcompartmental shifts, and increased renal losses.[3,44] Often, more than one of these mechanisms is active. Unless food intake is severely restricted, dietary intake and intestinal absorption of phosphorus are usually adequate. Intestinal absorption may be inhibited by administration of glucocorticoids, high dietary levels of magnesium, and hypothyroidism. Prolonged ingestion of antacids may also interfere with intestinal absorption. Antacids that contain aluminum hydroxide, aluminum carbonate, and calcium carbonate bind with phosphate, causing increased phosphate losses in the stool. Because of their ability to bind phosphate, calcium-based antacids are sometimes used therapeutically to decrease plasma phosphate levels in persons with chronic kidney disease.

Malnutrition increases phosphate excretion and phosphorus loss from the body. Refeeding of malnourished persons increases the incorporation of phosphorus into nucleic acids and phosphorylated compounds in the cell. The catabolic events that occur with diabetic ketoacidosis also deplete phosphorus stores. Usually the hypophosphatemia does not become apparent, however, until insulin and fluid replacement have reversed the dehydration and glucose has started to move back into the cell. Chronic alcohol use is a common cause of hypophosphatemia. Contributing factors include poor food intake and the effect that chronic alcohol use has on the renal threshold for phosphate reabsorption, causing more phosphate to be eliminated in the urine. Administration of hyperalimentation solutions without adequate phosphorus can cause a rapid influx of phosphorus into the body's muscle mass, particularly if treatment is initiated after a period of tissue catabolism. Respiratory alkalosis due to prolonged hyperventilation can produce hypophosphatemia through increased PTH levels and increased phosphate excretion. Clinical conditions associated with hyperventilation include sepsis, withdrawal from chronic alcoholism, fever, and primary hyperventilation.

Manifestations. Many of the manifestations of phosphorus deficiency result from a decrease in cellular energy stores associated with a deficiency in ATP and impaired oxygen transport due to a decrease in red blood cell 2,3-diphosphoglycerate (2,3-DPG).[3,44] The decrease in cellular energy can cause altered neural function, disturbed musculoskeletal function, and hematologic disorders (Table 8-7).

Red blood cell metabolism is impaired by phosphorus deficiency; causing the cells to become rigid, undergo increased hemolysis, and have diminished ATP and 2,3-DPG levels (see Chapter 14). The chemotactic and phagocytic functions of white blood cells and the hemostatic functions of the platelets are also impaired. Anorexia and dysphagia can occur. Neural manifestations (intention tremors, paresthesias, hyporeflexia, stupor, coma, and seizures) are uncommon but serious manifestations.

Chronic phosphorus depletion interferes with mineralization of newly formed bone matrix. In growing children, this process causes abnormal endochondral growth and clinical manifestations of rickets. In adults,

TABLE 8-7	Manifestations of Hypophosphatemia and Hyperphosphatemia
Hypophosphatemia	**Hyperphosphatemia**
Laboratory Values Serum phosphorus < 2.5 mg/dL (0.8 mmol/L)	***Laboratory Values*** Serum phosphorus >4.5 mg/dL (1.45 mmol/L)
Neural Manifestations Intentional tremor Ataxia Paresthesias Confusion, stupor, coma Seizures	***Neuromuscular Manifestations*** Paresthesias Tetany
Musculoskeletal Manifestions Joint stiffness Bone pain Osteomalacia	***Cardiovascular Effects*** Hypotension Cardiac arrhythmias
Blood Disorders Hemolytic anemia Platelet dysfunction with bleeding tendency Impaired white blood cell function	

the condition leads to joint stiffness, bone pain, and skeletal deformities consistent with osteomalacia (see Chapter 44).

Treatment. The treatment of hypophosphatemia is usually directed toward prophylaxis. This may be accomplished with dietary sources high in phosphorus (one glass of milk contains approximately 250 mg of phosphorus) or with oral or intravenous replacement solutions. Phosphorus supplements usually are contraindicated in hyperparathyroidism, chronic kidney disease, and hypercalcemia because of the increased risk of extracellular calcifications.

Hyperphosphatemia

Hyperphosphatemia represents a serum phosphorus concentration in excess of 4.5 mg/dL (1.45 mmol/L) in adults. Moderate hyperphosphatemia exists when serum phosphate is in the range of 4.6 to 6.0 mg/dL (1.49 to 1.94 mmol/L) and severe phosphatemia when serum phosphate levels are greater than 6.0 (1.94 mmol/L).[3]

Hyperphosphatemia can result from failure of the kidneys to excrete excess phosphate, rapid redistribution of intracellular phosphate to the ECF compartment, or high phosphate intake.[3,45] Because phosphorus is primarily eliminated by the kidneys, hyperphosphatemia due to impaired renal function is a common electrolyte disorder in persons with chronic kidney disease[3,46] (see Chapter 26). Release of intracellular phosphorus can result from conditions such as massive tissue injury, rhabdomyolysis (muscle dissolution), heat stroke, potassium deficiency, and seizures. The administration of excess phosphate-containing antacids, laxatives, or enemas can be another cause of hyperphosphatemia, especially when there is a decrease in vascular volume and a reduced glomerular filtration rate. Phosphate-containing laxatives and enemas predispose to hypovolemia and a decreased glomerular filtration rate by inducing diarrhea, thereby increasing the risk of hyperphosphatemia. Serious and even fatal hyperphosphatemia has reportedly resulted from administration of phosphate enemas.[47]

Manifestations. Many of the signs and symptoms of a phosphate excess are related to a calcium deficit (see Table 8-7). Because of the reciprocal relationship between calcium and phosphorus levels, a high serum phosphate level tends to lower serum calcium levels, which can lead to tetany and other signs of hypocalcemia.[3] Inadequately treated hyperphosphatemia in chronic kidney disease can lead to renal bone disease, and extraosseous calcifications in soft tissues (see Chapter 26). A secondary effect of hyperphosphatemia in chronic kidney disease is stimulation of nodular hyperplasia of the parathyroid glands that results in a secondary hyperparathyroidism.[46]

Treatment. The treatment of hyperphosphatemia is directed at the cause of the disorder. Dietary restriction of foods that are high in phosphorus may be used. Calcium-based phosphate binders are useful in chronic hyperphosphatemia. Sevelamer, a recently approved calcium- and aluminum-free phosphate binder, is as effective as a calcium-based binder, but lacks its adverse effects.[3] Hemodialysis is used to reduce phosphate levels in persons with chronic kidney disease.

Disorders of Magnesium Balance

Magnesium is the second most abundant intracellular divalent cation.[48–50] Although the average adult has approximately 24 g of magnesium distributed throughout the body, only an estimated 2% is distributed in the ECF.[50,51] The normal serum concentration of magnesium is 1.3 to 2.1 mg/dL (0.65 to 1.1 mmol/L).[3]

Regulation of Magnesium Balance

Magnesium is ingested in the diet, absorbed from the intestine, and excreted by the kidneys. Intestinal absorption is not closely regulated, and only about 30% to 50% of dietary magnesium is absorbed.[48] The kidney is the principal organ of magnesium regulation. The kidneys filter about 80% of the serum magnesium and only about 3% is excreted in the urine, although this amount can be influenced by other conditions and medications.[48] Renal reabsorption is stimulated by PTH and is decreased in the presence of increased serum levels of magnesium and calcium.

Magnesium is a cofactor in hundreds of metabolic reactions in the body. It is required for cellular energy metabolism, functioning of the Na^+/K^+-ATPase membrane pump, membrane stabilization, nerve conduction, and ion transport. It also acts as a cofactor in many intracellular enzyme reactions, including the transfer of high-energy phosphate groups in the generation of ATP from adenosine diphosphate (ADP). It is essential to all reactions that require ATP, for every step related to replication and transcription of DNA, and for translation of messenger RNA.[3,48–50]

Magnesium also participates in potassium and calcium channel activity. Magnesium blocks the outward movement of potassium in cardiac cells, preventing the development of cardiac arrhythmias.[51] It also acts as a smooth muscle relaxant by altering calcium levels that are responsible for muscle contraction. Because of its smooth muscle relaxing effect, there has been a recent interest in the use of magnesium in the treatment of severe bronchial asthma.[56] In addition, it has been suggested that magnesium may have an anticonvulsant effect. Currently, it is the first-line drug in the prevention and treatment of seizures associated with eclampsia in pregnant women (see Chapter 18).[52]

Hypomagnesemia

Magnesium deficiency refers to depletion of total body stores and hypomagnesemia to a low serum concentration of less than 1.3 mg/dL (0.65 mmol/L).[3] It is seen in conditions that limit intake or increase intestinal or renal losses, and it is a common finding in patients in emergency departments and critical care units.

Magnesium deficiency can result from insufficient intake, excessive losses, or movement between the ECF and ICF compartments.[3,53,54] It can result from conditions that directly limit intake, such as malnutrition, starvation, or prolonged use of magnesium-free parenteral nutrition. Other conditions, such as diarrhea, malabsorption syndromes, prolonged nasogastric suction, or laxative abuse, decrease intestinal absorption. Another common cause of magnesium deficiency is chronic alcoholism. Many factors contribute to hypomagnesemia in alcoholism, including low intake and gastrointestinal losses from diarrhea. There also have been recent reports of hypomagnesemia associated with prolonged use of proton-pump inhibitor medications, presumably due to decreased intestinal absorption of magnesium.[55]

Although the kidneys are able to defend against hypermagnesemia, they are less able to conserve magnesium and prevent hypomagnesemia. Urine losses are increased in diabetic ketoacidosis, hyperparathyroidism, and hyperaldosteronism. Some drugs increase renal losses of magnesium, including both loop and thiazide diuretics, nephrotoxic drugs such as aminoglycoside antibiotics, cyclosporine, cisplatin, and amphotericin B.[54]

Relative hypomagnesemia may also develop in conditions that promote movement of magnesium between the ECF and ICF compartments, including rapid administration of glucose, insulin-containing parenteral solutions, and alkalosis. Although transient, these conditions can cause serious alterations in body function.

Manifestations. Signs of magnesium deficiency are not usually apparent until the serum magnesium is less than 1.0 mEq/L (0.4 mmol/L).[3] Hypomagnesemia is characterized by an increase in neuromuscular excitability as evidenced by hyperactive deep tendon reflexes, paresthesias (i.e., numbness, pricking, tingling sensation), muscle fasciculations, and tetanic muscle contractions[3,50,53] (Table 8-8). A positive Chvostek or Trousseau sign may be present, especially if the abnormal serum magnesium level is associated with hypocalcemia. Other manifestations may include ataxia, vertigo, disorientation, depression, and psychotic symptoms.

Cardiovascular manifestations include tachycardia, hypertension, and ventricular arrhythmias.[51] There may be ECG changes such as widening of the QRS complex, appearance of peaked T waves, prolongation of the PR interval, T-wave inversion, and appearance of U waves. Ventricular arrhythmias, particularly in the presence of digitalis, may be difficult to treat unless magnesium levels are normalized.

Magnesium deficiency often occurs in conjunction with hypocalcemia and hypokalemia, producing a number of related neurologic and cardiovascular manifestations. Hypocalcemia is typical of severe hypomagnesemia. Most persons with hypomagnesemia-related hypocalcemia have decreased PTH levels, probably as a result of impaired magnesium-dependent mechanisms that control PTH synthesis and release. The resultant hypocalcemia is corrected with calcium replacement until the magnesium is normalized. Hypokalemia is also a typical feature of hypomagnesemia. It leads to a reduction in intracellular potassium and impairs the ability of the kidneys to conserve potassium. When hypomagnesemia is present, hypokalemia remains unresponsive to potassium replacement therapy.

Treatment. The treatment of hypomagnesemia consists of magnesium replacement.[3,50,54] The route of administration depends on the severity of the condition. Symptomatic moderate to severe magnesium deficiency is treated by parenteral administration. Treatment must be continued for several days to replace stored and serum levels. In conditions of chronic intestinal or renal loss, maintenance support with oral magnesium may be required.

Magnesium often is used therapeutically to treat cardiac arrhythmia, myocardial infarct, angina, bronchial asthma, and pregnancy complicated by preeclampsia or eclampsia. Caution is needed to prevent hypermagnesemia in persons with any degree of chronic kidney disease.

TABLE 8-8	Manifestations of Hypomagnesemia and Hypermagnesemia
Hypomagnesemia	**Hypermagnesemia**
Laboratory Values	***Laboratory Values***
Serum magnesium <1.3 mg/dL (0.65 mmol/L)	Serum magnesium >2.1 mg/dL (1.1 mmol/L)
Neural and Muscle Effects (increased)	***Neural and Muscle Effects (decreased)***
Paresthesias	Lethargy
Ataxia, dizziness,	Hyporeflexia
Muscle fasiculations, tetany	Confusion
Confusion, disorientation	Coma
Cardiovascular Effects	***Cardiovascular Effects***
Tachycardia	Hypotension
Hypertension	Cardiac arrhythmias
Cardiac arrhythmias	Cardiac arrest (severe hypomagnesemia)

Hypermagnesemia

Hypermagnesemia represents an increase in total body magnesium and a serum magnesium concentration in excess of 2.5 mg/dL (1.1 mmol/L).[3] Because of the ability of the normal kidney to excrete magnesium, hypermagnesemia is rare.

When hypermagnesemia does occur, it usually is related to renal insufficiency and the injudicious use of magnesium-containing medications such as antacids, mineral supplements, or laxatives.[3] The elderly are particularly at risk because they have age-related reductions in kidney function and tend to consume more magnesium-containing medications, including antacids and laxatives. Magnesium sulfate is used to treat toxemia of pregnancy and premature labor; in these cases, careful monitoring of serum magnesium levels and observation for signs of hypermagnesemia are essential. Neonatal hypermagnesemia may also occur, but usually the blood levels of magnesium are lower in the infant than in the mother.[52]

Manifestations. The signs and symptoms occur only when serum magnesium levels exceed 4.0 mg/dL (2.0 mmol/L).[35,52] Because magnesium tends to suppress PTH secretion, hypocalcemia may accompany hypermagnesemia.

Hypermagnesemia affects neuromuscular and cardiovascular function[3,50,53] (see Table 8-8). Increased levels of magnesium decrease acetylcholine release at the myoneural junction, causing hyporeflexia and muscle weakness. Cardiovascular effects are related to the calcium channel–blocking effects of magnesium. Blood pressure is decreased, and the ECG shows an increase in the PR interval, a shortening of the QT interval, T-wave abnormalities, and prolongation of the QRS and PR intervals. Severe hypermagnesemia is associated with muscle and respiratory paralysis, complete heart block, and cardiac arrest.

Treatment. The treatment of hypermagnesemia includes cessation of magnesium administration. Calcium is a direct antagonist of magnesium, and intravenous administration of calcium may be used. Peritoneal dialysis or hemodialysis may be required.

Disorders of Parathyroid Hormone

Both calcium and phosphate homeostasis are impacted by disorders of PTH. Parathyroid hormone is secreted by the four parathyroid glands located adjacent to the thyroid gland in the neck. The hormone is synthesized as a preprohormone, converted to a prohormone and then to PTH, and finally packaged into secretory granules for release into the circulation. The dominant regulator of PTH secretion is the serum calcium concentration (see Fig. 8-13). A unique ECF calcium-sensing receptor on the parathyroid cell membrane responds rapidly to changes in serum calcium levels.[1,2] When the serum calcium level is high, the secretion of PTH is inhibited, and serum calcium is deposited in the bones. When the level is low, PTH secretion is increased, and calcium is mobilized from the bones and released into the blood.

The synthesis and release of PTH from the parathyroid gland are also influenced by magnesium.[56] Magnesium serves as a cofactor in the generation of cellular energy and is important in the function of second messenger systems. Magnesium's effects on the synthesis and release of PTH are thought to be mediated through these mechanisms. Because of its function in regulating PTH release, severe and prolonged hypomagnesemia can markedly inhibit PTH levels.

The central function of PTH is to regulate ionized Ca^{++} levels through three target organs: bone, kidney, and intestine absorption. Parathyroid hormone stimulates the release of calcium from bone; and it increases calcium reabsorption by the kidney, while increasing the activation of vitamin D by the kidney; which in turn, increases the intestinal reabsorption of calcium.

Hypoparathyroidism

Hypoparathyroidism reflects deficient PTH secretion, resulting in low serum levels of ionized calcium. Parathyroid hormone deficiency may occur because of a congenital absence of all of the parathyroid glands, as in DiGeorge syndrome (see Chapter 16), or because of an acquired disorder due to inadvertent removal or irreversible damage to the glands during thyroidectomy, parathyroidectomy, or radical neck dissection for cancer.[35,56,57] A transient form of PTH deficiency may occur after thyroid surgery owing to parathyroid gland suppression. Hypoparathyroidism also may have an autoimmune origin. Antiparathyroid antibodies have been detected in some persons with hypoparathyroidism, particularly those with multiple autoimmune disorders such as type 1 diabetes mellitus or Graves disease. Other causes of hypoparathyroidism include heavy metal damage such as occurs with Wilson disease and metastatic tumors. Functional impairment of parathyroid function occurs with magnesium deficiency. Correction of the hypomagnesemia results in rapid disappearance of the condition.

Manifestations. Manifestations of acute hypoparathyroidism, which result from a decrease in serum calcium, include tetany with muscle cramps, carpopedal spasm, and convulsions (see section on hypocalcemia).[56,57] Paresthesias, such as tingling of the circumoral area and in the hands and feet, are almost always present. Low calcium levels may cause prolongation of the QT interval on the ECG, resistance to digitalis, hypotension, and refractory heart failure. Symptoms of chronic PTH deficiency include lethargy, an anxiety state, and personality changes. There may be blurring of vision because of cataracts, which develop over a number of years. Extrapyramidal signs, such as those seen with Parkinson disease, may occur because of calcification of the basal ganglia. Teeth may be defective if the disorder occurs during childhood.

Pseudohypoparathyroidism is a rare familial disorder characterized by target tissue resistance to PTH. It is characterized by hypocalcemia, increased parathyroid function, and a variety of congenital defects in the growth and development of the skeleton, including short stature and short metacarpal and metatarsal bones. There are variants of the disorder, with some persons having the pseudohypoparathyroidism along with the congenital defects and others having the congenital defects with normal calcium and phosphorus levels. The manifestations of the disorder are due primarily to chronic hypocalcemia.

Treatment. The goals of therapy focus on the control of symptoms while minimizing complications. Acute hypoparathyroid tetany, which usually occurs after surgery, is treated with intravenous calcium gluconate followed by oral administration of calcium salts and vitamin D. Magnesium supplementation is used when the disorder is caused by magnesium deficiency. Persons with chronic hypoparathyroidism are treated with oral calcium and vitamin D. Levels of serum calcium, phosphorus, and creatinine (to check kidney function) are monitored at regular intervals as a means of maintaining serum calcium within a slightly low but asymptomatic range.

Hyperparathyroidism

Hyperparathyroidism is characterized by increased levels of PTH. It can manifest as a primary disorder caused by hyperplasia or tumors of the parathyroid glands, as as a secondary disorder in persons with chronic kidney disease or chronic malabsorption of calcium.[58–61]

Manifestations. Primary hyperparathyroidism is a leading cause of hypercalcemia in the outpatient department. It is seen more commonly after 50 years of age and is more common in women than men.[58] Primary hyperparathyroidism causes an elevation in ionized serum calcium and increased urinary excretion of both calcium and phosphorus. The increased urinary concentration of calcium and phosphorus may prompt the development of kidney stones. Chronic bone resorption may produce diffuse demineralization, pathologic fractures, and cystic bone lesions.

Signs and symptoms of the disorder are related to skeletal abnormalities, exposure of the kidney to high calcium levels, and elevated serum calcium levels (see hypercalcemia). At the present time, primary hyperparathyroidism usually manifests as an asymptomatic disorder that is discovered in the course of routine biochemical testing. Although thought to be asymptomatic, these patents may experience nonspecific constitutional symptoms such as fatigue, weakness, anorexia, and bone pain.[60]

Secondary hyperparathyroidism involves hyperplasia of the parathyroid glands and occurs primarily in persons with chronic kidney disease.[59,60] In the early stages of chronic kidney disease, an increase in PTH results from decreased serum calcium and activated vitamin D levels. As the disease progresses, there is a decrease in

vitamin D and calcium receptors, making the parathyroid glands more resistant to feedback regulation by serum calcium and vitamin D levels. At this point, elevated phosphorus levels induce hyperplasia of the parathyroid glands independent of calcium and vitamin D levels. The bone disease seen in persons with secondary hyperparathyroidism due to chronic kidney disease is known as *renal osteodystrophy* (see Chapter 26).

Treatment. Treatment of hyperparathyroidism includes resolving the hypercalcemia with increased fluid intake. Whenever possible, the underlying cause of secondary hyperparathyroidism should be treated. Parathyroidectomy may be indicated in persons with symptomatic primary hyperparathyroidism. The goal of medical management is to normalize calcium levels. Calcitriol and other vitamin D analogs may be used to control parathyroid hyperplasia in chronic kidney disease. Persons with chronic kidney disease may also need phosphate binders to decrease intestinal absorption of phosphorus and prevent the skeletal disorders associated with the osteodystrophies (see Chapter 26). Calcimimetic agents, which act through the calcium-sensing receptor in the parathyroid gland, may be used to decrease PTH production in primary and secondary hyperparathyroidism.[59–61]

SUMMARY CONCEPTS

■ Calcium, phosphorus, and magnesium are the major divalent ions in the body. These divalent ions are directly or indirectly regulated by a number of factors including vitamin D and PTH.

■ Calcium is a major divalent cation with approximately 99% located in bone and less than 1% in the ECF compartment. Of the three forms of ECF calcium, only the ionized form can cross the cell membrane, contributing to neuromuscular function, blood clotting, and enzyme reactions. In *hypocalcemia*, decreased levels in ionized calcium produce an increase in neuromuscular excitability; and in *hypercalcemia* increased levels of ionized calcium produce a decrease in excitability.

■ Phosphorus is largely an ICF anion, being incorporated into nucleic acids, adenosine triphosphate (ATP), and 2,3-diphosphoglycerate in the red blood cells. *Hypophosphatemia*, which is associated with decreased intestinal absorption, transcompartmental shifts, and disorders of renal elimination, causes signs and symptoms of neural dysfunction, disturbed musculoskeletal function, and hematologic disorders. *Hyperphosphatemia*, which occurs with renal failure and PTH deficit, is associated with decreased plasma calcium levels.

- Magnesium, which is the second most abundant ICF cation, acts as a cofactor in many intracellular enzyme reactions and is required for cellular energy metabolism, functioning of the Na$^+$/K$^+$-ATPase membrane pump, nerve conduction, ion transport, and potassium and calcium channel activity. *Hypomagnesemia* produces a decrease in serum calcium due to suppression of PTH release and a decrease in serum potassium due to renal wasting, both of which contribute to an increase in neuromuscular exitability. *Hypermagnesemia* causes neuromuscular dysfunction with hyporeflexia, muscle weakness, and confusion.

- Parathyroid hormone disorders impact both calcium and phosphate homeostasis. Acute *hypoparathyroidism* causes hypocalcemia, manifested by signs of increased neuromuscular excitability such as muscle cramps and tetany. Chronic hypoparathyroidism is manifested by lethargy and fatigue. *Hyperparathyroidism* can occur as a primary disorder causing elevated serum calcium levels and increased urinary excretion of both calcium and phosphorus, which provides the potential for development of kidney stones. Secondary hyperparathyroidism, which associated with chronic kidney disease, exerts its effects on bone, causing renal osteodystrophies.

Acid–Base Balance

Metabolic activities of the body require precise regulation of acid–base balance as reflected in the pH of the ECF, which is normally maintained within a very narrow range of 7.35 to 7.45.[1–3] Membrane excitability, enzyme systems, and chemical reactions all depend on the pH being regulated within a narrow physiologic range to function in an optimal way.

Acid–Base Chemistry

Acids and bases have their own chemical properties and definitions. An *acid* is defined as a compound that can dissociate and release a hydrogen (H$^+$) ion and a *base* as a compound that can accept or combine with H$^+$.[1–3] For example, hydrochloric acid (HCl) dissociates in water to form H$^+$ and Cl$^-$ ions. The bicarbonate ion (HCO$_3^-$) is a base because it can combine with H$^+$ to form carbonic acid (H$_2$CO$_3$). Most of the body's acids and bases are weak; the most important are H$_2$CO$_3$, which is a weak acid derived from carbon dioxide (CO$_2$), and HCO$_3^-$, which is a weak base.

The concentration of H$^+$ in body fluids is low compared with other ions. For example, the Na$^+$ is present at a concentration approximately 3.5 million times that of the H$^+$. Because it is cumbersome to work with such a small number, the H$^+$ concentration is commonly expressed in terms of the *pH*. Specifically, pH represents the negative logarithm (log$_{10}$) of the H$^+$ concentration expressed in mEq/L. Since the pH is inversely related to the H$^+$ concentration, a low pH indicates a high concentration of H$^+$ and a high pH a low concentration of H$^+$.

Acid and Base Production

Acids are continuously generated as by-products of metabolic processes (Fig. 8-16). Physiologically, these acids fall into two groups: *volatile* H$_2$CO$_3$ and all other *nonvolatile* or *fixed acids* (e.g., sulfuric, hydrochloric, and

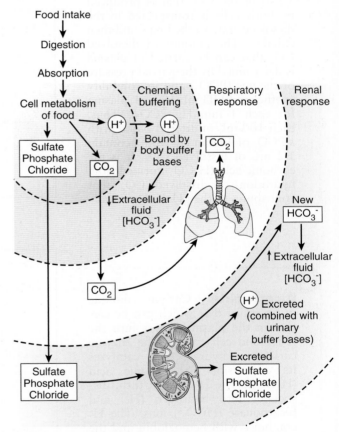

FIGURE 8-16. The maintenance of normal blood pH by chemical buffers, the respiratory system, and the kidneys. On a mixed diet, pH is threatened by the production of strong acids (sulfuric, hydrochloric, and phosphoric) mainly as the result of protein metabolism. These strong acids are buffered in the body by chemical buffer bases such as extracellular fluid (ECF) bicarbonate (HCO$_3^-$). The kidney eliminates hydrogen ions (H$^+$) combined with urinary buffers and anions in the urine. At the same time, they add new HCO$_3^-$ to the ECF to replace the HCO$_3^-$ consumed in buffering strong acids. The respiratory system disposes of carbon dioxide (CO$_2$). (From Rhoades RA, Bell DR. *Medical Physiology: Principles of Clinical Medicine.* 4th ed. Philadelphia, PA: Wolters Kluwer Health | Lippincott Williams & Wilkins; 2013:454.)

(*text continues on page 193*)

UNDERSTANDING → Carbon Dioxide

Body metabolism results in a continuous production of carbon dioxide (CO_2). As CO_2 is formed during the metabolic process, it diffuses out of body cells into the tissue spaces and then into the circulation. It is transported in the circulation in three forms: (1) dissolved in the plasma, (2) as bicarbonate, and (3) attached to hemoglobin.

1

Plasma. A small portion (about 10%) of the CO_2 that is produced by body cells is transported in the dissolved state to the lungs and then exhaled. The amount of dissolved CO_2 that can be carried in plasma is determined by the partial pressure of the gas (PCO_2) and its solubility coefficient (0.03 mL/100 mL plasma for each 1 mm Hg PCO_2). Thus, each 100 mL of arterial blood with a PCO_2 of 40 mm Hg would contain 1.2 mL of dissolved CO_2. It is the carbonic acid (H_2CO_3) formed from hydration of dissolved CO_2 that contributes to the pH of the blood.

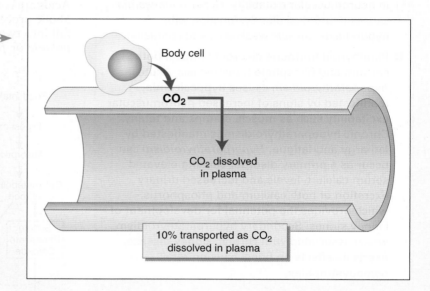

Body cell

CO_2

CO_2 dissolved in plasma

10% transported as CO_2 dissolved in plasma

2

Bicarbonate. Carbon dioxide in excess of that which can be carried in the plasma moves into the red blood cells, where the enzyme carbonic anhydrase (CA) catalyzes its conversion to carbonic acid (H_2CO_3). The H_2CO_3, in turn, dissociates into hydrogen (H^+) and bicarbonate (HCO_3^-) ions. The H^+ combines with hemoglobin and the HCO_3^- diffuses into plasma, where it participates in acid–base regulation. The movement of HCO_3^- into the plasma is made possible by a special transport system on the red blood cell membrane in which HCO_3^- ions are exchanged for chloride ions (Cl^-).

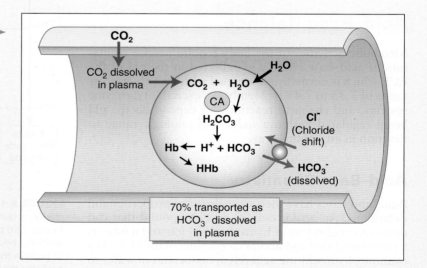

CO_2

CO_2 dissolved in plasma

H_2O

$CO_2 + H_2O$

CA

H_2CO_3

Cl^- (Chloride shift)

$Hb \leftarrow H^+ + HCO_3^-$

HHb

HCO_3^- (dissolved)

70% transported as HCO_3^- dissolved in plasma

Transport

3

Hemoglobin. The remaining CO_2 in the red blood cells combines with hemoglobin to form carbaminohemoglobin (HbCO$_2$). The combination of CO_2 with hemoglobin is a reversible reaction characterized by a loose bond, so that CO_2 can be easily released in the alveolar capillaries and exhaled from the lung.

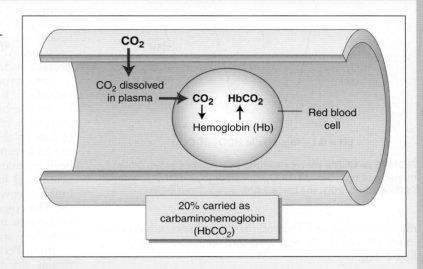

(text continued from page 191)

phosphoric acid). The difference between the two types of acids arises because H_2CO_3 is in equilibrium with dissolved CO_2, which is volatile and leaves the body by way of the lungs. The nonvolatile or fixed acids are not eliminated by the lungs. Instead, they are buffered by body proteins or extracellular buffers, such as HCO_3^-, and then eliminated by the kidney.

Carbon Dioxide and Bicarbonate Production. Carbon dioxide, which is the end product of aerobic metabolism, is transported in the circulation as a dissolved gas (i.e., PCO_2), as the HCO_3^- ion, or as CO_2 bound to hemoglobin in carbaminohemoglobin (see understanding carbon dioxide transport). Collectively, dissolved CO_2 and HCO_3^- account for approximately 77% of the CO_2 that is transported in the extracellular fluid; the remaining CO_2 travels as carbaminohemoglobin.[2] Although CO_2 is a gas and not an acid, a small percentage of the gas combines with water to form the weak H_2CO_3 acid. The reaction that generates H_2CO_3 from CO_2 and water is catalyzed by an enzyme called *carbonic anhydrase*, which is present in large quantities in red blood cells, renal tubular cells, and other tissues in the body. (see Understanding: Carbon Dioxide Transport)

Because it is almost impossible to measure H_2CO_3, carbon dioxide measurements are commonly used when calculating pH. The H_2CO_3 content of the blood can be calculated by multiplying the partial pressure of CO_2 (PCO_2) by its solubility coefficient, which is 0.03. This means that the concentration of H_2CO_3 in the arterial blood, which normally has a PCO_2 of approximately 40 mm Hg, is 1.20 mEq/L ($40 \times 0.03 = 1.20$), and that for venous blood, which normally has a PCO_2 of approximately 45 mm Hg, is 1.35 mEq/L.

Production of Nonvolatile Acids and Bases. The metabolism of dietary proteins and other substances results in the generation of nonvolatile acids and bases.[4] For example, the metabolism of sulfur-containing amino acids (e.g.,methonine and cysteine) results in the production of *sulfuric acid*; of arginine and lysine, *hydrochloric acid*; and of nucleic acids, *phosphoric acid*. Incomplete oxidation of glucose results in the formation of *lactic acid,* and incomplete oxidation of fats, the production of *ketoacids*. The major source of bases is the metabolism of amino acids such as aspartate and glutamate and the metabolism of certain organic anions (e.g., citrate, lactate, acetate).

Calculation of pH

The serum pH can be calculated using an equation called the *Henderson-Hasselbalch equation*. This equation uses the dissociation constant for the bicarbonate buffer system (which is 6.1) plus the log of the HCO_3^- - to - PCO_2 (used as a measure of H_2CO_3) ratio (normally 20:1) to determine the pH (i.e., pH = 6.1 + log of 20 = 7.4). Because the ratio is used, a change in either HCO_3^- or PCO_2 will have little or no effect on pH as long as there is an accompanying change in PCO_2 and HCO_3^- (Fig. 8-17). The pH will decrease when the ratio decreases and increase when the ratio increases.

Regulation of pH

The pH of body fluids is regulated by three major mechanisms: (1) chemical buffer systems in body fluids, which immediately combine with excess acids or bases to prevent large changes in pH; (2) the lungs, which control

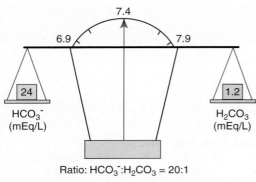

Ratio: $HCO_3^-:H_2CO_3 = 20:1$

$$pH = 6.1 + \log_{10} (\text{ratio } HCO_3^-:H_2CO_3)$$

FIGURE 8-17. The pH represented as a balance scale. When the ratio of bicarbonate (HCO_3) to carbonic acid (H_2CO_3, arterial $PCO_2 \times 0.30$) = 20:1, the pH is 7.4.

the elimination of CO_2; and (3) the kidneys, which eliminate H^+ and both reabsorb and generate HCO_3^- (see Fig. 8-16).

Chemical Buffer Systems

The moment-by-moment regulation of pH depends on chemical buffer systems in the ICF and ECF. The three major buffer systems that protect the pH of body fluids are the bicarbonate buffer system, the transcellular hydrogen–potassium exchange system, and body proteins.[1-3] Bone provides an additional buffering of body acids. These buffer systems are immediately available to combine with excess acids or bases and prevent large changes in pH from occurring during the time it takes for the respiratory and renal mechanisms to become effective.

The *bicarbonate buffer system*, which is the principal ECF buffer, uses H_2CO_3 as its weak acid and a bicarbonate salt such as sodium bicarbonate ($NaHCO_3$) as its weak base. It substitutes the weak H_2CO_3 for a strong acid such as hydrochloric acid or the weak bicarbonate base for a strong base such as sodium hydroxide. The bicarbonate buffer system is a particularly efficient system because its components can be readily added or removed from the body.[66] Metabolism provides an ample supply of CO_2, which can replace any H_2CO_3 that is lost when excess base is added, and CO_2 can be readily eliminated when excess acid is added. Likewise, the kidney can conserve or form new HCO_3^- when excess acid is added, and it can excrete HCO_3^- when excess base is added.

The *transcellular hydrogen/potassium exchange system* provides another important system for regulation of acid–base balance. Both H^+ and K^+ are positively charged, and both ions move freely between the ICF and ECF compartments (see Fig. 8-10). When excess H^+ is present in the ECF, it moves into the ICF in exchange for K^+, and when excess K^+ is present in the ECF, it moves into the ICF in exchange for H^+. Thus, alterations in potassium levels can affect acid–base balance, and changes in acid–base balance can influence potassium levels.[1]

Proteins are the largest buffer system in the body. Proteins are *amphoteric*, meaning that they can function either as acids or bases. They contain many ionizable groups that can release or bind H^+. The protein buffers are largely located within cells, and H^+ ions and CO_2 diffuse across cell membranes for buffering by intracellular proteins. Albumin and plasma globulins are the major protein buffers in the vascular compartment.

Bone represents an additional source of acid–base buffering.[3] Excess H^+ ions can be exchanged for Na^+ and K^+ on the bone surface, and dissolution of bone minerals with release of compounds such as sodium bicarbonate ($NaHCO_3$) and calcium carbonate ($CaCO_3$) into the ECF can be used for buffering excess acids. It has been estimated that as much as 40% of buffering of an acute acid load takes place in bone. The role of bone buffers is even greater in the presence of chronic acidosis. The consequences of bone buffering include demineralization of bone and predisposition to development of kidney stones due to increased urinary excretion of calcium. Persons with chronic kidney disease are at particular risk for reduction in bone calcium due to acid retention.

Respiratory Control Mechanisms

The respiratory system provides for the elimination of CO_2 into the air and plays a major role in acid–base regulation. Increased pulmonary ventilation increases CO_2 elimination, producing a decrease in arterial PCO_2; whereas decreased ventilation decreases CO_2 elimination, producing an increase in arterial PCO_2. Chemoreceptors in the brain stem and the peripheral chemoreceptors in the carotid and aortic bodies sense changes in the PCO_2 and pH of the blood and alter the ventilatory rate. The respiratory control of pH is rapid, occurring within minutes, and is maximal within 12 to 24 hours.[4] Although the respiratory response is rapid, it does not completely return the pH to normal and is only about 50% to 75% effective as a buffer system.[66]

Renal Control Mechanisms

The kidneys play a critical role in maintaining acid–base balance.[67] They accomplish this through the reabsorption of HCO_3^-, regulation of H^+ secretion, and generation of new HCO_3^-. The renal mechanisms for regulating acid–base balance cannot adjust the pH within minutes, as respiratory mechanisms can, but they continue to function for days until the pH has returned to normal or the near-normal range.

Hydrogen/Bicarbonate Exchange. The *hydrogen/bicarbonate exchange system* regulates pH through the secretion of excess H^+ and reabsorption of HCO_3^- by the renal tubules. Bicarbonate is freely filtered in the glomerulus and reabsorbed or reclaimed in the tubules.[2] Each HCO_3^- that is reclaimed requires the secretion of a H^+ ion, a process that is tightly coupled with Na^+ reabsorption. Another mechanism that the kidney uses in controlling HCO_3^- loss is the *chloride/bicarbonate* anion exchange that occurs in association with Na^+ reabsorption. Chloride is absorbed along with Na^+ throughout the tubules. In situations of volume depletion due to vomiting and Cl^- depletion, the kidney is forced to substitute HCO_3^- for the Cl^- anion, thereby increasing its absorption of HCO_3^-.

Both reabsorption of HCO_3^- and excretion of acid are accomplished through H^+ secretion as the urine filtrate moves through the tubular structure of the kidney. The epithelial cells of the proximal tubule, the thick ascending limb of Henle, and distal tubule all secrete H^+ nto the tubular fluid by the Na^+/H^+ counter-transport mechanism (see Chapter 24). The *potassium/hydrogen* exchange system in the collecting tubules functions in H^+ secretion by substituting the reabsorption of K^+ for excretion of H^+ Acidosis tends to increase H^+ elimination and decrease K^+ elimination, with a resultant increase in serum potassium levels, whereas alkalosis tends to decrease H^+ elimination and increase K^+ elimination, with a resultant decrease in serum potassium levels.[64–66]

Generation of New Bicarbonate. Another important but more complex buffer system that facilitates the excretion of H^+ and generation of new HCO_3^- is the *ammonia buffer system*. Renal tubular cells are able to use the amino acid glutamine to synthesize ammonia (NH_3) and secrete it into the tubular fluid. Hydrogen ions then combine with the NH_3 to form ammonium ions (NH_4^+). The NH_4^+ ions, in turn, combine with Cl^- ions that are present in the tubular fluid to form ammonium chloride (NH_4Cl), which is then excreted in the urine. Under normal conditions, the amount of H^+ ion eliminated by the ammonia buffer system is about 50% of the acid excreted and new HCO_3^- regenerated. However, with chronic acidosis, it can become the dominant mechanism for H^+ excretion and new HCO_3^- generation.

Phosphate Buffer System. Because extremely acidic urine (pH 4.0 to 4.5) would be damaging to structures in the urinary tract, the elimination of H^+ requires a buffer system. There are two important intratubular buffer systems: the phosphate buffer system and the previously described ammonia buffer system. The *phosphate buffer system* uses HPO_4^{2-} and $H_2PO_4^-$ that are present in the tubular filtrate to buffer H^+. Because HPO_4^{2-} and $H_2PO_4^-$ are poorly absorbed, they become more concentrated as they move through the tubules.

Laboratory Tests

Laboratory tests that are used in assessing acid–base balance include arterial blood gases and serum electrolytes, base excess or deficit, and anion gap. Although useful in determining whether acidosis or alkalosis is present, the pH measurements of the blood provide little information about the cause of an acid–base disorder.

Arterial blood gases provide a means of assessing the respiratory component of acid–base balance. H_2CO_3 levels are determined from arterial PCO_2 levels and the solubility coefficient for CO_2 (normal arterial PCO_2 is 38 to 42 mm Hg). Arterial blood gases are used because *venous blood gases* are highly variable, depending on metabolic demands of the various tissues that empty into the vein from where the sample is being drawn.

Laboratory tests are used to measure serum electrolytes, CO_2 content, and HCO_3^-. These measurements are determined by adding a strong acid to a blood sample and measuring the amount of CO_2 that is produced. More than 70% of the CO_2 in the blood is in the form of bicarbonate. The serum bicarbonate is then determined from the total CO_2 content of the blood. *Base excess or deficit* is a measure of the HCO_3^- excess or deficit. It describes the amount of a fixed acid or base that must be added to a blood sample to achieve a pH of 7.4 (normal ± 2.0 mEq/L).[60] A base excess indicates metabolic alkalosis, and a base deficit indicates metabolic acidosis.

The *anion gap* describes the difference between the serum concentration of the major measured cation (Na^+) and the sum of the measured anions (Cl^- and HCO_3^-). This difference represents the concentration of unmeasured anions, such as phosphates, sulfates, organic acids, and proteins (Fig. 8-18). Normally, the anion gap ranges between 8 and 12 mEq/L (a value of 16 mEq/L is normal if both Na^+ and K^+ concentrations are used in the calculation). The anion gap is increased in conditions such as lactic acidosis and ketoacidosis that result in a decrease in HCO_3, and it is normal in hyperchloremic acidosis, where Cl^- replaces the HCO_3^- anion.[1]

Disorders of Acid–Base Balance

The terms *acidosis* and *alkalosis* describe the clinical conditions that arise as a result of changes in dissolved CO_2 and HCO_3^- concentrations.[64] There are two types

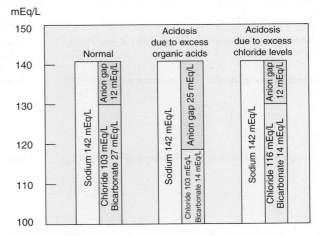

FIGURE 8-18. The anion gap in acidosis due to excess metabolic acids and excess serum chloride levels. Unmeasured anions such as phosphates, sulfates, and organic acids increase the anion gap because they replace bicarbonate. This assumes there is no change in sodium content.

of acid–base disorders: metabolic and respiratory (Table 8-9). *Metabolic disorders* produce an alteration in the serum HCO_3^- concentration and results from the addition or loss of nonvolatile acid or alkali to or from the extracellular fluids. A reduction in pH due to a decrease in HCO_3^- is called *metabolic acidosis*, and an elevation in pH due to increased HCO_3^- levels is called *metabolic alkalosis*. *Respiratory disorders* involve an alteration in the arterial PCO_2, reflecting an increase or decrease in alveolar ventilation. *Respiratory acidosis* is characterized by a decrease in pH, reflecting a decrease in ventilation and an increase in PCO_2. *Respiratory alkalosis* involves an increase in pH, resulting from an increase in alveolar ventilation and a decrease in PCO_2.

Primary Versus Compensatory Changes in pH

Acidosis and alkalosis typically involve a *primary* or *initiating event* and a *compensatory* or *adaptive state* that results from homeostatic mechanisms that attempt to correct or prevent large changes in pH. For example, a person may have a primary metabolic acidosis as a result of overproduction of ketoacids and respiratory alkalosis because of a compensatory increase in ventilation (see Table 8-9).

Compensatory mechanisms provide a means to control pH when correction is impossible or cannot be immediately achieved. Often, they are interim measures that permit survival while the body attempts to correct the primary disorder. Compensation requires the use of mechanisms different from those that caused the primary disorder. For example, the lungs cannot compensate for respiratory acidosis that is caused by lung disease, nor can the kidneys compensate for metabolic acidosis that occurs because of chronic kidney disease. The body can, however, use renal mechanisms to compensate for respiratory-induced changes in pH, and it can use respiratory mechanisms to compensate for metabolically induced changes in acid–base balance. Because compensatory mechanisms become more effective with time, there are often differences between the level of pH change that is present in acute and chronic acid–base disorders.

Single Versus Mixed Acid–Base Disorders

Thus far acid–base disorders have been discussed as if they existed as a single primary disorder such as metabolic acidosis, accompanied by a predicted compensatory response (i.e., hyperventilation and respiratory alkalosis). It is not uncommon, however, for persons to present with more than one primary disorder or a mixed disorder. For example, a person may present with a low serum HCO_3^- concentration due to metabolic acidosis and a high PCO_2 due to chronic lung disease.

Values for the predicted renal or respiratory compensatory responses can be used in the diagnosis of these mixed acid–base disorders (see Table 8-9).[1–3,64,65] If the values for the compensatory response fall outside the predicted values, it can then be concluded that more than one disorder (i.e., a mixed disorder) is present. Since the respiratory response to changes in HCO_3^- occurs almost immediately, there is only one predicted compensatory response for primary metabolic acid–base disorders. This is in contrast to the primary respiratory disorders,

TABLE 8-9	Summary of Single Acid–Base Disturbances and Their Compensatory Responses		
Acid–Base Imbalance	**Primary Disturbance**	**Respiratory Compensation and Predicted Response***	**Renal Compensation and Predicted Response*,†**
Metabolic acidosis	↓plasma pH and HCO_3^-	↑ventilation and ↓PCO_2 *1 mEq/L ↓HCO_3^- →* *1 to 1.5 mm Hg ↓PCO_2*	↑H^+ excretion and ↑HCO_3^- reabsorption if no renal disease
Metabolic alkalosis	↑plasma pH and HCO_3^-	↓ventilation and ↑PCO_2 *1 mEq/L ↑HCO_3^- →* *0.25 to 1.0 ↑PCO_2*	↓H^+ excretion and ↓HCO_3^- reabsorption if no renal disease
Respiratory acidosis	↓plasma pH and ↑PCO_2	None	↑H^+ excretion and ↑HCO_3^- reabsorption *Acute: 1 mm Hg ↑PCO_2→* *0.1 mEq/L ↑HCO_3^-* *Chronic: 1 mm Hg ↑PCO_2→* *0.4 mEq/L ↑HCO_3^-*
Respiratory alkalosis	↑plasma pH and ↓PCO_2	None	↑H^+ excretion and ↓HCO_3^- reabsorption *Acute: 1 mm Hg ↓PCO_2→* *0.2 mEq/L ↓HCO_3^-* *Chronic: 1 mm Hg ↓PCO_2→* *0.4 mEq/L ↓HCO_3^-*

Note: Predicted compensatory responses are in *italics*.

*If blood values are the same as predicted compensatory values, a single acid–base disorder is present; if values are different, a mixed acid–base disorder is present.[12]

†Acute renal compensation ≤48 hours, chronic renal compensation >48 hours.[12]

which have two ranges of predicted values, one for the acute and one for the chronic response. Renal compensation takes several days to become fully effective. The acute compensatory response represents the HCO_3^- levels before renal compensation has occurred and the chronic response after it has occurred. Thus, the values for the serum pH tend to become more normal in the chronic phase.

Metabolic Acidosis

Metabolic acidosis involves a decreased serum HCO_3^- concentration along with a decrease in pH. In metabolic acidosis, the body compensates for the decrease in pH by increasing the respiratory rate in an effort to decrease PCO_2 and H_2CO_3 levels.[1–3]

Metabolic acidosis can be caused by one or more of the following four mechanisms: (1) increased production of fixed metabolic acids or ingestion of fixed acids such as salicylic acid, (2) inability of the kidneys to excrete the fixed acids produced by normal metabolic processes, (3) excessive loss of bicarbonate by the kidneys or gastrointestinal tract, or (4) an increase in serum Cl^- concentration.[64] The anion gap is often useful in determining the cause of the metabolic acidosis[66] (Chart 8-2). The presence of excess metabolic acids produces an increase in the anion gap as sodium

---

CHART 8-2   **Serum Anion Gap in Differential Diagnosis of Metabolic Acidosis**

Decreased Anion Gap (<8 mEq/L)

Hypoalbuminemia (decrease in unmeasured anions)

Multiple myeloma (increase in unmeasured cationic IgG paraproteins)

Increased unmeasured cations (hyperkalemia, hypercalcemia, hypermagnesemia, lithium intoxication)

Increased Anion Gap (>12 mEq/L)

Presence of unmeasured metabolic anion
  Diabetic ketoacidosis
  Alcoholic ketoacidosis
  Lactic acidosis
  Starvation
  Renal insufficiency
Presence of drug or chemical anion
  Salicylate poisoning
  Methanol poisoning
  Ethylene glycol poisoning

Normal Anion Gap (8–12 mEq/L)

Loss of bicarbonate
  Diarrhea
  Pancreatic fluid loss
  Ileostomy (unadapted)
Chloride retention
  Renal tubular acidosis
  Ileal loop bladder
  Parenteral nutrition (arginine and lysine)

---

bicarbonate is replaced by the sodium salt of the offending acid (e.g., sodium lactate).

Increased Production of Metabolic Acids. Among the causes of metabolic acidosis are an accumulation of lactic acid and excess production of ketoacids. *Acute lactic acidosis*, which is one of the most common types of metabolic acidosis, develops when there is excess production or diminished removal of lactic acid from the blood.[60] Lactic acid is produced by the anaerobic metabolism of glucose. Most cases of lactic acidosis are caused by inadequate oxygen delivery, as in shock or cardiac arrest.[63] Such conditions not only increase lactic acid production, but also tend to impair lactic acid clearance because of poor liver and kidney perfusion. Lactic acidosis can also occur during periods of intense exercise in which the metabolic needs of the exercising muscles outpace their aerobic capacity for production of ATP, causing them to revert to anaerobic metabolism and the production of lactic acid. Lactic acidosis is also associated with disorders in which tissue hypoxia does not appear to be present. It has been reported in persons with leukemia, lymphomas and other cancers, poorly controlled diabetes, or severe liver failure. Mechanisms causing lactic acidosis in these conditions are poorly understood. Some conditions such as neoplasms may produce local increases in tissue metabolism and lactate production or they may interfere with blood flow to noncancerous cells.

Ketoacids (i.e., acetoacetic and β-hydroxybutyric acid), which are produced in the liver from fatty acids, are the source of fuel for many body tissues.[64,67] An overproduction of ketoacids occurs when carbohydrate stores are inadequate or when the body cannot use available carbohydrates as a fuel. The most common cause of ketoacidosis is uncontrolled diabetes mellitus, in which an insulin deficiency leads to the release of fatty acids from adipose cells with subsequent production of excess ketoacids[67] (see Chapter 33). Ketoacidosis may also develop as the result of fasting or food deprivation, during which the lack of carbohydrates produces a self-limited state of ketoacidosis.[68]

Decreased Renal Function. Chronic kidney disease is the most common cause of chronic metabolic acidosis. The kidneys normally conserve or generate HCO_3^- and secrete H^+ ions into the urine as a means of regulating acid–base balance. In chronic kidney disease, there is loss of both glomerular and tubular function, with retention of nitrogenous wastes and metabolic acids. In a condition called *renal tubular acidosis*, glomerular function is normal, but the tubular secretion of H^+ or reabsorption of HCO_3^- is abnormal (see Chapter 25).[75]

Increased Bicarbonate Losses. Increased HCO_3^- losses occur with the loss of bicarbonate-rich body fluids or with impaired conservation of HCO_3^- by the kidney. Intestinal secretions have a high HCO_3^- concentration.

Consequently, excessive loss of HCO_3^- occurs with severe diarrhea; small-bowel, pancreatic, or biliary fistula drainage; ileostomy drainage; and intestinal suction. In diarrhea of microbial origin, HCO_3^- is also secreted into the bowel as a means of neutralizing the metabolic acids produced by the microorganisms causing the diarrhea.

Hyperchloremic Acidosis. Hyperchloremic acidosis occurs when Cl^- levels are increased.[67] Because Cl^- and HCO_3^- are exchangeable anions, the serum HCO_3^- decreases when there is an increase in Cl^-. Hyperchloremic acidosis can occur as the result of abnormal absorption of Cl^- by the kidneys or as a result of treatment with chloride-containing medications (i.e., sodium chloride, amino acid–chloride hyperalimentation solutions, and ammonium chloride). With hyperchloremic acidosis, the anion gap remains within the normal range, while serum Cl^- levels are increased and HCO_3^- levels are decreased.

Manifestations. Metabolic acidosis is characterized by a decrease in serum pH (<7.35) and HCO_3^- levels (<24 mEq/dL[24 mmol/L]) due to H^+ gain or HCO_3^- loss. The manifestations of metabolic acidosis fall into three categories: signs and symptoms of the disorder causing the acidosis, changes in body function due to recruitment of compensatory mechanisms, and alterations in cardiovascular, neurologic, and musculoskeletal function resulting from the decreased pH[65-66] (Table 8-10).

Metabolic acidosis is seldom a primary disorder; it usually develops during the course of another disease. The manifestations of metabolic acidosis frequently are superimposed on the symptoms of the contributing health problem. With diabetic ketoacidosis, which is a common cause of metabolic acidosis, there is an increase in blood and urine glucose and a characteristic smell of ketones to the breath.[67] In metabolic acidosis that accompanies chronic kidney disease, blood urea nitrogen levels are elevated and other tests of renal function yield abnormal results.

Manifestations related to respiratory and renal compensatory mechanisms usually occur early in the course of metabolic acidosis.[65,66] In situations of acute metabolic acidosis, the respiratory system compensates for a decrease in pH by increasing ventilation to reduce PCO_2; this is accomplished through deep and rapid respirations. There may be complaints of difficulty breathing or dyspnea with exertion; with severe acidosis, dyspnea may be present even at rest. Respiratory compensation for acute metabolic acidosis tends to be somewhat greater than for chronic acidosis. When kidney function is normal, H^+ excretion increases promptly in response to acidosis, and the urine becomes more acid.

TABLE 8-10 Manifestations of Metabolic Acidosis and Alkalosis	
Metabolic Acidosis	**Metabolic Alkalosis**
Laboratory Tests	**Laboratory Tests**
pH decreased	pH increased
Bicarbonate (primary) decreased	Bicarbonate (primary) increased
PCO_2 (compensatory) decreased	PCO_2 (compensatory) increased
Signs of Compensation	**Signs of Compensation**
Increased respirations (rate and depth)	Decreased respirations (rate and depth) with various degrees of hypoxia
Hyperkalemia	and respiratory acidosis
Acid urine	
Increased ammonia in urine	
Gastrointestinal Effects	
Anorexia	
Nausea and vomiting	
Abdominal pain	
Nervous System Effects	**Nervous System Effects**
Weakness	Hyperactive reflexes
Lethargy	Tetany
Confusion	Confusion
Stupor	Seizures
Coma	
Depression of vital functions	
Cardiovascular Effects	**Cardiovascular Effects**
Peripheral vasodilation	Hypotension
Decreased cardiac output	Cardiac arrhythmias
Cardiac arrhythmias	
Skin	
Warm and flushed	
Skeletal System Effects	
Bone disease (chronic acidosis)	

Changes in pH have a direct effect on body function that can produce signs and symptoms common to most types of metabolic acidosis. A person with metabolic acidosis often complains of weakness, fatigue, general malaise, and a dull headache. They also may have anorexia, nausea, vomiting, and abdominal pain. Tissue turgor is decreased, and the skin is dry when fluid deficit accompanies acidosis. In persons with undiagnosed diabetes mellitus, the nausea, vomiting, and abdominal symptoms may be misinterpreted as being caused by gastrointestinal flu or another abdominal disease, such as appendicitis. Acidosis depresses neuronal excitability and as the condition progresses, the level of consciousness declines, and stupor and coma develop. The skin is often warm and flushed because blood vessels in the skin become less responsive to sympathetic nervous system stimulation and lose their tone.

When the pH falls to 7.0 to 7.1, cardiac contractility and cardiac output decrease, the heart becomes less responsive to catecholamines (i.e., epinephrine and norepinephrine), and arrhythmias, including fatal ventricular arrhythmias, can develop. A decrease in ventricular function may be particularly important in perpetuating shock-induced lactic acidosis, and partial correction of the acidemia may be necessary before tissue perfusion can be restored.[1]

Chronic acidemia, as in chronic kidney disease, can lead to a variety of musculoskeletal problems, some of which result from the release of calcium and phosphate during bone buffering of excess H^+ ions. Of particular importance is impaired growth in children. In infants and children, acidemia may be associated with a variety of nonspecific symptoms such as anorexia, weight loss, muscle weakness, and listlessness.[1] Muscle weakness and listlessness may result from alterations in muscle metabolism.

Treatment. The treatment of metabolic acidosis focuses on correcting the condition that is causing the disorder and restoring the fluids and electrolytes that have been lost from the body. For example, insulin administration and fluid replacement are frequently sufficient to correct a low pH in persons with diabetic ketosis (see Chapter 33).

The use of supplemental sodium bicarbonate ($NaHCO_3$) may be indicated in the treatment of some forms of normal anion gap acidosis. However, its use in treatment of metabolic acidosis with an increased anion gap is controversial, particularly in cases of impaired tissue perfusion.[70] In most patients with circulatory shock, cardiac arrest, or sepsis, impaired oxygen delivery is the primary cause of lactic acidosis. In these situations, the administration of large amounts of $NaHCO_3$ does not improve oxygen delivery and may produce hypernatremia, hyperosmolality, and decreased oxygen release by hemoglobin because of a shift in the oxygen dissociation curve.[70]

Metabolic Alkalosis

Metabolic alkalosis is a systemic disorder caused by an increase in serum pH due to a primary excess in HCO_3^-.[71] It is reported to be the second most common acid–base disorder in hospitalized adults, accounting for about 32% of all acid–base disorders. The disorder can be caused by factors that generate a gain of bicarbonate, a loss of fixed acids, or those that maintain the alkalosis by interfering with excretion of the excess bicarbonate by the kidneys.

Excess Bicarbonate Base. Because the normal kidney is extremely efficient at excreting bicarbonate, excess base intake is rarely a cause of significant chronic metabolic alkalosis. Transient acute alkalosis, on the other hand, is a rather common occurrence during or immediately following excess oral ingestion of bicarbonate-containing antacids (e.g., Alka-Seltzer) or intravenous infusion of $NaHCO_3$ or base equivalent (e.g., acetate in hyperalimentation solutions, lactate in Ringer lactate, and citrate in blood transfusions). As noted earlier, the *milk-alkali syndrome* is a condition in which the chronic ingestion of milk and/or calcium carbonate antacids leads to hypercalcemia and metabolic alkalosis.[42] In this case, the antacids raise the serum HCO_3^- concentration, while the hypercalcemia prevents the urinary excretion of HCO_3^-. The most common cause at present is the administration of calcium carbonate as a phosphate binder to persons with chronic kidney disease.[4]

Loss of Fixed Acids. The loss of fixed acids occurs mainly through the loss of acid from the stomach and through the loss of chloride in the urine. Vomiting and removal of gastric secretions through the use of nasogastric suction are common causes of metabolic alkalosis in acutely ill or hospitalized patients. Bulimia nervosa with self-induced vomiting also is associated with metabolic alkalosis.[71] Gastric secretions contain high concentrations of HCl and lesser concentrations of potassium chloride. As Cl^- is taken from the blood and secreted into the stomach, it is replaced by HCO_3^-. Under normal conditions, each mEq of H^+ that is secreted into the stomach generates 1 mEq of serum HCO_3^-.[72] Thus, the loss of gastric secretions through vomiting or gastric suction is a common cause of metabolic alkalosis. The accompanying ECF volume depletion, hypochloremia, and hypokalemia serve to maintain the metabolic alkalosis by increasing HCO_3^- reabsorption by the kidneys (Fig. 8-19).

Other factors that predispose persons to the development of metabolic alkalosis include the loss of potassium, such as that caused by the loop and thiazide diuretics and the presence of excessive adrenal cortical hormones (as in hyperaldosteronism and Cushing disease). Hypokalemia contributes to metabolic alkalosis through renal mechanisms that conserve K^+ while increasing H^+ elimination and through a cellular shift of K^+ into the ECF, while at the same time H^+ moves back into the cell.

Metabolic alkalosis can also occur with abrupt correction of respiratory acidosis in persons with chronic respiratory acidosis. Chronic respiratory acidosis is associated with a compensatory loss of H^+ and Cl^- in the urine along with HCO_3^- retention. When respiratory acidosis is corrected abruptly, as with mechanical

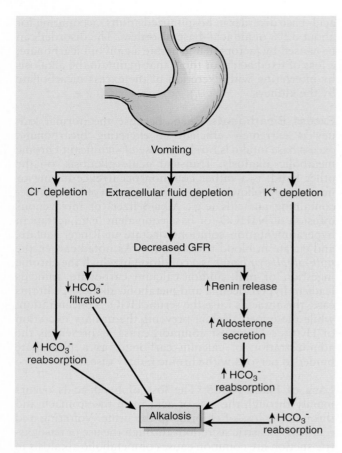

FIGURE 8-19. Renal mechanisms for bicarbonate (HCO₃⁻) reabsorption and maintenance of metabolic alkalosis following depletion of extracellular fluid volume, chloride (Cl⁻), and potassium (K⁺) due to vomiting. GFR, glomerular filtration rate.

ventilation, metabolic alkalosis may develop due to a rapid drop in PCO_2, while serum HCO_3^-, which must be eliminated through the kidney, remains elevated.

Maintenance of Metabolic Alkalosis. Maintenance of metabolic alkalosis resides within the kidney and its inability to rid the body of the excess HCO_3^-. Many of the conditions that accompany the development of metabolic alkalosis, such as contraction of the ECF volume, hypochloremia, and hypokalemia, also increase reabsorption of HCO_3^- by the kidney, thereby contributing to its maintenance.

Manifestations. Metabolic alkalosis is characterized by a serum pH above 7.45, serum HCO_3^- above 29 mEq/L (29 mmol/L), and base excess above 3.0 mEq/L (3 mmol/L). Persons with metabolic alkalosis often are asymptomatic or have signs related to ECF volume depletion or hypokalemia. The manifestations of metabolic alkalosis are summarized in Table 8-10.

Neurologic signs and symptoms (e.g., hyperexcitability) occur less frequently with metabolic alkalosis than with other acid–base disorders because HCO_3^- enters the cerebrospinal fluid (CSF) more slowly than CO_2. When neurologic manifestations do occur, as in acute

and severe metabolic alkalosis, they include mental confusion, hyperactive reflexes, tetany, and carpopedal spasm. Metabolic alkalosis also leads to a compensatory hypoventilation with development of various degrees of hypoxemia and respiratory acidosis. Significant morbidity occurs with severe metabolic alkalosis, including respiratory failure, arrhythmias, seizures, and coma.

Treatment. The treatment of metabolic alkalosis usually is directed toward correcting the cause of the condition. A chloride deficit requires correction. Potassium chloride usually is the treatment of choice when there is an accompanying potassium deficit. When potassium chloride is used as a therapy, the Cl⁻ anion replaces the HCO_3^- anion and the K⁺ corrects the potassium deficit, allowing the kidneys to retain H⁺ while eliminating K⁺. Fluid replacement is used in the treatment of volume contraction alkalosis.

Respiratory Acidosis

Respiratory acidosis represents a decrease in pH caused by an elevation in arterial PCO_2, usually due to conditions that impair alveolar ventilation. It can present as an acute or chronic condition, and can occur as the result of decreased ventilatory drive, lung disease, or disorders of the chest wall or respiratory muscles.[72,73] Less commonly, it results from excess CO_2 production.

Acute Disorders of Ventilation. Acute respiratory failure is associated with a rapid rise in arterial PCO_2 along with a minimal increase in serum HCO_3^- and a large decrease in pH. It can be caused by impaired function of the respiratory center in the medulla (as in narcotic overdose), lung disease, chest injury, weakness of the respiratory muscles, or airway obstruction. Almost all persons with acute respiratory acidosis become hypoxemic when breathing room air. In many cases, signs of hypoxemia develop prior to those of respiratory acidosis because CO_2 diffuses across the alveolar capillary membrane 20 times more rapidly than oxygen.[2,4]

Chronic Disorders of Ventilation. Chronic respiratory acidosis is characterized by a sustained increase in arterial PCO_2, resulting in renal adaptation with a more marked increase in serum HCO_3^- and a lesser decrease in pH.[72,73] It is a relatively common disturbance in persons with chronic obstructive pulmonary disease (COPD). In these persons, the persistent elevation of PCO_2 stimulates renal H⁺ secretion and HCO_3^- reabsorption. The effectiveness of these compensatory mechanisms can often return the pH to near-normal values as long as oxygen levels are maintained within a range that does not unduly suppress chemoreceptor control of respirations.

An acute episode of respiratory acidosis can develop in persons with chronic lung disease who receive oxygen therapy at a flow rate that raises their PO_2 to a level that produces a decrease in ventilation (see Chapter 23). In these persons, the medullary respiratory center has adapted to the elevated levels of CO_2 and no longer responds to increases in PCO_2. Instead, a decrease in the PO_2 becomes the major stimulus for respiration. If oxygen is administered at a flow rate that is sufficient to suppress this stimulus, the rate and depth of respiration decrease and PCO_2 increases. Thus, any person who is in need of additional oxygen should have it administered, but at a flow rate that does not depress the respiratory drive.

Increased Carbon Dioxide Production. Carbon dioxide is a product of the body's metabolic processes, generating a substantial amount of acid that must be excreted by the lungs or kidney to prevent acidosis. An increase in CO_2 production can result from numerous processes, including exercise, fever, sepsis, and burns. For example, CO_2 production increases by approximately 13% for each 1°C rise in temperature above normal.[72] Nutrition also affects the production of CO_2. A carbohydrate-rich diet produces larger amounts of CO_2 than one containing reasonable amounts of protein and fat. In healthy persons, the increase in CO_2 is usually matched by an increase in CO_2 elimination by the lungs, whereas persons with respiratory diseases may be unable to eliminate the excess CO_2.

Manifestations. Respiratory acidosis is associated with a serum pH below 7.35 and an arterial PCO_2 above 50 mm Hg. The signs and symptoms of respiratory acidosis depend on the rapidity of onset and whether the condition is acute or chronic (Table 8-11). Less severe forms of acidosis often are accompanied by warm and flushed skin, weakness, and tachycardia. Because respiratory acidosis often is accompanied by hypoxemia, the manifestations of respiratory acidosis often are intermixed with those of oxygen deficit. Carbon dioxide readily crosses the blood–brain barrier, exerting its effects by changing the pH of brain fluids. Elevated levels of CO_2 produce vasodilation of cerebral blood vessels, causing headache, blurred vision, irritability, muscle twitching, and psychological disturbances. If severe and prolonged, it can cause an increase in CSF pressure and papilledema. Impaired consciousness, ranging from lethargy to coma, develops as the PCO_2 rises to extreme levels. Paralysis of extremities may occur, and there may be respiratory depression.

Treatment. The treatment of acute and chronic respiratory acidosis is directed toward improving ventilation. In severe cases, mechanical ventilation may be necessary. The treatment of respiratory acidosis due to respiratory failure is discussed in Chapter 23.

Respiratory Alkalosis

Respiratory alkalosis is a systemic acid–base disorder characterized by a primary decrease in arterial PCO_2, which produces an elevation in pH and a subsequent decrease in HCO_3^-.[72] It is caused by hyperventilation or a respiratory rate in excess of that needed to maintain normal PCO_2 levels. It may occur as the result of central stimulation of the medullary respiratory center or stimulation of peripheral (e.g., carotid chemoreceptor) pathways to the medullary respiratory center. Because respiratory alkalosis can occur suddenly, a compensatory decrease in bicarbonate level may not occur before respiratory correction has already taken place.

Central stimulation of the medullary respiratory center occurs with anxiety, pain, pregnancy, febrile states, sepsis, encephalitis, and salicylate toxicity. One of the most common causes of respiratory alkalosis is

TABLE 8-11	Manifestations of Respiratory Acidosis and Alkalosis
Respiratory Acidosis	**Respiratory Alkalosis**
Laboratory Tests	*Laboratory Tests*
pH decreased	pH increased
PCO_2 (primary) increased	PCO_2 (primary) decreased
Bicarbonate (compensatory) increased	Bicarbonate (compensatory) decreased
Signs of Compensation	*Signs of Compensation*
Acid urine	Alkaline urine
Nervous System Effects	**Nervous System Effects**
Dilation of cerebral vessels and decreased neuronal activity	Constriction of cerebral vessels and increased neuronal activity
Headache	Dizziness, panic, light-headedness
Behavioral changes	Tetany
Confusion	Numbness and tingling of fingers and toes
Depression	Seizures (severe respiratory alkalosis)
Paranoia	
Hallucinations	
Weakness	
Tremors	
Paralysis	
Stupor and coma	
Skin	*Cardiovascular Effects*
Warm and flushed	Cardiac arrhythmias

hyperventilation syndrome, which is characterized by recurring episodes of overbreathing often associated with anxiety. Persons experiencing panic attacks frequently present in the emergency room with manifestations of acute respiratory alkalosis. Progesterone increases ventilation in women; during the progesterone phase of the menstrual cycle, normal women decrease their PCO_2 values by 2 to 4 mm Hg and increase their pH by 0.01 to 0.02.[74] Women can also develop substantial decrease in PCO_2 during pregnancy, most notably during the last trimester.[72]

Respiratory alkalosis has long been recognized as a common acid–base disorder in critically ill patients, and is a consistent finding in both septic shock and the systemic inflammatory response syndrome (see Chapter 20). Hypoxemia exerts its effect on pH through the peripheral chemoreceptors in the carotid bodies. Stimulation of peripheral chemoreceptors occurs in conditions that cause hypoxemia with relatively unimpaired CO_2 transport such as exposure to high altitudes.

Mechanical ventilation may produce respiratory alkalosis if the rate and tidal volume are set so that CO_2 elimination exceeds CO_2 production. Because carbon dioxide crosses the alveolar capillary membrane 20 times more rapidly than oxygen, the increased minute ventilation may be necessary to maintain adequate oxygen levels while producing a concomitant decrease in CO_2 levels. In some cases, respiratory alkalosis may be induced through mechanical ventilation as a means of controlling disorders such as severe intracranial hypertension.

Manifestations. Respiratory alkalosis manifests with a decrease in PCO_2 and a H_2CO_3 deficit. The pH is above 7.45, arterial PCO_2 is below 35 mm Hg, and serum HCO_3^- levels usually are below 24 mEq/L (24 mmol/L).

The signs and symptoms of respiratory alkalosis are associated with hyperexcitability of the nervous system and a decrease in cerebral blood flow[75] (see Table 8-11). A decrease in the CO_2 content of the blood causes constriction of cerebral blood vessels. CO_2 crosses the blood–brain barrier rather quickly; thus, the manifestations of acute respiratory alkalosis are usually of sudden onset. The person often experiences light-headedness, dizziness, tingling, and numbness of the fingers and toes. These manifestations may be accompanied by sweating, palpitations, panic, air hunger, and dyspnea. Chvostek and Trousseau signs may be positive, and tetany and convulsions may occur. Because CO_2 provides the stimulus for short-term regulation of respiration, short periods of apnea may occur in persons with acute episodes of hyperventilation.

Treatment. The treatment of respiratory alkalosis focuses on measures to correct the underlying cause. Hypoxia may be corrected by administration of supplemental oxygen. Changing ventilator settings may be used to prevent or treat respiratory alkalosis in persons who are being mechanically ventilated. Persons with hyperventilation syndrome may benefit from reassurance, rebreathing from a paper bag during symptomatic attacks, and attention to the psychological stress associated with the disorder.

SUMMARY CONCEPTS

- Normal body function depends on the precise regulation of acid–base balance. Metabolic processes produce the volatile carbonic acid (H_2CO_3) in equilibrium with dissolved carbon dioxide (PCO_2), which is eliminated through the lungs, and nonvolatile acids, which are excreted by the kidneys.

- Because of its low concentration in body fluids, the hydrogen (H^+) concentration is expressed as *pH*, or the negative log of the H^+ ion concentration. It is the ratio of the bicarbonate (HCO_3^-) concentration to H_2CO_3 (PCO_2), normally 20:1, that determines body pH.

- The ability of the body to maintain pH within the normal range depends on intracellular and extracellular buffers, as well as respiratory and renal compensatory mechanisms. The respiratory regulation of pH, which relies on pulmonary ventilation for release of CO_2 into the environment, is rapid but does not return the pH completely to normal. Renal mechanisms, which rely on the elimination of H^+ ions and conservation of HCO_3^- ions, take longer but return pH to normal or near-normal levels.

- Metabolic acid and base disorders reflect an decrease or increase in HCO_3^-. *Metabolic acidosis,* which reflects a decrease in pH due to a decrease in HCO_3^-, is caused by conditions that prompt an excessive production and accumulation of metabolic acids or excessive loss of HCO_3^-. *Metabolic alkalosis,* which reflects an increase in pH due to an increase in HCO_3^-, is caused by conditions that produce a gain in HCO_3^- or a decrease in H^+.

- Respiratory acid–base disorders reflect an increase or decrease in PCO_2 levels due to altered pulmonary ventilation. *Respiratory acidosis,* which reflects a decrease in pH due an increase in PCO_2 levels, is caused by conditions that produce hypoventilation. *Respiratory alkalosis,* which reflects an increase in pH due to a decrease in PCO_2 levels, is caused by conditions that produce hyperventilation.

REVIEW EXERCISES

1. A 40-year-old man with advanced acquired immunodeficiency syndrome (AIDS) presents with an acute chest infection. Investigations confirm a diagnosis of *Pneumocystis carinii* pneumonia. Although he is being treated appropriately, his serum sodium level is 118 mEq/L. Tests of adrenal function are normal.

   A. What is the likely cause of his electrolyte disturbance?
   B. What are the five cardinal features of this condition?

2. A 70-year-old woman who is taking furosemide (a loop diuretic) for congestive heart failure complains of weakness, fatigue, and cramping of the muscles in her legs. Her serum potassium is 2.0 mEq/L and her serum sodium is 140 mEq/L. She also complains that she notices a "strange heartbeat" at times.

   A. What is the likely cause of this woman's symptoms?
   B. An ECG shows a depressed ST segment and low T-wave changes. Explain the physiologic mechanism underlying these changes.
   C. What would be the treatment for this woman?

3. A 50-year-old woman presents with symptomatic hypercalcemia. She has a recent history of breast cancer treatment.

   A. How do you evaluate this person with increased serum calcium levels?
   B. What is the significance of the recent history of malignancy?
   C. What further tests may be indicated?

4. A 34-year-old woman with diabetes is admitted to the emergency room in a stuporous state. Her skin is flushed and warm, her breath has a sweet odor, her pulse is rapid and weak, and her respirations are rapid and deep. Her initial laboratory tests indicate a blood sugar of 320 mg/dL, serum HCO_3^- of 12 mEq/L (normal, 24 to 27 mEq/L), and a pH of 7.1 (normal, 7.35 to 7.45).

   A. What is the most likely cause of her lowered pH and bicarbonate levels?
   B. How would you account for her rapid and deep respirations?
   C. How would you explain her warm, flushed skin and stuporous mental state?

5. A 16-year-old girl is seen by her primary care provider because her parents are concerned about her binge eating and their recent discovery that she engages in self-induced vomiting. Initial laboratory tests reveal a serum K^+ of 3.0 mEq/L and Cl^- of 93.

   A. Explain her low K^+ and Cl^-.
   B. What type of acid–base abnormality would you expect her to have?

6. A 65-year-old man with chronic obstructive lung disease has been using low-flow oxygen therapy. He has recently developed a severe respiratory tract infection and has trouble breathing. He is admitted to the emergency room because his wife is having trouble arousing him. She relates that he had "turned his oxygen way up" because of difficulty breathing. His respirations are 12 breaths/minute. Arterial blood gases, drawn on admission to the emergency room, indicated a PO_2 of 85 mm Hg (normal, 90 to 95 mmHg) and a PCO_2 of 90 mm Hg (normal, 40 mm Hg). His serum HCO_3^- was 34 mEq/L (normal, 24 to 48 mEq/L). What is his pH?

   A. What is the most likely cause of this man's problem?
   B. How would you explain the lethargy and difficulty in arousal?
   C. What would be the main goal of treatment for this man in terms of acid–base balance?
   D. Explain the concurrent respiratory and metabolic acidosis that often occurs in persons with chronic respiratory acidosis.

REFERENCES

1. Rhoades RA, Bell DR. *Medical Physiology*. 4th ed. Philadelphia, PA: Wolter Kluwer Health | Lippincott Williams & Wilkins; 2013:20–33, 427–470, 282–287, 451–470.
2. Hall JE. *Guyton and Hall Textbook of Medical Physiology*. 12th ed. Philadelphia, PA: Saunders Elsevier; 2011:285–301, 177–189, 870–871, 355–360, 379–396, 955–967.
3. Metheney NM. *Fluid and Electrolyte Balance*. 5th ed. Sudbury, MA: Jones & Bartlett; 2012:3–12, 41–44, 45–67, 69–90, 91–109, 112–122, 123–126, 137–153.
4. Rose BD, Post TW. *Clinical Physiology of Acid–base and Electrolyte Disorders*. 5th ed. New York: McGraw-Hill; 2001:187–190, 478–479, 547, 682–692, 823–842, 896–897.
5. Demling RH. The burn edema process: Current concepts. *J Burn Care Rehabil*. 2005;26:207–227.
6. O'Brien JG, Chennubhotla RV. Treatment of edema. *Am Fam Physician*. 2005;71(11):2111–2117.
7. Koeppen BM, Stanton BA. *Berne & Levy Physiology*. 6th ed. Philadelphia, PA: Mosby Elsevier; 2010:346–353, 594–663, 699–705, 636–650.
8. Porth CM, Erickson M. Physiology of thirst and drinking. *Heart Lung*. 1992;21:273–284.
9. McKinley MJ, Johnson AK. The physiological regulation of thirst and fluid intake. *News Physiol Sci*. 2004;19:1–6.
10. Hodak SP, Verbalis JO. Abnormalities in water homeostasis in aging. *Endocrinol Metab Clin North Am*. 2005;34:1031–1046.
11. Dundas B, Harris M, Narasimhan M. Psychogenic polydipsia. *Curr Psychiatry Rep*. 2007;9(3):236–241.
12. Siegel AJ. Hyponatremia in psychiatric patients: Update on evaluation and management. *Harv Rev Psychiatry*. 2008;16(1):13–24.

13. Makaryus AN, McFarlane SI. Diabetes insipidus: Diagnosis and treatment of a complex disease. *Cleve Clin J Med.* 2006;73(1):65–71.

14. Ditorgi N, Napoli F, Allegri AEM. Diabetes insidus—diagnosis and management. *Horm Res Paediatr.* 2012;77:69–84.

15. Sands JM, Bichet DG. Nephrogenic diabetes insipidus. *Ann Intern Med.* 2006;144:186–194.

16. Behan LA, Phillips J, Thompson LT, et al. Neuroendocrine disorders after traumatic brain injury. *J Neurol Neurosurg Psychiatry.* 2008;79:753–759.

17. Alexander MP, Farag YM, Mattal BV, et al. Lithium toxicity: a double-edged sword. *Kidney Int.* 2008;73(2):233–237.

18. Robertson GL. Regulation of arginine vasopressin in the syndrome of inappropriate antidiuresis. *Am J Med.* 2006;119:S36–S42.

19. Hannon MJ, Thompson CJ. The syndrome of inappropriate antidiuretic hormone: prevalence, causes, and consequences. *Eur J Endocrinol.* 2010;162:S5–S12.

20. Sherlock M, Thompson CJ. The syndrome of inappropriate antidiuretic hormone: current and future management option. *Eur J Endocrinol.* 2010;162:S13–S18.

21. Adrogue HJ, Madias NE. Hyponatremia. *N Engl J Med.* 2000;343:1581–1589.

22. Adrogue HJ, Madias NE. The challenge of hyponatremia. *J Am Society Nephrol.* 2012;23:1140–1148.

23. Vaidya C, Warren H, Freda BJ. Management of hyponatremia: Providing treatment and avoiding harm. *Cleve Clin J Med.* 2010;27(10):715–726.

24. Mount DB. The brain in hyonatremia: both culprit and victim. *Semin Nephrol.* 2009;29(3):196–215.

25. Murase T, Sugimura Y, Takefuji S, et al. Mechanisms and therapy of osmotic demyelination. *Am J Med.* 2006;119(7A):S69–S73.

26. Adrogue HJ, Madias NE. Hypernatremia. *N Engl J Med.* 2000;342:1493–1499.

27. Sam R, Feizi I. Understanding hypernatremia. *Am J Nephrol.* 2012;36:97–104.

28. Al-Absi A, Gosmanova EO, Wall BM. The clinical approach to chronic hypernatremia. *Am J Kidney Dis.* 2012;60(6):1032–1038.

29. Rao MC. Oral rehydration therapy. *Annl Rev Physiol.* 2004;66:385–417.

30. Palmer BF, Dubose TD. Disorders of potassium metabolism. In: Scheir RW, ed. *Renal and Electrolyte Disorders.* 7th ed. Philadelphia, PA: Wolters Kluwer Health | Lippincott Williams & Wilkins; 2010:137–165.

31. Schaefer T, Wolford RW. Disorders of potassium. *Emerg Med Clin North Am.* 2005;23:723–747.

32. Palmer BF. A physiologic-based approach to the evaluation of a patient with hypokalemia. *Am J Kidney Dis.* 2010;56:1184–1190.

33. Pepin J, Shields C. Advances in diagnosis and management of hypokalemic and hyperkalemic emergencies. *Emerg Med Pract.* 2012;14(2):1–18.

34. Lehnhardt A, Kemper MJ. Pathogenesis, diagnosis and management of hyperkalemia. *Pediatr Nephrol.* 2011;26:377–384.

35. Moe SM. Disorders involving calcium, phosphorus, and magnesium. *Prim Care.* 2008;35(2):215–237.

36. Popovtzer MM. Disorders of calcium, phosphorus, vitamin D, and parathyroid hormone activity. In: Schrier RW, ed. *Renal and Electrolyte Disorders.* 7th ed. Philadelphia, PA: Wolters Kluwer Health | Lippincott Williams & Wilkins; 2010:166–228.

37. Peacock M. Calcium metabolism in health and disease. *Clin J Am Soc Nephrol.* 2010;5:S23–S30.

38. Fong J, Khan A. Hypocalcemia. *Can Fam Physician.* 2012;58:158–162.

39. Liamis G, Millionis H, Elisaf M. A review of drug-induced hypocalcemia. *J Bone Miner Metab.* 2009;27:635–642.

40. Assadi F. Hypercalcemia: an evidence-based approach to clinical cases. *Iran J Kidney Dis.* 2009;3(2):71–79.

41. Stewart AF. Hypercalcemia associated with cancer. *N Engl J Med.* 2005;353(4):373–379.

42. Medaroov BL. Milk-alkali syndrome. *Mayo Clin Proc.* 2009;84(8): 261–267.

43. Ziegler R. Hypercalcemia crisis. *J Am Soc Nephrol.* 2001;12: S3–S9.

44. Leaf DE, Wolf M. A physiologic-based approach to evaluation of a patient with hyperphosphatemia. *Am J Kidney Dis.* 2013;61(2):330–336.

45. Felsenfeld AJ, Levine BS. Approach to treatment of hypophosphatemia. *Am J Kidney Dis.* 2012;60(4):655–661.

46. Hruska KA, Mathew S, Lund R, et al. Hyperphosphatemia of chronic kidney disease. *Kidney Int.* 2008;74(2):148–157.

47. Hsu HJ, Wu MS. Extreme hyperphosphaemia and hypocalcemic coma associated with phosphate enema. *Intern Med.* 2008;47(7):643–648.

48. Musso CG. Magnesium metabolism in health and disease. *Int Urol Nephrol.* 2009;41:357–362.

49. Guerrera ME, Volpe S, Mao JJ. Therapeutic uses of magnesium. *Am Fam Physician.* 2009;80(2):157–162.

50. Speigel DM. Normal and abnormal magnesium metabolism. In: Schrier RW, ed. *Renal and Electrolyte Disorders.* 7th ed. Philadelphia, PA: Wolters Kluwer Health | Lippincott Williams & Wilkins; 2010:229–250.

51. Gums JG. Magnesium in cardiovascular and other disorders. *Am J Health Syst Pharm.* 2004;61:1569–1576.

52. Fogleman CD. Magnesium sulfate and other anticonvulsants for women with preeclampsia. *Am Fam Physician.* 2011;83(11):1269–1271.

53. Topf JM, Murray PT. Hypomagnesemia and hypermagnesemia. *Rev Endocr Metab Disord.* 2003;4:195–206.

54. Martin KJ, Gonzalez EA, Slatopolsky E. Clincial consequences and management of hypomagnesemia. *J Am Soc Nephrol.* 2009;20:2291–2295.

55. Hoom EJ, van der Hoek J, de Mart RA, et al. A series of proton pump inhibitor-induced hypomagnesemia. *Am J Kidney Dis.* 2010;56(1):112–116.

56. Shoback D. Primary hypoparathyroidism. *N Engl J Med.* 2008;359(4):391–403.

57. Bilezikian JP, Khan A, Potts JT Jr, et al. Hypoparathyroidism in the adult: Epidemiology, diagnosis, pathophysiology, target organ involvement, treatment, and challenges for the future. *J Bone Mineral Res.* 2011;26(10):2317–2337.

58. Mark SJ. Hypoparathyroid and hyperparathyroid disorders. *N Engl J Med.* 2000;343(25):1863–1875.

59. Taniegra ED. Hyperparathyroidism. *Am Family Physician.* 2004;69:333–339.

60. Ahmad R, Hammond JM. Primary, secondary, and tertiary hyperparathyroidism. *Otolaryngol Clin North Am.* 2004;17:703–713.

61. Marcocci C., Cetani F. Hyperparathyroidism. *N Engl J Med.* 2011;365(25):2389–2397.

62. Adrogue HE, Adrogue HJ. Acid–base physiology. *Respir Care.* 2001;46:328–341.

63. Koeppen BM. The kidney and acid–base balance. *Adv Physiol Educ.* 2009;33:275–281.

64. Whittier WL, Rutecki GW. Primer on clinical acid–base problem solving. *Dis Mon.* 2004;50:117–162.

65. Ralman S, Kaehny W, Shapiro JI. Pathogenesis of metabolic acidosis and alkalosis. In: Schrier RW, ed. *Renal and Electrolyte Disorders.* 7th ed. Philadelphia, PA: Wolters Kluwer Health | Lippincott Williams & Wilkins; 2010:86–121.

66. Kraut JA, Madas NE. Metabolic acidosis: Pathology, diagnosis, and management. *Nat Rev Nephrol.* 2010;6:274–285.

67. Trachtenbarg DE. Diabetic ketoacidosis. *Am Fam Physician.* 2005;71(9):1705–1714.

68. Toth HI, Greenbaum LA. Severe acidosis caused by starvation and stress. *Am J Kidney Dis.* 2003;42:E16–E19.

69. Soriano JR. Renal tubular acidosis. *J Am Soc Nephrol.* 2002;13:2160–2170.

70. Forsythe SM, Schmidt GA. Sodium bicarbonate for the treatment of lactic acidosis. *Chest.* 2000;117:260–267.

71. Galla JH. Metabolic alkalosis. *J Am Soc Nephrol.* 2000;11:369–375.

72. Kaehny WD. Pathogenesis and management of respiratory and mixed acid–base disorders. In: Schrier RW, ed. *Renal and Electrolyte Disorders.* 7th ed. Philadelphia, PA: Wolters Kluwer Health | Lippincott Williams & Wilkins; 2010:122–136.

73. Epstein SK, Singh N. Respiratory acidosis. *Resp Care.* 2001;46(4):366–383.

74. Laffey JH, Kavenaugh BP. Hypocapnia. *N Engl J Med.* 2002;347:43–53.

75. Palmer BF. Evaluation and treatment of respiratory alkalosis. *Am J Kidney Dis.* 2012;60(5):634–638.

Porth Essentials Resources

Explore these additional resources to enhance learning for this chapter:

- NCLEX-Style Questions and Other Resources on **the**Point, http://thePoint.lww.com/PorthEssentials4e
- Study Guide for Essentials of Pathophysiology
- Clinical Simulation Case Study
- Concepts in Action Animations
- Adaptive Learning | Powered by PrepU, http://thepoint.lww.com/prepu

Chapter 9

Stress and Adaptation

Stress, adaptation, and their relationship to health are a frequent topic of discussion. The human body and mind respond to stress by activating a complex repertoire of physiologic and behavioral adaptive responses which, if inadequate or excessive, may affect emotional behavior and have adverse effects on physiologic functioning. Stress may contribute directly to the production or exacerbation of a disease, or it may contribute to the development of behaviors such as smoking, overeating, and drug abuse that increase risk of disease.

The content in this chapter has been organized into two sections: the first focuses on stress and adaptation and the second on disorders of the stress response.

Stress and Adaptation

A variety of definitions have been ascribed to the phenomenon of stress. The concept of stress has been studied extensively by physiologists, psychologists, sociologists, and members of the health care professions. The nature of these disciplines and the individual work of their members have led to rather disparate bodies of knowledge about stress. Despite these disparities, the concept of stress is commonly viewed within the context of three major components: homeostasis, the stress response, and adaptation to stress.

Homeostasis

The concepts of stress and adaptation have their origin in the complexity of the human body and interactions between the body's cells and its many organ systems. These interactions require that a level of homeostasis or constancy be maintained during the many changes that occur in the internal and external environments. In effecting a state of constancy, homeostasis requires feedback control systems that regulate cellular function and integrate functions of the different body systems.

Constancy of the Internal Environment

The environment in which body cells live is not the external environment that surrounds the organism, but rather the local fluid environment that surrounds each cell. Claude Bernard, a 19th-century physiologist, was the first to clearly describe the central importance of a stable internal environment, which he termed the *milieu intérieur*.[1] Bernard recognized that body fluids surrounding cells and various organ systems provide a means for exchange between the external and internal environments. It is from this internal environment that body cells receive their nourishment, and it is into this fluid that they secrete their wastes. Even contents of the gastrointestinal tract and lungs do not become part of the internal environment until they have been absorbed into the extracellular fluid. A multicellular organism is able to survive only as long as the composition of the internal environment is compatible with the survival needs of the individual cells. For example, even a small change in the pH of body fluids can disrupt metabolic processes of individual cells.

The concept of a stable internal environment was supported by Walter B. Cannon, who proposed that this kind of stability, which he called *homeostasis,* was achieved through a system of carefully coordinated physiologic processes that oppose change.[2] Cannon proposed that these processes were largely automatic and emphasized that homeostasis involves resistance to both internal and external disturbances (Box 9-1).

In his book *The Wisdom of the Body,* published in 1939, Cannon presented four tentative propositions to describe general features of homeostasis.[2] Based upon this set of propositions, Cannon emphasized that when a factor is known to shift homeostasis in one direction, it is reasonable to expect mechanisms that have the opposite effect exist. For example, in the homeostatic regulation of

blood sugar, mechanisms that both raise and lower blood glucose play significant roles. As long as the responding mechanism to the initiating disturbance can recover homeostasis, body integrity and normality are retained.

Control Systems

The ability of the body to function and maintain homeostasis under conditions of change in the internal and external environment depends upon thousands of physiologic *control systems* that regulate body function. A homeostatic control system consists of a collection of interconnected components that function to keep a physical or chemical parameter of the body relatively constant. The body's control systems regulate cellular function, control life processes, and integrate functions of different organ systems.

Neuroendocrine control systems that influence behavior have recently been studied extensively. Biochemical messengers in our brain control nerve activity, information flow, and, ultimately, behavior.[3–5] These control systems mediate physical, emotional, and behavioral reactions to stressors. When taken together, these reactions are known as the *stress response.*

Most control systems in the body operate by *negative feedback mechanisms,* which function in a manner similar to the thermostat in a heating system. When the monitored function or value decreases below the set point of the system, feedback mechanisms cause the function or value to increase, and when the function or value is increased above the set point, the feedback mechanism causes it to decrease (Fig. 9-1). For example, in the negative feedback mechanism that controls blood glucose levels, an increase in blood glucose stimulates an increase in insulin, which enhances removal of glucose from the blood. When glucose has been taken up by cells and blood glucose levels fall, insulin secretion is inhibited and glucagon and other counter-regulatory mechanisms stimulate release of glucose from the liver, which causes blood glucose levels to return to normal.

Most physiologic control systems function under negative rather than *positive feedback mechanisms* because

---

BOX 9-1   Constancy of the Internal Environment

1. Constancy in an open system, such as our bodies represent, requires mechanisms that act to maintain this constancy. Cannon based this proposition on insights into the ways by which steady states such as glucose concentrations, body temperature, and acid-base balance were regulated.

2. Steady-state conditions require that any tendency toward change automatically meets with factors that resist change. An increase in blood sugar results in thirst as the body attempts to dilute the concentration of sugar in the extracellular fluid.

3. The regulating system that determines the homeostatic state consists of a number of cooperating mechanisms acting simultaneously or successively. Blood sugar is regulated by insulin, glucagon, and other hormones that control its release from the liver or its uptake by the tissues.

4. Homeostasis does not occur by chance, but is the result of organized self-government.

From THE WISDOM OF THE BODY, Revised Edition by Walter B. Cannon, M. D. Copyright 1932, 1939 by Walter B. Cannon, renewed © 1960, 1967, 1968 by Cornelia J. Cannon. Used by permission of W. W. Norton & Company, Inc.

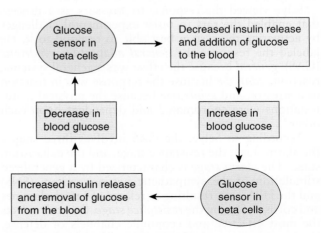

FIGURE 9-1. Illustration of negative feedback control mechanisms using blood glucose as an example.

a positive feedback mechanism interjects instability into a system, not stability. It produces a cycle in which the initiating stimulus produces more of the same response. For example, in a positive feedback system, exposure to an increase in environmental temperature would invoke compensatory mechanisms designed to increase body temperature rather than to decrease it.

The Stress Response

In the early 1930s, world-renowned endocrinologist Hans Selye was the first to describe a group of specific anatomic changes that occurred in rats that were exposed to a variety of different experimental stimuli.[6] He came to an understanding that these changes were manifestations of the body's attempt to adapt to stimuli. Selye described *stress* as "a state manifested by a specific syndrome of the body developed in response to any stimuli that made an intense systemic demand on it."[7] As a young medical student, Selye noticed that patients with diverse disease conditions had many signs and symptoms in common. He observed that "whether a man suffers from a loss of blood, an infectious disease, or advanced cancer, he loses his appetite, his muscular strength, and his ambition to accomplish anything; usually the patient also loses weight and even his facial expression betrays that he is ill."[8] Selye referred to this phenomenon as the "syndrome of just being sick."

In his early career as an experimental scientist, Selye noted that a triad of adrenal enlargement, thymic atrophy, and gastric ulcers appeared in rats he was using in his studies. These same three changes developed in response to many different or nonspecific experimental challenges. He assumed that the hypothalamic-pituitary-adrenal (HPA) axis played a pivotal role in development of this response. The primary effectors of the stress response are contained in the paraventricular nucleus of the hypothalamus, the anterior lobe of the pituitary gland, and the adrenal gland, making up the HPA axis.[9] In addition to the HPA axis, the brain stem noradrenergic neurons, sympathetic adrenomedullary circuits, and parasympathetic systems also play important roles in the regulation of adaptive responses to stress.[10]

Selye viewed the response to stressors as a process that enabled the rats to resist experimental challenges by activating the system best able to respond to it. He labeled the response the *general adaptation syndrome* (GAS): *general* because the effect was a general systemic reaction, *adaptive* because the response was in reaction to a stressor, and *syndrome* because the physical manifestations were coordinated and dependent upon each other.[7]

According to Selye, the GAS involves three stages: the alarm stage, the resistance stage, and the exhaustion stage. The *alarm stage* is characterized by a generalized stimulation of the sympathetic nervous system (SNS) and the HPA axis, resulting in release of catecholamines and cortisol. During the *resistance stage,* the body selects the most effective and economic channels of defense. During this stage, the increased cortisol levels present during the first-stage drop because they are no longer

needed. If the stressor is prolonged or overwhelms the ability of the body to defend itself, the *exhaustion stage* ensues, resulting in depletion of resources and emergence of signs of "wear and tear" or systemic damage.[11] Selye contended that many ailments, such as various emotional disturbances, mildly annoying headaches, insomnia, upset stomach, gastric and duodenal ulcers, certain types of rheumatic disorders, and cardiovascular and kidney diseases, appear to be initiated or encouraged by the "body itself because of its faulty adaptive reactions to potentially injurious agents."[8]

The events or environmental agents responsible for initiating the stress response were called *stressors.* According to Selye, stressors may be endogenous, arising from within the body, or exogenous, arising from outside the body.[8] In explaining the stress response, Selye proposed that two factors determine the nature of the stress response: properties of the stressor and conditioning of the person being stressed. Selye indicated that not all stress is detrimental; hence, he coined the terms *eustress* and *distress*.[11] He suggested that mild, brief, and controllable periods of stress may be perceived as positive stimuli to emotional and intellectual growth and development. Severe, protracted, and uncontrolled situations of psychological and physical distress are disruptive to health.[8] For example, the joy of becoming a new parent and the sorrow of losing a parent are completely different experiences, yet the effect of these stressors, the nonspecific demand for adjustment to a new situation, may be similar.

The brain appears central to development of the stress response, as it determines what is threatening and therefore potentially stressful.[12] Further, the brain elicits physiological and behavioral responses that can be either adaptive or harmful. It is becoming increasingly clear that the physiologic stress response is far more complicated than can be explained fully by classic stimulus–response mechanisms. These different responses occur in different persons, or in the same person at different times, indicating the influence of the adaptive capacity of the person, or what Selye called *conditioning factors.* These conditioning factors may be internal (e.g., genetic predisposition, age, gender) or external (e.g., exposure to environmental agents, life experiences, dietary factors, level of social support).[8] The relative risk for development of a stress-related pathologic process seems, at least in part, to depend on these factors.

Richard Lazarus was a well-respected psychologist who devoted his career to the study of stress and emotions. He considered "meanings and values to be at the center of human life and to represent the essence of stress, emotion, and adaptation."[13] Others described a "cognitive activation theory of stress" based on the belief that the stress response is dependent upon what a person expects to happen in a given situation based on previous learning experiences.[14] In other words, stimuli are filtered or evaluated before they reach a response system. Furthermore, there is evidence that the HPA axis, the adrenomedullary hormonal system, and the SNS are differentially activated depending on the type and intensity of the stressor.[15]

Neuroendocrine Responses

The stress response is mediated by anatomical structures found in both the central nervous system and peripheral tissues. Manifestations of the stress response are strongly influenced by both the nervous and endocrine systems.[9,16,17] The neuroendocrine systems integrate signals received along neurosensory pathways and from circulating mediators that are carried in the bloodstream. In addition, the immune system both affects and is affected by the stress response. Table 9-1 summarizes the action of hormones involved in the neuroendocrine responses to stress. Results of the coordinated release of these neurohormones include mobilization of energy, a sharpened focus and awareness, increased cerebral blood flow and glucose utilization, enhanced cardiovascular and respiratory functioning, redistribution of blood flow to the brain and muscles, modulation of the immune response, inhibition of reproductive function, and a decrease in appetite.[16,17]

The stress response is a normal, coordinated physiologic system intended to increase the probability of survival, but importantly, it also is designed to be an acute response. That is, optimally it is turned on when necessary to bring the body back to a stable state and turned off when the challenge to homeostasis abates. Therefore, under normal circumstances, the neural responses and hormones that are released during the response do not persist long enough to cause damage to vital tissues. Since the early 1980s, the term *allostasis* has been used by some investigators to describe the interactive physiologic changes in the neuroendocrine, autonomic, and immune systems that occur in response to either real or perceived challenges to homeostasis. More recently, others have proposed that allostasis is the body's attempt to maintain stability through change, thereby adequately or inadequately adapting to threatening or unpredictable stimuli.[18] The persistence or accumulation of these allostatic changes (e.g., immunosuppression, activation of the sympathetic nervous and renin-angiotensin-aldosterone systems) has been called an *allostatic load,* and this concept has been used to measure the cumulative effects of stress on humans.[16–21] Allostatic load can result in weakening a person's ability to respond to repeated stressors, and it may provide insight into how one might respond to future stressors. A number of indices have been suggested for measuring allostatic load, including blood pressure, cortisol, C-reactive protein, body mass index (BMI), and cholesterol.[22]

Integration of the components of the stress response, occurring at the level of the central nervous system (CNS), is complex and not completely understood.[23,24] It relies on communication along neuronal pathways of the cerebral cortex, limbic system, thalamus, hypothalamus, pituitary gland, and reticular activating system (RAS). The cerebral cortex is involved in vigilance, cognition, and focused attention, while the limbic system is associated with emotional components (e.g., fear, excitement, rage, anger) of the stress response (Fig. 9-2). The thalamus functions as the relay center and is important in receiving, sorting out, and distributing sensory input. The hypothalamus coordinates responses of the endocrine system and autonomic nervous system (ANS). The RAS modulates mental alertness, ANS activity, and skeletal muscle tone using input from other neural structures. The musculoskeletal tension that occurs during the stress response reflects increased activity of the RAS and its influence on reflex circuits that control muscle tone. Adding to the complexity of this system is the fact that individual brain circuits that participate in mediation of the stress response interact and regulate each other's activities. For example, reciprocal connections

---

TABLE 9-1   Hormones Involved in the Neuroendocrine Responses to Stress

Hormones Associated with the Stress Response	Source of the Hormone	Physiologic Effects
Catecholamines (norepinephrine, epinephrine)	Locus ceruleus, adrenal medulla	Produces a decrease in insulin release and an increase in glucagon release resulting in increased glycogenolysis, gluconeogenesis, lipolysis, proteolysis, and decreased glucose uptake by the peripheral tissues; an increase in heart rate, cardiac contractility, and vascular smooth muscle contraction; and relaxation of bronchial smooth muscle
Corticotropin-releasing factor (CRF)	Hypothalamus	Stimulates ACTH release from anterior pituitary and increased activity of neurons in locus ceruleus
Adrenocorticotropic hormone (ACTH)	Anterior pituitary	Stimulates the synthesis and release of cortisol
Glucocorticoid hormones (e.g., cortisol)	Adrenal cortex	Potentiates the actions of epinephrine and glucagon; inhibits the release and/or actions of the reproductive hormones and thyroid-stimulating hormone; and produces a decrease in immune cells and inflammatory mediators
Mineralocorticoid hormones (e.g., aldosterone)	Adrenal cortex	Increases sodium absorption by the kidney
Antidiuretic hormone (ADH, vasopressin)	Hypothalamus, posterior pituitary	Increases water absorption by the kidney; produces vasoconstriction of blood vessels; and stimulates the release of ACTH

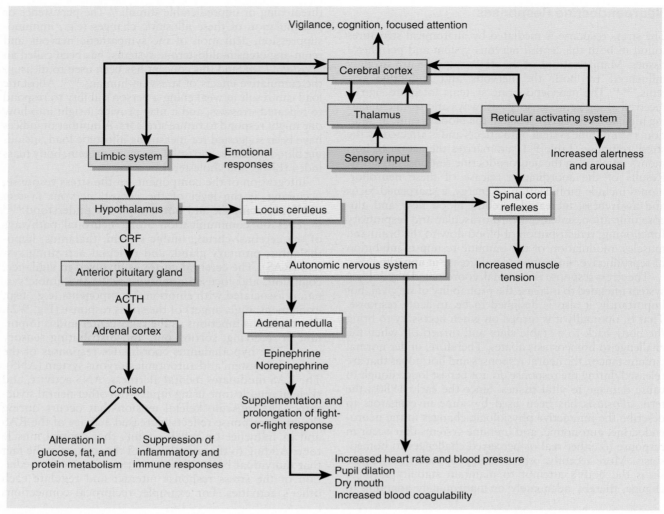

FIGURE 9-2. Neuroendocrine pathways and physiologic responses to stress. ACTH, adrenocorticotropic hormone; CRF, corticotropin-releasing factor.

exist between neurons in the hypothalamus that initiate release of corticotropin-releasing factor (CRF) and neurons in the locus ceruleus associated with release of norepinephrine. Thus, norepinephrine stimulates the secretion of CRF, and CRF stimulates the release of norepinephrine.[16,17]

Locus Ceruleus. Central to the neural component of the neuroendocrine response to stress is an area of the brain stem called the *locus ceruleus* (LC).[16,17] The LC is densely populated with neurons that produce norepinephrine (NE) and is thought to be the central integrating site for the ANS response to stressful stimuli (Fig. 9-3). The LC-NE system has afferent pathways to the hypothalamus, limbic system, hippocampus, and cerebral cortex.

The LC-NE system confers an adaptive advantage during a stressful situation. The SNS manifestation of the stress reaction has been called the *fight-or-flight response.*[2] This reaction is the most rapid of the stress responses and represents the basic survival response of our primitive ancestors when confronted with perils of the wilderness and its inhabitants. The increase in SNS

activity in the brain increases attention and arousal, and thus probably intensifies memory. Increased SNS arousal also results in heart and respiratory rate increases, moist hands and feet, dilated pupils, dry mouth, and reduced activity of the gastrointestinal tract.

Corticotropin-Releasing Factor. CRF is central to the endocrine component of the neuroendocrine response to stress, and it is the principal regulator of the HPA axis (see Fig. 9-3).[3,16,17] Corticotropin-releasing factor, also known as *corticotropin-releasing hormone,* is a small peptide hormone found in both the hypothalamus and extrahypothalamic structures, such as the limbic system and brain stem. It is both an important endocrine regulator of pituitary and adrenal activity, as well as a neurotransmitter involved in ANS activity, metabolism, and behavior. In response to stressors, CRF is released into the hypophysial portal vessels that enter the anterior pituitary gland. Receptors for CRF are distributed throughout the brain as well as many peripheral sites. Corticotropin-releasing factor from the hypothalamus binds to corticotropes, inducing secretion

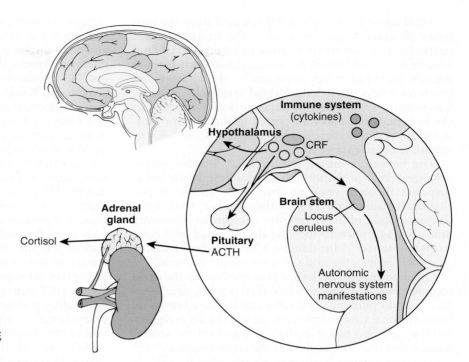

FIGURE 9-3. Neuroendocrine–immune system regulation of the stress response. ACTH, adrenocorticotropic hormone; CRF, corticotropin-releasing factor.

of adrenocorticotropic hormone (ACTH) from the anterior pituitary gland into the systemic circulation. Adrenocorticotropic hormone, in turn, stimulates the adrenal gland to synthesize and secrete glucocorticoid hormones (e.g., cortisol).[25]

Cortisol is the primary glucocorticoid in humans, representing a major subclass of steroid hormones that regulate metabolic, cardiovascular, immune, and behavioral responses. A glucocorticoid negative feedback system exists, whereby the HPA axis is subject to feedback inhibition from circulating glucocorticoids. These glucocorticoids have a number of direct or indirect physiologic effects that mediate the stress response, enhance the action of other stress hormones, or suppress other components of the stress system. In this regard, cortisol acts not only as a mediator of the stress response but also as an inhibitor so that overactivation of the stress response does not occur.[21,23] Cortisol maintains blood glucose levels and enhances the effect of catecholamines on the cardiovascular system. Blood glucose levels are elevated rapidly, in part by mobilization of glucose stores and by inhibition of further storage through the antagonizing effects of insulin.[21] Cortisol also suppresses osteoblast activity, hematopoiesis, protein and collagen synthesis, and immune responses. All of these functions are meant to protect the organism against the effects of a stressor and to focus energy on regaining balance in the face of an acute challenge to homeostasis.

Angiotensin II. Stimulation of the SNS also activates the peripheral renin-angiotensin-aldosterone system (RAAS), which mediates a peripheral increase in vascular tone and renal retention of sodium and water (see Chapter 18). These changes contribute to the physiologic alterations that occur with the stress response; if prolonged, they may contribute to pathologic changes. Angiotensin II,

peripherally delivered or locally produced, also has CNS effects; angiotensin II type 1 (AT_1) receptors are widely distributed in the hypothalamus and locus ceruleus. Through these receptors, angiotensin II enhances CRF formation and release, contributes to the release of ACTH from the pituitary, enhances stress-induced release of vasopressin from the posterior pituitary, and stimulates release of norepinephrine from the locus ceruleus. Results from animal studies on the effect of AT_1 receptor blockade suggest that receptor antagonists attenuate activation of the stress response and may be an effective treatment for chronic stimulation of the stress response.[26,27]

Other Hormones. A wide variety of other hormones, including growth hormone, thyroid hormone, and reproductive hormones, are responsive to stressful situations as well.[16,17,28] Systems responsible for reproduction, growth, and immunity are directly linked to the stress system, and hormonal effects of the stress response profoundly influence these systems.

Although growth hormone is initially elevated with the onset of stress, prolonged presence of cortisol leads to suppression of growth hormone, insulin-like growth factor 1 (IGF-1), and other growth factors, exerting a chronically inhibitory effect on growth. In addition, CRF directly increases somatostatin, which in turn inhibits growth hormone secretion. Although the connection is speculative, effects of stress on growth hormone may provide one of the vital links to understanding failure to thrive in children.

Stress-induced cortisol secretion also is associated with decreased levels of thyroid-stimulating hormone and inhibition of conversion of thyroxine (T_4) to the more biologically active triiodothyronine (T_3) in peripheral tissues (see Chapter 32). Both changes may serve as a means to conserve energy at times of stress.

Antidiuretic hormone (ADH) released from the posterior pituitary is also involved in the stress response, particularly in hypotensive stress or stress due to fluid volume loss. Antidiuretic hormone, also known as *vasopressin,* increases water retention by the kidneys and produces vasoconstriction of blood vessels. In addition, vasopressin, synthesized in paraventricular neurons of the hypothalamus and transported to the anterior pituitary, appears to synergize the capacity of the CRF to stimulate the release of ACTH.

The neurotransmitter serotonin or 5-hydroxytryptamine (5-HT) probably also plays a role in the stress response through neurons that innervate the hypothalamus, amygdala, and other limbic structures. Administration of 5-HT receptor agonists to laboratory animals was shown to increase the secretion of several stress hormones.[29,30] In addition, it has been demonstrated that CRF inhibits the firing of serotonergic neurons.

Other hormones that have a presumed role in the stress response include vasoactive intestinal peptide, neuropeptide Y, cholecystokinin, and substance P. These hormones have well-characterized physiologic roles in the periphery but they are also found in the CNS, and several studies suggest that they are involved in the stress response.[16,17,28]

The reproductive hormones are inhibited by CRF at the hypophyseal level and by cortisol at the pituitary, gonadal, and target tissue levels.[31] Sepsis and severe trauma can induce anovulation and amenorrhea in women and decreased spermatogenesis and decreased levels of testosterone in men.

Immune Responses

The hallmark of the stress response, as first described by Selye, is the endocrine–immune interactions (i.e., increased corticosteroid production and atrophy of the thymus) that are known to suppress the immune response. In concert, these two components of the stress system, through endocrine and neurotransmitter pathways, produce the physical and behavioral changes designed to adapt to acute stress. Much of the literature regarding stress and the immune response focuses on the causal role of stress in immune-related diseases. It also has been suggested that the reverse may occur; emotional and psychological manifestations of the stress response may be a reflection of alterations in the CNS resulting from the immune response (see Fig. 9-3). Immune cells such as monocytes and lymphocytes can penetrate the blood–brain barrier and take up residence in the brain, where they secrete chemical messengers called *cytokines* that influence the stress response.[24,32]

The exact mechanism by which stress produces its effect on the immune response is unknown and probably varies from person to person, depending on genetic endowment and environmental factors. The most significant arguments for interaction between the neuroendocrine and immune systems derive from evidence that the immune and neuroendocrine systems share common signal pathways (i.e., messenger molecules and receptors), that hormones and neuropeptides can alter the function of immune cells, and that the immune system and its mediators can modulate neuroendocrine function. Stress has the capacity to either enhance or suppress immune function.[33] Receptors for a number of CNS-controlled hormones and neuromediators reportedly have been found on lymphocytes. Among these are receptors for glucocorticoids, insulin, testosterone, prolactin, catecholamines, estrogens, acetylcholine, and growth hormone, suggesting that these hormones and neuromediators influence lymphocyte function. For example, cortisol is known to suppress immune function, and pharmacologic doses of cortisol are used clinically to suppress the immune response. There is evidence that the immune system, in turn, influences neuroendocrine function.[34] For example, it has been observed that the HPA axis is activated by cytokines such as interleukin-1, interleukin-6, and tumor necrosis factor that are released from immune cells (see Chapter 15).

A second possible route for neuroendocrine regulation of immune function is through the SNS and the release of catecholamines. The lymph nodes, thymus, and spleen are supplied with ANS nerve fibers. Centrally acting CRF activates the ANS through multisynaptic descending pathways, and circulating epinephrine acts synergistically with CRF and cortisol to inhibit the function of the immune system.

Not only is the quantity of immune expression changed because of stress, but the quality of the response is also changed. Stress hormones differentially stimulate proliferation of subtypes of T-lymphocyte helper cells. Because these T-helper cell subtypes secrete different cytokines, they stimulate different aspects of the immune response. One subtype tends to stimulate T lymphocytes and the cellular-mediated immune response, whereas a second type tends to activate B lymphocytes and humoral-mediated immune responses.[5]

Adaptation to Stress

The ability to adapt to a wide range of environments and stressors is not peculiar to humans. According to René Dubos (a microbiologist noted for his study of human responses to the total environment), "adaptability is found throughout life and is perhaps the one attribute that distinguishes most clearly the world of life from the world of inanimate matter."[35] Living organisms, no matter how primitive, do not submit passively to the impact of environmental forces. They attempt to respond adaptively, each in its own unique and most suitable manner. The higher the organism is on the evolutionary scale, the larger its repertoire of adaptive mechanisms and its ability to select and limit aspects of the environment to which it responds. The most fully evolved mechanisms are social responses through which individuals or groups modify their environments and/or habits in order to achieve a way of life that is best suited to their needs.

Control Mechanisms

Human beings, because of their highly developed nervous system and intellect, usually have alternative mechanisms for adapting and have the ability to control many aspects of their environment. Air conditioning and central heating limit the need to adapt to extreme changes in environmental temperature. Availability of antiseptic agents, immunizations, and antibiotics eliminates the need to respond to common infectious agents. At the same time, modern technology creates new challenges for adaptation and provides new sources of stress, such as increased noise, air pollution, exposure to harmful chemicals, and changes in biologic rhythms imposed by shift work and transcontinental air travel.

Of particular interest are differences in the body's response to events that threaten the integrity of the body's physiologic environment, and those influences that threaten the integrity of the person's psychosocial environment. Many of the body's responses to physiologic disturbances are controlled on a moment-by-moment basis by feedback mechanisms that limit their application and duration of action. For example, the baroreflex-mediated rise in heart rate that occurs when a person moves from the recumbent to standing position is almost instantaneous and subsides within seconds. Furthermore, the response to physiologic disturbances that threaten the integrity of the internal environment is specific to the threat; the body usually does not raise the body temperature when an increase in heart rate is needed. In contrast, the response to psychological disturbances is not regulated with the same degree of specificity and feedback control; instead, the effect may be inappropriate and sustained.

Adaptive Mechanisms

Adaptation implies that an individual has successfully created a new balance between the stressor and the ability to deal with it. The means used to attain this balance are called *coping strategies* or *coping mechanisms*. Coping mechanisms are the emotional and behavioral responses used to manage threats to our physiologic and psychological homeostasis. According to Lazarus, the coping strategies used for stressful events depend on how the events are perceived and interpreted.[36] Is the event perceived as a threat of harm or loss? Is the event perceived as a challenge rather than a threat? Physiologic and anatomic reserve, time, genetic endowment, age, health status, nutrition, sleep–wake cycles, hardiness, and psychosocial factors influence one's appraisal of a stressor and the coping mechanisms employed to adapt to the new situation (Fig. 9-4).

Physiologic and Anatomic Reserve. Adaptation is greatly influenced by an individual's physiologic and anatomic reserve. The safety margin for adaptation of most body systems is considerably greater than that needed for normal activities. Red blood cells carry more oxygen than tissues can use, the liver and fat cells store excess nutrients, and bone tissue stores calcium in excess of that needed for normal neuromuscular function. The ability of body systems to increase level of function, given the need to adapt, is known as the *physiologic reserve*. Many body organs, such as the lungs and kidney, are paired to provide anatomic reserve as well. Both organs are not needed to ensure the continued existence and maintenance of the internal environment. Many persons function normally with only one lung or one kidney.

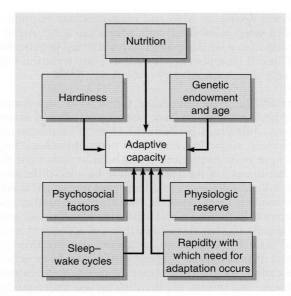

FIGURE 9-4. Factors affecting adaptation.

Time. Time is an essential element in adaptation. Adaptation is most efficient when changes occur gradually rather than suddenly. It is possible, for instance, to lose a liter or more of blood through chronic gastrointestinal bleeding over a week without manifesting signs of shock. However, a sudden hemorrhage that causes rapid loss of an equal amount of blood is likely to cause hypotension and shock.

Genetic Endowment. Genetic endowment is increasingly being viewed as a contributing factor in adaptation to stressful events, both physiological and psychological. Recent advances in the field of genetic research suggest that different variants of certain genes determine how an individual responds to stressful life experiences. For example, an inherited variant of the serotonin transporter gene is associated with a number of conditions such as alcoholism, and individuals who have the variant are more vulnerable to respond to stressful experiences by developing depressive disorders.[20] There also is evidence linking variants in the glucocorticoid receptor gene, which controls the body's response to cortisol during stressful situations, to the development of depressive disorders and posttraumatic stress disorder (PTSD).[37,38] It seems likely that recent advances in genetic research methodology will allow investigators to identify additional patterns of response to stressful events and their link to psychological and physical health problems.

Age. The capacity to adapt to stress is also influenced by age. The ability to adapt is impaired by the immaturity of an infant, much as it is by the decline in functional reserve that occurs with aging. For example, the infant has difficulty concentrating urine because of immature renal structures, and therefore an infant is less able than an adult to cope with decreased water intake or exaggerated water losses. A similar situation exists in the elderly, owing to age-related changes in renal function. Likewise, there is a reported decline in ANS and cardiovascular responsiveness to stress associated with advancing age.[39] Aging is also associated with impaired activation and proliferation of T and B lymphocytes, as well as poorer natural killer cell response to stimulatory cytokines.[40]

Gender. Within the last decade, primarily because females have been included in basic science and clinical investigations, differences between the sexes in cardiovascular, respiratory, endocrine, renal, and neurophysiologic function have been found, and it has been hypothesized that sex hormones are the basis of these biologic differences. Technological advances in cellular and molecular biology have made it clear, however, that there are fundamental differences in the locale and regulation of individual genes in the male and female genome that can account at a very basic level for differences in physiologic function and disease manifestation.[41] These differences have general implications for the prevention, diagnosis, and treatment of disease and specific implications for our understanding of the sex-based differences in response to life's stressors.

Given the nature of sex-based differences, it is not surprising that there are differences in the physiologic stress response in both the HPA axis and the ANS. For example, the male hypothalamus produces more CRF and more ACTH than the premenopausal female hypothalamus, in response to psychological stressors (e.g., public speaking).[42] However, secretion of arginine vasopressin (AVP), a hormone that has cardiovascular and renal effects and potentiates the release of ACTH, is greater in the female. Premenopausal women also tend to have a lower activation of the SNS than men in response to stressors. The phase of menstruation (luteal vs. follicular), as well as menopausal status, can alter these responses and need to be considered when studying these responses.[42] These sex-based differences in activation of the stress response may partially explain differences in susceptibility to diseases in which the stress response may play a causal role. These research results are not definitive, but they are intriguing and may serve as a foundation for further research.

Health Status. Physical and mental health status determine physiologic and psychological reserves, and they are strong determinants of one's ability to adapt. For example, persons with heart disease are less able to adjust to stressors that require recruitment of cardiovascular responses. Severe emotional stress often produces disruption of physiologic function and limits the ability to make appropriate choices related to long-term adaptive needs. Professionals who have worked with acutely ill persons have witnessed that the will to live often has a profound influence on survival during life-threatening illnesses.

Nutrition. There are 50 to 60 essential nutrients, including minerals, lipids, certain fatty acids, vitamins, and specific amino acids. Deficiencies or excesses of any of these nutrients can alter a person's health status and impair the ability to adapt. The importance of nutrition to enzyme function, immune response, and wound healing is well known. On a worldwide basis, malnutrition may be one of the most common causes of immunodeficiency.

Among problems associated with dietary excess are obesity and alcohol abuse. Obesity is a common problem. It predisposes an individual to a number of health problems, including atherosclerosis and hypertension. Alcohol is commonly used in excess. It acutely affects brain function, and with long-term use, can seriously impair function of the liver, brain, and other vital structures.

Sleep–Wake Cycles. Sleep is considered to be a restorative function, in which energy is restored and tissues are regenerated.[43] Sleep occurs in a cyclical manner, alternating with periods of wakefulness and increased energy use. Biologic rhythms play an important role in adaptation to stress, development of illness, and response to medical treatment. Many rhythms such as rest and activity, work and leisure, and eating and drinking oscillate with a frequency similar to that of the 24-hour light–dark solar day. The term *circadian*, from the Latin *circa* ("about") and *dies* ("day"), is used to describe these 24-hour diurnal rhythms.

Sleep disorders and alterations in the sleep–wake cycle have been shown to alter immune function, the normal circadian pattern of hormone secretion, and physical and psychological functioning.[44] The two most common manifestations of an alteration in the sleep–wake cycle are insomnia and sleep deprivation or increased somnolence. In some persons, stress may produce sleep disorders; in others, sleep disorders may lead to stress. Acute stress and environmental disturbances, loss of a loved one, recovery from surgery, and pain are common causes of transient and short-term insomnia. Air travel and jet lag constitute additional causes of altered sleep–wake cycles, as does shift work.

Hardiness. Studies by social psychologists have focused on individuals' emotional reactions to stressful situations and use of coping mechanisms in order to determine characteristics that help some people remain healthy despite being challenged by high levels of stressors. For example, the concept of *hardiness* describes a personality characteristic that includes a sense of having control over the environment, a sense of having a purpose in life, and an ability to conceptualize stressors as a challenge rather than a threat.[45] Lower levels of hardiness have been linked with greater reaction to stress, including suppressed pro-inflammatory cytokines (IL-12), increased anti-inflammatory cytokines (IL-4, IL-10), and lower neuropeptide-Y levels. Individuals with higher levels of psychological hardiness demonstrated more moderate and healthy immune and neuroendocrine responses to stress.[46]

Psychosocial Factors. Several studies have related social factors and life events to illness. Scientific interest in the social environment as a cause of stress has gradually broadened to include the social environment as a resource that modulates the relationship between stress and health. Presumably, persons who can mobilize strong supportive resources from within their social relationships are better able to withstand the negative effects of stress on their health. Studies suggest that social support has direct and indirect positive effects on health status and serves as a buffer or modifier of the physical and psychosocial effects of stress.[47]

Social networks contribute in a number of ways to a person's psychosocial and physical integrity.[20] The configuration of significant others that constitutes this network functions to mobilize resources of the person; these friends, colleagues, and family members share the person's tasks and provide monetary support, materials, and tools, as well as guidance in improving long-term problem-solving capabilities.

SUMMARY CONCEPTS

■ Physiologic and psychological adaptation involves the ability to maintain constancy of the internal environment (homeostasis) and behavior in the face of a wide range of changes in the internal and external environments. It involves negative feedback control systems that regulate cellular function, control life's processes, regulate behavior, and integrate functions of different body systems.

■ The stress response involves activation of several physiologic systems: the sympathetic nervous system (SNS), hypothalamic pituitary adrenal (HPA) axis, and immune system that work in a coordinated fashion to protect the body against damage from intense demands made upon it.

■ Selye, who referred to the stress response as the *general adaptation syndrome,* divided it into three stages: the *alarm stage,* with activation of the SNS and the HPA axis; the *resistance stage,* during which the body selects the most effective defenses; and the *exhaustion stage,* during which physiologic resources are depleted and signs of systemic damage appear.

■ Activation and control of the stress response are mediated by combined efforts of the nervous and endocrine systems. The neuroendocrine systems integrate signals received from neurosensory pathways and circulating mediators that are carried in the bloodstream. In addition, the immune system both affects and is affected by the stress response.

■ Adaptation implies that an individual has successfully created a new balance between the stressor and his or her ability to deal with it. Adaptation is affected by a number of factors, including experience and previous learning, the rapidity with which the need to adapt occurs, genetic endowment, age, health status, nutrition, sleep–wake cycles, hardiness, and psychosocial factors.

Disorders of the Stress Response

Stressors can assume a number of patterns in relation to time. They may be classified as acute time limited, chronic intermittent, or chronic sustained. An acute time-limited stressor is one that occurs over a short amount of time and does not recur; a chronic intermittent stressor is one to which a person is chronically exposed. The frequency or chronicity of circumstances to which the body is asked to respond often determines the availability and efficiency of the stress responses. The response of the immune system, for example, is more rapid and efficient on second exposure to a pathogen than it is on first exposure, but chronic exposure to a stressor can fatigue the system and impair its effectiveness.

Effects of Acute Stress

Generally, the stress response is meant to be acute and time limited. The time-limited nature of the process renders the accompanying catabolic and immunosuppressive effects advantageous. Reactions to acute stress are those associated with the ANS, the fight-or-flight response. Centrally, there is facilitation of neural pathways mediating arousal, alertness, vigilance, cognition, and focused attention, as well as appropriate aggression. For persons with limited coping abilities, either because of physical or mental illness, the acute stress response may be detrimental. For example, persons with preexisting heart disease who are faced with overwhelming sympathetic behaviors associated with the stress response may experience arrhythmias. In healthy individuals, the acute stress response may be detrimental as well, as it can redirect attention away from behaviors that promote health, such as attention to proper meals and getting adequate sleep. For persons with health problems, the stress response may result in interruption of compliance with medication regimens and exercise programs.

The acute physiologic stress associated with severe trauma, infection, and surgery can be extensive. Survival of such insults depends to a great extent upon the neuroendocrine component of the stress response, with activation of the HPA axis being one of the most important components of the response.[48–50] Cortisol, the primary glucocorticoid secreted by the adrenal cortex in response to activation of the HPA, has an important role in many of the physiologic functions during trauma and critical illness. The actions of cortisol include anti-inflammatory effects, as well as effects on blood glucose, vascular tone, endothelial integrity, and modulation of angiotensinogen synthesis.

Of recent concern has been the dramatic increase in blood glucose levels that occur during the acute stress response to critical injury and illness.[49,51,52] The causes of stress-induced hyperglycemia include enhanced release of glucose from glycogen stores, increased production of glucose from non-carbohydrate sources such as amino acids, and an accompanying state of insulin resistance that impairs glucose uptake into skeletal muscle. Clinical data suggest that hyperglycemia results in worse outcomes and recovery from acute coronary syndromes[51,53] (see Chapter 19), septic shock[52,54] (see Chapter 20), hemorrhagic shock,[49,55] and stroke[56] (see Chapter 36). These findings have led to a goal for strict control of blood glucose in most critically ill patients. This control is often accomplished through the use of low-dose insulin infusions. Insulin itself has been shown to produce anti-inflammatory, antioxidant, antithrombotic, and profibrinolytic effects, separate from those involved in reducing blood glucose levels.[51,53] The optimal level for regulation of blood glucose in the critical care setting, and the expediency of initiating insulin therapy, remain current areas of investigation.

Effects of Chronic Stress

The stress response is designed to be an acute self-limited response in which activation of the ANS and the HPA axis is controlled in a negative feedback manner. As with all negative feedback systems, pathophysiologic changes can occur in the stress response system. Function can be altered in several ways, including when a component of the system fails, when the neural and hormonal connections among components of the system are dysfunctional, and when the original stimulus for activation of the system is prolonged or of such magnitude that it overwhelms the ability of the system to respond appropriately. In these cases, the system may become overactive or underactive.

Chronicity and excessive activation of the stress response can result from chronic illnesses, and it can contribute to development of long-term health problems. It has been linked to a number of health disorders, including diseases of the cardiovascular, gastrointestinal, immune, and neurologic systems, as well as depression, chronic alcoholism and drug abuse, eating disorders, accidents, and suicide. Chronic activation of the stress response is also an important public health issue from both a health and an economic perspective. The National Institute for Occupational Safety and Health has declared stress as a hazard in the workplace.[57]

Occurrence of acute necrotizing gingivitis, an oral disease in which normal bacterial flora of the mouth become invasive, is known by dentists to be associated with acute stress, such as final examinations.[58] Similarly, herpes simplex virus type 1 infection (i.e., cold sores) often develops during periods of inadequate rest, fever, ultraviolet radiation, and emotional upset. The resident herpes virus is kept in check by body defenses, probably T lymphocytes, until a stressful event occurs that causes suppression of the immune system. Psychological stress is associated in a dose–response manner with an increased risk for development of the common cold, and this risk is attributable to increased rates of infection rather than frequency of symptoms after infection.[59]

The inflammatory phase of wound repair appears to be disrupted in the presence of chronic stress.[60] Skin blisters were induced on the forearms of 36 post-menopausal women. Women with greater stress produced significantly lower levels of IL-1α and IL-8, indicating a poorer response to the stressor. Lower cell-mediated immune response to influenza vaccination was observed in elderly participants experiencing chronic stress when compared with counterparts that were not experiencing chronic stress.[61] Chronic stress also has been linked to specific signaling pathways that impact cancer growth and metastasis.[62]

Posttraumatic Stress Disorder

Posttraumatic stress disorder (PTSD) is an example of chronic activation of the stress response to a traumatic event.[63–66] It was formerly called *battle fatigue* or *shell shock* because it was first characterized in men and women returning from combat. Although war is still a significant cause of PTSD, other major catastrophic events, such as weather-related disasters (hurricanes and floods), airplane crashes, terrorist bombings, rape or child abuse, or intimate partner violence also may result in development of the disorder. People who are exposed to such events are also at risk for development of major depression, panic disorder, generalized anxiety disorder, and substance abuse.[66] Frequently, bodily symptoms and physical illnesses such as hypertension, coronary heart disease, asthma, and chronic pain syndromes have been associated with PTSD.

Definition. The term *posttraumatic stress disorder* was originally defined in the third edition (1980) of the American Psychiatric Association's *Diagnostic and Statistical Manual of Mental Disorders* (DSM-III) as a gross stress reaction that was considered a temporary condition; however it could be changed to a neurotic condition if it persisted.[67] In the fourth edition of the *Diagnostic and Statistical Manual of Mental Disorders* (DSM-IV-TR) (1994), the diagnosis of acute stress disorder (ASD) was added to distinguish individuals with milder or more transient difficulties from those with PTSD.[68] In the fifth edition (DSM-5-TR) (2013), the traumatic event has been defined as exposure to actual or threatened death, serious injury, or sexual experience by directly experiencing, witnessing, learning that it happened to a close family member or friend, or being repeatedly exposed to the averse details of the event (e.g., first responders collecting human remains).[69]

According to the DSM-5, the essential features of PTSD include exposure to actual or perceived threat.[69,70] The exposure may not be as narrowly defined as previously thought, and it may include events such as rape, torture, combat, brutal assault, a difficult diagnosis, or sudden death of a loved one. A change in the DSM-5's criteria for diagnosis of PTSD is the removal of the necessity for the individual to experience an intense emotional response at the time of the exposure. This change was made because many individuals, particularly professionals that witness horrific events, reported feeling nothing at the time of the event—instead their professional training "kicked in."[71]

With PTSD, the threat results in a constellation of symptoms that are experienced as intrusion, avoidance, negative alterations in cognition and mood associated with the event, and marked alterations in arousal and reactivity associated with the event. *Intrusion* involves the recurrent involuntary distressing memories or "flashbacks" during waking hours or nightmares in which the past traumatic event is relived, often in vivid and frightening detail. In children, there may be frightening dreams without recognizable content. *Avoidance* refers to the attempt to avoid situations, including people, places, activities, and objects that arouse distressing memories. At least one avoidance symptom must be present for definitive diagnosis of PTSD. *Negative alterations in cognition and mood* involve an inability to remember an important aspect of the event (i.e., dissociative amnesia) that is not the result of a head injury, alcohol, or drugs. *Marked alterations in arousal and reactivity* replace the numbing symptom in DSM-IV, and it includes inability to experience positive emotions such as love, joy, pleasure, or satisfaction. In addition, distorted beliefs regarding blame of self or others about the causes or consequences of the traumatic event may occur. In addition, irritable and angry outbursts, reckless and destructive behavior, hypervigilance, problems with concentration, and sleep disturbances may occur. DSM-5 no longer includes immediate fear, helplessness, or horror following the event, as it did not improve diagnostic accuracy. Diagnosis of PTSD requires that the duration of disturbance persists for more than a month, causes clinically significant distress or impairment of social or other areas of functioning, and is not attributable to the effects of medication, alcohol, or other medical condition.

Pathophysiology. Although the pathophysiology of PTSD is not completely understood, there is increasing evidence that the disorder results from an exaggerated stress response and a failure of the stress response system to regain homeostasis. The SNS and the HPA axis are the major constituents of the body's neuroendocrine response to physical and physiological threat and stress. Normally, the SNS response is brief, followed by an HPA axis response that serves to reinstate homeostasis and induces long-lasting adaptive changes that contribute to stress recovery and resilience. This is mediated by glucocorticoids (i.e., cortisol), the product of the HPA axis.[72]

Initial research focused on an exaggerated and unrelenting extension of the normal sympathetic and HPA response to the stress associated with the traumatic event. More recent research has revealed that although persons with PTSD have been shown to have increased levels of the SNS activity, they have decreased cortisol levels and an enhanced negative feedback inhibition of cortisol release with the dexamethasone (a synthetic glucocorticoid) suppression test.[72] Cortisol's circadian rhythm, which is critically influenced by corticosteroid function, is altered with the progression of PTSD, suggesting a explanation for sleep disturbances that accompany the disorder.

Although neuroendocrine research suggests that lower cortisol levels are implicated in the pathophysiology of PTSD, emerging research findings suggest this may instead reflect pretraumatic stress vulnerability, explaining why some people develop the disorder and others do not. It has been suggested that genetic[73,74] and previous environmental/experiential factors[65,75,76] may predispose to subsequent development of PTSD.

In addition to the neuroendocrine changes that occur with PTSD, neuroanatomic studies have identified alterations in two brain structures (the amygdala and hippocampus) that occur in persons with PTSD. Positron emission tomography (PET) and functional magnetic resonance imaging (MRI) have shown increased reactivity of the amygdala and hippocampus and decreased reactivity of the anterior cingulate and orbitofrontal areas. These areas of the brain are involved in fear responses. The hippocampus also functions in memory processes. Differences in hippocampal function and memory processes suggest a neuroanatomic basis for the intrusive recollections and other cognitive problems that characterize PTSD.[77]

Diagnosis and Treatment. Although originally conceptualized as a mental disorder, PTSD is becoming increasingly recognized as a highly comorbid condition, much like hypertension, cardiovascular disease, chronic fatigue syndrome, fibromyalgia, and other diseases. For a number of reasons, including the stigma attached to mental illness, limited availability and high cost of treatment, and socioeconomic issues associated with the disorder, people with PTSD frequently do not seek specialized mental health treatment until the disorder has been present for a considerable amount of time.[78,79]

Initial treatment of PTSD focuses on reducing or eliminating the symptoms and signs of PTSD and any trauma-related comorbid conditions. Next, adaptive functioning must be improved, with an emphasis on returning the person to a psychological state of safety and trust. Finally, general treatment approaches focus on limiting any generalizations of the initial trauma and protecting the person with PTSD from subsequent relapse. Debriefing, or talking about the traumatic event at the time it happens, often is an effective therapeutic tool. Crisis teams are often among the first people to attend to the emotional needs of those caught in catastrophic events. Some people may need continued individual or group therapy. Selective serotonin reuptake inhibitors (SSRIs) are considered the first-line drug treatment for PTSD. Often concurrent pharmacotherapy with antidepressant, antianxiety, antipsychotic, and/or psychotropic agents are useful and may help the individual participate more fully in therapy.[80–82] In addition, exercise, participation in sports, and physical activity may be beneficial for persons with PTSD.[83]

Treatment of Stress Disorders

The treatment of stress should be directed toward helping people avoid coping behaviors that impose a risk to their health and providing them with alternative stress-reducing strategies. Purposeful priority setting and problem solving can be used by persons who are overwhelmed by the number of life stressors to which they have been exposed. Some popular evidence-based nonpharmacologic methods of stress reduction are progressive muscle relaxation, guided imagery, music therapy, massage, and biofeedback.

Progressive Muscle Relaxation Techniques

Practices for evoking the relaxation response are numerous. They are found in virtually every culture and credited with producing a generalized decrease in SNS activity and musculoskeletal tension. According to Herbert Benson, a physician, who worked on developing various relaxation strategies, four elements are integral to the various strategies: a repetitive mental device, a passive attitude, decreased mental tonus, and a quiet environment.[84] Benson incorporated these elements into a non-cultural method that is commonly used for achieving relaxation (Box 9-2). Progressive relaxation, also developed by Benson, is another method of relieving tension. This procedure, which has been modified by a number of therapists, consists of systematic contraction and relaxation of major muscle groups.[85,86] This procedure involves deliberate contraction, followed by relaxation, of 16 isolated muscle groups. Individuals are instructed to focus all of their attention on their muscles, focusing first on the sensations of tension associated with the muscle contractions, and then focusing on the sensations of warmth, softening, and relaxation when the tension is released. The contraction is to be held for approximately 5 to 7 seconds, and the relaxation is intended to last for approximately 30 seconds. The ultimate goal is to reduce or eliminate the tension in the body, both physical and mental.

The relaxation response has been shown to be an effective tool for treating stress-related disease processes, particularly certain immunologic, cardiovascular, and neurodegenerative disorders. It has been suggested that common underlying molecular mechanisms may exist that represent a connection between the stress response, pathophysiology of the stress-related diseases, and physiologic changes associated with the relaxation response.[87] Several molecular pathways have been suggested including those involving cortisol, norepinephrine/epinephrine, and nitric oxide signaling.

Guided Imagery

Guided imagery is another technique that can be used to achieve relaxation.[88,89] It can be used to control pain and anxiety, as a sleep aid, and as a means of coping with a stressful diagnosis or treatment regimens. It also can be used as a method for relieving anxiety in children. It has been reported that children are quick and eager to use imagery as means of relieving pain or relieving the anxiety associated with surgery.

Guided imagery is a mind–body technique intended to relieve stress and promote a sense of peace and tranquility during periods of stress or difficulty.[90] The individual is guided to focus on creating a specific mental image designed to bring about positive physical and/or emotional effects.[91] Instructions are given to focus on the present; if possible, it is desirable to tune out all outside thoughts and ideas. Frequently instructions include going to a "special place" in their minds, such as a secluded beach or a babbling brook. Sometimes visualization is used, in which the person is asked to sit back, close their eyes, and concentrate on a scene narrated by the therapist. Whenever possible, all five senses are involved: the person attempts to see, feel, hear, smell, and taste aspects of the visual experience. Guided imagery may be practiced with a coach using a script, or it can be used independently, with or without a recorded message.

Music Therapy

Music therapy is used for both its physiologic and psychological effects. It involves listening to selected pieces of music as a means of ameliorating anxiety or stress, reducing pain, decreasing feelings of loneliness and isolation, buffering noise, and facilitating expression of emotion.[92] Music is defined as having three components: rhythm, melody, and harmony. Rhythm is the order in the movement of the music. Rhythm is the most dynamic aspect of music, and particular pieces of music often are selected because they harmonize with body rhythms such as heart rhythm, respiratory rhythm, or gait. The melody is created by the musical pitch and the distance

---

BOX 9-2 The Relaxation Response

- Sit quietly in a comfortable position.

- Deeply relax all your muscles, beginning at your feet and progressing up to your face.

- Breathe through your nose. Become aware of your breathing. As you breathe out, say the word "one" silently to yourself. Continue for 20 minutes. When you have finished, sit quietly for several minutes, first with your eyes closed and then with them open.

- Do not worry about whether you are successful in achieving a deep level of relaxation. Maintain a positive attitude and permit the relaxation to occur at its own rate. Expect distracting thoughts, ignore them, and continue repeating "one" as you breathe out.

Modified from Benson H. Systemic hypertension and the relaxation response. *N Engl J Med.* 1977;296:1152.

(or interval) between the musical tones. The melody contributes to the listener's emotional response to the music. Harmony results from the way pitches are blended together, with the combination of sounds described as consonant or dissonant by the listener. Music usually is selected based on a person's musical preference and past experiences with music. Depending on the setting, headphones may be used to screen out other distracting noises. Radio and television music is inappropriate for music therapy because of the inability to control the selection of pieces that are played, the interruptions that occur (e.g., commercials and announcements), and the quality of the reception. Music therapy has been effective for reducing anxiety in many patient populations across the life span, including critical care,[93] palliative care,[94] and the perioperative arena.[95]

Massage Therapy

Massage is the manipulation of the soft tissues of the body to promote relaxation and relief of muscle tension. The technique that is used may involve a gentle stroking along the length of a muscle (effleurage), application of pressure across the width of a muscle (pétrissage), deep massage movements applied by a circular motion of the thumbs or fingertips (friction), squeezing across the width of a muscle (kneading), or use of light slaps or chopping actions (hacking).[96] Massage may be administered by practitioners who have received special training in its use, and it can be delivered by less prepared persons such as parents of small children[97] or caregivers of confused elders.[98] It often is used as a means of physiologic relaxation and stress relief in critically ill patients,[99,100] cancer patients,[101] and persons with dementia.[102]

Biofeedback

Biofeedback is a technique in which an individual learns to control physiologic functioning. It involves electronic monitoring of one or more physiologic responses to stress with immediate feedback of the specific response to the person undergoing treatment. Several types of responses are used: electromyographic (EMG), electrothermal, and electrodermal.[103] The EMG response involves the measurement of electrical potentials from muscles, usually the forearm extensor or frontalis. This technique is used to gain control over the contraction of skeletal muscles that occurs with anxiety and tension. The electrodermal sensors monitor skin temperature in the fingers or toes. The SNS exerts significant control over blood flow in the distal parts of the body such as the digits of the hands and feet. Consequently, anxiety often is manifested by a decrease in skin temperature in the fingers and toes. Electrodermal sensors measure conductivity of skin (usually the hands) in response to anxiety. Fearful and anxious people often have cold and clammy hands, which lead to a decrease in conductivity. Biofeedback has been used successfully to reduce anxiety in nursing students with test anxiety,[104] patients with functional constipation,[105] and those with cyclic vomiting syndrome.[106]

SUMMARY CONCEPTS

- Stress, in and of itself, is neither negative nor deleterious to health. The stress response is designed to be time limited and protective. However, in situations of prolonged activation of the response because of overwhelming or chronic stressors, it can be damaging to health. The acute stress reaction and stress-induced hyperglycemia are of particular concern in persons with critical injuries or illness.

- Post-traumatic stress disorder (PTSD) is an example of chronic activation of the stress response as a result of experiencing a traumatic event that involved actual or threatened death or serious injury. Essential features of PTSD include a constellation of symptoms that are experienced as states of intrusion (flashbacks of the event), avoidance (emotional numbing), and hyperarousal (intense activation of the neuroendocrine system).

- Treatment of stress should be aimed at helping people avoid coping behaviors that can adversely affect their health and providing them with other ways to reduce stress. Some popular evidence-based non-pharmacologic methods used in the treatment of stress include progressive muscle relaxation techniques, guided imagery, music therapy, massage therapy, and biofeedback.

REVIEW EXERCISES

1. A 21-year-old college student notices that she frequently develops "cold sores" during the stressful final exam week.

    A. What is the association between stress and the immune system?
    B. One of her classmates suggests that she listen to music or try relaxation exercises as a means of relieving stress. Explain how these interventions might work in relieving stress.

2. A 75-year-old woman with congestive heart failure complains that her condition gets worse when she worries and is under a lot of stress.

    A. Relate the effects stress has on the neuroendocrine control of cardiovascular function and its possible relationship to a worsening of the woman's congestive heart failure.
    B. She tells you that she dealt with much worse stresses when she was younger and never had any problems. How would you explain this?

3. A 30-year-old woman who was rescued from a collapsed building has been having nightmares recalling the event, excessive anxiety, and loss of appetite, and is afraid to leave her home for fear something will happen.

A. Given her history and symptoms, what is the likely diagnosis?

REFERENCES

1. Garcia J, Hankins WG, Rusiniak KW. Behavioral regulation of the milieu interne in man and rat. *Science.* 1974;185(4154):824–831.
2. Cannon WB. *The Wisdom of the Body.* New York: W.W. Norton; 1939:299–300.
3. Chrousos GP. Stressors, stress, and neuroendocrine integration of the adaptive response. *Ann N Y Acad Sci.* 1998;851:311–335.
4. Kassi EM, Chrousos GP. The central CLOCK system and the stress axis in health and disease. *Hormones.* 2013;12(2):172–191.
5. Wilcox RE, Gonzales RA. Introduction to neurotransmitters, receptors, signal transduction, and second messengers. In: Schatzberg AF, Nemeroff CB, eds. *Textbook of Psychopharmacology.* Washington, DC: American Psychiatric Press; 1995:3–29.
6. Selye H. A syndrome produced by diverse nocuous agents. *Nature.* 1936;138:32.
7. Selye H. *The Stress of Life*, rev. ed. New York: McGraw-Hill; 1976.
8. Selye H. The evolution of the stress concept. *Am Sci.* 1973;61:692–699.
9. Smith SM, Vale WW. The role of the hypothalamic-pituitary-adrenal axis in neuroendocrine responses to stress. *Dialogues Clin Neurosci.* 2006;8(4):383–395.
10. Habib KE, Gold PW, Chrousos GP. Neuroendocrinology of stress. *Endocrinol Metab Clin North Am.* 2001;30:695–728.
11. Selye H. *Stress Without Distress.* New York: New American Library; 1974:6.
12. McEwan BS. The brain as the central organ of stress and adaptation. *Neuroimage.* 2009;47(3):911–913.
13. Lazarus R. *Stress and Emotion: A New Synthesis.* New York: Springer; 1999:6.
14. Ursin H, Eriksen HR. The cognitive-activation theory of stress. *Psychoneuroendocrinology.* 2004;29:567–592.
15. Goldstein DS. Catecholamines and stress. *Endocr Regul.* 2003;37:69–80.
16. Carrasco GA, Van de Kar LD. Neuroendocrine pharmacology of stress. *Eur J Pharmacol.* 2003;463:235–272.
17. Charmandari E, Tsigos C, Chrous G. Endocrinology of the stress response. *Annu Rev Physiol.* 2005;67:259–284.
18. Romero LM, Dickens MJ, Cyr NE. The reactive scope model—a new model integrating homeostasis, allostasis, and stress. *Horm Behav.* 2009;55(3):375–399.
19. Karatsoreos IN, McEwen BS. Psychobiological allostasis: resistance, resilience, and vulnerability. *Trends Cogn Sci.* 2011;15(12):576–584.
20. McEwen BS. Physiology and neurobiology of stress and adaptation: central role of the brain. *Physiol Rev.* 2007;87:873–904.
21. Sapolsky RM, Romero LM, Munck AU. How do glucocorticoids influence stress responses? Integrating permissive, suppressive, stimulatory, and preparative actions. *Endocr Rev.* 2000;21:55–89.
22. Juster RP, McEwen BS, Lulpien SJ. Allostatic load biomarkers of chronic stress and impact on health and cognition. *Neurosci Biobehav Rev.* 2010;35(1):2–16.
23. de Kloet ER. Hormones, brain and stress. *Endocr Regul.* 2003;37:51–68.
24. Sternberg EM. Neural regulation of innate immunity: a coordinated nonspecific host response to pathogens. *Nat Rev Immunol.* 2006;6:318–328.
25. Bamberger CM, Schulte HM, Chrousos GP. Molecular determinants of glucocorticoid receptor function and tissue sensitivity to glucocorticoids. *Endocr Rev.* 1996;17:245–261.
26. Podowski M, Calvi C, Metzger S, et al. Angiotensin receptor blockade attenuates cigarette smoke-induced lung injury and rescues lung architecture in mice. *J Clin Invest.* 2012;122(1):229–240.
27. Whatley-Connell A, Habibi J, Rehmer N, et al. Renin inhibition and AT(1) blockade improve metabolic signaling, oxidant stress and myocardial tissue remodeling. *Metabolism.* 2013;62(6):861–872.
28. Motzer SA, Hertig V. Stress, stress response, and health. *Nurs Clin North Am.* 2004;39:1–17.
29. Conti LH. Interactions between corticotropin-releasing factor and the serotonin 1A receptor system on acoustic startle amplitude and prepulse inhibition of the startle response in two rat strains. *Neuropharmacology.* 2012;62(1):256–263.
30. Mentzelopoulos SD, Malachias S, Chamos C, et al. Vasopressin, steroids, and epinephrine and neurologically favorable survival after in-hospital cardiac arrest: a randomized clinical trial. *JAMA.* 2013;310(3):270–279.
31. Whirledge S, Cidlowski JA. A role for glucocorticoids in stress-impaired reproduction: beyond the hypothalamus and pituitary. *Endocrinology.* 2013;154(12):4450–4468.
32. Padgett DA, Glaser R. How stress influences the immune response. *Trends Immunol.* 2003;24(8):444–448.
33. Dhabhar FS, Malarkey WB, Neri E, et al. Stress-induced redistribution of immune cells—from barracks to boulevards to battlefields: a tale of three hormones. *Psychoneuroendocrinology.* 2012;37(9):1345–1368.
34. Woiciechowsky C, Schoning F, Lanksch WR, et al. Mechanisms of brain mediated systemic anti-inflammatory syndrome causing immunodepression. *J Mol Med.* 1999;77:769–780.
35. Dubos R. *Man Adapting.* New Haven, CT: Yale University Press; 1965:256, 258, 261, 264.
36. Lazarus R. Evolution of a model of stress, coping, and discrete emotions. In: Rice VH, ed. *Handbook of Stress, Coping, and Health.* Thousand Oaks, CA: Sage; 2012:199–225.
37. Hauer D, Weis F, Papassotiropoulos A, et al. Relationship of a common polymorphism of glucocorticoid receptor gene to traumatic memories and posttraumatic stress disorder in patients after intensive care therapy. *Crit Care Med.* 2001;39(4):643–650.
38. Menke A, Klengel T, Rubel J, et al. Genetic variation in FKBP5 associated with the extent of stress hormone dysregulation in major depression. *Genes Brain Behav.* 2013;12(3):289–296.
39. Smith JJ, Porth CM. Age and the response to orthostatic stress. In: Smith, JJ, ed. *Circulatory Response to the Upright Posture.* Boca Raton, FL: CRC Press; 1990:121–139.
40. Ogata K, Yokose N, Tamura H, et al. Natural killer cells in the late decades of human life. *Clin Immunol Immunopathol.* 1997;84(3):269–275.
41. Wizemann TM, Pardue ML, eds. *Exploring the Biological Contributions to Human Health: Does Sex Matter? Committee on Understanding the Biology of Sex and Gender Differences. Board on Health Sciences Policy, Institute of Medicine.* Washington, DC: National Academy Press; 2001.
42. Kajantie E, Phillips DI. The effects of sex and hormonal status on the physiological response to acute psychosocial stress. *Psychoneuroendocrinology.* 2006;31:151–178.

43. Adam K, Oswald I. Protein synthesis, bodily renewal and the sleep-wake cycle. *Clin Sci.* 1983;65:561–567.

44. Gillin JC, Byerley WF. The diagnosis and management of insomnia. *N Engl J Med.* 1990;322(4):239–248.

45. Ford-Gilboe M, Cohen JA. Hardiness: A model of commitment, challenge, and control. In: Rice VH, ed. *Handbook of Stress, Coping, and Health.* Thousand Oaks, CA: Sage; 2000: 425–436.

46. Sandvik AM, Bartone PT, Hystad SW, et al. Psychological hardiness predicts neuroimmunological responses to stress. *Psychol Health Med.* 2013;18(6):705–713.

47. Lehavot K, Der-Martirosian C, Simpson TL, et al. The role of military social support in understanding the relationship between PTSD, physical health, and healthcare utilization in women veterans. *J Trauma Stress.* 2013;26(6):772–775.

48. Arafah BM. Review: hypothalamic pituitary adrenal function during critical illness: limitations of current assessment methods. *J Clin Endocrinol Metab.* 2006;91:3725–3745.

49. Baranov D, Neligan P. Trauma and aggressive homeostasis management. *Anesthesiol Clin.* 2007;25:49–63.

50. Gibson SC, Hartman DA, Schenck JM. The endocrine responses to critical illness: update and implications for emergency medicine. *Emerg Med Clin North Am.* 2005;23:909–929.

51. Dandona P, Chaudhuri A, Ghanim H, et al. The effect of hyperglycemia and insulin in acute coronary syndromes. *Am J Cardiol.* 2007;99(suppl):12H–18H.

52. Marik PE, Raghavan M. Stress-hyperglycemia, insulin and immunomodulation in sepsis. *Intensive Care Med.* 2004;30:748–756.

53. Lipton J, Barendse R, VanDomburg R, et al. Hyperglycemia at admission and during hospital stay are independent risk factors for mortality in high risk cardiac patients admitted to an intensive care unit. *Eur Heart J Acute Cardiovasc Care.* 2013;2(4):306–313.

54. Schuetz P, Kennedy M, Lucas JM, et al. Initial management of septic patients with hyperglycemia in the noncritical care inpatient setting. *Am J Med.* 2012;125(7):670–678.

55. Neligan PJ, Baranov D. Trauma and aggressive homeostasis management. *Anesthesiol Clin.* 2013;31(1):21–31.

56. Harada S, Yamazaki Y, Nishioka H, et al. Neuroprotective effect through the cerebral sodium-glucose transporter on the development of ischemic damage in global ischemia. *Brain Res.* 2013;1541:61–68.

57. National Institute for Occupational Safety and Health. *Stress at work.* Publication no. 99-101, HE 20.7102: ST 8/4. Bethesda, MD: U.S. Department of Health and Human Services; 1999:1–26.

58. Dworkin SF. Psychosomatic concepts and dentistry: some perspectives. *J Periodontol.* 1969;40:647.

59. Takkouche B, Regueira C, Gestal-Otero JJ. A cohort study of stress and the common cold. *Epidemiology.* 2001;11:345–349.

60. Glaser R, Kiecot-Glaser JK, Marucha PT, et al. Stress-related changes in proinflammatory cytokine production in wounds. *Arch Gen Psychiatry.* 1999;56(5):450–456.

61. Wong SY, Wong CK, Chan FW, et al. Chronic psychosocial stress: does age modulate immunity to the influenza vaccine in Hong Kong Chinese elderly caregivers? *Age.* 2013;35(4):1479–1493.

62. Moreno-Smith M, Lutgendorf SK, Sood AK. Impact of stress on cancer metastasis. *Future Oncol.* 2010;6(12):1863–1881.

63. Edmondson D, Kronish IM, Shaffer JA, et al. Posttraumatic stress disorder and risk for coronary heart disease: a meta-analytic review. *Am Heart J.* 2013;166(5):806–814.

64. Galea S, Nandi A, Viahov D. The epidemiology of post-traumatic stress disorder after disasters. *Epidemiol Rev.* 2005;27:78–91.

65. McCloskey LA. Posttraumatic stress in children exposed to family violence and single event trauma. *J Am Acad Child Adolesc Psychiatry.* 2000;39:108–115.

66. Yehuda R. Post-traumatic stress disorder. *N Engl J Med.* 2002;346:108–114.

67. American Psychiatric Association. *Diagnostic and Statistical Manual of Mental Disorders,* 3rd ed., text rev. Washington, DC: American Psychiatric Society; 1980.

68. American Psychiatric Association. *Diagnostic and Statistical Manual of Mental Disorders,* 4th ed., text rev. Washington, DC: American Psychiatric Society; 1994.

69. American Psychiatric Association. *Diagnostic and Statistical Manual of Mental Disorders,* 5th ed., text rev. Washington DC: American Psychiatric Publishing.

70. Friedman MJ. Finalizing PTSD in DSM-5: getting from there and where to go next. *J Trauma Stress.* 2013;26(5):548–556.

71. Friedman MJ, Resick PA, Bryant RA, et al. Considering PTSD for DSM-5. *Depress Anxiety.* 2011;28(9):737–749.

72. Yehuda R. Biology of posttraumatic stress disorder. *J Clin Psychiatry.* 2000;61(suppl 7):14–21.

73. Logue MW, Solovieff N, Leussis MP, et al. The ankyrin-3 gene is associated with posttraumatic stress disorder and externalizing comorbidity. *Psychoneuroendocrinology.* 2013;38(10):2249–2257.

74. Xie P, Kranzler HR, Yang C, et al. Genome-wide association study identifies new susceptibility loci for posttraumatic stress disorder. *Biol Psychiatry.* 2013;74(9):656–663.

75. Cohen LR, Field C, Campbell AN, et al. Intimate partner violence outcomes in women with PTSD and substance use: a secondary analysis of NIDA Clinical Trials Network "Women and Trauma" Multi-site Study. *Addict Behav.* 2013;38(7):2325–2332.

76. Rosellini AJ, Coffey SF, Tracy M, et al. A person-centered analysis of posttraumatic stress disorder symptoms following a natural disaster: predictors of latent class membership. *J Anxiety Disord.* 2013;28(1):16–24.

77. Milad MR, Pitman RK, Ellis CB, et al. Neurobiological basis for failure to recall extinction memory in posttraumatic stress disorder. *Biol Psychiatry.* 2009;66(12):1075–1082.

78. Ben-Zeev D, Corrigan PW, Britt TW, et al. Stigma of mental illness and service use in the military. *J Ment Health.* 2010;21(3):264–273.

79. Mittal D, Blevins D, Corrigan P, et al. Stigma associated with PTSD: perceptions of treatment seeking combat veterans. *Psychiatr Rehabil J.* 2013;36(2):86–92.

80. American Psychiatric Association. Practice guidelines for the treatment of patients with acute stress disorder and posttraumatic stress disorder. *Am J Psychiatry.* 2004;161(suppl):1–31.

81. Cloitre M, Garvert DW, Brewin CR, et al. Evidence for proposed ICD-11 PTSD and complex PTSD: a latent profile analysis. *Eur J Psychotraumatol.* 2013;4. doi: 10.3402/ejpt.v4i0.20706.

82. Vieweg WVR, Julious DA, Fernandez A, et al. Posttraumatic stress disorder: clinical features, pathophysiology, and treatment. *Am J Med.* 2006;119(5):383–390.

83. Asmundson GJ, Fetzner MG, Deboer LB, et al. Let's get physical: a contemporary review of the anxiolytic effects of exercise for anxiety and its disorders. *Depress Anxiety.* 2013;30(4):362–373.

84. Benson H. Systemic hypertension and the relaxation response. *N Engl J Med.* 1977;296:1152–1154.

85. Jacobson E. *Progressive Relaxation.* Chicago, IL: University of Chicago Press; 1958.

86. Bernstein D, Borkovec T. *Progressive Muscle Relaxation: A Manual for the Helping Professionals.* Champaign, IL: Research Press; 1973.

87. Esch T, Fricchione GL, Stefano GB. The therapeutic use of relaxation response in stress-related diseases. *Med Sci Monit.* 2003;9(2):RA23–RA34.

88. Reed T. Imagery in the clinical setting: a tool for healing. *Nurs Clin North Am.* 2007;42:261–277.

89. Schaeffer L, Jallo N, Howland L, et al. Guided imagery: an innovative approach to improving maternal sleep quality. *J Perinat Neonatal Nurs.* 2013;27(2):151–159.

90. Tusek DL, Cwynar RE. Strategies for implementing a guided imagery program to enhance patient experience. *AACN Clin Issues.* 2000;11(1):68–76.

91. Kwekkeboom KL, Abbott-Anderson K, Wanta B. Feasibility of a patient-controlled cognitive-behavioral intervention for pain, fatigue, and sleep disturbance in cancer. *Oncol Nurs Forum.* 2010;37(3):E151–E159.

92. White JM. State of the science of music interventions. Critical care and perioperative practice. *Crit Care Nurs Clin North Am.* 2000;12(2):219–225.

93. Chlan LL, Weinert CR, Heiderscheit A, et al. Effects of patient-directed music intervention on anxiety and sedative exposure in critically ill patients receiving mechanical ventilatory support: a randomized clinical trial. *JAMA.* 2013;309(22):2335–2344.

94. Gutgsell KJ, Schluchter M, Margevicius S, et al. Music therapy reduces pain in palliative care patients: a randomized controlled trial. *J Pain Symptom Manage.* 2013;45(5):822–831.

95. Ko YL, Lin PC. The effect of using a relaxation tape on pulse, respiration, blood pressure and anxiety levels of surgical patients. *J Clin Nurs.* 2012;21(5–6):689–697.

96. Vickers A, Zollman C. ABC of complementary therapies: massage therapies. *Br Med J.* 1999;319:1254–1257.

97. Rusy LM, Weisman SJ. Complementary therapies for acute pediatric pain management. *Pediatr Clin North Am.* 2000;47:589–599.

98. Rowe M, Alfred D. The effectiveness of slow-stroke massage in diffusing agitated behaviors in individuals with Alzheimer's disease. *J Gerontol Nurs.* 1999;25(6):22–34.

99. Braun LA, Stanguts C, Casanelia L, et al. Massage therapy for cardiac surgery patients—a randomized trial. *J Thorac Cardiovasc Surg.* 2012;144(6):1453–1459.

100. Richards KC. Effect of back massage and relaxation intervention on sleep in critically ill patients. *Am J Crit Care.* 1998;7:288–299.

101. Jane SW, Chen SL, Wilkie DJ, et al. Effects of massage on pain, mood status, relaxation, and sleep in Taiwanese patients with metastatic bone pain: a randomized clinical trial. *Pain.* 2011;152(10):2432–2442.

102. Suzuki M, Tatsumi A, Otsuka T, et al. Physical and psychological effects of 6-week tactile massage on elderly patients with severe dementia. *Am J Alzheimers Dis Other Demen.* 2010;25(8):680–686.

103. McKee MG. Biofeedback: an overview in the context of heart-brain medicine. *Cleve Clin J Med.* 2008;75(2):S31–S34.

104. Prato CA, Yucha CB. Biofeedback-assisted relaxation training to decrease test anxiety in nursing students. *Nurs Educ Perspect.* 2013;34(2):76–81.

105. Ding M, Lin Z, Lin L, et al. The effect of biofeedback training on patients with functional constipation. *Gastroenterol Nurs.* 2012;35(2):85–92.

106. Slutsker B, Konichezky A, Gothelf D. Breaking the cycle: cognitive behavioral therapy and biofeedback training in a case of cyclic vomiting syndrome. *Psychol Health Med.* 2010;15(6):625–631.

Porth Essentials Resources

Explore these additional resources to enhance learning for this chapter:

- NCLEX-Style Questions and Other Resources on thePoint, http://thePoint.lww.com/PorthEssentials4e
- Study Guide for Essentials of Pathophysiology
- Adaptive Learning | Powered by PrepU, http://thepoint.lww.com/prepu

C h a p t e r **10**

Disorders of Nutritional Status

Nutritional status describes the condition of the body related to the availability and use of nutrients. Nutrients that are taken into the body can be used to provide the energy needed to perform various body functions or they can be stored for future use. The stability of body weight and composition of lean-to-fat tissue ratio over time requires that a person's energy intake is balanced with energy expenditure. Also, because different foods contain different amounts of proteins, fats, carbohydrates, vitamins, and minerals, appropriate amounts of these nutrients must be maintained to ensure that the body's metabolic systems are adequately supplied. This chapter discusses nutritional status, overnutrition and obesity, and undernutrition and eating disorders.

Energetics and Nutritional Status

The nutrients from the foods we eat are used by cells to provide the body with the energy needed to perform almost all cellular functions. Energy is measured in heat units called *calories*. A calorie, spelled with a small "c" and also called a *gram calorie*, is the amount of heat or energy required to raise the temperature of 1 g of water by 1°C. A *kilocalorie* (kcal), or *large calorie* (abbreviated as a capital C), is the amount of energy needed to raise the temperature of 1 kg of water by 1°C. Because a calorie is so small, kilocalories often are used in nutritional and physiologic studies.

Energy Metabolism

Metabolism is the organized process through which nutrients—carbohydrates, fats, and proteins—are broken down, transformed, or otherwise converted into cellular energy. The oxidation of carbohydrates and proteins provides 4 kcal/g, whereas fats yield 9 kcal/g.[1]

The process of metabolism is unique in that it enables the continual release of energy, and it couples this energy with physiologic functioning. For example, the energy used for muscle contraction is derived largely from energy sources that are stored in muscle cells and then released as the muscle contracts. Because most of our energy sources come from the nutrients in food that is eaten, the ability to store energy and control its release is important. Normally, energy utilization is balanced with energy expenditure. When the intake of food consistently exceeds energy expenditure, the excess energy is stored as fat, and the person becomes overweight. Conversely, when food intake does not meet energy expenditure, fat stores and other body tissues are broken down and the person loses weight.

More than 90% of body energy is stored as triglycerides in the fat cells of the body. The body has a limited ability to store dietary carbohydrates and proteins as energy sources. Dietary carbohydrates are largely converted to glucose, which is stored as glycogen in liver and skeletal muscle cells. Liver glycogen stores reach a maximum of approximately 200 to 300 g after a high-carbohydrate meal, after which the liver begins to convert some of the excess glucose to triglycerides for storage in fat cells. The amino acids from protein in the diet are stored mainly in the form of structural proteins, enzymes, nucleoproteins, and other types of cellular proteins. After all the cells have reached their limits, the excess amino acids are converted to glucose and used for energy or stored in the liver as glycogen or in adipose tissue as triglycerides.

Triglycerides, which contain no water, have the highest caloric content of all nutrients and are an efficient form of energy storage. When calorie intake is restricted for any reason, the triglycerides in fat cells are broken down, and their fatty acids and glycerol released as energy sources. Fat cells synthesize triglycerides from glucose and fatty acids. Insulin is required for fat storage. It promotes glucose transport through the cell membrane of fat cells. Some of the glucose is used to synthesize fatty acids, but more importantly it forms large amounts of α-glycerol phosphate. This compound supplies the glycerol that combines with fatty acids to form triglycerides. Therefore, in the absence of insulin, the storage of triglycerides in adipose tissue is almost blocked.

Fat cells, or *adipocytes*, are modified fibroblasts that store almost pure triglycerides in quantities as great as 80% to 95% of their total cell volume.[1] Adipocytes occur singly or in small groups in adipose connective tissue, entire regions of which are committed to triglyceride storage. Collectively, adipocytes constitute a large body organ that is metabolically active in the uptake, synthesis, storage, and mobilization of lipids. In addition, adipose tissue provides insulation for the body, fills body crevices, and protects body organs.[2]

Early studies suggested that fully differentiated adipocytes do not undergo further cell division, and thus that the number of fat cells is fixed in early childhood. This theory proposed that subsequent gains in adipose tissue represented increases in fat cell size. This is no longer considered to be true, since adipose tissue in adults is now known to contain *preadipocytes*, capable of forming new fat cells, and fat deposition can result from proliferation of these immature adipocytes.[3]

Some medications can also increase fat cell numbers. For example, the thiazolidinedione (TZD) class of antidiabetic drugs can stimulate the formation of new fat cells from the preadipocytes, allowing increased uptake of glucose into these cells (and storage as fat), resulting in the desired reduction in serum glucose levels but with unwanted weight gain.[4] In contrast, some drugs can cause loss of fat cells. This occurs in persons who are HIV-positive and are treated with highly active antiretroviral therapy (see Chapter 16). The mechanism of fat loss is not known; however, it may be due to increased apoptosis (programmed cell death) of the adipocytes.

There are two types of adipose tissue: white (unilocular) and brown (multilocular).[2] *White fat*, which despite its name is cream colored or yellow, is the predominant form of adipose tissue in adults. The adipocytes of white fat are large spherical cells that become polyhedral or oval when crowded in adipose tissue. The functions of white fat include energy storage, endocrine and adipocytokine secretion, insulation, and cushioning of vital organs. In the connective tissue under the skin, the white fat layer has significant insulating functions. Concentrations are found under the skin of the abdomen, buttocks, axilla, and thigh. Sex differences in the thickness of this fatty layer in different parts of the body account, in part, for the differences in body composition between males and females. Internally, white adipose tissue is preferentially located in the greater omentum, mesentery, and retroperitoneal space and is usually abundant around the kidney. It is also found in the orbits around the eyeballs, in the bone marrow, and between other tissues, where it fills spaces. It retains this structural function even during reduced caloric intake, when the lipid content of adipose tissue elsewhere has been depleted.[2]

Brown fat differs from white fat in terms of its thermogenic capacity (its ability to produce heat). The color of brown fat reflects the presence of iron in its abundant mitochondria. Brown fat mitochondria produce a specific protein called uncoupling protein-1 (UCP-1) that releases the energy generated from metabolism as heat. It is found abundantly in newborns, in whom thermogenesis is critical because of their proportionally greater heat loss as compared to adults and their reduced ability to shiver. Historically, adults were thought to have only a small amount of brown fat; however, recent studies have confirmed that moderate deposits of brown fat are commonly present in adults and can be stimulated by several factors including cold and the sympathetic nervous system.

Nutritional Status

The body obtains the energy needed to perform its various functions and maintain the integrity and health of its cells from the various foods that are consumed in the diet. Because different foods contain different proportions of proteins, carbohydrates, fats, minerals, and vitamins, appropriate balances must be maintained among these constituents so that all segments of the body's metabolic systems can be supplied with the prerequisite materials.

Dietary Reference Intakes

The Dietary Reference Intakes (DRIs) are a set of reference values that identify the level of nutrient intake an individual needs to maintain health and decrease the risk for disease.[5] They are published by the National Academy of Sciences and are periodically reviewed and updated by the Institute of Medicine's Food and Nutrition Board. A complete database of the DRIs is available online through the United States Department of Agriculture Food and Nutrition Information Center.[6]

The DRIs are a set of reference values that identify the recommended estimated average requirement, dietary allowance, adequate intake, tolerable upper intake level, and acceptable macronutrient distribution range, each of which has specific uses.[5] An Estimated Average Requirement (EAR) is the intake that meets the estimated nutrient need of half of the persons in a specific group. This figure is used as the basis for developing the Recommended Dietary Allowance (RDA), which defines the nutrient intakes that meet the needs of almost all healthy persons in a specific age and sex group.[5] The Adequate Intake (AI) is set when there is not enough scientific evidence to derive an EAR and therefore the RDA. The AI is derived from experimental or observational data that show a mean intake that appears to sustain a desired indicator of health. The Tolerable Upper Intake Level (UL) is the maximum intake that is judged unlikely to pose a health risk in almost all healthy persons in a specified group. It refers to the total intake from food, fortified food, and nutrient supplements. This value is not intended to be a recommended level of intake, and there is no established benefit for persons who consume nutrients above the RDA or AI levels. The Acceptable Macronutrient Distribution Range (AMDR) is a percentage of energy intake for carbohydrates, proteins, and fats, including the linoleic and α-linolenic essential fatty acids,

that is associated with good health. For example, the AMDR for protein is 10% to 35%; that is, no less than 10% and no more than 35% of the total energy (calorie) intake should come from proteins. Finally, the DRI for total energy is the estimated energy requirement (EER).

Food and supplement labels use the percent *Daily Value* (%DV), which is set by the Food and Drug Administration (FDA). The %DV tells the consumer what percent of an individual's daily need for a given nutrient one serving of a food or supplement supplies. Because individuals of different age and sex have different nutrient needs, the percent of DV is intended to be used as an example. It is based on a 2,000-calorie diet.

Calories

Energy requirements are greater during growth periods. Infants require approximately 115 kcal/kg of body weight at birth, 105 kcal/kg at 1 year of age, and 80 kcal/kg between 1 and 10 years of age. During adolescence, boys require 45 kcal/kg of body weight and girls require 38 kcal/kg. During pregnancy, a woman needs an extra 300 kcal/day above her usual requirement, and during the first 3 months of breast-feeding, she requires an additional 500 kcal.[5] Table 10-1 identifies the EER for healthy adults.[7]

Proteins, Fats, and Carbohydrates

Proteins, fats, and carbohydrates yield energy. They are referred to as macronutrients because the body requires them in relatively large amounts.

Proteins. Proteins are required for growth and maintenance of body tissues, enzymes and antibody formation, fluid and electrolyte balance, and nutrient transport. Proteins are composed of amino acids, nine of which

| TABLE 10-1 | Estimated Energy Requirements (EER) at Different Activity Levels for Men and Women 30 Years of Age With a Normal (<25), Overweight (25 to 29.9), and Obese (≥30) BMI |

BMI	Height m (in.)	Weight kg (lb)	Activity Level*	EER (kcal/d) Male	EER (kcal/d) Female
22.1 Normal	1.75 (69)	68 (150)	Rarely	2404	2055
			Low activity	2627	2285
			Active	2911	2571
			Very active	3378	2915
26.5 Overweight	1.75 (69)	77 (170)	Rarely	2620	2140
			Low activity	2867	2380
			Active	3182	2679
			Very active	3698	3038
31 Obese	1.75 (69)	95 (210)	Rarely	2837	2310
			Low activity	3108	2570
			Active	3452	2894
			Very active	4018	3284

*Activity level definitions:
  Sedentary = rarely exercises
  Low active = less 1 hour/day
  Active = about 1 hour/day
  Very active = more than 1 hour/day

Developed using "Adult Energy Needs and BMI Calculator" from USDA/ARS Children's Nutrition Center at Baylor College of Medicine. Available: http://www.bcm.edu/cnrc/caloriesneed.cfm. Accessed September 6, 2013.

are essential to the body. These are leucine, isoleucine, methionine, phenylalanine, threonine, tryptophan, valine, lysine, and histidine. The foods that provide these essential amino acids in adequate amounts are milk, eggs, meat, fish, and poultry. Dried peas and beans, nuts, seeds, and grains contain all the essential amino acids but in less than adequate proportions. These proteins need to be combined with each other or with complete proteins to meet the amino acid requirements for protein synthesis.

Unlike carbohydrates and fats, which are composed of hydrogen, carbon, and oxygen, proteins contain nitrogen; therefore, nitrogen excretion is an indicator of protein intake. The average protein contains about 16% nitrogen. About 90% of this is excreted in the urine as urea, uric acid, creatinine, and other less important nitrogen breakdown products, with the rest being excreted in the feces.[1] Therefore, the rate of protein breakdown can be estimated by measuring the amount of nitrogen in the urine. If the amount of nitrogen taken in by way of protein is equivalent to the nitrogen excreted, the person is said to be in nitrogen balance. A person is in positive nitrogen balance when the nitrogen consumed by way of protein is greater than the amount excreted. This occurs during growth, pregnancy, or healing after surgery or injury. A negative nitrogen balance often occurs with fever, illness, infection, trauma, or burns, when more nitrogen is excreted than is consumed.[1] It represents a state of tissue breakdown.

Fats. Dietary fats are composed primarily of triglycerides (i.e., a compound consisting of three fatty acid chains attached to a glycerol backbone). Saturated fatty acids have no double bonds between carbon atoms in the chains, whereas monounsaturated fatty acids have one double bond in the chain, and polyunsaturated fatty acids have two or more double bonds. The saturated fatty acids elevate blood cholesterol, whereas the monounsaturated and polyunsaturated fats lower blood cholesterol. Saturated fats are usually derived from animal sources and remain solid at room temperature. With the exception of coconut and palm oils (which are saturated), unsaturated fats are found in plant oils and usually are liquid at room temperature. *Trans fatty* acids are produced when unsaturated oils are partially hydrogenated and are called *artificial trans fats*. They are found primarily in vegetable shortenings and some margarines and foods. Small amounts of *natural trans fatty acids* are found in dairy products, some meats, and other animal-based foods. Although *trans* fatty acids tend to increase low-density lipoprotein (LDL) cholesterol and decrease high-density lipoprotein (HDL) cholesterol, the naturally occurring trans fats may have a beneficial effect.

Dietary fats provide energy, function as carriers for the fat-soluble vitamins, serve as precursors of prostaglandins, and are a source of the essential fatty acids, linoleic and alpha-linolenic acids.[7] Because vegetable oils are rich sources of linoleic acid, this level can be met by including two teaspoons per day of vegetable oil in the diet. Alpha-linolenic acid is found primarily in dark green, leafy vegetables, certain plant oils, soybeans, and walnuts. The ADMR for fat is 20% to 35% to prevent the fall of HDL cholesterol associated with very–low-fat diets.[7] Guidelines from the National Cholesterol Education Program recommend that 25% to 35% of the calories in the diet should come from fats.[8] The daily dietary recommendation for cholesterol is less than 300 mg. The American Heart Association recommends limiting saturated fat to less than 7% and trans fatty acids to less than 1% of calories daily.[9]

Carbohydrates. Dietary carbohydrates include simple sugars, such as glucose, sucrose, and fructose, as well as complex carbohydrates, which are commonly called starches. Fiber is an indigestible form of complex carbohydrate. It is recommended that the majority of carbohydrates consumed in the diet be complex carbohydrates, which are rich in fiber and a variety of vitamins and minerals. In contrast, simple sugars do not provide fiber and, unless fortified, usually contain few vitamins and minerals. Moreover, sucrose (i.e., table sugar) is implicated in the development of dental caries, and excessive dietary fructose (e.g., from high-fructose corn syrup in soft drinks and other sweetened foods and beverages) has been increasingly associated with childhood and adult obesity, diabetes, and cardiovascular disease.

The current RDA for adults is 130 g of carbohydrates per day. Some tissues, such as the nervous system, require glucose as an energy source. Although this need can be met by gluconeogenesis, in which amino acids are converted to glucose, a carbohydrate-deficient diet usually results in the loss of tissue proteins. The fatty acids from triglycerides can be converted to ketones and used for energy by other body tissues when glucose is inadequate; however, excessive ketone production can prompt the development of ketosis. Because protein and fat metabolism increases the production of osmotically active metabolic wastes that must be eliminated through the kidneys, there is also danger of dehydration and electrolyte imbalances. The minimum amount of carbohydrates needed to prevent tissue wasting and ketosis is 50 to 100 g/day. In practice, most of the daily energy requirement should be from dietary carbohydrate sources. This is because protein is an expensive source of calories, and it is recommended that dietary fat not exceed 35% of the calorie intake. The AMDR for carbohydrates intake is 45% to 65% of total calories to prevent a high intake of fat.[7]

Vitamins and Minerals

Vitamins are a group of organic compounds essential for numerous body functions. A compound cannot be classified as a vitamin unless it is shown that a deficiency causes disease. Contrary to popular belief, vitamins do not provide energy directly. Instead, many act as coenzymes, components of the enzyme systems required for the release of energy from protein, fat, and carbohydrates. Vitamins also are necessary for the formation of red blood cells, hormones, genetic materials, and the nervous system. They are essential for normal growth and development.

There are two types of vitamins: fat soluble and water soluble. The four fat-soluble vitamins are vitamins A, D,

E, and K. They require dietary fat for absorption and transport. The nine water-soluble vitamins are vitamin C and the B vitamins, which are thiamine, riboflavin, niacin, vitamin B_6, pantothenic acid, vitamin B_{12}, folate, and biotin. Because excess amounts of the water-soluble vitamins are excreted in the urine, it is less likely that they may become toxic to the body, but the fat-soluble vitamins are stored in adipose tissue and may reach toxic levels.

Minerals are inorganic elements, not compounds; however, they often function as components of certain enzyme systems, vitamins, and hormones. They are involved in energy metabolism, acid-base balance, maintenance of normal hemoglobin levels, and play a role in nervous system function, are involved in muscle contraction and skeletal development and maintenance, and are major components of bone tissue. Minerals that are present in relatively large amounts in the body are called *major minerals*. These include calcium, phosphorus, sodium, chloride, potassium, magnesium, and sulfur. The remainder are classified as *trace minerals*; they include iron, manganese, copper, iodine, zinc, cobalt, fluoride, chromium, molybdenum, and selenium.

Fiber

Fiber cannot be digested by the human gastrointestinal system and is not classified as a nutrient; however, it increases stool bulk and facilitates bowel movements. Soluble fiber, the type that produces a gel in the intestinal tract, binds with cholesterol and prevents it from being absorbed by the body. Soluble fiber also lowers blood glucose. More studies are needed to establish whether fiber prevents colon cancer and promotes weight loss. The adequate daily intake for fiber for adult men and women up to age 50 is 38 and 25 g, respectively. Adults over age 50 should consume 30 and 21 g, respectively, each day. The recommendation for children ranges from 19 to 31 g, and the recommendation for teenagers is similar to that for adults.[7]

Regulation of Food Intake

Stability of body weight and composition over time requires that energy intake matches energy utilization. Environmental, cultural, genetic, and psychological factors all influence food intake and energy expenditure. In addition, body weight is tightly controlled by various physiologic feedback control systems that contribute to the regulation of hunger and food intake.

Hunger, Appetite, and Satiety

Hunger and appetite are closely associated with food intake. The sensation of *hunger* is associated with several sensory perceptions, such as the rhythmic contractions of the stomach and that "empty feeling" in the stomach that stimulates a person to seek food. A person's *appetite* is the desire for a particular type of food. It is useful in helping the person determine the type of food that is eaten. *Satiety* is the feeling of fullness or decreased desire for food.

The hypothalamus contains the feeding center for hunger and satiety[1] (Fig. 10-1). It receives neural input from the gastrointestinal tract, which provides information about stomach distention, chemical signals from nutrients (glucose, amino acids, and fatty acids) in the blood, and input from the cerebral cortex regarding the smell, sight, and taste of the food. Centers in the hypothalamus also control the secretion of several hormones (e.g., thyroid and adrenocortical hormones) that regulate energy balance and metabolism.

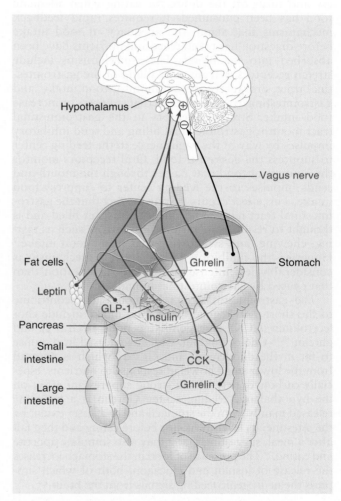

FIGURE 10-1. Feedback mechanisms for control of food intake. *Black lines* leading to – indicate feedback signals that decrease appetite and feeding, and *blue lines* with + indicate feedback signals that increase appetite and feeding. Stretch receptors in the stomach activate sensory afferent vagal pathways that inhibit food intake. Glucagon-like peptide-1 (GLP-1), cholecystokinin (CCK), and insulin are gastrointestinal hormones that are released by the ingestion of food and suppress further feeding. Ghrelin, which is released by the stomach and small intestine, especially during fasting, stimulates appetite. Leptin is a hormone produced by increasing amounts of fat cells as they increase in size; it inhibits food intake. (Modified from Guyton AC, Hall JE. *Textbook of Medical Physiology*. 11th ed. Philadelphia, PA: Elsevier Saunders; 2006:868.)

Regulatory Mechanisms

The control of food intake can be divided into short-term regulation, which is concerned with the amount of food that is consumed at a meal or snack, and intermediate and long-term regulation, which is concerned with the maintenance of constant stores of nutrients in the tissues, preventing them from becoming too low or too high.[1]

Short-Term Regulation. The short-term regulation of food intake provides a person with the feeling of satiety and turns off the desire for eating when adequate food has been consumed. It requires rapid feedback mechanisms that signal the adequacy of food intake before digestion has taken place and nutrients have been absorbed into the blood. These mechanisms include stretch receptors that monitor filling of the gastrointestinal tract, oral receptors that monitor food intake, and gastrointestinal tract hormones that suppress or increase food intake. Stretch receptors in the gastrointestinal tract monitor gastrointestinal filling and send inhibitory impulses by way of the vagus nerve to the feeding center to suppress the desire for food. Oral receptors monitor the amount of food that passes through the mouth and sends impulses to the feeding center to suppress food intake. This effect occurs despite the fact that the gastrointestinal tract has not become the least bit filled and is thought to result from various oral factors such as tasting, chewing, and swallowing that meter food intake.[1] However, the inhibition caused by this mechanism is considerably less intense and of shorter duration than that caused by gastrointestinal filling.

The gastrointestinal tract hormones that contribute to the short-term regulation of food intake include cholecytokinin (CCK), glucagon-like peptide 1 (GLP-1), and ghrelin.[10,11] Cholecytokinin, which is released in response to fat in the duodenum, and GLP-1, which is released from the lower small bowel in response to nutrients, especially carbohydrates, have a strong suppressant effect on the hypothalamic feeding center. Ghrelin is a hormone released mainly from the stomach and to a lesser extent by the intestine. Its levels peak just before eating and then fall after a meal, suggesting that it may also stimulate appetite and eating.[10] The presence of food in the stomach increases the release of insulin and glucagon, both of which suppress the neurogenic feeding signals from the brain.[1]

Intermediate and Long-Term Regulation. The intermediate and long-term regulation of food intake is determined by the amount of nutrients that are in the blood and in storage sites. It has long been known that a decrease in blood glucose causes hunger. In contrast, an increase in breakdown products of lipids such as ketoacids produces a decrease in appetite. A ketogenic weight loss diet (the Atkins diet) relies partly on the appetite suppressant effects of ketones in the blood.

Recent evidence suggests that the hypothalamus also senses the amount of energy through a hormone called *leptin* that is produced by fat cells.[1] The stimulation of leptin receptors in the hypothalamus has been shown to produce a decrease in appetite and food intake as well as an increase in metabolic rate and energy consumption. It also produces a decrease in insulin release from the beta cells of the pancreas, which decreases energy storage in fat cells.

Assessment of Energy Stores and Nutritional Status

The nutritional status of an individual can be assessed in a number of ways including a history of weight gain or loss, dietary intake, gastrointestinal symptoms that affect food intake, functional capacity, and physical signs of fat loss and muscle wasting. This information is usually combined with other objective measures of fat stores and skeletal muscle mass.

Anthropometric Measurements

Anthropometric measurements provide a means for assessing body composition, particularly fat stores and skeletal muscle mass.[12] This is done by measuring height, weight, body circumferences, and thickness of various skinfold areas. These measurements commonly are used to determine growth patterns in children and appropriateness of current weight in adults.

Body weight is the most frequently used method of assessing nutritional status; it should be used in combination with measurements of body height to establish whether a person is underweight or overweight. For weight measurement, subjects should ideally be in light clothing and bare feet, fasting, and with an empty bladder. Repeat measurements are best made at the same time of the day.

The body mass index (BMI) uses height and weight to determine healthy weight (Table 10-2). It is calculated by dividing the weight in kilograms by the height in meters squared (BMI = weight [kg]/height [m²]).[13] A BMI less than 18.5 is classified as being underweight and one between 25 and 29.9 is considered overweight.[13] A BMI at or greater than 30.0 is diagnosed as obesity and is furthered classified into classes I (BMI 30.0 to 34.9), II (BMI 35.0 to 39.9), and III or extreme obesity (BMI > 40). Body weight reflects both lean body mass and adipose tissue and cannot be used as a method for describing body composition or the percentage of fat tissue present. Statistically, the best percentage of body fat for men is between 12% and 20%, and for women, it is between 20% and 30%.[14] During physical training, body fat usually decreases, and lean body mass increases.

Among the methods used to estimate body fat are body circumferences, skinfold thickness, bioelectrical impedance, computed tomography (CT), and magnetic resonance imaging (MRI).[12] The measurement of *body circumferences* has received attention because excess visceral (or intra-abdominal) fat is closely associated with metabolic syndrome (i.e., a syndrome described by a collection of cardiovascular risk factors).[15,16] Measurements of *skinfold thickness* can provide a reasonable assessment of body fat, particularly if taken at

Classification of Overweight and Obesity by BMI, Waist Circumference, and Associated Disease Risk*

	BMI (kg/m²)	Obesity Class	Disease Risk* Relative to Normal Weight and Waist Circumference	
			Men ≤102 cm (≤40 in.) Women ≤88 cm (≤35 in.)	Men >102 cm (>40 in.) Women >88 cm (>35 in.)
Underweight	<18.5		—	—
Normal†	18.5–24.9		—	—
Overweight	25.0–29.9		Increased	High
Obesity	30.0–34.9	I	High	Very high
	35.0–39.9	II	Very high	Very high
Extreme obesity	≥40	III	Extremely high	Extremely high

BMI, body mass index.

*Disease risk for type 2 diabetes, hypertension, and cardiovascular disease.

†Increased waist circumference also can be a marker for increased risk, even in persons of normal weight.

Pi-Sunyer FX, Dietz WH, Becker DM, et al., for the NHLBI Obesity Education Initiative Expert Panel on the Identification, Evaluation, and Treatment of Overweight and Obesity in Adults. *Clinical Guidelines on the Identification, Evaluation, and Treatment of Overweight and Obesity in Adults.* 1998. NIH Publication No. 98–4083. Available at: http://www.nhlbi.nih.gov/guidelines/obesity/ob_gdlns.pdf

multiple sites. They can provide information about the location of the fat and can be used together with equations and tables to estimate the percentage of lean body mass and fat tissue. However, these measurements often are difficult to perform, are subject to considerable variation between clinicians, and do not provide information about abdominal and intramuscular fat.

Bioelectrical impedance involves the use of electrodes attached to the wrists and ankles to send a harmless current through the body. The flow of the current is affected by the amount of water in the body. Because fat-free tissue contains virtually all the water and current-conducting electrolytes, measurements of the resistance (i.e., impedance) can be used to estimate the percentage of body fat present.

Computed tomography and MRI can be used to provide quantitative pictures from which the thickness of fat can be determined. Computed tomography scans also can be used to provide quantitative estimates of regional fat and give a ratio of intra-abdominal to extra-abdominal fat. Another novel way of measuring body composition is the BOD POD. The subject sits inside the device, and air displacement is measured to determine body composition (i.e., fat vs. lean tissue). Because these methods are costly, they usually are reserved for research studies.

Laboratory Studies

Various laboratory tests can aid in evaluating nutritional status. Some of the most commonly performed tests are serum albumin and prealbumin to assess the protein status, total lymphocyte count and delayed hypersensitivity reaction to assess cellular immunity, and creatinine–height index to assess skeletal muscle protein. Vitamin and mineral deficiencies can be determined by measurements of their levels in blood, saliva, and other body tissues or by measuring nutrient-specific chemical reactions.

SUMMARY CONCEPTS

■ Nutritional status describes the condition of the body related to the availability and use of nutrients, which provide the energy and materials necessary for performing the activities of daily living and for the growth and repair of body tissues.

■ Metabolism is the organized process whereby nutrients such as carbohydrates, fats, and proteins are broken down, transformed, or otherwise converted to cellular energy, measured in kilocalories (kcal or C). *Carbohydrates* are the body's primary source of immediate energy. They supply 4 kcal/g, are stored in limited quantities as glycogen and can be converted to fatty acids. *Fats* are a concentrated water-free energy source. They contain 9 kcal/g and are stored in fat cells as triglycerides. *Proteins*, which are broken down into amino acids, generate 4 kcal/g. However, their main role is in building functional and structural body proteins. Excesses of any of the macronutrients will be stored as triglycerides in adipose tissue. Water, vitamins, and minerals are other essential nutrients.

■ Nutritional status can be assessed by evaluation of dietary intake; anthropometric measurements such as measurements of height and weight, body circumference, and skinfold thickness; and laboratory tests.

Overweight and Obesity

Overweight and obesity have become global health problems, increasing the risk of hypertension, hyperlipidemia, type 2 diabetes, coronary heart disease, and other health problems. According to recent worldwide estimates, 1.7 billion people are classified as overweight, more than 1 billion have hypertension, and more than 500 million have either diabetes or impaired glucose tolerance.[17]

Obesity is defined as having excess body fat, enlarged fat cells, and even an increased number of fat cells.[18] Clinically, obesity and overweight have been defined in terms of the BMI. Historically, various world bodies have used different BMI cutoff points to define obesity. In 1997, the World Health Organization (WHO) defined the various classifications of overweight (BMI $\geq$ 25) and obesity (BMI $\geq$ 30). This classification was subsequently adopted by the National Institutes of Health (NIH).[13] The use of a BMI cutoff of 25 as a measure of overweight raised some concern in that the BMI of some men might be increased due to muscle rather than fat weight. However, it has been shown that a BMI cutoff of 25 can sensitively detect most overweight people and does not erroneously detect overly lean people. An important caveat is that certain ethnicities (e.g., Asians), can develop complications from lower levels of BMI and waist circumference than Caucasians. This has resulted in ethnicity-specific definitions being adopted (e.g., overweight in Asians is defined as >23) by the WHO.

Obesity is associated with increased risk for developing many medical, psychosocial, and behavioral problems. In terms of health problems, many disorders occur more frequently in obese people (Fig. 10-2). The most important and common of these are hyperlipidemia, hypertension, coronary artery disease, stroke, and type 2 diabetes mellitus. The increased weight associated with obesity stresses the bones and joints, increasing the likelihood of osteoarthritis. Certain cancers (endometrial, prostate, colon, uterine, ovarian), thromboembolic disorders, and gastrointestinal tract disease (gastroesophageal reflux and gallbladder disease) are also more prevalent in the obese.[19] Other conditions associated with obesity include sleep apnea and pulmonary dysfunction, menstrual irregularities and complications of pregnancy, psychological distress, and nonalcoholic fatty liver disease (discussed in Chapter 30). Because some drugs are lipophilic and exhibit increased distribution in fat tissue, the administration of these drugs, including some anesthetic agents, can be more dangerous in obese persons. If surgery is required, obese persons heal slower and are at increased risk from anesthesia. Massive obesity, because of its close association with so many health problems, can be regarded as a disease in its own right. It is the second leading cause of preventable death.

Causes of Overweight and Obesity

Factors that are thought to lead to the development of overweight and obesity include the interaction of genotype and environmental factors, including diet and

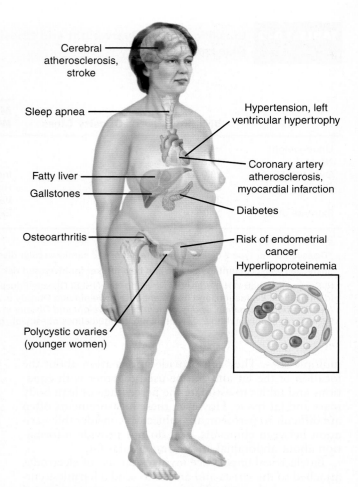

FIGURE 10-2. Clinical manifestations of obesity.

physical activity. Obesity is known to run in families, suggesting a hereditary component. The question that surrounds this observation is whether the disorder arises because of genetic endowment or environmental influences. Studies of twin and adopted children have provided evidence that heredity contributes to the disorder.[20] The most recent update of the human obesity gene map suggests that there are about 30 obesity candidate genes that might contribute to the risk of obesity in humans.[21] It is unknown what combinations of genes and mutations are involved in these risk factors and how environmental factors interact with them.

Although genetic factors may explain some of the individual variations in terms of excess weight, environmental influences are major contributors. These influences include family eating patterns, inactivity because of labor-saving devices and time spent on the computer and watching television, reliance on the automobile for transportation, easy access to food, energy density of food, increased consumption of sugar-sweetened beverages (especially fructose),[22] and increasing portion sizes.[23] The obese may be greatly influenced by the availability of food, the flavor of food, time of day, and other cues. The composition of the diet also may be a causal factor, and the percentage of dietary fat independent of total caloric intake may play a part in the development of obesity. Psychological factors include using food as a reward, comfort, or means of getting attention. Eating may be a way to cope with tension, anxiety, and mental fatigue.

Adipose Tissue

Adipose tissue is no longer simply viewed as a reservoir for energy storage. Adipose tissue is now known to express and secrete a variety of bioactive peptides, known as *adipocytokines* (e.g., leptin, tumor necrosis factor-α [TNF-α], interleukin-6 [IL-6]) that have autocrine, paracrine, and endocrine effects on the brain, liver, skeletal muscle, and other tissues of the body.[24] In addition, adipose tissue expresses numerous receptors that allow it to respond to afferent signals from traditional hormone systems as well as the central nervous system. Through this interactive network adipose tissue is integrally involved in coordinating a variety of physiologic processes including energy metabolism, neuroendocrine function, and immune function. It is the dysfunctional aspects of these processes that are implicated in the pathogenesis and adverse effects of adipose tissue excess or obesity.

Adipose Tissue as an Endocrine Organ

Adipose tissue is now recognized as an endocrine organ that produces several hormones, including *leptin*, an important mediator of body weight, and *adiponectin*, which regulates sensitivity to insulin and may be involved in the pathogenesis of type 2 diabetes.[24,25]

Leptin (from the Greek meaning "thin"), a peptide released from adipocytes, has led to renewed interest in the function of adipose tissue and its role in energy homeostasis. Leptin acts through binding to and activation of specific leptin receptors found in several peripheral tissues and in many areas of the brain, including specific regions of the hypothalamus. Receptors in these hypothalamic regions are known to be involved in appetite, food intake, sympathetic nervous system activity, temperature regulation, and insulin release by the pancreatic beta cells. Leptin levels rise following food intake, signaling the sensation of satiety, and fall during fasting, stimulating the sensation of appetite. Congenital leptin deficiency has been associated with hyperphagia (excessive eating) and obesity, impaired thermogenesis, insulin resistance, and hyperlipidemia, all reversed by leptin treatment.[25] The biology of leptin in normal individuals and its involvement in obesity and obesity-related diseases is uncertain.

Adipose tissue also secretes *adiponectin*, which regulates sensitivity to insulin and may be involved in the pathogenesis of type 2 diabetes.[24,25] Whereas dysfunctional adipose tissue increases the levels of certain other hormones and adipocytokines, the levels of adiponectin are decreased, leading to decreased insulin sensitivity, proatherosclerosis, and a proinflammatory milieu that can predispose the individual to *metabolic syndrome*

(see Chapter 33) and its associated complications (including type 2 diabetes and cardiovascular disease).[15,16]

Adipose Tissue and the Inflammatory Process

Recent evidence suggests that excess adipose tissue is also associated with a chronic inflammatory response, which is characterized by abnormal cytokine production; increased synthesis of acute-phase reactants, such as C-reactive protein; and activation of proinflammatory signaling pathways.[26] Systemic chronic inflammation has been proposed to have an important role in the pathogenesis of obesity-related insulin resistance and development of type 2 diabetes. It might also contribute to a state of endothelial dysfunction, an abnormal lipid profile, hypertension, and vascular inflammation, all of which promote the development of atherosclerotic cardiovascular disease.[26,27] Although there is evidence that the proinflammatory pathways are activated in adipose tissue in obesity, the source of the inflammatory mediators remains unclear. Besides adipocytes, adipose tissue contains a connective tissue matrix and macrophages, which may contribute to the production of inflammatory mediators.

Types of Obesity

Two types of obesity based on distribution of fat have been described: upper body and lower body obesity. *Upper body obesity* is also referred to as *central*, *abdominal*, or *visceral* obesity. Lower body obesity is also known as *peripheral* or *gluteal-femoral* obesity. Persons with upper body obesity are often referred to as being shaped like an "apple," compared with those with lower body obesity, who are more "pear" shaped (Fig. 10-3). The obesity type is determined by dividing the waist by the hip circumference. A waist-to-hip ratio greater than 1.0 in men and 0.8 in women indicates upper body obesity. Research suggests that fat distribution may be a more important factor for morbidity and mortality than overweight or obesity.

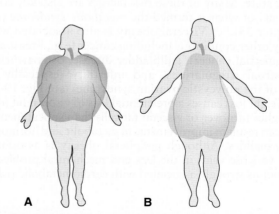

FIGURE 10-3. Distribution of adipose tissue in **(A)** upper body or central (visceral) obesity and **(B)** lower body or peripheral (subcutaneous) obesity. People with upper body obesity are often described as having an "apple-shaped" body and those with lower body obesity as having a "pear-shaped" body.

The presence of excess fat in the abdomen out of proportion to total body fat is an independent predictor of risk factors and mortality. Both BMI and waist circumference are positively correlated with total body adipose tissue, but waist circumference is a better predictor of abdominal or visceral fat content than BMI.[28] A waist circumference of 88 cm (35 inches) or greater in women and 102 cm (40 inches) or greater in men has been associated with increased health risk[13] (see Table 10-2). In general, men have more intra-abdominal fat and women more subcutaneous fat. As men age, the proportion of intra-abdominal fat to subcutaneous fat increases. After menopause, women tend to acquire more intra-abdominal fat. Increasing weight gain, alcohol, and low levels of activity are associated with central obesity.

Although central obesity is usually considered to be synonymous with visceral fat, CT or MRI scans can differentiate central obesity into visceral fat and subcutaneous fat. Visceral fat stores are believed to be more lipolytically active than subcutaneous fat and have a greater potential to affect liver metabolism, given the fact that the fatty acids in their venous drainage flow directly to the liver. In addition to their lipolytic effects, visceral adipocytes produce greater amounts of adipocytokines (e.g., TNF-α, IL-6), except adiponectin whose levels are decreased, resulting in a more insulin resistant, proinflammatory, and proatherosclerotic environment. These changes contribute to the development of systemic insulin resistance, hypertension, hyperlipidemia, and other features of the metabolic syndrome, and are thought to be associated with greater cardiometabolic risk.[15]

Cardiometabolic risk represents the overall risk of developing diabetes and/or atherosclerotic cardiovascular disease (e.g., myocardial infarction, stroke) due to a cluster of modifiable risk factors. These include abdominal obesity, dyslipidemia (elevated levels of triglycerides and low-density lipoproteins and decreased levels of high-density lipoproteins), hypertension, insulin resistance and elevated blood glucose levels, the presence of inflammatory cytokines, and smoking. Emerging risk factors include endothelial dysfunction and a prothrombotic state. Many of these risk factors are also key components of what is termed the *metabolic syndrome* (see Chapter 33).[15,16] Visceral obesity is also associated with many other conditions including cancer (e.g., breast and endometrial cancer), gallbladder disease, osteoarthritis, menstrual irregularities, and infertility (especially as part of the polycystic ovarian syndrome) (see Fig. 10-2).

Weight loss causes a preferential loss of visceral fat (due to higher turnover of visceral fat cells than subcutaneous) and can result in improvements in metabolic and hormonal abnormalities. Although peripheral obesity is associated with varicose veins in the legs and mechanical problems, it is not as strongly associated with cardiometabolic risk.

Prevention and Treatment of Obesity

Emphasis is being placed on the prevention of obesity. It has been theorized that obesity is preventable because the effect of hereditary factors is no more than moderate.

A more active lifestyle together with a low-fat diet (<30% of calories) is seen as the strategy for prevention. The target audience should be children, adolescents, and young adults.[29] Tools needed to achieve this goal include promotion of regular meals, increased intake of fruits and vegetables, substituting water for calorie-containing beverages, decreased television viewing time, a low-fat diet, and increased activity.[30] Other experts target the high-risk period from 25 to 35 years, menopause, and the year after successful weight loss.

The current recommendation is that treatment is indicated in all individuals who have a BMI of 30 or higher or who have a BMI of 25 to 29.9 or a high waist circumference plus two or more risk factors.[31] Treatment should focus on individualized lifestyle modification through a combination of a reduced-calorie diet, increased physical activity, and behavior therapy. Before treatment begins, an assessment should be made of the degree of overweight, the person's eating habits, the person's physical activity level, and the presence of obesity-associated risk factors and complications.[31] It also is advisable to determine the person's barriers and readiness to lose weight.

Dietary therapy should be individually prescribed based on the person's overweight status and risk profile.[30] The diet should be a personalized plan with realistic goals that are 500 to 1000 kcal/day less than the current intake. The aim should be for weight loss initially, followed by a strategy for weight maintenance. Many popular diets exist such as Atkins, Ornish, Weight Watchers, and South Beach. A recent study comparing several of these diets suggested that adherence to the diet, not the diet itself, is most closely associated with weight loss (i.e., the best diet is the one the person likes best).[32]

There is convincing evidence that increased physical activity decreases the risk of overweight and obesity. In addition, it reduces cardiovascular and diabetes risk beyond that achieved by weight loss alone. Although physical activity is an important part of weight loss therapy and helps with maintaining weight loss, it does not independently lead to a significant weight loss.[33] It may, however, help reduce abdominal fat, increase cardiorespiratory fitness, and prevent the decrease in muscle mass that often occurs with weight loss. Exercise should be started slowly with the duration and intensity increased independent of each other.

Techniques for changing behavior include self-monitoring of eating habits and physical activity, stress management, stimulus control, problem solving, contingency management, cognitive restructuring, social support, and relapse prevention.[30] Pharmacotherapy and surgery are available as adjuncts to lifestyle changes in individuals who meet specific criteria. Pharmacotherapy is usually considered only after combined diet, exercise, and behavioral therapy have been in effect for a reasonable period of time. Weight loss surgery is usually limited to persons with a BMI greater than 40, those with a BMI greater than 35 who have comorbid conditions and in whom efforts at medical therapy have failed, and those who have complications of extreme obesity. However, more recent studies have shown the potential benefit of offering surgery to patients with even lower levels of obesity (e.g., BMI >30 with comorbid conditions such as diabetes).[34]

 ## Childhood Obesity

Obesity is the most prevalent nutritional disorder affecting the pediatric population in industrialized countries in the world.[35,36] The definition for obesity in children is a BMI at or above the sex- and age-specific 95th percentile, while a BMI between the 85th and 95th percentile is defined as being overweight.[34] These criteria have been selected because they correspond to adult BMIs of 30 and 25, respectively.[37] The findings from the National Health and Nutrition Examination Survey (NHANES), conducted between 2008 and 2010, indicated that 16.9% of children and adolescents were obese.[35]

The major concern of childhood obesity is that obese children will grow up to become obese adults. Health care providers are now beginning to see hypertension, dyslipidemia, type 2 diabetes, and psychosocial stigma in obese children and adolescents. In North America, type 2 diabetes now accounts for half of all new diagnoses of diabetes (type 1 and type 2) in some populations of adolescents.[38] In addition, there is a growing concern that childhood and adolescent obesity may be associated with negative psychosocial consequences such as low self-esteem and discrimination by adults and peers.[34]

Childhood obesity is determined by a combination of hereditary and environmental factors. It is associated with obese parents, gestational diabetes and excessive weight gain during pregnancy, formula feeding, parenting style, parental eating habits, energy-dense food choices, erratic eating patterns, ethnicity, and sedentary lifestyle.[34–36,38,39] Children with overweight parents are at highest risk. One of the factors leading to childhood obesity is the increase in inactivity. Increasing perceptions that neighborhoods are unsafe has resulted in less time spent outside playing and walking and more time spent indoors engaging in sedentary activities such as television viewing and computer usage. Television viewing is associated with consumption of calorie-dense snacks and decreased indoor activity. Studies have shown a 10% decrease in obesity risk for each hour per day of moderate to vigorous physical activity, while the risk increased by 12% for each hour per day of television viewing.[38] Obese children also may have a deficit in recognizing hunger sensations, stemming perhaps from parents who use food as gratification. The impact of fast food, increased portion size, calorie density, sugar-sweetened soft drinks and foods (especially fructose),[22] and high-glycemic-index foods are likely contributing to the increased weights in children and adolescents.

Diagnosis and Treatment. Given the enormity of the problem of overweight and obesity in children, the American Medical Association (AMA), the Department of Health and Human Services' Health Resources and Services Administration (HRSA), and the Centers for Disease Control and Prevention (CDC) assembled an expert committee to develop recommendations for the assessment, prevention, and treatment of this public health problem.[37] Their recommendations include a yearly assessment of weight status in all children by measurement of height and weight to determine BMI for age and comparing it to standard growth charts. Children who are 2 to 18 years of age with a BMI greater than or equal to the 95th percentile for age and sex or a BMI greater than 30 (whichever is smaller) should be classified as obese. Those children with a BMI greater than or equal to the 85th percentile but less than the 95th percentile for age and sex should be placed in the overweight category.

Because adolescent obesity is predictive of adult obesity, treatment of childhood obesity is desirable.[36] The goals of therapy in uncomplicated obesity are directed toward healthy eating and activity, not achievement of ideal body weight. Families should be taught awareness of current eating habits, activity, and parenting behavior and how to modify them. In children with complications secondary to the obesity, the medical goal should be to improve that problem. The weight loss interventions should include all family members and caregivers; begin early at a point when the family is ready for change; and assist the family to learn to monitor eating and activity patterns and to make small and acceptable changes in these patterns.

Overweight and obese children should be treated using a staged method based on their age, BMI, and related comorbidities. Dietary goals should focus on well-balanced meals with a healthy approach to eating. Specific strategies can include reduction of specific high-calorie foods or an appropriate balance of foods that are low, medium, and high calorie. Commercial diets should be used with caution. Pharmacologic therapy and bariatric surgery should be reserved for children with complications and for severe obesity, respectively.

SUMMARY CONCEPTS

■ Obesity, which refers to excess body fat resulting from consumption of calories in excess of those expended for exercise and activities, reflects the influences of heredity; socioeconomic, cultural, and environmental factors; psychological influences; and activity levels.

■ Overweight and obesity are determined by measurements of body mass index (BMI) and waist circumference, which is used to determine the distribution of body fat in terms of upper or lower body obesity. In upper body or central (visceral) obesity, the adipocytes release free fatty acids and adipokines that increase cardiometabolic risk and produce many of the adverse effects of obesity.

(continued)

SUMMARY CONCEPTS *(continued)*

■ The risks associated with obesity include hyperlipidemia, insulin resistance, and hypertension, which together predispose to the development of type 2 diabetes mellitus and atherosclerotic cardiovascular disease (e.g., coronary artery disease, stroke). Obesity is also associated with gallbladder disease, infertility, osteoarthritis, sleep apnea, complications of pregnancy, menstrual irregularities, nonalcoholic fatty liver disease, thromboembolic disorders, and poor wound healing.

■ Childhood obesity is becoming an increasingly prevalent nutritional disorder that predisposes children and adolescents to hypertension, dyslipidemia, type 2 diabetes mellitus, and psychosocial stigma.

Undernutrition and Eating Disorders

Undernutrition continues to be a major health problem throughout the world.[40] Protein-energy malnutrition is most obvious in developing countries of the world, where it is indirectly responsible for half of all deaths of young children.[41] Even in developed nations, malnutrition remains a problem.

Malnutrition and Starvation

Malnutrition and starvation are conditions in which a person does not receive or is unable to use an adequate amount of nutrients for body function. An adequate diet should provide sufficient energy in the form of carbohydrates, fats, and proteins; essential amino acids and fatty acids for use as building blocks for synthesis of structural and functional proteins and lipids; and the necessary vitamins and minerals to function as coenzymes or hormones in vital metabolic processes or, as in the case of calcium and phosphate, as important structural components of bone.[42]

Among the many causes of malnutrition are poverty and lack of knowledge about nutritional needs, acute and chronic illness, and self-imposed dietary restrictions. Homeless people, the elderly, and the children of the poor often demonstrate the effects of protein and energy malnutrition, as well as vitamin and mineral deficiencies. Even the affluent may fail to recognize that infants, adolescents, and pregnant women have increased nutritional needs. Some types of malnutrition are caused by acute and chronic illnesses, such as

malabsorption disorders. In contrast, clinical eating disorders are caused by psychiatric illness.

Protein-Energy Malnutrition

Protein-energy malnutrition represents a depletion of the body's lean tissues caused by starvation or a combination of starvation and catabolic stress. The lean tissues are the fat-free, metabolically active tissues of the body, namely the skeletal muscles, viscera, and cells of the blood and immune system. Because lean tissues are the largest body compartment, their rate of loss is the main determinant of total body weight in most cases of protein energy malnutrion.

Much of the literature on malnutrition and starvation has dealt with infants and children in underdeveloped countries in which food deprivation results in an inadequate intake of protein and calories to meet the body's energy needs. Protein-energy malnutrition in this population commonly is divided into two distinct conditions: marasmus (protein and calorie deficiency) and kwashiorkor (protein deficiency). The pathologic changes for both types of malnutrition include humoral and cellular immunodeficiencies resulting from protein deficiency and lack of immune mediators. There is impaired synthesis of pigments of the hair and skin (e.g., hair color may change and the skin may become hyperpigmented) due to a lack of substrate (tyrosine) and coenzymes.

There are two functional compartments involved in the distribution of proteins within the body: the *somatic compartment*, represented by the skeletal muscles, and the *visceral compartment*, represented by protein stores in body organs, principally the liver.[42] These two compartments are regulated differently, with the somatic compartment being affected more severely in marasmus and the visceral compartment affected more severely in kwashiorkor.

Marasmus represents a progressive loss of muscle mass and fat stores due to inadequate food intake that is equally deficient in calories and protein.[42,43] It results in a reduction in body weight adjusted for age and size. The child with marasmus has a wasted appearance, with loss of muscle mass, stunted growth, and loss of subcutaneous fat; a protuberant abdomen (from muscular hypotonia); wrinkled skin; sparse, dry, and dull hair; and depressed heart rate, blood pressure, and body temperature. Diarrhea is common. Since immune function is impaired, concurrent infections occur and place additional stress on an already weakened body. An important characteristic of marasmus is growth failure; if sufficient food is not provided, these children will not reach their full potential stature.[43]

Kwashiorkor results from a deficiency in protein in diets that are relatively high in carbohydrates.[42,43] The term *kwashiorkor* comes from an African word meaning "the disease suffered by the displaced child," because the condition develops soon after a child is displaced from the breast after the arrival of a new infant and placed on a starchy gruel feeding. Kwashiorkor is a more severe form of malnutrition than marasmus. Unlike marasmus, severe protein deficiency is associated with severe loss of the visceral protein compartment with a resultant hypoalbuminemia that gives rise to generalized or dependent edema. The child with kwashiorkor usually presents with edema, desquamating skin, discolored hair, anorexia, and extreme apathy (Fig. 10-4). There are "flaky paint" lesions of the skin on the face (Fig.10-5), extremities, and perineum and the hair becomes a sandy or reddish color, with linear depigmentation (flag sign).[43] There is generalized growth failure and muscle wasting as in marasmus, but subcutaneous fat is normal, since calorie intake is adequate. Other manifestations include skin lesions, hepatomegaly and distended abdomen, cold extremities, and decreased cardiac output and tachycardia.

Marasmus-kwashiorkor is an advanced protein-calorie deficit together with increased protein requirement or loss. This results in a rapid decrease in anthropometric

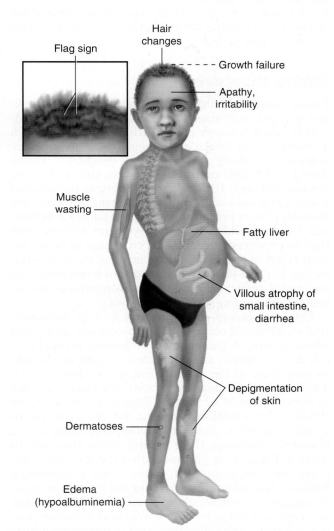

FIGURE 10-4. Clinical manifestations of Kwashiorkor.

Flag sign
Hair changes
Growth failure
Apathy, irritability
Muscle wasting
Fatty liver
Villous atrophy of small intestine, diarrhea
Depigmentation of skin
Dermatoses
Edema (hypoalbuminemia)

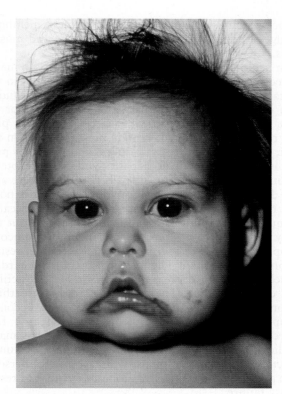

FIGURE 10-5. Infant with symptoms indicative of Kawashiokor, a dietary protein deficiency, as well as a vitamin B deficiency. (From the Centers for Disease Control and Prevention Public Health Image Library. No. 6180.)

measurements with obvious edema and wasting and loss of organ mass. One essential aspect of severe protein-energy malnutrition is fatty degeneration of such diverse organs as the heart and liver. This degeneration causes subclinical and overt cardiac dysfunction, especially when malnutrition is accompanied by edema. A second injurious aspect is the loss of subcutaneous fat, which markedly reduces the body's capacity for temperature regulation and water storage. As a consequence, malnourished children become dehydrated and hypothermic more quickly and more severely than normally nourished children.[40] Most children with severe protein-energy malnutrition have asymptomatic infections because their immune systems fail to respond appropriately.

Malnutrition in Trauma and Illness

In industrialized societies, protein-energy malnutrition most often occurs secondary to trauma or illness. Kwashiorkor-like secondary protein-energy malnutrition occurs most commonly in association with hypermetabolic acute illnesses, such as trauma, burns, and sepsis.[44] Marasmus-like secondary protein-energy malnutrition typically results from chronic illnesses such as chronic obstructive pulmonary disease (COPD), congestive heart failure, cancer, and HIV infection. Approximately half of all persons with cancer experience tissue wasting, in which the tumor induces metabolic changes leading to a loss of adipose tissue and muscle mass.[45]

In healthy adults, body protein homeostasis is maintained by a cycle in which the net loss of protein in the postabsorptive state is matched by a net postprandial gain of protein.[46] In persons with severe injury or illness, net protein breakdown is accelerated and protein rebuilding disrupted. Protein mass is lost from the liver, gastrointestinal tract, kidneys, and heart. As protein is lost from the liver, hepatic synthesis of proteins declines, and plasma protein levels decrease. There also is a decrease in immune cells. Wound healing is poor, and the body is unable to fight off infection because of multiple immunologic malfunctions throughout the body. The gastrointestinal tract undergoes mucosal atrophy with loss of villi in the small intestine, resulting in malabsorption. The loss of protein from cardiac muscle leads to a decrease in myocardial contractility and cardiac output. The muscles used for breathing become weakened, and respiratory function becomes compromised as muscle proteins are used as a fuel source. A reduction in respiratory function has many implications, especially for persons with burns, trauma, infection, or chronic respiratory disease and for persons who are being mechanically ventilated because of respiratory failure.

In hospitalized patients, malnutrition increases morbidity and mortality rates, incidence of complications, and length of stay. Malnutrition may present at the time of admission or develop during hospitalization. The hospitalized patient often finds eating a healthy diet difficult and commonly has restrictions on food and water intake in preparation for tests and surgery. Pain, medications, special diets, and stress can decrease appetite. Even when the patient is well enough to eat, being alone in a room where unpleasant treatments may be given is not conducive to eating. Although hospitalized patients may appear to need fewer calories because they are on bed rest, their actual need for caloric intake may be higher because of other energy expenditures. For example, more calories are expended during fever, when the metabolic rate is increased. There also may be an increased need for protein to support tissue repair after trauma or surgery.

Diagnosis

No single diagnostic measure is sufficiently accurate to serve as a reliable test for malnutrition. Techniques of nutritional assessment include evaluation of dietary intake, anthropometric measurements, clinical examination, and laboratory tests.[44] Evaluation of weight is particularly important. Body weight can be assessed in relation to height using the BMI. Evaluation of body composition can be performed by inspection or using anthropometric measurements such as skinfold thickness. Serum albumin and prealbumin are used in the diagnosis of protein-calorie malnutrition. Albumin, which has historically been used as a determinant of nutrition status, has a relatively large body pool and a

half-life of 20 days and is less sensitive to changes in nutrition than prealbumin, which has a shorter half-life and a relatively small body pool.[44]

Treatment

The treatment of severe protein-calorie malnutrition involves the use of measures to correct fluid and electrolyte abnormalities and replenish proteins, calories, and micronutrients.[44] Treatment is started with modest quantities of proteins and calories based on the person's actual weight. Concurrent administration of vitamins and minerals is needed. Either the enteral or parenteral route can be used. The treatment should be undertaken slowly to avoid complications. The administration of water and sodium with carbohydrates can overload a heart that has been weakened by malnutrition and result in congestive failure. Enteral feedings can result in malabsorptive symptoms due to abnormalities in the gastrointestinal tract. Refeeding edema is a benign dependent edema that results from renal sodium reabsorption and poor skin and blood vessel integrity. It is treated by elevation of the dependent area and modest sodium restrictions. Diuretics are ineffective and may aggravate electrolyte deficiencies.

Eating Disorders

Eating disorders, which include anorexia nervosa, bulimia nervosa, and binge-eating disorder and their variants to result from serious disturbances in eating, such as restriction of intake and binging, with an excessive concern over body shape or body weight.[47–50] Eating disorders typically occur in adolescent girls and young women, although 10% of cases of anorexia nervosa and bulimia nervosa occur in boys and men.[51] Binge-eating disorder is more prevalent in men than anorexia nervosa and bulimia combined. Compared with women, men tend to experience less pressure to engage in behaviors such as self-induced vomiting or laxative use when overeating, less of a sense of loss of control when binge eating, and a greater tendency to use compulsive exercise rather than purging for weight control.[51]

Eating disorders are more prevalent in industrialized societies and occur in all socioeconomic and major ethnic groups. A combination of genetic, neurochemical, developmental, and sociocultural factors is thought to contribute to the development of the disorders.[47,48] The American Psychiatric Association's *Diagnostic and Statistical Manual of Mental Disorders, Fifth Edition* (DSM-5) has established criteria for the diagnosis of anorexia nervosa, bulimia nervosa, and binge-eating disorder.[52] Although these criteria allow clinicians to make a diagnosis in persons with a specific eating disorder, the symptoms often occur along a continuum between those of anorexia nervosa and bulimia nervosa. Preoccupation with weight and excessive self-evaluation of weight and shape are common to both disorders, and persons with eating disorders may demonstrate a mixture of both disorders.[48] The female athlete triad, which includes low energy availability, menstrual dysfunction, such as amenorrhea, and low bone density,[53] does not meet the strict DSM-5 criteria for anorexia nervosa or bulimia nervosa, but shares many of the characteristics and therapeutic concerns (see Chapter 44). Persons with eating disorders may require concomitant evaluation for psychiatric illness because eating disorders often are accompanied by mood, anxiety, and personality disorders.

Anorexia Nervosa

Anorexia nervosa is an eating disorder that usually begins in adolescence and is characterized by determined dieting, often accompanied by compulsive exercise and, in a subgroup of persons, purging behavior with or without binge eating, resulting in sustained low weight.[54] Other features include a disturbed body image, a pervasive fear of becoming obese, and obsession with severely restricted caloric intake.

The causes of anorexia appear to be multifactorial, with determinants that include genetic influence, personality traits of perfectionism and compulsiveness, anxiety disorders, family history of depression and obesity, and peer, familial, and cultural pressures with respect to appearance.[54] Other psychiatric disorders often coexist with anorexia nervosa, including major depression or dysthymia and obsessive–compulsive disorder.

Many organ systems are affected by the malnutrition that occurs in persons with anorexia nervosa. The severity of the abnormalities tends to be related to the degree of malnutrition and is reversed by refeeding. The most frequent complication of anorexia is amenorrhea and loss of secondary sex characteristics with decreased levels of estrogen, which can eventually lead to osteoporosis. Bone loss can occur in young women after as short a period of illness as 6 months.[48] Symptomatic compression fractures and kyphosis have been reported. Constipation, cold intolerance and failure to shiver in cold, bradycardia, hypotension, decreased heart size, electrocardiographic changes, blood and electrolyte abnormalities, and skin with lanugo (i.e., increased amounts of fine hair) are common. Abnormalities in cognitive function may also occur. The brain loses both white and gray matter during severe weight loss; weight restoration results in return of white matter, but some loss of gray matter may persist.[54] Unexpected sudden deaths have been reported; the risk appears to increase as weight drops to less than 35% to 40% of ideal weight. It is believed that these deaths are caused by myocardial degeneration and heart failure rather than arrhythmias.

The most exasperating aspect of the treatment of anorexia is the inability of the person with anorexia to recognize there is a problem. Because anorexia is a form of starvation, it can lead to death if left untreated. A multidisciplinary approach appears to be the most effective method of treating persons with the disorder. The goals of treatment are eating and weight gain, and efforts to work on psychological, relationship, and emotional issues. Adults whose weight is more than 25% below the expected weight (or with less weight loss if there are coexisting medical or psychiatric conditions,

or both) and children or adolescents who are losing weight rapidly generally require hospitalization to ensure an adequate food intake and to limit physical activity.[54]

Bulimia Nervosa

Bulimia nervosa is defined by recurrent binge eating and activities including vomiting, fasting, excessive exercise, and use of diuretics, laxatives, or enemas to compensate for that behavior. Bulimia nervosa usually begins during adolescence, with a peak period of onset around 18 years of age.[55] In contrast to anorexia nervosa, which is characterized by a weight that is less than 85% of normal, most persons with bulimia nervosa are of normal weight. The disorder may be associated with other psychiatric disorders such as anxiety disorder or depression. There is also an association with substance abuse and risky and self-destructive behaviors.[55]

The complications of bulimia nervosa include those resulting from overeating, self-induced vomiting, and cathartic and diuretic abuse.[55-57] Among the complications of self-induced vomiting are dental disorders, parotitis, and fluid and electrolyte disorders. Dental abnormalities, such as sensitive teeth, increased dental caries, and periodontal disease, occur with frequent vomiting because the high acid content of the vomitus causes tooth enamel to dissolve. Esophagitis, dysphagia, and esophageal stricture are common. With frequent vomiting, there often is reflux of gastric contents into the lower esophagus because of relaxation of the lower esophageal sphincter. Vomiting may lead to aspiration pneumonia, especially in intoxicated or debilitated persons. Potassium, chloride, and hydrogen are lost in the vomitus, and frequent vomiting predisposes to metabolic acidosis with hypokalemia (see Chapter 8). An unexplained physical response to vomiting is the development of benign, painless parotid gland enlargement.

The weights of persons with bulimia nervosa may fluctuate, although not to the dangerously low levels seen in anorexia nervosa. Their thoughts and feelings range from fear of not being able to stop eating to a concern about gaining too much weight. They also experience feelings of sadness, anger, guilt, shame, and low self-esteem.

Treatment strategies include psychological and pharmacologic treatments. Cognitive-behavioral therapy is the psychosocial therapy predominately used.[56] This therapy is designed to help individuals become aware of other ways to cope with the feelings that precipitate the desire to purge and to try and correct maladaptive beliefs regarding their self-image. Unlike persons with anorexia nervosa, persons with bulimia nervosa are upset by the behaviors practiced and the thoughts and feelings experienced, and they are more willing to accept help. Pharmacotherapeutic agents include the tricyclic antidepressants, the selective serotonin reuptake inhibitors, and other antidepressant medications.[55]

Binge-Eating Disorder

Binge-eating disorder is characterized by eating too much in a short period of time, eating too fast, eating alone, eating when not hungry, and feeling uncomfortably full. Unlike bulimia nervosa, persons with binge eating do not engage in compensatory behaviors such as vomiting and laxative abuse. The great majority of persons with binge-eating disorder are overweight, and in turn, obese persons have a higher prevalence of binge-eating disorder than the nonobese populations.[56–59] The physical complications associated with binge-eating disorders are usually secondary to attendant obesity.

The primary goal of therapy for binge-eating disorders is to establish a regular, healthy eating pattern. Persons with binge-eating disorders who have been successfully treated for their eating disorder have reported that making meal plans, eating a balanced diet at three regular meals a day, avoiding high-sugar foods and other binge foods, recording food intake and binge-eating episodes, exercising regularly, finding alternative activities, and avoiding alcohol and drugs are helpful in maintaining their more healthful eating behaviors after treatment.

 SUMMARY CONCEPTS

■ Undernutrition, which can range from a selective deficiency of a single nutrient to starvation, is among the most widespread causes of morbidity and mortality in the world. Protein-energy malnutrition in this population is commonly divided into two distinct conditions: marasmus, (protein and calorie deficiency) in which there is a great loss of protein from the skeletal muscle compartment; and kwashiorkor (protein deficiency), in which there is a greater loss of visceral proteins, particularly those of the liver.

■ Malnutrition is also common during illness, recovery from trauma, and hospitalization. The effects of malnutrition and starvation on body function are widespread, including loss of muscle mass, impaired immunologic function and wound healing, decreased appetite, loss of calcium and phosphate from bone, anovulation and amenorrhea in women, and decreased testicular function in men.

■ Eating disorders, which include anorexia nervosa, bulimia, and binge-eating disorder, are psychiatric disorders characterized by severe disturbances in eating, such as willful restriction of intake and binge eating, as well as excessive concern over body weight and shape. Anorexia nervosa is characterized by a refusal to maintain a minimally normal body weight; bulimia nervosa is characterized by secretive episodes of binging followed by compensatory behaviors such as self-induced vomiting; and binge eating disorder is characterized by the consumption of unusually large quantities of food in a short period of time that is not followed by compensatory behaviors.

REVIEW EXERCISES

1. Stability of body weight and composition over time requires that energy (food) intake match energy utilization.

   A. Define the terms *hunger* and *appetite* and describe their role in regulating food intake.
   B. Differentiate between short- and long-term control of food intake and the neural and hormonal mechanisms involved in their regulation.

2. A 25-year-old woman is 65 inches (165 cm) tall and weighs 300 pounds (136 kg). She works as a receptionist in an office, brings her lunch to work with her, spends her evenings watching television, and gets very little exercise. She reports that she has been fat ever since she was a little girl, she has tried "every diet under the sun," and when she diets she loses some weight but gains it all back again.

   A. Calculate her BMI using the website referred to in Table 10-1.
   B. How would you classify her obesity?
   C. What are her risk factors for obesity?
   D. What would be one of the first steps in helping her develop a plan to lose weight?

3. A 16-year-old high school student is brought into the physician's office by her mother, who is worried because her daughter insists on dieting because she thinks she is too fat. The daughter is 67 inches tall and weighs 96 pounds. Her history reveals that she is a straight A student, plays in the orchestra, and is on the track team. She is given a tentative diagnosis of anorexia nervosa.

   A. What are the characteristic behaviors associated with anorexia nervosa?
   B. What are some of the physiologic manifestations of the malnutrition and severe weight loss associated with this disorder?

REFERENCES

1. Hall JE. *Guyton and Hall's Textbook of Medical Physiology*. 10th ed. Philadelphia, PA: W.B. Saunders; 2011:843–858, 859–866.
2. Ross MH, Pawlina W. *Histology*. 6th ed. Philadelphia, PA: Wolters Kluwer Health/Lippincott Williams & Wilkins; 2011:254–264.
3. Casteilla L, Dani C. Adipose tissue-derived cells: from physiology to regenerative medicine. *Diabetes Metab*. 2006;32(5 pt 1):393–401.

4. Chou FS, Wang PS, Kulp S, et al. Effects of thiazolidinediones on differentiation, proliferation, and apoptosis. *Mol Cancer Res.* 2007;5(6):523–530.

5. Otten JJ, Hellwig JP, Meyers LD. *Dietary Reference Intakes: The Essential Guide to Nutrient Requirements.* Washington, DC: National Academy Press; 2006.

6. U.S. Department of Agriculture. Food and Nutrition Center. Available at: http://fnic.nal.usda.gov/nal_display/index. php?info_center=4&tax_level=3&tax_subject=256&topic_ id=1342&level3_id=5140. Accessed September 6, 2013.

7. Trumbo P, Schlicker S, Yates AA, et al. Dietary reference intakes for energy, carbohydrate, fiber, fat, fatty acids, cholesterol, protein, and amino acids. *J Am Diet Assoc.* 2002;102:1621–1630.

8. National Institutes of Health Expert Panel. *Third Report of the National Cholesterol Education Program (NCEP) Expert Panel on Detection, Evaluation, and Treatment of High Blood Cholesterol in Adults (Adult Treatment Panel III).* NIH publication no. 02–5215. Bethesda, MD: National Institutes of Health; 2002.

9. Lichtenstein AL, Apple LJ, Brandis M, et al. AHA scientific statement. Diet and lifestyle recommendations revision 2006: a scientific statement from AHA Nutrition Committee. *Circulation.* 2006;114:82–96.

10. Murphy KG, Bloom SR. Gut hormones and the regulation of energy homeostasis. *Nature.* 2006;444:854–859.

11. Chaudhri OB, Salem V, Murphy KG, et al. Gastrointestinal satiety signals. *Annu Rev Physiol.* 2008;70:239–255.

12. Han TS, Sattar N, Lean M. Assessment of obesity and its clinical implications. *BMJ.* 2006;333:695–698.

13. Pi-Sunyer FX, Dietz WH, Becker DM, et al.; for the NHLBI Obesity Education Initiative Expert Panel on the Identification, Evaluation, and Treatment of Overweight and Obesity in Adults. *Clinical Guidelines on the Identification, Evaluation, and Treatment of Overweight and Obesity in Adults.* 1998. NIH Publication No. 98–4083. Available at: http://www.nhlbi.nih.gov/ guidelines/obesity/ob_gdlns.pdf

14. Abernathy RP, Black DR. Healthy body weight: an alternative perspective. *Am J Clin Nutr.* 1996;63(suppl):448S–451S.

15. Eckel R, Grundy S, Zimmet P. Metabolic syndrome. *Lancet.* 2005;365:1415–1428.

16. Scott M, Grundy JI, Cleeman SR, et al. Diagnosis and management of the metabolic syndrome: an American Heart Association/National Heart, Lung, and Blood Institute scientific statement. *Circulation.* 2005;112:2735–2752.

17. Hossain P, Kawar B, El Nahas M. Obesity and diabetes in the developing world—a growing challenge. *N Engl J Med.* 2007;356:213–215.

18. Bray GA. Obesity: the disease. *J Med Chem.* 2006;49:4001–4007.

19. Hellerstein MK, Parks EJ. Obesity and overweight. In: Gardner DG, Shoback D, eds. *Greenspan's Basic Endocrinology.* 8th ed. New York, NY: McGraw-Hill; 2007:796–808.

20. Soreneson TJ, Holst C, Stunkard AJ, et al. Correlations of body mass index of adult adoptees and their biological and adoptive relatives. *Int J Obes Relat Metab Disord.* 1992;16:227–236.

21. McCarthy M. Genomics, type 2 diabetes, and obesity. *N Engl J Med.* 2010;363:2339–2350.

22. Bray GB. Potential health risks from beverages containing fructose found in sugar or high-fructose corn syrup. *Diabetes Care.* 2013;36:11–12.

23. Young LR, Nestle M. The contribution of expanding portion sizes to U.S. obesity epidemic. *Am J Public Health.* 2002;92:246–249.

24. Kershaw EE, Flier JS. Adipose tissue as an endocrine organ. *J Clin Endocrinol Metab.* 2004;89:2548–2556.

25. Ahima R. Adipose tissue as an endocrine organ. *Obesity.* 2006;14:242S–248S.

26. Tilg H, Moschen AR. Adipocytokines: mediators linking adipose tissue, inflammation and immunity. *Nature.* 2006;5:772–782.

27. Greenberg AS, Obin MS. Obesity and the role of adipose tissue in inflammation and metabolism. *Am J Clin Nutr.* 2006;83(suppl):461S–465S.

28. Klein S, Allison DB, Heymsfield SB, et al. Waist circumference and cardiometabolic risk: a consensus statement from Shaping America's Health: Association for Weight Management and Obesity Prevention; NAASO, The Obesity Society; the American Society for Nutrition; and the American Diabetes Association. *Am J Clin Nutr.* 2007;85:1197–1202.

29. Task Force on Prevention and Treatment of Obesity. Towards prevention of obesity: research directives. *Obes Res.* 1994;2:571.

30. Avenell A, Sattar N, Lean M. Management: part 1–behaviour change, diet, and activity. *BMJ.* 2006;333:740–743.

31. U.S. Department of Health and Human Services. *The Practical Guide: Identification, Evaluation, and Treatment of Overweight and Obesity in Adults.* NIH publication no. 00–4084. Rockville, MD: U.S. Department of Health and Human Services, National Institute of Health; National Heart, Lung, and Blood Institute; North American Association of the Study of Obesity; 2000.

32. Dalsinger ML, Gleason JA, Griffith JL, et al. Comparison of the Atkins, Ornish, Weight Watchers, and Zone diets for weight loss and heart disease reduction. *JAMA.* 2005;293:43–53.

33. Jakicic JM, Marcus BH, Gallagher KI, et al. Effect of exercise duration and intensity on weight loss in overweight, sedentary women: a randomized trial. *JAMA.* 2003;290:1323–1330.

34. Wolfe BM, Purnell JQ, Belle SH. Treating diabetes with surgery. *JAMA.* 2013;309:2274–2275.

35. Ogden CL, Carroll MD, Curtin LR, et al. Prevalence of high body mass index in U.S. children and adolescents, 2007–2008. *JAMA.* 2010;303(3):242–249.

36. Centers for Disease Control and Prevention. *Childhood Overweight and Obesity.* 2007. Available at: http://www.cdc. gov/NCCDPHP/DNPA/obesity/childhood/index.htm. Accessed September 6, 2013.

37. Expert Committee Recommendations on the Assessment, Prevention, and Treatment of Child and Adolescent Overweight and Obesity. 2007. Available at: http://www.ama-assn.org/ama1/ pub/upload/mm/433/ped_obesity_recs.pdf. Accessed September 6, 2013.

38. Fagot-Campagna A, Pettitt DJ, Engelgau NM, et al. Type 2 diabetes among North American children and adolescents: an epidemiologic review and a public health perspective. *J Pediatr.* 2000;136:664–672.

39. Lakslakshmi L, Elks CE, Ong KK. Childhood obesity. *Circulation.* 2012;126(14):1770–1779.

40. Müller O, Krawinkel M. Malnutrition and health in developing countries. *CMAJ.* 2005;173(3):279–286.

41. Judge BS, Eisenga BH. Disorders of fuel metabolism: medical complications associated with starvation, eating disorders, dietary fads, and supplements. *Emerg Med Clin North Am.* 2005;23:789–813.

42. Kumar V, Abbas AK, Fausto N, et al., eds. *Robbins and Cotran Pathologic Basis of Disease.* 8th ed. Philadelphia, PA: Saunders Elsevier; 2010:438–443.

43. Strayer DS, Rubin E. Environmental and nutritional pathology. In: Rubin R, Strayer DE, eds. *Rubin's Pathology: Clinicopathologic Foundations of Medicine.* 6th ed. Philadelphia, PA: Wolters Kluwer Health/Lippincott Williams & Wilkins; 2012:319–320.

44. Baron RB. Nutritional disorders. In: McPhee SJ, Papadakis MA, eds. *Current Diagnosis and Treatment.* 52nd ed. New York, NY: McGraw-Hill; 2013:1252–1263.

45. Tisdale MJ. Wasting in cancer. *J Nutr.* 1999;129(IS suppl):43S–46S.

46. Biolo G, Gabriele T, Cicchi B, et al. Metabolic response to injury and sepsis: changes in protein metabolism. *J Nutr.* 1999;129(IS suppl):53S–57S.

47. Rome ES, Ammerman S, Rosen DS. Children and adolescents with eating disorders: the state of the art. *Pediatrics.* 2003;111:e98–e108.

48. Ricanati EHW, Rome ES. Eating disorders: recognizing early to prevent complications. *Cleve Clin J Med.* 2005;72(10): 895–906.

49. Treasure J, Claudino AM, Zucker N. Eating disorders. *Lancet.* 2010;375:583–593.

50. Goldstein MA, Dechant EJ, Beresin EV. Eating disorders. *Pediatr Rev.* 2011;32:508–520.

51. American Psychiatric Association. *Diagnostic and Statistical Manual of Mental Disorders, DSM-5.* 5th ed. Washington, DC: American Psychiatric Publishing; 2013:338–354.

52. Weltzin TE, Weisensel N, Francyk D, et al. Eating disorders in men. *J Men's Health Gender.* 2005;2(2):186–193.

53. Brunet M. Female athlete triad. *Clin Sports Med.* 2005;24:623–636.

54. Yager J, Anderson AE. Anorexia nervosa. *N Engl J Med.* 2005;353(14):1481–1488.

55. Zerbe KJ. *Women's Mental Health in Primary Care.* Philadelphia, PA: W.B. Saunders; 1999:109–137.

56. Mehler PS. Bulimia nervosa. *N Engl J Med.* 2003;349(9):875–881.

57. Kondo DG, Sokol MS. Eating disorders in primary care. *Postgrad Med.* 2006;119:59–65.

58. Sim LA, McAlpine DE, Grothe KB, et al. Identification and treatment of eating disorders in the primary care setting. *Mayo Clin Proc.* 2010;85(8):746–751.

59. Schneider M. Bulimia nervosa and binge-eating disorders in adolescents. *Adolesc Med.* 2003;14:119–131.

Porth Essentials Resources

Explore these additional resources to enhance learning for this chapter:

- NCLEX-Style Questions and Other Resources on the**Point**, http://thePoint.lww.com/PorthEssentials4e
- Study Guide for Essentials of Pathophysiology
- Concepts in Action Animations
- Adaptive Learning | Powered by PrepU, http://thepoint.lww.com/prepu

Chapter 11

Disorders of White Blood Cells and Lymphoid Tissues

The hematopoietic system and lymphoid tissues are responsible for the generation and regulation of the blood cells that function in the transport of oxygen, defense against microorganisms, and preservation of the integrity of the vascular system. This chapter is divided into two parts: the first provides an introduction to the hematopoietic system, lymphoid tissues, and the white blood cells; and the second focuses on disorders of the white blood cells, including those of nonneoplastic (neutropenia and infectious mononucleosis) and neoplastic (lymphomas, leukemias, and multiple myeloma) origin. The megakaryocytes and platelets are discussed in Chapter 12, the red blood cells in Chapter 13, and the immune system (lymphocytes and monocytes) in Chapter 15.

Hematopoietic and Lymphoid Tissues

Blood consists of blood cells (i.e., leukocytes or white blood cells, thrombocytes or platelets, and erythrocytes or red blood cells) and the plasma in which the cells are suspended. These cells all derive from a single pool of pluripotent stem cells in the bone marrow, which give rise to two types of multipotent stem cells: the hematopoietic stem cells, which remain in the bone marrow, and the lymphopoietic stem cells, which migrate to the thymus, lymph nodes, spleen, and mucosa-associated lymphoid tissues.

The Bone Marrow and Hematopoiesis

The bone marrow consists of hematopoietic or blood-forming cells and stromal tissue that provides support for the blood-forming cells. The blood-forming population of bone marrow is made up of three types of cells: pluripotent stem cells, multipotent stem cells, and committed progenitor cells that develop into the various types of blood cells[1-4] (Fig. 11-1). The pluripotent stem cells give rise to two types of multipotential stem cells, the common lymphoid and the common myeloid stem cells. The common lymphoid stem cells, in turn, differentiate into lineage-specific precursor cells that develop into T lymphocytes (T cells), B lymphocytes (B cells), and natural killer (NK) cells. From the common myeloid stem cells arise precursor cells capable of differentiating along the erythrocyte/megakaryocytic and granulocyte-monocyte pathways.

Several levels of differentiation lead to the development of committed unipotential cells, which are the progenitors for each of the blood cell types. These cells are referred to as *colony-forming units* (CFUs).[3] These progenitor cells only have a limited capacity for self-renewal but retain the potential to differentiate into lineage-specific precursor cells. These precursor cells have morphologic characteristics that permit them to be recognized as the first cell of a particular cell line. They have lost their ability for self-renewal but undergo cell division and differentiation, eventually giving rise to mature lymphocytes, monocytes, granulocytes, megakaryocytes, or erythrocytes.

Hematopoietic Growth Factors

Under normal conditions, the numbers and total mass for each type of circulating blood cell remain relatively constant. This regulation of blood cells is thought to be at least partially controlled by hormone-like growth factors called *cytokines*. The cytokines are a family of short-lived mediators that stimulate the proliferation, differentiation, and functional activation of the various blood cells.

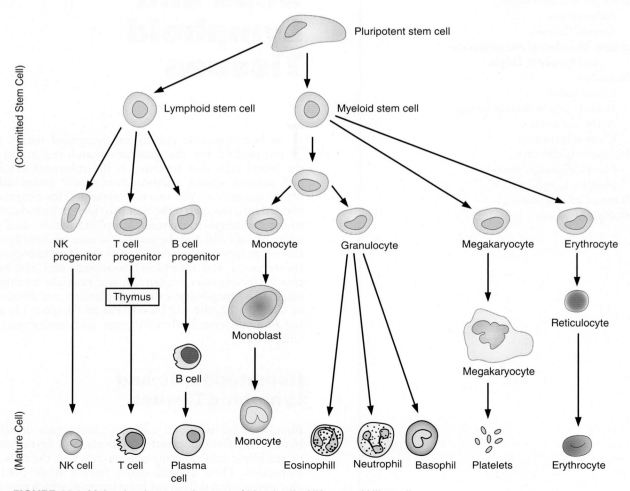

FIGURE 11-1. Major developmental stages of blood cells. NK, natural killer cell.

Many cytokines derived from lymphocytes or bone marrow stromal cells stimulate the growth and production of new blood cells. Several members of this family are called *colony-stimulating factors* (CSFs) because of their ability to promote the growth of hematopoietic cell colonies in the laboratory. The CSFs that act on committed progenitor cells include erythropoietin (EPO); thrombopoietin (TPO); *granulocyte-monocyte colony-stimulating factor* (GM-CSF), which stimulates progenitors for granulocytes, monocytes, erythrocytes, and megakaryocytes; *granulocyte colony-stimulating factor* (G-CSF), which promotes the proliferation of neutrophils; and *macrophage colony-stimulating factor* (M-CSF), which induces macrophage colonies.[3–5] Other cytokines, such as the interleukins, interferons, and tumor necrosis factor, support the proliferation of stem cells and the development of lymphocytes and act synergistically to aid the multiple functions of the CSFs.

The genes for most hematopoietic growth factors have been cloned and their recombinant proteins have been generated for use in a wide range of clinical conditions. The clinically useful factors include EPO, G-CSF, and GM-CSF.[5] They are used for treatment of bone marrow failure caused by chemotherapy or aplastic anemia, the anemia of kidney failure and cancer, hematopoietic neoplasms, infectious diseases such as acquired immunodeficiency syndrome (AIDS), and congenital and myeloproliferative disorders. Growth factors are used to increase peripheral stem cells for transplantation and to accelerate cell proliferation after bone marrow engraftment.

Leukocytes (White Blood Cells)

The leukocytes or white blood cells, which are the focus of this chapter, originate in the bone marrow and circulate throughout the lymphoid tissues of the body. Leukocytes are commonly classified into two groups based on the presence or absence of specific prominent granules in their cytoplasm.[1,2] Those containing specific granules (neutrophils, eosinophils, basophils) are classified as *granulocytes,* and those that lack granules (lymphocytes and monocytes) as *agranulocytes* (Fig. 11-2). The granulocytes and the agranular monocytes/macrophages are derived from the myeloid stem cells in the bone marrow and circulate in the blood (see Fig. 11-1). The lymphocytes originate from lymphoid stem cells in the bone marrow and migrate between the blood and the lymphatic system.

Granulocytes

Granulocytes are spherical and have distinctive multilobar nuclei. They are all phagocytic cells that are identifiable because of their cytoplasmic granules. They have two types of granules: *specific granules* that bind neutral, basic, or acidic dye components, and *azurophilic*

Granulocytes

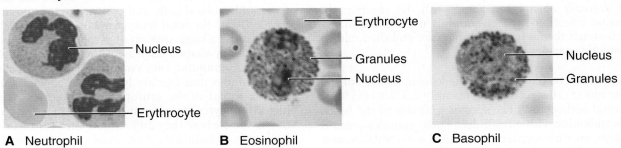

A Neutrophil   **B** Eosinophil   **C** Basophil

Agranulocytes

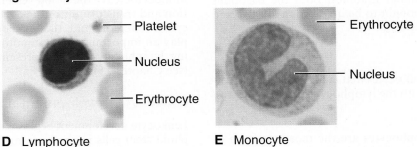

D Lymphocyte   **E** Monocyte

FIGURE 11-2. White blood cells. Granulocytes **(A–C)** and agranulocytes **(D, E)**. **(A)** The neutrophil has a large, segmented nucleus. **(B)** The eosinophil has many bright red–staining granules. **(C)** The basophil has large dark blue–staining granules. **(D)** The lymphocyte has a large undivided nucleus. **(E)** The monocyte is the largest of the leukocytes. (From Cohen BJ. *Memmler's The Human Body in Health and Disease*. 11th ed. Baltimore, MD: Wolters Kluwer Health I Lippincott Williams & Wilkins; 2009:284.)

granules. The azurophilic granules stain purple and are lysosomes. The granulocytes are divided into three types—neutrophils, eosinophils, and basophils—according to the staining properties of their specific granules.

Neutrophils.

The neutrophils, which constitute 60% to 65% of the total white blood cells, have specific granules that are neutral and do not stain with an acidic or a basic dye.[1] Because these white cells have nuclei that are divided into three to five lobes, they are often called *polymorphonuclear leukocytes* (PMNs).

The neutrophils are primarily responsible for maintaining normal host defenses against invading bacteria and fungi, cell debris, and a variety of foreign substances. After release from the marrow, the neutrophils spend only approximately 4 to 8 hours in the circulation before moving into the tissues. They survive in the tissues for approximately 4 to 5 days.[1] They die in the tissues by discharging their phagocytic function or from senescence. The pool of circulating neutrophils (i.e., those that appear in the blood count) is in a closely maintained equilibrium with a similar-sized pool of cells marginating along the walls of small blood vessels. These are the neutrophils that respond to chemotactic factors and migrate into the tissues toward the offending agent during an inflammatory reaction.

Eosinophils.

The specific cytoplasmic granules of the eosinophils stain red with the acidic dye eosin. These leukocytes constitute 1% to 3% of the total white blood cells and increase in number during allergic reactions and parasitic infections.[1] During allergic reactions, they are thought to release enzymes or chemical mediators that detoxify agents associated with the reaction. In parasitic infections, the eosinophils use surface markers to attach themselves to the parasite and then release hydrolytic enzymes that kill it.

Basophils.

The basophils are the least numerous of the white blood cells, accounting for only 0.3% to 0.5% of the total leukocytes.[1] The specific granules of the basophils stain blue with a basic dye. These granules contain heparin, an anticoagulant; histamine, a vasodilator; and other mediators of inflammation. The basophil, which is a blood cell, is related to the connective tissue mast cell that contains similar granules. Both the basophils and mast cells are thought to be involved in allergic and hypersensitivity reactions.

Agranulocytes

Agranulocytes are leukocytes that lack cytoplasmic granules. They include both the lymphocytes and monocytes/macrophages.

Lymphocytes.

Lymphocytes are the most common of the agranulocytes, accounting for approximately 30% of the total blood leukocytes.[1] They originate in the bone marrow from lymphoid stem cells and migrate through the peripheral lymphoid organs, where they recognize antigens and participate in immune responses.

There are three types of lymphocytes: B lymphocytes, T lymphocytes, and natural killer cells.[1,2] The *B lymphocytes* are so named because they were first recognized as a separate population in the bursa of Fabricius in birds and bursa-equivalent organs (e.g., bone marrow) in mammals. They differentiate to form antibody-producing plasma cells and are involved in humoral-mediated immunity. The *T lymphocytes* differentiate in the thymus. They activate other cells of the immune system (helper T cells) and are involved in cell-mediated immunity (cytotoxic T cells). *Natural killer cells* participate in innate or natural immunity and their function is to destroy foreign cells. The lymphocytes of the three different subsets have unique surface markers that can be identified and used to define their function and diagnose disease (discussed in Chapter 15).

Although all lymphocytes are morphologically similar, they comprise elements that vary in terms of lineage, cell membrane molecules and receptors, function, and response to antigen. These cells are often distinguished by surface proteins that can be identified using panels of monoclonal antibodies. These identified proteins are then correlated with cell functions. The standard nomenclature for these proteins is the "CD" (clusters of differentiation) numeric designation (CD4, CD8), which is used to delineate surface proteins that define a particular cell type or stage of cell differentiation and are recognized by a cluster or group of antibodies.[2] Although this nomenclature was originally developed for lymphocytes, it is now common practice to apply it to blood cells other than lymphocytes.

Monocytes/Macrophages.

Monocytes are the largest of the white blood cells and constitute approximately 3% to 8% of the total leukocyte count. They are distinguished by a large amount of cytoplasm and a darkly stained kidney-shaped nucleus. Although these cells are considered agranular, they contain small, dense, azurophilic granules that contain lysosomal enzymes similar to those found in the azurophilic granules of neutrophils. Monocytes travel from the bone marrow to the body tissues, where they differentiate into various tissue phagocytes including the *histiocytes* of loose connective tissue, *microglial cells* of the brain, *Kupffer cells* of the liver, and tissue macrophages. During inflammation, monocytes leave the blood vessel at the site of inflammation and transform into tissue macrophages that phagocytose bacteria and tissue debris. Macrophages also play an important role in immune responses by activating lymphocytes and by presenting antigen to T cells (see Chapter 15).

Leukocyte Developmental Stages

Leukocyte development begins with the myeloid and lymphoid stem cells in the bone marrow[2–4] (Fig. 11-3). The immature precursor cells for each of the cell lines are called *blast cells*. The names of the various leukocyte developmental stages are often used in describing blood cell changes that occur in hematopoietic disorders (e.g., acute lymphoblastic leukemia, chronic myelogenous leukemia).

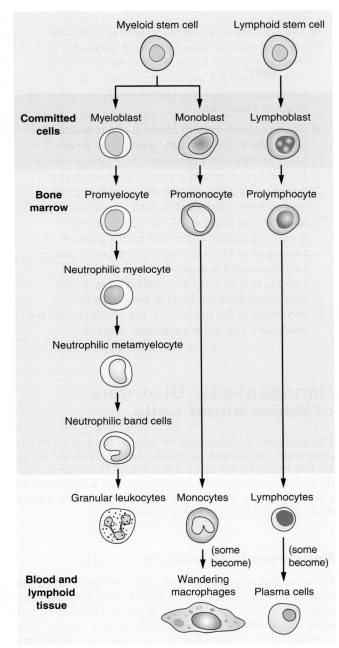

FIGURE 11-3. Leukocytes originate from multipotential stem cells in the bone marrow. Granular leukocytes (neutrophils, eosinophils, basophils) have their origin in the myeloid stem cells and develop through a sequence involving myeloblasts. Monocytes, like granulocytes, are progeny of the myeloid stem cell line, but develop along a pathway involving monoblasts. Only lymphocytes originate from the lymphoid stem cell line. They develop through a sequence involving lymphoblasts and are released from the bone marrow as prolymphocytes, which undergo further differentiation in the lymphoid organs.

The granulocytic precursor cells, which are called *myeloblasts*, have round to oval nuclei, with delicate chromatin and a blue to gray cytoplasm. During their next stage of development, the myeloblasts are transformed into *promyelocytes* with similar nuclei, but

with a cytoplasm containing many primary granules. In the subsequent *metamyelocyte* stage, the nuclei distort and become arclike, producing the band developmental stage. Maturation from metamyelocyte to mature neutrophil involves progressive condensation of nuclear chromatin, increasing nuclear lobulation, and the appearance of secondary (specific) granules. Eosinophils and basophils undergo similar developmental stages but develop different secondary granules. Like granulocytes, monocytes develop from the granulocyte-monocyte progenitor cell and progress through monoblast and promonocyte stages.

Lymphocytes derive from lymphoid stem cells and progress through the lymphoblast and prolymphocyte stages. The prolymphocytes leave the bone marrow and travel to the lymphoid tissues, where further differentiation into T and B lymphocytes occurs.

Lymphoid Tissues

The body's lymphatic system consists of the lymphatic vessels, lymphoid tissue and lymph nodes, thymus, and spleen (see Chapter 15). Although both precursor B and T lymphocytes begin their development in the bone marrow, they migrate to peripheral lymphoid structures to complete the differentiation process. B lymphocytes mature in the bone marrow, differentiate into plasma cells, and then move to the lymph nodes, where they continue to proliferate and produce antibodies. T lymphocytes leave the bone marrow as precursor T lymphocytes travel to the thymus, where they differentiate into CD4[+] helper T cells and CD8[+] cytotoxic T cells, after which many of them move to lymph nodes, where they undergo further proliferation.

Lymph nodes consist of organized collections of lymphoid tissue located along the lymphatic vessels.[2–4] Typically grayish white and ovoid or bean shaped, they range in diameter from 1 mm to 1 to 2 cm. A fibrous capsule and radiating trabeculae provide a supporting structure, and a delicate reticular network contributes to internal support (Fig. 11-4). The parenchyma of the lymph node is divided into an outer cortex and an inner medulla. The cortex contains well-defined B-cell and T-cell domains. The superficial outer cortex contains aggregates of cells called *follicles*. Follicles are the B-cell zones of the lymph nodes. There are two types of follicles: immunologically inactive follicles, called *primary follicles*, and active follicles that contain germinal centers, called *secondary follicles*. Germinal centers contain large lymphocytes (centroblasts) and small lymphocytes with cleaved nuclei (centrocytes). The mantle zone is the small layer of B cells surrounding the germinal centers. The cortex around the follicles is called the *paracortex*. This region contains most of the T cells in the lymph nodes. Like normal lymphocytes, malignant B and T cells tend to home to particular nodal sites, leading to characteristic patterns of involvement. For example, follicular lymphomas develop in the B-cell areas of the lymph node, whereas T-cell lymphomas typically grow in the paracortical T-cell zones.

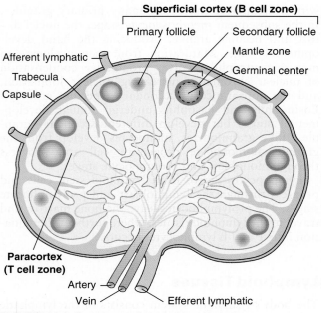

FIGURE 11-4. Structures of normal lymph node.

The alimentary canal, respiratory passages, and genitourinary systems are guarded by accumulations of lymphoid tissue that are not enclosed in a capsule. This form of lymphoid tissue is called *diffuse lymphoid tissue* or *mucosa-associated lymphoid tissue* (MALT) because of its association with mucous membranes. Lymphocytes are found in the subepithelium of these tissues. Lymphomas can arise from either MALT or lymph node tissue.

SUMMARY CONCEPTS

- The hematopoietic system consists of the different types of blood cells generated from the pluripotent stem cells in the bone marrow. These stem cells differentiate into committed cell lines that develop into red blood cells, platelets, and leukocytes. The development of the different types of blood cells is supported by chemical messengers, called *colony-stimulating factors,* other growth factors, and chemical mediators.

- White blood cells (leukocytes) development begins with myeloid stem cells that develop into granulocyte and monocyte cell lines, and lymphoid stem cells that develop into the lymphocyte cell line. The immature precursor cells for each of the cell lines are called *blast cells.* The blast cells progress through various maturational stages before becoming mature granulocytes, monocytes, or lymphocytes.

- The life span of white blood cells is relatively short so that constant renewal is necessary to maintain normal blood levels. Any conditions that decrease the availability of stem cells or hematopoietic growth factors produce a decrease in white blood cells.

- The lymphatic system consists of a network of lymphatic vessels, nodes, and tissues where B and T lymphocytes complete their differentiation. Lymph nodes, which are the site where many lymphomas originate, exhibit an outer cortex and an inner medulla. The cortex contains well-defined B-cell and T-cell domains. The B-cell–dependent superficial cortex consists of two types of follicles: immunologically inactive follicles, called *primary follicles,* and active follicles that contain germinal centers, called *secondary follicles.* Most of the T cells are contained in the paracortex, the area between the medullary and outer superficial cortices.

Nonneoplastic Disorders of White Blood Cells

The number of leukocytes, or white blood cells, in the peripheral circulation normally ranges from 4500 to 10,500 cells/μL (4.5 to 10.5 × 10⁹/L).[6] The nonneoplastic disorders of white blood cells include a deficiency of leukocytes (i.e., leukopenia) or proliferation of excess white blood cells (i.e., leukocytosis).

Neutropenia (Agranulocytosis)

The term *leukopenia* describes a decrease in the absolute number of leukocytes in the blood. The disorder may affect any of the specific types of white blood cells, but most often affects the neutrophils, which are the predominant type of granulocyte. *Agranulocytosis* denotes a virtual absence of neutrophils. In *aplastic anemia,* all of the myeloid stem cells are affected, resulting in anemia, thrombocytopenia, and agranulocytosis.

Neutropenia refers specifically to an abnormally low number of neutrophils and is commonly defined as a circulating neutrophil count of less than 1500/μL.[4,7–11] It can be further graded as mild (1000 to 1500/μL), moderate (500 to 1000/μL), or severe (<500/μL) based on an absolute number of neutrophils circulating in the blood. Since the neutrophil protects against bacterial infections, persons with neutropenia are prone to recurrent and sometimes severe bacterial infections.

Individuals of African descent and some ethnic groups from the Middle East have lower neutrophil counts without predisposition to bacterial infection, a condition referred to as *benign ethnic neutropenia.*[11]

Recent genetic studies in people of African descent have highlighted the role of the gene encoding the Duffy antigen receptor for chemokines (DARC). This genetic trait is strongly associated with protection against malaria.[11]

Pathogenesis

The reduction in the number of granulocytes in the blood (neutropenia) can be seen in a wide variety of conditions, including neoplasms, autoimmune disorders, and drug effect (Chart 11-1). Neutropenia is also a feature of a group of rare inherited disorders, such as Kostmann syndrome.[8]

Congenital Neutropenia. A decreased production of granulocytes is a feature of a group of hereditary hematologic disorders, including cyclic neutropenia and Kostmann syndrome.[9–11] *Periodic* or *cyclic neutropenia* is an autosomal dominant disorder with variable expression that begins in infancy and persists for decades. It is characterized by periodic neutropenia that develops approximately every 21 days and lasts approximately 2 or 3 days.[8] Although the cause is undetermined, it is thought to result from impaired feedback regulation of granulocyte production and release. Severe congenital neutropenia, also known as *Kostmann syndrome,* is a rare inherited form of neutropenia.[9–11] The condi-

---

CHART 11-1 | **Principal Causes of Neutropenia**

Congenital
Alloimmune neonatal neutropenia (transfer of maternal antibodies)
Cyclic neutropenia
Kostmann syndrome (severe congenital neutropenia)

Acquired
Autoimmune
    Primary (rare, usually occurs in children and runs a benign course)
Secondary
    Systemic lupus erythematosus
    Felty syndrome in persons with rheumatoid arthritis
Infection related
    Various infectious agents (most commonly viruses)
    Mechanisms include increased consumption of neutrophils, production of autoantibodies, direct infiltration of hematopoietic cells, bone marrow suppression
Drug related
    Immune-mediated reactions in which drugs act as haptens (e.g., penicillin, propylthiouracil, aminopyrine)
    Accelerated apoptosis (clozapine [antipsychotic agent])
    Bone marrow depression (i.e., vinblastine and other cancer chemotherapeutic agents)
Radiation therapy to bone marrow
Hematologic malignancies

---

tion occurs sporadically or as an autosomal recessive disorder, causing severe neutropenia while preserving the erythroid and megakaryocyte cell lineages that result in red blood cell and platelet production. The syndrome is usually recognized at birth or shortly thereafter. Infants with the syndrome have almost no neutrophils that develop beyond the promyelocyte stage (see Fig. 11-3). Treatment includes the administration of G-CSF. Before the advent of effective therapy, almost all patients died in early childhood.

Acquired Neutropenia. A number of conditions, including aplastic anemia and treatment with cancer chemotherapeutic drugs and irradiation, may cause suppression of bone marrow stem cells, with decreased production of all blood cell types.[8–10] Overgrowth of neoplastic cells in cases of nonmyelogenous leukemia and lymphoma also may suppress the function of neutrophil precursors. In splenomegaly, neutrophils may be trapped in the spleen along with other blood cells. Autoimmune disorders or idiosyncratic drug reactions may cause increased and premature destruction of neutrophils. In Felty syndrome, a variant of rheumatoid arthritis, there is increased destruction of neutrophils in the spleen. Infections by viruses or bacteria may drain neutrophils from the blood faster than they can be replaced, thereby depleting the neutrophil storage pool in the bone marrow.[8]

Many cases of neutropenia are drug related. Chemotherapeutic agents used in the treatment of cancer (e.g., alkylating agents, antimetabolites) cause predictable dose-dependent suppression of bone marrow function. The term *idiosyncratic* is used to describe drug reactions that are different from the effects observed in most persons and that cannot be explained in terms of allergy. A number of drugs, such as chloramphenicol (an antibiotic), phenothiazines (antipsychotic agents), propylthiouracil (used in the treatment of hyperthyroidism), and phenylbutazone (used in the treatment of arthritis), may cause idiosyncratic depression of bone marrow function.[7,8,10] Many idiosyncratic cases of drug-induced neutropenia are thought to be caused by immunologic mechanisms, with the drug or its metabolites acting as antigens (i.e., haptens) to incite the production of antibodies reactive against the neutrophils.

Clinical Course

The clinical features of neutropenia usually depend on the cause and severity of the disorder. Neutropenia from any cause places persons at risk for infection by gram-positive and gram-negative bacteria and by fungi. The risk of infection is related to the severity of the neutropenia. Persons with chronic benign neutropenia are often free of infection despite low neutrophil counts.

Neutrophils provide the first line of defense against organisms that inhabit the skin and gastrointestinal tract. Thus, skin infections and ulcerative necrotizing lesions of the mouth are common types of infection in neutropenia. The most frequent site of serious infection is the respiratory tract, a result of bacteria or fungi that frequently colonize the airways. Untreated infections can be rapidly fatal, particularly if the neutrophil count is less than 250/μL. In the presence of severe neutropenia, the usual signs of inflammatory response to infection may be absent. Nevertheless, fever in the person with neutropenia should always be assumed to be of infectious origin. A characteristic feature of bacterial infection in persons with neutropenia is the absence of pus, a purulent drainage containing leukocytes, dead cells, and tissue elements that have been liquefied by proteolytic enzymes elaborated by the neutrophils.[11]

Antibiotics are used to treat infections in those situations in which neutrophil destruction can be controlled or the neutropoietic function of the bone marrow can be recovered. Hematopoietic growth factors such as recombinant human G-CSF may be used to stimulate the maturation and differentiation of the granulocytic cell line.[8-11]

Infectious Mononucleosis

Infectious mononucleosis is a self-limiting lymphoproliferative disorder caused by the Epstein-Barr virus (EBV), a member of the herpesvirus family.[12-15] The term *EBV-associated infectious mononucleosis* is often used to designate infectious mononucleosis caused by EBV as opposed to non–EBV-associated clinical syndromes of infectious mononucleosis caused by other agents. Infectious mononucleosis may occur at any age, but occurs principally in adolescents and young adults in developed countries. Epstein-Barr virus is one of the viruses that is most successful in evading the immune system, infecting about 90% of humans and persisting for the lifetime of the person. Epstein-Barr virus spreads from person to person primarily through contact with infected oral secretions. Transmission requires close contact with infected persons. Thus, the virus spreads readily among young children in crowded conditions, where there is considerable sharing of oral secretions. Kissing is also an effective mode of transmission.[15]

Pathogenesis

Infectious mononucleosis is largely transmitted through oral contact with EBV-contaminated saliva. The virus initially penetrates the nasopharyngeal, oropharyngeal, and salivary epithelial cells. It then spreads to the underlying oropharyngeal lymphoid tissue and, more specifically, to B lymphocytes, all of which have receptors for EBV.[12-15] Infection of the B cells may take one of two forms—it may kill the infected B cell, or the virus may incorporate itself into the cell's genome. The B cells that harbor the EBV genome proliferate in the circulation and produce the well-known *heterophil* antibodies that are used for the diagnosis of infectious mononucleosis. A heterophil antibody is an immunoglobulin that reacts with antigens from another species—in this case, sheep red blood cells.

The normal immune response is important in controlling the proliferation of the EBV-infected B cells with the CD8+ cytotoxic T cells and NK cells playing the pivotal role. These virus-specific T cells appear as large, atypical lymphocytes that are characteristic of the infection (Fig. 11-5). In otherwise healthy persons, the humoral and cellular immune responses serve to control viral shedding by limiting the number of infected B cells rather than eliminating them.

Although infected B cells and free virions disappear from the blood after recovery from the disease, the virus remains in a few transformed B cells in the oropharyngeal region and is shed in the saliva. Once infected with the virus, persons remain asymptomatically infected for life, and a few such persons intermittently shed EBV. Immunosuppressed persons shed the virus more frequently. Asymptomatic shedding of EBV by healthy persons is thought to account for most of the spread of infectious mononucleosis, despite the fact that it is not a highly contagious disease.

Clinical Course

The onset of infectious mononucleosis usually is insidious. The incubation period from time of initial exposure to onset of symptoms is estimated at 4 to 8 weeks.[15] A prodromal period, which lasts for several days, follows and is characterized by malaise, anorexia, and chills. The prodromal period precedes the onset of fever, pharyngitis, and lymphadenopathy. Occasionally, the disorder comes on abruptly with a high fever. Most persons seek medical attention for severe pharyngitis, which usually is most severe on days 5 to 7 and persists for 7 to 14 days. The lymph nodes are typically enlarged throughout the body, particularly in the cervical, axillary, and groin areas. Hepatitis and splenomegaly are common manifestations of the disease and are thought to be immune mediated. Hepatitis is characterized by nausea, anorexia, hepatomegaly, and jaundice. Although discomforting, it usually is a benign condition that resolves without causing permanent liver damage. The spleen may be enlarged two to three times its

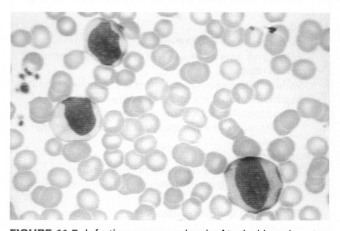

FIGURE 11-5. Infectious mononucleosis. Atypical lymphocytes are characteristic. (From Valdez R, Zutter M, Dulau FA, Rubin R. Hematopathology. In: Rubin R, Strayer DS, eds. *Rubin's Pathology: Clinicopathologic Foundations of Medicine*, 6th ed. Philadelphia, PA: Wolters Kluwer Health | Lippincott Williams & Wilkins; 2012:1002.)

normal size, and rupture of the spleen is an infrequent complication. In less than 1% of cases, mostly in the adult age group, complications of the central nervous system (CNS) develop. These complications include cranial nerve palsies, encephalitis, meningitis, transverse myelitis, and Guillain-Barré syndrome.

The peripheral blood usually shows an increase in the number of leukocytes, with a white blood cell count between 12,000 and 18,000 cells/μL, 60% of which are lymphocytes.[14] The rise in white blood cells begins during the first week, continues during the second week of the infection, and then returns to normal around the fourth week. Although leukocytosis is common, leukopenia may be seen in some persons during the first 3 days of illness. Atypical lymphocytes are common, constituting more than 20% of the total lymphocyte count. Heterophil antibodies usually appear during the second or third week and decline after the acute illness has subsided. They may, however, be detectable for up to 9 months after onset of the disease.

Most persons with infectious mononucleosis recover without incident. The acute phase of the illness usually lasts for 2 to 3 weeks, after which recovery occurs rapidly. Some degree of debility and lethargy may persist for 2 to 3 months. Treatment is primarily symptomatic and supportive. It includes bed rest and analgesics such as acetaminophen and nonsteroidal anti-inflammatory drugs (NSAIDs) to relieve the fever, headache, and sore throat. Although splenic rupture is rare, avoidance of contact sports for a minimum of 3 weeks after diagnosis is recommended.[15]

In persons with immunodeficiency disorders that lead to defects in cellular immunity (e.g., human immunodeficiency virus [HIV] infection, immunosuppressant-treated recipients of organ or bone marrow transplants), EBV infection may contribute to the development of lymphoproliferative disorders (e.g., non-Hodgkin lymphoma).[12] These persons have impaired T-cell immunity and are unable to control the proliferation of EBV-infected B cells.

SUMMARY CONCEPTS

■ Neutropenia, which represents a marked reduction in neutrophils, can occur as a congenital or acquired disorder. Because the neutrophil is essential to host defenses against bacterial and fungal infections, severe and often life-threatening infections are common in persons with neutropenia.

■ *Congenital neutropenia* consists primarily of cyclic neutropenia, which is characterized by cyclic oscillations of peripheral neutrophils, and severe congenital neutropenia or *Kostmann*

syndrome, which is associated with severe bacterial infections. The *acquired neutropenias* encompass a wide spectrum of etiologies, including immunologically mediated bone marrow suppression, neutrophil injury and destruction, infection-related processes, and drug-induced mechanisms—particularly those related to cancer chemotherapeutic agents.

■ Infectious mononucleosis is a self-limited lymphoproliferative disorder caused by the B-lymphotropic Epstein-Barr virus that is usually transmitted in the saliva. The disease is characterized by fever, sore throat, generalized lymphadenopathy, and the appearance of atypical lymphocytes and several antibodies in the blood, including the well-known heterophil antibodies commonly used in its diagnosis. Treatment is largely symptomatic and supportive and most people recover without incident.

Neoplastic Disorders of Hematopoietic and Lymphoid Origin

The neoplastic disorders of hematopoietic and lymphoid origin represent the most important of the white blood cell disorders. They can be divided into two broad categories based on the origin of the tumor cells: lymphoid neoplasms and myeloid neoplasms. The clinical features of these neoplasms are largely determined by their site of origin, the progenitor cell from which they originated, and the molecular events involved in their transformation into a malignant neoplasm.

Myeloid neoplasms arise from hematopoietic stem cells and normally give rise to monoclonal proliferations that replace normal bone marrow cells. They include the acute and chronic myelogenous leukemias.[4,7] The lymphoid neoplasms encompass a group of entities that vary widely in their clinical presentation and behaviors. They include the B- and T-cell leukemias and lymphomas (non-Hodgkin and Hodgkin lymphomas) that originate in peripheral lymphoid structures such as the lymph nodes, where B and T lymphocytes undergo differentiation and proliferation. The plasma cell dyscrasias originate in the lymph nodes, where B cells differentiate into plasma cells.

Leukemias

The leukemias are malignant neoplasms of cells originally derived from precursor myeloid or lymphoid tissue cells. The term *leukemia* (i.e., "white blood") was first used by Rudolf Virchow to describe a reversal of the usual ratio of red blood cells to white blood cells.[16]

Because blood cells circulate throughout the body, these neoplasms are often disseminated from the onset. The leukemic cells may also infiltrate the liver, spleen, lymph nodes, and other tissues throughout the body, causing enlargement of these organs.

Classification

The leukemias commonly are classified according to their predominant cell type (i.e., lymphocytic or myelocytic) and whether the condition is acute or chronic. Biphenotypic leukemias demonstrate characteristics of both lymphoid and myeloid lineages. The *lymphocytic leukemias* involve immature lymphocytes and their progenitors that originate in the bone marrow but infiltrate the spleen, lymph nodes, CNS, and other tissues. The *myelogenous leukemias,* which involve the pluripotent myeloid stem cells in bone marrow, interfere with the maturation of all blood cells, including the granulocytes, erythrocytes, and thrombocytes.

A rudimentary classification system divides leukemia into four types: acute lymphocytic leukemia (ALL), chronic lymphocytic leukemia (CLL), acute myelocytic leukemia (AML), and chronic myelocytic leukemia (CML).[4,7] Among children and adolescents, ALL is the most common type, accounting for 75% of leukemia cases. In adults 20 years of age and older, the most common types are CLL (38%) and AML (30%).[16]

Etiology and Molecular Biology

The causes of leukemia are largely unknown and likely differ among the different types of leukemia. The incidence of acute leukemia among persons who have been exposed to high levels of radiation is unusually high. Exposure to ionizing radiation, including medical radiation used in cancer treatment, increases the risk of leukemia.[16] Leukemia may occur as a second cancer after aggressive chemotherapy for other cancers, such as Hodgkin lymphoma. Some factors are associated with increased risk of certain types of leukemias.[16] Exposure to certain chemicals such as formaldehyde and benzene (a compound in cigarette smoke and gasoline) also increases the risk of AML. Family history is one of strongest risk factors for CLL. The existence of a genetic predisposition to development of acute leukemia is suggested by the increased leukemia incidence among a number of congenital disorders, including trisomy 21 (Down syndrome), neurofibromatosis, and Fanconi anemia.[7,16] In individuals with Down syndrome, the incidence of acute leukemia is 10 to 20 times that of the general population.

The molecular biology of leukemia suggests that the event or events causing the disorders exert their effects through disruption or dysregulation of genes that normally regulate blood cell development, blood cell homeostasis, or both. Most commonly, these are structural changes classified as *translocations,* in which a part of one chromosome becomes located on another chromosome and vice versa; *inversions,* in which part of a chromosome turns upside down and now is in reverse order but still attached to the original chromosome; and *deletions,* in which part of a chromosome has been lost (see Chapter 6). It is the disruption or dysregulation of specific genes and gene products occurring at the site of these chromosome aberrations that contributes to the development of leukemia.[17] In many instances, these genes and their products have been shown to be directly or indirectly involved in the normal development or maintenance of the hematopoietic system. Thus, it would appear that leukemia results, at least in part, from disruption in the activity of genes that normally regulate blood cell development. Advances in the understanding of the molecular biology of leukemia are beginning to provide a more complete understanding of the molecular complexity of this disorder for the purposes of diagnosis, classification, treatment, and monitoring of clinical outcomes.

One of the more studied translocations is the Philadelphia chromosome, which was the first chromosomal abnormality identified in cancer. The Philadelphia chromosome translocation represents a reciprocal translocation between the long arm of chromosome 22 and the long arm of chromosome 9.[17,18] During the translocation, a large portion of 22q is translocated to 9q, and a smaller piece of 9q is moved to 22q (Fig. 11-6). The portion of 9q that is translocated contains *ABL,*

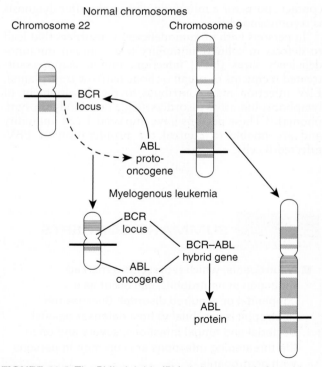

FIGURE 11-6. The Philadelphia (Ph) chromosome is formed by breaks at the ends of the long arms of chromosomes 9 and 22, allowing the *ABL* proto-oncogene on chromosome 9 to be translocated to the breakpoint cluster region (*BCR*) on chromosome 22. The result is a new fusion gene coding for the BCR–ABL protein, which is presumably involved in the pathogenesis of chronic myelogenous leukemia.

a proto-oncogene that is the cellular homolog of the Abelson murine leukemic virus. The *ABL* gene is received at a specific site on 22q called the *breakpoint cluster region* (BCR). The resulting *BCR–ABL* fusion gene codes for a novel protein that allows affected cells to bypass the regulated signals controlling normal cell growth and differentiation, and instead undergo malignant transformation to become leukemic cells. The Philadelphia chromosome translocation is found in more than 90% of persons with chronic myelogenous leukemia and in some persons with acute leukemia.[7] The recent development of tyrosine kinase inhibitors (e.g., imatinib mesylate) has contributed to the targeted approach for treatment of leukemias that display the Philadelphia chromosome translocation.[19]

Acute Leukemias

The acute leukemias are cancers of the hematopoietic progenitor cells. They usually have a sudden and stormy onset with signs and symptoms related to depressed bone marrow function.[19–29] There are two main forms of acute leukemia: acute lymphocytic (lymphoblastic) leukemia (ALL) and acute myeloid (myelogenous) leukemia (AML). Acute lymphocytic (lymphoblastic) leukemia is the most common form of leukemia in children. It accounts for three of four cases of childhood cancer, with AML accounting for most of the remaining cases.[22,23] Acute myeloid (myelogenous) leukemia is mainly a disease of older adults, but it is also seen in children and young adults.[24,29]

Acute lymphocytic (lymphoblastic) leukemia encompasses a group of neoplasms composed of precursor B (pre-B) or T (pre-T) lymphocytes referred to as *lymphoblasts* (see Fig. 11-3). Most cases (about 85%) of ALL are of pre–B-cell origin.[4,7] Approximately 90% of persons with ALL have numeric and structural changes in the chromosomes of their leukemic cells. They include hyperploidy (i.e., more than 50 chromosomes), polyploidy (i.e., three or more sets of chromosomes), and chromosomal translocations and deletions. Many of these chromosomal aberrations serve to dysregulate the expression and function of transcription factors required for normal hematopoietic cell development.

The AMLs are a diverse group of neoplasms affecting myeloid precursor cells in the bone marrow.[4,7] Most are associated with acquired genetic alterations that inhibit terminal myeloid differentiation. As a result, normal marrow elements are replaced by an accumulation of relatively undifferentiated blast cells. The result is suppression of the remaining progenitor cells and subsequent anemia, neutropenia, and thrombocytopenia. Specific chromosomal abnormalities, including translocations, are seen in a large number of AMLs. One subtype of AML, acute promyelocytic leukemia, which represents 10% of adult cases of AML, is associated with a (15;17) chromosomal translocation.[26] This translocation results in the fusion of the retinoic acid receptor α (RARA) gene on chromosome 17 with the promyelocytic leukemia (PML) gene on chromosome 15. This change in the retinoic acid receptor produces

a block in myeloid differentiation at the promyelocytic stage (see Fig. 11-3), probably by inhibiting the action of normal RARA receptors. This block can be overcome by pharmacologic preparations of retinoic acid (a vitamin A analog), causing the neoplastic promyelocytes to differentiate into neutrophils and die.

Manifestations. Although ALL and AML are distinct disorders, they typically present with similar clinical features. Both are characterized by an abrupt onset of symptoms, including fatigue resulting from anemia; low-grade fever, night sweats, and weight loss due to the rapid proliferation and hypermetabolism of the leukemic cells; bleeding due to a decreased platelet count; and bone pain and tenderness due to bone marrow expansion.[20–26] Infection results from neutropenia, with the risk of infection rising steeply as the neutrophil count falls below 500 cells/μL. Generalized lymphadenopathy, splenomegaly, and hepatomegaly caused by infiltration of leukemic cells occur in all acute leukemias but are more common in ALL.

In addition to the common manifestations of acute leukemia (i.e., fever, fatigue, weight loss, easy bruising), infiltration of malignant cells in the skin, gums, and other soft tissues is particularly common in the monocytic form of AML. The leukemic cells may also cross the blood–brain barrier and establish sanctuary in the CNS. Central nervous system involvement is more common in ALL than AML, and is more common in children than adults. Signs and symptoms of CNS involvement include cranial nerve palsies, headache, nausea, vomiting, papilledema, and occasionally seizures and coma.

Leukostasis is a condition in which the circulating blast count is markedly elevated (usually 100,000 cells/μL). The high number of circulating leukemic blasts increases blood viscosity and predisposes to the development of leukoblastic emboli with obstruction of small blood vessels in the pulmonary and cerebral circulations. Occlusion of the pulmonary vessels leads to vessel rupture and infiltration of lung tissue, resulting in sudden shortness of breath and progressive dyspnea. Cerebral leukostasis leads to diffuse headache and lethargy, which can progress to confusion and coma. Once identified, leukostasis requires immediate and effective treatment to lower the blast count rapidly. Initial treatment uses apheresis to remove excess blast cells, followed by chemotherapy to stop leukemic cell production in the bone marrow.[22]

Hyperuricemia occurs as the result of increased proliferation or increased breakdown of purine nucleotides (i.e., one of the components of nucleic acids) secondary to leukemic cell death that results from chemotherapy. It may increase before and during treatment. Prophylactic therapy with allopurinol, a drug that inhibits uric acid synthesis, is routinely administered to prevent renal complications secondary to uric acid crystallization in the urine filtrate.

Diagnosis and Treatment. A definitive diagnosis of acute leukemia is based on blood and bone marrow studies; it requires the demonstration of leukemic cells in the peripheral blood, bone marrow, or extramedullary tissue.[20–26] Bone marrow biopsy may be used to determine the molecular characteristics of the leukemia, the degree of bone marrow involvement, and the morphology and histology of the disease. Cytogenetic studies, which are used to determine chromosomal abnormalities, are one of the most powerful prognostic indicators in acute leukemia. In ALL, the staging includes a lumbar puncture to assess CNS involvement. Imaging studies that include computed tomography (CT) of the chest, abdomen, and pelvis may also be obtained to identify additional sites of disease.

Several types of treatment may be used for the management of ALL and AML with the primary treatment being chemotherapy. Treatment of ALL in childhood represents one of the great success stories in oncology. During the past decade, advances in ALL therapy have led to 5-year survival rates of greater than 80% in children.[19] Other age groups tend to do less well, with only about 30% to 40% of adults achieving long-term survival. Chemotherapy leads to remission in over 50% of persons with AML, but the overall survival rate is less than 30%.[4] Bone marrow or stem cell transplantation may be considered for persons with ALL and AML who have failed to respond to other forms of therapy.[17] Because of the risk of complications, bone marrow transplantation is not usually recommended for patients older than 50 to 55 years of age.

Chronic Leukemias

In contrast to acute leukemias, chronic leukemias are malignancies involving proliferation of more fully differentiated myeloid and lymphoid cells.[4,7] As with acute leukemia, there are two major types of chronic leukemia: chronic lymphocytic leukemia (CLL) and chronic myeloid (myelogenous) leukemia (CML). Chronic lymphocytic leukemia accounts for about one third of all leukemias and is mainly a disorder of older persons. The average age at time of diagnosis is approximately 72 years. It is rarely seen in people younger than 40 years of age, and is extremely rare in children.[30] Chronic myeloid (myelogenous) leukemia accounts for 10% to 15% of all leukemias. As with CLL, it is predominantly a disorder of older adults, with an average age of approximately 67 years at the time of diagnosis.

Chronic Lymphocytic Leukemia. Chronic lymphocytic leukemia, a clonal malignancy of B lymphocytes, is the most common form of leukemia in adults in the Western world. In the past, CLL was viewed as a homogeneous disease of immature, immune-incompetent, minimally self-renewing B cells, which accumulated because of faulty apoptotic mechanisms. Chronic lymphocytic leukemia is now becoming viewed as two related entities based on aggressiveness of the disease. Some persons with CLL survive for many years without therapy and eventually succumb to unrelated diseases, whereas others have a rapidly fatal disease despite aggressive therapy. The two entities are thought to reflect differences in the expression of cell surface CD markers (e.g., CD38) in immunoglobulin variable (V) gene mutations.[30–32]

This difference is rarely present in normal B cells but is found in persons with CLL. Persons whose CLL cells have mutated forms of the immunoglobulin gene generally have a more indolent form of the disease; these cells express low levels of the surface antigen.

The clinical signs and symptoms of CLL are largely related to the progressive infiltration of the bone marrow and lymphoid tissues by neoplastic lymphocytes and to secondary immunologic defects. Persons with the indolent form of CLL are often asymptomatic at the time of diagnosis, and the increase in lymphocytes is noted on a complete blood count obtained for another, unrelated disorder. As the disease progresses, lymph nodes gradually increase in size and new nodes are involved, sometimes in unusual areas such as the scalp, orbit, pharynx, pleura, gastrointestinal tract, liver, prostate, and gonads. Persons with the aggressive form of CLL experience a more rapid sequence of clinical deterioration characterized by increasing lymphadenopathy, hepatosplenomegaly, fever, abdominal pain, weight loss, progressive anemia, and thrombocytopenia, with a rapid rise in lymphocyte count.

Hypogammaglobulinemia is common in CLL, especially in persons with advanced disease. An increased susceptibility to infection reflects an inability to produce specific antibodies and abnormal activation of complement. The most common infectious organisms are those that require opsonization for bacterial killing, such as *Streptococcus pneumoniae*, *Staphylococcus aureus*, and *Haemophilus influenzae*.

The diagnostic hallmark of CLL is isolated increase in lymphocytes. The white blood cell count is usually greater than 20,000/μL and may be elevated to several hundred thousand. Usually, 75% to 98% are lymphocytes. Tests to determine the presence of mutated forms of the immunoglobulin gene (which currently can be detected only in research laboratories) and expression of the CD38 surface antigen may be used to determine whether the leukemia is the indolent or aggressive type.[31] Treatment of CLL usually depends on the presence of prognostic indicators.[31] Persons with the low-risk or indolent form of CLL usually do not require specific treatment for many years after diagnosis and eventually die of apparently unrelated causes. Many persons with intermediate-risk disease may remain stable for many years as well, whereas others may develop complications and need treatment within a few months. Most persons with high-risk CLL require combination chemotherapy at the time of diagnosis. In younger patients with aggressive disease, an allogeneic ablative (destruction of bone marrow cells by irradiation or chemotherapy) or nonmyeloablative stem cell transplant is a treatment option.

Chronic Myelogenous Leukemia. Chronic myeloid (myelogenous) leukemia is a disorder of the pluripotent hematopoietic progenitor cell. It is characterized by excessive proliferation of marrow granulocytes, erythroid precursors, and megakaryocytes.[4,7,33–38] The CML cells harbor a distinctive cytogenic abnormality, the previously described *Philadelphia chromosome*. It is generally believed that CML develops when a single, pluripotent hematopoietic stem cell acquires a Philadelphia chromosome. Although CML originates in the pluripotent stem cells, granulocyte precursors remain the dominant leukemic cell type.

The clinical course of CML is commonly divided into three phases: (1) a chronic phase of variable length, (2) a short accelerated phase, and (3) a terminal blast crisis phase. The onset of the chronic phase is usually slow, with nonspecific symptoms such as weakness and weight loss. The most characteristic laboratory finding at the time of presentation is leukocytosis with immature granulocyte cell types in the peripheral blood. Anemia and, eventually, thrombocytopenia develop. Anemia causes weakness, easy fatigability, and exertional dyspnea. Splenomegaly is often present at the time of diagnosis; hepatomegaly is less common; and lymphadenopathy is relatively uncommon. Persons in the early chronic phase of CML generally are asymptomatic, but without effective treatment most will enter the accelerated phase within 4 years.

The accelerated phase of CML is characterized by enlargement of the spleen and progressive symptoms. Splenomegaly often causes a feeling of abdominal fullness and discomfort. An increase in basophil count and more immature cells in the blood or bone marrow confirm transformation to the accelerated phase. During this phase, constitutional symptoms such as low-grade fever, night sweats, bone pain, and weight loss develop because of rapid proliferation and hypermetabolism of the leukemic cells. Bleeding and easy bruising may arise from dysfunctional platelets. Generally, the accelerated phase is short (6 to 12 months).

The terminal blast crisis phase of CML represents evolution to acute leukemia and is characterized by an increasing number of myeloid precursors, especially blast cells, in the blood (Fig. 11-7). Constitutional symptoms become more pronounced during this period, and splenomegaly may increase significantly. Isolated infiltrates of leukemic cells can involve the skin, lymph nodes, bones, and CNS. With very high blast counts (>100,000 cells/µL), symptoms of leukostasis may occur. The prognosis for patients who are in the blast crisis phase is poor, with a median survival of 3 months.

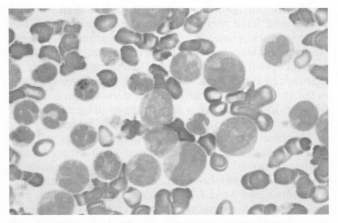

FIGURE 11-7. Peripheral blood showing blast crisis in chronic myelogenous leukemia. (From the Centers for Disease Control and Prevention Public Health Image Library. No. 6. Courtesy of Stacy Howard.)

A diagnostic feature of CML is an elevated white blood count, with a median count of 150,000/µL at the time of diagnosis, although in some cases it is only modestly increased. The hallmark of the disease is the presence of the BCR–ABL gene product, which can be detected in the peripheral blood. The treatment of CML is evolving rapidly. An inhibitor of the BCR–ABL tyrosine kinase, imatinib mesylate, induces complete remission in a high fraction of persons with stable-phase CML.[33,34] The only available curative treatment for CML is allogeneic bone marrow or stem cell transplantation.

Malignant Lymphomas

The lymphomas are a diverse group of solid tumors composed of neoplastic lymphoid cells that vary with respect to molecular features, genetics, clinical presentation, and treatment. Two groups of lymphomas are recognized: non-Hodgkin lymphomas (NHLs) and Hodgkin lymphoma (HL).[4,7,39]

Non-Hodgkin Lymphomas

The NHLs are one of the most common cancers in the United States, accounting for about 4% of all cancers. The average American has a risk of developing NHL during his or her lifetime of about 1 in 50. Personal risk factors that may affect the incidence level include gender, ethnicity, chemical or radiation exposure, and immune dysfunction.[40] Although some NHLs are common in children, more than 95% of cases occur in adults.[40] More than half of the people who develop NHLs are over age 65.[40]

As with most other malignancies, the cause of NHLs is largely unknown. However, impairment of the immune system and infectious agents may play a role. There is evidence of EBV infection in essentially all people with Burkitt lymphoma, which is endemic to some parts of Africa.[4,7] A second virus, the human T-cell lymphotropic virus (HTLV-1), which is endemic in the southwestern islands of Japan, has been associated with adult T-cell leukemia/lymphoma. The NHLs are also seen with increased frequency in persons infected with HIV, in those who have received chronic immunosuppressive therapy after organ transplantation, and in individuals with acquired or congenital immunodeficiencies.[40] There is also a reported association between chronic *Helicobacter pylori* infection and low-grade MALT lymphoma of the stomach.

Non-Hodgkin lymphomas can originate from malignant transformation of either the T or B cells during their differentiation in the peripheral lymphoid tissues.[4,7] Although the NHLs can originate in any of the lymphoid tissues, they most commonly originate in the lymph nodes. Like normal lymphocytes, transformed B and T cells tend to home into particular lymph node sites, leading to characteristic patterns of involvement. For example, B-cell lymphomas tend to proliferate in the B-cell areas of the lymph node, whereas T-cell lymphomas typically grow in the paracortical T-cell areas[4,7] (see Fig. 11-4). All have the potential to spread to various lymphoid tissues throughout the body, especially the liver, spleen, and bone marrow.

The classification of NHLs remains controversial and is still evolving. A commonly used classification is the World Health Organization (WHO) system[4,7,41] (Chart 11-2). The WHO system classifies lymphomas in terms of cell type (B or T cell), level of maturation (e.g., immature or mature), and anatomic sites (e.g., MALT lymphoma of the stomach).[4] The NHLs are actually a complex group of almost 40 distinct entities, based on the appearance of the lymphoma cells, the presence of surface markers (e.g., antigens, CD markers), and genetic features.[4,5,19] In addition, the specific types of lymphomas are sometimes grouped together into low-grade, aggressive, and very aggressive categories.

Mature B-Cell Lymphomas. Mature (peripheral) B-cell lymphomas are the most common type of lymphoma in the Western world. The most common of the mature B-cell lymphomas are the follicular lymphomas (22%) and diffuse large B-cell lymphomas (31%). Small lymphocytic lymphoma, mantle cell lymphoma, peripheral T-cell lymphoma, and MALT lymphoma together account for 28% of NHLs.[4]

Follicular lymphomas are derived from germinal center B cells and consist of a mixture of centroblasts and centrocytes. Follicular lymphomas are a particularly common neoplasm in the United States, where they constitute about one third of all adult NHLs, with a peak incidence at 60 years of age. The lymphoma predominantly affects lymph nodes. Other sites of involvement include the spleen, bone marrow, peripheral blood, head and neck region, gastrointestinal tract, and skin. Most persons have advanced disease at presentation and an indolent clinical course, with a median survival of 6 to 10 years.[7] Over time, approximately one of three follicular lymphomas transforms into a fast-growing diffuse large B-cell lymphoma.

Diffuse large B-cell lymphomas are a heterogeneous group of aggressive germinal or postgerminal center neoplasms. The disease occurs in all age groups but is most prevalent between 60 and 70 years of age. The cause of diffuse large B-cell lymphoma is unknown, but may involve EBV or HIV infections. It is a rapidly evolving, multifocal, nodal and extranodal tumor. Manifestations are typically seen at the time of presentation. As a group, diffuse large B-cell lymphomas are rapidly fatal if untreated.[42] However, with intensive combination chemotherapy, complete remission can be achieved in 60% to 80% of persons and approximately 40% to 50% remain disease free after several years and can be considered cured.[7]

Burkitt lymphoma, one of the most rapidly growing tumors of the NHLs, is also a disorder of germinal center B cells. Endemic Burkitt lymphoma is the most common childhood cancer (peak age 3 to 7 years) in Central Africa, often beginning in the jaw.[4] It occurs in regions of Africa where both EBV and malarial infections are common. Virtually 100% of patients with African Burkitt lymphoma have evidence of previous EBV infection, and their tumors carry the EBV genome and express EBV-encoded antigens.[4] Malarial infections in this population have been shown to cause T-cell immunodeficiencies, and it is postulated that this association may be the link between EBV infection and the development of lymphoma. A sporadic or nonendemic form of Burkitt lymphoma occurs less frequently in other parts of the world. The classic presentation of endogenous Burkitt lymphoma is a destructive tumor in the jaw and other facial bones (Fig. 11-8), whereas the sporadic form typically presents with abdominal masses. Both forms of Burkitt lymphoma respond to aggressive chemotherapy, with a cure rate of up to 90%.[4]

Mantle cell lymphomas constitute less than 10% of NHLs and have their origin in the naive B cell. After the precursor stage, B cells undergo immunoglobulin (Ig) gene rearrangements and develop into surface IgM- and IgD-positive naive B cells. These cells give rise to mantle cell lymphoma. Mantle cell lymphomas do not occur in children, but affect older persons (median age, 60 years).[4,7] They have a rapid rate of progression, and only one in five persons survives at least 5 years.

Marginal zone lymphomas involve late-stage memory B cells that reside in the marginal zone or outermost compartment of the lymph node follicle. Variants of marginal node lymphoma include splenic marginal zone lymphoma and MALT lymphomas of the stomach and other mucosal surfaces. *Mucosa-associated lymphoid tissue lymphomas* constitute 5% to 10% of all B-cell NHLs.[4] Most MALT lymphomas involve the stomach or other mucosal sites, including the respiratory system. Mucosa-associated lymphoid tissue lymphomas tend to

---

CHART 11-2 **WHO Classification of Selected Non-Hodgkin Lymphomas (most common)**

B-Cell Lymphomas

Precursor B-cell lymphomas
  B-cell lymphoblastic lymphoma
Mature B-cell lymphomas
  Diffuse large B-cell lymphoma
  Mediastinal large B-cell lymphoma
  Follicular lymphoma
  Small lymphocytic lymphoma
  Lymphoplasmacytic lymphoma
  Mantle cell lymphoma
  Mucosa-associated lymphoid tissue (MALT)
    lymphoma
  Burkitt lymphoma

T-Cell Lymphomas

Precursor T-cell lymphomas
  T-cell lymphoblastic lymphoma
Mature T- (and natural killer) cell lymphomas
  Anaplastic large cell lymphoma
  Peripheral T-cell lymphoma (unspecified)

Developed from the World Health Organization. Available at: http://www.who.int/classifications/apps/icd/meetings/tokyomeeting/B_6-3%20Annex1.pdf

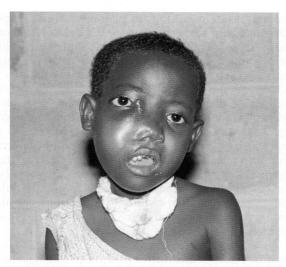

FIGURE 11-8. Burkitt lymphoma. A tumor of the jaw distorts this child's face. (From Valdez R, Zutter M, Dulau FA, et al. Hematopathology. In: Rubin R, Strayer DS, eds. *Rubin's Pathology: Clinicopathologic Foundations of Medicine.* 6th ed. Philadelphia, PA: Wolters Kluwer Health | Lippincott Williams & Wilkins; 2012:1012).

remain localized for prolonged periods and to follow an indolent course. Extranodal marginal B-cell lymphomas of the MALT type are curable by radiation or surgery when localized. Mucosa-associated lymphoid tissue lymphomas that occur in the stomach secondary to *H. pylori* infection often respond to treatment with appropriate antimicrobial agents.

Clinical Manifestations. The manifestations of NHLs depend on lymphoma type (i.e., indolent or aggressive) and the stage of the disease. Persons with indolent or slow-growing lymphomas usually present with painless lymphadenopathy, which may be isolated or widespread. Involved lymph nodes may be present in the retroperitoneum, mesentery, and pelvis. The indolent lymphomas are usually disseminated at the time of diagnosis, and bone marrow involvement is frequent. With or without treatment, the natural course of the disease may fluctuate over 5 to 10 or more years. Many low-grade lymphomas eventually transform into more aggressive forms of lymphoma/leukemia.

Persons with intermediate or more aggressive forms of lymphoma usually present with accompanying constitutional symptoms such as fever, drenching night sweats, or weight loss. Frequently, there is increased susceptibility to bacterial, viral, and fungal infections associated with hypogammaglobulinemia and a poor humoral antibody response, rather than the impaired cellular immunity seen with Hodgkin lymphoma. Because of their high growth fraction, these lymphomas tend to be sensitive to radiation and chemotherapy. Hence, with intensive combination chemotherapy, complete remission can be achieved in 60% to 80% of cases.[41]

Diagnosis and Treatment. A lymph node biopsy is used to confirm the diagnosis of NHLs and immu-

nophenotyping to determine the lineage and clonality. Lymphomas can be grouped according to surface markers or phenotypic markers (e.g., CD20).[43] Staging of the disease is important in selecting a treatment for persons with NHL. Bone marrow biopsy, blood studies, chest and abdominal CT scans, magnetic resonance imaging (MRI), positron emission tomography (PET), gallium scans, and bone scans may be used to determine the stage of the disease.[39] Newer technologies, such as deoxyribonucleic acid (DNA) microarray analysis, which identifies genes that are either overexpressed or underexpressed by tumor cells, may be used to further classify patients into distinct risk groups.

Treatment of NHLs depends on the histologic type, stage of the disease, and clinical status of the person.[40] For early-stage disease with single or limited node involvement, localized radiation may be used as a single treatment modality. However, because most people who present with indolent lymphomas have disseminated disease at the time of diagnosis, combination chemotherapy, combined adjuvant radiation therapy, or both are recommended. Persons with lymphomas that carry a risk of CNS involvement usually receive CNS prophylaxis with high doses of chemotherapeutic agents or cranial irradiation.

Hodgkin Lymphoma

Hodgkin lymphoma, previously known as *Hodgkin disease*, is a specialized form of lymphoma that features the presence of an abnormal cell called a *Reed-Sternberg cell*.[4,7,39,44] Because of improved treatment methods, death rates have decreased by more than 60% since the early 1970s. Distribution of the disease is bimodal; it occurs more frequently in two separate groups, the first in early adulthood (15 to 40 years) and the second in older adulthood (55 years of age or older).[39,44] About 10% to 15% of cases are diagnosed in children and teenagers.[44]

Hodgkin lymphoma differs from NHLs in many aspects. First, HL usually arises in a single node or chain of nodes and spreads first to anatomically contiguous lymphoid tissues, while NHLs frequently originates at extranodal sites and spreads in an unpredictable fashion. Therefore, the staging of HL is much more important in guiding therapy than it is for NHLs. Second, HL also has distinctive morphological features. It is characterized by the presence of large, atypical, mononuclear tumor cells, called *Reed-Sternberg cells* (Fig. 11-9). These cells release factors that induce the accumulation of reactive lymphocytes, macrophages, and granulocytes, which typically make up greater than 90% of the tumor cells.[7]

The origin of the neoplastic Reed-Sternberg cell of Hodgkin lymphoma has been difficult to study, in large part because these cells do not express many of the markers found on lymphocytes. It is only recently that methods have been developed that allow for the microanalysis of these cells and their variants. These studies have shown that the Reed-Sternberg cells of most individual cases harbor identical immunoglobulin genes that show evidence of mutation, establishing the cell of origin as a germinal center or postgerminal center B cell.

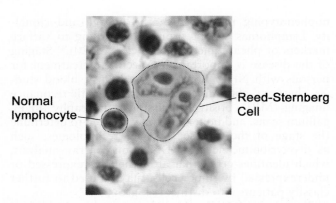

Normal lymphocyte — Reed-Sternberg Cell

FIGURE 11-9. Classic Reed-Sternberg cell; photograph shows normal lymphocyte compared with Reed-Sternberg cell. (From National Cancer Institute Visuals. No. CDR576466.)

As with NHL, the cause of Hodgkin lymphoma is largely unknown. Although exposure to carcinogens and viruses as well as genetic and immune mechanisms have been proposed as causes, none has been proven to be involved in the pathogenesis of the disease. It appears that people with a history of infectious mononucleosis are at increased risk for the development of Hodgkin lymphoma.[4,7,45]

Classification. The WHO classification proposed classifying Hodgkin lymphoma into two major categories: nodular lymphocyte-predominant Hodgkin lymphoma and classic Hodgkin lymphoma.[4,45] Nodular lymphocyte-predominant Hodgkin lymphoma represents only a small portion of all cases of HL and is a unique form that generally exhibits a nodular growth pattern, with or without diffuse areas and with rare Reed-Sternberg cells called "popcorn" or "L&H" (lymphohistiocytic) cells. It is often localized rather than disseminated at the time of diagnosis, exhibits a slowly progressive course, and has an overall survival rate greater than 80%.[4]

Classic Hodgkin lymphoma is characterized by clonal proliferation of typical mononuclear Hodgkin cells and multinucleated Reed-Sternberg cells with invariable expression of CD30. Four variants of classic Hodgkin lymphoma have been described: nodular sclerosing, mixed cellularity, lymphocyte rich, and lymphocyte depleted. The nodular sclerosing type is the most common and is often found in adolescent and young adult women, 15 to 35 years of age.[4] Lymphocyte-rich Hodgkin lymphoma is a newly defined entity, and lymphocyte-depleted Hodgkin lymphoma is rarely diagnosed. At present, all subtypes of classic Hodgkin lymphoma are treated in the same manner.[46]

Clinical Manifestations. Most persons with Hodgkin lymphoma present with painless enlargement of a single node or group of nodes. The initial lymph node involvement typically is above the level of the diaphragm (i.e., in the neck, supraclavicular area, or axilla). Mediastinal masses are frequent and are sometimes discovered on routine chest radiography. There may be complaints of chest discomfort with cough or dyspnea. Involvement of subdiaphragmatic lymph nodes at the time of

presentation is unusual and more common in elderly men. Additional symptoms that suggest Hodgkin lymphoma include fevers, chills, night sweats, and weight loss. Pruritus and intermittent fevers associated with night sweats are classic symptoms of Hodgkin lymphoma.

Other symptoms such as fatigue and anemia are indicative of disease spread. In the advanced stages of Hodgkin lymphoma, the liver, spleen, lungs, digestive tract, and, occasionally, CNS may be involved. As the disease progresses, the rapid proliferation of abnormal lymphocytes leads to an immunologic defect, particularly in cell-mediated responses, rendering the person more susceptible to viral, fungal, and protozoal infections. Anergy, or the failure to develop a positive response to skin tests such as the tuberculin test, is common early in the course of the disease.

Diagnosis and Treatment. A definitive diagnosis of Hodgkin lymphoma requires that the Reed-Sternberg cell be present in a biopsy specimen of lymph node tissue. Computed tomography scans of the chest and abdomen commonly are used to assess for involvement of mediastinal, abdominal, and pelvic lymph nodes.[44] If with initial screening the extent of lymph node involvement cannot be determined, PET imaging may be helpful.

Persons with Hodgkin lymphoma are staged according to the number of lymph nodes involved, whether the lymph nodes are on one or both sides of the diaphragm, and whether there is disseminated disease involving the bone marrow, liver, lung, or skin. The staging of Hodgkin lymphoma is of great clinical importance because the choice of treatment and the prognosis ultimately are related to the distribution of the disease. In addition, patients are designated stage A if they lack constitutional symptoms and stage B if 10% weight loss (over 6 months) or night sweats are present.

Irradiation and chemotherapy are used in treating the disease. Most people with localized disease are treated with radiation therapy[46,47] whereas a combined approach using radiation and chemotherapy is used in persons with advanced disease. As the accuracy of staging techniques, delivery of radiation, and curative efficacy of combination chemotherapy regimens have improved, the survival rate of people with Hodgkin lymphoma also has improved.

Plasma Cell Dyscrasias

Plasma cell dyscrasias are characterized by expansion of a single clone of immunoglobulin-producing plasma cells and a resultant increase in serum levels of a single monoclonal immunoglobulin or its fragments. The plasma cell dyscrasias include multiple myeloma, lymphoplasmacytic lymphoma, and monoclonal gammopathy of undetermined significance. *Monoclonal gammopathy of undetermined significance* (MGUS) is characterized by the presence of the monoclonal immunoglobulin in the serum without other findings of multiple myeloma. Monoclonal gammopathy of undetermined significance is considered a premalignant condition.[4,7] Approximately 2% per year of persons with MGUS will go on to develop a plasma cell dyscrasia (multiple myeloma or lymphoplasmacytic lymphoma). The strong link between MGUS and multiple myeloma suggests that a first oncogenic event produces MGUS and a second event results in multiple myeloma.[4]

Multiple Myeloma

Multiple myeloma is a B-cell malignancy of terminally differentiated plasma cells.[48–52] It accounts for 1% of all cancers in Western countries. Its incidence is higher in men and people of African-American descent.[4] It occurs most frequently in the elderly, with incidence peaking at the age of 63 to 70 years.

Pathogenesis. Multiple myeloma is characterized by proliferation of malignant plasma cells in the bone marrow and osteolytic bone lesions throughout the skeletal system. As with other hematopoietic malignancies, it is now recognized that multiple myeloma is associated with chromosomal abnormalities, including deletions of 13q and translocations involving the IgG locus on chromosome 14.[7] Changes also occur in the bone marrow microenvironment, including the induction of angiogenesis, the suppression of cell-mediated immunity, and the development of paracrine signaling loops involving cytokines such as IL-6 and vascular endothelial growth factor (VEGF). Other growth factors that are implicated in multiple myeloma include granulocyte-CSF, interferon-α, and IL-10.

One of the characteristic features resulting from the proliferating neoplastic plasma cells in multiple myeloma is the unregulated production of an abnormal monoclonal paraprotein referred to as the *M protein* because it is detected as an M spike on protein electrophoresis. In most cases the M protein is either IgG or IgA. In some cases, the plasma cells produce only the light chains of the immunoglobulin molecule. Because of their low molecular weight, the light chains are readily excreted in the urine, where they are termed *Bence Jones proteins*. More commonly, however, malignant plasma cells produce both complete immunoglobulins and free light chains; therefore, both M proteins and Bence Jones proteins are present. The excess light chains are directly toxic to renal tubular structures and are an important aspect of the pathophysiology of multiple myeloma.

Manifestations. The main sites involved in multiple myeloma are the bones and bone marrow (Fig. 11-10). In addition to the abnormal proliferation of marrow plasma cells, there is proliferation and activation of osteoclasts, which leads to bone resorption and destruction. This increased bone resorption predisposes the individual to pathologic fractures and hypercalcemia. Very high concentrations of paraproteins may cause a hyperviscosity of body fluids. The light-chain component may break down into amyloid, a proteinaceous substance deposited between cells, causing heart failure and nephropathy. Renal involvement, generally called *myeloma nephrosis*, is a distinctive feature

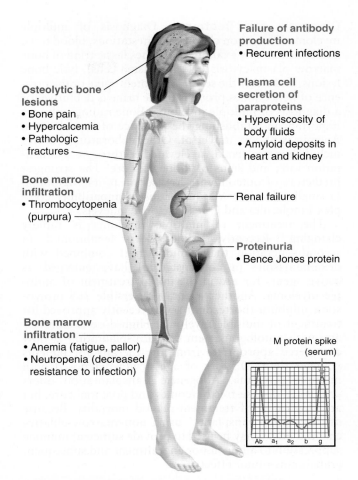

FIGURE 11-10. Clinical features of multiple myeloma.

of multiple myeloma. Although multiple myeloma is characterized by excessive production of monoclonal immunoglobulin, levels of normal immunoglobulins are usually depressed. This contributes to a general susceptibility to recurrent bacterial infections.

The malignant plasma cells also can form plasmacytomas (plasma cell tumors) in bone and soft tissue sites. The most common site of soft tissue plasmacytomas is the gastrointestinal tract. The development of plasmacytomas in bone tissue is associated with bone destruction and localized pain. Osteolytic lesions and compression fractures may be seen in the axial skeleton and proximal long bones. Occasionally, the lesions may affect the spinal column, causing vertebral collapse and spinal cord compression.

Bone pain is one of the first symptoms to occur in approximately three fourths of all individuals diagnosed with multiple myeloma. Bone destruction also impairs the production of erythrocytes, leukocytes, and thrombocytes. This predisposes the patient to anemia, recurrent infections, and thrombocytopenic purpura. Many patients experience weight loss and weakness. Renal insufficiency occurs in 50% of patients. Neurologic manifestations caused by neuropathy or spinal cord compression also may be present.

Diagnosis and Treatment. Diagnosis of multiple myeloma is based on clinical manifestations, blood tests, and bone marrow examination. The classic triad of bone marrow plasmacytosis (>10% plasma cells), lytic bone lesions, and either the serum M-protein spike or the presence of Bence Jones proteins in the urine is definitive for a diagnosis of multiple myeloma. Bone radiographs are important in establishing the presence of bone lesions. Anemia is almost universal. Other laboratory features include hypercalcemia, an elevated erythrocyte sedimentation rate, and signs of kidney failure. The strongest predictors of outcome are low serum β_2-microglobulin (a small subunit of the major histocompatibility complex I molecule) and C-reactive protein levels.

The treatment of multiple myeloma is rapidly changing.[49] Recently, thalidomide or lenalidomide (a second-generation thalidomide drug) combined with dexamethasone (a corticosteroid) have emerged as active agents for use in the initial treatment of multiple myeloma. Another agent, a reversible 26S proteosome inhibitor (bortezomib), was recently approved for treatment of multiple myeloma. High-dose chemotherapy with autologous stem cell transplantation is now considered appropriate front-line therapy for patients younger than 70 years of age newly diagnosed with multiple myeloma. Allogeneic transplantation offers prolonged disease-free outcomes and potential cure, but at a high cost of treatment-related mortality. Because of this, "mini-transplants" using non–marrow-ablative chemotherapy may be used to provide sufficient immune suppression to allow donor engraftment and subsequent graft-versus-tumor effect.

SUMMARY CONCEPTS

- The neoplastic disorders of hematopoietic and lymphoid origin include the leukemias, lymphomas, and multiple myeloma.

- The leukemias are malignant neoplasms arising from the transformation of a single blood cell line derived from hematopoietic stem cells in the bone marrow. Because leukemic cells are immature and poorly differentiated, they proliferate rapidly and have a long life span, they do not function normally, they interfere with the maturation of normal blood cells, and they circulate in the bloodstream, cross the blood–brain barrier, and infiltrate many body organs.

- Leukemias are classified according to cell type (i.e., lymphocytic or myelocytic) and whether the disease is acute or chronic. The *lymphocytic leukemias* involve immature lymphocytes and their progenitors that originate in the bone marrow but infiltrate the spleen, lymph nodes, CNS, and other tissues. The *myelogenous leukemias* involve the pluripotent myeloid stem cells in the bone marrow and interfere with the maturation of all blood cells, including the granulocytes, erythrocytes, and thrombocytes.

- The *acute leukemias* (i.e., ALL, which primarily affects children, and AML, which primarily affects adults) have a sudden and stormy onset with symptoms of depressed bone marrow function (anemia, fatigue, bleeding, and infections); bone pain; and generalized lymphadenopathy, splenomegaly, and hepatomegaly. The *chronic leukemias*, which largely affect adults, have a more insidious onset. Chronic lymphocytic leukemia often has the most favorable clinical course, with many persons living long enough to die of other, unrelated causes. The course of CML is slow and progressive, with transformation to a course resembling that of AML.

- The lymphomas (non-Hodgkin [NHL] and Hodgkin lymphoma) represent malignant neoplasms that arise in the peripheral lymphoid tissues. The NHLs, which usually originate in the lymph nodes, are multicentric in origin and spread early to various lymphoid tissues throughout the body, especially the liver, spleen, and bone marrow. Hodgkin lymphoma is a group of cancers characterized by Reed-Sternberg cells that begins as a malignancy in a single lymph node and then spreads to contiguous lymph nodes. Both types of lymphomas are characterized by manifestations related to uncontrolled lymph node and lymphoid tissue growth, bone marrow involvement, and constitutional symptoms (fever, fatigue, weight loss) related to the rapid growth of abnormal lymphoid cells and tissues.

- Multiple myeloma is a plasma cell dyscrasia characterized by expansion of a single clone of immunoglobulin-producing plasma cells and a resultant increase in serum levels of a single monoclonal immunoglobulin (paraprotein) or its fragments. The main sites involved in multiple myeloma are the bones and bone marrow. In addition to the abnormal proliferation of marrow plasma cells, there is proliferation and activation of osteoclasts, which leads to bone resorption and destruction and increased risk for pathologic fractures and development of hypercalcemia. Paraproteins secreted by the plasma cells may cause hyperviscosity of body fluids and may break down into amyloid, a proteinaceous substance deposited between cells that can cause heart failure and neuropathy.

REVIEW EXERCISES

1. Many of the primary immunodeficiency disorders, in which there is a defect in the development of immune cells of T- or B-lymphocyte origin, can be cured with allogeneic stem cell transplantation from an unaffected donor.

   A. Explain why stem cells are used rather than mature lymphocytes. You might want to refer to Figure 11-5.
   B. Describe how the stem cells would go about the process of repopulating the bone marrow.

2. A mother brings her 4-year-old son into the pediatric clinic because of irritability, loss of appetite, low-grade fever, pallor, and complaints that his legs hurt. Blood tests reveal anemia, thrombocytopenia, and an elevated leukocyte count with atypical lymphocytes. A diagnosis of acute lymphocytic leukemia (ALL) is confirmed with bone marrow studies.

   A. What is the origin of the anemia, thrombocytopenia, elevated leukocyte count, and atypical lymphocytes seen in this child?
   B. Explain the cause of the child's fever, pallor, increased bleeding, and bone pain.
   C. The parents are informed that the preferred treatment for ALL consists of aggressive chemotherapy with the purpose of achieving a remission. Explain the rationale for using chemotherapy to treat leukemia.
   D. The parents are told that the child will need intrathecal chemotherapy administered by a lumbar puncture. Why is this treatment necessary?

3. A 36-year-old man presents to his health care clinic with fever, night sweats, weight loss, and a feeling of fullness in his abdomen. Subsequent lymph node biopsy reveals a diagnosis of non-Hodgkin lymphoma (NHL).

   A. Although lymphomas can originate in any of the lymphoid tissues of the body, most originate in the lymph nodes, and most (80% to 85%) are of B-cell origin. Hypothesize as to why B cells are more commonly affected than T cells.
   B. A newly developed monoclonal antibody, rituximab, is being used in the treatment of NHL. Explain how this agent exerts its effect and why it is specific for B-cell lymphomas.

REFERENCES

1. Hall JE. *Guyton and Hall Textbook of Medical Physiology*. 12th ed. Philadelphia, PA: Elsevier Saunders; 2010:423–431.
2. Ross MH, Pawline W. *Histology: A Text and Atlas*. 5th ed. Philadelphia, PA: Lippincott Williams & Wilkins; 2006:275–286, 295–298.
3. Fey MF. Normal and malignant hematopoiesis. *Ann Oncol*. 2007;18(Suppl 1):9–13.
4. Valdez R, Zutter M, Dulau AE, et al. Hematopathology. In: Rubin R, Strayer DE, eds. *Rubin's Pathology: Clinicopathologic Foundations of Medicine*. 6th ed. Philadelphia, PA: Wolters Kluwer Health/Lippincott Williams & Wilkins; 2012:947–952, 986–1036.
5. Kaushansky K. Lineage-specific hematopoietic growth factors. *N Engl J Med*. 2006;354(19):2034–2045.
6. Fischbach F, Dunning MB III. *A Manual of Laboratory and Diagnostic Tests*. 8th ed. Philadelphia, PA: Wolters Kluwer Health/Lippincott Williams & Wilkins; 2009:67–91.
7. Kumar V, Abbas AK, Fausto N. *Robbins and Cotran Pathologic Basis of Disease*. 8th ed. Philadelphia, PA: Saunders Elsevier; 2010:589–638.
8. Schwartzberg LS. Neutropenia: etiology and pathogenesis. *Clin Cornerstone*. 2006;8(Suppl 5):S5–S11.
9. Boxer LA. How to approach neutropenia. *Hematology*. 2012:174–182.
10. Berliner N, Horwitz M, Loughran TP. Congenital and acquired neutropenia. *Hematology*. 2004:63–79.
11. Klein C. Congenital neutropenia. *Hematology*. 2009:344–350.
12. Cohen JI. Epstein-Barr virus infection. *N Engl J Med*. 2000;343:481–492.
13. McAdam AJ, Sharpe AH. Infectious diseases. In: Kumar V, Abbas AK, Fausto N, et al. *Robbins and Cotran Pathologic Basis of Disease*. 8th ed. Philadelphia, PA: Saunders Elsevier; 2010:355–357.
14. Schwartz DA. Infectious and parasitic diseases. In: Rubin R, Strayer DS, eds. *Rubin's Pathology: Clinicopathologic Foundations of Medicine*. 6th ed. Philadelphia, PA: Wolters Kluwer Health/Lippincott Williams & Wilkins; 2012:343–345.
15. Luzuiaga K, Sullivan JL. Infectious mononucleosis. *N Engl J Med*. 2010;362(21):1993–2000.
16. Kampen KR. The discovery and early understanding of leukemia. *Leuk Res*. 2012;36(1):6–13.
17. American Cancer Society. *Cancer Facts & Figures 2013*. Atlanta, GA: American Cancer Society; 2013.
18. Strayer DS, Rubin E. Neoplasia. In: Rubin R, Strayer DE, eds. *Rubin's Pathology: Clinicopathologic Foundations of Medicine*. 6th ed. Philadelphia, PA: Wolters Kluwer Health/Lippincott Williams & Wilkins; 2012:173–174.
19. Kurzrock R, Kantarjian HM, Druker BJ, et al. Philadelphia chromosome–positive leukemias: from basic mechanisms to molecular therapeutics. *Ann Intern Med*. 2003;138:819–830.
20. Pui C, Reiling MV, Downin JR. Acute lymphoblastic leukemia. *N Engl J Med*. 2004;350:1535–1548.
21. American Cancer Society. Acute lymphocytic leukemia (adults). 2013. Available at: http://www.cancer.org/acs/groups/cid/documents/webcontent/003109pdf.pdf. Accessed September 21, 2013.
22. Pieters R, Carroll WL. Biology and treatment of acute lymphocytic leukemia. *Hematol Oncol Clin North Am*. 2010;11:1–18.
23. Viole CS. Diagnosis, treatment, and nursing care of acute leukemia. *Semin Oncol Nurs*. 2003;19(2):98–108.
24. American Cancer Society. Childhood leukemia. 2012. Available at: http://www.cancer.org/acs/groups/cid/documents/webcontent/003095-pdf.pdf. Accessed September 21, 2013.
25. Belson M, Kingsley B, Holmes A. Risk factors for acute leukemia in children. *Environmental Health Perspectives*. 2007;115(1):138–145.
26. Rubnitz JE, Gibson B, Smith FO. Acute myeloid leukemia. *Hematol Oncol Clin North Am*. 2010;24:35–43.
27. Lo-Coco F, Ammatuna E. The biology of acute promyelocytic leukemia and its impact on diagnosis and treatment. *Hematology Am Soc Hematol Educ Program*. 2006:156–160.

28. American Cancer Society. Acute myeloid leukemia. 2013. Available at: http://www.cancer.org/acs/groups/cid/documents/webcontent/003110-pdf.pdf. Accessed September 21, 2013.

29. Krug U, Büchner T, Burdel WE, et al. The treatment of elderly patients with acute myeloid leukemia. *Dtsch Arziebi Int.* 2011;108(51–52):863–870.

30. American Cancer Society. Chronic lymphocytic leukemia. 2013. Available at: http://www.cancer.org/acs/groups/cid/documents/webcontent/003111-pdf.pdf. Accessed September 21, 2013.

31. Chiorazzi N, Rai KR, Farrarini M. Chronic lymphocytic leukemia. *N Engl J Med.* 2005;352:804–815.

32. Malayssi F, Deaglio S, Damie G. CD38 and chronic lymphocytic leukemia: a decade later. *Blood.* 2011;119(3):2470–3478.

33. American Cancer Society. Chronic myeloid leukemia. 2012. Available at: http://www.cancer.org/acs/groups/cid/documents/webcontent/003112-pdf.pdf. Accessed September 21, 2013.

34. Chen Y, Peng C, Sullivan C, et al. Critical molecular pathways in cancer stem cells of chronic myeloid leukemia. *Leukemia.* 2010;24(9):1545–1554.

35. Cervantes F, Mauro M. Practical management of chronic myeloid leukemia. *Cancer.* 2011;117:4343–4354.

36. Marin D. Initial choice of therapy among plenty for newly diagnosed chronic myeloid leukemia. *Hematology.* 2012:115–121.

37. Mahon F-X. Is going for a cure in chronic myeloid leukemia possible and justified. *Hematology.* 2012:122–128.

38. Goldman JM, Melo JV. Chronic myeloid leukemia: advances in biology and new approaches to treatment. *N Engl J Med.* 2003;349:1451–1464.

39. Rademaker J. Hodgkin's and non-Hodgkin's lymphoma. *Radiol Clin North Am.* 2007;45:69–83.

40. American Cancer Society. Non-Hodgkin lymphoma. 2013. Available at: http://www.cancer.org/acs/groups/cid/documents/webcontent/003126-pdf.pdf. Accessed September 21, 2013.

41. Armitage JO. Staging of non-Hodgkin lymphoma. *CA Cancer J Clin.* 2005;55:368–376.

42. Lenz C, Staudt LM. Aggressive lymphomas. *N Engl J Med.* 2010;362(15):1417–1429.

43. Reiser M, Diehl V. Current treatment of follicular non-Hodgkin's lymphoma. *Eur J Cancer.* 2002;38:1167–1172.

44. American Cancer Society. Hodgkin disease. 2012. Available at: http://www.cancer.org/acs/groups/cid/documents/webcontent/003105-pdf.pdf. Accessed September 21, 2013.

45. Yung L, Linch D. Hodgkin's lymphoma. *Lancet* 2003;361:943–951.

46. Conners JM. Hodgkin's lymphoma—the great teacher. *N Engl J Med.* 2011;365(3):264–265.

47. Armitage JO. Early-stage Hodgkin's lymphoma. *N Engl J Med.* 2010;363(7):653–662.

48. American Cancer Society. Multiple myeloma. 2013. Available at: http://www.cancer.org/acs/groups/cid/documents/webcontent/003126-pdf.pdf. Accessed September 21, 2013.

49. Palumbo A, Anderson K. Multiple myeloma. *N Engl J Med.* 2011;364(11):1046–1060.

50. Raab MS, Podar K, Breitkreutz I, et al. Multiple myeloma. *Lancet.* 2009;374:324–339.

51. Nau KC, Lewis WD. Multiple myeloma: diagnosis and treatment. *Am Fam Physician.* 2008;78(7):853–860.

52. Katzel JA. Multiple myeloma: charging toward a bright future. *CA Cancer J Clin.* 2007;57:301–318.

Porth Essentials Resources

Explore these additional resources to enhance learning for this chapter:

- NCLEX-Style Questions and Other Resources on thePoint, http://thePoint.lww.com/PorthEssentials4e
- Study Guide for Essentials of Pathophysiology
- Adaptive Learning | Powered by PrepU, http://thepoint.lww.com/prepu

Disorders of Hemostasis

Hemostasis is a multistep process that maintains the integrity of a closed high-pressure circulatory system after vessel injury. The normal process of hemostasis is regulated by a complex array of activators and inhibitors that maintain blood fluidity and prevent blood from leaving the vascular compartment. Hemostasis is normal when a blood vessel is sealed to prevent blood loss and hemorrhage. It is deemed abnormal when inappropriate blood clotting occurs or when clotting is insufficient to stop the flow of blood from the vascular compartment. Disorders of hemostasis fall into two main categories: the inappropriate formation of clots within the vascular system (thrombosis) and the failure of blood to clot in response to an appropriate stimulus (bleeding).

Hemostasis and Blood Coagulation

Hemostasis preserves vascular integrity by balancing the processes that maintain blood in a fluid state and prevent excessive bleeding following injury. The process involves the transformation of blood into a semisolid clot with erythrocytes trapped in its fibrin meshwork at the site of injury (Fig. 12-1).

Components of Hemostasis

Hemostasis is a multistep process that involves platelets, plasma clotting factors, naturally occurring anticoagulants, and the inherent properties of the endothelial lining of blood vessels.

Platelets

Platelets, also called *thrombocytes,* are large fragments from the cytoplasm of bone marrow cells called *megakaryocytes.*[1-5] There are normally 150,000 to 400,000 platelets in each microliter (μL) of blood[1] with an average platelet life span of 8 to 9 days. Platelets do not leave the blood as white blood cells do, but at any time about one third of them are stored in blood-filled spaces in the spleen and can be released into the circulation as needed. Platelet production is controlled by a protein

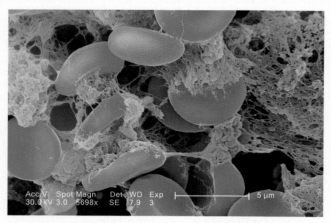

FIGURE 12-1. A scanning electron micrograph depicting a number of red cells enmeshed in a fibrinous matrix on the luminal surface of an indwelling catheter (magnification × 5698). (From the Centers for Disease Control and Prevention Public Health Images Library No. 7313. Courtesy of Janice Carr.)

called *thrombopoietin* that causes proliferation and maturation of megakaryocytes.[2] Thrombopoietin is produced in the liver, kidney, smooth muscle, and bone marrow. Its production and release are regulated by the number of platelets in the circulation.

Although platelets lack a nucleus, they have many of the structural and functional characteristics of a whole cell.[1-5] They contain an outer cell membrane, microtubular structures, and inner organelles (Fig. 12-2). The platelet cell membrane, which plays an important role in platelet adhesion and the coagulation process, is covered

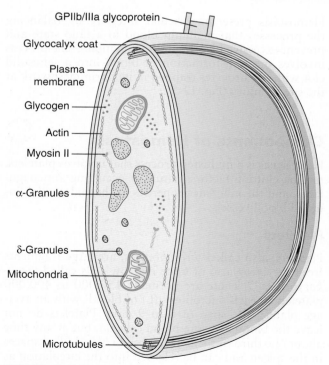

FIGURE 12-2. Platelet structure.

with a surface coat of glycocalyx, consisting of glycoproteins, glycosaminoglycans, and several coagulation factors adsorbed from the plasma.[2] One of the important glycoproteins is glycoprotein IIb/IIIa (gpIIb/IIIa), which binds fibrinogen (factor I) and acts to connect platelets together to form large aggregates. Phospholipids, which are also present in the platelet membrane, provide critical binding sites for calcium and coagulation factors in the intrinsic coagulation pathway.[2,3] The cell membrane is supported by a network of microtubules, actin filaments, myosin, and actin-binding proteins. They are arranged circumferentially and are responsible for maintaining the platelet's disk shape.

The central part of the platelet contains mitochondria, enzymes needed for synthesis of adenosine triphosphate (ATP) and the prostaglandin thromboxane A_2 (TXA$_2$), glycogen, and two specific types of granules (α- and δ-granules) that release mediators for hemostasis.[2-5] The α-granules contain fibrinogen, coagulation factors, plasminogen, plasminogen activator inhibitor, and platelet-derived growth factors. The contents of these granules play an important role in platelet aggregation, blood coagulation, and the initial phase of vessel repair. The release of growth factors causes vascular endothelial cells, smooth muscle cells, and fibroblasts to proliferate and grow. The δ-granules, or dense granules, mainly contain adenosine diphosphate (ADP), ATP, ionized calcium, serotonin, and histamine, which facilitate platelet adhesion and vasoconstriction at the site of vessel injury.

The Coagulation System

The coagulation system uses plasma proteins that are present as inactive procoagulation factors. Each of the procoagulation or coagulation factors, identified by Roman numerals, performs a specific step in the coagulation process. The activation of one procoagulant or proenzyme is designed to activate the next factor in the sequence (i.e., cascade effect). Because most of the inactive procoagulants are present in the blood at all times, the multistep process ensures that a massive episode of intravascular clotting does not occur by chance. It also means that abnormalities of the clotting process occur when one or more of the factors are deficient or when conditions lead to inappropriate activation of any of the steps.

Most of the coagulation factors are proteins synthesized in the liver. Vitamin K is necessary for the synthesis of factors VII, IX, and X; prothrombin (factor II); and proteins C and S. Calcium (factor IV) is required in all but the first two steps of the clotting process. The body usually has sufficient amounts of calcium for these reactions. Inactivation of the calcium ion prevents blood from clotting once removed from the body. The addition of citrate to blood stored for transfusion purposes prevents clotting by chelating ionized calcium.

A clot is not expected to be a permanent solution to vessel injury; thus, blood clotting is accompanied by processes designed to control the coagulation cascade and dissolve the clot once bleeding has been controlled.

Blood coagulation is regulated by several natural anticoagulants, such as antithrombin III and proteins C and S, which work by inactivating some of the clotting factors. The plasma also contains a plasma protein called *plasminogen* that gets activated and converted to plasmin, an enzyme capable of digesting the fibrin strands of the clot. In addition to removing clots that are no longer needed, plasmin scavenges continually to prevent clots from forming inappropriately.

Endothelium

The blood vessels themselves play an important role in preventing and controlling the formation of blood clots. Blood vessels are lined with endothelial cells that modulate several, frequently opposing stages of normal hemostasis. Under most circumstances endothelial cells maintain an environment that promotes blood flow by blocking platelet adhesion and activation, inhibiting the coagulation process, and lysing blood clots. It should be noted, however, that the endothelium can be activated by infectious agents, hemodynamic factors, plasma mediators, and cytokines that are liberated during an inflammatory reaction.

An intact endothelial surface prevents platelets and plasma coagulation factors from interacting with the underlying thrombogenic subendothelial extracellular matrix. Moreover, if platelets are activated, they are inhibited from adhering to the surrounding uninjured endothelium by endothelial prostacyclin (prostaglandin I_2 [PGI_2]) and nitric oxide (see Chapter 18). Both of these mediators are potent vasodilators and inhibitors of platelet aggregation. Endothelial cells also elaborate an enzyme called *adenosine diphosphatase* (ADP) that degrades and further inhibits platelet aggregation. The anticoagulant effects of endothelial cells are mediated by membrane-bound heparin and thrombomodulin, both of which inactivate thrombin (factor IIa). In addition, endothelial cells synthesize tissue plasminogen activator, promoting fibrinolytic activity that clears fibrin deposits from endothelial cell surfaces.

Although endothelial cells exhibit properties that inhibit blood clotting, they are also capable of exhibiting numerous procoagulant properties in response to injury and activation. An important function of activated endothelial cells is the synthesis of von Willebrand factor, which participates in platelet adhesion and blood clotting.

Clot Formation and Dissolution

Hemostasis is divided into five stages: (1) vessel spasm, (2) formation of the platelet plug, (3) blood coagulation or development of an insoluble fibrin clot, (4) clot retraction, and (5) clot dissolution.[1] During the process of hemostasis, hairlike fibrin strands glue the aggregated platelets together and intertwine to form the structural basis of the blood clot. In the presence of fibrin, plasma becomes gel-like and traps red blood cells and other formed elements in the blood (see Fig. 12-1). Hemostasis is complete when fibrous tissue grows into the clot and seals the hole in the vessel.

Vessel Spasm

Vessel spasm is initiated by endothelial injury and caused by local and humoral mechanisms. It is a transient event, usually lasting less than one minute, that results from neural reflexes and humoral factors released from platelets and traumatized tissue.[1] For smaller vessels, release of the vasoconstrictor TXA_2 is responsible for much of the vessel spasm.

Platelet Plug Formation

The platelet plug, the second line of defense, is initiated as platelets come in contact with the vessel wall. Small breaks in the vessel wall are often sealed with the platelet plug rather than with a blood clot. Platelet plug formation involves adhesion, granule release, and aggregation of platelets.[3] Platelets are attracted to a damaged vessel wall, become activated, and change from smooth disks to spiny spheres, exposing glycoprotein receptors on their surfaces. Platelet adhesion requires a protein molecule called *von Willebrand factor* (vWF). This factor is produced by both megakaryocytes and endothelial cells and circulates in the blood as a carrier protein for coagulation factor VIII. Adhesion to the vessel subendothelial layer occurs when the platelet membrane receptor binds to vWF at the injury site, linking the platelet to exposed collagen fibers.

Degranulation and release of the contents of both the α- and δ-granules occur soon after platelet adhesion. The δ-granule contents', including calcium, is required for the coagulation component of hemostasis.[3] The binding of ADP to the platelet membrane induces a conformation change of the gpIIb/IIIa receptors, allowing them to bind fibrinogen and form aggregates. Besides ADP, platelets secrete the prostaglandin TXA_2, which is an important stimulus for platelet aggregation. The combined actions of ADP and TXA_2 lead to the expansion of the enlarging platelet aggregate, which is called the *primary hemostatic platelet plug*. Conversion of the primary platelet plug into a definitive clot (known as a *secondary hemostatic plug*) occurs as the coagulation pathway is activated on the surface of the aggregated platelets and fibrinogen is converted to fibrin (factor Ia), thereby creating a fibrin meshwork that cements the platelets and other blood components together.

Platelet aggregation inhibitors, including aspirin, clopidogrel (Plavix), and ticlopidine (Ticlid), can be used to prevent platelet aggregation and clot formation in persons who are at risk for myocardial infarction, stroke, or peripheral artery disease.[6,7] Low-dose aspirin therapy inhibits prostaglandin synthesis, including TXA_2. Clopidogrel and ticlopidine achieve their antiplatelet effects by inhibiting the ADP pathway in platelets. Unlike aspirin, these drugs have no effect on prostaglandin synthesis. Drugs that act as gpIIb/IIIa receptor inhibitors (abciximab, eptifibatide, tirofiban) have been developed for use in the treatment of persons with acute coronary syndromes (see Chapter 19).[7]

(*text continues on page 266*)

UNDERSTANDING → Hemostasis

Hemostasis, which refers to the stoppage of blood flow, is divided into five stages: (1) vessel spasm, (2) formation of the platelet plug, (3) development of a blood clot (coagulation cascade), (4) clot retraction, and (5) clot dissolution. This multistep process involves the interaction of substrates, enzymes, protein cofactors, and calcium ions that circulate in the blood or are released from platelets and cells in the vessel wall.

1 **Vessel Spasm.** Injury to a blood vessel causes vascular smooth muscle in the vessel wall to contract and thus instantaneously reduce blood flow. Both local neural reflexes and local humoral factors such as thromboxane A_2 (TXA_2), which is released from platelets, contribute to the vasoconstriction.

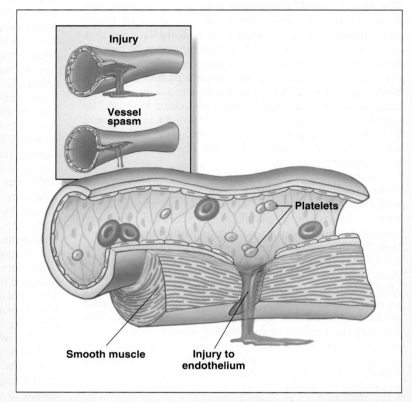

2 **Formation of the Platelet Plug.** Seconds after vessel injury, von Willebrand factor, released from the endothelium, binds to platelet receptors, causing adhesion of the platelets to the exposed collagen fibers (*inset*). As the platelets adhere to the collagen fibers on the damaged vessel wall, they become activated and release adenosine diphosphate (ADP) and TXA_2. The ADP and TXA_2 attract additional platelets, leading to platelet aggregation.

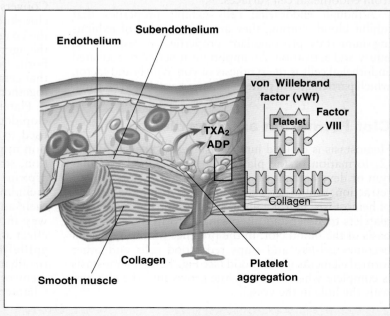

3 Blood Coagulation. Blood coagulation is a complex process involving the sequential activation of various factors in the blood. There are two coagulation pathways: (1) the intrinsic pathway which begins in the circulation and is initiated by activation of circulating factor XII, and (2) the extrinsic pathway which is activated by a cellular lipoprotein called *tissue factor* that becomes exposed when tissues are injured. Both pathways lead to the activation of factor X, conversion of prothrombin (II) to thrombin (IIa), and conversion of fibrinogen (I) to the insoluble fibrin (Ia) threads that hold the clot together.

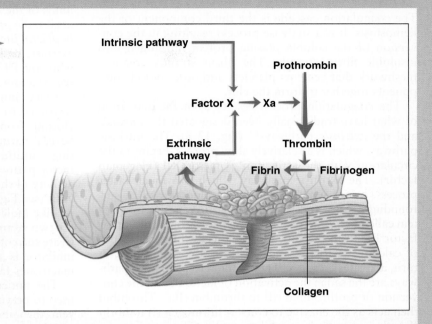

4 Clot Retraction. Within a few minutes after a clot is formed, the actin and myosin in the platelets that are trapped in the clot begin to contract in a manner similar to that in muscles. As a result, the fibrin strands of the clot are pulled toward the platelets, thereby squeezing serum (plasma without fibrinogen) from the clot and causing it to shrink.

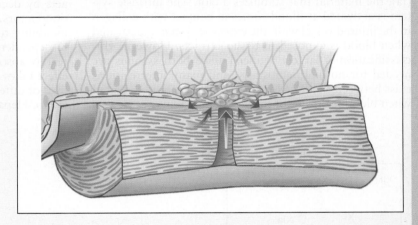

5 Clot Dissolution or Lysis. Clot dissolution begins shortly after a clot is formed. It begins with activation of plasminogen, an inactive precursor of the proteolytic enzyme, plasmin. When a clot is formed, large amounts of plasminogen are trapped in the clot. The slow release from injured tissues and vascular endothelium of a very powerful activator called tissue plasminogen activator (t-PA) converts plasminogen to plasmin, which digests the fibrin strands, causing the clot to dissolve.

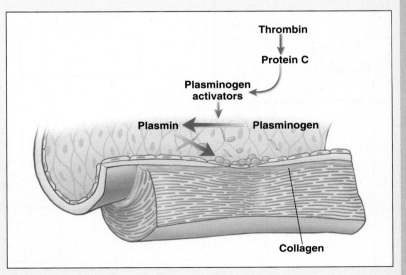

(text continued from page 263)

The Coagulation Cascade

The coagulation cascade is the third component of the hemostasis. It is a stepwise process resulting in the conversion of the soluble plasma protein fibrinogen into insoluble fibrin strands. The fibrin strands create a meshwork that cements platelets and other blood components together to form the clot.

The coagulation process results from the activation of what have traditionally been designated the *intrinsic* and the *extrinsic* pathways[1,3] (Fig. 12-3). The intrinsic pathway, which is a relatively slow process, begins in the circulation with the activation of factor XII (Hageman factor). The extrinsic pathway, which is a much faster process, begins with trauma to the blood vessel or surrounding tissues and the release of an adhesive lipoprotein called *tissue factor* (also known as thromboplastin or factor III) from the subendothelial cells. In the presence of calcium, factors V and VII form a complex that, in turn, activates factor X. The terminal steps in both pathways are the same: the activation of factor X and the conversion of prothrombin (II) to thrombin (IIa). Thrombin then acts as the enzyme to convert fibrinogen (I) to fibrin (Ia), the material that stabilizes a clot. The intrinsic system is activated as blood comes in contact with collagen in the injured vessel wall; the extrinsic system is activated when blood is exposed to tissue extracts. However, this classification is largely artificial since both systems are needed for normal hemostasis, and many interrelations exist between them.[8] Moreover, each system is activated when blood leaks out of the vascular system.

Clinical laboratories assess the function of the two limbs of the coagulation pathway through two standard assays: the *prothrombin time* (PT) and the *partial thromboplastin* time (PTT). The PT assesses the function of the extrinsic pathway (factors VII, X, V, II, and fibrinogen), while the PTT assesses the function of the intrinsic pathway (factors XII, XI, IX, VII, X, V, II, and fibrinogen).[3]

Once initiated, the coagulation cascade must be restricted to the local site of vascular injury to prevent clotting from occurring in the entire vascular system. Several natural anticoagulants function to control clotting—antithrombin III, proteins C and S, and tissue factor pathway inhibitor.[4] Antithrombin III inhibits the activity of thrombin (IIa) and factors IXa, Xa, XIa, and XIIa (see Fig. 12-3). It is activated by binding to heparin-like molecules on endothelial cells. Proteins C and S are two vitamin K–dependent plasma proteins that inactivate the cofactors Va and VIIIa. Tissue factor pathway inhibitor is a protein secreted by the endothelium that inactivates factor Xa and tissue factor VIIa complexes.

The anticoagulant drugs warfarin and heparin are used to prevent thromboembolic disorders, such as deep vein thrombosis and pulmonary embolism.[6] Warfarin acts by decreasing prothrombin and other procoagulation factors. It alters vitamin K in a manner that reduces its ability to participate in the synthesis of the vitamin K–dependent coagulation factors in the liver. Warfarin is readily absorbed after oral administration. Its maximum effect takes 36 to 72 hours because of the varying half-lives of different clotting factors that remain in the circulation. Heparin is naturally formed and released in small

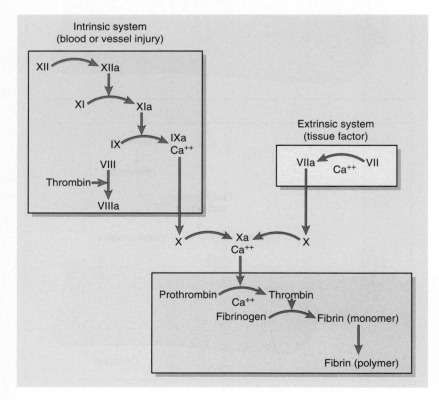

FIGURE 12-3. The intrinsic and extrinsic coagulation pathways. The terminal steps in both pathways is the same. Calcium, factor X, and platelet phospholipids combine to form prothrombin activator, which then converts prothrombin (II) to thrombin (IIa). This interaction causes conversion of fibrinogen (I) into the fibrin (Ia) strands that create the insoluble blood clot.

amounts by mast cells in connective tissue surrounding capillaries. Heparin binds to antithrombin III, causing a conformational change that increases the ability of antithrombin III to inactivate thrombin (IIa), factor Xa, and other clotting factors. By promoting the inactivation of clotting factors, heparin ultimately suppresses the formation of fibrin and therefore inhibits coagulation. Pharmacologic preparations of heparin are extracted from animal tissues. Heparin is unable to cross the membranes of the gastrointestinal tract and must be given by injection, usually by intravenous infusion. Low–molecular-weight heparins have been developed that inhibit activation of factor X, but have little effect on thrombin and other coagulation factors. The low–molecular-weight heparins are given by subcutaneous injection and require less-frequent administration and monitoring compared with the standard (unfractionated) heparin.

Clot Retraction

Clot retraction normally occurs within 20 to 60 minutes after a clot has formed, contributing to hemostasis by squeezing serum from the clot and joining the edges of the broken vessel. Platelets, through the action of their actin and myosin filaments, also contribute to clot retraction. Clot retraction therefore requires large numbers of platelets, and failure of clot retraction is indicative of a low platelet count.

Clot Dissolution

The dissolution of a blood clot begins shortly after its formation; this allows blood flow to be reestablished and permanent tissue repair to take place.[1] The process in which the strands of the clot are dissolved is called *fibrinolysis*. As with clot formation, clot dissolution requires a sequence of steps controlled by activators and inhibitors. Plasminogen, the proenzyme for the fibrinolytic process, normally is present in the blood in its inactive form. It is converted to its active form, plasmin, by plasminogen activators (PAs) formed in the vascular endothelium, liver, and kidneys. The plasmin formed from plasminogen digests the fibrin strands of the clot and certain clotting factors, such as fibrinogen (I), factor V, factor VIII, prothrombin (II), and factor XII. The most important of the plasminogen activators is *tissue-type plasminogen activator* (tPA), which is synthesized principally by endothelial cells and is most active when attached to fibrin. The affinity of tPA for fibrin makes it a useful therapeutic agent, since it largely confines its activity to sites of recent thrombosis.[3] Another plasminogen activator called *urokinase-type plasminogen activator* (uPA) is present in the tissues and can activate plasminogen in the fluid phase.

As with other potent physiologic systems, the activity of plasmin is tightly controlled. Excess circulating plasmin is rapidly inactivated by α_2-antiplasmin, which limits the fibrinolytic process to the local clot rather than allowing it to spread throughout the entire circulation.[3] Endothelial cells further modulate the coagulation/anticoagulation process by releasing PA inhibitors, which block fibrinolysis and confer an overall procoagulation effect. The PA inhibitors are increased by certain cytokines and probably play a role in the intravascular thrombosis accompanying severe inflammation.

SUMMARY CONCEPTS

- Hemostasis is an orderly multistep physiological process that preserves vascular integrity by balancing the processes that maintain blood in a fluid state and prevent excessive bleeding following injury.

- Hemostasis involves platelets, plasma clotting factors, naturally occurring anticoagulants, and the endothelial cells that line blood vessels, in order to transform blood into a semisolid clot with erythrocytes trapped in its fibrin meshwork.

- The process of hemostasis begins when a loss of endothelial integrity causes platelet activation. Upon activation, platelets undergo adhesion, granule release, and aggregation to form a primary platelet plug.

- The formation of the secondary hemostatic plug cements the platelet plug, forming an insoluble hemostatic clot. To occur, the formation of the definitive clot requires activation of the coagulation cascade, which terminates with thrombin converting fibrinogen into insoluble fibrin.

- The final step of the process involves fibrinolysis or clot dissolution, which involves the action of plasmin to dissolve the clot and allow blood flow to be reestablished and tissue healing to take place.

Hypercoagulability States

Hypercoagulability represents an exaggerated form of hemostasis that predisposes to thrombosis and blood vessel occlusion. There are two general forms of hypercoagulability states: conditions that create increased platelet function and conditions that cause accelerated activity of the coagulation system. Chart 12-1 summarizes conditions commonly associated with hypercoagulability states. Arterial thrombi are usually due to turbulence and composed largely of platelet aggregates, whereas venous thrombi are usually due to stasis of flow and composed largely of platelet aggregates and fibrin complexes that result from activation of the coagulation cascade.

Increased Platelet Function

Increased platelet function predisposes to platelet adhesion, formation of platelet clots, and the disruption of blood flow. The causes of increased platelet function

---

CHART 12-1 Conditions Associated with Hypercoagulability States

Increased Platelet Function
Increased platelet numbers
Reactive disorder (iron-deficiency anemia, splenectomy, cancer, chronic inflammatory conditions)
Myeloproliferative disorders (polycythemia vera)
Endothelial injury
Atherosclerosis
Elevated blood lipid and cholesterol levels
Smoking

Accelerated Activity of the Clotting System
Inherited disorders (primary)
Mutation in the factor V gene (factor V Leiden)
Mutation in the prothrombin gene
Acquired (secondary)
Prolonged bed rest or immobility
Oral contraceptive agents and pregnancy
Myocardial infarction
Heart failure
Malignant diseases
Antiphospholipid antibody syndrome

---

include an increase in platelet count and disturbances in blood flow, damage to the vascular endothelium, and increased sensitivity of platelets to factors that cause adhesiveness and aggregation.

The term *thrombocytosis* is used to describe elevations in the platelet count above 1,000,000/μL.[9] An increase in platelet count can occur as a reactive disorder associated with iron-deficiency anemia, especially in children; splenectomy; cancer; and chronic inflammatory conditions such as rheumatoid arthritis and Crohn disease. Usually the only clinically apparent signs are those of the underlying disease. Myeloproliferative disorders such as polycythemia vera (see Chapter 14) produce excess platelets that may predispose to thrombosis or, paradoxically, bleeding when the rapidly produced platelets are defective.

Atherosclerotic plaques disturb blood flow, causing endothelial damage and promoting platelet adherence. Platelets adhere to the vessel wall, release growth factors, cause proliferation of smooth muscle, and thereby contribute to the development of atherosclerosis (see Chapter 18). Smoking, elevated levels of blood lipids and cholesterol, hemodynamic stress, and diabetes mellitus predispose to vessel damage, platelet adherence, and eventual thrombosis.

Increased Clotting Activity

Thrombus formation due to activation of the coagulation system can result from primary (genetic) or secondary (acquired) disorders affecting the coagulation components of the blood clotting process (i.e., an increase in procoagulation factors or a decrease in anticoagulation factors).

Inherited Disorders

Of the inherited causes of hypercoagulability, mutations in the factor V and prothrombin genes are the most common.[4,10] In persons with inherited defects in factor V, the mutant factor Va cannot be inactivated by protein C; as a result, an important antithrombotic counterregulatory mechanism is lost. Approximately 2% to 5% of Caucasians carry a specific factor V mutation (referred to as the *Leiden mutation*, because of the Dutch city where it was first discovered).[3] The defect predisposes to venous thrombosis, and among persons with recurrent deep vein thrombosis, the frequency of the mutation may be as high as 60%.[3] It is one of the most common causes of primary and recurrent thromboembolism in pregnancy and is also associated with abruptio placentae (premature placental separation) and fetal growth disturbance.[10]

A single nucleotide change in the prothrombin gene, which affects 1% to 2% of the population, is associated with elevated prothrombin levels and an almost three-fold increase in venous thromboses.[4] Another hereditary defect results in high circulating levels of homocysteine, which predisposes to venous and arterial thrombosis by activating platelets and altering antithrombotic mechanisms.[4]

Acquired Disorders

Unlike the hereditary disorders, multiple conditions often predispose persons to acquired or secondary thrombotic disorders. Stasis of blood and accumulation of platelets and activated clotting factors are common in situations such as with prolonged bed rest and immobility. Hyperviscosity syndromes (e.g., polycythemia) and deformed red blood cells in sickle cell disease increase the resistance to flow and cause small vessel stasis. Hypercoagulability is associated with oral contraceptive use and the hyperestrogenic state of pregnancy, probably related to the increased synthesis of coagulation factors and reduced synthesis of antithrombin III.[11] The incidence of stroke, thromboemboli, and myocardial infarction is greater in women who use oral contraceptives, particularly those older than 35 years of age and those who smoke tobacco. In disseminated cancer, release of procoagulant tumor products predisposes to thrombosis. Smoking and obesity promote hypercoagulability for unknown reasons.

Antiphospholipid Syndrome. Another cause of increased venous and arterial thrombosis is the *antiphospholipid syndrome*. This condition is associated with a family of autoantibodies directed against several negatively charged phospholipids, causing an increase in coagulation activity. It is unclear how antiphospholipid antibodies lead to hypercoagulability, but possible explanations include direct platelet activation, endothelial cell activation or injury, or interference with the phospholipid-binding proteins involved in the regulation of blood coagulation (e.g., tissue factor, prothrombin, antithrombin III, and protein C).[12–14] Common features of the syndrome include recurrent thrombosis, repeated fetal loss, and thrombocytopenia. The disorder can manifest either as a primary condition occurring in isolation with signs of hypercoagulability or as a secondary condition most often associated with connective tissue disorders, particularly systemic lupus erythematosus (SLE).

Persons with the disorder present with a variety of clinical manifestations, typically those characterized by recurrent venous and arterial thrombi. Cardiac valvular vegetations associated with thrombi adherence and thrombocytopenia due to excessive platelet consumption may also occur. Venous thrombosis, especially in the deep leg veins, occurs in up to 50% of persons with the syndrome, half of whom develop pulmonary emboli. Arterial thromboses are less common than venous thromboses and most frequently manifest with features of ischemia and infarction. The cerebral arteries are the most commonly affected. Other sites for arterial thrombosis are the coronary arteries of the heart and the retinal, renal, and peripheral arteries. Women with the disorder commonly have a history of recurrent pregnancy losses after the 10th week of gestation because of ischemia and thrombosis of the placental vessels. These women also have increased risk of giving birth to a premature infant owing to pregnancy-associated hypertension and uteroplacental insufficiency.

In most persons with antiphospholipid syndrome, the thrombotic events occur as a single episode at one anatomic site. In some persons recurrences may occur months or years later and mimic the initial event. Occasionally, someone may present with multiple vascular occlusions involving many organ systems. This rapid-onset condition is termed *catastrophic antiphospholipid syndrome* and is associated with a high mortality rate.

Treatment of the syndrome focuses on removal or reduction in factors that predispose to thrombosis, including tobacco cessation and avoidance of estrogen-containing oral contraceptives by women. The acute thrombotic event is treated with anticoagulants (heparin and warfarin) and immune suppression in refractory cases. Aspirin and anticoagulant drugs may be used to prevent future thrombosis.[13]

SUMMARY CONCEPTS

■ Hypercoagulability states increase the risk of clot or thrombus formation in either the arterial or venous circulations. Arterial thrombi are associated with conditions that produce an increase in platelet numbers or turbulence in blood flow with platelet adhesion. Venous thrombi are associated with inherited or acquired conditions that cause a decrease in anticoagulation factors or produce a stasis of blood, thereby causing an increase in procoagulation factors.

■ Increased platelet function usually results from disorders such as atherosclerosis that damage the vascular endothelium and disturb blood flow, or from conditions such as smoking that increase sensitivity of platelets to factors that promote adhesiveness and aggregation.

■ Increased activity of the coagulation system results from hereditary (factor V Leiden mutation) or acquired disorders (immobility, hyperviscosity syndromes) causing alterations in the components of the coagulation system (i.e., an increase in procoagulation factors or a decrease in anticoagulation factors).

■ Thrombocytosis refers to an increase in the platelet count that can occur as an essential (primary thrombocytosis) or a reactive process (secondary thrombocytosis). The antiphospholipid syndrome, another cause of venous and arterial clotting, manifests as a primary or a secondary disorder associated with systemic lupus erythematosus. It is associated with antiphospholipid antibodies, which promote thrombosis throughout the body.

Bleeding Disorders

Bleeding disorders or impairment of blood coagulation can result from defects in any of the factors that contribute to hemostasis. Bleeding can occur as a result of disorders associated with platelet count, platelet function, coagulation factors, or blood vessel integrity.

Platelet Disorders

Bleeding due to platelet disorders reflects a failure of activated platelets to bring about hemostasis through the formation of a platelet plug at the site of injury to the blood vessel wall, an injury that causes physical and biochemical disruption of the endothelium.

Thrombocytopenia

Thrombocytopenia refers to a decrease in the number of circulating platelets to a level less than 100,000/μL.[15,16] The greater the decrease in the platelet count, the greater the risk of bleeding. However, spontaneous bleeding usually does not occur until the platelet count falls below 20,000/μL.

The anatomic sites of bleeding in persons with thrombocytopenia are the intercellular junctions in the postcapillary venules.[16] Key molecules in the junctions include adhesive proteins and associated intracellular binding components (see Chapter 1). Different vascular beds with varying functions require different types of junctions. For example, the regulatory control of capillary permeability in the skin and mucosal surfaces is far different from that in the brain. Common sites for spontaneous bleeding from platelet disorders are the skin and mucous membranes of the nose, mouth, gastrointestinal tract, and uterine cavity. Cutaneous bleeding is seen as purple areas of bruising (purpura) and pinpoint hemorrhages (petechiae) in dependent areas where the capillary pressure is higher. Petechiae are seen almost exclusively in conditions of platelet deficiency, not platelet dysfunction. They are also seen in conditions of poor collagen synthesis and impaired formation of capillary intercellular junctions[15] (Fig. 12-4). Because tight regulation of capillary permeability in the brain is essential to prevent intercellular leakage, nontraumatic intracranial bleeding is relatively rare, even in persons with severe thrombocytopenia.[16]

The major causes of thrombocytopenia are decreased platelet production, decreased platelet survival, splenic sequestration, and dilution.[3,4,16] Decreased platelet production due to loss of bone marrow function may occur because of congenital anemia (e.g., Wiskott-Aldrich syndrome [see Chapter 16]), acquired anemia (e.g., aplastic anemia [see Chapter 13]), bone marrow infiltration by malignant cells (e.g., leukemia), or bone marrow depression (e.g., radiation therapy, chemotherapy). Infection with human immunodeficiency virus (HIV) or cytomegalovirus may suppress the production of megakaryocytes, the platelet precursors.

Reduced platelet survival is caused by a variety of immune and nonimmune mechanisms. Platelet destruction may be caused by antiplatelet antibodies. These antibodies may be directed against platelet self-antigens or against antigens formed on the platelets from prior blood transfusions or pregnancy. In acute disseminated intravascular clotting or thrombotic thrombocytopenic purpura (TTP), excessive platelet consumption leads to a deficiency.

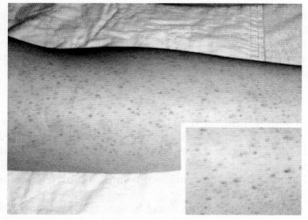

FIGURE 12-4. Leg of a 9-year-old boy with petechiae due to vitamin C deficiency. (From Duggan CP, Westra SJ, Rosenberg AE. Case 23–2007: A 9-year-old body with bone pain, rash, and gingival hyperplasia. *N Engl J Med.* 2007;357:395. Copyright © 2007. Massachusetts Medical Society.)

Production of platelets may be normal, but excessive pooling of platelets in the spleen may occur (splenic sequestration). When necessary, hypersplenic thrombocytopenia may be treated with splenectomy. Massive blood or plasma transfusions may cause a dilutional thrombocytopenia because blood stored for more than 24 hours has no viable platelets.

Immune Thrombocytopenic Purpura. Immune thrombocytopenic purpura (ITP) is an autoimmune disorder that results in platelet antibody formation and excess destruction of platelets.[7,18] The thrombocytopenia that occurs in ITP is thought to result from multiple mechanisms, including antiplatelet antibodies against glycoproteins (IIb/IIIa and Ib/IX) in the platelet membrane. The platelets are made more susceptible to phagocytosis because of the antibodies and are subsequently destroyed in the spleen. The disorder can occur in the absence of any known risk factors (primary or idiopathic ITP) or as a secondary disorder due to an underlying condition; it can also be classified as acute (duration of 6 months or less) or chronic. Secondary forms of ITP may be associated with acquired immunodeficiency syndrome (AIDS), systemic lupus erythematosus, antiphospholipid syndrome, chronic lymphocytic leukemia, lymphoma, hepatitis C, and drugs such as heparin and quinidine.

About half of the cases of ITP occur as an acute primary disorder in children, affecting both boys and girls.[18] The disorder occurs in young children (5 years of age), commonly following a viral infection. It is characterized by sudden onset of petechiae and purpura and is usually a self-limited disorder requiring no treatment. Most children recover in a few weeks. In contrast, primary ITP is often a chronic disorder in adults with an insidious onset that seldom follows an infection. Peak incidence is between the ages of 18 and 40 years, and is seen three times as often in women as in men.

Manifestations of ITP include a history of easy bruising, bleeding from gums, epistaxis, melena, and abnormal menstrual bleeding in those with moderately reduced platelet counts. Because the spleen is the site of platelet destruction, splenic enlargement may occur. The condition may be discovered incidentally or as a result of signs of bleeding, often into the skin (i.e., purpura and petechiae) or oral mucosa. About half of adults with primary ITP present with a platelet count of less than 10,000/μL and are at risk for internal hemorrhage.[18]

Diagnosis of ITP usually is based on severe thrombocytopenia (platelet counts <20,000 to 30,000/μL) and exclusion of other causes. Tests for the platelet-bound antibodies are available but lack specificity (e.g., they react with platelet antibodies from other sources). The secondary form of ITP sometimes mimics the idiopathic form of the disorder; therefore, the diagnosis is made only after excluding other known causes of thrombocytopenia.

The decision to treat ITP is based on the platelet count and the degree of bleeding. Many persons with

ITP do well without treatment. Corticosteroids are used as initial therapy; other effective initial treatment includes intravenous immune globulin. However, this treatment is expensive and the beneficial effect may last only one to two weeks. Because the spleen is the major site of antibody formation and platelet destruction, splenectomy is the traditional second-line treatment for persons who relapse or do not respond to medications.[18] Immunosuppressive therapy (i.e., azathioprine or cyclophosphamide) may be used in patients who are refractory to other forms of treatment.

Drug-Induced Thrombocytopenia. Some drugs, such as quinine, quinidine, and certain sulfa-containing antibiotics, may induce thrombocytopenia.[19] These drugs act as haptens to induce an antigen–antibody response and formation of immune complexes that cause platelet destruction by complement-mediated lysis (see Chapter 15). In persons with drug-associated thrombocytopenia, there is a fall in platelet count 7 or more days after initiating therapy with a given drug for the first time (i.e., the needed to mount an immune response) or 2 to 3 days after resuming therapy with the same drug. The platelet count rises rapidly after the drug is discontinued.

The anticoagulant drug heparin has been increasingly implicated in thrombocytopenia and, paradoxically, in thrombosis. The complications typically occur five days after the start of therapy and result from heparin-dependent antiplatelet antibodies that cause aggregation of platelets and their removal from the circulation. The antibodies often bind to vessel walls, causing complications such as deep vein thrombosis, pulmonary embolism, myocardial infarction, and stroke.[20] The treatment of heparin-induced thrombocytopenia (HIT) requires the immediate discontinuation of heparin therapy and the use of alternative anticoagulants (i.e., argatroban, fondaparinux) to prevent thrombosis recurrence. The use of low–molecular-weight heparin appears to have reduced the incidence of HIT, though there have only been a limited number of large, randomized, controlled studies.

Thrombotic Microangiopathies. The term *thrombotic microangiopathies* encompasses a spectrum of clinical syndromes that include thrombotic thrombocytopenic purpura (TTP) and hemolytic-uremic syndrome (HUS).[3] As originally described, TTP is associated with a combination of manifestations that includes fever, thrombocytopenia, microangiopathic hemolytic anemia, renal failure, and transient neurologic abnormalities. Hemolytic-uremic syndrome is also associated with microangiopathic hemolytic anemia and thrombocytopenia, but it is distinguished from TTP by the dominance of acute renal failure and absence of neurologic manifestations. Fundamental to both conditions is the widespread formation of hyaline thrombi in the microcirculation that are composed primarily of dense aggregates of platelets surrounded by fibrin. The consumption of platelets leads to thrombocytopenia, and the narrowing of the blood vessels by the platelet-rich thrombi results in the microangiopathic hemolytic anemia.

The pathogenesis of TTP is elusive but likely results from introduction of platelet-aggregating substances into the circulation. The underlying cause of many cases is the deficiency of an enzyme (ADAMTS 13, formerly known as vWF-cleaving protease) that degrades very high–molecular–weight multimers of vWF, allowing them to accumulate and cause platelet aggregation and adhesion to the endothelium.[3,4] The enzyme deficiency may be inherited or acquired as a result of antibody directed against the enzyme. Although TTP usually occurs in previously healthy persons, it may also complicate collagen vascular diseases (rheumatoid arthritis and systemic lupus erythematosus), drug-induced hypersensitivities, cancer chemotherapy, bone marrow transplantation, infections such as HIV, and pregnancy.[4]

Thrombotic thrombocytopenic purpura occurs at virtually every age, but is most common in women in their fourth or fifth decades. It can be chronic and recurrent, but more frequently the onset is abrupt and the outcome may be fatal. Widespread vascular occlusions result from thrombi in the arterioles and capillaries of many organs, including the heart, brain, and kidneys. The clinical manifestations include purpura, petechiae, vaginal bleeding, and neurologic symptoms ranging from headache to seizures and altered consciousness. Anemia is universal and may be marked. About half of patients have azotemia due to renal failure.[4]

Emergency treatment for TTP includes *plasmapheresis*, a procedure that involves removal of plasma from withdrawn blood and replacement with fresh-frozen plasma. Plasma infusion provides the deficient enzyme. With plasmapheresis and plasma infusion treatment, there is a complete recovery in 80% of cases.[4]

Although clinically similar to TTP, there is no underlying enzyme deficiency in HUS because ADAMTS 13 levels are normal. HUS in children and the elderly usually occurs following infectious gastroenteritis caused by *Escherichia coli* O157:H7[14] (see Chapter 29). The organism elaborates a toxin that damages endothelial cells, which initiates platelet activation and aggregation. Affected individuals often present with bloody diarrhea, which is followed a few days later by HUS. With supportive care and plasma exchange, recovery is possible, but irreversible renal damage and death can occur in severe cases.

Impaired Platelet Function

Impaired platelet function (also called *thrombocytopathia*) may result from inherited disorders of adhesion (e.g., von Willebrand disease) or acquired defects caused by drugs, disease, or surgery involving extracorporeal circulation (i.e., cardiopulmonary bypass). Defective platelet function is also common in uremia, presumably because of non-eliminated waste products.

The use of aspirin and other nonsteroidal anti-inflammatory drugs (NSAIDs) is the most common cause of platelet dysfunction. Aspirin produces irreversible acetylation of platelet cyclooxygenase activity, and consequently the synthesis of TXA_2, which is required for platelet aggregation. The effect of aspirin on platelet aggregation lasts for the life of the platelet—approximately 8 or 9 days. In contrast to the effects of aspirin, the inhibition of cyclooxygenase by other NSAIDs is reversible and lasts only for the duration of drug action. Aspirin (81 mg daily) commonly is used to prevent formation of arterial thrombi and thus reduce the risk of cardiovascular (i.e., myocardial infarction) or cerebrovascular (i.e., stroke) accidents.

Coagulation Disorders

Blood coagulation defects can result from deficiencies or impaired function of one or more of the clotting factors, including vWF. Deficiencies can arise because of inherited disease or because of defective synthesis or increased consumption of the clotting factors. Bleeding resulting from clotting factor deficiencies typically occurs after injury or trauma. Large bruises (ecchymoses), hematomas, and prolonged bleeding into the gastrointestinal or urinary tracts or joints are common.

Inherited Disorders

Hemophilia A and von Willebrand disease are two of the most common inherited disorders of bleeding.[21,22] Hemophilia A (factor VIII deficiency) affects 1 in 5000 male live births and von Willebrand disease about 1 in 1000 persons.[21] Hemophilia B (Factor IX deficiency) is clinically similar to hemophilia A and affects approximately 1 in 20,000 persons, accounting for 15% of people with hemophilia.[4]

Hemophilia A and von Willebrand disease are caused by defects involving the factor VIII–vWF complex. Von Willebrand factor, which is synthesized by the endothelium and megakaryocytes, is required for platelet adhesion to the subendothelial matrix of the blood vessel. It also serves as the carrier for factor VIII and it is important for the stability of factor VIII in the circulation by preventing its proteolysis. Factor VIII coagulant protein, the functional portion of factor VIII, is produced by the liver and endothelial cells. Thus, factor VIII and vWF, synthesized separately, come together and circulate in the plasma as a unit that serves to promote clotting and adhesion of platelets to the vessel wall.

Von Willebrand Disease. Von Willebrand disease is a relatively common hereditary bleeding disorder characterized by a deficiency or defect in vWF. It affects both men and women and is typically diagnosed in adulthood.[23,24] In most cases, it is transmitted as an autosomal dominant disorder, but several rare autosomal recessive variants have been identified.

As many as 20 variants of von Willebrand disease have been described.[4] These variants can be grouped into two categories: types 1 and 3, which are associated with reduced levels of vWF; and type 2, which is characterized by defects in vWF.[4] Type 1, an autosomal dominant disorder, accounts for approximately 75% of cases and is relatively mild. Type 2, also an autosomal dominant disorder, accounts for about 20% of cases and is associated with mild to moderate bleeding. Type 3, which is a relatively rare autosomal recessive disorder, is associated with extremely low levels of functional vWF and correspondingly severe clinical manifestations.

Persons with von Willebrand disease have a compound defect involving platelet function and the coagulation pathway. Clinical manifestations include spontaneous bleeding from the nose, mouth, and gastrointestinal tract; excessive menstrual flow; and a prolonged bleeding time in the presence of a normal platelet count. Most cases (i.e., types 1 and 2) are mild and the disorder is diagnosed when surgery or dental extraction results in prolonged bleeding. In severe cases (i.e., type 3), life-threatening gastrointestinal bleeding and joint hemorrhage may be similar to that seen in hemophilia.

The bleeding associated with von Willebrand disease is usually mild, and no treatment is routinely administered other than avoidance of aspirin. Desmopressin acetate (DDAVP), a synthetic analog of the hormone vasopressin, is used in the treatment of type 1 von Willebrand disease and for establishing hemostasis during surgical or dental procedures.[22,23] DDAVP stimulates the endothelial cells to release stored vWF and plasminogen activator. The drug is available as an intranasal spray. A vWF-containing factor VIII concentrate may be used for treatment of persons with excessive bleeding.[21]

Hemophilia A. Hemophilia A is an X-linked recessive disorder that primarily affects males.[3,4,22,24,25] Although it is a hereditary disorder, there is no family history of the disorder in approximately 30% of newly diagnosed cases, suggesting that it has arisen as a new mutation in the factor VIII gene. Approximately 90% of persons with hemophilia produce insufficient quantities of the factor and 10% produce a defective form. The percentage of normal factor VIII activity in the circulation depends on the genetic defect and determines the severity of hemophilia (i.e., 6% to 30% in mild hemophilia, 2% to 5% in moderate hemophilia, and 1% or less in severe forms of hemophilia). In mild or moderate forms of the disease, bleeding usually does not occur unless there is a local lesion or trauma such as surgery or a dental procedure. The mild disorder may not be detected in childhood. In severe hemophilia, bleeding usually occurs in childhood (e.g., it may be noticed at the time of circumcision) and is spontaneous and severe, often occurring several times a month.

Characteristically, bleeding occurs in soft tissues, the gastrointestinal tract, and the hip, knee, elbow, and ankle joints. Spontaneous joint bleeding usually begins when a child begins to walk, with the target joint often prone to recurrent incidences. The bleeding causes inflammation of the synovium, with acute pain and swelling. Without proper treatment, chronic bleeding and inflammation cause joint fibrosis and contractures, resulting in major disability. Muscle hematomas may be present in 30% of episodes, and intracranial hemorrhage, although uncommon, is an important cause of death.[22,26]

The prevention of trauma is important in persons with hemophilia. Aspirin and other NSAIDs that affect platelet function should be avoided. Factor VIII replacement therapy (either recombinant or heat-treated concentrates from human plasma) administered at home has reduced the typical musculoskeletal damage. It is initiated when bleeding occurs or as prophylaxis with repeated bleeding episodes. The newer recombinant products and continuous-infusion pumps may allow for prevention rather than therapy for hemorrhage. The development of inhibitory antibodies to recombinant factor VIII is still a major complication of treatment; 10% to 15% of treated persons produce high titers of antibodies that bind to and inhibit factor VIII. The rate of antibody production for plasma-derived products is approximately the same.

Current factor VIII products (both plasma derived and recombinant) are considered very safe as a result of technological advances over the last two decades.[27] Until the mid-1980s when routine screening of blood for HIV antibodies was instituted, thousands of patients with hemophilia received plasma-derived factor VIII that was contaminated with HIV, and many developed AIDS. Effective donor screening and development of purification and viral inactivation procedures now provide a safer product. A number of recombinant factor VIII preparations are available. These products were made with the use of blood-derived additives of human or animal origin, such as albumin. These additives were needed to keep the cells viable so they could produce the factor VIII protein. With mild hemophilia A, the person's endogenously produced factor VIII can be released by the administration of DDAVP.[27] In persons with moderate to severe factor VIII deficiency, the stored levels of factor VIII are insufficient, and DDAVP treatment is ineffective.

The cloning of the factor VIII gene and progress in gene delivery systems have led to the hope that hemophilia A may be cured by gene replacement therapy. Carrier detection and prenatal diagnosis can now be done by analysis of direct gene mutation or DNA linkage studies.

Acquired Disorders

Coagulation factors II, V, VII, IX, X, XI, and XII; prothrombin (II); and fibrinogen (I) are synthesized in the liver. In liver disease, synthesis of these clotting factors is reduced, and bleeding may result. Of the coagulation factors synthesized in the liver, factors II, VII, IX, and X and prothrombin require the presence of vitamin K for normal activity. In vitamin K deficiency, the liver produces the clotting factor, but in an inactive form. Vitamin K is a fat-soluble vitamin that is continuously being synthesized by intestinal bacteria. This means that a deficiency in vitamin K is not likely to occur unless intestinal synthesis is interrupted or absorption of the vitamin is impaired. Vitamin K deficiency can occur in the newborn infant before the establishment of the intestinal flora; it can also occur as a result of treatment with broad-spectrum antibiotics that destroy intestinal flora. Because vitamin K is a fat-soluble vitamin, its absorption requires bile salts. Vitamin K deficiency may also result from impaired fat absorption caused by liver or gallbladder disease.

Bleeding Associated with Vascular Disorders

Bleeding resulting from vascular disorders, sometimes called *nonthrombocytopenic purpura*, is relatively common and results in mild bleeding disorders.[3,4] These disorders may occur because of structurally weak vessel walls or because of damage to vessels by inflammation or immune responses. Most often they are characterized by easy bruising and the spontaneous appearance of petechiae and purpura of the skin and mucous membranes. In persons with bleeding disorders caused by vascular defects, the platelet count and results of other tests for coagulation factors are normal.

Among the vascular disorders that cause bleeding are hemorrhagic telangiectasia, vitamin C deficiency (scurvy), Cushing disease, and senile purpura. Hemorrhagic telangiectasia is an uncommon autosomal dominant disorder that is characterized by thin-walled, dilated capillaries and arterioles. Vitamin C is a reversible reducing agent that is an essential cofactor for the hydroxylation of proline in collagen synthesis. A severe vitamin C deficiency results in poor collagen synthesis and failure of capillary cells to be cemented together properly, which in turn causes a fragile vascular wall (see Fig. 12-4). Cushing disease causes protein wasting and loss of vessel tissue support because of excess cortisol (see Chapter 32). Senile purpura (i.e., bruising in elderly persons) is caused by impaired collagen synthesis due to the aging process.

Disseminated Intravascular Coagulation

Disseminated intravascular coagulation (DIC) is a paradox in the hemostatic sequence characterized by widespread coagulation and bleeding.[28–31] It is not a primary disease but a complication of many different disorders. Disseminated intravascular coagulation begins with massive activation of the coagulation sequence, which leads to fibrin deposition and formation of thrombi in the microcirculation of the body (Fig. 12-5). The widespread deposition of fibrin leads to tissue ischemia and hemolytic anemia from fragmentation of red cells as they squeeze through the narrowed microvasculature. As a consequence of the thrombotic process, there is consumption of platelets and coagulation factors and the activation of plasminogen that leads to a hemorrhagic diathesis.

The disorder can be initiated by activation of the intrinsic or extrinsic pathway, or both. Activation through the extrinsic pathway occurs with liberation of tissue factors and is associated with obstetric complications, trauma, bacterial sepsis, and cancer. The intrinsic pathway may be activated through extensive endothelial damage, with activation of factor XII. Endothelial damage may be caused by viruses, infections, immune mechanisms, stasis of blood, or temperature extremes. Impaired anticoagulation pathways are also associated with reduced levels of antithrombin and the protein C anticoagulant system in DIC. There is increasing

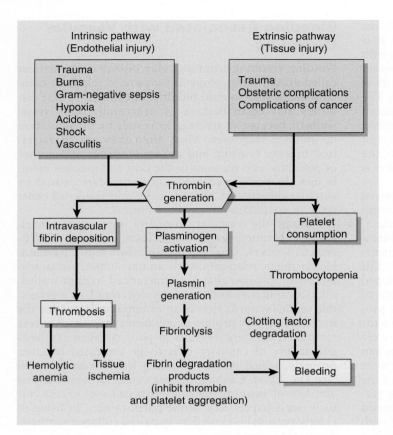

Intrinsic pathway
(Endothelial injury)

Extrinsic pathway
(Tissue injury)

Trauma
Burns
Gram-negative sepsis
Hypoxia
Acidosis
Shock
Vasculitis

Trauma
Obstetric complications
Complications of cancer

Thrombin
generation

Intravascular
fibrin deposition

Plasminogen
activation

Platelet
consumption

Thrombocytopenia

Plasmin
generation

Thrombosis

Clotting factor
degradation

Fibrinolysis

Hemolytic
anemia

Tissue
ischemia

Fibrin degradation
products
(inhibit thrombin
and platelet aggregation)

Bleeding

FIGURE 12-5. Pathophysiology of disseminated intravascular coagulation.

evidence that the underlying cause of DIC is infection or inflammation, and the cytokines (tumor necrosis factor, interleukin-1, and others) liberated in the process are the pivotal mediators.[29,30] These cytokines not only mediate inflammation, but can also increase the expression of tissue factor on endothelial cells and simultaneously decrease the expression of thrombomodulin. Thrombomodulin is a glycoprotein, present on the cell membrane of endothelial cells, that binds thrombin (IIa) and acts as an additional regulatory mechanism in coagulation. The net effect is a shift in balance toward a procoagulant state.[28]

Common clinical conditions that may cause DIC include obstetric disorders, accounting for 50% of cases; massive trauma; shock; sepsis; and malignant disease. Chart 12-2 summarizes the conditions associated with DIC. The factors involved in the conditions that cause DIC are often interrelated. In obstetric complications, tissue factors released from necrotic placental or fetal tissue or amniotic fluid may enter the circulation, inciting DIC. The hypoxia, shock, and acidosis that may coexist also contribute by causing endothelial injury. Gram-negative bacterial infections result in the release of endotoxins, which activate both the extrinsic pathway by release of tissue factor and the intrinsic pathway through endothelial damage. Endotoxins also inhibit the activity of protein C. Antigen–antibody complexes associated with infection can activate platelets through complement fragments.

Although coagulation and formation of microemboli characterize DIC, its acute manifestations usually

CHART 12-2 Conditions That Have Been Associated with Disseminated Intravascular Coagulation

Obstetric Conditions
Abruptio placentae
Dead fetus syndrome
Preeclampsia and eclampsia
Amniotic fluid embolism

Cancers
Metastatic cancer
Acute promyelocytic leukemia

Infections
Acute bacterial infections (e.g., meningococcal meningitis)
Histoplasmosis, Aspergillosis
Rickettsial infections (e.g., Rocky Mountain spotted fever)
Parasitic infections (e.g., malaria)
Sepsis/septic shock

Trauma or Surgery
Burns
Massive trauma
Surgery involving extracorporeal circulation
Snake bite
Heatstroke

Hematologic Conditions
Blood transfusion reactions

are more directly related to the bleeding problems that occur. The bleeding may be present as petechiae, purpura, oozing from puncture sites, or severe hemorrhage. Uncontrolled postpartum bleeding may indicate DIC. Microemboli may obstruct blood vessels and cause tissue hypoxia and necrotic damage to organ structures, such as the kidneys, heart, lungs, and brain. As a result, common clinical signs may be due to renal, circulatory, or respiratory failure; acute bleeding ulcers; or convulsions and coma. A form of hemolytic anemia may develop as red cells are damaged passing through vessels partially blocked by thrombus.

The treatment of DIC is directed toward managing the primary disease, replacing clotting components, and preventing further activation of clotting mechanisms. Transfusions of fresh-frozen plasma, platelets, or fibrinogen-containing cryoprecipitate may correct the clotting factor deficiency. Heparin may be given to decrease blood coagulation, thereby interrupting the clotting process. Heparin therapy is controversial, however, and the risk of hemorrhage may limit its use to severe cases. It typically is given as a continuous intravenous infusion that can be interrupted promptly if bleeding is accentuated. Tissue factor pathway inhibitors, antithrombin, protein C concentrates, and anti-inflammatory cytokines such as interleukin-10 are being evaluated in clinical trials as potential therapies.

SUMMARY CONCEPTS

■ Bleeding disorders or impairment of blood coagulation can result from defects in any of the factors that contribute to hemostasis: platelets, coagulation factors, or vascular integrity.

■ Disorders of platelet plug formation include a decrease in platelet numbers due to inadequate platelet production (bone marrow dysfunction), excess pooling of platelets in the spleen, excess platelet destruction (thrombocytopenia), abnormal platelet function (thrombocytopathia), or defects in von Willebrand factor.

■ Impairment of blood coagulation can result from deficiencies of one or more of the known clotting factors. Deficiencies can arise because of acquired disorders (i.e., liver disease or vitamin K deficiency) or inherited disorders (i.e., hemophilia A or von Willebrand disease).

■ Bleeding may also occur from structurally weak vessels that result from impaired synthesis of vessel wall components (i.e., vitamin C deficiency, excessive cortisol levels as in Cushing disease, or the aging process) or from damage by genetic mechanisms (i.e., hemorrhagic telangiectasia) or the presence of microthrombi.

■ Disseminated intravascular coagulation (DIC) is characterized by widespread coagulation and bleeding in the vascular compartment. It begins with massive activation of the coagulation cascade and generation of microthrombi that cause vessel occlusion and tissue ischemia. Clot formation consumes all available coagulation proteins and platelets, and severe hemorrhage may occur.

REVIEW EXERCISES

1. A 55-year-old man has begun taking one 81-mg aspirin tablet daily on the recommendation of his physician. The physician had told him that this would help to prevent heart attack and stroke.

   A. What is the action of aspirin in terms of heart attack and stroke prevention?
   B. The drug clopidogrel (Plavix) is often prescribed along with aspirin to prevent thrombosis in persons with severe atherosclerotic disease who are at risk for myocardial infarction or stroke. Explain the rationale for using the two drugs.

2. The drug desmopressin acetate (DDAVP), which is a synthetic analog of arginine vasopressin, increases the half-life of factor VIII and is sometimes used to treat bleeding in males with mild hemophilia.

   A. Explain.

3. A 29-year-old new mother, who delivered her infant three days ago, is admitted to the hospital with chest pain and is diagnosed as having venous thrombosis with pulmonary emboli.

   A. What factors would contribute to this woman's risk of developing thromboemboli?

4. The new mother is admitted to the intensive care unit and started on low–molecular-weight heparin and warfarin. She is told that she will be discharged in a day or two and will remain on the heparin for 5 days and the warfarin for at least 3 months.

   A. Use Figure 12-3 to explain the action of heparin and warfarin. Why is heparin administered for 5 days during the initiation of warfarin treatment?
   B. Anticoagulation with heparin and warfarin is not a definitive treatment for clot removal in pulmonary embolism, but a form of secondary prevention. Explain.

REFERENCES

1. Hall JE. *Guyton and Hall Textbook of Medical Physiology.* 12th ed. Philadelphia, PA: Elsevier Saunders; 2011:451–461.
2. Ross MH, Kaye G, Pawlina W. *Histology: A Text and Atlas.* 6th ed. Philadelphia, PA: Wolters Kluwer Health | Lippincott Williams & Wilkins; 2011:269–289, 271–272.
3. Kumar V, Abbas AK, Fausto N, et al. *Robbins and Cotran Pathologic Basis of Disease.* 8th ed. Philadelphia, PA: Saunders Elsevier; 2010:115–125, 666–675.
4. Valdez R, Zutter M, Flores AD, et al. Hematopathology. In: Rubin R, Strayer DS, eds. *Rubin's Pathology: Clinicopathologic Foundations of Medicine.* 6th ed. Philadelphia, PA: Wolters Kluwer Health | Lippincott Williams & Wilkins; 2012:947–998.
5. Weitz JI. Overview of hemostasis and thrombosis. In: Huffman R, Benz EJ Jr, Silverstein LE, et al. *Hoffman Hematology: Basic Principles and Practice.* 4th ed. London, UK: Elsevier Churchill Livingstone; 2013:1774–1783.
6. Messmore HL, Jeske WP, Wehrmacher W, et al. Antiplatelet agents: current drugs and future trends. *Hematol Oncol Clin North Am.* 2005;19:87–117.
7. Zehnder JL. Drugs used in disorders of coagulation. In: Katzung BG, ed. *Basic and Clinical Pharmacology.* 12th ed. New York, NY: McGraw-Hill; 2012:601–618.
8. Furie B, Furie BC. Mechanisms of thrombus formation. *N Engl J Med.* 2008;359(9):938–949.
9. Schafer AI. Thrombocytosis. *N Engl J Med.* 2004;350:1211–1219.
10. Bloomenthal D, von Dadelszen P, Liston R, et al. The effect of factor V Leiden carriage on maternal and fetal health. *Can Med Assoc J.* 2002;167:48–54.
11. Chrousos GP. The gonadal hormones and inhibitors. In: Katzung BG, ed. *Basic and Clinical Pharmacology.* 12th ed. New York, NY: McGraw-Hill; 2011;715–739.
12. Levine JS, Branch DW, Rausch J. The antiphospholipid syndrome. *N Engl J Med.* 2002;346:752–763.
13. Hanly JC. Antiphospholipid syndrome: an overview. *Can Med Assoc J.* 2003;168:1675–1682.
14. Lin W, Crowther MA, Eikelboom JW. Management of antiphospholipid antibody syndrome. *JAMA.* 2006;295:1050–1057.
15. Nachman RL, Rafii S. Platelets, petechiae, and preservation of the vascular wall. *N Engl J Med.* 2008;359(12):1261–1270.
16. Bromberg ME. Immune thrombocytopenia purpura: the changing therapeutic landscape. *N Engl J Med.* 2006;355: 1643–1645.
17. Cines DB, Blanchette VS. Immune thrombocytopenic purpura. *N Engl J Med.* 2002;346:995–1008.
18. van den Bemt PM, Meyboom RH, Egberts AC. Drug-induced immune thrombocytopenia. *Drug Saf.* 2004;27:1243–1252.
19. Franchini M. Heparin-induced thrombocytopenia: an update. *Thromb J.* 2005;3:14–18.
20. Mannucci PM, Tuddenham EGD. The hemophilias: from royal genes to gene therapy. *N Engl J Med.* 2001;344:1773–1779.
21. Carcoa M, Moorehead P, Lillicrap D. Hemophilia A and B. In: Huffman R, Benz EJ Jr, Silverstein LE, et al., eds. *Hoffman Hematology: Basic Principles and Practice.* 4th ed. London, UK: Elsevier Churchill Livingstone; 2013:1940–1960.
22. Lillicrap D. Von Willebrand disease: advances in pathogenetic understanding, diagnosis, and therapy. *Blood.* 2013;122:3735–3740.
23. Mannucci PM. Treatment of von Willebrand's disease. *N Engl J Med.* 2004;351:683–694.
24. Soliman DE, Broadman LM. Coagulation defects. *Anesthesiol Clin.* 2006;24:549–578.
25. Sadler JV. New concepts in von Willebrand disease. *Annu Rev Med.* 2005;56:173–180.
26. Klinge J, Ananyeva NM, Hauser C, et al. Hemophilia A: from basic science to clinical practice. *Semin Thromb Hemost.* 2002;28:309–322.
27. Mannucci PM. Desmopressin (DDAVP) in the treatment of bleeding disorders: the first 20 years. *Blood.* 1997;90:2515–2521.
28. Kitchens CS. Thrombocytopenia and thrombosis in disseminated intravascular coagulation (DIC). *Hematology.* 2009:240–246.
29. Franchini M, Lippi G, Manzato F. Recent acquisitions in the pathophysiology, diagnosis and treatment of disseminated intravascular coagulation. *Thromb J.* 2006;4:4–12.
30. Van der Poll T, Jonge E, Levi M. Regulatory role of cytokines in disseminated intravascular coagulation. *Semin Thromb Hemost.* 2001;27:639–651.
31. Levi M. Disseminated intravascular coagulation. *Crit Care Med.* 2007;35(9):2191–2195.

Porth Essentials Resources

Explore these additional resources to enhance learning for this chapter:

- NCLEX-Style Questions and Other Resources on thePoint, http://thePoint.lww.com/PorthEssentials4e
- Study Guide for Essentials of Pathophysiology
- Concepts in Action Animations
- Adaptive Learning | Powered by PrepU, http://thepoint.lww.com/prepu

Chapter 13

Disorders of Red Blood Cells

Although the lungs provide the means for gas exchange between the external and internal environments, it is the hemoglobin in the red blood cells that transports oxygen to the tissues. The red blood cells also function as carriers of carbon dioxide and participate in acid–base balance. The function of the red blood cells, in terms of oxygen transport, is discussed in Chapter 21, and acid–base balance is discussed in Chapter 8. This chapter focuses on the red blood cell, anemia, polycythemia, and age-related changes in the red blood cells.

The Red Blood Cell

The erythrocytes or mature red blood cells are the most common type of blood cell, being 500 to 1000 times more numerous than other blood cells. The erythrocyte is a nonnucleated, thin, biconcave disk (Fig. 13-1). This unique shape contributes in two ways to the oxygen transport function of the erythrocyte. The biconcave shape provides a larger surface area for oxygen diffusion than would a spherical cell of the same volume, and the thinness of the cell membrane enables oxygen to diffuse rapidly between the exterior and the interior of the cell[1-3] (Fig. 13-2A). Another structural feature that facilitates the transport function of the red blood cell is the flexibility of its membrane. The biconcave shape and flexibility of the red cell membrane are maintained by a complex network of fibrous proteins, especially one called *spectrin* (Fig. 13-3). Spectrin forms an attachment with another protein, called *ankyrin,* that resides on the inner surface of the membrane and is anchored to an integral protein that spans the membrane.[2] This unique arrangement of proteins imparts elasticity and stability to the red blood cell membrane and allows it to deform easily as it moves through narrow spaces in the vascular network.

The function of the red blood cell, facilitated by the hemoglobin molecule, is to transport oxygen to the tissues. Because oxygen is poorly soluble in plasma, about 95% to 98% is carried bound to hemoglobin. The hemoglobin molecule is composed of two pairs of structurally different alpha (α) and beta (β) polypeptide chains (see Fig. 13-2B). Each of the four polypeptide chains consists

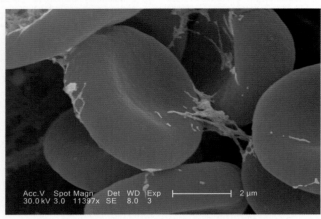

FIGURE 13-1. A highly magnified (× 11,397) electron micrograph of a number of red blood cells found enmeshed in a fibrinous matrix on the luminal surface of an indwelling vascular catheter. Note the biconcave shape of each erythrocyte, which increases the surface area of these hemoglobin-filled cells, thus promoting more effective gas exchange. (From the Centers for Disease Control and Prevention Public Health Images Library. No. 7315. Courtesy of Janice Carr.)

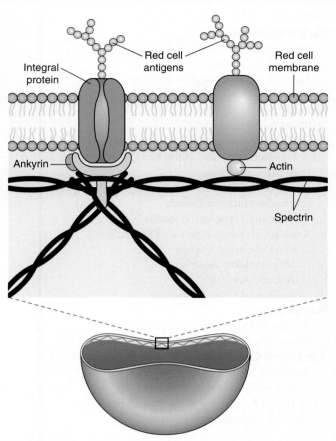

FIGURE 13-3. Cross-sectional side view of the biconcave structure of the red blood cell and diagram showing the cytoskeleton and flexible network of spectrin proteins that attach to the ankyrin protein, a transmembrane protein that resides on the inner surface of the membrane and is anchored to an integral protein that spans the membrane.

of a globin (protein) portion and a heme unit, which surrounds an atom of iron that binds oxygen.[1,3] Thus, each molecule of hemoglobin can carry four molecules of oxygen. Hemoglobin is a natural pigment; because of its iron content, it appears reddish when oxygen is attached and has a bluish cast when deoxygenated. The production of each type of globin chain is controlled by individual structural genes with five different gene loci. Mutations, which can occur anywhere in these five loci, have resulted in over 550 types of abnormal hemoglobin molecules.[1]

There are two major types of normal hemoglobin—adult hemoglobin (HbA) and fetal hemoglobin (HbF). Adult hemoglobin consists of a pair of α chains and a pair of β chains. Fetal hemoglobin is the predominant hemoglobin in the fetus from the third through the ninth months of gestation. It has a pair of gamma (γ) chains substituted for the α chains. Because of this chain substitution, HbF

has a higher affinity for oxygen than adult hemoglobin. This affinity facilitates the transfer of oxygen across the placenta from the HbA in the mother's blood to the HbF in the fetus's blood. HbF is replaced within 6 months of birth with HbA.

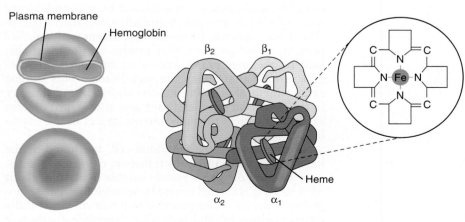

A Red blood cell   **B** Hemoglobin

FIGURE 13-2. (A) Biconcave structure of the red blood cell as shown in cross-section and in lateral surface view. **(B)** Hemoglobin molecule, showing the four iron (Fe)-containing heme subunits and their structure.

Hemoglobin Synthesis

The rate at which hemoglobin is synthesized depends on the availability of iron for heme synthesis. A lack of iron results in relatively small amounts of hemoglobin in the red blood cells. Body iron is found in several compartments. About 65% of iron is in the form of hemoglobin, with small amounts found in the myoglobin of muscle, the cytochromes, and iron-containing enzymes.[3] The remaining 15% to 30% is stored for later use, mainly in the liver but also in the reticuloendothelial cells of the bone marrow.[3] Iron in the hemoglobin compartment is recycled. When red blood cells age and are destroyed in the spleen, the iron from their hemoglobin is released into the circulation and returned to the bone marrow for incorporation into new red blood cells or to the liver and other tissues for storage.

Dietary sources help to maintain iron stores. Iron, principally derived from meat, is absorbed in the small intestine, especially the duodenum (Fig. 13-4). When body iron stores are diminished or erythropoiesis is stimulated, absorption is increased. In iron overload, excretion of iron is accelerated. Normally, some iron is sequestered in the intestinal epithelial cells and is lost in the feces as these cells slough off. The iron that is absorbed enters the circulation, where it immediately combines with a β-globulin, *apotransferrin,* to form *transferrin,* which is then transported in the plasma.[3] From the plasma, iron can be deposited in tissue cells such as the liver, where it is stored as *ferritin,* a protein–iron complex that is easily transferable back to the circulation. Serum ferritin levels can be measured in the laboratory to provide an index of body iron stores. Smaller quantities of iron are stored in cells in an extremely insoluble form called *hemosiderin.* This occurs when the total quantity of iron in the body is more than the ferritin storage pool can accommodate.

Red Cell Production

Erythropoiesis refers to the production of red blood cells. After birth, red cells are produced in the red bone marrow. Until 5 years of age, almost all bones produce red cells to meet the growth needs of a child, after which bone marrow activity gradually declines.[3] After 20 years of age, red cell production takes place mainly in the membranous bones of the vertebrae, sternum, ribs, and pelvis.[3] With this reduction in activity, the red bone marrow is replaced with fatty yellow bone marrow.

The red blood cells are derived from precursor cells called *proerythroblasts,* which are formed continuously from pluripotent stem cells in the bone marrow[3] (Fig. 13-5). The red cell precursors move through a series of divisions, each producing a smaller cell as they continue to develop into mature red blood cells. Hemoglobin synthesis begins at the early erythroblast stage and continues until the cell becomes a mature erythrocyte. During its transformation from normoblast to reticulocyte, the red blood cell accumulates hemoglobin as the nucleus condenses and is finally lost. The period from stem cell to emergence of the reticulocyte in the circulation normally takes approximately one week and maturation of reticulocyte to erythrocyte takes about 24 to 48 hours. During this process, the red cell loses its mitochondria and ribosomes, along with its ability to produce hemoglobin and engage in oxidative metabolism. Most maturing red cells enter the blood as reticulocytes.

Erythropoiesis is governed for the most part by tissue oxygen needs. Any condition that causes a decrease in the amount of oxygen that is transported in the blood ordinarily produces an increase in the rate of red cell production. The oxygen content of the blood does not act directly on the bone marrow to stimulate red blood cell production. Instead, the decreased oxygen content is sensed by the kidneys, which then produce a hormone called *erythropoietin.*[2,4] Normally, about 90% of all erythropoietin is produced by the kidneys, with the remaining 10% formed in the liver. Erythropoietin acts primarily in later stages of erythropoiesis to stimulate the production of proerythroblasts from stem cells in the bone marrow. In the absence of erythropoietin, as in kidney failure, hypoxia has little or no effect on red blood cell production. Human erythropoietin can be produced by recombinant deoxyribonucleic acid (DNA) technology. It is used for the management of anemia in cases of chronic kidney disease, for anemias induced by

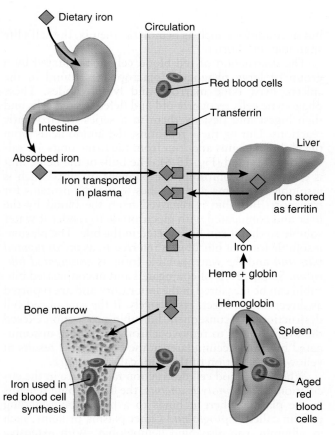

FIGURE 13-4. Diagrammatic representation of the iron cycle, including its absorption from the gastrointestinal tract, transport in the circulation, storage in the liver, recycling from aged red cells destroyed in the spleen, and use in the bone marrow synthesis of red blood cells.

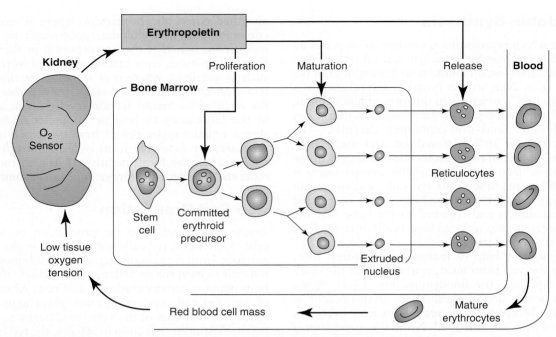

FIGURE 13-5. Red blood cell development involves the proliferation and differentiation of committed bone marrow cells through the erythroblast and normoblast stages to reticulocytes, which are released into the bloodstream and finally become erythrocytes.

chemotherapy in persons with malignancies, and in the treatment of anemia in human immunodeficiency virus (HIV)-infected persons treated with zidovudine.[4]

Because red blood cells are released into the blood as reticulocytes, the percentage of these cells is higher when there is a marked increase in red blood cell production. In some severe forms of anemia, the reticulocytes (normally about 1%) may account for as much as 30% of the total red cell count. In some situations, red cell production is so accelerated that numerous erythroblasts appear in the blood.

Red Cell Life Span and Destruction

Mature red blood cells have a life span of approximately 4 months, or 120 days.[3] Even though mature red cells do not have a nucleus, mitochondria, or endoplasmic reticulum, they have cytoplasmic enzymes that are capable of metabolizing glucose and forming small amounts of adenosine triphosphate (ATP). These enzymes also help to preserve the pliability of the cell membrane, maintain transmembrane transport of ions, keep the iron of the cell's hemoglobin in the reduced ferrous form that binds oxygen, and prevent oxidation of the proteins. Even so, the metabolic activity in the cell decreases as the red cell ages, and the cell membrane becomes more and more fragile, causing it to rupture as it passes through tight places in the circulation. Many of the aged red cells self-destruct in the spleen as they squeeze through spaces between the trabeculae of the red pulp, which are only about 3 mm wide, in comparison with the 8-mm width of the red cell.[3] The rate of red cell destruction (1% per day) normally is equal to the rate of red cell production,

but in conditions such as hemolytic anemia, the cell's life span may be shorter.

The destruction of red blood cells is facilitated by a group of large phagocytic macrophages found in the spleen, liver, bone marrow, and lymph nodes. These phagocytic cells recognize old and defective red cells and then ingest and destroy them in a series of enzymatic reactions. During these reactions, the amino acids from the globulin chains and iron from the heme units are salvaged and reused (Fig. 13-6). The bulk of the heme unit is converted to bilirubin, the pigment of bile, which is insoluble in plasma and attaches to plasma proteins for transport. Bilirubin is removed from the blood by the liver and conjugated with glucuronide to render it water soluble so that it can be excreted in the bile. The plasma-insoluble form of bilirubin is referred to as *unconjugated bilirubin* and the water-soluble form as *conjugated bilirubin*. Serum levels of conjugated and unconjugated bilirubin can be measured in the laboratory and are reported as direct and indirect, respectively. If the rate of red cell destruction and consequent bilirubin production exceed the liver's ability to remove it from the blood, unconjugated bilirubin accumulates in the blood. This results in yellow discoloration of the skin, called *jaundice*.

When red blood cell destruction takes place in the circulation, as in *hemolytic anemia*, the hemoglobin remains in the plasma where it binds to a hemoglobin-binding protein called *haptoglobin*.[1] Other plasma proteins, such as albumin, can also bind hemoglobin. With extensive intravascular destruction of red blood cells, hemoglobin levels may exceed the hemoglobin-binding capacity of haptoglobin and other plasma proteins. When this occurs, free hemoglobin appears in the blood (i.e., hemoglobinemia) and is excreted in the urine (i.e., hemoglobinuria).

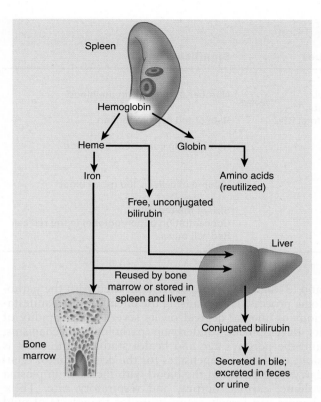

FIGURE 13-6. Destruction of red blood cells and fate of hemoglobin.

Because excessive red blood cell destruction can occur in hemolytic transfusion reactions, urine samples are tested for free hemoglobin after a transfusion reaction.

Laboratory Tests

Red blood cells can be studied by means of a sample of blood (Table 13-1). In modern clinical laboratories, specialized blood cell counters rapidly provide accurate measurements of red cell content and cell indices. The *red blood cell count* measures the total number of red blood cells in a microliter (μL) of blood. The *percentage of reticulocytes* (normally approximately 1%) provides an index of the rate of red cell production. The *hemoglobin* (grams per deciliter [dL] or 100 milliliters [mL] of blood) measures the hemoglobin content of the blood. The major components of blood are the red cell mass and plasma volume. The *hematocrit* measures the red cell mass in a 100-mL plasma volume. To determine the hematocrit, a sample of blood is placed in a glass tube, which is then centrifuged to separate the cells and the plasma. The hematocrit may be deceptive because it varies with the quantity of extracellular fluid, rising with dehydration and falling with overexpansion of extracellular fluid volume (Fig. 13-7).

Red cell indices are used to differentiate types of anemias by size or color of red cells. The *mean corpuscular volume* (MCV) reflects the volume or size of the red cells.[1] The MCV falls in microcytic (small cell) anemia and rises in macrocytic (large cell) anemia. Some anemias are normocytic (i.e., cells are of normal size or MCV). The *mean*

corpuscular hemoglobin concentration (MCHC) is the concentration of hemoglobin in each cell. Hemoglobin accounts for the color of red blood cells. Anemias are described as *normochromic* (normal color or MCHC) or *hypochromic* (decreased color or MCHC). *Mean cell hemoglobin* (MCH) refers to the mass of the red cell and is less useful in classifying anemias.

A stained blood smear provides information about the size, color, and shape of red cells and the presence of immature or abnormal cells. If blood smear results are abnormal, examination of the bone marrow may be indicated. Bone marrow commonly is aspirated with a special needle from the posterior iliac crest or the sternum. The aspirate is stained and observed for number and maturity of cells and abnormal types.

SUMMARY CONCEPTS

- The function of red blood cells (RBC), facilitated by the iron-containing hemoglobin molecule, is to transport oxygen from the lungs to the tissues. The biconcave shape of the red cell increases the surface area for diffusion of oxygen across the thin cell membrane. Each red cell has four hemoglobin moieties, each composed of two polypeptide chains consisting of a globin portion and a heme unit that surround an iron atom that reversibly combines with oxygen.

- *Erythropoiesis,* or production of RBC, occurs in the bone marrow and requires iron, vitamin B_{12}, and folate. RBC production is governed by tissue oxygen needs. The decrease in oxygen content in blood is sensed by the kidneys, which then produce a hormone called *erythropoietin.* Erythropoietin, in turn, stimulates the bone marrow to increase RBC production.

- The red blood cell has a life span of approximately 120 days and is broken down in the spleen, liver, or bone marrow. In the process of destruction, the heme portion of the hemoglobin molecule is converted to bilirubin. Bilirubin, which is insoluble in plasma, attaches to plasma proteins for transport in the blood. It is removed from the blood by the liver and conjugated to a water-soluble form so that it can be excreted in the bile.

- In the laboratory, automated blood cell counters rapidly provide accurate measurements of red blood cell count and cell indices. A stained blood smear provides information about the size, color, and shape of red cells and the presence of immature or abnormal cells. If blood smear results are abnormal, examination of the bone marrow may be indicated.

TABLE 13-1	Standard Laboratory Values for Red Blood Cells	
Test	**Normal Values**	**Significance**
Red blood cell count (RBC)		
Men	$4.2–5.4 \times 10^6/\mu L$	Number of red cells in the blood
Women	$3.6–5.0 \times 10^6/\mu L$	
Reticulocytes	1.0%–1.5% of total RBC	Rate of red cell production
Hemoglobin		
Men	14–16.5 g/dL	Hemoglobin content of the blood
Women	12–15 g/dL	
Hematocrit		
Men	40%–50%	Volume of cells in 100 mL of blood
Women	37%–47%	
Mean corpuscular volume	85–100 dL	Size of the red cell
Mean corpuscular hemoglobin concentration	31–35 g/dL	Concentration of hemoglobin in the red cell
Mean cell hemoglobin	27–34 pg/cell	Red cell mass

Anemia

Anemia is defined as an abnormally low number of circulating red blood cells or level of hemoglobin, or both, resulting in diminished oxygen-carrying capacity.[5,6] Anemia usually results from excessive loss (bleeding) or destruction (hemolysis) of red blood cells or deficient red blood cell production because of a lack of nutritional elements or bone marrow failure. These mechanisms serve as the basis for classifying anemia.

The effects of anemia can be grouped into three categories: (1) manifestations of impaired oxygen transport and the resulting compensatory mechanisms, (2) reduction in red cell indices and hemoglobin levels,

and (3) signs and symptoms associated with the pathologic process that is causing the anemia. The manifestations of anemia depend on its severity, the rapidity of its development, underlying pathologic mechanisms, and the person's age and health status. If the onset is slow, the body compensates for the decrease in oxygen-carrying capacity of the blood with increases in plasma volume, cardiac output, and respiratory rate. These changes can largely compensate for the effects of mild to moderate anemia in otherwise healthy individuals but are less effective in those with compromised respiratory or cardiac function.

The redistribution of the blood from cutaneous tissues or the lack of hemoglobin causes pallor of the skin, mucous membranes, conjunctivae, and nail beds. Tachycardia and palpitations may occur as the body tries to compensate with an increase in cardiac output. Anemias caused by premature destruction of red cells (hemolytic anemias) are associated with hyperbilirubinemia, jaundice, and pigment gallstones. Anemias that result from ineffective hematopoiesis (premature death of red blood cells in the bone marrow) are associated with inappropriately high levels of iron absorption from the gut, which can lead to iron overload and eventual damage to endocrine organs and the heart.

Laboratory tests are useful in determining the severity and cause of the anemia. The red cell count and hemoglobin levels provide information about the severity of the anemia, whereas red cell characteristics such as size (normocytic, microcytic, macrocytic), color (normochromic, hypochromic), and shape often provide information about the cause of anemia (Fig. 13-8).

Blood Loss Anemia

The clinical manifestations and red cell changes associated with blood loss anemia depend on the rate of hemorrhage and whether the bleeding loss is internal or external. With rapid blood loss, circulatory collapse may occur. With more slowly developing blood loss, the amount of red cell mass lost may reach 50% without the occurrence of signs and symptoms.[3]

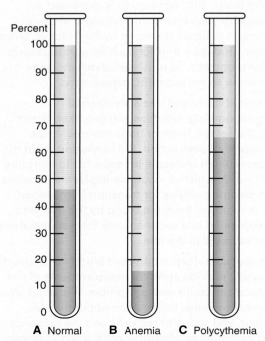

FIGURE 13-7. Hematocrit. The hematocrit measures the percentage of cells in 100 mL of plasma: **(A)** normal, **(B)** decreased in anemia, and **(C)** increased in polycythemia.

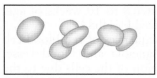
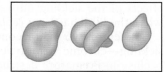

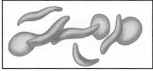
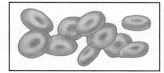

A Iron-deficiency anemia   **B** Megaloblastic anemia

C Sickle cell disease   **D** Normal

FIGURE 13-8. Red cell characteristics seen in different types of anemia: **(A)** microcytic and hypochromic red cells, characteristic of iron-deficiency anemia; **(B)** macrocytic and misshaped red blood cells, characteristic of megaloblastic anemia; **(C)** abnormally shaped red blood cells seen in sickle cell disease; and **(D)** normocytic and normochromic red blood cells, as a comparison.

The effects of acute blood loss are mainly due to loss of intravascular volume, which can lead to cardiovascular collapse and shock (see Chapter 20). A fall in the red blood cell count, and thus hemoglobin, is caused by hemodilution resulting from movement of fluid into the vascular compartment. Initially, the red cells are normal in size and color (normocytic, normochromic). The hypoxia that results from blood loss stimulates proliferation of committed erythroid stem cells in the bone marrow. It takes about 5 days for the progeny of hematopoietic stem cells to differentiate fully, an event that is marked by increased reticulocytes in the blood. If the bleeding is controlled and sufficient iron stores are available, the red cell concentration returns to normal within 3 to 4 weeks. External bleeding leads to iron loss and possible iron deficiency, which can hamper restoration of the red cell count.

Chronic blood loss does not affect blood volume but instead leads to iron-deficiency anemia with depleted iron stores. It is commonly caused by gastrointestinal bleeding and menstrual disorders. Because of compensatory mechanisms, persons are commonly asymptomatic until the hemoglobin level is less than 8 g/dL. The red cells that are produced have too little hemoglobin, giving rise to microcytic hypochromic anemia (see Fig. 13-8A).

Hemolytic Anemias

Hemolytic anemia is characterized by the premature destruction of red cells, the retention of iron and the other products of hemoglobin destruction, and a compensatory increase in erythropoiesis.[5,6] Almost all types of hemolytic anemia are distinguished by normocytic and normochromic red cells. Because of the red blood cell's shortened life span, the bone marrow usually is hyperactive, resulting in an increased number of reticulocytes in the circulating blood. As with other types of anemia, the person experiences easy fatigability, dyspnea, and other signs and symptoms of impaired oxygen transport.

Hemolytic anemias are commonly classified according to the red cell defect: intrinsic to the cell or due to some external factor.[5] Intrinsic factors have been described for all components of the red cell, including the cell membrane, enzyme systems, and hemoglobin, most of which are hereditary. Extrinsic or acquired factors include immune mechanisms, mechanical trauma, and infections.

Destruction of red cells can occur within the vascular compartment (intravascular) or within the phagocytic cells of the reticuloendothelial system (extravascular). Intravascular hemolysis is less common and occurs as a result of mechanical injury caused by defective cardiac valves, complement fixation in transfusion reactions, or exogenous toxic factors. Regardless of cause, intravascular hemolysis leads to hemoglobinemia, hemoglobinuria, and hemosiderinuria. The conversion of the heme pigment to bilirubin can result in unconjugated hyperbilirubinemia and jaundice. Massive intravascular hemolysis can lead to acute tubular necrosis (Chapter 25). Extravascular hemolysis, the most common type of red cell destruction, takes place largely within the phagocytic cells of the spleen and liver. Because extreme changes in shape are necessary for red cells to navigate the splenic sinusoids successfully, reduced deformability makes the passage difficult and leads to splenic sequestration, followed by phagocytosis. Extravascular hemolysis is not associated with hemoglobinemia or hemoglobinuria, but it often produces jaundice. It can also lead to the formation of bilirubin-rich gallstones, also called *pigment stones*.

Inherited Disorders of the Red Cell Membrane

Hereditary spherocytosis, in which the loss of membrane surface area relative to cytoplasmic contents causes the cell to become a tight sphere instead of a concave disk, is the most common inherited disorders of the red cell. The disorder, which transmitted as an autosomal dominant trait in about 75% of cases, is caused by disorders of the spectrin and ankyrin membrane proteins that lead to a loss of membrane surface. Although the spherical cell retains its ability to transport oxygen, it is poorly deformable and susceptible to destruction as it passes through the venous sinuses of the splenic circulation. Clinical signs are variable but typically include mild hemolytic anemia, jaundice, splenomegaly, and bilirubin gallstones. A life-threatening aplastic crisis may occur when a sudden disruption of red cell production (often from a viral infection) causes a rapid drop in the hemoglobin level. The disorder usually is treated with splenectomy to reduce red cell destruction, and with blood transfusions to support the circulation during a crisis.

Sickle Cell Disease

Sickle cell disease is an inherited disorder in which abnormal hemoglobin (hemoglobin S [HbS]) leads to chronic hemolytic anemia, pain, and organ failure. The HbS gene is transmitted by recessive inheritance and can manifest as sickle cell trait (i.e., heterozygote with one HbS gene) or sickle cell disease (i.e., homozygote with two HbS genes). Approximately 8% of African Americans are heterozygous for HbS and 0.1% to 0.2% are homozygous.[5] In parts of Africa, where malaria is endemic, the gene frequency approaches 30%, attributed to the slight protective effect it confers against *Plasmodium falciparum* malaria.[5]

The abnormal structure of HbS results from a point mutation in the β chain of the hemoglobin molecule, with an abnormal substitution of a single amino acid, valine, for glutamic acid (Fig. 13-9). In the heterozygote, only approximately 40% of the hemoglobin is HbS, but in the homozygote, 80% to 95% of the hemoglobin is HbS.[5] Variations in proportions exist, and the concentration of HbS correlates with the risk of sickling. HbS polymerizes when deoxygenated, creating a semisolid gel that makes the erythrocyte rigid, distorts its shape, and causes structural damage to the red cell membrane (see Figure 13-8C). The sickled cell may return to its normal shape with oxygenation in the lungs. However, after repeated episodes of deoxygenation, the cells remain permanently sickled. The person with sickle cell trait who has less HbS has little tendency to sickle and is virtually asymptomatic. Fetal hemoglobin (HbF) inhibits the polymerization of HbS; therefore, most infants with sickle cell disease do not begin to experience the effects of the sickling until after 8 to 10 weeks of age, when the HbF has been replaced by HbS.[6]

There are two major consequences of red blood cell sickling—chronic hemolytic anemia and blood vessel occlusion. Premature destruction of the cells due to the rigid, nondeformable membrane occurs in the spleen, causing hemolysis and anemia from a decrease in red cell numbers. Overall, the mean life span of red cells in persons with sickle cell disease averages only 20 days (one sixth of normal).[5] Vessel occlusion disrupts blood flow, causing tissue ischemia and a pain crisis. Recent evidence suggests that vessel occlusion is a complex process involving an interaction among the sickled cells, vessel endothelial cells, platelets, and other blood components.[7] The process is initiated by the adherence of sickled cells to the vessel endothelium, causing endothelial cell activation with liberation of inflammatory mediators and substances that increase platelet activation and promote blood coagulation.[5–7]

Factors associated with sickling and vessel occlusion include cold, stress, physical exertion, infection, and illnesses that cause hypoxia, dehydration, or acidosis. The rate of HbS polymerization is affected by the concentration of hemoglobin in the cell. Dehydration increases the hemoglobin concentration and contributes to the polymerization and resultant sickling. Acidosis reduces the affinity of hemoglobin for oxygen, resulting in more deoxygenated hemoglobin and increased sickling. Even such trivial incidents as reduced oxygen tension induced by sleep may contribute to the sickling process.

Clinical Course. Persons who are homozygous for the HbS gene experience severe hemolytic anemia, chronic hyperbilirubinemia, and vaso-occlusive crises. The hyperbilirubinemia that results from the breakdown products of hemoglobin often leads to jaundice and the formation of pigment gallstones.

The complications of sickle cell disease are numerous, with two of the most common being vaso-occlusive pain crisis and acute chest syndrome.[7–9] An acute pain episode results from tissue hypoxia due to vessel occlusion and can occur suddenly in almost any part of the body.[7–12] Common sites obstructed by sickled cells include the abdomen, chest, bones, and joints. Many areas may be affected simultaneously. Infarctions caused by sluggish blood flow may cause chronic damage to the liver, spleen, heart, kidneys, retinas, and other organs (Fig. 13-10). *Acute chest syndrome* is an atypical pneumonia resulting from pulmonary infarction. It is the second leading cause of hospitalization in persons with sickle cell disease and is characterized by pulmonary infiltrates, shortness of breath, fever, chest pain, and cough. The syndrome can cause chronic respiratory insufficiency and is a leading cause of death in sickle cell disease. Children may experience growth retardation and susceptibility to osteomyelitis. Painful bone crises may be caused by marrow infarcts of the bones of the hands and feet, resulting in swelling of those extremities. Another major complication is stroke. Approximately 25% of persons with sickle cell disease have neurologic complications, including stroke, related to vessel occlusion.[10]

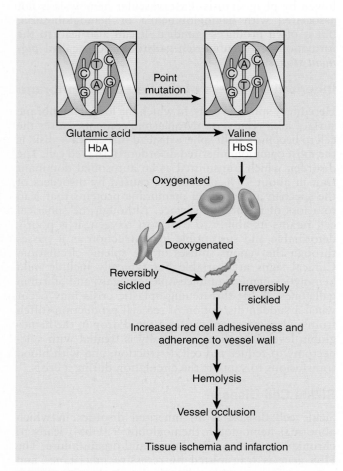

FIGURE 13-9. Mechanism of sickling and its consequences in sickle cell disease.

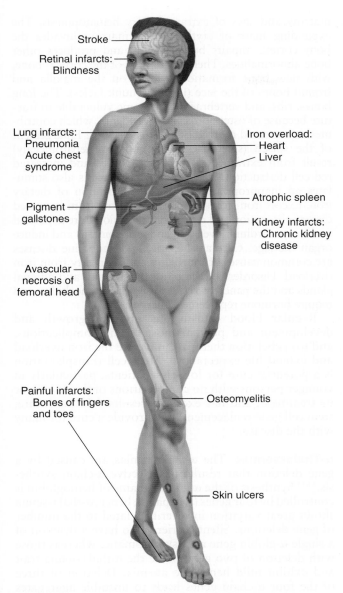

Stroke

Retinal infarcts:
Blindness

Lung infarcts:
Pneumonia
Acute chest
syndrome

Iron overload:
Heart
Liver

Pigment
gallstones

Atrophic spleen

Kidney infarcts:
Chronic kidney
disease

Avascular
necrosis of
femoral head

Painful infarcts:
Bones of fingers
and toes

Osteomyelitis

Skin ulcers

FIGURE 13-10. Clinical manifestations of sickle cell disease.

In addition to these crises, persons with sickle cell disease are prone to infections. Because of the spleen's sluggish blood flow and low oxygen tension, hemoglobin in red cells traversing the spleen becomes deoxygenated, causing ischemia. Splenic injury begins in early childhood, is characterized by intense congestion, and is usually asymptomatic. The congestion causes functional asplenia and predisposes the person to life-threatening infections by encapsulated organisms such as *Streptococcus pneumoniae, Haemophilus influenzae* type b, and *Klebsiella* species. Neonates and small children have not had time to create antibodies to these organisms and rely on the spleen for their removal. In the absence of specific antibody to the polysaccharide capsular antigens of these organisms, splenic activity is essential for removing these organisms when they enter the blood.

Diagnosis and Treatment. The signs and symptoms of sickle cell disease make their appearance during infancy. Neonatal diagnosis of sickle cell disease is made on the basis of clinical findings and hemoglobin solubility results, which are confirmed by hemoglobin electrophoresis. Prenatal diagnosis is done by the analysis of fetal DNA obtained by amniocentesis.[7]

In the United States, screening programs have been implemented to detect newborns with sickle cell disease and other hemoglobinopathies. Cord blood or heel-stick samples are subjected to electrophoresis to separate the HbF from the small amount of HbA and HbS. Other hemoglobins may also be detected and quantified by further laboratory evaluation. According to the National Newborn Screening and Genetics Resource Center (NNSGRC), all 50 states require screening of all newborns regardless of ethnic origin.

The clinical course of persons with sickle cell disease is highly variable. As a result of improvements in supportive care, an increasing number of persons are surviving into adulthood and producing offspring. Of particular importance is the early prophylactic treatment with penicillin to prevent pneumococcal infection. Treatment should begin as early as 2 months of age and continued until at least 5 years of age.[11] Maintaining full immunization, including the *H. influenzae* and hepatitis B vaccines, is recommended. The National Institutes of Health Committee on Management of Sickle Cell Disease also recommends administration of the 7-valent pneumococcal vaccine beginning at 2 to 6 months of age[11] (see Chapter 25). The 7-valent vaccine should be followed by immunization with the 23-valent pneumococcal vaccine at 24 months of age or later. Most recent recommendations (Advisory Committee on Immunization Practices 2013) have also included the use of the 13-valent pneumococcal conjugate vaccine in children ages 6 to 18 years old with immunocompromising conditions such as functional asplenia.

Hydroxyurea, an inhibitor of DNA synthesis, has been shown to reduce pain crises and prevent the complications of sickle cell disease. The drug produces an increase of HbF in red cells by decreasing the terminal differentiation of erythroid stem cells into HbS; acts as an anti-inflammatory agent by inhibiting the production of white blood cells; and is oxidized by heme groups to produce nitric oxide, a potent vasodilator and inhibitor of platelet aggregation.[5] Although the drug halves pain episodes and pulmonary complications, approximately 40% of persons do not respond.[12] Other therapies under investigation include drugs that affect globin gene expression; prevent hemoglobin polymerization, membrane damage, and cell dehydration; or inhibit sickle cell adhesion to endothelial cells.[12] Bone marrow or stem cell transplantation has the potential for cure in symptomatic children but carries the risk of graft-versus-host disease. Progress in gene therapy to treat sickle cell disease has been slow but promising, and may be a future option.

Thalassemias

The thalassemias are a heterogeneous group of inherited disorders caused by mutations that decrease the rate of synthesis of α- or β-globin chains. B-thalassemias are caused by deficient synthesis of the β chain and α-thalassemias by deficient synthesis of the α chain.[5,6,13–15] The defect is inherited as a Mendelian trait, and a person may be heterozygous (mild disease) or homozygous (severe disease) for the trait. Like sickle cell disease, the thalassemias occur with a high degree of frequency in certain populations. B-thalassemia, sometimes called *Cooley anemia* or *Mediterranean anemia*, is most common in the Mediterranean populations of southern Italy and Greece, whereas the α-thalassemias are more common among Asians. Both α- and β-thalassemias are more common in Africans and African Americans.

Two factors contribute to the anemia that occurs in thalassemia: a deficiency in hemoglobin due to the decreased synthesis of the affected chain, coupled with excess production of the unaffected chain. The reduced hemoglobin synthesis results in a hypochromic, microcytic anemia, whereas the accumulation of the unaffected chain interferes with normal red cell maturation and contributes to membrane changes that lead to hemolysis and anemia.

β-Thalassemias. The β-thalassemias result from a point mutation in the β-globin gene that directs β-chain synthesis.[13,14] Sequencing of the β-thalassemia genes has revealed more than 100 different mutations, the majority of which consist of single-base changes. The presence of one normal gene in heterozygous persons (thalassemia minor) usually results in sufficient normal hemoglobin synthesis to prevent severe anemia. Persons who are homozygous for the trait (thalassemia major) have severe, transfusion-dependent anemia that is evident at about 6 months of age when the hemoglobin switches from HbF to HbA. If transfusion therapy is not started early in life, severe growth retardation occurs in children with the disorder.

Two conditions contribute to the pathogenesis of the anemia in β-thalassemias: inadequate HbA formation due to reduced β-globin chain synthesis, and red cell hemolysis resulting from an unbalanced rate of β-globin and α-globin synthesis. The excess α-globin chains form insoluble aggregates (*Heinz bodies*) that precipitate within red cells and produce severe membrane damage that causes extravascular hemolysis. Erythroblasts in the bone marrow undergo a similar fate, which in severe β-thalassemia results in destruction of the majority of erythroid precursors before their maturation into red cells. In addition to anemia, persons with moderate to severe forms of the disease suffer from coagulation abnormalities. Thrombotic events (stroke and pulmonary embolism) appear to be related to altered platelet function, endothelial activation, and an imbalance of procoagulant and anticoagulant factors.[13]

In severe β-thalassemia, marked anemia produced by ineffective hematopoiesis and hemolysis leads to increased erythropoietin secretion and hyperplasia in the bone marrow and sites of extramedullary hematopoiesis. The expanding mass of erythropoietic marrow invades the bony cortex, impairs bone growth, and produces other bone abnormalities. There is thinning of the cortical bone, with new bone formation evident on the maxilla and frontal bones of the face (i.e., chipmunk facies). The long bones, ribs, and vertebrae may become vulnerable to fracture because of osteoporosis or osteopenia, which contributes to increased morbidity in older persons. Enlargement of the spleen (splenomegaly) and liver (hepatomegaly) result from extramedullary hematopoiesis and increased red cell destruction. Ineffective hematopoiesis also stimulates an inappropriate increase in absorption of dietary iron. Excess iron stores, which accumulate from increased dietary absorption and repeated transfusions, are deposited in the myocardium, liver, and endocrine organs and induce organ damage. Cardiac, hepatic, and endocrine diseases are common causes of morbidity and mortality from iron overload. Disorders of the pituitary, thyroid, and adrenal glands and the pancreas result in significant morbidity and require hormone replacement therapy.[14]

Regular blood transfusions improve growth and development and prevent most of the complications, and iron chelation therapy can reduce the iron overload and extend life expectancy.[14] Stem cell transplantation is a potential cure for low-risk patients, particularly in younger persons with no complications of the disease or its treatment, and has excellent results.[14] In the future, stem cell gene replacement may provide a cure for many with the disease.

α-Thalassemias. The α-thalassemias are caused by a gene deletion that results in defective α-chain synthesis.[13,15] Synthesis of the α-globin chains of hemoglobin is controlled by four genes (two pairs); hence, α-thalassemia shows great variation in severity related to the number of gene deletions. Silent carriers who have a deletion of a single α-globin gene are asymptomatic, whereas those with deletion of two genes have the α-thalassemia trait and exhibit mild hemolytic anemia. Deletion of three of the four α-chain genes leads to unstable aggregates of α chains called *hemoglobin H* (HbH). This disorder is the most important clinical form and is more common in Asians. The β chains are more soluble than the α chains, and their accumulation is less toxic to the red cells, so that senescent rather than precursor red cells are affected. Most persons with HbH have moderately severe hemolytic anemia but do not usually require transfusions.[13] The most severe form of α-thalassemia occurs in infants in whom all four α-globin genes are deleted. Such a defect results in a hemoglobin molecule (Hb Bart) that is formed exclusively from the chains of HbF. Hb Bart, which has an extremely high oxygen affinity, and cannot release oxygen in the tissues. This disorder usually results in death in utero or shortly after birth.[14]

Inherited Enzyme Defects

The red cell is vulnerable to injury by endogenous and exogenous oxidants, which are normally inactivated by the glucose-containing tripeptide *glutathione*, one of the body's principal means of preventing oxidative damage. Abnormalities of glutathione metabolism resulting from impaired enzyme function reduce the ability of red cells to protect against oxidative stress. The most common inherited enzyme defect that results in hemolytic anemia is a deficiency of glucose-6-phosphate dehydrogenase (G6PD). The gene that determines this enzyme is located on the X chromosome, and the defect is expressed only in males and homozygous females. There are several hundred variants of this gene, but only the G6PD A-variant, found in 10% to 15% of African Americans, and the G6PD Mediterranean variant are known to cause clinically significant hemolytic anemia.[5,6] The disorders are also associated with favism, a disorder of hemolysis due to consumption of fava beans.

Glucose-6-phosphate dehydrogenase deficiency makes red cells more vulnerable to oxidants. The disorder features direct oxidation of hemoglobin to methemoglobin, which cannot transport oxygen, and denaturing of the hemoglobin molecule to form Heinz bodies, which are precipitated in the red blood cell. Hemolysis usually occurs as the damaged red blood cells move through the narrow vessels of the spleen, causing hemoglobinemia, hemoglobinuria, and jaundice. The hemolysis is short-lived, occurring 2 to 3 days after the triggering event. In African Americans, the defect is mildly expressed and is not associated with chronic hemolytic anemia unless triggered by oxidant drugs, acidosis, or infection. In affected persons, the hemolysis can be triggered by exposure to oxidant drugs such as the antimalarial drug primaquine, quinine, the sulfonamides, and nitrofurantoin. Severe G6PD deficiency (as in Mediterranean variants) may produce a chronic hemolytic anemia. The disorder can be diagnosed through the use of a G6PD assay and other screening blood tests (complete blood count, bilirubin, and reticulocyte count). No treatment is necessary except to avoid known oxidant drugs.

Acquired Hemolytic Anemias

Several acquired factors exogenous to the red blood cell produce hemolysis by direct membrane destruction or antibody-mediated lysis. Various drugs, chemicals, toxins, venoms, and infections such as malaria destroy red cell membranes. Hemolysis can also be caused by mechanical factors such as prosthetic heart valves, vasculitis, and severe burns. Obstructions in the microcirculation, as in disseminated intravascular coagulation, thrombotic thrombocytopenic purpura, and renal disease, may traumatize the red cells by producing turbulence and changing pressure gradients.

Although commonly referred to as autoantibody anemia, the currently preferred designation is immunohemolytic anemia, since it may be initiated by an ingested drug. The antibodies that cause hemolysis are of two types: warm-reacting antibodies of the immunoglobulin G (IgG) class, which are maximally active at 37°C, and cold-reacting antibodies of the IgM type, which are optimally active at about 4°C.

In the warm-reacting antibody type, the most common form of immunohemolytic anemia, the antibodies react with antigens on the red cell membrane, causing destructive changes that lead to spherocytosis, with subsequent phagocytic destruction in the spleen or reticuloendothelial system. The antibodies lack specificity for the ABO antigens but may react with the Rh antigens. The hemolytic reactions usually have a rapid onset and may be severe and life-threatening. There are varied causes for this anemia: approximately 50% are idiopathic, and 50% are related to predisposing conditions such as lymphoid neoplasms, autoimmune disorders (particularly systemic lupus erythematosus), and exposure to drugs such as penicillin and the cephalosporins.[5,6] Some drugs, of which the antihypertensive drug α-methyldopa is the prototype, induce the production of antibodies against red cell antigens, particularly Rh antigens. About 10% of persons taking α-methyldopa develop antibodies, and about 10% develop clinically significant hemolysis.[5]

In the cold-reacting agglutinin type of hemolytic anemia, which is less common than the warm-reacting type, IgM antibodies bind red cells and cause agglutination and activate complement. Cold agglutinin antibodies sometimes appear transiently following certain infections (e.g., Epstein-Barr, influenza), in which case the condition is relatively benign. The condition may also develop as a chronic complication of B-cell neoplasms and as an idiopathic entity. Symptoms are variable and occur in parts of the body, such as the ears, fingers, and toes, where the temperature may fall below 30°C. They manifest due to vascular obstruction caused by agglutinated red cells resulting in pallor, cyanosis, and Raynaud phenomenon.

The diagnosis of immunohemolytic anemia requires use of the Coombs test to detect the presence of antibody or complement on the surface of red blood cells. The *direct Coombs test* uses antibodies specific for human immunoglobulins or complement to detect antibodies on red blood cells. It is positive in cases of autoimmune hemolytic anemia, Rh disease of the newborn, transfusion reactions, and drug-induced hemolysis. The *indirect Coombs test* uses commercially available red cells with known antigens to characterize the antigen target and temperature dependence of the responsible antigen.

Anemias of Deficient Red Cell Production

Anemia may result from the decreased production of erythrocytes by the bone marrow. This category includes anemias caused by a deficiency of substances that are needed for hematopoiesis, particularly iron, vitamin B_{12}, and folic acid. Other disorders that suppress erythropoiesis include those associated with bone marrow failure or replacement of the bone marrow by tumor or inflammatory cells.

Iron-Deficiency Anemia

Iron deficiency is a common worldwide cause of anemia affecting persons of all ages.[16] The anemia results from dietary deficiency, loss of iron through bleeding, or increased demands. Because iron is a component of heme, a deficiency leads to decreased hemoglobin synthesis and consequent impairment of oxygen delivery.

Body iron is used repeatedly. When red cells become senescent and are broken down, their iron is released and reused in the production of new red cells. Despite this efficient process, small amounts of iron are lost in the feces and need to be replaced by dietary uptake. Iron balance is maintained by the absorption of 0.5 to 1.5 mg daily to replace the 1 mg lost in the feces. The average Western diet supplies about 20 mg.[6] The absorbed iron is more than sufficient to supply the needs of most individuals, but may be barely adequate in toddlers, adolescents, and women of child-bearing age.

The usual reason for iron deficiency in adults in the Western world is chronic blood loss because iron cannot be recycled to the pool. In men and postmenopausal women, blood loss may occur from gastrointestinal bleeding because of peptic ulcer, intestinal polyps, hemorrhoids, or cancer. Excessive aspirin intake may cause undetected gastrointestinal bleeding. In women, menstruation may account for an average of 1.5 mg of iron lost per day, causing a deficiency.[16] Although cessation of menstruation removes a major source of iron loss in the pregnant woman, iron requirements increase during this time, and deficiency is common. The expansion of the mother's blood volume in addition to the growing fetus increase the total iron needs to about 1000 mg (27 mg/day) during pregnancy. In the postnatal period, lactation requires approximately 1 mg of iron daily.[16]

A child's growth places extra demands on the body. Blood volume increases, with a greater need for iron. Iron requirements are proportionally higher in infancy (3 to 24 months) than at any other age, although they are also increased in childhood and adolescence. In infancy, the two main causes of iron-deficiency anemia are low iron levels at birth because of maternal deficiency and a diet consisting mainly of cow's milk, which is low in absorbable iron. Adolescents are also susceptible to iron deficiency because of high requirements due to growth spurts, dietary deficiencies, and menstrual loss.[17]

Iron-deficiency anemia is characterized by low hemoglobin and hematocrit, decreased iron stores, and low serum iron and ferritin levels. The red cells are decreased in number and are microcytic and hypochromic (see Fig. 13-8). Poikilocytosis (irregular shape) and anisocytosis (irregular size) are also present. Laboratory values show reduced MCHC and MCV. Membrane changes may predispose to hemolysis, causing further loss of red cells.

The manifestations of iron-deficiency anemia are related to impaired oxygen transport and lack of hemoglobin. Depending on the severity of the anemia, pallor, easy fatigability, dyspnea, and tachycardia may occur. Epithelial atrophy is common and results in waxy pallor, brittle hair and nails, sometimes a spoon-shaped deformity of the fingernails, smooth tongue, sores in the corners of the mouth, and sometimes dysphagia and decreased acid secretion. A poorly understood symptom occasionally seen is pica, the bizarre, compulsive eating of ice, dirt, or other abnormal substances. Iron deficiency in infants may also result in long-term manifestations

such as poor cognitive, motor, and emotional function that may be related to effects on brain development and neurotransmitter function.[18]

Prevention of iron deficiency is a primary concern in infants and children. Avoidance of cow's milk, iron supplementation at 4 to 6 months of age in breast-fed infants, and use of iron-fortified formulas and cereals are recommended for infants younger than 1 year of age.[19] In the 2nd year, a diet rich in iron-containing foods and use of iron-fortified vitamins will help prevent iron deficiency. The treatment of iron-deficiency anemia in children and adults is directed toward controlling chronic blood loss, increasing dietary intake of iron, and administering supplemental iron. Ferrous sulfate, which is the usual oral replacement therapy, replenishes iron stores in several months. Parenteral iron therapy may be used when oral forms are not tolerated or are ineffective. Caution is required because of the possibility of severe hypersensitivity reactions.

Megaloblastic Anemias

Megaloblastic anemias are caused by impaired DNA synthesis that results in enlarged red cells (MCV > 100 fL) due to impaired maturation and division.[20] There are two principal causes of megaloblastic anemia: vitamin B_{12} and folic acid deficiencies. Because megaloblastic anemias develop slowly, there are often few symptoms until the anemia is far advanced.

Vitamin B_{12}–Deficiency Anemia. Vitamin B_{12}, also known as *cobalamin*, serves as a cofactor for two important reactions in humans. It is essential for DNA synthesis and nuclear maturation, which in turn leads to normal red cell maturation and division.[5,21] Vitamin B_{12} is also involved in a reaction that prevents abnormal fatty acids from being incorporated into neuronal lipids. This abnormality may predispose to myelin breakdown and produce some of the neurologic complications of vitamin B_{12} deficiency.[5]

Vitamin B_{12} is found in all foods of animal origin. Dietary deficiency is rare and usually found only in strict vegetarians who avoid all dairy products as well as meat and fish. Vitamin B_{12} is absorbed by a unique process. After release from the animal protein, it is bound to the intrinsic factor, a protein secreted by the gastric parietal cells (Fig. 13-11). The vitamin B_{12}–intrinsic factor complex protects vitamin B_{12} from digestion by intestinal enzymes. The complex travels to the ileum, where it binds to membrane receptors on the epithelial cells. Vitamin B_{12} is then separated from intrinsic factor and transported across the membrane into the circulation. There it is bound to its carrier protein, transcobalamin II, which transports vitamin B_{12} to its storage and tissue sites.

An important cause of vitamin B_{12} deficiency is pernicious anemia, resulting from atrophic gastritis (see Chapter 29). Pernicious anemia is believed to result from immunologically mediated, possibly autoimmune, destruction of the gastric mucosa. The resultant chronic atrophic gastritis is marked by loss of parietal

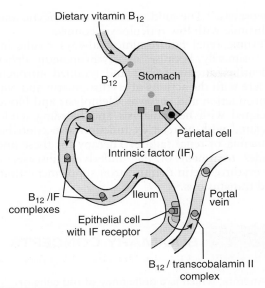

Dietary vitamin B₁₂

B₁₂

Stomach

Parietal cell

Intrinsic factor (IF)

B₁₂/IF complexes

Ileum

Portal vein

Epithelial cell with IF receptor

B₁₂/ transcobalamin II complex

FIGURE 13-11. Absorption of vitamin B_{12}.

cells and production of antibodies that interfere with binding of vitamin B_{12} to intrinsic factor. Other causes of vitamin B_{12} deficiency anemia include gastrectomy, ileal resection, inflammation or neoplasms in the terminal ileum, and malabsorption syndromes in which vitamin B_{12} and other B-vitamin compounds are poorly absorbed.

The hallmark of vitamin B_{12} deficiency is megaloblastic anemia. When vitamin B_{12} is deficient, the red cells that are produced are abnormally large because of excess cytoplasmic growth and structural proteins (see Fig. 13-8B). The cells have immature nuclei with evidence of cellular destruction and delicate membranes that are oval rather than biconcave. These oddly shaped cells have a short life span that can be measured in weeks rather than months. The loss of red cells results in moderate to severe anemia and mild jaundice. The MCV is elevated, and the MCHC is normal. As with other anemias, there is pallor, easy fatigability, and in severe cases dyspnea. The megaloblastic state also produces changes in mucosal cells, leading to glossitis (sore tongue), as well as other vague gastrointestinal disturbances such as anorexia and diarrhea. Vitamin B_{12} deficiency also leads to a complex neurologic syndrome caused by deranged methylation of myelin protein. Demyelination of the dorsal and lateral columns of the spinal cord causes symmetric paresthesias of the hands and feet, loss of vibratory and position sense, and eventual spastic ataxia. In more advanced cases, cerebral function may be altered with dementia and other neuropsychiatric changes preceding hematologic changes.

Diagnosis of vitamin B_{12} deficiency is made by finding an abnormally low serum vitamin B_{12} level. The diagnosis of pernicious anemia is usually made by the detection of parietal cell and intrinsic factor antibodies.[20] Lifelong treatment consisting of intramuscular injections or high oral doses of vitamin B_{12} reverses the anemia and prevents the neurologic changes.

Folic Acid–Deficiency Anemia. Folic acid is also required for DNA synthesis and red cell maturation, and its deficiency produces the same type of megaloblastic red cell changes that occur in vitamin B_{12}–deficiency anemia (i.e., increased MCV and normal MCHC).

Folic acid is readily absorbed from the intestine. It is found in vegetables (particularly the green leafy types), fruits, cereals, and meats. Much of the vitamin, however, is lost in cooking. The most common causes of folic acid deficiency are malnutrition or dietary lack, especially in the elderly or in association with alcoholism. Total body stores of folic acid amount to 2000 to 5000 μg with a 50 μg daily dietary requirement.[6] A dietary deficiency may result in anemia in a few months. Malabsorption of folic acid may be due to syndromes such as celiac disease or other intestinal disorders. Anti-epileptic medications such as primidone, phenytoin, phenobarbital, and the diuretic triamterene predispose to a deficiency by interfering with folic acid absorption. In neoplastic disease, tumor cells compete for folate, and deficiency is common. Methotrexate, a folic acid analog used in the treatment of cancer, impairs the action of folic acid by blocking its conversion to the active form. Because pregnancy increases the need for folic acid 5- to 10-fold, a deficiency commonly occurs. Poor dietary habits, anorexia, and nausea are other reasons for folic acid deficiency during pregnancy. Studies have shown an association between folate deficiency and neural tube defects (see Chapter 6).[20]

The features of folic acid deficiency are similar to those of vitamin B_{12} deficiency, with megaloblastic anemia and symptoms referable to changes in the mucosal surface of the gastrointestinal tract. However, there are essentially none of the neurologic abnormalities associated with B_{12} deficiency.

Aplastic Anemia

Aplastic anemia describes a disorder of pluripotential bone marrow stem cells that results in a reduction of all three hematopoietic cell lines—red blood cells, white blood cells, and platelets.[22,23] Pure red cell aplasia, in which only the red cells are affected, rarely occurs. Anemia results from the failure of the marrow to replace senescent red cells that are destroyed and leave the circulation, although the cells that remain are of normal size and color. At the same time, because the leukocytes, particularly the neutrophils, and the thrombocytes have a short life span, a deficiency of these cells usually is apparent before the anemia becomes severe.

The onset of aplastic anemia may be insidious, or it may strike with suddenness and great severity. It can occur at any age. The initial presenting symptoms include weakness, fatigability, and pallor caused by anemia. Petechiae (i.e., small, punctate skin hemorrhages [see Chapter 12, Fig. 12-4]) and ecchymoses (i.e., bruises) often occur on the skin, and bleeding from the nose, gums, vagina, or gastrointestinal tract may occur because of decreased platelet levels. The decrease in the number of neutrophils increases susceptibility to infection.

Causes of aplastic anemia include exposure to high doses of radiation, chemicals, and toxins that suppress hematopoiesis directly or through immune mechanisms. Chemotherapy and irradiation commonly result in bone marrow depression, which causes anemia, thrombocytopenia, and neutropenia. Identified toxic agents include benzene, the antibiotic chloramphenicol, and the alkylating agents and antimetabolites used in the treatment of cancer (see Chapter 7). Aplastic anemia caused by exposure to chemical agents may be an idiosyncratic reaction because it affects only certain susceptible persons. It typically occurs weeks after a drug is initiated. Such reactions often are severe and sometimes irreversible and fatal. It can also develop in the course of many infections and has been reported most often as a complication of viral hepatitis, mononucleosis, and other viral illnesses, including acquired immunodeficiency syndrome (AIDS). In two thirds of cases, the cause is unknown, a condition referred to as *idiopathic aplastic anemia*. The mechanisms underlying the pathogenesis of aplastic anemia are unknown. It is suggested that exposure to the chemicals, infectious agents, and other insults generates a cellular immune response resulting in production of cytokines by activated T cells. These cytokines (e.g., interferon, tumor necrosis factor [TNF]) then suppress hematopoietic stem cell growth and development.[5]

Therapy for aplastic anemia in the young and severely affected includes stem cell replacement by bone marrow or peripheral blood transplantation. Histocompatible donors supply the stem cells to replace the patient's destroyed marrow cells. Graft-versus-host disease, rejection, and infection are major risks of the procedure, yet 75% or more survive.[22] For those who are not transplantation candidates, immunosuppressive therapy with lymphocyte immune globulin (i.e., antithymocyte globulin) prevents suppression of proliferating stem cells, producing remission in up to 50% of patients.[22,23] Persons with aplastic anemia should avoid the offending agents and be treated with antibiotics for infection. Red cell transfusions to correct the anemia and platelets and corticosteroid therapy to minimize bleeding may also be required.

Anemia of Chronic Disease

Anemia often occurs as a complication of infections, inflammation, and cancer. The most common causes of chronic disease anemias are acute and chronic infections, including AIDS and osteomyelitis; cancers; autoimmune disorders such as rheumatoid arthritis, systemic lupus erythematosus, and inflammatory bowel disease; and chronic kidney disease.[24] It is theorized that the short red cell life span, deficient red cell production, a blunted response to erythropoietin, and low serum iron are caused by actions of cytokines and cells of the reticuloendothelial system. Microorganisms, tumor cells, and autoimmune dysregulation lead to T-cell activation and production of cytokines (e.g., interleukin-1, interferon, and TNF) that suppress the erythropoietin response, inhibit erythroid precursors, and cause changes in iron

homeostasis.[24] The mild anemia is normocytic and normochromic with low reticulocyte counts.

Chronic renal failure almost always results in anemia, primarily because of erythropoietin deficiency. Unidentified uremic toxins and retained nitrogen also interfere with the actions of erythropoietin and with red cell production and survival. Hemolysis and blood loss associated with hemodialysis and bleeding tendencies associated with platelet dysfunction also contribute to the anemia of renal failure. Therapy for these anemias includes treatment of the underlying disease, short-term erythropoietin therapy, iron supplementation, and blood transfusions.[24]

SUMMARY CONCEPTS

- Anemia, which is a deficiency of red cells or hemoglobin, results from excessive loss (blood loss anemia), increased destruction (hemolytic anemia), or impaired production of red blood cells (iron-deficiency, megaloblastic due to a Vitamin B$_{12}$ deficiency, and aplastic anemias).

- Blood loss anemia can be acute or chronic. With bleeding, iron and other components of the erythrocyte are lost from the body.

- Hemolytic anemia is characterized by the premature destruction of red cells, with body retention of iron and the other products of red cell destruction. It can be caused by defects in the red cell membrane, hemoglobinopathies (sickle cell disease or thalassemia), or inherited enzyme defects (G6PD deficiency). Acquired forms of hemolytic anemia are caused by agents extrinsic to the red blood cell, such as medications, bacterial and other toxins, antibodies, and physical trauma.

- Aplastic anemia is caused by bone marrow suppression and usually results in a reduction of white blood cells and platelets, as well as red blood cells.

- Chronic diseases such as inflammatory disorders (rheumatoid arthritis), cancers, and renal failure cause anemia through the production of inflammatory cytokines that interfere with erythropoietin production or response.

- The manifestations of anemia are caused by the decreased hemoglobin in the blood (pallor), tissue hypoxia due to deficient oxygen transport (weakness and fatigue), and recruitment of compensatory mechanisms (tachycardia and palpitations) designed to increase oxygen delivery to the tissues.

Polycythemia

Polycythemia represents an abnormally high total red blood cell count with a hematocrit greater than 50%.[25,26] It is categorized as *relative* or *absolute*. In *relative* polycythemia, the hematocrit rises because of a loss of plasma volume without a corresponding increase in red cells. This may occur with water deprivation, excess use of diuretics, or gastrointestinal losses. Relative polycythemia is corrected by increasing the vascular fluid volume. *Absolute* polycythemia is a rise in hematocrit due to an increase in total red cell mass and is classified as primary or secondary.

Primary Polycythemia

Primary polycythemia, or *polycythemia vera,* is a neoplastic disease of the pluripotent cells of the bone marrow characterized by an absolute increase in total red blood cell mass accompanied by elevated white cell and platelet counts. It most commonly is seen in men and may occur at any age with a median age of 62 years at the time of diagnosis.[25,26] In polycythemia vera, the manifestations are variable and are related to an increase in the red cell count, hemoglobin level, and hematocrit with increased blood volume and viscosity. Additional early findings include splenomegaly and depletion of iron stores.[25] Viscosity rises exponentially with the hematocrit and interferes with cardiac output and blood flow. Hypertension is common and there may be complaints of headache, dizziness, inability to concentrate, and some difficulty with hearing and vision because of decreased cerebral blood flow. Venous stasis gives rise to a dusky red or bluish skin color, particularly of the lips, fingernails, and mucous membranes. Because of the increased concentration of blood cells, the person may experience itching (abnormal histamine release) and pain in the fingers or toes, and the hypermetabolism may induce night sweats and weight loss. Thromboembolism and hemorrhage, due to hyperviscosity and platelet and neutrophil abnormal activation, are common complications that can be prevented by phlebotomy to reduce the hematocrit to less than 42% in women and less than 45% in men.[26]

The goal of treatment in primary polycythemia is to reduce blood viscosity. This can be done by withdrawing blood by periodic phlebotomy to reduce red cell volume. Low-dose aspirin may control the high platelet counts, and suppression of bone marrow function with medication (hydroxyurea) controls the elevated white cell count.[26]

Secondary Polycythemia

Secondary polycythemia results from a physiologic increase in the level of erythropoietin, commonly as a compensatory response to hypoxia. Conditions causing hypoxia include living at high altitudes, chronic heart and lung disease, and smoking. The resultant release of erythropoietin by the kidney causes the increased formation of red blood cells in the bone marrow. Neoplasms that secrete erythropoietin may also cause a secondary polycythemia. Kidney disease such as hydronephrosis or renal cysts may obstruct blood flow, cause hypoxia, and lead to an increase in erythropoietin as well. Treatment of secondary polycythemia focuses on relieving hypoxia. For example, continuous low-flow oxygen therapy can be used to correct the severe hypoxia that occurs in some persons with chronic obstructive pulmonary disease. This form of treatment is thought to relieve the pulmonary hypertension and polycythemia and to delay the onset of cor pulmonale (right heart failure due to lung disease).

> ## SUMMARY CONCEPTS
>
> ■ Polycythemia describes a condition of increased red blood cell (RBC) mass. It can present as a relative or absolute disorder, with the latter subcategorized as primary or secondary. Relative polycythemia results from a loss of vascular volume (i.e., diuretic use) and is corrected by fluid replacement.
>
> ■ Primary polycythemia, or polycythemia vera, is a proliferative disease of the bone marrow with an absolute increase in total RBC mass accompanied by elevated white cell and platelet counts. Secondary polycythemia results from increased erythropoietin levels caused by hypoxic conditions such as chronic heart and lung disease.
>
> ■ Many of the manifestations of polycythemia are related to increased blood volume and viscosity that lead to hypertension and stagnation of blood flow.

Age-Related Changes in Red Blood Cells

The red blood cell count and hemoglobin concentration are high at birth and decline with age. The process of aging and other health conditions often impair red cell development, with anemia being a common problem among the elderly.

Red Cell Changes in the Neonate

At birth, changes in the red blood cell indices reflect the transition to extrauterine life and the need to transport oxygen from the lungs (Table 13-2). Hemoglobin concentrations at birth are high, reflecting the high synthetic activity in utero to provide adequate oxygen delivery. Toward the end of the first postnatal week, hemoglobin concentration begins to decline, gradually falling to a minimum value at approximately age 2 months.

TABLE 13-2	Red Cell Values for Term Infants			
Age	**RBC × 10^6/mL Mean ± SD**	**Hb (g/dL)Mean ± SD**	**Hct (%)Mean ± SD**	**MCV (fL)Mean ± SD**
Days				
1	5.14 ± 0.7	19.3 ± 2.2	61 ± 7.4	119 ± 9.4
4	5.00 ± 0.6	18.6 ± 2.1	57 ± 8.1	114 ± 7.5
7	4.86 ± 0.6	17.9 ± 2.5	56 ± 9.4	118 ± 11.2
Weeks				
1–2	4.80 ± 0.8	17.3 ± 2.3	54 ± 8.3	112 ± 19.0
3–4	4.00 ± 0.6	14.2 ± 2.1	43 ± 5.7	105 ± 7.5
8–9	3.40 ± 0.5	10.7 ± 0.9	31 ± 2.5	93 ± 12.0
11–12	3.70 ± 0.3	11.3 ± 0.9	33 ± 3.3	88 ± 7.9

Hb, hemoglobin; Hct, hematocrit; MCV, mean corpuscular volume; RBC, red blood cell count.

Adapted from Matoth Y, Zaizov R, Varsano I. Postnatal changes in some red cell parameters. *Acta Paediatr Scand.* 1971;60:317.

The red cell count, hematocrit, and MCV likewise fall. The factors responsible for the decline include reduced red cell production and plasma dilution caused by increased blood volume with growth. Neonatal red cells also have a shorter life span of 50 to 70 days, and are thought to be more fragile than those of older persons. In addition, during the early neonatal period, there is a switch from HbF to HbA. The amount of HbF in term infants averages about 70% of the total hemoglobin and declines to trace amounts by 6 to 12 months of age.[27] The switch to HbA provides greater unloading of oxygen to the tissues because HbA has a lower affinity for oxygen compared with HbF. Infants who are small for gestational age, born to diabetic or smoking mothers, or who experienced hypoxia in utero have higher total hemoglobin levels, higher HbF levels, and a delayed switch to HbA.

Physiologic anemia of the newborn develops at approximately 2 months of age. It seldom produces symptoms and cannot be altered by nutritional supplements. Anemia of prematurity, an exaggerated physiologic response in infants with low birth weight, is thought to result from a poor erythropoietin response. A contributing factor is the frequent blood sampling often required in these infants. The hemoglobin level rapidly declines after birth to a low of 7 to 10 g/dL at approximately 6 weeks of age. Signs and symptoms include apnea, poor weight gain, pallor, decreased activity, and tachycardia. In infants born before 33 weeks gestation or those with hematocrits below 33%, the clinical features are more evident.

Anemia at birth, characterized by pallor, congestive heart failure, or shock, usually is caused by hemolytic disease of the newborn. Bleeding from the umbilical cord, internal hemorrhage, congenital hemolytic disease, or frequent blood sampling are other possible causes of anemia. The severity of symptoms and presence of coexisting disease may warrant red cell transfusion.

Hyperbilirubinemia in the Neonate

Hyperbilirubinemia, an increased level of serum bilirubin, is a common cause of jaundice in the neonate. A benign, self-limited condition, it most often is related to the developmental state of the neonate. Rarely, cases of hyperbilirubinemia are pathologic and may lead to serious brain damage.

In the 1st week of life, approximately 60% of term and 80% of preterm neonates are jaundiced.[28] This physiologic jaundice appears in term infants on the second or third day of life. Ordinarily, the indirect bilirubin in umbilical cord blood is 1 to 3 mg/dL and increases by no more than 5 mg/dL in 24 hours, giving rise to jaundice. The levels peak at 5 to 6 mg/dL between days 2 and 4 and decrease to less than 2 mg/dL by days 5 to 7.[28] The increase in bilirubin is related to the increased red cell breakdown and the inability of the immature liver to conjugate bilirubin for excretion. Premature infants exhibit a slower rise and longer duration of serum bilirubin levels, perhaps because of poor hepatic uptake and reduced albumin binding of bilirubin. Peak bilirubin levels of 8 to 12 mg/dL appear on days 5 to 7. Most neonatal jaundice resolves within 1 week and is untreated.

Many factors can contribute to elevated bilirubin levels in the neonate, including breast-feeding, hemolytic disease of the newborn, hypoxia, infections, and acidosis. Bowel or biliary obstruction and liver disease are less common causes. Associated risk factors include prematurity, Asian ancestry, and maternal diabetes. Breast milk jaundice occurs in approximately 2% of breast-fed infants.[28] These neonates accumulate significant levels of unconjugated bilirubin 7 days after birth, with maximum levels of 10 to 30 mg/dL reached in the 3rd week of life. It is thought that the breast milk contains fatty acids that inhibit bilirubin conjugation in the neonatal liver. A factor in breast milk is also thought to increase the absorption of bilirubin in the duodenum. This type of jaundice disappears if breast-feeding is discontinued. Nursing can be resumed in 3 to 4 days without any hyperbilirubinemia ensuing.

Hyperbilirubinemia places the neonate at risk for the development of a neurologic syndrome called *kernicterus*. This condition is caused by the accumulation of unconjugated bilirubin in brain cells. Unconjugated bilirubin is lipid soluble, crosses the permeable blood–brain barrier of the neonate, and is deposited in cells of the basal ganglia, causing brain damage. Asphyxia and hyperosmolality may also contribute by damaging the blood–brain barrier and allowing bilirubin to cross and enter the cells. The level of unconjugated bilirubin and the duration of exposure that will be toxic to the infant are unknown. The less-mature infant, however, is at greater risk for kernicterus.[28] The manifestations of kernicterus may appear 2 to 5 days after birth in term infants or by day 7 in premature infants. Lethargy, poor feeding, and short-term behavioral changes may be evident in mildly affected infants. Severe manifestations include rigidity, tremors, ataxia, and hearing loss. Extreme cases cause seizures and death. Most survivors are seriously damaged and by three years of age exhibit involuntary muscle spasms, seizures, mental retardation, and deafness.

Hyperbilirubinemia in the neonate is treated with phototherapy or exchange transfusion. Phototherapy is more commonly used to treat jaundiced infants and reduce the risk of kernicterus. Exposure to fluorescent light in the blue range of the visible spectrum (420- to 470-nm wavelength) reduces bilirubin levels. Bilirubin in the skin absorbs the light energy and is converted to a structural isomer that is more water soluble and can be excreted in the stool and urine. Effective treatment depends on the area of skin exposed and the infant's ability to metabolize and excrete bilirubin. Frequent monitoring of bilirubin levels, body temperature, and hydration is critical to the infant's care. Exchange transfusion is considered when signs of kernicterus are evident or hyperbilirubinemia is sustained or rising and unresponsive to phototherapy.

Hemolytic Disease of the Newborn

Erythroblastosis fetalis, or hemolytic disease of the newborn, occurs in Rh-positive infants of Rh-negative mothers who have been sensitized. The mother can produce anti-Rh antibodies from pregnancies in which the fetus is Rh positive or from blood transfusions of Rh-positive blood. The Rh-negative mother usually becomes sensitized during the first few days after delivery, when fetal Rh-positive red cells from the placental site are released into the maternal circulation. Because the antibodies take several weeks to develop, the first Rh-positive infant of an Rh-negative mother usually is not affected. Infants with Rh-negative blood have no antigens on their red cells to react with the maternal antibodies and are not affected.

After an Rh-negative mother has been sensitized, the Rh antibodies from her blood are transferred to subsequent infants through the placental circulation. These antibodies react with the red cell antigens of the Rh-positive fetus, causing agglutination and hemolysis. This leads to severe anemia with compensatory hyperplasia and enlargement of the blood-forming organs, including the spleen and liver, in the fetus. Liver function may be impaired, with decreased production of albumin causing massive edema, called *hydrops fetalis*. If blood levels of unconjugated bilirubin are abnormally high because of red cell hemolysis, there is a danger of kernicterus developing in the infant, resulting in severe brain damage or death.

Several advances significantly decreased the threat to infants born to Rh-negative mothers: prevention of sensitization, antenatal identification of the at-risk fetus, and intrauterine transfusion to the affected fetus. The injection of Rh immune globulin (i.e., γ-globulin containing Rh antibody) prevents sensitization in Rh-negative mothers who have given birth to Rh-positive infants if administered at 28 weeks gestation and within 72 hours of delivery, abortion, genetic amniocentesis, or fetal-maternal bleeding. After sensitization has developed, the immune globulin is of no value. Fetal Rh phenotyping can now be performed to identify at-risk fetuses in the first trimester using fetal blood or amniotic cells.[29] Hemolysis in these fetuses can be treated by intrauterine transfusions of red cells through the umbilical cord. Exchange transfusions are administered after birth by removing and replacing the infant's blood volume with type O Rh-negative blood. The exchange transfusion removes most of the hemolyzed red cells and some of the total bilirubin, treating the anemia and hyperbilirubinemia.

 ## Red Cell Changes in the Elderly

Anemia is an increasingly common health problem in the elderly, affecting approximately one fourth of all 80-year-olds and half of the chronically ill elderly.[30,31] Its prevalence is known to increase with age, with the highest incidence in men aged 85 years and older. Undiagnosed and untreated anemia can have severe consequences and is associated with increased risk of mortality, cardiovascular disease, lower functional ability, self-care deficits, cognitive disorders, and reduced bone density that increases the risk for fractures with falls.[30]

Hemoglobin levels decline after middle age. In studies of men older than 60 years of age, mean hemoglobin levels ranged from 15.3 to 12.4 g/dL, with the lowest levels found in the oldest persons. The decline is less in women, with mean levels ranging from 13.8 to 11.7 mg/dL.[30] In most asymptomatic elderly persons, lower hemoglobin levels result from iron deficiency and anemia of chronic disease.

As with other body systems, the capacity for red cell production changes with aging. The location of bone cells involved in red cell production shifts toward the axial skeleton, and the number of progenitor cells declines from approximately 50% at age 65 to approximately 30% at age 75.[32] Despite these changes, the elderly are usually able to maintain hemoglobin and hematocrit levels within a range similar to that of younger adults. However, during a stress situation such as bleeding, the red blood cells of the elderly are not replaced as promptly as those of their younger counterparts. This inability to replace red blood cells closely correlates with the increased prevalence of anemia in the elderly.

Although the age-associated decline in the hematopoietic reserve in the elderly is not completely understood, several factors seem to play a role, including a reduction in hematopoietic progenitors, reduced production of hematopoietic growth factors, and inhibition of erythropoietin or its interaction with its receptors.[29,32] Inflammatory cytokines, which have been found to increase with age, may mediate this reduced sensitivity to erythropoietin.

The diagnosis of anemia in the elderly requires a complete physical examination, a complete blood count, and studies to rule out comorbid conditions such as malignancy, gastrointestinal conditions that cause bleeding, and pernicious anemia. The complete blood count should include a peripheral blood smear and a reticulocyte count and index. If the reticulocyte index is appropriately increased for the level of anemia, then blood loss or red cell destruction should be suspected. If the reticulocyte index is inappropriately low, then decreased red cell production is presumed.[31,33]

The treatment of anemia in the elderly should focus on the underlying cause and correction of the red cell deficit. An important aspect of anemia of chronic disease is the inability to use and mobilize iron effectively.[30] Orally administered iron is poorly used in older adults, despite normal iron absorption.[31] Although erythropoietin remains the treatment of choice for anemias associated with cancer and renal disease, its potential use in treating anemias associated with aging remains to be established.

SUMMARY CONCEPTS

- The red blood count along with hemoglobin concentration changes from being high at birth, reflecting the in-utero need for oxygen, to declining in the elderly due to a decrease in the replacement ability of red cells.

- During the early neonatal period, there is a shift from fetal to adult hemoglobin. Many infants have physiologic jaundice because of hyperbilirubinemia during the 1st week of life, related to the increase in red blood cell breakdown and the inability of the infant's liver to conjugate bilirubin.

- Hemolytic disease of the newborn occurs in Rh-positive infants of Rh-negative mothers who have been sensitized. It involves hemolysis of an infant's red cells in response to maternal Rh antibodies that have crossed the placenta.

- Anemia is an increasingly common health problem in the elderly. Although most elderly persons are able to maintain their hemoglobin and hematocrit levels within a normal range, they are unable to replace their red cells as promptly as their younger counterparts during a stress situation such as bleeding.

REVIEW EXERCISES

1. A 29-year-old woman complains of generalized fatigue. Her physical examination reveals a heart rate of 115 beats/minute, blood pressure of 115/75 mmHg, and respiratory rate of 28 breaths/minute. Her skin and nail beds are pale. Her laboratory results include red blood cell count $3.0 \times 10^6/\mu L$, hemoglobin 9 g/dL, hematocrit 27%, and a decrease in serum ferritin levels.

   A. What disorder do you suspect this woman has?
   B. What additional data would be helpful in determining the etiology of her condition?
   C. Which of her signs reflect the body's attempt to compensate for the disorder?
   D. What is the significance of the low ferritin level, and how could it be used to make decisions related to her treatment?

2. A 65-year-old woman is seen in the clinic because of numbness in her lower legs and feet and difficulty walking. She has no other complaints. She takes a blood pressure pill, two calcium pills, and a multivitamin pill daily. Her laboratory results include red blood cell count $3.0 \times 10^6/\mu L$, hemoglobin 9 g/dL, hematocrit 20%, and a markedly elevated MVC.

   A. What type of anemia does she have?
   B. What is the reason for her neurologic symptoms?
   C. What type of treatment would be appropriate?

3. A 12-year-old boy with sickle cell disease presents in the emergency department with severe chest pain. His mother reports that he was doing well until he came down with a respiratory tract infection. She also states he insisted on playing basketball with the other boys in the neighborhood even though he wasn't feeling well.

   A. What is the most likely cause of pain in this boy?
   B. Infections and aerobic-type exercise produce sickling in persons who are homozygous for the sickle cell gene and have sickle cell disease, but not in persons who are heterozygous and have sickle cell trait. Explain.
   C. People with sickle disease experience anemia but not iron deficiency. Explain.

REFERENCES

1. Waite GN. Blood components. In: Rhoades RA, Bell DR, eds. *Medical Physiology.* 4th ed. Philadelphia, PA: Wolters Kluwer Health/Lippincott Williams & Wilkins; 2013:166–187.
2. Ross MH, Pawlina W. *Histology: A Text and Atlas.* 6th ed. Philadelphia, PA: Wolters Kluwer Health/Lippincott Williams & Wilkins; 2011:270–275.

3. Hall JE. *Guyton and Hall Textbook of Medical Physiology*. 12th ed. Philadelphia, PA: Saunders Elsevier; 2006:413–422.

4. Fisher JW. Erythropoietin: physiology and pharmacology update. *Exp Biol Med (Maywood)*. 2003;228:1–14.

5. Kumar V, Abbas AK, Fausto N, et al. *Robbins and Cotran Pathologic Basis of Disease*. 8th ed. Philadelphia, PA: Saunders Elsevier; 2010:639–675.

6. Valdez R, Zutter M, Florea AD, et al. Hematopathology. In: Rubin R, Strayer DS, eds. *Rubin's Pathology: Clinicopathologic Foundations of Medicine*. 6th ed. Philadelphia, PA: Wolters Kluwer Health/Lippincott Williams & Wilkins; 2012:948–972.

7. Meier ER, Miller JL. Sickle cell disease in children. *Drugs*. 2012;72(7):895–906.

8. Chiang EY, Frenette PS. Sickle cell vaso-occlusion. *Hematol Oncol Clin North Am*. 2005;19:771–784.

9. Gladwin MT, Vichinsky E. Pulmonary complications of sickle cell disease. *N Engl J Med*. 2008;359(21):2254–2265.

10. Stuart MJ, Nagel RL. Sickle-cell disease. *Lancet*. 2004;364:1343–1360.

11. National Institutes of Health. The management of sickle cell disease. *NIH publication no. 02–2117*. 2002. Available at: http://www.nhlbi.nih.gov/health/prof/blood/sickle/sc_mngt.pdf. Accessed August 20, 2013.

12. Rocs DC, Williams DN, Gladwin MT. Sickle cell disease. *Lancet*. 2010;376:2018–2031.

13. Giardina PJ, Rivella S. Thalasemai syndromes. In: Kleigman RM, Stanton BF, Gemelli JW, et al., eds. *Nelson Textbook of Pediatrics*. 19th ed. Philadelphia, PA: Elsevier Saunders; 2011:585e1–655e1.

14. Rund D, Rachmilewitz E. Thalassemia. *N Engl J Med*. 2005;353:1135–1146.

15. Muncie HL, Campbell JS. Alpha and beta thalassemia. *Am Fam Physician*. 2009;60(4):344–357.

16. Short MW, Dommagalshi JE. Iron deficiency anemia. *Am Fam Physician*. 2013;87(2):98–104.

17. Lerner NB. Anemia of inadequate production. In: Behrman RE, Kliegman RM, St. Gemelli JW, et al., eds. *Nelson Textbook of Pediatrics*. 19th ed. Philadelphia, PA: Elsevier Saunders; 2011:1650–1653.

18. Lozoff B, Beard J, Connor J, et al. Long-lasting neural and behavioral effects of iron deficiency in infancy. *Nutr Rev*. 2006;64:S34–S43.

19. Kazal LA. Prevention of iron deficiency in infants and toddlers. *Am Fam Physician*. 2002;66:1217–1224.

20. Aslinia F, Mazza JJ, Yale SH. Megaloblastic anemia and other causes of macrocytosis. *Clin Med Res*. 2006;3:236–241.

21. Langan RC, Zawistoski KJ. Update on vitamin B_{12} deficiency. *Am Fam Physician*. 2011;83(12):1425–1430.

22. Guinan EC. Diagnosis and management of aplastic anemia. *Hematology*. 2011;2011:76–81.

23. Young NS, Calada RT, Scheinberg P. Current concepts in the pathophysiology and treatment of aplastic anemia. *Blood*. 2006;108:2509–2519.

24. Weiss G, Goodnough LT. Anemia of chronic disease. *N Engl J Med*. 2005;352:1011–1023.

25. Stuart BJ, Viera AJ. Polycythemia vera. *Am Fam Physician*. 2004;69:2139–2144.

26. Tefferi A, Spivak JL. Polycythemia vera: scientific advances and current practice. *Semin Hematol*. 2005;42:206–220.

27. Christensen RD, Ohls RK. Development of the hematopoietic system. In: Kleigman RM, Stanton BF, St. Gemelli JW, et al., eds. *Nelson Textbook of Pediatrics*. 19th ed. Philadelphia, PA: Elsevier Saunders; 2011:1648e1–1648e5.

28. Almbalavanan N, Carlo WA. Jaundice and hyperbilirubinemia in the newborn. In: Kleigman RM, Stanton BF, St. Gemelli JW, et al., eds. *Nelson Textbook of Pediatrics*. 19th ed. Philadelphia, PA: Elsevier Saunders; 2011:603–612e5.

29. Kramer K, Cohen HJ. Antenatal diagnosis of hematologic disorders. In: Hoffman R, Benz EJ, Shattil SJ, et al., eds. *Hematology: Basic Principles and Practice*. 3rd ed. New York, NY: Churchill Livingstone; 2000:2495.

30. Eisenstaedt R, Pennix BW, Woodman RC. Anemia in the elderly: current understanding and emerging concepts. *Blood Rev*. 2006;20:213–226.

31. Bross MH, Soch K, Knuppel TS. Anemia in older persons. *Am Fam Physician*. 2010;82(5):480–487.

32. Rothstein G. Disordered hematopoiesis and myelodysplasia in the elderly. *J Am Geriatr Soc*. 2003;51(suppl 3):S22–S26.

33. Lipschitz D. Medical and functional consequences of anemia in the elderly. *J Am Geriatr Soc*. 2003;51(suppl 3):S10–S13.

Porth Essentials Resources

Explore these additional resources to enhance learning for this chapter:

- NCLEX-Style Questions and Other Resources on thePoint, http://thePoint.lww.com/PorthEssentials4e
- Study Guide for Essentials of Pathophysiology
- Adaptive Learning | Powered by PrepU, http://thepoint.lww.com/prepu

4 Infection and Immunity

C h a p t e r 14

Mechanisms of Infectious Disease

All living creatures share two basic objectives in life: survival and reproduction. This doctrine applies equally to bacteria, viruses, fungi, and protozoa. To satisfy these goals, organisms must extract from the environment essential nutrients for growth and proliferation; for countless microscopic organisms, that environment includes the human body.

The content in this chapter has been divided into four parts: (1) general concepts of infectious diseases, (2) epidemiology of infectious diseases, (3) general principles of diagnosis and treatment, and (4) new and emerging infectious diseases.

General Concepts of Infectious Diseases

Normally, the contact between humans and microorganisms is incidental and, in certain situations, may actually benefit both organisms. Under extraordinary circumstances, however, the invasion of the human body by microorganisms can produce harmful and potentially lethal consequences. The consequences of these invasions are collectively called *infectious diseases*.

Terminology

All scientific disciplines evolve with a distinct vocabulary, and the study of infectious diseases is no exception. The most appropriate way to approach this subject is

297

with a brief discussion of the terminology used to characterize interactions between humans and microbes.

Any organism capable of supporting the nutritional and physical growth requirements of another is called a *host*. Throughout this chapter, the term *host* most often refers to humans supporting the growth of microorganisms. Occasionally, *infection* and *colonization* are used interchangeably. However, the term *infection* describes the presence and multiplication within another living organism, with subsequent injury to the host, whereas *colonization* describes the act of establishing a presence, a step required in the multifaceted process of infection.

One common misconception should be dispelled from the start: not all interactions between microorganisms and humans are detrimental—in fact, most are beneficial. The internal and external exposed surfaces of the human body are normally and harmlessly inhabited by a multitude of bacteria, collectively referred to as the normal *microflora*. Although the colonizing bacteria acquire nutritional support from the host, the host is not adversely affected by the relationship. An interaction such as this is called *commensalism*, and the colonizing microorganisms are sometimes referred to as *commensal flora*. The term *mutualism* is applied to an interaction in which the microorganism and the host both derive benefits from the interaction. For example, certain inhabitants of the human intestinal tract extract nutrients from the host and secrete essential vitamin by-products of metabolism (e.g., vitamin K) that are absorbed and used by the host. A *parasitic relationship* is one in which only the infecting organism benefits from the relationship and the host either gains nothing from the relationship or sustains injury from the interaction. An *infectious disease* occurs if the host sustains injury in a parasitic relationship.

The severity of an infectious disease can range from mild to life-threatening depending on many variables, including the health of the host at the time of infection and the *virulence* (disease-producing potential) of the microorganism. A select group of microorganisms called *pathogens* are so virulent that they are rarely found in the absence of disease. Fortunately, there are few human pathogens in the microbial world. Most microorganisms are harmless *saprophytes*, free-living organisms obtaining their growth from dead or decaying organic material in the environment. However, all microorganisms, even saprophytes and members of the normal flora, can be *opportunistic pathogens* capable of producing an infectious disease when the health and immunity of the host have been severely weakened by illness, malnutrition, or medical therapy.

Agents of Infectious Disease

The agents of infectious disease include prions, viruses, bacteria, *Rickettsiaceae* and *Chlamydiaceae*, fungi, and parasites. A summary of the salient characteristics of these human microorganisms is provided in Table 14-1.

Prions

Can a protein alone cause a transmissible infectious disease? Prior to the discovery of prions, scientists assumed that all infectious agents must possess a genetic master plan (a genome of either ribonucleic acid [RNA] or deoxyribonucleic acid [DNA]) that codes for the production of the essential proteins and enzymes necessary for survival and reproduction. Prions, protein particles that lack any kind of a demonstrable genome, appear to be an exception to this rule. A number of prion-associated diseases have been identified, including Creutzfeldt-Jakob disease in humans, chronic wasting disease in deer and elk, scrapie in sheep, and bovine spongiform encephalopathy (BSE or mad cow disease) in cattle. The various prion-associated diseases produce very similar pathologic processes and symptoms in the hosts and are collectively called *transmissible neurodegenerative diseases*. All are characterized by a slowly progressive, noninflammatory neuronal degeneration, leading to loss of coordination (ataxia), dementia, and death over a period ranging from months to years.

TABLE 14-1	Comparison of Characteristics of Human Microbial Pathogens				
Organism	**Defined Nucleus**	**Genomic Material**	**Size***	**Intracellular or Extracellular**	**Motility**
Prions	No	Unknown	55 kDa	E	−
Viruses	No	DNA or RNA	0.02–0.3	I	−
Bacteria	No	DNA	0.5–15	I/E	±
Mycoplasmas	No	DNA	0.2–0.3	E	−
Spirochetes	No	DNA	6–15	E	+
Rickettsiaceae	No	DNA	0.2–2	I	−
Chlamydiaceae	No	DNA	0.3–1	I	−
Yeasts	Yes	DNA	2–60	I/E	−
Molds	Yes	DNA	2–15 (hyphal width)	E	−
Protozoans	Yes	DNA	1–60	I/E	+
Helminths	Yes	DNA	2 mm to >1 m	E	+

*Micrometers unless indicated.

The prion protein (PrP) is a human protein expressed on the cell surface. Its normal role is not well understood, but it is hypothesized to be involved in cell adhesion, cell binding, copper metabolism, or in synaptic function.

Recent studies have shown that the prion proteins in disease (called PrP^{SC}) are actually altered or mutated forms of a normal host protein called PrP^C. Differences in the posttranslational structure cause the two proteins to behave differently. The PrP^{SC} is resistant to the action of proteases (enzymes that degrade excess or deformed proteins) and aggregates in the cytoplasm of affected neurons as amyloid fibrils. The normal PrP^C is protease sensitive and appears on the cell surface.

Prion diseases present significant problems to the medical community because their method of replication is not clearly understood. Based on current models, it is believed that PrP^{SC} binds to the normal PrP^C on the cell surface, causing it to be processed into PrP^{SC}, which is released from the cell and then aggregates into amyloid-like plaques in the brain. The cell then replenishes the PrP^C and the cycle continues. As PrP^{SC} accumulates, it spreads within the axons of the nerve cells, causing progressively greater damage to host neurons and the eventual incapacitation of the host. In addition, because prions lack reproductive and metabolic functions, the currently available antimicrobial agents are useless against them.

Viruses

Viruses are the smallest obligate intracellular pathogens. They have no organized cellular structures but instead consist of a protein coat, or capsid, surrounding a nucleic acid core, or genome, of RNA or DNA—never both (Fig. **14-1**). Some viruses are enclosed within a lipoprotein envelope derived from the cell membrane of the parasitized host cell. Enveloped viruses include members of the herpesvirus group and paramyxoviruses, such as influenza and poxviruses. Certain viruses, enveloped in buds pinched from the cell membrane, are continuously shed from the infected cell surface.

The viruses of humans and animals have been categorized somewhat arbitrarily according to various characteristics. These include the type of viral genome (single-stranded or double-stranded DNA or RNA), physical characteristics (e.g., size, presence or absence of a membrane envelope), the mechanism of replication (e.g., retroviruses), the mode of transmission (e.g., arthropod-borne viruses, enteroviruses), target tissue, and the type of disease produced (e.g., hepatitis A, B, C, D, and E viruses), to name just a few.

Viruses are incapable of replication outside of a living cell. They must penetrate a susceptible living cell and use the biosynthetic machinery of the cell to produce viral progeny. The process of viral replication is shown in Figure 14-2. Not every viral agent causes lysis and death of the host cell during the course of replication. Some viruses enter the host cell and insert their genome into the host cell chromosome, where it remains in a latent state for long periods without causing disease. Under the appropriate stimulation, the virus undergoes

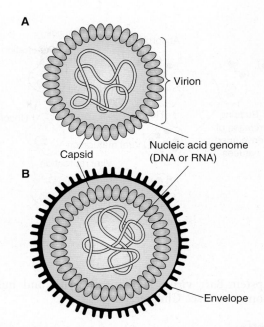

FIGURE 14-1. (A) The basic structure of a virus includes a protein coat surrounding an inner core of nucleic acid (DNA or RNA). **(B)** Some viruses may also be enclosed in a lipoprotein outer envelope.

active replication and produces symptoms of disease months to years later. Members of the herpesvirus group and adenovirus are the best examples of latent viruses. Herpesviruses include the viral agents of chickenpox and zoster (varicella-zoster), cold sores (herpes simplex virus [HSV], usually type 1), genital herpes (HSV, usually type 2), infectious mononucleosis (cytomegalovirus or Epstein-Barr virus), and Kaposi sarcoma (human herpesvirus 8). The resumption of the latent viral replication may produce symptoms of primary disease (e.g., genital herpes) or cause an entirely different symptomatology (e.g., shingles instead of chickenpox).

Since the early 1980s, members of the retrovirus group have received considerable attention after identification of the human immunodeficiency viruses (HIV) as the causative agent of acquired immunodeficiency syndrome (AIDS). The retroviruses have a unique mechanism of replication. After entry into the host cell, the viral RNA genome is first translated into DNA by a viral enzyme called *reverse transcriptase* (see Chapter 16). The viral DNA copy is then integrated into the host chromosome where it exists in a latent state, similar to the herpesviruses. Reactivation and replication require a reversal of the entire process. Some retroviruses lyse the host cell during the process of replication. In the case of HIV, the infected cells regulate the immunologic defense system of the host and their lysis leads to a permanent suppression of the immune response.

In addition to causing infectious diseases, certain viruses also have the ability to transform normal host cells into malignant cells during the replication cycle. This group of viruses is referred to as *oncogenic* and includes certain retroviruses and DNA viruses, such as

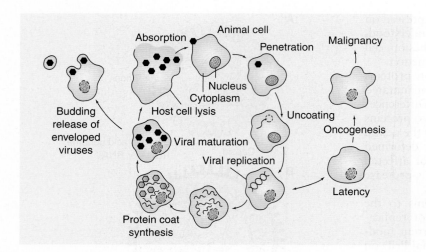

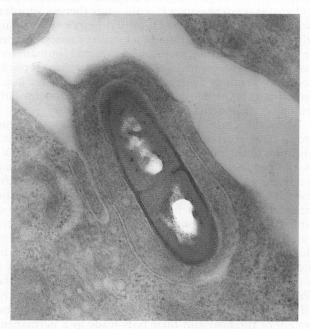

FIGURE 14-2. Schematic representation of the many possible consequences of viral infection of host cells, including cell lysis (poliovirus), continuous release of budding viral particles, or latency (herpesviruses) and oncogenesis (papovaviruses).

the Epstein-Barr virus, hepatitis B virus, and human papillomavirus (see Chapter 7).

Bacteria

Bacteria are autonomously replicating unicellular organisms known as *prokaryotes* because they lack an organized nucleus. Compared with nucleated eukaryotic cells (see Chapter 1), the bacterial cell is small and structurally primitive (Fig. 14-3). Similar to eukaryotic cells but unlike viruses, bacteria contain both DNA and RNA, although their genome is considerably smaller than eukaryotes and typically is encoded on a single

FIGURE 14-3. Electron micrograph of the rod-shaped, gram-positive bacterium *Listeria monocytogenes* showing the simple prokaryotic cell structure including the cytoplasm, the cytoplasmic membrane, and the rigid cell wall. (From the Centers for Disease Control and Prevention Public Health Images Library. No. 10828. Courtesy of Balasubr Swaminathan, Peggy Hayes.)

chromosome. Many bacteria transiently harbor smaller extrachromosomal pieces of circular DNA called *plasmids*. Occasionally, plasmids contain genetic information that increases the virulence or antibiotic resistance of the organism.

The prokaryotic cell is organized into an internal compartment called the *cytoplasm*, which contains the reproductive and metabolic machinery of the cell. The cytoplasm is surrounded by a flexible lipid membrane, called the *cytoplasmic membrane*. This in turn is enclosed within a rigid cell wall. The structure and synthesis of the cell wall determine the microscopic shape of the bacterium (e.g., spherical [cocci], helical [spirilla], or elongate [bacilli], Fig. 14-4). Most bacteria produce a cell wall composed of a distinctive polymer known as *peptidoglycan*. This polymer is produced only by prokaryotes and is therefore an attractive target for antibacterial therapy. For example, the penicillin antibiotics target the peptidoglycan cell wall. Several bacteria synthesize an extracellular capsule composed of protein or carbohydrate. The capsule protects the organism from environmental hazards such as the immunologic defenses of the host.

Certain bacteria are motile as the result of external whip-like appendages called *flagella*. The flagella rotate like a propeller, transporting the organism through a liquid environment. Bacteria can also produce hairlike structures projecting from the cell surface called *pili* or *fimbriae*, which enable the organism to adhere to surfaces such as mucous membranes or other bacteria.

Reproduction. Most prokaryotes reproduce asexually by simple cellular division. The manner in which an organism divides can influence the microscopic morphology. For instance, when the cocci divide in chains, they are called *streptococci*; in pairs, *diplococci*; and in clusters, *staphylococci* (Fig. 14-5). The growth rate of bacteria varies significantly among different species and depends greatly on physical growth conditions and the availability of nutrients. In the laboratory, a single bacterium placed in a suitable growth environment, such as an agar plate, reproduces to the extent that it forms a

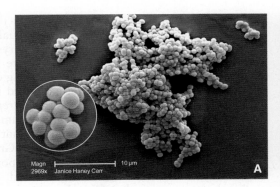

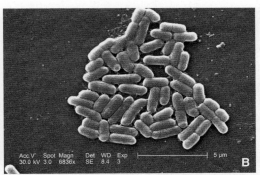

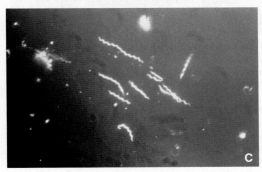

FIGURE 14-4. Microscopic morphology of bacteria demonstrating their variability in size and shape: **(A)** colorized scanning electron micrograph (SEM) of the spherical gram-positive β-hemolytic group C *Streptococcus* sp.; **(B)** colorized SEM of the rod-shaped gram-negative *Escherichia coli* of the strain O157:H7; and **(C)** corkscrew-shaped spirochete *Borrelia burgdorferi* (responsible for causing Lyme disease) shown using darkfield microscopy technique (magnified ×400). (From the Centers for Disease Control and Prevention Public Images Library. Nos. 10591, 10586, 10068, 6631. A and B courtesy of Janice Haney Carr.)

visible colony composed of millions of bacteria within a few hours.

In nature, however, bacteria rarely exist as single cells floating in an aqueous environment. Rather, bacteria prefer to stick to and colonize environmental surfaces, producing structured communities called *biofilms* (Fig. 14-6). The organization and structure of biofilms permit access to available nutrients and elimination of metabolic waste. Within the biofilm, individual organ-isms use chemical signaling as a form of primitive inter-cellular communication to represent the state of the environment. These signals inform members of the com-munity when sufficient nutrients are available for pro-liferation or when environmental conditions warrant dormancy or evacuation. Examples of biofilms abound in nature and are found on the surfaces of aquatic environments, in the human oral cavity, on indwelling medical devices, and on human cells. One has only to

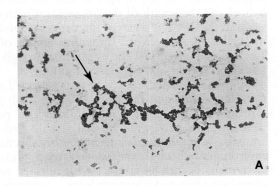

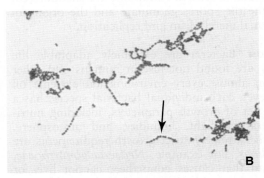

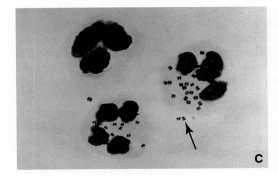

FIGURE 14-5. The manner in which microorganisms divide (*arrows*) can assist in their identification. Photomicrographs of gram-positive **(A)** *Staphylococcus aureus*, which divide in clusters; **(B)** *Streptococcus* spp. bacteria, which divide in chains; and **(C)** urethral exudate, which is diagnostic of gonococcal urethritis revealing intracellular (within polymorphonuclear leukocytes) and extracellular *Gonococci*, which divide in pairs. (From the Centers for Disease Control and Prevention Public Health Images Library. Nos. 2296, 2170, 4086. A courtesy of Richard Facklam; C courtesy of Norman Jacobs.)

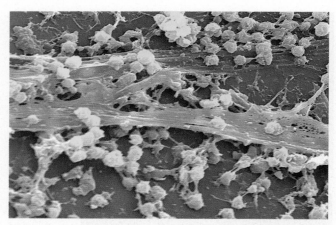

FIGURE 14-6. Electron micrograph depicting large numbers of *Staphylococcus aureus* bacteria, which were found on the luminal surface of an indwelling catheter. Of importance are the sticky-looking substances woven between the round cocci bacteria, which were composed of polysaccharides and are known as *biofilm*. This biofilm has been found to protect the bacteria that secrete the substance from attacks by antimicrobial agents such as antibiotics (magnified × 2363). (From the Centers for Disease Control and Prevention Public Health Images Library. No. 7488. Courtesy of Rodney M. Donlan, Janice Carr.)

disassemble a clogged sink drain to see a perfect example of a bacterial biofilm.

The physical appearance of a colony of bacteria grown on an agar plate can be quite distinctive for different species. Some produce pigments that give colonies a unique color. Some bacteria produce highly resistant spores when faced with an unfavorable environment. The spores can exist in a quiescent state almost indefinitely until suitable growth conditions are encountered, at which time the spores germinate and the organism resumes normal metabolism and replication.

Classification. Bacteria are extremely adaptable life forms. They are found not just in humans and other hosts, but in almost every environmental extreme on earth. However, each individual bacterial species has a well-defined set of growth parameters, including nutrition, temperature, light, humidity, and atmosphere. Bacteria with extremely strict growth requirements are called *fastidious*. For example, *Neisseria gonorrhoeae*, the bacterium that causes gonorrhea, cannot live for extended periods outside the human body. *Aerobes* are bacteria that require oxygen for growth and metabolism; *anaerobes* cannot survive in an oxygen-containing environment. An organism capable of adapting its metabolism to aerobic or anaerobic conditions is *facultatively anaerobic*. It is of interest to note that the vast majority of bacterial species found in humans and in the surrounding environment have not been cultivated on artificial media.

In the laboratory, bacteria are generally classified according to the microscopic appearance and staining properties of the cell. The Gram stain, originally developed in 1884 by Danish bacteriologist Christian Gram, is still the most widely used staining procedure. Bacteria

are designated as *gram-positive* organisms if they are stained purple by a primary basic dye (usually crystal violet); those that are not stained by the crystal violet but are counterstained red by a second dye (safranin) are called *gram-negative* organisms. Staining characteristics and microscopic morphology are used in combination to describe bacteria. For example, *Streptococcus pyogenes*, the agent of pharyngitis and rheumatic fever, is a gram-positive streptococcal organism that is spherical, grows in chains, and stains purple by Gram stain. *Legionella pneumophila*, the bacterium responsible for Legionnaires' disease, is a gram-negative rod.

Another means of classifying bacteria according to microscopic staining properties is the *acid-fast stain*. Because of the unique fatty acid content and composition of their cell membrane, certain bacteria are resistant to the decolorization of a primary stain (either carbol fuchsin or a combination of auramine and rhodamine) when treated with a solution of acid alcohol. These organisms are termed *acid-fast* and include a number of significant human pathogens, most notably *Mycobacterium tuberculosis* (the cause of tuberculosis) and other mycobacteria.

For purposes of taxonomy (i.e., identification and classification), each member of the bacterial kingdom is categorized into a small group of genetically related organisms called the *genus*, and further subdivided into distinct individuals within the genus called *species*. The genus and species assignment of the organism is reflected in its name (e.g., *Staphylococcus* [genus] *aureus* [species]).

Spirochetes. The spirochetes are an eccentric category of bacteria that are mentioned separately because of their unusual cellular morphology and distinctive mechanism of motility. Technically, the spirochetes are gram-negative rods but are unique in that the cell's shape is helical and the length of the organism is many times its width (Fig. 14-7). A series of filaments are wound about the cell wall and extend the entire length of the cell. These filaments propel the organism through an aqueous environment in a corkscrew motion.

Spirochetes are composed of four genera: *Leptospira, Borrelia, Treponema,* and *Brachyspira*. Each genus has saprophytic and pathogenic strains. The pathogenic leptospires infect a wide variety of wild and domestic animals. Infected animals shed the organisms into the environment through the urinary tract. Transmission to humans occurs by contact with infected animals or urine-contaminated surroundings. Leptospires gain access to the host directly through mucous membranes or breaks in the skin and can produce a severe and potentially fatal illness called *Weil syndrome*. In contrast, the borreliae are transmitted from infected animals to humans through the bite of an arthropod vector such as lice or ticks. (A vector is any organism that carries a pathogen from a source to a host.) Included in the genus *Borrelia* are the agents of relapsing fever (*Borrelia recurrentis*) and Lyme disease (*Borrelia burgdorferi*). Included in the genus *Borrelia* are the agents of relapsing fever (*Borrelia recurrentis*) and Lyme disease (*Borrelia burgdorferi* is the most common in North America).

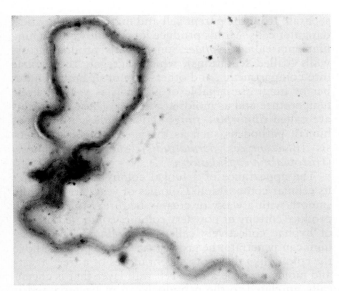

FIGURE 14-7. A photomicrograph of a *Treponema pallidum* bacterium that causes syphilis. This microscopic bacterium (spirochete) is a wormlike spiral-shaped microorganism that wiggles vigorously when viewed under the microscope. (From the Centers for Disease Control and Prevention Public Health Images Library. No. 2323.)

Pathogenic *Treponema* species require no intermediates and are spread from person to person by direct contact. The most important member of the genus is *Treponema pallidum*, the causative agent of syphilis.

Mycoplasmas. The mycoplasmas are unicellular prokaryotes capable of independent replication. These organisms are less than one-third the size of bacteria and contain a small DNA genome approximately one-half the size of the bacterial chromosome. The cell is composed of cytoplasm surrounded by a membrane, but, unlike bacteria, the mycoplasmas do not produce a rigid peptidoglycan cell wall. As a consequence, the microscopic appearance of the cell is highly variable, ranging from coccoid forms to filaments, and the mycoplasmas are resistant to cell wall–inhibiting antibiotics such as penicillins and cephalosporins.

The mycoplasmas affecting humans are divided into three genera: *Mycoplasma*, *Ureaplasma*, and *Acholeplasma*. The first two require cholesterol from the environment to produce the cell membrane; the acholeplasmas do not. In the human host, mycoplasmas are commensals. However, a number of species are capable of producing serious diseases, including pneumonia (*Mycoplasma pneumoniae*), genital infections (*Mycoplasma hominis* and *Ureaplasma urealyticum*), and maternally transmitted respiratory infections to infants with low birth weight (*U. urealyticum*).

Rickettsiaceae, Anaplasmataceae, Chlamydiaceae, and Coxiella

This interesting group of organisms combines the characteristics of viral and bacterial agents to produce disease in humans. All are obligate intracellular pathogens, like the viruses, but produce a rigid peptidoglycan cell wall, reproduce asexually by cellular division, and contain RNA and DNA, similar to the bacteria.

The *Rickettsiaceae* depend on the host cell for essential vitamins and nutrients, but the *Chlamydiaceae* appear to scavenge intermediates of energy metabolism such as adenosine triphosphate (ATP). The *Rickettsiaceae* infect but do not produce disease in the cells of certain arthropods such as fleas, ticks, and lice. The organisms are accidentally transmitted to humans through the bite of the arthropod (i.e., the vector) and produce a number of potentially lethal diseases, including Rocky Mountain spotted fever and epidemic typhus.

The *Chlamydiaceae* are slightly smaller than the *Rickettsiaceae* but are structurally similar and are transmitted directly between susceptible vertebrates without an intermediate arthropod host. Transmission and replication of *Chlamydiaceae* occur through a defined life cycle. The infectious form, called an *elementary body*, attaches to and enters the host cell, where it transforms into a larger *reticulate body*. This undergoes active replication into multiple elementary bodies, which are then shed into the extracellular environment to initiate another infectious cycle. Chlamydial diseases of humans include sexually transmitted genital infections (*Chlamydophila trachomatis*; see Chapter 41); ocular infections and pneumonia of newborns (*C. trachomatis*); upper and lower respiratory tract infections in children, adolescents, and young adults (*Chlamydophila pneumoniae*); and respiratory disease acquired from infected birds (*Chlamydophila psittaci*).

Organisms within the family *Anaplasmataceae* (including the reorganized genera *Ehrlichia*, *Anaplasma*, *Neorickettsia*, and *Wolbachia*) are also obligate intracellular organisms that resemble the *Rickettsiaceae* in structure and produce a variety of veterinary and human diseases, some of which have a tick vector. These organisms target host mononuclear and polymorphonuclear white blood cells for infection and, similar to the *Chlamydiaceae*, multiply in the cytoplasm of infected leukocytes within vacuoles called *morulae*. Unlike the *Chlamydiaceae*, however, the *Anaplasmataceae* do not have a defined life cycle and are independent of the host cell for energy production. The most common infections caused by *Anaplasmataceae* are human monocytic and granulocytic ehrlichiosis. Human monocytic ehrlichiosis is a disease caused by *Ehrlichia chaffeensis* that can easily be confused with Rocky Mountain spotted fever. Clinical disease severity ranges from mild to life-threatening. Manifestations include generalized malaise, anorexia and nausea, fever, and headache. Decreases in white blood cells (leukopenia) and platelets (thrombocytopenia) often occur. Severe sequelae include severe respiratory failure, encephalopathy, and acute renal failure. The disease is usually more severe in the elderly and persons with compromised immune function (e.g., those with HIV/AIDS). Human granulocytic ehrlichiosis is also transmitted by ticks, but is caused by *Anaplasma phagocytophilum*. The symptoms are similar to those seen with human monocytic ehrlichiosis.

The genus *Coxiella* contains only one species, *Coxiella burnetii*. Like its rickettsial counterparts, it is a gram-negative intracellular organism that infects a variety of animals, including cattle, sheep, and goats. In humans, *Coxiella* infection produces a disease called Q fever, characterized by a nonspecific febrile illness often accompanied by headache, chills, arthralgias, and mild pneumonia. The organism produces a highly resistant sporelike stage that is transmitted to humans when contaminated animal tissue is aerosolized (e.g., during meat processing) or by ingestion of contaminated milk.

Fungi

The fungi are free-living, eukaryotic saprophytes found in every habitat on earth. Some are members of the normal human microflora. Fortunately, few fungi are capable of causing diseases in humans, and most of these are incidental, self-limited infections of skin and subcutaneous tissue. Serious fungal infections are rare and usually initiated through puncture wounds or inhalation. Despite their normally harmless nature, fungi can cause life-threatening opportunistic diseases when host defense capabilities have been disabled.

The fungi can be separated into two groups, yeasts and molds, based on rudimentary differences in their morphology (Fig. 14-8). The yeasts are single-celled organisms, approximately the size of red blood cells that reproduce by a budding process. The buds separate from the parent cell and mature into identical daughter cells. Molds produce long, hollow, branching filaments called *hyphae*. Some molds produce crosswalls (called septations), which segregate the hyphae into compartments, and others do not. A limited number of fungi are capable of growing as yeasts at one temperature and as molds at another. These organisms are called *dimorphic fungi* and include a number of human pathogens such as the agents of blastomycosis (*Blastomyces dermatitidis*) and histoplasmosis (*Histoplasma capsulatum*).

The appearance of a fungal colony tends to reflect its cellular composition. Colonies of yeast are generally smooth with a waxy or creamy texture. Molds tend to produce cottony or powdery colonies composed of mats of hyphae collectively called a *mycelium*. The mycelium can penetrate the growth surface or project above the colony like the roots and branches of a tree. Yeasts and molds produce a rigid cell wall layer that is chemically unrelated to the peptidoglycan of bacteria and is therefore not susceptible to the effects of penicillin-like antibiotics.

Most fungi are capable of sexual or asexual reproduction. The former process involves the fusion of zygotes with the production of a recombinant zygospore. Asexual reproduction involves the formation of highly resistant spores called *conidia* or *sporangiospores*, which are borne by specialized structures that arise from the hyphae. Molds are identified in the laboratory by

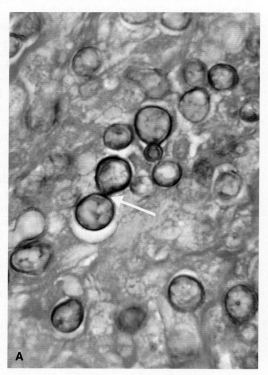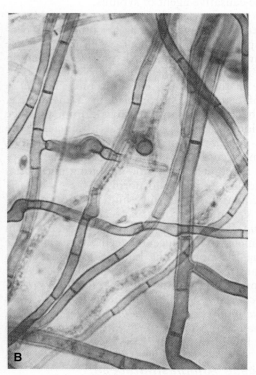

FIGURE 14-8. The microscopic morphology of fungal pathogens in humans. **(A)** Histopathologic changes seen in histoplasmosis due to *Histoplasma capsulatum var. duboisii.* Note the presence of typical yeast cells, some of which are undergoing replication by budding (*arrow*). **(B)** The molds produce long branched and unbranched filaments called *hyphae*. (A from the Centers for Disease Control and Prevention Public Health Images Library. No. 4221. Courtesy of Libero Ajello.)

the characteristic microscopic appearance of the asexual fruiting structures and spores.

Like the bacterial pathogens of humans, fungi can produce disease in the human host only if they can grow at the temperature of the infected body site. For example, a number of fungal pathogens called *dermatophytes* are incapable of growing at core body temperature (37°C), and the infection is limited to the cooler cutaneous surfaces. Diseases caused by these organisms, including ringworm, athlete's foot, and jock itch, are collectively called *superficial mycoses*. Systemic mycoses are serious fungal infections of deep tissues and, by definition, are caused by organisms capable of growth at 37°C. Yeasts such as *Candida albicans* are commensal flora of the skin, mucous membranes, and gastrointestinal tract and are capable of growth at a wider range of temperatures. Intact immune mechanisms and competition for nutrients provided by the bacterial flora normally keep colonizing fungi in check. Alterations in either of these components by disease states or antibiotic therapy can upset the balance, permitting fungal overgrowth and setting the stage for opportunistic infections.

Parasites

In a strict sense, any organism that derives benefits from its biologic relationship with another organism is a parasite. In the study of clinical microbiology, however, the term *parasite* has evolved to designate members of the animal kingdom that infect and cause disease in other animals and includes protozoa, helminths, and arthropods.

The protozoa are unicellular animals with a complete complement of eukaryotic cellular machinery, including a well-defined nucleus and organelles. Reproduction may be sexual or asexual, and life cycles may be simple or complicated, with several maturation stages requiring more than one host for completion. Most are saprophytes, but a few have adapted to the accommodations of the human environment and produce a variety of diseases, including malaria, amebic dysentery, and giardiasis. Protozoan infections can be passed directly from host to host through sexual contact, indirectly through contaminated water or food, or by way of an arthropod vector. Direct or indirect transmission results from the ingestion of highly resistant cysts or spores that are shed in the feces of an infected host. When the cysts reach the intestine, they mature into vegetative forms called *trophozoites*, which are capable of asexual reproduction or cyst formation. Most trophozoites are motile by means of flagella, cilia, or ameboid motion.

The helminths are a collection of wormlike parasites that include the nematodes or roundworms, cestodes or tapeworms, and trematodes or flukes. The helminths reproduce sexually within the definitive host, and some require an intermediate host for the development and maturation of offspring. Humans can serve as the definitive or intermediate host or, in certain diseases such as trichinosis, as both. Transmission of helminth diseases occurs primarily through the ingestion of fertilized eggs (ova) or the penetration of infectious larval stages through the skin—directly or with the aid of an arthropod vector. Helminth infections can involve many organ systems and sites, including the liver and lung, urinary and intestinal tracts, circulatory and central nervous systems, and muscle. Although most helminth diseases have been eradicated from the United States, they are still a major health concern of developing nations.

The parasitic arthropods of humans and animals include the vectors of infectious diseases (e.g., ticks, mosquitoes, biting flies) and the ectoparasites. The ectoparasites infest external body surfaces and cause localized tissue damage or inflammation secondary to the bite or burrowing action of the arthropod. The most prominent human ectoparasites are mites (scabies), chiggers, lice (head, body, and pubic), and fleas. Transmission of ectoparasites occurs directly by contact with immature or mature forms of the arthropod or its eggs found on the infested host or the host's clothing, bedding, or grooming articles such as combs and brushes. Many of the ectoparasites are vectors of other infectious diseases, including endemic typhus and bubonic plague.

SUMMARY CONCEPTS

- Throughout life, humans are continuously and harmlessly exposed to and colonized by a multitude of microscopic organisms. This relationship is kept in check by the intact defense mechanisms of the host (e.g., mucosal and cutaneous barriers, normal immune function) and the innocuous nature of most environmental microorganisms.

- The agents of infectious disease represent a diversity of microorganisms that are usually not visible to the human eye. The term *infection* describes the presence and injurious multiplication of an infectious agent within a human host, whereas *colonization* describes the act of establishing a presence, a step required in the multifaceted process of infection.

- Microorganisms can be separated into *eukaryotes* (fungi and parasites), organisms containing a membrane-bound nucleus; and *prokaryotes* (bacteria), organisms in which the nucleus is not separated. Both eukaryotes and prokaryotes are organisms because they contain all the biologic equipment necessary for replication and metabolism.

- Viruses, which are the smallest pathogens, have no organized cellular structure, but consist of a protein coat surrounding a nucleic acid core of DNA or RNA. Unlike eukaryotes and prokaryotes, viruses are incapable of replication outside of a living cell.

(continued)

Epidemiology of Infectious Diseases

Epidemiologists working in infectious disease study the factors, events, and circumstances that influence the transmission of infectious diseases among humans. The ultimate goal of epidemiologists is to devise strategies that interrupt or eliminate the spread of infectious agents. To accomplish this, they classify infectious diseases according to incidence, portal of entry and source, symptoms, disease course, site of infection, and virulence factors so that potential outbreaks may be predicted and averted or appropriately treated.

Mechanisms of Transmission

The outcomes of infections depend on the ability of microbes to breach host barriers and colonize and damage host tissues. Host barriers to infection prevent the microbes from entering the body and assist innate and adaptive immune defenses in eliminating the agent (see Chapter 15).

Portal of Entry

Microbes can enter the host by direct contact, ingestion, and inhalation. The portal of entry does not dictate the site of infection. Ingested pathogens may penetrate the intestinal mucosa, disseminate through the circulatory system, and cause diseases in other organs such as the lung or liver. Whatever the mechanisms of entry, the transmission of infectious agents is directly related to the number of infectious agents absorbed by the host.

Penetration. Any disruption in the integrity of the body's surface barrier—skin or mucous membranes—is a potential site for invasion of microorganisms. The break may be the result of an accidental injury causing abrasions, burns, or penetrating wounds; medical procedures such as surgery or catheterization; or a primary infectious process such as chickenpox or impetigo that produces surface lesions. Direct inoculation from intravenous drug use or an animal or arthropod bite also can occur.

Direct Contact. Some pathogens are transmitted directly from infected tissue or secretions to exposed, intact mucous membranes. This is especially true of certain sexually transmitted infections (STIs) such as gonorrhea, syphilis, chlamydia, and genital herpes, for which exposure of uninfected membranes to pathogens occurs during intimate contact (see Chapter 41).

The transmission of STIs is not limited to sexual contact. *Vertical transmission* of these agents, from mother to child, can occur across the placenta or during birth when the mucous membranes of the child come in contact with infected vaginal secretions of the mother. When an infectious disease is transmitted from mother to child during gestation or birth, it is classified as a *congenital infection.* The most frequently observed congenital infections include toxoplasmosis (caused by the parasite *Toxoplasma gondii*), syphilis, rubella, cytomegalovirus infection, and herpes simplex virus infections (the so-called TORCH infections, discussed in Chapter 6); varicella-zoster (chickenpox); parvovirus B19; group B streptococci (*Streptococcus agalactiae*); and HIV. Of these, cytomegalovirus is by far the most common cause of congenital infection in the United States, affecting nearly 1% of all newborns. However, with more than 500,000 babies contracting HIV from their mother and with a 25% to 30% chance of vertical transmission without appropriate antiretroviral treatment, HIV is rapidly gaining in stature as a congenitally transmitted infection (see Chapter 16).

Ingestion. The entry of pathogenic microorganisms or their toxins through the oral cavity and gastrointestinal tract represents one of the more efficient means of disease transmission in humans. Many bacterial, viral, and parasitic infections, including cholera, typhoid fever, dysentery (amebic and bacillary), food poisoning, traveler's diarrhea, cryptosporidiosis, and hepatitis A, are initiated through the ingestion of contaminated food and water. This mechanism of transmission necessitates that an infectious agent survive the low pH and enzyme activity of gastric secretions and the peristaltic action of the intestines in numbers sufficient to establish infection, deemed an infectious dose. Ingested pathogens also must compete successfully with the normal bacterial flora of the bowel for nutritional needs. Persons with reduced gastric acidity because of disease or medication are more susceptible to infection by ingestion because the number of ingested microorganisms surviving the gastric environment is greater. Ingested pathogens also must compete successfully for nutrients with the normal bacterial flora of the colon. Ingestion has also been postulated as a means of transmission of HIV infection from mother to child through breast-feeding.

Inhalation. The respiratory tract of a healthy person is equipped with a multilayered defense system to prevent potential pathogens from entering the lungs. The surface of the respiratory tree is lined with a layer of mucus that is continuously swept up and away from the lungs and toward the mouth by the beating motion of ciliated epithelial cells. Humidification of inspired air increases the size of aerosolized particles, which are effectively filtered by the mucous membranes of the upper respiratory tract. Coughing also aids in the removal of particulate matter from the lower respiratory tract. Respiratory secretions contain antibodies and enzymes capable of inactivating infectious agents. Particulate matter and microorganisms that ultimately reach the lungs are cleared by phagocytic cells.

Despite this impressive array of protective mechanisms, a number of pathogens can invade the human body through the respiratory tract, including agents of bacterial pneumonia (*Streptococcus pneumoniae, L. pneumophila*), meningitis (*Neisseria meningitidis, Haemophilus influenzae*), and tuberculosis, as well as the viruses responsible for measles, mumps, chickenpox, influenza, and the common cold. Defective pulmonary function or mucociliary clearance caused by noninfectious processes such as cystic fibrosis, emphysema, or smoking can increase the risk of inhalation-acquired diseases.

Source

The source of an infectious disease refers to the location, host, object, or substance from which the infectious agent was acquired: essentially the "who, what, where, and when" of disease transmission. The source may be endogenous (acquired from the host's own microbial flora, as would be the case in an opportunistic infection) or exogenous (acquired from sources in the external environment, such as the water, food, soil, or air). The source of the infectious agent can also be another human being, as from mother to child during gestation (congenital infections); an inanimate object; an animal; or a biting arthropod. Inanimate objects that carry an infectious agent are known as *fomites*. For example, rhinoviruses and many other nonenveloped viruses can be spread by contact with contaminated fomites such as handkerchiefs and toys. Zoonoses are a category of infectious diseases passed from other animal species to humans. Examples of zoonoses include cat-scratch disease, rabies, and Creutzfeldt-Jakob disease (vCJD). The spread of infectious diseases such as Lyme disease through biting arthropod vectors has already been mentioned.

Source can denote a place. For instance, infections that develop in patients while they are hospitalized are called *nosocomial* or *hospital acquired*, and those that are acquired outside of health care facilities are called *community acquired*. The source may also pertain to the body substance that is the most likely vehicle for transmission, such as feces, blood, body fluids, respiratory secretions, and urine. Infections can be transmitted from person to person through shared inanimate objects (fomites) contaminated with infected body fluids. An example of this mechanism of transmission would include the spread of the HIV and hepatitis B virus through the use of shared syringes by intravenous drug users. Infection can also be spread through a complex combination of source, portal of entry, and vector. Infection with hantavirus pulmonary syndrome is a prime example. This viral illness is transmitted from mice to humans by inhalation of dust contaminated with saliva, feces, and urine of infected rodents.

Mechanisms of Disease Production

Infectious agents establish infection and damage tissues by entering host cells and directly causing their death; by inducing host responses that, although directed against the invader, cause additional tissue damage; and by generating *virulence factors*, substances or products generated by infectious agents that enhance their ability to cause disease. Although a large number of microbial products fit this description, they can be grouped into four categories: toxins, adhesion factors, evasive factors, and invasive factors (Table 14-2).

Toxins

Toxins are substances that alter or destroy the normal function of the host or host's cells. Toxin production is a trait chiefly monopolized by bacterial pathogens, although certain fungal and protozoan pathogens also produce substances toxic to humans. Bacterial toxins have a diverse spectrum of activity and exert their effects on a wide variety of host target cells. For classification purposes, however, the bacterial toxins can be divided into two main types: *endotoxins* and *exotoxins*.

Bacterial endotoxins are lipopolysaccharides (LPS) found in the cell wall of gram-negative bacteria. Free LPS attaches to a circulating LPS-binding protein, and the complex then binds to specific leukocyte receptors that participate in activation of the innate immune system (see Chapter 15). The host response to low levels of LPS induces many important cytokines, as well as expression of costimulatory molecules, resulting in leukocyte recruitment and enhancement of T-lymphocyte activation. However, at high levels, LPS can precipitate septic shock, disseminated intravascular coagulation, and acute respiratory distress syndrome.

TABLE 14-2	Examples of Virulence Factors Produced by Pathogenic Microorganisms		
Factor	**Category**	**Organism**	**Effect on Host**
Cholera toxin	Exotoxin	*Vibrio cholerae* (bacterium)	Secretory diarrhea
Diphtheria toxin	Exotoxin	*Corynebacterium diphtheriae* (bacterium)	Inhibits protein synthesis
Lipopolysaccharide	Endotoxin	Many gram-negative bacteria	Fever, hypotension, shock
Toxic shock toxin	Enterotoxin	*Staphylococcus aureus* (bacterium)	Rash, diarrhea, vomiting, hepatitis
Hemagglutinin	Adherence	Influenza virus	Establishment of infection
Pili	Adherence	*Neisseria gonorrhoeae* (bacterium)	Establishment of infection
Leukocidin	Evasive	*S. aureus*	Kills phagocytes
IgA protease	Evasive	*Haemophilus influenzae* (bacterium)	Inactivates antibody
Capsule	Evasive	*Cryptococcus neoformans* (yeast)	Prevents phagocytosis
Collagenase	Invasive	*Pseudomonas aeruginosa* (bacterium)	Penetration of tissue
Protease	Invasive	*Aspergillus* (mold)	Penetration of tissue
Phospholipase	Invasive	*Clostridium perfringens* (bacterium)	Penetration of tissue
Botulinum toxin	Exotoxin	*Clostridium botulinum* (bacterium)	Neuroparalysis, inhibits acetylcholine release
Pneumolysin	Exotoxin	*Streptococcus pneumoniae* (bacterium)	Inhibition of respiratory ciliated and phagocytic cell function

Exotoxins are proteins released from the bacterial cell during growth. Bacterial exotoxins enzymatically inactivate or modify key aspects of host cell structure or function, leading to cell death or dysfunction. Diphtheria toxin, for example, inhibits protein synthesis; botulism toxin decreases the release of neurotransmitter from cholinergic neurons, causing flaccid paralysis; tetanus toxin decreases the release of neurotransmitter from inhibitory neurons, producing spastic paralysis; and cholera toxin induces fluid secretion into the lumen of the intestine, causing diarrhea. Bacterial exotoxins that produce vomiting and diarrhea are sometimes referred to as *enterotoxins*. There has been resurgent interest in streptococcal pyrogenic exotoxin A (SPEA), an exotoxin produced by certain strains of group A, β-hemolytic streptococci (*S. pyogenes*) that causes a life-threatening toxic shock–like syndrome. The syndrome, sometimes called *Henson disease* because this infection caused the death of famous puppeteer Jim Henson, is typified by invasion of the skin and soft tissues, acute respiratory distress syndrome, and renal failure. Other enterotoxins that have gained notoriety include the Shiga toxins produced by *Escherichia coli* O157:H7 (see Chapter 29). The ingestion of undercooked hamburger meat or unpasteurized fruit juices contaminated with this organism produces hemorrhagic colitis and a sometimes fatal illness called *hemolytic uremic syndrome* (HUS), characterized by vascular endothelial damage, acute renal failure, and thrombocytopenia. Hemolytic uremic syndrome occurs primarily in infants and young children who have not developed antibodies to the Shiga toxins.

Adhesion Factors

No interaction between microorganisms and humans can progress to infection or disease if the pathogen is unable to attach to and colonize the host. The process of microbial attachment may be site specific (e.g., mucous membranes, skin surfaces), cell specific (e.g., T lymphocytes, respiratory epithelium, intestinal epithelium), or nonspecific (e.g., moist areas, charged surfaces). In any of these cases, adhesion requires a positive interaction between the surfaces of host cells and the infectious agent.

After initial attachment, some bacterial agents become embedded in a gelatinous matrix of polysaccharides called a *slime* (or *mucous) layer*. The slime layer serves two purposes: it anchors the agent firmly to host tissue surfaces and it protects the agent from the immunologic defenses of the host.

Many viral agents, including influenza, mumps, measles, and adenovirus, produce hair-like appendages or spikes called *fimbriae*. Fimbriae are used by bacteria to attach to one another or attach to cell surfaces. On the distal tips of fimbriae, *hemagglutinins* recognize carbohydrate receptors on the surfaces of specific cells in the host, allowing the bacteria to attach to the host cell in a specific manner.

Evasion Factors

A number of factors produced by microorganisms enhance virulence by evading various components of the host's immune system. Extracellular polysaccharides, including capsules, slime, and mucous layers, discourage engulfment and killing of pathogens by the host's phagocytic white blood cells (i.e., neutrophils and macrophages). Encapsulated organisms such as *Cryptococcus neoformans*, *S. pneumoniae*, *N. meningitidis*, and *H. influenzae* type b (before the vaccine) are a cause of significant morbidity and mortality in neonates and children who lack protective anticapsular antibodies.

Some bacterial, fungal, and parasitic pathogens avoid phagocytosis by excreting leukocidin C toxins, which cause specific and lethal damage to the cell membrane of host neutrophils and macrophages. Other pathogens, such as the bacterial agents of salmonellosis, listeriosis, and Legionnaires' disease, are adapted to survive and reproduce within phagocytic white blood cells after ingestion, avoiding or neutralizing the usually lethal products contained within the lysosomes of the cell. *H. pylori*, the infectious cause of gastritis and gastric ulcers, produces a urease enzyme on its outer cell wall. The urease converts gastric urea into ammonia, thus neutralizing the acidic environment of the stomach and allowing the organism to survive in this hostile environment.

Other unique strategies used by pathogenic microbes to evade immunologic surveillance have evolved solely to avoid recognition by host antibodies. Strains of *S. aureus* produce a surface protein (protein A) that immobilizes immunoglobulin G (IgG), holding the antigen-binding region harmlessly away from the organisms. This pathogen also secretes a unique enzyme called *coagulase*. Coagulase converts soluble human coagulation factors into a solid clot, which envelops and protects the organism from phagocytic host cells and antibodies. *H. influenzae* and *N. gonorrhoeae* secrete enzymes that cleave and inactivate secretory IgA, neutralizing the primary defense of the respiratory and genital tracts at the site of infection. *Borrelia* species, including the agents of Lyme disease and relapsing fever, alter surface antigens during the disease course to avoid immunologic detection.

Invasion Factors

Infectious agents also produce invasive factors that facilitate the penetration of anatomic barriers and host tissue. Most invasive factors are enzymes capable of destroying cell membranes (e.g., phospholipases), connective tissue (e.g., elastases, collagenases), intercellular matrices (e.g., hyaluronidase), and structural protein complexes (e.g., proteases). The effects of the pathogen's invasive factors and toxins, combined with the antimicrobial and inflammatory substances released by host cells, mediate the tissue damage and pathophysiology of infectious diseases.

Clinical Presentation

The term *symptomatology* refers to the collection of signs and symptoms expressed by the host during the disease course. This is also known as the *clinical presentation* and can be characteristic of any given infectious agent. In terms of pathophysiology, symptoms are the outward expression of the struggle between invading organisms and the retaliatory inflammatory and immune responses of the host. The symptoms of an infectious disease may be specific and reflect the site of infection (e.g., diarrhea, rash, convulsions, hemorrhage, and pneumonia). Conversely, symptoms such as fever, myalgia, headache, and lethargy are relatively nonspecific and can be shared by a number of etiologic agents. The symptoms of a diseased host can be obvious, as in the case of chickenpox or measles. Other, covert symptoms, such as an increased white blood cell count, may require laboratory testing to detect. Accurate recognition and documentation of symptomatology can aid in the diagnosis of an infectious disease.

Site of Infection

Inflammation of an anatomic location is usually designated by adding the suffix *-itis* to the name of the involved tissue (e.g., bronchitis, inflammation of the bronchi and bronchioles; encephalitis, brain inflammation; carditis, inflammation of the heart). These are general terms, however, and they apply equally to inflammation from infectious and noninfectious causes. The suffix *-emia* is used to designate the presence of a substance in the blood (e.g., *bacteremia, viremia,* and *fungemia* describe the presence of these infectious agents in the bloodstream). The term *sepsis,* or *septicemia,* refers to the presence of a proven bloodstream infection combined with a systemic immune response.

The site of an infectious disease is ultimately determined by the type of pathogen, the portal of entry, and the competence of the host's immunologic defense system. Many pathogenic microorganisms are restricted in their capacity to invade the human body. *M. pneumoniae,* influenza viruses, and respiratory syncytial virus rarely cause disease outside the respiratory tract; infections caused by *N. gonorrhoeae* are generally confined to the genitourinary tract; and *Clostridium difficile,* shigellosis, and giardiasis seldom extend beyond the gastrointestinal tract. These are considered localized infectious diseases. The bacterium *Helicobacter pylori* is an extreme example of a site-specific pathogen. *H. pylori* is a significant cause of gastric ulcers but has not been implicated in disease processes elsewhere in the human body. Bacteria such as *N. meningitidis,* a prominent pathogen of children and young adults; *Salmonella typhi,* the cause of typhoid fever, and *B. burgdorferi,* the agent of Lyme disease, tend to disseminate from the primary site of infection to involve other locations and organ systems. These are examples of systemic pathogens disseminated throughout the body by the circulatory system.

An *abscess* is a localized pocket of infection composed of devitalized tissue, microorganisms, and the host's phagocytic white blood cells: in essence, a stalemate in the infectious process. In this case, the dissemination of the pathogen has been contained by the host, but white cell function within the toxic environment of the abscess is hampered, and the elimination of microorganisms is inhibited. Abscesses usually must be surgically drained to affect a complete cure. Similarly, infections of biomedical implants such as catheters, artificial heart valves, and prosthetic bone implants are seldom cured by the host's immune response and antimicrobial therapy. The infecting organism colonizes the surface of the implant, producing a dense matrix of cells, host proteins, and capsular material—a biofilm—necessitating the removal of the device.

Disease Course

The course of any infectious disease can be divided into several distinguishable stages after the point when the potential pathogen enters the host. These stages are the incubation period, the prodromal stage, the acute stage, the convalescent stage, and the resolution stage (Fig. 14-9). The stages are based on the progression and intensity of the host's symptoms over time. The duration of each phase and the pattern of the overall illness can be specific for different pathogens, thereby aiding in the diagnosis of an infectious disease.

The incubation period is the phase during which the pathogen begins active replication without producing recognizable symptoms in the host. The incubation period may be short, as in the case of salmonellosis (6 to 24 hours), or prolonged, such as that of hepatitis B (50 to 180 days) or HIV (months to years). The duration of the incubation period can be influenced by additional factors, including the general health of the host, the portal of entry, and the infectious dose of the pathogen.

The hallmark of the *prodromal stage* is the initial appearance of symptoms in the host, although the clinical presentation during this time may be only a vague sense of malaise. The host may experience mild fever, myalgia, headache, and fatigue. These are constitutional changes shared by a great number of disease processes. The duration of the prodromal stage can vary considerably from host to host.

The *acute stage* is the period during which the host experiences the maximum impact of the infectious process corresponding to rapid proliferation and dissemination of the pathogen. During this phase, toxic by-products of microbial metabolism, cell lysis, and the immune response mounted by the host combine to produce tissue damage and inflammation. The symptoms of the host are pronounced and more specific than in the prodromal stage, usually typifying the pathogen and sites of involvement.

The *convalescent period* is characterized by the containment of infection, progressive elimination of the pathogen, repair of damaged tissue, and resolution of associated symptoms. Similar to the incubation period, the time required for complete convalescence may be days, weeks, or months, depending on the type of pathogen and the voracity of the host's immune response. The *resolution* is the total elimination of a pathogen from the body without residual signs or symptoms of disease.

Several notable exceptions to the classic presentation of an infectious process have been recognized. Chronic infectious diseases have a markedly protracted and sometimes irregular course. The host may experience symptoms of the infectious process continuously or sporadically for months or years without a convalescent phase. In contrast, *subclinical* or *subacute illness* progresses from infection to resolution without clinically apparent symptoms. A disease is called *insidious* if the prodromal phase is protracted; a *fulminant* illness is characterized by abrupt onset of symptoms with little or no prodrome. Fatal infections are variants of the typical disease course.

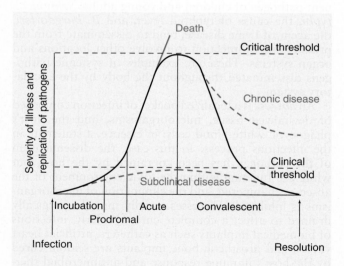

FIGURE 14-9. Stages of a primary infectious disease as they appear in relation to the severity of symptoms and numbers of infectious agents. The clinical threshold corresponds with the initial expression of recognizable symptoms, whereas the critical threshold represents the peak of disease intensity.

SUMMARY CONCEPTS

■ Epidemiology is the study of factors, events, and circumstances that influence the transmission of disease.

■ The outcomes of infections depend on the ability of microbes to breach host barriers and colonize and damage host tissues. Microbes can enter the host by direct contact, ingestion, and inhalation. The source of infection may be endogenous (acquired from the host's own microbial flora, as would be the case in an opportunistic infection) or exogenous (acquired from sources in the external environment, such as the water, food, soil, or air). It can also be another human being, as from mother to child during gestation (congenital infections); an inanimate object; an animal; or a biting arthropod.

■ The site of an infectious disease is determined ultimately by the type of pathogen, the portal of entry, and the competence of the host's immunologic defense system. It may be localized to the site of entry, disseminate from the primary site of infection to involve other locations and organ systems, or travel through the circulatory system to produce disseminated infection.

■ Virulence factors, which are substances or products generated by infectious agents that enhance their ability to cause disease, include toxins (endotoxins and exotoxins), adhesion factors, evasive factors, and invasive factors.

■ The natural history of an infectious disease includes its incubation period, as well as its prodromal, acute, convalescent, and resolution stages.

Diagnosis of Infectious Diseases

The diagnosis of an infectious disease requires two criteria: the recovery of a probable pathogen or evidence of its presence from the infected sites of a diseased host and accurate documentation of clinical signs and symptoms (symptomatology) compatible with an infectious process. In the laboratory, the diagnosis of an infectious agent is accomplished using three basic techniques: culture, serology, or the detection of characteristic antigens, genomic sequences, or metabolites produced by the pathogen.

Culture

Culture refers to the propagation of a microorganism outside of the body, usually on or in artificial growth media such as agar plates or broth (Fig. 14-10). The specimen from the host is inoculated into broth or onto the surface of an agar plate, and the culture is placed in a controlled environment such as an incubator until the growth of microorganisms becomes detectable. In the case of a bacterial pathogen, identification is based on microscopic appearance and Gram stain reaction, shape, texture, and color (i.e., morphology) of the colonies, by a panel of biochemical reactions that fingerprint salient biochemical characteristics of the organism, and by the organism's protein profile. Certain bacteria such as *Mycobacterium leprae*, the agent of leprosy, and *T. pallidum*, the syphilis spirochete, do not grow on artificial media and require additional methods of identification. Fungi and mycoplasmas are cultured in much the same way as bacteria, but with more reliance on microscopic and colonial morphology for identification.

Chlamydiaceae, *Rickettsiaceae*, and all human viruses are obligate intracellular pathogens. As a result, the propagation of these agents in the laboratory requires the inoculation of eukaryotic cells grown in culture (cell cultures). Cell culture is becoming more infrequent in modern clinical laboratories due to the extended time required for growth of viruses and reported poor sensitivity of culture. Diagnosis of viruses, *Chlamydiaceae*, and *Rickettsiaceae* now relies primarily on serology and nucleic acid detection, which will be discussed later in this chapter.

Although culture media have been developed for the growth of certain human-infecting protozoa and helminths in the laboratory, the diagnosis of parasitic infectious diseases has traditionally relied on microscopic or, in the case of worms, visible identification of organisms, cysts, or ova directly from infected patient specimens.

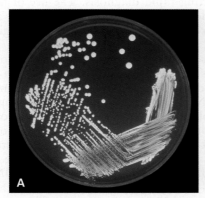
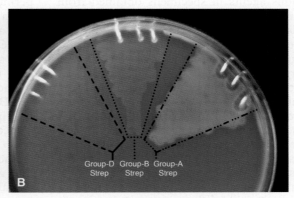

Group-D Strep   Group-B Strep   Group-A Strep

FIGURE 14-10. Use of agar culture for propagation and identification of microorganisms. **(A)** Photograph showing numerous *Legionella* species colonies that have been cultivated on an agar culture plate and illuminated using ultraviolet light. **(B)** Quantitative differences in hemolytic reactivity seen in trypticase soy agar culture plate containing 5% sheep's blood growing group D *Streptococci* (left wedge), group B *Streptococci* (middle wedge), and group A *Streptococci* (right wedge) bacteria. The plate was grown under normal atmospheric conditions, at 35°C, for a period of 18 hours. It is important to note that the group B *Streptococci* (GBS) in the center wedge produced a hemolytic reaction that is less than the reaction produced by group A *Streptococci* (GAS) in the right wedge of bacterial growth. Hemolysis, which results from destruction of red blood cells, is one of the traits used to help identify the bacteria. (From the Centers for Disease Control and Prevention Public Health Images Library. Nos. 7925, 10861. A courtesy James Gathany; B courtesy Richard Facklam.)

Serology

Serology—literally, "the study of serum"—is an indirect means of identifying infectious agents by measuring serum antibodies in the diseased host. A tentative diagnosis can be made if the antibody level, also called *antibody titer*, against a specific pathogen rises during the acute phase of the disease and falls during convalescence. Serologic identification of an infectious agent is not as accurate as culture, but it may be a useful adjunct, especially for the diagnosis of diseases caused by pathogens such as the hepatitis B virus that cannot be cultured or diagnosis of past diseases. The measurement of antibody titers has another advantage in that specific antibody types such as IgM and IgG are produced by the host during different phases of an infectious process. IgM-specific antibodies generally rise and fall during the acute phase of the disease, whereas the synthesis of the IgG class of antibodies increases during the acute phase and remains elevated until or beyond resolution.

Measurements of class-specific antibodies are also useful in the diagnosis of congenital infections. IgM antibodies do not cross the placenta, but certain IgG antibodies are transferred passively from mother to child during the final trimester of gestation. Consequently, an elevated level of pathogen-specific IgM antibodies in the serum of a neonate must have originated from the child and therefore indicates congenital infection. A similarly increased IgG titer in the neonate does not differentiate congenital from maternal infection.

The technology of *direct antigen detection* incorporates features of culture and serology but reduces to a fraction the time required for diagnosis. In principle, this method relies on purified antibodies to detect antigens of infectious agents in specimens obtained from the diseased host. Common sources of these antibodies are *hybridomas*, cell lines created by fusing normal antibody-producing spleen cells from an immunized animal with malignant myeloma cells. The resulting hybrid synthesizes large quantities of so-called *monoclonal antibodies* that are highly specific for a single antigen and a single pathogen.

The antibodies are labeled with a substance that allows microscopic or overt detection when bound to the pathogen or its products. In general, the three types of labels used for this purpose are fluorescent dyes, enzymes, and particles such as latex beads. Fluorescent antibodies allow visualization of an infectious agent with the aid of fluorescence microscopy. Depending on the type of fluorescent dye used, the organism may appear bright green or orange against a black background, making detection extremely easy. Enzyme-labeled antibodies function in a similar manner. The enzyme is capable of converting a colorless compound into a colored substance, thereby permitting detection of antibody bound to an infectious agent without the use of a fluorescent microscope. Particles coated with antibodies clump together, or agglutinate, when the appropriate antigen is present in

a specimen. Particle agglutination is especially useful when examining infected body fluids such as urine, serum, or spinal fluid.

Protein Detection

Mass spectrometry is a technique for determining the composition of a sample. It generates a protein-based profile or "fingerprint" from microbes that is unique to a given species. By analyzing the proteins that make up bacteria, yeast, or molds, clinical laboratories can quickly fingerprint these organisms and identify them based on the size and number of proteins detected. For example, analysis of bacteria such as *S. aureus* can often be accomplished by direct analysis of colony growth by the mass spectrometer within minutes of bacterial growth.

DNA and RNA Detection

Methods for identifying a pathogen by its unique DNA or RNA sequence are increasingly being used. Several techniques have been devised to accomplish this goal, each having different degrees of sensitivity regarding the number of organisms that need to be present in a specimen for detection.

The first of these methods is called *DNA probe hybridization*. Small fragments of DNA are cut from the genome of a specific pathogen and labeled with compounds (photo-emitting chemicals or antigens) that allow detection. The labeled DNA probes are added to specimens from an infected host. If the pathogen is present, the probe attaches to the complementary strand of DNA on the genome of the infectious agent, permitting rapid diagnosis. The use of labeled probes has allowed visualization of particular agents within and around individual cells in histologic sections of tissue.

A second and more sensitive method of DNA detection is the *polymerase chain reaction* (PCR). This method allows technicians to tag a segment of pathogen DNA—if present in the patient sample—and then multiply it to detectable levels. To perform the assay, a specimen containing the suspect pathogen is heated (Fig. 14-11). This causes the double-stranded DNA in the specimen to separate into single strands. It is then allowed to cool. Next, two short DNA sequences (usually less than 25 nucleotides long) called *primers* are added to the specimen. These primers locate and bind only to the complementary target DNA of the pathogen in question. Then, a heat-stable DNA polymerase—an enzyme that catalyzes the synthesis of DNA—is added. It begins to replicate the DNA from the point at which the primers attached, similar to two trains approaching each other on separate but converging tracks. After the initial cycle, DNA polymerization ceases at the point where the primers were located, producing two new strands of DNA. The specimen is heated again, and the process starts anew.

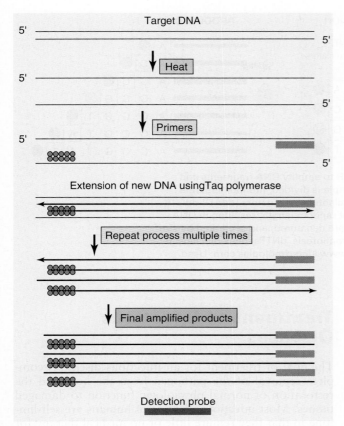

Target DNA

5' ——————————————————————
———————————————————————— 5'

↓ Heat

5' ——————————————————————

———————————————————————— 5'

↓ Primers

5' ——————————————————————

———————————————————————— 5'

Extension of new DNA usingTaq polymerase

↓ Repeat process multiple times

↓ Final amplified products

Detection probe

FIGURE 14-11. Polymerase chain reaction. The target DNA is first melted using heat (generally around 94°C) to separate the strands of DNA. Primers that *recognize* specific sequences in the target DNA are allowed to bind as the reaction cools. Using a unique, thermostable DNA polymerase called Taq and an abundance of deoxynucleoside triphosphates, new DNA strands are amplified from the point of the primer attachment. The process is repeated many times (called *cycles*) until millions of copies of DNA are produced, all of which have the same length (defined by the distance [in base pairs] between the primer binding sites). These copies are then detected by electrophoresis and staining or through the use of labeled DNA probes that, similar to the primers, recognize a specific sequence located in the amplified section of DNA.

After many cycles of heating, cooling, and polymerization, and only if the specific pathogen (or its DNA) is present in the specimen, millions of uniformly sized pathogen DNA fragments are produced. The polymerized DNA fragments are separated by electrophoresis and visualized with a dye or identified by hybridization with a specific probe.

A modification of PCR, known as *real-time PCR*, continues to revolutionize medical diagnostics. Real-time PCR uses the same principles as PCR, but includes a fluorescence-labeled probe that specifically binds a target DNA sequence between the oligonucleotide primers. As the DNA is replicated by the DNA polymerase, the level of fluorescence in the reaction is measured. If fluorescence increases beyond

a minimum threshold, the PCR is considered positive and indicates the presence of the target DNA in a specimen.

Several variations of molecular gene detection techniques in addition to PCR have been developed and incorporated into diagnostic kits for use in the clinical laboratory, including, transcription-mediated amplification (TMA), strand displacement amplification, hybrid capture assays, and DNA sequencing.

Many of the newer gene detection technologies have been adapted for quantitation of the target DNA or RNA in serum or plasma specimens of patients infected with viruses such as HIV and hepatitis C. If the therapy is effective, viral replication is suppressed and the viral load (level of viral genome) in the peripheral blood is reduced. Conversely, if mutations in the viral genome lead to resistant strains or if the antiviral therapy is ineffective, viral replication continues and the patient's viral load rises, indicating a need to change the therapeutic approach.

Molecular biology has revolutionized medical diagnostics. Using techniques such as PCR, laboratories now can detect as little as one virus or bacterium in a single specimen, allowing for the diagnosis of infections caused by microorganisms that are impossible or difficult to grow in culture. These methods have increased sensitivity while decreasing the time required to identify the etiologic agent of infectious disease. For example, using standard viral culture, it can take days to weeks to grow a virus and correlate the CPE with the virus. Using molecular biologic techniques, laboratories are able to complete the same work in a few hours.

DNA Sequencing

Originally described in 1976, DNA sequencing has gone through many modifications and has become one of the most powerful tools for laboratory diagnosis. The most common sequencing method is known as Sanger sequencing. Sanger sequencing uses nucleotides (similar to PCR) to build a chain of DNA. Terminator dyes that have been fluorescently labeled are inserted into the elongating fragment, causing the PCR reaction to stop at random lengths. The newly labeled double-stranded DNA fragments are broken apart, and separated by size (with a resolution of just one nucleotide) by gel or capillary electrophoresis. The resulting chart indicates the terminator color and the length of the fragment at termination (Fig. 14-12). Sanger sequencing has quickly become the "gold standard" for identification of microbes that cannot be identified by other routine methods. Sequencing has also become the most accurate method for classifying microbes into their taxonomic group (Genus and species).

While Sanger sequencing has improved diagnosis of infectious diseases, it is still limited to sequencing a very small section of the genome. Consider that Sanger sequencing was used in the first complete sequence of the human genome, which took more

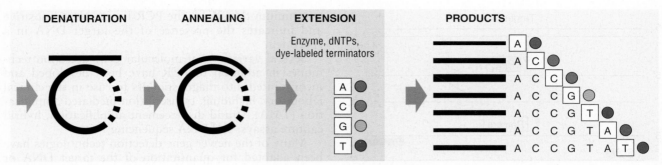

FIGURE 14-12. Sanger sequencing. Sanger sequencing uses PCR to amplify DNA fragments and labeled nucleotides as DNA elongation terminators. The DNA sample is divided into four separate sequencing reactions; to each reaction one of the four dideoxynucleotide terminators (ddATP, ddGTP, ddCTP, or ddTTP) are added to terminate DNA strand extension at random length, resulting in DNA fragments of varying lengths. The newly labeled DNA fragments are denatured, and separated by size (with a resolution of just one nucleotide) by gel or capillary electrophoresis. dNTPs, deoxynucleoside triphosphates. (Copyright © 2014 Life Technologies Corporation; www.lifetechnologies.com. Used under permission.)

than 10 years to complete at a cost of more than $3 billon. Today newer sequencing methods, collectively known as Next Generation Sequencing (NGS), have allowed laboratories to sequence whole genomes of bacteria, molds, mycobacteria, and even humans at a fraction of the cost and within days rather than decades. For infectious diseases, the applications of sequencing are exciting and impactful. In epidemiology, next-generation sequencing will likely replace our current laboratory methods. For example, in 2011 a new strain of *E. coli* was detected in an outbreak of serious foodborne illness beginning in northern Germany that ultimately affected nearly 4000 patients with 53 dead. Within 1 week of isolating the new strain of *E. coli*, clinical microbiologists had grown the organism, sequenced it, and identified the source of the outbreak. With powerful laboratory technologies like sequencing, epidemiologists will be better equipped to identify outbreaks early or even prevent them from occurring.

SUMMARY CONCEPTS

■ The diagnosis of infectious disease relies on the recovery of the probable pathogen or evidence of its presence from infected sites in the host and accurate documentation of signs and symptoms compatible with an infectious process.

■ In the laboratory, the diagnosis of an infectious agent is accomplished through the use of culture, serology, and DNA/RNA sequencing techniques.

Treatment of Infectious Diseases

The goal of treatment for an infectious disease is complete removal of the pathogen from the host and the restoration of normal physiologic function to damaged tissues. Most infectious diseases of humans are self-limiting in that they require little or no medical therapy for a complete cure. When an infectious process gains the upper hand and therapeutic intervention is essential, the choice of treatment may be medicinal through the use of antimicrobial agents or surgical by removing infected tissues. The decision about which therapeutic modality or combination of therapies to use is based on the extent, urgency, and location of the disease process; the pathogen; and the availability of effective antimicrobial agents.

Antibacterial Agents

Antibacterial agents are generally called *antibiotics*. Most antibiotics are actually produced by other microorganisms, primarily bacteria and fungi, as by-products of metabolism, and usually are effective only against other prokaryotic organisms. An antibiotic is considered *bactericidal* if it causes irreversible and lethal damage to the bacterial pathogen and *bacteriostatic* if its inhibitory effects on bacterial growth are reversed when the agent is eliminated. Antibiotics can be classified into families of compounds with related chemical structure and activity.

Not all antibiotics are effective against all pathogenic bacteria. Some agents are effective only against gram-negative bacteria, and others only gram-positive bacteria. The so-called *broad-spectrum antibiotics*, such as the newer cephalosporins, are active against a wide variety of gram-positive and gram-negative bacteria. The four basic mechanisms of antibiotic action are interference with a specific step in bacterial cell wall synthesis (e.g., penicillins, cephalosporins); inhibition of bacterial protein synthesis (e.g., aminoglycosides, tetracyclines); interruption of nucleic acid synthesis (e.g., fluoroquinolones, nalidixic acid); and interference with normal metabolism (e.g., sulfonamides, trimethoprim).

Of great concern is the increasing prevalence of bacteria resistant to the effects of antibiotics. The mechanisms by which bacteria acquire resistance to antibiotics include the production of enzymes that inactivate antibiotics, such as β-lactamases; genetic mutations that alter antibiotic binding sites; alternative metabolic pathways that bypass antibiotic activity; and changes in the filtration qualities of the bacterial cell wall that prevent access of antibiotics to the target site in the organism. It is the continuous search for a "better mousetrap" that makes anti-infective therapy such a fascinating aspect of infectious diseases.

Antiviral Agents

Until recently, few effective antiviral agents were available for treating human infections. The reason for this is host toxicity; viral replication requires the use of eukaryotic host cell enzymes, and the drugs that effectively interrupt viral replication are likely to interfere with host cell reproduction as well.

Almost all antiviral compounds are synthetic and, with few exceptions, their primary target is viral RNA or DNA synthesis. Like antibiotics, antiviral agents may be active against RNA viruses only, DNA viruses only, or occasionally both. A common class of antiviral drugs is the nucleoside analogs, which include agents such as acyclovir. These mimic the nucleoside building blocks of RNA and DNA. During active viral replication, the nucleoside analogs inhibit the viral DNA polymerase, preventing duplication of the viral genome and thus limiting the spread of infectious viral progeny to other susceptible host cells.

In response to the AIDS epidemic, there has been massive, albeit delayed, development of antiretroviral agents capable of targeting the replication of HIV, a retrovirus (see Chapter 16). These include the nucleoside analogs such as zidovudine as well as nonnucleoside inhibitors, which impair the synthesis of the HIV-specific enzyme reverse transcriptase. This key enzyme is essential for viral replication and has no counterpart in the infected eukaryotic host cells. Another class of antiviral agents developed solely for the treatment of HIV infections are the protease inhibitors. These drugs inhibit an HIV-specific enzyme that is necessary for late maturation events in the virus life cycle.

Antifungal Agents

The target site of the two most important families of antifungal agents is the cytoplasmic membranes of yeasts or molds. Fungal membranes differ from human cell membranes in that they contain the sterol ergosterol instead of cholesterol. The polyene family of antifungal compounds (e.g., amphotericin B, nystatin) preferentially binds to ergosterol and forms holes in the cell membrane, causing leakage of the fungal cell contents and, eventually, lysis of the cell. The imidazole class of drugs (e.g., fluconazole, itraconazole) inhibits the synthesis of ergosterol, thereby damaging the integrity of the fungal cytoplasmic membrane. Both types of drugs bind to a certain extent to the cholesterol component of host cell membranes and elicit a variety of toxic side effects in treated patients.

A new class of antifungal agents known as the echinocandins (e.g., caspofungin, micafungin, and anidulafungin) inhibit synthesis of the glucan in the cell wall, preventing the fungal cell wall from cross-linking. The lack of cross-linking causes the cell wall to become unstable and eventually lyse. The echinocandins are primarily active against *Candida* and *Aspergillus*.

Surgical Interventions

Before the discovery of antimicrobial agents, surgical removal of infected tissues, organs, or limbs was occasionally the only option available to prevent the demise of the infected host. Today, medicinal therapy with antibiotics and other anti-infective agents is an effective solution for most infectious diseases. However, surgical intervention is still an important option for cases in which the pathogen is resistant to available treatments. Surgical interventions may be used to hasten the recovery process by providing access to an infected site by antimicrobial agents (drainage of an abscess), cleaning the site (débridement), or removing infected organs or tissue (e.g., appendectomy). In some situations, surgery may be the only means to a complete cure, as in the case of endocarditis resulting in an infected heart valve, in which the diseased valve must be replaced with a mechanical or biologic valve to restore normal function. In other situations, surgical containment of a rapidly progressing infectious process such as gas gangrene may be the only means of saving a person's life.

SUMMARY CONCEPTS

■ The goal for treatment of infectious disease is complete removal of the infectious agent from the host and restoration of normal physiologic function to damaged tissues.

■ Treatment methods include the use of antimicrobial agents and, when necessary, surgical interventions that provide access to an infected site by antimicrobial agents (drainage of an abscess), clean the site (débridement), or remove infected organs or tissue (e.g., appendectomy).

New and Emerging Infectious Diseases

In recent years, the terms *emerging* (i.e., newly recognized) and *reemerging* (i.e., previously recognized) *infectious diseases* have entered the vocabulary of medical science. These infections also include deliberately emerging infections that are the result of bioterrorism.

Global Infectious Diseases

Aided by a global market and the ease of international travel, the end of the 20th century and the first years of the 21st century have witnessed the importation of a host of novel infectious diseases. Unexpected pathogens in the 1990s, such as the outbreak of the West Nile virus (WNV) in the New York City area, have become important reminders of emerging infections. In fact, WNV has become almost synonymous with mosquito-borne illness. Because WNV is a mosquito-borne disease and is transmitted to a number of susceptible avian (e.g., blue jays, crows, and hawks) and equine hosts, the potential for rapid and sustained spread of the disease across the United States was appreciated early. The disease ranges in intensity from a nonspecific febrile illness to fulminant meningoencephalitis. Efforts to prevent further spread of the disease are currently centered on surveillance of WNV-associated illness in birds, humans, and other mammals, as well as mosquito control.

In 2011, one of the largest foodborne outbreaks of *E. coli* emerged as a global threat. Beginning in May 2011, German public health authorities reported an outbreak of hemolytic-uremic syndrome. Within 3 weeks German authorities announced the source of the outbreak was cucumbers from Spain, a report later proven incorrect. As the investigation into the source of the outbreak continued, patients in surrounding countries also began to report illness. As the outbreak continued, epidemiologists focused their investigation on bean sprouts from a farm in Lower Saxony, Germany. They found that people who had eaten bean sprouts were 9 times more likely to develop bloody diarrhea versus those who had not consumed bean sprouts. Finally, more than one month following initiation of the outbreak, scientists at the Robert Koch Care institute isolated a novel strain of *E. coli*, known as O104:H4, from bean sprouts that had been contaminated with human feces. Interestingly, further study has demonstrated the O104:H4 strain of *E. coli* likely circulated in humans for 10 years prior to the outbreak.

As a result of the outbreak, Germany has implemented a policy to reduce the reporting time for potential outbreaks from 18 to 3 days. However, there are many obstacles to improving surveillance from reimbursement for medical tests, to communication between clinicians and public health authorities, to technologies for identification of relatedness among outbreak-causing diseases.

The worldwide movement of animals for commercial trade represents a substantial risk for translocation of zoonotic infections. In 2003, monkeypox, one of the orthopoxvirus family viruses, was introduced into the United States when a shipment of African Gambian giant rats was sold to dealers, one of whom housed the rats with prairie dogs intended for the pet market. The prairie dogs subsequently became ill and transmitted the infection to 71 humans, including prairie dog owners and veterinary staff caring for the animals.

These three scenarios highlight the rapidity with which novel or exotic diseases can be introduced into nonindigenous regions of the world and to a susceptible population. Although great strides in molecular microbiology have allowed for the rapid identification of new or rare microorganisms, the potential devastation in terms of human life and economic loss is great, underscoring the need to maintain resources for public health surveillance and intervention.

SUMMARY CONCEPTS

- The challenges associated with maintaining health throughout a global community are becoming increasingly apparent.

- Aided by a global market and the ease of international travel, the past decade has witnessed the importation and emergence of a host of novel infectious diseases. There is also the potential threat of the deliberate use of microorganisms as weapons of bioterrorism.

REVIEW EXERCISES

1. Newborn infants who have not yet developed intestinal flora are routinely given an intramuscular injection of vitamin K to prevent bleeding due to a deficiency in vitamin K–dependent coagulation factors.

   A. Use the concept of mutualism to explain why this is done.

2. Persons with human granulocytic ehrlichiosis may be coinfected with Lyme disease.

   A. Explain.

3. Persons with chronic lung disease are often taught to contact their health care provider when they notice a change in the color of their sputum (i.e., from white or clear to yellow or green tinged) because it might be a sign of a bacterial infection.

   A. Explain.

4. Microorganisms are capable of causing infection only if they can grow at the temperature of the infected body site.

A. Using this concept, explain the different sites of fungal infections due to the dermatophyte fungal species that cause tinea pedis (athlete's foot) and *Candida albicans*, which causes infections of the mouth (thrush) and female genitalia (vulvovaginitis).

BIBLIOGRAPHY

Centers for Disease Control and Prevention. Outbreak of West Nile-like viral encephalitis—New York, 1999. *MMWR Morb Mortal Wkly Rep.* 1999;48:845–849.

Centers for Disease Control and Prevention. Provisional surveillance summary of the West Nile virus epidemic—United States, January–November 2002. *MMWR Morb Mortal Wkly Rep.* 2002;51:1129–1133.

Centers for Disease Control and Prevention. Multistate outbreak of monkeypox—Illinois, Indiana, and Wisconsin, 2003. *MMWR Morb Mortal Wkly Rep.* 2003;52:537–540.

Centers for Disease Control and Prevention. Update: severe acute respiratory syndrome—Toronto, Canada, 2003. *MMWR Morb Mortal Wkly Rep.* 2003;52:547–550.

Centers for Disease Control and Prevention. Update: severe acute respiratory syndrome—worldwide and United States, 2003. *MMWR Morb Mortal Wkly Rep.* 2003;52:664–665.

Centers for Disease Control and Prevention. Ongoing multistate outbreak of *Escherichia coli* serotype O157:H7 infections associated with consumption of fresh spinach—United States, September 2006. *MMWR Morb Mortal Wkly Rep.* 2006;55(Dispatch):1–2.

Centers for Disease Control and Prevention. Epidemiology of HIV/AIDS—United States, 1981–2005. *MMWR Morb Mortal Wkly Rep.* 2006;55(21):589–592.

Drusano GL. Antimicrobial pharmacodynamics: Critical interactions of "bug and drug." *Nat Rev Microbiol.* 2004;2:289–300.

Dumler JS, Bakken JS. Ehrlichial diseases in humans: emerging tick-borne infections. *Clin Infect Dis.* 1995;20:1102–1110.

Dunne WM Jr. Bacterial adhesion: seen any good biofilms lately? *Clin Microbiol Rev.* 2002;15:155–166.

Grad YH, Lipsitch M, Feldgarden M, et al. Genomic epidemiology of the Escherichia coli O104:H4 outbreaks in Europe, 2011. *Proc Natl Acad Sci U S A.* 2012;109(8):3065–3070.

Jernigan DM, Raghunathan PL, Bell BP, et al. Investigation of bioterrorism-related anthrax, United States, 2001: epidemiologic findings. *Emerg Infect Dis.* 2002;8:1019–1028.

Lampiris HW, Maddix DS. Clinical use of antimicrobial agents. In: Katzung BG, Masters SB, Trevor A, eds. *Basic and Clinical Pharmacology.* 12th ed. New York, NY: McGraw-Hill Lange; 2007:901–913.

Marano N, Arquin PM, Pappaloanou M. Impact of globalization and animal trade in infection disease ecology. *Emerg Infect Dis.* 2007;13(12):1807–1808.

McFee RB. Global infections—Avian influenza and other significant emerging pathogens—an overview. *Dis Mon.* 2007;53:343–347.

Mellmann A, Harmsen D, Cummings CA, et al. Prospective genomic characterization of the German enterohemorrhagic *Escherichia coli* O104:H4 outbreak by rapid next generation sequencing technology. *PLoS One.* 2011;6(7):e22751.

Morens DM, Folkers GK, Fauci AS. The challenge of emerging and re-emerging diseases. *Nature.* 2004;430(6996):242–249.

Nolte FS, Caliendo AM. Molecular microbiology. In: Versalovic J, Carroll KC, Funke G, et al., eds. *Manual of Clinical Microbiology.* 10th ed. Washington, DC: American Society for Microbiology; 2011:27–59.

Prince AS. Biofilms, antimicrobial resistance, and airway infection. *New Engl J Med.* 2002;347:1110–1111.

Ryan ET, Wilson ME, Kain KC. Illness after international travel. *New Engl J Med.* 2002;347:505–516.

Stone JH, Dierberg K, Aram G, et al. Human monocytic ehrlichiosis. *JAMA.* 2004;292:2263–2270.

Turner M. Germany learns from *E. coli* outbreak: government plans to upgrade its disease-reporting processes. *Nature News* [online]. September 12, 2011. Available at http://www.nature.com/news/2011/110912/full/news.2011.530.html. Accessed January 6, 2014.

Tyler KL. Prions and prion diseases of the central nervous system (neurodegenerative diseases). In: Mandell GL, Bennett JE, Dolin R, eds. *Mandell, Douglas, and Bennett's Principles and Practice of Infectious Diseases.* 5th ed. Philadelphia, PA: Churchill Livingstone; 2000:1971–1985.

Writing Committee of the WHO Consultation on Clinical Aspects of Pandemic (H1N1) 2009 Influenza. Clinical aspects of pandemic 2009 Influenza A (H1N1) Infection. *New Engl J Med* 2010;362(18):1708–1719.

Porth Essentials Resources

Explore these additional resources to enhance learning for this chapter:

- NCLEX-Style Questions and Other Resources on the**Point**, http://thePoint.lww.com/PorthEssentials4e
- Study Guide for Essentials of Pathophysiology
- Adaptive Learning | Powered by PrepU, http://thepoint.lww.com/prepu

C h a p t e r 15

Innate and Adaptive Immunity

The immune system has evolved to defend against bacteria, viruses, and other foreign substances. Through recognition of molecular patterns, the immune system can distinguish itself from foreign substances and can discriminate potentially harmful from non-harmful agents. It also defends against abnormal cells and molecules that periodically develop. Although the immune response normally is protective, it also can produce undesirable effects such as when the response is excessive, as in allergies, or when it recognizes self-tissue as foreign, as in autoimmune disease. This chapter is divided into three parts: (1) introduction to the immune system, (2) innate immunity, (3) adaptive immunity, and (4) developmental aspects of the immune system.

Introduction to the Immune System

The term *immunity* has come to mean protection from disease and, more specifically, infectious disease. The collective, coordinated response of the cells and molecules of the immune system is called the *immune response*. Although the relationship between microbes and infectious diseases dates far back in history, it has only been within the last 30 to 40 years that an understanding of the cellular and biochemical mechanisms involved in the immune response has begun to emerge. Advances in cell culture techniques, immunochemistry, recombinant deoxyribonucleic acid (DNA) technology, and the creation of genetically altered animals, such as "transgenic" and "knockout" mice, have transformed immunology from a largely descriptive science to one of immune phenomena that can be explained in structural and biochemical terms.

Innate and Adaptive Immunity

There are two host defenses that cooperate to protect the body—the early, rapid responses of innate immunity, and the very effective but later responses of adaptive immunity. As the first line of defense, *innate* (also called *natural* or *native*) *immunity* consists of the physical, chemical, molecular, and cellular defenses that are in place before infection and can function immediately as an effective barrier to microbes. *Adaptive* (also called *specific* or *acquired*) *immunity* is the second major immune defense, responding less rapidly than innate immunity but more effectively. Adaptive immunity uses focused recognition of each unique type of foreign agent followed, in days, by an amplified and effective response.

The major components of innate immunity are the skin and mucous membranes, phagocytic leukocytes (mainly neutrophils and macrophages), specialized lymphocytes (the natural killer cells), and several plasma proteins, including the proteins of the complement system (Fig. 15-1). The innate immune system is able to distinguish self from nonself and is able to recognize and react against various classes of microbial agents. The response of the innate immune system is rapid, usually within minutes to hours, and prevents the establishment of infection and deeper tissue penetration of microorganisms. The effector responses used by the innate immune system to eliminate the microbes are very similar for different classes of microorganisms. Although most innate responses are very effective in controlling and destroying

the invading agent, pathogenic microbes have evolved several approaches to evade innate defenses. The microorganisms not controlled by innate immunity are usually controlled by the more specific approaches of adaptive immunity.

The adaptive immune system consists of two groups of lymphocytes and their products, including antibodies (see Fig. 15-1). Whereas the cells of the innate immune system recognize structures shared by classes of microorganisms, the cells of the adaptive immune system are capable of recognizing numerous microbial and noninfectious substances and developing a unique specific immune response for each substance. Substances that elicit adaptive immune responses are called *antigens*. A memory of the substance is also developed so that a repeat exposure to the same microbe or agent produces a quicker and more vigorous response.

There are two types of adaptive immune responses: humoral and cell-mediated immunity. *Humoral immunity* is mediated by molecules called *antibodies* that are produced by cells called *B lymphocytes*. Antibodies are secreted into the circulation and mucosal fluid, where they neutralize or eliminate extracellular microbes and microbial toxins. One of the important functions of

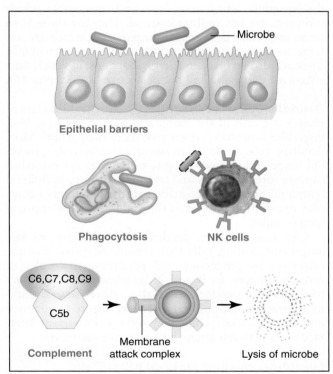

A   **Innate immunity**

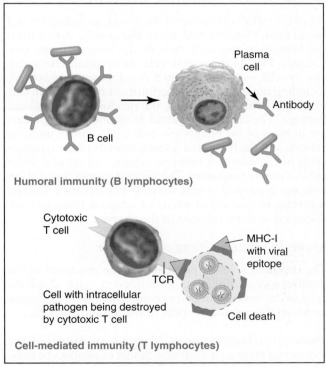

B   **Adaptive immunity**

FIGURE 15-1. Mechanisms of innate and adaptive immunity. **(A)** The major effectors of the innate immune system include the immediately available epithelial barriers, phagocytic leukocytes, natural killer (NK) cells, and complement system. These effectors are in place before an encounter with an infectious agent and provide rapid protection against infection. **(B)** Adaptive immunity develops later than innate immunity, is acquired through previous experience with a foreign agent, and is mediated by T and B lymphocytes and their products. Humoral immunity is provided by B lymphocytes that differentiate into antibody-producing plasma cells that interact with and protect against microbes that are present in the blood or on mucosal surfaces. Cell-mediated immunity is provided by cytotoxic T cells that destroy cells infected with intracellular pathogens. MHC-1, major histocompatibility complex-1; TCR, T-cell receptor.

humoral immunity is to stop microbes that are present on mucosal surfaces and in the blood from gaining access to and colonizing body tissues. *Cell-mediated immunity*, which defends against intracellular microbes such as viruses, is provided by cells called *T lymphocytes*. Some T lymphocytes activate phagocytes to destroy microbes that have been engulfed, whereas others kill any type of host cell that is harboring microbes.

Recent studies have shown that essential, cooperative interactions exist between innate and adaptive immunity. Innate immunity communicates to lymphocytes involved in adaptive immunity the characteristics of the pathogen and information about its intracellular or extracellular location. The innate immune response also stimulates and influences the nature of adaptive immune responses. At the effector stage of immunity, the adaptive immune response amplifies and increases its efficiency by recruitment and activation of additional phagocytes and molecules of the innate immune system. Both innate and adaptive immunity destroy the invading agent by using the effector responses of phagocytosis and the complement system. Thus, immunity is truly an interactive, cooperative effort.

Cells of the Immune System

All of the cellular elements of the blood, including the red blood cells, platelets, and white blood cells, derive from the hematopoietic stem cells in the bone marrow (see Chapter 11). As these stem cells differentiate, they give rise to cells with more limited developmental potential, including the immediate progenitors of the two main categories of white blood cells, the myeloid and lymphoid lineages. The common myeloid progenitor is the precursor of most of the phagocytic cells of the innate immune system, and the lymphoid lineage consists of the lymphocytes of the adaptive immune system and natural killer cells of innate immunity. The general properties of these cells are presented in this section, whereas their specific functions in relation to innate or adaptive immunity are discussed in those sections of the chapter.

Myeloid Lineage Phagocytic Cells

The common myeloid progenitor is the precursor of the monocytes/macrophages, granulocytes, and dendritic cells of the innate immune system. These three cell types make up the phagocytic cells of the immune system.

Monocytes/Macrophages. Macrophages are part of the monocytic phagocyte system, a family of phagocytic cells. They are resident in almost all tissues and are the mature form of monocytes, which circulate in the blood and continually migrate into tissues, where they differentiate into macrophages. Macrophages are relatively long-lived cells and perform several different functions during the innate and adaptive immune responses. One function is to engulf and kill invading microorganisms. In this phagocytic role they are an important first-line defense in innate immunity, and they dispose of pathogens and infected cells targeted for disposal by an adaptive immune response.

Although their primary role is in phagocytosis, macrophages also function as *antigen-presenting cells* of the adaptive immune response. That is, they process and present molecules of foreign antigens to the lymphocytes involved in adaptive immunity. Macrophages also help induce inflammation, and they secrete signaling proteins that activate other immune cells and recruit them into an immune response. In addition to these immune-system roles, macrophages act as general scavenger cells in the body, clearing dead cells and cell debris.

Granulocytes. The granulocytes are so called because they have densely staining granules in the cytoplasm. There are three types of granulocytes—neutrophils, eosinophils, and basophils—which are distinguished by the staining properties of their granules. Compared to the macrophages, they are relatively short-lived, surviving only a few days, and are produced in increased numbers during an immune response. Neutrophils, which are named for their neutral-staining granules, are the most numerous of the granulocytes and the most important cell in innate immunity. They take up a variety of microorganisms by phagocytosis and efficiently destroy them using degradative enzymes and other antimicrobial substances stored in their cytoplasmic granules. The protective functions of the basophils, which stain blue, and eosinophils, which stain red, are less well understood. They are thought to be an important defense against parasites, which are too large to be ingested by macrophages and neutrophils. They are also involved in allergic reactions, in which their effects are damaging and not protective (see Chapter 16).

Dendritic Cells. The dendritic cells are the third class of phagocytic cells of the immune system. They have long fingerlike processes, which give them their name. Most dendritic cells are found as immature cells under epithelial tissue and in most organs, where they are poised to capture foreign agents and transport them to peripheral lymphoid organs. Once activated, they undergo a complex maturation process as they migrate to the regional lymph nodes.

Like macrophages, dendritic cells function as key antigen-presenting cells that initiate adaptive immune responses by processing and presenting molecules of foreign antigens to B and T lymphocytes. Both macrophages and dendritic cells also release several communication molecules that direct the nature of adaptive immune responses. Thus, they serve as important intermediaries between innate and adaptive immunity.

Lymphocytes and Natural Killer Cells

The common lymphoid progenitor in the bone marrow gives rise to two types of antigen-specific lymphocytes—the B and T lymphocytes of the adaptive immune system—and a third type of lymphocyte, the natural killer cell, that does not respond to specific antigens but is considered part of the innate immune system. The B and T lymphocytes are the only cells that produce specific receptors for antigen and thus are the key mediators of adaptive immunity. A naive lymphocyte is a mature

B or T lymphocyte that has not previously encountered antigen or is not the progeny of an antigen-stimulated mature lymphocyte.

B lymphocytes (B cells) are the only cells capable of producing antibodies; therefore, they are the cells that mediate humoral immunity. B cells use membrane-bound antibodies to recognize a wide variety of proteins, polysaccharides, lipids, and small chemicals. These antigens may be expressed on microbial surfaces or they may be in soluble forms (toxins). In response to antigen and other signals, B cells differentiate into plasma cells which produce antibody. The secreted antibodies enter the circulation and mucosal fluids and bind to microbes before they have a chance to colonize body tissues.

T lymphocytes (T cells) are responsible for cell-mediated immunity. The antigen receptors of most T lymphocytes only recognize peptide fragments of protein antigens that are bound to specialized peptide display molecules called *major histocompatibility complex (MHC) molecules* on the surface of antigen-presenting cells. Among T lymphocytes are a subset of T cells called *helper T cells* that help B lymphocytes produce antibodies and help phagocytic cells destroy ingested pathogens, and another subset called *cytotoxic T cells* that kill or lyse intracellular microbes.

Although all lymphocytes are morphologically similar, they vary in terms of lineage, cell membrane molecules and receptors, function, and response to antigen. These cells are often distinguished by surface proteins. The standard nomenclature for these proteins is the CD (clusters of differentiation) numeric designation (CD4+, CD8+), which is used to delineate surface proteins that define a particular cell type or stage of cell differentiation and are recognized by a "cluster" of antibodies.

The CD classification is now widely used in clinical medicine and experimental immunology. In human immunodeficiency virus (HIV) infection, for example, a decline or rise in the CD4+ helper T-cell count is used to follow the progression of the disease and response to treatment. Further investigation of the CD molecules has shown that they are not merely phenotypic markers of cell type but are themselves involved in a variety of lymphocyte functions, including promotion of cell-to-cell adhesion and transduction of signals that lead to lymphocyte activation.

The third type of lymphocyte, the natural killer (NK) cell is part of the innate immune system and may be the first line of defense against viral infections. The NK cell also has the ability to recognize and kill tumor cells, abnormal body cells, and cells infected with *intracellular pathogens*, such as viruses and intracellular bacteria.

Organs and Tissues of the Immune System

The cells of the immune system are present in large numbers in the central and peripheral lymphoid organs. These organs and tissues are widely distributed in the body and provide different, but often overlapping, functions (Fig. 15-2). The lymphoid organs are connected by networks of lymph channels, blood vessels, and capillaries. The immune cells continuously circulate through the various tissues and organs to seek out and destroy foreign material.

Central Lymphoid Tissues

The central lymphoid tissues, the bone marrow and thymus gland, provide the environment for immune cell production and maturation (see Chapter 11). The specialized microenvironment of the bone marrow provides signals both for the development of lymphocyte progenitors from the hematopoietic stem cells and for the subsequent differentiation of B cells.

T-cell progenitors migrate from the bone marrow to the thymus where the process of maturation occurs. The thymus is an elongated, bilobed structure located in the neck region of the chest above the heart. The function of the thymus is central to the development of the immune system because it generates mature, immunocompetent T lymphocytes expressing appropriate receptors. The thymus is fully formed and functional at birth. It persists

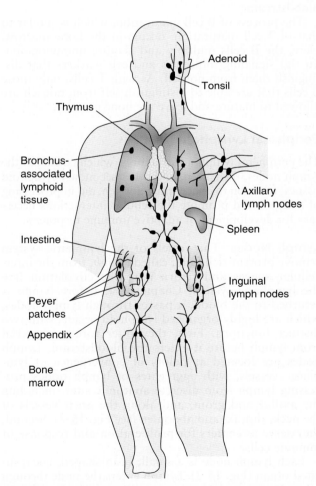

FIGURE 15-2. Central and peripheral lymphoid organs and tissues.

as a large organ until about the time of puberty, when T-cell development and proliferation are reduced and the thymus begins slowly regressing and is replaced by adipose tissue. Nevertheless, some thymus tissue persists and can be restimulated under conditions that demand rapid T-cell proliferation.

Precursor T (pre-T) cells enter the thymus as functionally and phenotypically immature T cells. They undergo cycles of proliferation and selection as they move from the cortical to medullary compartments of the thymus. Rapid cell multiplication, maturation, and selection occur in the cortex under the influence of the microenvironment, thymic hormones, and cytokines. As the T cells multiply and mature, they acquire T-cell receptors, surface markers that distinguish among the different types of T cells, and antigens that distinguish them from nonself. Only those T cells able to recognize foreign antigens and distinguish self from nonself are allowed to mature and leave the thymus. This process is called *thymic selection*. The thymus must be extremely thorough in eliminating self-reactive cells to ensure that autoimmune reactivity and disease do not result. Mature, immunocompetent T-helper and T-cytotoxic cells leave the thymus in 2 to 3 days and enter the peripheral lymphoid tissues through the bloodstream.

The process of B-cell maturation, which is similar to that of T-cell maturation, occurs in the bone marrow. Here, the B cells multiply and acquire immunoglobulin (Ig) signaling molecules and cell markers that distinguish them from nonself. As with T cells, only those B cells that are able to distinguish self from nonself are allowed to mature and leave the bone marrow.

Peripheral Lymphoid Tissues

The peripheral lymphoid structures, which consist of the lymph nodes, the spleen, and other secondary lymphoid tissues, function to concentrate antigen, aid in processing of antigen, and promote the cellular interactions necessary for development of adaptive immune responses.

Lymph Nodes. The vessels of the lymphatic system remove protein-rich fluid, called *lymph*, from the intercellular spaces and return it to the circulation (see the lymphatic system, Chapter 17). Before lymph is returned to the blood, it passes through lymph nodes, which are highly organized lymphoid organs with two distinct functions. First, they filter foreign material from lymph before it enters the bloodstream. Lymph nodes are located at points of convergence of lymphatic vessels, with aggregates of lymph nodes processing lymph from discrete anatomic sites, including the axillae and groin, and along the great vessels of the neck, thorax, and abdomen (see Fig. 15-2). Second, they serve as centers for proliferation and response of immune cells.

Each lymph node is a small, bean-shaped, encapsulated organ (Fig. 15-3). Lymph enters the node through afferent vessels that penetrate the capsule, and leaves through efferent vessels located in the deep indentation

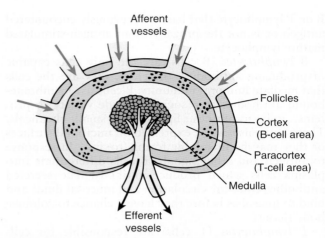

FIGURE 15-3. Structural features of a lymph node. Lymphocytes and macrophages flow slowly through the node, which allows for trapping and interactions of antigens and immune cells.

of the hilus. Lymphocytes and macrophages flow slowly through the node, which allows trapping and interaction of antigen and immune cells. As lymph passes through the lymph nodes, antigen-presenting cells in the nodes are able to sample the antigens that enter through the epithelia. In addition, microbes that bypass the epithelial barriers of the innate immune system are captured by resident dendritic cells and transported to draining lymph nodes.

A lymph node is divided into several specialized areas: an outer cortex, a paracortex, and an inner medulla. B lymphocytes are more abundant in the follicles located in the outer cortex. The T lymphocytes proliferate on antigenic stimulation and migrate to the follicles, where they interact with B lymphocytes. These activated follicles become germinal centers, containing macrophages, follicular dendritic cells, and maturing T and B cells. Activated B cells then migrate to the medulla, where they complete their maturation into plasma cells. These cells stay localized in the lymph node but release large quantities of antibodies into the circulation.

Spleen. The spleen is a large, ovoid secondary lymphoid organ located high in the left abdominal cavity. The spleen filters antigens from the blood and is important in the response to systemic infections. The spleen is composed of red and white pulp. The red pulp is well supplied with arteries and is the area where senescent and injured red blood cells are removed. The white pulp contains concentrated areas of B and T lymphocytes permeated by macrophages and dendritic cells. A sequence of activation events similar to that seen in the lymph nodes occurs in the spleen.

Other Secondary Lymphoid Tissues. Other secondary lymphoid tissues include the *mucosa-associated lymphoid tissues* (MALT). These nonencapsulated clusters of lymphoid tissues are located around membranes lining the respiratory, digestive, and urogenital tracts. These gateways into the body must harbor the immune cells needed to respond to a large and diverse population of microorganisms. In some tissues, the lymphocytes congregate in loose clusters, but in other tissues such as the tonsils, Peyer patches in the intestine, and the appendix, organized structures are evident (see Fig. **15-2**). These tissues contain all the necessary cell components (i.e., T cells, B cells, macrophages, and dendritic cells) for an immune response. Because of the continuous stimulation of the lymphocytes in these tissues by microorganisms constantly entering the body, large numbers of plasma cells are evident. Immunity at the mucosal layers helps to exclude many pathogens and thus protects the vulnerable internal organs.

Cytokines That Mediate and Regulate Immunity

Although cells of both the innate and adaptive immune systems communicate critical information by cell-to-cell contact, many interactions and effector responses depend on the secretion of short-acting soluble molecules called *cytokines*. The sources and properties of the main cytokines that participate in innate and adaptive immunity are summarized in Table 15-1.

General Properties of Cytokines

Cytokines are low–molecular-weight regulatory proteins that are produced by cells of the innate and adaptive immune systems and that mediate many of the actions of these cells. The names of specific types of cytokines were derived from the biologic properties first ascribed to them. For example, *interleukins* (ILs) were found to be made by leukocytes and to act on leukocytes, and *interferons* (IFNs) were found to interfere with virus multiplication.

Although cytokines have many diverse actions, all share several important properties. Most cytokines are released at cell-to-cell interfaces, where they bind to specific receptors on the membrane surface of their target cells. All cytokines are secreted in a brief, self-limited manner. They are not usually stored as preformed molecules and their synthesis is limited to new gene transcription resulting from cellular activation. The short half-life of cytokines ensures that excessive immune responses and systemic activation do not occur.

The actions of cytokines are often pleiotropic and redundant. *Pleiotropism* refers to the ability of a cytokine to act on different cell types. For example, IL-2, initially discovered as a T-cell growth factor, is also known to affect the growth of B cells and NK cells. Interferon-γ is the key macrophage-activating cytokine that functions in both innate and adaptive immune responses. Although pleiotropism allows cytokines to mediate diverse effects, it greatly limits their use for therapeutic purposes because of numerous unwanted side effects. *Redundancy* refers to the ability of different cytokines to stimulate the same or overlapping biologic functions. Because of this redundancy, antagonists against a single cytokine may not have functional consequences because other cytokines may compensate.

Not only are the actions of cytokines pleiotropic and redundant, but the same cytokines may be produced by several different cell types. For example, IL-1 can be produced by virtually all leukocytes, endothelial cells, and fibroblasts. Cytokines often influence the synthesis and actions of other cytokines. The ability of one cytokine to stimulate the production of others often leads to cascades in which the second and third cytokines may mediate the biologic effects of the first. Cytokines may also serve as antagonists to inhibit the action of another cytokine, or in some cases they may produce additive or greater than anticipated effects.

Cytokine actions may be local or systemic. Most cytokines act close to where they are produced, acting on the same cell that secreted the cytokine (autocrine mechanism), or they may influence the activity of nearby cells (paracrine mechanism). When produced in large amounts, cytokines may enter the bloodstream and exert their action on distant cells in an endocrine manner; the best examples are IL-1 and tumor necrosis factor-α (TNF-α), which produce the systemic acute-phase response during inflammation.

Chemokines

Chemokines are cytokines that stimulate the migration and activation of immune and inflammatory cells. There are two major subclasses, termed *CC chemokines* and *CXC chemokines,* which are distinguished by their amino acid sequence. The largest family, the CC chemokines, attracts mononuclear leukocytes to sites of chronic inflammation. The CXC chemokines attract neutrophils to sites of acute inflammation.

Chemokines are implicated in a number of acute and chronic diseases, including atherosclerosis, rheumatoid arthritis, inflammatory bowel disease (Crohn disease and ulcerative colitis), allergic asthma and chronic bronchitis, multiple sclerosis, systemic lupus erythematosus, and HIV infection. To enter target cells, HIV type 1 requires two distinct elements: the CD4 recognition molecule of the helper T cell and either the CXCR4 or CCR5 chemokine. The targeting of T cells and monocytes allows HIV-1 access to sanctuary sites throughout the body and also cripples the CD4$^+$ T-helper cell that orchestrates antiviral immunity (discussed in Chapter 16).

Colony-Stimulating Factors

Colony-stimulating factors (CSFs) are cytokines that stimulate bone marrow pluripotent stem and progenitor or precursor cells to produce large numbers of platelets, erythrocytes, lymphocytes, neutrophils, monocytes, eosinophils, basophils, and dendritic cells. The CSFs were named according to the type of target cell on which they act (see Table 15-1). Granulocyte-monocyte colony-stimulating factor (GM-CSF) acts on

TABLE 15-1	Cytokines of Innate and Adaptive Immunity	
Cytokines	**Source**	**Biologic Activity**
Interleukin-1 (IL-1)	Macrophages, endothelial cells, some epithelial cells	Wide variety of biologic effects; activates endothelium in inflammation; induces fever and acute-phase response; stimulates neutrophil production
Interleukin-2 (IL-2)	CD4+, CD8+ T cells	Growth factor for activated T cells; induces synthesis of other cytokines; activates cytotoxic T lymphocytes and NK cells
Interleukin-3 (IL-3)	CD4+ T cells	Growth factor for progenitor hematopoietic cells
Interleukin-4 (IL-4)	CD4+ T_H2 cells, mast cells	Promotes growth and survival of T, B, and mast cells; causes T_H2 cell differentiation; activates B cells and eosinophils and induces IgE-type responses
Interleukin-5 (IL-5)	CD4+ T_H2 cells	Induces eosinophil growth and development
Interleukin-6 (IL-6)	Macrophages, endothelial cells, T lymphocytes	Stimulates the liver to produce mediators of acute-phase inflammatory response; also induces proliferation of antibody-producing cells by the adaptive immune system
Interleukin-7 (IL-7)	Bone marrow stromal cells	Primary function in adaptive immunity; stimulates pre-B cells and thymocyte development and proliferation
Interleukin-8 (IL-8)	Macrophages, endothelial cells	Primary function in adaptive immunity; chemoattracts neutrophils and T lymphocytes; regulates lymphocyte homing and neutrophil infiltration
Interleukin-10 (IL-10)	Macrophages, some T-helper cells	Inhibitor of activated macrophages and dendritic cells; decreases inflammation by inhibiting T_H1 cells and release of IL-12 from macrophages
Interleukin-12 (IL-12)	Macrophages, dendritic cells	Enhances NK cell cytotoxicity in innate immunity; induces T_H1 cell differentiation in adaptive immunity
Type I interferons (IFN-α, IFN-β)	Macrophages, fibroblasts	Inhibit viral replication; activate NK cells; increase expression of MHC-I molecules on virus-infected cells
Interferon-γ (IFN-γ)	NK cells, CD4+ and CD8+ T lymphocytes	Activates macrophages in both innate immune responses and adaptive cell-mediated immune responses; increases expression of MHC-I and -II and antigen processing and presentation
Tumor necrosis factor-α (TNF-α)	Macrophages, T cells	Induces inflammation, fever, and acute-phase response; activates neutrophils and endothelial cells; kills cells through apoptosis
Chemokines	Macrophages, endothelial cells, T lymphocytes	Large family of structurally similar cytokines that stimulate leukocyte movement and regulate the migration of leukocytes from the blood to the tissues
Granulocyte-monocyte CSF (GM-CSF)	T cells, macrophages, endothelial cells, fibroblasts	Promotes neutrophil, eosinophil, and monocyte maturation and growth; activates mature granulocytes
Granulocyte CSF (G-CSF)	Macrophages, fibroblasts, endothelial cells	Promotes growth and maturation of neutrophils consumed in inflammatory reactions
Monocyte CSF (M-CSF)	Macrophages, activated T cells, endothelial cells	Promotes growth and maturation of mononuclear phagocytes

CSF, colony-stimulating factor; MHC, major histocompatibility complex; NK, natural killer; T_H1, T-helper type 1; T_H2, T-helper type 2.

the granulocyte-monocyte progenitor cells to produce monocytes, neutrophils, and dendritic cells; granulocyte colony-stimulating factor (G-CSF) specifically induces neutrophil proliferation; and macrophage colony-stimulating factor (M-CSF) directs the mononuclear phagocyte progenitor. Other cytokines, including IL-3, IL-7, and IL-11, also influence hematopoiesis. Recombinant CSF molecules are currently being used to increase the success rates of bone marrow transplantations. The availability of recombinant CSFs and cytokines offers the possibility of several clinical therapies where stimulation or inhibition of the immune response or cell production is desirable.

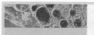 **SUMMARY CONCEPTS**

■ Immunity is the resistance to a disease that is provided by the immune system. *Innate immunity*, which is the first line of defense against microbial agents, can distinguish between self and nonself but not among specific pathogens. *Adaptive immunity*, which involves humoral and cell-mediated immune responses that react to a unique antigen, can distinguish self from nonself, and develop immunologic memory, allowing a prompt and heightened response on subsequent encounters with the same antigen.

■ The cellular components of innate and adaptive immunity include the phagocytic cells that are of myeloid lineage and the lymphocytes that are of lymphoid lineage. The phagocytic granulocytes, macrophages, and dendritic cells, along with the natural killer (NK) cells, participate in innate immune responses, and the B and T lymphocytes participate in adaptive immune responses.

■ The tissues of the immune system consist of the generative or central lymphoid organs in which B and T lymphocytes originate and mature and the peripheral lymphoid organs in which adaptive immune responses to microbes is initiated.

■ Cytokines are soluble proteins secreted by cells of both the innate and adaptive immune systems that mediate many of the functions of these cells. Some cytokines mediate inflammation or interfere with viral replication. Chemokines are cytokines that stimulate the migration and activation of immune and inflammatory cells. Colony-stimulating factors are cytokines that stimulate the growth and differentiation of bone marrow progenitors of immune cells.

Innate Immunity

The innate immune system consists of the epithelial barriers; phagocytic neutrophils, macrophages, dendritic cells, NK cells; and several plasma proteins, including those of the complement system. These mechanisms are present in the body before an encounter with an infectious agent and are rapidly activated by microbes before the development of adaptive immunity. The innate immune system also interacts with and directs adaptive immune responses.

With the ever-expanding wealth of information on immune system function, it is becoming clear that the innate immune system not only protects against microbial agents, but may also play a role in the pathogenesis of disease. Among the functions of the innate immune system is induction of a complex cascade of events known as the *inflammatory response* (discussed in Chapter 3). Recent evidence suggests that low-grade inflammation and activation of the innate immune system play a key role in the pathogenesis of a number of disorders, such as atherosclerosis and coronary artery disease, bronchial asthma, type 2 diabetes mellitus, rheumatoid arthritis, multiple sclerosis, and systemic lupus erythematosus.

Epithelial Barriers

Our outer body surfaces are protected by epithelia, which provide physical and chemical barriers between the internal environment and the pathogens of the external world. Epithelia include the epidermis of the skin and linings of the respiratory, gastrointestinal, and urogenital tracts. The intact skin is a formidable physical barrier because of its closely packed cells, multiple layers, continuous shedding of cells, and presence of the protective protein keratin. In addition to its barrier function, the skin has chemicals that create a salty and acidic environment, and antibacterial proteins, such as the enzyme lysozyme, that inhibit the colonization of microorganisms and aid in their destruction.

The mucous membrane linings of the gastrointestinal, respiratory, and urogenital tracts are protected by sheets of tightly packed epithelial cells that block the entry of microbes and destroy them by secreting antimicrobial enzymes, proteins, and peptides. Specialized cells in these linings secrete a viscous material called *mucus*. Mucus traps and washes away microorganisms, especially with the help of additional secretions such as saliva. Also in the lower respiratory tract, hairlike structures called *cilia* protrude through the epithelial cells. The synchronous action of the cilia moves many microbes trapped in the mucus toward the throat. The physiologic responses of coughing and sneezing further aid in their removal from the body.

Once microbes are trapped, various chemical defenses come into play. These include lysozyme, a hydrolytic enzyme capable of cleaving the walls of bacterial cells; complement, which binds and aggregates bacteria to increase their susceptibility to phagocytosis or disrupt their lipid membrane; and members of the *collectin* family of surfactant proteins (e.g., surfactants [SP]-A and SP-D) in the respiratory tract (see Chapter 21). The best-defined function of the surfactants is their ability to opsonize pathogens, including bacteria and viruses, and to facilitate phagocytosis by innate immune cells such as macrophages. In the stomach and intestines, death of microbes results from the action of digestive enzymes, acidic conditions, and secretions of *defensins*, small cationic peptides that rapidly kill many types of bacteria by disrupting their membrane.

Cells of Innate Immunity

Some pathogens can penetrate the epithelial barriers of the host and cause infection, particularly when the barrier has been breached as in wounds, burns, or loss of the body's internal epithelia. The subsequent innate immune response to the penetration of these invaders is initiated by several types of immune cells with receptors for recognition of general groups of microbes. The key cells of innate immunity include phagocytic leukocytes and NK cells.

Several types of phagocytic leukocytes recognize and kill infectious agents during an innate immune response. The early-responding phagocytic cell is the *neutrophil*, followed shortly by the more efficient, multifunctional *macrophage*. Phagocytes are activated to engulf and digest microbes that attach to their cell membrane. Once the cell is activated and the microbe ingested, the cell generates digestive enzymes and toxic oxygen and nitrogen intermediates (e.g., hydrogen peroxide or nitric oxide) that kill the pathogen. The phagocytic killing of microorganisms helps prevent the spread of infectious agents until adaptive immunity can be marshaled.

Dendritic cells, which are derived from bone marrow cells and related in lineage to the macrophage, also play important roles in the innate immune response to infections and in linking innate and adaptive immune responses (to be discussed in section on antigen-presenting cells). One subpopulation of dendritic cells governs the early response to viral infections. They recognize phagocytosed viruses and produce type 1 interferons that have potent antiviral actions.

NK cells are a class of lymphocytes that recognize infected and stressed cells and respond by killing these cells. Activation of NK cells triggers the release of cytoplasmic granules toward the infected cells. These NK granules contain molecules that form pores in the cell membrane and other molecules that induce apoptosis (programmed cell death). NK cells control their responses by using both activating and inhibitory receptors (Fig. 15-4). Their activating receptors (i.e., killer cell receptors) recognize altered host molecules expressed on stressed tissue cells that may be infected with intracellular microbes. The inhibitory receptors on NK cells recognize molecules on normal host cells and function to stop the killing response. This control ensures that normal body cells are not inappropriately destroyed. In contrast to the cytotoxic T lymphocytes of the adaptive immune system, which need to undergo amplification and maturation to become cytotoxic, the NK cell is directly programmed to kill foreign cells.

Pathogen Recognition

The ability of leukocytes and epithelial cells to participate in innate immunity depends on their first recognizing molecules that are a normal component of microbes but not host cells. These components are often essential for infectivity and cannot be mutated to allow the microbe to evade destruction. The receptors that the innate immune system uses to recognize and react against microbes are expressed on phagocytic leukocytes, NK cells, and other cells that participate in defense against various classes of microbes. These receptors are molecules that first tag the microbe and then bind it to the effector cell of the innate immune system. Microbial binding results in effector cell activation, phagocytosis, and subsequent killing of the microbe. Several classes of receptors have been identified that are specific for different types of microbial products including pattern receptors, Toll-like receptors, and serum proteins (e.g., complement proteins) that promote phagocytosis.

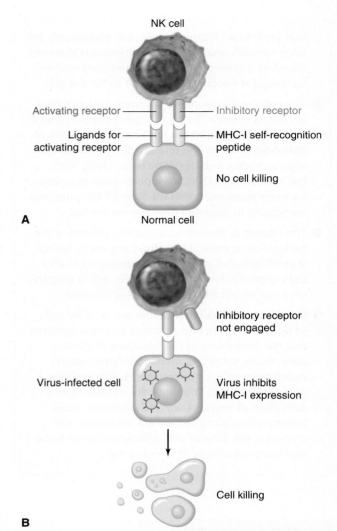

FIGURE 15-4. Natural killer (NK) cell receptors. **(A)** NK cells express activating receptors that respond to ligands from virus-infected or injured cells and inhibiting receptors that bind to the class I major histocompatibility complex (MHC-I) self-recognition molecules expressed by normal cells. Normal cells are not killed because inhibitory signals from normal MHC-I molecules override activating signals. **(B)** In virus-infected or tumor cells, increased expression of ligands for activating receptors and reduced expression or alteration of MHC molecules interrupts the inhibitory signals, allowing activation of NK cells and lysis of target cells.

Pattern Recognition

Microbes typically bear repeating patterns of molecular structure on their surface. The cell walls of Gram-negative and Gram-positive bacteria are composed of a matrix of sugars, lipid molecules, proteins, or patterns of modified nucleic acids. The lipopolysaccharides of the outer wall of Gram-negative bacteria, for example, are important recognition sites for the innate immune system. Other microbial components also have repetitive structures. Bacterial DNA contains unmethylated cysteine-guanine (CpG) sequences and viruses invariably express double-stranded RNA as part of their life cycle. These repetitive structures are generally known as *pathogen-associated molecular patterns* (PAMPs), and the receptors that recognize them as *pattern recognition receptors* (PRRs).

The recognized structures of PAMPs are essential to the functioning and infectivity of the microbe. The microbe cannot, therefore, evade innate immune recognition through mutation or a lack of production of the molecules because they would not survive. Humans inherit a limited number of germline genes for PRRs that effectively recognize major groups of microbes. One such receptor is the mannose-binding lectin (MBL), which is present as a free protein in the blood plasma. Pathogen recognition and discrimination of self from nonself by the MBL is due to the particular orientation and spacing of particular sugar residues, which are found only on microbes and not on host cells.

The phagocytic cells of the innate immune system are also equipped with several cell surface receptors that recognize pathogen surfaces directly. Among these is the macrophage-mannose receptor. This receptor binds certain sugars found on the surface of many bacteria and viruses, including HIV. A second set of phagocytic receptors, called the *scavenger receptors,* were originally defined as molecules that bind and mediate endocytosis of oxidized or acetylated low-density lipoproteins (LDLs) that do not interact with the conventional LDL receptor (see Chapter 18). Macrophage scavenger receptors bind a variety of microbes in addition to LDL particles.

Not all receptors that recognize pathogen-specific molecules are phagocytic receptors. The binding of pathogens to some receptors on leukocytes initiates a series of signaling events that lead to the tissue changes associated with acute inflammation. Stimulation of other pattern receptors leads macrophages and dendritic cells to display co-stimulatory molecules that enable them to act as antigen-presenting cells to lymphocytes and initiate an adaptive immune response.

Toll-Like Receptors

The best-defined activation pathway for the pathogen sensors of innate immunity is a family of transmembrane receptors called *Toll-like receptors* (TLRs). Interestingly,

the first protein to be identified in this family was the *Drosophila* Toll protein, which was found in the fruit fly *Drosophila*, where it functions in embryonic development as well as in protecting the fly from lethal fungal infections.

Eleven different TLRs have thus far been identified, each specific for different components of microbes (Table 15-2). Although most TLRs are found on the surface of the leukocytes, a few are intracellular, where they recognize viruses and intracellular pathogens such a *Mycobacterium*. Because there are only 11 recognized TLR genes, the Toll-like receptors have limited specificity compared with the antigen receptors of the adaptive immune system. Despite this limited diversity, they can recognize elements of most microorganisms.

Ligand binding to the TLR at the cell surface leads to an intracellular cascade of events which ultimately regulates the production of several proteins that are important components of innate immunity. Alterations in the structure of TLRs or mutations in the signaling system associated with TLRs have been suggested to play a pathologic role in disorders such as atherosclerosis, allergies, and certain autoimmune diseases.

Soluble Mediators of Innate Immunity

Although cells of the innate immune system can communicate critical information about microbial agents and self–nonself recognition through cell-to-cell contact, soluble mediators are essential for many other aspects of the response. Development of innate immunity and regulation of the behavior of effector cells both depend on the secretion of soluble mediators such as opsonins, cytokines, and proteins of the complement system.

Opsonins

Various soluble molecules can tag microorganisms for more efficient recognition by phagocytes. The coating of particles, such as microbes, is called *opsonization,*

(*text continues on page 330*)

TABLE 15-2 Types of Toll-Like Receptors (TLRs) and Their Recognized Ligands

TRLs	Ligands	Type of Microorganisms
TRL1	Lipopeptides	Mycobacteria
TRL2	Peptidoglycan	Gram-positive bacteria
	Lipoprotein	Mycobacteria
	Zymosan	Yeast and other fungi
TRL3	Double-stranded RNA	Viruses
TRL4	Lipopolysaccharide	Gram-negative bacteria
TRL5	Flagellin	Flagellated bacteria
TRL6	Lipopolypeptide	Mycobacteria
	Zymosan	Yeast and fungi
TRL7	Single-stranded RNA (ssRNA)	Viruses
TRL8	Single-stranded RNA (ssRNA)	Viruses
TRL9	CpG unmethylated dinucleotides	Bacterial DNA
TRLs 10,11	Unknown	

UNDERSTANDING ➤ The Complement System

The complement system provides one of the major effector mechanisms of both humoral and innate immunity. The system consists of a group of proteins (complement proteins C1 through C9) that are normally present in the plasma in an inactive form. Activation of the complement system is a highly regulated process, involving the sequential breakdown of the complement proteins to generate a cascade of cleavage products capable of proteolytic enzyme activity. This allows for tremendous amplification because each enzyme molecule activated by one step can generate multiple activated enzyme molecules at the next step. Complement activation is inhibited by proteins that are present on normal host cells; thus, its actions are limited to microbes and other antigens that lack these inhibitory proteins. The reactions of the complement system can be divided into three phases: (1) the initial activation phase, (2) the early-step inflammatory responses, and (3) the late-step membrane attack responses.

1

Initial Activation Phase. There are three pathways for recognizing microbes and activating the complement system: (1) the alternative pathway, which is activated by microbial cell surfaces in the absence of antibody and is a component of innate immunity; (2) the classical pathway, which is activated by certain types of antibodies bound to antigen and is part of humoral immunity; and (3) the lectin pathway, which is activated by a plasma lectin that binds to mannose on microbes and activates the classical system pathway in the absence of antibody.

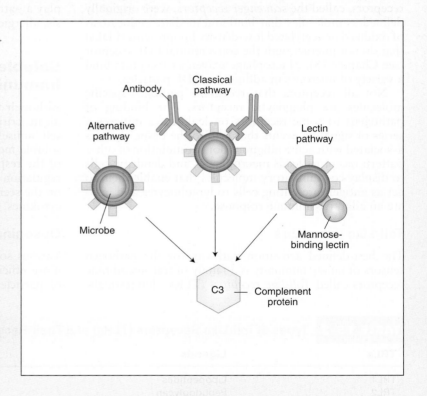

2

Early-Step Inflammatory Responses. The central component of complement for all three pathways is the activation of the complement protein C3 and its enzymatic cleavage into larger C3b fragments and smaller C3a fragments. The smaller 3a fragments stimulate inflammation by acting as a chemoattractant for neutrophils. The larger 3b fragment becomes attached to the microbe and acts as an opsonin for phagocytosis. They also act as an enzyme to cleave C5 (see next step).

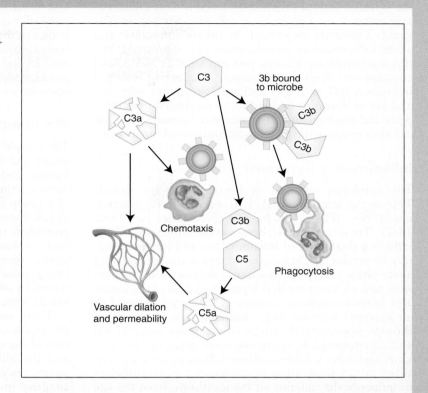

3

Late-Step Membrane Attack. In the late-step responses, C3b binds to other complement proteins to form an enzyme that cleaves C5, generating C5a and C5b fragments. C5a stimulates the influx of neutrophils and the vascular phase of acute inflammation. The C5b fragment, which remains attached to the microbe, initiates the formation of a complex of complement proteins C6, C7, C8, and C9 into a membrane attack complex protein, or pore, which allows fluids and ions to enter and cause cell lysis.

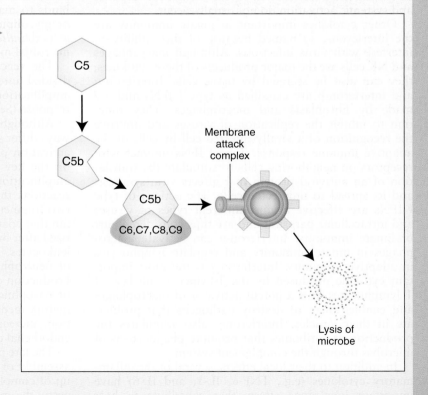

(text continued from page 327)

and the coating materials are called *opsonins*. Once the opsonin-coated microbe attaches to a complementary receptor on a phagocytic cell, phagocytosis is activated. Opsonins important in innate immunity and acute inflammation include acute-phase proteins, lectins (carbohydrate-binding proteins such as MBL), and complement. With the activation of adaptive humoral immunity, IgG and IgM antibodies can coat microbes and act as opsonins by binding to receptors on neutrophils and macrophages. The adaptive immune response can thus enhance the phagocytic function of innate cells.

Inflammatory Cytokines

The cytokines involved in innate immunity include TNF-α; the interleukins IL-1, IL-6, and IL-12; interferons (IFN-γ, IFN-α, IFN-β); and chemokines (see Table 15-1). These cytokines serve various functions. They influence the events of inflammation and innate immunity by producing chemotaxis of leukocytes, stimulating acute-phase protein production, inhibiting viral replication, and affecting the development of cells of the innate and adaptive immune systems. A leukocyte exposed to an external stimulus (e.g., bacteria) can be activated through appropriately triggered receptors (e.g., TLRs) and can respond by secreting small amounts of cytokines and other soluble mediators. If many cells are activated, the concentration of cytokines may be sufficient to influence the function of tissues distant from the site of infection, a true endocrine action. The short half-life of cytokines ensures that an excessive immune response and systemic activation do not usually occur.

Other cytokines important in innate immunity are the interferons, so named because of their ability to interfere with virus infections. Although macrophages and NK cells are the major producers of these cytokines, they can also be secreted by tissue cells. Interferon-α and interferon-β are classified as type I IFNs and are made by fibroblasts and macrophages. They function to inhibit the replication of viruses and improve the recognition of a virally infected cell by cells of the adaptive immune response. Type I IFNs interact with receptors on neighboring cells to stimulate the translation of an antiviral protein that affects viral synthesis and its spread to uninfected cells. The actions of type I IFNs are effective against different types of viruses and intracellular parasites and are thus considered part of innate immunity. Interferon-γ can activate macrophages in innate immunity and regulate lymphocytes in adaptive immunity. Interferon-γ is the most important cytokine produced by the T-helper 1 subclass of T lymphocytes. It is a potent activator of macrophages and enables them to destroy pathogens that proliferate in their vesicles. Interferon-γ also stimulates the production of antibodies that promote phagocytosis of microbes through the complement system.

In addition to their local effects, several of the inflammatory cytokines (e.g., TNF-α, IL-1, and IL-6) have important long-range effects that contribute to host defense. One of the most important of these is the initiation of the acute-phase response. This involves a shift

in the proteins synthesized by the liver into the plasma. Two of these, MBL and C-reactive protein (CRP), are of particular interest because they mimic the action of antibodies of the adaptive immune response, but unlike antibodies, these proteins have broad specificity for PAMPs and depend only on the presence of cytokines for their production. Mannose-binding lectin and CRP function as opsonins as well as activators of the complement system.

The Complement System

The complement system is an important effector of both innate and humoral immunity that enables the body to localize and destroy infectious pathogens. The complement system, like the blood coagulation system, consists of a group of proteins that are present in the circulation as functionally inactive precursors. These proteins, mainly proteolytic enzymes, make up 10% to 15% of the plasma proteins. For a complement reaction to occur, the complement components must be activated in the proper sequence. Uncontrolled activation of the complement system is prevented by inhibitor proteins and the instability of the activated complement proteins at each step of the process.

There are three parallel but independent pathways for recognizing microorganisms that result in activation of the complement system: the classical, the lectin, and the alternative pathways. The *classical pathway* recognizes complement-fixing antibodies (IgG, IgM) of adaptive immunity bound to the surface of a microbe or other structure. The *lectin pathway* uses a plasma protein called the *mannose-binding ligand* (MBL) that binds to mannose residues on microbial glycoproteins or glycolipids. It is a component of innate immunity, as is the *alternative pathway*, which recognizes certain microbial molecules in the absence of antibody.

The reactions of the complement systems can be divided into three phases: (1) initial activation, (2) amplification of inflammation, and (3) membrane attack response (See Understanding the Complement System).

Although the classical, lectin, and alternative pathways differ slightly in the proteins they use in the initial activation phase, all converge in the process by acting on the key complement protein C3, essential for the amplification phase. All generate a series of enzymatic reactions that prompt enzymatic cleavage of C3 into two fragments. The larger C3b fragment is a key opsonin that coats microbes and allows them to be phagocytized after binding to the type 1 complement receptor on leukocytes. The smaller C3a fragment triggers an influx of neutrophils to enhance the inflammatory response. Production of C3a and C5a also leads to the activation of basophils and mast cells and the release of inflammatory mediators that produce smooth muscle contraction, increased vascular permeability, and changes in endothelial cells to enhance migration of phagocytes.

The late phase of the complement cascade triggers the assembly of a membrane attack complex (MAC) made up of complement proteins C5 to C9. As its name suggests, the membrane attack complex leads to the lytic destruction of many kinds of cells, including bacteria and altered blood cells. The multiple functions of the complement system, including enhanced inflammatory responses, increased phagocytosis, and destruction and clearance of the pathogen from the body, make it an integral component of innate immunity and inflammation.

Role of Innate Immunity in Stimulating Adaptive Immunity

In addition to its role as a first-line defense in recognizing microbes and preventing infections, the innate immune response generates molecules that function as "second signals" together with antigens to activate the adaptive immune response. Full activation of antigen-specific B and T lymphocytes requires two signals. Antigen provides the first signal. Microbes, the response of the innate immune system to microbes, and host cells damaged by microbes all may provide the second signal. This requirement for a second microbe-initiated signal ensures that lymphocytes respond to microbes (the natural inducers of innate immunity) and not to harmless noninfectious substances. For the purpose of inducing immunity through vaccination, adaptive immune responses may be induced by antigens without microbes. In such instances, the antigens have to be administered with substances called *adjuvants* that elicit the same adaptive immune reactions as microbes do.

The second signals that are necessary for activation of the adaptive immune system can be generated by antigen-presenting dendritic cells and macrophages or by activation of the complement system. Microbes that breach the epithelial barriers of the innate immune system stimulate dendritic cells and macrophages to produce two types of second signals that activate T lymphocytes. First, the dendritic cells and macrophages express surface molecules called *co-stimulators*, which bind to receptors on naive T cells and function together with antigen recognition to activate T cells. Second, the dendritic cells and macrophages secrete cytokines that stimulate the differentiation of naive T cells into effector cells of cell-mediated adaptive immunity. Blood-borne microbes activate the complement system by the alternative pathway. One of the proteins produced by the complement system becomes covalently attached to the microbe, producing a second signal for activation of B lymphocytes.

SUMMARY CONCEPTS

- Innate immunity consists of the physical, cellular, chemical, and molecular defenses that are ready for activation and mediate rapid initial protection against infectious agents. Epithelial cells of the skin and mucous membranes, which are the first line of defense, block the entry of infectious agents and secrete antimicrobial molecules that can effectively kill a wide variety of microbes.

- The effector responses of innate immunity involve viral destruction by natural killer (NK) cells, phagocytosis of microbes by neutrophils and monocytes, initiation of the inflammatory response, and recruitment of the complement system.

- Development of innate immunity and regulation of effector cells depends on the secretion of soluble mediators, such as opsonins, cytokines, and acute-phase proteins. Opsonins bind to and tag microorganisms for more efficient recognition by phagocytes. Cytokines released from activated leukocytes regulate the activity of other cells, amplify inflammation, stimulate the production of *acute-phase proteins*, and aid in the initiation of an adaptive immune response.

- The *complement system*, which is a primary effector system for both the innate and adaptive immune systems, consists of a group of proteins that are activated by microbes and promote inflammation and destruction of the microbes. Recognition of microbes by complement occurs in three ways: by the *classical pathway*, an adaptive immune pathway which recognizes antibody bound to the surface of a microbe or other structure; by the *lectin pathway*, an innate pathway which uses a plasma protein called the *mannose-binding ligand* that binds to mannose residues on microbial glycoproteins or glycolipids; and by the *alternative pathway*, an innate pathway which recognizes certain microbial molecules.

Adaptive Immunity

The adaptive immune system is able to distinguish among different, even closely related, microbes and molecules and to "remember" the pathogen by quickly producing a heightened immune response on subsequent encounters with the same agent. The components of the adaptive immune system are lymphocytes and their products. Foreign substances that elicit specific responses are called *antigens*.

There are two types of adaptive immune responses: humoral and cell-mediated immunity. *Humoral immunity* is mediated by secreted molecules and is the principal defense against extracellular microbes and toxins. *Cell-mediated immunity*, or *cellular immunity*, is mediated by specific T lymphocytes and defends against intracellular microbes such as viruses.

Antigens

Before discussing the cells and responses inherent to adaptive immunity, it is important to understand the substances that elicit a response from the host. *Antigens*, also called *immunogens*, are substances foreign to the host that can stimulate an immune response. These foreign molecules are recognized by receptors on immune cells and by secreted proteins, called *antibodies* or *immunoglobulins*, made in response to the antigen. Antigens include bacteria, fungi, viruses, protozoa, and parasites. Nonmicrobial agents such as plant pollens, poison ivy resin, insect venom, and transplanted organs can also act as antigens. Although most antigens are macromolecules, such as proteins and polysaccharides, lipids and nucleic acids occasionally serve as antigens.

Antigens, which in general are large and chemically complex, are biologically degraded into smaller chemical units or peptides. These discrete, immunologically active sites on antigens are called *antigenic determinants,* or *epitopes.* It is the unique molecular shape of the epitope that is recognized by a specific immunoglobulin receptor found on the surface of a lymphocyte or by an antigen-binding site of a secreted antibody (Fig. 15-5). A single antigen may contain multiple antigenic determinants, each stimulating a distinct clone of T and B lymphocytes. For example, different proteins that comprise the influenza virus may function as unique antigens (A, B, C, H, and N antigens), each of which contains several antigenic determinants. Hundreds of antigenic determinants are found on structures such as the bacterial cell wall.

Smaller substances (molecular masses <10,000 daltons) usually are unable to stimulate an adequate immune response by themselves. When these low–molecular-weight compounds, known as *haptens,* combine with larger carrier molecules, they function as antigens. The hapten–carrier complex can stimulate the production of antibodies, some of which combine with the hapten portion of the complex. An allergic response to the antibiotic penicillin is an example of a medically important reaction due to hapten–carrier complexes. Penicillin (molecular mass of approximately 350 daltons) is

normally a nonantigenic molecule. However, in some individuals, it can chemically combine with body proteins to form larger complexes that can then generate a potentially harmful immune allergic response.

Cells and Molecules of Adaptive Immunity

B and T lymphocytes are the effector cells of the adaptive immune system that specifically recognize and respond to foreign antigens. Accessory cells, such as macrophages and dendritic cells, function as antigen-presenting cells by first processing a complex antigen into epitopes and then displaying the foreign and self-peptides on their membranes so that appropriate activation of lymphocytes occurs. We will begin with a discussion of the antigen-presenting cells, move to the lymphocytes, and end with the MHC molecules that display antigens for recognition by T lymphocytes.

Antigen-Presenting Cells

Macrophages are key members of the mononuclear phagocytic system that engulf and digest microbes and other foreign substances. The monocytes migrate from the blood to various tissues, where they mature into the major tissue phagocytes, the macrophages. As the general scavenger cells of the body, the macrophages can be fixed in a tissue or free to migrate from an organ to lymphoid tissues. The tissue macrophages are scattered in connective tissue or may be clustered in the lung (alveolar macrophages), liver (Kupffer cells), spleen, lymph nodes, peritoneum, or central nervous system (microglial cells).

Dendritic cells are found in most tissues where antigen enters the body and in the peripheral lymphoid tissues, where they function as potent antigen-presenting cells. In these environments, dendritic cells can acquire specialized functions and appearances, as do macrophages. Langerhans cells are specialized dendritic cells in the skin, whereas follicular dendritic cells are found in the lymph nodes. Langerhans cells are constantly surveying the skin for antigen and can transport foreign material to a nearby lymph node. Skin dendritic cells and macrophages also are involved in cell-mediated immune reactions of the skin such as allergic contact dermatitis.

Lymphocytes

Like other blood cells, B and T lymphocytes are generated from stem cells in the bone marrow. Undifferentiated, immature lymphocytes move to the central lymphoid tissues, where they develop into distinct types of mature lymphocytes (Fig. 15-6). B lymphocytes mature in the bone marrow and then move to the peripheral lymphoid tissues where they are exposed to antigen and stimulated to differentiate into antibody-producing plasma cells. T lymphocytes complete their maturation in the thymus and then move to the peripheral lymphoid tissues, where they function to produce cell-mediated immunity,

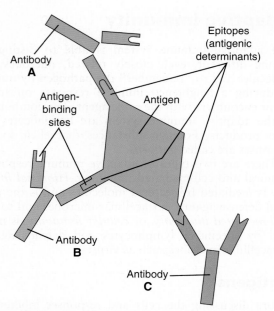

FIGURE 15-5. Multiple epitopes on a complex antigen being recognized by their respective (A, B, C) antibodies.

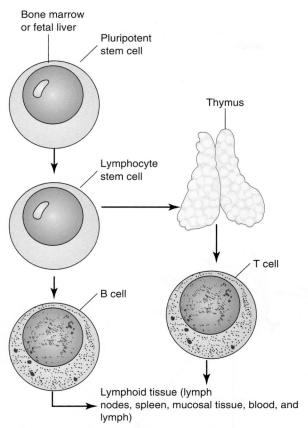

Bone marrow
or fetal liver

Pluripotent
stem cell

Thymus

Lymphocyte
stem cell

T cell

B cell

Lymphoid tissue (lymph
nodes, spleen, mucosal tissue, blood, and
lymph)

FIGURE 15-6. Pathway for T- and B-cell differentiation.

as well as aiding in antibody production. High concentrations of mature T and B lymphocytes are found in the lymph nodes, spleen, skin, and mucosal tissues, where they can respond to antigen.

B and T lymphocytes possess all of the key properties associated with the adaptive immune response—specificity, diversity, memory, and self–nonself recognition. These cells can exactly recognize and target a specific antigen and differentiate it from other substances that may be similar. The approximately 10^{12} lymphocytes in the body have tremendous diversity. They can respond to the millions of different kinds of antigens encountered daily. This diversity occurs because an enormous variety of lymphocyte populations have been programmed and selected during development, each to respond to a different antigen. After responding, they can acquire immunologic memory. The memory B and T lymphocytes that are generated remain in the body for a longer time and can respond more rapidly on repeat exposure than naive cells. Because of this heightened state of immune reactivity, the immune system usually can respond to commonly encountered microorganisms so efficiently that we are unaware of the response.

Adaptive immune responses are initiated when the antigen receptors of lymphocytes recognize antigens. The key trigger for the activation of B and T cells is the recognition of the antigen by unique surface receptors. B-cell antigen receptors (membrane-bound antibodies) and the antibodies that B cells secrete are able to recognize a broad range of structurally different molecules of varied sizes. This enables antibodies to detect diverse microbes and toxins. In contrast, the T-cell receptor recognizes only peptides, and only when these peptides are displayed on antigen-presenting cells bound to membrane proteins encoded by the MHC gene. Thus, T cells are only able to detect cell-associated microbes and antigens.

Activation of the lymphocytes depends on appropriate processing and presentation of antigen to T lymphocytes by antigen-presenting cells such as macrophages and dendritic cells (Fig. 15-7). On recognition of antigen and after additional stimulation by cytokines, the B and T lymphocytes divide several times to form clonal cell populations that continue to differentiate into effector and memory cells. After antigen binds to a B-cell receptor, the cell proliferates and differentiates into plasma cells that secrete antibodies that are a form of the B-cell receptor and have identical antigen specificity. Thus, the antigen that activates a given B cell becomes the target of the antibody produced by the cell's progeny. After a T cell is activated by its first encounter with an antigen, it proliferates and differentiates into helper or cytotoxic T cells. Helper T cells provide signals that activate antigen-stimulated B cells to differentiate and produce antibody. Some helper T cells also activate macrophages to become more efficient at killing engulfed pathogens. Cytotoxic T cells kill cells that are infected with viruses or other intracellular pathogens.

Major Histocompatibility Complex Molecules

Major histocompatibility complex molecules are membrane-bound proteins encoded by a MHC gene locus that display peptides for recognition by T lymphocytes. Although first identified as antigens that evoke rejection of transplanted organs, histocompatibility (i.e., tissue compatibility) molecules are now known to be extremely important for induction and regulation of immune responses. Recall that T cells (in contrast to B cells) can only recognize membrane-bound antigens, and hence histocompatibility molecules are critical to the induction of T-cell immunity. In humans, the genes encoding the most important MHC molecules are clustered on a small segment of chromosome 6.

The MHC molecules involved in self-recognition and cell-to-cell communication fall into two classes, class I and class II (Fig. 15-8). *Class I MHC* (MHC-I) molecules, which are expressed on all nucleated cells and platelets, are cell surface molecules that interact with the receptor–antigen peptide complex on CD8+ cytotoxic T cells. *Class II MHC* (MHC-II) molecules, which are expressed mainly on dendritic cells, macrophages, and B lymphocytes, communicate with the antigen receptor and the CD4 molecule on helper T cells.

Although the MHC-I and MHC-II proteins differ in subunit composition, they are similar in overall structure, and each contains a peptide-binding cleft on the extracellular portion of the molecule. The MHC-I molecule contains a cleft that accommodates a peptide fragment of antigen. Cytotoxic T cells can become activated only

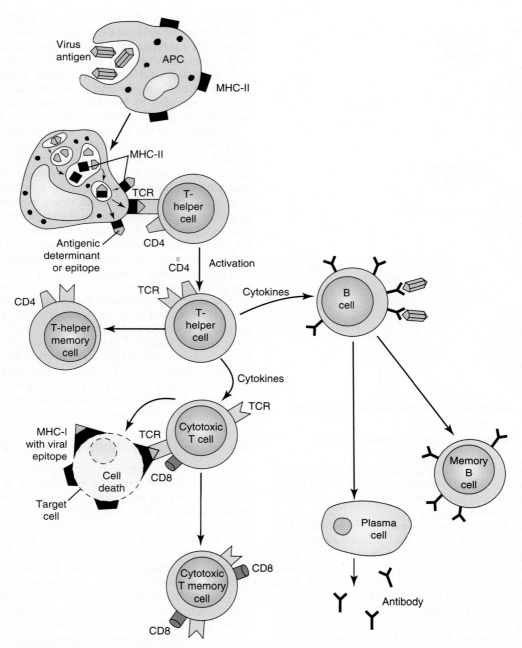

FIGURE 15-7. Pathway for immune cell participation in an adaptive immune response. APC, antigen-presenting cell; MHC, major histocompatibility complex; TCR, T-cell receptor.

when they are presented with the foreign antigen peptide associated with the class I MHC molecule. During a typical viral infection of a cell, small peptides from degraded viral proteins associate with MHC-I molecules and are then transported to the infected cell membrane. This complex communicates to the cytotoxic T cell that the cell must be destroyed for the overall survival of the host. The MHC-II molecule's binding cleft accommodates a fragment of antigen from pathogens that have been engulfed and digested by an antigen-presenting cell during the process of phagocytosis. The engulfed pathogen is degraded into peptides in cytoplasmic vesicles and

then complexed with the MHC-II molecule. Helper T cells recognize these complexes on the surface of antigen-presenting cells and become activated. These triggered helper T cells multiply quickly and direct other immune cells to respond to the invading pathogen through the secretion of cytokines.

Each individual has a unique collection of MHC proteins, and a variety of MHC molecules can exist in a population. Thus, MHC molecules are both polygenic and polymorphic. The MHC genes are the most polymorphic genes known. Because of the number of MHC genes and the possibility of several alleles for each gene, it is almost

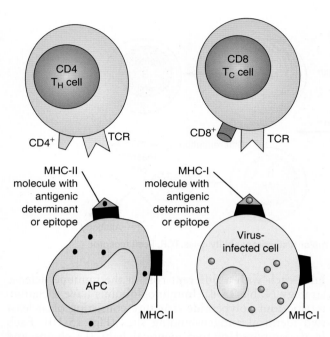

FIGURE 15-8. Recognition by a T-cell receptor (TCR) on a CD4+ helper T (T_H) cell of an epitope associated with a class II major histocompatibility complex (MHC) molecule on an antigen-presenting cell (APC), and by a TCR on a CD8+ cytotoxic T (T_C) cell of an epitope associated with a class I MHC molecule on a virus-infected cell.

expressed molecules are designated by a letter and numbers (e.g., HLA-B27).

Because the class I and II MHC genes are closely linked on one chromosome, the combination of HLA genes usually is inherited as a unit, called a *haplotype*. Each person inherits a chromosome from each parent and therefore has two HLA haplotypes. The identification or typing of HLA molecules is important in tissue or organ transplantation, forensics, and paternity evaluations. In organ or tissue transplantation, the closer the matching of HLA types, the greater the probability of identical antigens and the lower the chance of rejection.

B Lymphocytes and Humoral Immunity

Humoral immunity is mediated by antibodies, which are produced by B lymphocytes and their progeny. B lymphocytes can be identified by the presence of membrane immunoglobulin that functions as the antigen receptor, class II MHC proteins, complement receptors, and specific CD molecules. During the maturation process in the bone marrow, B-cell progenitors (pre-B cells) develop into mature or naive B cells. The mature B cell leaves the bone marrow, enters the circulation, and migrates to the various peripheral lymphoid tissues, where it is stimulated to respond to a specific antigen. Each of the stages of B-cell development are characterized by a specific pattern of immunoglobulin (Ig) gene expression and the expression of other cell surface proteins that serve as phenotypic markers of these maturational stages.

The commitment of a B-cell line to a specific antigen is evidenced by the expression of the membrane-bound Ig receptors that recognize antigen. B cells that encounter antigen complementary to their surface immunoglobulin receptor and receive T-cell help undergo a series of changes that transform them into antibody-secreting plasma cells or into memory B cells (Fig. 15-9). The antibodies produced by the plasma cells are released into the lymph and blood, where they bind and remove their unique antigen with the help of other immune effector cells and molecules. The longer-lived memory B cells are distributed to the peripheral tissues in preparation for subsequent antigen exposure.

impossible for any two individuals to have an identical MHC profile, unless they are identical twins. Major histocompatibility complex alleles affect immune responses as well as susceptibility to a number of diseases.

Human MHC proteins are called *human leukocyte antigens* (HLAs) because they were first detected on white blood cells. Because these molecules play a role in transplant rejection and are detected by immunologic tests, they are commonly called antigens. The classic human MHC-I molecules are divided into types called HLA-A, HLA-B, and HLA-C, and the MHC-II molecules are identified as HLA-DR, HLA-DP, and HLA-DQ (Table 15-3). Each of the gene loci that describe HLA molecules can be occupied by multiple alleles or alternative genes. For example, there are more than 350 possible alleles for the A locus, 650 alleles for the B locus, and 180 alleles for the C locus. The genes and their

TABLE 15-3	**Properties of Class I and II MHC Molecules**		
Properties	**HLA Antigens**	**Distribution**	**Functions**
Class I MHC	HLA-A, HLA-B, HLA-C	Nucleated cells and platelets	Present processed antigen to cytotoxic CD8+ T cells; restrict cytolysis to virus-infected cells, tumor cells, and transplanted cells
Class II MHC	HLA-DR, HLA-DP, HLA-DQ	Immune cells, antigen-presenting cells, B cells, and macrophages	Present processed antigenic fragments to CD4+ T cells; necessary for effective interaction among immune cells

HLA, human leukocyte antigen; MHC, major histocompatibility complex.

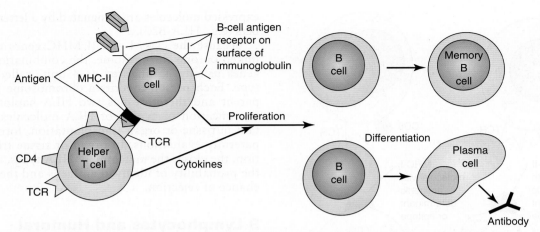

FIGURE 15-9. Pathway for B-cell differentiation. MHC, major histocompatibility class; TCR, T-cell receptor.

Immunoglobulins

Immunoglobulins, or antibodies, function as antigen receptors for B cells or as effector molecules of the humoral immune response. The immunoglobulins have been divided into five classes—IgG, IgA, IgM, IgD, and IgE—each with a different role in the immune defense strategy (Table 15-4). Immunoglobulins have a characteristic four-polypeptide structure consisting of at least two identical antigen-binding sites (Fig. 15-10). Each Ig is composed of two identical light (L) chains and two identical heavy (H) chains to form a "Y"-shaped

TABLE 15-4	Classes and Characteristics of Immunoglobulins		
Figure	**Class**	**Percentage of Total**	**Characteristics**
	IgG	75.0	Displays antiviral, antitoxin, and antibacterial properties; only Ig that crosses the placenta and thus responsible for protection of newborn; activates complement and binds to macrophages; prominent in the secondary immune response
	IgA	15.0	Predominant Ig in body secretions, such as saliva, nasal and respiratory secretions, and breast milk; protects mucous membranes
	IgM	10.0	Forms the natural antibodies such as those for ABO blood antigens; prominent in early immune responses; activates complement
	IgD	0.2	Found on B lymphocytes; needed for maturation of B cells
	IgE	0.004	Binds to mast cells and basophils; involved in parasitic infections and allergic and hypersensitivity reactions

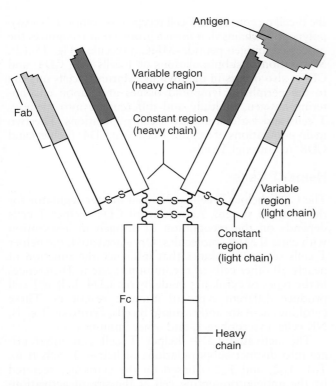

FIGURE 15-10. Schematic model of an immunoglobulin G (IgG) molecule showing the constant and variable regions of the light and heavy chains.

Labels in figure: Antigen, Variable region (heavy chain), Constant region (heavy chain), Fab, Variable region (light chain), Constant region (light chain), Fc, Heavy chain

molecule. The two forked ends bind antigen and are called *Fab* (i.e., antigen-binding) fragments. The tail of the molecule, which is called the *Fc fragment*, determines the biologic properties that are characteristic of a particular class of immunoglobulins.

The heavy and light chains show constant (C) regions and variable (V) regions. The *constant regions* have sequences of amino acids that vary little among the antibodies of a particular class of immunoglobulin. The constant regions are the basis for the separation of immunoglobulins into classes (e.g., IgM, IgG) and allow each class of antibody to interact with certain effector cells and molecules. The *variable regions* contain the antigen-binding sites of the molecule. The wide variation in the amino acid sequence of the variable regions seen from antibody to antibody allows this region to recognize its complementary antigenic determinant or epitope. A unique amino acid sequence in this region determines a distinctive three-dimensional pocket that is complementary to the antigen, allowing recognition and binding. Each B-cell clone produces antibody with one specific antigen-binding variable region or domain. During the course of the immune response, class switching (e.g., from IgM to IgG) can occur, causing the B-cell clone to produce one of the different immunoglobulin types.

Immunoglobulin G (gamma globulin) is the most abundant of the circulating immunoglobulins. It is present in body fluids and readily enters the tissues. Immunoglobulin G is the only immunoglobulin that crosses the placenta and can transfer immunity from the mother to the fetus. This class of immunoglobulin protects against bacteria, toxins, and viruses in body fluids and activates the complement system. This antibody can also bind to target cells and Fc receptors on NK cells and macrophages, leading to lysis of the target cell. There are four subclasses of IgG (i.e., IgG$_1$, IgG$_2$, IgG$_3$, and IgG$_4$), each of which has some restrictions in its response to certain types of antigens. For example, IgG$_2$ appears to be responsive to bacteria that are encapsulated with a polysaccharide layer, such as *Streptococcus pneumoniae, Haemophilus influenzae,* and *Neisseria meningitidis.*

Immunoglobulin A, a secretory immunoglobulin, is found in saliva, tears, breast milk, and bronchial, gastrointestinal, prostatic, and vaginal secretions. This dimeric secretory immunoglobulin is considered a primary defense against local infections in mucosal tissues. Immunoglobulin A prevents the attachment of viruses and bacteria to epithelial cells.

Immunoglobulin M is a macromolecule that forms a polymer of five basic immunoglobulin units. It cannot cross the placenta and thus does not transfer maternal immunity. It is the first circulating immunoglobulin to appear in response to an antigen and is the first antibody type made by a newborn. This is diagnostically useful because the presence of IgM suggests a current infection in the infant by a specific pathogen. The identification of newborn IgM rather than maternally transferred IgG to the specific pathogen is indicative of an in utero or newborn infection.

Immunoglobulin D is found primarily on the cell membranes of B lymphocytes. It serves as an antigen receptor for initiating the differentiation of B cells.

Immunoglobulin E is involved in inflammation, allergic responses, and combating parasitic infections. It binds to mast cells and basophils. The binding of antigen to mast cell– or basophil-bound IgE triggers these cells to release histamine and other mediators important in inflammation and allergies.

Humoral Immunity

Humoral immunity functions to eliminate extracellular microbes and microbial toxins. The combination of antigen with antibody can result in several effector responses, such as precipitation of antigen–antibody complexes, agglutination or clumping of cells, neutralization of bacterial toxins and viruses, lysis and destruction of pathogens or cells, adherence of antigen to immune cells, facilitation of phagocytosis, and complement activation. For example, antibodies can neutralize a virus by blocking the sites on the virus where it binds to the host cell, thereby negating its ability to infect the cell.

Two types of responses occur in the development of humoral immunity: primary and secondary (Fig. 15-11). A *primary immune response* occurs when the antigen is first introduced into the body. During the primary response, there is a latent period or lag before the antibody can be detected in the serum. This latent period involves the processing of antigen by the antigen-presenting cells and its recognition by CD4$^+$ helper T cells. After the antigen

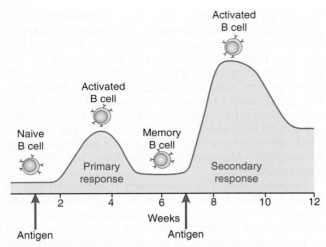

FIGURE 15-11. Primary and secondary or memory phases of the humoral immune response to the same antigen.

receptors on CD4+ helper T cells recognize the antigenic peptide–class II MHC molecules, the T cells become activated and produce cytokines to further stimulate and direct the immune system. In humoral immunity, activated CD4+ helper T cells trigger B cells to proliferate and differentiate into a clone of plasma cells that produce antibody. This activation process takes 1 to 2 weeks, but once generated, detectable antibody continues to rise for several weeks. Recovery from many infectious diseases occurs during the primary response when the antibody concentration is reaching its peak.

The *secondary* or *memory response* occurs on second or subsequent exposures to the antigen. During the primary response, a fraction of activated B cells does not differentiate into plasma cells but instead forms a pool of memory B cells. In a secondary response, the rise in antibody occurs sooner and reaches a higher level because of these available memory cells. The booster immunization given for some diseases, such as tetanus, makes use of the memory response. For a person who has been previously immunized, administration of a booster shot causes an almost immediate rise in antibody to a level sufficient to prevent development of the disease. Activated T cells can also generate primary and secondary cell-mediated immune responses.

T Lymphocytes and Cell-Mediated Immunity

T lymphocytes function in the activation of other T cells and B cells, in the control of intracellular viral infections, in the rejection of foreign tissue grafts, and in delayed hypersensitivity reactions (see Chapter 16). Collectively, these immune responses are referred to as *cell-mediated* or *cellular immunity.*

T lymphocytes arise from bone marrow stem cells, but unlike B cells, pre-T cells migrate to the thymus for their maturation. There the immature T lymphocytes undergo rearrangement of the genes needed for expression of a unique T-cell antigen receptor similar to but distinct from

the B-cell receptor. The T-cell receptor is composed of two polypeptide chains that form a groove that recognizes the processed antigen peptide–MHC molecules (Fig. 15-12). Maturation of subpopulations of T cells (i.e., CD4+ and CD8+) also occurs in the thymus. Mature T cells migrate to the peripheral lymphoid tissues and, upon encountering antigen, multiply and differentiate into memory T cells and various mature T-cell populations. The two main populations of mature T cells are CD4+ (helper) and CD8+ (cytotoxic) T cells.

Helper T Cells

The CD4+ helper T cell serves as a master regulator for the immune system. Activation of CD4+ helper T cells depends on the recognition of antigen in association with class II MHC molecules. Once activated, the helper T cells secrete cytokines that influence the function of nearly all other cells of the immune system. Differences in the types of cytokines made by the CD4+ helper T cell produce different types of immune responses. These cytokines activate and regulate B cells, cytotoxic T cells, NK cells, macrophages, and other immune cells.

The activated CD4+ helper T cell can differentiate into distinct subpopulations of helper T cells (e.g., T_H1, T_H2, and T_H17) based on the cytokines secreted by the antigen-presenting cell at the site of activation. The cytokine IL-12 produced by macrophages and dendritic cells directs the maturation of CD4+ helper T cells toward T_H1 cells. The cytokine IL-4 produced by mast cells and T cells induces differentiation toward T_H2 cells. The cytokines IL-6 and transforming growth factor-beta (TGF-β), notably in the absence of either IL-4 or IL-12, will induce differentiation toward T_H17 cells.

The distinct pattern of cytokines secreted by mature T_H1 and T_H2 cells defines these subpopulations of T cells and determines their functions. Activated T_H1 cells stimulate phagocyte-mediated ingestion and killing of microbes. T_H1 cells produce the cytokine IFN-γ,

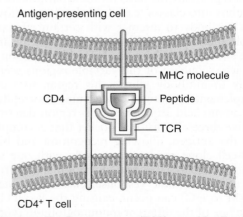

FIGURE 15-12. The T-cell receptor (TCR) on a CD4+ T cell and the interaction of the major histocompatibility complex (MHC) on the antigen-presenting cell. Note that the TCR recognizes the peptide fragment of antigen bound to the MHC class II molecule. The CD4 molecule binds to a portion of the MHC molecule, stabilizing the interaction.

which activates macrophages and stimulates B cells to produce IgG antibodies that activate complement and coat pathogens for phagocytosis. T_H2 cells produce IL-4, which stimulates B cells to differentiate into IgE-secreting plasma cells; IL-5, which activates eosinophils; and IL-13, which activates mucosal epithelial cells to secrete mucus and expel microbes. Differentiated $CD4^+$ T cells of the T_H1 subset recognize microbial peptides on macrophages and have the dual function of stimulating the production of IgG antibodies and eliminating cells infected with certain pathogenic intracellular microbes such as mycobacteria; whereas those of the T_H2 subset tend to recognize protein antigens or chemicals that stimulate the production of IgE and development of allergies. Activated T_H17 produces the cytokine IL-17, which promotes inflammation, and plays a role in the adaptive immune response and in some T cell–mediated inflammatory disorders.

In most immune responses, a balanced response of T_H1 and T_H2 cells occurs, but immunization or exposure to antigen can skew the response to one or the other subset. For example, the extensive exposure to an allergen in atopic individuals has been shown to shift the naive $CD4^+$ T cell toward a T_H2 response, with the production of the cytokines that influence IgE production and mast cell priming. An appreciation of these processes has led to clinical research that suggests that redirection of an allergic T_H2 response to a nonallergic T_H1 response can occur in atopic individuals through modified immunization protocols.

Cytotoxic T Cells

Activated $CD8^+$ lymphocytes become cytotoxic T cells after recognition of class I MHC–antigen complexes on target cell surfaces, such as body cells infected by viruses or transformed by cancer (Fig. 15-13). The recognition of class I MHC–antigen complexes on infected target cells ensures that neighboring uninfected host cells, which express class I MHC molecules alone or with self-peptide, are not indiscriminately destroyed. The $CD8^+$ cytotoxic T cells perform their killing function by injecting preformed cytotoxic proteins into target cells, thereby triggering apoptosis or programmed cell death (see Chapter 2). Cytotoxic T cells also produce and release cytokines, such as IFN-γ, which inhibits viral replication and is an important inducer of MHC class 1 molecule expression and macrophage activation. The $CD8^+$ cytotoxic T cells are especially important in controlling replicating viruses and intracellular bacteria because antibodies cannot readily penetrate the membrane of living cells.

Regulatory T Cells

A recently defined type of T lymphocyte is the *regulatory T cell,* which has CD4 and CD25 expressed on its cell membrane. Regulatory T cells, in contrast to $CD4^+$ helper T cells, suppress immune responses by inhibiting the proliferation of other potentially harmful self-reactive lymphocytes. The actions of regulatory T cells are antigen specific. Activation of a regulatory

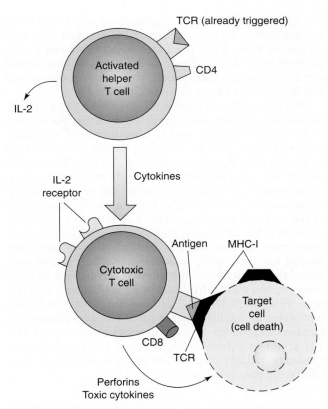

FIGURE 15-13. Destruction of target cell by cytotoxic T cell. Cytokines released from the activated helper T cell enhance the potential of the cytotoxic T cell in destruction of the target cell. IL, interleukin; MHC, major histocompatibility class; TCR, T-cell receptor.

T-cell receptor by the antigen prompts the secretion of the cytokine IL-10 and transforming growth factor-β (TGF-β). These cytokines inhibit the proliferation and activation of lymphocytes and macrophages. There is also recent evidence that regulatory $CD8^+$ T cells can selectively down-regulate T cells that are activated by either self or foreign antigens. These cells are thought to differentiate into effector cells during the primary immune response and function as suppressor cells during the secondary or memory phases of immunity, and are primarily involved in self–nonself discrimination. The potential clinical importance of regulatory T cells is suggested from animal studies showing inhibition of inflammatory bowel disease, experimental allergic encephalitis, and autoimmune diabetes by increased activity of regulatory T cells.

Cell-Mediated Immunity

Cell-mediated immunity functions against microbes, including bacteria, parasites, and all viruses that replicate inside cells where they cannot be destroyed by antibodies. Both $CD8^+$ and $CD4^+$ cells contribute to the response, with each having different effector mechanisms for the eradication of the infection.

The effector functions of $CD8^+$ cytotoxic T cells, which act against cells infected with viruses, are the most direct. Antigens derived from the virus multiply inside the infected cell and are displayed on the target cell's surface, where they are recognized by antigen receptors on the cytotoxic T cell (see Fig. 15-12). Cytotoxic T cells perform their killing function by releasing preformed cytotoxic proteins that induce apoptosis or programmed cell death of the target cell (see Chapter 2).

The principal function of CD4$^+$ cells of the T_H1 subset involves the defense against intracellular pathogens, such as mycobacteria, which grow primarily in phagosomes of macrophages, shielding them from the effects of both antibodies and cytotoxic T cells. These cells secrete the cytokine IFN-γ, a potent macrophage activator, which stimulates the induction of microbicidal substances in macrophages, leading to the destruction of the ingested microbes. CD4$^+$ T_H1 cells also produce a range of other cytokines, chemokines, and surface molecules that do not activate infected macrophages, but instead kill chronically infected senescent macrophages, stimulate the production of new macrophages in bone marrow, and recruit fresh macrophages to sites of infection. Thus, the CD4$^+$ T_H1 cell controls and coordinates host defenses against certain intracellular pathogens, a function that helps to explain why a decreased CD4$^+$ T_H1 count in persons with acquired immunodeficiency syndrome (AIDS) places them at high risk for intracellular pathogen infections.

Active Versus Passive Immunity

Adaptive, or specific, immune responses are designed to protect the body against potentially harmful foreign substances, infections, and other sources of non–self antigens. It is the specific protection that is acquired through exposure to antigens (active immunity) or through transfer of protective antibodies against an antigen (passive immunity).

Active immunity is acquired through immunization or actually having a disease. It is called *active immunity* because it depends on a response to the antigen by the person's immune system. Active immunity, although long lasting once established, requires a few days to weeks after a first exposure before the immune response is sufficiently developed to contribute to the destruction of the pathogen. However, the immune system usually is able to react within hours to subsequent exposure to the same agent because of the presence of memory B and T lymphocytes and circulating antibodies. The process of acquiring the ability to respond to an antigen after its administration by vaccine is known as *immunization*. An acquired immune response can improve on repeated exposures to an injected antigen or a natural infection.

Passive immunity is immunity transferred from another source. An infant receives passive immunity naturally from the transfer of antibodies from its mother in utero and through breast milk. Maternal IgG crosses the placenta and protects the newborn during the first few months of life. Normally, an infant has few infectious diseases during the first 3 to 6 months owing to the protection provided by the mother's antibodies. Passive immunity also can be artificially provided by the transfer of antibodies produced by other people or animals. Some protection against infectious disease can be provided by the injection of hyperimmune serum, which contains high concentrations of antibodies for a specific disease, or immune serum or gamma globulin, which contains a pool of antibodies from many individuals providing protection against many infectious agents. Passive immunity produces only short-term protection that lasts weeks to months.

Regulation of the Immune Response

Self-regulation is an essential property of the immune system. An inadequate immune response may lead to immunodeficiency, but an inappropriate or excessive response may lead to conditions varying from allergic reactions to autoimmune diseases. This regulation is not well understood and involves all aspects of the immune response—antigen, antibody, cytokines, regulatory T cells, and the neuroendocrine system.

With each exposure to antigen, the immune system must determine the branch of the immune system to be activated and the extent and duration of the immune response. After exposure to an antigen, the immune response to that antigen develops after a brief lag, reaches a peak, and then recedes. Normal immune responses are self-limited because the response eliminates the antigen, and the products of the response, such as cytokines and antibodies, have a limited life span and are secreted only for brief periods after antigen recognition. Evidence suggests that cytokine feedback from the helper T or regulatory T cells controls several aspects of the immune response.

Another facet of immune self-regulation is inhibition of immune responses by tolerance. The term *tolerance* is used to define the ability of the immune system to be nonreactive to self-antigens while producing immunity to foreign agents. Tolerance to self-antigens protects an individual from harmful autoimmune reactions (see Chapter 16). Exposure of an individual to foreign antigens may lead to tolerance and the inability to respond to potential pathogens that cause infection. Tolerance exists not only to self-tissues but also to maternal–fetal tissues. Special regulation of the immune system is evident in privileged sites such as the brain, testes, ovaries, and eyes. Immune damage in these areas could result in serious consequences to the individual and the species.

SUMMARY CONCEPTS

- The adaptive immune response involves a complex series of interactions between components of the immune system and the antigens of a foreign pathogen. It is able to distinguish between self and nonself, recognize and specifically react to large numbers of different microbes and pathogens, and remember the specific agents.

■ Antigens are substances foreign to the host that can stimulate an immune response. They have antigenic determinant sites or *epitopes*, which the adaptive immune system recognizes with specific receptors that distinguish the antigens as nonself.

■ The principal cells of the adaptive immune system are the T and B lymphocytes and antigen presenting cells. T lymphocytes differentiate into helper T and regulatory T cells and cytotoxic T cells and provide cell-mediated immunity. CD4+ helper T cells serve as a trigger for the immune response and are essential for the differentiation of B cells into antibody-producing plasma cells and the differentiation of T lymphocytes into CD8+ cytotoxic T cells. Antigen-presenting cells consist of macrophages and dendritic cells that process and present antigen peptides to CD4+ helper T cells.

■ Cell surface MHC molecules are key recognition molecules that the immune system uses in distinguishing self from nonself. *Class I MHC* molecules, which are present on all nucleated cells other than those of the immune system, interact with cytotoxic CD8+ T cells in the destruction of cells that have been affected by intracellular pathogens or cancer. *Class II MHC* molecules, found on antigen-presenting cells and B lymphocytes, aid in cell-to-cell communication between different cells of the immune system.

■ Humoral immunity consists of protection provided by the B lymphocyte–derived plasma cells, which produce immunoglobulins that travel in the blood and interact with circulating and cell surface antigens. The immunoglobulins have been divided into five classes, IgG, IgA, IgM, IgD, and IgE, each with a different role in immune defense.

■ Cell-mediated immunity consists of protection provided by cytotoxic T lymphocytes, which protect against virus-infected or cancer cells.

Developmental Aspects of the Immune System

Embryologically, the immune system develops in several stages, beginning at 5 to 6 weeks as the fetal liver becomes active in hematopoiesis. Development of the primary lymphoid organs (i.e., thymus and bone marrow) begins during the middle of the first trimester

and proceeds rapidly. Secondary lymphoid organs (i.e., spleen, lymph nodes, and mucosa-associated lymphoid tissues) develop soon after. These secondary lymphoid organs are rather small but well developed at birth and mature rapidly after exposure to microbes during the postnatal period. The thymus is fully formed and functional and is the largest lymphoid tissue relative to body size at birth.

Transfer of Immunity from Mother to Infant

Protection of a newborn against antigens occurs through transfer of maternal antibodies. Maternal IgG antibodies cross the placenta during fetal development and remain functional in the newborn for the first few months of life (Fig. 15-14). IgG is the only class of immunoglobulins to cross the placenta. Levels of maternal IgG decrease significantly during the first 3 to 6 months of life, while infant synthesis of immunoglobulins increases. Maternally transmitted IgG is effective against most microorganisms and viruses. The largest amount of IgG crosses the placenta during the last weeks of pregnancy and is stored in fetal tissues; therefore, infants born prematurely may be deficient. Because of the transfer of IgG antibodies to the fetus, an infant born to a mother infected with HIV will have a positive HIV antibody test result, although the child may not necessarily be infected with the virus.

Cord blood does not normally contain IgM or IgA. If present, these antibodies are of fetal origin and represent exposure to intrauterine infection. The infant begins producing IgM antibodies shortly after birth, in response to the immense antigenic stimulation of his or her new environment. Premature infants appear to be able to produce IgM as well as term infants. At approximately 6 days of age the IgM rises sharply, and this rise continues until approximately 1 year of age, when the adult level is achieved.

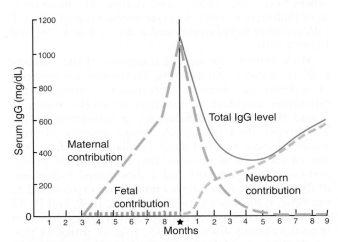

FIGURE 15-14. Maternal/neonatal serum immunoglobulin G levels. (From *J Pediatr*. 1968;72(2):276–290.)

Serum IgA normally is first detected at approximately 13 days after birth. The level increases during early childhood until adult levels are reached between the sixth and seventh years. Maternal IgA also is transferred to the infant in breast milk. These antibodies provide local immunity for the intestinal system and have been shown to decrease diarrheal infections. These evolutionary adaptations of the immune system have increased the survival of our species and optimized the development of other important organs in the early months of life.

Immune Response in the Elderly

Aging is characterized by a declining ability to adapt to environmental stresses. One of the factors thought to contribute to this problem is a decline in immune responsiveness. This includes changes in cell-mediated and humoral immune responses. Elderly persons tend to be more susceptible to infections, have more evidence of autoimmune and immune complex disorders than younger persons, and have a higher incidence of cancer. Experimental evidence suggests that vaccination is less successful in inducing immunization in older persons than in younger adults. However, the effect of altered immune function on the health of elderly persons is clouded by the fact that age-related changes or disease may affect the immune response.

The alterations in immune function that occur with advanced age are not fully understood. There is a decrease in the size of the thymus gland, which is thought to affect T-cell function. The size of the gland begins to decline shortly after sexual maturity, and by 50 years of age, it usually has diminished to 15% or less of its maximum size. There are conflicting reports regarding age-related changes in the peripheral lymphocytes. A suggested biologic clock in T cells that determines the number of times it divides may regulate cell number with age. Some researchers have reported a decrease in the absolute number of lymphocytes, and others have found little, if any, change. The most common finding is a slight decrease in the proportion of T cells to other lymphocytes and a decrease in CD4+ and CD8+ T cells.

More evident are altered responses of the immune cells to antigen stimulation; increasing proportions of lymphocytes become unresponsive, whereas the remainder continue to function relatively normally. T and B cells show deficiencies in activation. In the T-cell types, the CD4+ subset is most severely affected. Evidence indicates that aged T cells have a decreased rate of synthesis of the cytokines that drive the proliferation of lymphocytes and a diminished expression of the receptors that interact with those cytokines. For example, it has been shown that IL-2, IL-4, and IL-12 levels decrease with aging. Although B-cell function is compromised with age, the range of antigens that can be recognized is not diminished. If anything, the repertoire, including outgrowths of autoreactive B-cell clones, is increased to the extent that B cells begin to recognize some self-antigens as foreign antigens. This may be the basis for the increased incidence of autoimmune disease in the elderly.

SUMMARY CONCEPTS

■ Newborn infants are protected against antigens in early life by passive transfer of maternal antibodies through the placenta (IgG) and through breast feeding (IgA).

■ The largest amount of IgG crosses the placenta during the last weeks of pregnancy and is stored in fetal tissues; therefore, infants born prematurely may be deficient. Because of the transfer of IgG antibodies to the fetus, an infant born to a mother infected with HIV will have a positive HIV antibody test result, although the child may not necessarily be infected with the virus.

■ Aging is characterized by changes in immune responsiveness, including cell-mediated and humoral immune responses. Elderly persons tend to be more susceptible to infections, have more evidence of autoimmune and immune complex disorders than younger persons, and have a higher incidence of cancer.

REVIEW EXERCISES

1. The systemic manifestations (e.g., generalized muscle aches, chills and fever, loss of appetite) that accompany a severe sore throat or acute respiratory infection are stimulated by reactions to cytokines of the innate immune system rather than by the antibodies or cell-mediated responses of the adaptive immune response.

   A. Explain.

2. A nursing student is working in a community clinic as a volunteer. Each time she enters the clinic, she suffers bouts of sneezing and runny nose. She has a history of mold allergy and her younger brother has asthma. Analysis at the allergy clinic indicates a strong reaction to latex. She is advised to avoid exposure to all forms of latex.

   A. What class of immunoglobulin and what type of mediator cells are responsible for the symptoms expressed in this individual?

   B. What type of T-helper cell and cytokines direct the expression of this humoral immune response?

C. Is this an example of active or passive immunity? Is it a primary or secondary immune response?

3. A 5-month-old child presents with thrush, a yeast infection of the mouth. In the last 2 months, he has had recurrent bouts of otitis media. His tonsils are very small. Laboratory analysis indicates a low lymphocyte count and no T lymphocytes. Further analysis indicates a genetic mutation in the T-cell receptor that affects maturation of all T cells. The final diagnosis is severe combined immunodeficiency disease. A bone marrow transplant is being pursued with cells from his HLA-matched sibling.

A. Explain why infections were not present in the first few months of this child's life.

B. What would be the impact of an absence of T cells on both humoral and cell-mediated immunity?

BIBLIOGRAPHY

Abbas AK, Litchman AH, Pillai S. *Cellular and Molecular Immunology.* 7th ed. Philadelphia, PA: Elsevier Saunders; 2011.

Akashi-Takamura S, Miyake K. Toll-like receptors (TLRs) and immune disorders. *J Infect Chemother.* 2006;12:233–240.

Akira S, Uematsu S, Takeuchi O. Pathogen recognition and innate immunity. *Cell.* 2006;124:783–801.

Bryant CE, Monie TP. Mice, men and relatives: cross-species studies underpin innate immunity. *Open Biol.* 2005;2:1. Available at: http://rsob.royalsocietypublishing.org/content/2/4/120015. Accessed November 20, 2013.

Chapin DD. Overview of the human immune response. *J Allergy Clin Immunol.* 2010;125(suppl 2):S2–S23.

Clark R, Kupper T. Old meets new: the interaction between innate and adaptive immunity. *J Invest Dermatol.* 2005;125:629–637.

Goain A, Gamelli RL. A primer on cytokines. *J Burn Care Rehabil.* 2005;26:7–12.

Hajishengallis G. Too old to fight: aging and its toll on innate immunity. *Mol Oral Microbiol.* 2010;25(1):26–37.

Hoebe K, Janssen E, Beutler B. The interface between innate and adaptive immunity. *Nat Immunol.* 2004;5:971–974.

Iwasaki A, Medzhitov R. Regulation of adaptive immunity by the innate immune system. *Science.* 2010;327:291–295.

Jiang H, Chess L. Regulation of immune responses by T cells. *N Engl J Med.* 2006;354:1166–1176.

Jones SA. Directing transition from innate to acquired immunity. *J Immunol.* 2005;175:3463–3468.

Kawai T, Akira S. The role of pattern-recognition receptors in innate immunity. *Nat Immunol.* 2010;11(3):373–384.

Kumar H, Kawai T, AkiraS. Pathogen recognition by the innate immune system. *Int Rev Immunol.* 2011;30(1):16–34.

Lanier LL. NK cell recognition. *Annu Rev Immunol.* 2005;23:225–274.

Lasker MV, Nair SK. Intracellular TLR signaling: a structural perspective on human disease. *J Immunol.* 2006;177:11–16.

Murphy K, Travers P, Walport M. *Janeway's Immunobiology.* New York, NY: Garland; 2008.

Ooi EH, Psaltis AJ, Witterick EJ, et al. Innate immunity. *Otolaryngol Clin North Am.* 2010;43:473–487.

Rakoff-Nahoum S, Medzhitov R. Role of the innate immune system and host-commensal mutualism. *Curr Top Microbiol Immunol.* 2006;308:1–18.

Rossi M, Young JW. Human dendritic cells: potent antigen-presenting cells at the crossroads of innate and adaptive immunity. *J Immunol.* 2005;175:1373–1381.

Russell JH, Ley TJ. Lymphocyte mediated cytotoxicity. *Annu Rev Immunol.* 2002;20:323–370.

Sunyer JO, Boshra H, Lorenzo G, et al. Evolution of complement as an effector system in innate and adaptive immunity. *Immunol Res.* 2003;27:549–564.

Turvey SE, Broide DH. Chapter 2: innate immunity. *J Allergy Clin Immunol.* 2010;125(suppl 2):S24–S32.

Walport MJ. Complement: parts 1 and 2. *N Engl J Med.* 2001;344:1058–1066, 1141–1144.

Wright J. Immunoregulatory functions of surfactant proteins. *Nat Rev Immunol.* 2005;5:58–68.

Porth Essentials Resources

Explore these additional resources to enhance learning for this chapter:

- NCLEX-Style Questions and Other Resources on the**Point**, http://thePoint.lww.com/PorthEssentials4e
- Study Guide for Essentials of Pathophysiology
- Concepts in Action Animations
- Adaptive Learning | Powered by PrepU, http://thepoint.lww.com/prepu

Disorders of the Immune Response

The immune system is a multifaceted defense network that has evolved to protect against invading microorganisms, prevent the proliferation of cancer cells, and mediate the healing of damaged tissue. Under normal conditions, the immune response deters or prevents disease. Occasionally, however, the inadequate, inappropriate, or misdirected activation of the immune system can lead to debilitating or life-threatening illnesses, typified by allergic or hypersensitivity reactions, transplantation rejection, autoimmune disorders, and immunodeficiency states.

Hypersensitivity Disorders

Although activation of the immune system normally leads to production of antibodies and T-cell responses that protect the body against attack by microorganisms, it is also capable of causing tissue injury and disease. Disorders caused by immune responses are collectively referred to as *hypersensitivity reactions,* a term that arose from the observation that someone exposed to a particular antigen exhibited a detectable reaction or was "hypersensitive" to subsequent encounters with the same antigen.[1]

Hypersensitivity disorders are commonly classified into four groups according to the type of immune response causing the injury and the nature and location of the antigen that is the target of the response: type I, immediate hypersensitivity disorders; type II, antibody-mediated disorders; type III, immune complex–mediated disorders; and type IV, T-cell–mediated disorders[1–3] (Table 16-1).

Type I, Immediate Hypersensitivity Disorders

Type I hypersensitivity reactions are IgE-mediated reactions that begin rapidly, often within minutes of an antigen challenge. Often, they are referred to as allergic reactions and the antigens are called allergens. Typical

TABLE 16-1	**Classification of Hypersensitivity Responses**	
Type of Hypersensitivity	**Immune Mechanism**	**Mechanism of Injury**
Type I, immediate hypersensitivity	IgE antibody	Release of mast cell mediators
Type II, antibody-mediated	IgM, IgG antibodies against cell surface or extracellular matrix	Phagocytosis and opsonization of cells; complement- and receptor-mediated recruitment and activation of inflammatory cells (neutrophils, macrophages); abnormalities in cellular functioning (e.g., hormone receptor signaling)
Type III, immune complex–mediated	Formation of immune complexes involving circulating antigens and IgM or IgG antibodies	Complement-mediated recruitment and activation of inflammatory cells
Type IV, T-cell–mediated	CD4$^+$ T cells (delayed-type hypersensitivity) or CD8$^+$ cytotoxic T-cell–mediated cytolysis	Macrophage activation of cytokine-mediated inflammation; direct target cell killing, cytokine-mediated inflammation

IgE, immunoglobulin E; IgG, immunoglobulin G; IgM, immunoglobulin M.

allergens include the proteins in plant pollens, house dust mites, animal dander, foods, and chemicals like the antibiotic penicillin. Exposure to the allergen can be through inhalation, ingestion, injection, or skin contact. Depending on the portal of entry, type I reactions may be limited to merely annoying (e.g., seasonal rhinitis), severely debilitating (asthma), or systemic and potentially life-threatening (anaphylaxis).

Two types of cells are central to a type I hypersensitivity reaction: type 2 helper T (T_H2) cells and granule-containing cells, such as mast cells and/or basophils.[1-4] There are two subsets of helper T cells (T_H1 and T_H2) that develop from the same precursor CD4$^+$ T lymphocyte (see Chapter 15). T_H1 cells differentiate in response to microbes and stimulate the differentiation of B cells into IgM- and IgG-producing plasma cells. T_H2 cell differentiation occurs in response to allergens and helminths (intestinal parasites).[1] Cytokines secreted by T_H2 cells stimulate differentiation of B cells into IgE-producing plasma cells, act as growth factors for mast cells, and recruit and activate eosinophils.

The tissue-based mast cells and blood-based basophils are both derived from hematopoietic precursor cells in the bone marrow.[1] Mast cells are widely distributed in connective tissue, especially in areas beneath the skin and mucous membranes of the respiratory, gastrointestinal, and genitourinary tracts and adjacent to blood and lymph vessels.[5] This location places them near surfaces that are exposed to environmental antigens and parasites. Basophils, which share many features with mast cells, are granulocytes that circulate in the bloodstream and represent less than 1% of peripheral leukocytes (white blood cells). Both mast cells and basophils contain preformed mediators of inflammation that are stored in granules and released at the time of activation, and both have high-affinity receptors for IgE antibodies on their surface.

Type I hypersensitivity reactions begin with mast cell or basophil sensitization. During the sensitization or priming stage, allergen-specific IgE antibodies attach to receptors on the surface of mast cells and basophils.

With subsequent exposure, the sensitizing allergen binds to the cell-associated IgE and triggers a series of events that ultimately lead to degranulation of the sensitized mast cells or basophils, causing the release of their preformed mediators (Fig. 16-1). Mast cells are also the source of lipid-derived membrane products (e.g., prostaglandins and leukotrienes) and cytokines that participate in the continued response to the allergen.

Many type I hypersensitivity reactions, such as bronchial asthma, have two well-defined phases: (1) a primary or immediate-phase response characterized by vasodilation, vascular leakage, and smooth muscle contraction, and (2) a secondary or late-phase response characterized by more intense infiltration of tissues with eosinophils and other acute and chronic inflammatory cells, as well as tissue destruction in the form of epithelial cell damage.

The primary or immediate-phase response usually occurs within 5 to 30 minutes of exposure to antigen and subsides within 60 minutes. It is mediated by mast cell degranulation and the release of preformed mediators. These mediators include histamine, prostaglandins, leukotrienes, platelet activating-factor, interleukins, and enzymes such as chymase and trypsin that lead to the generation of kinins.[1] Histamine is a potent vasodilator that increases the permeability of capillaries and venules and causes smooth muscle contraction and bronchoconstriction. The kinins, which are a group of potent inflammatory peptides, require activation through enzymatic modification. Once activated, these peptide mediators (e.g., bradykinin) produce vasodilation and smooth muscle contraction.

The secondary or late-phase response occurs about 2 to 8 hours later and lasts for several days. It results from the action of lipid mediators and cytokines involved in the inflammatory response. The lipid mediators are derived from mast cell membrane phospholipids, which are broken down to form arachidonic acid. Arachidonic acid, in turn, is the parent compound from which the leukotrienes and prostaglandins are synthesized

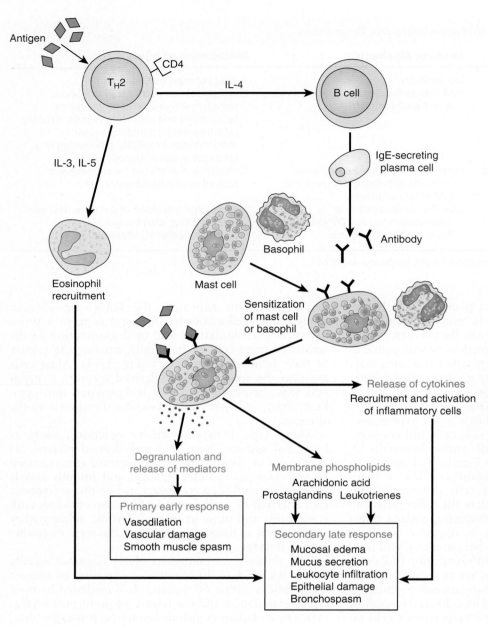

FIGURE 16-1. Type I, IgE-mediated hypersensitivity reaction. The stimulation of B-cell differentiation by an antigen-stimulated type 2 helper T (T$_H$2) cell leads to plasma cell production of IgE and mast cell or basophil sensitization. Subsequent binding of the antigen produces degranulation of the sensitized mast cell or basophil with release of preformed mediators that leads to a primary, or early-phase, response. T$_H$2 T-cell recruitment of eosinophils, along with the release of cytokines and membrane phospholipids from the mast cell, leads to a secondary, or late-phase, response. IgE, immunoglobulin E; IL, interleukin.

(see Chapter 3). The leukotrienes and prostaglandins produce responses similar to histamine, although their effects are delayed and prolonged by comparison. Mast cells also produce cytokines and chemotactic factors that prompt the influx of eosinophils and leukocytes to the site of allergen contact, additionally contributing to the inflammatory response.

At this point, it is important to note that not all IgE-mediated responses produce discomfort and disease. Type I hypersensitivity, particularly the late-phase response, plays a protective role in the control of parasitic intestinal infections. IgE antibodies directly damage the larvae of these parasites by recruiting inflammatory cells and causing antibody-dependent cell-mediated cytotoxicity. This type of type I

hypersensitivity reaction is particularly important in developing countries where much of the population is infected with intestinal parasites.

Systemic (Anaphylactic) Reactions

Anaphylaxis is a systemic life-threatening hypersensitivity reaction characterized by widespread edema, difficulty breathing, and vascular shock secondary to vasodilation[2,6-8] (see section on anaphylactic shock, Chapter 20). It results from the presence of antigen introduced by injection, insect sting, or absorption across the epithelial surface of the skin or gastrointestinal mucosa. The level of severity depends on the level of sensitization. Even small amounts of antigen, such as the presence of residual amounts of peanut that remain on equipment used for preparing foods containing peanuts, can be sufficient to cause anaphylaxis in an extremely sensitive person. Within minutes after exposure, itching, hives, and skin erythema develop, followed shortly by bronchospasm and respiratory distress. Vomiting, abdominal cramps, diarrhea, and laryngeal edema and obstruction follow, and the person may go into shock and die unless effective treatment is instituted.

The initial management of anaphylaxis focuses on the establishment of a stable airway and intravenous access, and the administration of epinephrine.[7,8] Epinephrine produces relaxation of bronchial smooth muscle and inhibits the immediate life-threatening cardiovascular effects of anaphylaxis. Persons with a history of anaphylaxis should be provided with preloaded epinephrine syringes and instructed in their use. They should also be instructed to seek immediate professional help regardless of the initial response to self-treatment. Family members and caregivers of young children should be trained to inject epinephrine. Prevention of exposure to potential triggers that cause anaphylaxis is particularly important. Finally, all persons with potential for anaphylaxis should be advised to wear or carry a medical alert bracelet, necklace, or other identification to inform emergency personnel of the possibility of anaphylaxis.

Local (Atopic) Reactions

Local or atopic reactions usually occur when the antigen is confined to a particular site by virtue of exposure. The term *atopic* refers to a genetically determined hypersensitivity to common environmental allergens mediated by an IgE–mast cell reaction. Persons with atopic disorders commonly are allergic to more than one (often many) environmental allergens. The most common atopic disorders are urticaria (hives), allergic rhinitis (hay fever), atopic dermatitis, food allergies, and some forms of asthma. The discussion in this section focuses on allergic rhinitis and food allergy. Allergic asthma is discussed in Chapter 23 and atopic dermatitis in Chapter 46.

The susceptibility to immediate hypersensitivity disorders tends to be inherited.[2] The genetic basis of atopy is unclear; however, linkage studies suggest an association with cytokine genes on chromosome 5q that regulate the expression of circulating IgE.[1] Persons with atopic allergic conditions tend to have high serum levels of IgE and increased numbers of basophils and mast cells. Although the IgE-triggered response is likely a key factor in the pathophysiology of atopic allergic disorders, it is not the only factor and may not be solely responsible for conditions such as atopic dermatitis and certain forms of asthma.

Allergic Rhinitis. Allergic rhinitis is characterized by symptoms of sneezing, itching, and watery discharge from the nose and eyes (rhinoconjunctivitis). Allergic rhinitis not only produces nasal symptoms but frequently is associated with other chronic airway disorders, such as sinusitis and bronchial asthma.[9,10] Severe attacks may be accompanied by malaise (general discomfort), fatigue, and muscle soreness from sneezing. Fever is absent. Sinus obstruction may cause headache. Typical allergens include pollens from ragweed, grasses, trees, and weeds; fungal spores; house dust mites; animal dander; and feathers. Allergic rhinitis can be divided into perennial and seasonal allergic rhinitis depending on the chronology of symptoms. Persons with the perennial type of allergic rhinitis experience symptoms throughout the year, whereas those with seasonal allergic rhinitis (e.g., hay fever) are plagued with intense symptoms in conjunction with periods of high allergen (e.g., pollens, fungal spores) exposure. Symptoms that become worse at night suggest a household allergen, and symptoms that improve or disappear on weekends suggest occupational exposure.

Diagnosis depends on a careful history and physical examination, microscopic identification of an increased number of eosinophils on a nasal smear, and skin or serum testing to identify the offending allergens. When possible, avoidance of the offending allergen is recommended. Treatment is symptomatic in most cases and includes the use of oral antihistamines and oral or topical decongestants. Intranasal corticosteroids often are effective when used appropriately. Intranasal cromolyn, a drug that stabilizes mast cells and prevents their degranulation, may be useful, especially when administered before expected contact with an offending allergen. A program of specific immunotherapy ("allergy shots") may be used when symptoms are particularly bothersome.[9,10] Desensitization involves frequent (often weekly) injections of the offending antigens. The antigens, which are given in increasing doses, stimulate production of high levels of IgG, which acts as a blocking antibody by combining with the antigen before it can combine with the cell-bound IgE antibodies.

Food Allergies. Virtually any food can produce atopic or nonatopic allergies. The primary target of food allergy may be the skin, the gastrointestinal tract, the respiratory system, or a combination thereof.[11,12] The foods most commonly causing these reactions are milk, eggs, peanuts, tree nuts, fish, and shellfish (i.e., crustaceans and mollusks). The allergenicity of a food may be changed by heating or cooking. A person may be allergic to drinking milk but may not have symptoms when milk is included in cooked foods. Both acute reactions (hives and anaphylaxis) and chronic reactions (asthma, atopic dermatitis, and gastrointestinal disorders) can occur. Anaphylaxis occurs as a multiorgan response associated with IgE-mediated hypersensitivity. The foods most responsible for anaphylaxis are peanuts,[13] tree nuts (e.g., walnuts, almonds, pecans, cashews, hazelnuts), and shellfish. One form of food-associated anaphylaxis occurs with exercise. It may occur when exercise follows ingestion of a particular food to which IgE sensitivity has been demonstrated, or it may occur after ingestion of any food. Exercise without ingestion of the incriminated food does not produce symptoms.

Food allergies can occur at any age but, similar to atopic dermatitis and rhinitis, they tend to manifest during childhood. The allergic response is thought to occur when there is contact between specific food allergens and sensitizing IgE in the intestinal mucosa, thereby causing local and systemic release of histamine and other mediators of the allergic response. In this disorder, allergens usually are food proteins and partially digested food products. Carbohydrates, lipids, or food additives, such as preservatives, colorings, or flavorings, also are potential allergens. Closely related food groups can contain common cross-reacting allergens. For example, some persons are allergic to all legumes (i.e., beans, peas, and peanuts).

Diagnosis of food allergies usually is based on a careful food history and through provocative diet testing. Provocative testing involves careful elimination of a suspected allergen from the diet for a period of time to see if the symptoms disappear and reintroducing the food to see if the symptoms reappear. Only one food should be tested at a time. Treatment focuses on avoidance of the food or foods responsible for the allergy. However, avoidance may be difficult for persons who are exquisitely sensitive to a particular food protein because foods may be contaminated with the protein during processing or handling of the food. As mentioned previously, contamination may occur when chocolate candies without peanuts are processed with the same equipment used for making candies with peanuts.

Type II, Antibody-Mediated Disorders

Type II (antibody-mediated) hypersensitivity reactions are mediated by IgG or IgM antibodies directed against target antigens on cell surfaces or in connective tissues.[2,3] The antigens may be endogenous antigens that are present on the membranes of body cells, or they may be exogenous antigens, such as drug metabolites, that are adsorbed on the membrane surface. Three different antibody-mediated mechanisms are involved in type II reactions: (1) complement- and antibody–mediated cell destruction, (2) complement- and antibody-mediated inflammation, and (3) antibody-mediated cellular dysfunction[2] (Fig. 16-2).

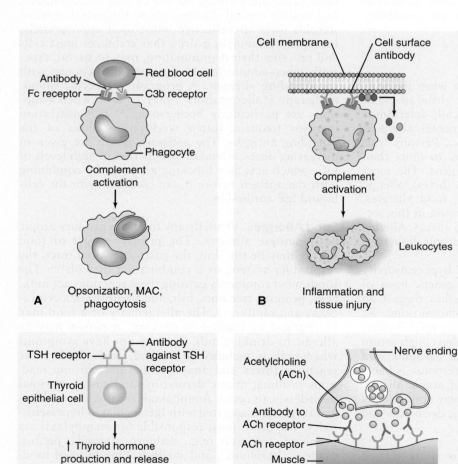

FIGURE 16-2. Type II, hypersensitivity reactions result from binding of antibodies to normal or altered surface antigens. **(A)** Opsonization and complement- or antibody receptor–mediated phagocytosis or cell lysis through membrane attack complex (MAC). **(B)** Complement- and antibody receptor–mediated inflammation resulting from recruitment and activation of inflammation-producing leukocytes (neutrophils and monocytes). Antibody-mediated cellular dysfunction, in which **(C)** antibody against the thyroid-stimulating hormone (TSH) receptor increases thyroid hormone production. **(D)** Antibody to acetylcholine receptor inhibits receptor binding of the neurotransmitter in myasthenia gravis.

Complement- and Antibody-Mediated Cell Destruction

The deletion of antibody-targeted cells can occur by way of the complement system or by antibody-dependent cell-mediated cytotoxicity (ADCC), which does not require complement.[2,3] Complement-mediated cell destruction can occur because the cells are coated with molecules (opsonized; see Fig. 16-2A) that make them attractive to phagocytes or because of the formation of membrane attack proteins that disrupt the integrity of the cell membrane and cause cell lysis (see Chapter 15, Understanding the Complement System). With ADCC destruction, cells that are coated with low levels of IgG antibody are killed by a variety of effector cells that bind to their target by their receptors for IgG, and cell lysis occurs without phagocytosis.

Examples of antibody-mediated cell destruction include mismatched blood transfusion reactions, hemolytic disease of the newborn due to ABO or Rh incompatibility (see Chapter 13), and certain drug reactions. In the latter, the binding of certain drugs or drug metabolites to the surface of red or white blood cells elicits an antibody response that lyses the drug-coated cell. Lytic drug reactions can produce transient anemia, leukopenia, or thrombocytopenia, which often are corrected by the removal of the offending drug.

Complement- and Antibody-Mediated Inflammation

When antibodies are deposited in extracellular tissue components, such as basement membranes and matrix, injury results from inflammation rather than phagocytosis or cell lysis (see Fig. 16-2B).[2,3] In this case, the deposited antibodies activate complement, generating chemotactic by-products that recruit and activate neutrophils and monocytes. The activated leukocytes release injurious substances, such as enzymes and reactive oxygen intermediates, that cause inflammation and tissue damage. Antibody-mediated inflammation is responsible for the tissue injury seen in some forms of glomerulonephritis, vascular rejection of organ grafts, and other diseases. In Goodpasture syndrome, for example, antibody binds to a major structural component of pulmonary and glomerular basement membranes, causing pulmonary hemorrhage and glomerulonephritis[3] (see Chapter 25).

Antibody-Mediated Cellular Dysfunction

In some type II reactions, antibody binding to specific target cell receptors does not lead to cell death, but to a change in cell function (see Figs. 16-2C, D). In Graves disease, for example, autoantibodies directed against thyroid-stimulating hormone (TSH) receptors on thyroid cells stimulates thyroxine production, leading to hyperthyroidism[2,3] (see Chapter 32). In myasthenia gravis, autoantibodies to acetylcholine receptors on the neuromuscular endplates either block the action of acetylcholine or mediate internalization or destruction of receptors, leading to decreased neuromuscular function (see Chapter 36).

Type III, Immune Complex–Mediated Disorders

Immune complex allergic disorders are mediated by the formation of insoluble antigen–antibody complexes, complement fixation, and localized inflammation[2,3] (Fig. 16-3). Immune complexes formed in the circulation produce damage when they come in contact with the vessel lining or are deposited in tissues, such as the renal glomerulus, skin venules, lung tissue, and joint synovium. Once deposited, the immune complexes elicit an inflammatory response by activating complement, thereby leading to chemotactic recruitment of neutrophils and other inflammatory cells. Activation of these inflammatory cells by immune complexes and complement, accompanied by the release of potent inflammatory mediators, is directly responsible for the injury.

Type III reactions are responsible for the vasculitis seen in certain autoimmune diseases such as systemic lupus erythematosus (SLE) or the kidney damage seen with acute glomerulonephritis. As with type I hypersensitivity reactions, type III immune complex disorders may present with systemic manifestations or as a local reaction.

Systemic Immune Complex Disorders

Serum sickness is a type III systemic immune complex disorder that is triggered by the deposition of insoluble antigen–antibody (IgM, IgG, and occasionally IgA)

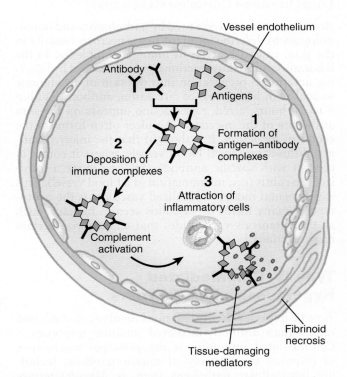

FIGURE 16-3. Type III, immune complex reactions involving complement-activating IgG or IgM immunoglobulins with (*1*) formation of blood-borne immune complexes that are (*2*) deposited in tissues. Complement activation at the site of immune complex deposition (*3*) leads to attraction of leukocytes that are responsible for vessel and tissue injury.

complexes in blood vessels, joints, and heart and kidney tissue.[2,3] The deposited complexes activate complement, increase vascular permeability, and recruit phagocytic cells, all of which can promote local tissue damage and edema. The term *serum sickness* was originally coined to describe a syndrome consisting of rash, lymphadenopathy, arthralgias, and occasionally neurologic disorders that appeared 7 or more days after injections of horse antiserum (used in protecting against tetanus). Although this therapy is not used today, the name remains. Currently, the most common causes of this allergic disorder include antibiotics (especially penicillin) and other drugs, various foods, and insect venoms.

The signs and symptoms of systemic immune complex disorders include urticaria, patchy or generalized rash, extensive edema (usually of the face, neck, and joints), and fever. In most cases, the damage is temporary, and symptoms resolve within a few days. However, a prolonged and continuous exposure to the sensitizing antigen can lead to irreversible damage. In previously sensitized persons, severe and even fatal forms of serum sickness may occur immediately or within several days after the sensitizing drug or serum is administered. Treatment usually is directed toward removal of the sensitizing antigen and providing symptomatic relief. This may include aspirin for joint pain and antihistamines for pruritus (itching). Epinephrine or systemic corticosteroids may be used for severe reactions.

Local Immune Complex Reactions

Arthus reaction is a term used by pathologists and immunologists to describe localized tissue necrosis (usually in the skin) caused by type III immune complexes. In the laboratory, an Arthus reaction can be produced by injecting an antigen preparation into the skin of an immune animal with high levels of circulating antibody. Within 4 to 10 hours, a red, raised lesion appears on the skin at the site of the injection.[2] An ulcer often forms in the center of the lesion. It is thought that the injected antigen diffuses into local blood vessels, where it comes in contact with specific antibody (IgG) to incite a localized vasculitis (i.e., inflammation of a blood vessel). This experimental model of localized vasculitis is the prototype of many forms of vasculitis seen in humans, such as the cutaneous vasculitides that characterize certain drug reactions.

Type IV, Cell-Mediated Hypersensitivity Disorders

Type IV hypersensitivity reactions involve cell-mediated rather than antibody-mediated immune responses.[2,3] Cell-mediated immunity is the principal mechanism of response to a variety of microorganisms, including intracellular pathogens such as *Mycobacterium tuberculosis* and viruses, as well as extracellular agents such as fungi, protozoa, and parasites. It can also lead to cell death and tissue injury in response to chemical antigens (contact dermatitis) or self-antigens (autoimmunity).

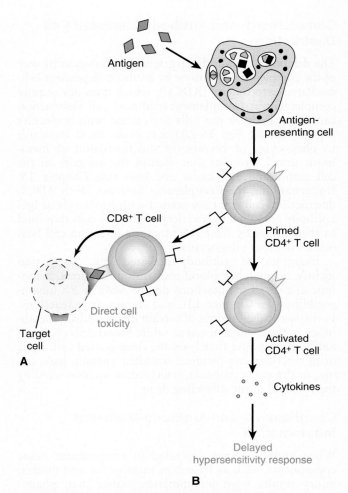

FIGURE 16-4. Type IV, cell-mediated hypersensitivity reactions, which include **(A)** direct cell-mediated cytotoxicity in which CD8+ T cells kill the antigen-bearing target cells, and **(B)** delayed-type hypersensitivity reactions in which presensitized CD4+ cells release cell-damaging cytokines.

Type IV hypersensitivity reactions, which are mediated by specifically sensitized T lymphocytes, can be divided into two basic types: direct cell-mediated cytotoxicity and delayed-type hypersensitivity (Fig. 16-4).

Direct Cell-Mediated Cytotoxicity

In direct cell-mediated cytotoxicity (see Fig. 16-4A), CD8+ cytotoxic T lymphocytes (CTLs) directly kill target cells that express peptides derived from cytosolic antigens that are presented in association with class I major histocompatibility complex (MHC) molecules (see Chapter 15). In viral infections, CTL responses can lead to tissue injury by killing infected target cells even if the virus itself has no cytotoxic effects.[2] Because CTLs cannot distinguish between cytopathic and noncytopathic viruses, they kill virtually all infected cells regardless of whether the infection is harmful. In certain forms of hepatitis, for example, the destruction of liver cells is due to the host CTL response and not the virus.

Delayed-Type Hypersensitivity Disorders

Delayed-type hypersensitivity (DTH) reactions (see Fig. 16-4B) occur in response to soluble protein antigens and primarily involve antigen-presenting cells such as macrophages and CD4+ helper T cells of the T_H1 type. During the reaction T_H1 cells are activated and secrete an array of cytokines that recruit and activate macrophages, lymphocytes, fibroblasts, and other inflammatory cells.[7] These T-cell–mediated responses require the synthesis of effector molecules and take 24 to 72 hours to develop, which is why they are called "delayed-type" hypersensitivity disorders.

The best-known DTH response is the reaction to the tuberculin test, in which inactivated tuberculin or purified protein derivative is injected under the skin. In a person who has been sensitized by previous infection, a local area of redness and induration develops within 8 to 12 hours, reaching a peak in 24 to 72 hours. The tuberculin reaction is characterized by perivascular accumulation of T_H1 cells and, to a lesser extent, macrophages. Local secretion of cytokines by these mononuclear inflammatory cells leads to increased microvascular permeability with local redness and swelling. The sequence of events in DTH, as demonstrated by the tuberculin reaction, begins with the first exposure to the tubercle bacilli (see Chapter 22). The T_H1 cells recognize the peptide antigens of the tubercle bacilli in association with class II MHC antigens on the surface of monocytes and antigen-presenting cells that have processed the mycobacterial antigens. This process leads to formation of sensitized T_H1 memory cells that remain in the circulation for years. Subsequent injection of tuberculin into such an individual results in the secretion of T_H1 cell cytokines that are ultimately responsible for the DTH response.

In addition to its beneficial protective role, DTH can also be the cause of disease, including allergic contact dermatitis and hypersensitivity pneumonitis. It also can be involved in transplant rejection and autoimmune disorders.

Allergic Contact Dermatitis. Allergic contact dermatitis denotes an inflammatory response confined to the skin that is initiated by re-exposure to an allergen to which a person had previously become sensitized (e.g., cosmetics, hair dyes, metals, topical drugs).[14,15] The most common form of this condition is the dermatitis that follows an encounter with poison ivy or poison oak antigens, although many other substances can trigger a reaction.

Contact dermatitis is characterized by erythematous, papular, and vesicular lesions associated with intense pruritus and weeping. The affected area often becomes swollen and warm, with exudation, crusting, and potentially the development of a secondary infection. The location of the lesions often provides a clue about the antigen causing the disorder. The severity of the reaction associated with contact dermatitis ranges from mild to intense, depending on the person and the allergen. Because this condition follows the mechanism of a DTH response, the reaction does not become apparent for at least 12 hours and usually more than 24 hours after exposure. Depending on the antigen and the duration of exposure, the reaction may last from days to weeks.

Diagnosis of contact dermatitis is made by observing the distribution of lesions on the skin surface and associating a particular pattern with exposure to possible allergens. If a particular allergen is suspected, a skin patch test can be used to confirm the suspicion. Treatment usually is limited to removal of the irritant and application of topical preparations (e.g., ointments, corticosteroid creams) to relieve symptomatic skin lesions and prevent secondary bacterial infections. Severe reactions may require systemic corticosteroid therapy.

Hypersensitivity Pneumonitis. Hypersensitivity pneumonitis, which is associated with exposure to inhaled organic dusts or related occupational antigens, is another example of a DTH reaction.[16] The disorder is thought to involve a susceptible host and activation of pulmonary T cells, followed by the release of cytokine mediators of inflammation. The inflammatory response that ensues (usually several hours after exposure) produces labored breathing, dry cough, chills, fever, headache, and malaise. The symptoms usually subside within hours after the sensitizing antigens are removed. A primary example of hypersensitivity pneumonitis is "farmer's lung," a condition resulting from exposure to moldy hay. Other sensitizing antigens include tree bark, sawdust, animal dander, and *Mycobacteria* that are occasionally found in humidifiers, hot tubs, and swimming pools. Exposure to small amounts of antigen for a long period may lead to chronic lung disease with minimal reversibility. This can occur in persons exposed to avian or animal antigens or a contaminated home air humidifier.

The most important element in the diagnosis of hypersensitivity pneumonitis is to obtain a good history (occupational and otherwise) of exposure to possible antigens. Treatment consists of first identifying and then avoiding the offending antigens. Severe forms of the disorder may be treated with systemic corticosteroid therapy.

SUMMARY CONCEPTS

- Hypersensitivity disorders are immune responses to environmental, food, or drug antigens that would not affect most of the population.

- *Type I hypersensitivity responses* are mediated by IgE and include anaphylactic shock, hay fever, and bronchial asthma;

- *Type II hypersensitivity responses* include antibody-mediated cell destruction (e.g., transfusion reactions, hemolytic disease of the newborn, and certain drug reactions), complement- and antibody-mediated inflammation (e.g., some forms of glomerulonephritis), and antibody-mediated cell dysfunction (e.g., Graves disease and myasthenia gravis).

- *Type III hypersensitivity reactions* involve the formation and deposition of insoluble antigen–

(continued)

Transplantation Immunopathology

Transplantation is the process of taking cells, tissues, or organs, called a *graft*, from one individual and placing them into another individual. Sometimes grafts are transplanted from another site in the same individual. The individual who provided the tissue is called the *donor*, and the individual who receives the graft is called either the *recipient* or the *host*. Transplantation rejection is discussed here because it involves several of the previously discussed immunologic reactions. A major barrier to transplantation is the process of rejection, in which the recipient's immune system recognizes the graft as foreign and attacks it.

The cell surface antigens that determine whether the tissue of transplanted organs is recognized as foreign are the MHC or *human leukocyte antigens* (HLA) that were discussed in Chapter 15. Transplanted tissue can be categorized as an *autologous* graft if the donor and recipient are the same person, *syngeneic* graft if the donor and recipient are identical twins, and *allogeneic* (genetic variations of the same gene within a given species) if the donor and recipient—whether related or not—share similar HLA types. The molecules that are recognized as foreign on allografts are called *alloantigens*. Donors of solid organ transplants can be living or dead (cadaver) and related or nonrelated (heterologous). Rejection of allografts is a response to MHC molecules, which are so polymorphic that no two individuals are likely to express the same MHC molecules, unless they are identical twins. The likelihood of rejection varies indirectly with the degree of MHC or HLA relatedness between the donor and recipient.

Immune Recognition of Allografts

Rejection of allografts is a complex process that involves cell-mediated immunity and circulating antibodies. Although many cells may participate in the process of acute transplant rejection, only the T lymphocytes seem to be absolutely required.[1-3] The recipient's T cells recognize allogeneic antigens in the graft by two pathways: the direct and indirect recognition pathways.[2]

In the *direct pathway*, T cells of the transplant recipient directly recognize donor MHC molecules of the surface of antigen-presenting cells in the graft.[1,2] Both the CD4+ and CD8+ cells of the transplant recipient are involved in the reaction. Recipient CD8+ T cells recognize donor class I MHC molecules and differentiate into mature CTLs that kill cells in the grafted tissue (see type IV hypersensitivity reactions). The CD4+ helper T-cell subset is triggered into proliferation and differentiation into T_H1 effector cells by recognition of donor class II MHC molecules. As with delayed hypersensitivity reactions, cytokines secreted by activated CD4+ cells cause increased vascular permeability and local accumulation and activation of macrophages, resulting in graft injury.

In the *indirect pathway*, recipient CD4+ T cells recognize donor MHC molecules after they have been picked up, processed, and presented by the recipient's own antigen-presenting cells.[1,2] Thus, the indirect pathway is similar to the physiologic processing and presentation of other foreign antigens. This form of recognition mainly activates DTH pathways of the type IV hypersensitivity reactions. This indirect pathway is also involved in the production of antibodies against graft alloantigens. If the alloantigens are proteins, they are picked up by host B cells and processed, and their peptides presented to helper T cells, which then stimulate antibody responses.[2]

Patterns and Mechanisms of Solid Organ Graft Rejection

The basic patterns of transplant rejection have historically been classified based on the time course of the response and the pathologic mechanisms involved.[1-3] Based on experience with kidney transplants, which have been done for a longer time and more often than any other organ, the patterns of response are called hyperacute, acute, and chronic. In actual practice, however, there is often an overlap in features. The diagnosis is further complicated by the effects of immunosuppressant drugs or the possible recurrence of the original disease.

Hyperacute Rejection

Hyperacute rejection occurs almost immediately after transplantation.[3] In kidney transplants, it can often be seen at the time of surgery. As soon as blood flow from the recipient to the donor kidney begins, it takes on a cyanotic, mottled appearance. At other times, the reaction may take hours or days to develop.

The hyperacute response is produced by existing recipient antibodies to graft antigens that initiate a type III, Arthus-type hypersensitivity reaction in the blood vessels of the graft. These antibodies usually have developed in response to previous blood transfusions, pregnancies in which the mother makes antibodies to fetal antigens, or infections with bacteria or viruses possessing antigens that mimic MHC antigens.

Acute Rejection

Acute rejection may occur within the first few days to weeks after transplantation, or it may occur suddenly months or even years later, after the discontinuation of immunosuppressants in the post-transplant period. Before modern immunosuppression, acute rejection would often begin several days to a few weeks after transplantation. The delayed time of onset of acute rejection reflects the time it takes for the recipient's immune system to generate T cells and antibodies against the graft.[1] In kidney transplantation it is characterized by abrupt onset of kidney failure, which may be associated with fever and graft tenderness.

Acute rejection most typically involves both cell-mediated and humoral mechanisms of tissue damage. In acute cell-mediated rejection the activated T cells cause direct lysis of graft cells and recruit and activate inflammatory cells that injure the graft. Acute antibody-mediated or humoral mechanisms involve blood vessel damage and intravascular thrombosis that leads to graft destruction.

Chronic Rejection

Chronic rejection develops insidiously over months and years and may or may not be preceded by episodes of acute rejection. In recent years, acute rejection has been significantly controlled by immunosuppressive therapy, and chronic rejection has emerged as an important cause of graft rejection. In kidney transplantation there are signs of progressive kidney failure.

The dominant lesion in chronic rejection is arterial occlusion resulting from the proliferation of vascular smooth muscle cells, with graft failure resulting from ischemic damage. These arterial changes are often referred to as graft vasculopathy or accelerated graft arteriosis.[1] The actual mechanism of this type of response is unclear but may include release of cytokines that stimulate proliferation of vascular endothelial and muscle cells; repair with fibrosis after repeated bouts of acute antibody-mediated or cellular rejection; and toxic effects of immunsuppressive drugs.[1]

Transplantation of Hematopoietic Cells

Bone marrow transplantation is increasingly being used as therapy for hematopoietic and some nonhematopoietic malignancies, aplastic anemia, and immunodeficiency disorders. Hematopoietic stem cells can be collected from donor bone marrow or peripheral blood. Stem cell aspiration from the bone marrow is the most common form of allograft collection. Peripheral blood offers a less-invasive method for obtaining stem cells. Hematopoietic growth factors, such as granulocyte colony-stimulating factor, often are used to induce stem cells to move out of the bone marrow into the blood. Before either bone marrow or peripheral blood stem cells are infused, recipients receive pretreatment conditioning regimens (e.g., total-body irradiation or treatment with cytotoxic drugs) to destroy malignant cells (e.g., in leukemia) and to create a graft bed. Rejection of the allogeneic bone marrow transplant appears to be mediated by a combination of reactive T cells and natural killer (NK) cells that are resistant to radiation therapy and chemotherapy.[2]

Graft-Versus-Host Disease

Graft-versus-host-disease (GVHD) occurs when immunologically competent cells or precursors are transplanted into recipients who are immunologically compromised.[17,18] Although GVHD occurs most often in persons who have undergone allogeneic bone marrow transplantation, it may also follow transplantation of organs rich in lymphoid tissue (e.g., the liver) or follow transfusions with nonirradiated blood.[2] Three basic requirements are necessary for GVHD to develop: (1) the transplant must have a functional cellular immune component, (2) the recipient tissue must bear antigens foreign to the donor tissue, and (3) recipient immunity must be compromised to the point that it cannot destroy the transplanted cells.[1,17,18] The primary agents of GVHD are the donor immunocompetent T cells derived from the donor marrow and the recipient tissue that they recognize as foreign and react against.[2] Graft-versus-host-disease results in activation of both CD4+ and CD8+ T cells, ultimately generating type IV cell-mediated DTH and CTL reactions. The greater the difference in tissue antigens between the donor and recipient, the greater the likelihood of GVHD.

Graft-versus-host-disease can occur as an acute or chronic reaction. *Acute GVHD*, which develops within days to weeks after transplantation, involves the epithelial cells of the skin, liver, and gastrointestinal tract.[2] The organ most commonly affected in acute GVHD is the skin. There is development of a pruritic, maculopapular rash, which begins on the palms and soles and frequently extends over the entire body, with subsequent desquamation (sloughing off skin). Involvement of the gastrointestinal tract usually parallels the development of skin and liver involvement. Gastrointestinal symptoms include nausea, bloody diarrhea, and abdominal pain. Graft-versus-host-disease of the liver is heralded by painless jaundice, hyperbilirubinemia, and abnormal liver function test results. Liver involvement can progress to development of veno-occlusive disease, drug toxicity, viral infection, iron overload, extrahepatic biliary obstruction, sepsis, and coma.[19]

Chronic GVHD may follow acute GVHD or it may develop insidiously. Persons in whom chronic GVHD develops are profoundly immunocompromised, and they develop skin lesions resembling systemic sclerosis (discussed in Chapter 44) and manifestations mimicking other autoimmune diseases. As a result of the severely compromised immune system, recurrent and life-threatening infections are common.

 SUMMARY CONCEPTS

■ Transplantation involves taking cells, tissues, or organs, called a *graft*, from one individual (a donor) and placing them into another individual (recipient). A major barrier to transplantation is the process of rejection in which the recipient's immune system recognizes the graft as foreign and attacks it.

(continued)

SUMMARY CONCEPTS *(continued)*

■ Destruction of the cells or tissues of the graft can result from direct action of the recipient's cytotoxic T cells, from T-cell–generated cytokines and a delayed hypersensitivity reaction, or from antibodies generated against antigens in the graft.

■ *Hyperacute rejection* occurs almost immediately after transplantation and is caused by existing recipient antibodies to graft antigens that initiate a type III, Arthus-type hypersensitivity reaction in the blood vessels of the graft. *Acute rejection* occurs within the first few weeks or months after transplantation and occurs when graft tissue or blood vessels are damaged by alloreactive T cells or antibodies. *Chronic rejection* occurs over a prolonged period and is caused by T-cell–generated cytokines that damage blood vessels, causing ischemic damage to graft tissue.

■ Graft-versus-host disease (GVHD), which occurs most often following bone marrow transplantation, develops when immunologically competent cells or precursors are transplanted into recipients who are immunologically compromised. Three basic requirements are necessary for GVHD to develop: (1) the transplant must have a functional cellular immune component, (2) the recipient tissue must bear antigens foreign to the donor tissue, and (3) recipient immunity must be compromised to the point that it cannot destroy the transplanted cells.

CHART 16-1 **Probable Autoimmune Disease***

Systemic
Mixed connective tissue disease
Polymyositis-dermatomyositis
Rheumatoid arthritis
Scleroderma
Sjögren syndrome
Systemic lupus erythematosus

Blood
Autoimmune hemolytic anemia
Autoimmune neutropenia and lymphopenia
Idiopathic thrombocytopenic purpura

Other Organs
Acute idiopathic polyneuritis
Atrophic gastritis and pernicious anemia
Autoimmune adrenalitis
Goodpasture syndrome
Hashimoto thyroiditis
Type 1 diabetes mellitus
Myasthenia gravis
Premature gonadal (ovarian) failure
Primary biliary cirrhosis
Sympathetic ophthalmia
Temporal arteritis
Thyrotoxicosis (Graves disease)
Crohn disease, ulcerative colitis

*Examples are not inclusive.

Autoimmune Disease

Autoimmune diseases represent a group of disorders that are caused by a breakdown in the ability of the immune system to differentiate between self- and nonself-antigens. They can affect almost any cell or tissue in the body. Some autoimmune disorders, such as Hashimoto thyroiditis, are tissue specific, whereas others, such as SLE, affect multiple organs and systems. Chart 16-1 lists some of the common autoimmune diseases. Many of these disorders are discussed elsewhere in this book.

Immunologic Tolerance

To function properly, the immune system must be able to differentiate foreign antigens from self-antigens in a process called *self-tolerance*.[1–3] It is the HLAs encoded by MHC genes that serve as recognition markers of self and nonself for the immune system (see Chapter 15). To elicit an immune response, an antigen must first be processed by an antigen-presenting cell (APC), such as a macrophage, which then presents the antigenic determinants along with an MHC II molecule to a CD4+ helper T cell. The dual recognition of the MHC–antigen complex by the T-cell receptor (TCR) of the CD4+ helper T cell acts like a security check. Similar recognition checks occur between CD8+ cytotoxic T cells and the MHC I–antigen complex of tissue cells that have been targeted for elimination. A number of chemical messengers (e.g., interleukins) and costimulatory signals are essential to the activation of immune responses and the preservation of self-tolerance.

Several mechanisms have been postulated to explain the tolerant state, including central tolerance and peripheral tolerance.[1,2,20–23] *Central tolerance* refers to the elimination of self-reactive T cells and B cells in the central lymphoid organs (i.e., the thymus for T cells and the bone marrow for B cells). *Peripheral tolerance* derives from the deletion or inactivation of autoreactive T cells or B cells that escaped elimination in the central lymphoid organs. *Anergy* represents the state of immunologic tolerance to specific antigens. It may take the form of diminished immediate hypersensitivity, delayed-type hypersensitivity, or both.

B-Cell Tolerance

Several mechanisms are available to filter autoreactive B cells out of the B-cell population: clonal deletion of immature B cells in the bone marrow; deletion of autoreactive B cells in the spleen or lymph nodes; functional inactivation or anergy; and receptor editing, a process that changes the specificity of a B-cell receptor when autoantigen is encountered.[20] There is increasing evidence that B-cell tolerance is predominantly due to help from T cells. Loss of self-tolerance with development of autoantibodies is characteristic of a number of autoimmune disorders. For example, hyperthyroidism in Graves disease is due to autoantibodies to the TSH receptor (see Fig. 16-2 and Chapter 32).

T-Cell Tolerance

The central mechanisms of T-cell tolerance involve the deletion of self-reactive T cells in the thymus (Fig. 16-5). T cells develop from bone marrow–derived progenitor cells that migrate to the thymus, where they encounter self-peptides bound to MHC molecules. T cells that display the host's MHC antigens and T-cell receptors for a nonself-antigen are allowed to mature in the thymus (i.e., positive selection). T cells that have a high affinity for host cells are sorted out and undergo apoptosis or cell death (i.e., negative selection). The deletion of self-reactive T cells in the thymus requires the presence of autoantigens. Because many autoantigens are not present in the thymus, self-reactive T cells may escape the thymus, so peripheral mechanisms that participate in T-cell tolerance are required.

Several mechanisms are available to control the responsiveness of self-reactive T cells in the periphery. Sometimes the host antigens are not available in the appropriate immunologic form or are separated from the T cells (e.g., by the blood–brain barrier) so that corresponding T cells remain *immunologically ignorant* of their presence.[20,21] In other cases, the autoreactive T cell encounters its corresponding antigen in the absence of

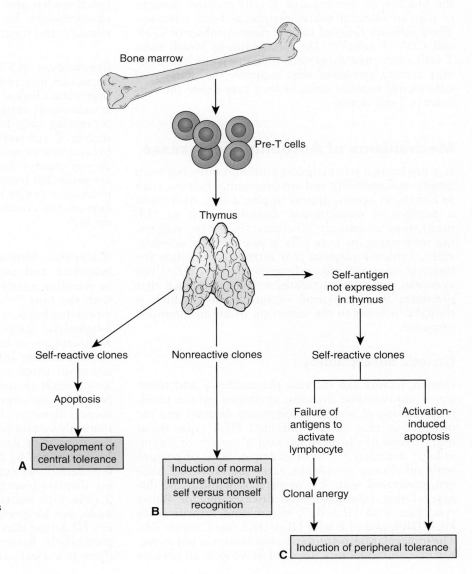

FIGURE 16-5. Development of immunologic T cell tolerance. **(A)** Development of central tolerance with deletion of self-reactive T lymphocytes in the thymus. **(B)** Nonreactive lymphocytes with development of normal immune function. **(C)** Induction of peripheral tolerance in self-reactive cells that are not eliminated in the thymus.

the costimulatory signals that are necessary for its activation. The peripheral activation of T cells requires two signals: recognition of the peptide antigen in association with the MHC molecules on the APCs, and a set of secondary costimulatory signals. Because costimulatory signals are not strongly expressed on most normal tissues, the encounter of the autoreactive T cells and their specific target antigens frequently results in anergy.[1,2]

Another self-tolerance mechanism involves the apoptotic death of autoreactive T cells.[20,21,24] This type of apoptosis is mediated by an apoptotic cell surface receptor (called Fas) that is present on the T cell and a soluble membrane messenger molecule (Fas ligand) that binds to the apoptotic receptor and activates the death program (see Chapter 2). The expression of the apoptotic Fas receptor is markedly increased in activated T cells; thus, coexpression of the Fas messenger molecule by the same cohort of activated autoreactive T cells may serve to induce their death.

Suppressor T cells with the ability to down-regulate the function of autoreactive T cells are also thought to play an essential role in peripheral T-cell tolerance. These cells are believed to be a distinct subset of CD4+ and CD8+ T cells.[25,26] The mechanism by which these T cells exert their suppressor function is unclear. They may secrete cytokines that suppress the activity of self-reactive immune cells, or they may delete the self-reactive T-cell clones.

Mechanisms of Autoimmune Disease

It is not known what triggers autoimmunity, but both genetic susceptibility and environmental factors, such as infectious agents, appear to play a role. Moreover, a number of autoimmune disorders such as SLE occur more commonly in women than men, suggesting that estrogens may play a role in their development. Evidence suggests that estrogens stimulate the immune response and androgens suppress it.[27,28] For example, estrogen stimulates a DNA sequence that promotes the production of interferon-γ, which is thought to assist in the induction of an autoimmune response.

Genetic Susceptibility

Genetic factors can increase the incidence and severity of autoimmune diseases, as shown by the familial clustering of several autoimmune diseases and the observation that certain inherited HLA types occur more frequently in persons with a variety of immunologic disorders.[2,22,23] For example, 90% of persons with ankylosing spondylitis carry the HLA-B27 antigen, compared with 7% of persons without the disease.[2] Other HLA-associated diseases include Reiter syndrome with HLA-B27, rheumatoid arthritis with HLA-DR4, and SLE with HLA-DR3 (see Chapter 44). The molecular basis for these associations is unknown. Because autoimmunity does not develop in all persons

with genetic predisposition, it appears that other factors—such as a "trigger event"—interact to precipitate the altered immune state. The event or events that trigger the development of an autoimmune response are unknown. It has been suggested that the "trigger" may be a virus or other microorganism, a chemical substance, or a self-antigen from a body tissue that has been hidden from the immune system during development.

Role of Infections

Viral and bacterial infections may contribute to the development and exacerbations of autoimmunity. In many persons, the onset of autoimmunity is associated with or preceded by infection. In most of these cases, the infectious microorganisms are not present in lesions or detectable when autoimmunity develops.[1-3] Therefore, the lesions of autoimmunity are not due to the infectious agent itself, but to the immune process that was triggered by the microbe. There are three proposed mechanisms through which infections can trigger autoimmunity: breakdown of T-cell anergy, molecular mimicry, and superantigens.

Breakdown of T-Cell Anergy. Infections of particular tissues may induce local innate immune responses that attract leukocytes into the tissue and result in the activation of antigen-presenting cells. These antigen-presenting cells begin to express costimulators and secrete T cell–activating cytokines, resulting in the breakdown of self-tolerance.[1,2] Most normal tissues do not express the costimulatory molecules and thus are protected from autoreactive T cells. However, this protection can be lost if the cells that do not normally express the costimulatory molecules are induced to do so.

Molecular Mimicry. One proposed link between infections and autoimmunity is *molecular mimicry*, in which a microbe shares an immunologic epitope with the host.[29,30] In rheumatic fever and acute glomerulonephritis, a protein in the cell wall of group A β-hemolytic streptococci has considerable similarity with antigens in heart and kidney tissue, respectively. After infection, antibodies directed against the microorganism cause a classic case of mistaken identity, which leads to inflammation of the heart or kidney. Not everyone exposed to group A β-hemolytic streptococci develops an autoimmune reaction. The reason that only certain persons are targeted for autoimmune reactions to a particular self-mimicry molecule may be determined by differences in HLA types. The HLA type determines exactly which fragments of a pathogen are displayed on the cell surface for presentation to T cells. One individual's HLA may bind self-mimicry molecules for presentation to T cells, whereas another's HLA type may not. In the spondyloarthropathies, particularly Reiter syndrome and reactive arthritis, there is a clear relationship between arthritis and a prior bacterial infection, combined with the inherited HLA-B27 antigens.

Superantigens. Superantigens are a family of related substances, including staphylococcal and streptococcal exotoxins, that can short-circuit the normal sequence of events in an immune response, leading to inappropriate activation of CD4+ helper T cells. Superantigens do not require the typical processing and presentation of antigen by APCs to induce a T-cell response.[31] Instead, they are able to interact with a T-cell receptor outside the normal antigen-binding site. This distinctive mode of activation, combined with the ability of superantigens to bind to a wide variety of MHC class II molecules, can lead to the activation of large numbers of T cells regardless of their MHC/peptide specificity. Superantigens are involved in several diseases, including food poisoning and toxic shock syndrome.

Release of Sequestered Antigens

Normally the body does not produce antibodies against self-antigens. Thus, any self-antigen that was completely sequestered during development and then reintroduced to the immune system is likely to be regarded as foreign. Among the sequestered tissues that could be regarded as foreign are spermatozoa and ocular antigens such as those found in uveal tissue. Posttraumatic uveitis and orchiditis after vasectomy may fall into this category.

Changes in antigen structure or release of hidden antigens may also account for the persistence of autoimmune disorders. Once an autoimmune disorder has been induced, it tends to be progressive, sometimes with sporadic relapses and remissions. A possible mechanism for the persistence and evolution of autoimmunity is the phenomenon called *epitope spreading*.[2] Infections, and even the initial autoimmune episode, may expose self-antigens that have been hidden from the immune system, resulting in continued activation of new lymphocytes that recognize the previously hidden epitopes.

Diagnosis and Treatment of Autoimmune Disease

Suggested criteria for determining whether a disorder is an autoimmune disease include the following: evidence of an autoimmune reaction, determination that the immunologic findings are not secondary to another condition, and no other identifiable causes for the disorder. Currently, the diagnosis of autoimmune disease is based primarily on clinical findings and serologic testing.

The basis for most serologic assays is the demonstration of antibodies directed against tissue antigens or cellular components. For example, an individual with a history of fever, arthritis, and a macular rash and who has high levels of antinuclear antibody has a probable diagnosis of SLE. The detection of autoantibodies in the laboratory usually is accomplished by one of three methods: indirect fluorescent antibody assay (IFA), enzyme-linked immunosorbent assay (ELISA), or particle agglutination of some kind. The rationale behind each of these methods is similar: the patient's serum is diluted and allowed to react with an antigen-coated surface (e.g., whole, fixed cells for the detection of antinuclear antibodies). In the case of IFA and ELISA, a second "labeled" antibody is added, which binds to the patient's antibody and can induce a visible reaction. Particle agglutination assays are much simpler—the binding of the patient's antibody to antigen-coated particles causes a visible agglutination reaction. For most serologic assays, the patient's serum is serially diluted until it no longer produces a visible reaction (e.g., 1:100 dilution). This is called a *positive titer*. Healthy persons sometimes have low titers of antibody against cellular and tissue antigens, but their titers usually are far lower than in patients with autoimmune disease.

Treatment of autoimmune disease is based on the tissue or organ that is involved, the effector mechanism involved, and the magnitude and chronicity of the effector processes. Ideally, treatment should focus on the mechanism underlying the autoimmune disorder. Corticosteroids and immunosuppressive drugs may be used to arrest or reverse the downhill course of some autoimmune disorders. Purging autoreactive cells from the immune repertoire through the use of plasmapheresis is also an option in some severe cases of autoimmunity.

Recent research has focused on the cytokines involved in the inflammatory response that accompanies many of the autoimmune disorders (e.g., interferon-β for multiple sclerosis and tumor necrosis factor-α [TNF-α] antibodies for rheumatoid arthritis and Crohn disease).

SUMMARY CONCEPTS

- Autoimmune diseases represent a disruption in self-tolerance that results in damage to body tissues by the immune system.

- Self-tolerance is maintained through central and peripheral mechanisms that delete autoreactive B or T cells or otherwise suppress or inactivate immune responses that would be destructive to host tissues. Defects in any of these mechanisms could impair self-tolerance and predispose to the development of autoimmune disease.

- Autoimmunity results from a failure of tolerance. Autoimmune disorders may be triggered by environmental stimuli, such as infections, in a genetically predisposed individual.

Immunodeficiency Disorders

Immunodeficiency can be defined as an abnormality in one or more components of the immune system that renders a person susceptible to diseases normally prevented by an intact immune system. These disorders can be broadly classified into two groups: primary and secondary.[1] The primary or congenital immunodeficiencies are genetic defects that result in increased susceptibility to infection that is frequently manifested early in life. Secondary or acquired immunodeficiency is not inherited but develops as a consequence of malnutrition, selective loss of immunoglobulins through the gastrointestinal or genitourinary tracts, treatment with immunosuppressant drugs, or human immunodeficiency virus (HIV), the etiologic agent of acquired immunodeficiency syndrome (AIDS). Regardless of the cause, primary and secondary deficiencies can produce the same spectrum of disease. The severity and symptomatology of the various disorders depend on the type and extent of the deficiency.

Primary Immunodeficiency Disorders

Until recently, little was known about the causes of primary immunodeficiency diseases. However, this has changed with recent advances in genetic technology.[1,32–35] To date, more than 180 primary immunodeficiency syndromes have been identified, and specific molecular defects have been identified in more than one third of these diseases.[1] Most are transmitted as recessive traits, caused by mutations in genes on the X chromosome or autosomal chromosomes. Many of these disorders have been traced to mutations affecting signaling pathways (e.g., cytokines and cytokine signaling, receptor subunits, and metabolic pathways) that dictate immune cell development and function. Furthermore, it has been shown that the immune system is a carefully balanced system that is designed to distinguish between self and nonself; therefore, symptoms of autoimmunity often are observed with primary immunodeficiency disease.

Early detection, which is possible for most primary immunodeficiency diseases, is critical for the success of some treatments and can be lifesaving. For infants with severe combined T- and B-cell immunodeficiency, early diagnosis is essential in terms of not only preventing life-threatening infections, but also preventing administration of live attenuated virus vaccines (e.g., measles, mumps, rubella, varicella), which could prove fatal.[35] The first clinical clue for the diagnosis of a primary immunodeficiency disease is usually a history of infections that are persistent, difficult to treat, or caused by unusual microbes. The Jeffrey Modell Foundation/Immune Deficiency Foundation has developed a set of warning signs that serve as an excellent tool for determining what should be considered abnormal (Chart 16-2).[36] Because these

---

CHART 16-2 Ten Warning Signs of Primary Immunodeficiency

- Four or more new ear infections within 1 year
- Two or more serious sinus infections within 1 year
- Two or more months on antibiotics with little effect
- Two or more pneumonias within 1 year
- Failure of an infant to gain weight or grow normally
- Recurrent, deep skin or organ abscesses
- Persistent thrush in mouth or fungal infections of the skin
- Need for intravenous antibiotics to clear infections
- Two or more deep-seated infections including septicemia
- A family history of primary immunodeficiency

These warning signs were developed by the Jeffrey Modell Foundation Medical Advisory Board. Consultation with primary immunodeficiency experts is strongly suggested. © Jeffrey Modell Foundation.

---

disorders are frequently inherited, a positive family history is also a key diagnostic tool. The type of infection can provide information regarding the type of defect that is present. Infections with bacterial organisms are frequently observed in cases of antibody deficiency, whereas severe viral, fungal, and opportunistic infections characterize T-cell deficiencies. Recurrent *Streptococcus pneumoniae* or *Neisseria* infections characterize persons with complement deficiencies, and recurrent infections with staphylococcal and other catalase-positive organisms indicate disorders of phagocytosis.

Humoral (B-Cell) Immunodeficiency Disorders

Of all the primary immunodeficiency diseases, those affecting antibody production and humoral immunity are the most common.[35] Antibody production depends on the differentiation of hematopoietic stem cells into mature B lymphocytes and the antigen-dependent generation of immunoglobulin-producing plasma cells[37,38] (Fig. 16-6). This maturation cycle initially involves the production of surface IgM, migration from the bone marrow to the peripheral lymphoid tissue, and switching to the production of specialized IgM-, IgA-, IgD-, IgE-, or IgG-secreting plasma cells after antigenic stimulation. Primary humoral immunodeficiency disorders can interrupt the production of one or all of the immunoglobulins.

Defects in humoral immunity increase the risk of recurrent pyogenic infections, including those caused by *S. pneumoniae, Haemophilus influenzae, Staphylococcus aureus,* and *Pseudomonas* species. Humoral immunity usually is not as important in defending against intracellular bacteria (mycobacteria), fungi, and protozoa. Viruses usually are handled normally, except for the enteroviruses that cause gastrointestinal infections.

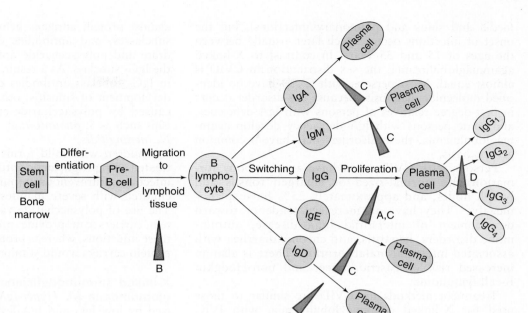

FIGURE 16-6. Stem cells to mature immunoglobulin-secreting plasma cells. *Arrows* indicate the stage of the maturation process that is interrupted in **(A)** transient hypogammaglobulinemia, **(B)** X-linked agammaglobulinemia, **(C)** common variable immunodeficiency, and **(D)** IgG subclass deficiency.

Transient Hypogammaglobulinemia of Infancy. During the first few months of life, infants are protected from infection by IgG antibodies that have been transferred from the maternal circulation during fetal life. Immunoglobulin A (IgA), IgM, IgD, and IgE do not normally cross the placenta. The presence of elevated levels of IgA or IgM in the infant cord blood suggests premature antibody production in response to an intrauterine infection. An infant's level of maternal IgG gradually declines over a period of approximately 6 months (see Chapter 15, Fig. 15-14). Concomitant with the loss of maternal antibody, the infant's immature humoral immune system begins to function, and between the ages of 1 and 2 years, the child's antibody production reaches adult levels.

Any abnormality that interferes with the production of immunoglobulin-producing plasma cells can produce a state of immunodeficiency. For example, certain infants may experience a delay in IgG production (IgM and IgA levels are normal) beyond 6 months of age. The total number and antigenic response of circulating B cells are normal, but the chemical communication between B and T cells that leads to clonal proliferation of antibody-producing plasma cells seems to be reduced.[35] This condition is referred to as *transient hypogammaglobulinemia of infancy.* The result of this condition usually is limited to repeated bouts of upper respiratory and middle ear infections. This condition usually resolves by 2 to 4 years of age.

X-Linked Agammaglobulinemia. X-linked (Bruton) agammaglobulinemia is a recessive trait that almost exclusively affects boys, as they have only one X chromosome.[32–35,37,39] As the name implies, persons with this disorder have essentially undetectable levels of all serum immunoglobulins. Therefore, they are susceptible to meningitis, recurrent otitis media, and sinopulmonary infections with organisms such as *S. pneumoniae, H. influenzae* type b, *S. aureus,* and *Neisseria meningitidis.*[33]

The abnormal gene in X-linked agammaglobulinemia that maps to the long arm of the X chromosome has a role in all stages of B-cell development. Mutation in the gene results in an absence of mature circulating B cells and plasma cells. T lymphocytes, however, are normal in number and function.

Most boys with the disorder remain asymptomatic until 6 to 9 months of age because of the presence of maternal antibodies. A clue to the presence of the disorder is the failure of an infection to respond completely and promptly to antibiotic therapy. Diagnosis is based on demonstration of low or absent serum immunoglobulins. Therapy consists of prophylaxis with intravenous immunoglobulin (IVIG) and prompt antimicrobial therapy for suspected infections. The prognosis for this condition depends on the prompt recognition and treatment of infections. Chronic pulmonary disease is an ever-present danger.

Common Variable Immunodeficiency. A similar disorder of B-cell maturation is a condition called *common variable immunodeficiency* (CVID). In this syndrome, the terminal differentiation of mature B cells to plasma cells is blocked.[35,37,38] More than 80% of persons with this disorder have a normal number of B lymphocytes, but they fail to differentiate into antibody-secreting cells when the lymphocytes are presented with antigen.[38] Some persons may also have increased apoptosis of helper T cells and decreased T-cell function and signaling.

The symptomatology of CVID is similar to that of X-linked agammaglobulinemia (i.e., recurrent otitis media and sinus and pulmonary infections), but the onset of infections occurs much later, usually between the ages of 15 and 35 years. In contrast to X-linked agammaglobulinemia, the sex distribution in CVID is almost equal. Most persons with CVID have no identified molecular diagnosis. Because the disorder occurs in first-degree relatives of persons with IgA deficiency, and some persons with IgA deficiency develop agammaglobulinemia, these disorders may have a common genetic basis.

Persons with CVID often have autoantibody formation and normal-sized or enlarged tonsils and lymph nodes, and approximately 25% have splenomegaly.[35] They have an increased tendency toward development of interstitial lung disease, autoimmune disorders, hepatitis, and chronic diarrhea with associated intestinal malabsorption. There is also an increased risk of gastric cancer and non-Hodgkin B-cell lymphoma.

Treatment methods for CVID are similar to those used for X-linked agammaglobulinemia, with IVIG being the cornerstone of therapy. Anaphylaxis to IgA in the IVIG can occur in persons with CVID who are IgA deficient. The use of IgA-depleted IVIG has greatly reduced this risk.

Selective Immunoglobulin A Deficiency. Selective IgA deficiency is the most common type of immunoglobulin deficiency.[2] The syndrome is characterized by moderate to marked reduction in levels of serum and secretory IgA, probably due to a block in the pathway that promotes terminal differentiation of mature B cells to IgA-secreting plasma cells. The occurrence of IgA deficiency in both men and women and in members of successive generations within families suggests autosomal inheritance with variable expressivity. The disorder has also been noted in persons treated with certain drugs (e.g., phenytoin, sulfasalazine), suggesting that environmental factors may trigger the disorder.[35]

Although an IgA deficiency can occur in apparently healthy persons, it is commonly associated with repeated infections in the respiratory, gastrointestinal, and urogenital systems. Persons with IgA deficiency also can develop antibodies against IgA, which can lead to severe anaphylactic reactions when blood components containing IgA are given.[5] Therefore, only specially washed erythrocytes from normal donors or erythrocytes from IgA-deficient donors should be used.

There is no specific treatment available for selective IgA deficiency unless there is a concomitant reduction in IgG levels. Administration of IgA immune globulin is of little benefit because IgA has a short half-life and is not secreted across the mucosa. There also is the risk of anaphylactic reactions associated with IgA antibodies in the immune globulin.

Immunoglobulin G Subclass Deficiency. An IgG subclass deficiency can affect one or more of the IgG subtypes, despite normal levels or elevated serum concentrations of IgG. In general, antibodies directed against protein antigens belong to the IgG_1 and IgG_3 subclasses, and antibodies directed against carbohydrate and polysaccharide antigens are primarily from the IgG_2 subclass. As a result, persons who are deficient in IgG_2 subclass antibodies can be at greater risk for development of sinusitis, otitis media, and pneumonia caused by polysaccharide-encapsulated microorganisms such as *S. pneumoniae, H. influenzae* type b, and *N. meningitidis.*

Children with mild forms of the deficiency can be treated with prophylactic antibiotics to prevent repeated infections. Intravenous immunoglobulin can be given to children with severe manifestations of this deficiency. The use of polysaccharide vaccines conjugated to protein carriers can provide protection against some of these infections, whereas protein vaccines conjugated to protein carriers would stimulate an IgG_1 response.

X-linked Immunodeficiency with Hyperimmunoglobulinemia M. *Hyper-IgM syndrome* is characterized by low IgG and IgA levels with normal or, more frequently, high IgM concentrations.[35] Being predominantly an X-linked recessive disorder, the disease is primarily seen in boys. Formerly classified as a B-cell defect, it now has been traced to a T-cell defect. The disorder results from the inability of T cells to signal B cells to undergo isotype switching to IgG and IgA; thus, they produce only IgM.[35,39]

Like those with X-linked agammaglobulinemia, affected individuals become symptomatic during the first and second years of life. They have recurrent pyogenic infections, including otitis media, sinusitis, tonsillitis, and pneumonia. Persons with the syndrome are also at increased risk for development of autoimmune diseases of the formed elements of the blood, including hemolytic anemia, thrombocytopenia, and recurrent severe neutropenia.[35,39]

Cellular (T-Cell) Immunodeficiency Disorders

Unlike B cells, in which a well-defined series of differentiation steps ultimately leads to the production of immunoglobulins, mature T lymphocytes consist of distinct subpopulations with diverse immunologic assignments.[39] They protect against fungal, protozoan, viral, and intracellular bacterial infections; control malignant cell proliferation; and are responsible for coordinating the overall immune response.

In general, persons with T-cell–mediated immunodeficiency disorders have infections or other clinical problems that are more severe than those seen with antibody disorders. Children with defects in this branch of the immune response rarely survive beyond infancy or childhood unless immunologic reconstitution is achieved.[35] However, exceptions are being recognized as newer T-cell defects, such as the X-linked hyper-IgM syndrome, are identified.[35] Other recently identified primary T-cell immunodeficiency disorders result from defective expression of the TCR complex, defective cytokine production, and defects in T-cell activation.

Thymic Hypoplasia: DiGeorge Syndrome. DiGeorge syndrome stems from an embryonic developmental defect.[35] The defect is thought to occur before the 12th week of gestation, when the thymus gland, parathyroid gland, and parts of the head, neck, and heart are developing. The disorder affects both males and females and is relatively more common than other T cell immunodeficiencies. Formerly thought to be caused by a variety of factors, including extrinsic teratogens, this defect has been traced to microdeletion of specific deoxyribonucleic acid (DNA) sequences from chromosome 22 (22q11).[1,35,39]

Infants born with this defect have partial or complete failure in development of the thymus and parathyroid glands and have congenital defects of the head, neck, and/or heart. The extent of immune and parathyroid abnormalities is highly variable, as are the other defects. In some children, the thymus is not absent but is in an abnormal location and is extremely small. These infants can have partial DiGeorge syndrome, in which hypertrophy of the thymus occurs with development of normal immune function. The facial disorders can include hypertelorism (increased distance between the eyes); micrognathia (abnormally small jaw); low-set, posteriorly angulated ears; split uvula; and high-arched palate (Fig. 16-7). Urinary tract abnormalities also are common. The most frequent presenting sign is hypocalcemia and tetany that develop within the first 24 hours of life. It is caused by the absence of the parathyroid gland and is resistant to standard therapy.

Children who survive the immediate neonatal period may have recurrent or chronic infections because of impaired T-cell immunity. Children also may have an absence of immunoglobulin production, caused by a lack of helper T-cell function. For children who do require treatment, thymus transplantation can be performed to reconstitute T-cell immunity. Bone marrow transplantation also has been successfully used to restore normal T-cell populations. If blood transfusions are needed, as during corrective heart surgery, special processing is required to prevent graft-versus-host disease.

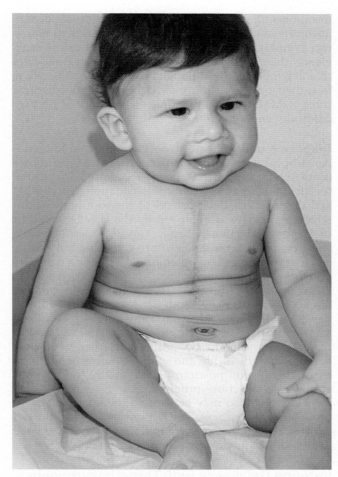

FIGURE 16-7. An infant with DiGeorge syndrome. The surgical scar on the chest indicates repair of heart disease caused by truncus arteriosus or interrupted aortic arch, which is common in this syndrome. The infant also has the facial features of a child with DiGeorge syndrome, as illustrated by hypertelorism, low-set ears, hypoplastic mandible, and bowing upward of the upper lip. (From Roberts R. Atlas of Infectious Diseases. Edited by Gerald Mandell [series editor], Catherine M. Wilfert. © 1998 Current Medicine, Inc. With kind permission of Springer Science + Business Media.)

Severe Combined Immunodeficiency Disorders

Severe combined immunodeficiency (SCID) is a syndrome of diverse genetic causes characterized by profound deficiencies in T- and B-cell function, and in some cases NK cells and function.[1,35] Mutations in 13 different genes have been found to cause the condition, which is usually fatal in the first 2 years of life unless reconstitution of the immune system can be accomplished. Although they appear normal at birth, affected infants begin to develop frequent episodes of diarrhea, pneumonia, otitis media, sepsis, and cutaneous lesions within the first few months of life. Growth may appear normal, but extreme wasting develops after infections and diarrhea begin. Exposure to live vaccines, nonirradiated blood products, and infections can prove life threatening.

Pathogenesis and Etiology. The most common form of SCID, accounting for about half of all cases in the United States, is X-linked, and hence is more common in boys than girls. These mutations are recessive so that heterozygous girls are usually normal carriers of the gene, whereas boys who inherit the abnormal chromosome manifest the disease.[40,41] The genetic defect in the X-linked form of SCID is due to a mutation in a transmembrane protein that is responsible for the survival and proliferation of T-lymphocyte precursors. T-cell numbers are greatly reduced in number and, although B cells are normal, antibody synthesis is greatly impaired because of a T–cell help. There may also be a deficiency in NK cells.

The remaining cases of SCID show an autosomal recessive pattern of inheritance, with the most common cause being mutations in the gene encoding adenosine deaminase (ADA), an enzyme involved in purine metabolism.[41] A deficiency in ADA leads to deoxy-adenosine and its derivatives, which are toxic to immature lymphocytes, especially those of the T-cell lineage. Hence there is a greater reduction in T lymphocytes than B lymphocytes. Although the number of NK cells is low, their function is normal. Other distinguishing features of ADA deficiency include the presence of rib cage deformity and numerous skeletal deformities.

Diagnosis and Treatment. Severe combined immunodeficiency is a pediatric emergency. Because the disorder is not apparent at birth and early recognition is essential for lifesaving treatment, a recommendation to add SCID and other severe T-cell defects to the routine newborn screening panel was approved by the U.S. Department of Health and Human Services in 2010.[42] All infants who test positive on the newborn screening test should receive rapid referral to an immunologist for a complete immune evaluation.

Bone marrow transplant is the mainstay treatment for all forms of SCID. Both HLA-identical and T-cell depleted HLA-haploidentical hematopoietic stem cell transplants have been very effective in reconstitution of the immune system, especially if performed within the first 3.5 months of life and without pretransplantation chemotherapy or posttransplantation drugs for graft-versus-host rejection prophylaxis.[35] Enzyme replacement therapy also may be used in the management of persons ADA-deficient SCID. However, it should not be used if bone marrow transplantation is anticipated because it can predispose to graft rejection.[35,40]

Immune Deficiency with Thrombocytopenia and Eczema

Immune deficiency with thrombocytopenia and eczema (Wiskott-Aldrich syndrome) is an X-linked recessive disorder characterized by thrombocytopenia, eczema, and marked susceptibility to bacterial infections.[2,43] Bleeding episodes or symptoms due to infection usually begin within the first 6 months of life. Abnormalities of humoral immunity include decreased serum levels of IgM and markedly elevated serum IgA and IgE concentrations. T-cell dysfunction initially is mild but progressively deteriorates, and children with the disorder become increasingly susceptible to the development of malignancies of the mononuclear phagocytic system, including Hodgkin lymphoma and leukemia. Children with Wiskott-Aldrich syndrome typically are unable to produce antibody to polysaccharide antigens and therefore are susceptible to infections caused by encapsulated microorganisms, including septicemia and meningitis. Varicella infection can be lethal to children with this condition.

Management of children with Wiskott-Aldrich syndrome focuses on treatment of eczema, control of infections, and management of bleeding episodes. Bone marrow transplantation has been successful in children with Wiskott-Aldrich syndrome. Splenectomy, sometimes recommended for children with thrombocytopenia, effectively stops the bleeding episodes but increases the risk of septicemia.[43]

Acquired Immunodeficiency Syndrome

Acquired immunodeficiency syndrome is a disease caused by infection with human immunodeficiency virus (HIV) and is characterized by profound immunosuppression with associated opportunistic infections, malignancies, wasting, and central nervous system degeneration. HIV is a retrovirus that selectively attacks the CD4+ T lymphocytes, the immune cells responsible for orchestrating and coordinating the immune response to infection. As a consequence, persons with HIV infection have a deteriorating immune system, and thus are more susceptible to severe infections from ordinarily harmless organisms.

As a national and global epidemic, the degree of morbidity and mortality caused by HIV, as well as its impact on health care resources and the economy, is tremendous and unrelenting. In 2011, it was estimated that there were nearly 34 million people worldwide living with HIV/AIDS and 1.7 million people died of HIV-related causes.[44] During the same year, 2.5 million people were newly infected with HIV. Because the reporting of cases is not uniform throughout the world, many countries may not be accurately represented in this number.[44]

Transmission of HIV Infection

Human immunodeficiency virus is transmitted through conditions that facilitate the exchange of blood or body fluids that contain the virus or virus-infected cells, the major routes being sexual contact; contaminated blood, either through sharing needles or syringes used for illicit drugs; or passage from infected mothers to their newborns.[2,3,45,46] It is estimated that more than 90% of children living with HIV acquired the virus in utero, during the birth process, or through breast-feeding.[47] Human immunodeficiency virus is not transmitted through casual contact. Several studies involving more than 1000 uninfected, nonsexual household contacts with persons with HIV infection (including siblings, parents, and children) have shown no evidence of casual transmission.[48]

Sexual contact is the most frequent mode of HIV transmission. There is a risk of transmitting HIV when semen or vaginal fluids come in contact with a part of the body that lets them enter the bloodstream. This can include the vaginal mucosa, anal mucosa, and wounds or sores on the skin. Thus, the risk of infection is increased in the presence of ulcerative sexually transmitted infections (STIs) such as syphilis, herpes simplex virus infection, and chancroid; however, it is also increased with nonulcerative STIs such as gonorrhea, chlamydial infection, and trichomoniasis.[46] Condoms are highly effective in preventing the transmission of HIV. Unprotected sex between men is still the main mode of transmission in both Canada and the United States (48% of new HIV cases in Canada in 2011[49] and 63% in the United States in 2010.[50]) During the same years, 25% of newly diagnosed HIV/AIDS cases in the United States[50] and 30% of newly diagnosed cases in Canada were attributable to high-risk heterosexual intercourse.[49]

Transfusions of whole blood or blood products before 1985 resulted in the transmission of HIV. Since 1985, all blood donations in the United States have been screened for HIV, dramatically reducing the transmission risk to an extremely small number.[2] Currently, all donated blood and plasma are screened for HIV-associated antigen and antibodies to HIV. Screening tests may be negative in the so-called *window period*, the 1 to 6 months following a new HIV infection and before seroconversion, the point at which HIV antibodies can be detected in the blood. Therefore, the U.S. Food and Drug Administration (FDA) requires blood collection centers to screen potential donors through interviews designed to identify behaviors known to present a risk for HIV infection. In addition, nucleic acid amplification testing (NAAT) of blood donors has reduced the risk of transfusion transmission of both HIV and hepatitis C virus to approximately 1 in 2 million blood units.[51]

Occupational HIV infection among health care workers is uncommon. Universal blood and body fluid precautions should be used in encounters with all patients in the health care setting because HIV status is not always known. Occupational risk of infection for health care workers most often is associated with percutaneous inoculation (e.g., needle stick) of blood from a patient with HIV infection. Transmission is associated with the size of the needle, amount of blood present, depth of the injury, type of fluid contamination, stage of illness of the patient, and viral load of the patient. The average risk for HIV infection from percutaneous exposure to HIV-infected blood is about 0.3%, and about 0.09% after mucous membrane exposure.[52,53]

The HIV-infected person is infectious even when no symptoms are present. The point at which an infected person converts from being negative for the presence of HIV antibodies in the blood to being positive is called *seroconversion*. Seroconversion typically occurs within 1 to 3 months after exposure to HIV, but rarely can take as long as 6 months. Recent data suggest that 50% of transmissions occur during primary HIV infection and early HIV infection.[54] The time after infection and before seroconversion is known as the *window period*. During the window period, a person's HIV antibody test result will be negative but he or she can still transmit the virus.

Molecular and Biologic Features of HIV Infection

The primary etiologic agent of AIDS is HIV, an enveloped ribonucleic acid (RNA) retrovirus that carries its genetic material in RNA rather than DNA. Two genetically different but antigenically related forms of HIV—HIV-1 and HIV-2—have been isolated in people with AIDS.[1-3] Human immunodeficiency virus-1 is the type most commonly associated with AIDS in the United States, Europe, and central Africa, whereas HIV-2 causes a similar disease principally in western Africa. Human immunodeficiency virus-2 spreads more slowly and causes disease more slowly than HIV-1. Specific tests are now available for HIV-2, and blood collected

for transfusion is routinely screened for HIV-2. The remaining discussion focuses on HIV-1, but the information is generally applicable to HIV-2 as well.

HIV infects a limited number of cell types in the body, including CD4+ T lymphocytes, macrophages, and dendritic cells (see Chapter 15). The CD4+ T cells are necessary for recognition of foreign antigens, activating antibody-producing B lymphocytes, and orchestrating cell-mediated immunity, in which cytotoxic CD8+ T cells and NK cells directly destroy virus-infected cells, tubercle bacilli, and foreign antigens. The phagocytic function of monocytes and macrophages is also influenced by CD4+ T cells.

The HIV is spherical and contains an electron-dense core surrounded by a lipid envelope[1-3] (Fig. 16-8A). The core contains an outer shell, or capsid, made up primarily of a protein called p24; two copies of the genomic RNA; and three viral enzymes (protease, reverse transcriptase, and integrase). The viral core is surrounded by a matrix protein called *p17*, which lies beneath the viral envelope, a structure studded with two viral glycoproteins, gp120 and gp41, which are critical for the infection of cells.

Replication of HIV occurs in eight steps[2,3] (see Fig. 16-8B). Each of these steps provides insights into the development of methods used for preventing or treating the infection. The *first step* involves the binding of the virus to the CD4+ T cell. Once HIV has entered the bloodstream, it attaches to the surface of a CD4+ T cell by binding to the CD4 molecule, which acts as a high-affinity receptor for the virus. This process is known as *attachment*. However, attaching to the CD4 molecule is not sufficient for infection; the virus must also bind with other surface molecules (chemokine coreceptors, such as CCR5 and CXCR4) that bind the gp120 and gp41 envelope glycoproteins. The chemokine coreceptors are critical components of the HIV infection process: the virus can only infect cells expressing CD4+ and the coreceptors. People with defective coreceptors are more resistant to development of HIV infection, despite repeated exposure.[55] Research aimed at developing coreceptor-targeted viral entry inhibitors raises new hope for bridging the gap toward a cure of HIV infection.

The *second step* of the replication process allows for internalization of the virus. After attachment, the viral envelope peptides fuse to the CD4+ T-cell membrane. Fusion results in an *uncoating* of the virus, allowing the contents of the viral core (the two single strands of viral RNA and the reverse transcriptase, integrase, and protease enzymes) to enter the host cell. The *third step* consists of DNA synthesis. In order for HIV to reproduce, it must change its RNA into DNA. It does this using the *reverse transcriptase* enzyme. Reverse transcriptase makes a copy of the viral RNA, and then in reverse makes a complementary DNA (cDNA) strand. The result is a double-stranded DNA that carries instructions for viral replication.

The *fourth step* is called *integration*. In dividing cells, the cDNA enters the nucleus and, with the help of the enzyme integrase, is inserted into the cell's original DNA. The integrated virus is called a *provirus*. In quiescent

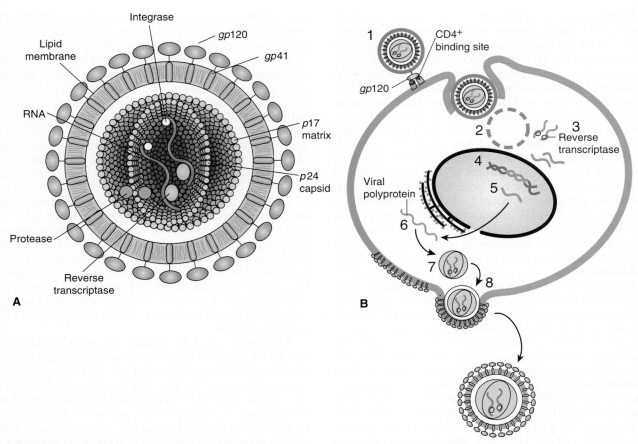

FIGURE 16-8. (A) Structure of the human immunodeficiency virus (HIV). RNA, ribonucleic acid. **(B)** Life cycle of HIV-1. (*1*) Attachment of the HIV virus to CD4+ T-cell receptor; (*2*) internalization and uncoating of the virus with viral RNA and reverse transcriptase; (*3*) reverse transcription, which produces a mirror image of the viral RNA and double-stranded DNA molecule; (*4*) integration of viral DNA into host DNA using the integrase enzyme; (*5*) transcription of the inserted viral DNA to produce viral messenger RNA; (*6*) translation of viral messenger RNA to create viral polyprotein; (*7*) cleavage of viral polyprotein into individual viral proteins that make up the new virus; and (*8*) assembly and release of the new virus from the host cell.

T cells, the proviral cDNA may remain in the cytoplasm in a linear extrachromosomal form. The *fifth step* involves *transcription* of the double-stranded viral DNA to form a single-stranded messenger RNA (mRNA) with the instructions for building new viruses. Transcription involves activation of the T cell and induction of host cell transcription factors. Alternatively, the provirus may remain nontranscribed within infected cells for months or years, hidden from the host's immune system and even from antiviral therapies. Long-lived reservoirs of HIV are established within the first month of acute infection.[46] These reservoirs of latent infected cells do not spontaneously produce virus unless activated. Their long life span constitutes one of the main barriers to HIV eradication by current antiviral therapies.

The *sixth step* includes translation of the viral mRNA. During *translation*, ribosomal RNA (rRNA) uses the instructions in the mRNA to create a chain of proteins and enzymes called a *polyprotein*. These polyproteins contain the components needed for the next stages in the construction of new viruses. The *seventh step* is called *cleavage*. During cleavage, the protease enzyme cuts the polyprotein chain into the individual proteins that will make up the new viruses. Finally, during the *eighth step*, the core proteins migrate to the cell membrane, where they acquire a lipid envelope that buds off from the cell membrane. Productive infections, associated with extensive viral budding, lead to cell death.[2] It is important to note that although HIV can infect resting cells, the initiation of transcription and viral replication occurs only when the infected cell is activated by exposure to antigens or cytokines.

Within 72 hours of a transmission event, local virus replication occurs at the site of infection and the draining lymph nodes.[46] Infection becomes systemic by the end of the first week, as the virus disseminates to other lymphoid tissue compartments. By day 10 after infection, most circulating CD4+ T cells either have been infected with or have interacted with HIV. The availability and rapid consumption of targets during this early period leads to massive viral replication, accounting in part for the high levels of viremia and genital shedding achieved by the end of the first month. Once infection has become truly systemic, viral loads grow exponentially, with a doubling time of approximately 0.3 days during the first 2 to 3 weeks of infection.

The problem is that, over years, the CD4+ T-cell count gradually decreases through this process, and the number of viruses detected in the blood of persons infected with HIV increases. The depletion of CD4+ T cells after infection is due to the cytopathic effect of the virus, resulting from production of viral particles, as well as death of unaffected cells. Other infected cells, such as macrophages and dendritic cells, may also die, resulting in destructive changes in the lymphoid organs. Until the CD4+ T-cell count falls to a very low level, a person infected with HIV can remain asymptomatic, although active viral replication is still taking place and serologic tests can identify antibodies to HIV. These antibodies, unfortunately, do not convey protection against the virus. Although symptoms are not evident, the infection proceeds on a microbiologic level, including the invasion and selective destruction of CD4+ T cells. The continual decline of CD4+ T cells, which are pivotal cells in the immune response, strips the HIV-infected person of protection against common organisms and cancerous cells.

Classification and Stages of HIV Infection

The definitions and classification systems for HIV and AIDS have been evolving, due in part to improvements in diagnostic and therapeutic capabilities, including increased use of new HIV-testing technologies. In 1993, the Centers for Disease Control and Prevention (CDC) developed a classification system that emphasized the clinical importance of the CD4+ T-cell count along with a list of AIDS-defining conditions (Chart 16-3).[56] The 1993 classification system, which was revised in 2008, highlights the central importance of the CD4+ T-cell count and percentages, which are objective measures of immunosuppression routinely used in the care of HIV-infected persons[57] (Table 16-2). It distinguishes three stages of HIV infection based on CD4+ T-cell counts and total T-cell percentages: stage one >500 cells/μL (29%); stage two 200 to 499 cells/μL (14% to 28%); and stage three (AIDS) <200 cells/μL (<14%). An undetermined stage has also been included.

Clinical Course. The typical course of HIV infection is characterized by three phases, which usually occur over a period of 8 to 12 years. These are the primary infection phase, chronic asymptomatic or latency phase, and overt AIDS phase (Fig. 16-9).[56]

When initially infected with HIV, many persons have an acute mononucleosis-like syndrome known as *primary infection*. This acute phase (stage 1) may include fever, fatigue, myalgias, sore throat, night sweats, gastrointestinal problems, lymphadenopathy, maculopapular rash, and headache. Fever and malaise are the symptoms most commonly associated with primary infection.[46,57] During primary infection, there is an increase in viral replication, which leads to very high viral loads, sometimes greater than 1,000,000 copies/mL, and a decrease in the CD4+ T-cell count. The signs

CHART 16-3	Conditions Included in the 1993 AIDS Surveillance Case Definition

Candidiasis of bronchi, trachea, or lungs
Candidiasis, esophageal
Cervical cancer, invasive*
Coccidioidomycosis, disseminated or extrapulmonary
Cryptococcosis, extrapulmonary
Cryptosporidiosis, chronic intestinal (>1 month duration)
Cytomegalovirus disease (other than liver, spleen, or nodes)
Cytomegalovirus retinitis (with loss of vision)
Encephalopathy, HIV related
Herpes simplex: chronic ulcer(s) (>1 month duration) or bronchitis, pneumonitis, or esophagitis
Histoplasmosis, disseminated or extrapulmonary
Isosporiasis, chronic intestinal (>1 month's duration)
Kaposi sarcoma
Lymphoma, Burkitt (or equivalent term)
Lymphoma, immunoblastic (or equivalent term)
Lymphoma, primary, of brain
Mycobacterium avium-intracellulare complex or *Mycobacterium kansasii,* disseminated or extrapulmonary
Mycobacterium tuberculosis, any site (pulmonary* or extrapulmonary)
Mycobacterium, other species or unidentified species, disseminated or extrapulmonary
Pneumocystis jiroveci pneumonia
Pneumonia, recurrent*
Progressive multifocal leukoencephalopathy
Salmonella septicemia, recurrent
Toxoplasmosis of the brain
Wasting syndrome due to HIV

*Added to the 1993 expansion of the AIDS surveillance case definition.

From Centers for Disease Control and Prevention. 1993 Revised classification system for HIV infection and expanded surveillance case definition for AIDS among adolescents and adults. *MMWR Recomm Rep.* 1992;41(RR-17):19.

and symptoms of primary HIV infection usually appear 1 to 4 weeks after exposure to HIV, and have an average duration of 7 to 10 days.[57] After several weeks, the immune system acts to control viral replication and reduces the viral load to a lower level, where it often remains for several years. This relatively stable level of virus is referred to as the set point. People who are diagnosed with HIV infection while they are in the primary infection phase may have a unique opportunity for treatment. Some experts hypothesize that treatment, if started early, may reduce the number of HIV-infected CD4+ memory T cells; protect the functioning of HIV-infected CD4+ T cells and cytotoxic T cells; and potentially help to maintain a homogeneous viral population that will be better controlled by antiretroviral therapy and the immune system.[46,58]

TABLE 16-2	The Revised CDC Classification System for Human Immunodeficiency Virus (HIV) Infection in Adults and Adolescents Aged 13 Years.*		
Stage	**CD4⁺ T-cell Count Cells/µL (CD4⁺ T-cell Percentage)**		**AIDS-defining Conditions (ADC)**
Stage 1	≥500 (29%)		No ADC
Stage 2	200–499 (14%–28%)		No ADC
Stage 3	<200 (<14%)		No documented ADC
Stage undetermined	No information		No information

*A confirmed case meets the laboratory diagnosis of HIV infection and one of the four stages. Although cases with no information on AIDS-defining characteristics can be classified as stage unknown, every effort should be made to obtain CD4⁺ T-cell counts and percentages and the presence of AIDS-defining conditions at the time of diagnosis.

Developed from Schneider E, Whitmore S, Glynn KM, et al., for the Centers for Disease Control and Prevention (CDC). Revised case definitions for HIV infections among adults, adolescents, and children aged <18 months and for children aged 18 months to <13 years—United States, 2008. *MMWR Recomm Rep.* 2008;57(RR-10):1–12.

The primary stage is followed by a latent period (stage 2) during which the person has no signs or symptoms of illness. The median time of the latent period is about 10 years. During this time, the CD4⁺ T-cell count falls gradually from the normal range of 800 to 1000 cells/µL to 200 to 499 cells/µL (14% to 28%). More recent data suggest that the CD4⁺ T-cell decline may not fall in an even slope based on HIV RNA levels, and factors related to the variability in the decline in CD4⁺ T cells are under investigation.[59] Lymphadenopathy (i.e., swollen lymph nodes) for more than 3 months in at least two locations (not including the groin) develops in some persons with HIV infection during this phase. The lymph nodes may be sore or visible externally.

Stage 3 (overt AIDS) occurs when a person has a CD4⁺ T-cell count of less than 200 cells/µL (<14%) or an AIDS-defining illness.[60] Without antiretroviral therapy, this phase can lead to death within 2 to 3 years. The risk of opportunistic infections and death increases significantly when the CD4⁺ T-cell count falls below 200 cells/µL.

The clinical course of HIV varies from person to person. In the absence of treatment, most people with HIV infection progress to AIDS after 7 to 10 years.[2,60] These people are the *chronic* or *typical progressors*. Another 10% to 20% are *rapid progressors* who develop AIDS within 2 to 3 years after primary infection. The final 5% to 15% are *long-term nonprogressors*, who remain asymptomatic for 10 years or more after seroconversion, with stable CD4⁺ T-cell counts and low plasma HIV RNA levels. A subset of these long-term nonprogressors, called *elite controllers*, have plasma HIV RNA levels that are below the level of detection. Studies of these individuals have helped to identify host and viral factors that influence disease progression.[2] One factor found to be important in elite control is a mutation in the genes coding for CCR5, a coreceptor used for HIV entry. Mutations in both genes result in CD4⁺ cells with a defective CCR5, thereby preventing HIV entry into those cells. Research in this area is ongoing.

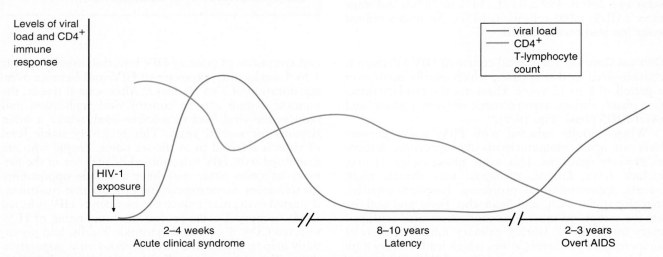

FIGURE 16-9. Viral load and CD4⁺ cell count during the phases of HIV infection. AIDS, acquired immunodeficiency syndrome; HIV, human immunodeficiency virus.

Opportunistic Infections

Opportunistic infections involve common organisms that do not typically produce infection unless there is impaired immune function. As the number of CD4⁺ T cells declines, the risk of these infections increases. In addition, the baseline HIV RNA level contributes and serves as an independent risk factor.[2,3]

Opportunistic infections are most often categorized by the type of organism (e.g., fungal, protozoal, bacterial and mycobacterial, viral). Bacterial and mycobacterial opportunistic infections include bacterial pneumonia, salmonellosis, bartonellosis, *Mycobacterium tuberculosis* (TB), and *Mycobacterium avium* complex (MAC). Fungal opportunistic infections include candidiasis, coccidioidomycosis, cryptococcosis, histoplasmosis, penicilliosis, and pneumocystosis. Protozoal opportunistic infections include cryptosporidiosis, microsporidiosis, isosporiasis, and toxoplasmosis. Viral infections include those caused by cytomegalovirus (CMV), herpes simplex and zoster viruses, human papillomavirus, and JC virus, a virus that is the causative agent of progressive multifocal leukoencephalopathy (PML).

Respiratory Tract Infections. The most common causes of respiratory disease in persons with HIV infection are bacterial pneumonia, *Pneumocystis jiroveci* pneumonia, and pulmonary tuberculosis. Other organisms that cause opportunistic pulmonary infections in persons with AIDS include CMV, MAC, *Toxoplasma gondii*, and *Cryptococcus neoformans*.[2] Pneumonia also may be caused by more common bacterial pulmonary pathogens, including *S. pneumoniae*, *Pseudomonas aeruginosa*, and *H. influenzae*. Some persons may become infected with multiple organisms, causing a polymicrobial infection. Kaposi sarcoma (to be discussed) also can occur in the lungs.

P. jiroveci (formerly known as *P. carinii*) pneumonia (PCP) was the most common presenting manifestation of AIDS during the first decade of the epidemic. *P. jiroveci* is an organism common in soil, houses, and many other places in the environment, and in healthy persons does not cause infection or disease. In persons with HIV infection, *P. jiroveci* can multiply quickly in the lungs and cause pneumonia. As the disease progresses, the alveoli become filled with a foamy exudate that forms cup-shaped cyst walls within the exudate (Fig. 16-10). Since highly active antiretroviral therapy (HAART) and prophylaxis for PCP were instituted, the incidence of PCP has decreased.[61] *P. jiroveci* (formerly known as *P. carinii*) pneumonia still is common in people unaware of their HIV-infected status, in those who choose not to treat their HIV infection or take prophylaxis, and in those with poor access to health care. The best predictor of PCP is a CD4⁺ cell count below 200 cells/μL,[61] and it is at this point that antimicrobial prophylaxis with trimethoprim-sulfamethoxazole or an alternative agent (in the case of adverse reactions to

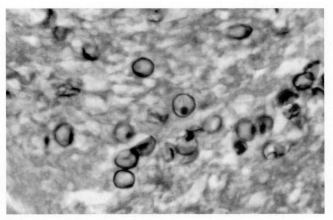

FIGURE 16-10. *Pneumocystis jiroveci* pneumonia. Histopathology of lung shows characteristic cysts with cup forms and dotlike wall thickening (methenamine silver stain). (From the Centers for Disease Control and Prevention Public Health Image Library. No. 960. Courtesy of Edwin P. Ewing, Jr.)

sulfa drugs) is strongly recommended. The symptoms of *P. jiroveci* pneumonia may be acute or gradually progressive. Patients may present with complaints of a mild cough, fever, shortness of breath, and weight loss. Diagnosis is made by identifying the organism in pulmonary secretions.

Tuberculosis (TB) is the leading cause of death for people with HIV infection worldwide, and is often the first manifestation of HIV infection. In 2011, 23% of those with TB tested positive for HIV.[44] In the United States, the number of TB cases decreased from the 1950s to 1985; then, in 1986, the number began to increase (see Chapter 22).[62] Several factors contributed to this increase, but the most profound factor was HIV infection. The lungs are the most common site of *M. tuberculosis* infection, but extrapulmonary infection of the kidney, bone marrow, and other organs also occurs in people with HIV infection. Whether a person has pulmonary or extrapulmonary TB, most persons present with fever, night sweats, cough, and weight loss. Persons infected with both HIV and TB are more likely to have a rapidly progressive form of TB, and usually have an increase in viral load, which decreases the success of TB therapy. They also have an increased number of other opportunistic infections and an increased mortality rate.

Since the late 1960s, most persons with TB have responded well to therapy. However, in 1991, there were outbreaks of multidrug-resistant (MDR) TB. Since the original outbreak of MDR TB in the early 1990s, new cases of MDR TB have declined, largely because of improved infection control practices and the expansion of directly observed therapy programs.

Gastrointestinal Manifestations. Diseases of the gastrointestinal tract are some of the most frequent complications of HIV infection and AIDS. Esophageal candidiasis, CMV infection, and herpes simplex virus infection commonly cause esophagitis in people with

HIV infection.[63] Aphthous ulcers presumed secondary to HIV are also common. Persons experiencing these infections usually complain of painful swallowing or retrosternal pain. Endoscopy or barium esophagography is required for definitive diagnosis.

Diarrhea or gastroenteritis is a common complaint in persons with HIV infection. Although diarrhea is often a side effect of medications used to treat HIV, it should be evaluated for the same common causes as in the general population. The most common protozoal opportunistic infection that causes diarrhea is *Cryptosporidium parvum*. Clinical features of cryptosporidiosis can range from mild diarrhea to severe, watery diarrhea with a loss of up to several liters of water per day, as well as malabsorption, electrolyte disturbances, dehydration, and weight loss. Other organisms that cause gastroenteritis and diarrhea are *Salmonella*, CMV, *Clostridium difficile*, *Escherichia coli*, *Shigella*, *Giardia*, and microsporidia.[63] These organisms are identified by examination of stool cultures or endoscopy.

Nervous System Manifestations. Human immunodeficiency virus infection, particularly in the late stages of severe immunocompromise, leaves the nervous system vulnerable to an array of neurologic disorders, including neurocognitive disorders, toxoplasmosis, and progressive multifocal leukoencephalopathy.

HIV-associated neurocognitive disorders (HANDs) is a syndrome of cognitive impairment with motor dysfunction or behavioral/psychosocial symptoms associated with HIV infection itself.[64] In 2007, the National Institute of Mental Health and National Institute of Neurologic Diseases and Stroke developed a new classification with standardized diagnostic criteria for HANDs. The three conditions comprising HANDs are HIV-associated asymptomatic neurocognitive impairment, HIV-associated mild neurocognitive disorder, and HIV-associated dementia, formerly known as *AIDS dementia complex*.[64] The clinical features of HIV-associated dementia, which is usually a late complication of HIV infection, include impairment of attention and concentration, slowing of mental and motor speed and agility, and apathetic behavior. There is no specific treatment for HAND, but HAART comprised of medications which penetrate the blood-brain barrier is considered the best therapeutic option at this time.

Toxoplasmosis is a common opportunistic infection in persons with AIDS. The organism responsible, *T. gondii*, is a parasite that most often affects the CNS.[65] Toxoplasmosis usually is a reactivation of a latent *T. gondii* infection that has been dormant in the CNS. The typical presentation includes fever, headaches, and neurologic dysfunction, including confusion and lethargy, visual disturbances, and seizures. Computed tomography scans or, preferably, magnetic resonance imaging (MRI) should be performed immediately to detect the presence of neurologic lesions. Prophylactic treatment with trimethoprim-sulfamethoxazole or an alternative agent, which is also used for prevention of *P. jiroveci* pneumonia, is effective against *T. gondii*.

Progressive multifocal leukoencephalopathy (PML) is a demyelinating disease of the white matter of the brain caused by the JC virus, a DNA papovavirus that attacks the oligodendrocytes.[66] PML advances slowly, and is characterized by progressive limb weakness, sensory loss, difficulty controlling the digits, visual disturbances, subtle alterations in mental status, hemiparesis, ataxia, diplopia, and seizures.[66] The mortality rate is high, and the average survival time is 2 to 4 months after diagnosis. Diagnosis is suspected based on clinical findings and an MRI, and confirmed by the presence of the JC virus in the cerebrospinal fluid.[66] There is no proven cure for PML, but improvement can occur after starting effective HAART.

Malignancies

Persons with AIDS have a high incidence of certain malignancies, especially Kaposi sarcoma (KS), non-Hodgkin lymphoma, and noninvasive cervical carcinoma. The increased incidence of malignancies probably is a function of impaired cell-mediated immunity. As persons with HIV infection are living longer, there has been increasing incidence of age- and gender-specific malignancies.[67] Non–AIDS-defining malignancies account for more morbidity and mortality than AIDS-defining malignancies in the HAART era.

Kaposi sarcoma is a malignancy of the endothelial cells that line small blood vessels.[68] An opportunistic cancer, KS occurs in immunosuppressed persons (e.g., transplant recipients or persons with AIDS). Kaposi sarcoma was one of the first and most common opportunistic cancers associated with AIDS. Since the introduction of HAART, the incidence of KS has decreased dramatically but has not reached zero. There is evidence linking KS to a herpesvirus (herpesvirus 8 [HHV-8], also called *KS-associated herpes virus* [KSHV]).[68] The virus is readily transmitted through homosexual and heterosexual activities; however, there is a disproportionately higher incidence of KS in men who have sex with men compared with women and other men. Maternal–infant transmission also can rarely occur. The virus has been detected in saliva from infected persons, and other nonsexual modes of transmission are suspected.

The lesions of KS can be found on the skin and on any mucosal surface in the oral cavity, gastrointestinal tract, and lungs. More than 50% of people with skin lesions also have gastrointestinal lesions. The disease usually begins as one or more macules, papules, or violet skin lesions that enlarge and become darker (Fig. 16-11). Tumor nodules frequently are located on the trunk, neck, and head, especially the tip of the nose. They usually are painless in the early stages, but discomfort may occur as the tumor develops. Invasion of internal organs, including the lungs, gastrointestinal tract, and lymphatic system, commonly occurs. Gastrointestinal tract KS is often asymptomatic, but can cause pain, bleeding, or obstruction.[68]

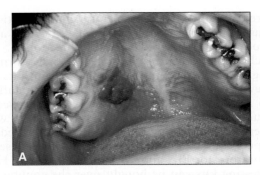

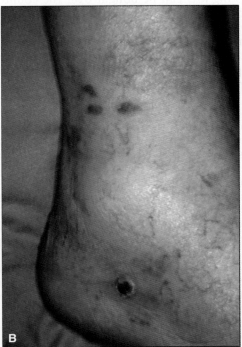

FIGURE 16-11. Kaposi sarcoma. **(A)** Intraoral Kaposi sarcoma of the hard palate secondary to HIV infection. **(B)** Cutaneous brown Kaposi sarcoma lesions located over the medial left ankle and foot. (From the Centers for Disease Control and Prevention Public Health Image Library. Nos. 6070, 5515. A courtesy of Sol Silverman, Jr; B courtesy of Steve Kraus.)

Pulmonary KS usually is a late development of the disease and causes dyspnea, cough, and hemoptysis (coughing up blood).[68]

With prolonged survival, the number of persons with AIDS who develop *non-Hodgkin lymphoma* has increased steadily.[2] The clinical features are nonspecific and include fever, night sweats, and weight loss (see Chapter 11). Because the manifestations of non-Hodgkin lymphoma are similar to those of other opportunistic infections, diagnosis often is difficult. Diagnosis can be made by biopsy of the affected tissue.

The high prevalence of human papillomavirus (HPV) infection in persons with AIDS has been linked to the development of *cervical carcinoma* and anal carcinoma in both HIV-positive men and women.[2]

Gynecologic examination with cervical cytologic analysis for HPV should be part of the routine evaluation of HIV-infected women. Since HPV can also cause anal dysplasia, a precursor of anal carcinoma, cytologic evaluations of the anal canal are also recommended for both HIV-infected men and women. A quadrivalent vaccine to prevent HPV infection became available in 2007. The safety and immunogenicity of this vaccine among HIV-infected men and women are being studied.[69]

Wasting Syndrome and Metabolic Disorders

Wasting Syndrome. The wasting syndrome, which is an AIDS-defining illness, is characterized by involuntary weight loss of at least 10% of baseline body weight in the presence of diarrhea, more than two stools per day, or chronic weakness and a fever.[70] This diagnosis is made when no other opportunistic infections or neoplasms can be identified as causing these symptoms. Factors that contribute to wasting are anorexia, metabolic abnormalities, endocrine dysfunction, malabsorption, and cytokine dysregulation. Treatment for wasting includes nutritional interventions such as oral supplements or enteral or parenteral nutrition, as well as pharmacologic agents, including appetite stimulants, cannabinoids, and megestrol acetate.

Metabolic Disorders. A wide range of metabolic and morphologic disorders are associated with HIV infection, including insulin resistance and diabetes, lipodystrophy, hyperlipidemia, and mitochondrial disorders.[71] It is not known why insulin resistance appears to be increased in people with HIV infection; however, most experts believe it is secondary to dysregulation of metabolic pathways or to indirect effects through mitochondrial toxicity linked to adipocyte toxicity.[72] Moreover, metabolic complications among people with HIV infection have been increasing since the introduction of potent HAART.

The term *lipodystrophy* is frequently used to describe the body composition changes with or without the other metabolic derangements. Lipodystrophy related to HIV infection includes symptoms that fall into two categories: changes in body composition and metabolic changes.[73] The alterations in body appearance are an increase in abdominal girth, buffalo hump development (abnormal distribution of fat in the dorsoclavical area), wasting of fat from the face and extremities, and breast enlargement in men and women. Most individuals experience either lipohypertrophy or lipoatrophy. Mixed patterns of fat changes are less common.[74] The metabolic changes include elevated serum cholesterol, low HDL cholesterol, elevated triglyceride levels, and insulin resistance. Originally attributed solely to the use of protease inhibitors, the pathogenesis of these metabolic derangements is complex and there may be multiple confounding factors.[75]

The mitochondria control many of the oxidative chemical reactions that release energy from glucose and other organic molecules and transform it into adenosine triphosphate (ATP), which cells use as an energy source. In the absence of normal mitochondrial function, cells revert to anaerobic metabolism, generating lactic acid. The mitochondrial disorders seen in persons with HIV infection are attributed to a class of drugs called the *nucleoside/nucleotide analog reverse transcriptase inhibitors* (NRTIs), particularly the thymidine analogs.[76] The most common presentations are lipoatrophy and peripheral neuropathy, although patients may not experience both. Patients may also present with nonspecific gastrointestinal symptoms, including nausea, vomiting, and abdominal pain. They may develop altered liver function and lactic acidosis. Since the recognition of the ascending polyneuropathy syndrome and reports of hepatic failure due to combination therapy with stavudine and didanosine, reports of life-threatening events due to mitochondrial toxicities have dramatically decreased.

Diagnosis and Treatment

A diagnosis of HIV infection may be prompted by a number of scenarios, including positive results of a screening test, accompanying signs and symptoms of an acute HIV infection, or manifestations of an immunodeficiency state. Unfortunately, there are approximately 250,000 persons living with HIV infection in the United States who are not aware of their infection or their risk of transmitting it, and therefore are missing the opportunity to benefit from early treatment.

Diagnostic Methods. The most accurate and inexpensive method for identifying HIV infection is the HIV antibody test. The first commercial assays for HIV were introduced in 1985 to screen donated blood. Since then, use of antibody detection tests has been expanded to include evaluating persons at increased risk for HIV infection. The HIV antibody test procedure consists of screening with an *enzyme immunoassay* (EIA), also known as *enzyme-linked immunosorbent assay* (ELISA), followed by a confirmatory test such as the *Western blot assay,* which is performed if the EIA is positive.[77] The EIA detects antibodies produced in response to HIV infection. In an EIA, antibodies to HIV in the blood sample bind to HIV antigens in the test material.[56] The Western blot is a more sensitive assay than the EIA that looks for the presence of antibodies to specific viral antigens.[56] In the case of a false-positive EIA result, the Western blot test can identify the person as uninfected. *Polymerase chain reaction* (PCR) is a technique for detecting HIV DNA (see Chapter 14). Polymerase chain reaction detects the presence of the virus rather than the antibody to the virus, which the EIA and Western blot tests detect. Polymerase chain reaction is useful in diagnosing HIV infection in infants born to infected mothers because these infants have their mothers' HIV antibodies regardless of whether the children are infected. Polymerase chain reaction is also useful in determining acute HIV infection as the antibody tests are negative in early infection.

Technologic advances have led to new forms of testing, such as the oral test, home testing kits, and the new rapid blood test. Oral fluids contain antibodies to HIV. In the late 1990s, the FDA approved the OraSure test. The OraSure uses a cotton swab, which is inserted into the mouth for 2 minutes, placed in a transport container with preservative, and then sent to a laboratory for EIA and Western blot testing. Home HIV testing kits can be bought over the counter. The kits, approved by the FDA, allow persons to collect their own blood sample through a finger-stick process, mail the specimen to a laboratory for EIA and confirmatory Western blot tests, and receive results by telephone in 3 to 7 days. In November 2002, the FDA approved the Ora Quick Rapid HIV-1 Antibody Test.[78] The Ora Quick uses a whole-blood specimen from a fingerstick and can provide results in about 20 minutes. Reactive, or positive, test results require confirmation using Western blot testing on the serum. Persons with a reactive result need to be told that the preliminary test was positive and that they need a confirmatory test. The use of a rapid test should facilitate people receiving the results of their HIV test more regularly because they do not need to return for their test results 2 weeks later unless it is positive or there is concern that the person may be in the window period before seroconversion. The newest development in HIV testing is a combined antigen-antibody test (p24 antigen, HIV antibodies), which has the advantage of early detection of HIV, potentially within 2 weeks of infection.

Treatment. Currently, there is no cure for HIV infection. The medications that are currently available to treat HIV infection decrease the amount of virus in the body, but they do not eradicate HIV.[79] The treatment of HIV infection is one of the most rapidly evolving fields in medicine.

There currently are five different classes of HIV antiretroviral medications: nucleoside and nucleotide analog reverse transcriptase inhibitors; nonnucleoside reverse transcriptase inhibitors; protease inhibitors; entry inhibitors; and the newest class, integrase inhibitors. Each class of agents attempts to interrupt the life cycle of the HIV at different points (see Fig. 16-8). *Reverse transcriptase inhibitors* inhibit HIV replication by acting on the enzyme reverse transcriptase. *Nucleoside analog reverse transcriptase inhibitors* and *nucleotide reverse transcriptase inhibitors* act by blocking the elongation of the DNA chain by stopping more nucleosides from being added. *Nonnucleoside reverse transcriptase inhibitors* work by binding to the reverse transcriptase enzyme so it cannot copy the virus's RNA into DNA. *Protease inhibitors* bind to the protease enzyme and inhibit its action. This inhibition prevents cleavage of the polypeptide chain into individual proteins, which would be used to construct a new virus.

Two new classes of antiretroviral therapy are the *entry inhibitors* and *integrase inhibitors*. The entry inhibitors prevent HIV from entering or fusing with the CD4+ cell, thus blocking the virus from inserting its genetic information into the CD4+ T cell. The integrase inhibitors block the integration step of the viral cycle, thus preventing the HIV genome from integrating into the host's genome.

Because different drugs act at different stages of the replication cycle, optimal treatment includes a combination of at least three antiretroviral drugs, referred to as *highly active antiretroviral therapy* (HAART). The goal of HAART is a sustained suppression of HIV replication, resulting in an undetectable viral load and increasing CD4+ cell count. In general, antiviral therapies are prescribed to slow the progression of AIDS and improve the overall quality of life and survival time of persons with HIV infection.

Preventive and therapeutic vaccines for HIV are also being investigated.[80] The preventive vaccine would be given to someone who is HIV negative, with the goal of preventing infection if exposed to HIV. The therapeutic vaccine would be used in people who are already infected with HIV as a way to control HIV replication. In trials to date, these vaccines have not proven beneficial.

A new preventive strategy has been approved by the FDA in the United States. PrEP—pre-exposure prophylaxis—involves consistently taking antiretroviral medication that may interrupt infection if exposed to HIV in high-risk settings. It is not 100% effective at preventing HIV infection; routine counseling on reducing risky behaviors and routine evaluations for sexually transmitted infections are still paramount. Individuals taking PrEP also need to be routinely monitored for efficacy and side effects of the medication.

HIV Infection in Pregnancy and in Infants and Children

Transmission from mother to infant is the most common way that children become infected with HIV. Human immunodeficiency virus may be transmitted from infected women to their offspring in utero, during labor and delivery, or through breast-feeding.[81] Most transmissions from mother to child occur during childbirth when the mother's infected blood in the birth canal infects the baby. Breast-feeding, particularly in poor countries, can account for one third to one half of all mother-to-child transmission. Screening programs for pregnant women and antiretroviral prophylaxis are available for preventing mother-to-child transmission in HIV-positive women. Epidemiologic estimates suggest that coverage for antiviral prophylaxis to HIV-positive women for prevention of mother-to-child transmission in low- to middle-income countries increased from 9% in 2004 to 33% in 2007 to 57% in 2011.[44,47]

Diagnosis and Treatment. Diagnosis of HIV infection in children born to HIV-infected mothers is complicated by the presence of maternal anti-HIV IgG antibody, which crosses the placenta to the fetus.[82] Consequently, infants born to HIV-infected women can be HIV antibody positive by ELISA up until 18 months of age even though they are not infected with HIV. Polymerase chain reaction testing for HIV DNA is used most often to diagnose HIV infection in infants younger than 18 months of age. Two positive PCR tests are needed for diagnosis. Children born to mothers with HIV infection are considered uninfected if they become HIV antibody negative after 18 months of age, have no other laboratory evidence of HIV infection, and have not met the case definition criteria for AIDS in children.

The landmark Pediatric AIDS Clinical Trials Group (PACTG) 076 study reported that perinatal transmission could be lowered by two-thirds, from 26% to 8%, by administering zidovudine to the mother during pregnancy and labor and delivery and to the infant when it is born.[83] The U.S. Public Health Service therefore recommends that HIV counseling and testing should be offered to all pregnant women.[84] The recommendations also stress that women who test positive for HIV antibodies should be informed of the perinatal prevention benefits of zidovudine therapy and offered HAART, which often includes zidovudine. This is done because it has been found that women receiving antiretroviral therapy who also have a viral load less than 1000 copies/mL have very low rates of perinatal transmission. Efavirenz, a non-nucleoside reverse transcriptase inhibitor, has the potential for causing neural tube defects within the first 6 weeks of pregnancy. HIV-infected women of child-bearing age should be tested for pregnancy and counseled regarding the potential adverse effects prior to initiating HAART with efavirenz. If a woman is taking an efavirenz-based regimen and pregnancy is determined after 6 weeks, then she may continue the regimen as long as virologic suppression is maintained and the pregnancy is monitored.[79] Benefits of voluntary testing for mothers and newborns include reduced morbidity because of intensive treatment and supportive health care, the opportunity for early antiretroviral therapy for mother and child, and information regarding the risk of transmission from breast milk.

Clinical Manifestations. Children may have a different clinical presentation of HIV infection than adults.[82] Failure to thrive, CNS abnormalities, and developmental delays are the most prominent primary manifestations of HIV infection in children. Children born with HIV infection usually weigh less and are shorter than noninfected infants. A major cause of early mortality for HIV-infected children is *P. jiroveci* pneumonia, which occurs early in children, with the peak age of onset at 3 to 6 months. For this reason, prophylaxis with trimethoprim-sulfamethoxazole should be started beginning at 4 to 6 weeks for all infants born to HIV-infected mothers, regardless of their CD4+ cell count or infection status.[85]

SUMMARY CONCEPTS

■ Immunodeficiency is an absolute or partial loss of the normal immune response, which places a person at increased risk for development of infections or malignant complications. It can be classified as primary (i.e., congenital or inherited) or secondary (i.e., due to another disease or condition).

■ Immunodeficiency can affect the humoral or cellular components of the adaptive immune system. Defects in humoral immunity increase the risk of recurrent pyogenic infections but have less effect on the defense against intracellular bacteria (mycobacteria), fungi, protozoa, and viruses (except for the enteroviruses that cause gastrointestinal infections). Defects in cellular immunity increase the risk of developing fungal, protozoan, viral, and intracellular bacterial infections, and malignant cell proliferation.

■ Acquired immunodeficiency syndrome (AIDS), the most common type of secondary immunodeficiency, is caused by infection with the human immunodeficiency virus (HIV), a retrovirus that infects the body's $CD4^+$ T cells and macrophages. Destruction of $CD4^+$ cells constitutes an attack on the entire immune system because this subset of lymphocytes exerts critical regulatory and effector functions that involve both humoral and cellular immunity.

■ The clinical course of HIV infection can be divided into three phases: a primary phase that occurs shortly after infection and is usually manifested by mononucleosis-like symptoms, a latency phase that may last for years, and an overt AIDS phase that is characterized by a marked decrease in $CD4^+$ T cells and the development of opportunistic infections, malignancies, wasting syndrome, and metabolic disorders. There is no cure for AIDS. Treatment largely involves the use of drugs that interrupt the replication of HIV and prevention or treatment of complications such as opportunistic infections.

■ Women who are infected with HIV may transmit the virus to their offspring in utero, during labor and delivery, or through breast milk. Diagnosis of HIV infection in children born to HIV-infected mothers is complicated by the presence of maternal HIV antibody, which crosses the placenta to the fetus. This antibody usually disappears within 18 months in uninfected children.

REVIEW EXERCISES

1. A 32-year-old man presents in the allergy clinic with complaints of allergic rhinitis or hay fever. His major complaints are those of nasal pruritus (itching), nasal congestion with profuse watery drainage, sneezing, and eye irritation. The physical examination reveals edematous and inflamed nasal mucosa and redness of the ocular conjunctiva. He relates that this happens every fall during "ragweed season."

   A. Explain the immunologic mechanisms that are responsible for this man's symptoms.
   B. What type of diagnostic test might be used?
   C. What type(s) of treatment might be used to relieve his symptoms?

2. Persons with intestinal parasites and those with allergies may both have elevated levels of eosinophils in their blood.

   A. Explain.

3. A 20-year-old woman has been diagnosed with IgA deficiency. She has been plagued with frequent bouts of bronchitis and sinus infections.

   A. Why are these types of infections particularly prominent in persons with an IgA deficiency?
   B. She has been told that she needs to be aware that she could have a severe reaction when given unwashed blood transfusions. Explain.

4. Persons with impaired cellular immunity may not respond to the tuberculin test, even when infected with *Mycobacterium tuberculosis*.

   A. Explain.

5. A 29-year-old woman presents to the clinic for her initial obstetric visit about 10 weeks into her pregnancy.

   A. This woman is in a monogamous relationship. Should an HIV test be a part of her initial blood work? Why?
   B. The woman's HIV test comes back positive. What should be done to decrease the risk of transmitting HIV to her child?
   C. The infant is born, and its initial antibody test is positive. Does this mean the infant is infected? How is the diagnosis of HIV infection in a child younger than 18 months made, and why is this different than the diagnosis for adults?

6. A 40-year-old man presents to the clinic very short of breath, and after a radiograph and an examination, he is diagnosed with PCP. His provider does an HIV test, which is positive. Upon further testing, the man's $CD4^+$ cell count is found to be 100 cells/μL and his viral load is 250,000 copies/mL.

A. Why did the provider do an HIV test after the man was diagnosed with PCP?

B. Is there a way to prevent PCP?

C. What classification does this man fall into based on his CD4⁺ count and symptomatology, and why?

REFERENCES

1. Abbas AK, Lichtman AH, Pillai S. *Cellular and Molecular Immunology*. 7th ed. Philadelphia, PA: Elsevier Saunders; 2012:319–344, 365–388, 407–424, 445–470.

2. Kumar V, Abbas AK, Fautso N, et al. *Robbins and Cotran Pathologic Basis of Disease*. 8th ed. Philadelphia, PA: Saunders Elsevier; 2010:183–249.

3. Warren JS, Strayer DS. Immunopathology. In: Rubin R, Strayer DS, eds. *Rubin's Pathology: Clinicopathologic Foundations of Medicine*. 6th ed. Philadelphia, PA: Lippincott Williams & Wilkins; 2012:115–156.

4. Kay AB. Allergy and allergic disease (parts 1 and 2). *N Engl J Med*. 2001;344:(1,2)30–37, 109–113.

5. Galli SJ. New concepts about the mast cell. *N Engl J Med*. 1993;328:257–265.

6. Arnold JJ, Williams PAM. Anaphylaxsis: recognition and management. *Am Fam Physician*. 2011;84(10):1111–1118.

7. Lieberman P. Anaphylaxis. *Med Clin North Am*. 2006;90:77–95.

8. Lieberman P, Kemp SF, Oppenheimer J, et al.; Chief Editors for the Joint Task Force on Practice Parameters, Joint Counsel of Allergy, Asthma and Immunology. The diagnosis and management of anaphylaxis: an updated practice parameter. *J Allergy Clin Immunol*. 2005;115(3 suppl):S483–S523.

9. Mucci T, Govindaraj S, Tversky J. Allergic rhinitis. *Mt Sinai J Med*. 2011;78(5):634–644.

10. Steinsvaag SK. Allergic rhinitis: an updated overview. *Curr Allergy Asthma Rep*. 2012;12:99–103.

11. Sicherer SH, Sampson HA. Food allergy. *J Allergy Clin Immunol*. 2010;125:S116–S125.

12. Masilamani M, Commins S, Shreffler W. Determinants of food allergy. *Immunol Allergy Clin North Am*. 2012;33:11–33.

13. Sampson HA. Peanut allergy. *N Engl J Med*. 2002;346:1294–1299.

14. Berke RC, Singh A, Guralnice M. Atopic dermatitis: an overview. *Am Fam Physician*. 2012;86:35–42.

15. Mark BJ, Slavin RG. Allergic contact dermatitis. *Med Clin North Am*. 2006;90:169–185.

16. Ohshimo S, Bonella F, Guzman J, et al. Hypersensitivity pneumonitis. *Immunol Allergy Clin North Am*. 2012;32:537–556.

17. Gilliam AC. Update on graft versus host disease. *J Invest Dermatol*. 2004;123:251–257.

18. Choi SW, Levine JE, Ferrara JLM. Pathogenesis and management of graft-versus-host disease. *Immunol Allergy Clin North Am*. 2010;30:75–101.

19. Crawford JM. The liver and biliary tract. In: Kumar V, Abbas AK, Fausto N, eds. *Robbins and Cotran Pathologic Basis of Disease*. 7th ed. Philadelphia, PA: Elsevier Saunders; 2005:919–920.

20. Yin Y, Yili L, Maniuzza RA. Structural basis for self-recognition by autoimmune T-cell receptors. *Immunol Rev*. 2012;250(1):32–48.

21. Davidson A, Diamond B. Autoimmune disease. *N Engl J Med*. 2001;345:340–350.

22. Rioux JD, Abbas AK. Paths to understanding the genetic basis of autoimmune disease. *Nature*. 2005;435:584–589.

23. Goodnow CC, Sprent J, de St Groth BF, et al. Cellular and genetic mechanisms of self tolerance and autoimmunity. *Nature*. 2005;435:590–597.

24. Navratil JS, Sabatine JM, Ahearn JM. Apoptosis and immune responses to self. *Rheum Dis Clin North Am*. 2004;30:193–212.

25. Jiang H, Chess L. Regulation of immune responses by T cells. *N Engl J Med*. 2006;354:166–176.

26. Kronberg M, Rudensky A. Regulation of immunity by self-reactive T cells. *Nature*. 2005;435:598–604.

27. Zandman-Goddard G, Peeva E, Shoenfeld Y. Gender and autoimmunity. *Autoimmun Rev*. 2007;6:366–372.

28. Cutolo M, Sulli A, Seriolo S, et al. Estrogens, the immune response and autoimmunity. *Clin Exp Rheumatol*. 1995;13:217–226.

29. Cusick MF, Libbey JE, Fujinami RS. Molecular mimicry as a mechanism of autoimmune disease. *Clin Rev Allergy Immunol*. 2012;42:102–111.

30. Anders H-J, Zecher D, Pawar RD, et al. Molecular mechanisms of autoimmunity triggered by microbial infection. *Arthritis Res Ther*. 2005;7:215–224.

31. Llewelyn M, Cohen J. Superantigen antagonist peptides. *Crit Care*. 2001;5:53–55.

32. Verbsky JW, Grossman WJ. Cellular and genetic basis of primary immune deficiencies. *Pediatr Clin North Am*. 2006;53:649–684.

33. Bonilla FA, Geha RS. Update on primary immunodeficiency diseases. *J Allergy Clin Immunol*. 2006;117(2 suppl):S435–S441.

34. Parvaneh N, Casanova J-L, Notarangelo LD. Primary immunodeficiencies: a rapidly evolving story. *J Allergy Clin Immunol*. 2013;131:314–323.

35. Buckley R. Evaluation of suspected immunodeficiency. In: Kliegman RM, Stanton BF, St Gemelli JW, et al. *Nelson Textbook of Pediatrics*. 19th ed. Piladelphia, PA: Elsevier Saunders, 2011:714–722.e1.

36. The Jeffrey Modell Foundation Medical Advisory Board. *Ten Warning Signs of Primary Immunodeficiency*. 2009. Available at: http://www.info4pi.org/aboutPI/index.cfm?section=aboutPI&content=warningsigns. Accessed August 26, 2013.

37. Sorensen RU, Moore C. Antibody deficiency syndromes. *Pediatr Clin North Am*. 2000;47:1225–1252.

38. Rose ME, Lang DM. Evaluating and managing hypogammaglobulinemia. *Cleve Clin J Med*. 2006;73:133–144.

39. Elder ME. T-cell immunodeficiencies. *Pediatr Clin North Am*. 2000;47:1253–1274.

40. Buckley RH. Molecular defects in human severe combined immunodeficiency and approaches to immune reconstitution. *Annu Rev Immunol*. 2004;22:625–655.

41. Rudd CE. Disabled receptor signaling and new primary immunodeficiency disorders. *N Engl J Med*. 2006;354:1874–1877.

42. Buckley RH. The long quest for neonatal screening for severe combined immunodeficiency. *J Allergy Clin Immunol*. 2012;129(3):597–604.

43. Ochs HD, Thrasher AJ. The Wiskott-Aldrich syndrome. *J Allergy Clin Immunol*. 2006;117:725–738.

44. UNAIDS. *2012 UNAIDS Report on the Global AIDS Epidemic, November 2012*. Available at: http://www.unaids.org/en/resources/publications/2012/name,76121,en.asp. Accessed August 26, 2013.

45. Karim SSA, Karim QA, Gouws E, et al. Global epidemiology of HIV-AIDS. *Infect Dis Clin North Am*. 2007;21:1–17.

46. Zetola NM, Pilcher CD. Diagnosis and management of acute HIV infection. *Infect Dis Clin North Am*. 2007;21:19–48.

47. UNAIDS. *2008 Report on Global AIDS Epidemic, August 2008*. Available at: http://www.unaids.org/en/KnowledgeCentre/HIVData/GlobalReport/2008/2008_Global_report.asp. Accessed August 26, 2013.

48. Gershon RRM, Vlahov D, Nelson KE. The risk of transmission of HIV-1 through non-percutaneous, non-sexual modes: a review. *AIDS*. 1990;4:645–650.

49. Public Health Agency of Canada. *Summary: Estimation of HIV prevalence and incidence in Canada, 2011*. 2012. Available at: http://www.phac-aspc.gc.ca/aids-sida/publication/survreport/2011/dec/index-eng.php. Accessed August 26, 2013.

50. Centers for Disease Control and Prevention. Estimated HIV incidence in the United States, 2007–2010. *HIV Surveillance Supplemental Report*. December 2012;17(4). Available at: http://www.cdc.gov/hiv/topics/surveillance/resources/reports/#supplemental. Accessed August 26, 2013.

51. Stramer SL, Glynn SA, Kleinman SH, et al. Detection of HIV-1 and HCV infections among antibody-negative blood donors by nucleic acid-amplification testing. *N Engl J Med.* 2004;351:760–768.

52. Centers for Disease Control and Prevention. *Occupational HIV transmission among healthcare workers.* 2011. Available at: http://www.cdc.gov/hiv/resources/factsheets/ hcwprev.htm. Accessed August 26, 2013.

53. Kuhar DT, Henderson DK, Struble KA, et al.; for the USPHS Writing Group. Updated U.S. Public Health Service guidelines for the management of occupational exposures to human immunodeficiency virus and recommendations for postexposure prophylaxis. *Infect Control Hosp Epidemiol.* 2013;34(9):875–892.

54. Brenner BG, Roger M, Routy JP, et al. Amplified transmission in early HIV infection. *J Infect Dis.* 2007;195:951–959.

55. Trecarichi EM, Tumbarello M, de Gaetano Donati K, et al. Partial protective effect of CCR5-delta 32 heterozygosity in a cohort of heterosexual Italian HIV-1 exposed uninfected individuals. *AIDS Res Ther.* 2006;3:22.

56. Centers for Disease Control and Prevention. 1993 Revised classification system for HIV infection and expanded surveillance case definition for AIDS among adolescents and adults. *Morb Mortal Wkly Rep.* 1992;41(RR-17):1–23.

57. Schneider E, Whitmore S, Glynn MK, et al. Revised surveillance case definitions for HIV infections among adults, adolescents, and children aged <18 months and for children aged 18 months to <13 years–United States, 2008. *MMWR Recomm Rep.* 2008;57(RR-10),1–8.

58. Hecht FM, Wang L, Collier A. A multicenter observational study of potential benefits of initiating combination antiretroviral therapy during acute infection. *J Infect Dis.* 2006;194:725–733.

59. Rodriguez B, Sethi AK, Cheruvu VK. Predictive value of plasma HIV RNA level on rate of CD4 T-cell decline in untreated HIV infection. *JAMA.* 2006;296:1498–1506.

60. Casaa C, Solomba S, Rauch A, et al. Host and viral genetic correlates of clinical definitions of HIV-1 progression. *PLoS One.* 2010;5(6):e11079.

61. Kaplan JE, Hanson D, Dworkin MS, et al. Epidemiology of HIV associated opportunistic infections in the United States in the era of highly active antiretroviral therapy. *Clin Infect Dis.* 2000;30(suppl 1):S5–S14.

62. UNAIDS. *Frequently asked questions about tuberculosis.* 2006. Available at: http://data.unaids.org/pub/factsheet/2006/tb_ hiv_ qa.pdf. Accessed August 26, 2013.

63. Wilcox CM. Gastrointestinal manifestations of AIDS. *Nutr Clin Pract.* 2004;19:356–364.

64. Antinori A, Arendt G, Becker JT. Updated research nosology for HIV-associated neurocognitive disorders. *Neurology.* 2007;69:1789–1799.

65. Dedicoat M, Livesley N. Management of toxoplasmic encephalitis in HIV-infected adults (with an emphasis on resource-poor settings). *Cochrane Database Syst Rev.* 2006;19(3):CD005420.

66. Berger JR, Houff S. Progressive multifocal leukoencephalopathy: lessons from AIDS and natalizumab. *Neurol Res.* 2006;28:299–305.

67. Silverberg MJ, Abrams DI. AIDS-defining and non-AIDS-defining malignancies: cancer occurrence in the antiretroviral therapy era. *Curr Opin Oncol.* 2007;19:446–451.

68. Antman K, Chang Y. Kaposi's sarcoma. *N Engl J Med.* 2000;342:1027–1038.

69. De Vuyst H, Franceschi S. Human papillomavirus vaccines in HIV-positive men and women. *Curr Opin Oncol.* 2007;19:470–475.

70. Polsky B, Kotler D, Steinhart C. Treatment guidelines for HIV-associated wasting. *HIV Clin Trials.* 2004;5:50–61.

71. Umeh OC, Currier JS. Lipids, metabolic syndrome, and risk factors for future cardiovascular disease among HIV-infected patients. *Curr HIV/AIDS Rep.* 2005;2:132–139.

72. Brown TT, Cole SR, Li X, et al. Antiretroviral therapy and the prevalence and incidence of diabetes mellitus in the multicenter AIDS cohort study. *Arch Intern Med.* 2005;165:1179–1184.

73. Tershakovec AM, Frank I, Rader D. HIV-related lipodystrophy and related factors. *Atherosclerosis.* 2004;174:1–10.

74. Mulligan K, Parker RA, Komarow L, et al. Mixed patterns of changes in central and peripheral fat following initiation of antiretroviral therapy in a randomized trial. *J Acquir Immune Defic Syndr.* 2006;41:590–597.

75. Grinspoon S, Carr A. Cardiovascular risk and body-fat abnormalities in HIV-infected adults. *N Engl J Med.* 2005;352:48–62.

76. McComsey G, Lonergan JT. Mitochondrial dysfunction: patient monitoring and toxicity management. *J Acquir Immune Defic Syndr.* 2004;37(suppl 1):S30–S35.

77. Aberg JA, Kaplan JE, Libman H, et al. Primary care guidelines for the management of persons infected with human immunodeficiency virus: 2009 update by the HIV Medicine Association of the Infectious Diseases Society of America. *Clin Infect Dis.* 2009;49(5):651–681.

78. Delaney KP, Branson BM, Uniyal A, et al. Performance of an oral rapid HIV-1/2 test experience with four CDC studies. *AIDS.* 2006;20:1655–1660.

79. Panel on Antiretroviral Guidelines for Adults and Adolescents. Guidelines for the use of antiretroviral agents in HIV-1-infected adults and adolescents. *Department of Health and Human Services.* Updated February 12, 2013; 1–161. Available at: http:// www.aidsinfo.nih.gov/ContentFiles/Adultand AdolescentGL.pdf. Accessed August 26, 2013.

80. Maplanka C. AIDS: is there an answer to the global pandemic? The immune system in HIV infection and control. *Viral Immunol.* 2007;20:331–342.

81. McIntyre J. Managing pregnant patients. In: Dolin R, Masur H, Saag M, eds. *AIDS Therapy.* 3rd ed. London, UK: Churchill Livingston; 2008:595–597.

82. Yogev R, Chadwick EG. Acquired immunodeficiency syndrome (human immunodeficiency virus). In: Behrman RE, Kliegman RM, Jenson HB, et al., eds. *Nelson Textbook of Pediatrics.* 18th ed. Philadelphia, PA: Saunders Elsevier; 2007:1427–1443.

83. Connor EM, Sperling RS, Gelber R, et al. Reduction of maternal-infant transmission of human immunodeficiency virus type 1 with zidovudine treatment. *N Engl J Med.* 1994;33:1173–1180.

84. Panel on Treatment of HIV-Infected Pregnant Women and Prevention of Perinatal Transmission. *Recommendations for use of antiretroviral drugs in pregnant HIV-1-infected women for maternal health and interventions to reduce perinatal HIV transmission in the United States.* 2012. Available at: http:// AIDSinfo.nih.gov/contentfiles/lvguidelines/perinatalgl.pdf. Accessed August 26, 2013.

85. Centers for Disease Control and Prevention, the National Institutes of Health, the HIV Medicine Association of Infectious Diseases Society of America, the Pediatric Infectious Disease Society, and the American Academy of Pediatrics. *Guidelines for Prevention and Treatment of Opportunistic Infections Among HIV-Exposed and HIV-Infected Children.* 2009. Available at: http://aidsinfo.nih.gov/contentfiles/lvguidelines/oi_guidelines_ pediatrics.pdf. Accessed August 26, 2013.

Porth Essentials Resources

Explore these additional resources to enhance learning for this chapter:

- NCLEX-Style Questions and Other Resources on **thePoint**, http://thePoint.lww.com/PorthEssentials4e
- Study Guide for Essentials of Pathophysiology
- Concepts in Action Animations
- Adaptive Learning | Powered by PrepU, http://thepoint.lww.com/ prepu

C h a p t e r 17

Control of Cardiovascular Function

The main function of the cardiovascular or circulatory system, which consists of the heart and blood vessels, is transport. The circulatory system transports and distributes oxygen and nutrients needed for metabolic processes to the tissues, carries waste products from cellular metabolism to the kidneys and other excretory organs for elimination, and circulates fluids, electrolytes, and hormones needed to regulate body function. This process is carried out with exquisite precision so that oxygen and nutrient delivery is exactly matched to meet tissue needs.

Organization of the Circulatory System

The circulatory system can be divided into two parts: the *pulmonary* (or *central*) *circulation,* which moves blood through the lungs and creates a link with the gas exchange function of the respiratory system, and the *systemic* (or *peripheral*) *circulation*, which moves blood throughout all the other tissues of the body (Fig. 17-1).

Pulmonary and Systemic Circulations

The pulmonary circulation consists of the right side of the heart, the pulmonary arteries and arterioles, the pulmonary capillaries, and the pulmonary veins. The large pulmonary vessels are unique in that the

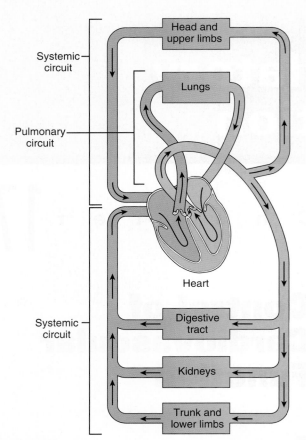

Systemic circuit

Pulmonary circuit

Systemic circuit

FIGURE 17-1. Systemic and pulmonary circulations. The right side of the heart pumps blood to the lungs, and the left side of the heart pumps blood to the systemic circulation.

vessels in the lungs, and the left heart, which propels blood through the vessels that supply all the other tissues in the body. Both sides of the heart are further divided into two chambers, an *atrium* and a *ventricle*. The atria function as collection chambers for blood returning to the heart and as auxiliary pumps that assist in filling the ventricles. The ventricles are the main pumping chambers of the heart. The right ventricle pumps blood through the pulmonary artery to the lungs and the left ventricle pumps blood through the aorta into the systemic circulation. The ventricular chambers of the right and left heart have inlet and outlet valves that act reciprocally (i.e., one set of valves is open while the other is closed) to control the direction of blood flow through the cardiac chambers and out into the arteries.

Because the circulatory system is a closed system, both sides of the heart must pump the same amount of blood over time. If the output of the left heart were to fall below that of the right heart, blood would accumulate in the pulmonary circulation. Likewise, if the right heart were to pump less effectively than the left heart, blood would accumulate in the systemic circulation. However, the left and right heart seldom eject exactly the same amount of blood with each beat. This is because blood return to the heart is affected by activities such as taking a deep breath or moving from the seated to standing position. These beat-by-beat variations in stroke volume (amount of blood pumped with each beat) are accommodated by the large storage capabilities of the venous system that allow for temporary changes in blood volume. The accumulation of blood occurs only when the storage capacity of the venous system has been exceeded.

Volume and Pressure Distribution

Blood flow in the systemic circulatory system depends on a blood volume that is sufficient to fill the blood vessels in the systemic circulation and a pressure difference that provides the force needed to move blood forward. As shown in Figure 17-2, approximately 4% of the blood at any given time is in the left heart, 16% is in the arteries and arterioles, 4% is in the capillaries, 64% is in the venules and veins, and 4% is in the right heart. The arteries and arterioles, which have thick, elastic walls and function as a distribution system, have the highest pressure. The capillaries are small, thin-walled vessels that link the arterial and venous sides of the circulation. They serve as an exchange system where transfer of gases, nutrients, and wastes take place. Because of their small size and large surface area, the capillaries contain the smallest amount of blood. The venules and veins, which contain the largest amount of blood, are thin-walled, distensible vessels that function as a reservoir to collect blood from the capillaries and return it to the right heart.

Because the pulmonary and systemic circulations are connected and function as a closed system, blood can be shifted from one circulation to the other.

pulmonary artery is the only artery that carries deoxygenated venous blood and the pulmonary veins are the only veins that carry oxygenated arterial blood. The systemic circulation consists of the left side of the heart, the aorta and its branches, the capillaries that supply the brain and peripheral tissues, and the systemic venous system and the vena cava. The veins from the lower portion of the body merge to form the inferior vena cava and those from the head and upper extremities form the superior vena cava, both of which empty into the right heart.

Although the pulmonary and systemic circulations function similarly, they have some important differences. The pulmonary circulation, which is the smaller of the two, is located in the chest near the heart and functions as a low-pressure system (mean arterial pressure of approximately 12 mm Hg). This low pressure allows blood to move through the lungs more slowly, providing more time for gas exchange. Because the systemic circulation must transport blood to distant parts of the body, often against the effects of gravity, it functions as a high-pressure system, with a mean arterial pressure of 90 to 100 mm Hg.

The heart, which propels blood through the circulatory system, consists of two pumps in series—the right heart, which propels blood through the gas exchange

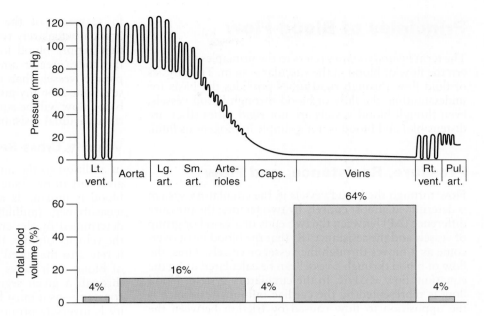

FIGURE 17-2. Pressure and volume distribution in the systemic circulation. The graphs show the inverse relation between internal pressure and volume in different portions of the circulatory system. (From Smith JJ, Kampine JP. *Circulatory Physiology: The Essentials.* 3rd ed. Baltimore, MD: J.B.Lippincott; 1990.)

In the pulmonary circulation, the blood volume (approximately 450 mL in the adult) can vary from as low as 50% of normal to as high as 200% of normal. An increase in intrathoracic pressure, such as occurs when exhaling against a closed glottis, impedes venous return to the right heart. This can produce a transient shift from the pulmonary to the systemic circulation of as much as 250 mL of blood as blood backs up in the vena cava and large veins. Body position also affects the distribution of blood volume. In the recumbent position, approximately 25% to 30% of the total blood volume is in the pulmonary circulation. On standing, gravity causes a rapid displacement of this blood to the lower part of the body. Because the volume of the systemic circulation is approximately seven times that of the pulmonary circulation, a shift of blood from one system to the other has a much greater effect on the pulmonary than on the systemic circulation.

The movement of blood from the arterial to the venous side of the circulation depends on a pressure difference or gradient, moving from an area of higher pressure to one of lower pressure. The pressure distribution in different parts of the circulation is almost an inverse of the volume distribution (see Fig. 17-2). The pressure in the arterial side of the circulation, which contains only approximately one sixth of the blood volume, is much higher than the pressure on the venous side of the circulation, which contains approximately two thirds of the blood. This pressure and volume distribution is due in large part to the structure and relative elasticity of the arteries and veins. The pressure difference between the arterial and venous sides of the circulation (approximately 84 mm Hg) provides the driving force for the flow of blood in the systemic circulation. The pulmonary circulation has a similar arterial–venous pressure difference, albeit it of a lesser magnitude, that facilitates blood flow.

SUMMARY CONCEPTS

■ The cardiovascular or circulatory system, which consists of a pump (heart), a series of distributing (arteries and arterioles) and collecting (veins and venules) blood vessels, and an extensive system of exchange vessels (capillaries), functions mainly as a transport system that circulates nutrients and other materials to and removes waste products from tissues throughout the body.

■ The circulatory system can be divided into two parts: the right heart and pulmonary circulation, which moves blood through the lungs and creates a link with the gas exchange function of the respiratory system; and the left heart and systemic circulation, which moves blood throughout all the other tissues of the body.

■ Blood flow in the circulatory system depends on a blood volume that is sufficient to fill the blood vessels and a pressure difference across the system that provides the force that is needed to move blood forward. The venous system, which is a low pressure system designed to collect and return blood to the heart, contains about two-thirds of the blood; the arterial system, which is a high pressure distributive system, contains about one-sixth of the blood; and the capillaries, which have the lowest pressure and function as an exchange system for gases, nutrients, and wastes, contain the least amount of blood.

Principles of Blood Flow

The term *hemodynamics* refers to the principles that govern the flow of blood in the vascular system. The physics of fluid flow through rigid tubes provides the basis for understanding the flow of blood through blood vessels, even though blood vessels are not rigid tubes (they are distensible) and blood is not a simple homogenous fluid.

Pressure, Resistance, and Flow

Flow through the blood vessels in the circulatory system is determined almost entirely by two factors: the pressure difference (ΔP) between the two ends of a vessel or group of vessels and the resistance (R) that the blood must overcome as it moves through the vessel or vessels. Thus, the flow of blood through a vessel can be calculated using the equation: flow = $\Delta P/R$. In the circulatory system, blood flow is represented by the cardiac output. Resistance is the opposition to flow caused by friction between the moving blood components and the stationary vessel wall. In the peripheral circulation, the collective resistance of all the vessels in that part of the circulation is referred to as the *total peripheral vascular resistance*.

The relationship between pressure and resistance can be quantified by what has become known as *Poiseuille's law*. In the 1840s, Louis Poiseuille determined that the flow of fluid was determined by the pressure difference between the two ends of a tube ($P_1 - P_2$), the fourth power of the radius (r^4) of the tube, the viscosity (η) of the fluid, the tube length (l), and two constants (π and 8) using the following equation: flow = $\pi \Delta P\ r^4/8\eta l$. Simplifying the equation (i.e., flow = $\Delta P\ r^4/\eta$) by deleting the constants π and 8 along with the length, which usually does not change, makes it clear that flow will increase as the pressure gradient and vessel radius increase and decrease as the blood viscosity increases. Note particularly that the rate of flow is directly related to the *fourth power of the radius,* emphasizing the importance of vessel diameter in determining the rate of flow through the vessel. For example, if the pressure remains constant, the rate of flow is 16 times greater in a vessel with a radius of 2 mm ($2 \times 2 \times 2 \times 2 = 16$) than in a vessel with a radius of 1 mm ($1 \times 1 \times 1 \times 1 = 1$).

Viscosity generates resistance to flow by producing friction between the molecules of a liquid. Unlike water that flows through plumbing pipes, blood is a nonhomogeneous liquid. It contains blood cells, platelets, fat globules, and plasma proteins that increase its viscosity. It is mainly the hematocrit or percentage of suspended red cells in the blood that determines viscosity.

Flow in Series and Parallel Vessels

The interaction between pressure and resistance is determined by whether blood vessels are arranged in series or in parallel. In vessels such as arteries, arterioles, capillaries, venules, and veins, which are collectively arranged in series, flow through each vessel at any given pressure is the same; therefore, the total resistance is equal to the sum of the resistances (R) of each vessel ($R_1 + R_2 + R_3$).

In segments of the circulation where blood vessels branch extensively to form parallel circuits, as in those that supply blood to the many organs and tissues of the body, greater amounts of blood will flow through parallel vessels than through any of the individual vessels. Thus, for any given pressure, the total resistance to blood flow will be equal to the sum of the reciprocals of the individual resistances ($1/R_1 + 1/R_2 + 1/R_3$).

Velocity, Cross-Sectional Area, and Flow

In addition to the amount of blood flowing through a given organ or tissue, the rate or velocity at which the blood is moving is also important. *Flow* is a volume measurement (milliliters [mL] per second [sec]) that is determined by the cross-sectional area of a vessel and the velocity of flow. *Velocity* is a distance measurement; it refers to the speed or linear movement per unit time of blood as it flows through a vessel. When the flow through a given segment of the circulatory system is constant—as it must be for continuous flow—the velocity is inversely proportional to the cross-sectional area of the vessel (i.e., the smaller the cross-sectional area, the greater is the velocity of flow).

The linear velocity of blood flow in the circulatory system varies widely from 30 to 35 cm/second in the aorta to 0.2 to 0.3 mm/second in the capillaries. This is because even though each individual capillary is very small, the total cross-sectional area of all the systemic capillaries greatly exceeds the cross-sectional area of other parts of the circulation. As a result of this large surface area, the slower movement of blood allows ample time for exchange of nutrients, gases, and metabolites between the tissues and the blood.

Laminar Versus Turbulent Flow

Ideally, blood flow should be *laminar* or *streamlined,* with the blood components arranged in layers so that the plasma is adjacent to the smooth, slippery endothelial lining of the blood vessel, and the blood elements, including the platelets, are in the center or *axis* of the bloodstream. This arrangement reduces friction by allowing the blood layers to slide smoothly over one another, with the axial layer having the most rapid rate of flow.

Under certain conditions, however, blood flow can switch from laminar to turbulent. In *turbulent flow* the laminar stream is disrupted and the flow becomes mixed, moving both radially (crosswise) and axially (lengthwise). Turbulent flow can be caused by a number of factors, including high velocity of flow, change in vessel diameter, and low blood viscosity. The tendency for turbulence to occur is increased in direct proportion to the velocity of flow.

Because energy is used in propelling blood both radially and axially, more energy (pressure) is required to drive turbulent flow than laminar flow. Turbulence is often accompanied by vibrations of the blood and surrounding cardiovascular structures. Some of these vibrations are in the audible range and can be heard using a stethoscope. For example, a heart murmur results from turbulent flow through a diseased heart valve.

Wall Tension, Radius, and Pressure

In a blood vessel, *wall tension* is the force in the vessel wall that opposes the distending pressure inside the vessel. French astronomer and mathematician Pierre de Laplace described the relationship between wall tension, pressure, and the radius of a vessel or sphere more than 200 years ago. This relationship, which has come to be known as the *law of Laplace,* can be expressed by the Equation P = T/r, in which T is the wall tension, P is the intraluminal pressure or pressure within the vessel, and r is the vessel radius (Fig. 17-3A). Accordingly, the internal pressure expands the vessel until it is exactly balanced by the tension in the vessel wall. The smaller the radius, the greater is the pressure needed to balance the wall tension. The law of Laplace can also be used to express the effect of the vessel radius on wall tension (T = P × r). This correlation can be compared with a partially inflated balloon (Fig. 17-3B). Because the pressure is equal throughout, the tension in the part of the balloon with the smaller radius is less than the tension in the section with the larger radius. The same holds true for an arterial aneurysm in which the tension and risk of rupture increase as the aneurysm grows in size (see Chapter 18).

The law of Laplace was later expanded to include wall thickness (T = P × r/wall thickness). Wall tension is inversely related to wall thickness, such that the thicker the vessel wall, the lower the tension, and vice versa. In hypertension, for example, arterial vessel walls hypertrophy and become thicker, thereby reducing the tension and minimizing wall stress. The law of Laplace can also be applied to the pressure required to maintain the patency of small blood vessels. Provided that the thickness of a vessel wall remains constant, it takes more pressure to overcome wall tension and keep a vessel open as its radius decreases in size. The *critical closing pressure* refers to the point at which vessels collapse so that blood can no longer flow through them. In circulatory shock, for example, there is a decrease in blood volume and vessel radii, along with a drop in blood pressure. As a result, many of the small vessels collapse as the blood pressure drops to the point where it can no longer overcome the wall tension. The collapse of peripheral veins often makes it difficult to insert venous lines that are needed for fluid and blood replacement.

Vascular Distensibility

Distensibility refers to the ability of a blood vessel to be stretched and accommodate an increased volume of blood. It is normally expressed as the fractional increase in volume for each millimeter of mercury (mm Hg) increase in pressure. *Vascular compliance* or *capacitance* refers to the *total quantity* of blood that can be stored in a given portion of the circulation for each millimeter of mercury rise in pressure. Both compliance and capacitance can be used to as a measure of the distensibility or flexibility of a blood vessel. The most distensible of all vessels are the veins, which can increase their volume with only slight changes in pressure, allowing them to function as a reservoir for storing large quantities of blood that can be returned to the circulation when it is needed. Although arteries have a thicker muscular wall than veins, their distensibility allows them to store some of the blood that is ejected from the heart during systole, providing for continuous flow through the capillaries as the heart relaxes during diastole.

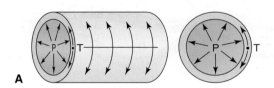

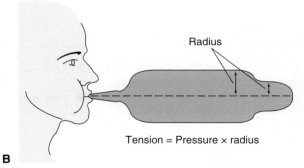

Tension = Pressure × radius

FIGURE 17-3. The law of Laplace relates pressure (P), tension (T), and radius (r) to a cylindrical blood vessel. **(A)** The pressure expanding the vessel is equal to the wall tension divided by the vessel radius. **(B)** Effect of the radius on tension in a cylindrical balloon. In a balloon, the tension in the wall is proportional to the radius because the pressure is the same everywhere inside the balloon. The tension is lower in the portion of the balloon with the smaller radius. (From Rhoades RA, Tanner GA. *Medical Physiology.* Boston, MA: Little, Brown; 1996:627.)

SUMMARY CONCEPTS

■ Blood flow is determined largely by the pressure difference between the two ends of a vessel or group of vessels and the resistance that the blood must overcome as it moves through the vessel or vessels. The resistance or opposition to blood flow, which is directly related to the viscosity of the blood as determined by the percentage of red blood cells and inversely related to the fourth power of the vessel radius, increases as the viscosity of the blood increases and decreases as the radius of a vessel increases and vice versa.

■ The relationship between the wall tension of a vessel, its intraluminal pressure, and its radius can be described using the law of Laplace (wall tension = pressure × radius). Thus, at any given

(*text continues on page 382*)

UNDERSTANDING → Hemodynamics of

The term *hemodynamics* is used to describe factors such as (1) pressure and resistance, (2) vessel radius, (3) cross-sectional area and velocity of flow, and (4) laminar versus turbulent flow that affect blood flow through the blood vessels in the body.

① Pressure, Resistance, and Flow. The flow of fluid through a tube, such as blood through a blood vessel, is directly related to a pressure difference ($P_1 - P_2$) between the two ends of the tube and inversely proportional to the resistance (R) that the fluid encounters as it moves through the tube.

The resistance to flow, in peripheral resistance units (PRUs), is determined by the blood viscosity, vessel radius, and whether the vessels are aligned in series or in parallel. In vessels aligned in series, blood travels sequentially from one vessel to another such that the resistance becomes additive (e.g., 2 + 2 + 2 = 6 PRU). In vessels aligned in parallel, such as capillaries, the blood is not confined to a single channel but can travel through each of several parallel channels such that the resistance becomes the reciprocal of the total resistance (i.e., 1/R). As a result, there is no loss of pressure, and the total resistance (e.g., 1/2 + 1/2 + 1/2 = 3/2 PRU) is less than the resistance of any of the channels.

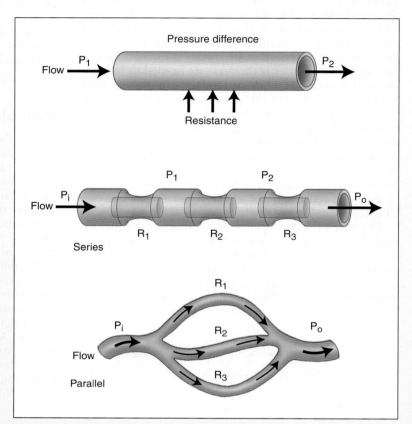

Pi, pressure in; Po, pressure out.

② Vessel Radius. In addition to pressure and resistance, the rate of blood flow through a vessel is affected by the fourth power of its radius (the radius multiplied by itself four times). Thus, blood flow in vessel B with a radius of 2 mm will be 16 times greater than in vessel A with a radius of 1 mm.

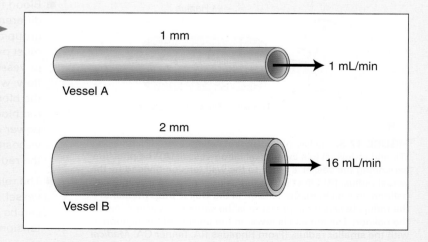

Blood Flow

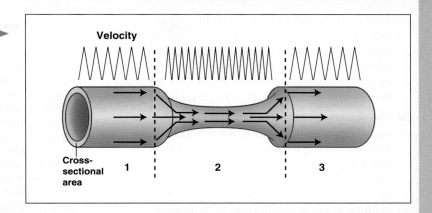

3

Cross-Sectional Area and Velocity of Flow. The velocity or rate of forward movement of the blood is affected by the cross-sectional area of a blood vessel. As the cross-sectional area of a vessel increases (Sections 1 and 3), blood must flow laterally as well as forward to fill the increased area. As a result, the mean forward velocity decreases. In contrast, when the cross-sectional area is decreased (Section 2), the lateral flow decreases and the mean forward velocity is increased.

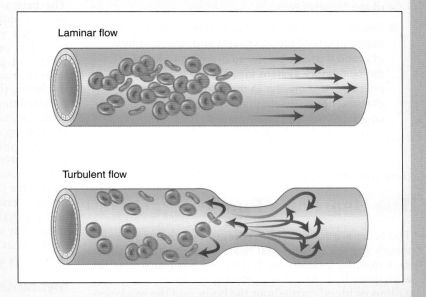

4

Laminar and Turbulent Flow. Blood flow is normally laminar, with platelets and blood cells remaining in the center or axis of the bloodstream. Laminar blood flow can be described as layered flow in which a thin layer of plasma adheres to the vessel wall, while the inner layers of blood cells and platelets shear against this motionless layer. This allows each layer to move at a slightly faster velocity, with the greatest velocity occurring in the central part of the bloodstream.

Turbulent blood flow is flow in which the blood elements do not remain confined to a definite lamina or layer, but develop vortices (i.e., a whirlpool effect) that push blood cells and platelets against the wall of the vessel. More pressure is required to force a given flow of blood through the same vessel (or heart valve) when the flow is turbulent rather than laminar. Turbulence can result from an increase in velocity of flow, a decrease in vessel diameter, or low blood viscosity. Turbulence is usually accompanied by vibrations of the fluid and surrounding structures. Some of these vibrations in the cardiovascular system are in the audible frequency range and may be detected as murmurs or bruits.

SUMMARY CONCEPTS *(continued)*

intraluminal pressure, wall tension becomes greater as the radius of a vessel increases; and more pressure will be needed to overcome the contractile tension in a vessel wall as the diameter decreases. Wall tension is also affected by wall thickness, increasing as the wall becomes thinner and decreasing as it becomes thicker.

■ The velocity or speed of blood flow through a vessel is greatly affected by its cross-sectional area, increasing as the cross-sectional area decreases and decreasing as it increases. High velocity can create turbulent blood flow, in which the blood moves crosswise and lengthwise in blood vessels; as opposed to laminar or layered flow, in which the blood components are arranged so that the plasma is adjacent to the smooth surface of the inner lining of the vessel wall and the blood components are in the center of the bloodstream.

■ Vascular compliance or capacitance reflects the distensibility of blood vessels and total quantity of blood that can be stored in a given part of the circulatory system for a given change in pressure. It is greater in the thin-walled vessels of the venous system than in the thick-walled vessels of the arterial system.

(text continued from page 379)

The Heart as a Pump

The heart is a four-chambered muscular pump approximately the size of a fist that beats an average of 70 times each minute, 24 hours each day, 365 days each year for a lifetime. In 1 day, this pump moves more than 1800 gallons of blood throughout the body, and the work performed by the heart over a lifetime would lift 30 tons to a height of 30,000 ft.

Functional Anatomy of the Heart

The heart, which is enclosed in a loose-fitting sac called the *pericardium*, is located between the lungs in the mediastinal space of the intrathoracic cavity. It is located posterior to the sternum and anterior to the vertebral column and extends about 5 inches from the second to fifth vertebrae (Fig. 17-4A). The heart is suspended by the great vessels, with its broader side (i.e., base) facing upward and its tip (i.e., apex) pointing downward, forward, and to the left. The heart is positioned obliquely, so that the right side of the heart is almost fully in front of the left side of the heart, with only a small portion of the lat-

eral left ventricle on the frontal plane of the heart (Fig. 17-4B). When the hand is placed on the thorax, the main impact of the heart's contraction is felt against the chest wall at a point between the fifth and sixth ribs, a little below the nipple and approximately 3 inches to the left of the midline. This is called the *point of maximum impulse*.

The wall of the heart is composed of an outer epicardium, which lines the pericardial cavity; the myocardium or muscle layer; and the smooth endocardium, which lines the chambers of the heart (Fig. 17-5). A fibrous skeleton separates the atria and ventricles and forms a rigid support for attachment of the heart valves. The interatrial and interventricular septa divide the heart into a right and a left pump, each composed of two muscular chambers: a thin-walled atrium, which serves as a reservoir for blood coming into the heart, and a thick-walled ventricle, which pumps blood out of the heart. The increased thickness of the left ventricular wall compared to the right ventricle (Fig. 17-4C) results from the additional work this ventricle is required to perform.

Pericardium

The pericardium forms a fibrous covering around the heart, holding it in a fixed position in the thorax and providing physical protection and a barrier to infection. The pericardium consists of a tough outer fibrous layer and a thin inner serous layer. The outer fibrous layer is attached to the great vessels that enter and leave the heart, the sternum, and the diaphragm. The fibrous pericardium is highly resistant to distention; it prevents acute dilatation of the heart chambers and exerts a restraining effect on the left ventricle. The inner serous layer consists of a visceral layer and a parietal layer. The visceral layer, also known as the visceral pericardium or *epicardium*, covers the entire heart and great vessels and then folds over to form the parietal layer that lines the fibrous pericardium (see Fig. 17-5). Between the visceral and parietal layers is the *pericardial cavity*, a potential space that contains 30 to 50 mL of serous fluid. This fluid acts as a lubricant to minimize friction between the two layers as the heart contracts and relaxes.

Myocardium

The myocardium, or muscular portion of the heart, forms the walls of the atria and ventricles. Cardiac muscle cells, like skeletal muscle, are striated and composed of *sarcomeres* that contain actin and myosin filaments (see Chapter 1). They are smaller and more compact than skeletal muscle cells and contain many large mitochondria, reflecting their continuous energy needs.

The contractile properties of cardiac muscle are similar to those of skeletal muscle, except the contractions are involuntary and the duration of contraction is much longer. Unlike the orderly longitudinal arrangement of skeletal muscle fibers, cardiac muscle cells are arranged as an interconnecting latticework, with their fibers dividing, recombining, and then dividing again (Fig. 17-6A). The fibers are separated from neighboring cardiac muscle cells by dense structures called *intercalated disks*. The intercalated disks, which are unique to cardiac muscle,

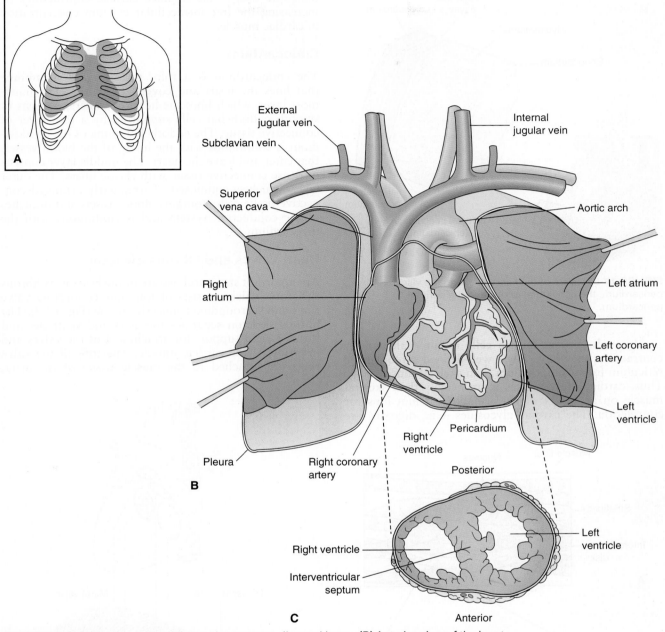

FIGURE 17-4. (A) The heart in relation to the sternum, ribs, and lungs. **(B)** Anterior view of the heart and great vessels (note that the lungs, which normally fold over part of the heart's anterior, have been pulled back). **(C)** Cross-section of the heart showing the increased thickness of the left ventricle compared to the right.

contain gap junctions that serve as low-resistance pathways for passage of ions and electrical impulses from one cardiac cell to another (Fig. 17-6B). Thus, the myocardium behaves as a single unit, or *syncytium*, rather than as a group of isolated units, as does skeletal muscle. When one myocardial cell becomes excited, the impulse travels rapidly so the heart can beat as a unit.

As in skeletal muscle, cardiac muscle cells contain actin and myosin filaments, which interact and slide along one another during muscle contraction.

A number of important proteins regulate the interaction between the actin and myosin filaments. These include the tropomyosin and the troponin complex, which consists of three subunits (troponin T, troponin I, and troponin C) that regulate calcium-mediated muscle contraction (see Chapter 1, Fig. 1-19). In clinical practice, the serum levels of specific cardiac forms of troponin T and troponin I, released from injured heart muscle, are used in the diagnosis of myocardial infarction (see Chapter 19).

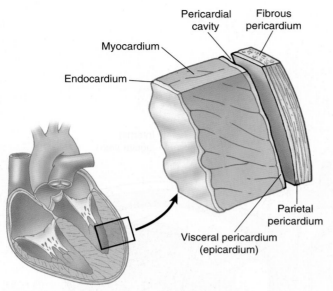

FIGURE 17-5. Layers of the heart, showing the visceral pericardium, the pericardial cavity, and the parietal pericardium.

Although cardiac muscle cells require calcium for contraction, they have a less well-defined sarcoplasmic reticulum for storing calcium than skeletal muscle cells. Thus, cardiac muscle relies more heavily than skeletal muscle on an influx of extracellular calcium ions for contraction. The cardiac glycosides (e.g., digoxin) are inotropic drugs that enhance cardiac contractility by increasing the free intracellular calcium concentration in cardiac muscle.

Endocardium

The endocardium is a thin, three-layered membrane that lines the heart and covers the valves. The innermost layer, which lines the heart chambers, consists of smooth endothelial cells supported by a thin layer of connective tissue. The endothelial lining of the endocardium is continuous with the lining of the blood vessels that enter and leave the heart. The middle layer consists of dense connective tissue with elastic fibers. The outer layer, which is composed of irregularly arranged connective tissue cells, contains blood vessels and branches of the conduction system and is continuous with the myocardium.

Heart Valves and Fibrous Skeleton

An important structural feature of the heart is its fibrous skeleton, which consists of four interconnecting valve rings and surrounding connective tissue (Fig. 17-7). The fibrous skeleton separates the atria and ventricles and forms a rigid support for attachment of the valves and insertion of the cardiac muscle. The tops of the valve rings are attached to the muscle tissue of the atria,

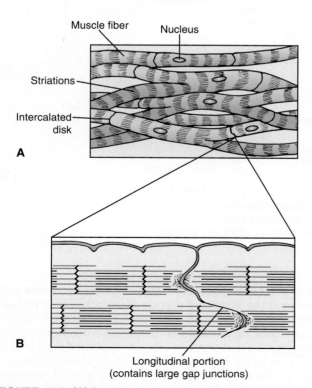

FIGURE 17-6. (A) Cardiac muscle fibers showing their branching structure. **(B)** Area indicated where cell junctions lie in the intercalated disks.

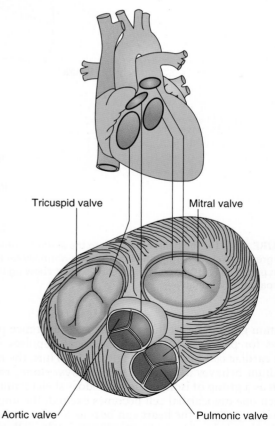

FIGURE 17-7. Fibrous skeleton of the heart, which forms the four interconnecting valve rings and support for attachment of the valves and insertion of cardiac muscle.

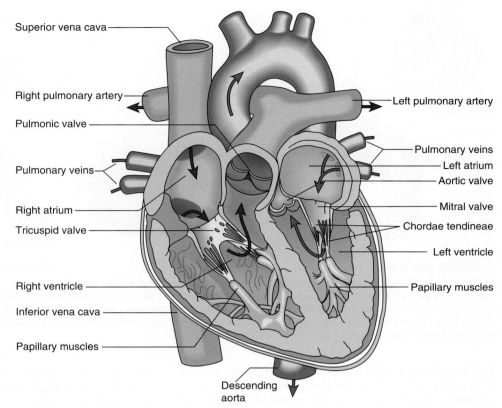

Superior vena cava

Right pulmonary artery

Pulmonic valve

Pulmonary veins

Right atrium

Tricuspid valve

Right ventricle

Inferior vena cava

Papillary muscles

Left pulmonary artery

Pulmonary veins
Left atrium
Aortic valve

Mitral valve

Chordae tendineae

Left ventricle

Papillary muscles

Descending aorta

FIGURE 17-8. Valvular structures of the heart. The atrioventricular valves are in an open position, and the semilunar valves are closed. There are no valves to control the flow of blood at the inflow channels (i.e., vena cava and pulmonary veins) to the heart.

pulmonary trunks, and aorta. The bottoms are attached to the ventricular walls. For the heart to function effectively, blood must flow in one direction only, moving forward through the chambers of the right heart to the lungs and then through the chambers of the left heart to the systemic circulation. This unidirectional flow is provided by the heart's paired atrioventricular (i.e., tricuspid and mitral) valves and two semilunar (i.e., pulmonic and aortic) valves (Fig. 17-8).

The atrioventricular (AV) valves control the flow of blood between the atria and the ventricles (Fig. 17-9). The thin edges of the AV valves form cusps, two on the left side of the heart (i.e., *bicuspid* or *mitral valve*) and three on the right side (i.e., *tricuspid valve*). The AV valves are supported by the papillary muscles, which project from the wall of the ventricles, and the chordae tendineae, which attach to the valve. Contraction of the papillary muscles at the onset of systole ensures closure by producing tension on the leaflets of the AV valves before the full force of ventricular contraction pushes against them. The chordae tendineae are cordlike structures that support the AV valves and prevent them from everting into the atria during systole.

The *aortic* and *pulmonic* valves control the movement of blood out of the ventricles (Fig. 17-10). The pulmonic valve, which is located between the right ventricle and the pulmonary artery, controls the flow of blood into the pulmonary circulation; and the aortic valve, located between the left ventricle and the aorta, controls the flow of blood into the systemic circulation. Because their flaps are shaped like half-moons, they are often referred to as

the *semilunar* valves (Fig. 17-10B). The semilunar valves have three cuplike cusps that are attached to the valve rings. These cuplike structures collect the *retrograde*, or backward, flow of blood that occurs toward the end of systole, enhancing closure. For the development of a perfect seal along the free edges of the semilunar valves, each valve cusp must have a triangular shape, which is

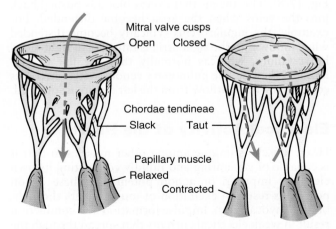

Mitral valve cusps
Open   Closed

Chordae tendineae
Slack   Taut

Papillary muscle
Relaxed
Contracted

A Mitral valve open   **B** Mitral valve closed

FIGURE 17-9. The mitral atrioventricular valve showing the papillary muscles and chordae tendineae. **(A)** The open mitral valve with relaxed papillary muscles and slack chordae tendineae. **(B)** The closed mitral valve with contracted papillary muscles and taut chordae tendineae that prevent the valve cusps from everting into the atria.

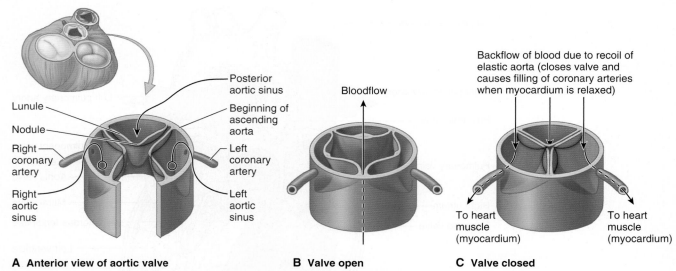

Posterior aortic sinus
Lunule
Nodule
Right coronary artery
Beginning of ascending aorta
Left coronary artery
Right aortic sinus
Left aortic sinus

A Anterior view of aortic valve

Bloodflow

B Valve open

Backflow of blood due to recoil of elastic aorta (closes valve and causes filling of coronary arteries when myocardium is relaxed)

To heart muscle (myocardium)
To heart muscle (myocardium)

C Valve closed

FIGURE 17-10. Aortic valve, aortic sinuses, and coronary arteries. **(A)** Like the pulmonary valve, the aortic valve has three semilunar cusps: right, posterior, and left. **(B)** Blood ejected from the left ventricle forces the cusps open. **(C)** When the valve closes, the valve edges and nodules meet in the center. (From Moore KL, Dalley AF, Agur AMR. *Clinically Oriented Anatomy.* 6th ed. Philadelphia, PA: Wolters Kluwer Health | Lippincott Williams & Wilkins; 2010:144.)

facilitated by a nodular thickening at the apex of each leaflet (Fig. 17-10C). Immediately behind each of the semilunar cusps, the walls the pulmonary trunk and aorta are slightly dilated, forming a sinus (Fig. 17-10A). In these sinuses, eddy currents develop that tend to keep the valve cusps away from the vessel wall. The opening for the right coronary artery is located in right aortic sinus, and the opening for the left coronary artery is located in left aortic sinus. Were it not for the presence of the sinuses and eddy currents, the coronary artery openings would be blocked by the valve cusps.

There are no valves at the atrial sites (i.e., venae cavae and pulmonary veins) where blood enters the heart (see Fig. 17-8). This means that excess blood is pushed back into the veins when the atria become distended. For example, the jugular veins typically become distended when inflow into the right atria is impeded in right-sided heart failure, whereas normally they are flat or collapsed. Likewise, the pulmonary venous system becomes congested when outflow from the left atrium is impeded.

Electrical Activity of the Heart

Heart muscle is unique among other muscles in that it is capable of generating and rapidly conducting its own electrical impulses or action potentials. These action potentials result in excitation of muscle fibers throughout the myocardium. Impulse formation and conduction result in weak electrical currents that spread through the entire body.

Cardiac Conduction System

In certain areas of the heart, the myocardial cells have been modified to form the specialized cells of the conduction system (Fig. 17-11). Although most myocardial cells are capable of initiating and conducting impulses, it is this specialized conduction system that maintains the pumping efficiency of the heart. Specialized pacemaker cells generate impulses at a faster rate than other myocardial cells, and the cells of the conduction system transmit impulses at a faster rate than other myocardial cells. Because of these properties, the conduction system normally controls the rhythm of the heart.

The conduction system consists of (1) the sinoatrial (SA) node, where the rhythmic impulse is generated; (2) the internodal pathways, which conduct the impulse from the SA node to the AV node; (3) the AV node, in which the impulse from the atria is delayed before passing to the ventricles; (4) the AV bundle, which conducts the impulse from the atria to the ventricles; and the (5) left and right bundles of the Purkinje system, which conduct the impulses to all parts of the ventricles.

The SA node has the fastest intrinsic rate of firing (60 to 100 beats per minute) and normally functions as the pacemaker of the heart. From the SA node, the impulse travels radially throughout the right atrium, ultimately reaching the AV node. A special pathway, the anterior interatrial pathway, conducts the impulse to the left atrium.

The heart essentially has two conduction systems: one that controls atrial activity and one that controls ventricular activity. The AV node connects the two systems and normally provides for a one-way conduction between the atria and ventricles. Within the AV node, atrial fibers connect with very small junctional fibers in the node itself. Because of these connections, the zone surrounding and including the AV node and the adjacent atrial and ventricular conduction pathways is often referred to as the *AV junctional area.* The velocity of conduction through these fibers is very slow (approximately one-half that of normal cardiac muscle), which greatly

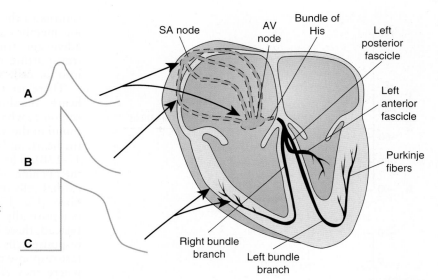

FIGURE 17-11. Conduction system of the heart and action potentials. **(A)** Action potential of sinoatrial (SA) and atrioventricular (AV) nodes. **(B)** Atrial muscle action potential. **(C)** Action potential of ventricular muscle and Purkinje fibers.

delays impulse transmission. A further delay occurs as the impulse travels through the transitional fibers and into the AV bundle, also known as the *bundle of His*. This delay provides a mechanical advantage whereby the atria can complete their ejection of blood before ventricular contraction begins. Under normal circumstances, the AV node provides the only connection between the atrial and ventricular conduction systems. The atria and ventricles would beat independently of each other if the transmission of impulses through the AV node were blocked.

The *Purkinje system*, which supplies the ventricles, has large specialized fibers that allow for rapid conduction and almost instantaneous excitation of both the right and left ventricles. This rapid rate of conduction is necessary for the swift and efficient ejection of blood from the heart. Fibers of the Purkinje system originate in the AV node and then travel downward in the AV bundle into the ventricular septum, where they divide to form the *right* and *left bundle branches* that lie beneath the endocardium on the two respective sides of the ventricular septum. The main trunk of the left bundle branch extends for approximately 1 to 2 cm before fanning out as it enters the septal area and divides further into two segments: the *left posterior* and *anterior fascicles*.

The AV nodal fibers, when not stimulated, discharge at an intrinsic rate of 45 to 50 times a minute, and the Purkinje fibers discharge at 15 to 40 times per minute. Although the AV node and Purkinje system have the ability to control the rhythm of the heart, they do not normally do so because the discharge rate of the SA node is considerably faster. Each time the SA node discharges, its impulses are conducted into the AV nodal and Purkinje fibers, causing them to fire. Should the SA node fail to discharge, the AV node can assume the pacemaker function of the heart, and the Purkinje system can assume the pacemaker function of the ventricles should the AV junction fail to conduct impulses from the atria to the ventricles. Under these circumstances, the heart rate reflects the intrinsic firing rate of the prevailing structures.

Action Potentials

An action potential represents the sequential change in electrical potential that occurs across a cell membrane when excitation occurs (see Chapter 1, "Understanding Membrane Potentials"). Action potentials can be divided into three parts: the *resting* or *unexcited* state during which the membrane is polarized (positive on the outside and negative on the inside of the membrane), *depolarization* or change in the direction of polarity (positive on the inside and negative on the outside), and *repolarization* or reestablishment of polarity of the resting membrane potential. The sodium (Na^+), potassium (K^+), and calcium (Ca^{++}) ions are the major electrical charge carriers in cardiac muscle cells. Disorders of the ion channels along with disruption in the flow of these current-carrying ions are increasingly being linked to the generation of cardiac arrhythmias and conduction disorders.

The action potential of cardiac muscle is divided into five phases: *phase 0*—the upstroke or rapid depolarization; *phase 1*—early repolarization; *phase 2*—the plateau; *phase 3*—rapid repolarization; and *phase 4*—the resting membrane potential (Fig. 17-12A). Cardiac muscle has three types of membrane ion channels that contribute to the voltage changes that occur during these phases of the action potential. They are the (1) fast sodium (Na^+) channels, (2) slow calcium (Ca^{++}) channels, and (3) potassium (K^+) channels.

During *phase 0* in atrial and ventricular muscle and in the Purkinje conduction system, opening of the fast Na^+ channels for a few ten-thousandths of a second is responsible for the spikelike onset of the action potential. The point at which the Na^+ gates open is called the *depolarization threshold*. When the cell has reached this threshold, a rapid influx of Na^+ to the interior of the cell membrane causes the membrane potential to shift from a resting membrane potential of approximately –90 mV to +20 mV.

Phase 1 occurs at the peak of the action potential and signifies inactivation of the fast Na^+ channels with an

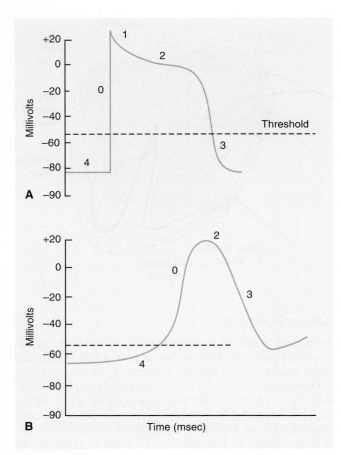

FIGURE 17-12. Phases in an action potential recorded from **(A)** a fast response in a cardiac muscle cell and **(B)** a slow response recorded in the sinoatrial and atrioventricular nodes. The phases of the action potential are identified by numbers: phase 4, resting membrane potential; phase 0, depolarization; phase 1, brief period of repolarization; phase 2, plateau; phase 3, repolarization. The slow response is characterized by a slow, spontaneous rise in the phase 4 membrane potential to threshold levels; it has a lesser amplitude and shorter duration than the fast response. Increased automaticity **(B)** occurs when the rate of phase 4 depolarization is increased.

abrupt decrease in Na$^+$ permeability. *Phase 2* represents the plateau of the action potential. It is caused primarily by the slower opening of the Ca^{++} channels, which lasts for a few tenths of a second. Calcium ions entering the muscle during this phase of the action potential play a key role in the contractile process of the cardiac muscle fibers. These unique features of the phase 2 plateau cause the action potential of cardiac muscle to last 3 to 15 times longer than that of skeletal muscle and cause a corresponding increased period of contraction.

Phase 3 reflects the final rapid repolarization phase and begins with the downslope of the action potential. During the phase 3 repolarization period, the slow Ca^{++} channels close and the influx of Ca^{++} and Na$^+$ cease. There is a sharp rise in K$^+$ permeability, contributing to the rapid outward movement of K$^+$ and reestablishment of the resting membrane potential (-90 mV). At the conclusion of phase 3, the distribution of Na$^+$ and K$^+$

returns to the normal resting state. *Phase 4* is the resting membrane potential. During phase 4, the Na$^+$–K$^+$ adenosine triphosphate (ATPase) pump is activated, transporting Na$^+$ out of the cell and moving K$^+$ back into the cell.

There are two main types of action potentials in the heart—the slow response and the fast response. The *slow response,* which is initiated by the slow Ca^{++} channels, is found in the SA node, which is the natural pacemaker of the heart, and the conduction fibers of the AV node (Fig. 17-12B). The *fast response,* which is characterized by the opening of the fast Na$^+$ channels, occurs in the myocardial cells of the atria, the ventricles, and the Purkinje fibers (Fig. 17-12A). The fast-response cardiac cells do not normally initiate cardiac muscle action potentials. Instead, these impulses originate in the specialized slow-response cells of the SA node and are conducted to the fast-response myocardial cells in the atria and ventricles, where they effect a change in membrane potential to the threshold level. On reaching threshold, the voltage-dependent Na$^+$ channels open to initiate the rapid upstroke of the phase 1 action potential. The amplitude and rate of rise in the action potential during phase 1 are important to the conduction velocity of the fast response.

The hallmark of the pacemaker cells in the SA and AV nodes is a spontaneous phase 4 depolarization. The membrane permeability of these cells allows a slow inward leak of current to occur through the slow channels during phase 4. This leak continues until the threshold for firing is reached, at which point the cell spontaneously depolarizes. The rate of pacemaker cell discharge varies with the resting membrane potential and the slope of phase 4 depolarization (Fig. 17-12B). The catecholamines, the sympathetic nervous system neurotransmitters epinephrine and norepinephrine, increase the heart rate by increasing the slope or rate of phase 4 depolarization. Acetylcholine, the parasympathetic neurotransmitter released during vagal stimulation of the heart, slows the heart rate by decreasing the slope of phase 4.

Absolute and Relative Refractory Periods

There is a period in the action potential curve during which no stimuli can generate another action potential (Fig. 17-13). This period, which is known as the *absolute refractory period,* includes phases 0, 1, 2, and part of phase 3. During this time, the cell cannot depolarize again under any circumstances. In skeletal muscle, the refractory period is very short compared with the duration of muscle contraction such that a second contraction can be initiated before the first is over, resulting in a summated tetanized contraction. In cardiac muscle, the absolute refractory period is almost as long as the contraction and a second contraction cannot be stimulated until the first is over. The longer length of the absolute refractory period of cardiac muscle is important in maintaining the alternating contraction and relaxation that are essential to the pumping action of the heart and for the prevention of fatal arrhythmias. When repolarization has returned the membrane potential to a level below

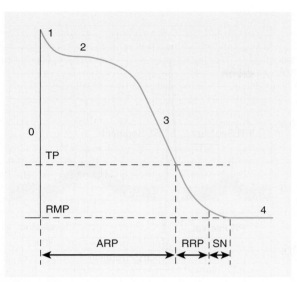

FIGURE 17-13. Diagram of an action potential of a ventricular muscle cell, showing the threshold potential (TP), resting membrane potential (RMP), absolute refractory period (ARP), relative refractory period (RRP), and supernormal (SN) period.

the threshold potential, but not to the resting membrane potential, the cell is capable of responding to a greater than normal stimulus. This part of the action potential is referred to as the *relative refractory period*. After the relative refractory period there is a short period, called the *supernormal excitatory period,* during which a weak stimulus can evoke a response. It is during this period that many cardiac arrhythmias develop.

Arrhythmias and Conduction Disorders

Arrhythmias represent disorders of cardiac rhythm. Cardiac arrhythmias are commonly divided into two categories: supraventricular and ventricular arrhythmias. The supraventricular arrhythmias include those that originate in the SA node, atria, AV node, and junctional tissues. The ventricular arrhythmias include those that originate in the ventricular conduction system and ventricular muscle. Because the ventricles are the pumping chambers of the heart, ventricular arrhythmias (e.g., ventricular tachycardia and fibrillation) are the most serious in terms of immediate life-threatening events.

Conduction disorders disrupt the flow of impulses through the conduction system of the heart. *Heart block* occurs when the conduction of impulses is blocked, often in AV nodal fibers. Under normal conditions, the AV node provides the only connection for transmission of impulses between the atrial and ventricular conduction systems; in complete heart block, the atria and ventricles beat independently of each other. The most serious effect of some forms of AV block is a slowing of heart rate to the extent that circulation to the brain is compromised.

An *ectopic pacemaker* is an excitable focus outside the normally functioning SA node. A *premature ventricular complex* (PVC) occurs when an ectopic ventricular pacemaker initiates a beat. The occurrence of frequent

PVCs in the diseased heart predisposes to the development of other more serious arrhythmias, including ventricular tachycardia and ventricular fibrillation.

Fibrillation is the result of disorganized current flow within the atria (atrial fibrillation) or ventricle (ventricular fibrillation). Fibrillation interrupts the normal contraction of the atria or ventricles. In ventricular fibrillation, the ventricles quiver but do not contract. Thus, there is no cardiac output, and there are no palpable or audible pulses. Ventricular fibrillation is a fatal event unless treated with immediate defibrillation.

Electrocardiography

The electrocardiogram (ECG) is a recording of the electrical activity of the heart. The electrical currents generated by the heart spread through the body to the skin, where they can be sensed by appropriately placed electrodes, amplified, and viewed on an oscilloscope or chart recorder. Figure 17-14 depicts the electrical activity of the conduction system on an ECG tracing. The deflection points of an ECG are designated by the letters P, Q, R, S, and T. Sinoatrial node depolarization does not have sufficient current to be revealed on the ECG. The P wave represents atrial depolarization; the QRS comples (i.e., beginning of the Q wave to the end of the S wave), ventricular depolarization; and the T wave, ventricular repolarization. Atrial repolarization occurs during ventricular depolarization and is hidden in the QRS complex.

On the horizontal axis of the ECG, the unit of measurement is time in seconds, and on the vertical axis the unit of measurement is the amplitude of the impulse in millivolts (mV). The vertical lines are time calibration lines, with five 0.04-second vertical lines representing 0.20 seconds (see Fig. 17-14). The horizontal lines are arranged so that five lines of upward or downward deflection in the ECG tracing represent 0.50 mV.

The ECG records the potential difference in charge between two electrodes as the depolarization and repolarization waves move through the heart and are conducted to the skin surface. The shape of the tracing is determined by the direction in which the impulse spreads through the heart muscle in relation to electrode placement. A depolarization wave that moves toward the recording electrode registers as a positive, or upward, deflection. Conversely, if the impulse moves away from the recording electrode, the deflection is downward, or negative. When there is no flow of charge between electrodes, the potential is zero, and a straight line is recorded at the baseline of the chart.

Conventionally, 12 leads or electrodes are used for recording a diagnostic ECG, each providing a unique view of the electrical forces of the heart from a different position on the body's surface. Six limb leads view the electrical forces as they pass through the heart on the frontal or vertical plane. The electrodes for the limb leads are attached to the four extremities or representative areas on the body near the shoulders and lower chest or abdomen. Chest electrodes provide a view of the electrical forces as they pass through the heart on the

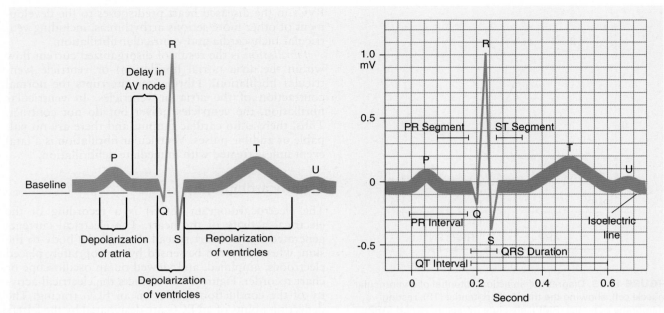

FIGURE 17-14. Diagram of the electrocardiogram (lead II) and representative depolarization and repolarization of the atria and ventricles. The P wave represents atrial depolarization, the QRS complex ventricular depolarization, and the T wave ventricular repolarization. Atrial repolarization occurs during ventricular depolarization and is hidden under the QRS complex. AV, atrioventricular.

horizontal plane. They are applied to different positions on the chest, including the right and left sternal borders and the left anterior surface. When indicated, additional electrodes may be applied to other areas of the body, such as the posterior or right anterior chest.

Cardiac Cycle

The term *cardiac cycle*, which is used to describe the rhythmic pumping action of the heart, is divided into two parts: *systole,* the period during which the ventricles are contracting, and *diastole,* the period during which the ventricles are relaxed and filling with blood. Simultaneous changes occur in atrial pressure, ventricular pressure, aortic or pulmonary artery pressure, ventricular volume, the ECG, and heart sounds that occur during the cardiac cycle (Fig. 17-15). Four heart sounds are usually generated by closure of the heart valves during the cardiac cycle, but only two (the first and second) are ordinarily heard through a stethoscope. The first heart sound is initiated at the onset of systole and reflects the closure of AV valves. The second heart sound occurs at the end of systole with abrupt closure of the semilunar valves.

Ventricular Systole and Diastole

Ventricular systole is divided into two periods: the isovolumetric (*iso,* meaning same) contraction period and the ejection period. The *isovolumetric contraction period,* which begins with the closure of the AV valves and occurrence of the first heart sound, heralds the onset of systole (see Fig. 17-15A). Immediately after closure of the AV valves, there is an additional 0.02- to 0.03-second period during

which the pulmonic and aortic valves remain closed. During this period, the ventricular volume remains the same while the ventricles contract, producing an abrupt increase in pressure. The ventricles continue to contract until left ventricular pressure is slightly higher than aortic pressure and right ventricular pressure is higher than pulmonary artery pressure. At this point, the aortic and pulmonic valves open, signaling the onset of the *ejection period.* Approximately 60% of the stroke volume is ejected during the first quarter of systole, and the remaining 40% is ejected during the next two quarters of systole. Little blood is ejected from the heart during the last quarter of systole, although the ventricles remain contracted. At the end of systole, the ventricles relax, causing a precipitous fall in intraventricular pressures. As this occurs, blood from the large arteries flows back toward the ventricles, causing the aortic and pulmonic valves to snap shut—an event that is marked by the second heart sound.

The aortic pressure reflects changes in the ejection of blood from the left ventricle. There is a rise in pressure and stretching of the elastic fibers in the aorta as blood is ejected into the aorta at the onset of the ejection period. The aortic pressure continues to rise and then begins to fall during the last quarter of systole as blood flows out of the aorta into the peripheral vessels. The incisura, or notch, in the aortic pressure tracing represents closure of the aortic valve. The aorta is highly elastic and as such stretches during systole to accommodate the blood that is being ejected from the left heart during systole. During diastole, recoil of the elastic fibers in the aorta serves to maintain the arterial pressure.

Diastole is marked by ventricular relaxation and filling. After closure of the semilunar valves, the ventricles continue to relax for another 0.03 to 0.06 second.

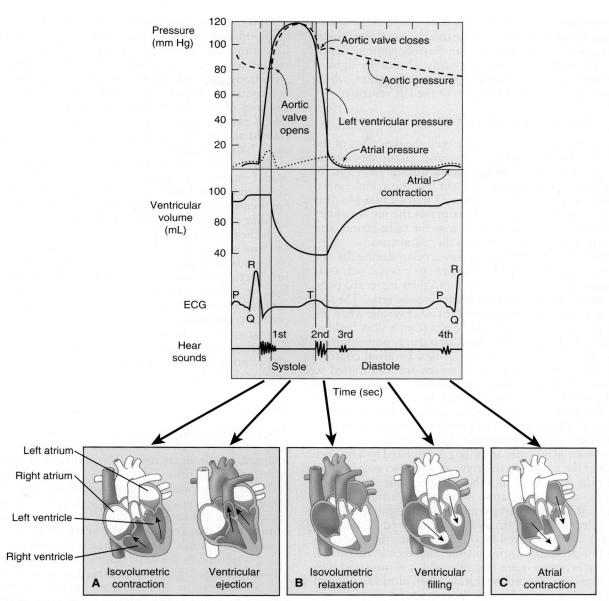

FIGURE 17-15. (*Top*) Events in the left side of the heart, showing changes in aortic pressure, left ventricular pressure, atrial pressure, left ventricular volume, the electrocardiogram (ECG), and heart sounds during the cardiac cycle. (*Bottom*) Position of the atrioventricular valves during (**A**) the isovolumetric contraction and ejection phases of ventricular systole, (**B**) the isovolumetric relaxation and ventricular filling phases during early diastole, and (**C**) atrial contraction.

During this time, which is called the *isovolumetric relaxation period,* ventricular volume remains the same but ventricular pressure drops until it becomes less than atrial pressure (see Fig. 17-15B). As this occurs, the AV valves open, and the blood that has been accumulating in the atria during systole flows into the ventricles. Most of ventricular filling occurs during the first third of diastole, which is called the *rapid filling period.* During the middle third of diastole, inflow into the ventricles is almost at a standstill. The last third of diastole is marked by atrial contraction, which gives an additional thrust to ventricular filling. When audible, the third heart sound is heard at the end of the rapid filling period

due to vibrations that are caused by the abrupt cessation of ventricular distention and by the deceleration of blood entering the ventricles. A third heart sound is sometimes heard in children with thin chest walls and in persons with a distended or noncompliant ventricle. A fourth heart sound, when present, occurs during the last third of diastole as the atria contract (see Fig. 17-15C).

During diastole, the ventricles increase their volume to approximately 120 mL (i.e., the *end-diastolic volume*), and at the end of systole, approximately 50 mL of blood (i.e., the *end-systolic volume*) remains in the ventricles. The difference between the end-diastolic and end-systolic volumes (approximately 70 mL) is called the *stroke volume.* The *ejection fraction,* which is the stroke volume divided by the end-diastolic volume, represents the fraction or percentage of the diastolic volume that is ejected from the heart during systole. One of the signs of heart failure is a decrease in the ejection fraction, which reflects the diminished function of the left ventricle.

Atrial Filling and Contraction

Because there are no valves between the junctions of the central veins (i.e., venae cavae and pulmonary veins) and the atria, atrial filling occurs during both systole and diastole. During normal quiet breathing, right atrial pressure usually varies between −2 and +2 mm Hg. It is this low atrial pressure that maintains the movement of blood from the systemic veins into the right atrium and from the pulmonary veins into the left atrium.

Three main atrial pressure waves occur during the cardiac cycle (see Fig. 17-15). The first, or *c wave,* occurs as the ventricles begin to contract and their increased pressure causes the AV valves to bulge into the atria. The second, or *v wave,* occurs toward the end of systole when the AV valves are still closed and results from a slow buildup of blood in the atria. The third, or *a wave,* occurs during the last part of diastole and is caused by atrial contraction. The right atrial pressure waves are transmitted to the internal jugular veins as pulsations. These pulsations can be observed visually and may be used to assess cardiac function. For example, exaggerated a waves occur when the volume of the right atrium is increased because of impaired emptying into the right ventricle.

Right atrial pressure and filling is regulated by a balance between the ability of the right ventricle to move blood out of the right heart and the pressures that move blood from the venous circulation into the right atrium (venous return). When the heart pumps strongly, right atrial pressure is decreased and atrial filling is enhanced. Right atrial pressure is also affected by changes in intrathoracic pressure. It is decreased during inspiration when intrathoracic pressure becomes more negative, and it is increased during coughing or forced expiration when intrathoracic and right atrial pressures become more positive.

Although the main function of the atria is to store blood as it enters the heart, these chambers also act as pumps that aid in ventricular filling. Atrial contraction occurs during the last third of diastole. Atrial contraction becomes more important during periods of increased activity when the diastolic filling time is decreased because of an increase in heart rate or when heart disease impairs ventricular filling. In these two situations, the cardiac output would fall drastically were it not for the action of the atria. It has been estimated that atrial contraction can contribute as much as 30% to cardiac reserve during periods of increased need, while having little or no effect on cardiac output during rest.

Regulation of Cardiac Performance

The efficiency and work of the heart as a pump often is measured in terms of *cardiac output* or the amount of blood the heart pumps each minute. The cardiac output (CO) is the product of the stroke volume (SV) or amount of blood that the heart ejects with each beat and the heart rate (HR) or number of times the heart beats each minute (i.e., CO = SV x HR). The cardiac output varies with body size and the metabolic needs of the tissues. It increases with physical activity and decreases during rest and sleep. The average cardiac output in normal adults ranges from 3.5 to 8.0 L/minute. In the highly trained athlete, this value can increase to levels as high as 32 L/minute during maximum exercise.

The *cardiac reserve* refers to the maximum percentage of increase in cardiac output that can be achieved above the normal resting level. The normal young adult has a cardiac reserve of approximately 300% to 400%. Cardiac performance is influenced by the work demands of the heart and the ability of the coronary circulation to meet its metabolic needs. The heart's ability to increase its output according to body needs mainly depends on four factors: the *preload* or ventricular filling, the *afterload* or resistance to ejection of blood from the heart, *cardiac contractility,* and the *heart rate.* Heart rate and cardiac contractility are strictly cardiac factors, meaning they originate in the heart, although they are controlled by various neural and humoral mechanisms. Preload and afterload, on the other hand, are mutually dependent on the behavior of both the heart and blood vessels.

Preload

The preload represents the volume work of the heart. It is called the *preload* because it is the work or load imposed on the heart before the contraction begins. It is the amount of blood that the heart must pump with each beat and represents the volume of blood stretching the ventricular muscle fibers at the end of diastole (i.e., end-diastolic volume). It is determined by the amount of the blood that remains in the ventricle at the end of systole (end-systolic volume) plus the amount of venous blood returning to the heart during diastole.

The increased force of contraction that accompanies an increase in ventricular end-diastolic volume is referred to as the *Frank-Starling mechanism* or Starling law of the heart (Fig. 17-16). The anatomic arrangement of the actin and myosin filaments in the myocardial muscle fibers is such that the tension or force of contraction is greatest when the muscle fibers are optimally stretched just before the heart begins to contract. The maximum force of contraction and cardiac output is achieved when the muscle fibers are stretched about two and one-half times their normal resting length. When the muscle fibers are stretched to this degree, there is optimal overlap of the actin and myosin filaments needed for maximal contraction.

The Frank-Starling mechanism allows the heart to adjust its pumping ability to accommodate various levels of venous return. Cardiac output is less when decreased filling causes excessive overlap of the actin and myosin filaments or when excessive filling causes the filaments to be pulled too far apart. The Frank-Starling mechanism also plays an important role in balancing the output of the two ventricles.

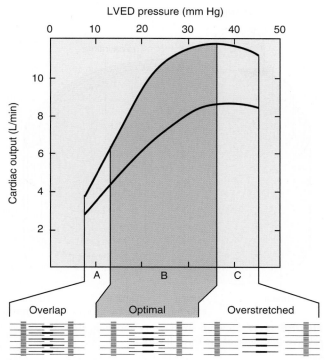

FIGURE 17-16. The Frank-Starling ventricular function curve. (*Lower curve*) The effect of diastolic filling and left ventricular end-diastolic (LVED) pressure on cardiac output by means of the Frank-Starling mechanism: **(A)** decreased filling with excessive overlap of actin and myosin filaments; **(B)** maximum force of contraction when the muscle fibers are stretched about two and one-half times their resting length; and **(C)** increased filling with overstretching of muscle fiber. Upper and lower curves represent the effect of cardiac contractility on cardiac output, with an increase in contractility (*upper curve*) producing and increase in cardiac output without a change in diastolic filling or LVED pressure.

Afterload

The afterload is the pressure or tension work of the heart. It is the pressure that the heart must generate to move blood into the aorta. It is called the *afterload* because it is the work presented to the heart after the contraction has commenced. The systemic arterial blood pressure is the main source of afterload work for the left heart, and the pulmonary arterial pressure is the main source of afterload work for the right heart. The afterload work of the left ventricle is also increased with narrowing (i.e., stenosis) of the aortic valve.

Cardiac Contractility

Cardiac contractility refers to the ability of the heart to change its force of contraction without changing its resting or diastolic length (see Fig. 17-16 upper curve). The contractile state of the myocardial muscle is determined by biochemical and biophysical properties that govern the interaction between the actin and myosin filaments in the myocardial cells. It is strongly influenced by the number of calcium ions that are available to participate in the contractile process.

An *inotropic* influence is one that modifies the contractile state of the myocardium independent of the Frank-Starling mechanism. For example, sympathetic stimulation produces a positive inotropic effect by increasing the calcium that is available for interaction between the actin and myosin filaments. Hypoxia exerts a negative inotropic effect by interfering with the generation of ATP, which is needed for muscle contraction.

Heart Rate

The heart rate influences cardiac output and the work of the heart by determining the frequency with which the ventricles contract and blood is ejected from the heart. Heart rate also determines the time spent in diastolic filling. Although systole and the ejection period remain fairly constant across heart rates, the time spent in diastole and filling of the ventricles becomes shorter as the heart rate increases. This leads to a decrease in stroke volume and, at high heart rates, may produce a decrease in cardiac output. One of the dangers of ventricular tachycardia is a reduction in cardiac output because the heart does not have time to fill adequately.

SUMMARY CONCEPTS

■ The heart is a four-chambered pump consisting of two atria (the right atrium, which receives blood returning to the heart from the systemic circulation, and the left atrium, which receives oxygenated blood from the lungs) and two ventricles (a right ventricle, which pumps blood into the pulmonary circulation, and a left ventricle, which pumps blood into the systemic circulation).

■ The myocardium or muscle layer of the atria and ventricles produces the pumping action of the heart and the heart valves control the directional flow of blood, with the AV valves controlling flow between the atria to the ventricles; the pulmonic valve, flow between the right side of the heart to the lungs; and the aortic valve, flow between the left side of the heart and the systemic circulation.

■ Specialized cells in the heart's conduction system control the rhythmic contraction and relaxation of the heart. The SA node, which has the fastest inherent rate of impulse generation, acts as the pacemaker of the heart. Impulses from the SA node travel through the atria to the AV node, then to the ventricular Purkinje system. Disorders of the cardiac conduction system include arrhythmias and conduction defects. Ventricular arrhythmias are generally more serious than atrial arrhythmias because they afford the potential for disrupting the pumping ability of the heart.

(continued)

■ The cardiac cycle, which describes the pumping action of the heart, is divided into two parts: systole, during which the ventricles contract and blood is ejected from the heart; and diastole, during which the ventricles relax and allow for filling to occur. The cardiac output, or amount of blood that the heart pumps each minute, represents the stroke volume, or amount of blood pumped with each beat; and the heart rate, the number of times the heart beats each minute. Cardiac reserve refers to the maximum percentage of increase in cardiac output that can be achieved above the normal resting level.

■ The heart's ability to increase its output according to body needs depends on: (1) the preload, or filling of the ventricles (i.e., end-diastolic volume); (2) the afterload, or resistance to ejection of blood from the heart; (3) cardiac contractility, which is determined by the interaction of the actin and myosin filaments of cardiac muscle fibers; and (4) the heart rate, which determines the frequency with which blood is ejected from the heart.

The Systemic Circulation and Control of Blood Flow

The systemic vascular system is a closed system of vessels that distributes blood from the heart to the tissues and returns blood to the heart. Its three divisions include the arterial system, which delivers blood to the tissues; the venous system, which returns blood to the heart; and the capillaries of the microcirculation, which separate the arterial and venous systems and is the site where nutrients and gas exchange take place.

Blood Vessels

All blood vessels, except the capillaries, have walls composed of three layers, or coats, called *tunicae* (Fig. 17-17). The outermost layer of a vessel, called the *tunica externa* or *tunica adventitia*, is composed primarily of loosely woven collagen fibers that protect the blood vessel and anchor it to the surrounding structures. The middle layer, the *tunica media*, is largely a smooth muscle layer that constricts to regulate and control the diameter of the vessel. Larger arteries have an external elastic lamina that separates the tunica media from the tunica externa. The innermost layer, the *tunica intima*, consists of a single layer of flattened endothelial cells with minimal underlying subendothelial connective tissue. The endothelial layer provides a smooth and

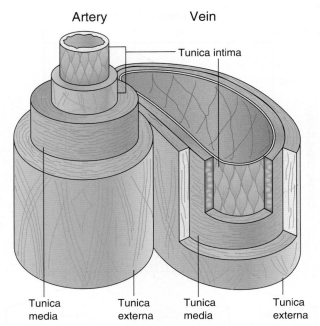

FIGURE 17-17. Medium-sized artery and vein, showing the relative thickness of the three layers.

slippery inner surface for the vessel that prevents platelet adherence and blood clotting.

The layers of the different types of blood vessels vary with vessel function. The walls of the arterioles, which control blood pressure, have large amounts of smooth muscle. Veins are thin-walled, distensible, and collapsible vessels. Capillaries are single-cell–thick vessels designed for the exchange of gases, nutrients, and waste materials.

Vascular smooth muscle cells, which form the predominant cellular layer in the tunica media, produce vasoconstriction or dilation of blood vessels. Smooth muscle contracts slowly and generates high forces for long periods with low energy requirements; using only 1/10 to 1/300 the energy of skeletal muscle. These characteristics are important in blood vessels that must maintain their tone day in and day out.

Compared with skeletal and cardiac muscle, smooth muscle has a less–well-developed sarcoplasmic reticulum for storing intracellular calcium, and it has very few fast sodium channels. Therefore, depolarization of smooth muscle relies largely on extracellular calcium, which enters through calcium channels in the muscle membrane. Sympathetic nervous system control of vascular smooth muscle tone occurs by way of receptor-activated opening and closing of the calcium channels. In general, α-adrenergic receptors are excitatory, in that they causing the channels to open and produce vasoconstriction, and β-adrenergic receptors are inhibitory, in that they causing the channels to close and produce vasodilation. Calcium channel–blocking drugs cause vasodilation by blocking calcium entry through the calcium channels.

Smooth muscle contraction and relaxation also occur in response to local tissue factors such as lack of oxygen, increased hydrogen ion concentrations, and excess carbon dioxide. Nitric oxide (formerly known as the *endothelial relaxing factor*) acts locally to produce smooth muscle relaxation and regulate blood flow. These factors are discussed more fully in the section on local control of blood flow.

Arterial System

The arterial system consists of the large and medium-sized arteries and the arterioles. Arteries are thick-walled vessels with large amounts of elastic fibers. The elasticity of these vessels allows them to stretch during cardiac systole, when the heart contracts and blood is ejected into the circulation, and to recoil during diastole, when the heart relaxes. The arterioles, which are predominantly smooth muscle, serve as resistance vessels for the circulatory system. They act as control valves through which blood is released as it moves into the capillaries. Changes in the activity of sympathetic fibers that innervate these vessels cause them to constrict or relax as needed to maintain blood pressure. The regulation of arterial blood pressure is discussed further in Chapter 18.

The delivery of blood to the tissues of the body is dependent on pressure pulsations or waves of pressure that are generated by the intermittent ejection of blood from the left ventricle into the distensible aorta and large arteries of the arterial system. The arterial pressure pulse represents the energy that is transmitted from molecule to molecule along the length of the vessel (Fig. 17-18). In the aorta, this pressure pulse is transmitted at a velocity of 4 to 6 m/second, which is approximately

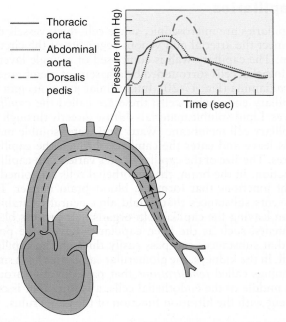

FIGURE 17-18. Amplification of the arterial pressure wave as it moves forward in the peripheral arteries. This amplification occurs as a forward-moving pressure wave merges with a backward-moving reflected pressure wave. (*Inset*) The amplitude of the pressure pulse increases in the thoracic aorta, abdominal aorta, and dorsalis pedis.

20 times faster than the flow of blood. Therefore, the pressure pulse has no direct relation to blood flow and could occur if there were no flow at all. When taking a pulse, it is the pressure pulses that are felt, and it is the pressure pulses that produce the Korotkoff sounds heard during blood pressure measurement. The tip or maximum deflection of the pressure pulsation coincides with the systolic blood pressure, and the minimum point of deflection coincides with the diastolic pressure. The pulse pressure is the difference between systolic and diastolic pressure. If all other factors are equal, the magnitude of the pulse pressure reflects the volume of blood ejected from the left ventricle in a single beat.

Both the pressure values and the conformation of the pressure wave change as it moves though the peripheral arteries, such that the systolic and pulse pressures are higher in the large arteries than in the aorta (see Fig. 17-18). The increase in pulse pressure in the "downstream" arteries is due to the fact that immediately following ejection from the left ventricle, the pressure wave travels at a higher velocity than the blood itself, augmenting the downhill pressure. Furthermore, at branch points of arteries, the forward-moving pressure waves are reflected backward, which also tends to augment the pressure. With peripheral arterial disease, there is a delay in the transmission of the reflected wave so that the pulse decreases rather than increases in amplitude.

After its initial amplification, the pressure pulse becomes smaller and smaller as it moves through the smaller arteries and arterioles, until it disappears almost entirely in the capillaries. This dampening of the pressure pulse is caused by the resistance and distensibility characteristics of these vessels. The increased resistance of these small vessels impedes the transmission of the pressure waves, whereas their distensibility is great enough so that any small change in flow does not cause a pressure change. Although the pressure pulses usually are not transmitted to the capillaries, there are situations in which this does occur. For example, injury to a finger or other area of the body often results in a throbbing sensation. In this case, extreme dilatation of the small vessels in the injured area produces a reduction in the dampening of the pressure pulse.

Venous System

The venous system is a low-pressure system that returns blood to the heart. The venules collect blood from the capillaries, and the veins transport blood back to the right heart. Blood from the systemic veins flows into the right atrium of the heart; therefore, the pressure in the right atrium is called the *central venous pressure*. Right atrial pressure is regulated by the ability of the right ventricle to pump blood into the pulmonary circulation and the tendency of blood to flow from the peripheral veins into the right atrium. The normal right atrial pressure is about 0 mm Hg, which is equal to atmospheric pressure. It can increase to 20 to 30 mm Hg in conditions such as right heart failure or when the rapid infusion of blood or intravenous fluids greatly increases the total blood volume and causes blood to accumulate in the systemic veins and right heart.

The veins and venules are thin-walled, distensible, and collapsible vessels. The veins are capable of enlarging and storing large quantities of blood, which can be made available to the circulation as needed. Even though the veins are thin walled, they are muscular. This allows them to contract or expand to accommodate varying amounts of blood. Veins are innervated by the sympathetic nervous system. When blood is lost from the circulation, the veins constrict as a means of maintaining the circulating blood volume.

Because the venous system is a low-pressure system, blood flow must oppose the effects of gravity. In a person in the standing position, the weight of the blood in the vascular column causes an increase of 1 mm Hg in pressure for every 13.6 mm of distance below the level of the heart. Were it not for the valves in the veins and the action of the skeletal muscles, the venous pressure in the feet would be about +90 mm Hg in the standing adult. Gravity has no effect on the venous pressure in a person in the recumbent position because the blood in the veins is then at the level of the heart.

Valves in the veins of extremities counteract the effects of gravity (Fig. 17-19), and with the help of skeletal muscles that surround and intermittently compress the leg veins in a milking manner, move blood forward to the heart. This pumping action is known as the *venous* or *muscle pump* and is efficient enough that under normal circumstances, the pressure in the feet of a walking

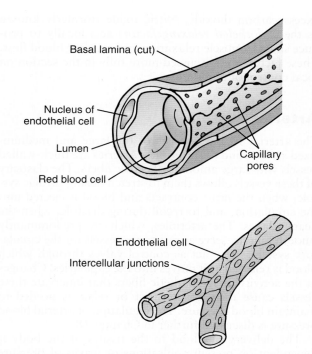

FIGURE 17-20. Endothelial cells and intercellular junctions in a section of capillary.

adult remains less than 20 mm Hg. There are no valves in the abdominal or thoracic veins, and blood flow in these veins is heavily influenced by the pressure in the abdominal and thoracic cavities, respectively.

Capillaries

Capillaries are microscopic, single-cell–thick vessels that connect the arterial and venous segments of the circulation. The capillary wall is composed of a single layer of endothelial cells surrounded by a basement membrane or basal lamina (Fig. 17-20). Intercellular junctions join the capillary endothelial cells; these are called the *capillary pores*. Lipid-soluble materials diffuse directly through the capillary cell membrane. Water and water-soluble materials leave and enter the capillary through the capillary pores. The size of the capillary pores varies with capillary function. In the brain, the endothelial cells are joined by tight junctions that form the blood–brain barrier. This prevents substances that would alter neural excitability from leaving the capillary. In organs that process blood contents, such as the liver, capillaries have large pores so that substances can pass easily through the capillary wall. In the kidneys, the glomerular capillaries have small openings called *fenestrations* that pass directly through the middle of the endothelial cells, a feature that is consistent with the filtration function of the glomerulus.

Lymphatic System

The lymphatic system, commonly called the *lymphatics*, represents an accessory route through which fluid can flow through the tissue spaces into the blood and then

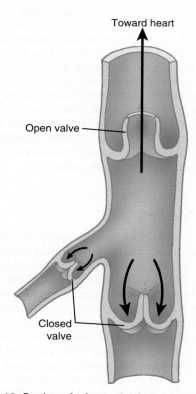

FIGURE 17-19. Portion of a femoral vein opened, to show the valves. The direction of flow is upward. Backward flow closes the valve.

back to the heart. Importantly, the lymphatics can carry proteins and large particulate matter away from the tissue spaces, neither of which can be removed by absorption into the venous system. The lymphatic system is also the main route for absorption of fats and fat soluble vitamins from the gastrointestinal tract.

The lymphatic system is made up of vessels similar to those of the blood vessels in the circulatory system. These vessels commonly travel along with an arteriole or venule or with a companion artery and vein. The terminal lymphatic vessels are made up of a single layer of connective tissue with an endothelial lining and resemble blood capillaries. The lymphatic vessels lack tight junctions and are loosely anchored to the surrounding tissues by fine filaments (Fig. 17-21). The loose junctions permit the entry of large particles, and the filaments hold the vessels open under conditions of edema, when the pressure of the surrounding tissues would otherwise cause them to collapse. The lymph capillaries drain into larger lymph vessels that ultimately empty into the right and left thoracic ducts (Fig. 17-22). The thoracic ducts empty into the circulation at the junctions of the subclavian and internal jugular veins.

Although the divisions are not as distinct as in the circulatory system, the larger lymph vessels show evidence of having intimal, medial, and adventitial layers similar to those of blood vessels. Contraction of the smooth muscle in the medial layer of the larger collecting lymph channels assists in propelling lymph fluid toward the thorax. External compression of the lymph channels by active and passive movements of body parts also aids in forward propulsion of lymph fluid. The rate of flow through the lymphatic system by way of all of the various lymph channels, approximately 120 mL/hour, is determined by the interstitial fluid pressure and the activity of lymph pumps.

The Microcirculation

The most important function of the circulatory system occurs in the microcirculation, which consists of the arterioles, capillaries, and venules. It is here that the transport of nutrients to the tissues and removal of metabolites takes place. Blood enters the microcirculation through an arteriole, passes through the capillaries, and leaves by way of a small venule (Fig. 17-23). Small cuffs of smooth muscle, the precapillary sphincters, are positioned at the arterial end of the capillary. The smooth muscle tone of the arterioles, precapillary sphincters, and venules controls blood flow through the capillary bed. Depending on venous pressure, blood flows through the capillary channels when the precapillary sphincters are open.

An important aspect of the circulatory system, which occurs at the level of the microcirculation, is the ability of organs and tissues to regulate their blood flow based on metabolic needs. Local control is particularly important in tissues such as skeletal muscle and in the heart, organs in which the metabolic activity and need for blood flow vary extensively; and in the brain where metabolic activity and need for blood flow remain relatively constant.

Autoregulation of Blood Flow

Autoregulation is a local control mechanism that automatically adjusts tissue blood flow independent of systemic factors. For example, blood flow to organs such as the heart, brain, and kidneys remains relatively constant, although blood pressure may vary over a range of 60 to 180 mm Hg. In contrast to the mean arterial pressure, which is controlled by systemic mechanisms that adjust the cardiac output to maintain that pressure, changes in blood flow to the individual body tissues are controlled intrinsically by modifying the diameter of local arterioles feeding the capillaries.

There are two mechanisms that control autoregulation: metabolic and myogenic. In most tissues, declining levels of nutrients, particularly oxygen, are the strongest stimuli for autoregulation. Substances released by metabolically active tissues (such as potassium and hydrogen ions, lactic acid, and adenosine, which is a breakdown product of ATP) serve as autoregulation stimuli. Whatever the precise stimuli, the net result is an immediate vasodilation of the arterioles serving the capillaries of the metabolically deprived tissues. Inadequate blood perfusion to an organ is quickly followed by a decline in its metabolic rate and, if prolonged, death of its cells. Likewise, excessively high arterial pressure and tissue perfusion can be dangerous because it may damage the more fragile blood vessels. The *myogenic* (myo = muscle; gen = organ) control mechanisms rely on stretch of the vascular smooth muscle in the vessel wall.

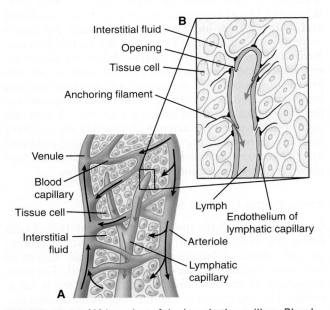

FIGURE 17-21. (A) Location of the lymphatic capillary. Blood from the arterial side of the capillary moves into the interstitial spaces and is reabsorbed in the venous side of the capillary bed. **(B)** Details of the lymphatic capillary with its anchoring filaments and overlapping edges that serve as valves and can be pushed open, allowing the inflow of interstitial fluids and suspended particles.

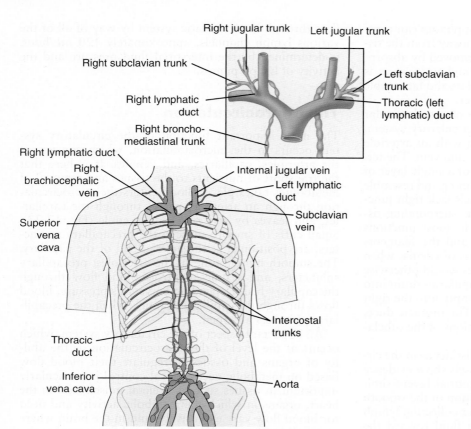

FIGURE 17-22. Lymphatic system showing the thoracic duct and position of the left and right lymphatic ducts (*inset*).

Therefore, it has been proposed that when the arterial pressure stretches the vessel, this in turn causes reactive vascular constriction that reduces the blood flow nearly back to normal. Conversely, at low pressures, the degree of stretch of the vessel is less, so that the smooth muscle relaxes, reducing vascular resistance and helping to return blood flow toward normal.

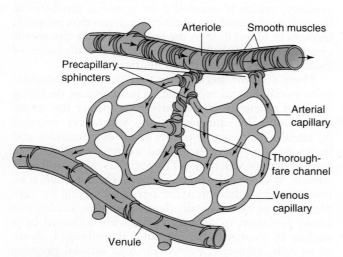

FIGURE 17-23. Capillary bed. Precapillary sphincters control the flow of blood through the capillary network. Thoroughfare channels (i.e., arteriovenous shunts) allow blood to move directly from the arteriole into the venule without moving through nutrient channels of the capillary.

A phenomenon called *reactive hyperemia* is a manifestation of local metabolic regulation of blood flow. When the blood supply to an area has been occluded and then restored, local blood flow through the tissues increases within seconds to restore the metabolic equilibrium of the tissues. This increased flow is called reactive hyperemia. The transient redness seen on an arm after leaning on a hard surface is an example of reactive hyperemia. Local control mechanisms rely on a continuous flow from the main arteries; therefore, hyperemia cannot occur when the arteries that supply the capillary beds are narrowed. For example, if a major coronary artery becomes occluded, the opening of channels supplied by that vessel cannot restore blood flow.

Endothelial Control of Blood Flow

One of the important functions of the endothelial cells lining the arterioles and small arteries is the synthesis and release of factors that can affect the degree of relaxation or contraction of the arterial wall. The most important of the *endothelial relaxing factors* is *nitric oxide*. The normal endothelium maintains a continuous release of nitric oxide, which is synthesized from the amino acid arginine and oxygen and reduction of inorganic nitrate. The production of nitric oxide can be stimulated by a variety of endothelial agonists, including acetylcholine, bradykinin, histamine, and thrombin. Shear stress on the endothelium resulting from an increase in blood flow or blood pressure also stimulates nitric oxide production and vessel relaxation. Nitric oxide also inhibits platelet aggregation and secretion of platelet contents, many of which cause vasoconstriction. Nitroglycerin, a drug used in treatment of angina, produces its effects by releasing nitric oxide in vascular smooth muscle of the target tissues.

The endothelium also produces a number of vasoconstrictor substances, including *angiotensin II*, vasoconstrictor prostaglandins, and a family of peptides called *endothelins*. There are at least three endothelins. Endothelin-1 is the most potent endogenous vasoconstrictor known.

Humoral Control of Blood Flow

Humoral control of blood flow involves the effect of vasodilator and vasoconstrictor substances in the blood. Some of these substances are formed by special glands and transported in the blood throughout the entire circulation. Others are formed in local tissues and aid in the local control of blood flow. Among the most important of the humoral factors are norepinephrine and epinephrine, angiotensin II, histamine, serotonin, bradykinin, and the prostaglandins.

Norepinephrine and Epinephrine. Norepinephrine is an especially powerful vasoconstrictor hormone; epinephrine is less so and in some tissues (e.g., skeletal muscle) even causes mild vasodilation. Stimulation of the sympathetic nervous system during stress or exercise causes local constriction of veins and arterioles due to the release of norepinephrine from sympathetic nerve endings. In addition, sympathetic stimulation causes the adrenal medullae to secrete both norepinephrine and epinephrine into the blood. These hormones then circulate in the blood, causing direct sympathetic stimulation of blood vessels in all parts of the body.

Angiotensin II. Angiotensin II, another powerful vasoconstrictor, is produced as a part of the renin-angiotensin-aldosterone system. It normally acts on many arterioles at the same time to increase the peripheral vascular resistance, thereby increasing the arterial blood pressure (discussed in Chapter 18).

Histamine. Histamine has a powerful vasodilator effect on arterioles and has the ability to increase capillary permeability, allowing leakage of both fluid and plasma proteins into the tissues. Histamine is largely derived from mast cells in injured tissues and basophils in the blood. In certain tissues, such as skeletal muscle, the activity of the mast cells is mediated by the sympathetic nervous system; when sympathetic control is withdrawn, the mast cells release histamine.

Serotonin. Serotonin, which is liberated from aggregating platelets during the clotting process, causes vasoconstriction and plays a major role in control of bleeding. Serotonin is found in brain and lung tissues, and there is some speculation that it may be involved in the vascular spasm associated with some allergic pulmonary reactions and migraine headaches.

Bradykinin. The kinins (i.e., kallidins and bradykinin) are small polypeptides that are liberated from the globulin kininogen, which is present in body fluids. They cause powerful vasodilation when formed in the blood and tissue fluids of organs. Bradykinin causes intense dilation of arterioles, increased capillary permeability, and constriction of venules. It is thought that the kinins play special roles in regulating blood flow and capillary leakage in inflamed tissues. It is also believed that bradykinin plays a major role in regulating blood flow in the skin as well in the salivary and gastrointestinal glands.

Prostaglandins. Prostaglandins are synthesized from constituents of the cell membrane (i.e., the long-chain fatty acid *arachidonic acid*). Tissue injury incites the release of arachidonic acid from the cell membrane, which initiates prostaglandin synthesis (see Chapter 3, Fig. 3-4). There are several prostaglandins (e.g., E2, F2, D2), which are subgrouped according to their solubility; some produce vasoconstriction and some produce vasodilation. As a general rule, those in the E group are vasodilators and those in the F group are vasoconstrictors. The corticosteroid hormones produce an anti-inflammatory response by blocking the release of arachidonic acid, thereby preventing prostaglandin synthesis.

Collateral Circulation

Collateral circulation is a mechanism for the long-term regulation of local blood flow. In the heart and other vital structures, anastomotic channels exist between some of the smaller arteries. These channels permit perfusion of an area by more than one artery. When one artery becomes occluded, these anastomotic channels increase in size, allowing blood from a patent artery to perfuse the area supplied by the occluded vessel. For example, persons with extensive obstruction of a coronary blood vessel may rely on collateral circulation to meet the oxygen needs of the myocardial tissue normally supplied by that vessel. As with other long-term compensatory mechanisms, the recruitment of collateral circulation is most efficient when the obstruction to flow is gradual, rather than sudden.

Neural Control of Blood Flow

The neural control of the circulation occurs primarily through the *sympathetic* and *parasympathetic* divisions of the autonomic nervous system (ANS). The ANS contributes to the control of cardiovascular function through modulation of cardiac function (i.e., heart rate and cardiac contractility) and peripheral vascular resistance.

The neural control centers for the integration and modulation of cardiac function and blood pressure are located bilaterally in the medulla oblongata of the brain. The medullary cardiovascular neurons are grouped into three distinct pools that lead to sympathetic innervation of the heart and blood vessels and parasympathetic innervation of the heart. The first two, which control sympathetic-mediated acceleration of heart rate and blood vessel tone, are called the *vasomotor center*. The third, which controls parasympathetic-mediated slowing of heart rate, is called the *cardioinhibitory center*. These brain stem centers receive information from many areas of the nervous system, including the hypothalamus. The arterial baroreceptors and chemoreceptors provide the medullary cardiovascular center with continuous information regarding changes in blood pressure (see Chapter 18).

The sympathetic nervous system serves as the final common pathway for controlling the smooth muscle tone of the blood vessels. Most of the sympathetic preganglionic fibers that control vessel function originate in the vasomotor center of the brain stem, travel down the spinal cord, and exit in the thoracic and lumbar (T1 to L2) segments. The sympathetic neurons that supply the blood vessels maintain them in a state of tonic activity, so that even under resting conditions, the blood vessels are partially constricted. Vessel constriction and relaxation are accomplished by altering this basal input. Increasing sympathetic activity causes constriction of some vessels, such as those of the skin, the gastrointestinal tract, and the kidneys. Blood vessels in skeletal muscle are supplied by both vasoconstrictor and vasodilator fibers. Activation of sympathetic vasodilator fibers causes vessel relaxation and provides the muscles with increased blood flow during exercise. Although the parasympathetic nervous system contributes to the regulation of heart function, it has little or no control over blood vessels.

The actions of the ANS are mediated by chemical neurotransmitters. *Acetylcholine* is the postganglionic neurotransmitter for parasympathetic neurons and *norepinephrine* is the main postganglionic neurotransmitter for sympathetic neurons. Sympathetic neurons also respond to epinephrine, which is released into the bloodstream by the adrenal medulla. The neurotransmitter *dopamine* can also act as a neurotransmitter for some sympathetic neurons. The synthesis, release, and inactivation of the autonomic neurotransmitters are discussed in Chapter 34.

- The arterial system is a high-pressure system that delivers blood to the tissues. It relies on the intermittent ejection of blood from the left ventricle and the generation of arterial pressure pulsations that move blood toward the capillaries where the exchange of gases, nutrients, and wastes occur.

- The venous system is a low-pressure system that collects blood from the capillaries. It relies on the presence of valves in the veins of the extremities to prevent retrograde flow and on the milking action of the skeletal muscles that surround the veins to return blood to the right heart.

- The arterioles, capillaries, and venules of the microcirculation facilitate the exchange of gases, nutrients, and metabolic waste-products between body tissues and the circulatory system. Local control of blood flow in the microcirculation is governed largely by the metabolic needs of the tissues and is regulated by local tissue factors such as lack of oxygen and the accumulation of metabolites, endothelial-derived vasodilators and vasoconstrictors, and humoral factors such as histamine, bradykinin, and the prostaglandins.

- Collateral circulation, which involves the development of collateral channels between smaller arteries, is a mechanism for long-term regulation of blood flow in areas where larger vessels have become occluded.

- Neural control of the circulation is vested in the autonomic nervous system, with both the sympathetic and parasympathetic nervous systems exerting control over heart rate and the sympathetic nervous system controlling cardiac contractility and blood vessel tone.

SUMMARY CONCEPTS

- The systemic circulation consists of arteries and arterioles, capillaries, and venules and veins. The walls of the blood vessels, except the capillaries, are composed of three layers: an outer layer, the *tunica externa*, composed of large collagen fibers that protect the vessel and anchor it to the surrounding structures; a middle layer, the *tunica media*, composed of smooth muscle that constricts to regulate vessel diameter; and an inner layer, the *tunica intima*, of flattened endothelial cells that provide a smooth and slippery surface for blood flow.

REVIEW EXERCISES

1. In persons with atherosclerosis of the coronary arteries, symptoms of myocardial ischemia do not usually occur until the vessel has been 75% occluded. Use Poiseuille law to explain.

2. Once an arterial aneurysm has begun to form, it will continue to enlarge as the result of the increased tension in its wall.

   A. Explain the continued increase in size using the law of Laplace.
   B. Using information related to cross-sectional area and velocity of flow, explain why there is stasis of blood flow with the tendency to form clots in aneurysms with a large cross-sectional area.

3. Use events in the cardiac cycle depicted in Figure 17-11 to explain:

A. The effect of hypertension on the isovolumetric contraction period.

B. The effect of an increase in heart rate on the time spent in diastole.

C. The effect of an increase in the isovolumetric relaxation period on the diastolic filling of the ventricle.

4. Use the Frank-Starling ventricular function curve depicted in Figure 17-16 to explain the changes in cardiac output that occur with the following changes in respiratory effort:

A. What happens to cardiac output during increased inspiratory effort in which a marked decrease in intrathoracic pressure produces an increase in venous return to the right heart?

B. What happens to cardiac output during increased expiratory effort in which a marked increase in intrathoracic pressure produces a decrease in venous return to the right heart?

C. Given these changes in cardiac output that occur during increased respiratory effort, what would you propose as one of the functions of the Frank-Starling curve?

BIBLIOGRAPHY

Balger P, Segal SS. Regulation of blood flow in the microcirculation: role of conducted vasodilation. *Acta Physiol (Oxf)*. 2011;202(3):271–284.

Ellis CG, Jagger J, Sharpe M. The microcirculation as a functional system. *Crit Care*. 2005;9:S3–S8.

Hall JE. *Guyton and Hall Textbook of Medical Physiology*. 12th ed. Philadelphia, PA: Elsevier Saunders; 2011:157–254.

Klabunde RE. *Cardiovascular Physiology Concepts*. 2nd ed. Philadelphia, PA: Wolters Kluwer Health/Lippincott Williams & Wilkins; 2012.

Levy MN, Pappano AJ. *Cardiovascular Physiology*. 9th ed. Philadelphia, PA: Mosby Elsevier; 2007.

Norton JM. Toward consistent definitions for preload and afterload. *Adv Physiol Educ*. 2001;25(1):53–61.

Rhoades RS, Bell DR. *Medical Physiology: Principles of Clinical Medicine*. 4th ed. Philadelphia, PA: Wolters Kluwer Health/Lippincott Williams & Wilkins; 2013:212–325.

Koeppen BM, Stanton BA. *Berne & Levy Physiology*. 6th ed. Philadelphia, PA: Mosby Elsevier; 2010:287–414.

Ross MH, Pawlina W. *Histology: A Text and Atlas*. 5th ed. Philadelphia, PA: Wolters Kluwer Health/Lippincott Williams & Wilkins; 2011:400–430.

Segal SS. Regulation of blood flow in the microcirculation. *Microcirculation*. 2005;12(1):33–45.

Sherwood L. *Human Physiology: From Cells to Systems*. 8th ed. Belmont, CA: Brooks/Cole; 2013:304–333.

Smith JJ, Kampine JP. *Circulatory Physiology*. 3rd ed. Baltimore, MD: J.B.Lippincott; 1989.

Toda N, Okamura T. The pharmacology of nitric oxide in the peripheral nervous system of blood vessels. *Pharmacol. Rev.* 2003;55(2):271–324.

Porth Essentials Resources

Explore these additional resources to enhance learning for this chapter:

- NCLEX-Style Questions and Other Resources on thePoint, http://thePoint.lww.com/PorthEssentials4e
- Study Guide for Essentials of Pathophysiology
- Concepts in Action Animations
- Adaptive Learning | Powered by PrepU, http://thepoint.lww.com/prepu

C h a p t e r 18

Disorders of Blood Flow and Blood Pressure

Disorders of the blood vessels are directly or indirectly responsible for many human diseases. Arterial diseases, such as stroke and coronary heart disease, are responsible for more morbidity and mortality than any other type of disease. Hypertension, or elevation of the arterial blood pressure, is probably the most common of all health problems in adults and is the leading risk factor for cardiovascular disorders. Although venous diseases are less common, they also cause clinically significant problems. The discussion in this chapter is organized into four parts: blood vessel structure and function, disorders of the arterial circulation, disorders of the arterial blood pressure, and disorders of the venous circulation.

Blood Vessel Structure and Function

The walls of arteries and veins are composed of three layers called tunica: an outer layer called the *tunica externa*, a middle layer called the *tunica media*, and an inner layer called the *tunica intima* (Fig. 18-1). The tunica externa is composed primarily of loosely woven collagen fibers that protect the blood vessel and anchor it to the surrounding structures. It is infiltrated with nerve fibers and, in larger vessels, a system of tiny blood vessels called the *vasa vasorum*. The tunica media is composed mainly of circularly arranged smooth muscle cells and sheets of elastin. Larger arteries have an external elastic lamina that separates the tunica media from the tunica externa. The tunica intima consists of a single layer of flattened endothelial cells with minimal underlying subendothelial connective tissue. As the main cellular component of the blood vessel wall, the endothelial and smooth muscle cells play an important role in the pathogenesis of many blood vessel diseases.

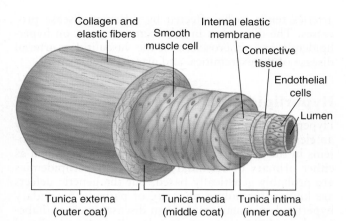

Collagen and
elastic fibers   Smooth
muscle cell   Internal elastic
membrane   Connective
tissue   Endothelial
cells   Lumen

Tunica externa
(outer coat)   Tunica media
(middle coat)   Tunica intima
(inner coat)

FIGURE 18-1. Diagram of a typical artery showing the tunica externa, tunica media, and tunica intima.

Endothelial Cells

Endothelial cells form a continuous lining for the entire vascular system called the *endothelium*. Once thought to be nothing more than a lining for blood vessels, it is now known that the endothelium is a versatile, multifunctional tissue that plays an active role in controlling vascular function[1-4] (Table 18-1). As a selectively permeable monolayer, the endothelium controls the transfer of molecules across the vessel wall. The endothelium also plays a role in the modulation of blood flow and vascular resistance; control of platelet adhesion and blood clotting; metabolism of hormones; regulation of immune and inflammatory reactions; and elaboration of factors that influence the growth of other cell types, especially vascular smooth muscle cells.

Structurally intact endothelial cells respond to various abnormal stimuli by adjusting their usual functions and by expressing newly acquired functions.[1] The term *endothelial dysfunction* describes several types of potentially reversible changes in endothelial function that occur in response to environmental stimuli. Endothelial cell dysfunction has been implicated in a number of pathologies including thrombosis, atherosclerosis, and hypertensive vascular lesions.[3,4] There is also evidence that the dysfunction contributes to conditions such as erectile dysfunction, disorders of the retina, kidney disease, pulmonary hypertension, and septic shock.

Inducers of endothelial dysfunction include cardiovascular risk factors such as smoking, hyperlipidemia, hypertension, insulin resistance and diabetes, and aging that contribute to the development of atherosclerosis. Dysfunctional endothelial cells, in turn, produce proinflammatory cytokines, growth factors (e.g., vascular endothelial growth factor), reactive oxygen species, procoagulant or anticoagulant substances, and a variety of other disease-producing products. They also influence the reactivity of underlying smooth muscle cells through production of both relaxing factors (e.g., nitric oxide) and contracting factors (e.g., endothelins; see Chapter 17).

Vascular Smooth Muscle Cells

Vascular smooth muscle cells, which form the predominant cellular layer in the tunica media, produce vasoconstriction or vasodilation. A network of vasomotor nerves of the sympathetic component of the autonomic nervous system supplies the smooth muscle in the blood vessels. These nerves are responsible for constriction of the vessel walls. Because they do not enter the tunica media of the blood vessel, the nerves do not synapse directly on the smooth muscle cells. Instead, they release the neurotransmitter norepinephrine, which diffuses into the media and acts on the nearby smooth muscle cells. The resulting impulses are propagated along the smooth muscle cells, causing contraction of the entire smooth muscle cell layer and thus reducing the radius of the vessel lumen.

TABLE 18-1	**Endothelial Cell Properties and Functions**
Major Properties	**Associated Functions/Factors**
Maintenance of a selectively permeable barrier	Controls the transfer of small and large molecules across the vessel wall
Regulation of thrombosis	Elaboration of pro- and antithrombotic molecules (von Willebrand factor, plasminogen activator) and antithrombotic molecules (prostacyclin, heparin-like molecules, plasminogen activator)
Modulation of blood flow and vascular reactivity	Elaboration of vasodilators (nitric oxide, prostacyclin) and vasoconstrictors (endothelins, angiotensin-converting enzyme)
Regulation of cell growth, particularly smooth muscle cells	Production of growth-stimulating factors (platelet-derived growth factor, hematopoietic colony-stimulating factor) and growth-inhibiting factors (heparin, transforming growth factor-β)
Regulation of inflammatory/immune responses	Expression of adhesion molecules that regulate leukocyte migration and release of inflammatory and immune system mediators (e.g., interleukins, interferons)
Maintenance of the extracellular matrix	Synthesis of collagen, laminin, proteoglycans
Involvement in lipoprotein metabolism	Oxidation of very low density lipoproteins, low density lipoproteins, and cholesterol

Data from Schoen FJ. Blood vessels. In: Kumar V, Abbas AK, Fausto N, et al; eds. *Robbins and Cotran Pathologic Basis of Disease*, 8th ed. Philadelphia, PA: Saunders Elsevier; 2010:490–491; Ross MH, Pawlina W. Histology: *A Text and Atlas*, 6th ed. Philadelphia, PA: Wolters Kluwer | Lippincott Williams & Wilkins; 2011:412–414.

Vascular smooth muscle cells also synthesize collagen, elastin, and other components of the extracellular matrix; elaborate growth factors and cytokines; and after vascular injury migrate into the intima and proliferate.[1] Thus, smooth muscle cells are important in both normal vascular repair and pathologic processes such as atherosclerosis. The migratory and proliferative activities of vascular smooth muscle cells are stimulated by growth promoters and inhibitors, such as platelet-derived growth factor, thrombin, fibroblast growth factor, cytokines, and nitric oxide.

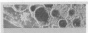

SUMMARY CONCEPTS

- The walls of blood vessels are composed of an inner layer of endothelial cells, a middle layer of vascular smooth muscle, and an outer layer of loosely woven collagen tissue.

- The endothelium, which forms a continuous lining for the entire vascular system, controls the transfer of molecules across the vascular wall and plays a role in the control of platelet adhesion and blood clotting, modulation of blood flow and vascular resistance, metabolism of hormones, regulation of immune and inflammatory reactions, and elaboration of factors that influence the growth of other cell types, particularly the smooth muscle cells.

- The term *endothelial dysfunction* describes changes in endothelial function that occur in response to stimuli derived from cardiovascular risk factors such as smoking, hyperlipidemia, hypertension, insulin resistance and diabetes, and obesity.

- Vascular smooth muscle cells, which form the middle layer of blood vessels, control the dilation and constriction of blood vessels, elaborate growth factors, and synthesize collagen, elastin, and other components of the extracellular matrix that are important in both normal vascular repair and pathologic processes such as atherosclerosis.

Disorders of the Arterial Circulation

The arterial system distributes blood to all the tissues in the body. There are three types of arteries: large elastic arteries, including the aorta and its distal branches; medium-sized arteries, such as the coronary and renal arteries; and small arteries and arterioles that pass through the tissues. Each of these different types of arteries tends to be affected by different disease processes. The discussion in this section focuses on hyperlipidemia and atherosclerosis, the vasculitides, arterial disease of the extremities, and arterial aneurysms.

Hyperlipidemia

Hyperlipidemia is a medical condition characterized by an elevation of any or all lipid profiles and/or lipoproteins in the blood. Hyperlipidemias can be classified as either primary or secondary.[5] Primary hyperlipidemias are probably genetically based, but the genetic defects are known for only a minority of patients. Secondary hyperlipidemia may result from diseases such as diabetes, thyroid disease, renal disorders, liver disorders, and Cushing syndrome, as well as obesity, alcohol consumption, estrogen administration, and other drug-associated changes in lipid metabolism. Besides the primary and secondary hyperlipidemia subtypes, hyperlipidemia is also classified according to the type of lipid that is elevated—hypercholesterolemia, hypertriglyceridemia, or both in combined hyperlipidemia. The condition, specifically hypercholesteremia, is strongly associated with the development of atherosclerosis, which causes more morbidity and mortality in the Western world than any other disorder. By the year 2025, it is predicted that cardiovascular mortality will likely exceed that of every other major disease group including infections, cancer, and trauma.[6]

Lipoprotein Metabolism and Transport

Because lipids, namely cholesterol and triglycerides, are insoluble in plasma, they are encapsulated by special fat-carrying proteins called lipoproteins for transport in the blood. There are five main types of lipoproteins, classified by their protein content or densities: chylomicrons, very–low-density lipoprotein (VLDL), intermediate-density lipoprotein (IDL), low-density lipoprotein (LDL), and high-density lipoprotein (HDL). Thus, VLDLs carry large amounts of triglycerides and much less cholesterol and protein. Low-density lipoprotein is the main carrier of cholesterol, whereas HDL is about 50% protein and carries less cholesterol and little triglyceride (Fig. 18-2).

Lipoproteins are macromolecules made up of a hydrophobic core of insoluble cholesterol esters and triglycerides, surrounded by a hydrophilic outer shell of soluble phospholipids, and nonesterified cholesterol[7] (Fig. 18-3). In addition, the shell contains a variety of apolipoproteins, proteins that bind lipids, thereby increasing the stability and water solubility of the resulting lipoprotein. The apolipoproteins also activate certain enzymes required for normal lipoprotein metabolism, and they serve as reactive sites that specific receptors on peripheral tissues can recognize and use in the endocytosis and metabolism of the lipoproteins. Apolipoproteins can be grouped into two classes: exchangeable and nonexchangeable. Exchangeable apolipoproteins (e.g., apoA-I, apoC-II, and apoE) are able to dissociate from one lipoprotein and associate with another, whereas the nonexchangeable apolipoproteins (e.g., apoB-48 and

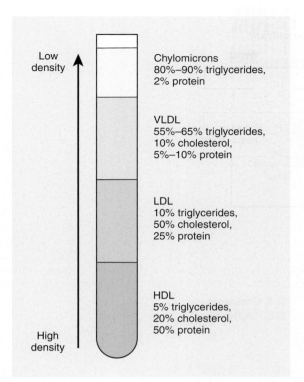

FIGURE 18-2. Lipoproteins are named based on their protein content, which is measured in density. Because fats are less dense than proteins, as the proportion of triglycerides decreases, the density increases. HDL, high-density lipoprotein; LDL, low-density lipoprotein; VLDL, very–low-density lipoprotein.

apoB-100) remain attached to the same lipoprotein particle from biosynthesis to breakdown.[8]

There are two pathways involved in the generation and transport of lipoproteins: the exogenous intestinal and endogenous hepatic pathways.[1,2,7,9] The exogenous pathway is involved in the transport of dietary

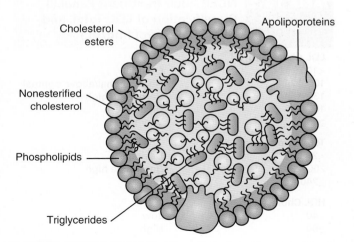

FIGURE 18-3. General structure of a lipoprotein. The cholesterol esters and triglycerides are located in the hydrophobic core of the macromolecule, surrounded by an outer hydrophilic shell of phospholipids, nonesterified lipoproteins, and apolipoproteins.

cholesterol and triglycerides from the intestine to the liver. The endogenous pathway involves the processing of triglycerides and cholesterol by the liver and their distribution throughout the body (Fig. 18-4).

Exogenous Pathway. The exogenous pathway involves the chylomicron transport of dietary triglycerides and cholesterol from the intestines to the liver. The chylomicrons, which are the largest of the lipoprotein molecules, are synthesized in the wall of the small intestine. These triglyceride-rich lipoproteins transfer their triglycerides to peripheral tissues, especially adipose tissue and skeletal muscle, for energy and storage. The remnant chylomicron particles, which contain cholesterol, are then taken up by the liver and the cholesterol is used in the synthesis of VLDL or excreted in the bile.

Endogenous Pathway. The liver is the central site for handling of lipids: it is able to store glycerols and fats in its cells; synthesize triglycerides; and use esterified cholesterol and triglycerides to form VLDL. Like chylomicrons, VLDLs carry their triglycerides to fat and muscle cells, where the triglycerides are removed. The resulting IDL particles, which are reduced in triglyceride content and enriched in cholesterol, are then taken to the liver and recycled to form VLDL or converted to LDL.

Low-Density Lipoproteins

Sometimes called *bad cholesterol*, LDL is the main carrier of cholesterol. Low-density lipoprotein particles are rich in cholesterol and cholesterol esters. Approximately 60% of the LDL is transported back to the liver, where its apoB-100 binds to specific LDL receptors on liver cells, allowing the particles to be internalized.[2,7,9] The remaining 40% of LDL particles are carried to extrahepatic tissues, such as those of the adrenal cortex and gonads, which also have apoB-100 receptors that allow them to internalize the LDL particles and use the cholesterol in the synthesis of their cell membranes and steroid hormones.

There are different types of LDL, and some people with markedly elevated LDL do not develop atherosclerotic vascular disease, whereas other people with only modest elevations in LDL develop severe disease. This can be partially explained by the quality and size of the LDL particles. Small, dense LDL is more toxic or atherogenic to the endothelium than large, buoyant LDL. It is more likely to enter the vessel wall, become oxidized, and trigger the atherosclerotic process.

High-Density Lipoproteins

Often referred to as the *good cholesterol*, HDL is synthesized by several pathways, including direct secretion by the intestine and liver and transfer of lipid constituents released during lipolysis of lipoproteins that contain apoB100. It participates in reverse cholesterol transport (see Fig. 18-4)—that is, carrying cholesterol from the peripheral tissues back to the liver. Epidemiologic studies show an inverse relation between HDL levels and the development of atherosclerosis.[6] It is thought that HDL, which is low in cholesterol and rich in surface phospholipids,

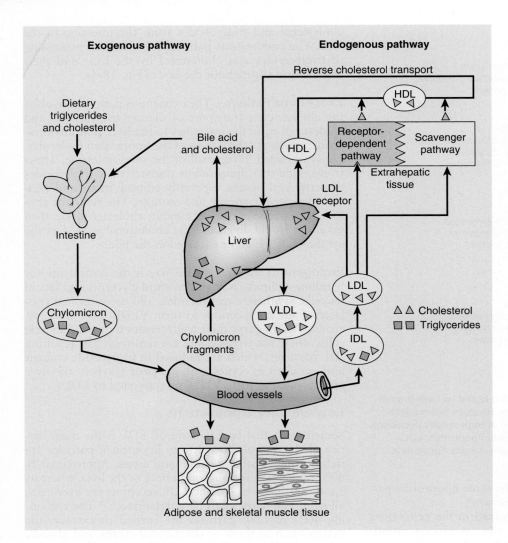

Exogenous pathway

Endogenous pathway

Reverse cholesterol transport

Dietary triglycerides and cholesterol

Bile acid and cholesterol

Intestine

Liver

Chylomicron

Chylomicron fragments

VLDL

Blood vessels

HDL

Receptor-dependent pathway

Scavenger pathway

Extrahepatic tissue

LDL receptor

LDL

IDL

△ △ Cholesterol
▢ ▢ Triglycerides

Adipose and skeletal muscle tissue

FIGURE 18-4. Schematic representation of the exogenous and endogenous pathways for triglyceride and cholesterol transport. HDL, high-density lipoprotein; IDL, intermediate-density lipoprotein; LDL, low-density lipoprotein; VLDL, very–low-density lipoprotein.

facilitates the clearance of cholesterol from atheromatous plaques and transports it to the liver, where it may be excreted rather than reused in the formation of VLDL. The mechanism whereby HDL takes up cholesterol from peripheral cells has recently been elucidated. A lipid transporter (adenosine triphosphate [ATP]–binding cassette transporter A class 1, or ABCA1) promotes the movement of cholesterol from peripheral cells to the lipid-poor HDL cholesterol.[7,9] Defects in this system (resulting from mutations in the ABCA1 transporter gene) are responsible for a condition called *Tangier disease*, which is characterized by accelerated atherosclerosis and little or no HDL cholesterol.[9]

Hypercholesterolemia

Hypercholesterolemia refers to increased levels of cholesterol in the blood. The Third Report of the National Cholesterol Educational Program (NCEP) Expert Panel on Detection, Evaluation, and Treatment of High Blood Cholesterol in Adults classification system describes optimal to very high levels of LDL cholesterol and triglycerides, and low and high levels of HDL cholesterol[10] (Table 18-2).

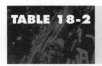

TABLE 18-2 **NCEP Adult Treatment Panel III Classification of LDL, Total, and HDL Cholesterol (mg/dL)**

LDL Cholesterol

<100	Optimal
100–129	Near optimal/above optimal
130–159	Borderline high
160–189	High
≥190	Very high

Total Cholesterol

<200	Desirable
200–239	Borderline high
≥240	High

HDL Cholesterol

<40	Low
≥60	High

From National Institutes of Health Expert Panel. *Third Report of the National Cholesterol Education Program [NCEP] Expert Panel on Detection, Evaluation, and Treatment of High Blood Cholesterol in Adults [Adult Treatment Panel III].* NIH Publication No. 01-3670. Bethesda, MD: National Institutes of Health; 2001.

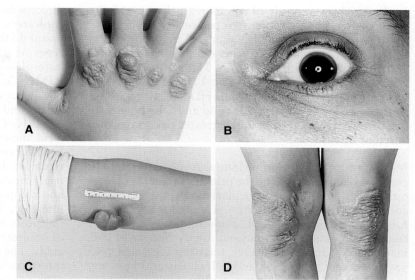

FIGURE 18-5. Xanthomas in the skin and tendons **(A, C, D)**. Arcus lipoides represents the deposition of lipids in the peripheral cornea **(B)**. (From Gotlieb AI, Lui A. Blood vessels. In: Rubin R, Strayer DS, eds. *Rubin's Pathology: Clinicopathologic Foundations of Medicine*, 6th ed. Philadelphia, PA: Wolters Kluwer Health/Lippincott Williams & Wilkins; 2012:459.)

Several factors, including nutrition, genetics, comorbid conditions, medications, and metabolic diseases, can raise blood lipid levels. Most cases of elevated levels of cholesterol are probably multifactorial. Hypercholesterolemia can be divided into two types: primary or secondary. In primary hypercholesteremia elevated cholesterol levels develop independent of other causes. Secondary hypercholesterolemia is associated with other health problems and behaviors.

Many types of primary hypercholesterolemia have a genetic basis. There may be a defective synthesis of the apolipoproteins, a lack of lipoprotein receptors, defective receptors, or defects in the handling of cholesterol in the cell that are genetically determined.[1,2,9] For example, the LDL receptor is deficient or defective in the genetic disorder known as *familial hypercholesterolemia (type 2A)*. This autosomal dominant type of hyperlipidemia results from a mutation in the gene specifying the receptor for LDL. It is one of the most common of all Mendelian disorders, with heterozygotes having one defective gene representing about 1 in 500 persons in the general population.[1,2,9] Because most of the circulating cholesterol is removed by receptor-dependent mechanisms, blood cholesterol levels are markedly elevated in persons with this disorder. Plasma LDL levels in heterozygotes range between 250 and 500 mg/dL, whereas in homozygotes LDL cholesterol levels may rise to 1000 mg/dL. Although heterozygotes commonly have an elevated cholesterol level from birth, the disorder does not typically manifest until adult life, when *xanthomas* (i.e., cholesterol deposits) develop along the tendons, and atherosclerosis appears (Fig. 18-5). Myocardial infarction before 40 years of age is common. Homozygotes are much more severely affected; they have cutaneous xanthomas in childhood and may experience myocardial infarction by as early as 1 to 2 years of age.

Secondary causes of hypercholesterolemia include obesity with high-calorie intake, sedentary lifestyle, and diabetes mellitus.[9,11] High-calorie diets increase the production of VLDL, with triglyceride elevation and high conversion of VLDL to LDL. Excess ingestion of cholesterol may reduce the formation of LDL receptors and thereby decrease LDL removal from the blood. Diets that are high in saturated fats increase cholesterol synthesis and suppress LDL receptor activity. A sedentary lifestyle influences interactions among lipids and lipoproteins. Diabetes mellitus and the metabolic syndrome are associated with elevated triglycerides, low HDL, and minimal or modest elevation of LDL. Other systemic disorders that can elevate lipids include hypothyroidism, the nephrotic syndrome, and obstructive liver disease. Medications such as beta-blockers, estrogens, and protease inhibitors (used in the treatment of human immunodeficiency virus [HIV] infection) can also increase lipid levels.

Diagnosis of Hyperlipidemia. Diagnosis of hyperlipidemia depends on a person's complete lipid profile (total cholesterol, LDL, HDL, and triglyceride levels) after an overnight fast.[9,11] Most clinical laboratories measure the total serum cholesterol, total triglycerides, and the amount of cholesterol carried in the HDL fraction. The LDL is then estimated by subtracting the HDL from the total serum cholesterol and the triglycerides divided by 5* (i.e., LDL [mg/dL] = total cholesterol [mg/dL] – HDL [mg/dL] – triglycerides [mg/dL]/5). The relationship between the different lipid fractions can then be used as a means for determining an individual's risk for developing coronary heart disease and other atherosclerosis-related diseases. Cholesterol is carried in the blood as VLDL, LDL, and HDL, with the total serum cholesterol being equal to the sum of these three components.[11,12] Thus, total serum cholesterol levels may

---

* When using SI units (expressed in mmol/L), the triglycerides are divided by 2.2.

be elevated as a result of an increase in any of the lipoproteins. For example, two persons with the same total serum cholesterol of 275 mg/dL may have very different lipid profiles.[11] One person may have a favorable lipid profile with an HDL of 110 mg/dL, a triglyceride level of 175 mg/dL, and an LDL of 130 mg/dL, whereas another person with an HDL of 40 mg/dL, a triglyceride level of 150 mg/dL, and an LDL cholesterol of 205 mg/dL would be at much greater risk for cardiovascular disease.

Management of Hyperlipidemia. A reduction in LDL cholesterol continues to be the primary target for cholesterol-lowering therapy, particularly in people at risk for coronary artery disease (CAD). The major risk factors for CAD, exclusive of LDL cholesterol levels, include cigarette smoking, hypertension, family history of premature CAD in a first-degree relative, age (men ≥45 years; women ≥55 years), an HDL cholesterol level less than 40 mg/dL, and diabetes mellitus.[6,11,12] Guidelines recommend that persons with none of the major risk factors should have an LDL cholesterol goal of 160 mg/dL or less; those with two or more of the major risk factors should have an LDL cholesterol goal of less than 130 mg/dL; persons with *high-risk* factors (i.e., those with CAD, other forms of atherosclerotic disease, or diabetes) should have an LDL cholesterol goal of less than 100 mg/dL; and persons with *very–high-risk* factors (i.e., acute coronary syndromes or CAD with other risk factors) should have an LDL cholesterol goal of less than 70 mg/dL.[13] It is also recommended that persons with a greater than 20% 10-year risk of experiencing myocardial infarction or coronary death, as determined by the risk assessment tool developed from Framingham Heart Study data, should have an LDL cholesterol goal of less than 100 mg/dL (to calculate a risk score, go to http://hp2010.nhlbihin.net/atpIII/calculator.asp?usertype=prof)

The management of hypercholesterolemia focuses on dietary and therapeutic lifestyle changes; when these are unsuccessful, pharmacologic treatment may be necessary. Therapeutic lifestyle changes include an increased emphasis on physical activity, dietary measures to reduce LDL levels, smoking cessation, and weight reduction for people who are overweight.

Several dietary elements affect cholesterol and its lipoprotein fractions: (1) excess calorie intake, (2) saturated and trans fats, and (3) cholesterol.[12] Excess calories consistently lower HDL and less consistently elevate LDL. Saturated fats in the diet can strongly influence cholesterol levels. Depending on individual differences, they raise VLDL and LDL levels. Trans fats, which are manufactured from vegetable oils and are used to enhance the taste and extend the shelf life of fast foods, are more atherogenic than saturated fats. Dietary cholesterol tends to increase LDL cholesterol.

Lipid-lowering drugs work in several ways, including decreasing cholesterol production, decreasing cholesterol absorption from the intestine, and removing cholesterol from the bloodstream. Drugs that act to directly decrease cholesterol levels also indirectly lower cholesterol levels by stimulating the production of additional LDL receptors. There currently are five major types of medications available for treating hypercholesterolemia: 3-hydroxy-3-methyl-glutaryl coenzyme A (HMG-CoA) reductase inhibitors (statins), bile acid–binding resins, cholesterol absorption inhibitor agents, niacin and its congeners, and the fibrates.[9,12] Inhibitors of HMG-CoA reductase, a key enzyme in the cholesterol biosynthetic pathway, can reduce or block the hepatic synthesis of cholesterol and are the cornerstone of LDL-reducing therapy. Statins also reduce triglyceride levels. The bile acid–binding resins bind and sequester cholesterol-containing bile acids in the intestine. This leads to increased production of LDL receptors by the liver, with resulting increased removal of cholesterol from the blood for synthesis of new bile acids. The cholesterol absorption inhibitor (ezetimibe) interferes with the absorption of cholesterol. Nicotinic acid, a niacin congener, blocks the synthesis and release of VLDL by the liver, thereby lowering not only VLDL levels but also IDL and LDL levels. Nicotinic acid also increases HDL concentrations up to 30%. The fibrates decrease the synthesis of VLDL by the liver and also enhance the clearance of triglycerides from the circulation.

Atherosclerosis

Atherosclerosis is a condition in which an artery wall thickens as a result of the accumulation of fatty materials. The term atherosclerosis, which comes from the Greek words atheros ("gruel" or "paste") and sclerosis ("hardness"), denotes the formation of fibrous plaque in the intimal lining of the large and medium-sized arteries such as the aorta and its branches, the coronary arteries, and the cerebral arteries that supply the brain (Fig. 18-6). The disorder, which remains a leading cause of coronary artery disease, stroke, and peripheral artery disease, can begin in the late teens, but usually takes decades to cause symptoms. Some people experience rapidly progressing atherosclerosis during their 30s, others during their 50s or 60s.

Epidemiology and Risk Factors

Atherosclerosis is a complex disorder. Although its exact cause is unknown, epidemiologic studies have identified predisposing risk factors (Chart 18-1).[1,2,6,11] Some of these are constitutional and cannot be changed, but others are affected by lifestyle and can be modified. The major risk factor, hypercholesterolemia, has both constitutional and lifestyle components.

Constitutional risk factors such as increasing age, male gender, and family history of premature coronary artery disease cannot be changed. The tendency toward the development of atherosclerosis appears to run in families. Persons who come from families with a strong history of heart disease or stroke due to atherosclerosis are at greater risk for developing atherosclerosis than those with a negative family history. Several genetically

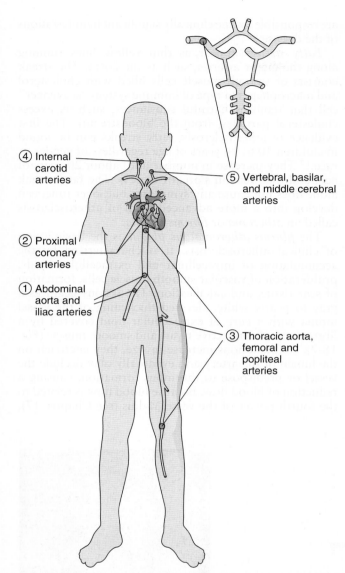

④ Internal carotid arteries

⑤ Vertebral, basilar, and middle cerebral arteries

② Proximal coronary arteries

① Abdominal aorta and iliac arteries

③ Thoracic aorta, femoral and popliteal arteries

FIGURE 18-6. Sites of severe atherosclerosis in order of frequency. (From Gotlieb AI, Lui A. Blood vessels. In: Rubin R, Strayer DS, eds. *Rubin's Pathology: Clinicopathologic Foundations of Medicine*, 6th ed. Philadelphia, PA: Wolters Kluwer Health/Lippincott Williams & Wilkins; 2012:452.)

CHART 18-1	**Risk Factors for Atherosclerosis**

Nonmodifiable
- Increasing age
- Male gender
- Genetic disorders of lipid metabolism
- Family history of premature coronary artery disease

Potentially Modifiable
- Cigarette smoking
- Obesity
- Hypertension
- Hyperlipidemia with elevated low-density lipoprotein and low high-density lipoprotein cholesterol
- Diabetes mellitus

Additional Nontraditional
- Inflammation marked by elevated C-reactive protein levels
- Hyperhomocysteinemia
- Increased lipoprotein (a) levels

cardiovascular risk factors. Smoking affects atherosclerosis by several mechanisms other than its unfavorable effects on blood pressure, sympathetic vascular tone, and reduction in myocardial oxygen supply.[6] It has adverse hemostatic and inflammatory effects and it may enhance the oxidation of LDL cholesterol, causing damage to the endothelial lining of blood vessels. Obesity, type 2 diabetes, high blood pressure, high blood triglycerides and low HDL levels (all components of the metabolic syndrome; see Chapter 33) often can be controlled with a change in health care behaviors and medications.

However, not all cases of atherosclerosis can be explained by the established genetic and environmental risk factors. Other so-called nontraditional risk factors have been associated with increased risk for development of atherosclerosis, including C-reactive protein (CRP), serum homocysteine, and lipoprotein (a).[6] There also has been increased interest in the possible connection between infectious agents (e.g., *Chlamydia pneumoniae*, herpesvirus, cytomegalovirus) and the development of vascular disease.[2] Genomic evidence of these organisms has been found in atherosclerotic lesions, but whether they are causally associated with lesions or simply enter the diseased vessel is unknown.[2]

Considerable interest in the role of inflammation in the etiology of atherosclerosis has emerged over the past two decades. C-reactive protein is an acute-phase reactant synthesized in the liver that is a marker for systemic inflammation (see Chapter 3). A number of population-based studies have demonstrated that baseline CRP levels can predict future cardiovascular events among apparently healthy individuals.[1] High-sensitivity CRP (hs-CRP) may be a better predictor of cardiovascular risk than lipid measurement alone.[6] Because CRP is an acute inflammatory phase reactant, major infections, trauma, or acute hospitalization can elevate CRP levels (usually 100-fold or more). Thus, CRP levels to determine cardiovascular risk should be performed when the person is clinically stable.

determined alterations in lipoprotein and cholesterol metabolism have been identified, and it seems likely that others will be identified in the future.[2] The incidence of atherosclerosis increases with age. Other factors being equal, men are at greater risk for the development of CAD than are premenopausal women, probably because of the protective effects of natural estrogens. After menopause, the incidence of atherosclerosis-related diseases in women increases, and by the seventh to eighth decade of life, the frequency of myocardial infarction in the two genders tends to equalize.[1]

The major risk factors that can be modified by a change in health care behaviors include cigarette smoking, obesity, hypertension, hyperlipidemia and elevated LDL cholesterol, and diabetes mellitus, all of which are traditional

Homocysteine is derived from the metabolism of dietary methionine, an amino acid that is abundant in animal protein. Homocysteine inhibits elements of the anticoagulant cascade and is associated with endothelial damage, which is thought to be an important first step in the development of atherosclerosis.[1,6] The normal metabolism of homocysteine requires adequate folate and vitamin B_6 intake, although the jury is still out on whether supplemental folate and vitamin B_6 can reduce the incidence of cardiovascular disease.[1] Homocystinuria, due to rare hereditary errors of metabolism, results in elevated homocysteine levels and premature cardiovascular disease.[1]

Lipoprotein(a) (Lp[a]), which is an altered form of LDL that contains apoB-100 linked to apoA, is considered to be an independent risk factor for the development of atherosclerosis.[1,2] Lp(a) enhances cholesterol delivery to injured blood vessels, suppresses the generation of plasmin, and promotes smooth muscle proliferation. Lipoprotein(a) levels are heritable and are not altered by most cholesterol-lowering drugs.[2]

Pathogenesis and Mechanisms of Development

The lesions associated with atherosclerosis are of three different stages or subtypes: fatty streaks, fibrous atheromatous plaques, and complicated lesions. The latter two are responsible for the clinically significant manifestations of the disease.[1,2,14]

Fatty streaks appear as thin yellow lines running along the major arteries, such as the aorta. The streak consists of smooth muscle cells filled with cholesterol and macrophages (a type of immune system "scavenger" cell that removes harmful substances, such as excess cholesterol particles, from the bloodstream). The first evidence of atherosclerosis, fatty streaks can be found in children 10 to 14 years of age regardless of gender or race.[1,2] They increase in number until about 20 years of age, and then remain static or regress. The fatty streak alone does not cause any symptoms but, over time, can develop into a more advanced form of atherosclerosis called an *atheroma* or *fibrous plaque*.

The *fibrous atheromatous plaque* is the basic lesion of clinical atherosclerosis. It is characterized by the accumulation of intracellular and extracellular lipids, proliferation of vascular smooth muscle cells, formation of scar tissue, and calcification. The lesions begin as a gray to pearly white, elevated thickening of the vessel intima with a core of extracellular lipid covered by a fibrous cap of connective tissue and smooth muscle (Fig. 18-7). As the lesions increase in size, they encroach on the lumen of the artery and eventually may occlude the vessel or predispose to thrombus formation, causing a reduction of blood flow. Because blood flow is related to the fourth power of the vessel radius (see Chapter 17),

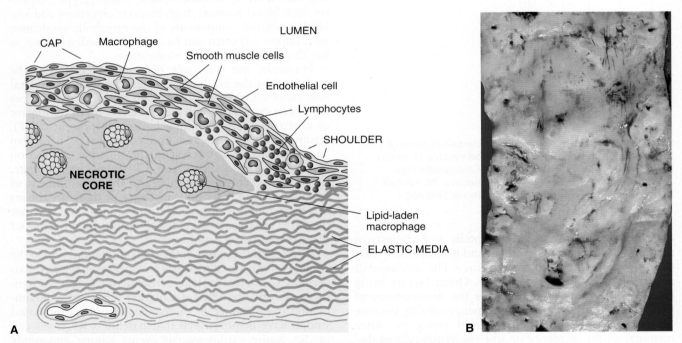

FIGURE 18-7. Fibrofatty plaque of atherosclerosis. **(A)** In this fully developed fibrous plaque, the core contains lipid-filled macrophages and necrotic smooth muscle cell debris. The "fibrous" cap is composed largely of smooth muscle cells, which produce collagen, small amounts of elastin, and glycosaminoglycans. Also shown are infiltrating macrophages and lymphocytes. Note that the endothelium over the surface of the fibrous cap frequently appears intact. **(B)** The aorta shows discrete raised, tan plaques. Focal plaque ulcerations are also evident. (From Gotlieb AI, Lui A. Blood vessels. In: Rubin R, Strayer DS, eds. *Rubin's Pathology: Clinicopathologic Foundations of Medicine*, 6th ed. Philadelphia, PA: Wolters Kluwer Health/Lippincott Williams & Wilkins; 2012:447–448.)

the reduction in blood flow becomes increasingly greater as the disease progresses.

Complicated atherosclerotic lesions develop when the fibrous plaque breaks open, producing hemorrhage, ulceration, and scar tissue deposits. Thrombosis is the most important complication of atherosclerosis. It is caused by slowing and turbulence of blood flow in the region of the plaque and ulceration of the plaque.

Although the risk factors associated with atherosclerosis have been identified through epidemiologic studies, many unanswered questions remain regarding the mechanisms that contribute to the development of atherosclerotic lesions. The vascular endothelial layer, which consists of a single layer of cells with cell-to-cell attachments, normally serves as a selective barrier that protects the subendothelial layers by interacting with blood cells and other blood components. One hypothesis of plaque formation suggests that injury to the endothelial vessel layer is the initiating factor.[1,2] A number of factors are regarded as possible injurious agents, including products associated with smoking, immune mechanisms, and mechanical stress such as that associated with hypertension. The fact that atherosclerotic lesions tend to form where vessels branch or where there is turbulent flow suggests that hemodynamic factors may also play a role.

Hyperlipidemia, particularly elevated LDL, is also believed to play an active role in the pathogenesis of the atherosclerotic lesion. Interactions between the endothelial layer of the vessel wall and white blood cells, particularly the monocytes (blood macrophages), normally occur throughout life; these interactions increase when blood cholesterol levels are elevated. One of the earliest responses to elevated cholesterol levels is the attachment of monocytes to the endothelium. The monocytes have been observed to move through the cell-to-cell attachments of the endothelial layer into the subendothelial spaces, where they are transformed into macrophages.

Activated macrophages release free radicals that oxidize LDL, which in turn is toxic to the endothelium, causing endothelial cell loss and exposure of the subendothelial tissue to blood components. This leads to platelet adhesion and aggregation and fibrin deposition. Platelets and activated macrophages release various factors that are thought to modulate the proliferation of smooth muscle cells and the deposition of extracellular matrix in the lesions.[1,2,14] Activated macrophages also ingest the oxidized LDL to become foam cells, which are present in all stages of atherosclerotic plaque formation. Some of these cells die in place, releasing their fat and cholesterol-laden membranes into the intercellular space. This attracts more macrophages. Lipids released from necrotic foam cells accumulate to form unstable plaques (also known as vulneral plaque). Unstable plaques typically are characterized histologically by a large central lipid core, an inflammatory infiltrate, and a thin fibrous cap. These vulnerable plaques are at risk of rupture, often at the shoulder of the plaque (see Fig. 18-7A) where the fibrous cap is thinnest and the mechanical stresses highest.[2,14]

Clinical Manifestations

Atherosclerosis usually doesn't cause signs and symptoms until it severely narrows or totally blocks an artery. Many people don't know they have the disease until they have a medical emergency, such as a heart attack or stroke. Signs and symptoms will depend on the vessels involved and the extent of vessel obstruction. Atherosclerotic lesions produce their effects through narrowing of the vessel and production of ischemia; sudden vessel obstruction due to plaque hemorrhage or rupture; thrombosis and formation of emboli resulting from damage to the vessel endothelium; and aneurysm formation due to weakening of the vessel wall.[1,2] In larger vessels, such as the aorta, the important complications are those of thrombus formation and weakening of the vessel wall. In medium-sized arteries, such as the coronary and cerebral arteries, ischemia and infarction due to vessel occlusion are more common. Although atherosclerosis can affect any organ or tissue, the arteries supplying the heart, brain, kidneys, lower extremities, and small intestine are most frequently involved (see Fig. 18-6).

Vasculitis

The vasculitides are a group of vascular disorders that cause inflammatory injury and necrosis of the blood vessel wall.[1,2,15,16] Vessels of any type in virtually any organ can be affected, resulting in a broad spectrum of signs and symptoms. Because they may affect veins and capillaries, the terms *vasculitis, angiitis,* and *arteritis* often are used interchangeably. Besides the finding referable to the specific tissue or organ involved, the clinical manifestations typically include constitutional signs and symptoms such as fever, myalgia, arthralgia, and malaise.

The two most common pathogenic mechanisms of vasculitis are direct invasion of the vascular wall by an infectious agent and immune-mediated inflammation.[1] The most common mechanisms that initiate noninfectious vasculitis are pathological immune responses that result in endothelial activation, with subsequent vessel obstruction, and ischemia of the dependent tissue. In almost all forms of vasculitis, the triggering event initiating and driving the inflammatory process is unknown.[2,16]

A number of persons with vasculitis have circulating antibodies called *antineutrophil cytoplasmic antibodies* (ANCAs) that react with antigens in the cytoplasm of neutrophils.[1] Although the precise pathologic mechanism is unknown, these antibodies may serve to initiate an inflammatory state that continually recruits and stimulates neutrophils to release reactive oxygen species and proteolytic enzymes.[1] Serum ANCA titers, which can correlate with disease activity, may serve as a useful quantitative diagnostic marker for ANCA-associated vasculitides.

The vasculitides are commonly classified based on etiology, pathologic findings, and prognosis. One

(*text continues on page 414*)

UNDERSTANDING → Development of

Atherosclerosis is characterized by the development of atheromatous lesions within the intimal lining of the large- and medium-sized arteries that protrude into and can eventually obstruct blood flow. The development of atherosclerotic lesions is a progressive process involving (1) endothelial cell injury, (2) migration of inflammatory cells, (3) smooth muscle cell proliferation and lipid deposition, and (4) gradual development of the atheromatous plaque with a lipid core.

1

Endothelial Cell Injury. The vascular endothelium consists of a single layer of cells with cell-to-cell attachments, which normally resist attachment of the white blood cells and other blood components streaming past them. Agents such as smoking, elevated low-density lipoprotein (LDL) levels, immune mechanisms, and mechanical stress associated with hypertension share the potential for causing endothelial injury with adhesion of monocytes and platelets.

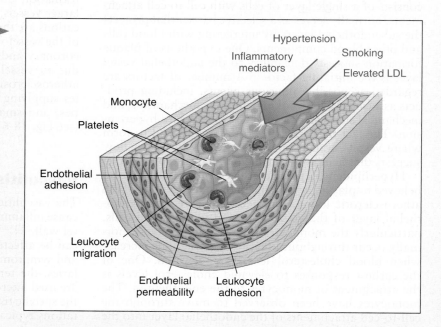

2

Migration of Inflammatory Cells. Early in the development of atherosclerotic lesions, endothelial cells begin to express selective adhesion molecules that capture monocytes and other inflammatory cells that initiate the development of atherosclerotic lesions. After monocytes adhere to the endothelium, they migrate between the endothelial cells to localize in the intima, transform into macrophages, and engulf lipoproteins, largely LDL particales.

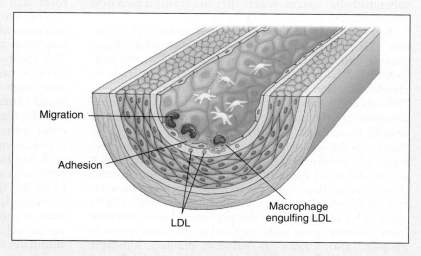

Atherosclerosis

3 **Lipid Accumulation and Smooth Muscle Cell Proliferation.** Although the recruitment of monocytes to the arterial wall and their subsequent differentiation into activated macrophages that remove LDL from the circulation is protective, it also contributes to the development of atherosclerosis. Activated macrophages release toxic oxygen species that oxidize LDL. The oxidized LDL is then aggressively ingested by the macrophages through scavenger receptors on their plasma membrane, resulting in the formation of foam cells, which are the primary component of atherosclerotic lesions. Activated macrophages also produce growth factors that contribute to the migration and proliferation of smooth muscle cells (SMCs) and the elaboration of extracellular matrix (ECM).

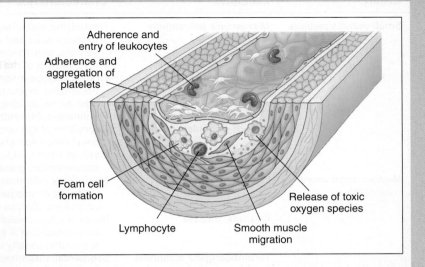

4 **Plaque Structure.** Atherosclerotic plaques consist of an aggregation of SMCs, macrophages, and other leukocytes; ECM, including collagen and elastic fibers; and intracellular and extracellular lipids. Typically, the superficial fibrous cap is composed of SMCs and dense ECM. Immediately beneath and to the side of the fibrous cap is a cellular area (the shoulder) consisting of macrophages, SMCs, and lymphocytes. Below the fibrous cap is a central core of lipid-laden foam cells and fatty debris. Rupture, ulceration, or erosion of an unstable or vulnerable fibrous cap may lead to hemorrhage into the plaque or thrombotic occlusion of the vessel lumen.

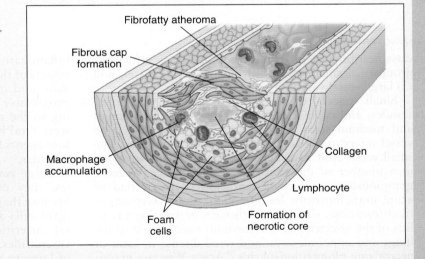

TABLE 18-3	**Classification of the Vasculitides**	
Group	**Examples**	**Characteristics**
Small vessel vasculitis	Microscopic polyangiitis	Necrotizing vasculitis with few or no immune deposits affecting medium-sized and small blood vessels, including capillaries, venules, and arterioles; necrotizing glomerulonephritis and involvement of the pulmonary capillaries is common
	Wegener granulomatosis	Granulomatous inflammation involving the respiratory tract and necrotizing vasculitis affecting capillaries, venules, arterioles, and arteries; necrotizing glomerulonephritis is common, associated with antineutrophil cytoplasmic antibodies (ANCA)
	Henoch–Schönlein purpura	Deposition of IgA-containing immune complexes; inflammation of small blood vessels; form of Type III hypersensitivity
	Churg-Strauss syndrome	Involves arteries of lung and skin; may be generalized, vascular and extravascular; granulomatosis; medium-sized and small vessels
Medium-sized vessel vasculitis	Polyarteritis nodosa	Necrotizing inflammation of medium-sized or small arteries without vasculitis in arteries, capillaries, or venules; usually associated with underlying disease or environmental agents
	Kawasaki disease	Involves large, medium-sized, and small arteries (frequently the coronaries) and is associated with mucocutaneous lymph node syndrome; usually occurs in small children
	Thromboangiitis obliterans	Segmental, thrombosing, acute, and chronic inflammation of the medium-sized and small arteries, principally the tibial and radial arteries but sometimes extending to the veins and nerves of the extremities; occurs almost exclusively in men who are heavy smokers
Large vessel vasculitis	Giant cell (temporal) arteritis	Granulomatous inflammation of the aorta and its major branches with predilection for extracranial vessels of the carotid artery; infiltration of vessel wall with giant cells and mononuclear cells; usually occurs in people older than 50 years of age and is often associated with polymyalgia rheumatica
	Takayasu arteritis	Granulomatous inflammation of the aorta and its branches; usually occurs in people younger than 50 years of age

(text continued from page 411)

classification system divides the conditions into three groups: (1) small vessel, (2) medium-sized vessel, and (3) large vessel vasculitides (Table 18-3).[1,2]

Small vessel refers to small arteries, arterioles, venules, and capillaries; medium vessel refers to small and medium–sized arteries and arterioles; and large vessel refers to the aorta and its major tributaries. The small vessel ANCA-associated vasculitides are involved in a number of different diseases, including Wegener granulomatosis, which is characterized by a triad of acute granulomatous lesions of the upper respiratory tract (ear, nose, sinuses, and throat), necrotizing vasculitis of the affected small to medium sized vessels of the lungs and upper airways, and renal disease in form of necrotizing glomerulonephritis.[1] Acute Wegener granulomatosis is potentially life-threatening and requires initial treatment with corticosteroids combined with a cytotoxic agent.

Medium-sized vessel vasculitides produce necrotizing damage to medium-sized muscular arteries of major organ systems. This group includes polyarteritis nodosa, Kawasaki disease (discussed in Chapter 19), and thromboangiitis obliterans (discussed in the section on arterial disease of the extremities). Polyarteritis nodosa is an uncommon, acute multisystem inflammatory disease of small and medium-sized blood vessels of the kidney, liver, intestine, peripheral nerves, skin, and muscle. The usual course of the disease is progressive with various signs and symptoms according to the pattern of organ involvement. Most cases were fatal before corticosteroid and immunosuppressant agents became available for use in treatment of the disorder.[1]

Large vessel vasculitides involve large elastic arteries; they commonly are called *giant cell arterides* because they involve infiltration of the vessel wall with giant cells and mononuclear cells. Giant cell (temporal) arteritis, the most common of the large vessel vasculitides, is an acute and chronic inflammation of large to small arteries. It mainly affects arteries of the head—especially the temporal arteries—but may include the vertebral and ophthalmic arteries. About half of persons with the disease have accompanying pain and stiffness of the shoulder and hip (polymyalgia rheumatica; see Chapter 44). The most common clinical presentation is headache and tenderness over the superficial temporal artery. Diagnosis followed by treatment with corticosteroid drugs is important because involvement of the ophthalmic artery can cause blindness.[1,2]

Arterial Disease of the Extremities

Disorders of the circulation in the extremities often are referred to as *peripheral vascular disorders*.[17] In many respects, the disorders that affect arteries in the extremities are the same as those affecting the coronary and cerebral arteries in that they produce ischemia, pain, impaired function, and in some cases infarction and tissue necrosis. Not only are the effects similar, but the pathologic conditions that impair circulation in the extremities are also identical. This section focuses on peripheral arterial disease, thromboangiitis obliterans, and Raynaud phenomenon.

Peripheral Arterial Disease

Peripheral artery disease (PAD) refers to the obstruction of large arteries that supply the body's peripheral structures rather than its central structures such as the heart or brain. Often PAD is a term used to refer to atherosclerotic blockages found in the lower extremities. Peripheral artery disease can result from atherosclerosis, inflammatory processes leading to stenosis, embolism, or thrombus formation. It causes either acute or chronic ischemia. The disease is seen most commonly in men in their 60s and 70s. The risk factors for PAD are similar to those for coronary artery disease. Cigarette smoking and diabetes mellitus are the strongest risk factors, with more than 80% of persons with the disorder being current or former smokers.[17]

As with atherosclerosis in other locations, the signs and symptoms of vessel occlusion are gradual. The primary symptom of chronic obstructive arterial disease is pain with walking or *claudication* (from the Latin verb claudicare, "to limp").[18] Typically, persons with the disorder complain of calf pain because the gastrocnemius muscle has the highest oxygen consumption of any muscle group in the leg during walking. Some persons may complain of a vague aching feeling or numbness, rather than pain. Other activities such as swimming, bicycling, and climbing stairs use other muscle groups and may not incite the same degree of discomfort as walking. Other signs of ischemia include atrophic changes and thinning of the skin and subcutaneous tissues of the lower leg and diminution in the size of the leg muscles. The foot often is cool, and the popliteal and pedal pulses are weak or absent. Limb color blanches with elevation of the leg because of the effects of gravity on perfusion pressure and becomes deep red when the leg is in the dependent position because of an autoregulatory increase in blood flow and a gravitational increase in perfusion pressure.

When blood flow is reduced to the extent that it no longer meets the minimal needs of resting muscle and nerves, ischemic pain at rest, ulceration, and gangrene develop. As tissue necrosis develops there typically is severe pain in the region of skin breakdown, which is worse at night with limb elevation and is improved with standing.

Diagnostic methods include inspection of the limbs for signs of chronic low-grade ischemia such as subcutaneous atrophy, brittle toenails, hair loss, pallor, coolness, or dependent rubor. Palpation of the femoral, popliteal, posterior tibial, and dorsalis pedis pulses allows for an estimation of the level and degree of obstruction. The ratio of ankle to arm (i.e., tibial and brachial arteries) systolic blood pressure is used to detect significant obstruction, with a ratio of less than 0.9 indicating occlusion. Blood pressures may be taken at various levels on the leg to determine the level of obstruction. A Doppler ultrasound stethoscope may be used for detecting pulses and measuring blood pressure. Ultrasound imaging, magnetic resonance imaging (MRI) arteriography, spiral computed tomographic (CT) arteriography, and invasive contrast angiography also may be used as diagnostic methods.[17,18]

Treatment includes measures directed at protection of the affected tissues and preservation of functional capacity. Walking (slowly) to the point of claudication usually is encouraged because it increases collateral circulation. Avoidance of injury is important because tissues of extremities affected by atherosclerosis are easily injured and slow to heal. It is important to address other cardiovascular risk factors such as smoking, hypertension, hyperlipidemia, and diabetes. Drug therapy includes antiplatelet therapy (e.g., aspirin or clopidogrel). Other medications that are useful include statins, cilostazol (a vasodilator with antiplatelet properties), and pentoxifylline (an antiplatelet agent that decreases blood viscosity and improves erythrocyte flexibility). Percutaneous or surgical intervention is typically reserved for the patient with disabling claudication or limb-threatening ischemia. Surgery (i.e., femoropopliteal bypass grafting using a section of saphenous vein) may be indicated in severe cases. Percutaneous transluminal angioplasty and stent placement, in which a balloon catheter is inserted into the area of stenosis and the balloon inflated to increase vessel diameter, is another form of treatment.[17,18]

Thromboangiitis Obliterans

Thromboangiitis obliterans, also known as *Buerger disease*, is a recurring progressive, nonatherosclerotic inflammation and thrombosis of small and medium-sized arteries and veins, usually the plantar and digital vessels in the foot and lower leg.[1,2,19,20] Arteries in the arm and hand also may be affected. Although primarily an arterial disorder, the inflammatory process often extends to involve adjacent veins and nerves. Usually it is a disease of young, heavy cigarette smokers, occurring before the age of 35. The pathogenesis of Buerger disease remains elusive, though cigarette smoking and in some instances tobacco chewing seem to be involved. It has been suggested that the tobacco may trigger an immune response in susceptible persons or it may unmask a clotting defect, either of which could incite an inflammatory reaction of the vessel wall.[19] It is more common in the Mediterranean region, Middle East, and Asia.[1,2]

Pain is the predominant symptom of the disorder. It usually is related to distal arterial ischemia. During the early stages of the disease, there is intermittent claudication in the arch of the foot and the digits. In severe cases, pain is present even when the person is at rest.

The impaired circulation increases sensitivity to cold. The peripheral pulses are diminished or absent, and there are changes in the color of the extremity. In moderately advanced cases, the extremity becomes cyanotic when the person assumes a dependent position, and the digits may turn reddish-blue even when in a nondependent position. With lack of blood flow, the skin becomes thin and shiny, hair growth slows, and nail growth is impaired. Chronic ischemia causes thick, malformed nails. If the disease continues to progress, tissues eventually ulcerate and gangrenous changes arise that may necessitate amputation[2] (Fig. 18-8).

Diagnostic methods are similar to those for atherosclerotic disease of the lower extremities. It is essential that the person stop smoking cigarettes or using tobacco. Even passive smoking and nicotine replacement therapy should be eliminated. Other treatment measures are of secondary importance and focus on methods for producing vasodilation and preventing tissue injury. Sympathectomy, or excision of a segment of a sympathetic nerve, may be done to alleviate the vasospastic manifestations of the disease. As the distal arterial tree is occluded, revascularization is not possible. If smoking cessation is not achieved, then the prognosis is generally poor, with amputation of both lower and upper extremities the eventual outcome.

Raynaud Phenomenon

Raynaud phenomenon is a functional disorder caused by intense vasospasm of the arteries and arterioles in the fingers and, less often, the toes.[1,2,21,22] The disorder is divided into primary and secondary types.

Primary Raynaud phenomenon is seen in otherwise healthy young women, and it often is precipitated by exposure to cold or by strong emotions and usually is limited to the fingers. The cause of vasospasm in primary Raynaud phenomenon is unknown or idiopathic.

Hyperreactivity of the sympathetic nervous system has been suggested as a contributing cause. Secondary Raynaud phenomenon is associated with previous vessel injury, such as frostbite, occupational trauma associated with the use of heavy vibrating tools, collagen diseases, neurologic disorders, chronic arterial occlusive disorders, and drugs, such as bleomycin. Another occupation-related cause is the exposure to alternating hot and cold temperatures such as that experienced by butchers and food preparers. Raynaud phenomenon often is the first symptom of collagen diseases. It occurs in almost all persons with scleroderma and can precede the diagnosis of scleroderma by many years.[22]

The ischemic phase of Raynaud phenomenon is manifested by changes in skin color that progress from pallor to cyanosis, a sensation of cold, and changes in sensory perception, such as numbness and tingling. The color changes usually are first noticed in the tips of the fingers, later moving into one or more of the distal phalanges (Fig. 18-9). After the ischemic episode, there is a period of hyperemia with intense redness, throbbing, and paresthesias. The period of hyperemia is followed by a return to normal color. Primary Raynaud phenomenon attacks typically involve all fingers in a symmetric fashion and are associated with minimal pain, whereas asymmetric finger involvement and intense pain suggest secondary Raynaud phenomenon.[21,22] In severe progressive cases, trophic skin changes may develop. The nails may become brittle, and the skin over the tips of the affected fingers may thicken. Ulceration and superficial gangrene of the fingers, although infrequent, may occur.

The initial diagnosis is based on a history of vasospastic attacks supported by other evidence of the disorder. Immersion of the hand in cold water may be used to initiate an attack as an aid to diagnosis. Laser Doppler flow velocimetry may be used to quantify digital blood flow during changes in temperature. Primary Raynaud phenomenon is differentiated from secondary Raynaud

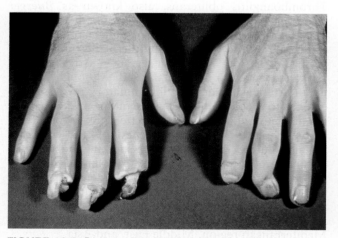

FIGURE 18-8. Buerger disease. Hand showing necrosis of the tips of the fingers. Temporal arteritis. (From Gotlieb AI, Lui A. Blood vessels. In: Rubin R, Strayer DS, eds. *Rubin's Pathology: Clinicopathologic Foundations of Medicine*, 6th ed. Philadelphia, PA: Wolters Kluwer Health/Lippincott Williams & Wilkins; 2012:446.)

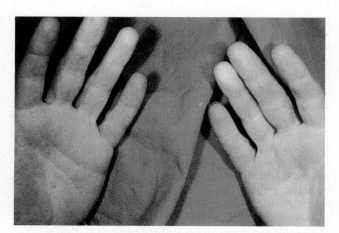

FIGURE 18-9. Raynaud phenomenon. The tips of the fingers show marked pallor. (From Gotlieb AI, Lui A. Blood vessels. In: Rubin R, Strayer DS, eds. *Rubin's Pathology: Clinicopathologic Foundations of Medicine*, 6th ed. Philadelphia, PA: Wolters Kluwer Health/Lippincott Williams & Wilkins; 2012:463.)

phenomenon by excluding other disorders known to cause vasospasm.

Treatment measures are directed toward eliminating factors that cause vasospasm and protecting the digits from trauma during an ischemic episode. Abstinence from smoking and protection from cold are priorities. The entire body must be protected from cold, not just the extremities. Avoidance of emotional stress is another important factor in controlling the disorder because anxiety and stress may precipitate a vascular spasm in predisposed persons. Vasoconstrictor medications, such as the decongestants contained in allergy and cold preparations, should be avoided. Treatment with vasodilator drugs may be indicated, particularly if episodes are frequent, because frequency encourages the potential for development of thrombosis and gangrene. A recent advancement in the treatment of Raynaud phenomenon therapy is phosphodiesterase inhibitors (e.g., sildenafil, tadalfil, vardenafil) that produce arterial vasodilation. Surgical interruption of sympathetic nerve pathways (sympathectomy) may be used for persons with severe symptoms.[21]

Aneurysms and Dissection

Aneurysm is a pathological outpouching or sac-like dilatation in the wall of a blood vessel usually caused by weakening of the vessel wall. Aneurysms can occur in arteries and veins, but they are most common in the arteries. There are two types of aneurysms.[1,23] A *true aneurysm* is bounded by a complete vessel wall. The blood in a true aneurysm remains within the vascular compartment. A *false aneurysm* represents a localized dissection or tear in the inner wall of the artery with formation of an extravascular hematoma that causes vessel enlargement (Fig. 18-10B). Unlike true aneurysms, false aneurysms are bounded only by the outer layers of the vessel wall or supporting tissues.

Aneurysms can assume several forms and may be classified according to their cause, location, and anatomic features (Fig. 18-10). A *berry aneurysm* consists of a small, spherical dilation of the vessel at a bifurcation (Fig. 18-10A).[1,2] This type of aneurysm usually is found in the circle of Willis in the cerebral circulation. A *fusiform aneurysm* involves the entire circumference of the vessel and is characterized by a gradual and progressive dilation of the vessel (Fig. 18-10C). These aneurysms, which vary in diameter (up to 20 cm) and length, may involve the entire ascending and transverse portions of the thoracic aorta or may extend over large segments of the abdominal aorta. A *saccular aneurysm* extends over part of the circumference of the vessel and appears saclike. A *dissecting aneurysm* is a false aneurysm resulting from a tear in the intimal layer of the vessel that allows blood to enter the vessel wall, dissecting its layers to create a blood-filled cavity.

The weakness that leads to aneurysm formation may be caused by a number of factors, including congenital defects, trauma, infections, and atherosclerosis. Once initiated, the aneurysm grows larger as the tension in

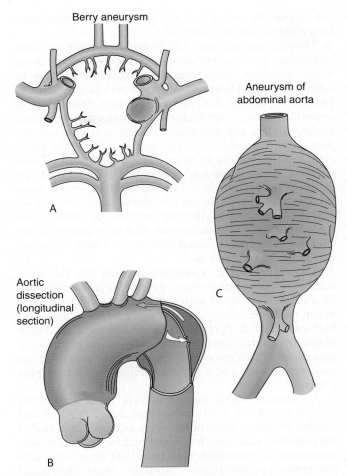

FIGURE 18-10. Three forms of aneurysms: **(A)** berry aneurysm in the circle of Willis, **(B)** aortic dissection, and **(C)** fusiform-type aneurysm of the abdominal aorta.

the vessel increases. This is because the tension in the wall of a vessel is equal to the pressure multiplied by the radius (i.e., tension = pressure × radius; see Chapter 17). In this case, the pressure in the segment of the vessel affected by the aneurysm does not change but remains the same as that of adjacent portions of the vessel. As an aneurysm increases in diameter, the tension in the wall of the vessel increases in direct proportion to its increased size. If untreated, the aneurysm may rupture because of the increased tension. Even an unruptured aneurysm can cause damage by exerting pressure on adjacent structures and interrupting blood flow.

Aortic Aneurysms

Aortic aneurysms may involve any part of the aorta: the ascending aorta, aortic arch, descending aorta, thoracoabdominal aorta, or abdominal aorta. Multiple aneurysms may be present. The signs and symptoms of aortic aneurysms depend on the size and location. With both thoracic and abdominal aneurysms, the most dreaded complication is rupture. The likelihood of rupture correlates with increasing aneurysm size. The risk of rupture rises from less than 2% for small abdominal aneurysms

(<4 cm in diameter) to 11% per year for aneurysms larger than 5 cm in diameter.[1]

Thoracic aneurysms, which are less common than abdominal aortic aneurysms, may involve one or more aortic segments. Most thoracic aneurysms are due to atherosclerosis. Disorders of connective tissue, such as Marfan syndrome (Chapter 6), are rare causes but of important clinical significance. The majority of thoracic aneurysms are asymptomatic. When symptoms occur, they depend largely on the size and position of the aneurysm. Substernal, back, or neck pain may occur. There may be dyspnea, stridor, or a brassy cough caused by pressure on the trachea. Hoarseness may result from pressure on the recurrent laryngeal nerve, and there may be difficulty swallowing because of pressure on the esophagus.[23] The aneurysm also may compress the superior vena cava, causing distention of neck veins and edema of the face and neck.

Abdominal aortic aneurysms, which are the most common type of aneurysm, usually develop after age 50 and are associated with severe atherosclerosis. They occur more frequently in men than women, and over half of affected persons are hypertensive. Although abdominal aortic aneurysms usually occur in the context of atherosclerosis, it is thought that other factors such as smoking and a genetic predisposition may play a role.[2,24]

Abdominal aortic aneurysms are most commonly located below the level of the renal artery (>90%) and involve the bifurcation of the aorta and proximal end of the common iliac arteries.[1,2] They can involve any part of the vessel circumference (saccular) or extend to involve the entire circumference (fusiform). Most abdominal aneurysms are asymptomatic. Because an aneurysm is of arterial origin, a pulsating mass may provide the first evidence of the disorder. Typically, aneurysms larger than 4 cm are palpable. The mass may be discovered during a routine physical examination or the affected person may complain of its presence. Calcification, which frequently exists on the wall of the aneurysm, may be detected during abdominal radiologic examination. Pain may be present and varies from mild midabdominal or lumbar discomfort to severe abdominal and back pain. As the aneurysm expands, it may compress the lumbar nerve roots, causing lower back pain that radiates to the posterior aspects of the legs. The aneurysm may extend to and impinge on the renal, iliac, or mesenteric arteries, or to the vertebral arteries that supply the spinal cord. An abdominal aneurysm also may cause erosion of vertebrae. Stasis of blood favors thrombus formation along the wall of the vessel (Fig. 18-11), and peripheral emboli may develop, causing symptomatic arterial insufficiency.

Diagnostic methods include ultrasonography, echocardiography, CT scans, and MRI. Unruptured aneurysms are generally asymptomatic and are often diagnosed incidentally during clinical examination. Measures to slow aneurysm growth and lower the risk of rupture include risk factor modification. Hypercholesterolemia and high blood pressure should be controlled and smoking discontinued. Surgical repair,

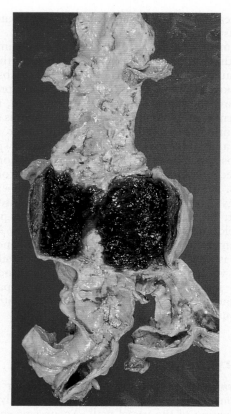

FIGURE 18-11. Atherosclerotic aneurysm of the abdominal aorta. The aneurysm has been opened longitudinally to reveal a large thrombus in the lumen. The aorta and common iliac arteries display complicated lesions of atherosclerosis. (From Gotlieb AI, Lui A. Blood vessels. In: Rubin R, Strayer DS, eds. *Rubin's Pathology: Clinicopathologic Foundations of Medicine*, 6th ed. Philadelphia, PA: Wolters Kluwer Health/Lippincott Williams & Wilkins; 2012:471.)

in which the involved section of the aorta is replaced with a synthetic graft of woven Dacron, frequently is the treatment of choice.[23,24]

Aortic Dissection

Aortic dissection (dissecting aneurysm) is an acute, life-threatening condition.[1,2,28] It involves hemorrhage into the vessel wall with longitudinal tearing of the vessel wall to form a blood-filled channel (see Fig. 18-10B). Unlike atherosclerotic aneurysms, aortic dissection often occurs without evidence of previous vessel dilation. The dissection can originate anywhere along the length of the aorta but most often involves the ascending aorta.

Aortic dissection is caused by conditions that weaken or cause degenerative changes in the elastic and smooth muscle layers of the aorta. There are two risk factors that predispose to aortic dissection: hypertension and degeneration of the medial layer of the vessel wall. It is most common in 40- to 60-year-old men with an antecedent history of hypertension.[1] Aortic dissection also is associated with connective tissue diseases, such as

Marfan syndrome. It also may occur during pregnancy because of changes in the aorta that occur during this time. Other factors that predispose to dissection are congenital defects of the aortic valve (i.e., bicuspid or unicuspid valve structures) and aortic coarctation.

Aortic dissections are commonly classified into two types, A and B, as determined by the level of dissection.[1,25] Type A aneurysms, which involve the proximal aorta (ascending aorta only or both the ascending and the descending aorta), are the most common and potentially serious in terms of complications. Type B aneurysms usually begin distal to the subclavian artery and do not involve the ascending aorta. Dissections usually extend distally from the intimal tear. When the ascending aorta is involved, expansion of the wall of the aorta may impair closure of the aortic valve. There also is the risk of aortic rupture with blood moving into the pericardium and compressing the heart. Although the length of dissection varies, it is possible for the abdominal aorta to be involved with progression into the renal, iliac, or femoral arteries. Partial or complete occlusion of the arteries that arise from the aortic arch or the intercostal or lumbar arteries may lead to stroke, ischemic peripheral neuropathy, or impaired blood flow to the spinal cord.

A major symptom of a dissecting aneurysm is the abrupt presence of excruciating pain, described as tearing or ripping.[1,2,25] Pain associated with dissection of the ascending aorta frequently is located in the anterior chest, and pain associated with dissection of the descending aorta often is located in the back. In the early stages, blood pressure typically is moderately or markedly elevated. Later, the blood pressure and pulse rate become unobtainable in one or both arms as the dissection disrupts arterial flow to the arms. Syncope, hemiplegia, or paralysis of the lower extremities may occur because of occlusion of blood vessels that supply the brain or spinal cord. Heart failure may develop when the aortic valve is involved.

Diagnosis of aortic dissection is based on history and physical examination. Aortic angiography, transesophageal echocardiography, CT scans, and MRI studies aid in the diagnosis. The treatment of dissecting aortic aneurysm may be medical or surgical. Aortic dissection is a life-threatening emergency; persons with a probable diagnosis are stabilized medically even before the diagnosis is confirmed. Two important factors that participate in propagating the dissection are high blood pressure and the steepness of the pulse wave. Without intervention, these forces produce continued extension of the dissection. Medical treatment therefore focuses on control of hypertension and the use of drugs that lessen the force of systolic blood ejection from the heart.[25] Two commonly used drugs, often given in combination, are an intravenous β-adrenergic blocking drug and sodium nitroprusside (a vasodilator). Adequate pain control is necessary to alleviate anxiety and relieve sympathetic stimulation, which will raise blood pressure. Surgical treatment consists of resection of the involved segment of the aorta and replacement with a prosthetic graft. Despite recent advances in diagnosis and treatment, the mortality rate in acute aortic dissection remains high.

SUMMARY CONCEPTS

- Disorders of the arterial circulation produce ischemia due to narrowing and obstruction of blood vessels, thrombus formation associated with platelet adhesion, and weakening of the vessel wall with development of an aneurysm.

- Cholesterol and triglycerides are transported within lipoproteins, macromolecules made up of a hydrophobic lipid core surrounded by an apoprotein-containing outer shell. The high-density lipoproteins (HDLs), which are protective, remove cholesterol from the tissues and carry it back to the liver for disposal. The low-density lipoproteins (LDLs) carry cholesterol to the liver and extrahepatic tissues to be removed from the blood. Low-density lipoproteins that are not removed from the blood are taken up by phagocytic scavenger cells in the arterial wall, leading to an accumulation of cholesterol-laden macrophages and development of atherosclerosis.

- Atherosclerosis is a progressive arterial disease characterized by the formation of fibrofatty plaques in the inner lining of large and medium-sized arteries, including the aorta, coronary arteries, and cerebral vessels. The major risk factors for development of atherosclerosis are hypercholesterolemia and inflammation.

- The vasculitides are a group of vascular disorders characterized by inflammation and necrosis of the blood vessels in various tissues and organs of the body. The inflammatory process may be initiated by direct injury, infectious agents, or immune mechanisms.

- The peripheral arterial disorders, such as Raynaud phenomenon and Buerger disease, interrupt arterial flow of blood and interfere with the delivery of oxygen and nutrients to the tissues. Occlusion of flow can result from a thrombus or emboli, vessel compression, vasospasm, or structural changes in the vessel.

- Aneurysms are localized areas of vessel dilation caused by weakness of the arterial wall. A berry aneurysm is a small spherical dilation usually found in the circle of Willis in the cerebral circulation. The most serious consequence of thoracic and abdominal aortic aneurysms is rupture. A dissecting aneurysm is an acute, life-threatening condition. It involves tearing (dissection) of the tunica intima, which allows formation of a blood-filled channel between the layers of the vessel and reduces blood flow through the vessel's true lumen.

Disorders of Arterial Blood Pressure

The arterial blood pressure reflects the rhythmic ejection of blood from the left ventricle into the aorta.[26] It rises as the left ventricle contracts and falls as it relaxes. In healthy adults, the highest pressure, called the *systolic pressure,* is ideally less than 120 mm Hg and the lowest pressure, called the *diastolic pressure,* is less than 80 mm Hg (Fig. 18-12). The difference between the systolic and diastolic pressure is called the *pulse pressure* (approximately 40 mm Hg). The pulse pressure reflects the pulsatile nature of arterial blood flow. It rises when the stroke volume is increased and falls when the resistance to outflow is decreased. The *mean arterial pressure* represents the average pressure (approximately 90 to 100 mm Hg) in the arterial system during ventricular contraction and relaxation and is a good indicator of tissue perfusion. Mean arterial pressure can be estimated using the following equation: mean arterial pressure = 1/3 systolic + 2/3 diastolic pressures.

The systolic and diastolic components of blood pressure are determined by cardiac output and total peripheral vascular resistance and can be expressed as the product of the two (blood pressure = cardiac output × total peripheral resistance). The cardiac output is the product of the stroke volume (amount of blood ejected from the heart with each beat) and the heart rate: cardiac ouput = stroke volume × heart rate. The total peripheral resistance reflects changes in the radius of the arterioles as well as the viscosity or thickness of the blood. The arterioles often are referred to as the *resistance vessels* because they can selectively constrict or relax to control the resistance to outflow of blood into the capillaries. The body maintains its blood pressure by adjusting the cardiac output to compensate for changes in peripheral vascular resistance, and it changes the peripheral vascular resistance to compensate for changes in cardiac output.

In hypertension and disease conditions that affect blood pressure, changes in blood pressure usually are described in terms of the systolic and diastolic pressures, pulse pressure, and mean arterial pressure. These pressures are influenced by the stroke volume, the rapidity with which blood is ejected from the heart, the elastic properties of the aorta and large arteries and their ability to accept various amounts of blood as it is ejected from the heart, and the properties of the resistance blood vessels that control the runoff of blood into the smaller vessels and capillaries that connect the arterial and venous circulations.

Mechanisms of Blood Pressure Regulation

An adequate systemic arterial pressure is perhaps the single most important requirement for proper functioning of the cardiovascular system. Although different tissues in the body are able to regulate their own blood flow, without sufficient arterial pressure the brain and the heart do not receive adequate blood flow, no matter what adjustments are made in their vascular resistance by local control mechanisms. The mechanisms used to regulate the arterial pressure depend on whether short-term or long-term adaptation is needed[29] (Fig. 18-13).

Short-Term Regulation

The mechanisms for short-term regulation of blood pressure, those acting over seconds or minutes, are intended to correct temporary imbalances in blood pressure, such as occur during physical exercise and changes in body position. These mechanisms also are responsible for maintenance of blood pressure at survival levels during life-threatening situations such as during an acute hemorrhagic incident. The short-term regulation of blood pressure relies mainly on neural and humoral mechanisms, the most rapid of which are the neural mechanisms.

Neural Mechanisms. The neural control of blood pressure is vested in centers that are located in the reticular formation of the medulla and lower third of the pons, where integration and modulation of autonomic nervous system (ANS) responses occur.[26] This area of the brain contains the vasomotor and cardiac control centers and is often collectively referred to as the *cardiovascular center.* The cardiovascular center transmits parasympathetic impulses to the heart through the vagus nerve and sympathetic impulses to the heart and blood vessels through the spinal cord and peripheral sympathetic nerves. Parasympathetic stimulation of the heart produces a slowing of heart rate, whereas sympathetic

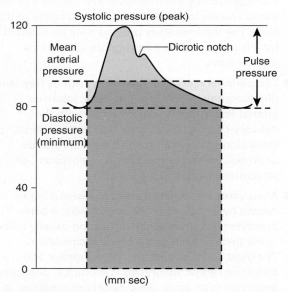

FIGURE 18-12. Intra-arterial pressure tracing made from the brachial artery. Pulse pressure is the difference between systolic and diastolic pressures. The darker area represents the mean arterial pressure, which can be calculated using the formula of mean arterial pressure = diastolic pressure + pulse pressure/3.

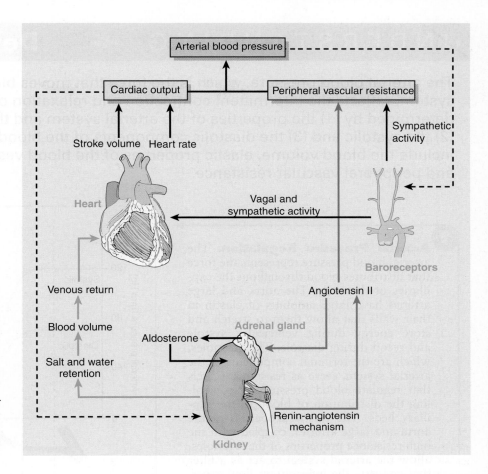

FIGURE 18-13. Mechanisms of blood pressure regulation. The *solid lines* represent the mechanisms for renal and baroreceptor control of blood pressure through changes in cardiac output and peripheral vascular resistance. The *dashed lines* represent the stimulus for regulation of blood pressure by the baroreceptors and the kidneys.

stimulation produces an increase in heart rate and cardiac contractility. Blood vessels are mainly innervated by the sympathetic nervous system, which produces constriction of the small arteries and arterioles with a resultant increase in peripheral vascular resistance.

The ANS control of blood pressure is mediated through both intrinsic and extrinsic cardiovascular reflexes, as well as higher neural control centers.[26] The *intrinsic reflexes,* including the baroreceptor and chemoreceptor reflexes, respond to stimuli originating from within the cardiovascular system and are essential to rapid and short-term regulation of blood pressure. The *extrinsic reflexes* mediate the cardiovascular response to stimuli originating from outside the cardiovascular system. They mediate blood pressure responses associated with factors such as pain and temperature changes. The neural pathways for these reactions are more diffuse, and their responses are less consistent than those of the intrinsic reflexes. Many of these responses are channeled through the hypothalamus, which plays an essential role in the control of sympathetic nervous system responses.

The baroreceptors are pressure-sensitive receptors located in the walls of blood vessels and the heart. They can be classified as high-pressure and low-pressure baroreceptors based on the type of blood vessel in which they are located. The high-pressure carotid and aortic

baroreceptors are located in strategic position between the heart and the brain (Fig. 18-14). They respond to changes in the stretch of the vessel wall by sending impulses to cardiovascular centers in the brain stem to effect appropriate changes in heart rate and vascular smooth muscle tone. For example, the fall in blood pressure that occurs on moving from the lying to the standing position produces a decrease in the stretch of the baroreceptors with a resultant increase in heart rate and sympathetically induced vasoconstriction that produces an increase in peripheral vascular resistance. The low-pressure baroreceptors, which are located in large systemic veins, pulmonary vessels, and walls of the right atrium and ventricles of the heart, have both circulatory and renal effects. They produce changes in antidiuretic hormone (ADH) secretion, resulting in profound effects on the retention of salt and water.

The arterial chemoreceptors are cells that monitor the oxygen, carbon dioxide, and hydrogen ion content of the blood. They are located in the carotid bodies, which lie in the bifurcation of the two common carotids, and in the aortic bodies of the aorta[26] (see Fig. 18-14). Because of their location, these chemoreceptors are always in close contact with the arterial blood. Although the main function of the chemoreceptors is to regulate ventilation, they also communicate

(*text continues on page 423*)

UNDERSTANDING ➡ Determinants of

The arterial blood pressure, which is the force that moves blood through the arterial system, reflects the intermittent contraction and relaxation of the left ventricle. It is determined by (1) the properties of the arterial system and the factors that maintain (2) the systolic and (3) the diastolic components of the blood pressure. These factors include the blood volume, elastic properties of the blood vessels, cardiac output, and peripheral vascular resistance.

1 Arterial Pressure Regulation. The arterial blood pressure represents the force that distributes blood throughout the capillaries of the body. The aorta and large arteries have large amounts of elastin in their walls that allow them to stretch and store energy during ventricular systole and recoil during diastole. The arterioles, which are the terminal components of the arterial system, serve as resistance vessels that regulate blood pressure by controlling the distribution of blood to the capillary beds. The elastic properties of the aorta and large arteries, coupled with the high resistance properties of the arterioles, allow the arterial system to act as a filter that converts the intermittent flow generated by the heart to virtually steady flow in the capillaries. The low-pressure venous system collects blood from the capillaries and returns it to the heart as a means of maintaining the cardiac output needed to sustain the arterial pressure.

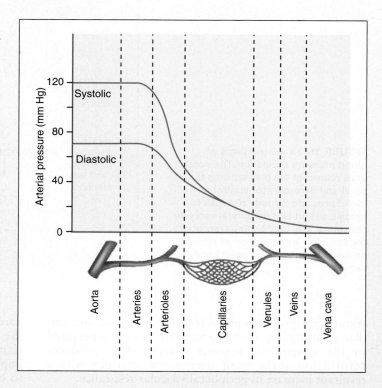

2 Systolic Pressure. The systolic blood pressure reflects the amount of blood (stroke volume) that is ejected from the heart with each beat, the rate and force with which it is ejected, and the elasticity or compliance of the aorta and large arteries. The blood that is ejected from the heart during systole does not move directly through the circulation. Instead, a substantial fraction of the stroke volume is stored in large arteries. Because the walls of these vessels are elastic, they can be stretched to accommodate a large volume of blood without an appreciable change in pressure. The systolic pressure often increases with aging as the aorta and large arteries lose their elasticity and become more rigid.

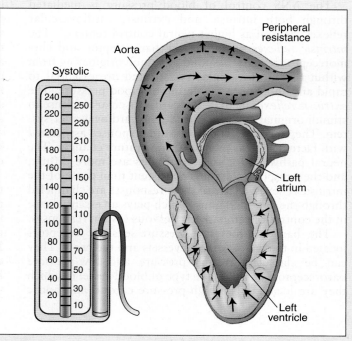

Blood Pressure

3 **Diastolic Pressure.** The diastolic blood pressure reflects the closure of the aortic valve, the energy that has been stored in the elastic fibers of the large arteries during systole, and the resistance to flow through arterioles into the capillaries. Closure of the aortic valve at the onset of diastole and recoil of the elastic fibers in the aorta and large arteries continue to drive the blood forward, even though the heart is not pumping. These effects, largely restricted to the elastic vessels, convert the discontinuous systolic flow in the ascending aorta into a continuous flow in the peripheral arteries.

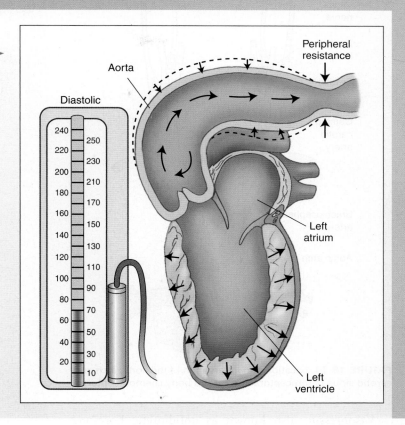

(text continued from page 421)

with cardiovascular centers in the brain stem and can induce widespread vasoconstriction. Whenever the arterial pressure drops below a critical level, the chemoreceptors are stimulated because of diminished oxygen supply and a buildup of carbon dioxide and hydrogen ions. In persons with chronic lung disease, systemic and pulmonary hypertension may develop because of hypoxemia (see Chapter 23). Persons with sleep apnea may also experience an increase in blood pressure because of the hypoxemia that occurs during the apneic periods.

Humoral Mechanisms. The *humoral control* of blood pressure relies on a number of mechanisms, including the *renin-angiotensin-aldosterone* system and *vasopressin*.[26] Other humoral substances, such as epinephrine, a sympathetic neurotransmitter released from the adrenal gland, have the effect of directly producing an increase in heart rate, cardiac contractility, and vascular tone.

The *renin-angiotensin-aldosterone system* plays a central role in blood pressure regulation. Renin is an enzyme that synthesized and stored by the juxtaglomerular cells of the kidney and released in response to an increase in sympathetic nervous system activity or a decrease in blood pressure, extracellular fluid volume, or extracellular sodium concentration.[26] Most of the renin that is released leaves the kidney and enters the bloodstream, where it acts enzymatically to convert an inactive circulating plasma protein called *angiotensinogen* to angiotensin I (Fig. 18-15). Angiotensin I is then converted to angiotensin II. This conversion occurs almost entirely in the small vessels of the lung, catalyzed by an enzyme called the *angiotensin-converting enzyme* that is present in the endothelium of the lung vessels. Although angiotensin II has a half-life of only several minutes, renin persists in the circulation for 30 minutes to 1 hour and continues to cause production of angiotensin II during this time.

Angiotensin II functions in both the short- and long-term regulation of blood pressure. It is a strong vasoconstrictor, particularly of arterioles and, to a lesser extent, of veins. Constriction of the arterioles increases the peripheral vascular resistance, thereby contributing to the short-term regulation of blood pressure. Angiotensin II also reduces sodium excretion by increasing sodium reabsorption by the proximal tubules of the kidney. A second major function of angiotensin II, stimulation of aldosterone secretion from the adrenal gland, contributes to the long-term regulation of blood pressure by increasing salt and water retention by the kidney.

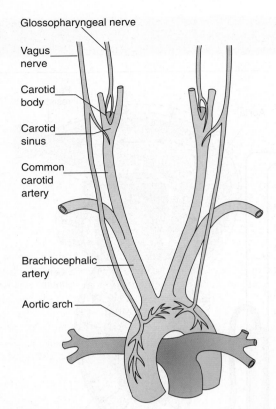

FIGURE 18-14. Location and innervation of the aortic arch and carotid sinus baroreceptors and carotid body chemoreceptors.

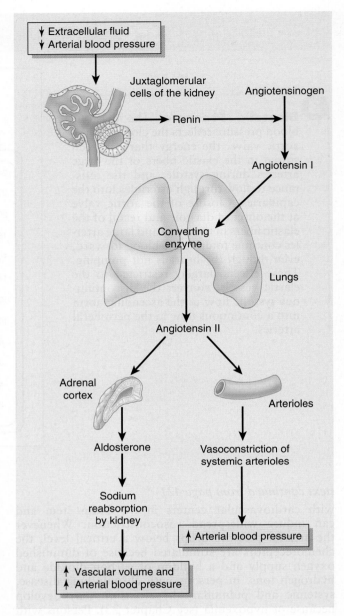

FIGURE 18-15. Control of blood pressure by the renin-angiotensin-aldosterone system. Renin enzymatically converts the plasma protein angiotensinogen to angiotensin I; angiotensin-converting enzyme in the lung converts angiotensin I to angiotensin II; and angiotensin II produces vasoconstriction and increases salt and water retention through direct action on the kidney and through increased aldosterone secretion by the adrenal cortex.

Vasopressin, also known as antidiuretic hormone (ADH), is released from the posterior pituitary gland in response to decreases in blood volume and blood pressure, an increase in the osmolality of body fluids, and other stimuli.[26] The antidiuretic actions of vasopressin are discussed in Chapter 8. Vasopressin has a direct vasoconstrictor effect, particularly on the vessels of the splanchnic circulation that supplies the abdominal viscera. However, long-term increases in vasopressin cannot maintain an increase in blood pressure, and vasopressin does not enhance hypertension produced by sodium-retaining hormones or other vasoconstricting substances. It has been suggested that vasopressin plays a permissive role in hypertension through its water-retaining properties or as a neurotransmitter that serves to modify ANS function.

Long-Term Regulation

Long-term mechanisms, which are responsible for the hourly, daily, weekly, and monthly regulation of blood pressure, are largely vested in the kidneys and their role in regulation of extracellular fluid volume.[26] These mechanisms function largely by regulating the blood pressure around an equilibrium point, which represents the normal pressure for a given individual. Accordingly, when the body contains too much extracellular fluid, the arterial pressure rises and the rate at which water (i.e., *pressure diuresis*) and sodium (i.e., *pressure natriuresis*) are excreted by the kidney is increased.[26,27] When

blood pressure returns to its equilibrium point, water and sodium excretion return to normal. A fall in blood pressure due to a decrease in extracellular fluid volume has the opposite effect. In persons with hypertension, renal control mechanisms are often altered such that the equilibrium point for blood pressure regulation is maintained at a higher level of sodium and water elimination.

There are two general mechanisms by which an increase in fluid volume can elevate blood pressure—

through a direct effect on cardiac output, or indirectly from the autoregulation of blood flow and its effect on peripheral vascular resistance. Autoregulatory mechanisms function in distributing blood flow to the various tissues of the body according to their metabolic needs (see Chapter 17). When the blood flow to a specific tissue bed is excessive, local blood vessels constrict, and when the flow is deficient, the local vessels dilate. In situations of increased extracellular fluid volume and a resultant increase in cardiac output, all of the tissues of the body are exposed to the same increase in flow. This results in a generalized constriction of arterioles and an increase in peripheral vascular resistance and blood pressure.

The role that the kidneys play in long-term regulation of blood pressure is emphasized by the fact that many antihypertensive medications produce their blood pressure–lowering effects by increasing sodium and water elimination.

Measurement of Blood Pressure

The diagnosis of blood pressure disorders is facilitated by blood pressure measurements, which should be obtained with a well-calibrated sphygmomanometer. Accuracy of the measurements requires that persons taking the pressure are adequately trained in blood pressure measurement, the equipment is properly maintained, and the cuff bladder is appropriate for the upper arm size.[28] The width of the bladder should be at least 40% of arm circumference and the length at least 80% of arm circumference. Undercuffing (using a cuff with a bladder that is too small) can cause an overestimation of blood pressure. This is because a cuff that is too small results in an uneven distribution of pressure across the arm, such that a greater cuff pressure is needed to occlude blood flow. Likewise, overcuffing (using a cuff with a bladder that is too large) can cause an underestimation of blood pressure. Readings should be taken after the person is

relaxed and has rested for at least 5 minutes and has not smoked or ingested caffeine within 30 minutes. At least two measurements should be made on each occasion in the same arm while the person is seated in a chair (rather than on the examination table) with the feet on the floor and the arm supported at heart level.[28] Both the systolic and diastolic pressures should be recorded.

Hypertension

Hypertension, or high blood pressure, is probably the most common of all health problems in adults and is the leading risk factor for cardiovascular disorders. It affects approximately 50 million individuals in the United States and approximately 1 billion persons worldwide.[29] Hypertension is more common in younger men compared with younger women in the United States, in blacks compared with whites, in persons from lower socioeconomic groups, and in older persons. Men have higher blood pressures than women up until the time of menopause, at which point women quickly lose their protection. The prevalence of hypertension increases with age. Thus, the problem of hypertension can be expected to become even greater with the aging of the "baby-boomer" population.

Hypertension commonly is divided into the categories of primary and secondary hypertension. In primary, or *essential*, hypertension, the chronic elevation of blood pressure occurs without evidence of other disease conditions. Primary hypertension accounts for approximately 90% to 95% of all cases of hypertension.[30] In secondary hypertension, the elevation of blood pressure results from some other disorder, such as kidney disease.

Hypertension is diagnosed when the systolic pressure is consistently elevated above 140 mm Hg, or the diastolic blood pressure is 90 mm Hg or higher.[29] Hypertension is further divided into stages 1 and 2 based on systolic and diastolic blood pressure measurements (Table 18-4).

TABLE 18-4	Classification of Blood Pressure for Adults and Recommendations for Follow-up		
Blood Pressure Classification	**Systolic Blood Pressure (mm Hg)**	**Diastolic Blood Pressure (mm Hg)**	**Follow-up Recommendations for Initial Blood Pressure*,†**
Normal	<120	And <80	Recheck in 2 years
Prehypertensive	120–139	or 80–89	Recheck in 1 year†
Stage 1 hypertension	140–159	or 90–99	Confirm within 2 months‡
Stage 2 hypertension	≥160	or ≥100	Evaluate or refer to source of care within 1 month
			For those with higher pressure (e.g., >180/110 mm Hg), evaluate and treat immediately or within 1 week, depending on clinical situation and complications

*Initial blood pressure: If systolic and diastolic categories are different, follow recommendations for shorter follow-up (e.g., 160/86 mm Hg should be evaluated or referred to source of care within 1 month).

†Follow-up blood pressure: Modify the scheduling of follow-up according to reliable information about past blood pressure measurements, other cardiovascular risk factors, or target-organ disease.

‡Provide advice about lifestyle modification.

Modified from the National Heart, Lung, and Blood Institute. *The Seventh Report of the National Committee on Detection, Evaluation, and Treatment of High Blood Pressure*. NIH publication No. 04-5230. Bethesda, MD: National Institutes of Health; 2004.

A systolic pressure of less than 120 mm Hg and a diastolic pressure of less than 80 mm Hg are normal, and systolic pressures between 120 and 139 mm Hg and diastolic pressures between 80 and 89 mm Hg are considered prehypertensive. For adults with diabetes mellitus, the blood pressure goal has been lowered to less than 130/80 mm Hg.[31] A single elevated blood pressure reading is not sufficient to make a diagnosis of hypertension. Rather, the diagnosis depends on a series of measurements, since readings can vary from time to time.

Systolic hypertension has been defined as a systolic pressure of 140 mm Hg or greater and a diastolic pressure of less than 90 mm Hg.[29] Historically, diastolic hypertension was thought to confer a greater risk for cardiovascular events than systolic hypertension. However, there is mounting evidence that elevated systolic blood pressure is at least as important, if not more so.[32] There are two aspects of systolic hypertension that confer increased risk for cardiovascular events—one is the actual elevation in systolic pressure and the other is the disproportionate rise in pulse pressure. Elevated pressures during systole favor the development of left ventricular hypertrophy, increased myocardial oxygen demands, and eventual left heart failure. At the same time, the absolute or relative lowering of diastolic pressure is a limiting factor in coronary perfusion because coronary perfusion is greatest during diastole. Elevated pulse pressures produce greater stretch of arteries, causing damage to the elastic elements of the vessel and thus predisposing to aneurysms and development of the intimal damage that leads to atherosclerosis and thrombosis.

Primary (Essential) Hypertension

Essential (primary) hypertension is the term applied to hypertension for which no cause can be identified. Although the cause or causes of essential hypertension are largely unknown, both constitutional and lifestyle factors have been implicated, either singly or collectively, as contributing factors.

Constitutional Risk Factors. Constitutional risk factors include family history of hypertension, race, and age-related increases in blood pressure.[29,33] The inclusion of heredity as a contributing factor in the development of hypertension is supported by the fact that hypertension is seen most frequently among persons with a family history of hypertension. The inherited predisposition does not seem to rely on other risk factors, but when they are present, the risk apparently is additive. Hypertension not only is more prevalent in blacks than whites, but also is more severe, tends to occur earlier, and often is not treated early enough or aggressively enough.[34] Blacks also tend to experience greater cardiovascular and renal damage at any level of pressure.

Maturation and growth are known to cause predictable increases in blood pressure. For example, the arterial blood pressure in the newborn is approximately 50 mm Hg systolic and 40 mm Hg diastolic.[35] Sequentially, blood pressure increases with physical growth from a value of 78 mm Hg systolic at 10 days of age to 120 mm Hg at the end of adolescence. Diastolic pressure increases until 50 years of age and then declines from the sixth decade onward, whereas systolic blood pressure continues to rise with age.[35]

Another factor that is thought to contribute to the development of hypertension is insulin resistance and the hyperinsulinemia that occurs in persons with diabetes.[36] This clustering of cardiovascular risk factors has been named the *insulin resistance syndrome, cardiometabolic syndrome,* or *metabolic syndrome* (see Chapter 33).

Lifestyle Risk Factors. Lifestyle factors can contribute to the development of hypertension by interacting with other risk factors. These lifestyle factors include high salt intake, excessive calorie intake and obesity, and excessive alcohol consumption. Although stress can raise blood pressure acutely, there is less evidence linking it to chronic elevations in blood pressure. Smoking and a diet high in saturated fats and cholesterol, although not identified as primary risk factors for hypertension, are independent risk factors for coronary heart disease and should be avoided.

Increased sodium intake has long been suspected as an etiologic factor in the development of hypertension, although just how it contributes to the development of hypertension is still unclear.[37,38] It may be that sodium causes an elevation in blood volume, increases the sensitivity of cardiovascular or renal mechanisms to sympathetic nervous system influences, or exerts its effect through some other mechanism such as the renin-angiotensin-aldosterone system. Regardless of the mechanism, numerous studies have shown that a reduction in salt intake can lower blood pressure.

Excessive weight commonly is associated with hypertension. It has been suggested that fat distribution might be a more critical indicator of hypertension risk than actual overweight. The waist-to-hip ratio commonly is used to differentiate central or upper body obesity, with fat deposits located in the abdomen and viscera, from peripheral or lower body obesity, with fat deposits in the buttocks and legs (see Chapter 10).[39,40] Abdominal or visceral fat seems to be more insulin resistant than fat deposited over the buttocks and legs. The mechanisms involved in obesity-related hypertension are complex and involve multiple organ systems. They include increased sympathetic nervous system activation, increased activity of the angiotensin-aldosterone system, and insulin resistance.[40] Recent evidence indicates that leptin, an adipocyte-derived hormone, may represent a link between adiposity and increased cardiovascular sympathetic activity. Besides its effect on appetite and metabolism, leptin is thought to act on the hypothalamus to increase blood pressure through activation of the sympathetic nervous system.[40] High levels of circulating free fatty acids in obese people also appear to participate in activation of the sympathetic nervous system. There is also research supporting activation of the renin-angiotensin-aldosterone system by adipocyte-derived angiotensinogen and the ability of adipose tissue to increase aldosterone levels through the production of factors that induce aldosterone production.[40]

Regular alcohol consumption plays a role in the development of hypertension.[41] The effect is seen with different types of alcoholic drinks, in men and women, and in a variety of ethnic groups. One of the first reports of a link between alcohol consumption and hypertension came from the Oakland–San Francisco Kaiser Permanente Medical Care Program study that correlated known drinking patterns and blood pressure levels of 84,000 persons.[42] This study revealed that the regular consumption of three or more drinks per day increases the risk for hypertension. Systolic pressures were more markedly affected than diastolic pressures. Blood pressure may improve or return to normal when alcohol consumption is decreased or eliminated.

Secondary Hypertension

Secondary hypertension, which describes an elevation in blood pressure due to another disease condition, accounts for 5% to 10% of hypertension cases.[43] Unlike essential hypertension, many of the conditions causing secondary hypertension can be corrected or cured by surgery or specific medical treatment. Secondary hypertension tends to be seen in persons younger than 30 and older than 50 years of age. Among the most common causes of secondary hypertension are kidney disease (i.e., renovascular hypertension), adrenal cortical disorders, pheochromocytoma, and coarctation of the aorta. Oral contraceptive agents are also implicated as a cause of secondary hypertension. Cocaine, amphetamines, and other illicit drugs can also cause a significant elevation in blood pressure, as can sympathomimetic agents (decongestants, anorectics), erythropoietin, and licorice (including some chewing tobaccos with licorice as an ingredient). Obstructive sleep apnea is an independent risk factor for secondary hypertension.

Renal Hypertension. With the dominant role that the kidney assumes in blood pressure regulation, it is not surprising that the largest single cause of secondary hypertension is renal disease. Most acute kidney disorders result in decreased urine formation, retention of salt and water, and hypertension. This includes acute glomerulonephritis, acute renal failure, and acute urinary tract obstruction. Hypertension also is common among persons with chronic pyelonephritis, polycystic kidney disease, diabetic nephropathy, and end-stage kidney disease, regardless of cause. In older persons, the sudden onset of secondary hypertension often is associated with atherosclerotic disease of the renal blood vessels.

Renovascular hypertension refers to hypertension caused by reduced renal blood flow and activation of the renin-angiotensin-aldosterone mechanism. It is the most common cause of secondary hypertension, accounting for 1% to 2% of all cases of hypertension.[44] The reduced renal blood flow that occurs with renovascular disease causes the affected kidney to release excessive amounts of renin, increasing circulating levels of angiotensin II. Angiotensin II, in turn, acts as a vasoconstrictor to increase peripheral vascular resistance and as a stimulus for increased aldosterone levels and sodium retention by the kidney. One or both of the kidneys may be affected. When the renal artery of only one kidney is involved, the unaffected kidney is subjected to the detrimental effects of the elevated blood pressure.

There are two major types of renovascular disease: (1) atherosclerosis of the proximal renal artery, and (2) fibromuscular dysplasia, a noninflammatory vascular disease that affects the renal arteries and branch vessels.[44,45] Atherosclerotic stenosis of the renal artery accounts for 70% to 90% of cases and is seen most often in older persons, particularly those with diabetes, aortoiliac occlusive disease, coronary artery disease, or hypertension.[44] Fibromuscular dysplasia is more common in women and tends to occur in younger age groups, often persons in their third decade.[45] Genetic factors may be involved, and the incidence tends to increase with risk factors such as smoking and hyperlipidemia.

Diagnostic tests for renovascular hypertension may include studies to assess overall renal function, physiologic studies to assess the renin-angiotensin system, perfusion studies to evaluate renal blood flow, and imaging studies to identify renal artery stenosis.[44] Renal arteriography remains the definitive test for identifying renal artery disease. Duplex ultrasonographic scanning, contrast-enhanced CT scans, and magnetic resonance angiography (MRA) are other tests that can be used to screen for renovascular hypertension.[44]

The goal of treatment for renal hypertension is to control the blood pressure and stabilize renal function. Angioplasty or revascularization has been shown to be an effective long-term treatment for the disorder. Angiotensin-converting enzyme (ACE) inhibitors may be used in medical management of renal stenosis. However, these agents must be used with caution because of their ability to produce marked hypotension and renal dysfunction.

Disorders of Adrenocortical Hormones. Increased levels of adrenocortical hormones also can give rise to hypertension. Primary hyperaldosteronism (excess production of aldosterone due to adrenocortical hyperplasia or adenoma) and excess levels of glucocorticoid (Cushing disease or syndrome) tend to raise the blood pressure[30,46] (see Chapter 32). These hormones facilitate sodium and water retention by the kidney; the hypertension that accompanies excessive levels of either hormone probably is related to this factor. For patients with primary hyperaldosteronism, a sodium-restricted diet often produces a reduction in blood pressure. Because aldosterone acts on the distal renal tubule to increase sodium absorption in exchange for potassium elimination in the urine, persons with hyperaldosteronism usually have decreased potassium levels. Screening tests for primary hyperaldosteronism involve the determination of plasma aldosterone concentration and plasma renin activity. Computed tomography and magnetic resonance imaging scans are used to localize the lesion. Persons with solitary adenomas are usually treated surgically. Potassium-sparing diuretics, such as spironolactone, which is an aldosterone antagonist, often are used in the medical management of persons with bilateral hyperplasia.

Pheochromocytoma. Pheochromocytomas are rare catecholamine-secreting tumors of adrenal chromaffin cells.[30] They can occur at any age, including infancy, but are uncommon after 60 years of age. They can occur as part of hereditary syndromes, but most are sporadic. Of the sporadic tumors, about 10% are malignant.[46]

Like adrenal medullary cells, the tumor cells of a pheochromocytoma produce and secrete the catecholamines epinephrine and norepinephrine. The hypertension that develops is a result of the massive release of these catecholamines. Their release may be paroxysmal rather than continuous, causing periodic episodes of headache, excessive sweating, and palpitations. Headache is the most common symptom and can be quite severe. Nervousness, tremor, facial pallor, weakness, fatigue, and weight loss occur less frequently. Marked variability in blood pressure between episodes is typical.

Diagnostic methods include urinary and blood assays for catecholamines and their metabolites and CT and MRI studies to locate tumors and possible metastases. Surgical removal of the tumor or tumors is the treatment of choice. If the tumor is not resectable, treatment with drugs that block the action or synthesis of catecholamines can be used. When correctly diagnosed and treated, most pheochromocytomas are curable. When they are undiagnosed or improperly treated, they can be fatal.[30–46]

Coarctation of the Aorta. Coarctation of the aorta or aortic coarctation is a congenital condition in which a narrowing or constriction of the lumen of the aorta exists.[47] In the adult form, narrowing most commonly occurs just distal to the origin of the subclavian (see Chapter 19). The ejection of a large stroke volume into a narrowed aorta results in an increase in systolic blood pressure and blood flow to the upper part of the body. Blood pressure in the lower extremities may be normal, although it frequently is low. It has been suggested that the increase in cardiac output and maintenance of the blood pressure to the lower part of the body is achieved through the renin-angiotensin-aldosterone mechanism in response to a decrease in renal blood flow.

Coarctation of the aorta should be considered as a cause of secondary hypertension in young people with an elevation in blood pressure. Because the aortic capacity is diminished in coarctation of the aorta, there usually is a marked increase in pressure (measured in the arms) during exercise, when the stroke volume and heart rate are exaggerated. Pulse pressure in the legs almost always is narrowed, and the femoral pulses are weak. It is important that blood pressure be measured in both arms and one leg when coarctation of the aorta is suspected. A pressure in the arms 20 mm Hg or more higher than in the legs suggests coarctation of the aorta.

Treatment consists of surgical repair or balloon angioplasty. Although balloon angioplasty is a relatively recent form of treatment, it has been used in children

and adults with good results. However, there are few data on long-term follow-up.

Oral Contraceptive Drugs. The use of oral contraceptive pills is probably the most common cause of secondary hypertension in young women. Women taking oral contraceptives should have their blood pressure taken regularly.[30] The cause of the increased blood pressure is largely unknown, although it has been suggested that the probable cause is volume expansion because both estrogens and synthetic progesterones used in oral contraceptive pills cause sodium retention. Various contraceptive drugs contain different amounts and combinations of estrogen and progestational agents, and these differences may contribute to the occurrence of hypertension in some women but not others. Fortunately, the hypertension associated with oral contraceptives usually disappears after the drug has been discontinued, although it may take as long as 3 months for this to occur. However, in some women the blood pressure may not return to normal, and they may be at risk for development of hypertension. The risk for hypertension-associated cardiovascular complications is found primarily in women older than 35 years of age and in those who smoke.

Target-Organ Damage

Hypertension is typically an asymptomatic disorder. When symptoms do occur, they are usually related to the long-term effects of hypertension on other organ systems, termed *target organs*, such as the kidneys, heart, eyes, and blood vessels[29] (Chart 18-2). The excess morbidity and mortality related to hypertension is progressive over the whole range of systolic and diastolic pressures, with target-organ damage varying markedly among persons with similar levels of hypertension.

Hypertension is a major risk factor for atherosclerosis; it predisposes to all major atherosclerotic cardiovascular disorders, including coronary heart disease, heart failure, stroke, and peripheral artery disease. The risk for coronary artery disease and stroke depends to a great extent on other risk factors, such as obesity, smoking, and elevated cholesterol levels. In clinical

---

CHART 18-2 Target-Organ Damage

Heart
- Left ventricular hypertrophy
- Angina or prior myocardial infarction
- Prior coronary revascularization
- Heart failure

Brain
- Stroke or transient ischemic attack

Chronic kidney disease

Peripheral vascular disease

Retinopathy

From the National Heart, Lung, and Blood Institute. *The Seventh Report of the National Committee on Detection, Evaluation, and Treatment of High Blood Pressure.* Publication No. 03–5233. Bethesda, MD: National Institutes of Health; 2003.

trials, antihypertensive therapy has been associated with reductions in stroke incidence averaging 30% to 40%; myocardial infarction, 20% to 25%; and heart failure, more than 50%.[29]

Hypertension increases the workload of the left ventricle by increasing the pressure against which the heart must pump as it ejects blood into the systemic circulation.[30] As the workload of the heart increases, the left ventricular wall hypertrophies to compensate for the increased pressure work. Despite its adaptive advantage, left ventricular hypertrophy is a major risk factor for coronary heart disease, cardiac arrhythmias, sudden death, and congestive heart failure. Hypertensive left ventricular hypertrophy regresses with therapy. Regression is most closely related to systolic pressure reduction and does not appear to reflect the particular type of medication used.

Chronic hypertension can lead to nephrosclerosis, a common cause of chronic kidney disease (see Chapter 25). Hypertensive kidney disease is more common in blacks than whites. Hypertension also plays an important role in accelerating the course of other types of kidney disease, particularly diabetic nephropathy. Because of the risk for diabetic nephropathy, the American Diabetes Association recommends that persons with diabetes maintain their blood pressure at levels less than 130/80 mm Hg[31] (see Chapter 33).

Dementia and cognitive impairment occur more commonly in persons with hypertension.[29] Hypertension, particularly systolic hypertension, is a major risk factor for ischemic stroke and intracerebral hemorrhage[30] (see Chapter 37). Narrowing and sclerosis of small penetrating arteries in the subcortical regions of the brain are common findings on autopsy in persons with chronic hypertension.[29] These changes are thought to contribute to hypoperfusion, loss of autoregulation of blood flow, and impairment of the blood–brain barrier, ultimately leading to subcortical white matter demyelination. Magnetic resonance imaging studies have revealed more extensive white matter lesions and brain atrophy in hypertensive versus normotensive persons. Effective antihypertensive therapy strongly reduces the risk of development of significant white matter changes; however, existing white matter changes, once established, do not appear to be reversible.[29]

Diagnosis and Treatment

Unlike disorders of other body systems that are diagnosed by methods such as radiography and tissue examination, hypertension and other blood pressure disorders are determined by repeated blood pressure measurements. Laboratory tests, x-ray films, and other diagnostic tests usually are done to exclude secondary hypertension and determine the presence or extent of target-organ damage.

The increased availability of hypertensive screening clinics provides one of the best means for early detection. Because blood pressure in many individuals is highly variable, unless the pressure is extremely elevated or associated with symptoms it should be measured on different occasions over a period of several months before a diagnosis of hypertension is made.

Ambulatory and self/home measurement of blood pressure may provide valuable information outside the clinician's office regarding a person's blood pressure and response to treatment. Self/home measurement can help detect "white coat hypertension," a condition in which the blood pressure is consistently elevated in the health care provider's office but normal at other times; it can also be used to assess the response to treatment measure, motivate adherence to treatment regimes, and eventually reduce health care costs.[29,30]

The main objective for treatment of hypertension is to achieve and maintain arterial blood pressure below 140/90 mm Hg, with the goal of preventing morbidity and mortality. In persons with hypertension and diabetes or renal disease, the goal is blood pressure below 130/80 mm Hg. Treatment methods include lifestyle modification and, when necessary, pharmacologic agents to achieve and maintain blood pressure within an optimal range.[29]

Lifestyle Modification. Lifestyle modification has been shown to reduce blood pressure, enhance the effects of antihypertensive drug therapy, and prevent cardiovascular risk. Major lifestyle modifications shown to lower blood pressure include weight reduction in persons who are overweight or obese, regular physical activity, reduction of dietary sodium intake, and limitation of alcohol intake to no more than two drinks per day for most men and one drink for women and persons of lighter weight.[48]

Pharmacologic Treatment. The decision to initiate pharmacologic treatment is based on the severity of the hypertension, the presence of target-organ disease, and the existence of other conditions and risk factors.[29,48] Drug selection is based on the stage of hypertension. Among the drugs used in the treatment of hypertension are diuretics, β-adrenergic receptor inhibitors, ACE inhibitors or angiotensin II receptor blockers, calcium channel blockers, central α_2-adrenergic agonists, α_1-adrenergic receptor blockers, and vasodilators.

The physiologic mechanisms whereby the different antihypertension drugs produce a reduction in blood pressure differ among agents. *Diuretics* lower blood pressure initially by decreasing vascular volume (by suppressing renal reabsorption of sodium and increasing sodium and water excretion) and cardiac output. With continued therapy, a reduction in peripheral resistance becomes a major mechanism of blood pressure reduction. The β-*adrenergic receptor inhibitors* are effective in treating hypertension because they decrease heart rate, cardiac output, and renin release by the kidney. The *ACE inhibitors* act by inhibiting the conversion of angiotensin I to angiotensin II, thus decreasing angiotensin II levels and reducing its effect on vasoconstriction, aldosterone levels, intrarenal blood flow, and glomerular filtration rate. The *calcium channel blockers* decrease peripheral vascular resistance by inhibiting the movement of calcium into arterial smooth muscle cells. The centrally acting α₂-*adrenergic receptor agonists* act in a negative-feedback manner to decrease sympathetic outflow from the central nervous system. The α₁-*adrenergic receptor antagonists* block α₁ receptors on vascular smooth muscle, causing vasodilatation and a reduction in peripheral vascular resistance. The direct-acting smooth muscle *vasodilators* promote a decrease in peripheral vascular resistance by producing relaxation of vascular smooth muscle, particularly of the arterioles.

Pharmacologic treatment of hypertension usually follows a stepwise approach.[29,48] It is usually initiated with a low dose of a single drug. The dose is slowly increased at a schedule dependent on the person's age, needs, and desired response. If the response to the initial drug is not adequate, one of three approaches can be used: the dose can be increased if the initial dose was below the maximum recommended; a drug with a different mode of action can be added; or the initial drug can be discontinued and another substituted. Combining drugs with different modes of action often allows smaller doses to be used to achieve blood pressure control while minimizing the dose-dependent side effects from any one drug.

Hypertensive Crisis

A small number of persons with hypertension develop an accelerated or severe form of hypertension.[30,49,50] *Hypertensive crisis* is defined as a systolic pressure greater than 180 or a diastolic pressure greater than 120 mm Hg.[49,50] Hypertensive crisis can be further classified as hypertensive urgency or a hypertensive emergency depending on end-organ involvement including cardiac, renal, or neurologic injury. *Hypertensive urgency* is defined by a markedly elevated blood pressure, usually in the same range seen in a hypertension emergency, but without the rapid progression of target-organ involvement.

Hypertensive emergency occurs when elevated blood pressure is responsible for symptoms, signs, or laboratory evidence of end-organ damage, such as mental status changes (hypertensive encephalopathy), intracranial hemorrhage, retinopathy, aortic dissection, cardiac ischemia or congestive heart failure, or acute renal failure. The central nervous system is particularly susceptible to high blood pressure. The effects of extreme elevations in blood pressure include intense arterial spasm of the cerebral arteries with hypertensive encephalopathy. Cerebral vasoconstriction probably is an exaggerated homeostatic response designed to protect the brain from excesses of blood pressure and flow. The regulatory mechanisms often are insufficient to protect the capillaries, and cerebral edema frequently develops. As it advances, papilledema (i.e., swelling of the optic nerve at its point of entrance into the eye) ensues, giving evidence of the effects of pressure on the optic nerve and retinal vessels. The person may have headache, restlessness, confusion, stupor, motor and sensory deficits, and visual disturbances. In severe cases, convulsions and coma follow.

The complications associated with a hypertensive crisis demand immediate and rigorous medical treatment in an intensive care unit with continuous monitoring of arterial blood pressure.[49,50] Because chronic hypertension

is associated with autoregulatory changes in coronary artery, cerebral artery, and kidney blood flow, care should be taken to avoid excessively rapid decreases in blood pressure, which can lead to hypoperfusion and ischemic injury. Therefore, the goal of initial treatment measures should be to obtain a partial reduction in blood pressure to a safer, less critical level, rather than to normotensive levels.

Hypertension in Special Populations

High Blood Pressure in Pregnancy

Hypertensive disorders complicate 5% to 10% of pregnancies and remain a major cause of maternal and neonatal morbidity and morality in the United States and worldwide.[51,52] In 2000, the National Institutes of Health Working Group on High Blood Pressure in Pregnancy published a revised classification system for high blood pressure in pregnancy that included preeclampsia–eclampsia, gestational hypertension, chronic hypertension, and preeclampsia superimposed on chronic hypertension.[51] Most adverse events are attributable directly to the preeclampsia syndrome, characterized by new-onset hypertension with proteinuria that develops in the last half of pregnancy. Women with chronic hypertension can also manifest adverse events.

Preeclampsia–Eclampsia. Preeclampsia–eclampsia is a pregnancy-specific syndrome with both maternal and fetal manifestations.[51–55] It is defined as an elevation in blood pressure (systolic blood pressure >140 mm Hg or diastolic pressure >90 mm Hg) and proteinuria (≥300 mg in 24 hours) developing after 20 weeks of gestation. The presence of a systolic blood pressure of 160 mm Hg or higher or a diastolic pressure of 110 mm Hg or higher, proteinuria greater than 2 g in 24 hours, serum creatinine greater than 1.2 mg/dL, platelet counts less than 100,000 cells/mm³, elevated liver enzymes (alanine aminotransferase [ALT] or aspartate aminotransferase [AST]), persistent headache or cerebral or visual disturbances, and persistent epigastric pain serve to reinforce the diagnosis.[55] Preeclampsia occurs primarily during first pregnancies and during subsequent pregnancies in women with multiple fetuses, diabetes mellitus, collagen vascular disease, or underlying kidney disease.[51] It is also associated with a condition called a *hydatidiform mole,* an abnormal mass of cysts that develops due to an abnormal pregnancy caused by a pathologic ovum. Women with chronic hypertension who become pregnant have an increased risk for preeclampsia and adverse neonatal outcomes, particularly when associated with proteinuria early in pregnancy. *Eclampsia* is the occurrence, in a woman with preeclampsia, of seizures that cannot be attributed to other causes.

The cause of pregnancy-induced hypertension is largely unknown. Considerable evidence suggests that the placenta is a key factor in all the manifestations because delivery is the only definitive cure for this disease. Pregnancy-induced hypertension is thought to involve a decrease in placental blood flow leading to the release of toxic mediators that alter the function of endothelial cells in blood vessels throughout the body, including those of the kidney, brain, liver, and heart. The endothelial changes result in signs and symptoms of preeclampsia and, in more severe cases, of intravascular clotting and hypoperfusion of vital organs.

Gestational Hypertension. *Gestational hypertension* is defined as the development of new hypertension without proteinuria occurring after 20 weeks' gestation, which resolves within 12 weeks of termination of the pregnancy.[51] The final diagnosis of gestational hypertension is made only postpartum. Women with gestational hypertension progress to preeclampsia in 15% to 45% of cases and often require early delivery. Surveillance for development of preeclampsia and close fetal monitoring are recommended.

Chronic Hypertension. Chronic hypertension in pregnancy is considered to be hypertension that is unrelated to the pregnancy. It is defined as a blood pressure of 140/90 or greater on two separate occasions before 20 weeks' gestation or persisting beyond 12 weeks postpartum.[51] In women with chronic hypertension, blood pressure often decreases in early pregnancy and increases during the last trimester (3 months) of pregnancy, resembling preeclampsia. Consequently, women with undiagnosed chronic hypertension who do not present for medical care until the later months of pregnancy may be incorrectly diagnosed as having preeclampsia.

Preeclampsia Superimposed on Chronic Hypertension. Women with chronic hypertension are at increased risk for the development of preeclampsia, in which case the prognosis for the mother and fetus tends to be worse than for either condition alone. Superimposed preeclampsia should be considered in women with hypertension before 20 weeks of gestation who develop new-onset proteinuria, women with hypertension and proteinuria before 20 weeks of gestation, women with previously well-controlled hypertension who experience a sudden increase in blood pressure, and women with chronic hypertension who develop thrombocytopenia or an increase in serum ALT or AST to abnormal levels.[51]

Diagnosis and Treatment. Early prenatal care is important in the detection of high blood pressure during pregnancy. It is recommended that all pregnant women, including those with hypertension, refrain from alcohol and tobacco use. A low-sodium diet usually is not recommended during pregnancy because pregnant women with hypertension tend to have lower plasma volumes than normotensive pregnant women, and because the severity of hypertension may reflect the degree of volume contraction. The exception is women with preexisting hypertension who have been following a low-sodium diet.

In women with preeclampsia, delivery of the fetus is curative. The timing of delivery becomes a difficult decision in preterm pregnancies because the welfare of both the mother and the infant must be taken into account.

Bed rest is a traditional therapy. Antihypertensive medications, when required, must be carefully chosen because of their potential effects on uteroplacental blood flow and on the fetus. For example, the ACE inhibitors can cause injury and even death of the fetus when given during the second and third trimesters of pregnancy.

High Blood Pressure in Children and Adolescents

High blood pressure in children and adolescents is a growing health problem. In persons 3 to 18 years of age, the prevalence of hypertension is 3% to 4% in the United States.[56] This may be due in part to increasing prevalence of obesity and other lifestyle factors, such as decreased physical activity and increased intake of foods that are high in calories and sodium content.[56–58]

Normative Values. Blood pressure is known to increase from infancy to late adolescence. The average systolic pressure at 1 day of age is approximately 70 mm Hg and increases to approximately 85 mm Hg at 1 month of age. Systolic blood pressure continues to increase with physical growth to about 120 mm Hg at the end of adolescence. During the preschool years, blood pressure begins to follow a pattern that tends to be maintained as the child grows older. This pattern continues into adolescence and adulthood, suggesting that the roots of primary hypertension have their origin early in life. A familial influence on blood pressure often can be identified early in life. Children of parents with high blood pressure tend to have higher blood pressures than do children with normotensive parents.

Blood pressure norms for children are based on age-, height-, and gender-specific percentiles[59] (Table 18-5). The National High Blood Pressure Education Program (NHBPEP) first published its recommendations in 1977. The fourth task force report (revised in 2005) recommended classification of blood pressure (systolic or diastolic) for age, height, and gender into four categories: normal (less than the 90th percentile), high normal (between the 90th and 95th percentiles), stage 1 hypertension (between the 95th and 99th percentiles plus 5 mm Hg), and stage 2 hypertension (greater than the 99th percentile plus 5 mm Hg).[58] The height percentile is determined using the revised Centers for Disease Control and Prevention (CDC) growth charts.[59] As with the seventh report of the Joint National Committee on Detection, Evaluation, and Treatment of High Blood Pressure (JNC 7) of the National Institutes of Health, high normal is now considered to be "prehypertensive" and is an indication for lifestyle modification. Children and adolescents with hypertension should be evaluated for target-organ damage.[58]

Pathogenesis and Risk Factors. Secondary hypertension is the most common form of high blood pressure in infants and children. In later childhood and adolescence, essential hypertension is more common. Approximately 75% to 80% of secondary hypertension in children is caused by kidney abnormalities.[60] Coarctation of the

		Height Percentile for Boys				**Height Percentile for Girls**			
Blood Pressure Percentile	**Age (yrs)**	**5th**	**25th**	**75th**	**95th**	**5th**	**25th**	**75th**	**95th**
Systolic Pressure									
90th	1	94	97	100	103	97	98	101	103
95th		98	101	104	106	100	102	105	107
90th	3	100	103	107	109	100	102	104	106
95th		104	107	110	113	104	105	108	110
90th	6	105	108	111	113	104	106	109	111
95th		109	112	115	117	108	110	113	115
90th	10	111	114	117	119	112	114	116	118
95th		115	117	121	123	116	117	120	122
90th	13	117	120	124	126	117	119	122	124
95th		121	124	128	130	121	123	126	128
90th	16	125	128	131	134	121	123	126	128
95th		129	132	135	137	125	127	130	132
Diastolic Pressure									
90th	1	49	51	53	54	52	53	55	56
95th		54	55	58	58	56	57	59	60
90th	3	59	60	62	63	61	62	64	65
95th		63	64	66	67	65	66	68	69
90th	6	68	69	71	72	68	69	70	72
95th		72	73	75	76	72	73	74	76
90th	10	73	74	76	78	73	73	75	76
95th		77	79	81	82	77	77	79	80
90th	13	75	76	78	79	76	76	78	79
95th		79	80	82	83	80	80	82	83
90th	16	78	79	81	82	78	79	81	82
95th		82	83	85	87	82	83	85	86

TABLE 18-5 The 90th and 95th Percentiles of Systolic and Diastolic Blood Pressure for Boys and Girls 1 to 16 Years of Age by Percentiles for Height

The height percentile is determined using the newly revised CDC growth charts. Blood pressure levels are based on data from the 1999–2000 National Health and Nutritional Examination Survey (NHANES) that have been added to the childhood BP database.

From the National High Blood Pressure Education Program Working Group on High Blood Pressure in Children and Adults. Fourth report on the diagnosis, evaluation, and treatment of high blood pressure in children and adolescents. *Pediatrics*. 2004;114:555–576.

aorta is another cause of hypertension in children and adolescents. Endocrine causes of hypertension, such as pheochromocytoma and adrenal cortical disorders, are rare. Hypertension in infants is most commonly associated with high umbilical catheterization and renal artery obstruction caused by thrombosis.[65] Most cases of essential hypertension are associated with obesity or a family history of hypertension.

A number of drugs of abuse, therapeutic agents, and toxins also may increase blood pressure.[60] Alcohol should be considered as a risk factor in adolescents. Oral contraceptives may be a cause of hypertension in adolescent girls. The nephrotoxicity of the drug cyclosporine, an immunosuppressant used in transplant therapy, may cause hypertension in children (and adults) after bone marrow, heart, kidney, or liver transplantation. The coadministration of corticosteroid drugs appears to increase the incidence of hypertension.

Diagnosis and Treatment. Children 3 years of age through adolescence should have their blood pressure taken once each year.[58] The auscultatory method using a cuff of an appropriate size for the child's upper arm is recommended.[58] Repeated measurements over time, rather than a single isolated determination, are required to establish consistent and significant observations. Children with high blood pressure should be referred for medical evaluation and treatment as indicated. Treatment includes nonpharmacologic methods and, if necessary, pharmacologic therapy.

High Blood Pressure in the Elderly

The prevalence of hypertension increases with advancing age to the extent that half of people aged 60 to 69 years and approximately three fourths of people 70 years and older are affected.[29] The age-related rise in systolic blood pressure is primarily responsible for the increase in hypertension that occurs with increasing age.

Pathogenesis and Risk Factors. Among the aging processes that contribute to an increase in blood pressure are a stiffening of the large arteries, particularly the aorta; decreased baroreceptor sensitivity; increased peripheral vascular resistance; and decreased renal blood flow.[61,62] Systolic blood pressure rises almost linearly between 30 and 84 years of age, whereas diastolic pressure rises until 50 years of age and then levels off or decreases.[63] This rise in systolic pressure is thought to be related to increased stiffness of the large arteries. With aging, the elastin fibers in the walls of the arteries are gradually replaced by collagen fibers that render the vessels stiffer and less compliant.[61] Differences in the central and peripheral arteries relate to the fact that the larger vessels contain more elastin, whereas the peripheral resistance vessels have more smooth muscle and less elastin. Because of increased wall stiffness, the aorta and large arteries are less able to buffer the increase in systolic pressure that occurs as blood is ejected from the left heart, and they are less able to store the energy needed to maintain the diastolic pressure. As a result, the systolic pressure increases, the diastolic pressure remains unchanged or actually decreases, and the pulse pressure or difference between the systolic pressure and diastolic pressure widens.

Isolated systolic hypertension (systolic pressure ≥140 mm Hg and diastolic pressure <90 mm Hg) is recognized as an important risk factor for cardiovascular morbidity and mortality in older persons.[29] The treatment of hypertension in the elderly has beneficial effects in terms of reducing the incidence of cardiovascular events such as stroke. Studies have shown a reduction in stroke, coronary heart disease, and congestive heart failure in persons who were treated for hypertension compared with those who were not.[61]

Diagnosis and Treatment. The recommendations for measurement of blood pressure in the elderly are similar to those for the rest of the population.[64] Blood pressure varies among older persons, so it is especially important to obtain multiple measurements on different occasions to establish a diagnosis of hypertension. The effects of food, position, and other environmental factors are also exaggerated in older persons. Although sitting has been the standard position for blood pressure measurement, it is recommended that blood pressure also be taken in the supine and standing positions in the elderly. In some elderly persons with hypertension, a silent interval, called the *auscultatory gap*, may occur between the end of the first and beginning of the third phases of the Korotkoff sounds, providing the potential for underestimating the systolic pressure, sometimes by as much as 50 mm Hg. Because the gap occurs only with auscultation, it is recommended that a preliminary determination of systolic blood pressure be made by palpation and the cuff be inflated 30 mm Hg above this value for auscultatory measurement of blood pressure. In some older persons, the indirect measurement using a blood pressure cuff and the Korotkoff sounds has been shown to give falsely elevated readings compared with the direct intra-arterial method. This is because excessive cuff pressure is needed to compress the rigid vessels of some older persons. Pseudohypertension should be suspected in older persons with hypertension in whom the radial or brachial artery remains palpable but pulseless at higher cuff pressures.

The treatment of hypertension in the elderly is similar to that for younger people. However, blood pressure should be reduced slowly and cautiously. When possible, appropriate lifestyle modification measures should be tried first. Antihypertensive medications should be prescribed carefully because the older person may have impaired baroreflex sensitivity and renal function. Usually, medications are initiated at smaller doses, and doses are increased more gradually. There is also the danger of adverse drug interactions in older persons, who may be taking multiple medications, including over-the-counter drugs.

Orthostatic Hypotension

Orthostatic hypotension refers to an abnormal drop in blood pressure that occurs when a person stands after having been in the seated or supine position After the assumption of the upright posture from the supine position, approximately 500 to 700 mL of blood is momentarily shifted to the lower part of the body, with an accompanying decrease in central blood volume and arterial pressure.[65] Normally, this decrease in blood pressure is transient, lasting through several cardiac cycles, because the baroreceptors located in the thorax and carotid sinus area sense the decreased pressure and initiate reflex constriction of the veins and arterioles and an increase in heart rate, which brings the blood pressure back to normal. Within a few minutes of a change to the standing position, blood levels of the sympathetic neuromediators and antidiuretic hormone increase as a secondary means of ensuring maintenance of normal blood pressure in the standing position. Muscle movement in the lower extremities also aids venous return to the heart by pumping blood out of the legs.

Orthostatic or *postural hypotension* is defined as a decrease in systolic blood pressure of at least 20 mm Hg or diastolic blood pressure of at least 10 mm Hg within 3 minutes of standing.[65–67] Alternatively, the diagnosis can be made by head-up tilt of 60° on a tilt table. When the standing position is assumed in the absence of normal circulatory reflexes or blood volume, blood pools in the lower part of the body; cardiac output falls, blood pressure drops, and blood flow to the brain is inadequate (Fig. 18-16). Dizziness, syncope (fainting), or both may occur.

Etiology

A wide variety of conditions, acute and chronic, are associated with orthostatic hypotension. These include reduced blood volume, drug-induced hypotension, altered vascular responses associated with aging, bed rest, and autonomic nervous system dysfunction.

Reduced Blood Volume. Orthostatic hypotension often is an early sign of reduced blood volume or fluid deficit. When blood volume is decreased, the vascular compartment is only partially filled; although cardiac

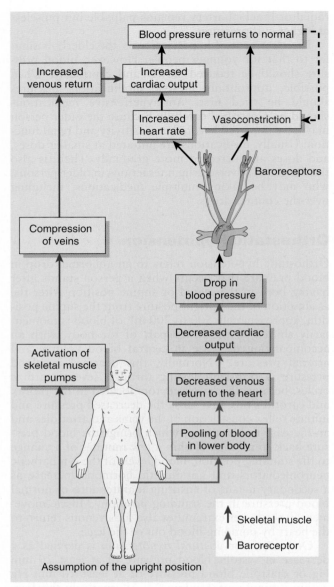

FIGURE 18-16. Skeletal muscle pump (blue) and baroreceptor mechanism (red) for blood pressure control on assumption of the upright posture.

output may be adequate when a person is in the recumbent position, it often decreases to the point of causing weakness and fainting when the person assumes the standing position. Common causes of orthostatic hypotension related to hypovolemia are excessive use of diuretics, excessive diaphoresis, loss of gastrointestinal fluids through vomiting and diarrhea, and loss of fluid volume associated with prolonged bed rest.

Drug-Induced Hypotension. Antihypertensive drugs and psychotropic drugs are a common cause of chronic orthostatic hypotension. In most cases, the orthostatic hypotension is well tolerated. If postural hypotension is severe enough to cause light-headedness or dizziness, it is recommended that the dosage of the drug be reduced or a different drug be used.

Aging. Weakness and dizziness on standing are common complaints of elderly persons. Orthostatic tolerance is usually well maintained until the age of 70 years, after which there is an increasing tendency toward arterial pressure instability and postural hypotension. Although orthostatic hypotension may be either systolic or diastolic, hypertensoin associated with aging seems more often to be systolic.[68] Several deficiencies in the circulatory response may predispose the elderly to this problem, including diminished ability to produce an adequate increase in the heart rate, ventricular stroke volume, or peripheral vascular resistance; decreased function of the skeletal muscle pumps; and decreased blood volume. Because cerebral blood flow primarily depends on systolic pressure, persons with impaired cerebral circulation may experience symptoms of weakness, ataxia, dizziness, and syncope when their arterial pressure falls even slightly. This may occur in older persons who are immobilized for even brief periods or whose blood volume is decreased owing to inadequate fluid intake or overzealous use of diuretics.

Postprandial blood pressure often decreases in elderly persons.[68,69] The greatest postprandial changes occur after a high-carbohydrate meal. Although the mechanism responsible for these changes is not fully understood, it is thought to result from glucose-mediated impairment of baroreflex sensitivity and increased splanchnic blood flow mediated by insulin and vasoactive gastrointestinal hormones.

Bed Rest and Immobility. Prolonged bed rest promotes a reduction in plasma volume, a decrease in venous tone, failure of peripheral vasoconstriction, and weakness of the skeletal muscles that support the veins and assist in returning blood to the heart. Physical deconditioning follows even short periods of bed rest. After 3 to 4 days, the blood volume is decreased. Loss of vascular and skeletal muscle tone is less predictable but often becomes maximal after approximately 2 weeks of bed rest. Orthostatic intolerance is a recognized problem of space flight—a potential risk after reentry into the earth's gravitational field.

Disorders of Autonomic Nervous System Function. The sympathetic nervous system plays an essential role in adjustment to the upright position. Sympathetic stimulation increases heart rate and cardiac contractility and causes constriction of peripheral veins and arterioles. Orthostatic hypotension caused by altered ANS function is common in peripheral neuropathies associated with diabetes mellitus, after injury or disease of the spinal cord, or as the result of a cerebral vascular accident in which sympathetic outflow from the brain stem is disrupted. The American Autonomic Society and the American Academy of Neurology have distinguished three forms of primary ANS dysfunction: (1) pure autonomic failure, which is defined as a sporadic, idiopathic cause of persistent orthostatic hypotension and other manifestations of autonomic failure such as urinary retention, impotence, or decreased sweating; (2) Parkinson disease with autonomic failure; and (3) multiple-system atrophy (Shy-Drager syndrome).[70] The Shy-Drager syndrome usually develops in middle to late life as orthostatic hypotension associated with uncoordinated movements, urinary incontinence, constipation, and other signs of neurologic deficits referable to the corticospinal, extrapyramidal, corticobulbar, and cerebellar systems.

Diagnosis and Treatment

Orthostatic hypotension can be assessed with the auscultatory method of blood pressure measurement. A reading should be made when the person is supine, immediately after assumption of the seated or upright position, and 3 minutes after assumption of the standing position. A tilt table also can be used for this purpose. When the table is tilted, the recumbent person can be moved to a head-up position without voluntary movement. The tilt table also has the advantage of rapidly and safely returning persons with a profound postural drop in blood pressure to the horizontal position. Persons with a drop in blood pressure to orthostatic levels should be evaluated to determine the cause and seriousness of the condition. A history should be taken to elicit information about symptoms, particularly dizziness and history of syncope and falls; medical conditions, particularly those such as diabetes mellitus that predispose to orthostatic hypotension; use of prescription and over-the-counter drugs; and symptoms of ANS dysfunction, such as impotence or bladder dysfunction. A physical examination should document blood pressure in both arms and the heart rate while the person is in the supine, sitting, and standing positions and note the occurrence of symptoms. Noninvasive, 24-hour ambulatory blood pressure monitoring may be used to determine blood pressure responses to other stimuli of daily life, such as food ingestion and exertion.

Treatment of orthostatic hypotension usually is directed toward alleviating the cause, or if this is not possible, toward helping the person learn to cope with the disorder and prevent falls and injuries. Medications that predispose to postural hypotension should be avoided. Correcting the fluid deficit and trying a different antihypertensive medication are examples of measures designed to correct the cause. Measures designed to help persons prevent symptomatic orthostatic drops in blood pressure include gradual ambulation to allow the circulatory system to adjust (i.e., sitting on the edge of the bed for several minutes and moving the legs to initiate skeletal muscle pump function before standing); avoidance of situations that encourage excessive vasodilation (e.g., drinking alcohol, exercising vigorously in a warm environment); and avoidance of excess diuresis (e.g., use of diuretics), diaphoresis, or loss of body fluids. Tight-fitting elastic support hose or an abdominal support garment may help prevent pooling of blood in the lower extremities and abdomen.

Pharmacologic treatment may be used when non-pharmacologic methods are unsuccessful. A number of types of drugs can be used for this purpose.[68]

Mineralocorticoids (e.g., fludrocortisone) can be used to reduce salt and water loss and probably increase α-adrenergic sensitivity. Vasopressin-2–receptor agonists (desmopressin as a nasal spray) may be used to reduce nocturnal polyuria. Sympathomimetic drugs that act directly on the resistance vessels (e.g., phenylephrine, clonidine) or on the capacitance vessels (e.g., dihydroergotamine) may be used. Many of these agents have undesirable side effects.

SUMMARY CONCEPTS

■ Arterial blood pressure reflects the rhythmic ejection of blood from the left ventricle, rising as the ventricle contracts and falling as it relaxes; with the *systolic blood pressure* or highest pressure representing the amount of blood that is ejected from the heart with each beat and the *diastolic pressure* or lowest pressure representing the energy that has been stored in the large arteries during systole.

■ Hypertension, which represents an elevation in systolic and/or diastolic blood pressure, is one of the most common health problems. It may occur as a primary disorder or as a sign of some other disorder, such as kidney disease (i.e., secondary hypertension).

■ The pathogenesis of primary hypertension is thought to include constitutional and environmental factors involving the kidney and its role in regulating extracellular fluid volume, intracellular sodium and calcium levels, sympathetic nervous system activity, and regulation of the renin-angiotensin-aldosterone system.

■ Uncontrolled hypertension increases the risk of heart disease, renal complications, retinopathy, and stroke. Treatment of primary hypertension focuses on nonpharmacologic methods such as weight reduction, reduction of sodium intake, and regular physical activity.

■ Hypertension that occurs during pregnancy can be divided into four categories: preeclampsia–eclampsia, gestational hypertension, chronic hypertension, and chronic hypertension with superimposed preeclampsia–eclampsia. Preeclampsia–eclampsia is hypertension that develops after 20 weeks' gestation and is accompanied by proteinuria, posing a particular threat to the mother and the fetus. Chronic hypertension is hypertension that is present before 20 weeks' gestation.

(continued)

SUMMARY CONCEPTS *(continued)*

■ Blood pressure is known to increase from infancy through late adolescence. Among infants and children, secondary hypertension is the most common form of high blood pressure. In later childhood and adolescence, essential hypertension is more common.

■ Isolated systolic hypertension, the most common type of hypertension in the elderly, represents the effects of aging on the distensibility of the aorta and its ability to stretch and accommodate blood being ejected from the left heart during systole. Untreated systolic hypertension is recognized as an important risk factor for stroke and other cardiovascular morbidity and mortality in older persons.

■ Orthostatic hypotension, which is an abnormal decrease in systolic and diastolic blood pressures that occurs on assumption of the upright position, is an important consideration in the occurrence of dizziness and syncope. Among the factors that contribute to its occurrence are decreased fluid volume, medications, aging, defective function of the autonomic nervous system, and the effects of immobility. Treatment includes correcting the reversible causes and assisting the person to compensate for the disorder and prevent falls and injuries.

Disorders of the Venous Circulation

Veins are low-pressure, thin-walled vessels that rely on the ancillary action of skeletal muscle pumps and changes in abdominal and intrathoracic pressure to return blood to the heart. Unlike the arterial system, the venous system is equipped with valves that prevent retrograde flow of blood (see Chapter 17). Although its structure enables the venous system to serve as a storage area for blood, it also renders the system susceptible to problems related to stasis and venous insufficiency. This section focuses on three common problems of the venous system: varicose veins, venous insufficiency, and venous thrombosis.

Venous Circulation of the Lower Extremities

The venous system in the lower extremities consists of two components: the superficial veins (i.e., saphenous vein and its tributaries) and the deep venous channels (Fig. 18-17A). Perforating or communicating veins connect these two systems. Blood from the skin and subcutaneous tissues in the leg collects in the superficial veins

and is then transported across the communicating veins into the deeper venous channels for return to the heart. Venous valves prevent the retrograde flow of blood and play an important role in the function of the venous system. Although these valves are irregularly located along the length of the veins, they almost always are found at junctions where the communicating veins merge with the larger deep veins and where two veins meet. The number of venous valves differs somewhat from one person to another, as does their structural competence, factors that may help explain the familial predisposition to development of varicose veins.

The action of the leg muscles assists in moving venous blood from the lower extremities back to the heart.[26] When a person walks, the action of the leg muscles serves to increase flow in the deep venous channels and return venous blood to the heart (Fig. 18-18). The function of the so-called *muscle pump,* located in the gastrocnemius and soleus muscles of the lower extremities, can be compared with the pumping action of the heart.[75] During muscle contraction, which is similar to systole, valves in the communicating channels close to prevent backward flow of blood into the superficial system, as blood in the deep veins is moved forward by the action of the contracting muscles. During muscle relaxation, which is similar to diastole, the communicating valves open, allowing blood from the superficial veins to move into the deep veins.

Varicose Veins and Venous Insufficiency

The venous system of the lower limbs is associated with a wide clinical spectrum of disorders ranging from cosmetic problems of superficial varicose veins to severe symptoms, including ulceration.

Varicose Veins

Varicose, or dilated, tortuous veins of the lower extremities are common and often lead to secondary problems of venous insufficiency[71-75] (see Fig. 18-17B). The prevalence of varicose veins in Western populations is about 25% to 30% in women and 10% to 20% in men. The condition is more common after 50 years of age and in obese persons, and it occurs more often in women, probably because of venous stasis caused by pregnancy.[2]

Varicose veins are described as being primary or secondary. Primary varicose veins originate in the superficial saphenous veins, and secondary varicose veins result from impaired flow in the deep venous channels. Approximately 80% to 90% of venous blood from the lower extremities is transported through the deep channels. The development of secondary varicose veins becomes inevitable when flow in these deep channels is impaired or blocked. The most common cause of secondary varicose veins is deep vein thrombosis. Other causes include congenital or acquired arteriovenous fistulas, congenital venous malformations, and pressure on the abdominal veins caused by pregnancy or a tumor.

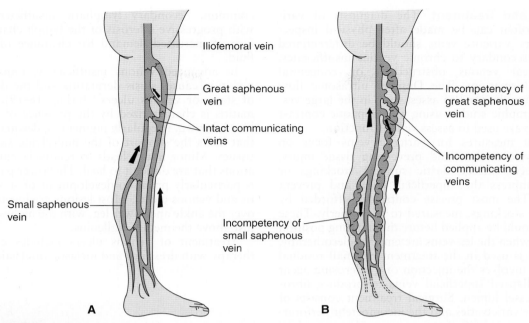

FIGURE 18-17. Superficial and deep venous channels of the leg. **(A)** Normal venous structures and flow patterns. **(B)** Varicosities in the superficial venous system are the result of incompetent valves in the communicating veins. The *arrows* in both views indicate the direction of blood flow. (Modified from Abramson DI. *Vascular Disorders of the Extremities*, 2nd ed. New York, NY: Harper & Row; 1974.)

Etiology. Prolonged standing and increased intra-abdominal pressure are important contributing factors in the development of primary varicose veins.[71-75] Because there are no valves in the inferior vena cava or common iliac veins, blood in the abdominal veins must be supported by the valves located in the external iliac or femoral veins. When intra-abdominal pressure increases, as it does during pregnancy, or when the valves in these two veins are absent or defective, the stress on the saphenofemoral junction is increased. The high incidence of varicose veins in women who have been pregnant also suggests a hormonal effect on venous smooth muscle contributing to venous dilation and valvular incompetence. Lifting also increases intra-abdominal pressure and decreases flow of blood through the abdominal veins. Occupations that require repeated heavy lifting predispose to development of varicose veins.

Prolonged exposure to increased pressure causes the venous valves to become incompetent so they no longer close properly. When this happens, the reflux of blood causes further venous enlargement, pulling the valve leaflet apart and causing more valvular incompetence in sections of adjacent distal veins. Another consideration in the development of varicose veins is the fact that the superficial veins have only subcutaneous fat and superficial fascia for support, whereas the deep venous channels are supported by muscle, bone, and connective tissue. Obesity reduces the support provided by the superficial fascia and tissues, increasing the risk for development of varicose veins.

Clinical Manifestations. The signs and symptoms associated with primary varicose veins vary. Most women with superficial varicose veins complain of their unsightly appearance. In many cases, aching in the lower extremities and edema, especially after long periods of standing, may occur. The edema usually subsides at night when the legs are elevated. When the communicating veins are incompetent, symptoms are more common.

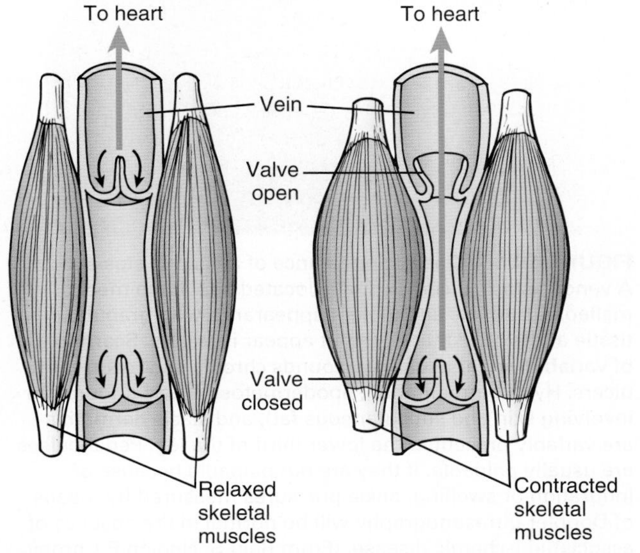

FIGURE 18-18. The skeletal muscle pumps and their function in promoting blood flow in the deep and superficial calf vessels of the leg.

Diagnosis and Treatment. The diagnosis of varicose veins often can be made after physical inspection. Primary varicose veins should be differentiated from those secondary to chronic venous insufficiency, retroperitoneal venous obstruction, or congenital venous malformations. The Doppler ultrasonic flow probe also may be used to assess flow in the large vessels. Angiographic studies using a radiopaque contrast medium also are used to assess venous function.

Treatment measures for varicose veins focus on improving venous flow and preventing tissue injury. When correctly fitted, elastic support stockings or leggings compress the superficial veins and prevent distention. The most precise control is afforded by prescription stockings, measured to fit properly. These stockings should be applied before the standing position is assumed, when the leg veins are empty. Sclerotherapy, which often is used in the treatment of small residual varicosities, involves the injection of a sclerosing agent into the collapsed superficial veins to produce fibrosis of the vessel lumen. Surgical treatment consists of removing the varicosities and the incompetent perforating veins, but it is limited to persons with patent deep venous channels.

Chronic Venous Insufficiency

Chronic venous disease of the lower extremities is manifested by venous hypertension and a range of signs, the most obvious of which are varicose veins and venous ulcers due to venous insufficiency.[74,75] Venous hypertension represents a sustained increase in venous blood pressures.

Etiology. Chronic venous insufficiency is most commonly caused by reflux through incompetent veins, but can also be caused by venous outflow obstruction and impaired function of the skeletal muscle pumps. Pressure in the veins of the legs is determined by two components: a *hydrostatic component* related to the weight of a column of blood below the level of the heart, and a *hydrodynamic component* related to the action of the skeletal muscle pump. Prolonged standing increases venous pressure and causes dilation and stretching of the vessel wall. When a person is in the erect position, the full weight of the venous columns of blood is transmitted to the leg veins. The effects of gravity are compounded in persons who stand for long periods without using their leg muscles to assist in pumping blood back to the heart.

Clinical Manifestations. Chronic venous insufficiency is characterized by signs and symptoms associated with impaired venous blood flow. In contrast to the ischemia caused by arterial insufficiency, venous insufficiency leads to tissue congestion, edema, and eventual impairment of tissue nutrition. The edema is exacerbated by long periods of standing. Necrosis of subcutaneous fat deposits occurs, followed by skin atrophy. Brown pigmentation of the skin caused by hemosiderin deposits resulting from the breakdown of red blood cells is common. Secondary lymphatic insufficiency occurs, with progressive sclerosis of the lymph channels in the face of increased demand for clearance of interstitial fluid.

In advanced venous insufficiency, impaired tissue nutrition causes stasis dermatitis and the development of stasis or venous ulcers[74,76] (Fig. 18-19). Stasis dermatitis is characterized by the presence of thin, shiny, bluish brown, irregularly pigmented, desquamative skin that lacks the support of the underlying subcutaneous tissues. Minor injury leads to relatively painless ulcerations that are difficult to heal. The lower part of the leg is particularly prone to development of stasis dermatitis and venous ulcers. Most lesions are located medially over the ankle and lower leg, with the highest frequency just above the medial malleolus.

Treatment of venous ulcers includes compression therapy with dressings and inelastic or elastic bandages.

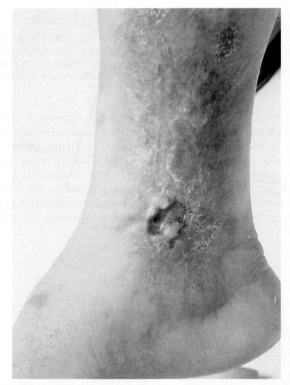

FIGURE 18-19. Classic appearance of a venous stasis ulcer. A venous stasis ulcer is usually located above the medial malleolus and has an indolent appearance with granulation tissue at the base that does not appear ischemic. Scarring of variable extent usually surrounds chronic and recurrent ulcers. Hyperpigmentation, lipodermatosclerosis (induration involving skin and subcutaneous fat), and stasis dermatitis are variably present in the lower third of the leg. Pedal pulses are usually palpable. If they are not palpable because of induration or swelling, ankle pressures measured by means of Doppler ultrasonography will be normal in the absence of associated ischemic disease. (From Raju S, Neglén P. Chronic venous insufficiency and varicose veins. *N Engl J Med.* 2009;360(22):2322. Copyright © 2009. Massachusetts Medical Society.)

Occasionally skin grafting is required for large or slow-healing venous ulcers. Growth factors (which are administered topically or by perilesional injection) may also be warranted.[76]

Venous Thrombosis

The term *venous thrombosis,* or *thrombophlebitis,* describes the presence of thrombus in a vein and the accompanying inflammatory response in the vessel wall.[77,78] Thrombi can develop in the superficial or the deep veins. Deep venous thrombosis (DVT) most commonly occurs in the lower extremities. Deep venous thrombosis of the lower extremity is a serious disorder, complicated by pulmonary embolism (see Chapter 23), recurrent episodes of DVT, and development of chronic venous insufficiency. Isolated calf thrombi often are asymptomatic. If left untreated, they may extend to the larger, more proximal veins, with an increased risk of pulmonary emboli (up to 50% risk from proximal DVTs).

Etiology

In 1846, German pathologist Rudolf Virchow described the triad that has come to be associated with venous thrombosis: stasis of blood, increased blood coagulability, and vessel wall injury.[79] Risk factors for venous thrombosis are summarized in Chart 18-3. Stasis of

---

CHART 18-3   Risk Factors Associated with Venous Thrombosis*

Venous Stasis
Bed rest
Immobility
Spinal cord injury
Acute myocardial infarction
Congestive heart failure
Shock
Venous obstruction

Hyperreactivity of Blood Coagulation
Genetic factors
Stress and trauma
Pregnancy
Childbirth
Oral contraceptive and hormone replacement use
Dehydration
Cancer
Antiphospholipid syndrome
Hyperhomocysteinemia

Vascular Trauma
Indwelling venous catheters
Surgery
Massive trauma or infection
Fractured hip
Orthopedic surgery

*Many of these disorders involve more than one mechanism.

---

blood occurs with immobility of an extremity or the entire body. Bed rest and immobilization are associated with decreased blood flow, venous pooling in the lower extremities, and increased risk of DVT. Persons who are immobilized by a hip fracture, joint replacement, or spinal cord injury are particularly vulnerable to DVT. The risk of DVT is increased in situations of impaired cardiac function. This may account for the relatively high incidence in persons with acute myocardial infarction and congestive heart failure. Elderly persons are more susceptible than younger persons, probably because disorders that produce venous stasis occur more frequently in older persons. Long airplane travel poses a particular threat in persons predisposed to DVT because of prolonged sitting and increased blood viscosity due to dehydration.[80]

Hypercoagulability is a homeostatic mechanism designed to increase clot formation, and conditions that increase the concentration or activation of clotting factors predispose to DVT. Thrombosis also can be caused by inherited or acquired deficiencies in certain plasma proteins that normally inhibit thrombus formation, such as antithrombin III, protein C, and protein S. However, the most common inherited risk factors are the factor V Leiden and prothrombin gene mutations (see Chapter 12). The postpartum state is associated with increased levels of fibrinogen, prothrombin, and other coagulation factors. The use of oral contraceptives and hormone replacement therapy appear to increase coagulability and predispose to venous thrombosis, a risk that is further increased in women who smoke. Certain cancers are associated with increased clotting tendencies, and although the reason for this is largely unknown, substances that promote blood coagulation may be produced by the tumor cells or released from the surrounding tissues in response to the cancerous growth. Immune interactions with cancer cells can result in the release of cytokines that can cause endothelial damage and predispose to thrombosis. When body fluid is lost because of injury or disease, the resulting hemoconcentration causes clotting factors to become more concentrated. Other important risk factors include the antiphospholipid syndrome (discussed in Chapter 12) and hyperhomocysteinemia.

Vessel injury can result from a trauma situation or from surgical intervention. It also may occur secondary to infection or inflammation of the vessel wall. Persons undergoing hip surgery and total hip replacement are at particular risk because of trauma to the femoral and iliac veins and, in the case of hip replacement, thermal damage from heat generated by the polymerization of the acrylic cement that is used in the procedure. Venous catheters are another source of vascular injury.

Clinical Manifestations

Many persons with venous thrombosis are asymptomatic, probably because the vein is not totally occluded or because of collateral circulation.[81–83] When present, the most common signs and symptoms of venous thrombosis are those related to the inflammatory process: pain, swelling, and deep muscle tenderness. Fever, general malaise, and an elevated white blood cell count and erythrocyte sedimentation rate are accompanying indications of inflammation. There may be tenderness and pain along the vein. Swelling may vary from minimal to maximal. As many as 50% of persons with DVT are asymptomatic.

The site of thrombus formation determines the location of the physical findings. The most common site is in the venous sinuses in the soleus muscle and posterior tibial and peroneal veins. Swelling in these cases involves the foot and ankle, although it may be slight or absent. Calf pain and tenderness are common. Femoral vein thrombosis produces pain and tenderness in the distal thigh and popliteal area. Thrombi in ileofemoral veins produce the most profound manifestations, with swelling, pain, and tenderness of the entire extremity. With DVT in the calf veins, active dorsiflexion produces calf pain (i.e., Homans' sign).

Diagnosis and Treatment

The risk of pulmonary embolism emphasizes the need for early detection and treatment of DVT.[81] Several tests are useful for this purpose: ascending venography, ultrasonography (e.g., real time, B mode, duplex), and plasma D-dimer (a degradation product of fibrin) assessment[84] (see Chapter 23).

Whenever possible, venous thrombosis should be prevented in preference to being treated. Early ambulation after childbirth and surgery is one measure that decreases the risk of thrombus formation. Exercising the legs and wearing support stockings improve venous flow. A further precautionary measure is to avoid assuming body positions that favor venous pooling. Antiembolism stockings of the proper fit and length should be used routinely in persons at risk for DVT. Another strategy used for immobile persons at risk for development of DVT is a sequential pneumatic compression device. This consists of a plastic sleeve that encircles the legs and provides alternating periods of compression on the lower extremity. When properly used, these devices enhance venous emptying to augment flow and reduce stasis.

The objectives of treatment of venous thrombosis are to prevent the formation of additional thrombi, prevent extension and embolization of existing thrombi, and minimize venous valve damage.[83,84] Anticoagulation therapy (i.e., warfarin and low–molecular-weight warfarin) is used to treat and prevent venous thrombosis (see Chapter 12). A 15- to 20-degree elevation of the legs prevents stasis. It is important that the entire lower extremity or extremities be carefully extended to avoid acute flexion of the knee or hip. Heat often is applied to the leg to relieve venospasm and to aid in the resolution of the inflammatory process. Bed rest usually is maintained until local tenderness and swelling have subsided. Gradual ambulation with elastic support is then permitted. Standing and sitting increase venous pressure and are to be avoided. Elastic support is needed for 3 to 6 months to permit recanalization and collateralization and to prevent venous insufficiency.

SUMMARY CONCEPTS

■ Veins are thin-walled, distensible vessels that collect blood from the tissues and return it to the heart. The venous system is a low-pressure system that relies on the pumping action of the skeletal muscles to move blood forward and the presence of venous valves to prevent retrograde flow.

■ The storage function of the venous system renders it susceptible to venous insufficiency, stasis, and thrombus formation. Disorders of the venous system produce congestion of the affected tissues and predispose to clot formation because of stagnation of flow and activation of the clotting system.

■ Varicose veins are dilated and tortuous veins that result from a sustained increase in pressure that causes the venous valves to become incompetent, allowing for reflux of blood and vein engorgement.

■ Venous insufficiency, which is associated with stasis dermatitis and venous ulcers, reflects chronic venous stasis resulting from valvular incompetence.

■ Thrombophlebitis refers to thrombus formation in a vein and the accompanying inflammatory response in the vessel wall as a result of conditions that obstruct or slow blood flow, increase the activity of the coagulation system, or cause vessel injury. Deep vein thrombosis may be a precursor to pulmonary embolism.

REVIEW EXERCISES

1. The Third Report of the NCEP Expert Panel on Detection, Evaluation, and Treatment of High Blood Cholesterol in Adults recommends that a person's high density lipoprotein (HDL) should be above 40 mg/dL.

A. Explain the role of HDL in prevention of atherosclerosis.

2. A 55-year-old man presents at the emergency department of his local hospital with complaints of excruciating, "ripping" pain in his upper back. He has a history of poorly controlled hypertension. His radial pulse and blood pressure, which on admission were 92 and 140/80 mm Hg, respectively, become unobtainable in both arms. A transesophageal echocardiogram reveals a dissection of the descending aorta. Aggressive blood pressure control is initiated with the goal of reducing the systolic pressure and pulsatile blood flow (pulse pressure).

A. Explain how aortic dissection differs from a thoracic aortic aneurysm.

B. Explain the role of poorly controlled hypertension as an etiologic factor in dissecting aneurysms.

C. Why did the patient's radial pulse and blood pressure become unobtainable?

D. Explain the need for aggressive control of aortic pressure and pulsatile blood flow.

3. A 34-year-old, otherwise healthy woman complains of episodes lasting several hours in which her fingers become pale and numb. This is followed by a period during which the fingers become red, throbbing, and painful.

A. What do you think is causing this woman's problem?

B. She relates that the episodes often occur when her fingers become cold or when she becomes upset. Explain the possible underlying mechanisms.

C. What types of measures could be used to treat this woman?

4. A 47-year-old African-American man who is an executive in a law firm has his blood pressure taken at a screening program and is told that his pressure is 142/90 mm Hg. His father and older brother have hypertension, and his paternal grandparents had a history of stroke and myocardial infarction. The man enjoys salty foods and routinely uses a salt shaker to add salt to meals his wife prepares, drinks about four beers while watching television in the evening, and has gained 15 pounds in the past year. Although his family has encouraged him to engage in physical activities with them, he states he is either too busy or too tired.

A. According to the JNC 7 guidelines, into what category does the patient's blood pressure fall?

B. What are his risk factors for hypertension?

C. Explain how an increased salt intake might contribute to his increase in blood pressure.

D. What lifestyle changes would you suggest to the patient? Explain the rationale for your suggestions.

5. A 36-year-old woman enters the clinic complaining of headache and not feeling well. Her blood pressure is 175/90 mm Hg. Her renal test results are abnormal, and follow-up tests confirm that she has a stricture of the left renal artery.

A. Would this woman's hypertension be classified as primary or secondary?

B. Explain the physiologic mechanisms underlying her blood pressure elevation.

6. A 75-year-old woman residing in an extended care facility has multiple health problems, including diabetes, hypertension, and heart failure. Lately, she has been feeling dizzy when she stands up, and she has almost fallen on several occasions. Her family is concerned and wants to know why this is happening and what they can do to prevent her from falling and breaking her hip.

A. How would you go about assessing this woman for orthostatic hypotension?

B. What are the causes of orthostatic hypotension in elderly persons?

C. How might this woman's medical conditions and their treatment contribute to her orthostatic hypotension?

D. The woman tells you that she feels particularly dizzy after she has eaten, yet staff members insist that she sit up and socialize with the other residents even though she would rather lie down and rest until the dizziness goes away. Explain the possible reason for her dizziness and what measures might be used to counteract the dizziness.

E. The woman recently had an episode of vomiting and diarrhea on an extremely hot day. She told her family that she was so dizzy that she was sure she would fall. Explain why her dizziness was more severe under these conditions and what might be done to alleviate the situation.

REFERENCES

1. Kumar V, Abbas AK, Fausto N, et al. *Robbins and Cotran Pathologic Basis of Disease*, 8th ed. Philadelphia, PA: Saunders Elsevier; 2010:147–149, 487–520.
2. Gottlieb AI, Liu A. Blood vessels. In: Rubin R, Strayer DS, et al., eds. *Pathology: Clinicopathologic Foundations of Medicine*, 6th ed. Philadelphia, PA: Wolters Kluwer Health/Lippincott Williams & Wilkins; 2012:435–478.
3. Deanfield JE, Halcox JP, Rabelink TJ. Endothelial function and dysfunction. *Circulation*. 2007;115:1285–1295.
4. Hirase T, Node K. Endothelial dysfunction as a cellular mechanism for vascular failure. *Am J Physiol Heart Circ Physiol*. 2012;302:H409–H505.
5. Chait A, Brunzell JD. Acquired hyperlipidemia (secondary dyslipoproteinemias). *Endocrinol Metab Clin North Am*. 1990;19(2):259–278.
6. Ridker PM, Libby P. Risk factors for atherosclerotic disease. In: Bonow RO, Mann DL, Zipes DP, et al., eds. *Braunwald's Heart Disease*, 9th ed. Philadelphia, PA: Elsevier Saunders; 2012:914–935.
7. Smith C, Marks AD, Lieberman M, et al. *Marks' Basic Medical Biochemistry*, 4th ed. Philadelphia, PA: Wolters Kluwer Health/Lippincott Williams & Wilkins; 2011:587–624, 627–662.
8. Sunaram M, Yao Z. Intrahepatic role of exchangeable apolipoproteins in lipoprotein assembly and secretion. *Arterioscler Thromb Vasc Biol*. 2012;32:1073–1978.
9. Genest J, Libby P. Lipoprotein disorders and cardiovascular disease. In: Bonow RO, Mann DL, Zipes DP, et al., eds. *Braunwald's Heart Disease*, 9th ed. Philadelphia, PA: Elsevier Saunders; 2012:975–996.

10. National Institute of Health Expert Panel. *Third Report of the National Cholesterol Education Program (NCEP) Expert Panel on Detection, Evaluation, and Treatment of High Blood Cholesterol in Adults (Adult Treatment Panel III)*. NIH publication No. 01-3670. Bethesda, MD: National Institutes of Health; 2002.

11. Baron RB. Lipid disorders. In: McPhee SJ, Papadakis MA, eds. *Current Medical Diagnosis and Treatment*, 52nd ed. New York, NY: McGraw-Hill Medical; 2013:1245–1256.

12. Fletcher B, Berra K, Ades P. Managing abnormal blood lipids. *Circulation*. 2005;112:3184–3209.

13. Grundy SM, Cleeman JI, Merz CN, et al. Implications of recent clinical trials for the National Cholesterol Education Program (NCEP) Adult Treatment Panel III guidelines. *Circulation*. 2004;110:227–239.

14. Libby P. The vascular pathology of atherosclerosis. In: Libby L, Bonow RO, Mann DL, et al., eds. *Braunwald's Heart Disease*, 9th ed. Philadelphia, PA: Saunders Elsevier; 2011:985–1002.

15. Sharma P, Sharma S, Baltaro R. Systemic vasculitis. *Am Fam Physician*. 2011;83(5):556–565.

16. Guillevin L, Dörner T. Vasculitis: mechanisms involved and clinical manifestations. *Arthritis Res Ther*. 2007;9(suppl 2):2–9.

17. Sontheimer DL. Peripheral vascular disease: diagnosis and treatment. *Am Fam Physician*. 2006;73:1971–1976.

18. White C. Intermittent claudication. *N Engl J Med*. 2007;356:1241–1250.

19. Olin JW. Thromboangiitis obliterans (Buerger's disease). *N Engl J Med*. 2000;343:864–869.

20. Piazzo G, Creager MA. Thromboangiitis obliterans. *Circulation*. 2010;121(16):1858–1861.

21. Bakst R, Merola JE, Franks AG, et al. Raynaud's phenomenon. *J Am Acad Dermatol*. 2008;59:633–653.

22. Herrick AL. The pathogenesis, diagnosis and treatment of Raynaud phenomenon. *Nat Rev Rheumatol*. 2012;8:469–479.

23. Sakalihasen N. Abdominal aortic aneurysms. *Lancet*. 2005;365:1577–1589.

24. Isselbacher EM. Thoracic and abdominal aortic aneurysm. *Circulation*. 2005;111:816–828.

25. Kamalakannan D, Rosman HS, Eagle KA. Acute aortic dissection. *Crit Care Clin*. 2007;23:779–800.

26. Hall JE. *Guyton and Hall Textbook of Medical Physiology*, 12th ed. Philadelphia, PA: *Elsevier Saunders*; 2010:171–176, 213–228.

27. Dorrington KL, Pandit JJ. The obligatory role of the kidney in long-term arterial pressure control: extending Guyton's model of the circulation. *Anesthesia*. 2009;64:1218–1228.

28. Ogedegbe G, Pickering T. Principles and techniques of blood pressure measurement. *Cardiol Clin*. 2010;28(4):571–586.

29. National Heart, Lung, and Blood Institute. *The Seventh Report of the Joint National Committee on Detection, Evaluation, and Treatment of High Blood Pressure*. U.S. Department of Health and Human Services (NIH publication 04-5230). 2004. Available at: http://www.nhlbi.nih.gov/guidelines/hypertension/jnc7full.pdf. Accessed December 28, 2013.

30. Victor RG. Systemic hypertension: mechanisms and diagnosis. In: Bonow RO, Mann DL, Zipes DP, et al., eds. *Braunwald's Heart Disease: Textbook of Cardiovascular Medicine*, 9th ed. Philadelphia, PA: Elsevier Saunders; 2012:935–954.

31. American Diabetes Association. Standards of medical care in diabetes: 2009. *Diabetes Care*. 2009;32(suppl 1):28.

32. Griffith TF, Klassen PS, Franklin SS. Systolic hypertension: an overview. *Am Heart J*. 2005;149:769–775.

33. Staesen JA, Wang J, Bianchi G, et al. Essential hypertension. *Lancet*. 2003;361:1629–1641.

34. Gadegbeku CA, Lea JP. Update on disparities in the pathophysiology and management of hypertension: focus on African Americans. *Med Clin North Am*. 2005;89:921–933.

35. Burt VL, Whelton P, Roccella EJ, et al. Prevalence of hypertension in the U.S. population: results from the Third National Health and Nutrition Examination Survey, 1988–1991. *Hypertension*. 1995;25:305–313.

36. Natali A, Ferrannini E. Hypertension, insulin resistance, and the metabolic syndrome. *Endocrinol Metab Clin North Am*. 2004;33:417–429.

37. Whelton PK, Appel LJ, Sacco RL, et al. Sodium, blood pressure, and cardiovascular disease: further evidence supporting the American Heart Association sodium reduction recommendations. *Circulation* 2012;126:2880–2889.

38. Kotchen TA, Cowley AW, Froehlich ED. Salt in health and disease—a delicate balance. *N Engl J Med*. 2013;368(13):1229–1237.

39. Mathieu P, Poirier P, Pibarot P, et al. Visceral obesity: the link among inflammation, hypertension, and cardiovascular disease. *Circulation*. 2009;53:577–584.

40. Kurukulasuriya R, Stas S, Lasta G, et al. Hypertension and obesity. *Med Clin North Am*. 2011;95:903–917.

41. Beilin LJ, Puddey IB. Alcohol and hypertension: an update. *Hypertension*. 2006;47:1035–1038.

42. Klatsky AL, Freidman GD, Siegelaub AB. Alcohol consumption and blood pressure. *N Engl J Med*. 1977;296:1194–1200.

43. Taler SJ. Secondary causes of hypertension. *Prim Care*. 2008;35:489–500.

44. Textor SC. Current approaches to renovascular hypertension. *Med Clin North Am*. 2009;93:7717–723.

45. Prisant LM, Szerlip HM, Mulloy LL. Fibromuscular dysplasia: an uncommon cause of secondary hypertension. *J Clin Hypertens*. 2006;81:894–898.

46. Merino MJ, Quezado Q. The endocrine system. In: Rubin R, Strayer DS, et al., eds. *Pathology: Clinicopathologic Foundations of Medicine*, 6th ed. Philadelphia, PA: Wolters Kluwer Health/Lippincott Williams & Wilkins; 2012:1074–1076.

47. Hager A. Hypertension in coarctation of the aorta. *Minerva Cardioangiol*. 2009;57:733–742.

48. Kaplan NM. Systemic hypertension: therapy. In: Bonow RO, Mann DL, Zipes DP, et al., eds. *Braunwald's Heart Disease: Textbook of Cardiovascular Medicine*, 9th ed. Philadelphia, PA: Elsevier Saunders; 2012:955–975.

49. Rodriquez MA, Kumar SK, DeCaro M. Hypertensive crisis. *Cardiol Rev*. 2010;18(2):102–107.

50. Johnson W, Nguyen M-L. Hypertensive crises in the Emergency Department. *Cardiol Clin*. 2008;30:533–543.

51. Gifford RW Jr, Roberts JM, August PA, et al.; for the National High Blood Pressure Education Program. *Working Group Report on High Blood Pressure in Pregnancy*. NIH publication No. 00-3029. Bethesda, MD: National Institutes of Health; 2000.

52. Vest AR, Cho L. Hypertension in pregnancy. *Cardiol Clin*. 2012;30:407–423.

53. Kesk TM, Moskovitz JB. Hypertension and pregnancy. *Emerg Med Clin North Am*. 2012;30:903–917.

54. Mustafa R, Ahmed A, Gupta A, et al. A comprehensive review of hypertension in pregnancy. *J Pregnancy*. 2012;11:1–19.

55. Sibai B, Dekker G, Kupfemic M. Pre-eclampsia. *Lancet*. 2005;365:785–799.

56. Riley MR, Bluhm B. High blood pressure in children and adolescents. *Am Fam Physician*. 2012;85(7):693–700.

57. Mitsnefes MM. Hypertension in children and adolescents. *Pediatr Clin North Am*. 2006;53:493–512.

58. National High Blood Pressure Education Program Working Group on High Blood Pressure in Children and Adolescents. *The Fourth Report on the Diagnosis, Evaluation, and Treatment of High Blood Pressure in Children and Adolescents*. NIH Publication 05-5267. 2005. Available at: http://www.nhlbi.nih.gov/health/prof/heart/hbp/hbp_ped.pdf Accessed August 31, 2013.

59. National Center for Health Statistics. *2000 CDC Growth Charts: United States.* 2000. Available at: http://www.cdc.gov/growthcharts. Accessed December 28, 2013.

60. Lando MB. Systemic hypertension. In: Kliegman RM, Stanton BF, St. Gemilli JW, et al. eds. *Nelson Textbook of Pediatrics*, 19th ed. Philadelphia, PA: Saunders Elsevier; 2011:1639–1649.

61. Maddens M, Imam K, Ashkar A. Hypertension in the elderly. *Prim Care Clin Office Pract.* 2005;32:723–753.

62. Acelajado MC, Oparil S. Hypertension in the elderly. *Clin Geriatr Med.* 2009;25:391–412.

63. Chobanian AV. Isolated systolic hypertension in the elderly. *N Engl J Med.* 2007;357(8):789–796.

64. Dickerson LM, Gibson MV. Management of hypertension in older persons. *Am Fam Physician.* 2005;71:469–476.

65. Smith JJ, Porth CJM. Age and the response to orthostatic stress. In: Smith JJ, ed. *Circulatory Response to the Upright Posture.* Boca Raton, FL: CRC Press; 1990:121–138.

66. Lanier JB, Mott MB, Clay EC. Evaluation and management of orthostatic hypotension. *Am Fam Physician.* 2011;84(5):527–536.

67. Calkins H, Zipes DP. Hypotension and syncope. In: Bonow RO, Mann DL, Zipes DP, et al., eds. *Braunwald's Heart Disease: Textbook of Cardiovascular Medicine*, 9th ed. Philadelphia, PA: Elsevier Saunders; 2012:885–995.

68. Gupta V, Lipsitz LA. Orthostatic hypotension in the elderly: diagnosis and treatment. *Am J Med.* 2007;120:841–847.

69. Jansen RWMM, Lipsitz LA. Postprandial hypotension: epidemiology, pathophysiology, and clinical management. *Ann Intern Med.* 1995;122:286–295.

70. American Autonomic Society and American Academy of Neurologists. Consensus statement of the definition of orthostatic hypotension, pure autonomic failure, and multiple system atrophy. *Neurology.* 1996;46:1470.

71. Bergen JJ, Schmid-Schönein GW, Smith PDC, et al. Chronic venous disease. *N Engl J Med.* 2006;355(5):485–498.

72. Brown KR, Rossi PJ. Superficial venous disease. *Surg Clin North Am.* 2013;93:963–982.

73. Jones RH, Carek PJ. Management of varicose veins. *Am Fam Physician.* 2008;78(11):1289–1294.

74. Raju S, Neglén P. Chronic venous insufficiency and varicose veins. *N Engl J Med.* 2009;360:2319–2327.

75. Eberhardt RT, Raffeno JD. Chronic venous insufficiency. *Circulation.* 2005;111:2398–2409.

76. Nelson EA, Cullun N, Jones J. Venous leg ulcers. *Clin Evid.* 2006;15:657–660.

77. López JA, Kearon C, Lee AYY. Deep venous thrombosis. *Hematology.* 2004;2004:439–455.

78. Wakefield TW, Myers DD, Henke PK. Mechanisms of venous thrombosis and resolution. *Arterioscler Thromb Vasc Biol.* 2008;28:387–391.

79. Virchow R. Weinere untersuchungen uber die verstropfung der lungenrarterie und ihre folgen. *Beitr Exp Pathol Physiol.* 1846;2:21.

80. Schurr JH, Machin SJ, Bailey-King S, et al. Frequency and prevention of symptomless deep-vein thrombosis in long-haul flights. *Lancet.* 2001;357:1485-1489.

81. Wilbur J, Shian B. Diagnosis of deep venous thrombosis and pulmonary embolism. *Am Fam Physician.* 2012;86(11):913–919.

82. Galioto NJ, Danley DL, Van Maanen RJ. Recurrent venous thromboembolism. *Am Fam Physician.* 2011;83(3):293–500.

83. Burnett B. Management of venous thromboembolism. *Prim Care Clin Office Pract.* 2013;48:73–90.

84. Merti GJ. Treatment of venous thromboembolism. *Am J Med.* 2008;121(11A):52

Porth Essentials Resources

Explore these additional resources to enhance learning for this chapter:

- NCLEX-Style Questions and Other Resources on thePoint, http://thePoint.lww.com/PorthEssentials4e
- Study Guide for Essentials of Pathophysiology
- Concepts in Action Animations
- Adaptive Learning | Powered by PrepU, http://thepoint.lww.com/prepu

C h a p t e r 19

Disorders of Cardiac Function

Heart disease affects persons of all ages and ethnicities and remains the leading cause of death in developed countries, including the United States. Heart disease accounts for approximately 30% of deaths worldwide, including nearly 40% in high-income countries and approximately 28% in low- and middle-income countries.[1] Experts predict that heart disease will become the leading cause of death worldwide by 2020 and will surpass death rates from infectious diseases as a result of economic advances, social structures, and demographics.[1]

In an attempt to focus on common health problems that affect persons of all age groups, the chapter has been organized into five sections: coronary artery disease, endocardial and valvular disorders, disorders of the pericardium, cardiomyopathies, and heart disease in infants and children.

Coronary Artery Disease

Coronary artery disease (CAD) describes heart disease caused by impaired coronary blood flow. Diseases of the coronary arteries can cause a spectrum of ischemic disorders ranging from angina to myocardial infarction (i.e., heart attack), as well as conduction defects, heart failure, and sudden cardiac death.

Coronary Circulation

The coronary arteries and coronary veins comprise the blood vessels of the heart that carry blood to and from most of the myocardium (Fig. 19-1). The coronary vessels lay across the surface of the heart and are embedded in adipose tissue just under the epicardium.

There are two main coronary arteries, the left and the right, which arise from the aortic sinus. The *left main coronary artery* extends approximately 4 cm and then divides into the left anterior descending and circumflex branches.[2,3] The *left anterior descending artery* passes through the groove between the two ventricles, giving off diagonal branches, which supply the anterior wall of the left ventricle, and perforating branches, which supply the anterior portion of the interventricular septum

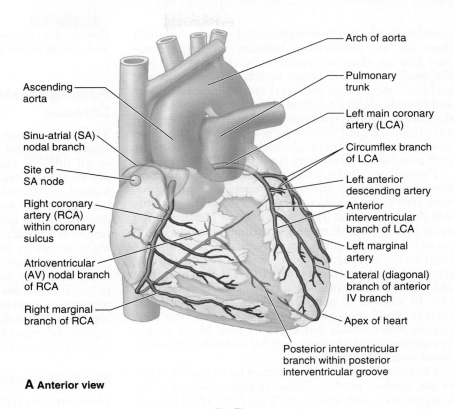

A Anterior view

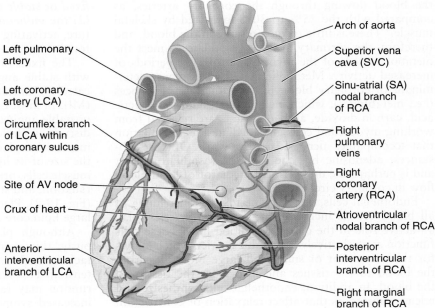

B Posteroinferior view

FIGURE 19-1. Coronary circulation.
(A) Anterior view of the coronary arteries.
(B) Posterior view of the coronary arteries and coronary sinus veins. (From Moore KL, Dalley AF, Agur AMR. *Clinically Oriented Anatomy.* 6th ed. Philadelphia, PA: Wolters Kluwer Health | Lippincott Williams & Wilkins; 2010:146.)

and the anterior papillary muscle of the left ventricle. The *circumflex branch* of the left coronary artery passes to the left and moves posteriorly in the groove that separates the left atrium and ventricle, giving off branches that supply the left lateral wall of the left ventricle. The *right coronary artery* lies in the right atrioventricular groove, and its branches supply the right ventricle. The right coronary artery usually crosses to the back of the

heart, where this vessel forms the *posterior descending artery,* which, in most individuals, supplies the posterior portion of the heart, interventricular septum, sinoatrial (SA) and atrioventricular (AV) nodes, and posterior papillary muscle.[4-6]

The right and left coronary arteries or epicardial arteries branch into smaller intramyocardial arteries, which penetrate the myocardium before merging with a network or plexus of subendocardial vessels. Although there are no connections between the large coronary arteries, there are anastomotic channels that join the small arteries. If larger vessels gradually become occluded, the smaller collateral vessels increase in size and provide alternative channels for blood flow. One of the reasons individuals with CAD may not experience any symptoms until the disease is advanced is due to the development of collateral channels occurring in concert with atherosclerotic changes (see Chapter 18).

Physical, metabolic, and neural factors control blood flow in the coronary arteries. The openings for the coronary arteries originate in the root of the aorta just outside the aortic valve. Thus, aortic blood pressure is the main factor controlling the perfusion pressure in the coronary arteries; aortic pressure is generated by the heart itself. Myocardial blood flow, in turn, is largely regulated by the metabolic activity of the myocardium and autoregulatory mechanisms that control vessel dilation. In addition to generating the aortic pressure that propels blood through the coronary vessels, the contracting heart muscle influences its own blood supply by compressing the intramyocardial and subendocardial blood vessels during systole.

Coronary blood flow is regulated by oxygen demand of the cardiac muscle. Under resting conditions, the heart extracts and utilizes 60% to 80% of oxygen in the blood flowing through the coronary arteries, as compared with the 25% to 30% extracted by skeletal muscle.[4] There is little oxygen reserve in the blood, and therefore, the coronary arteries vasodilate to meet the metabolic needs of the myocardium during periods of increased activity. Metabolic activity is a major determinant of coronary blood flow. Numerous substances (i.e., metabolites), which include potassium ions, lactic acid, carbon dioxide, and adenosine, are released from working myocardial cells and mediate the vasodilation that accompanies increased cardiac work. Of these substances, adenosine has the greatest vasodilator effect and is perhaps the most critical mediator of local blood flow in coronary circulation.[4]

Endothelial cells, which make up the inner lining of all blood vessels including the coronary arteries, play an active role in the control of blood flow. These cells function as a selectively permeable barrier, which allows for the movement of small and large molecules from the blood to the tissues and also from the tissues to the blood. In addition, endothelial cells synthesize and release substances that affect relaxation or constriction of the vascular smooth muscle cells in the arterial wall. Potent vasodilators produced by the endothelium include nitric oxide (NO), prostacyclin, and endothelium-dependent hyperpolarizing factor (EDHF). The most important of these is nitric oxide. Most vasodilating stimuli exert their effects through nitric oxide pathways.[7,8] The endothelium also is the source of endothelium-dependent constricting factors, the best known of which are the endothelins. Coagulation factors (e.g., thrombin), inflammatory mediators (e.g., histamine), and mechanical factors (e.g., increased shear force exerted on the vessel wall) and ischemia contribute to

flow-mediated vasodilation, and stimulate the synthesis and release of nitric oxide.[5]

Pathogenesis of Coronary Artery Disease

The most common cause of CAD is atherosclerosis (discussed in Chapter 18). Atherosclerosis may affect one or all three of the major epicardial coronary arteries and their branches. Clinically significant lesions may be located anywhere in these vessels, but tend to predominate in the first several centimeters of the left anterior descending and left circumflex artery or along the entire length of the right coronary artery.[6] In some cases the major secondary branches also are involved.

Coronary heart disease is commonly divided into two broad disorders: acute coronary syndromes and chronic ischemic heart disease. The acute coronary syndromes represent a spectrum ranging from unstable angina to myocardial infarction that is caused by acute plaque disruption, whereas chronic ischemic heart disease is caused by atherosclerosis or vasospasm of the coronary arteries.

Plaque Disruption and Thrombus Formation

There are two types of atherosclerotic lesions: (1) the *fixed* or *stable plaque*, which obstructs blood flow, and (2) the *vulnerable* or *unstable* plaque, which can rupture, activating a cascade of events leading to thrombus formation.

The fixed or stable plaque is commonly associated with stable angina, and the unstable plaque is implicated in unstable angina and myocardial infarction (MI). In most cases the myocardial ischemia underlying unstable angina and acute MI is precipitated by plaque disruption, followed by thrombosis. The major determinants of plaque vulnerability to disruption include the size of its lipid-rich core, lack of stabilizing smooth muscle cells, presence of inflammation with plaque degradation, and stability and thickness of its fibrous cap[6,9] (Fig. 19-2). Plaques with a thin fibrous cap overlying a large lipid core are at high risk for rupture.[10]

Although plaque disruption may occur spontaneously, this event is often triggered by hemodynamic factors, such as blood flow characteristics and vessel tension. For example, an elevated risk for plaque disruption may result from physiologic events including increased sympathetic activity elicited by rising blood pressure, heart rate, or cardiac contractility.[6] Plaque disruption is also associated with diurnal variation, which commonly occurs within an hour of rising. This phenomenon suggests that physiologic factors (e.g., coronary artery tone and blood pressure) may promote atherosclerotic plaque disruption and subsequent platelet deposition.[6] The elevated sympathetic activity associated with wakefulness and being active may promote platelet aggregation and fibrinolytic activity that favor plaque disruption and thrombosis.

Local thrombosis occurring after plaque disruption results from a complex interaction among the contents

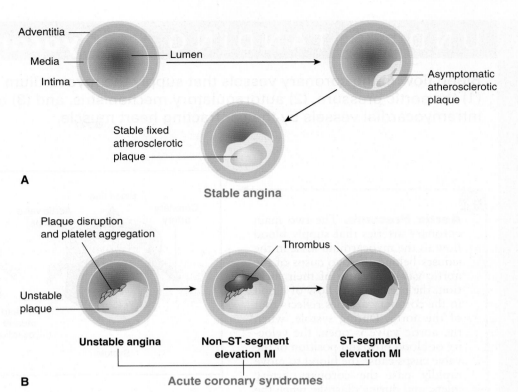

FIGURE 19-2. Atherosclerotic plaque. **(A)** Stable fixed atherosclerotic plaque in stable angina and **(B)** unstable plaque with plaque disruption and platelet aggregation in the acute coronary syndromes.

of the lipid core, smooth muscle cells, macrophages, and collagen. The lipid core provides a stimulus for platelet aggregation and thrombus formation.[6] Both smooth muscle and foam cells in the lipid core contribute to the expression of tissue factor in unstable plaques. Once exposed to blood, tissue factor initiates the extrinsic coagulation pathway, resulting in the local generation of thrombin and deposition of fibrin (see Chapter 12).

Platelets are critical to the events following plaque disruption in acute CAD. Platelets adhere to the endothelium and release substances (i.e., adenosine diphosphate [ADP], thromboxane A_2, and thrombin) that promote further aggregation of platelets and thrombus formation. Glycoprotein receptors expressed on the platelet surface bind fibrinogen and cross-link platelets, contributing to thrombus formation. Platelet adhesion and aggregation occurs in several steps. First, release of ADP, thromboxane A_2, and thrombin initiates the aggregation process. Second, activation of glycoprotein IIb/IIIa receptors on the platelet surface occurs. Third, fibrinogen binds to the activated glycoprotein receptors, forming bridges between adjacent platelets.

Acute Coronary Syndrome

Acute coronary syndrome (ACS) represents a spectrum of acute ischemic heart diseases ranging from unstable ischemia to acute MI based on the presence or absence of an ST-segment elevation or depression on the ECG.[11,12] This criterion allows for immediate classification of risk and guides whether a person should be considered for acute reperfusion therapy. The evaluation of serum

biomarkers (e.g., troponin I) is then used to determine whether an acute MI has occurred.

Electrocardiographic Changes

The classic ECG changes that occur with ACS include ST-segment elevation, T-wave inversion, and development of an abnormal Q wave[11,12] (Fig. 19-3). These changes may not be present immediately after the onset of symptoms and vary considerably depending on the duration of the ischemic event (acute versus evolving), its extent (subendocardial versus transmural), and its location (anterior versus inferior posterior). Because these changes usually occur over time and are seen on the ECG leads that view the involved area of the myocardium, provision for continuous and serial 12-lead ECG monitoring is indicated.

The T wave and ST segment, which represent the ventricular repolarization phase of the cardiac action potential on the ECG, are usually the first to be involved during myocardial ischemia and injury.[13] During myocardial ischemia, repolarization is altered as the involved area becomes ischemic. This leads to T wave abnormalities, such as T-wave inversion. ST-segment changes also occur with acute ischemic myocardial injury. Normally, the ST segment of the ECG is nearly isoelectric (i.e., does not deviate from the baseline) because healthy myocardial cells attain the same resting membrane potential during early repolarization. Acute ischemia reduces the resting membrane potential and shortens the duration of the action potential of the cells within the ischemic area. The voltage difference in the cell membranes between the normal and ischemic areas of the myocardium leads to a "current of injury" between these regions.

(*text continues on page 449*)

U N D E R S T A N D I N G ➡ **Myocardial Blood**

Blood flow in the coronary vessels that supply the myocardium is influenced by (1) the aortic pressure, (2) autoregulatory mechanisms, and (3) compression of the intramyocardial vessels by the contracting heart muscle.

①

Aortic Pressure. The two main coronary arteries that supply blood flow to the myocardium arise in the sinuses behind the two cusps of the aortic valve. Because of their location, the pressure and flow of blood in the coronary arteries reflects that of the aorta. During systole, when the aortic valve is open, the velocity of blood flow and position of the valve cusps cause the blood to move rapidly past the coronary artery inlets, and during diastole, when the aortic valve is closed, blood flow and the aortic pressure are transmitted directly into the coronary arteries.

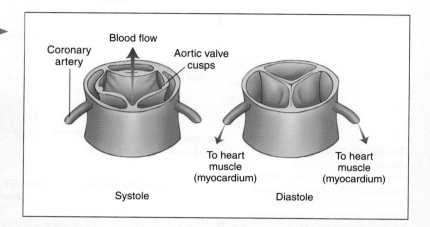

②

Autoregulatory Mechanisms. The heart normally extracts 60% to 80% of the oxygen in the blood delivered to it, leaving little in reserve. Accordingly, oxygen delivery during periods of increased metabolic demand depends on autoregulatory mechanisms that regulate blood flow through a change in vessel tone and diameter. During increased metabolic demand, vasodilation produces an increase in blood flow; during decreased demand, vasoconstriction or return of vessel tone to normal produces a reduction in flow. The mechanisms that link the metabolic activity of the heart to changes in vessel tone result from vasoactive mediators released from myocardial cells and the vascular endothelium.

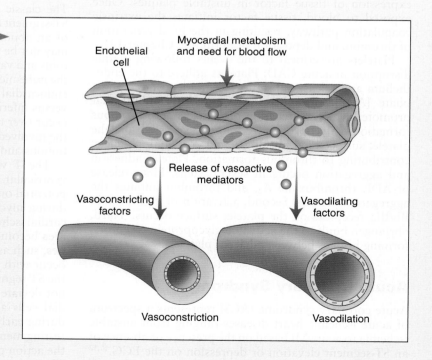

Flow

3 **Vessel Compression.** The large coronary arteries lie on the epicardial surface of the heart, with the smaller intramyocardial vessels branching off and moving through the myocardium before merging with a plexus of vessels that supply the subendocardial muscle with blood. During systole, the contracting cardiac muscle has a squeezing effect on the intramyocardial vessels while at the same time producing an increase in intraventricular pressure that pushes against and compresses the subendocardial vessels. As a result, blood flow to the subendocardial muscle is greatest during diastole. Because the time spent in diastole becomes shortened as the heart rate increases, myocardial blood flow can be greatly reduced during sustained periods of tachycardia.

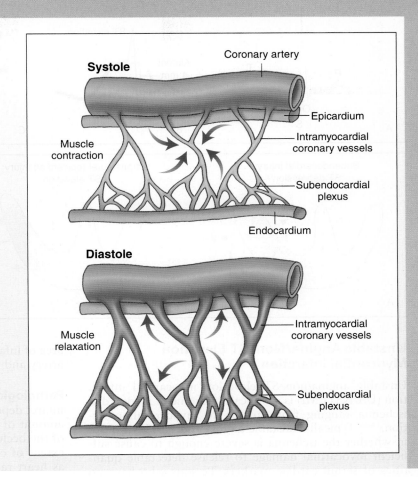

(text continued from page 447)

These currents of injury are represented as a deviation of the ST segment on the ECG. When the acute injury is transmural, the overall ST vector is shifted in the direction of the outer epicardium, resulting in an elevation of the ST segment (see Fig. 19-3). When the injury is confined primarily to the subendocardium, the ST vector is shifted toward the inner ventricular layer, resulting in an overall depression of the ST segment. Additional ventricular depolarization (QRS) changes may follow the T-wave and ST-segment abnormalities.[11,13] With actual infarction, depolarization (QRS) changes often follow the T-wave and ST-segment abnormalities.

Serum Biomarkers

Serum biomarkers for ACS, referred to as a cardiac panel, include cardiac-specific troponin I (TnI) and troponin T (TnT), creatine kinase MB (CK-MB), and myoglobin.[12,14] As myocardial cells become necrotic, their intracellular contents diffuse into the surrounding interstitium and into the blood. The rate at which the enzymes appear in the blood depends on their intracellular location, molecular weight, and local blood flow. For example, they may appear at an earlier-than-predicted time in patients who have undergone successful reperfusion therapy.

The *troponin assays* have high specificity for myocardial tissue and are the primary biomarker tests for the diagnosis of MI. The troponin complex, which is part of the actin filament, consists of three subunits (i.e., TnC, TnT, and TnI) that regulate the calcium-mediated actin–myosin contractile process in striated muscle (see Chapter 1, Fig. 1-19). Troponin I and troponin T, which are present in cardiac muscle, begin to rise within 3 hours after the onset of myocardial infarction and may remain elevated for 7 to 10 days after the event. This is especially useful in the late diagnosis of MI.[12] *Creatine kinase* is an intracellular enzyme found in muscle cells. There are three isoenzymes of CK, with the MB isoenzyme being highly specific for injury to myocardial tissue. Serum levels of CK-MB exceed normal ranges within 4 to 8 hours of myocardial injury and decline to normal within 2 to 3 days.[12] *Myoglobin* is an oxygen-carrying protein, similar to hemoglobin, expressed in cardiac and skeletal muscle. This small molecule is released quickly from infarcted myocardial tissue, and elevated levels can be detected in the blood within 1 hour after myocardial cell death with peak levels reached within 4 to 8 hours.[12] Because myoglobin is present in both cardiac and skeletal muscle, this molecule is not specific to cardiac injury.

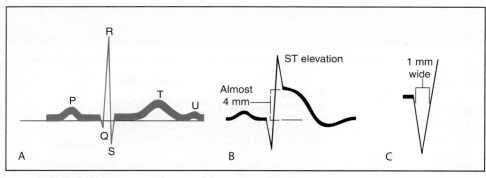

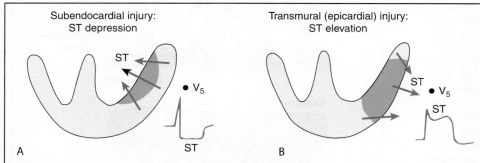

FIGURE 19-3. (*Top*)
(A) Electrocardiogram tracing showing normal P, Q, R, S, and T waves. **(B)** ST-segment elevation with acute ischemia. **(C)** Q wave with acute myocardial infarction. (*Bottom*) Current-of-injury patterns with acute ischemia. **(A)** With predominant subendocardial ischemia, the resultant ST segment is directed toward the inner layer of the affected ventricle and the ventricular cavity. Overlying leads therefore record ST-segment depression. **(B)** With ischemia involving the outer ventricular layer (transmural or epicardial injury), the ST vector is directed outward. Overlying leads record ST-segment elevation. (Bottom from Zipes DP, Bonow RO, Mann DL, et al., eds. *Heart Disease: A Textbook of Cardiovascular Medicine.* 8th ed. Philadelphia, PA: Saunders Elsevier; 2008:174.)

Unstable Angina/Non–ST Elevation Myocardial Infarction

Unstable angina/non–ST elevation myocardial infarction (UA/NSTEMI) is a clinical syndrome of myocardial ischemia ranging from angina to myocardial infarction.[14–16] Typically, unstable angina and NSTEMI differ in whether the ischemia is severe enough to cause sufficient myocardial damage to release detectable quantities of serum cardiac markers. Persons who have no evidence of serum markers for myocardial damage are considered to have unstable angina, whereas a diagnosis of NSTEMI is indicated when there are detectable serum markers of myocardial injury.

The pain associated with unstable angina typically has a persistent and severe course and is characterized by at least one of three features: (1) it occurs at rest (or with minimal exertion), usually lasting more than 20 minutes if untreated (i.e., without nitroglycerine); (2) it is severe and described as frank pain and of new onset (i.e., within 1 month); and (3) it is more severe, prolonged, or frequent than previously experienced.[16]

The risk of acute MI in an individual diagnosed with UA/NSTEMI is classified as low, intermediate, or high based upon the clinical history, ECG pattern, and serum biomarkers. The ECG pattern associated with in NSTEMI may display normal or ST-segment depression (or transient ST-segment elevation) and T-wave changes. The degree of ST-segment deviation from baseline is an important measure of ischemia and indicator of prognosis.

ST Elevation Myocardial Infarction

Acute ST elevation MI (STEMI) is characterized by the necrosis of myocardial tissue and a consequence of atherosclerotic disease of the coronary arteries. The specific area of infarction is determined by the affected coronary artery and its distribution of blood flow (Fig. 19-4).

Pathologic Changes. The size and pattern of the infarct depends on the location and extent of occlusion, amount of heart tissue supplied by the vessel, duration of the occlusion, metabolic needs of the affected tissue, extent of collateral circulation, and other factors such as heart rate, blood pressure, and cardiac rhythm. An infarct may involve the endocardium, myocardium, or epicardium, or a combination of these tissue layers.[6] Transmural infarcts involve the full thickness of the ventricular wall and most commonly occur when there is obstruction of a single artery (Fig. 19-5). Subendocardial infarcts involve the inner one third to one half of the ventricular wall and occur more frequently in the presence of severely narrowed but still patent arteries.

The principal biochemical consequence of MI is the conversion from aerobic to anaerobic metabolism with inadequate production of energy to sustain normal myocardial function.[18] As a result, a striking loss of contractile function occurs within 60 seconds of onset.[6] Changes in cell structure (i.e., glycogen depletion and mitochondrial swelling) develop within several minutes. These early changes are reversible if blood flow is restored. Although gross tissue changes are not apparent for hours after the onset of MI, the ischemic area ceases to function within a matter of minutes, and damage to cells occurs in approximately 40 minutes. Irreversible myocardial cell death (necrosis) occurs after 20 to 40 minutes of severe ischemia[6] (Fig. 19-6).

The term *reperfusion* refers to the reestablishment of blood flow using fibrinolytic therapy or revascularization procedures. Early reperfusion after onset of occlusion can prevent necrosis and improve myocardial perfusion in the infarct zone. Reperfusion after a

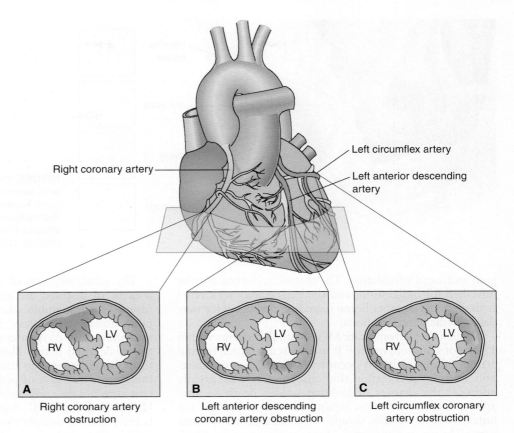

FIGURE 19-4. Areas of the heart affected by occlusion of the **(A)** right coronary artery, **(B)** left anterior descending coronary artery, and **(C)** left circumflex coronary artery. LV, left ventricle; RV, right ventricle.

Right coronary artery

Left circumflex artery

Left anterior descending artery

A Right coronary artery obstruction

B Left anterior descending coronary artery obstruction

C Left circumflex coronary artery obstruction

longer interval can salvage some ischemic myocardial cells. Reestablishing blood flow may also prevent the microvascular injury that occurs over a longer period.

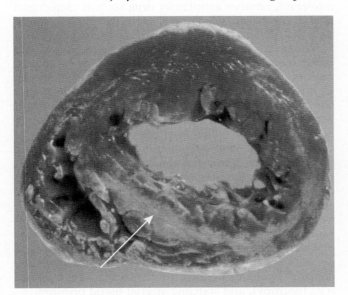

FIGURE 19-5. Acute myocardial infarct. A cross-section of the ventricles of a man who died a few days after the onset of severe chest pain shows a transmural infarct in the posterior and septal regions of the left ventricle. The necrotic myocardium is soft, yellowish, and sharply demarcated. (From Rubin E, Farber JL. *Rubin's Pathology: Clinicopathologic Foundations of Medicine.* 3rd ed. Philadelphia, PA: Lippincott Williams & Wilkins; 1999:558.)

Even though much of the viable myocardium existing at the time reperfusion recovers, critical abnormalities in biochemical function may persist, and these changes can lead to chronic impairment of ventricular function. The recovering area of the heart is often referred to as a *stunned myocardium*. Because myocardial function is lost before cell death occurs, a stunned myocardium may not be capable of sustaining life, and persons with large areas of dysfunctional myocardium may require supportive care until the stunned regions regain their function.[6]

The onset of STEMI involves abrupt and significant chest pain. The pain typically is severe, often described as being constricting, suffocating, and crushing. Substernal pain that radiates to the left arm, neck, or jaw is common, although it may be experienced in other areas of the chest and back. Unlike that of angina, the pain associated with MI is more prolonged and not relieved by rest or nitroglycerin; this pain frequently requires morphine for relief. Some persons may not describe it as "pain," but as "discomfort." Women may experience atypical ischemic-type chest pain, whereas the elderly may complain of shortness of breath more frequently than chest pain.[17] Complaints of fatigue and weakness, especially of the arms and legs, are common. Pain and elevated sympathetic activity invoke tachycardia, anxiety, and restlessness, as well as emotional responses (e.g., a feeling of impending doom). Impairment of myocardial function may lead to hypotension and shock. In addition, gastrointestinal complaints are common with acute MI. There may be a sensation of epigastric distress; nausea and vomiting may occur. These symptoms are thought to be related to the severity of the

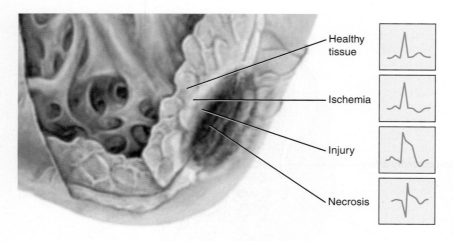

Healthy tissue

Ischemia

Injury

Necrosis

FIGURE 19-6. Zone of myocardial infarction with associated ECG changes. (Adapted from Anatomical Chart Company. *Atlas of Pathophysiology.* 3rd ed. Philadelphia, PA: Wolters Kluwer Health | Lippincott Williams & Wilkins; 2010:63.)

pain and vagal stimulation. The epigastric distress may be mistaken for indigestion, and the person may seek relief with antacids or other home remedies; this behavior may delay medical interventions.

Sudden death from acute MI is death that occurs within 1 hour of symptom onset.[12] It usually is attributed to fatal arrhythmias, which may occur without evidence of infarction. Early hospitalization after onset of symptoms greatly improves the chances of averting sudden death because appropriate resuscitation equipment and personnel are immediately available should a ventricular arrhythmia occur. The recent distribution of automatic external defibrillators in multiple public arenas highlights the importance of early defibrillation in the survival of patients with STEMI.

Diagnosis and Treatment. Because STEMI diagnosis can be challenging before biomarkers and ECG data are available, the immediate management of unstable angina/NSTEMI and STEMI is similar.[12,14] Acute coronary syndrome prognosis is associated with the risk of two general complications—arrhythmias and mechanical (pump) failure. The majority of deaths from ACS are due to sudden cardiac death related to the development of ventricular fibrillation. Therefore, seeking prompt medical care is a critical element in the effective management of persons with ACS. The immediate deployment of an emergency medical team capable of resuscitation procedures—specifically defibrillation and expeditious transport to a hospital equipped to initiate reperfusion therapy, manage arrhythmias, and provide advanced cardiac life support—is crucial.[12]

The emergency department goals for management of ACS include rapid identification of persons who are candidates for reperfusion therapy. Evaluation of the person's chief complaint, typically chest pain, along with other associated symptoms is essential in differentiating ACS from other diagnoses. For any person presenting with symptoms of ACS, providers should perform a 12-lead ECG and continuous ECG monitoring. Treatment regimens also include administration of oxygen, aspirin, nitrates, morphine, antiplatelet and anticoagulant therapy, β-adrenergic blocking agents (beta blockers), and an angiotensin-converting enzyme (ACE) inhibitor.[12,14]

The administration of oxygen augments the oxygen content of inspired air and increases the oxygen saturation of hemoglobin. Arterial oxygen levels may fall precipitously after acute MI, and oxygen administration maintains oxygen content of the blood perfusing the myocardial tissue. Platelets play a major role in the thrombotic response to atherosclerotic plaque disruption; therefore, inhibition of platelet aggregation is an important aspect in the early treatment of both unstable angina/NSTEMI and STEMI. Aspirin (i.e., acetylsalicylic acid) is the preferred antiplatelet agent for preventing platelet aggregation in persons with ACS. Aspirin, which acts by inhibiting synthesis of the prostaglandin thromboxane A_2, is thought to promote reperfusion and reduce the likelihood of re-thrombosis. For patients who are aspirin-intolerant, another antiplatelet drug such as clopidogrel may be prescribed. Clopidogrel exerts its effects by inhibiting the ADP pathway in platelets[18] (see Chapter 12).

The severe pain of acute MI gives rise to anxiety and recruitment of autonomic nervous system responses, both of which increase the work demands on the heart. Control of pain in acute MI is accomplished through a combination of nitrates, analgesics (e.g., morphine), and beta-blocking agents.[12] Nitroglycerin is administered because of its vasodilating effect and ability to relieve coronary pain. The vasodilating effects of the drug decrease venous return (i.e., reduce preload) and arterial blood pressure (i.e., reduce afterload), thereby reducing oxygen consumption. Although a number of analgesic agents have been used to treat the pain of acute MI, morphine is usually the drug of choice to be given intravenously for rapid onset of action.[11] Beta antagonists block β-receptor–mediated functions of the sympathetic nervous system and thus decrease myocardial oxygen demand by reducing heart rate, cardiac contractility (i.e., inotropy), and systemic arterial blood pressure.

Immediate reperfusion therapy through use of pharmacologic agents (fibrinolytic therapy), percutaneous coronary intervention, or coronary artery bypass grafting is usually indicated for persons with ECG evidence of STEMI. *Fibrinolytic drugs* degrade blood and platelet clots, and their use is associated with positive outcomes such as reduced mortality and incidence of lethal arrhythmias, limited infarct size, improved infarct healing, and myocardial remodeling.[12] These agents interact with plasminogen to generate plasmin, which lyses fibrin clots and digests clotting factors V and VIII, prothrombin, and fibrinogen (see Chapter 12). The person must be at low risk for complications caused by bleeding, with no intracranial hemorrhage or significant trauma within the last 3 months.[14]

Percutaneous coronary intervention (PCI) is indicated as an early invasive procedure for patients with unstable angina/NSTEMI.[19] Percutaneous coronary intervention includes percutaneous transluminal coronary angioplasty (PTCA) and stent implantation. *Balloon PTCA* involves dilating the coronary artery with an inflatable balloon positioned at the narrowing of stenotic atherosclerotic plaque within the vessel (Fig. 19-7). Similar to an angiogram, the procedure is performed under local anesthesia in the cardiac catheterization laboratory. Balloon PTCA is almost exclusively used in conjunction with coronary stenting. The addition of *coronary stenting* significantly improved short- and long-term outcomes for patient with ACS compared with PTCA alone but patients remain at risk for restenosis and thrombosis following the procedure. Persons undergoing stent procedures must be treated with antiplatelet and anticoagulant drugs to prevent thrombosis and restenosis. Drug-eluting stents that provide sustained delivery of an antiproliferative pharmacologic agent may be used to decrease the risk of thrombosis.[19]

Coronary artery bypass grafting (CABG) may be the treatment of choice for people with significant CAD who do not respond to medical treatment and who are not suitable candidates for PCI. It may also be indicated as an emergent treatment for STEMI, in which case the surgery should be done within 4 to 6 hours

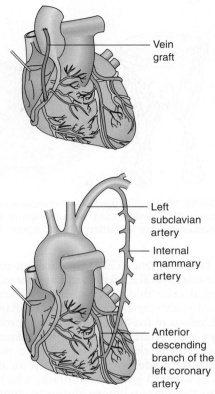

FIGURE 19-8. Coronary artery revascularization. (*Top*) Saphenous vein bypass graft. The vein segment is sutured to the ascending aorta and the right coronary artery at a point distal to the occluding lesion. (*Bottom*) Mammary artery bypass graft. The mammary artery is anastomosed to the descending branch of the left coronary artery, bypassing the obstructing lesion.

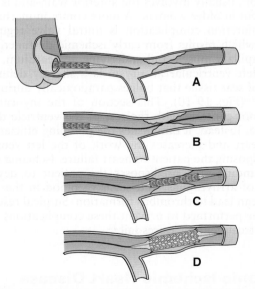

FIGURE 19-7. Balloon-expandable stent insertion. **(A)** Insertion of a guide catheter with a collapsed balloon-expandable stent mounted over a guide wire into a coronary artery. **(B)** Advancement of guide wire across the coronary lesion. **(C)** Positioning of the balloon-expandable stent across the lesion. **(D)** Balloon inflation with deployment of the stent. Once the stent is expanded, the balloon system is removed.

of symptom onset if possible. The procedure involves revascularization of the affected myocardium by attaching a saphenous vein graft between the aorta and the affected coronary artery distal to the site of occlusion, or by using the internal mammary artery to revascularize the left anterior descending artery or its branches (Fig. 19-8). This procedure often involves one to five distal anastomoses. Using emergent or urgent CABG as a reperfusion strategy is indicated in situations such as failed PCI with persistent pain or hemodynamic instability, or for patients who are not candidates for PCI or fibrinolytic therapy.

Myocardial Postinfarction Recovery Period. After a MI, there usually are three zones of tissue damage: a zone of myocardial tissue that becomes necrotic because of an absolute lack of blood flow; a surrounding zone of injured or hypoxic cells, some of which will recover; and an outer zone in which cells are ischemic and can be salvaged if blood flow can be reestablished. The boundaries of these zones may change with respect to the timeliness of treatment to successfully reestablish blood flow. If blood flow can be restored within 20 to 40 minutes, loss of cell viability is minimized.[6] The process of ischemic necrosis usually begins in the subendocardial area of the

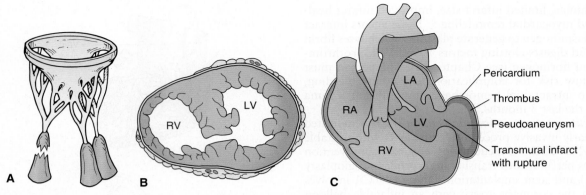

FIGURE 19-9. Acute mechanical complications of myocardial infarction. **(A)** Papillary muscle rupture. **(B)** Interventricular septum rupture. **(C)** Rupture of the free wall of the left ventricle with pseudoaneurysm formation. LA, left atrium; LV, left ventricle; RA, right atrium; RV, right ventricle.

heart and extends through the myocardium to involve more of the transmural thickness of the ischemic zone.

Myocardial cells that undergo necrosis are gradually replaced with scar tissue. An acute inflammatory response develops in the area of necrosis approximately 2 to 3 days after infarction.[6] Thereafter, macrophages begin phagocytizing the damaged necrotic tissue; the infarcted area is gradually replaced with an ingrowth of highly vascularized granulation tissue, which in turn becomes less vascular and more fibrous in composition. At approximately 3 to 7 days, the center of the infarcted area remains soft and yellow; therefore, if rupture of the ventricle, interventricular septum, or valve structures occurs, it will usually happen at this time. Replacement of the necrotic myocardial tissue usually is complete by the 7th week. Importantly, areas of the myocardium that have been replaced with scar tissue lack the ability to contract and initiate or conduct action potentials.

The stages of recovery from MI are closely related to the size of the infarct. Fibrous scar tissue lacks the contractile, elastic, and conductive properties of normal myocardial cells; the residual effects and the complications of the MI are determined essentially by the extent and location of the injury. Among the numerous complications of MI are life-threatening arrhythmias, pericarditis, stroke, thromboemboli, and mechanical defects (e.g., mitral valve regurgitation, ventricular septal rupture, left ventricular wall rupture, and left ventricular aneurysm). Depending on its severity, MI has the potential for compromising cardiac contractility resulting in cardiogenic shock or heart failure (see Chapter 20). These serious complications are discussed later.

Pericarditis tends to occur in patients with large infarcts, a lower ejection fraction, and a higher occurrence of heart failure. It may appear as early as the 2nd or 3rd day postinfarction or up to several weeks later.[12] Pericarditis that occurs weeks to months after MI or Dessler syndrome is thought to be mediated by autoimmune mechanisms. In contrast to the pain associated with MI, the pain with pericarditis is sharp and stabbing, and this pain increases with inspiration. The pain may be relieved by positional changes. Because of reperfusion therapy, this complication has been greatly reduced.

Mechanical defects result from changes that occur in the necrotic and subsequently inflamed myocardium and include rupture of the ventricular septum, papillary muscle, or free ventricular wall (Fig. 19-9).[6,12] Partial or complete rupture of a papillary muscle is a rare but often fatal complication of transmural myocardial infarction. It is detected by the presence of a new systolic murmur and clinical deterioration, often with pulmonary edema. Ventricular septal rupture occurs less frequently than in the past because of reperfusion therapy. Previously thought to require surgical intervention only in symptomatic patients, surgical repair is now recommended for all patients with ventricular septal rupture. Complete rupture of the free wall of the infarcted ventricle occurs in up to 10% of patients and usually results in immediate death.[12] It usually occurs 3 to 7 days postinfarction, usually involves the anterior wall, and is more frequent in older women.[6] A more common mechanical postinfarction complication is mitral valve regurgitation, which results from early ischemic dysfunction of the papillary muscle and underlying myocardium.

A left ventricular aneurysm is a sharply delineated area of scar tissue that bulges paradoxically during systole[6,12] (Fig. 19-10). This section of the myocardium does not contract with the rest of the ventricle during systole. Instead, it diminishes the pumping efficiency of the heart and increases the work of the left ventricle, predisposing the patient to heart failure. Ischemia in the surrounding area predisposes the patient to development of arrhythmias, and stasis of blood in the aneurysm can lead to thrombus formation. Surgical resection may be performed to prevent these complications when other treatment measures fail.[12]

Chronic Ischemic Heart Disease

Myocardial ischemia is defined as the inability of the coronary arteries to supply blood to meet the metabolic demands of the heart. Most often limitations in coronary blood flow are the result of atherosclerosis, but vasospasm may serve as an initiating or contributing factor.[20,21] Coronary artery disease is divided into three

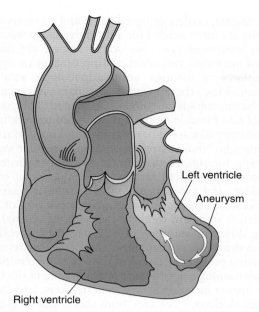

FIGURE 19-10. Paradoxical movement of a left ventricular aneurysm during systole.

classifications: chronic stable angina, silent myocardial ischemia, and variant or vasospastic angina.

Chronic Stable Angina

Angina pectoris is a symptomatic paroxysmal chest pain or pressure sensation associated with transient myocardial ischemia. Chronic stable angina is associated with a fixed coronary obstruction that produces an imbalance between coronary blood flow and the metabolic demands of the myocardium. Stable angina is the initial manifestation of ischemic heart disease in approximately half of persons with CAD.[21,22] Although most persons with stable angina have atherosclerotic heart disease, angina is not a clinical manifestation in a considerable number of persons with advanced coronary atherosclerosis. Some persons may not report severe pain, perhaps because they are physically inactive, have collateral circulation, or do not feel pain due to neuropathy.

Angina pectoris usually is precipitated by situations that increase the work demands of the heart, such as physical exertion, exposure to cold, and emotional stress. The pain is typically described as a steady constricting, squeezing, or a suffocating sensation, increasing in intensity only at the onset and end of the episode. This pain is commonly located in the precordial or substernal area of the chest; it is similar to sensations associated with myocardial infarction in that it may radiate to the left shoulder, jaw, arm, or other areas of the chest or back (Fig. 19-11). In some persons, the arm or shoulder pain may be confused with arthritis; in others, epigastric pain is confused with indigestion. Angina commonly is categorized according to whether it occurs with physical activity, occurs during rest, is of new onset, or is of increasing severity.

Typically, chronic stable angina is provoked by exertional activity or emotional stress and relieved within minutes by rest or by nitroglycerin. A delay of more than 5 to 10 minutes before relief is obtained suggests that the symptoms result from severe ischemia. Angina that occurs at rest, is of new onset, or is increasing in intensity or duration denotes an increased risk for myocardial infarction and should be evaluated using the criteria for ACS.

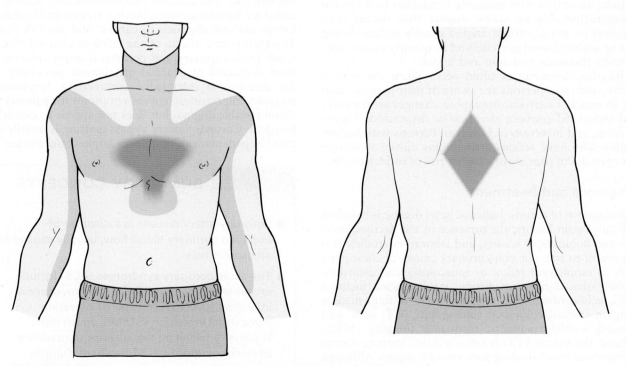

FIGURE 19-11. Areas of pain due to Angina including anterior and posterior views.

Silent Myocardial Ischemia

Silent myocardial ischemia occurs in the absence of anginal pain. The factors associated with asymptomatic ischemia appear to be the same as those responsible for angina: impaired blood flow from the effects of coronary atherosclerosis or vasospasm. Silent myocardial ischemia affects three populations—persons who are asymptomatic without other evidence of CAD, persons who have had a myocardial infarct and continue to have episodes of silent ischemia, and persons with angina who also have episodes of silent ischemia.[21] The reason for the painless episodes of ischemia is unclear. The ischemic episodes may be shorter and involve less myocardial tissue than those producing pain. Another explanation is that persons with silent angina have defects in pain threshold or pain transmission, or an autonomic neuropathy with sensory denervation. For example, asymptomatic ischemia is observed in persons with diabetes mellitus, probably the result of autonomic neuropathy, which is a common complication of diabetes.[21] Silent myocardial ischemia makes up a significant proportion of all STEMIs in the elderly.

Variant (Vasospastic) Angina

Variant angina, also known as *vasospastic* or *Prinzmetal angina,* is caused by coronory artery spasm. The causes of variant angina are not completely understood, but a combination of pathologic processes may be responsible. Endothelial dysfunction, hyperactive sympathetic nervous system responses, defective handling of calcium by vascular smooth muscle, or altered nitric oxide production may all contribute.[21] In some persons it is associated with hypercontractility of vascular smooth muscle, as well as with migraine headaches or Raynaud phenomenon. Unlike stable angina that occurs with exertion or stress, variant angina usually occurs during rest or with minimal exercise and frequently occurs nocturnally (between midnight and 8 AM).

Rhythm disturbances often occur when the pain is severe, and most persons are aware of their presence during an attack. Electrocardiographic changes are transient and include ST-segment elevation or depression, T-wave peaking, and inversion of U waves. Persons with variant angina who have serious arrhythmias during spontaneous episodes of pain are at a higher risk of sudden death.[23]

Diagnosis and Treatment

The diagnosis of chronic ischemic heart disease is based on a detailed pain history, the presence of risk factors, invasive and noninvasive studies, and laboratory studies. It is important to rule out non-coronary causes of chest pain, such as esophageal reflux or musculoskeletal disorders. Noninvasive testing for chronic stable angina includes ECG, echocardiography, exercise stress testing, nuclear imaging studies, computed tomography (CT) scan, and possibly cardiac magnetic resonance imaging (MRI). Because the resting ECG is often normal, exercise testing is important for evaluating persons with angina. Although noninvasive testing is valuable in the diagnosis of chronic stable angina, cardiac catheterization and coronary arteriography are often needed for a definitive diagnosis.[21]

The treatment goals for stable angina are directed toward symptom reduction and prevention of myocardial infarction through nonpharmacologic strategies, pharmacologic therapy, and coronary interventions. Nonpharmacologic methods are aimed at symptom control and lifestyle modifications to reduce risk factors for coronary disease. They include smoking cessation in persons who smoke, stress reduction, a regular exercise program, limiting dietary intake of foods high in cholesterol and saturated fats, weight reduction if obesity is present, and avoidance of cold or other stresses that produce vasoconstriction. Immediate cessation of activity often is sufficient to abort the onset of anginal pain. Sitting down or standing quietly may be preferable to lying down because these positions decrease preload by producing pooling of blood in the lower extremities.

Pharmacologic agents used in the treatment of chronic stable angina include nitrates, beta blockers, and calcium channel blockers.[22] Nitrates, both short- and long-acting, are vasodilators used in the treatment of chronic stable angina and in silent myocardial ischemia. Nitrates exert their effect mainly through a decrease in venous return to the heart with a resultant decrease in intraventricular volume. Arterial pressure also decreases. Decreased intraventricular pressure and volume are associated with decreased wall tension and myocardial oxygen requirement. Although they are not vasodilators, beta blockers are extremely useful in management of angina associated with effort. The benefits of beta blockers are due primarily to their hemodynamic effects—decreased heart rate, blood pressure, and myocardial contractility—which decrease myocardial oxygen requirements at rest and during exercise. The calcium channel–blocking agents, also called *calcium antagonists*, block activated and inactivated L-type calcium channels in cardiac and smooth muscle. The therapeutic effects of the calcium channel blockers result from coronary and peripheral artery dilation and from decreased myocardial metabolism associated with the decrease in myocardial contractility. Percutaneous coronary intervention relieves symptoms for patients with chronic stable angina, but does not appear to extend the life span. Coronary artery bypass grafting is usually indicated in patients with double- or triple-vessel disease.[22]

SUMMARY CONCEPTS

■ Coronary artery disease is a disorder of impaired coronary blood flow, usually caused by atherosclerosis.

■ The acute coronary syndromes (ACS) include unstable angina/non-ST elevation myocardial infarction (UA/NSTEMI) and ST elevation myocardial infarction (STEMI), which differ in severity based on the absence or presence of electrocardiograph ST segment changes.

Serum biomarkers, which are useful tools for predicting the extent and progress of MI, represent intracellular contents of necrotic cells that have diffused into the blood.

■ Unstable angina/NSTEMI is an accelerated form of angina that is caused by subtotal or intermittent coronary occlusion.

■ Acute STEMI, also known as *heart attack*, refers to the ischemic death of myocardial tissue associated with obstructed blood flow in the coronary arteries, potentially fatal arrhythmias, and other adverse cardiac events.

■ The chronic ischemic heart diseases include chronic stable angina, variant (vasospastic) angina, and silent myocardial ischemia. *Chronic stable angina* is associated with a fixed atherosclerotic obstruction and pain that is precipitated by increased work demands on the heart and relieved by rest. *Variant angina* results from spasms of the coronary arteries or other dysfunctions. *Silent myocardial* ischemia occurs without symptoms.

Endocardial and Valvular Disorders

The endocardium, which lines the heart and covers the heart valves, is continuous with the tunica intima of the blood vessels entering and leaving the heart. It is composed of an inner endothelium, consisting of endothelial cells and subendothelial connective tissue; a middle layer of connective tissue and smooth muscle cells; and a deeper layer of loose connective tissue, called the subendocardial layer, which is continuous with the connective tissue of the myocardium. The subendocardium contains small blood vessels, nerves, and Purkinje fibers from the cardiac conduction system.

Disorders of the Endocardium

Among the disorders that affect the endocardium are infective endocarditis, rheumatic fever, and valvular heart disorders.

Infective Endocarditis

Infective endocarditis (IE) is a serious and potentially life-threatening infection of the inner surface of the heart including the cardiac valves. Although rare in most contemporary population surveys (annual incidence 3 to 7 per 100,000 persons),[24,25] IE is associated with significant mortality.[26] Infective endocarditis is characterized by colonization or invasion of the valves and the mural endocardium by a microbial agent, leading to vegetations and destruction of underlying cardiac tissues.[6] Although other microorganisms, such as fungi, can cause endocarditis, the vast majority of cases are caused by bacteria.

Infective endocarditis is commonly classified into acute or subacute–chronic forms, depending on the onset, etiology, and severity of the disease.[27] The onset of acute IE is usually rapid and occurs in patients with previously normal cardiac valves who are healthy and perhaps have a history of intravenous drug abuse, whereas subacute-chronic IE evolves over months, usually in persons who have underlying heart valve abnormalities.[28]

Etiology and Pathogenesis. Two factors contribute to the development of IE: a portal of entry by which the organism gains access to the circulatory system and a damaged endocardial surface. The portal of entry into the bloodstream may be an obvious infection, a dental or surgical procedure that causes transient bacteremia, intravenous injection of a contaminated substance directly into the blood, or an occult source such as the oral cavity, gut, or a subcutaneous injury.[6] Although infective endocarditis can develop in individuals with normal heart valves, persons with structural abnormalities of the values, such as mitral valve prolapse or congenital heart disease, are at significantly higher risk. Host factors such as neutropenia, immunodeficiency, malignancy, therapeutic immunosuppression, diabetes, and alcohol or intravenous drug use are predisposing factors.[6] Infections may also be associated with cardiovascular prostheses and devices, such as pacemakers, defibrillators, and left ventricular assist devices.

Staphylococcal infections are the leading cause of IE, with streptococci and enterococci as the other two most common infectious agents. Other bacterial agents include the so-called HACEK group (*Haemophilus* species, *Actinobacillus actinomycetemcomitans*, *Cardiobacterium hominis*, *Eikenella corrodens*, and *Kingella kingae*), all commensals in the oral cavity.[6,27] Less commonly, gram-negative bacteria and fungi are involved. The causative agents differ somewhat in high-risk groups. For example, *Staphylococcus aureus* is the major offender in intravenous drug users, whereas prosthetic heart valve infective endocarditis tends to be caused by coagulase-negative staphylococci (e.g., *Staphylococcus epidermidis*).[6]

In both acute and subacute–chronic forms of IE, friable, bulky, and potentially destructive vegetative lesions form on the heart valves (Fig. 19-12). The aortic and mitral valves are the most common sites of infection, although the right heart may also be involved, particularly in intravenous drug abusers. The vegetative lesions consist of a collection of infectious organisms and cellular debris enmeshed in the fibrin strands of clotted blood. The lesions may be singular or multiple, may grow as large as several centimeters, and usually are found loosely attached to the free edges of the valve surface.[6] The infectious loci continuously release bacteria into the bloodstream and are a source of persistent bacteremia, sometimes contributing to pericarditis.

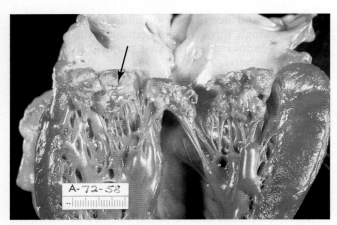

FIGURE 19-12. Gross pathology of subacute bacterial endocarditis involving the mitral valve. Left ventricle of the heart has been opened to show mitral valve fibrin vegetations due to infection with *Haemophilus parainfluenza*. Autopsy. (From the Centers for Disease Control and Prevention Public Health Images Library No. 851. Courtesy of Edwin P. Ewing Jr.)

As the lesions grow, they cause valve destruction and dysfunction such as regurgitation, ring abscesses with heart block, and perforation. The loose organization of these lesions permits the organisms and fragments of the lesions to form emboli and travel in the bloodstream, causing cerebral, systemic, or pulmonary emboli. The fragments may lodge in small blood vessels, causing small hemorrhages, abscesses, and infarction of tissue. The bacteremia also can initiate immune responses thought to be responsible for skin manifestations, polyarthritis, glomerulonephritis, and other immune disorders.[6,27]

Manifestations. Signs and symptoms of IE can include fever and signs of systemic infection, development of a new heart murmur, change in the character of an existing heart murmur, and evidence of embolic distribution of the vegetative lesions.[27] In the acute form, the person is likely to develop a high fever accompanied by chills. In the subacute form, the fever usually is low grade, of gradual onset, and frequently accompanied by other systemic signs of inflammation, such as anorexia, malaise, and lethargy. Small petechial hemorrhages frequently result when emboli lodge in the small vessels of the skin, nail beds, and mucous membranes. Splinter hemorrhages (i.e., dark red lines) under the nails of the fingers and toes are common.[27] Cough, dyspnea, arthralgia or arthritis, diarrhea, and abdominal or flank pain may occur as the result of systemic emboli.

Diagnosis and Treatment. Infective endocarditis continues to pose major challenges in terms of diagnosis and treatment.[27–31] The blood culture remains the most definitive diagnostic procedure and is essential for guiding the treatment. However, the indiscriminate use of antibiotics has made identifying the causative organism much more difficult. Negative blood cultures can occur in up to 30% of cases of IE, delaying diagnosis and

treatment and consequently having a profound effect on outcome.[29] This may result from the prior administration of antibiotics, because the infection is growing slowly, or because it is challenging to culture in a laboratory (i.e., the organism requires a special culture medium). Transthoracic and transesophageal echocardiography are the primary techniques for detection of vegetation and cardiac complications resulting from IE and are important tools in the diagnosis and management of the disease.[27]

Treatment of IE focuses on identifying and eliminating the causative microorganism, minimizing the residual cardiac effects, and treating the pathologic effect of emboli. The choice of antimicrobial therapy depends on the organism cultured and whether the infection involves a native or prosthetic valve. The widespread emergence of multidrug-resistant organisms, including *S. aureus*, poses a serious challenge in the treatment of IE. In addition to antibiotic therapy, surgery may be needed for unresolved infection, severe heart failure, and significant emboli.

Prevention of IE through the use of prophylactic antibiotics is controversial. The current recommendations conclude that only a very small number of IE cases might be prevented by antibiotic prophylaxis for dental procedures. Therefore, prophylaxis is recommended only for patients with predisposing congenital or valvular disorders undergoing select dental and surgical procedures.[31,32]

Rheumatic Heart Disease

Rheumatic fever (RF) is an immune-mediated, multisystem inflammatory disease (involving heart, skin, and connective tissue) that occurs a few weeks after a group A (β-hemolytic) streptococcal (GAS) pharyngitis (sore throat) in children and young adults. It rarely occurs with streptococcal infections at other sites (e.g., skin).[6] Acute rheumatic heart disease (RHD) is the cardiac manifestation of RF and is associated with inflammation of all three layers of the heart (myocardium, pericardium, and endocardium including the heart valves). Chronic deformity and impairment of one or more of the heart valves is the most important consequence of RHD. Although RF and RHD are rare in developed countries, the disorders continue to be major health problems in underdeveloped countries, where inadequate health care, poor nutrition, and crowded living conditions still prevail.[33] Data from recent studies that used echocardiography to screen for RHD indicate that the prevalence of RHD is increasing in these regions. As a result, there has been an increased awareness and interest in RF and RHD.[34]

Pathogenesis. The pathology of RF does not involve direct bacterial infection of the heart. Rather, the time frame for development of symptoms relative to the onset of pharyngitis and the presence of antibodies to the GAS organism strongly suggests an immunologic response.[33–35] It is thought that antibodies directed against the M protein of certain strains of streptococci cross-react with glycoprotein antigens in the heart, joints, and other tissues to produce an autoimmune response through a phenomenon called *molecular mimicry*[33] (see Chapter 16). Although only a small percentage of persons with untreated GAS pharyngitis develop RF, the incidence of recurrence with a subsequent untreated infection is substantially greater. These observations and more recent studies suggest a genetic predisposition to development of the disease.[6]

Clinical Features. Rheumatic fever can manifest as an acute, recurrent, or chronic disorder. The acute stage of rheumatic fever includes a history of an initiating streptococcal infection and subsequent development of discrete inflammatory lesions seen on histopathologic exam within the connective tissue elements of the heart, blood vessels, joints, and subcutaneous tissues. Within the heart these lesions are called Aschoff bodies.[6] The recurrent phase usually involves extension of the cardiac effects of the disease. The chronic phase is characterized by permanent deformity of the heart valves. Chronic rheumatic heart disease usually does not appear until at least 10 years after the initial attack, sometimes decades later.

Most persons with rheumatic fever have a history of sore throat, headache, fever, abdominal pain, nausea, vomiting, swollen glands (usually at the angle of the jaw), and other signs and symptoms of streptococcal infection. Other clinical features are related to the acute inflammatory process and the structures involved in the disease process. The course of the disease is characterized by a constellation of findings that includes carditis, migratory polyarthritis of the large joints, erythema marginatum, subcutaneous nodules, and Sydenham chorea.[6,35]

Acute *rheumatic carditis*, which complicates the acute phase of rheumatic fever, is a pancarditis involving all three layers of the heart. In some cases, the myocardium can be so severely affected that the resulting cardiac dilation causes functional mitral insufficiency and even heart failure. Clinical features include pericardial friction rubs, arrhythmias, and a new heart murmur. Usually, both the pericarditis and myocarditis are self-limited manifestations of the acute stage of the rheumatic fever. Involvement of the endocardium and valvular structures produces the permanent and disabling effects of disease. Although any of the four valves can be involved, the mitral and aortic valves are affected most often. During the acute inflammatory stage, the valvular structures become red and swollen, and small vegetative lesions develop on the valve leaflets. These changes gradually proceed to the development of fibrous scar tissue, which tends to contract and cause permanent deformity of the valve leaflets and shortening of the chordae tendineae. In some cases, the edges or commissures of the valve leaflets fuse together as healing occurs.

Polyarthritis is the most common manifestation of rheumatic fever. It may be the only major diagnostic criterion in adolescents and adults. The arthritis most often involves larger joints, particularly the knees and ankles, and is almost always migratory, affecting one joint and then moving to another. Untreated, it lasts approximately 4 weeks, but it typically responds within 48 hours to salicylates. Polyarthritis usually heals completely.

Erythema marginatum lesions are commonly seen on the trunk or inner aspects of the upper arm and thigh, but never on the face. These transitory skin lesions occur early in the course of a rheumatic attack and usually with subcutaneous nodules, which are hard, painless, and freely movable masses that usually occur over the extensor muscles of the wrist, elbow, ankle, and knee joints.

Chorea (i.e., Sydenham chorea) is the major central nervous system manifestation of rheumatic fever. It is rarely seen after 20 years of age. The onset is typically insidious: the child often is fidgety, cries easily, drops things, and walks clumsily. The choreiform movements are spontaneous, rapid, jerking movements that interfere with voluntary activities. Facial grimaces are common, and speech may be affected. The chorea is self-limited, usually running its course within a matter of weeks or months, but recurrences are not uncommon.

Diagnosis. Diagnosis of acute rheumatic fever is made using serologic evidence of GAS infection along with a consideration of the cardinal symptoms and clinical manifestations or Jones criteria, which were developed to assist in standardizing the diagnosis of RF. Serologic tests for streptococcal antibodies (antistreptolysin O and antideoxyribonuclease B) can provide retrospective confirmation of recent streptococcal infection in persons thought to have rheumatic fever. Laboratory markers of acute inflammation include an elevated white blood cell count, erythrocyte sedimentation rate (ESR), and C-reactive protein (CRP). The Jones criteria divide the clinical features of RF into major and minor categories, based on prevalence and specificity.[34,36] The presence of two major signs (i.e., carditis, polyarthritis, chorea, erythema marginatum, and subcutaneous nodules) or one major and two minor signs (i.e., arthralgia, fever, elevated ESR, CRP, or leukocyte count and prolonged PR interval on EKG), accompanied by evidence of a preceding GAS infection (antistreptolysin 0 antibodies, positive throat culture for GAS) indicates a high probability of RF.

The use of echocardiography has enhanced the understanding of both acute and chronic RHD. It is useful in assessing the severity of valvular stenosis and regurgitation, chamber size and ventricular function, and the presence and size of pleural effusions. Doppler ultrasonography may be useful in identifying cardiac lesions in persons who do not show typical signs of cardiac involvement during an attack of RF.[34,36]

Treatment and Prevention. It is important that GAS infections be promptly diagnosed and treated to prevent RF. The gold standard for detecting a GAS infection is a throat culture. However, it takes 24 to 48 hours to produce a result, which may delay treatment. Rapid tests for direct detection of GAS antigens are highly specific for GAS infection but are limited in terms of their sensitivity (i.e., the person may have a negative test result but have a streptococcal infection). Thus a negative antigen test result should be confirmed with a throat culture when a streptococcal infection is suspected.[36]

Treatment of acute RF is designed to control the acute inflammatory response and prevent cardiac complications and recurrence of the disease. During the acute phase, antibiotics, anti-inflammatory drugs, and selective restriction of activities are prescribed. Penicillin, or another antibiotic in penicillin-sensitive patients, is the treatment of choice.[36] Salicylates and corticosteroids can be used to suppress the inflammatory response, but should not be given until the diagnosis of RF is confirmed. Surgery, including valve repair and replacement, is indicated for chronic rheumatic valve disease and is determined by the severity of the symptoms or cardiac dysfunction.

Persons who had RF are at high risk for recurrence after subsequent GAS throat infections. Penicillin is the treatment of choice for secondary prophylaxis, but sulfadiazine or erythromycin may be used in those who are allergic to penicillin. The duration of prophylaxis depends on whether residual valvular disease is present or absent. It is recommended that persons with persistent valvular disease receive low-dose antibiotic prophylaxis for at least 5 years after the acute episode of RF or until age 21 years if there is no evidence of carditis.[35]

Valvular Heart Disease

The past several decades have brought remarkable advances in the treatment of valvular heart disease. This is undoubtedly due to improved methods for noninvasive monitoring of ventricular function, improvement in prosthetic valves, advances in valve reconstruction, and the development of guidelines to improve the timing of surgical interventions.[37] Nevertheless, valvular heart disease continues to produce considerable mortality and morbidity.

Hemodynamic Derangements

The function of the heart valves is to promote unidirectional flow of blood through the chambers of the heart. Dysfunction of the valves can result from a number of disorders including congenital defects, trauma, ischemia, degenerative changes, and inflammation. Although any of the heart valves can become diseased, the most commonly involved are the mitral and aortic valves. Disorders of the pulmonary and tricuspid valves are less common, probably because of the low pressure in the right side of the heart.

The heart valves consist of thin leaflets of tough, flexible, endothelium-covered fibrous tissue firmly attached at the base to the fibrous valve rings (see Chapter 17). The leaflets of the heart valves may be damaged or inflamed, which can deform their line of closure. Healing of the valve leaflets is associated with increased collagen content and scarring, causing the leaflets to shorten and stiffen. Another problem is that the edges of the healing valve leaflets can fuse together so that the valve does not open or close properly.

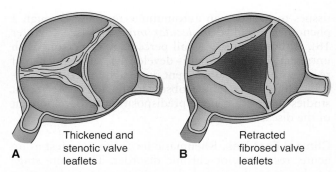

A — Thickened and stenotic valve leaflets
B — Retracted fibrosed valve leaflets

FIGURE 19-13. Disease of the aortic valve as viewed from the aorta. **(A)** Stenosis of the valve opening. **(B)** An incompetent or regurgitant valve that is unable to close completely.

Two types of mechanical disruption occur with valvular heart disease: narrowing of the valvular opening, so it does not open properly, and distortion of the valve, so it does not close properly (Fig. 19-13). *Stenosis* refers to a narrowing of the valve orifice and failure of the valve leaflets to open normally (Fig. 19-14). Significant narrowing of the valve orifice increases the resistance to blood flow through the valve, converting the normally smooth laminar flow to a less efficient turbulent flow. This increases the work and volume of the chamber emptying through the narrowed valve—the left atrium in the case of mitral stenosis and the left ventricle in aortic stenosis. An *incompetent* or *regurgitant* valve does not close properly, thereby permitting the backward flow of blood to occur when the valve should be closed. When the aortic valve is affected, blood flows back into the left ventricle during diastole. When the mitral valve is affected, blood flows back into the left atrium during systole. Stenosis and regurgitation can occur in pure forms, or these abnormalities may exist in the same valve. Alterations in hemodynamic function that accompany aortic and mitral valve stenosis and regurgitation are illustrated in Figure 19-15.

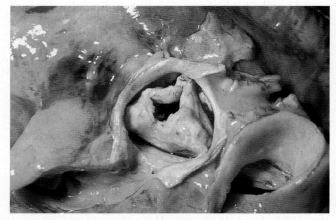

FIGURE 19-14. Gross pathology of rheumatic heart disease: aortic stenosis. Fused aortic valve leaflets and opened coronary arteries from above. (From the Centers for Disease Control and Prevention Public Health Images Library No. 848. Courtesy of Edwin P. Ewing, Jr.)

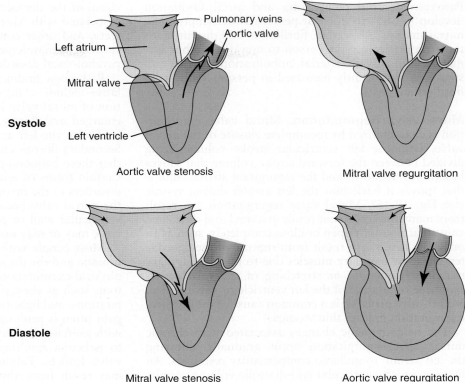

Systole

Pulmonary veins
Aortic valve
Left atrium
Mitral valve
Left ventricle

Aortic valve stenosis

Mitral valve regurgitation

Diastole

Mitral valve stenosis

Aortic valve regurgitation

FIGURE 19-15. Alterations in hemodynamic function that accompany aortic valve stenosis, mitral valve regurgitation, mitral valve stenosis, and aortic valve regurgitation. The *thin arrows* indicate direction of normal flow, and *thick arrows* the direction of abnormal flow. Expand description.

The effects of valvular heart disease depend on the valve involved, the degree of involvement, the rapidity of onset, and the rate and adequacy of compensatory mechanisms. For example, sudden destruction of an aortic valve cusp by infection can cause massive regurgitation and rapid heart failure, whereas rheumatic mitral stenosis usually develops over years without obvious symptoms. Abnormal turbulent flow through diseased valves typically produces abnormal heart sounds called *murmurs.*

Mitral Valve Disorders

The mitral or left atrioventricular (AV) valve controls the directional flow of blood between the left atrium and the left ventricle. The edges or cusps of both AV valves, which are thinner than those of the semilunar (i.e., pulmonic and aortic) valves, are anchored to the papillary muscles by the chordae tendineae. During much of systole, the mitral valve is subjected to the high pressure generated by the left ventricle as it pumps blood into the systemic circulation. During this period of increased pressure, the chordae tendineae prevent the eversion of the valve leaflets into the left atrium.

Mitral Valve Stenosis. Mitral valve stenosis represents the incomplete opening of the mitral valve during diastole, with left atrial distension and impaired filling of the left ventricle (see Fig. 19-15). Mitral valve stenosis is most commonly the result of rheumatic fever.[37,38] Less frequently, the defect is congenital and manifests during infancy or early childhood or calcification in elderly

patients. Mitral valve stenosis is a continuous, progressive, lifelong disorder consisting of a slow, stable course in the early years and progressive acceleration in later years.

Mitral valve stenosis is characterized by fibrous replacement of valvular tissue, along with stiffness and fusion of the valve apparatus (see Fig. 19-14). Typically, the mitral cusps fuse at the edges and the chordinae tendinae thicken and shorten pulling the valvular structures into the ventricles. As the resistance to flow through the valve increases, the left atrium dilates and left atrial pressure increases. The increased left atrial pressure eventually is transmitted to the pulmonary venous system, causing pulmonary congestion. A characteristic auscultatory finding in mitral stenosis is an opening snap following the second heart sound, which is caused by the stiff mitral valve. As the stenosis worsens, there is a localized low-pitched diastolic murmur that increases in duration with the severity of the stenosis.

The clinical presentation of mitral valve stenosis depends on the severity of the obstruction or the degree of reduction in the valve area—the more severe the stenosis, the greater the symptoms. Manifestations are related to the elevation in left atrial pressure and pulmonary congestion such as dyspnea with exertion, decreased cardiac output owing to impaired left ventricular filling, and left atrial enlargement with the development of atrial arrhythmias and mural thrombi. More severe stenosis is associated with symptoms of pulmonary congestion, including paroxysmal nocturnal dyspnea (PND) and orthopnea. Palpitations, chest pain, weakness, and fatigue are common complaints.

Paroxysmal atrial tachycardia and atrial fibrillation develop in 30% to 40% of persons with symptomatic mitral stenosis.[38] Together, fibrillation and distention of the atria predispose the person to mural thrombus formation. The risk of arterial embolization, particularly stroke, is significantly increased in persons with atrial fibrillation.

Mitral Valve Regurgitation. Mitral valve regurgitation is characterized by incomplete closure of the mitral valve, with the left ventricular stroke volume being divided between the forward stroke volume that moves blood into the aorta and the regurgitant stroke volume that moves it back into the left atrium during systole (see Fig. 19-15). Mitral valve regurgitation can result from many processes that result in a rigid and thickened valve that does not open or close completely, such as IE or RHD. It can also result from rupture of the chordae tendineae or papillary muscles due to an MI, papillary muscle dysfunction, or stretching of the valve structures due to dilation of the left ventricle or valve orifice. Mitral valve prolapse is a common cause of mitral valve regurgitation in lean, thin women.

The hemodynamic changes associated with chronic mitral valve regurgitation occur gradually, allowing the left atrium to undergo compensatory responses. An increase in left ventricular end-diastolic volume permits an increase in total stroke volume, with restoration of forward flow into the aorta. Augmented preload and reduced or normal afterload (provided by unloading the left ventricle into the left atrium) facilitate left ventricular ejection. At the same time, a gradual increase in left atrial size allows for accommodation of the regurgitant volume at a lower filling pressure. A characteristic feature of mitral valve regurgitation is an enlarged or hypertrophied left ventricle, a hyperdynamic left ventricular impulse, and a pansystolic (throughout systole) heart murmur. Mitral regurgitation, like mitral stenosis, predisposes to atrial fibrillation.

The increased volume work associated with mitral regurgitation is relatively well tolerated, and many persons with the disorder remain asymptomatic for many years, developing symptoms between 6 and 10 years after diagnosis. The severity of regurgitation reflects the degree of left ventricular enlargement and may correlate with murmur intensity[39] and typically correlates with the patients' symptoms.[38] As the disorder progresses, left ventricular function becomes impaired, the forward (aortic) stroke volume decreases, and the left atrial pressure increases, with the subsequent development of pulmonary congestion. It is usually recommended that valve surgery be performed before the onset of these symptoms.

Mitral Valve Prolapse. Sometimes referred to as floppy mitral valve syndrome, mitral valve prolapse occurs in 1% to 2.5% of the general population.[37] The disorder is seen more frequently in thin women, and there may be a familial basis. Familial mitral valve prolapse is transmitted as an autosomal dominant trait, and several chromosomal loci have been identified. Although the exact cause of the disorder usually is unknown, it has been associated with Marfan syndrome, osteogenesis imperfecta, and other connective tissue disorders, and with cardiac, hematologic, neuroendocrine, metabolic, and psychological disorders.

Pathologic findings in persons with mitral valve prolapse include a myxedematous (mucinous) degeneration of mitral valve leaflets that causes them to become enlarged and floppy so that they prolapse or balloon back into the left atrium during systole[37] (Fig. 19-16). Secondary fibrotic changes reflect the stresses and injury that these ballooning movements impose on the valve. Certain forms of mitral valve prolapse may arise from disorders of the myocardium that place undue stress on the mitral valve because of abnormal movement of the ventricular wall or papillary muscle. Mitral valve prolapse may or may not cause mitral regurgitation.

Most people with mitral valve prolapse are asymptomatic and the disorder is discovered during a routine physical examination. A minority of people have symptoms such as chest pain, dyspnea, fatigue, anxiety, palpitations, and light-headedness. Unlike angina, the chest pain often is prolonged, ill defined, and not associated with exercise or exertion. The pain has been attributed to ischemia resulting from traction of the prolapsing valve leaflets. Palpitations, arrhythmias, and anxiety may result from abnormal autonomic nervous system function that commonly accompanies the disorder. Rare cases of sudden death have been reported for persons with mitral valve prolapse, mainly those with a family history of similar occurrences.

The disorder is characterized by a spectrum of auscultatory findings, ranging from a silent form to one or more midsystolic clicks followed by a late systolic or pansystolic murmur heard best at the apex. The clicks are caused by the sudden tensing of the mitral valve

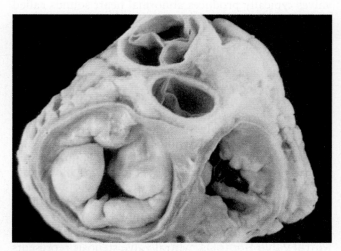

FIGURE 19-16. Mitral valve prolapse. A view of the mitral valve from the left atrium shows redundant and deformed leaflets that billow into the left atrial cavity. (From Saffitz JE. The heart. In: Rubin E, Strayer DS, eds. *Rubin's Pathology: Clinicopathologic Foundations of Medicine.* 6th ed. Philadelphia, PA: Wolters Kluwer Health | Lippincott Williams & Wilkins; 2012:518.)

apparatus as the leaflets prolapse. Two-dimensional and Doppler echocardiography is used to diagnose mitral valve prolapse.

The treatment of mitral valve prolapse focuses on the relief of symptoms and the prevention of complications.[38] Persons with palpitations and mild tachyarrhythmias or increased adrenergic symptoms, and those with chest discomfort, anxiety, and fatigue often respond well to therapy with beta blockers. In many cases, the cessation of stimulants such as caffeine, alcohol, and cigarettes may be sufficient to control symptoms. Although infective endocarditis is an uncommon complication in persons with a murmur, antibiotic prophylaxis may be recommended before extensive dental or surgical procedures associated with bacteremia. Transient ischemic attacks occur more frequently in persons with mitral valve prolapse. Therefore, daily aspirin therapy is recommended in persons with documented events who have a sinus rhythm and no atrial thrombi. Persons with severe valve dysfunction may require valve surgery.

Aortic Valve Disorders

The aortic valve, which is located between the left ventricle and aorta, has three cuplike cusps and sometimes is referred to as the *aortic semilunar valve* because its leaflets are crescent or moon shaped. The aortic valve has no chordae tendineae. Although their structures are similar, the edges of the aortic valve leaflets are thicker than those of the mitral valve, particularly at the middle of the leaflet (see Chapter 17, Fig. 17-10). The mechanism of action of the aortic valve is also different from that of the mitral valve. During ventricular systole when the ventricles contract and blood is being ejected into the aorta, the cusps of the valve are flattened against the aortic wall and blood rushes past them; when the ventricles relax and the blood (no longer propelled forward by the pressure of ventricular contraction) begins to flow backward toward the heart, it fills the cusps and this closes the valve.

An important feature of the aortic valve is the location of the orifices for the two main coronary arteries, which are located behind the valve and at right angles to the direction of blood flow. It is the lateral pressure in the aorta that propels blood into the coronary arteries. During the ejection phase of the cardiac cycle, the lateral pressure is diminished by conversion of potential energy to kinetic energy as blood moves forward into the aorta. This process is grossly exaggerated in aortic valve stenosis because of the high flow velocities.

Aortic Valve Stenosis. Aortic valve stenosis is characterized by narrowing of the valve orifice with increased resistance to ejection of blood from the left ventricle into the aorta (see Fig. 19-15). The most common causes of aortic valve stenosis are congenital valve malformations and acquired calcification of a normal aortic valve. Congenital malformations may result in unicuspid, bicuspid, or misshapen valve leaflets. Acquired aortic stenosis is usually the consequence of calcification associated with age-related degenerative changes or the normal "wear and tear" of either previously normal aortic valves or congenitally bicuspid valves with which approximately 1% of the population are born.[9] The incidence of acquired aortic valve stenosis is increasing with the rising average age of the population.[6,40]

The progression of calcific aortic stenosis is usually slow and varies widely among individuals. It usually becomes clinically evident in the sixth and seventh decades in persons with bicuspid aortic valves, and not until the eighth and ninth decades in those with previously normal valves. Valve changes range from mild thickening without obstruction to severe calcification with impaired leaflet motion and obstructed left ventricular outflow.[41] Processes in the development of calcific aortic valve disease have been shown to be similar to those in CAD. Both conditions are more common in men, older persons, and persons with hypercholesteremia, and both derive in part from an active inflammatory process.[40]

Early lesions of aortic sclerosis show focal subendothelial plaquelike lesions, similar to the initial phases of an atherosclerotic lesion. Aortic sclerosis is distinguished from aortic stenosis by the degree of valve impairment. In aortic sclerosis the valve leaflets are abnormally thickened, but the obstruction to outflow is minimal, whereas in aortic stenosis the functional area of the valve has decreased enough to cause measurable obstruction to outflow. Calcification of the aortic valve progresses from the base of the cusps to the leaflets. This reduces leaflet motion and effective valve area, but without commissural fusion. As calcification progresses, the leaflets become more rigid, there is worsening of obstruction to left ventricular outflow, and fusion of the commissures leads to aortic stenosis.

Because aortic stenosis usually develops gradually, the left ventricle has time to adapt. With increased systolic pressure from obstruction, the left ventricular wall becomes thicker, or hypertrophies, but a normal chamber volume is maintained. With this increase in wall thickness, called concentric remodeling, the left ventricular ejection fraction is maintained within normal limits. Hemodynamic variables remain stable even though the valve opening area is reduced to half of its normal size. However, an additional reduction in the valve opening area from one half to one fourth of its normal size produces severe obstruction to flow and a progressive increase in the pressure overload on the left ventricle. At this point, the increased work of the heart begins to exceed the coronary blood flow reserve, causing both systolic and diastolic dysfunction and signs of heart failure.[38,40,41]

Aortic stenosis is usually first diagnosed with auscultation of a loud systolic ejection murmur or a single or paradoxically split-second heart sound. Eventually, the classic symptoms of advanced aortic stenosis such as angina, syncope, and heart failure develop, although more subtle signs of a decrease in exercise tolerance or exertional dyspnea should be monitored closely. Angina occurs in approximately two thirds of persons with advanced aortic stenosis and is similar to that observed in CAD. Dyspnea, marked fatigability, peripheral cyanosis, and other signs of heart failure usually are not prominent until late in the course of the disease. Syncope (fainting) is most commonly due to the reduced cerebral circulation that occurs during exertion when the arterial pressure declines consequent to vasodilation in the presence of a fixed cardiac output.

Aortic Valve Regurgitation. Aortic valve regurgitation or aortic insufficiency is the result of an incompetent aortic valve that allows blood to flow back to the left ventricle during diastole (see Fig. 19-15). As a result, the left ventricle increases its stroke volume to accommodate blood entering from the pulmonary veins in addition to the volume of blood leaking back through the regurgitant valve. This defect may result from conditions that cause scarring of the valve leaflets or from enlargement of the valve orifice to the extent that the valve leaflets no longer meet. There are various causes of aortic regurgitation, including rheumatic fever, idiopathic dilation of the aorta, congenital abnormalities, infective endocarditis, and Marfan syndrome. Other causes include hypertension, trauma, and failure of a prosthetic valve.

Acute aortic regurgitation is characterized by a sudden, large regurgitant volume to a left ventricle of normal size that has not had time to adapt to the volume overload. It is caused by disorders such as infective endocarditis, trauma, or aortic dissection. Using the Frank-Starling mechanism, the heart responds by increasing heart rate, but the compensatory mechanisms fail to maintain the cardiac output. As a result, there is severe elevation in left ventricular end-diastolic pressure, which is transmitted to the left atrium and pulmonary veins, culminating in pulmonary edema. A decrease in cardiac output leads to sympathetic activation and a resultant increase in heart rate and peripheral vascular resistance that cause the regurgitation to worsen. Death from pulmonary edema, ventricular arrhythmias, or circulatory collapse is common in severe acute aortic regurgitation.

Chronic aortic regurgitation, which usually has a gradual onset, represents a condition of combined left ventricular volume and pressure overload. As the valve deformity increases, regurgitant flow into the left ventricle increases, diastolic blood pressure falls, and the left ventricle progressively enlarges or eccentrically hypertrophies. Hemodynamically, the increase in left ventricular volume results in the ejection of a large stroke volume that usually is adequate to maintain the forward cardiac output until late in the course of the disease. Most persons remain asymptomatic during this compensated phase, which may last decades. The only sign for many years may be a soft systolic aortic murmur.

As the disease progresses, signs and symptoms of left ventricular failure begin to appear. These include exertional dyspnea, orthopnea, and paroxysmal nocturnal dyspnea. In aortic regurgitation, failure of aortic valve closure during diastole causes an abnormal drop in diastolic pressure. Because coronary blood flow is greatest during diastole, the drop in diastolic pressure produces a decrease in coronary perfusion. Although angina is rare, it may occur when the heart rate and diastolic pressure fall to low levels. Persons with severe aortic regurgitation often complain of an uncomfortable awareness of heartbeat, particularly when lying down, and chest discomfort due to pounding of the heart against the chest wall. Tachycardia, occurring with emotional stress or exertion, may produce palpitations, head pounding, and premature ventricular contractions.

The major physical findings relate to the widening of the arterial pulse pressure, a hallmark of chronic aortic regurgitation. The pulse has a rapid rise and fall (Corrigan pulse), with an elevated systolic pressure and low diastolic pressure owing to the large stroke volume and rapid diastolic runoff of blood back into the left ventricle. Korotkoff sounds may persist to zero, even though intra-arterial pressure rarely falls below 30 mm Hg.[37] The large stroke volume and wide pulse pressure may result in prominent carotid pulsations in the neck, throbbing peripheral pulses, and a left ventricular impulse that causes the chest to move with each beat. The hyperkinetic pulse of more severe aortic regurgitation, called a *water-hammer pulse,* is characterized by distention and quick collapse of the artery. On auscultation, the turbulence of flow across the aortic valve during diastole produces a high-pitched or blowing sound.

Diagnosis and Treatment

Valvular defects usually are detected through cardiac auscultation (i.e., heart sounds). Echocardiography provides a means of visualizing valvular motion, patterns of flow, and closure patterns. Pulsed Doppler ultrasonography provides a semiquantitative or qualitative estimation of the severity of transvalvular gradients, right ventricular systolic pressure, and valvular regurgitation. Color flow Doppler provides a visual pattern of flow velocities over the anatomic 2-D echocardiographic image. This allows for demonstration of turbulence from stenotic and regurgitant valves. Transesophageal echocardiography with Doppler ultrasonography is used to obtain echocardiographic data when surface sound transmission is poor, particularly of the AV valves and prosthetic heart valves. Cardiac catheterization may be used to further describe the effects of the defect.

The treatment of valvular defects consists of medical management of heart failure and associated problems and surgical valve repair or replacement, if warranted by the extent of deformity. Valvular replacement with a prosthetic device or a homograft usually is reserved for severe disease because the ideal substitute valve has not as yet been developed. Percutaneous balloon valvuloplasty involves the opening of a stenotic valve by guiding an inflated balloon through the valve orifice. The procedure is done in the cardiac catheterization laboratory and involves the insertion of a balloon catheter into the heart through a peripheral blood vessel.

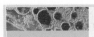

SUMMARY CONCEPTS

■ Infective endocarditis involves the invasion of the endocardium by pathogens that produce vegetative lesions on the endocardial surface. The loose organization of these lesions permits the organisms and fragments of the lesions to be disseminated throughout the systemic circulation. Although several organisms can cause the condition, staphylococci have become the leading cause. Treatment of infective endocarditis focuses on identifying and eliminating the causative microorganism, minimizing the residual cardiac effects, and treating the pathologic effect of emboli.

■ Rheumatic fever, an immune-mediated, multisystem inflammatory disease associated with group A (β-hemolytic) streptococcal (GAS) pharyngitis, can result in serious and disabling impairment of the heart valves. Primary and secondary prevention strategies focus on appropriate antibiotic therapy.

■ Dysfunction of the heart valves can result from a number of disorders, including congenital defects, rheumatic heart disease, trauma, ischemic heart disease, degenerative changes, and inflammation. Valvular heart disease causes disturbances of blood flow. A stenotic valvular defect is one that causes a decrease in blood flow through a valve, resulting in impaired emptying and increased work demands on the heart chamber that pushes blood across the diseased valve. A regurgitant valve permits blood flow to continue despite closure of the valve. Valvular heart disorders produce blood flow turbulence and often are detected through heart sound heard during cardiac auscultation.

Disorders of the Pericardium

The pericardium is a double-layered fibroserous sac that encircles the heart. It isolates the heart from other thoracic structures, maintains its position in the thorax, prevents it from overfilling, and serves as a barrier to infection. The pericardium consists of two layers: a thin inner layer, called the visceral pericardium, adheres to the epicardium; and an outer fibrous layer, called the parietal pericardium, is attached to the great vessels that enter and leave the heart (see Chapter 17, Fig. 17-15). The two layers of the pericardium are separated by a thin layer of serous fluid, which prevents frictional forces from developing as the heart contracts and relaxes. Although the fibrous tissue outer layer of the pericardium allows for moderate changes in cardiac size, it cannot stretch sufficiently to accommodate rapid dilation of the heart or accumulation of pericardial fluid without increasing pericardial and intracardiac pressures.

The pericardium is subject to many of the same pathologic processes (e.g., congenital disorders, infections, trauma, and immune mechanisms) that affect other structures of the body. Pericardial disorders frequently are associated with other diseases in the heart or surrounding structures (Chart 19-1). The most common disorder of the pericardium is acute pericarditis.

Acute Pericarditis

Acute pericarditis, defined as signs and symptoms resulting from pericardial inflammation of less than 2 weeks' duration, may result from an infection or noninfectious disease. Viral infections (especially infections with coxsackieviruses and echoviruses) are the most common cause of pericarditis and probably are responsible for many cases of idiopathic or pericarditis of unknown etiology. Other causes of acute pericarditis include bacterial or

| CHART 19-1 | Classification of Disorders of the Pericardium* |

Idiopathic (no identifiable cause of disease)
■ Infectious
Viral (echovirus, coxsackievirus, and others)
Bacterial (e.g., *Staphylococcus, Streptococcus*, Lyme disease, tuberculosis)
Fungal (Hisplasmosis, candida)

■ Autoimmune and collagen disorders
Rheumatic fever
Rheumatoid arthritis
Systemic lupus erythematosus

■ Metabolic disorders
Uremia and dialysis
Myxedema

■ Ischemia and tissue injury
Myocardial infarction
Cardiac surgery
Chest trauma (blunt and penetrating)

■ Physical and drug-induced
Radiation therapy
Hydralazine, procainamide, and anticoagulants

Neoplastic Disease
■ Primary (mesothelioma, fibrosarcoma)
■ Secondary (e.g., carcinoma of the lung or breast, lymphoma)

Congenital Disorders
■ Complete or partial absence of the pericardium
■ Congenital pericardial cysts

*Chronic inflammatory pericarditis can be associated with some agents causing an acute inflammatory response.

mycobacterial infections, connective tissue diseases (e.g., systemic lupus erythematosus, rheumatoid arthritis), uremia, postcardiac surgery, neoplastic invasion of the pericardium, radiation, trauma, drug toxicity, and contiguous inflammatory processes of the myocardium or lung.[42,43]

Similar to other inflammatory processes, acute pericarditis is associated with local vasodilation, increased capillary permeability, and accumulation of white blood cells. The capillaries that supply the serous pericardium become permeable, allowing plasma proteins, including fibrinogen, to exit the capillaries and enter the pericardial space. This results in an exudate that varies in composition and amount according to the causative agent. Acute pericarditis frequently is associated with an exudate containing protein and fibrin and heals by resolution or progresses to form scar tissue and adhesions between the layers of the serous pericardium.

The manifestations of acute pericarditis include a triad of chest pain, an auscultatory pericardial friction rub, and electrocardiographic (ECG) changes. The clinical findings may vary according to the causative agent. Nearly all persons with acute pericarditis have chest pain and fever. The pain usually is sharp and abrupt in onset, occurring in the precordial area, and may radiate to the neck, back, abdomen, or side. Pain in the scapular area may result from irritation of the phrenic nerve. The pain typically is pleuritic (aggravated by inspiration and coughing) and positional (decreases with sitting and leaning forward) because of changes in venous return and cardiac filling. These pain characteristics differentiate pericarditis from acute myocardial infarction or pulmonary embolism. A pericardial friction rub (auscultated through the diaphragm of a stethoscope), often described as "leathery" or "close to the ear," results from the rubbing and friction between the inflamed pericardial surfaces.[43]

Diagnosis of acute pericarditis is based on clinical manifestations, ECG, chest radiography, and echocardiography, with laboratory tests being used to confirm the diagnosis. Treatment depends on the cause. When an infection is present, antibiotics specific for the causative agent are prescribed. Aspirin and other non-steroidal anti-inflammatory drugs (NSAIDs) may be given to minimize the inflammatory response and the accompanying undesirable effects.

Recurrent pericarditis can occur in up to 30% of persons with acute pericarditis who responded satisfactorily to treatment.[42] A minority of these develop recurrent bouts of pericardial pain, which can sometimes be chronic and debilitating. The process commonly is associated with autoimmune disorders, such as lupus erythematosus, rheumatoid arthritis, scleroderma, and myxedema, but may also occur following viral pericarditis. Treatment includes the use of anti-inflammatory medications such as NSAIDs, corticosteroids, or colchicine.

Pericardial Effusion

Pericardial effusion is the accumulation of fluid in the pericardial cavity, usually as a result of an inflammatory or infectious process that includes pericarditis. It may also develop with neoplasms, cardiac surgery, or trauma. Pericardial effusion exerts its effects through compression of the heart chambers. The normal pericardial space contains about 15 to 50 mL of fluid. Increases in the volume of this fluid, the rapidity with which it accumulates, and the elasticity of the pericardium determine the effect that the effusion has on cardiac function. Small pericardial effusions may produce no symptoms or abnormal clinical findings. Even a large effusion that develops slowly may cause few or no symptoms, provided the pericardium is able to stretch and avoid compressing the heart. However, a sudden accumulation of even 200 mL may raise intracardiac pressure to levels that significantly limit venous return of blood to the heart. Symptoms of cardiac compression also may occur with relatively small accumulations of fluid if the pericardium has become thickened by scar tissue or neoplastic infiltrations and loses its elasticity.

The echocardiogram is a rapid, accurate, and widely used noninvasive method of evaluating pericardial effusion. Treatment depends on the extent of the effusion. In small pericardial effusions, diuretics are given to remove the fluid, and NSAIDs, colchicine, or corticosteroids may minimize fluid accumulation. Pericardiocentesis, or removal of fluid from the pericardial sac, often with the aid of echocardiography, is the initial treatment of choice for larger effusions. Aspiration of fluid with laboratory evaluation of the pericardial fluid may be used to identify the causative agent.

Cardiac Tamponade

Pericardial effusion can lead to or may initially present as a condition called cardiac tamponade, in which there is compression of the heart due to the accumulation of fluid or blood in the pericardial sac. This life-threatening condition can be caused by bleeding into the pericardial sac after blunt or penetrating trauma, rupture of the heart following myocardial infarction, complications during percutaneous cardiac procedures or device placement, or retrograde bleeding during aortic dissection.[42,43]

Cardiac tamponade results in increased intracardiac pressure, progressive limitation of ventricular diastolic filling, and reductions in stroke volume and cardiac output. In other words, the heart cannot fill properly with blood. The severity of the condition depends on the volume of fluid present and the rate at which it accumulates. Rapid accumulation results in an elevated central venous pressure, jugular vein distention, a fall in systolic blood pressure, narrowed pulse pressure, and signs of circulatory shock. The heart sounds may become muffled because of the insulating effects of the pericardial fluid and reduced cardiac function. Persons with slowly developing cardiac tamponade usually appear acutely ill, but not to the extreme seen in those with rapidly developing tamponade.

A significant accumulation of fluid in the pericardium results in increased sympathetic nervous system stimulation, which leads to tachycardia and increased cardiac contractility. A key diagnostic finding in cardiac tamponade is pulsus paradoxus, or an exaggeration of the normal variation in the systolic blood pressure. Pulsus paradoxus is defined as a 10 mm Hg or more fall in the systolic blood pressure that occurs with inspiration.[42,43] Normally, the decrease in intrathoracic pressure that occurs during inspiration accelerates venous flow, increasing right atrial and right ventricular filling. This causes the interventricular septum to bulge to the left, producing a slight decrease in left ventricular filling, stroke volume output, and systolic blood pressure. In cardiac tamponade, the left ventricle is compressed from within by movement of the interventricular septum and from without by fluid in the pericardium (Fig. 19-17). This produces a marked decrease in left ventricular filling and left ventricular stroke volume output following inspiration.

Computed tomography (CT) and magnetic resonance imaging (MRI) are useful adjuncts to echocardiography in cardiac tamponade. The ECG often reveals nonspecific T-wave changes and low QRS voltage. Usually only moderate to large effusions can be detected by chest radiography.

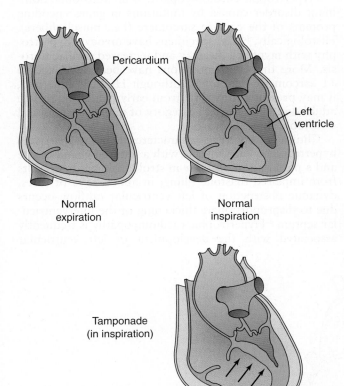

Normal
expiration

Normal
inspiration

Tamponade
(in inspiration)

FIGURE 19-17. Effects of respiration and cardiac tamponade on ventricular filling and cardiac output. During inspiration, venous flow into the right heart increases, causing the interventricular septum to bulge into the left ventricle. This produces a decrease in left ventricular volume, with a subsequent decrease in stroke volume output. In cardiac tamponade, the fluid in the pericardial sac produces further compression of the left ventricle, causing an exaggeration of the normal inspiratory decrease in stroke volume and systolic blood pressure.

Closed pericardiocentesis, in which fluid is removed from the pericardial sac through a needle inserted through the chest wall, may be an emergency lifesaving measure in severe cardiac tamponade. Open pericardiocentesis may be used for recurrent or loculated effusions (i.e., those confined to one or more pockets in the pleural space), during which biopsies can be obtained and pericardial windows created. As with pericardial effusion, laboratory evaluation of the pericardial fluid may be used to identify the causative agent.

Constrictive Pericarditis

In constrictive pericarditis, fibrous scar tissue develops between the visceral and parietal layers of the serous pericardium. In time, the scar tissue contracts and interferes with diastolic filling of the heart, at which point cardiac output and cardiac reserve become fixed. It is most commonly associated with inflammation resulting from infections, mediastinal radiation, or cardiac surgical trauma.

The condition is characterized by high venous pressure, low cardiac output, narrow pulse pressure, and fluid retention.[44] Ascites is a prominent early finding and may be accompanied by pedal edema, dyspnea on exertion, fatigue, and jugular venous distention. The Kussmaul sign is an inspiratory distention of the jugular veins (opposite of normal physiology) caused by the inability of the right atrium, encased in its rigid pericardium, to accommodate the increase in venous return that occurs with inspiration. Exercise intolerance, muscle wasting, and weight loss develop in end-stage constrictive pericarditis. Surgical removal or resection of the pericardium (i.e., pericardiectomy) is the treatment of choice.

SUMMARY CONCEPTS

■ The major threat of pericardial disorders, which include acute and chronic or recurrent pericarditis, pericardial effusion, cardiac tamponade, and constrictive pericarditis, is compression of the heart chambers.

■ Acute pericarditis may be infectious in origin or it may be due to systemic diseases. It is characterized by pleuritic chest pain, fever, ECG changes, and pericardial friction rub. Recurrent pericarditis, which is usually associated with autoimmune disorders, often produces few symptoms.

■ Pericardial effusion, either acute or chronic, refers to the accumulation of fluid or exudate in the pericardial cavity. It can increase intracardiac pressure, compress the heart, and interfere with venous return to the heart. The amount of fluid

(continued)

SUMMARY CONCEPTS *(continued)*

or exudate, how quickly it accumulates, and the elasticity of the pericardium determine the effect the effusion has on cardiac function.

■ Cardiac tamponade represents a life-threatening compression of the heart resulting from excess fluid in the pericardial sac. It may be caused by bleeding into the pericardial sac due to conditions such as chest trauma or rupture of the heart following myocardial infarction.

■ In constrictive pericarditis, scar tissue develops between the visceral and parietal layers of the serous pericardium. In time, the scar tissue contracts and interferes with cardiac filling.

Cardiomyopathies

Cardiomyopathies are disorders of the heart muscle. They are usually associated with disorders of myocardial performance, which may be mechanical (e.g., heart failure) or electrical (e.g., life-threatening arrhythmias). The definition and classification of the cardiomyopathies have evolved tremendously with the advance of molecular genetics. The American Heart Association's classification system divides the cardiomyopathies into two major groups: primary cardiomyopathies, which are confined to the myocardium, and secondary cardiomyopathies, which are associated with other disease conditions.[45]

Primary Cardiomyopathies

The primary cardiomyopathies are classified as genetic, mixed, or acquired, based on their etiology.[45] The genetic cardiomyopathies include hypertrophic cardiomyopathy and arrhythmogenic right ventricular dysplasia. The mixed cardiomyopathies, which include dilated and restrictive cardiomyopathy, are of both genetic and nongenetic origin. Acquired cardiomyopathies include those that have their origin in the inflammatory process (e.g., myocarditis), pregnancy (peripartum cardiomyopathy), and stress (takotsubo cardiomyopathy). In many cases the cause is unknown, and in these cases it is referred to as an idiopathic cardiomyopathy.

Hypertrophic Cardiomyopathy

Hypertrophic cardiomyopathy (HCM) is characterized by unexplained left ventricular hypertrophy with disproportionate thickening of the ventricular septum, abnormal diastolic filling, cardiac arrhythmias, and, in some cases, intermittent left ventricular outflow obstruction (Fig. 19-18). It is one of the most common types of cardiomyopathy, occurring in approximately 1 out of 500 persons in the general population.[46] Hypertrophic cardiomyopathy is the most common cause of sudden cardiac death in young athletes.[47]

Hypertrophic cardiomyopathy is an autosomal dominant disorder caused by mutations in genes encoding proteins of the cardiac sarcomere (i.e., muscle fibers). Histologically, HCM specimens have myocyte hypertrophy with myofibril disarray and increased cardiac fibrosis. More than 400 mutations have been identified in 11 sarcomeric genes.[46–48] Although HCM is inherited, it may present at any time from early childhood to late adulthood with a broad category of manifestations and a variable clinical course.

Clinically, HCM is characterized by a massively hypertrophied left ventricle with a reduced chamber size and a paradoxical decrease in stroke volume that results from impaired diastolic filling; in about 25% of cases, dynamic obstruction of left ventricular outflow occurs due to disproportionate thickening of the interventricular septum.[6] Hypertrophic cardiomyopathy is frequently associated with the development of left ventricular

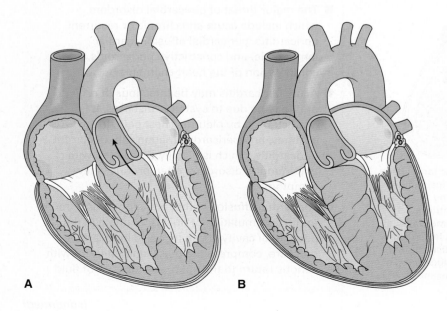

A **B**

FIGURE 19-18. Normal heart **(A)** and hypertrophic cardiomyopathy **(B)** in which disproportionate thickening of the intraventicular septum causes intermittent left ventricular outflow obstruction.

outflow obstruction that is caused by systolic anterior motion of the mitral valve and midsystolic contact with the ventricular septum. The obstruction is worsened by factors that increase myocardial contraction (e.g., sympathetic stimulation or exertion) or decrease left ventricular filling (e.g., Valsalva maneuver, peripheral vasodilation).

Clinical Manifestations. The clinical manifestations of HCM are highly variable and may progress to end-stage heart failure with left ventricular remodeling and systolic dysfunction. The most frequent symptoms of HCM are dyspnea and chest pain in the absence of coronary artery disease. Syncope (fainting) is also common and is typically post-exertional, when diastolic filling diminishes and outflow obstruction increases. Atrial fibrillation can occur as a long-term consequence of elevated left atrial pressures. Ventricular arrhythmias are also common and sudden death may occur, often in athletes after extensive exertion. Risk factors for sudden cardiac death among patients with HCM include a family history of syncope or sudden cardiac death, certain gene mutations, and extreme hypertrophy of the left ventricle.

Diagnosis and Treatment. Diagnosis of HCM is frequently established with 2D echocardiography, ECG, and continuous ambulatory monitoring. Cardiac MRI can also be helpful. Genetic testing, through bidirectional deoxyribonucleic acid (DNA) sequence analysis, is important for identifying gene mutations and making diagnoses, although with some limitations.[48] In many patients with HCM, physical examination results are normal.

Medical management of HCM is primarily focused on symptom management. The first-line approach to relief of symptoms is pharmacologic therapy designed to block the effects of catecholamines that exacerbate outflow obstruction and to slow heart rate to enhance diastolic filling. In the majority of cases of symptomatic HCM, beta blockers are the initial choice for therapy. Calcium channel blockers, especially verapamil, can also be used in patients who do not respond to beta blockers. Calcium channel blockers can, however, exacerbate left ventricular outflow obstruction and are not recommended for persons with severe outflow obstruction and pronounced symptoms.

Dual-chamber and biventricular pacing may be used to prevent progression of hypertrophy and obstruction. In obstructive HCM that is refractory to drug therapy, septal myotomy–myectomy (surgical excision of part of the outflow myocardial septum) or alcohol ablation of the interventricular septum can be used. An implantable cardioverter–defibrillator should be considered for persons with HCM who have sustained ventricular tachycardia or ventricular fibrillation and are receiving optimal medical therapy.[46]

Arrhythmogenic Right Ventricular Dysplasia

Arrhythmogenic right ventricular dysplasia (ARVD) also called arrhythmogenic right ventricular cardiomyopathy (ARVC), is a heart muscle disease that primarily affects the right ventricle, leading to various rhythm disturbances, particularly ventricular tachycardia, and potentially to heart failure.[49] It ranks second, after HCM, as the leading cause of sudden cardiac death in young athletes. The incidence of ARVD varies from about 1 in 2000 to 1 in 5000, affecting men more frequently than women.[49]

Arrhythmogenic right ventricular dysplasia is inherited as an autosomal dominant trait in greater than 50% of cases, although often with incomplete penetrance and variable expression. Although multiple gene mutations have been identified (mapping to chromosomes 1, 2, 3, 14, and 17),[50] the pathogenesis of the disorder remains undefined.

Clinical Manifestations. The disorder is characterized by progressive loss of myocytes, with partial or complete replacement of the right ventricular muscle with adipose or fibrofatty tissue. These changes are associated with reentrant ventricular tachyarrhythmias of right ventricular origin that are often precipitated by an exercise-induced discharge of catecholamines. Clinical manifestations include palpitations, syncope, or cardiac arrest, usually in young or middle-aged men. Other symptoms may include abdominal pain and mental confusion.

Diagnosis and Treatment. Diagnosis of ARVD is based on clinical, ECG, echocardiographic, and histologic findings. Personal and family history, including first- and second-degree relatives, is important. Treatment for ARVD is aimed at prevention of sudden cardiac death, prevention or delay. Although ARVD cannot be cured, the goal of treatment is to prevent and control the arrhythmias with antiarrhythmic agents.[49] Radiofrequency ablation may be used in cases that are refractory to drug therapy, although it is completely successful in only 30% to 65% of cases, with multiple ablations sometimes needed. An implantable cardioverter–defibrillator is also indicated for drug-refractory cases and for those who have survived a sudden cardiac death episode. Final options for treatment include ventriculotomy and heart transplantation.[49] There are no randomized trials evaluating ARVD treatment modalities at this time.

Dilated Cardiomyopathy

Dilated cardiomyopathy (DCM) is a common cause of heart failure and the leading indication for heart transplantation. Up to 35% of cases are reported as familial; however, that proportion may be even higher, but due to incomplete penetrance it is difficult to identify early or latent disease in family members.[6,51] Most familial cases appear to be transmitted as an autosomal dominant trait, but autosomal recessive, X-linked recessive, and mitochondrial inheritance patterns have been identified. Other causes include infections (i.e., viral, bacterial, fungal, mycobacterial, parasitic), toxins, alcoholism, chemotherapeutic agents, metals, and multiple other disorders. Often no cause is found, in which case it is often referred to as idiopathic DCM.

Dilated cardiomyopathy is characterized by progressive cardiac dilation and contractile (systolic) dysfunction, usually with concurrent hypertrophy.[6,51]

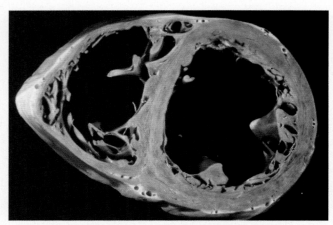

FIGURE 19-19. Idiopathic dilated cardiomyopathy. A transverse section of the enlarged heart reveals conspicuous dilation of both ventricles. Although the ventricular wall appears thinned, the increased mass of the heart indicates considerable hypertrophy. (From Saffitz JE. The heart. In: Rubin E, Strayer DS, eds. *Rubin's Pathology: Clinicopathologic Foundations of Medicine.*, 6th ed. Philadelphia, PA: Wolters Kluwer Health | Lippincott Williams & Wilkins; 2012:525.)

The heart is enlarged (two to three times its normal weight) and flabby with dilation of all four chambers (Fig. 19-19). Because of wall thinning that accompanies dilation, the ventricular thickness may be less than, equal to, or greater than normal. The histologic abnormalities in DCM are nonspecific. Microscopically, most myocytes are hypertrophied with enlarged nuclei, but many are thinned, stretched, and irregular or atrophied.

Clinical Manifestations. The most common clinical manifestations of DCM are those related to heart failure, such as dyspnea, orthopnea, and reduced exercise capacity. In the end stages, persons with DCM often have ejection fractions of less than 25% (normal ejection fraction 50% to 65%).[6] As the disease progresses, stasis of blood in the walls of the heart chambers can lead to thrombus formation and systemic emboli. Secondary mitral valve regurgitation and abnormal cardiac rhythms are common. Death is usually due to heart failure or arrhythmias and can occur suddenly.

Treatment. The treatment of DCM is directed toward relieving the symptoms of heart failure, reducing the work of the heart, and preventing atrial and ventricular dysrhythmias. Pharmacologic agents include diuretics to reduce preload, beta blockers to reduce heart rate and myocardial oxygen demand, afterload-reducing agents to decrease left ventricular filling pressures, and angiotensin converting enzyme (ACE) inhibitors to prevent vasoconstriction. Anticoagulant and antiarrhythmic drugs (e.g., amiodarone for atrial fibrillation) may be used. Other treatments may include a biventricular pacemaker, an implantable cardioverter–defibrillator for chronic symptomatic DCM with reduced systolic function, and in cases that are refractory to treatment, cardiac transplantation. The prognosis for patients with DCM who do not undergo cardiac transplantation is poor with the average 5-year survival rate being less than 50%. Removing or avoiding causative agents (if identified); avoiding myocardial depressants, including alcohol; and spacing rest with asymptomatic levels of exercise or activity are also important.

Primary Restrictive Cardiomyopathy

Restrictive cardiomyopathy is a rare form of heart muscle disease in which ventricular filling is restricted because of excessive rigidity (but not necessarily thickening) of the ventricular walls, although the contractile properties or systolic function of the heart remain relatively normal.[6] Restrictive cardiomyopathy can be idiopathic or associated with other conditions that affect the myocardium, principally radiation fibrosis, amyloidosis, sarcoidosis, or metastatic tumors. Genetics may also play a role because familial forms of restrictive cardiomyopathy have been reported.[46]

Symptoms of restrictive cardiomyopathy include dyspnea, PND, orthopnea, peripheral edema, ascites, fatigue, and weakness. The manifestations of restrictive cardiomyopathy resemble those of constrictive pericarditis. In the advanced form of the disease, all the signs of heart failure are present except cardiomegaly.

Myocarditis

Myocarditis, or inflammatory cardiomyopathy, can be defined as an inflammation of the heart.[6,51,52] The clinical spectrum of the disease is broad: at one end, the disease is asymptomatic with full recovery, and at the other end it has a precipitous onset of heart failure or arrhythmias, occasionally with sudden cardiac death.

An acquired cardiomyopathy, myocarditis is associated with a number of etiologies; however, it is usually caused by a viral infection, most commonly an enterovirus (coxsackievirus group B).[6,52–54] In young children adenovirus and parvovirus are the most likely causative agents. Other etiologies include bacterial or fungal infections, hypersensitivity to certain drugs, and autoimmune diseases, such as systemic lupus erythematosus. Myocarditis is a frequent pathologic cardiac finding in persons with acquired immunodeficiency syndrome (AIDS), although it is unclear whether it is due to the human immunodeficiency virus infection itself or to secondary infections.

The pathogenesis of myocarditis is one of cardiac injury, followed by an immunologic response. Myocardial injury due to infectious agents is thought to result from necrosis caused by direct invasion of the offending organism, toxic effects of exotoxins or endotoxins produced by a systemic pathogen, or destruction of cardiac tissue by immunologic mechanisms initiated by the infectious agent. The immunologic response may be directed at foreign antigens of the infectious agent that share molecular characteristics with those of the host cardiac myocytes (i.e., molecular mimicry; see Chapter 16), providing a continuous stimulus for the immune response even after the infectious agent has been cleared from the body.

Clinical Manifestations. The signs and symptoms of myocarditis vary from person to person.[53] Some persons may present with fever, chills, nausea, vomiting, arthralgia, and myalgia, occurring up to 6 weeks before the diagnosis of myocarditis. Other persons may present with heart failure without antecedent symptoms. The onset of heart failure may be gradual or abrupt and fulminant. Emboli may occur because of the procoagulant effect of inflammatory cytokines combined with decreased myocardial contractility. At times, the presentation may mimic ACS, with ST-segment and T-wave changes, positive serum cardiac biomarkers, and regional wall motion abnormalities despite normal coronary arteries. Viral myocarditis in children or young adults is often nonspecific, with symptoms such as fever and poor eating.

Diagnosis and Treatment. The diagnosis of myocarditis can be suggested by clinical manifestations. Methods used in confirming the diagnosis include the ECG, chest radiography, serum cardiac biomarkers (i.e., creatinine phosphokinase, troponin I), and echocardiography. Endomyocardial biopsy findings, obtained through cardiac catheterization, remain the gold standard for establishing the diagnosis of acute myocarditis, despite limited accuracy.[52–54]

Many cases of myocarditis are mild and self-limiting, so first-line treatment remains largely supportive.[52–54] Initial treatments include supplemental oxygen, bed rest, and antibiotics, if needed. In persons with more severe myocarditis, arrhythmia suppression and hemodynamic support with vasopressors and positive inotropic agents may be needed. Persons with severe fulminant myocarditis may require aggressive short-term support with an intra-aortic balloon pump or left ventricular assist devices.[52] Immunosuppressive therapy continues to be investigated. Although treatment of myocarditis is successful in many persons, some progress to heart failure. For these patients, cardiac transplantation is an important intervention.

 Peripartum Cardiomyopathy

Peripartum cardiomyopathy is a dilated cardiomyopathy that occurs in the last month of pregnancy or within 5 months after delivery.[55] It is manifested by signs of systolic dysfunction and heart failure for which there is no identifiable cause or evidence prior to the last month of pregnancy.[55–57] The incidence is greater in black, multiparous, or older women, and in women with twin fetuses, preeclampsia, or using tocolytic therapy to prevent premature labor and delivery.[56,57]

Although the etiology of peripartum cardiomyopathy is unknown, several causes have been proposed, including infectious, immunologic, nutritional, drug-induced, and genetic factors. Some women exhibit inflammatory cells in heart biopsies taken during the symptomatic phase of the disorder, suggesting a disordered immune response.

Management of peripartum cardiomyopathy includes standard therapy for heart failure. However, potential teratogenic effects and the excretion of drugs during breast-feeding need to be considered. Prognosis depends on resolution of the heart failure. About half of women with peripartum cardiomyopathy spontaneously recover normal cardiac function; the other half are left with persistent left ventricular dysfunction or progress to develop heart failure.[57]

Stress or "Takotsubo" Cardiomyopathy

First described in Japan in 1991, takotsubo-like left ventricular dysfunction is named after the fishing pot used to trap octopus that has a narrow neck and wide base, a shape similar to that of the affected ventricle.[58,59] The term transient left ventricular apical ballooning has also been used to describe this syndrome.

An acquired disorder, stress cardiomyopathy has been identified in the clinical setting as a transient, reversible left ventricular dysfunction in response to profound psychological or emotional stress. The syndrome occurs primarily in middle-aged women who present with acute STEMI but who, on cardiac catheterization, have no evidence of CAD. There is, however, impaired myocardial contractility characterized by left ventricular apical ballooning with hypercontractility of the basal left ventricle.

The mechanism for myocardial stunning in stress cardiomyopathy is unclear, although some theories suggest ischemia from coronary artery spasm, microvascular spasm, or direct myocyte injury. When catecholamine levels return to normal, the interventricular gradient resolves and left ventricular function recovers.[60]

Treatment of stress cardiomyopathy is the same as that for heart failure, and most patients with takotsubo cardiomyopathy demonstrate rapid improvement and an excellent prognosis.

Secondary Cardiomyopathies

Secondary cardiomyopathy is a heart muscle disease in the presence of a multisystem disorder. The conditions most commonly associated with secondary cardiomyopathies are identified in Chart 19-2. Some of these disorders produce accumulation of abnormal substances between myocytes (extracellular), whereas others produce accumulation of abnormal substances within myocytes (intracellular).

Almost 100 distinct myocardial diseases can result in the clinical features of DCM. They include cardiomyopathies associated with drugs, diabetes mellitus, muscular dystrophy, autoimmune disorders, and cancer treatment agents (radiation and cancer drugs).[59] Alcoholic cardiomyopathy is the single most common identifiable cause of DCM in the United States and Europe. Doxorubicin (Adriamycin) and other anthracycline drugs used in the treatment of cancer, are potent agents whose usefulness is limited by cumulative dose-dependent cardiac toxicity. Another cancer chemotherapeutic agent with cardiotoxic potential is cyclophosphamide (Cytoxan). Unlike the primary myocyte injury that occurs with doxorubicin, the principal insult with cyclophosphamide appears to be vascular, leading to myocardial hemorrhage.

CHART 19-2 **Conditions Associated with Secondary Cardiomyopathies***

Autoimmune Disorders
Systemic lupus erythematosus
Rheumatoid arthritis
Scleroderma
Polyarteritis nodosa

Endocrine Disorders
Acromegaly
Diabetes mellitus
Hypothyroidism and hyperthyroidism
Hyperparathyroidism

Familial Storage Diseases
Glycogen storage disease
Mucopolysaccharidoses
Hemochromatosis

Infiltrative Disorders
Amyloidosis
Sarcoidosis
Radiation-induced fibrosis

Neuromuscular/Neurologic Disorders
Friedreich ataxia
Muscular dystrophy
Neurofibromatosis

Nutritional Deficiencies
Thiamine (beriberi)
Protein (kwashiorkor)

Toxins
Alcohol and its metabolites
Arsenic
Chemotherapeutic agents (anthracyclines [doxorubicin, daunorubicin], cyclophosphamide)
Catecholamines
Hydrocarbons

*Not intended to be inclusive.

SUMMARY CONCEPTS

■ The cardiomyopathies, which involve both mechanical and electrical etiologies of myocardial dysfunction, are classified as either primary or secondary based on whether they are confined to the myocardium or are associated with other disease conditions. Symptoms related to most cardiomyopathies, whether primary or secondary, are those associated with heart failure and sudden cardiac death. Treatment focuses on symptom management and prevention of lethal arrhythmias.

■ The primary cardiomyopathies include genetic, mixed, or acquired types. The genetic cardiomyopathies include hypertrophic cardiomyopathy and arrhythmogenic right ventricular dysplasia. The mixed cardiomyopathies, which include dilated and restrictive cardiomyopathies, are of both genetic and acquired origin. Acquired cardiomyopathies include those that have their origin in the inflammatory process (e.g., myocarditis), stress (takotsubo cardiomyopathy), or pregnancy (peripartum cardiomyopathy). In many cases the cause is unknown, in which case it is referred to as an idiopathic cardiomyopathy.

■ The secondary cardiomyopathies are heart diseases in which myocardial involvement occurs as part of a multisystem disorder. They include cardiomyopathies associated with drugs, diabetes mellitus, muscular dystrophy, autoimmune disorders, and cancer treatment agents (radiation and chemotherapeutic drugs).

Heart Disease in Infants and Children

Heart disease in children encompasses both congenital and acquired disorders. Approximately 1 of every 125 infants born has a congenital heart defect, making this the most common form of structural birth defect.[61] Advances in diagnostic methods and surgical treatment have greatly increased the long-term survival and positive outcomes for children born with congenital heart defects. Although thousands of infants born each year will have a congenital heart disease, other children will develop an acquired heart disease, such as Kawasaki disease. Other acquired disorders that affect children, the cardiomyopathies and rheumatic fever, were discussed earlier in the chapter.

Fetal and Perinatal Circulation

The fetal circulation is different anatomically and physiologically from the postnatal circulation. Before birth, oxygenation of blood occurs through the placenta; after birth it occurs through the lungs. The fetus is maintained in a low-oxygen state (PO_2 30 to 35 mm Hg; hemoglobin O_2 saturation 60% to 70%). To compensate, fetal cardiac output is higher than at any other time in life (400 to 500 mL/kg/minute) and fetal hemoglobin has a higher affinity for oxygen.[62] Also, the pulmonary vessels in the fetus are markedly constricted because of the fluid-filled lungs and the heightened hypoxic stimulus for vasoconstriction that is present in the fetus.

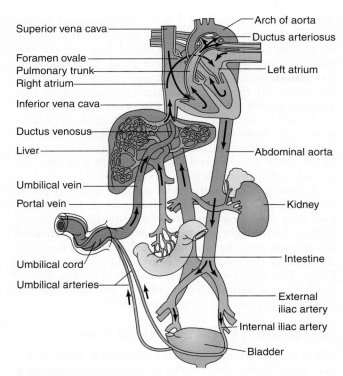

FIGURE 19-20. Fetal circulation.

As a result, blood flow through the lungs is less than at any other time in life.

In the fetus, blood enters the circulation through the umbilical vein and returns to the placenta through the two umbilical arteries[62–64] (Fig. 19-20). A vessel called the *ductus venosus* allows the majority of blood from the umbilical vein to bypass the hepatic circulation and pass directly into the inferior vena cava. From the inferior vena cava, blood flows into the right atrium, where approximately 40% of the blood volume moves through the foramen ovale into the left atrium. It then passes into the left ventricle and is ejected into the ascending aorta to perfuse the head and upper extremities. In this way, the best-oxygenated blood from the placenta is used to perfuse the brain. At the same time, venous blood from the head and upper extremities returns to the right side of the heart through the superior vena cava, moves into the right ventricle, and is ejected into the pulmonary artery. Because of the very high pulmonary vascular resistance that is present, almost 90% of blood ejected into the pulmonary artery gets diverted through the ductus arteriosus into the descending aorta. This blood perfuses the lower extremities and is returned to the placenta by the umbilical arteries.

At birth, the infant takes its first breath and switches from placental to pulmonary oxygenation of the blood. The most dramatic alterations in the circulation after birth are the elimination of the low-resistance placental vascular bed and the marked pulmonary vasodilation that is produced by initiation of ventilation. Within minutes of birth, pulmonary blood flow increases from 35 mL/kg/minute to 160 to 200 mL/kg/minute.[62]

The pressure in the pulmonary circulation and the right side of the heart falls as fetal lung fluid is replaced by air and as lung expansion decreases the pressure transmitted to the pulmonary blood vessels. With lung inflation, the alveolar oxygen tension increases, causing reversal of the hypoxemia-induced pulmonary vasoconstriction of the fetal circulation. Cord clamping and removal of the low-resistance placental circulation produce an increase in systemic vascular resistance and a resultant increase in left ventricular pressure. The resultant decrease in right atrial pressure and increase in left atrial pressure produce closure of the foramen ovale flap valve. Reversal of the fetal hypoxemic state also produces constriction of ductal smooth muscle, contributing to closure of the ductus arteriosus. The foramen ovale and the ductus arteriosus normally close within the 1st day of life, effectively separating the pulmonary and systemic circulations.

After the initial precipitous fall in pulmonary vascular resistance, a more gradual decrease occurs during the first 2 to 9 weeks of life, related to regression of the medial smooth muscle layer in the pulmonary arteries. By the time a healthy, term infant is several weeks old, the pulmonary vascular resistance has fallen to adult levels. Several factors, including alveolar hypoxia, prematurity, lung disease, and congenital heart defects, may affect postnatal pulmonary vascular development. Much of the development of the smooth muscle layer in the pulmonary arterioles occurs during late gestation; as a result, infants born prematurely have less medial smooth muscle; therefore, the muscle layer may regress in a shorter time. The pulmonary vascular smooth muscle in premature infants also may be less responsive to hypoxia. For these reasons, a premature infant may demonstrate a larger decrease in pulmonary vascular resistance resulting in shunting of blood from the aorta through the ductus arteriosus to the pulmonary artery within hours of birth.

Alveolar hypoxia may also delay or prevent the normal decrease in pulmonary vascular resistance that occurs during the first few weeks of life. During this period, the pulmonary arteries remain highly reactive and can constrict in response to hypoxia, acidosis, hyperinflation of the alveoli, and hypothermia.

Congenital Heart Defects

The major development of the fetal heart occurs between the 4th and 7th weeks of gestation, and most congenital heart defects arise during this time. The development of the heart can be altered by environmental, genetic, or chromosomal influences. Most congenital heart defects are thought to be multifactorial in origin, resulting from an interaction between a genetic predisposition toward development of a heart defect and environmental influences.

Knowledge about the genetic basis of congenital heart defects has grown dramatically in recent years. This area of research is particularly important as more individuals with congenital heart disease survive into adulthood and consider having children of their own. Recent evidence suggests that the genetic contribution to congenital heart disease has been underestimated in the past.[65,66] Some heart defects, such as aortic stenosis, atrial septal defect of the secundum type, pulmonary valve stenosis, tetralogy of Fallot, and certain ventricular septal defects, have a stronger familial predisposition than others. Chromosomal abnormalities are also associated with congenital heart defects, as evidenced by the observation that as many as 30% of children with congenital heart disease have an associated chromosomal abnormality. Heart disease is found in nearly 100% of children with trisomy 18, 50% of those with trisomy 21, and 35% of those with Turner syndrome.[66]

Congenital heart diseases are commonly classified according to their anatomic site (atrial septal or ventricular septal defects), the hemodynamic alterations caused by the anatomic defects (left-to-right or right-to-left shunts), and their effect on pulmonary blood flow and tissue oxygenation (cyanotic or noncyanotic defects).

Shunting

Shunting of blood refers to the diversion of blood flow from one system to the other—from the arterial to the venous system (i.e., left-to-right shunt) or from the venous to the arterial system (i.e., right-to-left shunt).[64] The shunting of blood in congenital heart defects is determined by the presence of an abnormal opening between the right and left circulations and the degree of resistance to flow through the opening. The shunting of blood can affect both the oxygen content of the blood and the volume of blood being delivered to the vessels in the pulmonary circulation.

The direction of shunting (right-to left or left-to-right) is largely determined by the vascular resistance of the systemic and pulmonary circulations. Due to the high pulmonary vascular resistance in the neonate, atrial and ventricular septal defects usually do not produce a significant shunt during the 1st weeks of life. As the pulmonary vascular smooth muscle regresses in the neonate, the resistance in the pulmonary circulation falls below that of the systemic circulation, causing a left-to-right shunt in uncomplicated atrial or ventricular septal defects. In more complicated ventricular septal defects, increased resistance to outflow may affect the pattern of shunting. For example, defects that increase resistance to aortic outflow (e.g., aortic valve stenosis, coarctation of the aorta, hypoplastic left heart syndrome) increase left-to-right shunting, whereas defects that obstruct pulmonary outflow (e.g., pulmonary valve stenosis, tetralogy of Fallot) increase right-to-left shunting. Crying, defecating, or even the stress of feeding may increase pulmonary vascular resistance and cause an increase in right-to-left shunting in infants with septal defects.

Cyanosis, a bluish color of the skin most notable in the nail beds and mucous membranes, develops when sufficient deoxygenated blood from the right side of the heart mixes with oxygenated blood in the left side of the heart.[67] Abnormal color becomes obvious when the oxygen saturation falls below 80% in the capillaries (equal to 5 g of deoxygenated hemoglobin). Defects that result in a right-to-left shunting or obstruction of pulmonary blood flow are categorized as cyanotic disorders and those involving left-to-right shunting are usually categorized as acyanotic disorders. Of the congenital defects discussed in this chapter, patent ductus arteriosus, atrial and ventricular septal defects, endocardial cushion defects, pulmonary valve stenosis, and coarctation of the aorta are considered acyanotic; tetralogy of Fallot, transposition of the great vessels, and single-ventricle anatomy are considered cyanotic defects.

A right-to-left shunt results in deoxygenated blood moving from the right side of the heart to the left side and then being ejected into the systemic circulation. With a left-to-right shunt, oxygenated blood intended for ejection into the systemic circulation is recirculated through the right side of the heart and back through the lungs. This increased volume distends the right side of the heart and pulmonary circulation and increases the workload placed on the right ventricle.[68]

Alterations in Pulmonary Blood Flow

Many of the complications of congenital heart disorders result from a decrease or an increase in pulmonary blood flow. Defects that reduce pulmonary blood flow (e.g., pulmonary stenosis) typically cause symptoms of fatigue, dyspnea, and failure to thrive. In contrast to the arterioles in the systemic circulation, the arterioles in the pulmonary circulation are normally thin-walled vessels that can accommodate the various levels of stroke volume that are ejected from the right heart. The thinning of the pulmonary vessels occurs during the 1st weeks after birth, during which the vessel media thin and pulmonary vascular resistance decreases. In a term infant who has a congenital heart defect that produces markedly increased pulmonary blood flow (e.g., ventricular septal defect), the increased flow stimulates pulmonary vasoconstriction and delays or reduces the normal involutional thinning of the small pulmonary arterioles. In most cases pulmonary vascular resistance is only slightly elevated during early infancy, and the major contribution to pulmonary hypertension is the increased blood flow. However, in some infants with a large right-to-left shunt, the pulmonary vascular resistance never decreases.

Congenital heart defects that persistently increase pulmonary blood flow or pulmonary vascular resistance have the potential of causing pulmonary hypertension and producing irreversible pathologic changes in the pulmonary vasculature. When shunting of systemic blood flow into the pulmonary circulation threatens permanent injury to the pulmonary vessels, a surgical procedure should be done to reduce the flow temporarily or permanently. Pulmonary artery banding consists of placing a constrictive band around the main pulmonary artery, thereby increasing resistance to outflow from the right ventricle. The banding technique is a temporary measure to alleviate symptoms and protect the pulmonary vasculature in anticipation of later surgical repair of the defect.

General Manifestations, Diagnosis, and Treatment

It is increasingly common for congenital heart defects to be diagnosed prenatally.[69] In this case, the infant can be evaluated shortly after birth to confirm the diagnosis and develop a treatment plan. Reliable transabdominal diagnostic images of the fetal heart can be obtained as early as 16 weeks of gestation, and recently, accurate trans-vaginal images have been obtained as early as 11 to 14 weeks of gestation. Among the disorders that can be diagnosed with certainty by fetal echocardiography are AV septal defects, hypoplastic left heart syndrome, aortic valve stenosis, hypertrophic cardiomyopathy, pulmonic valve stenosis, and transposition of the great arteries. Disorders that result in an abnormal four-chamber view, an image typically obtained during routine prenatal ultrasonography, are the most likely to be detected.[69]

In the postnatal period, congenital heart defects may present with numerous signs and symptoms, most commonly a murmur audible on auscultation. Some defects, such as patent ductus arteriosus and small ventricular septal defects, close spontaneously. In other less-severe defects, there may be no obvious signs and symptoms and the disorder may be discovered during a routine health examination. Cyanosis, pulmonary congestion, cardiac failure, and decreased peripheral perfusion are the major concerns in children with more severe defects. Such defects often cause problems immediately after birth or early in infancy. The child may exhibit cyanosis, respiratory difficulty, and fatigability, and is likely to have difficulty with feeding and failure to thrive. Heart failure manifests itself as tachypnea or dyspnea at rest or on exertion. For the infant, this most commonly occurs during feeding. Recurrent respiratory infections and excessive sweating may also be reported.[70] The infant whose peripheral perfusion is markedly decreased may be in a shocklike state.

A generalized cyanosis that persists longer than 3 hours after birth suggests congenital heart disease. An oxygen challenge (administration of 100% oxygen for 5 to 10 minutes) can help to determine whether congenital heart disease is present in a cyanotic newborn.[70] Because infant cyanosis may appear as duskiness, it is important to assess the color of the mucous membranes, fingernails, toenails, tongue, and lips. Several programs have instituted routine pulse oximetry screening for all newborns.[71] Pulmonary congestion in the infant causes an increase in respiratory rate, orthopnea, grunting, wheezing, coughing, and crackles. A chest radiograph can quickly differentiate infants who have reduced pulmonary vascular markings (densities) from those who have normal or increased markings.

The treatment plan usually includes supportive therapy (e.g., digoxin, diuretics, and feeding supplementation) designed to help the infant compensate for the limitations in cardiac reserve and to prevent complications. Surgical intervention often is required for severe defects. It may be done in the early weeks of life or, conditions permitting, delayed until the child is older. Children with structural congenital heart disease and those who have had corrective surgery may have a higher-than-expected risk for development of infective endocarditis. Prophylactic antibiotic therapy before dental procedures or other periods of increased risk for bacteremia is suggested for children with certain types of heart defects or surgical procedures.[72]

Children with congenital heart disease also experience a higher than expected incidence of developmental delays.[73,74] A characteristic pattern of combined disabilities in the areas of visual motor integration, language, motor skills, attention, executive function and behavior has been described in multiple research studies.[73–75] In an effort to promote early detection of developmental delays and appropriate intervention, the American Heart Association and the American Academy of Pediatrics issued a joint guideline statement in 2012 suggesting systematic surveillance, screening, and evaluation throughout childhood to assess academic, behavioral, psychosocial and adaptive functioning.[76] Early detection of developmental problems will direct interventions which can prevent or reduce long-term issues known to have a profoundly negative impact on quality of life and ability to achieve optimum potential in adulthood.[77]

Types of Defects

Congenital heart defects can affect almost any of the cardiac structures or central blood vessels (Fig. 19-21). Defects include communication between heart chambers, interrupted development of the heart chambers or valve structures, malposition of heart chambers and great vessels, and altered closure of fetal communication channels. The particular defect reflects the embryo's stage of development at the time it occurred. It is common for multiple defects to be present in one child and for some congenital heart disorders, such as tetralogy of Fallot, to involve several defects.

Patent Ductus Arteriosus. Patent ductus arteriosus results from persistence of the fetal ductus beyond the prenatal period.[78] In fetal life, the ductus arteriosus is the vital link by which blood from the right side of the heart bypasses the lungs and enters the systemic circulation (Fig. 19-21G). After birth, this passage no longer is needed, and it usually closes during the first 24 to 72 hours of life. The physiologic stimulus and mechanisms associated with permanent closure of the ductus are not entirely known, but the fact that infant hypoxia predisposes to a delayed closure suggests that the increase in arterial oxygen levels that occurs immediately after birth plays a role. Additional factors that contribute to closure are a fall in endogenous levels of prostaglandins and adenosine and the release of vasoactive substances. After constriction, the lumen of the ductus becomes permanently sealed with fibrous tissue within 2 to 3 weeks. Ductal closure may be delayed or prevented in very premature infants, probably as a result of a combination of factors, including decreased medial smooth muscle in the ductus wall, decreased vasoconstriction response to oxygen, and increased circulating levels of prostaglandins,

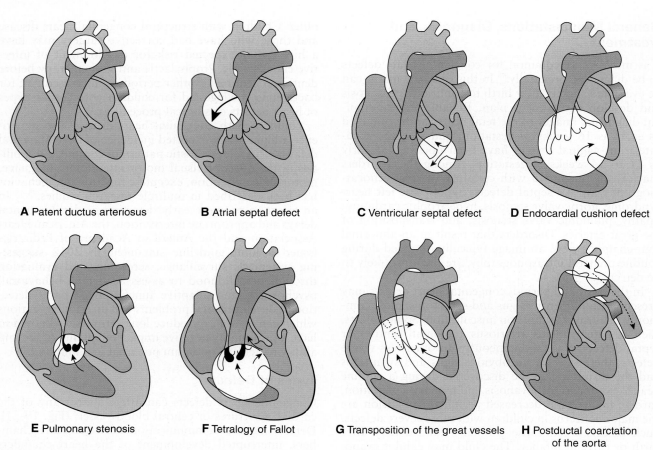

A Patent ductus arteriosus   **B** Atrial septal defect   **C** Ventricular septal defect   **D** Endocardial cushion defect

E Pulmonary stenosis   **F** Tetralogy of Fallot   **G** Transposition of the great vessels   **H** Postductal coarctation of the aorta

FIGURE 19-21. Congenital heart defects. **(A)** Patent ductus arteriosus. The high-pressure blood of the aorta is shunted back to the pulmonary artery. **(B)** Atrial septal defect. Blood is shunted from left to right. **(C)** Ventricular septal defect. Blood is usually shunted from left to right. **(D)** Endocardial cushion defect. Blood flows between the chambers of the heart. **(E)** Pulmonary stenosis, with decreased pulmonary blood flow and right ventricular hypertrophy. **(F)** Tetralogy of Fallot. This involves a ventricular septal defect, dextroposition of the aorta, right ventricular outflow obstruction, and right ventricular hypertrophy. Blood is shunted from right to left. **(G)** Transposition of the great vessels. The pulmonary artery is attached to the left side of the heart and the aorta to the right side. **(H)** Postductal coarctation of the aorta.

which have a vasodilating effect. Ductal closure also may be delayed in infants with congenital heart defects that produce a decrease in oxygen tension.[78]

Persistent patency of the ductus arteriosus is defined as a duct that remains open beyond 3 months in the full-term infant. The size of the persistent ductus and the difference between the systemic and pulmonary vascular resistance determine its clinical manifestations. Blood typically shunts across the ductus from the higher-pressure left side (systemic circulation) to the lower-pressure right side (pulmonary circulation). After the infant's pulmonary vascular resistance falls, the patent ductus arteriosus provides for a continuous runoff of aortic blood into the pulmonary artery. With a large patent ductus, the runoff is continuous, resulting in increased pulmonary blood flow, pulmonary congestion, and increased resistance against which the right side of the heart must pump. Increased pulmonary venous return and increased work demands may lead to left ventricular failure.[79]

Spontaneous closure of the ductus seldom occurs after infancy. In the full-term infant or older child, closure can be achieved with either surgical ligation or device occlusion. In children with a small patent ductus, closure is done to prevent infective endocarditis or other complications. In children with a moderate to large patent ductus, closure is accomplished to treat heart failure, prevent the development of pulmonary vascular disease, or both.[78] Drugs that inhibit prostaglandin synthesis (e.g., indomethacin) may be used to induce closure of a patent ductus in preterm newborns. Indomethacin works best if it is used in infants younger than 13 days of age; it is not effective later than 4 to 6 weeks of age.[78]

Although closure of a patent ductus is uniformly recommended when it is present as an isolated lesion, deliberate maintenance of ductal patency can be a lifesaving therapy for children with complex forms of congenital heart disease who have ductal-dependent pulmonary or systemic blood flow, or those with obligatory mixing of the arterial and venous circulations (i.e., transposition of the great arteries). Intravenous infusion of prostaglandin E_1 (PGE_1) has proved extremely effective in maintaining ductal patency or reopening the ductus in newborns. Today, this therapy is routinely administered to newborns with suspected congenital heart defects until they can be transported to a specialized center where a diagnosis can be confirmed.[80]

Atrial Septal Defects. In atrial septal defects, an opening in the atrial septum persists as a result of improper septal formation[81] (see Fig. 19-21A). Partitioning of the atria takes place during the 4th and 5th weeks of development and occurs in two stages, beginning with the formation of a thin, crescent-shaped membrane called the *septum primum* followed by the development of a second membrane called the *septum secundum*. As the septum secundum develops, it gradually overlaps an opening in the upper part of the septum primum, forming an oval opening with a flap-type valve called the *foramen ovale* (Fig. 19-22). The foramen ovale, which closes shortly after birth, allows blood from the umbilical vein to pass directly into the left heart, bypassing the lungs.

Atrial septal defects may be single or multiple and vary from a small, asymptomatic opening to a large, symptomatic opening. The type of defect is determined by its position and may include an abnormal opening in the septum primum (ostium primum defects), the septum secundum (ostium secundum defects), or a patent foramen ovale. An ostium secundum atrial septal defect in the region of the foramen ovale is the most common defect. The defect may be single or multiple (fenestrated atrial septum). Most atrial septal defects are small and young children with these defects are often asymptomatic, with the defects discovered inadvertently during a routine physical examination at a few years of age.[81] In the case of an isolated septal defect large enough to

allow shunting, the flow of blood usually is from the left side to the right side of the heart because of the more compliant right ventricle and because the pulmonary vascular resistance is lower than the systemic vascular resistance. This produces right ventricular volume overload and increased pulmonary blood flow. In most cases there is a moderate shunt resulting in dilation of the right heart chambers and overperfusion of the pulmonary circulation.

Children with undiagnosed atrial defects are at risk for pulmonary vascular disease, although this is a rare occurrence before 20 years of age. Rarely, infants with a large shunt may develop congestive heart failure and failure to thrive, prompting early intervention to close the defect.[81] Adolescents and young adults may experience atrial flutter or atrial fibrillation and palpitations because of atrial dilatation. Larger symptomatic defects are usually treated surgically or by transcatheter device closure. Smaller defects may be observed for spontaneous closure in the young child.

Ventricular Septal Defects. A ventricular septal defect is an opening in the ventricular septum that results from an incomplete separation of the ventricles during early fetal development (see Fig. 19-21B). These defects may be single or multiple and may occur in any position along the ventricular septum. Ventricular septal defects are the most common form of congenital heart defect, accounting for 25% to 30% of congenital heart disorders.[82] A ventricular septal defect may be the only cardiac defect, or it may occur in association with multiple cardiac anomalies.

The ventricular septum originates from two sources: the interventricular groove of the folded tubular heart that gives rise to the muscular part of the septum, and the endocardial cushions that extend to form the membranous portion of the septum. The upper membranous portion of the septum is the last area to close, typically by the 7th week of gestation, and it is here that most defects occur.

Depending on the size of the opening and the pulmonary vascular resistance, the signs and symptoms of a ventricular septal defect may range from an asymptomatic murmur to congestive heart failure.[82] If the defect is small, it allows a small shunt and small increases in pulmonary blood flow. These defects produce few symptoms, and approximately one third close spontaneously. With medium-sized defects, a larger shunt occurs, producing a larger increase in pulmonary blood flow. Most of the children with such defects are asymptomatic and have a low risk for development of pulmonary vascular disease.

In children with large nonrestrictive defects, right and left ventricular pressure is equalized and the degree of shunting is determined by the ratio of pulmonary to systemic vascular resistance. Pulmonary vascular resistance normally falls rapidly after birth, owing to the onset of ventilation and subsequent release of hypoxic pulmonary vasoconstriction. This process is often delayed in infants with large ventricular septal defects. As a result, the pulmonary vascular resistance remains somewhat

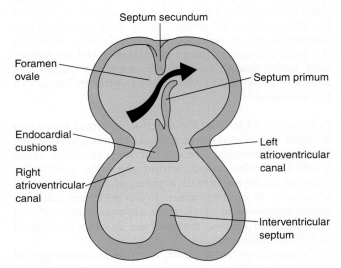

FIGURE 19-22. Development of the endocardial cushions, right and left atrioventricular canals, interventricular septum, and septum primum and septum secundum of the foramen ovale. Note that blood from the right atrium flows through the foramen ovale to the left atrium.

higher than normal, and thus the size of the left-to-right shunt may initially be limited. As the pulmonary vascular resistance falls during the first few weeks after birth, the size of the left-to right shunt increases. Eventually, a large left-to-right shunt develops, and clinical symptoms (e.g., tachypnea; diaphoresis, especially with feeding; and failure to thrive) become apparent. In most cases pulmonary vascular pressure is only slightly elevated during infancy, and the major contributor to pulmonary hypertension is an increase in pulmonary blood flow. However, in some infants with a large septal defect, pulmonary arteriolar thickness never decreases. With continued exposure to high pulmonary blood flow, pulmonary vascular disease develops. In untreated patients, the pulmonary vascular resistance can eventually exceed the systemic resistance. In this case, a reversal of shunt flow occurs and the child demonstrates progressive cyanosis as deoxygenated blood moves from the right to the left side of the heart. These symptoms, coupled with irreversible changes in the pulmonary vasculature, represent an end-stage form of congenital heart disease called *Eisenmenger syndrome*, a condition that is quite rare today due to advances in diagnosis and treatment.

The treatment of a ventricular septal defect depends on the size of the defect, accompanying hemodynamic derangements, and symptomatology. Children with small or medium-sized defects may be followed without intervention if they remain free from signs of congestive heart failure or pulmonary hypertension. Ventricular defects do not increase in size, and some spontaneously close over time.[22] Prophylactic antibiotic therapy is given during periods of increased risk for bacteremia. The management of infants with large ventricular defects aims to control heart failure and prevent the development of pulmonary vascular disease. Symptomatic infants may require feeding supplements or tube feeding to promote growth and development. In the symptomatic infant in whom complete repair cannot be achieved because of size or other complicating lesions, a palliative procedure may be performed to reduce symptoms. Placement of a synthetic band around the main pulmonary artery (pulmonary artery banding) can reduce pulmonary blood flow until complete repair can be accomplished. Surgical closure of the defect is completed by placement of a synthetic or autologous patch effectively to close the shunt across the ventricular septum. These procedures are typically done electively in the infant or young child and are associated with low morbidity and mortality rates.

Endocardial Cushion Defects. The endocardial cushions form the AV canals, the upper part of the ventricular septum, and the lower part of the atrial septum. The endocardial cushions surround this canal and contribute tissue to the lower part of the atrial septum, the upper part of the ventricular septum, the septal leaflet of the tricuspid valve, and the anterior leaflet of the mitral valve.[83] Any flaw in the development of these tissues results in an endocardial cushion defect. Endocardial cushion defects are responsible for approximately 2% of all congenital heart defects. As many as 30% of children with Down syndrome have endocardial cushion defects.[66]

Because the endocardial cushions contribute to multiple aspects of heart development, several variations of endocardial cushion defects are possible. The defect may be described as *partial* or *complete*. The anatomy of the AV valve determines the classification. In partial AV canal defects, the two AV valve rings are complete and separate. The most common type of partial AV canal defect is an ostium primum defect, often associated with a cleft in the mitral valve. In a complete canal defect, there is a common AV valve orifice along with defects in both the atrial and ventricular septal tissue (see Fig. 19-21E). Other cardiac defects may be associated with endocardial cushion defects and most commonly include cardiac malposition defects and tetralogy of Fallot.[83]

Physiologically, endocardial cushion defects result in abnormalities similar to those described for atrial or ventricular septal defects. The direction and magnitude of a shunt in a child with an endocardial cushion defect are determined by the combination of defects and the child's pulmonary and systemic vascular resistance. The hemodynamic effects of an isolated ostium primum defect are those of the previously described atrial septal defect. These children are largely asymptomatic during childhood. With a complete AV canal defect, pulmonary blood flow is increased after the pulmonary vascular resistance falls because of left-to-right shunting across both the ventricular and atrial septal defects. Children with complete defects often have effort intolerance, easy fatigability, failure to thrive, recurrent infections, and other signs of congestive heart failure, particularly when the shunt is large. Pulmonary hypertension and increased pulmonary vascular resistance result if the lesion is left untreated.

The timing of treatment for endocardial cushion defects is determined by the severity of the defect and symptoms. With an ostium primum defect, surgical repair usually is planned on an elective basis before the child reaches school age. Corrective surgery is required for all complete AV canal defects. Infants with severe symptoms may require a palliative procedure in which the main pulmonary artery is banded to reduce pulmonary blood flow. This typically improves the infant's ability to grow and develop until a complete repair can be performed.[83]

Pulmonary Stenosis. Obstruction of blood flow from the right ventricle to the pulmonary circulation is termed *pulmonary stenosis*. The obstruction can occur as an isolated valvular lesion, within the right ventricular chamber, in the pulmonary arteries, or as a combination of stenoses in multiple areas. It is a relatively common defect, estimated to account for approximately 10% of all congenital cardiac disease, and is often associated with other abnormalities.[84]

Pulmonary valvular defect, the most common type of disorder, usually produces some impairment of pulmonary blood flow and increases the workload imposed on the right side of the heart (see Fig. 19-21D). Most children with pulmonic valve stenosis have mild stenosis that does not increase in severity. These children are largely asymptomatic and are diagnosed by the presence of a systolic murmur. Moderate or greater stenosis has been shown to progress over time, particularly before 12 years of age, so these children require careful follow-up. Critical pulmonary stenosis in the neonate is evidenced by cyanosis due to right-to-left atrial-level shunting and right ventricular hypertension. These infants require prostaglandin E_1 to maintain circulation to the lungs through the ductus arteriosus.[84]

Pulmonary valvotomy is the treatment of choice for all valvular defects with pressure gradients from the right ventricle to the pulmonary circulation greater than 30 mm Hg. Transcatheter balloon valvuloplasty has been quite successful in this lesion. Stenosis in the peripheral pulmonary arteries can also be effectively treated with balloon angioplasty, with or without stent placement.[84]

Tetralogy of Fallot. Tetralogy of Fallot is the most common cyanotic congenital heart defect, accounting for approximately 5% to 7% of all congenital heart defects.[85] As the name implies, tetralogy of Fallot consists of four associated defects: (1) a ventricular septal defect involving the membranous septum and the anterior portion of the muscular septum; (2) dextroposition (shifting to the right of the aorta) so that it overrides the right ventricle and is in communication with the septal defect; (3) obstruction or narrowing of the pulmonary outflow channel, including pulmonic valve stenosis, a decrease in the size of the pulmonary trunk, or both; and (4) hypertrophy of the right ventricle because of the increased work required to pump blood through the obstructed pulmonary channels[86] (see Fig. 19-21C). Variations of the defect can include complete atresia of the pulmonary valve or absence of pulmonary valve tissue altogether.

Most children with tetralogy of Fallot display some degree of cyanosis that is caused by a right-to-left shunt across the ventricular septal defect. The degree of cyanosis is determined by the restriction of blood flow into the pulmonary bed. Right ventricular outflow obstruction causes deoxygenated blood from the right ventricle to shunt across the ventricular septal defect and be ejected into the systemic circulation. The degree of obstruction may be dynamic and can increase during periods of stress, causing hypercyanotic attacks ("tet spells"). These spells typically occur in the morning during crying, feeding, or defecating. These activities increase the infant's oxygen requirements. Crying and defecating may further increase pulmonary vascular resistance, thereby increasing right-to-left shunting and decreasing pulmonary blood flow. With the hypercyanotic spell, the infant becomes acutely cyanotic, hyperpneic, irritable, and diaphoretic. Later in the spell, the infant becomes limp and may lose consciousness. Placing the infant in the knee–chest position increases systemic vascular resistance, which increases pulmonary blood flow and decreases right-to-left shunting. During a hypercyanotic spell, toddlers and older children may spontaneously assume the squatting position, which functions like the knee–chest position to relieve the spell.

Total surgical correction is required for all children with tetralogy of Fallot. Early definitive repair in infancy is currently advocated in most centers experienced in intracardiac surgery in infants.[86]

Transposition of the Great Arteries. In complete transposition of the great arteries, the aorta arises from the right ventricle, and the pulmonary artery arises from the left ventricle (see Fig. 19-21F). The defect is more common in infants whose mothers have diabetes and is two to three times more common in boys.[87]

Cyanosis is the most common presenting symptom, resulting from an anomaly that allows the systemic venous return to be circulated through the right heart and ejected into the aorta, and the pulmonary venous return to be recirculated to the lungs through the left ventricle and main pulmonary artery. In infants born with this defect, survival depends on communication between the right and left sides of the heart in the form of a patent ductus arteriosus or septal defect. Ventricular septal defects are present in 50% of infants with transposition of the great arteries at birth and may allow effective mixing of blood. Prostaglandin E_1 should be administered to neonates when this lesion is suspected in an effort to maintain the patency of the ductus arteriosus. Balloon atrial septostomy may be done to increase the blood flow between the two sides of the heart. In this procedure, a balloon-tipped catheter is inserted into the heart through the vena cava and then passed through the foramen ovale into the left atrium. The balloon is then inflated and pulled back through the foramen ovale, enlarging the opening as it goes.

Corrective surgery is essential for long-term survival. An arterial switch procedure, which corrects the relation of the systemic and pulmonary blood flows, is the current procedure of choice, and has survival rates greater than 90%.[87] This procedure is preferably performed in the first 2 to 3 weeks of life, before the postnatal reduction in pulmonary vascular resistance occurs. The coronary arteries are moved to the left-sided great artery and any ventricular septal defects are closed during the same operation. Complications of the arterial switch procedure may include coronary insufficiency, supravalvar pulmonary stenosis, neoaortic regurgitation, and rhythm abnormalities.[87]

Coarctation of the Aorta. Coarctation of the aorta consists of a localized narrowing of the aorta. It can occur proximal to (preductal) (see Fig. 19-21H), distal to (postductal), or opposite of (juxtaductal) the entry of the ductus arteriosus. Approximately 98% of coarctations are juxtaductal. The defect is frequently associated with other congenital cardiac lesions, most commonly bicuspid aortic valve, and occurs in approximately 10% of subjects with Turner syndrome, suggesting a genetic linkage[88] (see Chapter 6).

The classic sign of coarctation of the aorta is a disparity in pulsations and blood pressures in the arms and legs. The femoral, popliteal, and dorsalis pedis pulsations are weak or delayed compared with the bounding pulses of the arms and carotid vessels. Normally, the systolic blood pressure in the legs obtained by the cuff method is 10 to 20 mm Hg higher than in the arms.

In coarctation, the pressure in the legs is lower and may be difficult to obtain. Patients with coarctation are often identified during a diagnostic workup for hypertension. Most patients with moderate coarctation remain otherwise asymptomatic owing to collateral vessels that form around the area of narrowing. Left untreated, however, coarctation will result in left ventricular hypertension and hypertrophy and significant systemic hypertension (see Chapter 18). Infants with severe coarctation demonstrate early symptoms of heart failure and may present in critical condition upon ductal closure. Reopening of the duct with prostaglandin E_1, if possible, and emergent surgery are needed in this subgroup.[88]

Children with coarctation causing a blood pressure gradient between the arms and legs of 20 mm Hg or greater should ideally be treated by 2 years of age to reduce the likelihood of persistent hypertension.[88] A surgical approach typically involves resection of the narrowed segment of the aorta and end-to-end anastomosis of healthy tissue. This can usually be accomplished without cardiopulmonary bypass, with a mortality rate near zero. Balloon angioplasty with or without stent placement has also been used, although the presence of residual gradients and the reliability of the surgical approach have limited this technique.[88]

Functional Single-Ventricle Anatomy. Several forms of complex congenital heart disease result in only one functional ventricle. Functional single-ventricle anatomy is the most common form of congenital heart disease diagnosed on routine prenatal ultrasonography. There may be a single right or a single left ventricle, or a ventricle of indeterminate morphology.[89–92] Hypoplastic left heart syndrome, a term used to describe a group of closely related cardiac anomalies characterized by underdevelopment of the left cardiac chambers, is the most common form of this disorder.[92] Several other forms of double-inlet ventricle have been described; however, all forms of this disease result in similar pathologic effects and follow a common pathway of intervention.[89–93]

All forms of single-ventricle anatomy result in a common mixing chamber of pulmonary and systemic venous return and cause varying degrees of cyanosis (Fig. 19-23). The single ventricle must pump blood to both the pulmonary and systemic circulations, and thus the flow to each circulation is determined by the resistance in each system.[89–92] As pulmonary vascular resistance falls, flow to the pulmonary circulation will be preferential and systemic circulation will be compromised. In some defects, such as hypoplastic left heart syndrome, systemic flow depends on a patent ductus arteriosus. Neonates with this lesion typically present with extreme cyanosis and symptoms of heart failure as the ductus begins to close.[92]

Although functional single-ventricle anatomy cannot be completely repaired, the surgical palliation of these defects has been one of the most innovative interventions for congenital heart disease. The goal of surgical palliation is to redirect systemic venous return directly to the pulmonary arteries and allow the single ventricle to deliver oxygenated blood to the systemic circulation.

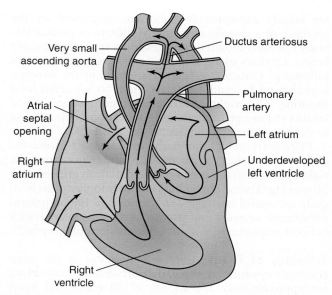

FIGURE 19-23. Functional single-ventricle anatomy with an underdeveloped left ventricle and small ascending aorta. Because of the markedly decreased left ventricular compliance, most of the pulmonary venous blood returning to the left atrium shunts left to right at the atrial level. Pulmonary arterial blood flows into the pulmonary arteries as well as right to left across a patent ductus arteriosus into the aorta.

This is accomplished in a series of two to three staged surgical palliation interventions during the child's first years of life. Stage one palliation is designed to ensure unobstructed systemic blood flow and adequate flow to the pulmonary circulation. Stage two, a bidirectional cavopulmonary shunt, redirects systemic venous return from the superior vena cava directly to the pulmonary arteries. Stage three connects flow from the inferior vena cava directly into the pulmonary arteries so that the pulmonary and systemic circulations are effectively separated.[93] Cardiac transplantation is also used as an intervention for the most complex forms of single-ventricle congenital heart disease.

Survival rates for children with complex forms of single-ventricle heart disease have improved markedly, but long-term outcomes remain uncertain. Ventricular dysfunction, arrhythmias, and thromboses plague this population of patients. Defining the optimal medical and surgical management strategies for these patients remains an active area of research in pediatric cardiology and cardiac surgery.[89–93]

Kawasaki Disease

Kawasaki disease is an acute vasculitis (i.e., inflammation of the blood vessels) with potential for involvement of the coronary arteries. The disease occurs predominantly in young children; about 80% of patients are younger than 5 years of age.[94,95] First described in Japan in 1967 by Dr. Tomisaku Kawasaki, the disease is the leading cause of acquired heart disease in North America and Japan.[35,36,67,68] Although most common in

Japan, the disease affects children of many races, occurs worldwide, and is increasing in frequency.

The disease is characterized by a vasculitis that begins in the small vessels (i.e., arterioles, venules, and capillaries) and progresses to involve some of the larger arteries, such as the coronaries. The exact etiology and pathogenesis of the disease remain unknown, but it is thought to be of immunologic origin.[94,95] Immunologic abnormalities, including increased activation of helper T cells and increased levels of immune mediators and antibodies that destroy endothelial cells, have been detected during the acute phase of the disease. It has been hypothesized that some unknown antigen, possibly a common infectious agent, triggers the immune response in a genetically predisposed child.

Manifestations and Clinical Course

The course of the disease is triphasic and includes an acute febrile phase that lasts approximately 7 to 14 days, a subacute phase that follows the acute phase and lasts from days 10 through 24, and a convalescent phase that follows the subacute stage and continues until the signs of the acute-phase inflammatory response have subsided and the signs of the illness have disappeared.[34,35,67–69]

The *acute phase* begins with an abrupt onset of fever, followed by bilateral conjunctivitis, usually without exudates; erythema of the oral and pharyngeal mucosa with "strawberry tongue" and dry, fissured lips; redness and swelling of the hands and feet; rash of various forms; and enlarged cervical lymph nodes. The fever typically is high, reaching 40°C (104°F) or more; has an erratic spiking pattern; is unresponsive to antibiotics; and persists for 5 or more days.[94] The conjunctivitis begins shortly after the onset of fever, persists throughout the febrile course of the disease, and may last as long as 3 to 5 weeks.

The *subacute phase* begins with abatement of the fever and lasts until all signs of the disease have disappeared. During the subacute phase, desquamation (i.e., peeling) of the skin of the fingers and toe tips begins and progresses to involve the entire surface of the palms and soles. Patchy peeling of skin areas other than the hands and feet may occur in some children. The convalescent stage persists from the complete resolution of symptoms until all signs of inflammation have disappeared. This usually takes approximately 8 weeks.

In addition to the major manifestations that occur during the acute stage of the illness, there are several associated, less specific characteristics of the disease, including arthritis, urethritis and pyuria, gastrointestinal manifestations (e.g., diarrhea, abdominal pain), and hepatitis. Arthritis is more common in girls and may occur early in the illness along with the fever and other acute manifestations of the disease or during the 2nd or 3rd week, generally affecting the hands, knees, ankles, or toes.[96,97] Central nervous system involvement occurs in almost all children and is characterized by pronounced irritability and lability of mood.

Cardiac involvement is the most important manifestation of Kawasaki disease. Coronary artery abnormalities develop in approximately 20% of children,

manifested by coronary artery dilation and aneurysm formation as seen on 2D echocardiography.[96,97] The manifestations of coronary artery involvement include signs and symptoms of myocardial ischemia or, rarely, overt myocardial infarction or rupture of a coronary aneurysm. Pericarditis, myocarditis, endocarditis, heart failure, and arrhythmias also may develop.

Diagnosis and Treatment

No specific diagnostic test for Kawasaki disease is available; therefore, the diagnosis is made on clinical grounds following published guidelines.[98] The guidelines specify fever persisting at least 5 days or more without another source in association with at least four principal features, including oral changes that may include erythema or cracking of the lips, strawberry tongue, and erythema of the oral mucosa; bilateral, nonexudative conjunctivitis; rash of various forms (maculopapular, erythema multiforme, or scarlatiniform) with accentuation in the groin region; erythema and swelling of the hands or feet with desquamation of fingers and toes 1 to 3 weeks after onset of illness; and cervical lymphadenopathy, often unilateral, with at least one node that is 1.5 cm in size.[98] Chest radiographs, ECG tests, and 2D echocardiography are used to detect coronary artery involvement and follow its progress. Coronary angiography may be used to determine the extent of coronary artery involvement.

Intravenous gamma globulin and aspirin are considered the best therapies for prevention of coronary artery abnormalities in children with Kawasaki disease. During the acute phase of the illness, aspirin usually is given in larger doses (80 to 100 mg/kg/day divided in four doses) for its anti-inflammatory and antipyretic effects. After the fever is controlled, the aspirin dose is lowered (3 to 5 mg/kg/day, single dose), and the drug is given for 6 to 8 weeks for its anti–platelet-aggregating effects.[95,98]

Recommendations for cardiac follow-up evaluation (i.e., stress testing and sometimes coronary angiography) are based on the level of coronary artery changes. Anticoagulant therapy may be recommended for children with multiple or large coronary aneurysms. Some restrictions in activities such as competitive sports may be advised for children with significant coronary artery abnormalities.[95]

SUMMARY CONCEPTS

■ Congenital heart defects arise during fetal heart development, which occurs during weeks 3 through 8 after conception, and reflect the stage of development at the time the causative event occurred. Several factors contribute to the development of congenital heart defects, including genetic and chromosomal influences, viruses, and environmental agents such as drugs and radiation.

(continued)

SUMMARY CONCEPTS (continued)

- Congenital heart defects are commonly classified according to anatomic site (e.g., atrial or ventricular septal), hemodynamic alterations (shunting of blood), and their effect on pulmonary blood flow and tissue oxygenation (noncyanotic, cyanotic).

- Hemodynamic alterations may produce shunting of blood from the right to the left or from the left to the right side of the heart, with the direction and degree of shunt depending on the size and position of the defect that connects the two sides of the heart and the difference in resistance between the two sides of the circulation. Left-to-right shunts typically increase the volume of the right side of the heart and pulmonary circulation, and right-to-left shunts transfer deoxygenated blood from the right side of the heart to the left side, diluting the oxygen content of blood that is being ejected into the systemic circulation and causing cyanosis.

- Kawasaki disease is an acute vasculitis of young children that affects the skin, brain, eyes, joints, liver, lymph nodes, and heart. The disease can produce aneurysmal disease of the coronary arteries and is the most common cause of acquired heart disease in young children.

REVIEW EXERCISES

1. A 40-year-old man presents in the emergency department complaining of substernal chest pain that is also felt in his left shoulder. He is short of breath and nauseated. His blood pressure is 148/90 mm Hg and his heart rate is 110 beats/minute. His ECG shows an ST-segment elevation with T-wave inversion. He is given aspirin, morphine, and oxygen. Blood tests reveal elevated CK-MB and troponin I.

   A. What is the probable cause of the man's symptoms?
   B. Explain the origin of the left arm pain, nausea, and increased heart rate.
   C. What is the significance of the ST-segment changes and elevation in CK-MB and troponin I?
   D. Relate the actions of aspirin, morphine, and oxygen to the treatment of this man's condition.

2. A 50-year-old woman presents with complaints of paroxysmal nocturnal dyspnea and orthopnea, palpitations, and fatigue. An echocardiogram demonstrates a thickened, immobile mitral valve

with anterior and posterior leaflets moving together; slow early diastolic filling of the ventricle; and left atrial enlargement.

   A. What is the probable cause of this woman's symptoms?
   B. Explain the pathologic significance of the slow early diastolic filling, distended left atrium, and palpitations.
   C. Given the echocardiographic data, what type of cardiac murmur would you expect to find in this woman?
   D. Which circulation (systemic or pulmonary) would you expect to be affected as this woman's mitral valve disorder progresses?

3. A 4-month-old male infant is brought into the pediatric clinic by his mother. She reports that she noted over the past several weeks that her baby's lips and mouth and his fingernails and toenails have become a bluish-gray color. She also states that he seems to tire easily and that even nursing seems to wear him out. Lately, he has had several spells where he has suddenly turned blue, has had difficulty breathing, and has been very irritable. During one of these spells he turned limp and seemed to have passed out for a short time. An echocardiogram reveals a thickening of the right ventricular wall with overriding of the aorta, a large subaortic ventricular septal defect, and narrowing of the pulmonary outflow with stenosis of the pulmonary valve.

   A. What is this infant's probable diagnosis?
   B. Describe the shunting of blood that occurs with this disorder and its relationship to the development of cyanosis.
   C. The mother is instructed to place the infant in the knee–chest position when he has one of the spells in which he becomes blue and irritable. How does this position help to relieve the cyanosis and impaired oxygenation of tissues?
   D. The surgical creation of a shunt between the aorta and pulmonary artery may be performed as a palliative procedure for infants with marked hypoplasia of the pulmonary artery, with corrective surgery performed later in childhood. Explain how this procedure increases blood flow to the lungs.

REFERENCES

1. Gaziano TA, Gaziano JM. Global burden of cardiovascular disease. In: Bonow R, Mann DL, Zipes DP, et al., eds. *Braunwald's Heart Disease: A Textbook of Cardiovascular Medicine.* 9th ed. Philadelphia, PA: Saunders Elsevier; 2012:1–22.
2. Moore KL, Dalley AF, Agur AMR. *Clinically Oriented Anatomy.* 6th ed. Philadelphia, PA: Wolters Kluwer Health | Lippincott Williams & Wilkins; 2010:144–148.

3. Waller BF, Orr CM, Slack JD, et al. Anatomy, histology, and pathology of coronary arteries: a review relevant to new interventional and imaging techniques–Part IV. *Clin Cardiol.* 1992;15(9):675–687.

4. Guyton A, Hall JE. *Textbook of Medical Physiology.* 12th ed. Philadelphia, PA: Elsevier Saunders; 2011:246–253.

5. Canty JM. Coronary blood flow and myocardial ischemia. In: Bonow R, Mann DL, Zipes DP, et al., eds. *Braunwald's Heart Disease: A Textbook of Cardiovascular Medicine.* 9th ed. Philadelphia, PA: Saunders Elsevier; 2012:1049–1075.

6. Schoen FJ, Mitchell RN. The heart. In: Kumar V, Abbas AK, Fausto N, et al., eds. *Robbins and Cotran Pathologic Basis of Disease.* 8th ed. Philadelphia, PA: Saunders Elsevier; 2010:529–587.

7. Bryan NS, Bian K, Murad F. Discovery of the nitric oxide signaling pathway and targets for drug development. *Front Biosci (Landmark Ed).* 2009;14:1–18.

8. Vanhoutte PM, Shimokawa H, Tang EH, et al. Endothelial dysfunction and vascular disease. *Acta Physiol (Oxf).* 2009;196(2):193–222.

9. Forrester JS. Role of plaque rupture in acute coronary syndromes. *Am J Cardiol.* 2000;86(suppl):15J–23J.

10. Libby P. The molecular mechanisms of the thrombotic complications of atherosclerosis. *J Intern Med.* 2008;263(5):517–527.

11. Smith SW, Whitwam W. Acute coronary syndromes. *Emerg Med Clin North Am.* 2006;24:53–89.

12. Antman EM, Morrow DA. ST-elevation myocardial infarction: pathology, pathophysiology, and clinical features. In: Libby P, Bonow R, Mann DL, et al., eds. *Braunwald's Heart Disease: A Textbook of Cardiovascular Medicine.* 9th ed. Philadelphia, PA: Saunders Elsevier; 2012:1111–1078.

13. Mirvis DM, Goldberger AL. Electrocardiography. In: Bonow R, Mann DL, Zipes DP, et al., eds. *Braunwald's Heart Disease: A Textbook of Cardiovascular Medicine.* 9th ed. Philadelphia, PA: Saunders Elsevier; 2012:126–167.

14. Bhatheja R, Mukherjee D. Acute coronary syndromes: unstable angina/non-ST elevation myocardial infarction. *Crit Care Clin.* 2007;23:709–735.

15. Makki N, Brennan TM, Girota S. Acute coronary syndrome. *J Intensive Care Med.* 2013;28(5).

16. Cannon CP, Braunwald E. Unstable angina and non-ST elevation myocardial infarction. In: Bonow R, Mann DL, Zipes DP, et al., eds. *Braunwald's Heart Disease: A Textbook of Cardiovascular Medicine.* 9th ed. Philadelphia, PA: Saunders Elsevier; 2012:1319–1351.

17. Cannon CP, Lee TH. Approach to the patient with chest pain. In: Bonow R, Mann DL, Zipes DP, et al., eds. *Braunwald's Heart Disease: A Textbook of Cardiovascular Medicine.* 9th ed. Philadelphia, PA: Saunders Elsevier; 2012:1076–1088.

18. Rhee J-W, Sabatine MS, Lilly LS. Ischemic heart disease. In: Lilly LS, ed. *Pathophysiology of Heart Disease: A Collaborative Project of Medical Students and Faculty.* 5th ed. Philadelphia, PA: Wolters Kluwer Health/Lippincott Williams & Wilkins; 2011:135–160.

19. Lischke S, Schneider DJ. Recent developments in the use of antiplatelet agents to prevent cardiovascular events. *Future Cardiol.* 2011;7(3):403–413.

20. Popma JI, Bhatt DL. Percutaneous coronary intervention. In: Bonow R, Mann DL, Zipes DP, et al., eds. *Braunwald's Heart Disease: A Textbook of Cardiovascular Medicine.* 9th ed. Philadelphia, PA: Saunders Elsevier; 2012:1270–1300.

21. Morrow DA, Boden WE. Stable ischemic heart disease. In: Bonow R, Mann DL, Zipes DP, et al., eds. *Braunwald's Heart Disease: A Textbook of Cardiovascular Medicine.* 9th ed. Philadelphia, PA: Saunders Elsevier; 2012:1210–1269.

22. Fraker TD Jr, Fihn SD; for the 2002 Chronic Stable Angina Writing Committee. 2007 chronic angina focused update of the ACC/AHA 2002 guidelines for the management of patients with chronic stable angina. *Circulation.* 2007;116:2762–2772.

23. Miller DD, Waters DD, Szlachcic J, et al. Clinical characteristics associated with sudden death in patients with variant angina. *Circulation.* 1982;66(3):588–592.

24. Duval X, Delahaye F, Alla F, et al. Temporal trends in infective endocarditis in the context of prophylaxis guideline modifications: three successive population-based surveys. *J Am Coll Cardiol.* 2012;59(22):1968–1976.

25. Correa de Sa DD, Tleyjeh IM, Anavekar NS, et al. Epidemiological trends of infective endocarditis: a population-based study in Olmsted County, Minnesota. *Mayo Clin Proc.* 2010;85(5):422–426.

26. Murray CJ, Vos T, Lozano R, et al. Disability-adjusted life years (DALYs) for 291 diseases and injuries in 21 regions, 1990–2010: A systematic analysis for the Global Burden of Disease Study. *Lancet.* 2010;380(9859):2197–2223.

27. Mylonakis E, Calderwood SB. Infective endocarditis in adults. *New Engl J Med.* 2001;345:1318–1330.

28. Holcomb S. Infective endocarditis guidelines assist in early identification. *Nurse Pract.* 2005;30(11):7–17.

29. Baddour LM, Wilson WR, Bayer AS, et al. Infective endocarditis: Diagnosis, antimicrobial therapy, and management of complications. *Circulation.* 2005;111:394–434.

30. Devlin RK, Andrews MM, von Reyn CF. Recent trends in infective endocarditis: Influence of case definitions. *Curr Opin Cardiol.* 2004;19:134–139.

31. Prendergast BD. The changing face of infective endocarditis. *Heart.* 2006;92:879–885.

32. Wilson W, Taubert KA, Gewitz M, et al. Prevention of infective endocarditis: Guidelines from the American Heart Association. *Circulation.* 2007;115:1656–1658.

33. Guilherme L, Cury P, Demarchi LMF, et al. Rheumatic heart disease. *Am J Pathol.* 2004;165:1583–1591.

34. World Health Organization. *Rheumatic Fever and Rheumatic Heart Disease: Report of WHO Expert Consultation.* WHO Technical Report Series 923. Geneva: World Health Organization; 2004.

35. Radju BS, Turi ZG. Rheumatic fever. In: Libby P, Bonow RO, Mann DL, et al., eds. *Braunwald's Heart Disease: A Textbook of Cardiovascular Medicine.* 8th ed. Philadelphia, PA: Elsevier Saunders; 2008:2079–2086.

36. Ferrieri P; for the Jones Criteria Working Group. Proceedings of the Jones criteria workshop. *Circulation.* 2002;106:2521–2527.

37. Otto CM, Bonow RO. Valvular heart disease. In: Bonow R, Mann DL, Zipes DP, et al., eds. *Braunwald's Heart Disease: A Textbook of Cardiovascular Medicine.* 9th ed. Philadelphia, PA: Elsevier Saunders; 2012:1625–1712.

38. Bonow RO, Carabello BA, Chatterjee K, et al. ACC/AHA 2006 guidelines for the management of patients with valvular heart disease. *Circulation.* 2006;114:e84–e231.

39. Desjardins VA, Enriquez-Sarano M, et al. Intensity of murmurs correlates with severity of valvular regurgitation. *Am J Med.* 1996;100(2):149–156.

40. Carabello BA. Aortic stenosis. *New Engl J Med.* 2004;346:677–682.

41. Freeman RV, Otto CM. Spectrum of calcific aortic valve disease: Pathogenesis, disease progression, and treatment strategies. *Circulation.* 2005;111:3316–3326.

42. LeWinter MM, Tischler MD. Pericardial diseases. In: Bonow R, Mann DL, Zipes DP, et al., eds. *Braunwald's Heart Disease: A Textbook of Cardiovascular Medicine.* 9th ed. Philadelphia, PA: Saunders Elsevier; 2012:1651–1671.

43. Lange RA, Hillis L. Acute pericarditis. *New Engl J Med.* 2004;351:2195–2202.

44. Little WC, Freeman GL. Pericardial disease. *Circulation.* 2006;113:1622–1632.

45. Maron BJ, Towbin JA, Thiene G, et al. Contemporary definitions and classification of the cardiomyopathies. *Circulation*. 2006;113:1807–1816.

46. Nishimura RA, Holmes DR. Hypertrophic obstructive cardiomyopathy. *New Engl J Med*. 2004;350:1320–1327.

47. Moran BJ. Hypertrophic cardiomyopathy. In: Bonow R, Mann DL, Zipes DP, et al., eds. *Braunwald's Heart Disease: A Textbook of Cardiovascular Medicine*. 9th ed. Philadelphia, PA: Saunders Elsevier; 2012:1582–1594.

48. Ho CY, Seidman CE. A contemporary approach to hypertrophic cardiomyopathy. *Circulation*. 2006;113:858–862.

49. Anderson EL. Arrhythmic right ventricular dysplasia. *Am Fam Physician*. 2006;73:1391–1398.

50. Thiene G, Basso C, Calabrese F, et al. Pathology and pathogenesis of arrhythmogenic right ventricular cardiomyopathy. *Herz*. 2000;25(3):210–215.

51. Saffitz JE. The heart. In: Rubin E, Strayer DE, eds. *Rubin's Pathology: Clinicopathologic Foundations of Medicine*, 5th ed. Philadelphia, PA: Wolters Kluwer Health/Lippincott Williams & Wilkins; 2012:479–536.

52. Liu PP, Baughman KL. Myocarditis. In: Bonow R, Mann DL, Zipes DP, et al., eds. *Braunwald's Heart Disease: A Textbook of Cardiovascular Medicine*. 9th ed. Philadelphia, PA: Saunders Elsevier; 2012:1595–1610.

53. Feldman AM, McNammara D. Myocarditis. *New Engl J Med*. 2000;343:1387–1398.

54. Magnani JW, Dec GW. Myocarditis: Current trends in diagnosis and treatment. *Circulation*. 2006;113:876–890.

55. Newby LK, Douglas PS. Cardiovascular disease in women. In: Bonow R, Mann DL, Zipes DP, et al., eds. *Braunwald's Heart Disease: A Textbook of Cardiovascular Medicine*. 9th ed. Philadelphia, PA: Saunders Elsevier; 2012:1757–1769.

56. Ro A, Frishman WH. Peripartum cardiomyopathy. *Cardiol Rev*. 2006;14(1):35–42.

57. Pearson GD, Veille JC, Rahimtoola S, et al. Peripartum cardiomyopathy: National Heart, Lung, and Blood Institute and Office of Rare Diseases (National Institutes of Health) Workshop recommendations and review. *JAMA*. 2000;283:1183–1188.

58. Gianni M, Dentali F, Grandi AM, et al. Apical ballooning syndrome or takotsubo cardiomyopathy: a systematic review. *Euro Heart J*. 2006;27:1523–1529.

59. Maron BJ. Sudden death in hypertrophic cardiomyopathy. *J Cardiovasc Transl Res*. 2009;2(4):368–380.

60. Merli E, Sutcliffe S, Gori M, et al. Tako-tsubo cardiomyopathy: New insights into the possible underlying pathophysiology. *Eur J Echocardiogr*. 2006;7:53–61.

61. American Heart Association. Understand your risk for congenital heart defects. http://www.heart.org/HEARTORG/Conditions/CongenitalHeartDefects/UnderstandYourRiskforCongenitalHeartDefects/Understand-Your-Risk-for-Congenital-Heart Defects_UCM_001219_Article.jsp. Updated 2013. Accessed December 21, 2013.

62. Freed MD. Fetal and transitional circulation. In: Keane J, Lock J, Fyler D, eds. *Nadas' Pediatric Cardiology*. 2nd ed. Philadelphia, PA: Elsevier Saunders; 2006:75–79.

63. Gardiner H. Physiology of the developing heart. In: Anderson R, Baker E, Penny D, et al., eds. *Paediatric Cardiology*. 3rd ed. Philadelphia, PA: Churchill Livingstone/Elsevier; 2010:73–90.

64. Bernstein D. Cardiac development. In: Kleigman R, Stanton B, Schor N, et al., eds. *Nelson Textbook of Pediatrics*. 19th ed. Philadelphia, PA: Elsevier; 2011:1527–1528.

65. Sander TL, Klinkner DB, Tomita-Mitchell A, et al. Molecular and cellular basis of congenital heart disease. *Pediatr Clin North Am*. 2006;53(5):989–1009.

66. Goldmuntz E, Crenshaw ML, Lin AE. Genetic aspects of congenital heart disease. In: Allen HD, Driscoll DJ, Shaddy RE, et al., eds. *Moss and Adams' Heart Disease in Infants, Children, and Adolescents*, vol. I, 8th ed. Philadelphia, PA: Wolters Kluwer Health | Lippincott Williams & Wilkins; 2013:617.

67. Edwards WD, Maleszewski JJ. Classification and terminology of cardiovascular anomalies. In: Allen HD, Driscoll DJ, Shaddy RE, et al., eds. *Moss and Adams' Heart Disease in Infants, Children, and Adolescents*, vol I, 8th ed. Philadelphia, PA: Wolters Kluwer Health | Lippincott Williams & Wilkins; 2013:32.

68. Nadas A, Fyler D. Hypoxemia. In: Keane J, Lock J, Fyler D, eds. *Nadas' Pediatric Cardiology*. 2nd ed. Philadelphia, PA: Elsevier Saunders; 2006:97–101.

69. Kleinman CS, Glickstein JS, Krishnamurthy G, et al. Fetal echocardiography and fetal cardiology. In: Allen HD, Driscoll DJ, Shaddy RE, et al., eds. *Moss and Adams' Heart Disease in Infants, Children, and Adolescents*, vol. I, 8th ed. Philadelphia, PA: Wolters Kluwer Health | Lippincott Williams & Wilkins; 2013:644.

70. Cassidy SC, Allen HD, Phillips JR. History and physical examination. In: Allen HD, Driscoll DJ, Shaddy RE, et al., eds. *Moss and Adams' Heart Disease in Infants, Children, and Adolescents*, vol. I, 8th ed. Philadelphia, PA: Wolters Kluwer Health | Lippincott Williams & Wilkins; 2013:82–92.

71. Thangaratinam S, Brown K, Zamora J, et al. Pulse oximetry screening for critical congenital heart defects in asymptomatic newborn babies: A systematic review and meta-analysis. *Lancet*. 2012;379(9835):2459–2464.

72. Wilson W, Taubert KA, Gewitz M, et al. Prevention of infective endocarditis: guidelines from the American Heart Association: a guideline from the American Heart Association Rheumatic Fever, Endocarditis and Kawasaki Disease Committee, Council on Cardiovascular Disease in the Young, and the Council on Clinical Cardiology, Council on Cardiovascular Surgery and Anesthesia, and the Quality of Care and Outcomes Research Interdisciplinary Working Group. *J Am Dent Assoc*. 2008;139(Suppl):3S–24S.

73. Snookes SH, Gunn JK, Eldridge BJ, et al. A systematic review of motor and cognitive outcomes after early surgery for congenital heart disease. *Pediatrics*. 2010;125(4):e818–e827.

74. Tabbutt S, Gaynor JW, Newburger JW. Neurodevelopmental outcomes after congenital heart surgery and strategies for improvement. *Curr Opin Cardiol*. 2012;27(2):82–91.

75. Gaynor JW, Gerdes M, Nord AS, et al. Is cardiac diagnosis a predictor of neurodevelopmental outcome after cardiac surgery in infancy? *J Thorac Cardiovasc Surg*. 2010;140(6):1230–1237.

76. Marino BS, Lipkin PH, Newburger JW, et al. Neurodevelopmental outcomes in children with congenital heart disease: Evaluation and management: A scientific statement from the American Heart Association. *Circulation*. 2012;126(9):1143–1172.

77. Bellinger DC, Wypij D, Rivkin MJ, et al. Adolescents with d-transposition of the great arteries corrected with the arterial switch procedure: Neuropsychological assessment and structural brain imaging. *Circulation*. 2011;124(12):1361–1369.

78. Moore P, Brook MM. Patent ductus arteriosus and aortopulmonary window. In: Allen HD, Driscoll DJ, Shaddy RE, et al., eds. *Moss and Adams' Heart Disease in Infants, Children, and Adolescents*, vol. I, 8th ed. Philadelphia, PA: Wolters Kluwer Health | Lippincott Williams & Wilkins; 2013:722–745.

79. Redington AN. Cardiopulmonary and right-left heart interactions. In: Allen HD, Driscoll DJ, Shaddy RE, et al., eds. *Moss and Adams' Heart Disease in Infants, Children, and Adolescents*, vol. I, 8th ed. Philadelphia, PA: Wolters Kluwer Health | Lippincott Williams & Wilkins; 2013:546–551.

80. Hoffman TM, Welty SE. Physiology of the preterm and term infant. In: Allen HD, Driscoll DJ, Shaddy RE, et al., eds. *Moss and Adams' Heart Disease in Infants, Children, and Adolescents*, vol. I, 8th ed. Philadelphia, PA: Wolters Kluwer Health | Lippincott Williams & Wilkins; 2013:473–482.

81. Sachdeva R. Atrial septal defects. In: Allen HD, Driscoll DJ, Shaddy RE, et al., eds. *Moss and Adams' Heart Disease in Infants, Children, and Adolescents*, vol. I, 8th ed. Philadelphia, PA: Wolters Kluwer Health | Lippincott Williams & Wilkins; 2013:672.

82. Rubio AE, Lewin MB. Ventricular septal defects. In: Allen HD, Driscoll DJ, Shaddy RE, et al., eds. *Moss and Adams' Heart Disease in Infants, Children, and Adolescents*, vol. I, 8th ed. Philadelphia, PA: Wolters Kluwer Health | Lippincott Williams & Wilkins; 2013:713.

83. Cetta F, Minich LL, Maleszewski JJ, et al. Atrioventricular septal defects. In: Allen HD, Driscoll DJ, Shaddy RE, et al., eds. *Moss and Adams' Heart Disease in Infants, Children, and Adolescents*, vol. I, 8th ed. Philadelphia, PA: Wolters Kluwer Health | Lippincott Williams & Wilkins; 2013:691.

84. Prieto LR, Latson LA. Pulmonary stenosis. In: Allen HD, Driscoll DJ, Shaddy RE, et al., eds. *Moss and Adams' Heart Disease in Infants, Children, and Adolescents*, vol. II, 8th ed. Philadelphia, PA: Wolters Kluwer Health | Lippincott Williams & Wilkins; 2013:913–938.

85. McCrindle BW. Prevalence of congenital cardiac disease. In: Anderson R, Baker E, Penny D, et al., eds. *Paediatric Cardiology*. 3rd ed. Philadelphia, PA: Churchill Livingstone/Elsevier; 2010:143–160.

86. Roche SL, Greenway SC, Redington AN. Tetralogy of fallot with pulmonary stenosis and tetralogy of fallot with absent pulmonary valve. In: Allen HD, Driscoll DJ, Shaddy RE, et al., eds. *Moss and Adams' Heart Disease in Infants, Children, and Adolescents*, vol. II, 8th ed. Philadelphia, PA: Wolters Kluwer Health | Lippincott Williams & Wilkins; 2013:969.

87. Wernovsky G. Transposition of the great arteries. In: Allen HD, Driscoll DJ, Shaddy RE, et al., eds. *Moss and Adams' Heart Disease in Infants, Children, and Adolescents*, vol. II, 8th ed. Philadelphia, PA: Wolters Kluwer Health | Lippincott Williams & Wilkins; 2013:1097.

88. Beekman RH. Coarctation of the aorta. In: Allen HD, Driscoll DJ, Shaddy RE, et al., eds. *Moss and Adams' Heart Disease in Infants, Children, and Adolescents*, vol. II, 8th ed. Philadelphia, PA: Wolters Kluwer Health | Lippincott Williams & Wilkins; 2013:1044–1060.

89. Wernovsky G, Dominguez TE, Gruber PJ, et al. Hypoplasia of the left heart. In: Anderson R, Baker E, Penny D, et al., eds. *Paediatric Cardiology*. 3rd ed. Philadelphia, PA: Churchill Livingstone/Elsevier; 2010:625–646.

90. Daubeney PEF. Hypoplasia of the right ventricle. In: Anderson R, Baker E, Penny D, et al., eds. *Paediatric Cardiology*. 3rd ed. Philadelphia, PA: Churchill Livingstone/Elsevier; 2010:647–664.

91. Penny DJ, Anderson RH. Other forms of functionally univentricular hearts. In: Anderson R, Baker E, Penny D, et al., eds. *Paediatric Cardiology*. 3rd ed. Philadelphia, PA: Churchill Livingstone/Elsevier; 2010:665–686.

92. Tweddell JS, Hoffman GM, Ghanayem NS, et al. Hypoplastic left heart syndrome. In: Allen HD, Driscoll DJ, Shaddy RE, et al., eds. *Moss and Adams' Heart Disease in Infants, Children, and Adolescents*, vol. II, 8th ed. Philadelphia, PA: Wolters Kluwer Health | Lippincott Williams & Wilkins; 2013:1061–1096.

93. Hutter D, Redington AN. The principles of management, and outcomes for, patients with functionally univentricular hearts. In: Anderson R, Baker E, Penny D, et al., eds. *Paediatric Cardiology*. 3rd ed. Philadelphia, PA: Churchill Livingstone/Elsevier; 2010:687–696.

94. Bayers S, Shulman ST, Paller AS. Kawasaki disease: Part I. Diagnosis, clinical features, and pathogenesis. *J Am Acad Dermatol*. 2013;69(4):501.e1–501.e11; quiz 511–512.

95. De Ferranti SD, Newburger JW. Kawasaki disease (mucocutaneous lymph node syndrome). In: Allen HD, Driscoll DJ, Shaddy RE, et al., eds. *Moss and Adams' Heart Disease in Infants, Children, and Adolescents*, vol. II, 8th ed. Philadelphia, PA: Wolters Kluwer Health/Lippincott Williams & Wilkins; 2013:1287–1302.

96. Lue HC, Chen LR, Lin MT, et al. Epidemiological features of Kawasaki disease in Taiwan, 1976–2007: results of five nationwide questionnaire hospital surveys. *Pediatr Neonatol*. 2013;55(2):93–96.

97. Bayers S, Shulman ST, Paller AS. Kawasaki disease: Part II. Complications and treatment. *J Am Acad Dermatol*. 2013;69(4):513.e1–513.e8; quiz 521–522.

98. Newburger JW, Takahashi M, Gerber MA, et al., Committee on Rheumatic Fever, Endocarditis, and Kawasaki Disease, Council on Cardiovascular Disease in the Young, and American Heart Association. Diagnosis, treatment, and long-term management of Kawasaki disease: A statement for health professionals from the Committee on Rheumatic Fever, Endocarditis, and Kawasaki Disease, Council on Cardiovascular Disease in the Young, American Heart Association. *Pediatrics*. 2004;114(6):1708–1733.

Porth Essentials Resources

Explore these additional resources to enhance learning for this chapter:

- NCLEX-Style Questions and Other Resources on thePoint, http://thePoint.lww.com/PorthEssentials4e
- Study Guide for Essentials of Pathophysiology
- Adaptive Learning | Powered by PrepU, http://thepoint.lww.com/prepu

Heart Failure and Circulatory Shock

Adequate perfusion of body tissues depends on the pumping ability of the heart, a vascular system to transport blood to the tissues of the body and back to the heart, sufficient blood to fill the circulatory system, and tissues that are able to extract and to use oxygen and nutrients from the blood. Heart failure and circulatory shock are different conditions that reflect an impairment of the circulatory system; however both conditions involve many of the same compensatory mechanisms even though they differ in terms of pathogenesis and causes.

Heart Failure

Heart failure is a complex syndrome resulting from functional or structural impairment of ventricular filling or ejection of blood into the circulation.[1,2] It may result from disorders of the pericardium, myocardium, endocardium, cardiac valves, or great vessels, or from metabolic abnormalities. Among the most common causes of heart failure are coronary artery disease, hypertension, dilated cardiomyopathy, and valvular heart disease.[1] Heart failure can occur in any age group but primarily affects the elderly; however, African Americans are disproportionately affected at a younger age.[3] Although morbidity and mortality rates from other cardiovascular diseases have decreased over the past several decades,[4] the incidence of heart failure is increasing at an alarming rate.[1] This change undoubtedly reflects improved treatment methods and increased survival from other forms of heart disease. Mortality rates from heart failure are variable (5% to 75% annually).[4] Once the initial diagnosis of heart failure is made, the survival rate is approximately 50% within 5 years.[1]

Heart failure is associated with either a reduced or preserved left ventricular ejection fraction. Heart failure was traditionally defined as a syndrome with impaired ability of the ventricles to contract and eject blood (systolic failure with a reduced ejection fraction) or impaired ventricular relaxation (diastolic failure with a reduced end-diastolic volume). It is now recognized that heart failure can occur even when the ejection fraction is normal or preserved. Persons with symptoms or below normal ejection fractions are classified as having heart failure with a reduced ejection fraction, while those with a normal or near-normal ejection fraction are classified as having heart failure with a preserved ejection fraction.

Pathophysiology of Heart Failure

In *heart failure*, the heart does not adequately pump and/or fill with blood, which results in the inability to meet the metabolic needs of the body.[1] The efficiency of the heart as a pump is determined by the volume of blood that it ejects each minute. The volume of blood ejected is dependent upon the ability of the ventricles to relax and fill.[5,6] The heart has the amazing capacity to adjust its output to meet the varying needs of the body. During sleep, the output declines, and during exercise, it increases markedly. The ability of the heart to increase its output during increased activity is called the *cardiac reserve*. For example, competitive swimmers and long-distance runners have large cardiac reserves. During exercise, the cardiac output of these athletes rapidly increases to as much as five to six times their resting level.[6] In sharp contrast with healthy athletes, persons with heart failure often use their cardiac reserve at rest. For them, just climbing a flight of stairs or even walking[7] may cause shortness of breath because they exceed their cardiac reserve.

Cardiac Performance and Output

The cardiac cycle consists of diastole and systole. During diastole, normal filling of the ventricles increases the volume of each to about 110 to 120 mL.[6] Then, as the ventricles contract during systole, blood is ejected from the heart, and the volume decreases by about 70 mL, which is called the *stroke volume*. The fraction of the end-diastolic volume that is ejected is called the *ejection fraction* (usually about 60% in a healthy person).[6]

Cardiac output, which is the major determinant of cardiac performance, reflects how often the heart beats each minute (heart rate) and how much blood it ejects with each beat (stroke volume). Cardiac output is expressed as the product of the heart rate and stroke volume (i.e., cardiac output = heart rate × stroke volume). The heart rate is regulated by a balance between the activity of the sympathetic nervous system, which produces an increase in heart rate, and the parasympathetic nervous system, which slows it down, whereas the stroke volume is a function of preload, afterload, and myocardial contractility.[5,6]

Preload and Afterload. The ability of the heart to eject blood that has returned to the ventricles during diastole is determined largely by the loading conditions, or what are called the *preload* and *afterload*.

Preload reflects the volume of blood that stretches the ventricle at the end of diastole, just before the onset of systole. It is determined by the venous return to the heart. Also known as the *end-diastolic volume*, preload increases the length of the myocardial muscle fibers. Within limits, as preload increases, the stroke volume increases in accord with the Frank-Starling mechanism.[6]

Afterload represents the force that the contracting heart muscle must generate to eject blood from the filled ventricles. The main components of afterload are the systemic (peripheral) vascular resistance and ventricular wall tension. When the systemic vascular resistance is elevated, as with arterial hypertension, an increased left intraventricular pressure must be generated to first open the aortic valve and then to eject blood out of the ventricle and into the systemic circulation. This increased pressure equates to an increase in ventricular wall stress or tension.[6]

Myocardial Contractility

Myocardial contractility, also known as *inotropy*, refers to the contractile performance of the heart, or the ability of the contractile elements (actin and myosin filaments) of the heart muscle to interact and shorten against a load[5,6,8] (see Chapter 1, Fig. 1-18). Contractility increases cardiac output independent of preload and afterload. The interaction between the actin and myosin filaments during cardiac muscle contraction (i.e., cross-bridge attachment and detachment) requires the use of energy supplied by the breakdown of adenosine triphosphate (ATP) and the presence of calcium ions (Ca^{++}).[8]

As with skeletal muscle, calcium is released from the sarcoplasmic reticulum of cardiac muscle during an action potential (Fig. 20-1). This calcium, in turn, diffuses into the myofibrils and catalyzes the chemical reactions that promote the sliding of the actin and myosin filaments along one another to produce muscle shortening. In addition to the calcium released from the sarcoplasmic reticulum at the time of an action potential, a large quantity of extracellular calcium diffuses into the sarcoplasm through voltage-dependent L-type calcium channels located in the T tubules and myocardial cell membrane. Without the extra calcium that enters through the L-type calcium channels, the strength of the cardiac contraction would be considerably weaker. Opening of the L-type calcium channels is facilitated by the second messenger cyclic adenosine monophosphate (cAMP), the formation of which is coupled to β-adrenergic receptors. The catecholamines (norepinephrine and epinephrine) exert their inotropic effects by binding to these adrenergic receptors. The L-type calcium channel also contains several other types of receptors. Blockade of L-type calcium channels by drugs that bind to these receptors (i.e., calcium channel-blocking drugs) results in a selective reduction in cardiac contractility.[9]

Another mechanism that can modulate inotropy is the increased activity of the sodium ion (Na^+)/Ca^{++} exchange pump and the ATPase-dependent Ca^{++} pump in the myocardial cell membrane (see Fig. 20-1). These pumps transport calcium out of the cell, thereby preventing the cell from becoming overloaded with calcium. If calcium efflux is inhibited, the rise in intracellular calcium produces an increased inotropy. Digitalis and related

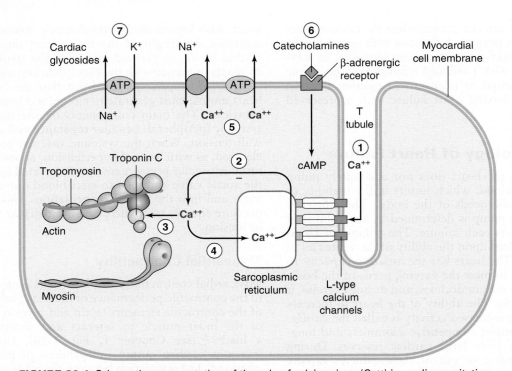

FIGURE 20-1. Schematic representation of the role of calcium ions (Ca++) in cardiac excitation–contraction coupling. The influx (site 1) of extracellular Ca++ through the L-type Ca++ channels in the T tubules during excitation triggers (site 2) release of Ca++ by the sarcoplasmic reticulum. This Ca++ binds to troponin C (site 3). The Ca++–troponin complex interacts with tropomyosin to unblock active sites on the actin and myosin filaments, allowing cross-bridge attachment and contraction of the myofibrils (systole). Relaxation (diastole) occurs as a result of calcium reuptake by the sarcoplasmic reticulum (site 4) and extrusion of intracellular Ca++ by the Na+/Ca++ exchange transporter or, to a lesser extent, by the Ca++ adenosine triphosphatase (ATPase) pump (site 5). Mechanisms that raise systolic Ca++ increase the level of developed force (inotropy). Binding of catecholamines to β-adrenergic receptors (site 6) increases Ca++ entry by phosphorylation of the Ca++ channels through a cyclic adenosine monophosphate (cAMP)–dependent second messenger mechanism. The cardiac glycosides (site 7) increase intracellular Ca++ by inhibiting the Na+/K+-ATPase pump. The elevated intracellular Na+ reverses the Na+/Ca++ exchange transporter (site 5), so less Ca++ is removed from the cell. (Modified from Klabunde RE. *Cardiovascular Physiology Concepts*. Philadelphia, PA: Lippincott Williams & Wilkins; 2005:46.)

cardiac glycosides are inotropic agents that exert their effects by inhibiting the Na+/potassium ion (K+)-ATPase pump in the myocardial cell membrane, thereby leading to an increase in intracellular calcium handling through the Na+/Ca++ exchange pump.[8]

Compensatory Mechanisms

In heart failure, the cardiac reserve is largely maintained through compensatory mechanisms such as the Frank-Starling mechanism, activation of neurohumoral influences such as the sympathetic nervous system reflexes, the renin-angiotensin-aldosterone mechanism, natriuretic peptides, locally produced vasoactive substances, and myocardial hypertrophy and remodeling[5,10] (Fig. 20-2). The first two of these adaptations occur rapidly over minutes to hours of myocardial dysfunction and may be adequate to maintain the overall pumping performance of the heart at relatively normal levels. Myocardial hypertrophy and remodeling occur slowly over weeks to months and play an important role in the long-term adaptation to hemodynamic overload. In the failing heart, early decreases in cardiac function may go unnoticed because these compensatory mechanisms maintain the cardiac output. However, these mechanisms contribute not only to the adaptation of the failing heart but also to the pathophysiology of heart failure.[11]

Length-Tension/Frank-Starling Mechanism

The Frank-Starling mechanism describes the process whereby the heart increases its stroke volume through an increase in end-diastolic volume or preload (Fig. 20-3). With increased diastolic filling, there is increased stretching of the myocardial fibers, more optimal approximation of the actin and myosin filaments, and a resultant increase in the force of the next contraction (see Chapter 17). As illustrated in Figure 20-3, there is no single Frank-Starling curve.[6] An increase in contractility will increase cardiac output at any end-diastolic volume, causing the curve to move up and to the left, whereas a decrease in contractility will cause the curve to move down and to the right.

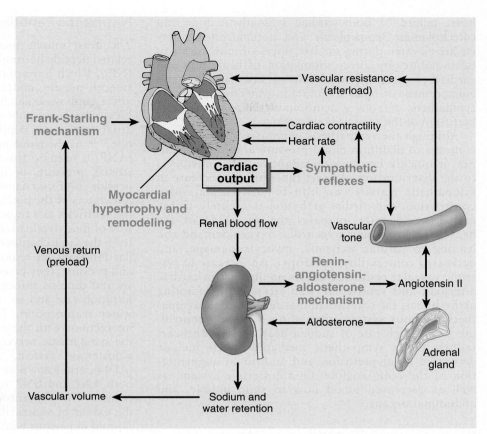

FIGURE 20-2. Compensatory mechanisms in heart failure. The Frank-Starling mechanism, sympathetic reflexes, renin-angiotensin-aldosterone mechanism, and myocardial hypertrophy function in maintaining cardiac output for the failing heart.

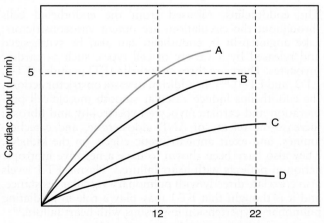

FIGURE 20-3. Left ventricular length-tension (Frank-Starling) function curves. *Curve A:* Normal function curve, with a normal cardiac output and optimal left ventricular end-diastolic (LVED) filling pressure. *Curve B:* Compensated heart failure with normal cardiac output at higher LVED pressures. *Curve C:* Decompensated heart failure with a decrease in cardiac output and elevated LVED pressures, with eventual elevation of pulmonary capillary pressure and development of pulmonary congestion. *Curve D:* Cardiogenic shock, with an extreme decrease in cardiac output and marked increase in LVED pressures.

In heart failure with a reduced ejection fraction, a decrease in cardiac output and renal blood flow leads to increased sodium and water retention by the kidney with a resultant increase in vascular volume and venous return to the heart, and an increase in ventricular end-diastolic volume. Within limits, as preload and ventricular end-diastolic volume increase, there is a resultant increase in cardiac output. Although this may preserve the resting cardiac output, the resulting chronic elevation of left ventricular end-diastolic pressure is transmitted to the atria and the pulmonary circulation, causing pulmonary congestion.

An increase in cardiac muscle stretch, as occurs with the Frank-Starling mechanism, also produces an increase in ventricular wall tension with a resultant increase in myocardial oxygen consumption. Because increased wall tension increases myocardial oxygen requirements, it can produce ischemia and contribute to further impairment of cardiac function. The use of diuretics in persons with heart failure helps to reduce vascular volume and ventricular filling, thereby unloading the heart and reducing ventricular wall tension.

Sympathetic Nervous System

Stimulation of the sympathetic nervous system plays an important role in the compensatory response to decreased cardiac output and in the pathogenesis of heart failure.[5,6,8] Both cardiac sympathetic tone and catecholamine (epinephrine and norepinephrine) levels are elevated during the late stages of most forms of heart failure. By direct stimulation of heart rate and cardiac contractility, regulation of vascular tone, and enhancement of renal sodium and water retention, the sympathetic nervous system initially helps to maintain perfusion of the various body organs.

Although the sympathetic nervous system response is meant to maintain blood pressure and cardiac output, it quickly becomes maladaptive and contributes to the deterioration of heart function. An increase in sympathetic activity can lead to tachycardia, vasoconstriction, and cardiac arrhythmias. Acutely, tachycardia significantly increases the workload of the heart, thus increasing myocardial oxygen demand and leading to cardiac ischemia, myocyte damage, and decreased contractility (inotropy). An increase in systemic vascular resistance causes an increase in cardiac afterload and ventricular wall stress. By promoting arrhythmias, the catecholamines released with sympathetic nervous system stimulation also may contribute to the high rate of sudden death seen with heart failure. Other sympathetic mediated effects include decreased renal perfusion and additional augmentation of the renin-angiotensin-aldosterone system, as well as decreased blood flow to skin, muscle, and abdominal organs.[12]

Renin-Angiotensin-Aldosterone Mechanism

One of the most important effects of lowered cardiac output in heart failure is a reduction in renal blood flow and glomerular filtration rate, which leads to sodium and water retention by way of aldosterone production. With decreased renal blood flow, there is a progressive increase in renin secretion by the kidneys with parallel increases in circulating levels of angiotensin II.[10–13] The increased concentration of angiotensin II contributes directly to generalized and excessive vasoconstriction, as well as facilitating norepinephrine release and inhibiting reuptake of norepinephrine by the sympathetic nervous system.[8] Angiotensin II also provides a powerful stimulus for aldosterone production by the adrenal cortex (see Chapter 18).

Aldosterone increases tubular reabsorption of sodium, with an accompanying increase in water retention. Because aldosterone is metabolized in the liver, its levels are further increased when heart failure causes liver congestion. Angiotensin II also increases the level of antidiuretic hormone (ADH), which serves as a vasoconstrictor and inhibitor of water excretion (see Chapter 8). In addition to their individual effects on sodium and water balance, angiotensin II and aldosterone are also involved in regulating the inflammatory and reparative processes that follow tissue injury.[10] However, the sustained expression of aldosterone may stimulate fibroblast and collagen deposition, resulting in ventricular hypertrophy as well as fibrosis within the vasculature and myocardium, and thereby contributing to reduced vascular compliance and increased ventricular stiffness.[10]

Natriuretic Peptides

The heart muscle produces and secretes a family of related peptide hormones, called the *natriuretic peptides* (NPs), which have potent diuretic, natriuretic, vascular smooth muscle, and other neurohumoral actions that affect cardiovascular function. Two of the four known NPs most commonly associated with heart failure are atrial natriuretic peptide and B-type natriuretic peptide.[10,14] As the name indicates, atrial natriuretic peptide (ANP) is released from atrial cells in response to atrial stretch, pressure, or fluid overload. B-type natriuretic peptide (BNP), so named because it was originally found in extracts of the porcine brain, is primarily secreted by the ventricles as a response to increased ventricular pressure or fluid overload. Although the NPs are not secreted from the same chambers in the heart, they have very similar functions. In response to increased chamber stretch and pressure, they promote rapid and transient natriuresis and diuresis through an increase in the glomerular filtration rate and an inhibition of tubular sodium and water reabsorption. The NPs also facilitate complex interactions with the neurohormonal system, inhibiting the sympathetic nervous system, the renin-angiotensin-aldosterone system, and the antidiuretic hormone (ADH), also known as vasopressin. Circulating levels of both ANP and BNP are elevated in persons with heart failure. The concentrations are well correlated with the extent of ventricular dysfunction, increasing up to 30-fold in persons with advanced heart disease.[14] Assays of BNP are used clinically in the diagnosis of heart failure and to predict the severity of the condition.

Endothelins

The endothelins, released from the endothelial cells throughout the circulation, are potent vasoconstrictors. Like angiotensin II, endothelin can also be synthesized and released by a variety of cell types, such as cardiac myocytes. There are three endothelin (ET) peptides (ET-1, ET-2, and ET-3).[10,15] In addition to vasoconstrictor actions, the endothelins induce vascular smooth muscle cell proliferation and cardiac myocyte hypertrophy and fibrosis; increase the release of ANP, aldosterone, and catecholamines; and exert antinatriuretic effects on the kidneys. They also have been shown to have a negative inotropic action in patients with heart failure.[15] Plasma ET-1 levels also correlate directly with pulmonary vascular resistance, and it is thought that ET-1 may play a role in mediating pulmonary hypertension in persons with heart failure.[10]

Myocardial Hypertrophy and Remodeling

The development of myocardial hypertrophy constitutes one of the principal mechanisms by which the heart compensates for an increase in workload.[10,16] Although ventricular hypertrophy improves the work performance of the heart, it is also an important risk factor for subsequent cardiac morbidity and mortality. Inappropriate hypertrophy and remodeling can result in changes in structure (i.e., muscle mass, chamber dilation) and cardiac function (i.e., impaired systolic or diastolic function) that often lead to further pump dysfunction and hemodynamic overload.

Myocardial hypertrophy and remodeling involve a series of complex events at both the molecular and cellular levels. The myocardium is composed of myocytes, or muscle cells, and nonmyocytes. The myocytes are the functional units of cardiac muscle. The nonmyocytes include cardiac macrophages, fibroblasts, vascular smooth muscle, and endothelial cells. These cells, which are present in the interstitial space, remain capable of an increase in cell number and provide support for the myocytes. The nonmyocytes also determine many of the inappropriate changes that occur during myocardial hypertrophy. For example, uncontrolled fibroblast growth is associated with increased synthesis of collagen fibers, myocardial fibrosis, and ventricular wall stiffness.

Recent research has focused on understanding the type of hypertrophy that develops in persons with heart failure. At the cellular level, cardiac muscle cells respond to stimuli from stress placed on the ventricular wall by pressure and volume overload by initiating several different processes that lead to hypertrophy. These include stimuli that produce a *symmetric hypertrophy* with a proportionate increase in muscle length and width, as occurs in athletes; *concentric hypertrophy* with an increase in wall thickness, as occurs in hypertension; and *eccentric hypertrophy* with a disproportionate increase in muscle length, as occurs in dilated cardiomyopathy[16] (Fig. 20-4). When the primary stimulus for hypertrophy is *pressure overload,* the increase in wall stress leads to parallel replication of myofibrils, thickening of the individual myocytes, and concentric hypertrophy. Concentric hypertrophy may preserve systolic function for a time, but eventually the work performed by the ventricle exceeds the vascular reserve, predisposing to ischemia. With *ventricular volume overload,* the increase in wall stress leads to replication of myofibrils in series, elongation of the cardiac muscle cells, and eccentric hypertrophy. Eccentric hypertrophy leads to a decrease in ventricular wall thickness or thinning of the wall with an increase in diastolic volume and wall tension.

Types of Heart Failure

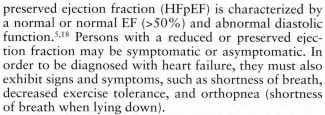

Heart failure is commonly classified by the ejection fraction (reduced or preserved) or as left-sided or right-sided failure.[17] Heart failure with a reduced ejection fraction (HFrEF) is defined as the inability of the ventricle to eject an adequate cardiac output despite a normal blood pressure with an EF ≤ 40% .[1,18] Heart failure with a

preserved ejection fraction (HFpEF) is characterized by a normal or normal EF (>50%) and abnormal diastolic function.[5,18] Persons with a reduced or preserved ejection fraction may be symptomatic or asymptomatic. In order to be diagnosed with heart failure, they must also exhibit signs and symptoms, such as shortness of breath, decreased exercise tolerance, and orthopnea (shortness of breath when lying down).

Over the last decade, there has been growing recognition that approximately 50% of adult persons with heart failure have normal or near normal ejection fractions.[18–20] These people are as a group older, more commonly female, and more frequently have systolic hypertension (associated with large artery stiffness) than those with a reduced ejection fraction. Most people with HFpEF do not complain of symptoms at rest, but rather with physical exercise. When present, the signs and symptoms of heart failure are related to which ventricle is dysfunctional: left or right.

Reduced versus Preserved Ejection Fraction

Heart failure can result from pump failure and an impaired ability to eject blood at a rate commensurate with the metabolic needs of the tissues (systolic failure), or it can occur because of resistance to filling of one or both ventricles leading to symptoms of congestion (diastolic failure).[17]

Reduced Ejection Fraction Heart Failure. Heart failure with a reduced ejection fraction or systolic heart failure is defined as an EF of less than 40%.[21–23] It may result from conditions that impair the contractile performance of the heart (e.g., ischemic heart disease and cardiomyopathy), produce a volume overload (e.g., valvular insufficiency and anemia), or generate a pressure overload (e.g., hypertension and valvular stenosis) on the heart.

Along with the decreased EF and cardiac output that occurs with systolic failure, there is a resultant increase in end-systolic and end-diastolic volumes, ventricular dilation and wall tension, and a rise in ventricular end-diastolic pressure.[17,22] This increased volume, in addition to the normal venous return, leads to an increase in ventricular preload. The rise in preload may represent a compensatory response to maintain stroke volume through the Frank-Starling mechanism despite a reduction in EF. Increased preload, however, can also lead to an excessive accumulation of blood in the atria and the pulmonary venous system, which causes pulmonary congestion.

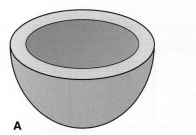
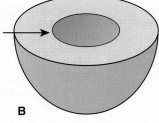
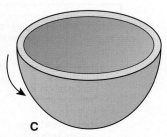

FIGURE 20-4. Different types of myocardial hypertrophy. **(A)** Normal symmetric hypertrophy with proportionate increases in myocardial wall thickness and length. **(B)** Concentric hypertrophy with a disproportionate increase in wall thickness. **(C)** Eccentric hypertrophy with a disproportionate decrease in wall thickness and ventricular dilation.

The cardinal symptoms of systolic failure are dyspnea, fatigue, and peripheral edema. Other symptoms include orthopnea and paroxysmal nocturnal dyspnea, signs of jugular venous distention and cardiac enlargement.[22]

Preserved Ejection Fraction Heart Failure. Although heart failure is commonly associated with impaired systolic function, in approximately half of the cases systolic function is preserved (EF > 50%) and heart failure results from an inability of the left ventricle to fill sufficiently during diastole.[23–25] Hypertension remains the leading cause of diastolic dysfunction. Other conditions that cause diastolic dysfunction include those that impede filling of the ventricle (e.g., pericardial effusion, constrictive pericarditis), increase ventricular wall thickness and reduce chamber size (e.g., myocardial hypertrophy, hypertrophic cardiomyopathy), or delay diastolic relaxation of the ventricle (e.g., aging, hypertension).[25] The prevalence of diastolic failure increases with age and is higher in women than men, and in persons with obesity, hypertension, and diabetes. Aging is often accompanied by a delay in relaxation of the heart during diastole such that diastolic filling begins while the ventricle is still stiff and resistant to stretching. A similar delay in filling occurs in myocardial ischemia, resulting from a lack of energy to break the bonds that form between the actin and myosin filaments and to pump calcium out of the cytosol and back into the sarcoplasmic reticulum.[23]

With diastolic dysfunction, ventricular relaxation and distensibility are impaired leading to an increase in intraventricular pressure at any given volume.

The elevated pressures are transmitted backward from the left ventricle into the left atrium and pulmonary venous system, causing pulmonary congestion and a decrease in lung compliance, which increases the work of breathing and evokes symptoms of dyspnea. Cardiac output is decreased, not because of a reduced ventricular EF as seen with systolic dysfunction but because of a decrease in ventricular filling. Diastolic function is further influenced by the heart rate, which determines how much time is available for ventricular filling. An increase in heart rate shortens the diastolic filling time. Thus, diastolic dysfunction can be aggravated by tachycardia and improved by a reduction in heart rate, which allows the heart to fill over a longer period of time.

Left-sided versus Right-sided Heart Dysfunction

The clinical manifestations of heart failure depend upon which heart chamber (i.e., the left or right) is dysfunctional (Fig. 20-5). An important feature of the circulatory system is the fact that the left and right ventricles function as two pumps that are connected in series. To function effectively, the left and right ventricles must maintain equal outputs. Although the initial event that leads to heart failure may be primarily left or right ventricular in origin, heart failure usually progresses over time to involve both ventricles.

Left Ventricular Dysfunction. The clinical features of heart failure affecting the left ventricle result from a diminished cardiac output with a resultant decrease in

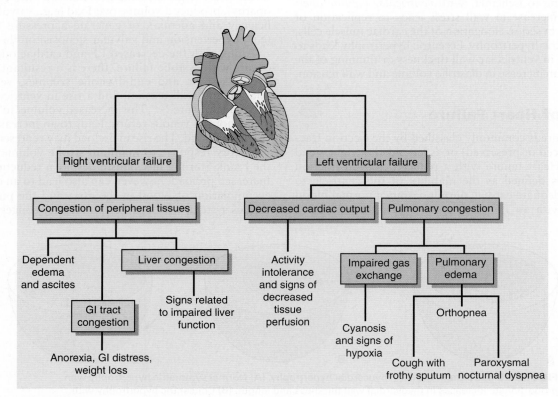

FIGURE 20-5. Manifestations of right and left ventricular failure. GI, gastrointestinal.

peripheral blood flow and a progressive accumulation of blood in the pulmonary circulation (see Fig. 20-5). With impairment of left ventricular function, there is a decrease in the ejection of blood into the systemic circulation, an increase in left ventricular and left atrial end-diastolic pressures, and congestion of the pulmonary circulation. When the filtration pressure in the pulmonary capillaries (normally approximately 10 mm Hg) exceeds the capillary osmotic pressure (normally approximately 25 mm Hg), there is a shift of intravascular fluid into the interstitium of the lung and development of pulmonary edema (Fig. 20-6). An episode of pulmonary edema often occurs at night, after the person has been reclining for some time and the gravitational forces have been removed from the circulatory system. It is then that the excess fluid that had been sequestered in the lower extremities during the day is returned to the vascular compartment and redistributed to the pulmonary circulation, causing what is called *paroxysmal nocturnal dyspnea.*

The most common causes of left ventricular dysfunction are hypertension and acute myocardial infarction. Left ventricular heart failure and pulmonary congestion can develop very rapidly in persons with acute myocardial infarction (see Chapter 19). Even when the infarcted area is small, there may be a surrounding area of ischemic tissue. This may result in large areas of ventricular wall hypokinesis or akinesis and rapid onset of pulmonary congestion and edema. Another cause of left heart failure is valvular defects such as stenosis or regurgitation of the aortic or mitral valve. These valvular defects increase the work of the left heart and eventually lead to heart failure if untreated.

Right Ventricular Dysfunction. Dysfunction of the right ventricle is often the consequence of disease of the left ventricle; an increase in pulmonary blood volume eventually produces an increased burden on the right side of the heart. Isolated dysfunction of the right ventricle is less common and occurs in persons with intrinsic lung disease or pulmonary hypertension.[26] It can also occur in persons with pulmonic or tricuspid valvular disease, right ventricular infarction, and cardiomyopathy. Congenital heart defects with right-to-left cardiac shunt can cause isolated right ventricular dysfunction as well (see Chapter 19). When right ventricular dysfunction occurs in response to chronic pulmonary disease, it is referred to as cor pulmonale (see Chapter 23).[27]

Dysfunction of the right ventricle impairs the ability to move blood from the systemic venous circulation into the pulmonary circulation. Consequently, when the right ventricle fails, there is a reduction in the amount of blood that is delivered to the left side of the heart. This causes an increase in right ventricular end-diastolic, right atrial, and systemic venous pressures. A major consequence is the development of peripheral edema (see Fig. 20-5). Because of the effects of gravity, the edema is most pronounced in the dependent parts of the body—in the lower extremities when the person is in the upright position and in the area over the sacrum when the person is supine. The accumulation of fluid may be evidenced by a gain in weight (edema or effusion). Daily measurement of weight can be used as a means of assessing fluid accumulation in a patient with chronic heart failure.

Failure of the right ventricle also causes congestion of the viscera. As venous distention progresses, blood backs up in the hepatic veins that drain into the inferior vena cava and the liver becomes engorged. This may cause hepatomegaly and pain in the right upper quadrant, and in time, liver function may become significantly impaired. Congestion of the portal circulation also may lead to engorgement of the spleen and the development of ascites. Congestion of the gastrointestinal tract may interfere with digestion and absorption of nutrients, causing anorexia and abdominal discomfort. When severe, the external jugular veins become distended and can be visualized when the person is sitting up or standing.

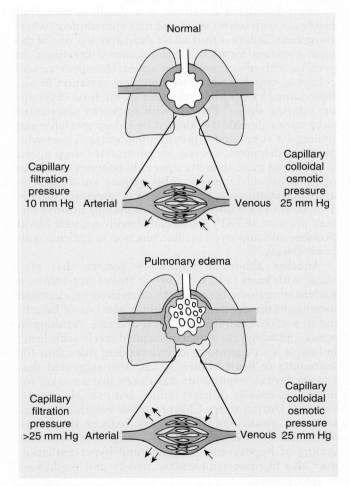

Normal

Capillary filtration pressure 10 mm Hg   Arterial   Venous   Capillary colloidal osmotic pressure 25 mm Hg

Pulmonary edema

Capillary filtration pressure >25 mm Hg   Arterial   Venous   Capillary colloidal osmotic pressure 25 mm Hg

FIGURE 20-6. Mechanisms of respiratory symptoms in left-sided heart dysfunction. In the normal exchange of fluid in the pulmonary capillaries (*top*), the capillary filtration pressure that pushes fluid out of the capillary into the lung is less than the colloidal osmotic pressure that pulls fluid back into the capillary. Development of pulmonary edema (*bottom*) occurs when the capillary filtration pressure that pushes fluid out of the capillary is greater than the colloidal osmotic pressure that pulls it back into the capillary.

Manifestations of Heart Failure

The manifestations of heart failure depend on the extent and type of cardiac dysfunction that is present and the rapidity with which it develops. A person with previously stable compensated heart failure may develop signs of heart failure for the first time when the condition has advanced to a critical point, such as with a progressive increase in pulmonary hypertension in a person with mitral valve regurgitation. Heart failure also may be precipitated by conditions such as infection, emotional stress, uncontrolled hypertension, or fluid overload.[28] Many persons with serious underlying heart disease, regardless of whether they have previously experienced heart failure, may be relatively asymptomatic as long they carefully adhere to their treatment regimen. A dietary excess of sodium may be a cause of sudden cardiac decompensation.

The signs and symptoms of heart failure reflect the physiologic effects of the impaired pumping ability of the heart, decreased renal blood flow, and activation of sympathetic compensatory mechanisms. They include fluid retention and edema, shortness of breath and other respiratory manifestations, fatigue and limited exercise tolerance, cachexia and malnutrition, and cyanosis.

Fluid Retention and Edema

Many of the manifestations of heart failure result from the increased capillary pressures (increased hydrostatic pressures) that develop in the peripheral and pulmonary circulations. The increased capillary pressure reflects an overfilling of the vascular system because of increased sodium and water retention and venous congestion, resulting from impaired cardiac output.[28] *Nocturia* is a nightly increase in urine output that occurs relatively early in the course of heart failure. It occurs because of the increased cardiac output, renal blood flow, and glomerular filtration rate that follow the increased blood return to the heart when the person is in a supine position. *Oliguria,* which is a decrease in urine output, is a late sign related to severely reduced cardiac output and resultant renal failure.

Transudation of fluid into the pleural cavity (pleural effusion or hydrothorax) or the peritoneal cavity (ascites) may occur in persons with advanced heart failure. Because the pleural veins drain into both the systemic and pulmonary venous beds, hydrothorax is observed more commonly in persons with hypertension involving both venous systems.[28] Pleural effusion occurs as the excess fluid in the lung interstitial spaces crosses the visceral pleura, which in turn overwhelms the capacity of the pulmonary lymphatic system. Ascites can occur in persons with increased pressure in the hepatic and peroneal veins. It usually reflects right ventricular failure and long-standing elevation of systemic venous pressure.[28]

Respiratory Manifestations

Dyspnea due to congestion of the pulmonary circulation is one of the major manifestations of heart failure. Dyspnea related to activity is called exertional dyspnea;

however, patients with advanced heart failure may experience dyspnea even at rest. Orthopnea is shortness of breath that occurs when a person is supine. Gravitational forces cause fluid to become sequestered in the lower legs and feet when the person is standing or sitting. When the person assumes the recumbent position, fluid from the legs and dependent parts of the body is mobilized and redistributed to an already distended pulmonary circulation. Paroxysmal nocturnal dyspnea is a sudden attack of dyspnea that occurs during sleep. It disrupts sleep, and the person awakens with a feeling of extreme suffocation that resolves when he or she sits up.

A subtle and often overlooked symptom of heart failure is a chronic dry, nonproductive cough that becomes worse when the person is lying down. Bronchospasm due to congestion of the bronchial mucosa may cause wheezing and difficulty in breathing. This condition is sometimes referred to as *cardiac asthma.*[28]

Sleep-disordered breathing is a common comorbid condition with heart failure and may contribute to worsening heart failure. Obstructive sleep apnea is one of the most common forms of sleep-disordered breathing. In persons with obstructive sleep apnea, the upper airway collapses, which leads to the complete cessation of airflow (apnea) or partial cessation of air flow (hypoapnea) during sleep.[29] Persons with suspected obstructive sleep apnea should be evaluated by a sleep specialist and undergo a sleep study (polysomnography). Those who meet the diagnostic criteria for obstructive sleep apnea (i.e., exhibit more than five apneas/hypoapneas per hour of sleep caused by airway obstruction) are treated by applying continuous positive airway pressure (usually 5 to 10 cm H_2O) during sleep. Continuous positive airway pressure (CPAP) is associated with reduced blood pressure and improved cardiac function in patients with heart disease.[29]

Another abnormal respiratory pattern that may occur with heart failure is *Cheyne-Stokes respiration,* a pattern of periodic breathing characterized by a gradual increase in the depth and sometimes the rate of breathing to a maximum, followed by a decrease, resulting in apnea. Although no longer associated solely with heart failure, it is recognized as an independent risk factor for worsening of heart failure. It has been suggested that Cheyne-Stokes respirations may not be just a marker for increasing severity of heart failure, but may also aggravate it.[30] During sleep, Cheyne-Stokes breathing causes recurrent awakening and thereby reduces slow-wave and rapid eye movement (REM) sleep. The recurrent cycling of hypoventilation/apnea and hyperventilation may also increase sympathetic activity and predispose to arrhythmias.

Fatigue, Weakness, and Cognitive Impairment

Fatigue and weakness often accompany diminished output from the left ventricle. Cardiac fatigue is different from general fatigue in that it usually is not present in the morning but appears and progresses as activity increases during the day. In acute or severe failure of the left ventricle, cardiac output may fall to levels that are insufficient for providing the brain with adequate oxygen, causing cognitive impairment and disturbed behavior. Confusion, impairment of memory, anxiety, restlessness, and insomnia are common in elderly persons with advanced heart failure, particularly in those with cerebral atherosclerosis. These symptoms may confuse the diagnosis of heart failure in the elderly because of other possible causes associated with aging.

Cachexia and Malnutrition

Cardiac cachexia is a condition of malnutrition and tissue wasting that occurs in persons with end-stage heart failure.[31] A number of factors probably contribute to its development, including fatigue and depression that interfere with food intake, and congestion of the liver and gastrointestinal structures that impairs digestion and absorption and produces feelings of fullness. Other factors are circulating toxins and mediators released from poorly perfused tissues that impair appetite and contribute to tissue wasting.

Cyanosis

Cyanosis, or a bluish discoloration of the skin and mucous membranes, is caused by excess desaturated hemoglobin in the blood. It is often a late sign of heart failure, and may be visible especially around the lips and in the peripheral parts of the extremities.

Cyanosis may be central or peripheral. Central cyanosis develops when impaired pulmonary gas exchange reduces oxygenation of the arterial blood in conditions such as pulmonary edema, left heart failure, or right-to-left cardiac shunting. Peripheral cyanosis develops as a consequence of venous desaturation resulting from extensive extraction of oxygen at the capillary level. It is caused by conditions such as low-output failure that result in delivery of poorly oxygenated blood to the peripheral tissues, or by conditions such as peripheral vasoconstriction that cause excessive removal of oxygen from the blood. Central cyanosis is best monitored by assessing the lips and mucous membranes because these areas are not subject to environmental conditions, such as cold temperatures, that cause peripheral constriction and cyanosis.

Arrhythmias and Sudden Cardiac Death

Both atrial and ventricular arrhythmias can occur in persons with heart failure. Atrial fibrillation is the most common arrhythmia (see Chapter 17). Manifestations associated with atrial fibrillation are related to loss of atrial contraction, tachycardia, irregular heart rate, and symptoms related to a drop in blood pressure.[32] There is also strong evidence that persons with heart failure are at increased risk for sudden cardiac arrest; that is, unwitnessed death or death that occurs within 1 hour of symptom onset. In persons with ventricular dysfunction, sudden death is caused most commonly by ventricular tachycardia or ventricular fibrillation.[1]

Acute Heart Failure Syndromes

The acute heart failure syndromes (AHFS) are defined as "gradual or rapid change in heart failure signs and symptoms resulting in a need for urgent therapy."[33] These signs and symptoms are primarily the result of severe pulmonary edema due to elevated left ventricular filling pressures, with or without a low cardiac output.[33–35] The AHFS are among the most common disorders seen in emergency departments. A worsening of chronic heart failure, often complicated by episodes of acute decompensation, is the most common cause of the syndrome.

The AHFS are thought to encompass three different types of conditions: (1) worsening of chronic systolic or diastolic dysfunction that appears to respond to treatment; (2) new-onset acute heart failure that occurs secondary to a precipitating event such as a large myocardial infarction or a sudden increase in blood pressure superimposed on a noncompliant left ventricle; and (3) worsening of end-stage/advanced heart failure that is refractory to treatment, with predominantly left ventricular systolic dysfunction associated with a low-output state.[34] The difference between new-onset AHFS and AHFS caused by chronic heart failure is in the degree of physiologic response, which is more pronounced in the new-onset AHFS and more subtle in chronic heart failure because of the compensatory pathophysiology. For example, with new-onset AHFS, the person will have a strong sympathetic response such as tachycardia with enhanced pulmonary vascular permeability causing rapid and dramatic symptoms of pulmonary edema. Because many compensatory mechanisms operate in persons with chronic heart failure, they tolerate higher pulmonary vascular pressures. Chronic changes in neurohormonal regulation lead to a strong activation of the angiotensin-aldosterone system with a resultant volume overload, and venous congestion in both the systemic and pulmonary circulations.[35]

Acute pulmonary edema is the most dramatic symptom of AHFS. It is a life-threatening condition in which capillary fluid moves into the alveoli.[28] The accumulated fluid in the alveoli and airways causes lung stiffness, makes lung expansion more difficult, and impairs the gas exchange function of the lung. With the decreased ability of the lungs to oxygenate the blood, the hemoglobin leaves the pulmonary circulation without being fully oxygenated, resulting in shortness of breath and cyanosis.

The person with severe pulmonary edema is usually seen sitting and gasping for air. The pulse is rapid, the skin is moist and cool, and the lips and nail beds are cyanotic. As the pulmonary edema worsens and oxygen supply to the brain drops, confusion and stupor appear. Dyspnea and air hunger are accompanied by a productive cough with frothy (resembling beaten egg whites) and often blood-tinged sputum—the effect of air mixing with the serum albumin and red blood cells that have moved into the alveoli. The movement of air through the alveolar fluid produces fine crepitant sounds called *crackles,* which can be heard with a stethoscope on chest auscultation. As fluid moves into the larger airways, the crackles become louder and coarser.

Diagnosis

Diagnostic methods in heart failure are directed toward establishing the cause of the disorder and determining the extent of the dysfunction.[1,2] Because heart failure represents the failure of the heart as a pump and can occur in the course of a number of heart diseases or other systemic disorders, the diagnosis of heart failure often is based on signs and symptoms related to the failing heart itself, such as dyspnea and fatigue. Functional classification systems from the New York Heart Association (NYHA) and the American College of Cardiology Foundation/American Heart Association (ACCF/AHA) provide important information about the presence and severity of HF (Table 20-1). The NYHA functional classification system is subjective, meaning the patient describes their level of activity and symptoms. It is widely used in clinical practice and research settings. The ACCF/AHA classification system is more recent and emphasizes the progression of the disease along with risk factors associated with HF, such as hypertension (Stages A and B).

The methods used in the diagnosis of heart failure include history and physical examination, laboratory studies, electrocardiography, chest radiography, and echocardiography. The history should include information

related to dyspnea, cough, nocturia, generalized fatigue, exercise intolerance and other signs and symptoms of heart failure. A complete physical examination includes assessment of heart rate and rhythm, heart sounds, blood pressure, jugular veins for venous congestion, lungs for signs of pulmonary congestion, and lower extremities for edema. Pulse oximetry can be used to measure the percentage of hemoglobin oxygen saturation.

Laboratory tests are used in the diagnosis of anemia and electrolyte imbalances and to detect signs of chronic liver congestion. Measurements of BNP are recommended to confirm the diagnosis of heart failure; to evaluate the severity of left ventricular compromise, estimate the prognosis, and evaluate the effectiveness of treatment. BNP may not be as sensitive in persons with heart failure who are obese or have renal failure.[1,36]

Echocardiography plays a key role in assessing ejection fraction, right and left ventricular wall motion (normal, akinesis, or hypokinesis), wall thickness, ventricular chamber size, valve function, heart defects and pericardial disease. Radionuclide ventriculography and cardiac angiography are recommended if there is reason to suspect coronary artery disease or ischemia as the underlying cause for heart failure. Chest radiographs provide information about the size and shape of the heart and pulmonary vasculature, and also can indicate the relative severity of the failure by revealing if pulmonary edema is predominantly vascular or interstitial or has advanced to the alveolar and bronchial stages. Cardiac magnetic resonance imaging and cardiac computed tomography

TABLE 20-1	Comparison of ACCF/AHA Stages of HF and NYHA Functional Classification		
ACCF/AHA Stages of HF[a]		**NYHA Functional Classification[b]**	
A	At high risk for HF but without structural heart disease or symptoms of HF	None	
B	Structural heart disease but without signs or symptoms of HF	I	No limitation of physical activity. Ordinary physical activity does not cause symptoms of HF.
C	Structural heart disease with prior or current symptoms of HF	I	No limitation of physical activity. Ordinary physical activity does not cause symptoms of HF.
		II	Slight limitation of physical activity. Comfortable at rest, but ordinary physical activity causes symptoms of HF.
		III	Marked limitation of physical activity. Comfortable at rest, but less-than-ordinary physical activity causes symptoms of HF.
D	Refractory HF requiring specialized interventions	IV	Unable to carry on any physical activity without symptoms of HF, or symptoms of HF at rest.

[a]From Hunt SA, Abraham WT, Chin MH, et al. 2009 focused update incorporated into the ACC/AHA 2005 guidelines for the diagnosis and management of heart failure in adults: A report of the American College of Cardiology Foundation/American Heart Association Task Force on Practice Guidelines. *J Am Coll Cardiol.* 2009;53:e1–e90.

[b]The Criteria Committee of the New York Heart Association. *Nomenclature and Criteria for Diagnosis of Diseases of the Heart and Great Vessels.* Boston, MA: Little & Brown; 1994.

From Yancy CW, Jessup M, Bozkurt B, et al. 2013 ACCF/AHA guideline for the management of heart failure: a report of the American College of Cardiology Foundation/American Heart Association Task Force on Practice Guidelines. *Circulation.* 2013;128(16):e240–e319.

are used to document ejection fraction, ventricular pre-load, and regional wall motion.

Invasive hemodynamic monitoring may be used for assessment in acute, life-threatening episodes of heart failure.[37] These monitoring methods include central venous pressure (CVP), pulmonary artery pressure monitoring, measurements of cardiac output, and intra-arterial measurements of blood pressure. Central venous pressure reflects the amount of blood returning to the right side of the heart. Measurements of CVP are best obtained by a catheter inserted into the right atrium through a peripheral vein or by the right atrial port (opening) in a pulmonary artery catheter.

Ventricular volume pressures are obtained indirectly, such as by means of a flow-directed, balloon-tipped pulmonary artery catheter. This catheter is introduced through a peripheral or central vein and then advanced into the right atrium. The balloon is then inflated with air, enabling the catheter to float through the right ventricle into the pulmonary artery until it becomes wedged in a small pulmonary vessel. With the balloon inflated, the catheter monitors pulmonary capillary pressures (i.e., *pulmonary capillary wedge pressure* or *pulmonary artery occlusion pressure*), which reflect pressures from the left ventricle. The pulmonary capillary pressures provide a means of assessing the pumping ability of the left ventricle. One type of pulmonary artery catheter is equipped with a thermistor probe to obtain *thermodilution measurements* of cardiac output. Catheters with oximeters built into their tips that permit continuous monitoring of oxygen saturation (SvO_2) also are available. Intra-arterial blood pressure monitoring provides a means for continuous monitoring of blood pressure. It is used in persons with acute heart failure who need continuous blood pressure monitoring, such as when aggressive intravenous medication therapy or a mechanical assist device is required.

Treatment

The goals of treatment for heart failure are determined by the rapidity of onset and severity of the heart failure. Persons with acute heart failure require urgent therapy directed at stabilizing and correcting the cause of the cardiac dysfunction. For persons with chronic heart failure, the goals of treatment are directed toward relieving the symptoms, improving the quality of life, and treating or reducing or eliminating risk factors (hypertension, diabetes, or obesity) with the long-term goal of slowing, halting, or reversing the cardiac dysfunction.[1,2]

Treatment measures for both acute and chronic heart failure include pharmacologic and nonpharmacologic approaches. Mechanical support devices, including the aortic balloon pump (for short-term acute failure) and ventricular assist devices (VADs), can be used to sustain life in persons with severe heart failure. Heart transplant or a VAD remains an option for some people with end-stage heart disease.

It is important to note that current guideline-directed therapies only target HF patients with a reduced ejection fraction. Therapies specific to patients with a preserved ejection fraction or HFpEF have not been established.

Nonpharmacologic Methods

Exercise intolerance is typical of persons with chronic heart failure. Consequently, individualized exercise training is important to maximize muscle conditioning. Persons who are not accustomed to exercise and those with more severe heart failure are started at a lower intensity and shorter duration than those who are largely asymptomatic. Sodium and fluid restriction and weight management are important for all persons with heart failure, with the level of sodium and fluid restriction individualized to the severity of sodium intake, and diuretic therapy facilitates the excretion of edema fluid. Counseling, health teaching, and ongoing evaluation programs assist persons with heart failure to self-manage and cope with their treatment regimen.[38]

Pharmacologic Treatment

Once heart failure becomes moderate to severe, polypharmacy becomes a management standard. First line therapies for patients with a reduced ejection fraction include β-adrenergic inhibitors, angiotensin-converting enzyme (ACE)/angiotensin receptor inhibitors, and diuretics. But for patients who are intolerant to these drugs or who remain symptomatic despite guideline-directed therapies, additional agents may be used, such as aldosterone antagonists or digoxin.[1,2,39] The choice of pharmacologic agents is determined by problems caused by the disorder (i.e., systolic or diastolic dysfunction), those brought about by activation of compensatory mechanisms (e.g., excess fluid retention, inappropriate activation of sympathetic mechanisms), and the person's comorbidities.[40] *Diuretics* are among the most frequently prescribed medications for symptoms of volume overload.[13] They promote the excretion of fluid and help to sustain cardiac output and tissue perfusion by reducing preload and allowing the heart to operate at a more optimal part of the Frank-Starling curve. In emergencies, such as acute pulmonary edema, loop diuretics such as furosemide (Lasix) can be administered intravenously. When given intravenously, these medications act quickly to reduce venous return through vasodilation so that right ventricular output and pulmonary vascular resistance are decreased. This response to intravenous administration is extrarenal and precedes the onset of diuresis.

The *ACE inhibitors*, which prevent the conversion of angiotensin I to angiotensin II, have been used effectively in the treatment of chronic heart failure.[40] The renin-angiotensin-aldosterone system is activated early in the course of heart failure and plays an important role in its progression. It results in an increase in angiotensin II, which causes vasoconstriction, unregulated ventricular remodeling, and increased aldosterone production with a subsequent increase in sodium and water retention by the kidneys. Angiotensin-converting enzyme inhibitors have been shown to limit these harmful complications. The *angiotensin II receptor blockers* appear to have similar but more limited beneficial effects. They have the advantage of not causing a cough, which is a troublesome side effect of the ACE inhibitors for many persons. *Aldosterone receptor antagonists* may be used in combination with other agents for persons with heart failure. Hyperkalemia is a potential side effect of aldosterone antagonism that requires additional monitoring.[1]

β-*Adrenergic receptor blocking drugs* are used to decrease left ventricular dysfunction associated with activation of the sympathetic nervous system.[40] Large clinical trials have shown that long-term therapy with β-adrenergic receptor blocking agents reduces morbidity and mortality in persons with chronic heart failure. The mechanism of this benefit remains unclear, but it is likely that chronic elevation of catecholamines and sympathetic nervous system activity causes progressive myocardial damage, leading to a worsening of left ventricular function and a poorer prognosis in persons with heart failure.

Digitalis has been a recognized treatment for heart failure for over 200 years. The various forms of digitalis are called *cardiac glycosides*. They improve cardiac function by increasing the force and strength of ventricular contractions. Digitalis and related cardiac glycosides are inotropic agents that exert their effects by inhibiting the Na^+/K^+-ATPase membrane pump, which increases intracellular sodium; this in turn leads to an increase in intracellular calcium through the Na^+/Ca^+ exchange pump[40] (see Fig. 20-1). The cardiac glycosides also decrease sinoatrial node activity and decrease conduction through the atrioventricular node, thereby slowing the heart rate and increasing diastolic filling time.

Vasodilator agents such as isosorbide dinitrate and hydralazine may be added to other standard medications for African-American patients with chronic heart failure.[1] Agents such as nitroglycerin, nitroprusside, and nesiritide (B-type natriuretic peptide) are used in AHFSs to improve left heart performance by decreasing the preload (through vasodilation) or reducing the afterload (through arteriolar dilation), or both.

Oxygen Therapy

Oxygen therapy increases the oxygen content of the blood and is often used in patients with acute episodes of heart failure. Noninvasive ventilation using continuous positive airway pressure (CPAP) may be used to relieve dyspnea, respiratory distress, and/or pulmonary edema.[34] Continuous positive airway pressure by face mask reduces the need for endotracheal intubation and has minimal adverse effects or complications. Because CPAP increases intrathoracic pressure, it also has the potential for decreasing venous return and left ventricular preload, thereby improving the cardiac ejection fraction and stabilizing the hemodynamic status in persons with severe heart failure.[40] Noninvasive ventilation can also be provided by bilevel ventilation (BiPAP), which delivers positive pressure during both inspiration and expiration.

Advanced Therapies

Individuals with heart failure are at significant risk of sudden cardiac death from ventricular fibrillation or ventricular tachycardia. Implantation of a cardioverter–defibrillator is indicated in selected patients with heart failure to prevent sudden cardiac death.[1,2] A cardioverter–defibrillator is a programmable implanted device that monitors the cardiac rhythm. It has the capacity to pace the heart and deliver electric shocks to terminate lethal arrhythmias.

Refractory heart failure reflects deterioration in cardiac function that is unresponsive to medical or surgical interventions. Since the early 1960s, significant progress has been made in improving the efficacy of *ventricular assist devices* (VADs), which are mechanical pumps used to support ventricular function.[41] VADs are used to decrease the workload of the myocardium while maintaining cardiac output and systemic arterial pressure. This decreases the workload on the ventricle and allows it to rest and recover. Most VADs require an invasive open chest procedure for implantation. They may be used in patients who fail or have difficulty being weaned from cardiopulmonary bypass after cardiac surgery, those who develop cardiogenic shock after myocardial infarction, those with end-stage cardiomyopathy, and those who are awaiting cardiac transplantation. Earlier and more aggressive use of VADs as a bridge to transplantation and destination therapy (permanent support) has been shown to increase survival.[41,42] Ventricular assist devices that allow the patient to be mobile and managed at home are sometimes used for long-term or permanent support for treatment of end-stage heart failure, rather than simply as a bridge to transplantation. Ventricular assist devices can be used to support the function of the left ventricle, right ventricle, or both.[42]

Heart transplantation is the preferred treatment for many persons with end-stage cardiac failure and otherwise good life expectancy.[1,2] Despite the overall success of heart transplantation, donor availability remains a key problem, and thousands are denied transplantation each year. Left ventricular remodeling is a surgical procedure designed to restore the size and shape of the ventricle, and in a subset of patients with severe left ventricular dysfunction this procedure may provide an alternative to cardiac transplantation.[43]

Heart Failure in the Elderly

Heart failure is one of the most common causes of disability in the elderly and is the most frequent hospital discharge diagnosis for the elderly. Among the factors that have contributed to the increased numbers of older people with heart failure are the improved therapies for ischemic and hypertensive heart disease.[44] Thus, persons who would have died from acute myocardial disease 20 years ago are now surviving, but with residual heart damage. Advances in treatment of other diseases have also contributed indirectly to the rising prevalence of heart failure in the older population. In contrast to the etiology in middle-aged persons with heart failure, factors other than systolic failure contribute to heart failure in the elderly. Preserved left ventricular function may be seen in 40% to 80% of older persons with heart failure.[44]

There are four changes associated with aging that contribute to the development of heart failure in the elderly.[44-46] First, reduced responsiveness to β-adrenergic stimulation limits the heart's capacity to maximally increase heart rate and contractility during an increase in activity or stress. A second major effect of aging is increased vascular stiffness, which leads to a progressive increase in systolic blood pressure with advancing age, which in turn contributes to the development of left ventricular hypertrophy and altered diastolic filling. Third, in addition to increased vascular stiffness, the heart itself becomes stiffer and less compliant with age. The changes in diastolic stiffness result in important alterations in diastolic filling and atrial function. A reduction in ventricular filling not only affects cardiac output, but also produces an elevation in diastolic pressure that is transmitted back to the left atrium, where it stretches the muscle wall and predisposes to atrial ectopic beats and atrial fibrillation. Fourth, aging alters myocardial metabolism at the level of the mitochondria. Although older mitochondria may be able to generate sufficient ATP to meet the normal energy needs of the heart, they may be less able to respond under stress.

Clinical Manifestations

The manifestations of heart failure in the elderly often are masked by other disease.[1,2] Nocturia or nocturnal incontinence is an early heart failure symptom but may be caused by other conditions such as prostatic hypertrophy. Lower extremity edema may reflect venous insufficiency. Impaired perfusion of the gastrointestinal tract is a common cause of anorexia and profound loss of lean body mass. Loss of lean body mass may be masked by edema. Exertional dyspnea, orthopnea, and impaired exercise tolerance are cardinal symptoms of heart failure in both younger and older persons with heart failure. However, with increasing age, which is often accompanied by a more sedentary lifestyle, exertional dyspnea becomes less prominent.

Physical signs of heart failure such as elevated jugular venous pressure, hepatic congestion, and pulmonary crackles are less common in the elderly, in part because of the increased incidence of diastolic failure, in which the signs of right ventricular failure are late manifestations and a third heart sound is typically absent.[45] Instead, behavioral changes and altered cognition such as short-term memory loss and impaired problem solving are more common. With exacerbation of heart failure, the elderly may present with acute delirium, dementia, and restlessness. Depression is common in the elderly with heart failure and shares the symptoms of sleep disturbances, cognitive changes, and fatigue.

The elderly also maintain a precarious balance between the managed symptom state and acute symptom exacerbation. During the managed symptom state, they are relatively symptom free while adhering to their treatment regimen. Acute symptom exacerbation, often requiring emergency medical treatment, can be precipitated by seemingly minor conditions such as poor adherence to sodium restriction, infection, or stress. Failure to promptly seek medical care is a common cause of progressive acceleration of symptoms.

Diagnosis and Treatment

The diagnosis of heart failure in the elderly is based on the history, physical examination, chest radiograph, and echocardiographic findings.[1,47] However, the presenting symptoms of heart failure often are difficult to evaluate and differentiate from changes associated with aging and other co-morbidities. Symptoms of dyspnea on exertion are often interpreted as a sign of "getting older" or attributed to deconditioning from other diseases. Ankle edema is not unusual in the elderly because of decreased skin turgor and the tendency of the elderly to be more sedentary with the legs in a dependent position.

Treatment of heart failure in the elderly involves many of the same methods as in younger persons, with medication dose adaptations to reduce age-related adverse and toxic events. ACE inhibitors may be particularly beneficial to preserve cognitive and functional capacities. Activities are restricted to a level that is commensurate with the cardiac reserve. Seldom is bed rest recommended or advised. Bed rest causes rapid deconditioning of skeletal muscles and increases the risk of complications such as orthostatic hypotension and thromboemboli. Instead, carefully prescribed exercise programs can help to maintain activity tolerance. Even walking around a room usually is preferable to continuous bed rest.

SUMMARY CONCEPTS

■ Heart failure occurs when the heart fails to deliver sufficient blood to meet the metabolic needs of body tissues.

■ The pathophysiology of heart failure reflects the interplay between a decrease in cardiac output that accompanies heart failure and the compensatory mechanisms that preserve the cardiac reserve. Compensatory mechanisms include the Frank-Starling mechanism, sympathetic nervous system activation, the renin-angiotensin-aldosterone mechanism, natriuretic peptides, endothelins, and myocardial hypertrophy and remodeling. In the failing heart, early decreases in cardiac function may go unnoticed because these compensatory mechanisms maintain the cardiac output.

■ Heart failure may be described in terms of ejection fraction (reduced vs preserved). Clinical manifestation depends upon which ventricle is dysfunctional. With a reduced ejection fraction,

(continued)

SUMMARY CONCEPTS *(continued)*

there is impaired ejection of blood from the heart during systole; with diastolic dysfunction, there is impaired filling of the heart during diastole. Left ventricular dysfunction is characterized by congestion in the pulmonary circulation and impaired blood flow in the peripheral circulation, and right ventricular dysfunction by congestion in the peripheral circulation.

■ The manifestations of heart failure include fluid retention and edema, shortness of breath, fatigue and impaired exercise tolerance, impaired gastrointestinal function and malnutrition, and cyanosis. When performance of the right ventricle is impaired, there is dependent edema of the lower parts of the body, engorgement of the liver, and ascites. With failure of the left ventricle, pulmonary congestion with shortness of breath and chronic, nonproductive cough are common.

■ The acute heart failure syndromes represent a gradual or rapid change in heart failure signs and symptoms, indicating the need for urgent therapy. These symptoms are primarily the result of pulmonary congestion due to elevated left ventricular filling pressures with or without a low cardiac output.

■ The diagnostic methods in heart failure are directed toward establishing the cause and extent of the syndrome. Treatment is directed toward correcting the cause whenever possible, improving cardiac function, maintaining the fluid volume within a compensatory range, and developing an activity pattern consistent with individual limitations in cardiac reserve. Among the medications used in the treatment of heart failure are diuretics, digitalis, ACE inhibitors and angiotensin receptor blocking agents, β-adrenergic receptor blockers, vasodilators, and aldosterone blockers.

■ Among the devices used to treat heart failure patients with a reduced ejection fraction are an implantable cardiac defibrillator and ventricular assist devices. Heart transplantation remains the treatment of choice for many persons with end-stage heart failure.

■ The manifestations of heart failure in the elderly often are different and superimposed on other disease conditions; therefore, heart failure often is more difficult to diagnose in the elderly than in younger persons. Because the elderly are more susceptible to adverse and toxic medication reactions, medication doses need to be adapted and more closely monitored.

Circulatory Failure (Shock)

Circulatory shock can be described as an acute failure of the circulatory system to supply the peripheral tissues and organs of the body with an adequate blood supply, resulting in cellular hypoxia.[48,49] Most often hypotension and hypoperfusion are present, but shock may occur in the presence of normal vital signs. Shock is not a specific disease but a syndrome that can occur in the course of many life-threatening traumatic conditions or disease states. Moreover, no single classification system exists; rather, shock can be classified by the cause, primary pathophysiological derangement, or clinical manifestations. Generally each type of shock has certain distinguishing features; nonetheless, all types of shock reflect an imbalance between oxygen supply and demand. As a result, all shock states share common derangements, such as inadequate peripheral tissue perfusion, alterations in cellular metabolism and function, and impaired organ perfusion, and all share common compensatory mechanisms in response to these derangements.

Pathophysiology of Shock

Circulatory failure results in hypoperfusion of organs and tissues, which in turn results in an insufficient supply of oxygen and nutrients for cellular function and the accumulation of waste products.[6] The cellular injury created by an inadequate delivery of oxygen and substrates also induces the production and release of inflammatory mediators that further compromise perfusion through functional and structural changes within the microvascular circulation. This leads to a vicious cycle in which impaired perfusion is responsible for cellular injury, which causes maldistribution of blood flow, further compromising cellular perfusion, and can culminate in irreversible end-organ damage.

Cellular Responses

Shock ultimately exerts its effect at the cellular level, with failure of the circulation to supply body cells with the oxygen and nutrients needed for production of ATP. Cells require ATP for a number of functions, including operation of the Na^+/K^+–ATPase membrane pump that moves sodium out of the cell and returns potassium to the inside of the cell. The cell uses two pathways to convert nutrients to ATP (see Chapter 1). The first is the anaerobic (non–oxygen-dependent) glycolytic pathway, located in the cytoplasm, which converts glucose to ATP and pyruvate. The second is the aerobic (oxygen-dependent) pathway, which is located in the mitochondria. When oxygen is available, pyruvate from the anaerobic pathway moves into the mitochondria and enters the aerobic pathway, where it is transformed into ATP and the metabolic by-products carbon dioxide and water. When oxygen is lacking, pyruvate is converted to lactic acid.

As a shock state progresses, cellular metabolism becomes anaerobic because of the decreased availability of oxygen. Excess amounts of lactic acid accumulate in the cellular and extracellular compartments, and limited amounts of ATP are produced. Without sufficient energy production, normal cell function cannot be maintained. The Na^+/K^+-ATPase membrane pump function is impaired, resulting in intracellular accumulation of sodium and loss of potassium. The increase in intracellular sodium results in cellular edema and increased cell membrane permeability. Mitochondrial activity becomes severely depressed and lysosomal membranes may rupture, resulting in the release of enzymes that cause further cellular destruction. This is followed by cell death and the release of intracellular contents into the extracellular space. The extent of the cell injury and organ dysfunction is primarily determined by the degree and duration of the shock state.

Compensatory Mechanisms

The clinical manifestations of shock are at least partly due to the body's compensatory responses to hypoperfusion. The most immediate of the compensatory mechanisms are those of the sympathetic nervous system and the renin-angiotensin mechanism, which maintain cardiac output and blood pressure. Often blood is shunted from the kidneys to other vital organs.

The sympathetic nervous system provides important reflexive mechanisms that are essential to the support of the circulatory system during shock, particularly hypovolemic shock.[6] These reflexes increase heart rate and stimulate constriction of blood vessels throughout the body. There are two types of adrenergic receptors for the sympathetic nervous system: alpha (α) and beta (β). The β receptors which are further divided into subtypes β_1 and β_2 receptors. Stimulation of the α receptors causes vasoconstriction; stimulation of β_1 receptors cause an increase in heart rate and force of myocardial contraction; and of β_2 receptors, vasodilation of the skeletal muscle beds and relaxation of the bronchioles. In shock, there is an increase in sympathetic outflow that results in increased epinephrine and norepinephrine release and activation of both α and β receptors (Chapter 34). Thus, increases in heart rate and vasoconstriction occur in most types of shock (cardiac output = stroke × heart rate). The arterioles constrict in most parts of the systemic circulation, thereby increasing the peripheral vascular resistance, and the veins and venous reservoirs constrict, thereby helping to maintain adequate venous return to the heart.

There also is an increase in renin release, leading to an increase in angiotensin II, which augments vasoconstriction and leads to an aldosterone-mediated increase in sodium and water retention by the kidneys. In addition, there is a local release of vasoconstrictors as well as norepinephrine, angiotensin II, vasopressin, and endothelin, which contribute to arterial and venous vasoconstriction.

The compensatory mechanisms that the body recruits cannot be sustained over the long term and become detrimental when the shock state is prolonged. This intense vasoconstriction causes a decrease in tissue perfusion and insufficient supply of oxygen. Cellular metabolism is impaired, vasoactive inflammatory mediators such as

histamine are released, production of oxygen free radicals is increased, and excessive lactic acid and hydrogen ions result in intracellular acidity and accompanying metabolic acidosis.[6] Each of these factors promotes cellular dysfunction or death. If circulatory function is reestablished, whether the shock is irreversible or if the patient will survive is determined largely at the cellular level regardless of the type of shock.

Types of Shock

In general, shock states are distinguished by clinical signs and symptoms, history, and physical exam. Circulatory shock can be caused by a decrease in blood volume (hypovolemic shock), an alteration in cardiac function, obstruction of blood flow through the circulatory system (obstructive shock), or excessive vasodilation with maldistribution of blood flow (distributive shock). The main types of shock are summarized in Chart 20-1 and depicted in Figure 20-7.

Hypovolemic Shock

Hypovolemic shock occurs when there is an acute loss of 15% or more of the circulating blood volume. The decrease may be caused by a loss of whole blood, plasma, extracellular fluid or excessive dehydration (Chart 20-1). Hypovolemic shock also can result from an internal hemorrhage or from third-space losses, when extracellular fluid is shifted from the vascular compartment to the interstitial space.

Hypovolemic shock, which has been the most widely studied type of shock, is often used as a prototype in

---

CHART 20-1	**Classification of Circulatory Shock**

Hypovolemic
Loss of whole blood
Loss of plasma
Loss of extracellular fluid

Cardiogenic
Myocardial damage (myocardial infarction, contusion)
Sustained arrhythmias
Acute valve damage, ventricular septal defect
Cardiac surgery

Obstructive
Inability of the heart to fill properly (cardiac tamponade)
Obstruction to outflow from the heart (pulmonary embolus, cardiac myxoma, pneumothorax, or dissecting aneurysm)

Distributive
Loss of sympathetic vasomotor tone (neurogenic shock)
Presence of vasodilating substances in the blood (anaphylactic shock)
Presence of inflammatory mediators (septic shock)

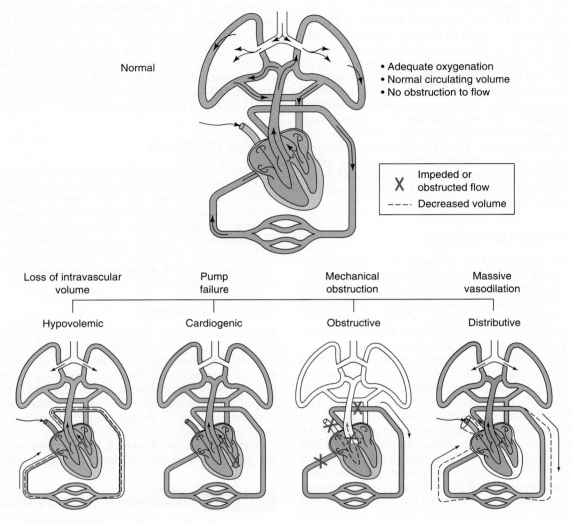

Normal

- Adequate oxygenation
- Normal circulating volume
- No obstruction to flow

X	Impeded or obstructed flow
----	Decreased volume

Loss of intravascular volume	Pump failure	Mechanical obstruction	Massive vasodilation
Hypovolemic	Cardiogenic	Obstructive	Distributive

FIGURE 20-7. Types of shock.

discussions of the manifestations of shock. Approximately 10% of the total blood volume can be lost or shifted without changing cardiac output or arterial pressure. The average blood donor loses approximately 500 mL or 10% of his or her blood without experiencing adverse effects.[6] However, as increasing amounts of blood (15% to 30% or 750 to 1500 mL) are removed, compensatory mechanisms are triggered.[50,51] The most immediate of these compensatory mechanisms are the sympathetic-mediated responses designed to maintain cardiac output and blood pressure (Fig. 20-8). Shortly after the onset of hemorrhage or the loss of fluid volume, tachycardia, increased cardiac contractility, vasoconstriction, and other signs of sympathetic and adrenal medullary activity appear.

The sympathetic vasoconstrictor response also mobilizes blood that has been stored in the venous side of the circulation as a means of increasing venous return to the heart. There is considerable capacity for blood storage in the large veins of the abdomen, and approximately 350 mL of blood that can be mobilized in shock is stored in the liver.[6] Sympathetic stimulation does not initially cause constriction of the cerebral and coronary

vessels, and blood flow to the heart and brain is maintained at essentially normal levels as long as the mean arterial pressure remains above 70 mm Hg.[6] Without (and, at times, despite) compensatory mechanisms to maintain cardiac output and blood pressure, the loss of vascular volume results in a rapid progression from the initial to the progressive, and finally to the irreversible stages of shock (more than 40% volume loss).[51]

Compensatory mechanisms designed to restore blood volume (i.e., draw volume into the intravascular space) include absorption of fluid from the interstitial spaces, conservation of sodium and water by the kidneys, and thirst. Extracellular fluid is distributed between the interstitial spaces and the vascular compartment. When there is a loss of vascular volume, capillary pressures decrease and water is drawn into the vascular compartment from the interstitial spaces. The maintenance of vascular volume is further enhanced by renally mediated humoral mechanisms that conserve fluid. A decrease in renal blood flow and glomerular filtration rate results in activation of the renin-angiotensin-aldosterone mechanism, which produces an increase in sodium reabsorption by

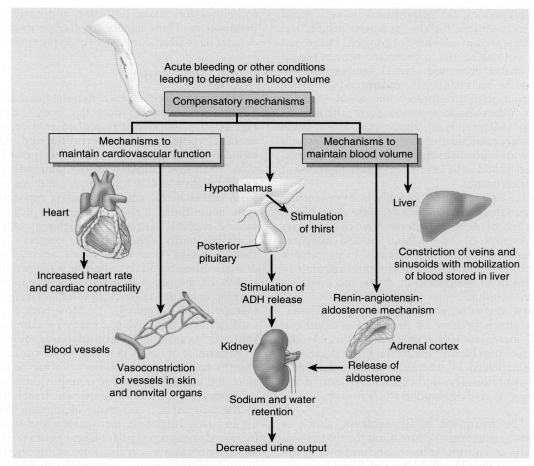

FIGURE 20-8. Compensatory mechanisms used to maintain circulatory function and blood volume in hypovolemic shock. ADH, antidiuretic hormone.

the kidneys. The decrease in blood volume also stimulates centers in the hypothalamus that regulate antidiuretic hormone (ADH) release and thirst. Antidiuretic hormone, also known as vasopressin, constricts the peripheral arteries and veins and greatly increases water retention by the kidneys. Although the mechanism of ADH is more sensitive to changes in serum osmolality, a decrease of 10% to 15% in blood volume serves as a strong stimulus for ADH and thirst.[6]

During the early or initial stages of hypovolemic shock, vasoconstriction decreases the size of the vascular compartment and increases systemic vascular resistance. This response usually is all that is needed when the injury is slight and blood loss is minimal (e.g., 10% or less). As hypovolemic shock progresses, vasoconstriction of the blood vessels that supply the skin, skeletal muscles, kidneys, and abdominal organs becomes more severe, with a further decrease in blood flow and conversion to anaerobic metabolism resulting in cellular injury.

Manifestations. The signs and symptoms of hypovolemic shock depend on its severity and are closely related to low peripheral blood flow and excessive sympathetic stimulation. They include thirst, increased heart rate, cool and clammy skin, decreased arterial blood pressure, oliguria (decreased urine output), and changes in mentation.[50,51] Laboratory tests of hemoglobin and hematocrit provide information regarding the severity of blood loss or hemoconcentration due to dehydration. Serum lactate levels and arterial pH provide information about the severity of acidosis due to anaerobic metabolism.[52]

Early signs of hypovolemic shock include tachycardia, peripheral vasoconstriction, and a slight increase or decrease in blood pressure, as the body tries to maintain cardiac output despite the decrease in stroke volume. Thirst is an early symptom in hypovolemic shock.

In moderate to severe shock arterial blood pressure is decreased. However, controversy exists over the value of blood pressure measurements in the early diagnosis and management of shock. This is because compensatory mechanisms tend to preserve blood pressure until shock is relatively far advanced.[51] Furthermore, a normal arterial pressure does not ensure adequate tissue perfusion and oxygenation of vital organs at the cellular level. This does not imply that blood pressure should not be closely monitored in patients at risk for development of shock, but it does indicate the need for other assessment measures.

As shock progresses, the respirations become rapid and deep to compensate for the increased production of acid and decreased availability of oxygen. Decreased intravascular volume results in decreased venous return to the heart and a decreased central venous pressure (CVP). The pulse becomes weak and thready, indicating vasoconstriction and reduced filling of the vascular compartment. When shock becomes severe, the peripheral veins may collapse. Sympathetic stimulation leads to intense vasoconstriction of the skin vessels, which results in cool and mottled skin. In hemorrhagic shock, the loss of red blood cells results in pallor of the skin and mucous membranes.

Urine output decreases very quickly in hypovolemic shock. Compensatory mechanisms decrease renal blood flow as a means of diverting blood flow to the heart and brain. Oliguria of 20 mL/hour or less indicates inadequate renal perfusion. Continuous measurement of urine output is essential for assessing the circulatory and volume status of the person in shock and monitoring the response to fluid replacement.

Restlessness, agitation, and apprehension are common in early shock because of increased sympathetic outflow and increased levels of epinephrine. As the shock progresses and blood flow to the brain decreases, restlessness is replaced by altered arousal and mentation. Loss of consciousness and coma may occur if the person does not receive or respond to treatment.

Treatment. The treatment of hypovolemic shock is directed toward correcting or controlling the underlying cause (replacing or shifting volume) and improving tissue perfusion. Ongoing loss of blood must be corrected, such as in surgery. Oxygen is administered to increase oxygen delivery to the tissues. Medications usually are administered intravenously. Frequent measurements of heart rate and cardiac rhythm, blood pressure, and urine output are used to assess the severity of circulatory compromise and to monitor treatment.

Restoration of vascular volume can be accomplished through intravenous administration of fluids, blood and blood products.[52] The crystalloids (e.g., isotonic saline and Ringer lactate) are readily available and effective, at least temporarily. Colloids or plasma volume expanders (e.g., pentastarch and colloidal albumin) have a high molecular weight, do not necessitate blood typing, and remain in the vascular space for longer periods than crystalloids such as dextrose and saline, but are considerably more expensive.[52,53] Blood or blood products (packed or frozen red cells) are administered based on hematocrit and hemodynamic findings. Fluids and blood are best administered based on volume indicators such as CVP and urine output.

Vasoactive medications are agents capable of constricting or dilating blood vessels. Considerable controversy exists about the advantages or disadvantages related to the use of these drugs. As a general rule, vasoconstrictor agents are not used as a primary form of therapy in hypovolemic shock, and may be detrimental.[54] Replacing volume is the first priority but vasopressor and inotropic agents may be used as an adjunct to help restore tissue perfusion and normalize cellular metabolism. These agents are given only when volume deficits have been corrected yet hypotension persists.

Cardiogenic Shock

Cardiogenic shock occurs when the heart fails to pump blood sufficiently to meet the body's demands (see Fig. 20-7). Clinically, it is defined as decreased cardiac output, hypotension, hypoperfusion, and indications of tissue hypoxia despite an adequate intravascular volume.[55,56] Cardiogenic shock most commonly occurs from an acute myocardial infarction,[57] but may also occur from non-ischemic causes including myocardial contusion, acute mitral valve regurgitation due to papillary muscle rupture, sustained arrhythmias, severe dilated cardiomyopathy, and cardiac surgery. Cardiogenic shock can also occur with other types of shock because of inadequate coronary blood flow. Approximately 3% to 6% of the patients with ST elevation MI (STEMI) develop cardiogenic shock despite receiving reperfusion therapy (see Chapter 19).[55-57] Most patients who die of cardiogenic shock have had extensive damage to the left ventricle because of a recent infarct or reinfarction.

Regardless of cause, in persons with cardiogenic shock there is failure to eject blood from the heart, hypotension, and inadequate cardiac output. Compensatory neurohumoral responses take place, which include activation of the sympathetic and renin-angiotensin systems leading to vasoconstriction, tachycardia, and fluid retention. Increased systemic vascular resistance often contributes to the deterioration of cardiac function by increasing afterload or the resistance to ventricular systole. Preload, the filling pressure, also is increased as blood returning to the heart is added to blood that previously was not pumped forward, resulting in an increase in end-systolic ventricular volume. Increased resistance to ventricular systole (i.e., afterload) combined with decreased myocardial contractility causes an increase in end-systolic ventricular volume and preload, further complicating cardiac status.

Manifestations. The signs and symptoms of cardiogenic shock are consistent with those of end-stage heart failure. The lips, nail beds, and skin may become cyanotic because of stagnation of blood flow and increased extraction of oxygen from the hemoglobin as it passes through the capillary bed. Mean arterial and systolic blood pressures decrease due to poor stroke volume, and there is a narrow pulse pressure and near-normal diastolic blood pressure because of arterial vasoconstriction. Urine output decreases because of lower renal perfusion pressures and the increased release of aldosterone. Elevated preload is reflected in a rise in CVP and pulmonary capillary wedge pressure of at least 15 mm Hg. Neurologic changes, such as alterations in cognition or consciousness, may occur because of low cardiac output and poor cerebral perfusion.

Treatment. Treatment of cardiogenic shock requires striking a precarious balance between improving cardiac output, reducing the workload and oxygen needs of the myocardium, and increasing coronary perfusion.[56,58] Fluid volume must be regulated within a level that optimizes the filling pressure and stroke volume. Pulmonary edema and arrhythmias should be corrected or prevented to increase stroke volume and decrease the oxygen demands of the heart. Coronary artery perfusion is increased by promoting coronary artery vasodilation, increasing blood pressure, decreasing ventricular wall tension, and decreasing intracardiac pressures. Currently there are two therapeutic options for patients with cardiogenic shock to support the circulation—pharmacologic therapy and mechanical support.

The goal of pharmacologic treatment is to increase cardiac contractility without increasing heart rate. Dopamine, dobutamine and norepinephrine are the most commonly used inotropic and vasopressor agents.[56,58,59] Dopamine is often the drug of choice because it acts both as an inotrope as well as a vasoconstrictor. Dobutamine, an inotropic agent with arterial vasodilator properties, can be used in persons with less severe hypotension. Catecholamines, such as norepinephrine, increase cardiac contractility but also result in arterial constriction and tachycardia, which worsens the imbalance between myocardial oxygen supply and demand. Overall, these drugs must be used with caution as they have been associated with dysrhythmias, myocardial injury, and increased mortality.[56,58]

Mechanical support using an intra-aortic balloon pump or extracorporeal membrane oxygenation can help to increase systemic blood flow and stabilize the patient.[60] The percutaneous intra-aortic balloon pump, also referred to as counterpulsation, enhances coronary and systemic perfusion yet decreases afterload and myocardial oxygen demands.[56,60] The device, which pumps in synchrony with the heart, consists of a balloon that is inserted through a catheter into the descending aorta (Fig. 20-9). The balloon is timed to inflate during ventricular diastole and deflate just before ventricular systole. Diastolic inflation creates a pressure wave in the ascending aorta that increases coronary artery blood flow and a less intense wave in the lower aorta that enhances organ perfusion. The abrupt balloon deflation at the onset of systole results in a displacement of blood volume that lowers the resistance to ejection of blood from the left ventricle. Thus, the heart's pumping efficiency is increased, myocardial oxygen supply is increased, and myocardial oxygen consumption is decreased.

Obstructive Shock

The term obstructive shock describes circulatory shock that results from mechanical obstruction of the flow of blood through the central circulation (great veins, heart, or lungs; see Fig. 20-7). It is also referred to as extracardiac shock. Obstructive shock may be caused by a number of conditions, including dissecting aortic aneurysm, cardiac tamponade, pneumothorax, atrial myxoma, and evisceration of abdominal contents into the thoracic cavity because of a ruptured hemidiaphragm.[6] The most frequent cause of obstructive shock is pulmonary embolism.

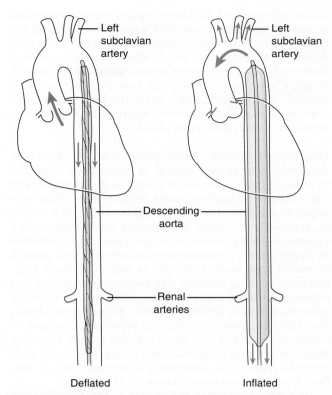

FIGURE 20-9. Aortic balloon pump placed in the descending aorta. (With permission from the Division of Cardiac Surgery; Department of Surgery; Medical University Graz, Austria.)

The primary physiologic result of obstructive shock is elevated right heart pressure due to right ventricular dysfunction. Pressures are increased despite impaired venous return to the heart. Signs of right ventricular dysfunction occur, including elevation of CVP and jugular venous distention. Treatment modalities focus on correcting the cause of the disorder, frequently requiring a procedure to remove or correct the obstruction; for example, surgical interventions such as pulmonary embolectomy, pericardiocentesis (i.e., removal of fluid from the pericardial sac) for cardiac tamponade, or the insertion of a chest tube for correction of a pneumothorax or hemothorax. In severe or massive pulmonary embolus, fibrinolytic drugs may be used to break down the clots causing the obstruction. Once the obstruction to blood flow is removed then normal blood flow can be re-established.

Distributive Shock

Distributive or vasodilatory shock is characterized by loss of blood vessel tone, enlargement of the peripheral vascular compartment, and displacement of the vascular volume away from the heart and central circulation.[61] In distributive shock, the capacity of the vascular compartment expands to the extent that a normal volume of blood does not fill the circulatory system (see Fig. 20-7). Therefore, this type of shock is also referred to as normo-volemic shock. There are two main causes of the loss of vascular tone: a decrease in the sympathetic control of vasomotor tone, or the release of excessive vasodilator substances. It can also occur as a complication of vessel damage resulting from prolonged and severe hypotension due to hemorrhage, known as irreversible or late-stage hemorrhagic shock.[61] Three shock states share the basic circulatory pattern of distributive shock: neurogenic shock, anaphylactic shock, and septic shock.

Neurogenic Shock. Neurogenic shock is caused by decreased sympathetic control of blood vessel tone due to a defect in the vasomotor center in the brain stem or the sympathetic outflow to the blood vessels.[6] The term spinal shock describes the neurogenic shock that occurs in persons with spinal cord injury (see Chapter 36). Output from the vasomotor center can be interrupted by brain injury, the depressant action of drugs, general or spinal anesthesia, hypoxia, or lack of glucose (e.g., insulin reaction). Fainting due to emotional causes is a transient form of impaired sympathetic outflow. Many general anesthetic agents can cause a neurogenic shock-like reaction, especially during induction, because of interference with sympathetic nervous system function. Spinal anesthesia or spinal cord injury above the midthoracic region can interrupt the transmission of outflow from the vasomotor center.

In contrast to other shock states, the heart rate in neurogenic shock often is slower than normal, and the skin is dry and warm. These findings are considered the cardinal signs of neurogenic shock. This type of distributive shock is rare and usually transitory.[62]

Anaphylactic Shock. Anaphylaxis is a clinical syndrome that represents the most severe systemic allergic reaction.[63] Anaphylactic shock results from an immunologically mediated reaction in which vasodilator substances such as histamine are released into the blood. These substances cause vasodilation of arterioles and venules along with a marked increase in capillary permeability. The vascular response in anaphylaxis is often accompanied by life-threatening laryngeal edema and bronchospasm, circulatory collapse, contraction of gastrointestinal and uterine smooth muscle, and urticaria (hives) or angioedema.[63]

Among the most frequent causes of anaphylactic shock are reactions to medications, such as penicillin; foods, such as nuts and shellfish; and insect venoms. The most common cause is stings from insects of the order Hymenoptera (i.e., bees, wasps, and fire ants). Latex allergy causes life-threatening anaphylaxis in a growing segment of the population (see Chapter 16). Health care workers and others who are exposed to latex are developing latex sensitivities that range from mild urticaria, contact dermatitis, and mild respiratory distress to anaphylactic shock.[64] Children with spina bifida also are at extreme risk for this serious and increasingly common allergy.[64]

The onset and severity of anaphylaxis depend on the sensitivity of the person and the rate and quantity of antigen exposure. Signs and symptoms associated with impending anaphylactic shock include abdominal cramps; apprehension; warm or burning sensation of the skin, itching, and urticaria (i.e., hives); and respiratory distress such as coughing, choking, wheezing, chest tightness, and difficulty in breathing. After blood begins to pool peripherally, there is a precipitous drop in blood pressure and the pulse becomes so weak that it is difficult to detect. Life-threatening airway obstruction may ensue as a result of laryngeal angioedema or bronchial spasm. Early signs appear with a more severe reaction. Anaphylactic shock often develops suddenly; death can occur within minutes unless appropriate medical intervention is promptly instituted.

Treatment includes immediate discontinuation of the inciting agent or action to decrease its absorption (e.g., application of ice to the site of an insect bite); close monitoring of cardiovascular and respiratory function; and maintenance of respiratory gas exchange, cardiac output, and tissue perfusion. Epinephrine, which stimulates alpha and beta receptors, is given in an anaphylactic reaction because it causes systemic vasoconstriction and relaxes the smooth muscle in the bronchioles, thus restoring cardiac and respiratory function.[65] Other treatment measures include the administration of oxygen, antihistamine drugs, corticosteroids, and bronchodilators. The person should be placed in a supine position because the sitting position can produce a severe decrease in venous return.[65]

The prevention of anaphylactic shock is preferable to treatment. Once a person has been sensitized to an antigen, the risk of repeated anaphylactic reactions with subsequent exposure is high. All health care providers should question patients regarding previous drug reactions and inform patients as to the name of the medication they are to receive before it is administered or prescribed. Persons with known hypersensitivities should wear MedicAlert jewelry and carry an identification card to alert medical personnel if they become unconscious or unable to relate this information. Persons who are at risk for anaphylaxis should be provided with emergency medications (e.g., epinephrine autoinjector), instructed to avoid the allergen, and given procedures to follow in case they are inadvertently exposed to the offending antigen.[65]

Sepsis and Septic Shock. Septic shock, which is the most common type of distributive shock, is associated with the systemic immune response to severe infection (Fig. 20-10).[66] The nomenclature related to sepsis and septic shock has been evolving. Sepsis has been defined as a suspected or proven infection plus the clinical manifestations of what has been termed the systemic inflammatory response (e.g., fever, tachycardia, and elevated white blood cell count [leukocytosis]).[66] Severe sepsis is sepsis plus evidence of sepsis-induced organ dysfunction or tissue hypoxia (e.g., hypotension, hypoxemia, oliguria, metabolic acidosis, thrombocytopenia).[67,68] Septic shock is defined as severe sepsis with hypotension, despite fluid resuscitation.[67–69]

Severe sepsis accompanied by acute organ dysfunction is a frequently occurring condition in critically ill patients. The growing incidence has been attributed to

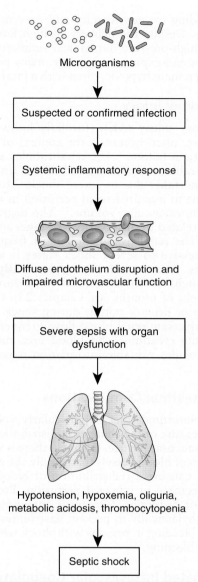

Microorganisms

Suspected or confirmed infection

Systemic inflammatory response

Diffuse endothelium disruption and
impaired microvascular function

Severe sepsis with organ
dysfunction

Hypotension, hypoxemia, oliguria,
metabolic acidosis, thrombocytopenia

Septic shock

FIGURE 20-10. Pathogenic mechanisms leading from
infection to septic shock.

enhanced awareness of the diagnosis, increased number
of resistant organisms, growing number of immunocompromised and elderly persons, and greater use of invasive procedures.[69] With early intervention and advances
in treatment methods, the mortality rate has decreased;
however, the number of deaths has increased because of
the increased prevalence.

The pathogenesis of sepsis involves a complex process
of cellular activation resulting in release of proinflammatory mediators such as cytokines; recruitment of neutrophils and monocytes; involvement of neuroendocrine
reflexes; and activation of complement, coagulation, and
fibrinolytic systems.[66] Initiation of the response begins
with activation of the innate immune system and release
of a number of proinflammatory and anti-inflammatory
mediators (Chapter 15). Two of these mediators, tumor
necrosis factor (TNF)-α and interleukin-1, are involved

in leukocyte adhesion, local inflammation, neutrophil
activation, generation of fever, tachycardia, lactic acidosis, ventilation–perfusion abnormalities, and other signs
of sepsis. Although activated neutrophils kill microorganisms, they also injure the endothelium (endothelial
dysfunction) by releasing mediators that increase vascular permeability. In addition, injured endothelial cells
release an excess of nitric oxide, a potent vasodilator
that acts as a key mediator of septic shock.

Another important aspect of sepsis that is also
related to endothelial dysfunction is an alteration of
the procoagulation–anticoagulation balance with an
increase in procoagulation factors and a decrease in
anticoagulation factors. Lipopolysaccharide on the surface of microorganisms stimulates endothelial cells lining blood vessels to increase their production of tissue
factor, thus activating coagulation[67] (see Chapter 12).
Fibrinogen is then converted to fibrin, leading to the
formation of microvascular thrombi that further
amplify tissue injury. In addition, sepsis lowers levels of
protein C, protein S, antithrombin III, and tissue factor
pathway inhibitor, substances that modulate and inhibit
coagulation.[67]

Sepsis and septic shock are typically manifested by
hypotension and warm, flushed skin. Whereas other
forms of shock (i.e., cardiogenic, hypovolemic, and
obstructive) are characterized by a compensatory
increase in systemic vascular resistance, septic shock
often presents with a decrease in systemic vascular
resistance. Hypovolemia is due to arterial and venous
dilatation, plus leakage of plasma into the interstitial
spaces. Abrupt changes in cognition or behavior are
due to reduced cerebral blood flow and may be early
indications of septic shock. Regardless of the underlying cause, fever and increased leukocytes are present. An
elevated serum lactate or metabolic acidosis indicates
anaerobic metabolism due to tissue hypoxia or cellular
dysfunction and altered cellular metabolism.[70] Tissue
hypoxia produces continued production and activation
of inflammatory mediators, resulting in further increases
in vascular permeability, impaired vascular regulation,
and altered hemostasis. As sepsis continues, organ system failure can occur. Multiple organ dysfunction is the
major cause of death in sepsis.

Early recognition of the signs and symptoms of conditions that could lead to sepsis is key to optimizing
outcomes and decreasing sepsis-related mortality. The
treatment of sepsis and septic shock focuses on control of the causative agent, support of the circulation
and the failing organ systems.[68] The administration of
antibiotics that are specific for the infectious agent is
essential. However, antibiotics do not treat inflammation; thus, the cardiovascular status of the patient must
be supported to increase oxygen delivery to the cells
and prevent further cellular injury. Swift and aggressive
fluid administration is needed to compensate for third
spacing, though which type of fluid is optimal remains
controversial.[71] Equally aggressive use of vasopressor
agents, such as norepinephrine or epinephrine, is needed
to counteract the vasodilation caused by inflammatory
mediators.[67]

Persons with severe sepsis and hyperglycemia (two consecutive blood glucose readings > 180 mg/dL) should receive insulin therapy following a protocol to maintain their blood glucose levels at a target level of ≤180 mg/dL.[67] Ongoing assessment of CVP, mixed venous or arterial oxygen saturation, mean arterial pressure, urinary output, and laboratory measurements of blood chemistries, serum lactate, base deficit, and pH are used to evaluate the progression of sepsis and adequacy of treatment as well as the need for other supportive therapies. This group of interventions lists the sepsis "bundle" that when implemented together produce better outcomes than when implemented individually.[67,68]

Complications of Shock

As the late Carl Wiggers, a noted circulatory physiologist, once stated, "shock not only stops the machine, but it wrecks the machinery."[72] Many body systems are wrecked by severe shock. Five major complications of severe shock are lung injury, acute kidney failure, gastrointestinal complications, disseminated intravascular coagulation, and multiple organ dysfunction syndrome. These complications of shock are serious and often fatal.

Acute Lung Injury/Acute Respiratory Distress Syndrome

Acute lung injury/acute respiratory distress syndrome (ALI/ARDS) is a potentially lethal form of pulmonary injury that may be either the cause or result of shock (see Chapter 23). Acute lung injury/acute respiratory distress syndrome represents a spectrum of acute respiratory failure with ARDS being the more severe form, associated with greater hypoxemia and mortality.

Acute lung injury/acute respiratory distress syndrome is marked by the rapid onset of profound dyspnea that usually occurs after an initiating event, such as trauma, aspiration, or pancreatitis. The respiratory rate and effort of breathing increase. Arterial blood gas analysis establishes the presence of profound hypoxemia that is refractory to supplemental oxygen. The hypoxemia results from impaired matching of ventilation and perfusion and from the greatly reduced diffusion of blood gases across the thickened alveolar membranes.[6]

The exact cause of ALI/ARDS is unknown. Neutrophils are thought to play a key role in its pathogenesis. A cytokine-mediated activation and accumulation of neutrophils in the pulmonary vasculature and subsequent endothelial and epithelial injury are thought to cause leaking of fluid and plasma proteins into the interstitium and alveolar spaces.[73] The fluid leakage causes atelectasis, impairs gas exchange, and makes the lung stiff (poor compliance) and more difficult to inflate. Abnormalities in the production, composition, and function of surfactant may contribute to alveolar collapse and gas exchange abnormalities. Inappropriate vasodilation and vasoconstriction worsen the ventilation and perfusion mismatch.

Interventions for ALI/ARDS focus on increasing the oxygen concentration in the inspired air and supporting ventilation mechanically to optimize gas exchange while avoiding oxygen toxicity and preventing further lung injury. Despite the delivery of high levels of oxygen using high-pressure mechanical ventilatory support and positive end-expiratory pressure, many persons with ALI/ARDS remain hypoxic, often with a fatal outcome.[74]

Acute Kidney Injury

Acute kidney injury (AKI), formerly known as acute renal failure, often occurs in the context of sepsis and multiple organ failure.[75] The renal tubules are particularly vulnerable to ischemia, and AKI is an important factor in mortality due to severe shock. Most cases of AKI are due to impaired renal perfusion in response to decreased intravascular volume.[75] The degree of renal damage is related to the severity (or stage) and duration of shock. The renal dysfunction most frequently seen with progressive to severe shock states is acute tubular necrosis. Acute tubular necrosis usually is reversible, although return to normal renal function may require weeks or months (see Chapter 25). Continuous monitoring of urinary output during shock provides a means of assessing renal blood flow. Frequent monitoring of serum creatinine and blood urea nitrogen levels also provides valuable information regarding renal status.

Gastrointestinal Complications

The gastrointestinal tract is particularly vulnerable to ischemia because of the changes in distribution of blood flow to its mucosal surface. In shock, there is widespread constriction of blood vessels that supply the gastrointestinal tract, causing a redistribution of blood flow and a severe decrease in mucosal perfusion. Proton pump inhibitors or histamine 2–receptor antagonists may be given prophylactically to prevent gastrointestinal ulcerations and bleeding in persons with shock who have risk factors for bleeding.[67]

Disseminated Intravascular Coagulation

Disseminated intravascular coagulation (DIC) is characterized by widespread activation of the coagulation system with resultant formation of fibrin clots and thrombotic occlusion of small and mid-sized vessels (see Chapter 12). The systemic formation of fibrin results from increased generation of thrombin, the simultaneous suppression of physiologic anticoagulation mechanisms, and the delayed removal of fibrin as a consequence of impaired fibrinolysis. Clinically overt DIC is reported to occur in as many as 30% to 50% of persons with Gram negative sepsis.[76] As with other systemic inflammatory responses, the derangement of coagulation and fibrinolysis is thought to be mediated by inflammatory mediators and cytokines.

The contribution of DIC to morbidity and mortality in sepsis depends on the underlying clinical condition and the intensity of the coagulation disorder. Depletion of the platelets and coagulation factors increases the risk of bleeding. Deposition of fibrin in the vasculature of organs contributes to ischemic damage and organ failure.

In a number of clinical trials, the occurrence of DIC appeared to be associated with an unfavorable outcome and was an independent predictor of mortality. The mortality rates for persons admitted to the intensive care unit who developed DIC were 45% to 78%.[76] However, it remains uncertain whether DIC was a predictor of unfavorable outcome or merely a marker of the seriousness of the underlying condition causing the DIC.

The management of sepsis-induced DIC focuses on treatment of the underlying disorder and measures to interrupt the coagulation process. Anticoagulation therapy and administration of platelets and plasma may be used. Clinical trials have shown modest to marked reductions in mortality based on the dose of antithrombin III used.

Multiple Organ Dysfunction Syndrome

Multiple organ dysfunction syndrome (MODS) represents the presence of altered organ function in an acutely ill patient such that homeostasis cannot be maintained without intervention.[77,78] As the name implies, MODS commonly affects multiple organ systems, including the kidneys, lungs, liver, brain, and heart. Multiple organ dysfunction syndrome is a particularly life-threatening complication of shock, especially septic shock. It has been reported as the most frequent cause of death in the noncoronary intensive care unit. Mortality rates vary from 30% to 100%, depending on the number of organs involved.[77] A high mortality rate is associated with failure of the brain, liver, kidneys, and lungs. The pathogenesis of MODS is not clearly understood, and current management therefore is primarily supportive. Major risk factors for the development of MODS are severe trauma, sepsis, prolonged periods of hypotension, hepatic dysfunction, infarcted bowel, advanced age, and alcohol abuse. Interventions for multiple organ failure are focused on support of the affected organs.

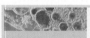 **SUMMARY CONCEPTS**

- Circulatory shock is a life-threatening condition in which body tissues are deprived of oxygen and cellular nutrients or are unable to use these materials in their metabolic processes. The clinical presentation varies and is dependent upon the length of time tissue perfusion has been compromised.

- The manifestations of circulatory shock reflect both the impaired perfusion of body tissues and the body's attempt to maintain tissue perfusion through conservation of water by the kidney, translocation of fluid from the extracellular to the intravascular compartment, and activation of sympathetic nervous system mechanisms that increase heart rate and divert blood from less essential to more essential body tissues.

- Circulatory shock can result from insufficient volume within the vascular compartment (i.e., hypovolemic shock), failure of the heart as a pump (cardiogenic shock), obstruction of blood flow or venous return to the heart (i.e., obstructive shock), or a maldistribution of blood due to expanded vascular space as a result of excessive vasodilation (i.e., distributive shock).

- Hypovolemic shock, which serves as a prototype for circulatory shock, is characterized as low peripheral blood flow and excessive compensatory sympathetic stimulation. Decreased intravascular volume produces thirst, changes in skin temperature, decreased blood pressure, increased heart rate, decreased venous pressure, decreased urine output, and changes in the sensorium. The intense vasoconstriction that serves to maintain blood flow to the heart and brain causes a decrease in tissue perfusion, impaired cellular metabolism, excessive production of lactic acid, and, eventually, cell death. Whether the shock is irreversible or the patient will survive is determined largely by changes that occur at the cellular level.

- Cardiogenic shock occurs when the heart suddenly fails to pump blood sufficiently to meet the body's demands. It most commonly occurs from an acute myocardial infarction, but may occur with other types of shock because of inadequate coronary blood flow.

- Obstructive shock results from mechanical obstruction of the flow of blood through the central circulation (great veins, heart, or lungs) that can be caused by a number of conditions, including dissecting aortic aneurysm, cardiac tamponade, pneumothorax, atrial myxoma, and evisceration of abdominal contents into the thoracic cavity because of a ruptured hemidiaphragm.

- There are three types of distributive shock that share the same basic circulatory pattern: neurogenic shock, anaphylactic shock, and septic shock. Septic shock, which is the most common of the three types, is a complex process that is associated with impaired tissue perfusion and an imbalance in the inflammatory response. Sepsis and septic shock have a high mortality rate.

- The complications of shock result from the continued deprivation of blood flow to vital organs or systems. Acute lung injury/acute

(continued)

SUMMARY CONCEPTS *(continued)*

respiratory distress syndrome (ALI/ARDS) is characterized by changes in the permeability of the alveolar–capillary membrane with development of interstitial edema and severe hypoxemia that is refractory to oxygen therapy. The renal tubules are particularly vulnerable to ischemia, and acute kidney injury is an important complication of shock. Gastrointestinal ischemia may lead to gastrointestinal bleeding and increased vascular permeability to intestinal bacteria, which can cause further sepsis and shock. Disseminated intravascular coagulation (DIC) is characterized by formation of small clots in the circulation. Multiple organ dysfunction syndrome (MODS), perhaps the most ominous complication of shock, rapidly depletes the body's ability to compensate and ultimately recover from the shock state.

REVIEW EXERCISES

1. A 75-year-old woman with long-standing hypertension and angina due to coronary heart disease presents with ankle edema, nocturia, increased shortness of breath with activity, and a chronic nonproductive cough. Her blood pressure is 170/80 and her heart rate 92. Electrocardiography and chest radiography indicate the presence of left ventricular hypertrophy.

   A. Relate the presence of uncontrolled hypertension and coronary artery disease to the development of heart failure in this woman.
   B. Explain the significance of left ventricular hypertrophy in terms of both a compensatory mechanism and a pathologic mechanism in the progression of heart failure.
   C. Use Figure 20-2 to explain this woman's symptoms, including shortness of breath and nonproductive cough.

2. A 26-year-old man is admitted to the emergency department after an automobile injury with excessive blood loss. He is alert and anxious, his skin is cool and moist, his heart rate is 135, and his blood pressure is 100/85. He is receiving intravenous fluids, which were started at the scene of the accident by an emergency medical technician. He has been typed and cross-matched for blood transfusions and a urinary catheter has been inserted to monitor his urinary output. His urinary output has been less than 10 mL since admission and his blood pressure has dropped to 85/70. Efforts to control his bleeding have been unsuccessful and he is being prepared for emergency surgery.

   A. Use information regarding the compensatory mechanisms in circulatory shock to explain this man's presenting symptoms, including urinary output.
   B. Use Figure 20-8 to hypothesize about this man's blood loss and maintenance of blood pressure.
   C. The treatment of hypovolemic shock is usually directed at maintaining the circulatory volume through fluid resuscitation rather than maintaining the blood pressure through the use of vasoactive medications. Explain.

REFERENCES

1. Yancy CW, Jessup M, Bozkurt B, et al. 2013 ACCF/AHA guideline for the management of heart failure: a report of the American College of Cardiology Foundation/American Heart Association Task Force on practice guidelines. *Circulation.* 2013;128(16):e240–e327.
2. Arnold JMO, Liu P, Demers C, et al. Canadian Cardiovascular Society consensus conference recommendations on heart failure 2006: diagnosis and management. *Can J Cardiol.* 2006;22:23–45.
3. Bibbins-Domingo K, Pletcher MJ, Lin F, et al. Racial differences in incident heart failure among young adults. *N Engl J Med.* 2009;360(12):1179–1190.
4. Mozaffarian D, Anker SD, Anand I, et al. Prediction of mode of death in heart failure: the seattle heart failure model. *Circulation.* 2007;116(4):392–398.
5. Opie LH, Hassenfuss G. Mechanisms of cardiac contraction and relaxation. In: Bonow R, Mann DL, Zipes DP, et al., eds. *Braunwald's Heart Disease: A Textbook of Cardiovascular Medicine.* 9th ed. Philadelphia, PA: Elsevier Saunders; 2012:459–486.
6. Guyton AC, Hall JE. *Textbook of Medical Physiology.* 11th ed. Philadelphia, PA: Elsevier Saunders; 2011:106, 255–254, 273–282.
7. Vuckovic KM, Fink AM. The 6-min walk test: is it an effective method for evaluating heart failure therapies? *Biol Res Nurs.* 2012;14(2):147–159.
8. Klabunde RE. *Cardiovascular Physiology Concepts.* Philadelphia, PA: Wolters Kluwer Health | Lippincott Williams & Wilkins; 2011.
9. Piano MR, Bondmass M, Schwertz DW. The molecular and cellular pathophysiology of heart failure. *Heart Lung.* 1998;27(1):3–19.
10. Mann DL. Pathophysiology of heart failure. In: Bonow R, Mann DL, Zipes DP, et al., eds. *Braunwald's Heart Disease: A Textbook of Cardiovascular Medicine.* 9th ed. Philadelphia, PA: Elsevier Saunders; 2012:487–504.
11. Piano MR, Law WR. Cardiovascular physiology: the myocardium. In: Moser DK, Riegel B, eds. *Cardiac Nursing: A Companion to Braunwald's Heart Disease.* Philadelphia, PA: Elsevier Saunders; 2007.
12. Thomas GD. Neural control of the circulation. *Adv Physiol Educ.* 2011;35(1):28–32.
13. Ronco C, Kaushik M, Valle R, et al. Diagnosis and management of fluid overload in heart failure and cardio-renal syndrome: the "5B" approach. *Semin Nephrol.* 2012;32(1):129–141.
14. Levin ER, Gardner DG, Samson WK. Natriuretic peptides. *N Engl J Med.* 1998;339:321–328.
15. Spieker LE, Lüscher TF. Will endothelin receptor antagonists have a role in heart failure? *Med Clin N Am.* 2003;87:459–474.

16. Hunter JJ, Chien KR. Signaling pathways for cardiac hypertrophy and failure. *N Engl J Med.* 1999;341(17):1276–1283.

17. Chatterjee K. Pathophysiology of systolic and diastolic failure. *Med Clin North Am.* 2012;96:891–899.

18. Brouwers FB, Hillege HL, van Gist WH, et al. Comparing new onset heart failure with reduced ejection fraction and new onset heart failure with preserved heart failure. *Curr Heart Fail Rep.* 2012;9:363–368.

19. Redfield M. Heart failure with normal ejection fraction. In: Bonow R, Mann DL, Zipes DP, et al., eds. *Braunwald's Heart Disease: A Textbook of Cardiovascular Medicine.* 9th ed. Philadelphia, PA: Elsevier Saunders; 2012:586–600.

20. Bortaug BA, Paulus WJ. Heart failure with preserved ejection fraction: pathophysiology, diagnosis, and treatment. *Eur Heart J.* 2011;32:670–679.

21. Fletcher L, Thomas D. Congestive heart failure: understanding the pathophysiology and management. *J Am Acad Nurse Pract.* 2001;13,249–257.

22. McMurray JJV. Systolic heart failure. *N Engl J Med.* 2010;362(3):228–238.

23. Wu EB, Yu CM. Management of diastolic heart failure: a practical review of pathophysiology and treatment trial data. *Int J Clin Pract.* 2005;59:1239–1246.

24. Aurigemma GP, Gaasch WH. Diastolic heart failure. *N Engl J Med.* 2004;351:1095–1105.

25. Haney S, Sur D, Xu Z. Diastolic heart failure: a review and primary care perspective. *J Am Board Fam Pract.* 2005;18:189–195.

26. Guglin M, Verma S. Right side of heart failure. *Heart Fail Rev.* 2012;17:511–527.

27. Budev MM, Arroliga AC, Wiedemann HP, et al. Cor pulmonale: an overview. *Semin Respir Crit Care Med.* 2003;23:233–243.

28. Greenberg B, Kahn AM. Clinical assessment of heart failure. In: Bonow R, Mann DL, Zipes DP, et al., eds. *Braunwald's Heart Disease: A Textbook of Cardiovascular Medicine.* 9th ed. Philadelphia, PA: Elsevier Saunders; 2012:505–516.

29. Calvin AD, Albuquerque FN, Adachi T, et al. Obstructive sleep apnea and heart failure. *Curr Treat Options Cardiovasc Med.* 2009;11(6):447–454.

30. Brack T. Cheyne-Stokes respiration in patients with congestive heart failure. *Swiss Med Wkly.* 2003;133:605–610.

31. Pureza V, Florea VG. Mechanisms for cachexia in heart failure. *Curr Heart Fail Rep.* 2013;10(4):307–314.

32. Crijns HJ, Tjeerdsma G, DeKam PJ, et al. Prognostic value of the presence and development of atrial fibrillation in patients with advanced chronic HF. *Eur Heart J.* 2000;21:1238–1245.

33. Gheorghiade M, Zannad F, Sopko G, et al. Acute heart failure syndrome: current state and framework for future research. *Circulation.* 2005;112:3958–3968.

34. Mebazaa A, Gheorghliade M, Piña IL. Practical recommendations for prehospital and early in-hospital management of patients presenting with acute heart failure syndromes. *Crit Care Med.* 2008;36(1 suppl):S129–S139.

35. Chen HH, Schrier RW. Pathophysiology of volume overload in acute heart failure syndromes. *Am J Med.* 2006;119(12A):S11–S26.

36. Kale P, Fang JC. Devices in acute heart failure. *Crit Care Med.* 2008;36(1 suppl):S121–S128.

37. Clerico A, Vittorini S, Passino C. Circulating forms of the B-type natriuretic peptide prohormone: pathophysiologic and clinical considerations. *Adv Clin Chem.* 2012;58:31–44.

38. Bridges EJ. Hemodynamic monitoring. In: Woods SL, Froelicher ESS, Motzer SU, et al., eds. *Cardiac Nursing.* 5th ed. Philadelphia, PA: Lippincott Williams & Wilkins; 2005:478–526.

39. Riegel B, Moser DK, Anker SD, et al. State of the science: promoting self-care in persons with heart failure: a scientific statement from the American Heart Association. American Heart Association Council on Cardiovascular Nursing; American Heart Association Council on Cardiovascular Nursing; American Heart Association Council on Clinical Cardiology; American Heart Association Council on Nutrition, Physical Activity, and Metabolism; American Heart Association Interdisciplinary Council on Quality of Care and Outcomes Research. *Circulation.* 2009;120(12):1141–1163.

40. Katzung BG. Drugs used in heart failure. In: Katzung BG, Masters SB, Trevor AJ, eds. *Basic & Clinical Pharmacology.* 12th ed. New York, NY: McGraw-Hill; 2012.

41. Slaughter MS, Pagani FD, Rogers JG. Clinical management of continuous-flow left ventricular assist devices in advanced heart failure. *J Heart Lung Transplant.* 2010;29:S1–S39.

42. Wheeldon DR. Mechanical circulatory support: state of the art and future perspectives. *Perfusion.* 2003;8:233–243.

43. Patel ND, Barreiro CJ, Williams JA, et al. Surgical ventricular remodeling for patients with clinically advanced congestive HF and severe left ventricular dysfunction. *J Heart Lung Transplant.* 2005;24:2202–2210.

44. Thomas S, Rich MW. Epidemiology, pathophysiology, and prognosis of heart failure in the elderly. *Clin Geriatr Med.* 2007;23:1–10.

45. Rich MW. Heart failure in older adults. *Med Clin North Am.* 2006;90:863–885.

46. Schwartz JB, Zipes DP. Cardiovascular disease in the elderly. In: Bonow RO, Mann DL, Zipes DP, et al., eds. *Braunwald's Heart Disease: A Textbook of Cardiovascular Medicine.* 9th ed. Philadelphia, PA: Elsevier Saunders; 2012:1727–1756.

47. Abdelhafiz AH. Heart failure in older people: causes, diagnosis, and treatment. *Age Ageing.* 2002;31:29–36.

48. Holmes CL, Walley KR. The evaluation and management of shock. *Clin Chest Med.* 2003;24:775–789.

49. Graham CA, Parke TRJ. Critical care in the emergency department: shock and circulatory support. *Emerg Med J.* 2005;22:17–21.

50. Guly HR, Bouamra O, Spiers M, et al. Vital signs and estimated blood loss in patients with major trauma: testing the validity of the ATLS classification of hypovolaemic shock. *Resuscitation.* 2011;82:556–559.

51. Dutton RP. Current concepts in hemorrhagic shock. *Anesthesiol Clin.* 2007;25:23–34.

52. Reinhart K, Perner A, Sprung CL, et al. Consensus statement of the ESICM task force on colloid volume therapy in critically ill patients. *Intensive Care Med.* 2012;3:368–383.

53. Perel P, Roberts I, Ker K. Colloids versus crystalloids for fluid resuscitation in critically ill patients. *Cochrane Database Syst Rev.* 2013;2:CD000567.

54. Hollenberg SM. Vasoactive drugs in circulatory shock. *Am J Respir Crit Care Med.* 2011;183:847–855.

55. Buerke M, Lemm H, Dietz K. Pathophysiology, diagnosis, and treatment of infarction-related cardiogenic shock. *Herz.* 2011;36:73–83.

56. Antman EM, Morrow DA. ST-elevation myocardial infarction: management. In: Bonow RO, Mann DL, Zipes DP, et al., eds. *Braunwald's Heart Disease: A Textbook of Cardiovascular Medicine.* 9th ed. Philadelphia, PA: Elsevier Saunders; 2012:1111–1170.

57. Goldberg RJ, Spencer FA, Gore JM, et al. Thirty-year trends (1975 to 2005) in the magnitude of, management of, and hospital death rates associated with cardiogenic shock in patients with acute myocardial infarction: a population-based perspective. *Circulation.* 2009;119:1211–1219.

58. Abdel-Qadir HM, Ivanov J, Austin PC, et al. Temporal trends in cardiogenic shock treatment and outcomes among Ontario patients with myocardial infarction between 1992 and 2008. *Circ Cardiovasc Qual Outcomes.* 2011;4:440–447.

59. Topalian S, Ginsberg F, Parrillo JE. Cardiogenic shock. *Crit Care Med.* 2008;36(1):S66–S74.

60. Ouweneel DM, Henriques JPS. Percutaneous cardiac support devices for cardiogenic shock: current indications and recommendations. *Heart.* 2012;98:1246–1254.

61. Landry DW, Oliver JA. The pathogenesis of vasodilatory shock. *N Engl J Med.* 2001;345:588–595.

62. Popa C, Popa F, Grigorean VT, et al. Vascular dysfunctions following spinal cord injury. *J Med Life.* 2010;3:275–285.

63. Lee JK, Vadas P. Anaphylaxis: mechanisms and management. *Clin Exp Allergy.* 2011;41:923–938.

64. Taylor JS, Erkek E. Latex allergy: diagnosis and management. *Dermatol Ther.* 2004;17:289–301.

65. Brown SGA. The pathophysiology of shock in anaphylaxis. *Immunol Allergy Clin N Am.* 2007;27:165–175.

66. Annane D, Bellissant E, Cavaillon JM. Septic shock. *Lancet.* 2005;365:63–78.

67. Dellinger RP, Levy MM, Rhodes A, et al. Surviving sepsis campaign: International guidelines for management of severe sepsis and septic shock. *Crit Care Med.* 2013;39:165–228.

68. Kleinpell R, Aitken L, Schorr CA. Implications of the new international sepsis guidelines for nursing care. *Am J Crit Care.* 2013;22:212–222.

69. Angus DC, van der Poll T. Severe sepsis and septic shock. *Crit Care Med.* 2013;369(9):840–851.

70. Vincent JL, Taccone F, Schmit X. Classification, incidence, and outcomes of sepsis and multiple organ failure. *Contrib Nephrol.* 2007;156:64–74.

71. Zhong Z, Wei D, Pan HF, et al. Colloid solutions for fluid resuscitation in patients with sepsis: systematic review of randomized controlled trials. *J Emerg Med.* 2013;45(4):485–495.

72. Smith JJ, Kampine JP. *Circulatory Physiology.* Baltimore, MD: J.B. Lippincott; 1980:298.

73. Shafeeq H, Lat I. Pharmacotherapy for acute respiratory distress syndrome. *Pharmacotherapy.* 2012;10:943–957.

74. Rubenfeld GD, Herridge MS. Epidemiology and outcomes of acute lung injury. *Chest.* 2007;131:554–562.

75. Bonventre JV, Yang L. Cellular pathophysiology of ischemic acute kidney injury. *J Clin Invest.* 2011;121(11):4210–4221.

76. Singh B, Hanson AC, Alhurani R, et al. Trends in the incidence and outcomes of disseminated intravascular coagulation in critically ill patients (2004–2010): a population-based study. *Chest.* 2013;143:1235–1242.

77. Balk RA. Pathogenesis and management of multiple organ dysfunction or failure in acute sepsis and septic shock. *Crit Care Clin.* 2000;16:337–352.

78. Tsukamoto T, Chanthaphavong RS, Pape H-C. Current theories on the pathophysiology of multiple organ failure. *Injury.* 2010;41:21–26.

Porth Essentials Resources

Explore these additional resources to enhance learning for this chapter:

- NCLEX-Style Questions and Other Resources on the**Point**, http://thePoint.lww.com/PorthEssentials4e
- Study Guide for Essentials of Pathophysiology
- Concepts in Action Animations
- Adaptive Learning | Powered by PrepU, http://thepoint.lww.com/prepu

Chapter 21

Control of Respiratory Function

The primary function of the respiratory system is gas exchange, with oxygen from the air being transferred to the blood and carbon dioxide from the blood being eliminated into the atmosphere. In addition to gas exchange, the lungs serve as a host defense by providing a barrier between the external environment and the inside of the body. And finally, the lungs are metabolic organs that synthesize and break down different substances.

The content in this chapter focuses on the structure and function of the respiratory system as it relates to the exchange of gases. The function of the red cell in the transport of oxygen is discussed in Chapter 13.

Structural Organization of the Respiratory System

The respiratory system consists of the air passages, the two lungs and the blood vessels that supply them, and the respiratory muscles involved in moving air into and out of the lungs. Functionally, the respiratory system can be divided into two parts: the *conducting airways*, through which air moves as it passes between the atmosphere and the lungs, and the *respiratory airways* of the lungs, where gas exchange takes place.

The lungs are soft, spongy, cone-shaped organs located side by side in the chest cavity (Fig. 21-1). They are separated from each other by the *mediastinum* (i.e., the space between the lungs) and its contents—the heart,

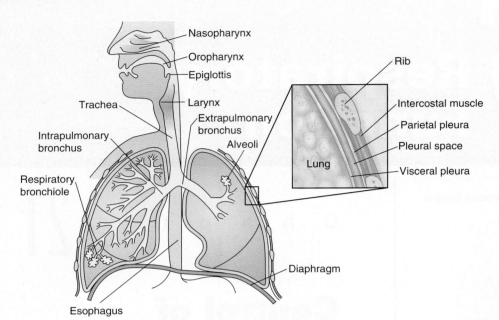

FIGURE 21-1. Structures of the respiratory system. The structures of the pleura are shown in the *inset*.

blood vessels, lymph nodes, nerve fibers, thymus gland, and esophagus. Each lung is suspended in its own pleural cavity and connected to the mediastinum by vascular and bronchial structures. The upper part of the lung, which lies against the top of the thoracic cavity, is called the *apex*, and the lower part, which lies against the diaphragm, is called the *base*.

Conducting Airways

The conducting airways consist of the nasal passages, mouth and pharynx, larynx, trachea, bronchi, and bronchioles (see Fig. 21-1). The air we breathe is warmed and moistened as it moves through these structures. Heat is transferred to the air from the blood flowing through the walls of the respiratory passages, and water from the mucous membranes is used to moisten the air.

Except for the vocal cords, which are covered with stratified epithelium, the walls of the conducting airways, including the larynx, trachea, and bronchioles, are lined by pseudostratified columnar epithelium, containing a mosaic of mucus-secreting glands, ciliated cells with hairlike projections, and serous glands that secrete a watery fluid containing antibacterial enzymes. In addition, some less common cell types are interspersed in different parts of the airway.

The mucus produced by the epithelial cells in the conducting airways forms a layer called the *mucociliary blanket* that protects the respiratory tract by entrapping dust, bacteria, and other foreign particles that enter the airways. The cilia, which constantly are in motion, propel the mucociliary blanket with its entrapped particles in an escalator-like fashion toward the oropharynx, from which it is expectorated or swallowed. The function of the cilia in clearing the lower airways and alveoli is optimal at normal oxygen levels and is impaired in situations of low and high oxygen levels. It is also impaired by drying conditions, such as breathing heated

but unhumidified indoor air during the winter months. Cigarette smoking slows down or paralyzes the motility of the cilia. This slowing allows the residue from tobacco smoke, dust, and other particles to accumulate in the lungs, decreasing the efficiency of this pulmonary defense system. As discussed in Chapter 23, these changes are thought to contribute to the development of chronic bronchitis and emphysema.

The air in the conducting airways is kept moist by water contained in the mucous layer of the upper airways and tracheobronchial tree. The capacity of the air to contain water vapor without condensation increases as the temperature rises. Thus, the air in the alveoli, which is maintained at body temperature, usually contains considerably more water vapor than the atmospheric-temperature air that we breathe. The difference between the water vapor contained in the air we breathe and that found in the alveoli is drawn from the moist surface of the mucous membranes that line the conducting airways and is a source of insensible water loss (see Chapter 8). Under normal conditions, approximately 1 pint of water is used each day to humidify the air we breathe. During fever, the water vapor in the lungs increases, causing more water to be lost through the respiratory tract. In addition, fever usually is accompanied by an increase in respiratory rate so that more air passes through the airways, withdrawing moisture from its mucosal surface. As a result, respiratory secretions thicken, preventing free movement of the cilia and impairing the protective function of the mucociliary defense system. This is particularly true in persons whose water intake is inadequate.

Nasopharyngeal Airways

The nose is the preferred route for the entrance of air into the respiratory tract during normal breathing. As air passes through the nasal passages, it is filtered, warmed, and humidified. The outer nasal passages are lined with coarse hairs, which filter and trap dust and other large particles from the air. The upper portion of the nasal cavity, which is lined with a mucous membrane that contains a rich network of small blood vessels, supplies both warmth and moisture to the air we breathe.

The mouth serves as an alternative airway when the nasal passages are plugged or when there is a need for the exchange of large amounts of air, as occurs during exercise. The oropharynx, which extends posteriorly from the soft palate to the epiglottis, is the only opening between the nose, mouth, and lungs. Both swallowed food on its way to the esophagus and air on its way to the larynx pass through it. Obstruction of the oropharynx leads to immediate cessation of ventilation.

Neural control of the tongue and pharyngeal muscles may be impaired in coma and certain types of neurologic disease. In these conditions, the tongue falls back into the pharynx and obstructs the airway, particularly if the person is lying on his or her back. Swelling of the pharyngeal structures caused by injury, infection, or severe allergic reaction also predisposes a person to airway obstruction, as does the presence of a foreign body.

Laryngotracheal Airways

The larynx, or voice box, connects the oropharynx with the trachea. The walls of the larynx are supported by rigid cartilaginous structures that prevent collapse during inspiration. The functions of the larynx can be divided into two categories: those associated with speech and those associated with protecting the lungs from substances other than air. The larynx is located in a strategic position between the upper airways and the lungs and sometimes is referred to as the "watchdog of the lungs."

The cavity of the larynx is divided into two pairs of two-by-two folds of mucous membrane stretching from front to back with an opening in the middle (Fig. 21-2).

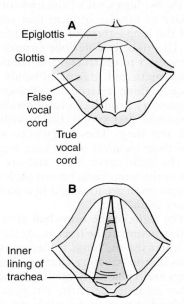

FIGURE 21-2. Epiglottis and vocal cords viewed from above with **(A)** glottis closed and **(B)** glottis open.

The upper pair of folds, called the vestibular folds or *false vocal cords*, have a protective function. The lower pair of folds, which have cordlike margins, are termed the vocal folds or *vocal cords* because their vibrations are required for making vocal sounds. The true vocal cords and the elongated opening between them make up the *glottis*. A complex set of muscles and ligaments control the opening and closing of the glottis. Speech involves the intermittent release of expired air and opening and closing of the glottis. The epiglottis, which is located above the vocal folds, is a large, leaf-shaped piece of cartilage that is covered with epithelium. During swallowing, the free edges of the epiglottis move downward to cover the larynx, thus routing liquids and foods into the esophagus.

In addition to opening and closing the glottis for speech, the vocal folds of the larynx can perform a sphincter function in closing off the airways. When confronted with substances other than air, the laryngeal muscles contract and close off the airway. At the same time, the cough reflex helps in removing the foreign substance from the airway. If the muscles that control the swallowing mechanism are partially or totally paralyzed, food and fluids can enter the airways instead of the esophagus when a person attempts to swallow. These substances are not easily removed, and when they are pulled into the lungs, they can cause a serious inflammatory condition called *aspiration pneumonia*.

Tracheobronchial Airways

The tracheobronchial airways, which consist of the trachea, bronchi, and bronchioles, can be viewed as a system of branching tubes (Fig. 21-3A). They are similar to a tree whose branches become smaller and more numerous as they divide. There are approximately 23 levels of branching, beginning with the conducting airways and ending with the respiratory airways, where gas exchange takes place (Fig. 21-3B).

The trachea, or windpipe, can be viewed as a continuous tube that connects the larynx and the major bronchi of the lungs. The wall of the trachea consists of four distinct layers: a mucosa layer of ciliated pseudostratified epithelium, a submucosal layer of dense connective tissue, a cartilaginous layer, and an outer layer of connective tissue that binds the trachea to the adjacent structures. A unique feature of the trachea is the presence of a series of horseshoe- or C-shaped rings of hyaline cartilage that prevent it from collapsing when the pressure in the thorax becomes negative (Fig. 21-4). The open part of the C-shaped ring, which abuts the esophagus, is connected by smooth muscle. Since this portion of the trachea is not rigid, the esophagus can expand anteriorly as swallowed food passes through it.

The trachea divides into two branches, forming the right and left main or primary bronchi, as it moves into the thorax (Fig. 21-5A). Between the main bronchi is a keel-like ridge called the *carina* (Fig. 21-5B). The mucosa of the carina is highly sensitive, producing violent coughing, when a foreign object (e.g., suction catheter) makes contact with it. Initially, the bronchi have

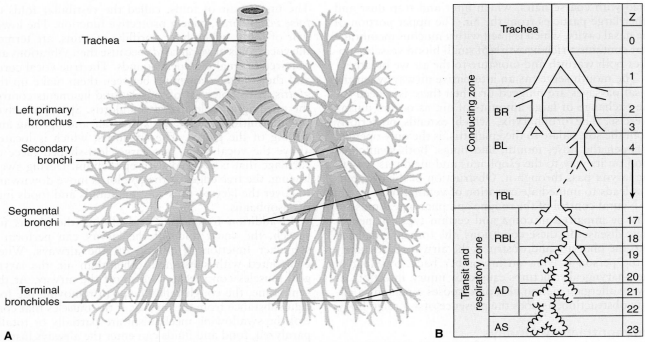

FIGURE 21-3. (A) Conducting and respiratory air pathways inferior to the larynx. (From Anatomic Chart Company. *Atlas of Human Anatomy.* Springhouse, PA: Springhouse; 2001:175.) **(B)** Idealization of the human airways. The first 16 generations of branching (Z) make up the conducting airways, and the last seven constitute the respiratory zone (or transitional and respiratory zone). AD, alveolar ducts; AS, alveolar sacs; BL, bronchiole; BR, bronchus; RBL, respiratory bronchiole; TBL, terminal bronchiole. (From Wei bei ER. *Morphometry of the Human Lung.* Berlin: Springer-Verlag;1962:111.)

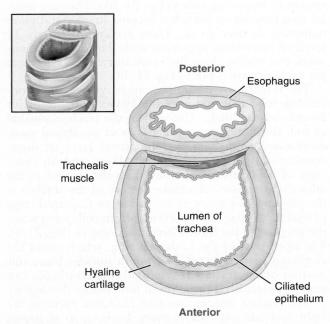

FIGURE 21-4. Cross-section of the trachea, illustrating its relationship to the esophagus, the position of the supporting hyaline cartilage rings in its wall, and the trachealis muscle connecting the free ends of the cartilage rings.

the same basic structure as the trachea. Each primary bronchus, accompanied by the pulmonary arteries, veins, and lymph vessels, enters the lung through a slit called the *hilus*.

On entering the lungs, each primary bronchus divides into secondary or lobular bronchi that supply each of the lobes of the lung—three in the right lung and two in the left. The right middle lobe bronchus, which is particularly subject to obstruction, is relatively small in diameter and length and sometimes bends sharply near its bifurcation, making it particularly subject to obstruction. The secondary bronchi, in turn, divide to form the segmental bronchi that supply the bronchopulmonary segments of the lung. These segments are identified according to their location in the lung (e.g., the apical segment of the right upper lobe) and are the smallest named units in the lung. Lung lesions such as atelectasis and pneumonia often are localized to a particular bronchopulmonary segment.

Initially, the walls of the bronchial airways have the same general structure as the trachea. At the point where the bronchi enter the the lungs to become the intrapulmonary bronchi, the structure changes (Fig. 21-6). The cartilage rings are replaced by cartilage plates of irregular shape that encircle the entire circumference of the airway. A second change that is observed in the wall of

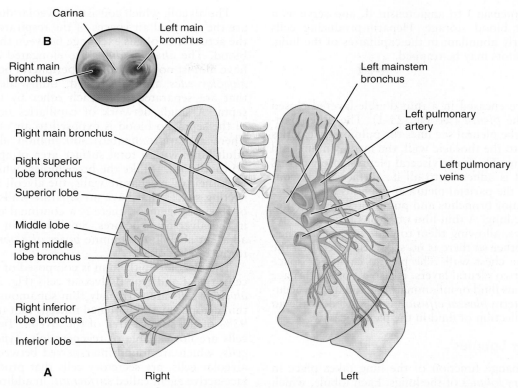

FIGURE 21-5. (A) Anterior view of respiratory structures including the lobes of the lung, the larynx, the trachea, and the main bronchi on the left and the main pulmonary artery and vein on the right. **(B)** The carina that is located at the bifurcation of right and left mainstem bronchi.

the intrapulmonary bronchus is the addition of a circumferential ring of smooth muscle.

The segmental bronchi continue to branch, forming smaller bronchi, until they become the terminal bronchioles, the smallest of the conducting airways. As these bronchi branch and become smaller, their wall structure changes. The cartilage gradually decreases and there is an increase in smooth muscle and elastic tissue with respect to the thickness of the wall. By the time the bronchioles are reached, there is no cartilage present and their walls are composed mainly of smooth muscle and elastic fibers. Bronchospasm, or contraction of these muscles, causes narrowing of the bronchioles

and impairs air flow. The elastic fibers, which radiate from the outer surface of the bronchial wall and connect with elastic fibers arising from other parts of the bronchial tree, exert tension on the bronchial walls; by pulling uniformly in all directions, they help maintain airway patency.

Lungs and Respiratory Airways

The lungs are the functional structures of the respiratory system. In addition to their gas exchange function, they inactivate vasoactive substances such as bradykinin,

FIGURE 21-6. Airway wall structure: bronchus, bronchiole, and alveolus. The bronchial wall contains pseudostratified epithelium, smooth muscle cells, mucous glands, connective tissue, and cartilage. In smaller bronchioles, a simple epithelium is found, cartilage is absent, and the wall is thinner. The alveolar wall is designed for gas exchange, rather than structural support.

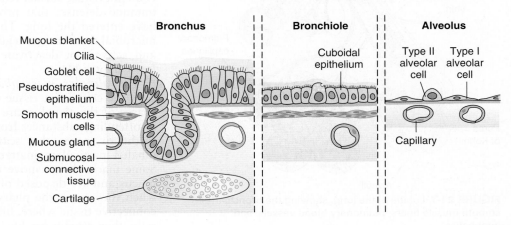

convert angiotensin I to angiotensin II, and serve as a reservoir for blood storage. Heparin-producing cells are particularly abundant in the capillaries of the lung, where small clots may be trapped.

Pleura

The lungs are encased in a thin double-layered closed sac, called the *pleura* (see Fig. 21-1). The outer parietal layer of the pleural sac lines the pulmonary cavities and adheres to the thoracic wall, the mediastinum, and the diaphragm. The inner visceral pleura closely covers the lung and is adherent to all its surfaces. It is continuous with the parietal pleura at the hilus of the lung, where the major bronchus and pulmonary vessels enter and leave the lung. A thin film of serous fluid separates the two layers, allowing them to glide over each other, yet hold together so there is no separation between the lungs and the chest wall. The pleural cavity, or space between the two pleural layers, is also a potential space in which serous fluid or inflammatory exudate can accumulate. The term *pleural effusion* is used to describe an abnormal collection of fluid in the pleural cavity.

Respiratory Lobules

The gas exchange function of the lung takes place in the *respiratory lobules* of the lungs. Each lobule, which is the smallest functional unit of the lung, is supplied by a terminal bronchiole, alveoli, and pulmonary blood vessels (Fig. 21-7). Blood enters the lobules through a pulmonary artery and exits through a pulmonary vein. Lymphatic structures surround the lobule and aid in the removal of plasma proteins and other particles from the interstitial spaces.

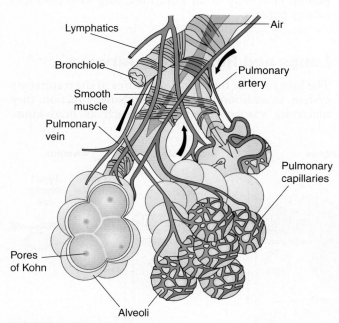

FIGURE 21-7. Lobule of the lung, showing the bronchial smooth muscle fibers, pulmonary blood vessels, and lymphatics.

The alveoli, which consist of alveolar ducts and sacs, are the terminal air spaces of the respiratory tract and the actual sites of gas exchange between the air and the blood. The *alveolar ducts* are elongated airways that have almost no walls at their peripheral boundary. The *alveolar sacs* are cup-shaped, thin-walled structures that are separated from each other by thin alveolar septa. A single network of capillaries occupies most of the septa, so blood is exposed to air on both sides. There are approximately 300 million alveoli in the adult lung, with a total surface area of approximately 50 to 100 m². Unlike the bronchioles, which are tubes with their own separate walls, the alveoli are interconnecting spaces that have no separate walls. As a result of this arrangement, there is a continual mixing of air in the alveolar structures. Small holes in the walls of adjacent alveoli, the minute *pores of Kohn*, contribute to the mixing of air.

The alveolar epithelium is composed of two types of cells: type I and type II alveolar cells (Fig. 21-8). *Type I alveolar cells* are extremely thin squamous cells with a thin cytoplasm and flattened nucleus that occupy about 95% of the surface area of the alveoli. Type I alveolar cells are not capable of regeneration. *Type II alveolar cells,* which are found interspersed between the type I alveolar cells, are secretory cells that produce the surface-active agent called *surfactant*. In addition to secreting surfactant, type II alveolar cells are the progenitor cells for type I cells. Following lung injury, they proliferate and restore both type I and type II alveolar cells. The alveoli also contain brush cells and macrophages. The brush cells, which are few in number, are thought to act as receptors that monitor the air quality of the lungs.

The *surfactant molecules* produced by the type II alveolar cells reduce the surface tension at the air-epithelium interface, and they modulate the immune functions of the lung. Recent research has identified four types of surfactant, each with a different molecular structure: surfactant proteins A, B, C, and D. Surfactants B and C serve to reduce the surface tension at the air-epithelium interface and increase lung compliance and ease of lung inflation. Surfactant B is particularly important to the generation of the surface-reducing film that makes lung expansion possible (to be discussed). Surfactants A and D do not reduce surface tension, but contribute to innate immune defenses that protect against pathogens that have entered the lung. They bind pathogens, damage microbial membranes, regulate microbial phagocytosis, and activate or deactivate the inflammatory response (see Chapter 16).

The *alveolar macrophages*, which are present in both the connective tissue of the septum and in the air spaces of the alveolus, are responsible for the removal of offending substances from the alveoli (see Fig. 21-8). In the air spaces, they scavenge the surface to remove inhaled particulate matter, such as dust and pollen. Some macrophages move up the bronchial tree in the mucus and are disposed of by swallowing or coughing when they reach the pharynx. Others enter the septal connective tissue where, filled with phagocytosed materials, they remain for life. Thus, at autopsy, the lungs

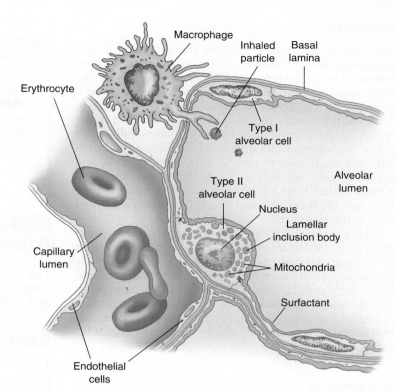

FIGURE 21-8. Schematic illustration of type I and type II alveolar cells and their relationship to the alveoli and pulmonary capillaries. Type I alveolar cells comprise most of the alveolar surface. The type II alveolar cells, which produce surfactant, are located at the corners between adjacent alveoli. Also shown are the endothelial cells, which line the pulmonary capillaries, and an alveolar macrophage.

of urban dwellers, as well as smokers, usually show many alveolar macrophages filled with carbon and other polluting particles from the environment. The alveolar macrophages also phagocytose insoluble infectious agents such as *Mycobacterium tuberculosis*. The activated macrophages then aggregate to form a fibrin-encapsulated granuloma, called a *tubercle*, which serves to contain the infection (see Chapter 23).

Pulmonary and Bronchial Circulations

The lungs are provided with a dual blood supply: the pulmonary and bronchial circulations. The pulmonary circulation arises from the pulmonary artery and provides for the gas exchange function of the lungs (see Fig. 21-7). Deoxygenated blood leaves the right heart through the pulmonary artery, which divides into a left pulmonary artery that enters the left lung and a right pulmonary artery that enters the right lung. Return of oxygenated blood to the heart occurs by way of the pulmonary veins, which empty into the left atrium. It is important to note that this is the only part of the circulation in which arteries carry deoxygenated blood and veins carry oxygenated blood.

The pulmonary circulation serves several important functions in addition to gas exchange. It removes thromboemboli (blood clots) from the circulation, functions as a metabolic organ, and serves as a blood reservoir for the left side of the heart. Small pulmonary vessels trap thromboemboli, and endothelial cells lining the vessels release fibrolytic substances that help dissolve them. Vasoactive hormones are metabolized in the pulmonary circulation. Angiotensin I is activated and converted to angiotensin II by the angiotensin-converting enzyme (ACE) located on the surface of the pulmonary capillary endothelial cells. Pulmonary endothelial cells also inactivate bradykinin, serotonin, and some of the prostaglandins. As a blood reservoir, the pulmonary circulation contains approximately 500 mL of the total blood volume. During a hemorrhagic event, some of this blood can be mobilized to improve cardiac output.

The bronchial circulation provides the blood supply for the conducting airways and the supporting structures of the lung. It also has a secondary function of warming and humidifying incoming air as it moves through the conducting airways. The bronchial arteries arise from the thoracic aorta and enter the lungs with the major bronchi, dividing and subdividing along with the bronchi as they move out into the lung, supplying them and other lung structures with oxygen. The blood from the capillaries in the bronchial circulation drains into the bronchial veins, with the blood from the larger bronchial veins emptying into the vena cava and blood from the smaller bronchial veins draining into the pulmonary veins. Because the bronchial circulation does not participate in gas exchange, this blood is deoxygenated. As a result, it dilutes the oxygenated blood returning to the left side of the heart by way of the pulmonary veins.

The bronchial blood vessels are the only ones that can undergo angiogenesis (formation of new vessels) and develop collateral circulation when vessels in the pulmonary circulation are obstructed, as in pulmonary embolism. The development of new blood vessels helps to keep lung tissue alive until the pulmonary circulation can be restored.

Innervation

The lung is innervated by both the sympathetic and parasympathetic divisions of the autonomic nervous system. The parasympathetic fibers, which are derived from vagal nerves, and the sympathetic fibers, which originate in the upper thoracic and cervical ganglia, form the pulmonary plexuses that enter the lung in the region of the hilus. Fibers from the plexus follow the major bronchi and blood vessels into the lung to innervate bronchial smooth muscle cells, blood vessels, and epithelial cells (including the goblet and submucosal glands). There is no voluntary motor innervation of the lung, nor are there any pain fibers. Pain fibers are found only in the pleura.

The parasympathetic (cholinergic) fibers are excitatory neurons that respond to acetylcholine. Stimulation of the parasympathetic nervous system is responsible for airway constriction, blood vessel dilation, and increased glandular secretion. The sympathetic nervous system, which responds to the catecholamines norepinephrine and epinephrine, produces bronchodilation, blood vessel constriction, and inhibition of glandular secretion.

■ Innervation of the lungs occurs by way of the sympathetic and parasympathetic divisions of the autonomic nervous system. Parasympathetic innervation produces airway constriction and an increase in respiratory secretions; whereas sympathetic innervation produces bronchodilation and a decrease in respiratory tract secretions.

SUMMARY CONCEPTS

■ The primary function of the respiratory system is gas exchange, with oxygen from the air being transferred to the blood and carbon dioxide from the blood being eliminated into the atmosphere.

■ Functionally, the respiratory system can be divided into two parts: the conducting airways (nasopharynx, oropharynx, larynx, trachea, and bronchi and bronchioles), through which air moves as it passes between the atmosphere and the lungs, and the respiratory airways of the lungs (terminal bronchioles and alveoli), where gas exchange takes place.

■ There are two types of alveolar cells: type I and type II. Type I alveolar cells provide the surface area for the gas exchange function of the lung. Type II alveolar cells secrete surface-active surfactants that serve to decrease alveolar surface tension (surfactants B and C) and mediate the immune destruction of pathogens that have entered the lung (surfactants A and D).

■ The lungs are provided with a dual blood supply: the pulmonary circulation, which provides for the gas exchange function of the lungs; and the bronchial circulation, which supplies blood to the conducting airways and supporting structures of the lung.

Exchange of Gases Between the Atmosphere and the Lungs

The exchange of gases between the atmosphere and the lungs occurs along a pressure gradient, moving from an area of higher pressure to one of lower pressure.

Basic Properties of Gases

The air we breathe is made up of a mixture of gases, mainly nitrogen and oxygen. These gases exert a combined pressure called the *atmospheric pressure*. The pressure at sea level is defined as 1 atmosphere, which is equal to 760 millimeters of mercury (mm Hg) or 14.7 pounds per square inch (PSI). Respiratory pressures—the pressures within the alveoli and other respiratory structures—are always expressed relative to atmospheric pressure, which is assigned a value of 0 mm Hg. This means that a respiratory pressure of +15 mm Hg is 15 mm Hg above atmospheric pressure, and a respiratory pressure of –15 mm Hg is 15 mm Hg less than atmospheric pressure. Respiratory pressures often are expressed in centimeters of water (cm H_2O) because of the small pressures involved (1 mm Hg = 1.35 cm H_2O pressure).

The pressure exerted by a single gas in a mixture is called the *partial pressure*. The capital letter "P" followed by the chemical symbol of the gas (e.g., PO_2) is used to denote its partial pressure. The law of partial pressures states that the total pressure of a mixture of gases, as in the atmosphere, is equal to the sum of the partial pressures of the different gases in the mixture. If the concentration of oxygen at 760 mm Hg (1 atmosphere) is 21%, its partial pressure is 160 mm Hg (760 × 0.21).

Water vapor is different from other types of gases; its partial pressure is affected by temperature but not atmospheric pressure. The relative humidity refers to the percentage of moisture in the air compared with the amount that the air can hold without causing condensation (100% saturation). Warm air holds more moisture than cold air. This is the reason that precipitation in the form of rain or snow commonly occurs when the relative humidity is high and there is a sudden drop in atmospheric temperature. The air in the alveoli, which remains 100% saturated at normal body temperature, has a water vapor pressure of 47 mm Hg, which must be included in the sum of the total pressure of the gases.

Pulmonary Ventilation

Ventilation refers to the exchange of gases within the respiratory system. There are two types of ventilation: pulmonary and alveolar. *Pulmonary ventilation* refers to the total exchange of gases between the atmosphere and the lungs, and *alveolar ventilation* to the transfer of gases within the gas exchange portion of the lungs.

Pulmonary ventilation relies on a system of open airways and a change in pressure that is created as the respiratory muscles change the size of the chest cage. The degree to which the lungs inflate and deflate depends on the movement of the chest cage and pressures created by respiratory muscles, the resistance that the air encounters as it moves through the airways, and the compliance or ease with which the lungs can be inflated.

Respiratory Pressures

The pressure inside the airways and alveoli of the lungs is called the *intrapulmonary pressure* or *alveolar pressure*. The gases in the lungs are in communication with atmospheric air pressure (Fig. 21-9). When the glottis is open and air is not moving into or out of the lungs, as occurs just before inspiration or expiration, the intrapulmonary pressure is zero or equal to atmospheric pressure.

The pressure in the pleural cavity is called the *intrapleural pressure*. The intrapleural pressure is always negative in relation to alveolar pressure in the normally inflated lung. The lungs are elastic structures that would collapse and expel all their air were it not for the negative intrapleural pressure (normally about −4 mm Hg between breaths) that holds them against the chest wall. During inspiration, expansion of the chest cage pulls

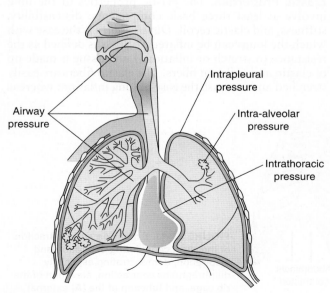

FIGURE 21-9. Partitioning of respiratory pressures.

outward on the lungs to increase the negative pressure so air can move into the lungs; and during expiration, the pressures are reversed causing air to move out of the lung. Although the intrapleural pressure of the inflated lung is always negative in relation to alveolar pressure, it may become positive in relation to atmospheric pressure (e.g., as during forced expiration and coughing).

The *intrathoracic pressure* is the pressure in the thoracic cavity. It is essentially equal to intrapleural pressure and is the pressure to which the lungs, heart, and great vessels are exposed. Forced expiration against a closed glottis (Valsalva maneuver) compresses the air in the thoracic cavity and produces marked increases in both the intrathoracic and intrapleural pressures.

Chest Cage and Respiratory Muscles

The *chest cage* is a closed compartment bounded on the top by the neck muscles and at the bottom by the diaphragm. The outer walls of the chest cage are formed by 12 pairs of ribs, the sternum, the thoracic vertebrae, and the intercostal muscles that lie between the ribs. The lungs and major airways share the inner chest cavity with the heart, great vessels, and esophagus. Mechanically, ventilation or the act of breathing depends on the fact that the chest cavity is a closed compartment whose only opening to the exterior is the trachea.

Air moves between the atmosphere and the lungs because of a pressure difference or gradient. According to the laws of physics, the pressure of a gas varies inversely with the volume of its container, with the pressure of the same quantity of gas in a smaller container being greater than that in a larger container. The movement of gases is always from the container with the greater pressure to the one with the lesser pressure. The chest cavity can be likened to a volume container in which the pressure becomes more negative during inspiration as the chest cavity expands, and becomes more positive during expiration as the chest cage contracts. Because of the change in size and pressure of the chest cage, air moves into the lungs during inspiration and out of the lungs during expiration (Fig. 21-10).

The diaphragm is the principal muscle of inspiration. When the diaphragm contracts, the abdominal contents are forced downward and the chest expands from top to bottom (see Fig. 21-10). During normal levels of inspiration, the diaphragm moves approximately 1 cm, but this can be increased to 10 cm on forced inspiration. The diaphragm is innervated by the phrenic nerve roots, which arise from the cervical level of the spinal cord, mainly from C4 but also from C3 and C5. Persons with spinal cord injury above this level require mechanical ventilation. Paralysis of one side of the diaphragm causes the chest to move up on that side rather than down during inspiration because of the negative pressure in the chest. This is called *paradoxical movement*.

The external intercostal muscles, which aid in inspiration, connect to the adjacent ribs and slope downward and forward (Fig. 21-11). When they contract, they raise the ribs and rotate them slightly so that the sternum is pushed forward, enlarging the chest from side

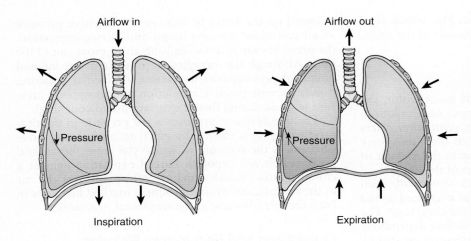

FIGURE 21-10. Movement of the diaphragm and changes in chest volume and pressure during inspiration and expiration. During inspiration, contraction of the diaphragm and expansion of the chest cavity produce a decrease in intrathoracic pressure, causing air to move into the lungs. During expiration, relaxation of the diaphragm and chest cavity produces an increase in intrathoracic pressure, causing air to move out of the lungs.

to side and from front to back. The external intercostal muscles receive their innervation from nerves that exit the central nervous system (CNS) at the thoracic level of the spinal cord. Paralysis of these muscles usually does not have a serious effect on respiration because of the effectiveness of the diaphragm.

The accessory muscles of inspiration include the scalene muscles and the sternocleidomastoid muscles. The scalene muscles elevate the first two ribs, and the sternocleidomastoid muscles raise the sternum to increase the size of the chest cavity. These muscles contribute little to quiet breathing but contract vigorously during exercise. For the accessory muscles to assist in ventilation, they must be stabilized in some way. Persons with bronchial asthma often brace their arms against a firm object during an attack as a means of stabilizing their shoulders so that the attached accessory muscles can exert their full effect on ventilation. The head commonly is bent backward so that the scalene and sternocleidomastoid muscles can elevate the ribs more effectively. Other muscles that play a minor role in inspiration are the alae nasi, which produce flaring of the nostrils during obstructed breathing.

Expiration is largely passive. It occurs as the elastic components of the chest wall and lung structures that were stretched during inspiration recoil, causing air to leave the lungs as the intrathoracic pressure increases. When needed, the abdominal and the internal intercostal muscles can be used to increase expiratory effort (see Fig. 21-11B). The increase in intra-abdominal

pressure that accompanies the forceful contraction of the abdominal muscles pushes the diaphragm upward and results in an increase in intrathoracic pressure. The internal intercostals pull the ribs downward and inward, assisting in exhalation.

Lung Compliance

Lung compliance refers to the ease with which the lungs can be inflated. Compliance can be appreciated by comparing the ease of blowing up a balloon that has been previously inflated with a new balloon that is stiff and noncompliant. Specifically, lung compliance is a measure of the change in lung volume that occurs with a change in intrapulmonary pressure.

Lung compliance is determined by the elastic properties of the lung and alveolar surface tension. It also depends on the compliance of the thoracic or chest cage. It is diminished in conditions that reduce the natural elastic properties of the lung, increase the surface tension in the alveoli, or impair the flexibility of the chest cage.

Elastic Properties. The elastic properties of the lung involve at least three basic components: distensibility, stiffness, and elastic recoil. *Distensibility* is the ease with which the lungs can be inflated *Stiffness* is defined as the resistance to stretch or inflation. Lung tissue is made up of elastin and collagen fibers. The elastin fibers are easily stretched and increase the ease of lung inflation, whereas

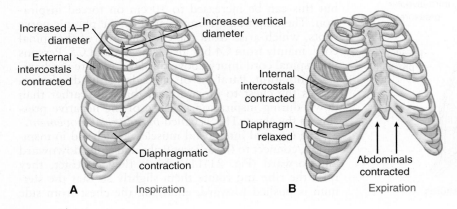

FIGURE 21-11. Expansion and contraction of the chest cage during expiration and inspiration, demonstrating especially diaphragmatic contraction, elevation of the rib cage, and function of the **(A)** external and **(B)** internal intercostals.

the collagen fibers resist stretching and make lung inflation more difficult. In lung diseases such as interstitial lung disease and pulmonary fibrosis, the lungs become stiff and noncompliant as the elastin fibers are replaced with the collagen fibers of scar tissue. Pulmonary congestion and edema produce a reversible decrease in pulmonary compliance by increasing the water content of the lung.

Elastic recoil describes the ability of the elastic components of the stretched or inflated lung to return to their original position after having been stretched. Overstretching lung tissues, as occurs with emphysema, causes the elastic components of the lung to lose their recoil, making the lung more compliant and easier to inflate but more difficult to deflate because of its inability to recoil.

Surface Tension. An important factor in lung compliance is the *surface tension* in the alveoli. The alveoli are lined with a thin film of liquid, and it is at the interface between this liquid film and the alveolar air that surface tension develops. This can be explained by the fact that the forces that hold the liquid molecules together are stronger than those that hold the air molecules together. In the alveoli, excess surface tension causes the liquid film to contract, making lung inflation more difficult.

The relationship between the pressure within a sphere such as an alveolus and the tension in the wall can be described using the law of Laplace (pressure = 2 × surface tension/radius). If the surface tension were equal throughout the lungs, the alveoli with the smallest radii would have the greatest pressure, and this would cause them to empty into the larger alveoli (Fig. 21-12A). The reason this does not occur is because of the surface tension-lowering molecules, called *surfactant*, that line the inner surface of the alveoli.

Pulmonary surfactants, particularly surfactant B, exert several important effects on lung inflation. They decrease alveolar surface tension, thereby increasing lung compliance and ease of inflation. Without this, lung inflation would be extremely difficult. In addition, surfactant helps to keep the alveoli dry and prevents the development of pulmonary edema. This is because water is pulled out of the pulmonary capillaries into the alveoli when increased surface tension causes the alveoli to recoil.

Surfactants also stabilize alveolar inflation by changing their density in relation to alveolar size, with the surfactant molecules becoming more tightly compressed in the small alveoli with their higher surface tension and less compressed in the larger alveoli with their lower surface tension (Fig. 21-12B). At low lung volumes, the molecules become tightly packed, and at higher lung volumes they spread out to cover the alveolar surface. In surgical patients and bed-ridden persons, shallow and quiet breathing often impairs the spreading of surfactant. Encouraging these persons to cough and deep breathe enhances the spreading of surfactant, allowing for a more even distribution of ventilation and prevention of atelectasis (incomplete expansion of a portion of the lung).

The type II alveolar cells that produce surfactant do not begin to mature until the 26th to 27th week

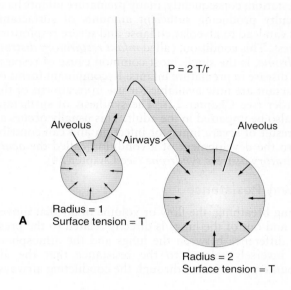

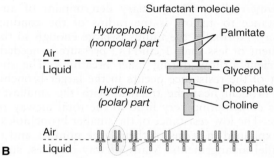

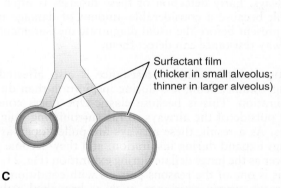

FIGURE 21-12. (A) The effect of the surface tension (forces generated at the fluid-air interface) and radius on the pressure and movement of gases in the alveolar structures. According to the law of Laplace (P = 2 T/r, P = pressure, T = tension, r = radius), the pressure generated within the sphere is inversely proportional to the radius. Air moves from the alveolus with a small radius and higher pressure to the alveolus with the larger radius and lower pressure. **(B)** The surfactant molecules with their hydrophilic heads (that attach to the fluid lining of the alveolus) and their hydrophobic tails (that are oriented toward the air interface). **(C)** The surfactant molecules form a monolayer (shaded in *blue*) that disrupts the intermolecular forces and lowers the surface tension more in the smaller alveolus with its higher concentration of surfactant than in the larger alveolus with its lower concentration of surfactant.

of gestation; consequently, many premature infants have difficulty producing sufficient amounts of surfactant. This can lead to alveolar collapse and severe respiratory distress. This condition, called *infant respiratory distress syndrome*, is the single most common cause of respiratory disease in premature infants. Recombinant forms of surfactant are now available for use in treatment of the disorder (see Chapter 22). The synthesis of surfactant can also be impaired in the adult. This usually occurs as the result of severe injury or infection and can contribute to the development of a condition called the *acute respiratory distress syndrome* (see Chapter 24).

Airway Resistance

During breathing, the flow or volume of air that moves into and out of the lungs is directly related to the pressure difference between the lungs and the atmosphere and inversely related to the resistance that the air encounters as it moves through the conducting airways.

Airway radius. The primary determinant of airway resistance to airflow is the radius of the conducting airway. Normally, the radius is large enough so that a gradient of less than 1 cm/H_2O pressure is needed for sufficient airflow during quiet breathing. The site of most of the resistance occurs in the larger bronchioles and bronchi near the trachea, with the smallest airways contributing very little to the total airway resistance. The low resistance of the smaller bronchioles can be explained in terms of their large number and their parallel arrangements. Many airway diseases, such as emphysema and chronic bronchitis, begin in the small airways. Early detection of these diseases is often difficult because a considerable amount of damage must be present before the usual diagnostic measurements of airway resistance can detect them.

Lung Volume. Airway resistance is also affected by lung volume, being less during inspiration than during expiration. This is because elastic-type fibers connect the outside of the airways to the surrounding lung tissues. As a result, these airways are pulled open as the lungs expand during inspiration, and they become narrower as the lungs deflate during expiration (Fig. 21-13). This is one of the reasons persons with conditions that increase airway resistance, such as bronchial asthma, usually have less difficulty during inspiration than during expiration.

Neural and Local Control of Airway Diameter. Constriction of bronchial smooth muscle, which controls airway diameter, also contributes to airway resistance. The smooth muscles in the airways are under autonomic nervous system control. Stimulation of the parasympathetic nervous system produces bronchial constriction as well as increased mucus secretion, whereas sympathetic stimulation has the opposite effect. Parasympathetic nerves can be stimulated by reflexes that originate in the lungs, most of which begin with irritation of the epithelial cells by cigarette smoke, dust, noxious gases, or

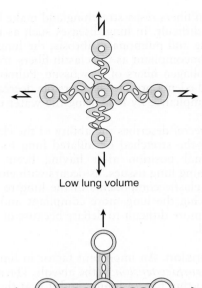

Low lung volume

High lung volume

FIGURE 21-13. Interaction of tissue forces on airways during low and high lung volumes. At low lung volumes, the tissue forces promote folding or collapsing and place less tension on the airways, which become smaller; during high lung volumes, the tissue forces stretch and pull the airways open.

bronchial infections. Inflammatory mediators such as the leukotrienes, histamine, and prostaglandins released by resident mast cells and airway epithelial cells can also cause bronchial constriction.

Many of the drugs used in the treatment of bronchial asthma and other respiratory conditions that produce bronchial constriction act at the level of the autonomic nervous system or inflammatory mediators to relieve airway obstruction. For example, β-adrenergic stimulants are often used to achieve short-term relief of asthma symptoms. Anti-inflammatory agents, such as the corticosteroids or leukotriene antagonists, are used to achieve long-term relief (see Chapter 3, Fig. 3-4).

Laminar and Turbulent Airflow. Depending on the velocity and pattern of flow, airflow can be laminar or turbulent. *Laminar*, or *streamlined*, *airflow* occurs at low flow rates in which the air stream is parallel to the sides of the airway. With laminar flow, the air at the periphery must overcome the resistance to flow; and as a result, the air in the center of the airway moves faster. In the bronchial tree with its many branches, laminar airflow probably occurs only in the very small airways, where the velocity of flow is low. Because the small airways contribute little resistance to airflow, they constitute a silent zone in terms of respiratory sounds.

Turbulent airflow is disorganized flow in which the molecules of the gas move laterally, collide with one another, and change their velocities. Whether turbulence develops depends on the radius of the airways, the interaction of the gas molecules, and the velocity of airflow. It is most likely to occur when the radius of the airways is large and the velocity of flow is high. Turbulent flow occurs regularly in the trachea. Turbulence of airflow accounts for the respiratory sounds that are heard during chest auscultation (i.e., listening to chest sounds using a stethoscope).

Airway Compression During Forced Expiration.
Airway resistance does not change considerably during normal quiet breathing, but is significantly increased during forced expiration, such as occurs during vigorous exercise. The marked changes that occur during forced expiration are the result of airway compression. Airflow through the collapsible airways in the lungs depends on the distending airway (intrapulmonary) pressures that hold the airways open and the external (intrathoracic) pressures that surround and compress the airways. The difference between these two pressures (airway minus intrathoracic pressure) is called the *transpulmonary pressure*. For airflow to occur, the distending pressure inside the airways must be greater than the compressing pressure outside the airways.

During forced expiration, the transpulmonary pressure is decreased because of a disproportionate increase in the intrathoracic pressure compared with airway pressure. The resistance that air encounters as it moves out of the lungs causes a further drop in airway pressure. If this drop in airway pressure is sufficiently great, the surrounding intrathoracic pressure will compress the collapsible airways that lack cartilaginous support, causing airflow to be interrupted and air to be trapped in the terminal airways (Fig. 21-14).

Although this type of airway compression usually is seen only during forced expiration in persons with normal respiratory function, it may occur during normal breathing in persons with lung diseases. For example, in conditions that increase airway resistance, such as asthma or chronic obstructive lung disease, the pressure drop along the smaller airways is magnified, and an increase in intra-airway pressure is needed to maintain airway patency. Measures such as pursed-lip breathing increase airway pressure and improve expiratory flow rates in persons with obstructive lung diseases (discussed in Chapter 23). This is also the rationale for using positive end-expiratory pressure in persons who are being mechanically ventilated. Infants who are having trouble breathing often grunt to increase their expiratory airway pressures and keep their airways open.

Lung Volumes and Pulmonary Function Studies

Lung volumes, or the amount of air exchanged during ventilation, can be subdivided into three components: (1) the tidal volume, (2) the inspiratory reserve volume, and (3) the expiratory reserve volume. The tidal volume (TV), usually about 500 mL, is the amount of air that moves into and out of the lungs during a normal breath (Fig. 21-15). The inspiratory reserve volume (IRV) is the maximum amount of air that can be inspired in excess of the normal TV, and the expiratory reserve volume (ERV) is the maximum amount that can be exhaled in excess of the normal TV. Approximately 1200 mL of air remains in the lungs after forced expiration; this air is the *residual volume* (RV). The RV increases with age because there is more trapping of air in the lungs at the end of expiration.

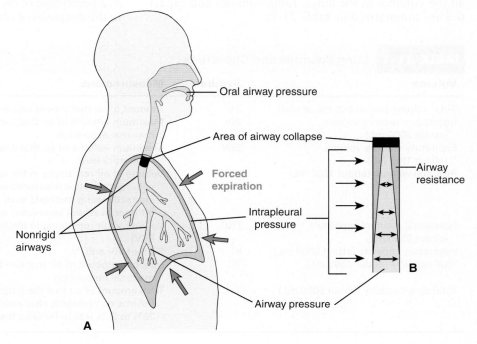

FIGURE 21-14. Mechanism that limits maximal expiratory flow rate. **(A)** Airway patency and airflow in the nonrigid airways of the lungs rely on a transpulmonary pressure gradient in which airway pressure is greater than intrapleural pressure. **(B)** Airway resistance normally produces a drop in airway pressure as air moves out of the lungs. The increased intrapleural pressure that occurs with forced expiration produces airway collapse in the nonrigid airways at the point where intrapleural pressure exceeds airway pressure.

Oral airway pressure

Area of airway collapse

Forced expiration

Airway resistance

Intrapleural pressure

Nonrigid airways

Airway pressure

A

B

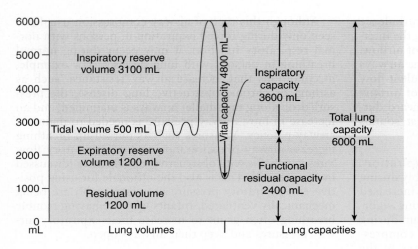

FIGURE 21-15. Spirometry recording of respiratory volumes (*left*) and diagram of lung capacities (*right*). The tidal volume (TV, yellow) is the volume of air inhaled and exhaled during normal breathing; the inspiratory reserve volume (IRV, pink), the maximal volume of air that can be forcefully inhaled in excess of the TV; the expiratory reserve volume (ERV, blue), the maximal volume of air that can be exhaled in excess of the TV; and the residual volume (RV, green), the air that continues to remain in the lung after maximal respiratory effort. The functional residual capacity (FRC) is the sum of the ERV and the RV. The vital capacity is the IRV, TV, and ERV.

Many of these volumes can be measured using an instrument called a *spirometer*. The person is asked first to breathe normally into the spirometer, during which the tidal volume is measured, and then to inhale and exhale maximally, during which the IRV and ERV are measured. The RV cannot be measured with the spirometer because this air cannot be expressed from the lungs. It is measured by indirect methods, such as the helium dilution methods, the nitrogen washout methods, or body plethysmography.

Lung capacities include two or more lung volumes. The *vital capacity* (VC) equals the IRV plus the TV and the ERV and is the amount of air that can be exhaled from the point of maximal inspiration. The *inspiratory capacity* (IC) equals the TV plus the IRV. It is the amount of air a person can breathe in beginning at the normal expiratory level. The *functional residual capacity* (FRC) is the sum of the RV and ERV; it is the volume of air that remains in the lungs at the end of normal expiration. The *total lung capacity* (TLC) is the sum of all the volumes in the lungs. Lung volumes and capacities are summarized in Table 21-1.

The previously described lung volumes and capacities are anatomic and static measurements, determined by spirometry and recorded without relation to time. The spirometer also is used to measure dynamic lung volumes (i.e., ventilation with respect to time); these tests often are used in assessing pulmonary function (Table 21-2). The *maximum voluntary ventilation* measures the volume of air that a person can move into and out of the lungs during maximum effort lasting for a specific period of time. This measurement usually is converted to liters per minute. Two other useful tests are the forced vital capacity and the forced expiratory volume. The *forced vital capacity* (FVC) involves full inspiration to total lung capacity followed by forceful maximal expiration. Obstruction of airways produces an FVC that is lower than that observed with more slowly performed vital capacity measurements. The *forced expiratory volume* (FEV) is the expiratory volume achieved in a given time period. The $FEV_{1.0}$ is the forced expiratory volume that can be exhaled in 1 second. The $FEV_{1.0}$ frequently is expressed as a percentage of the FVC. The $FEV_{1.0}$ and FVC are used in the diagnosis of obstructive lung disorders.

TABLE 21-1 Lung Volumes and Capacities

Volume	Symbol	Measurement
Tidal volume (about 500 mL at rest)	TV	Amount of air that moves into and out of the lungs with each breath
Inspiratory reserve volume (about 3000 mL)	IRV	Maximum amount of air that can be inhaled from the point of maximal expiration
Expiratory reserve volume (about 1100 mL)	ERV	Maximum volume of air that can be exhaled from the resting end-expiratory level
Residual volume (about 1200 mL)	RV	Volume of air remaining in the lungs after maximal expiration. This volume cannot be measured with the spirometer; it is measured indirectly using methods such as the helium dilution method, the nitrogen washout technique, or body plethysmography.
Functional residual capacity (about 2300 mL)	FRC	Volume of air remaining in the lungs at end-expiration (sum of RV and ERV)
Inspiratory capacity (about 3500 mL)	IC	Sum of IRV and TV
Vital capacity (about 4600 mL)	VC	Maximal amount of air that can be forcibly exhaled from the point of maximal inspiration
Total lung capacity (about 5800 mL)	TLC	Total amount of air that the lungs can hold; it is the sum of all the volume components after maximal inspiration. This value is about 20% to 25% less in females than in males.

TABLE 21-2 **Pulmonary Function Tests**

Test	Symbol	Measurement*
Maximal voluntary ventilation	MVV	Maximum amount of air that can be breathed in a given time
Forced vital capacity	FVC	Maximum amount of air that can be rapidly and forcefully exhaled from the lungs after full inspiration. The expired volume is plotted against time.
Forced expiratory volume achieved in 1 s	$FEV_{1.0}$	Volume of air expired in the first second of FVC
Percentage of forced vital capacity	$(FEV_{1.0}/FVC\%)$ $\times 100$	Volume of air expired in the first second, expressed as a percentage of FVC
Forced midexpiratory flow rate	$FEF_{25\%-75\%}$	The forced midexpiratory flow rate determined by locating the points on the volume-time curve recording obtained during FVC corresponding to 25% and 75% of FVC and drawing a straight line through these points. The slope of this line represents the average midexpiratory flow rate.
Forced inspiratory flow rate	$FIF_{25\%-75\%}$	FIF is the volume inspired from RV at the point of measurement. $FIF_{25\%-75\%}$ is the slope of a line between the points on the volume pressure tracing corresponding to 25% and 75% of the inspired volume.

*By convention, all the lung volumes and rates of flow are expressed in terms of body temperature and pressure and saturated with water vapor (BTPS), which allows for a comparison of the pulmonary function data from laboratories with different ambient temperatures and altitudes.

Efficiency and Work of Breathing

The efficiency of breathing is determined by matching the TV and respiratory rate in a manner that provides an optimal minute volume while minimizing the work of breathing. The *minute volume*, or total ventilation, is the amount of air that is exchanged in 1 minute (TV multiplied by the respiratory rate). It is determined by the metabolic needs of the body, which during normal activity are about 6000 mL (500 mL TV × respiratory rate of 12 breaths/min).

The work of breathing is determined by the amount of effort required to move air through the conducting airways and by the ease of lung expansion. Because expansion of the lungs is difficult for persons with stiff and noncompliant lungs, they usually find it easier to breathe if they keep their TV low and breathe at a more rapid rate (e.g., 300 mL × 20 breaths/min = 6000 mL/min) to achieve their minute volume and meet their oxygen needs. In contrast, persons with obstructive airway disease usually find it less difficult to inflate their lungs but expend more energy in moving air through the airways. As a result, these persons tend to take deeper breaths and breathe at a slower rate (e.g., 600 mL × 10 breaths/min = 6000 mL) to achieve their oxygen needs.

SUMMARY CONCEPTS

■ Breathing involves the movement of atmospheric air into and out of the alveolar structures in the lungs. It requires a system of open airways and alternating pressure changes resulting from the action of the respiratory muscles in changing the volume of the chest cage.

■ Lung compliance or ease with which the lungs can be inflated reflects the elastic forces of the lung tissue and the surface tension in the alveoli. Surfactant molecules, produced by type II alveolar cells, reduce the surface tension in the lungs, thereby increasing lung compliance and ease of inflation.

■ Airway resistance refers to the impediment to flow that the air encounters as it moves through the airways. It varies with airway radius and lung volume, being greatest in the bronchi with medium-sized radii and lowest in the bronchioles with their smaller radii. Airway resistance decreases as the lungs expand and pull the airways open during inspiration and it increases as the lungs deflate during expiration.

■ Lung volumes reflect the amount of air that is exchanged during normal and forced breathing. The minute volume (tidal volume [TV] multiplied by the respiratory rate) is determined by the metabolic needs of the body.

■ The efficiency of breathing is determined by matching the TV and respiratory rate in a manner that provides an optimal minute volume while minimizing the work of breathing. Persons with stiff and noncompliant lungs usually find it easier to keep their TV low and breathe at a more rapid rate, whereas those with increased airway resistance usually find it less difficult to inflate their lungs and increase their TV, while breathing at a slower rate.

Exchange of Gases Within the Lungs

The primary functions of the lungs are oxygenation of the blood and removal of carbon dioxide. Pulmonary gas exchange is conventionally divided into three processes: (1) ventilation or the flow of gases into and out of the alveoli of the lungs, (2) perfusion or flow of blood in the adjacent pulmonary capillaries, and (3) diffusion or transfer of gases between the alveoli and the pulmonary capillaries.

Alveolar Ventilation

The ultimate importance of the alveolar ventilation is to continually renew the air in the gas exchange areas of the lungs where the air is in close proximity to the blood. These areas include the alveoli, alveolar sacs, alveolar ducts, and respiratory bronchioles. It is affected by body position and lung volume as well as by disease conditions that affect the heart and respiratory system.

Distribution of Alveolar Ventilation

The distribution of ventilation between the base (bottom) and apex (top) of the lung varies with body position and reflects the effects of gravity on intrapleural pressure and lung compliance. Compliance reflects the change in volume that occurs with a change in intrapleural pressure. It is lower in fully expanded alveoli, which have difficulty accommodating more air, and greater in alveoli that are less inflated and can more easily expand to accommodate more air. In the seated or standing position, gravity exerts a downward pull on the lung, causing intrapleural pressure at the apex of the lung to become more negative. As a result, the alveoli at the apex of the lung are more fully expanded and less compliant than those at the base of the lung. The same holds true for lung expansion in the dependent portions of the lung in the supine or lateral position. In the supine position, ventilation in the lowermost (posterior) parts of the lung exceeds that in the uppermost (anterior) parts. In the lateral position (i.e., lying on the side), the alveoli in the dependent lung is better ventilated.

The distribution of ventilation also is affected by lung volumes. During full inspiration (high lung volumes) in the seated or standing position, the airways are pulled open and air moves into the more compliant portions of the lower lung. At low lung volumes, the opposite occurs. At functional residual capacity, the intrapleural pressure at the base of the lung exceeds airway pressure, compressing the airways so that ventilation is greatly reduced. In contrast, the airways in the apex of the lung remain open, and the alveoli in this area of the lung are well ventilated.

Even at low lung volumes, some air remains in the alveoli of the lower portion of the lungs, preventing their collapse. According to the law of Laplace (discussed previously), the pressure needed to overcome the tension in the wall of a sphere or an elastic tube is inversely related to its radius; therefore, the small airways close first, trapping some air in the alveoli. This trapping of air may be increased in older persons and persons with chronic lung disease owing to a loss in the elastic recoil properties of the lungs. In these persons, airway closure occurs at the end of normal instead of low lung volumes, trapping larger amounts of air that cannot participate in gas exchange.

Dead Air Space

Dead space refers to the air that must be moved with each breath but does not participate in gas exchange. The movement of air through dead space contributes to the work of breathing but not to gas exchange. Some of the air that enters the respiratory tract during breathing fails to reach the alveoli. This volume (about 150 to 200 mL), which remains in the conducting airways of the nose, pharynx, trachea, bronchi, and bronchioles and does not participate in gas exchange, is referred to as *anatomic dead space*. A second type of dead space, *physiological dead space,* consists of the total amount of air that does not participate in gas exchange. It includes the anatomic dead space plus the dead space in alveoli that are perfused, but not ventilated. Physiologic dead space tends to be the same as anatomic dead space in persons with normal respiratory function, but can be considerably larger in the presence of lung disease.

Perfusion

The term *perfusion* is used to describe the flow of blood through the gas exchange portion of the lung. Deoxygenated blood enters the lung through the pulmonary artery, which has its origin in the right side of the heart and enters the lung at the hilus, along with the primary bronchus. The pulmonary arteries branch in a manner similar to that of the airways. The small pulmonary arteries accompany the bronchi as they move down the lobules and branch to supply the capillary network that surrounds the alveoli (see Fig. 21-7). The oxygenated capillary blood is collected in the small pulmonary veins of the lobules, and then it moves to the larger veins to be collected in the four large pulmonary veins that empty into the left atrium.

The pulmonary blood vessels are thinner, more compliant, and offer less resistance to flow than those in the systemic circulation, and the pressures in the pulmonary system are much lower (e.g., 22/8 mm Hg versus 120/70 mm Hg). The low pressure and low resistance of the pulmonary circulation accommodate the delivery of varying amounts of blood from the systemic circulation without producing signs and symptoms of congestion. The volume in the pulmonary circulation is approximately 500 mL, with approximately 100 mL of this volume located in the pulmonary capillary bed. When the input of blood from the right heart and output of blood to the left heart are equal, pulmonary blood flow remains constant. Small differences between input and output can result in large changes in pulmonary volume if the differences continue for many heartbeats.

The movement of blood through the pulmonary capillary bed requires that the mean pulmonary arterial pressure be greater than the mean pulmonary venous pressure.

Distribution of Pulmonary Blood Flow

As with ventilation, the distribution of pulmonary blood flow is affected by body position and gravity. In the upright position, the distance of the upper apices of the lung above the level of the heart may exceed the perfusion capabilities of the mean pulmonary arterial pressure (approximately 12 mm Hg); therefore, blood flow in the upper part of the lungs is less than that in the base. In the supine position, the lungs and the heart are at the same level, and blood flow to the apices and base of the lungs becomes more uniform. In this position, however, blood flow to the posterior or dependent portions (e.g., bottom of the lung when lying on the side) exceeds flow in the anterior or nondependent portions of the lungs.

The alveolar concentration of oxygen also affects pulmonary blood flow. When the concentration of oxygen in air of the alveoli decreases below normal blood, the adjacent blood vessels constrict in an effort to distribute blood where it will be most effectively oxygenated. When alveolar oxygen levels drop below 60 mm Hg, marked vasoconstriction occurs, and at very low oxygen levels, the local flow may be almost abolished. In regional hypoxia, as occurs with a localized airway obstruction (e.g., atelectasis), vasoconstriction is localized to a specific region of the lung. Generalized hypoxia, such as occurs at high altitudes causes vasoconstriction throughout all of the vessels of the lung.

Shunt

Shunt refers to blood that moves from the right to the left side of the circulation without being oxygenated. As with dead air space, there are two types of shunts: anatomic and physiologic. In an *anatomic shunt*, blood moves from the venous to the arterial side of the circulation without moving through the lungs. Anatomic shunting of blood is most commonly due to congenital heart defects (see Chapter 19). In a *physiologic shunt*, there is mismatching of ventilation and perfusion within the lung, resulting in insufficient ventilation to provide the oxygen needed to oxygenate the blood flowing through the alveolar capillaries. Physiologic shunting of blood usually results from destructive lung disease that impairs ventilation or from heart failure that interferes with movement of blood through sections of the lungs.

Mismatching of Ventilation and Perfusion

The gas exchange properties of the lung depend on matching ventilation and perfusion, ensuring that equal amounts of air and blood are entering the respiratory portion of the lungs. Both dead air space and shunt produce a mismatching of ventilation and perfusion, as depicted in Figure 21-16. With shunt (depicted on the

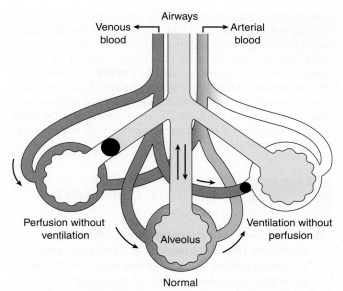

FIGURE 21-16. Matching of ventilation and perfusion. (*Center*) Normal matching of ventilation and perfusion; (*left*) perfusion without ventilation (i.e., shunt); (*right*) ventilation without perfusion (i.e., dead air space).

left), there is perfusion without ventilation, resulting in a low ventilation-perfusion ratio. It occurs in conditions such as atelectasis in which there is airway obstruction (see Chapter 23). With dead air space (depicted on the right), there is ventilation without perfusion, resulting in a high ventilation–perfusion ratio. It occurs with conditions such as pulmonary embolism, which impairs blood flow to a part of the lung. The arterial blood leaving the pulmonary circulation reflects mixing of blood from normally ventilated and perfused areas of the lung as well as areas that are not perfused (dead air space) or ventilated (shunt). Many of the conditions that cause mismatching of ventilation and perfusion involve both dead air space and shunt. In chronic obstructive lung disease, for example, there may be impaired ventilation in one area of the lung and impaired perfusion in another area.

Diffusion

Diffusion takes place in the respiratory portions of the lung and refers to the movement of gases across the alveolar–capillary membrane. Diffusion of gases in the lung is affected by (1) difference in the pressure of the gas on either side of the membrane, (2) the surface area that is available for diffusion, (3) the thickness of the alveolar–capillary membrane through which the gas must pass, and (4) the diffusion characteristics of the gas. Administration of high concentrations of oxygen increases the difference in partial pressure between the two sides of the membrane and increases the diffusion of the gas. Diseases that destroy lung tissue and the surface area for diffusion and those that increase the thickness of the alveolar–capillary membrane adversely influence the diffusing capacity of the lungs.

For example, the removal of one lung reduces the diffusing capacity by one half. The thickness of the alveolar–capillary membrane and the distance for diffusion are increased in persons with pulmonary edema or pneumonia. The characteristics of the gas and its molecular weight and solubility determine how rapidly the gas diffuses through the respiratory membranes. Carbon dioxide, for example, diffuses 20 times more rapidly than oxygen because of its greater solubility in the respiratory membranes.

SUMMARY CONCEPTS

- The primary function of the lungs, which is gas exchange, requires matching of ventilation and perfusion so that equal amounts of air and blood enter the respiratory portion of the lungs.

- Dead air space refers to areas of the lungs that are ventilated but not perfused. The *anatomic dead air space* represents the volume of air that moves through the conducting airways, but does not participate in air exchange. The *physiologic dead space* is the total volume of dead air space, including the anatomic dead space and dead space associated with ventilated but unperfused alveoli.

- Shunt refers to blood that moves from the left to the right side of the circulation without being oxygenated. In an *anatomic shunt,* blood moves directly from the venous to the arterial side of the circulation without moving through the lungs. In a *physiologic shunt,* there is an absence of ventilation in a perfused portion of the lung.

- Diffusion or movement of gases across the alveolar–capillary membranes of the lung is influenced by the: (1) difference in the partial pressures of the gas on either side of the membrane; (2) surface area available for diffusion; (3) diffusion characteristics of the gas; and (4) thickness of the alveolar-capillary membrane.

Oxygen and Carbon Dioxide Transport

Although the lungs are responsible for the exchange of gases with the external environment, it is the blood that transports these gases between the lungs and body tissues. The blood carries oxygen and carbon dioxide in the physically dissolved state and in combination with hemoglobin. Carbon dioxide also is converted to bicarbonate and transported in that form.

Dissolved oxygen and carbon dioxide exert a partial pressure that is designated in the same manner as the partial pressure in the gas state. In the clinical setting, blood gas measurements are used to determine the partial pressure of oxygen (PO_2) and carbon dioxide (PCO_2) in the blood. Arterial blood commonly is used for measuring blood gases. Venous blood is not used because venous levels reflect the metabolic demands of the tissues rather than the gas exchange function of the lungs. The PO_2 of arterial blood normally is above 80 mm Hg, and the PCO_2 is in the range of 35 to 45 mm Hg. Normally, the arterial blood gases are the same or nearly the same as the partial pressure of the gases in the alveoli. The arterial PO_2 often is written PaO_2, and the alveolar PO_2 as PAO_2, with the same types of designations being used for PCO_2. This text uses PO_2 and PCO_2 to designate both arterial and alveolar levels of the gases.

Oxygen Transport

Oxygen is transported both in the dissolved state and in chemical combination with hemoglobin. Hemoglobin carries about 97% of oxygen in the blood and is the main transporter of oxygen. The remaining 3% of the oxygen is carried in plasma in the dissolved state. Only the dissolved form of oxygen (i.e., PO_2) passes through the cell membranes and makes itself available for use in tissue metabolism. The *oxygen content* of the blood (measured as mL of O_2 per deciliter [dL] or 100 mL of blood) includes both the oxygen carried by hemoglobin and in the dissolved state.

Hemoglobin Transport

Hemoglobin is a highly efficient carrier of oxygen. Hemoglobin with bound oxygen is called *oxyhemoglobin*, and when oxygen is removed, it is called *deoxygenated* or *reduced hemoglobin*. Each gram of hemoglobin carries approximately 1.34 mL of oxygen when it is fully saturated. This means that a person with a hemoglobin level of 14 g/dL carries 18.8 mL of oxygen per dL (i.e., 1.34 × 14 g/dL hemoglobin) of blood.

In the lungs, oxygen moves across the alveolar-capillary membrane, through the plasma, and into the red blood cell, where it forms a loose and reversible bond with the hemoglobin molecule. In normal lungs, this process is rapid, so that even with a fast heart rate, the hemoglobin is almost completely saturated with oxygen during the short time it spends in the pulmonary capillaries. As the oxygen moves out of the capillaries in response to the needs of the tissues, the hemoglobin saturation, which usually is approximately 95% to 97% as the blood leaves the left side of the heart, drops to approximately 75% as the mixed venous blood returns to the right side of the heart.

The efficiency of the hemoglobin transport system depends on the ability of the hemoglobin molecule to bind oxygen in the lungs and release it as it is needed in the tissues. Oxygen that remains bound to hemoglobin cannot participate in tissue metabolism.

The term *affinity* refers to hemoglobin's ability to bind oxygen. Hemoglobin binds oxygen more readily when its affinity is increased and releases it more readily when its affinity is decreased.

The hemoglobin molecule is composed of four polypeptide chains with an iron-containing heme group (see Chapter 14, Fig. 14-2). Because oxygen binds to the iron atom, each hemoglobin molecule can bind four molecules of oxygen when it is fully saturated. Oxygen binds cooperatively with the heme groups on the hemoglobin molecule. After the first molecule of oxygen binds to a heme group, the hemoglobin molecule undergoes a change in shape. As a result, the second and third molecules of oxygen bind more readily, and binding of the fourth molecule is even easier. In a like manner, the unloading of the first molecule of oxygen enhances the unloading of the next molecule and so on. Thus, the affinity of hemoglobin for oxygen changes with hemoglobin saturation.

Hemoglobin's affinity for oxygen is also influenced by pH, carbon dioxide concentration, and body temperature. It binds oxygen more readily under conditions of increased pH (alkalosis), decreased carbon dioxide concentration, and decreased body temperature and it releases it more readily under conditions of decreased pH (acidosis), increased carbon dioxide concentration, and fever. For example, increased tissue metabolism generates carbon dioxide and metabolic acids and thereby decreases the affinity of hemoglobin for oxygen. Heat also is a by-product of tissue metabolism, explaining the effect of fever on oxygen binding.

Red blood cells contain a metabolic intermediate called *2,3-diphosphoglycerate (2,3-DPG)* that also affects the affinity of hemoglobin for oxygen. An increase in 2,3-DPG enhances unloading of oxygen from hemoglobin at the tissue level. Conditions that increase 2,3-DPG include exercise, hypoxia that occurs at high altitude, and chronic lung disease.

Plasma Transport

The partial pressure (PO_2) of oxygen represents the level of dissolved oxygen in plasma. The amount of dissolved oxygen that is carried in the plasma depends on its partial pressure and its solubility in the plasma. The PO_2 of the arterial blood normally ranges from 85 to 100 mm Hg when breathing room air at 1 atmosphere (760 mm Hg). The solubility of oxygen in plasma is fixed and very small. For every 1 mm Hg of PO_2 present, 0.03 mL of oxygen becomes dissolved in 1 dL of plasma. This means that at a normal arterial PO_2 of 95 mm Hg, about 0.29 mL of oxygen is dissolved in every dL of plasma. Therefore, the amount of oxygen transported in the dissolved state is very small, only about 3% of the total, as compared with the 97% transported by the hemoglobin.

Although the amount of oxygen carried in plasma under normal conditions is small, it can become a life-saving mode of transport in cases of carbon monoxide poisoning, when most of the hemoglobin sites are occupied by carbon monoxide and are unavailable for transport of oxygen. Carbon monoxide, which combines

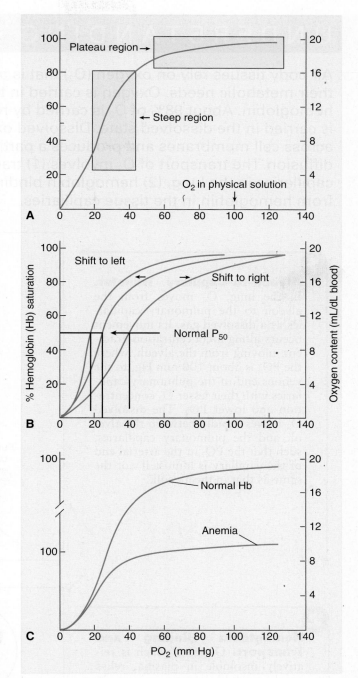

FIGURE 21-17. Oxygen-hemoglobin dissociation curve. **(A)** Left boxed area represents the steep portion of the curve where oxygen is released from hemoglobin (Hb) to the tissues, and the top boxed area on the plateau of the curve where oxygen is loaded onto hemoglobin in the lung. P_{50} is the partial pressure of oxygen required to saturate 50% of hemoglobin with oxygen. **(B)** The effect of body temperature, arterial PCO_2, and pH on hemoglobin affinity for oxygen as indicated by a shift in the curve and position of the P_{50}. A shift of the curve to the right due to an increase in temperature or PCO_2 or a decrease in pH favors release of oxygen to the tissues. A decrease in temperature or PCO_2 or an increase in pH shifts the curve to the left. **(C)** Effect of anemia on the oxygen-carrying capacity of blood. The hemoglobin can be completely saturated, but the oxygen content of the blood is reduced. (Adapted from Rhoades RA, Tanner GA. *Medical Physiology.* Boston, MA: Little, Brown; 1996.)

(*text continues on page 533*)

UNDERSTANDING ➡ Oxygen Transport

All body tissues rely on oxygen (O_2) that is transported in the blood to meet their metabolic needs. Oxygen is carried in two forms: dissolved and bound to hemoglobin. About 98% of O_2 is carried by hemoglobin and the remaining 2% is carried in the dissolved state. Dissolved oxygen is the only form that diffuses across cell membranes and produces a partial pressure (PO_2), which, in turn, drives diffusion. The transport of O_2 involves (1) transfer from the alveoli to the pulmonary capillaries in the lung, (2) hemoglobin binding and transport, and (3) the dissociation from hemoglobin in the tissue capillaries.

1

Alveoli-to-Capillary Transfer. In the lung, O_2 moves from the alveoli to the pulmonary capillaries as a dissolved gas. Its movement occurs along a concentration gradient, moving from the alveoli, where the PO_2 is about 100 mm Hg, to the venous end of the pulmonary capillaries with their lesser O_2 concentration and lower PO_2. The dissolved O_2 moves rapidly between the alveoli and the pulmonary capillaries, such that the PO_2 at the arterial end of the capillary is almost if not the same as that in the alveoli.

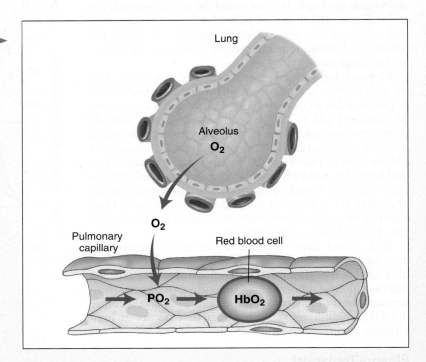

2

Hemoglobin Binding and Transport. Oxygen, which is relatively insoluble in plasma, relies on hemoglobin for transport in the blood. Once oxygen has diffused into the pulmonary capillary, it moves rapidly into the red blood cells and reversibly binds to hemoglobin to form HbO_2. The hemoglobin molecule contains four heme units, each capable of attaching an oxygen molecule. Hemoglobin is 100% saturated when all four units are occupied and is usually about 97% saturated in the systemic arterial blood. The capacity of the blood to carry O_2 is dependent both on hemoglobin levels and the ability of the lungs to oxygenate the hemoglobin.

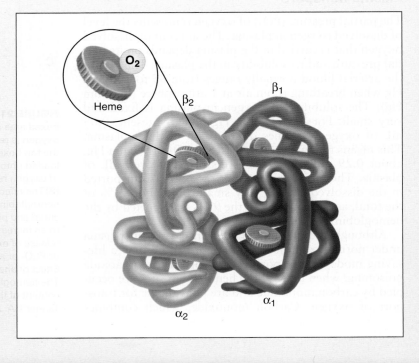

3 **Oxygen Dissociation in the Tissues.** The dissociation or release of O_2 from hemoglobin occurs in the tissue capillaries where the PO_2 is less than that of the arterial blood. As oxygen dissociates from hemoglobin, it dissolves in the plasma and then moves into the tissues where the PO_2 is less than that in the capillaries. The affinity of hemoglobin for O_2 is influenced by the carbon dioxide (PCO_2) content of the blood and its pH, temperature, and 2,3-diphosphoglycerate (2,3-DPG), a by-product of glycolysis in red blood cells. Under conditions of high metabolic demand, in which the PCO_2 is increased and the pH is decreased, the binding affinity of hemoglobin is decreased, and during decreased metabolic demand, when the PCO_2 is decreased and the pH is increased, the affinity is increased.

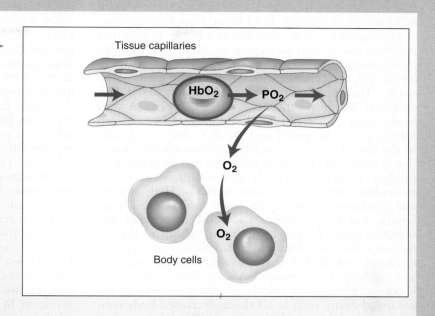

(text continued from page 531)

with hemoglobin at the same site as oxygen, has a binding tenacity that is 250 times that of oxygen. Therefore, small concentrations of carbon monoxide in the air (less than 1 part per thousand of air) can be lethal. Even though the oxygen content of the blood is greatly reduced in carbon monoxide poisoning, the PO_2 may be normal, making detection difficult because the blood is bright red and there are no obvious signs of hypoxemia, such as a bluish discoloration of the lips or fingertips. The use of a hyperbaric chamber, in which 100% oxygen can be administered at high atmospheric pressures (e.g., 3 ATM), increases the PO_2, or the amount of oxygen carried in the dissolved form, to life-saving levels.

Oxygen–Hemoglobin Dissociation Curve

The relationship between the oxygen carried in combination with hemoglobin and the PO_2 of the blood is described by the *oxygen–hemoglobin dissociation curve*, depicted in Figure 21-17. The *x* axis of the graph depicts the PO_2 or dissolved oxygen. It reflects the partial pressure of oxygen in the lungs (i.e., the PO_2 ranges from 95 to 100 mm Hg when breathing room air, but can rise to 200 mm Hg or higher when oxygen-enriched air is breathed). The *y* axis on the left depicts hemoglobin saturation or the amount of oxygen that is carried by hemoglobin. The right *y* axis depicts oxygen content or total amount of oxygen (i.e., mL O_2/dL) that is being carried in the blood.

The S-shaped oxygen dissociation curve reflects the effect that oxygen saturation has on the conformation of the hemoglobin molecule and its affinity for oxygen. Its flat upper-right portion represents the binding of oxygen to hemoglobin in the lungs (see Fig. 21-17A). Notice that this plateau occurs at approximately 100 mm Hg PO_2, at which point the hemoglobin is approximately 98% saturated. Increasing the alveolar PO_2 above this level does not increase hemoglobin saturation. Even at high altitudes, when the partial pressure of oxygen is considerably decreased, the hemoglobin remains relatively well saturated. At 60 mm Hg PO_2, for example, the hemoglobin is still approximately 89% saturated.

The steeper lower-left portion of the dissociation curve—between 60 and 40 mm Hg—represents the removal of oxygen from hemoglobin as it moves through the tissue capillaries. This portion of the curve reflects the fact that there is considerable transfer of oxygen from hemoglobin to the tissues with only a small drop in PO_2, thereby ensuring a gradient for oxygen to move into body cells. The tissues normally remove approximately 5 mL of oxygen per dL of blood, and the hemoglobin of mixed venous blood is approximately 75% saturated as it returns to the right side of the heart. In this portion of the dissociation curve (saturation <75%), the rate at which oxygen is released from hemoglobin is determined largely by tissue uptake. During strenuous exercise, for example, the muscle cells may remove as much as 15 mL of oxygen per dL of blood from hemoglobin.

Hemoglobin can be regarded as a buffer system that regulates the delivery of oxygen to the tissues. In order to function as a buffer system, the affinity of hemoglobin for oxygen must change with the metabolic needs of the tissues. This change is represented by a shift to the right or left in the dissociation curve (Fig. 21-17B). A shift to the right indicates that the affinity of hemoglobin for oxygen is decreased and the PO_2 that is available to the tissues at any given level of hemoglobin saturation is increased. It usually is caused by conditions that produce an increase in tissue metabolism, such as fever or acidosis, or by an increase in PCO_2. High altitude and conditions such as pulmonary insufficiency, heart failure, and severe anemia also cause the oxygen dissociation curve to shift to the right. A shift to the left indicates that the affinity of hemoglobin for oxygen is increased and the PO_2 that is available to the tissues at any given level of hemoglobin saturation is decreased. It occurs in situations associated with a decrease in tissue metabolism, such as alkalosis, decreased body temperature, and decreased PCO_2 levels. The degree of shift can be determined by the P_{50}, or the partial pressure of oxygen that is needed to achieve a 50% saturation of hemoglobin. Returning to Figure 22-17B, the dissociation curve on the left has a P_{50} of approximately 20 mm Hg; the normal curve, a P_{50} of 26; and the curve on the right, a P_{50} of 39 mm Hg.

The oxygen content (measured in mL/dL) of blood represents the total amount of oxygen that is carried in the blood, including the dissolved oxygen and that carried by the hemoglobin. It is the oxygen content rather than the PO_2 or hemoglobin saturation that determines the amount of oxygen that is carried in the blood and delivered to the tissues. Thus, an anemic person may have a normal PO_2 and hemoglobin saturation level but decreased oxygen content because of the decreased amount of hemoglobin that is available for binding of oxygen (Fig. 21-17C).

Carbon Dioxide Transport

Carbon dioxide is transported in the blood in three forms: dissolved in plasma (10%), attached to hemoglobin (30%), and as bicarbonate (60%). Acid–base balance is influenced by the amount of dissolved carbon dioxide and the bicarbonate level in the blood (see Chapter 8, Understanding Carbon Dioxide Transport).

As carbon dioxide is formed during metabolism, it diffuses out of cells into the tissue spaces and then into the capillaries. The amount of dissolved carbon dioxide that can be carried in plasma is determined by the partial pressure of the gas and its solubility coefficient (0.3 mL/dL blood/mm Hg PCO_2). Carbon dioxide is 20 times more soluble in plasma than oxygen. Thus, the dissolved state plays a greater role in transport of carbon dioxide compared with oxygen.

Most of the carbon dioxide diffuses into the red blood cells, where it either forms carbonic acid or combines with hemoglobin. *Carbonic acid* (H_2CO_3) is formed when carbon dioxide combines with water ($CO_2 + H_2O = H^+ + HCO_3^-$). The process is catalyzed by an enzyme called *carbonic anhydrase*, which is present in large quantities in red blood cells. Carbonic anhydrase increases the rate of the reaction between carbon dioxide and water approximately 5000-fold. Carbonic acid readily ionizes to form bicarbonate (HCO_3^-) and hydrogen (H^+) ions. The hydrogen ions combine with hemoglobin, which is a powerful acid–base buffer, and the bicarbonate ion diffuses into plasma in exchange for a chloride (Cl^-) ion. This exchange is made possible by a special bicarbonate-chloride carrier protein in the red blood cell membrane. As a result of the bicarbonate-chloride shift, the chloride and water content of the red blood cell is greater in venous blood than in arterial blood.

In addition to the carbonic anhydrase-mediated reaction with water, carbon dioxide reacts directly with hemoglobin to form *carbaminohemoglobin*. The combination of carbon dioxide with hemoglobin is a reversible reaction that involves a loose bond, which allows transport of carbon dioxide from tissues to the lungs, where it is released into the alveoli for exchange with the external environment. The release of oxygen from hemoglobin in the tissues enhances the binding of carbon dioxide to hemoglobin; in the lungs, the combining of oxygen with hemoglobin displaces carbon dioxide.

SUMMARY CONCEPTS

- Although the lungs are responsible for the exchange of gases with the environment, it is the blood that transports oxygen from the lungs to the tissues and returns carbon dioxide to the lungs. Most of the oxygen (97% to 99%) in the blood is carried in chemical combination with hemoglobin in red blood cells, with the remaining 1% to 3% being carried in the plasma as a dissolved gas.

- The oxygen dissociation curve is S shaped with a plateau area, above which an increase in dissolved oxygen (PO_2) has minimal or no effect on hemoglobin saturation. This insures adequate hemoglobin saturation over a wide range of dissolved oxygen values.

- The oxygen content or amount of oxygen that is carried in the blood is equal to amount of oxygen that is carried bound to hemoglobin plus the dissolved form. Since each gram of hemoglobin carries approximately 1.34 mL oxygen, it is the hemoglobin content of the blood rather than the hemoglobin saturation that determines the amount of oxygen that the blood can carry.

> ■ Carbon dioxide is transported in the blood:
> (1) as the dissolved gas (10%), (2) attached to
> hemoglobin (30%), and (3) as bicarbonate (60%).
> The reversible action of carbon dioxide with water
> to form bicarbonate is catalyzed by the enzyme
> carbonic anhydrase within red cells and is the
> major pathway for generation of bicarbonate.

Control of Breathing

Unlike the heart, which has inherent rhythmic properties and can beat independently of the nervous system, the muscles that control respiration require continuous input from the nervous system. Movement of the diaphragm, intercostal muscles, sternocleidomastoid, and other accessory muscles that control ventilation is integrated by neurons located in the pons and medulla. These neurons are collectively referred to as the *respiratory center* (Fig. 21-18).

Respiratory Center

The respiratory center consists of two dense, bilateral aggregates of respiratory neurons involved in initiating inspiration and expiration and incorporating afferent impulses into motor responses of the respiratory muscles. The first, or dorsal, group of neurons is concerned primarily with inspiration. These neurons control the activity of the phrenic nerves that innervate the diaphragm and drive the second, or ventral, group of respiratory neurons. They are thought to integrate sensory input from the lungs and airways into the ventilatory response. The second group of neurons, which contains inspiratory and expiratory neurons, controls the spinal motor neurons of the intercostal and abdominal muscles.

The pacemaker properties of the respiratory center in the medulla result from the cycling of two groups of neurons: the *pneumotaxic center* in the upper pons and the *apneustic center* in the lower pons (see Fig. 21-18). The apneustic center has an excitatory effect on inspiration, tending to prolong inspiration. The pneumotaxic center switches inspiration off, assisting in the control of the respiratory rate and inspiratory volume. Brain injury, which damages the connections between the pneumotaxic and apneustic centers, results in an irregular breathing pattern that consists of prolonged inspiratory gasps interrupted by expiratory efforts.

Axons from the neurons in the respiratory center cross in the midline and descend in the ventrolateral columns of the spinal cord. The tracts that control expiration and inspiration are spatially separated in the cord, as are the tracts that transmit specialized reflexes (i.e., coughing and hiccupping) and voluntary control of ventilation. Only at the level of the spinal cord are the respiratory impulses integrated to produce a reflex response.

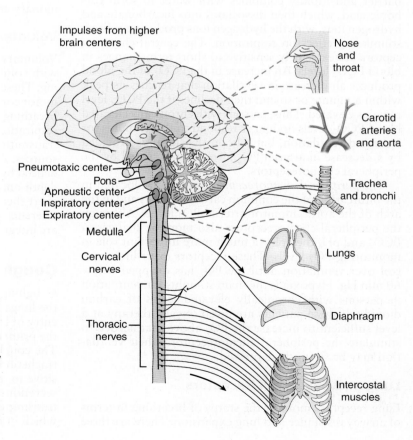

FIGURE 21-18. Schematic representation of activity in the respiratory center. Impulses traveling over afferent neurons (*dashed lines*) communicate with central neurons, which activate efferent neurons that supply the muscles of respiration. Respiratory movements can be altered by a variety of stimuli.

Regulation of Breathing

The control of breathing has both automatic and voluntary components. Automatic regulation involves afferent input from two types of sensors or receptors: chemoreceptors and lung and chest wall receptors.

Chemoreceptors

Chemoreceptors monitor blood levels of oxygen, carbon dioxide, and pH and adjust ventilation to meet the changing metabolic needs of the body. Input from these sensors is transmitted to the respiratory center, and ventilation is adjusted to maintain the arterial blood gases within a normal range. There are two types of chemoreceptors: central chemoreceptors, located in the brain stem, and peripheral chemoreceptors, located in the carotid arteries and aorta.

Central chemoreceptors are located near the respiratory center in the medulla and are bathed in cerebrospinal fluid (CSF). They are exquisitely sensitive to changes in the PCO_2 of the blood perfusing them. Although the central chemoreceptors monitor carbon dioxide levels, the actual stimulus for these receptors is provided by hydrogen ions in the CSF. The CSF is separated from the blood by the blood–brain barrier, which permits free diffusion of carbon dioxide but not hydrogen ions. For this reason, changes in the pH of the blood have considerably less effect in stimulating ventilation than carbon dioxide, which stimulates the central chemoreceptors indirectly by changing the hydrogen ion concentration of the CSF. This occurs as carbon dioxide crosses the blood–brain barrier and rapidly combines with water to form carbonic acid, which then dissociates into bicarbonate and hydrogen ions, with the hydrogen ions producing a direct stimulating effect on respiration. The central chemoreceptors are extremely sensitive to short-term changes in blood PCO_2 levels. An increase in the PCO_2 of the blood produces an increase in ventilation that reaches its peak within a minute or so and then declines if the PCO_2 level remains elevated. Thus, persons with chronically elevated blood PCO_2 levels no longer respond to this stimulus for increased ventilation, but rely on the stimulus provided by a decrease in arterial PO_2 levels that is sensed by the peripheral chemoreceptors.

The *peripheral chemoreceptors*, which are located in the bifurcation of the common carotid arteries and in the arch of the aorta, monitor arterial PO_2 levels. Although the peripheral chemoreceptors also monitor changes in PCO_2 and pH, they play a much more important role in monitoring PO_2 levels. These receptors exert little control over ventilation until the PO_2 has dropped below 60 mm Hg. Hypoxia is the main stimulus for ventilation in persons with chronically elevated levels of carbon dioxide. If these patients are given oxygen therapy at a level sufficient to increase the PO_2 above that needed to stimulate the peripheral chemoreceptors, their ventilation may be seriously depressed.

Lung and Chest Wall Receptors

Lung receptors monitor the status of breathing in terms of airway resistance and lung expansion. There are three types of lung receptors: stretch, irritant, and juxtacapillary receptors. Receptors in the joints, tendons, and muscles of the chest wall structures may also play a role in breathing, particularly when quiet breathing is called for or when breathing efforts are opposed by increased airway resistance or reduced lung compliance.

Stretch receptors are located in the smooth muscle layers of the conducting airways. They respond to changes in pressure in the walls of the airways. When the lungs are inflated, these receptors inhibit inspiration and promote expiration. They are important in establishing breathing patterns and minimizing the work of breathing by adjusting respiratory rate and TV to accommodate changes in lung compliance and airway resistance.

The *irritant receptors* are located between the airway epithelial cells. They are stimulated by noxious gases, cigarette smoke, inhaled dust, and cold air. Stimulation of the irritant receptors leads to airway constriction and a pattern of rapid, shallow breathing. This pattern of breathing probably protects respiratory tissues from the damaging effects of toxic inhalants. It also is thought that the mechanical stimulation of these receptors may ensure more uniform lung expansion by initiating periodic sighing and yawning. It is possible that these receptors are involved in the bronchoconstriction response that occurs in some persons with bronchial asthma.

The *juxtacapillary* or *J receptors* are located in the alveolar wall, close to the pulmonary capillaries. It is thought that these receptors sense lung congestion. These receptors may be responsible for the rapid, shallow breathing that occurs with pulmonary edema, pulmonary embolism, and pneumonia.

Voluntary Regulation of Ventilation

Voluntary regulation of ventilation integrates breathing with voluntary acts such as speaking, blowing, and singing. These acts, which are initiated by the motor and premotor cortex, cause a temporary suspension of automatic breathing. The automatic and voluntary components of respiration are regulated by afferent impulses that are transmitted to the respiratory center from a number of sources. Afferent input from higher brain centers is evidenced by the fact that a person can consciously alter the depth and rate of respiration. Fever, pain, and emotion exert their influence through lower brain centers. Vagal afferents from sensory receptors in the lungs and airways are integrated in the dorsal area of the respiratory center.

Cough Reflex

Coughing is a neurally mediated reflex that protects the lungs from the accumulation of secretions and from entry of irritating and destructive substances. It is one of the primary defense mechanisms of the respiratory tract. The cough reflex is initiated by receptors located in the tracheobronchial wall, receptors that are extremely sensitive to irritating substances and the presence of excess secretions. Afferent impulses from these receptors are transmitted through the vagus to the medullary center, which integrates the cough response.

Coughing requires the rapid inspiration of a large volume of air (usually about 2.5 L), followed by rapid closure of the glottis and forceful contraction of the abdominal and expiratory muscles. As these muscles contract, intrathoracic pressures are elevated to levels of 100 mm Hg or more. The rapid opening of the glottis at this point leads to an explosive expulsion of air.

A number of conditions interfere with the cough reflex and its protective function. The reflex is impaired in persons whose abdominal or respiratory muscles are weak. This problem can be caused by disease conditions that lead to muscle weakness or paralysis, by prolonged inactivity, or as an outcome of surgery involving these muscles. Bed rest interferes with expansion of the chest and limits the amount of air that can be taken into the lungs in preparation for coughing, making the cough weak and ineffective. Disease conditions that prevent effective closure of the glottis and laryngeal muscles interfere with production of the marked increase in intrathoracic pressure that is needed for effective coughing. For example, the presence of a nasogastric tube may prevent closure of the upper airway structures and may fatigue the receptors for the cough reflex that are located in the area. The cough reflex also is impaired when there is depressed function of the medullary centers in the brain that integrate the cough reflex.

Although the cough reflex is a protective mechanism, frequent and prolonged coughing can be exhausting and painful and can have undesirable effects on the cardiovascular and respiratory systems and on the elastic tissues of the lungs. This is particularly true in young children and elderly persons.

Dyspnea

Dyspnea is the perceived shortness of breath or difficulty breathing. It may occur at rest or with exertion, be continuous or intermittent, or have a pattern of acute or chronic occurrences. Dyspnea may occur in otherwise healthy persons, as during exercise or exposure to low ambient levels of oxygen. It is a common complaint of persons with primary lung diseases such as pneumonia, asthma, and emphysema; heart disease that is characterized by pulmonary congestion; and neuromuscular disorders such as myasthenia gravis and muscular dystrophy that affect the respiratory muscles.

The physiological mechanisms underlying the sensation of dyspnea remain elusive. Dyspnea is not a single phenomenon. There are at least three varieties of breathing difficulty—air hunger, labored breathing, and chest tightness. The sensation of *air hunger* is thought to be mediated by transmission of excessive chemoreceptor stimulation of the medullary respiratory center to sensory centers in the forebrain. *Labored breathing*, a sensation of working hard to breathe, is a common complaint of persons with weakened respiratory muscles. It is thought to be mediated by excessive input from stretch receptors in the chest muscles or chest wall. The sensation of *chest tightness*, an early symptom of an asthmatic attack, appears to be related to input from

lung receptors that monitor bronchial constriction. In contrast, the dyspnea that accompanies pulmonary congestion due to heart failure appears to be related to input from lung receptors that monitor vascular distention (i.e., the previously described J receptors). More than one mechanism may be responsible for the dyspnea seen in a particular disease state. For example, severe flow limitations in chronic pulmonary disease can produce stimuli that give rise to the sensation of increased breathing difficulty, and the presence of hypoxia and/or hypercapnia may produce the sensation of air hunger.

Like other subjective symptoms, such as fatigue and pain, dyspnea is difficult to quantify because it relies on a person's perception of the problem. Like pain, dyspnea is also a multidimensional sensation, involving the sensation of both sensory intensity (i.e., work of breathing) and unpleasantness (i.e., air hunger or chest tightness). A commonly used method for assessing dyspnea is a retrospective determination of the level of daily activity at which dyspnea is experienced. The visual analog scale may be used to assess breathing difficulty that occurs with a given activity, such as walking a certain distance. The visual analog scale consists of a line (often 10 cm in length) with descriptors such as "easy to breathe" on one end and "very difficult to breathe" on the other.

The treatment of dyspnea depends on the cause. For example, persons with impaired respiratory function may require oxygen therapy, and those with pulmonary edema may require measures to improve heart function. Methods to decrease anxiety, breathing retraining, and energy conservation measures may be used to decrease the subjective sensation of dyspnea.

SUMMARY CONCEPTS

- Pulmonary ventilation or the act of breathing involves movement of the diaphragm, intercostal muscles, and other respiratory muscles. These muscles are controlled by neurons of respiratory centers in the pons and medulla with input from higher brain centers and peripheral receptors.

- Control of breathing has both automatic and voluntary components. The automatic regulation of ventilation is controlled by two types of receptors: chemoreceptors, which monitor blood levels of carbon dioxide, oxygen, and pH; and lung receptors, which monitor the status of breathing in terms of airway resistance and lung expansion. Voluntary respiratory control is needed for integrating breathing and actions such as speaking, blowing, and singing. These acts, which are initiated by the motor and premotor cortex, cause temporary suspension of automatic breathing.

(continued)

SUMMARY CONCEPTS (continued)

■ The cough reflex protects the lungs from the accumulation of secretions and from the entry of irritating and destructive substances; it is one of the primary defense mechanisms of the respiratory tract.

■ Dyspnea is a subjective sensation of difficulty in breathing that is seen in cardiac, pulmonary, and neuromuscular disorders. It can present as *air hunger* brought about by inadequate ventilation, *labored* or *difficulty breathing* due to weakened respiratory muscles, or *chest tightness* that occurs with bronchoconstriction.

REVIEW EXERCISES

1. Relate the efficiency and work of breathing to changes in the tidal volume and respiratory rate observed in persons with:

   A. Decreased lung compliance in fibrotic lung disease
   B. Increased airway resistance in emphysema.

2. Use the solubility coefficient for oxygen and the oxygen-hemoglobin dissociation curve depicted in Figure 22-17 to answer the following questions:

   A. What is the hemoglobin saturation at a high altitude in which the barometric pressure is 500 mm Hg (consider oxygen to represent 21% of the total gases)?
   B. It is usually recommended that the hemoglobin saturation of persons with chronic lung disease be maintained at about 89% when they are receiving supplemental low-flow oxygen. What would their PO_2 be at this level of hemoglobin saturation, and what is the rationale for keeping the PO_2 at this level?
   C. Why are measures of hemoglobin saturation not necessarily a good measure of the oxygen-carrying capacity of blood?
   D. What is the oxygen content of a person with carbon monoxide poisoning who is receiving 100% oxygen at 3 atmospheres pressure in a hyperbaric chamber? Consider that most of the person's hemoglobin is saturated with carbon dioxide.

3. Describe the receptor/s (peripheral and central), afferent pathways, central integration, and efferent neural pathways that:

   A. Determine the tidal volume and respiratory rate of the minute volume
   B. Participate in the cough reflex
   C. Contribute to the breathlessness that accompanies intensive exercise and the dyspnea that accompanies lung disease.

BIBLIOGRAPHY

Burke NK, Lu-Yuan L. Mechanisms of dyspnea. *Chest.* 2010;135(5):1196–1201.

Canning BJ. Afferent nerves regulating the cough reflex: mechanisms and mediators of cough in disease. *Otolaryngol Clin North Am.* 2010;43(1):1–14.

Chroneos ZC, Zvezdana S-C, Shepard VL. Pulmonary surfactant: an immunological perspective. *Cell Physiol Biochem.* 2010;25:13–26.

Crapo RO. Pulmonary function testing. *N Engl J Med.* 1994;331:25–30.

DeTroyer A, Kirkwood PA, Wilson TA. Respiratory action of inspiratory muscles. *Physiol Rev.* 2005;85:717–756.

Hall JE. *Guyton and Hall Textbook of Medical Physiology.* 12th ed. Philadelphia, PA: Saunders Elsevier; 2011:465–523.

Koeppen BM, Stanton BA. *Berne and Levy Physiology.* 6th ed. Philadelphia, PA: Mosby Elsevier; 2010:417–444.

Lansing RW, Gracely RH, Banzett RD. The multiple dimensions of dyspnea: review and hypothesis. *Respir Physiol Neurobiol.* 2009;167(1):53–60.

Moore KL, Dalley AF, Agur AMR. *Clinically Oriented Anatomy.* 6th ed. Philadelphia, PA: Wolters Kluwer Health/Lippincott Williams & Wilkins; 2009:107–127.

O'Donnell DE, Banzett RB, Carrieri-Kohlman V, et al. Pathophysiology of dyspnea in chronic obstructive lung disease: a roundtable. *Proc Am Thorac Soc.* 2007;4(2):145–168.

Prabhakar NR, Peng Y-J. Peripheral chemoreceptors in health and disease. *J Applied Physiol.* 2004;96:359–366.

Rhoades RA, Bell DR. *Medical Physiology: Principles of Clinical Medicine.* 4th ed. Philadelphia, PA: Wolters Kluwer Health/ Lippincott Williams & Wilkins; 2013: 326–398.

Ross MH, Pawlina W. *Histology: A Text and Atlas.* 6th ed. Philadelphia, PA: Wolters Kluwer Health/Lippincott Williams & Wilkins; 2011:664–684.

West JB. *Respiratory Physiology: The Essentials.* 8th ed. Philadelphia, PA: Wolters Kluwer Health/Lippincott Williams & Wilkins; 2008.

Porth Essentials Resources

Explore these additional resources to enhance learning for this chapter:

• NCLEX-Style Questions and Other Resources on thePoint, http://thePoint.lww.com/PorthEssentials4e
• Study Guide for Essentials of Pathophysiology
• Concepts in Action Animations
• Adaptive Learning | Powered by PrepU, http://thepoint.lww.com/prepu

Respiratory Tract Infections, Neoplasms, and Childhood Disorders

Respiratory illnesses represent one of the more common reasons for visits to the physician, admission to the hospital, and forced inactivity among all age groups. The common cold, although not usually serious, results in missed work and school days. Pneumonia and influenza are ranked as the eighth leading cause of death in the United States.[1] Tuberculosis remains one of the deadliest diseases in the world. In addition to microbial pathogens, cigarette smoking contributes significantly to disorders of the respiratory tract, including lung cancer. The content in this chapter is divided into three sections: respiratory tract infections, cancer of the lung, and respiratory disorders in children.

Respiratory Tract Infections

Respiratory tract infections can involve the upper respiratory tract (i.e., nose, oropharynx, and larynx), the lower respiratory tract (i.e., lower airways and lungs), or both. The discussion in this section of the chapter focuses on the common cold, rhinosinusitis, influenza, pneumonia, tuberculosis, and fungal infections of the lung. For the most part, the signs and symptoms of respiratory tract infections depend on the function of the structure involved, the severity of the infectious process, and the person's general health status and age. Acute respiratory infections in children are discussed in the last section of the chapter.

Viruses are the most frequent cause of respiratory tract infections. They can cause infections ranging from a self-limited cold to life-threatening pneumonia. Moreover, viral infections can damage the bronchial epithelium, obstruct airways, and lead to secondary bacterial infections. Each viral species has its own pattern of respiratory tract involvement. The rhinoviruses grow best at 33°C and remain strictly confined to the upper respiratory tract.[2] The influenza virus can infect both the upper and lower respiratory tracts. Bacteria can infect the nose and sinuses, and both bacteria and fungi can produce infections of the lung, many of which cause significant morbidity and mortality.

The Common Cold

The common cold is a viral infection of the upper respiratory tract. It occurs more frequently than any other respiratory tract infection. Most adults have two to three colds per year, whereas the average school child may have up to 12 per year.[3] The condition usually begins with a sore and scratchy throat followed by profuse and watery rhinorrhea, nasal congestion, sneezing, and coughing. Other cold symptoms include malaise, fatigue, headache, hoarseness, sinus congestion, and myalgia. Fever is a common sign in children but is an infrequent finding in adults.[3] The disease process is self-limited, usually lasting up to 10 days.

Initially thought to be caused by either a single "cold virus" or group, the common cold is now recognized to be associated with many different viruses.[3,4] The most common are the rhinoviruses, parainfluenza viruses, respiratory syncytial virus, coronaviruses, and adenoviruses. Of these, the rhinoviruses are the most common cause of colds in persons between 5 and 40 years of age. In children younger than 3 years of age, infections from the respiratory syncytial virus and parainfluenza viruses are most common.

The "cold viruses" are rapidly spread from person to person. Children are the main source of infection often acquiring a new strain of the virus from another child in school or day care. The fingers are the greatest source of spread, and the nasal mucosa and conjunctival surface of the eyes are the most common portals for entry of the virus. The most highly contagious period is during the first 3 days after the onset of symptoms, and the incubation period is approximately 5 days. Cold viruses have been found to survive for more than 5 hours on the skin and hard surfaces, such as plastic countertops.[4,5] Aerosol spread of colds through coughing and sneezing is much less important than the spread by fingers picking up the virus from contaminated surfaces and carrying it to the nasal membranes and eyes.[5] This suggests that careful attention to hand washing is one of the most important preventive measures for avoiding the common cold.

Because the common cold is an acute and self-limited illness in persons who are otherwise healthy, symptomatic treatment with rest and antipyretic drugs is usually all that is needed. Antibiotics are ineffective against viral infections and are not recommended.[6] Over-the-counter (OTC) remedies are available for treating the symptoms of a common cold. Antihistamines are popular OTC drugs because of their action in drying nasal secretions. Although they do not work as a monotherapy, a first-generation antihistamine in combination with a decongestant may be slightly beneficial in relieving general symptoms, nasal congestion, and cough.[6] However, there is no evidence that they shorten the duration of the cold. They are not recommended for use in children. Decongestant drugs (i.e., sympathomimetic agents) are available in OTC nasal sprays, drops, and oral cold medications. These drugs constrict the blood vessels in the nasal mucosa and reduce nasal swelling. Rebound nasal swelling can occur with indiscriminate or chronic use of nasal drops and sprays. Oral preparations containing decongestants may cause systemic vasoconstriction and elevation of blood pressure when given in doses large enough to relieve nasal congestion, and they should be avoided in persons with hypertension, heart disease, hyperthyroidism, diabetes mellitus, or other health problems.[3]

Rhinosinusitis

The term *rhinitis* refers to an inflammation of the nasal passages and *sinusitis* to an inflammation of the paranasal sinuses.[7–12] Although it has not been universally accepted, the suggestion has been made that the term *rhinosinusitis* is a more accurate term for what is commonly referred to as *sinusitis*, because the mucosa of the nasal cavities and paranasal sinuses are lined with a continuous mucous membrane layer and sinusitis rarely occurs in the absence of infectious or allergic rhinitis.

The paranasal sinuses are air-filled extensions of the respiratory part of the nasal cavities into the frontal, ethmoid, sphenoid, and maxilla bones (Fig. 22-1A). The sinuses, which are named for the bones in which they are found, are connected by narrow openings or *ostia* with the superior, middle, and inferior nasal turbinates of the nasal cavity. The anterior ethmoid, frontal, and maxillary sinuses all drain into the nasal cavity through a relatively convoluted and narrow passage called the *ostiomeatal complex* (see Fig. 22-1B). The *sphenoidal sinuses* drain from a separate complex between the septum and the superior turbinate (see Fig. 22-1C).

The most common causes of rhinosinusitis are conditions that obstruct the narrow ostia that drain the sinuses. Most commonly, rhinosinusitis develops when a viral upper respiratory tract infection or allergic rhinitis obstructs the ostiomeatal complex and impairs the mucociliary clearance mechanism. Nasal polyps also can obstruct the sinus openings and facilitate sinus infection. Infections associated with nasal polyps can be self-perpetuating because constant irritation from the infection can facilitate polyp growth. Barotrauma caused by changes in barometric pressure, as occurs in airline pilots and flight attendants, may lead to impaired sinus ventilation and clearance of secretions. Swimming, diving, and abuse of nasal decongestants are other causes of sinus irritation and impaired drainage. Maxillary sinusitis may result from dental infection, and teeth that are tender should be carefully examined for signs of an abscess.

Clinical Features

Rhinosinusitis can be classified as acute, subacute, or chronic.[7,8] Acute viral rhinosinusitis may last from 5 to 7 days and acute bacterial rhinosinusitis up to 4 weeks. Subacute rhinosinusitis lasts from 4 weeks to less than 12 weeks, whereas chronic rhinosinusitis lasts beyond 12 weeks.

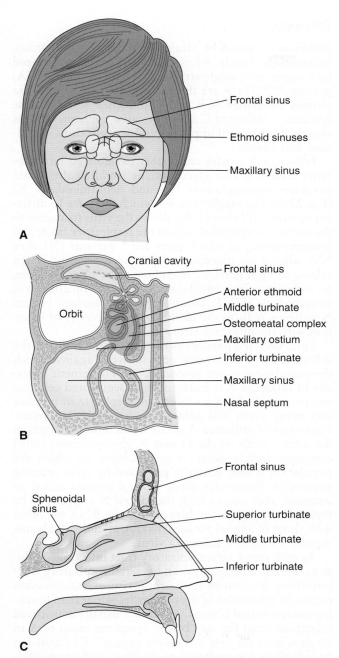

FIGURE 22-1. Paranasal sinuses. **(A)** Frontal view showing the frontal, ethmoid, and maxillary sinuses. **(B)** Cross-section of nasal cavity (anterior view). The shaded area is the osteomeatal complex, which is the final common pathway for drainage of the anterior ethmoid, frontal, and maxillary sinuses. **(C)** Lateral wall, left nasal cavity showing the frontal sphenoidal sinuses and the superior, middle, and inferior turbinates.

Acute rhinosinusitis may be of viral, bacterial, or viral–bacterial etiology. In most cases, bacterial infection is preceded by a viral upper respiratory infection, which in turn leads to inflammation and obstruction of the ostiomeatal complex. Rhinovirus is the most common viral pathogen. *Haemophilus influenzae, Streptococcus pneumoniae,* and *Moraxella catarrhalis* make up the majority of community-acquired bacterial pathogens.

In contrast to acute infections, the pathogens found in chronic rhinosinusitis are usually a mixture of aerobic and anaerobic bacteria, including *Staphylococcus aureus,* coagulase-negative *Staphylococcus,* and anaerobic gram-negative bacilli. Although the mechanisms that contribute to the chronicity of the disorder are uncertain, mucociliary dysfunction, mucostasis, hypoxia, and release of microbial products are thought to play a role. Allergies may also play an important role in the pathogenesis of chronic rhinosinusitis. In immunocompromised persons, such as those with human immunodeficiency virus (HIV) infection, the sinuses may become infected with gram-negative species and opportunistic fungi. In persons in this group, particularly those with leukopenia, the disease may have a fulminant and even fatal course.

Manifestations. The symptoms of acute viral rhinosinusitis often are similar to those of the common cold and allergic rhinitis[7–12] (discussed in Chapter 16). They include facial pain, headache, purulent nasal discharge, decreased sense of smell, and fever. A history of a preceding common cold and the presence of purulent nasal drainage, pain on bending, unilateral maxillary pain, and pain in the teeth are common findings with involvement of the maxillary sinuses. The symptoms of acute viral rhinosinusitis usually resolve within 5 to 7 days without medical treatment. Acute bacterial rhinosinusitis is suggested by symptoms that worsen after 5 to 7 days or persist beyond 10 days, or symptoms that are out of proportion to those usually associated with a viral upper respiratory tract infection. Persons who are immunocompromised, such as those with leukemia, aplastic anemia, bone marrow transplant, or HIV infection, may present with fever of unknown origin, rhinorrhea, or facial edema. Often, other signs of inflammation such as purulent drainage are absent.

In persons with chronic rhinosinusitis, the only symptoms may be nasal obstruction, a sense of fullness in the ears, postnasal drip, hoarseness, chronic cough, and loss of taste and smell. Sinus pain often is absent; instead, the person may complain of a headache that is dull and constant. Persons with chronic rhinosinusitis may have superimposed bouts of acute rhinosinusitis. The mucosal changes that occur during acute and subacute forms of rhinosinusitis as usually reversible; whereas, those that occur during chronic rhinosinusitis may be irreversible.

Diagnosis. The diagnosis of rhinosinusitis usually is based on symptom history and a physical examination that includes inspection of the nose and throat. Headache due to sinusitis needs to be differentiated from other types of headache. Sinusitis headache usually is exaggerated by bending forward, coughing, or sneezing. Physical examination findings in acute bacterial sinusitis include turbinate edema, nasal crusts, purulent drainage, and failure of transillumination of the maxillary sinuses. Transillumination is done in a completely darkened room by placing a flashlight against the skin overlying the infraorbital rim, directing the light inferiorly, having the person open his or her mouth, and observing the hard palate for light transmission. Sinus radiographs and computed tomography (CT) scans may be used. CT scans usually are reserved for diagnosis of chronic rhinosinusitis or to exclude complications.[7,8] Magnetic resonance imaging (MRI) is expensive and usually reserved for cases of suspected neoplasms or fungal sinusitis.

Treatment. Treatment of rhinosinusitis depends on the cause and includes appropriate use of antibiotics, intranasal corticosteroids, mucolytic agents, and symptom relief measures.[7–12] Antibiotics are usually reserved for persons with severe or persistent symptoms and specific findings of bacterial infection. The treatment of acute rhinosinusitis includes measures to promote adequate drainage by reducing nasal congestion. The topical α-adrenergic decongestants may be used on a short-term (3 days) basis in older children and adults for this purpose. The use of antihistamines is controversial, particularly for acute rhinosinusitis, because they can dry up secretions and thereby decrease drainage. Mucolytic agents such as guaifenesin may be used to thin secretions. Intranasal corticosteroids reduce inflammation and edema of the nasal mucosa, nasal turbinates, and sinus ostia. They may be used as an initial treatment in persons with acute rhinosinusitis and in those with both allergies and rhinosinusitis.[7,8] Nonpharmacologic measures include saline nasal sprays and steam inhalation.

Surgical intervention directed at correcting obstruction of the ostiomeatal openings may be indicated in persons with chronic rhinosinusitis that is resistant to other forms of therapy. Indications for surgical intervention include obstructive nasal polyps and obstructive nasal deformities.

Complications. Because of the sinuses' proximity to the brain and orbital wall, sinusitis can lead to intracranial and orbital wall complications. Intracranial complications are seen most commonly with infection of the frontal and ethmoid sinuses because of their proximity to the dura and drainage of the veins from the frontal sinus into the dural sinus. Orbital complications can range from edema of the eyelids to orbital cellulitis and subperiosteal abscess formation. Facial swelling over the involved sinus, abnormal extraocular movements, protrusion of the eyeball, periorbital edema, or changes in mental status may indicate intracranial complications and require immediate medical attention.

Influenza

Influenza is one of the most important causes of acute upper respiratory tract infection in humans. Until the advent of acquired immunodeficiency syndrome (AIDS), influenza was the last uncontrolled, potentially fatal pandemic. In the United States, epidemics of influenza typically occur during the winter months, accounting for over 35,000 deaths annually.[13] Rates of infection are highest among children, but rates of serious illness and death are highest among persons who are 65 years of age or older.

Etiology

Influenza is caused by viruses belonging to the Orthomyxoviridae family, whose members are characterized by a segmented, single-stranded ribonucleic acid (RNA) genome.[13–15] There are three distinct types of influenza viruses, designated A, B, and C. Influenza A and B cause epidemics. Influenza C does not cause epidemics, but is responsible for mild upper respiratory infections in children and adults.

Influenza A viruses are further categorized into subtypes based on two glycoproteins studding their lipid envelope: hemagglutinin (H) and neuraminidase (N) (Fig. 22-2). Hemagglutinin, for which there are 16 different variants (H1 thru H16), allows the virus to anchor to the surface of epithelial cells in the respiratory tract; and neuraminidase, of which there are 9 variants (N1 thru N9), allows for digestion of host secretion and, later, release of viral particles from host cells.[15] For example, an influenza virus circulating worldwide in 2013 was identified as H3N2. Immunity to the surface H and N antigens reduces the likelihood and severity of infection with the influenza virus.

Epidemics and pandemics result from the ability of the influenza virus to develop new subtypes against which the population is not protected.[13–15] The genetic diversity of influenza A is fostered by its segmented genomic structure and ability to infect and replicate in humans and many avian and animal species, including swine. Epidemics of influenza A occur when minor changes in the amino acids of the H and N glycoproteins, called *antigenic drift,* generate a new subtype to which the population is only partially protected by cross-reacting antibodies. Pandemics occur when a process called an *antigenic shift* causes both the H and N antigens to be replaced through recombination of the RNA segments with those of animal viruses, making all individuals susceptible to the new influenza virus.

As with many viral respiratory tract infections, influenza is more contagious than bacterial respiratory tract infections. In contrast to the rhinoviruses, transmission occurs by inhalation of droplet nuclei rather than touching contaminated objects. Adults are usually considered infectious from the day before symptom onset to 5 to 10 days after the first symptoms appear.[15] Children can be infectious for greater than 10 days, and young children can shed virus for up to 6 days before their illness onset. Severely immunocompromised persons can shed virus for weeks or months.

Pathogenesis

The influenza viruses can cause three types of infections: an uncomplicated upper respiratory infection (rhinotracheitis), viral pneumonia, and a respiratory viral infection followed by a bacterial infection. Influenza initially establishes upper airway infection. In doing this, the virus first targets and kills mucus-secreting, ciliated, and other epithelial cells, leaving gaping holes between the underlying basal cells and allowing extracellular fluid to escape. This is the reason for the rhinorrhea or "runny nose" that is characteristic of this phase of the infection.

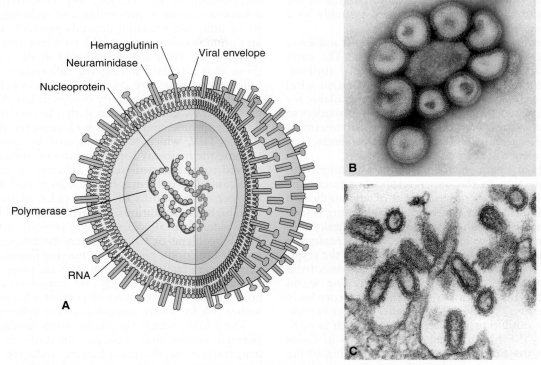

FIGURE 22-2. Influenza type A virus. **(A)** Model of the RNA influenza A virus, showing the hemagglutinin and neuraminidase envelope glycoproteins that provide access to host cells. **(B)** Negative-stained transmission electron micrograph (TEM) depicting the ultrastructural details of a number of influenza viral particles, or "virions." **(C)** TEM revealing ultrastructural features of the 1918 influenza pandemic virus virions. (B and C from the Centers for Disease Control and Prevention Public Health Image Library. Nos. 8432, 8996. B courtesy of F.A. Murphy; C courtesy of Cynthia Goldsmith.)

If the virus spreads to the lower respiratory tract, the infection can cause severe shedding of bronchial and alveolar cells. In addition to compromising the natural defenses of the respiratory tract, influenza infection promotes bacterial adhesion to epithelial cells.

Manifestations

In the early stages, the symptoms of influenza often are indistinguishable from other viral infections. There is an abrupt onset of fever and chills; malaise; muscle aching; headache; profuse, watery nasal discharge; nonproductive cough; and sore throat.[15–17] One distinguishing feature of an influenza viral infection is the rapid onset, sometimes in as little as minutes, of profound malaise. The symptoms of uncomplicated rhinotracheitis usually peak by days 3 to 5 and disappear by days 7 to 10. Weakness, cough, and malaise may persist for weeks after clinical resolution of influenza. Young children with influenza viral infection can have initial symptoms mimicking bacterial sepsis with high fevers and febrile convulsions.

Viral pneumonia occurs as a complication of influenza, most frequently in the elderly or in persons with cardiopulmonary disease, but has been reported in pregnant women and in healthy, immunocompetent people.[18] It typically develops within 1 day after onset of influenza and is characterized by rapid progression of fever, tachypnea, tachycardia, cyanosis, and hypotension. The clinical course of influenza pneumonia progresses rapidly. It can cause hypoxemia and death within a few days of onset. Survivors often develop diffuse pulmonary fibrosis.

Secondary complications typically include sinusitis, otitis media, bronchitis, and bacterial pneumonia.[15] Persons who develop secondary bacterial pneumonia usually report that they were beginning to feel better when they experienced a return of fever, shaking chills, pleuritic chest pain, and productive cough. The most common causes of secondary bacterial pneumonia are *S. pneumoniae, S. aureus, H. influenzae,* and *M. catarrhalis.* This form of pneumonia commonly produces less cyanosis and tachypnea and is usually milder than primary influenza pneumonia. Influenza-related deaths can result from pneumonia as well as exacerbations of cardiopulmonary conditions and other disease. Reye syndrome (fatty liver with encephalitis) is a rare complication of influenza, particularly in young children who have been given aspirin as an antipyretic agent.[15]

Diagnosis and Treatment

Diagnosis is based on symptoms such as sudden onset of fever, cough, weakness, and myalgias. The probability of influenza varies with the prevalence of the disease in the community and with the vaccination status of the person. Nationally, influenza-like illnesses usually hit a peak between January and March.

The appropriate treatment of people with influenza depends on accurate and timely diagnosis. The early diagnosis can reduce the inappropriate use of antibiotics and provide the opportunity for use of an antiviral drug.[15-17] Rapid diagnostic tests, which are available for use in outpatient settings, allow health care providers to diagnose influenza more accurately, consider treatment options more carefully, and monitor the influenza type and its prevalence in their community.[18]

The goals of treatment for influenza are designed to limit the infection to the upper respiratory tract. The symptomatic approach for treatment of uncomplicated influenza rhinotracheitis focuses on rest, keeping warm, and drinking large amounts of liquids. Analgesics and cough medications can also be used. Rest decreases the oxygen requirements of the body and reduces the respiratory rate and the chance of spreading the virus from the upper to lower respiratory tract. Keeping warm helps maintain the respiratory epithelium at a core body temperature of 37°C (98.6°F) or higher if fever is present, thereby inhibiting viral replication, which is optimal at 35°C (96°F). Drinking large amounts of fluids ensures that the function of the epithelial lining of the respiratory tract is not further compromised by dehydration. Antiviral medications may be indicated in some persons. Antibacterial antibiotics should be reserved for bacterial complications. The use of aspirin to treat fever should be avoided in children because of the risk of Reye syndrome.

Two antiviral drugs are available for treatment of influenza: Zanamivir (Relenza) and oseltamivir (Tamiflu) are inhibitors of neuraminidase, the glycoprotein necessary for viral replication and release. These drugs, which have been approved for treatment of acute uncomplicated influenza infection, are effective against both influenza A and B viruses. Zanamivir is administered intranasally and oseltamivir is administered orally. Zanamivir can cause bronchospasm and is not recommended for persons with asthma or chronic obstructive lung disease. To be effective, the antiviral drugs should be initiated within 36 hours after onset of symptoms.[15,16]

Influenza Immunization

Because influenza is so highly contagious, prevention relies primarily on vaccination. Currently, a trivalent inactivated influenza vaccine (TIIV) and a live attenuated influenza vaccine (LAIV3) are available.[19] A quadrivalent live attenuated influenza vaccine (LAIV4), which contains an additional B-type strain of the virus, is expected to replace the trivalent formulation. A quadrivalent inactivated influenza vaccine will also be available, in addition to the trivalent vaccine.[19]

The formulation of the vaccines must be changed yearly in response to antigenic changes in the influenza virus. The Centers for Disease Control and Prevention (CDC) Advisory Committee on Immunization Practices (ACIP) annually updates its recommendations for the composition of the vaccine. The effectiveness of the influenza vaccine in preventing and reducing the severity of influenza infection depends primarily on the age and immunocompetence of the recipient and the match between the virus strains included in the vaccine and those that circulate during the influenza season. The influenza vaccines are contraindicated in persons with anaphylactic hypersensitivity to eggs or to other components of the vaccine, persons with a history of Guillain-Barré syndrome, and persons with acute febrile illness.[19]

The TIIV, which is administered by injection, has become the mainstay for prevention of influenza. It has proved to be inexpensive and effective in reducing illness caused by influenza. Immunization may be used for any person 6 months of age or older, including those with high-risk conditions. It is recommended for all persons older than 50 years of age, persons with chronic health problems or who have immunodeficiencies (such as HIV infection), residents of nursing homes and other chronic-care facilities, women who are pregnant during the influenza season, health care providers, and household contacts or caregivers of persons who put them at higher risk for severe complications of influenza.[19]

The LAIVs, which are administered nasally, are cold-adapted viruses that replicate efficiently in the 25°C temperatures of the nasopharynx, inducing protective immunity against viruses included in the vaccine, but replicate inefficiently at the 38°C to 39°C temperature of the lower airways. Live attenuated influenza vaccine is an option for vaccination of healthy, nonpregnant persons, 2 to 49 years who do not have a medical condition that predisposes them to medical complications from influenza.[19]

Pneumonias

The term *pneumonia* describes inflammation of the parenchymal structures of the lung, such as the alveoli and bronchioles. Although antibiotics have significantly reduced the mortality rate from pneumonias, these diseases remain a leading cause of morbidity and mortality worldwide, particularly among the elderly and those with debilitating diseases. Etiologic agents include both infectious and noninfectious agents.

Classification

Pneumonias can be commonly classified according to the type of agent (typical or atypical) causing the infection, and distribution of the infection (lobar pneumonia or bronchopneumonia). Because of the overlap in symptomatology and changing spectrum of infectious organisms involved, pneumonias are increasingly being classified as community-acquired and hospital-acquired (nosocomial) pneumonias, depending on the setting in which they occur. Persons with compromised immune function constitute a special concern in both categories.

Typical pneumonias result from infection by bacteria that multiply extracellularly in the alveoli and cause inflammation and exudation of fluid into the air-filled alveolar spaces (Fig. 22-3A). *Atypical pneumonias* are caused by viral and mycoplasma infections that invade

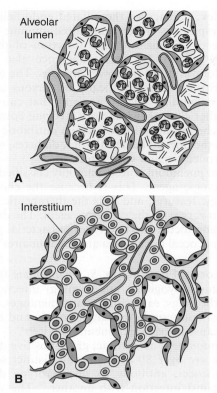

FIGURE 22-3. Location of inflammatory processes in **(A)** typical and **(B)** atypical forms of pneumonia.

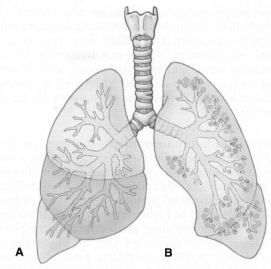

FIGURE 22-4. Distribution of lung involvement in **(A)** lobar pneumonia and **(B)** bronchopneumonia.

the alveolar septum and the interstitium of the lung (Fig. 22-3B). They produce less striking symptoms and physical findings than bacterial pneumonia; there is a lack of alveolar infiltration and purulent sputum, leukocytosis, and lobar consolidation on the radiograph. Acute bacterial pneumonias can be classified as lobar pneumonia or bronchopneumonia, based on their anatomic pattern of distribution.[14] In general, *lobar pneumonia* refers to consolidation of a part or all of a lung lobe, and *bronchopneumonia* signifies a patchy consolidation involving more than one lobe (Fig. 22-4).

Community-Acquired Pneumonia. The term *community-acquired pneumonia* is used to describe infections from organisms found in the community rather than in the hospital or nursing home. It is defined as an infection that begins outside the hospital or is diagnosed within 48 hours after admission to the hospital in a person who has not resided in a long-term care facility for 14 days or more before admission.[20–23] Community-acquired pneumonia may be further categorized according to risk of mortality and need for hospitalization based on age, presence of coexisting disease, and severity of illness, using physical examination, laboratory, and radiologic findings.

Community-acquired pneumonia may be either bacterial or viral.[14,20–23] The most common cause of infection in all categories is *S. pneumoniae*. Other common pathogens include *H. influenzae*, *S. aureus*, and gram-negative bacilli. Less common agents are *Mycoplasma pneumoniae*, *Chlamydia* species, and viruses, sometimes called *atypical agents*. Common viral causes of community-acquired pneumonia include the influenza virus, respiratory syncytial virus, adenovirus, and parainfluenza virus.

The methods used in the diagnosis of community-acquired pneumonia depend on age, coexisting health problems, and the severity of illness. In persons younger than 65 years of age and without coexisting disease, the diagnosis usually is based on history and physical examination, chest radiographs, and knowledge of the microorganisms currently causing infections in the community. Sputum specimens may be obtained for staining procedures and culture. Blood cultures may be done for persons requiring hospitalization.

Treatment involves the use of appropriate antibiotic therapy. Empiric antibiotic therapy, based on knowledge regarding an antibiotic's spectrum of action and ability to penetrate bronchopulmonary secretions, often is used for persons with community-acquired pneumonia who do not require hospitalization. Hospitalization and more intensive care may be required depending on the person's age, preexisting health status, and severity of the infection.

Hospital-Acquired Pneumonia. Hospital-acquired, or nosocomial, pneumonia is defined as a lower respiratory tract infection that was not present or incubating on admission to the hospital. Usually, infections occurring 48 hours or more after admission are considered hospital acquired.[14,24,25] Persons requiring intubation and mechanical ventilation are particularly at risk, as are those with compromised immune function, chronic lung disease, and airway instrumentation, such as endotracheal intubation or tracheotomy. Ventilator-associated pneumonia is pneumonia that develops in mechanically ventilated patients more than 48 hours after intubation.

Most hospital-acquired infections are bacterial. The organisms differ from those responsible for community-acquired pneumonias, and reflect those present in the hospital environment. Gram-negative rods (*Enterobacteriaceae and Pseudomonas* species) *and S. aureus are the most common isolates.*[14] Many of these organisms have acquired antibiotic resistance and are thus difficult to treat.

Pneumonia in Immunocompromised Persons. Pneumonia in immunocompromised persons remains a major source of morbidity and mortality. Although almost all types of microorganisms can cause pulmonary infection in immunocompromised persons, certain types of immunologic defects tend to favor certain types of infections.[14] Defects in humoral immunity predispose to bacterial infections against which antibodies play an important role, whereas defects in cellular immunity predispose to infections caused by viruses, fungi, mycobacteria, and protozoa. Neutropenia and impaired granulocyte function, as occur in persons with leukemia or bone marrow depression as well as persons undergoing chemotherapy, predispose to infections caused by *S. aureus, Aspergillus,* gram-negative bacilli, and *Candida.* The time course of infection often provides a hint to the type of agent involved. A fulminant pneumonia usually is caused by bacterial infection, whereas an insidious onset usually is indicative of a viral, fungal, protozoal, or mycobacterial infection.

Acute Bacterial (Typical) Pneumonia

Bacterial pneumonias remain an important cause of mortality among the elderly and debilitated. The lung below the main bronchi is normally sterile despite frequent entry of microorganisms into the air passages by inhalation during ventilation or aspiration of nasopharyngeal secretions. Most people unknowingly aspirate small amounts of organisms that have colonized their upper airways, particularly during sleep. These organisms do not normally cause infection because of the small number that are aspirated and because the respiratory tract's defense mechanisms prevent them from entering the distal air passages (Table 22-1). Loss of the cough reflex, damage to the ciliated endothelium that lines the respiratory tract, or impaired immune defenses predispose to colonization and infection of the lower respiratory system. Bacterial adherence also plays a role in colonization of the lower airways. The epithelial cells of critically and chronically ill persons are more receptive to binding microorganisms that cause pneumonia. Other clinical risk factors favoring colonization of the tracheobronchial tree include antibiotic therapy that alters the normal bacterial flora, diabetes, smoking, chronic bronchitis, and viral infection.

Bacterial pneumonias are commonly classified according to etiologic agent. This is because the clinical and morphologic features, and thus the therapeutic implications, often vary with the causative agent. The discussion in this section focuses on two types of bacterial pneumonia: pneumococcal pneumonia and Legionnaires' disease.

Pneumococcal Pneumonia. *S. pneumoniae (pneumococcus)* causes pyogenic (pus-forming) infections, primarily of the lungs, ears, sinuses, and meninges. It is one of the most common bacterial pathogens and the most common cause of bacterial pneumonia.[14,26,27]

S. pneumoniae is an aerobic, gram-positive diplococcus. There are over 80 antigenically distinct serotypes of pneumococci; antibody to one serotype does not protect against infection with another.[26] The virulence of *S. pneumoniae* is a function of its polysaccharide capsule, which prevents or delays digestion by phagocytes. The polysaccharide is an antigen that primarily elicits a B-cell response with antibody production. In the absence of antibody, clearance of the pneumococci from the body relies on the reticuloendothelial system, with the macrophages in the spleen playing a major role in elimination of the organism. This, along with the spleen's role in antibody generation, increases the risk for pneumococcal bacteremia in persons who are anatomically or functionally asplenic, such as children with sickle cell disease.

The initial step in the pathogenesis of pneumococcal infection is the attachment and colonization of the organism to the mucus and cells of the nasopharynx. Colonization does not equate with signs of infection.

TABLE 22-1 Respiratory Defense Mechanisms and Conditions That Impair Their Effectiveness

Defense Mechanism	Function	Factors That Impair Effectiveness
Glottic and cough reflexes	Protect against aspiration into tracheobronchial tree	Loss of cough reflex due to stroke or neural lesion, neuromuscular disease, abdominal or chest surgery, depression of the cough reflex due to sedation or anesthesia, presence of a nasogastric tube (tends to cause adaptation of afferent receptors)
Mucociliary blanket	Removes secretions, microorganisms, and particles from the respiratory tract	Smoking, viral diseases, chilling, inhalation of irritating gases
Phagocytic and bactericidal action of alveolar macrophages	Removes microorganisms and foreign particles from the lung	Tobacco smoke, chilling, alcohol, oxygen intoxication
Immune defenses (IgA and IgG and cell-mediated immunity)	Destroy microorganisms	Congenital and acquired immunodeficiency states

Perfectly healthy people can be colonized and carry the organism without evidence of infection. The spread of particular strains of pneumococci, particularly antibiotic-resistant strains, is largely by healthy, colonized individuals.

The signs and symptoms of pneumococcal pneumonia vary widely, depending on the age and health status of the infected person.[14,26,27] In previously healthy persons, the onset usually is sudden and is characterized by malaise; severe, shaking chills; and fever. The temperature may go as high as 106°F (41°C). During the initial or congestive stage, coughing brings up watery sputum and breath sounds are limited, with fine crackles. As the disease progresses, the character of the sputum changes; it may be blood tinged or rust colored to purulent. Pleuritic pain, a sharp pain that is more severe with respiratory movements, is common. With antibiotic therapy, fever usually subsides in approximately 48 to 72 hours, and recovery is uneventful. Elderly persons are less likely to experience marked elevations in temperature; in these persons, the only sign of pneumonia may be a loss of appetite and deterioration in mental status.

Treatment includes the use of antibiotics that are effective against *S. pneumoniae*. In the past, *S. pneumoniae* was uniformly susceptible to penicillin. However, penicillin-resistant and multidrug-resistant strains have been emerging in the United States and other countries.

The prevalence and intrinsic virulence of the pneumococci and their resistance to antimicrobial therapy has emphasized the need for vaccination. Two vaccine formulations are currently available: the pneumococcal conjugate vaccine (PCV13) and the pneumococcal polysaccharide vaccine (PPSV23).[28] The PCV13 protects against 13 types of pneumococcal bacteria. It is recommended for use in infants and young children and for all adults 50 years of age and older who have conditions that weaken the immune system such as HIV infection, organ transplantation, leukemia, lymphoma, and severe kidney disease.[28] The PPSV23 vaccine consists of the 23 most common capsular serotypes that cause the most common invasive pneumococcal disease.[27] It is recommended for all adults 65 years of age and older and for those 2 years of age and older who are at high risk for the disease. It is also recommended for adults who smoke or have asthma.[28]

Legionnaires' Disease. Legionnaires' disease is a form of bronchopneumonia caused by a gram-negative rod, *Legionella pneumophila*.[14,26,29] Transmission from person to person has not been documented; instead, the infection typically occurs when water that contains the pathogen is aerosolized into appropriately sized droplets and is inhaled or aspirated by a susceptible host. Although healthy persons can contract the infection, the risk is greater among persons with chronic diseases and those with impaired cell-mediated immunity.

Legionella pneumonia may present subacutely for days or a week, but more typically presents acutely with malaise, weakness, lethargy, fever, and dry cough.[29] Other manifestations include disturbances of central nervous system function, gastrointestinal tract involvement, arthralgias, and elevation in body temperature, sometimes to more than 40°C (104°F). The presence of pneumonia along with diarrhea, hyponatremia, and confusion is characteristic of *Legionella* pneumonia. The disease causes consolidation of lung tissues and impairs gas exchange. Another characteristic of the disease is a lack of a normal pulse-temperature relationship in which a fever is not accompanied by an appropriate rise in heart rate.[28] For example, a temperature of 102°F is normally accompanied by a heart rate of 110 beats/min; in *Legionella* pneumonia it is often less than 100 beats/min.[29]

Diagnosis is based on clinical manifestations, radiologic studies, and specialized laboratory tests to detect the presence of the organism. Urine antigen tests and sputum fluorescent antibody tests allow for rapid detection of *L. pneumophila* serotype 1, but are less sensitive than culture for identifying other serotypes. Treatment consists of administration of antibiotics that are known to be effective against *L. pneumophila*. Delay in instituting antibiotic therapy significantly increases mortality rates; therefore, antibiotics known to be effective against *L. pneumophila* should be included in the treatment regimen for severe community-acquired pneumonia.[29]

Primary Atypical Pneumonia

The atypical pneumonias are characterized by patchy involvement of the lung, largely confined to the alveolar septum and pulmonary interstitium. The term *atypical* denotes a lack of lung consolidation, production of moderate amounts of sputum, moderate elevation of white blood cell count, and lack of alveolar exudate.[14] These pneumonias are caused by a variety of agents, the most common being *Mycoplasma pneumoniae*. Mycoplasma infections are particularly common among children and young adults. Other etiologic agents include viruses (e.g., influenza virus, respiratory syncytial virus, adenoviruses, rhinoviruses, rubella [measles] and varicella [chickenpox] viruses) and *Chlamydia pneumoniae*.[14] In some cases, the cause is unknown.

The agents that cause atypical pneumonias damage the respiratory tract epithelium and impair respiratory tract defenses, thereby predisposing to secondary bacterial infections. The sporadic form of atypical pneumonia is usually mild with a low mortality rate. It may, however, assume epidemic proportions with intensified severity and greater mortality, as occurred in the influenza pandemic of 1918.

The clinical course among persons with mycoplasma and viral pneumonias varies widely from a mild infection that masquerades as a chest cold to a more serious and even fatal outcome. The symptoms may remain confined to fever, headache, and muscle aches and pains. Cough, when present, is characteristically dry, hacking, and nonproductive. The diagnosis is usually made based on history, physical findings, and chest radiographs.

Tuberculosis

Pulmonary tuberculosis remains one of the deadliest diseases in the world. It is estimated that, if better methods to control infection are not developed, by the year 2020 nearly 1 billion people worldwide will be newly infected with tuberculosis, over 150 million will become clinically ill, and 36 million will die of the disease.[30] With the introduction of antibiotics in the 1950s, the United States and other Western countries enjoyed a long period of decline in the number of infections. However, since the mid-1980s the rate of infection has increased, particularly among HIV-infected people. In the United States, the biggest increase in new cases was from 1985 to 1993, after which the number of reported cases has again declined.[29] In part, this decline reflects the impact of resources committed to assist state and local control efforts, wider screening and prevention programs, and increased support for prevention programs among HIV-infected persons.

Tuberculosis is more common among foreign-born persons from countries with a high incidence of tuberculosis and among residents of high-risk congregate settings such as correctional facilities, drug treatment facilities, and homeless shelters. Outbreaks of a drug-resistant form of tuberculosis have emerged, complicating the selection of drugs and affecting the duration of treatment.

Etiology

Tuberculosis is an airborne infection caused by the *M. tuberculosis* mycobacterium. The mycobacteria are slender, rod-shaped, aerobic bacilli that do not form spores[2,31–33] (Fig. 22-5). They are similar to other bacteria except for a waxy cell wall that is responsible for many of the bacteria's characteristics including its slow growth, antigenicity, and resistance to detergents, disinfectants, and antibiotics. It also renders the bacteria resistant to common laboratory stains. Once stained,

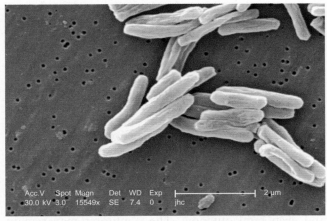

FIGURE 22-5. Scanning electron micrograph (SEM) depicting some of the ultrastructural details seen in the cell wall configuration of a number of gram-positive *Mycobacterium tuberculosis* bacteria. (From the Centers for Disease Control and Prevention Public Health Image Library. No. 9997. Courtesy of Ray Butler.)

the dye cannot be discolored with acid solution, hence the name acid-fast bacilli. Although *M. tuberculosis* can infect practically any organ of the body, the lungs are most frequently involved.

Tuberculosis is an airborne infection spread by minute, invisible particles, called *droplet nuclei,* that are harbored in the respiratory secretions of persons with active tuberculosis.[32,33] Coughing, sneezing, and talking all create respiratory droplets; these droplets evaporate, leaving the organisms (droplet nuclei), which remain suspended in the air and are circulated by air currents. Thus, living in crowded and confined conditions increases the risk for spread of the disease.

Pathogenesis

The pathogenesis of tuberculosis in a previously unexposed, immunocompetent person is centered on the development of a cell-mediated immune response that confers resistance to the organism and development of tissue hypersensitivity to the tubercular antigens.[2,32,33] The destructive features of the disease result from a cell-mediated hypersensitivity response (see Chapter 16) rather than the destructive capabilities of the tubercle bacillus.

Macrophages are the primary cell infected with *M. tuberculosis.* Inhaled droplet nuclei pass down the bronchial tree without settling on the epithelium and are deposited in the alveoli. Soon after entering the lung, the bacilli are phagocytosed by alveolar macrophages, but resist destruction. Although the macrophages that first ingest *M. tuberculosis* cannot kill the organisms, they initiate a cell-mediated immune response that eventually contains the infection. As the tubercle bacilli multiply, the infected macrophages degrade them and present their antigens to helper (CD4+) T lymphocytes. The sensitized helper T cells, in turn, stimulate the macrophages to increase their concentration of lytic enzymes. This boosts their ability to kill the bacilli; however, when released, these lytic enzymes also damage lung tissue. The development of a population of activated cytotoxic (CD8+) T cells and macrophages capable of ingesting and destroying the bacilli constitutes the cell-mediated immune response, a process that takes about 3 to 6 weeks to become effective.

In immunocompetent persons, the cell-mediated immune response results in the development of a gray-white, circumscribed granulomatous lesion, called a *Ghon focus,* that contains the tubercle bacilli, modified macrophages, and other immune cells.[2,13] It is usually located in the subpleural area of the upper segments of the lower lobes or in the lower segments of the upper lobe. When the number of organisms is high, the hypersensitivity reaction causes the central portion of the Ghon focus to undergo necrosis, producing a soft, whitish core of dead cells referred to as a caseous (cheeselike) necrosis. During this same period, tubercle bacilli, free or inside macrophages, drain along the lymph channels to the tracheobronchial lymph nodes of the affected lung and there evoke the formation of caseous granulomas. The combination of the primary lung lesion and lymph

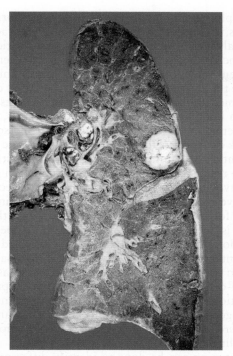

FIGURE 22-6. Primary tuberculosis. A healed Ghon complex is represented by a subpleural nodule and involved hilar lymph nodes. (From Beasley MB, Travis WD, Rubin E. The respiratory system. In: Rubin R, Strayer DS, eds. *Rubin's Pathology: Clinicopathologic Foundations of Medicine*. 6th ed. Philadelphia, PA: Wolters Kluwer Health | Lippincott Williams & Wilkins; 2012:550.)

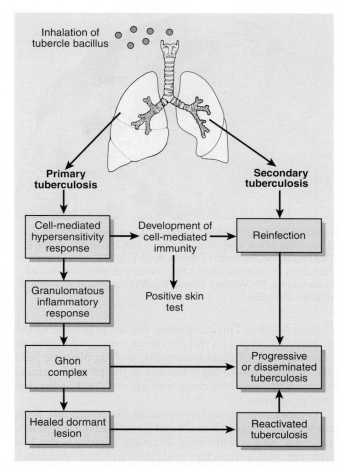

FIGURE 22-7. Pathogenesis of tuberculosis infection.

node granulomas is called a *Ghon complex* (Fig. 22-6). The Ghon complex eventually heals, undergoing shrinkage, fibrous scarring, and calcification, the last of these being visible radiographically. However, small numbers of organisms may remain viable for years. Later, if immune mechanisms decline or fail, latent tuberculosis infection has the potential to develop into secondary tuberculosis.

Primary Tuberculosis

Primary tuberculosis is a form of the disease that develops in previously unexposed, and therefore unsensitized, persons.[2,13,32,33] It typically is initiated as a result of inhaling droplet nuclei that contain the tubercle bacillus (Fig. 22-7). Most people with primary tuberculosis are asymptomatic and go on to develop *latent tuberculosis infection* in which T lymphocytes and macrophages surround the organism in granulomas that limit their spread. Individuals with latent tuberculosis do not have active disease and cannot transmit the organism to others.[34]

In approximately 5% of newly infected people, the immune response is inadequate; these people go on to develop progressive primary tuberculosis with continued destruction of pulmonary tissue and spread to multiple sites within the lung.[2,32,33] This usually occurs in young children, whose immune systems are immature, or in adults with HIV infection or other immunodeficiency

disorders. Sometimes the onset of symptoms is abrupt, with high fever, pleuritis, and lymphadenitis. As the disease spreads, the organism gains access to the sputum, allowing the person to infect others.

In rare instances, tuberculosis may erode into a blood vessel, giving rise to hematogenic dissemination. *Miliary tuberculosis* describes minute lesions, resembling millet seeds, resulting from this type of dissemination that can involve almost any organ, particularly the brain, meninges, liver, kidney, and bone marrow.

Secondary Tuberculosis

Secondary tuberculosis represents either reinfection from inhaled droplet nuclei or reactivation of a previously healed primary lesion[2] (see Fig. 22-7). It often occurs in situations of impaired body defense mechanisms. The partial immunity that follows primary tuberculosis normally affords protection against reinfection and helps localize the disease should reactivation occur. After the development of hypersensitivity, the infection becomes quiescent in the majority of patients. Cavities are formed as a result of the immune response walling off the infection. These cavities may coalesce to a size of up to 10 to 15 cm in diameter (Fig. 22-8). In vulnerable patients such as the very young or immunocompromised adults, the primary infection can progress into

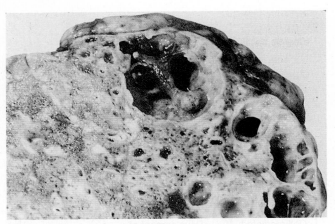

FIGURE 22-8. Cavitary tuberculosis in the apex of the left upper lobe of the lung. (From Beasley MB, Travis WD, Rubin E. The respiratory system. In: Rubin R, Strayer DS, eds. *Rubin's Pathology: Clinicopathologic Foundations of Medicine.* 6th ed. Philadelphia, PA: Wolters Kluwer Health | Lippincott Williams & Wilkins; 2012:550.)

clinical disease. This commonly occurs at the site of the primary lesion or at a distant site as a result of hematogenous spread. Clinical symptoms, such as pleuritic pain due to extension of the infection to the pleural surfaces between the lung and chest wall are common as the disease progresses.

Persons with secondary tuberculosis commonly present with low-grade fevers, night sweats, easy fatigability, anorexia, and weight loss.[2] A cough initially is dry but later becomes productive with purulent and sometimes blood-tinged sputum. Dyspnea and orthopnea develop as the disease advances.

Diagnosis

A definitive diagnosis of active pulmonary tuberculosis requires identification of the organism from cultures or DNA amplification techniques.[33,35] Culture remains the gold standard for laboratory confirmation of infection and is required for drug sensitivity testing. Culture specimens may be obtained from early morning sputum specimens, gastric aspirations, or bronchial washings obtained during fiber-optic bronchoscopy. Because *M. tuberculosis* grows slowly, cultures in liquid media require several days, and cultures on solid media require up to 12 weeks. Several nucleic acid amplification [NAA] tests are available. These permit the diagnosis of tuberculosis in as quickly as several hours.[35] However, their applicability is limited by variable sensitivity and high cost. Chest radiographs are used to determine the extent of lung involvement. In patients with secondary tuberculosis, CT scanning may also be performed.

The tuberculin skin test, which measures the delayed hypersensitivity response to an intradermal injection of tuberculin, a sterile liquid containing proteins derived from the tubercle bacillus, is used for tuberculosis screening. The test is recommended for high-risk populations, including persons who are in close contact with someone who has confirmed active tuberculosis, residents

and employees in congregate settings (e.g., corrections facilities, homeless shelters, long-term care facilities), and health care workers with high-risk patients.[32,35] The tuberculin test cannot distinguish between active and latent infection, and has several other limitations. Because the hypersensitivity response to the test depends on cell-mediated immunity, false-negative test results can occur in immunocompromised persons; that is, a negative tuberculin test result can mean that the person has a true lack of exposure to tuberculosis or is anergic (unable to mount a normal immune response to the test). False-positive results can also occur; for example, in persons who have nontuberculosis mycobacteria infection or who have received the Bacillus Calmette-Guérin (BCG) vaccine for tuberculosis prevention. Although the BCG vaccine is not used in the United States for tuberculosis prevention, many immigrants will have received it.

Recently, two interferon gamma release assays have come on the market. These tests are in vitro assays of CD4[+] T-cell-interferon gamma release in response to stimulation by specific *M. tuberculosis* antigens. Since the antigens are absent from all BCG strains and most nontuberculous mycobacteria, the test is superior to the tuberculin skin test.[16,34]

Genotyping can be done to identify different strains of *M. tuberculosis* in persons who have been diagnosed with active tuberculosis. It can be used to evaluate second episodes of tuberculosis to determine whether the second episode was due to relapse or reinfection. Genotyping also permits the evaluation of isolates with different patterns of drug susceptibility.[35] In addition, it is useful in investigating outbreaks of infection and determining sites and patterns of *M. tuberculosis* transmission in communities.

Treatment

The goals of therapy are to treat infected individuals by eliminating the tubercle bacilli while preventing the spread of infection and development of drug-resistant forms of the disease. The tubercle bacillus is an aerobic organism that multiplies slowly and remains relatively dormant in oxygen-poor caseous material. However, it undergoes a high rate of mutation and tends to acquire resistance to any one drug. For this reason, multidrug regimens are used for treating persons with active tuberculosis, and treatment typically continues for 6 months or longer. Treatment duration is prolonged due to the slow-growing nature of the tuberculosis bacteria that impairs the effectiveness of antibiotics that target actively replicating organisms.

The basic principles of tuberculosis treatment are: (1) to administer multiple drugs to which the organisms are susceptible, (2) to add at least two new drugs when treatment failure is suspected, (3) to provide the safest and most effective therapy in the shortest period of time, and (4) to ensure adherence to therapy.[16] Adherence to treatment can be improved by providing detailed education about the disease and its treatment in addition to a case manager who supervises all aspects of an individual's care. Direct observed therapy (DOT), which requires that a health care worker physically observe the person's ingestion of the medications, also improves adherence to the program.[16]

The primary drugs used are isoniazid (INH), ethambutol, pyrazinamide, and rifampin. In addition to persons with active tuberculosis, persons who have had contact with cases of active tuberculosis and who are at risk for development of an active form of the disease are treated.[35–38] Prophylactic treatment is also used for persons who have latent tuberculosis infection but do not have active disease. These persons are considered to harbor a small number of microorganisms and usually are treated with INH.[34]

Persons with drug-resistant *M. tuberculosis* infection require careful supervision and more extensive drug regimens.[36–38] Drug susceptibility tests are used to guide treatment. Tuberculosis in persons with concomitant HIV infection requires management by experts in both tuberculosis and HIV.

Fungal Infections

Although most fungal infections are asymptomatic, they can be severe or even fatal in persons who have experienced a heavy exposure, have underlying immune deficiencies, or develop progressive disease that is not recognized or treated. The host's cell-mediated immune response is paramount in controlling such infections; thus, immunocompromised persons, particularly those with HIV infection, are particularly prone to development of severe or fatal infection.

Pathologic fungi generally induce a delayed cell-mediated hypersensitivity response to their chemical constituents (see Chapter 15). Cellular immunity is mediated by antigen-specific T lymphocytes and cytokine-activated macrophages that assume fungicidal properties. The primary pulmonary lesions consist of aggregates of macrophages stuffed with organisms, with similar lesions developing in the lymph nodes that drain the area. These lesions develop into granulomas complete with giant cells and may develop central necrosis and calcification resembling that of primary tuberculosis.

Types of Infections

Fungi are classified as yeasts and molds. Yeasts are round and grow by budding. Molds form tubular structures called *hyphae* and grow by branching and forming spores (see Chapter 14). Some fungi are *dimorphic,* meaning that they grow as yeasts at body temperatures and as molds at room temperatures.

A simple classification of mycoses (diseases caused by fungi) divides them into superficial, cutaneous, subcutaneous, or deep (systemic) mycoses. The superficial, cutaneous, or subcutaneous mycoses cause disease of the skin, hair, and nails. Deep fungal infections may produce pulmonary and systemic infections and are sometimes fatal. They are caused by virulent fungi that live freely, typically in soil or decaying organic matter and frequently in specific geographic regions. The most

common of these are the dimorphic fungi, *Histoplasma capsulatum, Coccidioides immitis,* and *Blastomyces dermatitidis.*[39,40] These fungi form infectious spores, which enter the body through the respiratory system. Most people who become infected with these fungi develop only minor symptoms or none at all—only a small minority develop serious disease.

Each of the dimorphic fungi has a typical geographic distribution. *H. capsulatum,* which is the etiologic agent in *histoplasmosis,* is endemic along the major river valleys of the central and eastern United States (i.e., Ohio, Missouri, Mississippi river valleys), eastern Canada, Mexico, Central and South America, Africa, and southeast Asia.[40,41] The organism grows in areas that have been enriched with bird excreta: old chicken houses, pigeon lofts, barns, and trees where birds roost. The infection is acquired by inhaling the fungal spores that are released when the dirt or dust from the infected areas is disturbed. *C. immitis,* which causes *coccidioidomycosis,* is most prevalent in the southwestern United States, principally in California, Arizona, and Texas; Mexico; and Central and South America.[40,42] Because of its prevalence in the San Joaquin Valley, the disease is sometimes referred to as *San Joaquin fever* or *valley fever. C. immitis* lives in soil, and events that disturb soil, such as dust storms and digging during construction, have been associated with increased incidence of the disease. *B. capsulatum,* the agent causing *blastomycosis,* is most commonly found in the south-central and northwestern United States and Canada.[40,43]

Clinical Features

Depending on the host's resistance and immunocompetence, the diseases usually take one of three forms: (1) an acute primary disease, (2) a chronic (cavitary) pulmonary disease, or (3) a disseminated infection. The lesions of fungal infections consist of epithelioid cell granulomatous containing aggregates of macrophages with engulfed microorganisms. Similar nodules develop in the regional lymph nodes. There is a striking similarity to the primary lesions of tuberculosis. The clinical manifestations often consist of a mild, self-limited flulike syndrome.

In the vulnerable host, chronic cavitary lesions develop, with a predilection for the upper lobe of the lung, resembling the secondary form of tuberculosis. The most common manifestations are productive cough, fever, night sweats, and weight loss. Disseminated disease most often develops as an acute and fulminating infection in the very old or the very young or in persons with compromised immune function. Although the macrophages of the reticuloendothelial system can remove the fungi from the bloodstream, they are unable to destroy them. Characteristically, this form of the disease presents with a high fever, generalized lymph node enlargement, hepatosplenomegaly, muscle wasting, anemia, leukopenia, and thrombocytopenia. There may be hoarseness, ulcerations of the mouth and tongue, nausea, vomiting, diarrhea, and abdominal pain. Often, meningitis becomes a dominant feature of the disease. Persons with blastomycosis may experience cutaneous infections that induce pseudoepitheliomatous hyperplasia, which may be mistaken for squamous cell carcinoma.

Skin tests similar to the tuberculin test can be used to detect exposure to *Histoplasma* and *Coccidioides*. There is no reliable skin test for *Blastomyces*. The diagnosis of acute infection is usually made by direct visualization of the organism in tissue sections or sputum culture. Serologic tests that detect antibodies against the specific fungi are available, but lack sensitivity and specificity.

Treatment depends on the severity of infection. General symptomatic therapy is given as needed for disease that is limited to the chest with no evidence of progression. The oral or intravenous antifungal drugs are used in the treatment of persons with progressive disease.

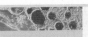

SUMMARY CONCEPTS

■ Viruses are the most frequent cause of respiratory tract infections, including the common cold and infection with the influenza virus. The common cold occurs more frequently than any other respiratory infection. The fingers are the usual source of transmission, and the most common portals of entry are the nasal mucosa and the conjunctiva of the eye. The influenza virus causes three syndromes: an uncomplicated rhinotracheitis, a respiratory viral infection followed by a bacterial infection, and viral pneumonia. The contagiousness of influenza results from the ability of the virus to mutate and form subtypes against which the population is unprotected.

■ Pneumonias are respiratory disorders involving inflammation of the lung structures, such as the alveoli and bronchioles. They are caused by infectious agents such as bacteria and viruses. They are commonly classified according to the type of organism causing the infection (typical or atypical), location of the infection (lobar pneumonia or bronchopneumonia), and setting in which it occurs (community or hospital acquired).

■ Tuberculosis is a chronic respiratory infection caused by the bacterium *M. tuberculosis*. The destructiveness of the disease results from the cell-mediated hypersensitivity response that the bacillus evokes rather than its inherent destructive capabilities. The treatment of tuberculosis, which focuses on eliminating the tuberculosis bacilli from infected persons and eliminating its spread, requires multiple medications and has been complicated by outbreaks of drug-resistant forms of the disease.

■ Infections caused by the fungi *H. capsulatum* (histoplasmosis), *C. immitis* (coccidioidomycosis), and *B. dermatitidis* (blastomycosis) produce pulmonary manifestations that resemble tuberculosis. These infections are common but seldom serious unless they produce progressive destruction of lung tissue or the infection disseminates to organs and tissues outside the lungs.

Cancer of the Lung

Cancer of the lung is currently the leading cause of cancer-related death in the United States and worldwide.[13,14,44-48] The incidence and rates of death from the disease rose dramatically in the 20th century, correlating with an increase in cigarette smoking. This epidemic of lung cancer deaths is now receding in countries where tobacco control has reduced smoking, but it is rapidly rising in others. Because lung cancer often is far advanced before it is discovered, the prognosis is generally poor. The overall 5-year survival rate is 16%, a dismal statistic that has changed little in the past 50 years.

Carcinogenic chemicals in tobacco smoke trigger genetic changes that convert normal bronchial cells to cancer cells. Other influences may act in concert with smoking or may by themselves be responsible for some lung cancers. For example, there is increased incidence of lung cancer in asbestos workers and workers exposed to dusts containing arsenic, chromium, nickel, and vinyl chloride.[14] Lung cancer is also a disease of aging, with 60% of cases diagnosed in persons older than 65 years of age.[44]

Types of Lung Cancer

Four histologic types account for most primary lung cancers: adenocarcinoma (males 37%, females 47%), squamous cell lung carcinoma (males 32%, females 25%), large cell carcinoma (males 18%, females 10%), and small cell carcinoma (males 14%, females 18%).[14] For therapeutic purposes such as staging and treatment, lung cancers are further identified as non–small cell lung cancer (NSCLC) and small cell lung cancer (SCLC).[13,14] One of the key reasons for this classification is that SCLC has usually metastasized by the time of diagnosis and hence is not typically amenable to surgery. It is usually best treated with chemotherapy, with or without radiation.

Non–Small Cell Lung Cancers

The NSCLCs include squamous cell carcinomas, adenocarcinomas, and large cell carcinomas.[13,14] *Squamous cell carcinoma* is most commonly found in men and is closely correlated with a smoking history. Squamous cell

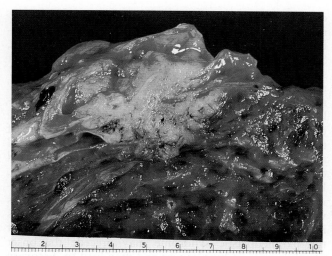

FIGURE 22-9. Squamous cell carcinoma of the lung in which the tumor grows within the lumen of a bronchus and invades the adjacent intrapulmonary lymph node. (From Beasley MB, Travis WD, Rubin E. The respiratory system. In: Rubin R, Strayer DS, eds. *Rubin's Pathology: Clinicopathologic Foundations of Medicine.* 6th ed. Philadelphia, PA: Wolters Kluwer Health | Lippincott Williams & Wilkins; 2012:595.)

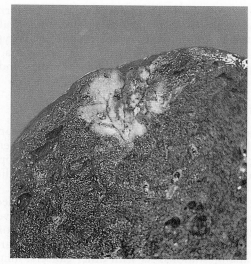

FIGURE 22-10. Adenocarcinoma of the lung. A peripheral tumor is located in the upper right lobe of the lung. (From Beasley MB, Travis WD, Rubin E. The respiratory system. In: Rubin R, Strayer DS, eds. *Rubin's Pathology: Clinicopathologic Foundations of Medicine.* 6th ed. Philadelphia, PA: Wolters Kluwer Health | Lippincott Williams & Wilkins; 2012:595.)

carcinoma tends to originate in the central bronchi as an intraluminal growth and is thus more amenable to early detection through cytologic examination of the sputum than other forms of lung cancer.[13] It tends to spread centrally into major bronchi and adjacent intrapulmonary lymph nodes (Fig 22-9). Central cavitation of the tumor is frequent.

Currently, *adenocarcinoma* is the most common subtype of lung cancer in North America.[13,14] Its association with cigarette smoking is weaker than for squamous cell carcinoma. It is the most common type of lung cancer in women and nonsmokers. Adenocarcinoma is a malignant epithelial cell tumor with glandular differentiation or mucin production by the tumor cells. These tumors tend to be located more peripherally than squamous cell sarcomas and are often associated with pleural fibrosis and scarring (Fig. 22-10). In general, adenocarcinomas have a poorer stage-for-stage prognosis than squamous cell carcinomas.

Large cell carcinomas have large, polygonal cells. They constitute a group of neoplasms that are highly anaplastic and difficult to categorize as squamous cell carcinoma or adenocarcinoma. They tend to occur in the periphery of the lung, invading subsegmental bronchi and larger airways. They have a poor prognosis because of their tendency to spread to distant sites early in their course.[13,14]

Small Cell Lung Cancer

Small cell lung cancer is characterized by a distinctive cell type—small round to oval cells that are approximately the size of a lymphocyte.[13,14,49,50] The cells grow in clusters that exhibit neither glandular nor squamous organization. The tumors are thought to arise from the neuroendocrine cells of the bronchial epithelium, and some of the tumor cells may be able to secrete hormonally active products. This cell type is associated with several types of paraneoplastic syndrome (signs and symptoms caused by secretions of or immune response to tumor cells), including the syndrome of inappropriate antidiuretic hormone secretion (SIADH; see Chapter 8). This type of cancer has the strongest association with cigarette smoking and is rarely observed in someone who has not smoked.

Small cell lung cancer is highly malignant, tends to infiltrate widely, disseminate early, and is rarely resectable. About 70% of the cancers have detectable metastases at the time of diagnosis; the rest are assumed to have micrometastases. Brain metastases are particularly common with SCLC and may provide the first evidence of the tumor. Response rates for treatment with chemotherapy (cisplatin and etoposide) are excellent, with 50% to 60% complete response in persons with limited disease and 15% to 20% complete response in those with extensive disease.[47] However, remissions tend to be short-lived with a mean duration of 6 to 8 months. Once the disease has recurred, the mean survival length is 3 to 4 months. Overall the 2-year survival is 20% to 40% in limited-stage disease and less than 5% in extensive disease.

Clinical Features

Lung cancers are aggressive, locally invasive, and widely metastasizing tumors. Squamous cell and adenocarcinomas usually begin as small mucosal lesions that may follow one of several patterns of growth. They may form intraluminal masses that invade the bronchial mucosa and infiltrate the peribronchial connective tissue, or they may form large, bulky masses that extend into the adjacent lung tissue. Some large tumors undergo central necrosis and acquire local areas of hemorrhage, and some invade the pleural cavity and chest wall and spread to adjacent intrathoracic structures.[15] All types of lung cancer, especially small cell lung carcinoma, have the capacity to synthesize bioactive products and produce paraneoplastic syndromes.

Manifestations

The manifestations of lung cancer are extremely variable, depending on the location of the tumor, the presence of distant metastasis, and the occurrence of paraneoplastic syndromes. Often the malignancy develops insidiously, giving little or no warning of its presence.[46–50]

The manifestations of lung cancer can be divided into three categories based on: (1) those due to involvement of the lung and adjacent structures; (2) the effects of local spread and metastasis; and (3) nonmetastatic paraneoplastic manifestations. As with other cancers, lung cancer also causes nonspecific symptoms such as anorexia and weight loss. Because its symptoms are similar to those associated with smoking and chronic bronchitis, they often are disregarded. Metastases already exist in many patients presenting with evidence of lung cancer. The most common sites of these metastases are the brain, bone, and liver. Many of the manifestations of lung cancer result from local irritation and obstruction of the airways and from invasion of the mediastinum and pleural space. The earliest symptoms usually are chronic cough, shortness of breath, and wheezing because of airway irritation and obstruction. Hemoptysis (i.e., blood in the sputum) occurs when the lesion erodes into blood vessels. Pain receptors in the chest are limited to the parietal pleura, mediastinum, larger blood vessels, and peribronchial afferent vagal fibers. Dull, intermittent, poorly localized retrosternal pain is common in tumors that involve the mediastinum. Pain becomes persistent, localized, and more severe when the disease invades the pleura. Brain metastasis, which occurs in 10% of NSCLC (most commonly with adenocarcinoma) and 20% to 30% of SCLC, may present with headache, nausea, vomiting, seizures, dizziness, and altered mental status.[46]

Tumors that invade the mediastinum may cause hoarseness because of the involvement of the recurrent laryngeal nerve and cause difficulty in swallowing because of compression of the esophagus. An uncommon complication called the *superior vena cava syndrome* occurs in some persons with mediastinal involvement. Interruption of blood flow in this vessel usually results from compression by the tumor or involved lymph nodes. The disorder can interfere with venous drainage from the head, neck, and chest wall. The outcome is determined by the speed with which the disorder develops and the adequacy of the collateral circulation. Tumors adjacent to the visceral pleura often insidiously produce pleural effusion. This effusion can compress the lung and cause atelectasis and dyspnea. It is less likely to cause fever, pleural friction rub, or pain than pleural effusion resulting from other causes.

Paraneoplastic syndromes are incompletely understood patterns of organ dysfunction related to immune-mediated or secretory effects neoplasia (see Chapter 7). They include hypercalcemia from secretion of parathyroid-like peptide, Cushing syndrome from ACTH secretion, SIADH, neuromuscular syndromes (e.g., Eaton-Lambert syndrome), and hematologic disorders (e.g., migratory thrombophlebitis, nonbacterial endocarditis, disseminated intravascular coagulation). Neurologic or muscular symptoms can develop 6 months to 4 years before the lung tumor is detected. One of the more common of these problems is weakness and wasting of the proximal muscles of the pelvic and shoulder girdles, with decreased deep tendon reflexes but without sensory changes. Hypercalcemia is most often seen in persons with squamous cell carcinoma, hematologic syndromes in persons with adenocarcinomas, and the remaining syndromes in persons with small cell neoplasms. Manifestations of the paraneoplastic syndrome may precede the onset of other signs of lung cancer and may lead to discovery of an occult tumor.

Diagnosis and Treatment

The diagnosis of lung cancer is based on a careful history and physical examination and on other tests such as chest radiography, bronchoscopy, cytologic studies (Papanicolaou [Pap] test) of the sputum or bronchial washings, percutaneous needle biopsy of lung tissue, and scalene lymph node biopsy. Computed tomographic scans, MRI studies, and ultrasonography are used to locate lesions and evaluate the extent of the disease. Positron emission tomography (PET) is a noninvasive alternative for identifying metastatic lesions in the mediastinum or distant sites. Persons with SCLC should also have a CT scan or MRI of the brain for detection of metastasis. Annual screening of some high-risk groups with low-dose computed tomography (LDCT) has been proposed as a method for reducing the lung cancer mortality rate by detecting the disease at an earlier stage.[45]

Like other cancers, lung cancer is classified according to extent of disease. Non-small cell lung cancers are usually classified according to cell type (i.e., squamous cell carcinoma, adenocarcinoma, and large cell carcinoma) and staged according to the 2009 revised Tumor, Node, Metastasis (TNM) staging system.[48,49] Initial clinical staging involves a CT scan of the chest that includes the adrenal gland to determine tumor size, invasion, and local and regional lymph node involvement. Small cell lung cancers are not staged using the TNM system because micrometastases are assumed to be present at the time of diagnosis. Instead, they are usually classified as limited disease, when the tumor is limited to the unilateral hemithorax, or extensive disease, when it extends beyond these boundaries.[15]

Treatment methods for NSCLC include surgery, radiation therapy, and systemic chemotherapy.[48,49] These treatments may be used singly or in combination. Surgery is used for the removal of small, localized NSCLC tumors. It can involve a lobectomy, pneumonectomy, or segmental resection of the lung. Radiation therapy can be used as a definitive or main treatment modality, as part of a combined treatment plan, or for palliation of symptoms. Because of the frequency of metastases, chemotherapy often is used in treating lung cancer. Combination chemotherapy, which uses a regimen of several drugs, is often employed for lung cancer treatment. New targeted treatments are under development with the goal of increasing survival and ultimately providing a cure for this type of cancer.

Therapy for SCLC is based on chemotherapy and radiation therapy.[50,51] Advances in the use of combination chemotherapy, along with thoracic irradiation, have improved the outlook for persons with SCLC. Because SCLC may metastasize to the brain, prophylactic cranial irradiation is often indicated. In most persons who achieve a complete remission from SCLC, the brain is the most frequent site of relapse. About half of such persons develop clinical metastasis within 3 years. Newer combination chemotherapy regimens and targeted therapies are being developed in hopes of providing treatment alternatives that increase survival and produce fewer treatment liabilities.

SUMMARY CONCEPTS

■ Cancer of the lung is a leading cause of death worldwide, with cigarette smoking being implicated in the majority of cases. Environmental hazards, such as exposure to asbestos, increase the risk for development of lung cancer. Because the disease develops insidiously, it often is far advanced before it is diagnosed, a fact that explains the poor 5-year survival rate.

■ For purposes of staging and treatment, lung cancer is divided into nonsmall cell and small cell carcinoma. The main reason for this is that almost all small cell lung cancers have metastasized at the time of diagnosis and are not amenable to surgical resection.

■ The manifestations of lung cancer can be attributed to the involvement of the lung and adjacent structures, the effects of local spread and metastasis, and paraneoplastic syndromes involving endocrine, neurologic, and hematologic disorders. As with other cancers, lung cancer causes nonspecific symptoms such as anorexia and weight loss. Treatment methods for lung cancer include surgery, irradiation, and chemotherapy.

Respiratory Disorders in Children

Acute respiratory diseases are the most common cause of illness in infancy and childhood. This section focuses on (1) lung development, with an emphasis on the developmental basis for lung disorders in children; (2) respiratory disorders in the neonate; and (3) respiratory infections in children. A discussion of bronchial asthma in children and cystic fibrosis is included in Chapter 23.

Lung Development

Although other body systems are physiologically ready for extrauterine life as early as 25 weeks of gestation, the lungs take much longer to mature. Immaturity of the respiratory system is a major cause of morbidity and mortality in infants born prematurely. Even in infants born at term, the lungs are not fully mature, and additional growth and maturation continue well into childhood.

Lung development may be divided into four characteristic stages: the embryonic, pseudoglandular, canalicular, saccular, and alveolar stages. It is generally accepted that weeks 0 to 6 of gestation comprise the *embryonic stage*; weeks 6 to 16, the *pseudoglandular stage*; weeks 16 to 26, the *canalicular* stage; weeks 24 to birth, the *terminal sac (saccular)* stage; and 32 weeks to 8 years, the alveolar stage.[52,53] The first three stages are devoted to development of the conducting airways and the last two stages to development of the gas exchange portion of the lung. By the 25th to 28th weeks, sufficient terminal sacs are present to permit survival. Before this time, the premature lungs are incapable of adequate gas exchange. Development of the pulmonary circulation occurs in parallel with lung development. The vessels increase in length and diameter. By the 20th week of gestation, the full number of pre-acinar vessels is present in each segment.[53] During the terminal saccular stage of development, the saccular epithelium becomes very thin and the pulmonary capillaries begin to bulge into these sacs to form the alveoli of the lung.

By 28 weeks, the terminal sacs are lined with squamous epithelial cells or type I alveolar cells, across which gas exchange takes place. Scattered among the squamous epithelial cells are rounded secretory epithelial cells–type II alveolar cells. Type II alveolar cells begin to develop at approximately 24 weeks. These cells produce surfactant, a substance capable of lowering the surface tension of the air–alveoli interface (see Chapter 21). By the 26th to 30th weeks, sufficient amounts of surfactant are available to prevent alveolar collapse when breathing begins.

Although transformation of the lungs from glandlike structures to highly vascular, alveoli-like organs occurs during the late fetal period, mature alveoli do not form for some time after birth. The growth of the lung during infancy and early childhood involves an increase in the number rather than the size of the alveoli. Only about one sixth of the adult number of alveoli is present in the lungs of a full-term infant. By the 8th year of life, the adult complement of alveoli is present.[52]

Ventilation in the Neonate

Effective ventilation requires coordinated interaction between the muscles of the upper airways, including those of the pharynx and larynx, the diaphragm, and the intercostal muscles of the chest wall. In the infant, the diaphragm inserts more horizontally than in the adult. As a result, contraction of the diaphragm tends to draw the lower ribs inward, especially if the infant is placed in the horizontal position.[54] The intercostal muscles, which normally lift the ribs during inspiration, are not fully developed in the infant. Instead, they function largely to stabilize the chest. Under circumstances such as crying, the intercostal muscles of the neonate function together with the diaphragm to splint the chest wall and prevent its collapse.

The chest wall of the neonate is highly compliant.[54] A striking characteristic of neonatal breathing is the paradoxical inward movement of the upper chest during inspiration, especially during active sleep. Normally, the infant's lungs also are compliant, which is advantageous to the infant with its compliant chest cage because it takes only small changes in inspiratory pressure to inflate a compliant lung. However, with respiratory disorders that decrease lung compliance, the diaphragm must generate more negative pressure; as a result, the compliant chest wall structures are sucked inward. *Inspiratory retractions* are abnormal inward movements of the chest wall during inspiration; they may occur intercostally (between the ribs), in the substernal or epigastric area, and in the supraclavicular spaces (Fig. 22-11).

Airway Resistance

Normal lung inflation requires uninterrupted movement of air through the extrathoracic airways (i.e., nose, pharynx, larynx, and upper trachea) and intrathoracic airways (i.e., bronchi and bronchioles). The neonate (0 to 4 weeks of age) breathes predominantly through the nose and does not adapt well to mouth breathing. Any obstruction of the nose or nasopharynx may increase upper airway resistance and increase the work of breathing.

The airways of the infant and small child are much smaller than those of the adult. Because the resistance to airflow is inversely related to the fourth power of the radius (resistance = $1/\text{radius}^4$), relatively small amounts of mucus secretion, edema, or airway constriction can produce marked changes in airway resistance and

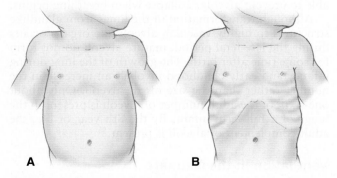

FIGURE 22-11. (A) Normal inspiratory appearance of the chest during unobstructed breathing in the neonate. **(B)** Sternal and intercostal retractions during obstructed breathing in the neonate.

airflow. Nasal flaring (enlargement of the nares) is a method that infants use to take in more air. This method of breathing increases the size of the nares and decreases the resistance of the small airways.

Normally, the extrathoracic airways (i.e., those extending from the nose to the thoracic inlet) in the infant narrow during inspiration and widen during expiration, and the intrathoracic airways (i.e., those located within the thorax) widen during inspiration and narrow during expiration.[54] This occurs because the pressure inside the extrathoracic airways reflects the intrapleural pressures that are generated during breathing, whereas the pressure outside the airways is similar to atmospheric pressure. Thus, during inspiration, the pressure inside becomes more negative, causing the airways to narrow, and during expiration it becomes more positive, causing them to widen. In contrast to the extrathoracic airways, the pressure outside the intrathoracic airways is equal to the intrapleural pressure. These airways widen during inspiration as the surrounding intrapleural pressure becomes more negative and pulls them open, and they narrow during expiration as the surrounding pressure becomes more positive.[54,55] These changes are exaggerated in conditions that cause airway obstruction, particularly in infants with their softer and more compliant airways.

Lung Volumes and Gas Exchange

The functional residual capacity, which is the air left in the lungs at the end of normal expiration, plays an important role in the infant's gas exchange. In the infant, the functional residual capacity occurs at a higher lung volume than in the older child or adult.[53,55] This higher end-expiratory volume results from a more rapid respiratory rate, which leaves less time for expiration. However, the increased residual volume is important to the neonate for several reasons: (1) it holds the airways open throughout all phases of respiration, (2) it favors the reabsorption of intrapulmonary fluids, and (3) it maintains more uniform lung expansion and enhances gas exchange. During active sleep, the tone of the upper airway muscles is reduced, so that the time spent in expiration is shorter and the intercostal activity that stabilizes the chest wall is less. This results in a lower end-expiratory volume and less optimal gas exchange during active sleep.

Control of Ventilation

Fetal arterial oxygen pressures (PO_2) normally range from 25 to 30 mm Hg, and carbon dioxide pressures (PCO_2) range from 45 to 50 mm Hg, independent of any respiratory movements. Any decrease in oxygen levels induces quiet sleep in the fetus with subsequent cessation of breathing movements, both of which lead to a decrease in oxygen consumption. At birth, switching to oxygen derived from the aerated lung causes an immediate increase in arterial PO_2 to approximately 50 mm Hg; within a few hours, it increases to approximately 70 mm Hg.[55] These levels, which greatly exceed fetal levels, cause the chemoreceptors that sense arterial PO_2 levels to become silent for several days. Although the infant's arterial PO_2 may fluctuate during this critical time, the chemoreceptors do not respond appropriately. It is not until several days after birth that the chemoreceptors "reset" their PO_2 threshold; only then do they become the major controller of breathing. However, the response seems to be biphasic, with an initial hyperventilation followed by a decreased respiratory rate and even apnea. In normal infants, especially those born prematurely, breathing patterns and respiratory reflexes depend on the arousal state.[54] Periodic breathing and apnea are characteristic of premature infants and reflect patterns of fetal breathing. The fact that they occur with sleep and disappear during wakefulness underscores the importance of arousal.

Alterations in Breathing Patterns

Most respiratory disorders in the infant or small child produce a decrease in lung compliance or an increase in airway resistance manifested by changes in breathing patterns, rib cage distortion (retractions), audible respiratory sounds, and use of accessory muscles.[55]

Children with restrictive lung disorders, such as pulmonary edema or respiratory distress syndrome, breathe at faster rates, and their respiratory excursions are shallow. *Grunting* is an audible noise emitted during expiration. An expiratory grunt is common as the child tries to raise the end-expiratory pressure to maintain airway patency and prolong the period of oxygen and carbon dioxide exchange across the alveolar–capillary membrane.

Increased airway resistance can occur in either the extrathoracic or intrathoracic airways. When the obstruction is in the extrathoracic airways, inspiration is more prolonged than expiration. *Nasal flaring* helps reduce the nasal resistance and maintain airway patency. It can be a sign of increased work of breathing and is a significant finding in an infant. *Inspiratory retractions* are often observed with airway obstruction in infants and small children (see Fig. 22-11). In conditions such as croup, the pressures distal to the point of obstruction must become more negative to overcome the resistance; this causes collapse of the distal airways, and the increased turbulence of air moving through the obstructed airways produces an audible crowing sound called *stridor* during inspiration.

When the obstruction is in the intrathoracic airways, as occurs with bronchiolitis and bronchial asthma, expiration is prolonged and the child makes use of the accessory expiratory muscles (abdominals). Rib cage retractions may also be present. Intrapleural pressure becomes more positive during expiration because of air trapping; this causes collapse of intrathoracic airways and produces an audible wheezing or whistling sound during expiration.

Respiratory Disorders in the Neonate

The neonatal period is one of transition from placental dependency to air breathing. This transition requires functioning of the surfactant system, conditioning of the respiratory muscles, and establishment of parallel pulmonary and systemic circulations. Respiratory disorders develop in infants who are born prematurely or who have other problems that impair this transition. Among the respiratory disorders of the neonate are respiratory distress syndrome, bronchopulmonary dysplasia, and persistent fetal circulation (i.e., delayed closure of the ductus arteriosus and foramen ovale; see Chapter 19).

Respiratory Distress Syndrome

Respiratory distress syndrome (RDS), also known as *hyaline membrane disease,* is one of the most common causes of respiratory disease in premature infants.[55,56] In these infants, pulmonary immaturity, together with surfactant deficiency, leads to alveolar collapse (Fig. 22-12). The type II alveolar cells that produce surfactant do not begin to mature until approximately the 25th to 28th weeks of gestation; consequently, many premature infants are born with poorly functioning type II alveolar cells and have difficulty producing sufficient amounts of surfactant. The incidence of RDS is higher among preterm male infants,

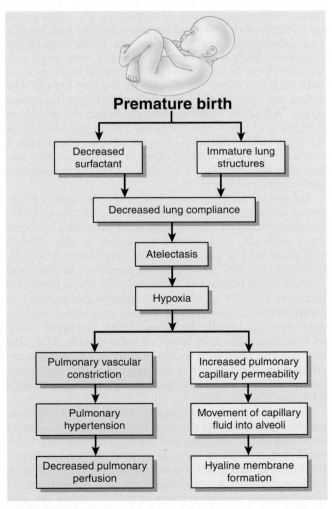

FIGURE 22-12. Pathogenesis of respiratory distress syndrome (RDS) in the infant.

white infants, infants of diabetic mothers, and those subjected to asphyxia, cold stress, precipitous deliveries, and delivery by cesarean section (when performed before the 38th week of gestation).

Surfactant synthesis is influenced by several hormones, including insulin and cortisol. Insulin tends to inhibit surfactant production; this explains why infants of insulin-dependent diabetic mothers are at increased risk for development of RDS. Cortisol can accelerate maturation of type II cells and formation of surfactant. The reason that premature infants born by cesarean section presumably are at greater risk for development of RDS is that they are not subjected to the stress of vaginal delivery, which is thought to increase the infants' cortisol levels. These observations have led to administration of corticosteroid drugs before delivery to mothers with infants at high risk for development of RDS.[55]

Surfactant reduces the surface tension in the alveoli, thereby equalizing the retractive forces in the large and small alveoli and reducing the amount of pressure needed to inflate and hold the alveoli open. Without surfactant, the large alveoli remain inflated, whereas the small alveoli become difficult to inflate. At birth, the first breath requires high inspiratory pressures to expand the lungs. With normal levels of surfactant, the lungs retain up to 40% of the residual volume after the first breath, and subsequent breaths require far lower inspiratory pressures. With a surfactant deficiency, the lungs collapse between breaths, making the infant work as hard with each successive breath as with the first breath. The airless portions of the lungs become stiff and noncompliant. A hyaline membrane forms inside the alveoli as protein- and fibrin-rich fluids are pulled into the alveolar spaces. The fibrin–hyaline membrane constitutes a barrier to gas exchange, leading to hypoxemia and carbon dioxide retention, a condition that further impairs surfactant production.

Infants with RDS present with multiple signs of respiratory distress, usually within the first 24 hours of birth. Central cyanosis is a prominent sign. Breathing becomes more difficult, and retractions occur as the infant's soft chest wall is pulled in as the diaphragm descends. Grunting sounds accompany expiration. As the tidal volume drops because of atelectasis, the respiratory rate increases (usually to 60 to 120 breaths per minute) in an effort to maintain normal minute ventilation. Fatigue may develop rapidly because of the increased work of breathing. The stiff lungs of infants with RDS also increase the resistance to blood flow in the pulmonary circulation. As a result, a hemodynamically significant patent ductus arteriosus may develop in infants with RDS (see Chapter 19).

The basic principles of treatment for infants with suspected RDS focus on the provision of supportive care, including gentle handling and minimal disturbance.[55] An incubator or radiant warmer is used to prevent hypothermia and increased oxygen consumption. Continuous cardiorespiratory monitoring is needed. Monitoring of blood glucose and prevention of hypoglycemia are also recommended. Oxygen levels can be assessed through an arterial (umbilical) line or by a transcutaneous oxygen sensor. Treatment includes administration of supplemental oxygen, continuous positive airway pressure through nasal prongs, and often, assisted mechanical ventilation.

Exogenous surfactant therapy is used to prevent and treat RDS. The surfactants are suspended in saline and administered into the airways, usually through an endotracheal tube. The treatment often is initiated soon after birth in infants who are at high risk for RDS.

Bronchopulmonary Dysplasia

Bronchopulmonary dysplasia (BPD) is a chronic lung disease that occurs in infants, usually preterm infants treated with mechanical ventilation or prolonged oxygen supplementation.[57-59] Bronchopulmonary dysplasia is primarily a disease of infants weighing less than 1000 g born at less than 28 weeks' gestation, many of whom have little or no lung disease at birth but develop progressive respiratory failure over the first few weeks of life. Although the disorder is most often associated with preterm birth, it can occur in term infants who require aggressive ventilator therapy for severe, acute lung disease.

Morphologic features of BPD include alveolar hypoplasia, variable alveolar wall fibrosis, and minimal airway disease.[55,57-59] The histopathology of BPD indicates interference with normal lung maturation, which may prevent subsequent lung growth and development. This pathogenesis is thought to be multifactorial and affect both the lungs and the heart. Mechanical ventilation and oxygen produce lung injury through their effect on alveolar and vascular development. Oxygen induces injury by producing free radicals that cannot be metabolized by the immature antioxidant systems of the preterm infant. Several clinical features, including immaturity, acquired infections, and malnutrition, may contribute to the development of BPD.

Bronchopulmonary dysplasia is characterized by chronic respiratory distress, persistent hypoxemia when breathing room air, reduced lung compliance, increased airway resistance, and severe expiratory flow limitation. There is a mismatching of ventilation and perfusion with development of hypoxemia and hypercapnia. Acute lung injury also impairs growth, structure, and function of the developing pulmonary circulation after premature birth. Pulmonary vascular resistance may be increased and pulmonary hypertension and cor pulmonale (i.e., right heart failure associated with lung disease) may develop. The infant with BPD often demonstrates tachycardia, rapid and shallow breathing, chest retractions, cough, and poor weight gain. Clubbing of the fingers occurs in children with severe disease. Hepatomegaly and periorbital edema may develop in infants with right heart failure.

The treatment of BPD includes nutritional support, maintenance of adequate oxygenation, and prompt treatment of infections.[55,57] Severe BPD requires mechanical ventilation and administration of supplemental oxygen. Weaning from ventilation is accomplished gradually, and some infants may require ventilation at home. Rapid lung growth occurs during the first year of life, and lung function usually improves. Adequate nutrition is essential for recovery of infants with BPD. There has been an interest in the protective effect of polyunsaturated fatty acids, vitamin A, and other nutrients such as inositol (a sulfur-containing amino acid) and selenium in preventing lung injury in high-risk premature infants.[57]

Most adolescents and young adults who had severe BPD during infancy have some degree of pulmonary dysfunction, consisting of airway obstruction, airway hyperreactivity, or hyperinflation.

Respiratory Infections in Children

In children, respiratory tract infections are common, and although they are troublesome, they usually are not serious. Frequent infections occur because the immune systems of infants and small children have not been exposed to many common pathogens; consequently, they tend to contract infections with each new exposure. Although most of these infections are not serious, they can impair airflow because of the small size of the child's airways. For example, an infection that causes only sore throat and hoarseness in an adult may result in serious airway obstruction in a small child.

Upper Airway Infections

In infants and children, obstruction of the upper airways because of infection tends to exert its greatest effect during the inspiratory phase of respiration. Movement of air through an obstructed upper airway, particularly the vocal cords in the larynx, causes stridor. Impairment of the expiratory phase of respiration also can occur, causing wheezing. With mild to moderate obstruction, inspiratory stridor is more prominent than expiratory wheezing because the airways tend to dilate with expiration. When the swelling and obstruction become severe, the airways no longer can dilate during expiration, and both stridor and wheezing occur.

Cartilaginous support of the trachea and the larynx is poorly developed in infants and small children. These structures are soft and tend to collapse when the airway is obstructed and the child cries, causing the inspiratory pressures to become more negative. When this happens, the stridor and inspiratory effort are increased. The phenomenon of airway collapse in the small child is analogous to what happens when a thick beverage, such as a milkshake, is pulled through a soft paper or plastic straw. The straw collapses when the negative pressure produced by the sucking effort exceeds the flow of liquid through the straw.

Common upper airway infections in infants and small children include croup (laryngotracheobronchitis) and epiglottitis.[60,61] Croup is the more common and usually is benign and self-limited. Epiglottitis is a rapidly progressive and life-threatening condition. The site of involvement is illustrated in Figure 22-13, and the characteristics of both infections are compared in Table 22-2.

Croup. Croup is characterized by inspiratory stridor, hoarseness, and a barking cough. The British use the term *croup* to describe the cry of the crow or raven, and this is undoubtedly how the term originated.

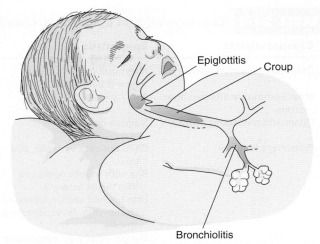

FIGURE 22-13. Location of airway obstruction in epiglottitis, acute laryngotracheobronchitis (croup), and bronchiolitis. (Courtesy of Carole Russell Hilmer, C.M.)

Croup is usually caused by viruses.[60-65] The parainfluenza virus (types 1 to 3) accounts for approximately 75% all cases, with the remaining 25% being caused by adenoviruses, respiratory syncytial virus, and influenza A and B.[63] Viral croup usually is seen in children 3 months to 5 years of age. The condition may affect the entire laryngotracheal tree, but because the subglottic area is the narrowest part of the respiratory tree in this age group, the obstruction usually is greatest in this area.

Although the respiratory manifestations of croup may appear suddenly, they usually are preceded by upper respiratory infections that cause rhinorrhea (i.e., runny nose), coryza (i.e., common cold), hoarseness, and a low-grade fever. In most children, the manifestation of croup advances only to stridor and slight dyspnea before they begin to recover. The symptoms usually subside when the child is exposed to moist air. For example, letting the bathroom shower run and then taking the child into the bathroom often brings prompt and dramatic relief of symptoms. Exposure to cold air also seems to relieve the airway spasm; often, the severe symptoms are relieved simply because the child is exposed to cold air on the way to the hospital emergency department. Viral croup does not respond to antibiotics; expectorants, bronchodilating agents, and antihistamines are not helpful. The child should be disturbed as little as possible and carefully monitored for signs of respiratory distress.

Airway obstruction may progress in some children. As the obstruction increases, the stridor becomes continuous and is associated with nasal flaring with substernal and intercostal retractions. Agitation and crying aggravate the signs and symptoms, and the child prefers to sit up or be held upright. In the cyanotic, pale, or obstructed child, any manipulation of the pharynx, including use of a tongue depressor, can cause cardiorespiratory arrest and should be done only in a medical setting that has the facilities for emergency airway management. Other treatments may be required when a humidifier or mist tent is ineffective. One method is to administer a racemic

TABLE 22-2 Characteristics of Epiglottitis, Croup, and Bronchiolitis in Small Children

Characteristics	Epiglottitis	Croup	Bronchiolitis
Common causative agent	*Haemophilus influenzae* type B bacterium	Mainly parainfluenza virus	Respiratory syncytial virus
Most commonly affected age group	2 to 7 y (peak 3 to 5 y)	3 mo to 5 y	<2 y (most severe in infants younger than 6 mo)
Onset and preceding history	Sudden onset	Usually follows symptoms of a cold	Preceded by stuffy nose and other signs
Prominent features	Child appears very sick and toxic	Stridor and a wet, barking cough	Breathlessness; rapid, shallow breathing; wheezing; cough; and retractions of lower ribs and sternum during inspiration
	Sits with mouth open and chin thrust forward	Usually occurs at night	
	Low-pitched stridor, difficulty swallowing, fever, drooling, anxiety	Relieved by exposure to cold or moist air	
	Danger of airway obstruction and asphyxia		
Usual treatment	Hospitalization	Mist tent or vaporizer	Supportive treatment, administration of oxygen and hydration
	Intubation or tracheotomy	Administration of oxygen	
	Treatment with appropriate antibiotic		

mixture of epinephrine (L-epinephrine and D-epinephrine) by positive-pressure breathing through a face mask.[60,63] Establishment of an artificial airway may become necessary in severe airway obstruction.

Spasmodic Croup. Spasmodic croup manifests with symptoms similar to those of acute viral croup. Because the child is afebrile and lacks other manifestations of the viral prodrome, it is thought that it may have an allergic origin. Spasmodic croup characteristically occurs at night and tends to recur with respiratory tract infections. The episode usually lasts several hours and may recur several nights in a row.[60]

Most children with spasmodic croup can be effectively managed at home. An environment of high humidification (i.e., cold-water room humidifier or taking the child into a bathroom with a warm, running shower) lessens irritation and prevents drying of secretions.

Epiglottitis. Acute epiglottitis is a dramatic, potentially fatal condition characterized by inflammatory edema of the supraglottic area, including the epiglottis and pharyngeal structures[60,65,66] (see Fig. 22-13), that comes on suddenly, bringing the danger of airway obstruction and asphyxia.[60] In the past, the *H. influenzae* type B bacterium was the most commonly identified etiologic agent. It is seen less commonly since the widespread use of immunization against *H. influenzae* type B. Therefore, other agents such as *Streptococcus pyogenes*, *S. pneumoniae*, and *S. aureus* now represent the most common causes of pediatric epiglottitis.[65]

Epiglottitis typically presents with an acute onset of sore throat and fever.[60,65] The child appears pale, toxic, and lethargic and assumes a distinctive position—sitting up with the mouth open and the chin thrust forward. Symptoms rapidly progress to difficult swallowing,

a muffled voice, drooling, and extreme anxiety. Moderate to severe respiratory distress is evident. There is inspiratory and sometimes expiratory stridor, flaring of the nares, and inspiratory retractions of the suprasternal notch and supraclavicular and intercostal spaces. Within a matter of hours, epiglottitis may progress to complete obstruction of the airway and death unless adequate treatment is instituted. Epiglottitis is a medical emergency and immediate establishment of an airway by endotracheal tube or tracheostomy is usually needed. If epiglottitis is suspected, the child should never be forced to lie down because this causes the epiglottis to fall backward and may lead to complete airway obstruction. Examination of the throat with a tongue blade or other instrument may cause airway spasm and cardiopulmonary arrest and should be done only by medical personnel experienced in intubation of small children. It also is unwise to attempt any procedure, such as drawing blood, which would heighten the child's anxiety because this also could precipitate airway spasm and cause death. Recovery from epiglottitis usually is rapid and uneventful after an adequate airway has been established and appropriate antibiotic therapy initiated.

Lower Airway Infections

Lower airway infections produce air trapping with prolonged expiration. Wheezing results from bronchospasm, mucosal inflammation, and edema. The child presents with increased expiratory effort, increased respiratory rate, and wheezing. If the infection is severe, there also are marked intercostal retractions and signs of impending respiratory failure.

Acute bronchiolitis is a viral infection of the lower airways, most commonly caused by the respiratory syncytial virus.[66–72] Other viruses, such as parainfluenza-3 virus and some adenoviruses, as well as mycoplasmas, also are causative. The infection produces inflammatory obstruction of the small airways and necrosis of the cells lining the lower airways. It usually occurs during the first 2 years of life, with a peak incidence between 3 and 6 months of age. The source of infection usually is a family member with a minor respiratory illness. Older children and adults tolerate bronchiolar edema much better than infants and do not manifest the clinical picture of bronchiolitis. Because the resistance to airflow in a tube is inversely related to the fourth power of the radius, even minor swelling of bronchioles in an infant can produce profound changes in airflow.

Most affected infants in whom bronchiolitis develops have a history of a mild upper respiratory tract infection. These symptoms usually last several days and may be accompanied by fever and diminished appetite. There is then a gradual development of respiratory distress, characterized by a wheezy cough, dyspnea, and irritability. The infant usually is able to take in sufficient air but has trouble exhaling it. Air becomes trapped in the lung distal to the site of obstruction and interferes with gas exchange. Hypoxemia and, in severe cases, hypercapnia may develop. Airway obstruction may produce air trapping and hyperinflation of the lungs or collapse of the alveoli. Infants with acute bronchiolitis have a typical appearance, marked by breathlessness with rapid respirations, a distressing cough, and retractions of the lower ribs and sternum. Crying and feeding exaggerate these signs. Wheezing and crackles may or may not be present, depending on the degree of airway obstruction. In infants with severe airway obstruction, wheezing decreases as the airflow diminishes. Usually, the most critical phase of the disease is the first 48 to 72 hours. Cyanosis, pallor, listlessness, and sudden diminution in or absence of breath sounds indicate impending respiratory failure. The characteristics of bronchiolitis are described in Table 22-2.

Infants with respiratory distress usually are hospitalized. Treatment is largely supportive. Hypoxic children should receive humidified oxygen.[70] Elevation of the head facilitates respiratory movements and avoids airway compression. Handling is kept at a minimum to avoid tiring. Because the infection is viral, antibiotics are not effective and are given only for a secondary bacterial infection. The use of bronchodilators (i.e., epinephrine) and corticosteroids remains controversial.[67] Dehydration may occur as the result of increased insensible water losses because of the rapid respiratory rate and feeding difficulties, and measures to ensure adequate hydration are needed. Recovery usually begins after the first 48 to 72 hours and usually is rapid and complete. Adequate hand washing is essential to prevent the nosocomial spread of respiratory syncytial virus.

Signs of Impending Respiratory Failure

Respiratory problems of infants and small children often originate suddenly, and respiratory failure can develop rapidly from obstructive disorders such as

---

CHART 22-1	Signs of Respiratory Distress and Impending Respiratory Failure in the Infant and Small Child

Severe increase in respiratory effort, including severe retractions or grunting, decreased chest movement
Cyanosis that is not relieved by administration of oxygen (40%)
Heart rate of 150 per minute or greater and increasing bradycardia
Very rapid breathing (rate 60 per minute from birth to 6 months of age, or above 30 per minute in children 6 months to 2 years)
Very depressed breathing (rate 20 per minute or below)
Retractions of the supraclavicular area, sternum, epigastrium, and intercostal spaces
Extreme anxiety and agitation
Fatigue
Decreased level of consciousness

---

epiglottitis or lung infection such as bronchiolitis. Children with impending respiratory failure due to airway or lung disease have rapid breathing; exaggerated use of the accessory muscles; retractions, which are more pronounced in the child than in the adult because of higher chest compliance; nasal flaring; and grunting during expiration.[73] The signs and symptoms of impending respiratory failure are listed in Chart 22-1.

SUMMARY CONCEPTS

■ Although other body systems are physiologically ready for extrauterine life as early as 25 weeks of gestation, the lungs take much longer to mature. Type II alveolar cells, which produce surfactant, a substance capable of lowering the surface tension at the air–alveoli interface, begin to develop at approximately 24 weeks, and by the 26th to 30th weeks produce sufficient amounts of surfactant to prevent alveolar collapse.

■ Respiratory distress syndrome is one of the most common causes of respiratory disease in premature infants. In these infants, pulmonary immaturity, together with surfactant deficiency, lead to alveolar collapse.

■ Normally, both an infant's chest wall and lungs are compliant, allowing for small changes in inspiratory pressure to inflate the lung. In respiratory disorders that decrease lung compliance, the diaphragm must generate more negative pressure; as a result, the compliant chest wall structures are sucked inward, producing abnormal inward movements of the chest wall during inspiration called *retractions*.

(continued)

SUMMARY CONCEPTS (continued)

■ Children with restrictive lung disorders, such as pulmonary edema or respiratory distress syndrome, breathe at faster rates, and their respiratory excursions are shallow. *Grunting* is an audible noise emitted during expiration. An expiratory grunt is common as the child tries to raise the end-expiratory pressure to maintain airway patency and prolong the period of oxygen and carbon dioxide exchange across the alveolar–capillary membrane.

■ Because of the small size of the airway of infants and children, respiratory tract infections in these groups often are more serious. Infections that may cause only a sore throat and hoarseness in the adult may produce serious obstruction in the child. Among the respiratory tract infections that affect small children are croup, bronchiolitis, and epiglottitis, a life-threatening supraglottic infection that may cause airway obstruction and asphyxia.

REVIEW EXERCISES

1. It is flu season, and although you had a flu shot last year, you have not had one this year. Imagine yourself experiencing an abrupt onset of fever, chills, malaise, muscle aching, and nasal stuffiness.

   A. Which of these symptoms would lead you to believe you are coming down with the flu?
   B. Because you hate to miss classes, you decide to go to the student health center to get an antibiotic. After being seen by a health professional, you are told that antibiotics are ineffective against the flu virus, and you are instructed not to attend classes but instead to go home, take acetaminophen for your fever, go to bed and stay warm, and drink a lot of fluids. Explain the rationale for each of these recommendations.
   C. Explain why last year's flu shot did not protect you during this year's flu season.
   D. There is concern about the possibility of an influenza pandemic such as the one that occurred during the 1917–1918 season. What is the rationale for this concern?

2. Bacterial (e.g., *S. pneumoniae*) pneumonia is commonly manifested by a cough productive of sputum, whereas with atypical (e.g., *M. pneumoniae*) pneumonia, the cough is usually nonproductive or absent.

   A. Explain.

3. A 4-month-old infant is admitted to the pediatric intensive care unit with a diagnosis of bronchiolitis. The infant is tachypneic, with wheezing, nasal flaring, and retractions of the lower sternum and intercostal spaces during inspiration.

   A. What is the usual pathogen in bronchiolitis? Would this infection be treated with an antibiotic?
   B. Explain the physiologic mechanism involved in the retraction of the lower sternum and intercostal spaces during inspiration.
   C. What would be the signs of impending respiratory failure in this infant?

REFERENCES

1. American Lung Association. 2013. *Pneumonia fact sheet*. [Online]. Available at: http://www.lung.org/lung–disease/influenza/in–depth–resources/pneumonia–fact–sheet.html. Accessed October 11, 2013.
2. McAdams AJ, Sharpe AH. Infectious diseases. In: Kumar V, Abbas AK, Fausto N, et al., eds. *Robbins and Cotran Pathologic Basis of Disease*. 8th ed. Philadelphia, PA: Elsevier Saunders; 2010:366–372.
3. Covington TR, Henkin R, Miller S, et al. Treating the common cold. *Am J Nurse Pract*. 2004;811:77–88.
4. Heikkinen T, Järvinsen A. The common cold. *Lancet*. 2003;361:51–59.
5. Goldman DA. Transmission of viral respiratory tract infections in the home. *Pediatr Infect Dis J*. 2000;19:S97–S107.
6. Fashner J, Erickson K, Werner S. Treatment of the common cold in children and adults. *Am Fam Physician*. 2012;862:153–159.
7. Aring AM, Chan MM. Acute rhinosinusitis in adults. *Am Fam Physician*. 2011;839:1057–1063.
8. Meltzer EO, Hamilos DL. Rhinosinusitis diagnosis and management for the clinician: a synopsis of recent consensus guidelines. *Mayo Clin Proc*. 2011;865:427–443.
9. Brook I. Acute and chronic bacterial sinusitis. *Infect Dis Clin North Am*. 2007;21:427–446.
10. Leung RS, Katial R. The diagnosis and management of acute and chronic sinusitis. *Prim Care*. 2007;35:11–24.
11. Piccirillo JF. Acute bacterial sinusitis. *N Engl J Med*. 2004;351:902–910.
12. Slavin RG, Spector SL, Bernstein IL, et al, chief editors; American Academy of Allergy, Asthma and Immunology; American College of Allergy, Asthma and Immunology; Joint Council of Allergy, Asthma and Immunology. The diagnosis and management of sinusitis: a practice parameter update. *J Allergy Clinical Immunol*. 2005;116(Suppl 6):S13–S17.
13. Beasley MB, Travis WD, Rubin E. The respiratory system. In: Rubin R, Strayer D, eds. *Rubin's Pathology: Clinicopathologic Foundations of Medicine*. 6th ed. Philadelphia, PA: Wolters Kluwer Health/Lippincott Williams & Wilkins; 2012:537–604.
14. Husain AN. The lung. In Kumar V, Abbas AK, Fausto N, et al., eds. 2010. *Robbins and Cotran Pathologic Basis of Disease*. 8th ed. Philadelphia, PA: Elsevier Saunders; 2010:710–731.
15. Labella AM, Merel SE. Influenza. *Med Clin North Am*. 2013;97:621–645.
16. Chestnut MS, Prendergast J, Tavan ET. Pulmonary disorders. In: McPhee SJ, Papadakis MA, eds. *Current Medical Diagnosis and Treatment*. 52nd ed. New York, NY: McGraw–Hill Medical; 2013:270–292.

17. Centers for Disease Control. 2009. *Clinical signs and symptoms of influenza*. [Online]. Available at: http://www.cdc.gove/flu/professionals/acip/clinical.htm. Accessed December 28, 2013.

18. Harper SA, Bradley JS, England JA, et al. Seasonal influenza in adults and children—Diagnosis, treatment, chemoprophylaxis, and institutional outbreak management: clinical practice guidelines of the Infectious Diseases Society of America. *Clin Infect Dis.* 2009;488:1003–1032.

19. Grobskopf LA, Shay DK, Shimabukuro TT, et al. Prevention and control of seasonal influenza with vaccines: recommendations of the Advisory Committee on Immunization Practices—United States, 2013–2014. *MMWR Recomm Rep.* 2013;627:1–43.

20. Moran GJ, Talan DA, Abrahamian FM. Diagnosis and management of pneumonia in the emergency department. *Infect Dis Clin North Am.* 2008;22:53–72.

21. Waterer GW, Relio J, Wunderink RG. Management of community-acquired pneumonia in adults. *Am J Respir Crit Care Med.* 2011;1832:157–164.

22. Watkins RR, Lemonovich TL. Diagnosis and management of community-acquired pneumonia. *Am Fam Physician.* 2011;83(11):1299–1306.

23. Nair G, Niederman MS. Community-acquired pneumonia: an unfinished battle. *Med Clin North Am.* 2011;95:1143–1181.

24. Kieninger AN, Lipsett PA. Hospital-acquired pneumonia: pathophysiology, diagnosis, and treatment. *Surg Clin North Am.* 2009;89:439–461.

25. Labelle A, Kollef MH. Healthcare-associated pneumonia: approach to management. *Clin Chest Med.* 2011;32:507–515.

26. Schwartz DA. Infectious and parasitic diseases. In: Rubin R, Strayer D, eds. *Rubin's Pathology: Clinicopathologic Foundations of Medicine.* 6th ed. Philadelphia, PA: Wolters Kluwer Health/Lippincott Williams & Wilkins; 2012:351–352, 364, 386–389.

27. van der Poll T, Opal SM. Pathogenesis, treatment, and prevention of pneumococcal pneumonia. *Lancet.* 2009;374:3543–3556.

28. Centers for Disease Control. Pneumococcal vaccination. 2013. Available at: http://www.cdc.gov/VACCINES/vpd-vac/pneumo/default.htm. Accessed December 30, 2013.

29. Cunha BA. Legionnaires' disease: clinical differentiation from typical and other forms of atypical pneumonias. *Infect Dis Clin North Am* 2010;24:73–105.

30. American Lung Association. *Tuberculosis.* [Online]. Available at: http://www.lung.org/about-us/our-impact/top-stories/tuberculosis–still–lurking–and–evolving.html. Accessed October 11, 2013.

31. Murray PR, Rosenthal KS, Pfalle MA. *Medical Microbiology.* 7th ed. Philadelphia, PA: Elsevier Saunders; 2013:235–247.

32. Zuma A, Raviglione H, Hafner R, et al. Tuberculosis. *N Engl J Med.* 2013;3688:745–755.

33. Schossberg D. Acute tuberculosis. *Infect Dis Clin North Am.* 2010;24:139–146.

34. Horsburgh CR, Rubin EJ. Latent tuberculosis in the United States. *N Engl J Med.* 2011;364(15):1441–1448.

35. Keshavjee S, Farmer PE. Tuberculosis, drug resistance, and the history of modern medicine. *N Engl J Med.* 2012;367(10):931–936.

36. Nahid P, Pai M, Hopewell PC. Advances in the diagnosis and treatment of tuberculosis. *Proc Am Thorac Soc.* 2006;3:103–110.

37. Nathanson E, Nunn P, Uptekar M, et al. MDR tuberculosis—Critical steps for prevention and control. *N Engl J Med.* 2010;349(12):1149–1156.

38. Ingle LD, Wilson JW. Update on the treatment of tuberculosis. *Am Fam Physician.* 2008;784:457–465, 469–470.

39. Shelburne SA, Hamill RJ. Mycotic infections. In: McPhee SJ, Papadakis MA, eds. *Current Medical Diagnosis and Treatment.* 52nd ed. New York, NY: McGraw–Hill Medical; 2013:1529–1542.

40. Kauffman CA. Endemic mycoses: blastomycosis, histoplasmosis, and sporotrichosis. *Infect Dis Clin North Am.* 2006;20:645–662.

41. Wheat LJ, Kauffman CA. Histoplasmosis. *Infect Dis Clin North Am.* 2003;17:1–19.

42. Anstead GM, Grayhill JR. Coccidioidomycosis. *Infect Dis Clin North Am.* 2006;20:621–643.

43. Bradsher RW, Chapman SW, Pappas PG. Blastomycosis. *Infect Dis Clin North Am.* 2003;17:21–40.

44. deGroot P, Munden RF. Lung cancer epidemiology, risk factors, and prevention. *Radiol Clin North Am.* 2012;45:21–43.

45. Wender R, Fontham ETH, Barrera E, et al. American Cancer Society lung cancer screening guidelines. *CA Cancer J Clin.* 2013;63:107–117.

46. Wang S. Lung cancer. In: McPhee SJ, Papadakis MA, eds. *Current Medical Diagnosis and Treatment.* 52nd ed. New York, NY: McGraw–Hill Medical; 2013:1595–1602.

47. Molina JR, Yang P, Cassivi SD, et al. Non–small cell cancer: Epidemiology, risk factors, treatment, and survivorship. *Mayo Clin Proc.* 2008;83(5):584–594.

48. Carr LL, Finigan JH, Kern JA. Evaluation and treatment of patients with non–small cell lung cancer. *Med Clin North Am.* 2011;95(6):1041–1054.

49. Reck M, Heigener DF, Mak T, et al. Management of non-small-cell lung cancer: recent developments. *Lancet* 2013;382:709–719.

50. van Meerbeeck JP, Fennell DA, De Ruysscher DKM. Small-cell lung cancer. *Lancet.* 2011;378:741–755.

51. Sher T, Dy GK, Adjei AA. Small cell lung cancer. *Mayo Clin Proc.* 2008;83(3):355–367.

52. Moore K, Persaud TVN, Torchia MG. *The Developing Human.* 9th ed. Philadelphia, PA: Elsevier Saunders; 2013:199–211.

53. Smith LJ, McKay KO, VanAsperen PP, et al. Normal development of the lung and premature birth. *Paediatr Respir Rev* 2010;113:135–142.

54. Sarnaik AP, Heidemann SM. Respiratory development and function. In: Kliegman RM, Stanton BF, St. Geme JW, et al., eds. *Nelson Textbook of Pediatrics.* 19th ed. Philadelphia, PA: Elsevier Saunders; 2011:1419–1455.

55. Carlo WA. Respiratory tract disorders. In: Kliegman RM, Stanton BF, St. Geme JW, et al., eds. *Nelson Textbook of Pediatrics.* 19th ed. Philadelphia, PA: Elsevier Saunders; 2011:579–599.

56. Edwards MO, Kotecha SJ, Kotecha S. Respiratory distress of the term newborn infant. *Paediatr Respir Rev.* 2013;14(1):29–36.

57. Ambalavanan N, Carlo WA. Bronchopulmonary dysplasia. *Clin Perinatol.* 2004;31:613–628.

58. Kinsella JP, Greenough A, Abman SH. Bronchopulmonary dysplasia. *Lancet.* 2006;367:1421–1430.

59. Kair LR, Leonard DT, Anderson JM. Bronchopulmonary dysplasia. *Pediatr Rev.* 2012;33:255–263.

60. Roosevelt GE. Acute inflammatory upper airway obstruction. In: Kliegman RM, Stanton BF, St. Geme JW, et al., eds. *Nelson Textbook of Pediatrics.* 19th ed. Philadelphia, PA: Elsevier Saunders; 2011:1445–1449.

61. Shah S, Sharieff GQ. Pediatric respiratory infections. *Emerg Med Clin North Am.* 2007;25(4):961–979.

62. Knutson D, Arling A. Viral croup. *Am Fam Physician.* 2004;69:535–540.

63. Zoorob T, Sidani M, Murray J. Croup. *Am Fam Physician.* 2011;839:1067–1073.

64. Everard ML. Acute bronchiolitis and Croup. *Pediatr Clin North Am.* 2009;56:119–133.

65. Sobol SE, Zapata S. Epiglottitis and croup. *Otolaryngol Clin North Am.* 2008;41:551–566.

66. Garibaldi BT, Danoff SK. Bronchiolitis. *Immunol Allergy Clin North Am.* 2012;32:601–619.

67. Zorc JJ, Hall CB. Bronchiolitis: recent evidence on diagnosis and management. *Pediatrics*. 2010;125:342–349.

68. Zentz SE. Care of infants and children with bronchiolitis: a systematic review. *J Pediatr Nurs*. 2011;26:519–529.

69. Wainwright C. Acute viral bronchiolitis in children—a very common condition with few therapeutic options. *Paediatr Respir Rev*. 2010;11:35–45.

70. Watts KD, Goodman DM. Wheezing, bronchiolitis, and bronchitis. In Kliegman RM, Stanton BF, St. Geme JW, et al., eds. *Nelson Textbook of Pediatrics*. 19th ed. Philadelphia, PA: Elsevier Saunders; 2011:1458–1460.

71. Smyth RL, Openshaw PJM. Bronchiolitis. *Lancet*. 2006;368: 312–322.

72. American Academy of Pediatrics Subcommittee on Diagnosis and Management of Bronchiolitis. Diagnosis and management of bronchiolitis. *Pediatrics*. 2006;118:1774–1793.

73. Sarnak AP, Clark JA. Respiratory distress and failure. In Kliegman RM, Stanton BF, St. Geme JW, et al., eds. *Nelson Textbook of Pediatrics*. 19th ed. Philadelphia, PA: Elsevier Saunders; 2011:314–321.

Porth Essentials Resources

Explore these additional resources to enhance learning for this chapter:

- NCLEX-Style Questions and Other Resources on **the**Point, http://thePoint.lww.com/PorthEssentials4e
- Study Guide for Essentials of Pathophysiology
- Adaptive Learning | Powered by PrepU, http://thepoint.lww.com/prepu

C h a p t e r 23

Disorders of Ventilation and Gas Exchange

The major function of the lungs is to oxygenate the blood and remove carbon dioxide as a means of supporting the metabolic functions of the body's tissues. Many types of disease are capable of disrupting the normal gas exchange function of the lungs. In some cases the disruption is temporary and in other cases it is marked and disabling. This chapter focuses on disorders that disrupt ventilation and pulmonary gas exchange. It is divided into six sections: the physiologic effects of altered ventilation and gas exchange, disorders of lung inflation, obstructive airway disorders, chronic interstitial lung disorders, disorders of the pulmonary circulation, and acute respiratory disorders.

Physiologic Effects of Ventilation and Diffusion Disorders

The primary function of the respiratory system is gas exchange between the atmospheric air in the alveoli and the blood in the pulmonary circulation.[1-3] In the process, oxygen (O_2) from air in the alveoli diffuses into the blood in the pulmonary capillaries and carbon dioxide (CO_2) moves from the blood in pulmonary capillaries into the alveoli (discussed in Chapter 21). This section provides a brief overview of two abnormal states (hypoxemia and hypercapnia) that develop as the result of impaired ventilation and gas exchange that occur with many of the disorders discussed in the chapter.

Respiration can be divided into three parts: ventilation, perfusion, and diffusion. *Ventilation* involves the movement of air into the lungs. However, not all inspired air reaches the alveoli where gas exchange takes place. Of each 500 mL of air, which is the typical volume of air that is inhaled by the average-sized adult, about 150 mL remains behind in the airways, with the remainder (350 mL) moving into the alveoli. This is called *alveolar ventilation* and represents the portion of ventilation that participates in gas exchange. The actual movement or *diffusion* of O_2 and CO_2 takes place in the lung driven by the partial pressure (P) of the gases. Thus, oxygen moves from the alveoli, where the partial pressure of oxygen (PO_2) averages 104 mm Hg when breathing room air, to the blood in the pulmonary capillaries, where the average PO_2 is only 40 mm Hg.[1] Carbon dioxide moves in the opposite direction, from the blood in the pulmonary capillaries, where the partial pressure of carbon dioxide (PCO_2) is 45 mm Hg, to the alveolar air, where the PCO_2 is 40 mm Hg.[1] These values vary with tissue metabolism and the oxygen content of the inspired air.

Perfusion involves the movement of blood through the pulmonary circulation, including the pulmonary capillaries, where gas exchange takes place. Adequate oxygenation of the blood and removal of CO_2 depend on perfusion or movement of blood through the pulmonary blood vessels and appropriate contact between ventilated alveoli and perfused capillaries of the pulmonary circulation (ventilation and perfusion matching).

Hypoxemia

Hypoxemia refers to a reduction in the PO_2 of the arterial blood. It can result from an inadequate amount of O_2 in the air, disease of the respiratory system, dysfunction of the neurologic system, or alterations in circulatory function. The mechanisms whereby respiratory disorders lead to a significant reduction in PO_2 are hypoventilation, impaired diffusion of gases, inadequate circulation of blood through the pulmonary capillaries, and mismatching of ventilation and perfusion[2,3] (see Chapter 21). Often, more than one mechanism contributes to hypoxemia in persons with respiratory or cardiac disease.

Hypoxemia produces its effects through tissue hypoxia and the compensatory mechanisms that the body uses to adapt to the lowered oxygen level. Body tissues vary considerably in their vulnerability to hypoxia; those with the greatest need are the brain and heart. If the PO_2 in these organs falls below a critical level, aerobic metabolism ceases and anaerobic metabolism takes over, with formation and release of lactic acid. This results in increased serum lactate levels and a metabolic acidosis (see Chapter 8).

Mild hypoxemia or reduction in the PO_2 of arterial blood produces few manifestations. Recruitment of sympathetic nervous system compensatory mechanisms produces an increase in heart rate, peripheral vasoconstriction, and a mild increase in blood pressure.[3] This is because hemoglobin saturation is still approximately 90% when the PO_2 is only 60 mm Hg (see Chapter 21, Fig. 21-22). More pronounced hypoxemia may produce personality changes, restlessness, uncoordinated muscle movements, euphoria, impaired judgment, delirium, and, eventually, stupor and coma.

Cyanosis refers to the bluish discoloration of the skin and mucous membranes resulting from an excessive concentration of reduced or deoxygenated hemoglobin in the small blood vessels. It usually is most pronounced in the lips, nail beds, ears, and cheeks. The degree of cyanosis is modified by the amount of cutaneous pigment, skin thickness, and the state of the cutaneous capillaries. Cyanosis is more difficult to distinguish in persons with dark skin and in areas of the body with increased skin thickness. Although cyanosis may be evident in persons with respiratory failure, it often is a late sign. A deoxygenated hemoglobin concentration of approximately 5 g/dL of deoxygenated hemoglobin is required in the circulating blood for cyanosis to occur.[1] The absolute quantity of reduced hemoglobin, rather than the relative quantity, is important in producing cyanosis. Persons with anemia are less likely to exhibit cyanosis because they have less hemoglobin to transport oxygen even though their cardiac output and lung function are normal. A person with a high hemoglobin level because of polycythemia may be cyanotic in the absence of hypoxia.

Cyanosis can be divided into two types: central and peripheral. *Central cyanosis* is evident in the tongue and lips. It is caused by an increased amount of deoxygenated hemoglobin in the arterial blood. *Peripheral cyanosis* occurs in the extremities and on the tip of the nose or ears. It is caused by slowing of blood flow to an area of the body, with increased extraction of oxygen from the blood. It results from vasoconstriction and diminished peripheral blood flow, as occurs with cold exposure, shock, heart failure, or peripheral vascular disease.

The manifestations of chronic hypoxemia may be insidious in onset and attributed to other causes, particularly in persons with chronic lung disease. The body compensates for chronic hypoxemia with increased ventilation, pulmonary vessel vasoconstriction, and increased production of red blood cells. Pulmonary vasoconstriction occurs as a local response to alveolar hypoxia; it increases pulmonary arterial pressure and improves the matching of ventilation and perfusion. Increased production of red blood cells results from the release of erythropoietin from the kidneys in response to hypoxia (see Chapter 13). Other adaptive mechanisms include a shift to the right in the oxygen dissociation curve, which increases O_2 release to the tissues (see Chapter 21).

Diagnosis of hypoxemia is based on clinical observation and diagnostic tests that measure PO_2 levels. The analysis of arterial blood gases provides a direct measure of the O_2 content of the blood and is the best indicator of the ability of the lungs to oxygenate the blood. Mixed venous oxygen saturation (SvO_2; i.e., oxygen saturation of hemoglobin in venous blood) reflects the body's extraction at the tissue levels. Venous blood samples can be obtained either through a pulmonary artery catheter or central line.

Noninvasive measurements of arterial O_2 saturation of hemoglobin can be obtained using pulse oximetry.[4,5] Reusable clip probes (finger, nasal, ear) and single-use adhesive probes (finger and forehead) are available.[5] Advantages of the reusable clip probe include the rapidity with which measurements can be obtained and cost-effectiveness. The adhesive probes allow for more secure placement and ability to monitor sites other than those used by the clip probes.

Pulse oximetry uses light-emitting diodes and combines plethysmography (i.e., changes in light absorbance and vasodilation) with spectrophotometry.[4,5] Spectrophotometry uses a red-wavelength light that passes through oxygenated hemoglobin and is absorbed by deoxygenated hemoglobin, and an infrared-wavelength light that is absorbed by oxygenated hemoglobin and passes through deoxygenated hemoglobin. The pulse oximeter cannot distinguish between oxygen–carrying hemoglobin and carbon monoxide–carrying hemoglobin. In addition, the pulse oximeter cannot detect elevated levels of methemoglobin. Although pulse oximetry is not as accurate as arterial blood gas measurements, it provides the means for noninvasive and continuous monitoring of O_2 saturation, which is a useful indicator of respiratory and circulatory status.

Treatment of hypoxemia is directed toward correcting the cause of the disorder and increasing the gradient for diffusion through the administration of supplemental oxygen. Oxygen may be delivered by nasal cannula or mask or administered directly into an endotracheal or tracheostomy tube in persons who are mechanically ventilated.[3] A high-flow administration system is one in which the flow rate and reserve capacity are sufficient to provide all the inspired air. A low-flow administration system delivers less than the total inspired air. The concentration of O_2 being administered (usually determined by the flow rate) is based on the PO_2. A high flow rate must be carefully monitored in persons with chronic lung disease because increases in alveolar oxygen concentration above the person's baseline may suppress the hypoxia-induced ventilatory drive. Although oxygen is necessary and vital to life, there also is the danger of oxygen toxicity with concentrations above 60%. Continuous breathing of oxygen at high concentrations can lead to diffuse parenchymal lung injury due to oxygen free radicals. Persons with healthy lungs begin to experience respiratory symptoms such as cough, sore throat, substernal distress, nasal congestion, and painful inspiration after breathing pure oxygen for 24 hours.[2]

Hypercapnia

Hypercapnia refers to an increase in the carbon dioxide content of the arterial blood.[3,6] The PCO_2 is proportional to carbon dioxide production and inversely related to alveolar ventilation. The diagnosis of hypercapnia is based on physiologic manifestations and arterial blood gas levels.

Hypercapnia can occur in a number of disorders that cause hypoventilation or mismatching of ventilation and perfusion.[3,6] The diffusing capacity of carbon dioxide is 20 times that of oxygen; therefore, hypercapnia without hypoxemia is usually observed only in situations when supplemental oxygen is provided. In cases of ventilation–perfusion mismatching, hypercapnia is usually accompanied by a decrease in arterial PO_2 levels. Conditions that increase carbon dioxide production, such as an increase in metabolic rate or a high-carbohydrate diet, can contribute to the degree of hypercapnia that occurs in persons with impaired respiratory function. Changes in the metabolic rate resulting from an increase in activity, fever, or disease can have profound effects on carbon dioxide production. Alveolar ventilation usually rises proportionally with these changes, and hypercapnia occurs only when this increase is inappropriate or a compensatory rise in alveolar ventilation is inadequate.

Hypercapnia affects a number of body functions, including acid–base balance, as well as kidney, nervous system, and cardiovascular function. Elevated levels of PCO_2 produce respiratory acidosis (see Chapter 8). The body normally compensates for an increase in PCO_2 by increasing renal bicarbonate (HCO_3^-) retention, which results in an increase in serum HCO_3^- and pH levels. As long as the pH is within normal range, the main complications of hypercapnia are those resulting from the accompanying hypoxia. Because the body adapts to chronic increases in blood levels of carbon dioxide, persons with chronic hypercapnia may not have symptoms until the PCO_2 becomes markedly elevated, causing respiratory depression and altered mental status.

The treatment of hypercapnia is directed at decreasing the work of breathing and improving the ventilation–perfusion balance. The use of intermittent rest therapy, such as nocturnal negative-pressure ventilation, in persons with chronic obstructive pulmonary disease or chest wall disease may be effective in increasing the strength and endurance of the respiratory muscles and improving the PCO_2. Respiratory muscle retraining aimed at improving the respiratory muscles, their endurance, or both has been used to improve exercise tolerance and diminish the likelihood of respiratory fatigue. Mechanical ventilation may become necessary in situations of acute hypercapnia.

SUMMARY CONCEPTS

■ The primary functions of the respiratory system are to remove appropriate amounts of carbon dioxide from the blood entering the pulmonary circulation and provide adequate amount of oxygen to blood leaving the pulmonary circulation. This is accomplished through the process of ventilation, in which air moves into and out of the lungs, and diffusion, in which gases move between the alveoli and the pulmonary capillaries. Although both affect gas exchange, oxygenation of the blood largely depends on diffusion, while removal of carbon dioxide depends on ventilation.

■ Hypoxemia refers to a decrease in blood oxygen levels that results in a decrease in tissue oxygenation. Hypoxemia can occur as the result of hypoventilation, diffusion impairment, shunt, and ventilation–perfusion abnormalities. Acute hypoxemia is manifested by increased respiratory effort (increased respiratory and heart rates), cyanosis, and impaired sensory and neurologic function. The body compensates for chronic hypoxemia by increased ventilation, pulmonary vasoconstriction, and increased production of red blood cells.

(continued)

Disorders of Lung Inflation

Air entering through the airways inflates the lung, and the negative pressure in the pleural cavity keeps the lung from collapsing. Disorders of lung inflation are caused by conditions that obstruct the airways, cause lung compression, or produce lung collapse. There can be compression of the lung by an accumulation of fluid in the intrapleural space; complete collapse of an entire lung, as in pneumothorax; or collapse of a segment of the lung due to airway obstruction, as in atelectasis.

Disorders of the Pleura

The pleura is a thin, double-layered serous membrane that encases the lungs.[7,8] The outer parietal layer lines the thoracic wall and superior aspect of the diaphragm. It continues around the heart and between the lungs, forming the lateral walls of the mediastinum. The inner visceral layer covers the lung and is adherent to all its surfaces. The pleural cavity or space between the two layers contains a thin film of serous fluid that lubricates the pleural surfaces and allows the parietal and visceral pleurae to slide smoothly over each other during breathing movements.[1] The pressure in the pleural cavity, which is negative in relation to atmospheric pressure, holds the lungs against the chest wall and keeps them from collapsing. Disorders of the pleura include pleuritis, pleural effusion, and pneumothorax.

Pleuritis

Pleuritis (also called *pleurisy*) refers to inflammation of the parietal pleura that typically results in characteristic pleural pain.[9] Since the visceral pleura does not contain pain receptors, pleural pain results from somatic pain fibers that innervate the parietal pleura. The pain is usually unilateral and abrupt in onset, and is usually made worse by chest movements such as deep breathing and coughing that exaggerate pressure changes in the pleural cavity and increase movement of the inflamed or injured pleural surfaces. Because deep breathing is painful, tidal volumes usually are kept small, and breathing becomes more rapid to maintain the minute ventilation. Reflex splinting of the chest muscles may occur, causing a lesser respiratory expansion on the affected side.

There are numerous causes of pleuritis and pleuritic pain. The setting in which it occurs provides useful diagnostic information. In young, healthy individuals, it is commonly caused by viral infections or pneumonia. The presence of pleural effusion or air in the pleural cavity requires further diagnostic information.

It is important to differentiate pleural pain from pain produced by other conditions, such as musculoskeletal strain of the chest muscles, bronchial irritation, and myocardial disease. Musculoskeletal pain may occur as the result of frequent, forceful coughing. This type of pain usually is bilateral and located in the inferior portions of the rib cage, where the abdominal muscles insert into the anterior rib cage. It is made worse by movements associated with contraction of the abdominal muscles. The pain associated with irritation of the bronchi usually is substernal and dull in character rather than sharp. It is made worse with coughing but is not affected by deep breathing. Myocardial pain, which is discussed in Chapter 19, usually is located in the substernal area and is not affected by respiratory movements.

Treatment of pleuritis consists of treating the underlying disease and inflammation. Analgesics and nonsteroidal anti-inflammatory drugs (NSAIDs; e.g., indomethacin) may be used for pleuritic pain. Although these agents reduce inflammation, they may not entirely relieve the discomfort associated with deep breathing and coughing.

Pleural Effusion

Pleural effusion refers to an abnormal collection of fluid in the pleural cavity.[8,10,11] Like fluid developing in other transcellular spaces in the body, pleural effusion occurs when the rate of fluid formation exceeds the rate of its removal (see Chapter 8). Normally, fluid enters the pleural space from capillaries in the parietal pleura and is removed by their lymphatics. Fluid can also enter from the interstitial spaces of the lung through the visceral pleura or from small holes in the diaphragm. The lymphatics have the capacity to reabsorb about 20 times the fluid that is formed.[1] Accordingly, fluid may accumulate when there is excess fluid formation (from the interstitium of the lung, the parietal pleura, or the peritoneal cavity) or when there is decreased removal by the lymphatics.

The fluid that accumulates in a pleural effusion may be a transudate or exudate, purulent (containing pus), chyle, or sanguineous (bloody).[8,10,11] The accumulation of a serous transudate (clear fluid) in the pleural cavity often is referred to as *hydrothorax*. The condition may be unilateral or bilateral. The most common cause of hydrothorax is congestive heart failure.[8] Other causes are renal failure, nephrosis, liver failure, and malignancy. An *exudate* is a pleural fluid that has a specific gravity greater than 1.020 and often contains inflammatory cells.

Transudative and exudative pleural effusions are distinguished by measuring the lactate dehydrogenase (LDH) and protein levels in the pleural fluid.[8,11] Lactate dehydrogenase is an enzyme that is released from inflamed and injured pleural tissue. Exudative pleural effusions are characterized by the presence of proteins and/or elevated LDH levels in the pleural fluid, whereas transudates have none of these features. Because measurements of LDH are easily obtained from a sample of pleural fluid, it is a useful marker for diagnosis of exudative pleural disorders. Conditions that produce exudative pleural effusions are bacterial pneumonia, viral infection, pulmonary infarction, and malignancies.

Empyema refers to an infection in the pleural cavity that results in exudate containing glucose, proteins, leukocytes, and debris from dead cells and tissue.[3] The infection may be caused by invasion from an adjacent bacterial pneumonia or a subdiaphragmatic infection, by rupture of a lung abscess into the pleural space, or by trauma.

Chylothorax is the effusion of lymph in the thoracic cavity.[12] Chyle, a milky fluid containing chylomicrons, is found in the lymph fluid drained by lacteals in the villi of the small intestine. The thoracic duct transports chyle to the central circulation. Chylothorax results from trauma, inflammation, or malignant infiltration obstructing chyle transport from the thoracic duct into the central circulation. It is the most common cause of pleural effusion in the fetus and neonate, resulting from congenital malformation of the thoracic duct or lymph channels. Chylothorax also can occur as a complication of intrathoracic surgical procedures and use of the great veins for total parenteral nutrition and hemodynamic monitoring.

Hemothorax is the presence of blood in the pleural cavity. Bleeding may arise from chest injury, a complication of chest surgery, malignancies, or rupture of a great vessel such as an aortic aneurysm. It is usually diagnosed by the presence of blood in the pleural fluid. Hemothorax usually requires drainage, and if the bleeding continues, surgery to control the bleeding may be required.

The manifestations of pleural effusion vary with the cause.[7,8,10,11] Fluid in the pleural cavity acts as a space-occupying mass, causing a decrease in lung expansion on the affected side that is proportional to the amount of fluid collected. Characteristic signs of pleural effusion are dullness to percussion and diminished breath sounds. Hypoxemia may occur because of decreased surface area for diffusion and usually is corrected with supplemental oxygen. Dyspnea, the most common symptom, occurs when fluid in the pleural cavity compresses the lung, resulting in increased effort or rate of breathing. Pleuritic pain usually occurs only when inflammation is present, although constant discomfort may be felt with large effusions.

Diagnosis of pleural effusion is based on chest radiographs, chest ultrasonography, and computed tomography (CT).[8] Thoracentesis (aspiration of fluid from the pleural space) can be used to obtain a sample of pleural fluid for diagnosis. The treatment of pleural effusion is directed at the cause of the disorder.[8] With large effusions, thoracentesis may be used to remove fluid from the intrapleural space and allow for reexpansion of the lung. A palliative method used for treatment of pleural effusions caused by a malignancy is the injection of a sclerosing agent into the pleural cavity. This method of treatment causes obliteration of the pleural space and prevents the reaccumulation of fluid. Chest tube drainage may be necessary in cases of continued effusion.

Pneumothorax

Pneumothorax refers to the presence of air in the pleural space. Pneumothorax causes partial or complete collapse of the affected lung. Pneumothorax can occur without an obvious cause or injury (i.e., spontaneous pneumothorax) or as a result of direct injury to the chest or major airways (i.e., traumatic pneumothorax).[7,8] Tension pneumothorax describes a life-threatening condition in which increased pressure within the pleural cavity impairs both respiratory and cardiac function.

Spontaneous Pneumothorax. Spontaneous pneumothorax is hypothesized to occur due to the rupture of an air-filled bleb, or blister, on the surface of the lung.[8,10,13,14] Rupture of these blebs allows atmospheric air from the airways to enter the pleural cavity (Fig. 23-1). Because alveolar pressure normally is greater than pleural pressure, air flows from the alveoli into the pleural space, causing the involved portion of the lung to collapse as a result of its own recoil. Air continues to flow into the pleural space until a pressure gradient no longer exists or the decline in lung size causes the leak to seal. Spontaneous pneumothoraces can be divided into primary and secondary pneumothoraces.[8,13,14] Primary pneumothorax occurs in otherwise healthy persons, whereas secondary pneumothorax occurs in persons with underlying lung disease.

In primary spontaneous pneumothorax, the blebs usually are located at the top of the lungs. The condition is seen in persons who are tall and thin. It has been suggested that the difference in pleural pressure from the top to the bottom of the lung is greater in tall persons and that this difference in pressure may contribute to the development of blebs. Smoking is another factor that has been associated with primary spontaneous pneumothorax. Inflammation of the small airways related

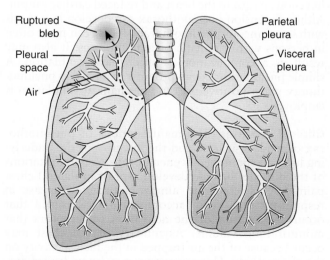

FIGURE 23-1. Mechanism for development of spontaneous pneumothorax, in which an air-filled bleb on the surface of the lung ruptures, allowing atmospheric air from the airways to enter the pleural space.

to smoking is thought to contribute to the condition, and cessation of smoking may reduce the chance of recurrence.

Secondary spontaneous pneumothoraces usually are more serious because they occur in persons with lung disease. They are associated with many different types of lung conditions that cause trapping of gases and destruction of lung tissue, including asthma, tuberculosis, cystic fibrosis, sarcoidosis, bronchogenic carcinoma, and metastatic pleural diseases. The most common cause of secondary spontaneous pneumothorax is emphysema. Secondary spontaneous pneumothorax may be life-threatening because of the underlying lung injury and poor compensatory reserves.

Traumatic Pneumothorax. Traumatic pneumothorax may be caused by penetrating or nonpenetrating chest injuries, most commonly fractured or dislocated ribs that penetrate the pleura. Hemothorax may accompany these injuries.[8,13] Pneumothorax also may accompany fracture of the trachea or major bronchus or rupture of the esophagus. Persons with pneumothorax due to chest trauma frequently have other complications and may require chest surgery. Medical procedures such as transthoracic needle aspirations, central line insertion, intubation, and positive-pressure ventilation occasionally may cause pneumothorax. Traumatic pneumothorax also can occur as a complication of cardiopulmonary resuscitation.

Tension Pneumothorax. Tension pneumothorax occurs when the intrapleural pressure exceeds atmospheric pressure.[8,13] It is a life-threatening condition and occurs when injury to the chest or respiratory structures allows air to enter but not leave the pleural space (Fig. 23-2). This results in a rapid increase in pressure within the chest that causes compression of the unaffected lung, a shift in the mediastinum to the opposite side of the chest, and compression of the vena cava, which results in a decrease in venous return to the heart and reduced cardiac output. Although tension pneumothorax can develop in persons with spontaneous pneumothoraces, it is seen most often in persons with traumatic pneumothoraces. It also may result as a complication of mechanical ventilation. A simple pneumothorax can progress to a tension pneumothorax when positive-pressure mechanical ventilation is employed.

Clinical Features. The manifestations of pneumothorax depend on its size and the integrity of the underlying lung. In spontaneous pneumothorax, manifestations of the disorder include development of ipsilateral chest pain.[7,8,13,14] There is an almost-immediate increase in respiratory rate, often accompanied by dyspnea that occurs as a result of the activation of receptors that monitor lung volume. Asymmetry of the chest may occur because of the air trapped in the pleural cavity on the affected side. This asymmetry may be evidenced during inspiration as a lag in the movement of the affected side, with inspiration delayed until the unaffected lung reaches the same level of pressure as the lung with the

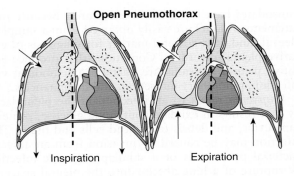

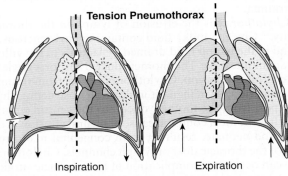

FIGURE 23-2. Open or communicating pneumothorax (*top*) and tension pneumothorax (*bottom*). In an open pneumothorax, air enters the chest during inspiration and exits during expiration. There may be slight inflation of the affected lung because of a decrease in pressure as air moves out of the chest. In tension pneumothorax, air can enter but not leave the chest. As the pressure in the chest increases, the heart and great vessels are compressed and the mediastinal structures are shifted toward the opposite side of the chest. The trachea is pushed from its normal midline position toward the opposite side of the chest, and the unaffected lung is compressed.

air trapped in the pleural space. Percussion of the chest produces a more hyperresonant sound, and breath sounds are decreased or absent over the area of the pneumothorax.

With tension pneumothorax, the trachea deviates toward the opposite side of the chest along with the structures in the mediastinal space (see Fig. 23-2). The position of the trachea can be used as a means of assessing for a mediastinal shift. Because of the increase in intrathoracic pressure, stroke volume or the amount of blood that the heart ejects with each beat is reduced to such an extent that cardiac output is decreased despite an increase in heart rate. There may be distention of the neck veins, subcutaneous emphysema (i.e., presence of air in the subcutaneous tissues of the chest and neck), and clinical signs of shock due to impaired cardiac function.

Hypoxemia usually develops immediately after a large pneumothorax, followed by vasoconstriction of the blood vessels in the affected lung, causing the blood flow to shift to the unaffected lung. In persons with primary spontaneous pneumothorax, this mechanism usually returns oxygen saturation to normal within 24 hours. Hypoxemia usually is more serious in persons with underlying lung disease in whom secondary spontaneous pneumothorax develops or in persons with underlying heart disease who are unable to compensate with an increase in heart rate and stroke volumes. Regardless of etiology, the hypoxemia caused by the partial or total loss of lung function can be life-threatening. Without immediate intervention, the increased thoracic pressure will further impair both cardiac and pulmonary function, resulting in severe hypoxemia and hypotension.

Diagnosis of pneumothorax can be confirmed by chest radiograph, CT scan, or ultrasonography.[8,13,14] Pulse oximetry and blood gas analysis may be done to determine the effect on blood oxygen levels. Treatment of pneumothorax varies with the cause and extent of the disorder. In small spontaneous pneumothoraces, the air usually reabsorbs spontaneously, and only observation and follow-up chest radiographs are required. Supplemental oxygen may be used to correct the hypoxemia until the air is reabsorbed. In larger pneumothoraces, the air is removed by needle aspiration or a closed drainage system used with or without suction. This type of drainage system uses a one-way valve to allow air to exit the pleural space and prevent it from reentering the chest.

Emergency treatment of tension pneumothorax involves the prompt insertion of a large-bore needle or chest tube into the affected side of the chest along with one-way valve drainage or continuous chest suction to aid in lung reexpansion.[8,13] Sucking chest wounds, which allow air to pass in and out of the chest cavity, should be treated by promptly covering the area with an airtight covering. Chest tubes are inserted as soon as possible.

Atelectasis

Atelectasis refers to an incomplete expansion of a lung or portion of a lung.[15,16] It can be caused by airway obstruction, lung compression such as occurs in pneumothorax or pleural effusion, or increased recoil of the lung due to loss of pulmonary surfactant (see Chapter 21). The disorder may be present at birth (i.e., primary atelectasis) or develop during the neonatal period or later in life (i.e., acquired or secondary atelectasis).

Primary atelectasis of the newborn implies that the lung has never been inflated. It is seen most frequently in premature and high-risk infants. A secondary form of atelectasis can occur in infants who established respiration and subsequently experienced impairment of lung expansion. Among the causes of secondary atelectasis in the newborn is the respiratory distress syndrome associated with lack of surfactant and airway obstruction due to aspiration of amniotic fluid or blood.

Acquired atelectasis occurs mainly in adults. It most commonly results from airway obstruction, for example, by a mucus plug in the airway or by external compression of the airway from fluid, a tumor mass, exudate, or other matter in the pleural cavity or area surrounding the

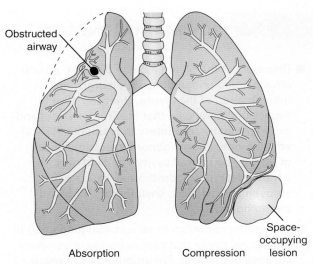

FIGURE 23-3. Atelectasis caused by airway obstruction and absorption of air from the involved lung area (*left*) and by compression of lung tissue (*right*).

airway (Fig. 23-3). Portions of alveoli, a small segment of lung, or an entire lung lobe may be involved. Complete obstruction of an airway is followed by the absorption of air from the dependent alveoli and collapse of that portion of the lung. Breathing high concentrations of oxygen increases the rate at which gases are absorbed from the alveoli and predisposes to atelectasis. The danger of obstructive atelectasis increases after surgery.[15] Anesthesia, pain, administration of narcotics, and immobility tend to promote retention of viscid bronchial secretions and airway obstruction. The encouragement of coughing and deep breathing, frequent change of position, adequate hydration, and early ambulation decrease the risk for atelectasis.

The clinical manifestations of atelectasis include tachypnea, tachycardia, dyspnea, cyanosis, signs of hypoxemia, diminished chest expansion, absence of breath sounds, and intercostal retractions. Both chest expansion and breath sounds are decreased on the affected side. There may be intercostal retraction (pulling in of the intercostal spaces) over the involved area during inspiration. Signs of respiratory distress are proportional to the extent of lung collapse. If the collapsed area is large, the mediastinum and trachea shift to the affected side. In compression atelectasis, the mediastinum shifts away from the affected lung.

The diagnosis of atelectasis is based on signs and symptoms. Chest radiographs are used to confirm the diagnosis. Computed tomography scans may be used to show the exact location of the obstruction. Treatment depends on the cause and extent of lung involvement. It is directed at reducing the airway obstruction or lung compression and at reinflation of the collapsed area of the lung. Ambulation, deep breathing, and body positions that favor increased lung expansion are used when appropriate. Administration of oxygen may be needed to correct the hypoxemia. Bronchoscopy may be used as both a diagnostic and treatment method.

SUMMARY CONCEPTS

- Disorders of the pleura include pleuritis, pleural effusion, and pneumothorax. Pleuritis, or inflammation of the pleura, characteristically causes unilateral pain that is abrupt in onset and exaggerated by respiratory movements. Pleural effusion refers to the abnormal accumulation of fluid in the pleural cavity. The fluid may be a transudate (i.e., hydrothorax), exudate (i.e., empyema), chyle (i.e., chylothorax), or blood (hemothorax).

- Pneumothorax refers to an accumulation of air in the pleural cavity that causes partial or complete collapse of the lung. Pneumothorax can result from rupture of an air-filled bleb on the lung surface or from penetrating or nonpenetrating injuries. A tension pneumothorax is a life-threatening event in which air accumulates in the thorax, collapsing the lung on the injured side and progressively shifting the mediastinum to the opposite side of the thorax, producing severe cardiac and respiratory impairment.

- Atelectasis refers to an incomplete expansion of the lung. Primary atelectasis occurs most often in premature and high-risk infants. Acquired atelectasis occurs mainly in adults and is caused most commonly by a mucus plug in the airway or by external compression by fluid, tumor mass, exudate, or other matter in the area surrounding the airway.

Obstructive Airway Disorders

Obstructive airway disorders are caused by conditions that limit expiratory airflow. Bronchial asthma represents an acute and reversible form of airway disease caused by narrowing of the airways due to bronchospasm, inflammation, and increased airway secretions. Chronic obstructive disorders include a variety of airway diseases, such as bronchial asthma, chronic obstructive pulmonary disease, bronchiectasis, and cystic fibrosis.

Physiology of Airway Disease

Air moves through the upper airways (i.e., trachea and major bronchi) into the lower or pulmonary airways (i.e., bronchi and alveoli), which are located in the lung.[1,2] In the pulmonary airways, the cartilaginous layer that provides support for the trachea and major bronchi gradually disappears and is replaced with crisscrossing strips of smooth muscle (see Chapter 21).

The contraction and relaxation of the smooth muscle layer, which is innervated by the autonomic nervous system, controls the diameter of the bronchial airways and consequent resistance to airflow. Parasympathetic stimulation through the vagus nerve and cholinergic receptors produces bronchoconstriction, whereas sympathetic stimulation, through β_2-adrenergic receptors, produces bronchodilation. At rest, a slight vagal-mediated bronchoconstrictor tone predominates. When there is need for increased airflow, as during exercise, the bronchodilator effects of the sympathetic nervous system are stimulated and the bronchoconstrictor effects of the parasympathetic nervous system are inhibited. Bronchial smooth muscle also responds to inflammatory mediators, such as histamine, that act directly on bronchial smooth muscle cells to produce bronchoconstriction.

Bronchial Asthma

Bronchial asthma is a common obstructive airway disease that affects adults and children and occurs in all populations and locations throughout the world. It has been estimated that 25.7 million people in the United States suffer from asthma, 7.0 million of them children under 18 years of age.[17,18] The disease continues to be costly, both in terms of emergency room visits and lost work days. Close to 2.1 million emergency room visits were attributed to asthma in 2009, and in 2008 it accounted for an estimated 14.2 million lost work days for adults.[18]

Asthma is a chronic inflammatory disease of the airways involving recurring symptoms of airflow obstruction and bronchial hyper-responsiveness.[19–22] Airway obstruction is characterized by episodic wheezing, difficulty breathing, feeling of chest tightness, and a cough that often is worse at night and in the early morning. These episodes, which usually are reversible either spontaneously or with treatment, also cause an associated increase in bronchial responsiveness to a variety of stimuli.

Etiology and Pathogenesis

Asthma is commonly categorized into two types: extrinsic or allergic, due to a type I hypersensitivity reaction, and intrinsic or *non-atopic*, that occurs without an allergic component. In either type, episodes of bronchospasm can be triggered by diverse nonimmune mechanisms, including respiratory tract infections, exercise, ingestion of aspirin, emotional upset, and exposure to bronchial irritants such as cigarette smoke.[15,16] Asthma may also be classified according to the agents or events that trigger an attack. These include seasonal, exercise-induced, drug-induced (e.g., aspirin), and occupational asthma.

The common denominator underlying all forms of asthma is an exaggerated hypersensitivity response to a variety of stimuli. After exposure to an inciting factor (allergens, drugs, cold, or exercise), inflammatory mediators released by activated macrophages, eosinophils, mast cells, and basophils induce bronchoconstriction, increased vascular permeability, and mucus production.[15,16] In some persons, persistent changes in airway structures occur, including injury to epithelial cells, smooth muscle hypertrophy, and blood vessel proliferation.

Recent research has focused on the role of T lymphocytes in the pathogenesis of bronchial asthma. It is now known that there are two subsets of T-helper cells (T_H1 and T_H2) that develop from the same precursor $CD4^+$ T lymphocyte (see Chapter 15).[15] T_H1 cells differentiate in response to microbes and stimulate the differentiation of B cells into immunoglobulin (Ig) M and IgG-producing plasma cells. T_H2 cells, on the other hand, respond to allergens by stimulating B cells to differentiate into IgE-producing plasma cells that bind to mucosal mast cells. Subsequent IgE-mediated reactions to inhaled allergens elicit an asthmatic attack (see Chapter 16, Fig. 16-1). In persons with allergic asthma, T-cell differentiation appears to be skewed toward T_H2 cells. Although the molecular basis for this preferential differentiation is unclear, it seems likely that both genetic and environmental factors play a role.

Atopic Asthma. Atopic asthma is typically initiated by a type I hypersensitivity reaction induced by exposure to an extrinsic antigen or allergen.[15,16] It usually has its onset in childhood or adolescence and is seen in persons with a family history of atopic allergy (see Chapter 16). Persons with atopic asthma often have other allergic disorders, such as hay fever, urticaria, and eczema. Attacks are related to exposure to specific allergens. Among air-borne allergens implicated in perennial (year-round) asthma are house dust mite allergens, cockroach allergens, animal danders, and *Alternaria* (a fungus).

The mechanisms of response to allergens in atopic asthma can be described in terms of the early-phase and the late-phase responses[15,16] (Fig. 23-4). The symptoms of the *early-phase response* (also called the *acute-phase response*), which usually develop within 10 to 20 minutes of exposure to the allergen, are caused by the release of chemical mediators from presensitized IgE-coated mast cells. In the case of air-borne antigens, the reaction occurs when antigen binds to previously sensitized mast cells on the mucosal surface of the airways (Fig. 23-5A). Mediator release results in the infiltration of inflammatory cells, opening of the mucosal intercellular junctions, and increased access of antigen to the more prevalent submucosal mast cells. In addition, there is bronchospasm caused by stimulation of parasympathetic receptors, mucosal edema caused by increased vascular permeability, and increased mucus secretions. The acute response usually can be inhibited or reversed by bronchodilators, such as β_2-agonists, but not by the anti-inflammatory actions of corticosteroids.

The *late-phase response,* which develops 4 to 8 hours after exposure to an asthmatic trigger, involves inflammation and increased airway responsiveness that

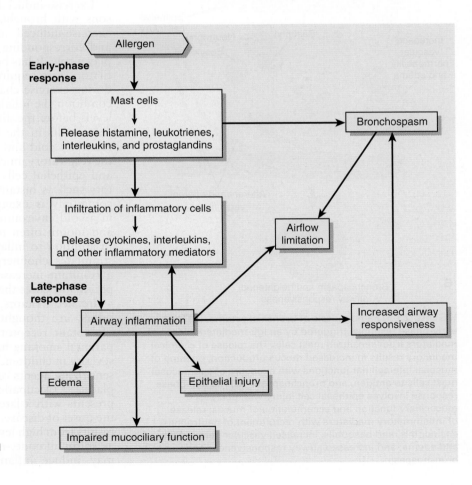

FIGURE 23-4. Mechanisms of early- and late-phase IgE-mediated bronchospasm.

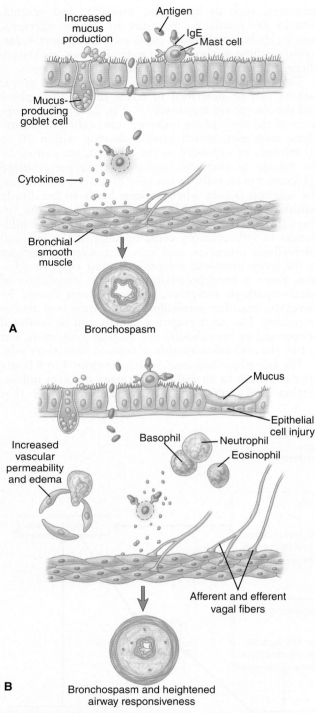

A Bronchospasm

B Bronchospasm and heightened
airway responsiveness

FIGURE 23-5. Pathogenesis of bronchial asthma. **(A)** The early-phase response triggered by an IgE-mediated release of mediators from sensitized mast cells. The release of chemical mediators results in increased mucus production, opening of mucosal intercellular junctions with exposure of submucosal mast cells to antigen, and bronchospasm. **(B)** The late-phase response involves epithelial cell injury with decreased mucociliary function and accumulation of mucus; release of inflammatory mediators with recruitment of neutrophils, eosinophils, and basophils; increased vascular permeability and edema; and increased airway responsiveness and bronchospasm.

prolong the asthma attack and set into motion a vicious cycle of exacerbations.[18] Typically, the response reaches a maximum within a few hours and may persist for 12 to 24 hours or longer. An initial trigger in the late-phase response causes the release of inflammatory mediators from mast cells, macrophages, and epithelial cells. These substances induce the migration and activation of other inflammatory cells (e.g., basophils, eosinophils, neutrophils), which then produce epithelial injury and edema, changes in mucociliary function, reduced clearance of respiratory tract secretions, and increased airway responsiveness (see Fig. 23-5B). Chronic inflammation can lead to airway remodeling, in which case airflow limitations may be only partially reversible.[19]

Nonatopic Asthma. Intrinsic or nonatopic asthma triggers include respiratory tract infections, exercise, hyperventilation, cold air, drugs and chemicals, hormonal changes and emotional upsets, air-borne pollutants, and gastroesophageal reflux. Respiratory tract infections, especially those caused by viruses, may produce their effects by causing epithelial damage and stimulating the production of IgE antibodies directed toward the viral antigens. In addition to precipitating an asthmatic attack, viral respiratory infections increase airway responsiveness to other asthma triggers. This hyperresponsiveness may persist for weeks beyond the original infection.

Exercise-induced asthma occurs in a number of persons with bronchial asthma.[23] Although the cause of exercise-induced asthma is unclear, hyperventilation and corresponding changes in airway physiology may play a role. It has been suggested that the increased ventilatory rate required to meet higher oxygen demands during exercise challenges the ability of the airways to condition the inhaled air to the correct moist and heat levels before the air reaches the alveoli. Vigorous exercise results in the inhalation of increased volumes of relatively cold and dry air and loss of body heat from the respiratory mucosa, which in turn induces mast cells and epithelial cells to release proinflammatory mediators such as histamine and leukotrienes. The response commonly is exaggerated when the person exercises in a cold environment. Wearing a mask over the nose and mouth often minimizes the attack or prevents it. In addition to inflammatory cytokines, airway cooling stimulates cholinergic receptors in the airways, with a resultant increase in airway resistance. A warm-up period alleviates the symptoms for some persons.

Inhaled irritants, such as tobacco smoke and strong odors, are thought to induce bronchospasm by way of irritant receptors and a vagal reflex. Exposure to parental smoking has been reported to increase asthma severity in children.[24] Occupational asthma is caused by sensitizing agents or irritants encountered in the workplace.[25,26] Occupational asthma from sensitizers usually presents with a latent period of exposure, followed by the onset of disease. Irritant or nonimmunologic asthma results from high levels of exposure to irritant gases such as sulfur dioxide, nitrogen dioxide, and ozone, which may induce inflammatory exacerbations of airway responsiveness (e.g., smog-related asthma). A group of chemicals that can provoke an asthmatic attack are the sulfites used in food processing and as preservatives added to beer, wine, and fresh vegetables.

There is a small group of persons in whom aspirin and other NSAIDs evoke the clinical triad of nasal polyps, chronic rhinosinusitis, and bronchial asthma.[15,16,27] The mechanism of the hypersensitivity reaction is complex and not fully understood, but most evidence points toward an abnormality in arachidonic acid (AA) metabolism in which aspirin inhibits the bronchodilating cyclooxygenase pathway without affecting the lipoxygenase pathway, thereby shifting the balance toward the bronchoconstrictor leukotrienes (see Chapter 3, Fig. 3-4). Avoidance of aspirin and all NSAIDs is a necessary part of the treatment program.

Both emotional factors and changes in hormone levels are thought to contribute to an increase in asthma symptoms. Emotional factors produce bronchospasm by way of vagal pathways. They can act as a bronchospastic trigger, or they can increase airway responsiveness to other triggers through noninflammatory mechanisms. Reproductive hormones may play a role in asthma in women. Up to 40% of women with asthma report a premenstrual increase in asthma symptoms.[28] Female reproductive hormones have a regulatory role on β_2-adrenergic function, and it has been suggested that abnormal regulation may be a possible mechanism for premenstrual asthma.

Symptoms of gastroesophageal reflux are common in both adults and children with asthma, suggesting that reflux of gastric secretions may act as a bronchospastic trigger. Reflux during sleep can contribute to nocturnal asthma.[19]

Manifestations

Persons with asthma exhibit a wide range of signs and symptoms ranging from episodes of wheezing and feelings of chest tightness to acute immobilizing attacks. The attacks differ from person to person, and between attacks, many persons are symptom free. Attacks may occur spontaneously or in response to various triggers, respiratory infections, emotional stress, or weather changes. Asthma is often worse at night. Studies of nocturnal asthma suggest that there is a circadian and sleep-related variation in hormones and respiratory function.[29] The greatest decrease in respiratory function occurs at about 4:00 AM, at which time cortisol levels are low, melatonin levels high, and eosinophil activity increased.[30]

During an asthmatic attack, the airways narrow because of bronchospasm, edema of the bronchial mucosa, and mucus plugging. Expiration becomes prolonged because of progressive airway obstruction.[19–22] The amount of air that can be forcibly expired in 1 second (forced expiratory volume in 1 second [$FEV_{1.0}$]) and the peak expiratory flow rate (PEF), measured in liters per second, are decreased.

During a prolonged attack, air becomes trapped behind the occluded and narrowed airways, causing hyperinflation of the lungs. This produces an increase in the residual volume (RV) along with a decrease in the inspiratory reserve capacity (tidal volume + inspiratory reserve volume [IRV]) and forced vital capacity (FVC), such that the person breathes close to his or her functional residual capacity (residual volume + expiratory reserve volume; see Chapter 21, Fig. 21-17). As a result, more energy is needed to overcome the tension already present in the lungs, and the accessory muscles (e.g., sternocleidomastoid muscles) are required to maintain ventilation and gas exchange. This increased work of breathing further increases oxygen demands and causes dyspnea and fatigue. Because air is trapped in the alveoli and inspiration is occurring at higher residual lung volumes, the cough becomes less effective. As the condition progresses, the effectiveness of alveolar ventilation declines, and mismatching of ventilation and perfusion occurs, causing hypoxemia and hypercapnia. Pulmonary vascular resistance may increase as a result of the hypoxemia and hyperinflation, leading to a rise in pulmonary arterial pressure and increased work demands on the right heart.

The physical signs of bronchial asthma vary with the severity of the attack. A mild attack may produce a feeling of chest tightness, a slight increase in respiratory rate with prolonged expiration, and mild wheezing. A cough may accompany the wheezing. More severe attacks are accompanied by use of the accessory muscles, distant breath sounds due to air trapping, and loud wheezing. As the condition progresses, fatigue develops, the skin becomes moist, and anxiety and apprehension ensue. Sensations of shortness of breath may be severe, and often the person is able to speak only one or two words before taking a breath. At the point at which airflow is markedly decreased, breath sounds become inaudible, wheezing diminishes, and the cough becomes ineffective despite being repetitive and hacking.[19] This point often marks the onset of respiratory failure. A common error on physical examination is the absence of wheezing which signifies severe bronchospasm and represents the lack of air movement. With appropriate treatment, wheezing can be unmasked as air movement improves.

Diagnosis and Treatment

The diagnosis of asthma is based on a careful history and physical examination, laboratory findings, and pulmonary function studies (see Chapter 21).[19–22] Spirometry provides a means for measuring FVC, FEV1.0, PEF, tidal volume, expiratory reserve volume, and inspiratory reserve volume. The FEV1.0/FVC ratio can then be calculated. The level of airway responsiveness can be measured by inhalation challenge tests using methacholine (a cholinergic agonist), histamine, or exposure to a nonpharmacologic agent such as cold air. The Expert Panel of the National Asthma Education and Prevention Program (NAEPP) has developed classification systems intended for use in identifying persons at high risk for development of life-threatening asthma attacks and directing asthma treatment[19] (Table 23-1).

Small, inexpensive, portable meters that measure PEF are available. Although not intended for use in the

TABLE 23-1	Classification of Asthma Severity		
Asthma Severity	Symptoms, Interference with Normal Activities, and Frequency of Short-Acting β_2-Agonist Use	Nighttime Awakenings	Lung Function
Mild intermittent	Symptoms ≤2 days a week No interference with normal activity Short-acting β_2-agonist use <2 days a week	<2 times a month	Normal $FEV_{1.0}$ between exacerbations $FEV_{1.0}$ >80% predicted $FEV_{1.0}$/FVC normal
Mild persistent	Symptoms 2 days a week but not daily Minor limitation in normal activity Short-acting β_2-agonist use ≥2 days a week but not daily	3–4 times a month	$FEV_{1.0}$ >80% predicted $FEV_{1.0}$/FVC normal
Moderate persistent	Symptoms daily Some limitation in normal activity Short-acting β_2-agonist daily	>1 time a week but not nightly	$FEV_{1.0}$ >60% normal but <80% predicted $FEV_{1.0}$/FVC reduced 5%
Severe persistent	Symptoms throughout the day Extreme limitation in normal activity Short-acting β_2-agonist several times a day	Often 7 times a week	$FEV_{1.0}$ <60% normal $FEV_{1.0}$/FVC reduced >5%

$FEV_{1.0}$, forced expiratory volume in 1 second; FVC, forced vital capacity.

Adapted from National Lung, Heart, and Blood Institute National Asthma Education and Prevention Program. *Expert Panel Report 3: Guidelines for Diagnosis and Management of Asthma*. Bethesda, MD: National Institutes of Health; 2007.

diagnosis of asthma, they can be used in clinics and physicians' offices and by persons in their home to provide frequent measures of flow rates. Day–night (circadian) variations in asthma symptoms and PEF variability can be used to indicate the severity of bronchial hyperresponsiveness. The person's best performance is established from readings taken over several weeks. This often is referred to as the individual's *personal best* and is used as a reference to indicate changes in respiratory function. A PEF below 40% of the predicted or personal best during an acute asthmatic attack indicates a severe exacerbation and the need for immediate intervention, and a PEF below 25% of the predicted or personal best indicates a life-threatening attack.[19]

Successful management of bronchial asthma requires control of factors contributing to asthma severity and pharmacologic treatment. Control measures are aimed at prevention of exposure to allergens and irritants. They include education of the person and family regarding known triggers; therefore, a careful history is needed to identify all contributory factors. Annual influenza vaccination is recommended for persons with persistent asthma.

A program of desensitization may be undertaken in persons with persistent asthma who react to allergens, such as house dust mites, that cannot be avoided. This involves the injection of selected antigens (based on skin tests) to stimulate the production of IgG antibodies that block the IgE response. A course of allergen immunotherapy is typically of 3 to 5 years' duration.[19]

Traditionally, drugs used to treat asthma were categorized according to their predominant mechanism of action—relaxation of bronchial smooth muscle (bronchodilator) and suppression of airway inflammation (anti-inflammatory drugs). A more recent classification divides asthma medications into two general categories according to their roles in the overall management of asthma symptoms (quick-relief or long-term maintenance medications).[19]

Quick-relief Medications. The *quick-relief medications* include the short-acting β_2-agonists, anticholinergic agents, and systemic corticosteroids.[19,21,31] The short-acting β_2-agonists relax bronchial smooth muscle and provide prompt relief of symptoms, usually within 30 minutes. They are administered by inhalation (i.e., metered-dose inhaler [MDI] or nebulizer).

The anticholinergic agents block cholinergic receptors and reduce intrinsic vagal tone that causes bronchoconstriction. These medications, which are administered by inhalation, produce bronchodilation by direct action on the large airways but do not change the composition or viscosity of the bronchial mucus. It is thought that they may provide some additive benefit for treatment of asthma exacerbations when administered with inhaled β_2-agonists.

A short course of systemic corticosteroids, administered orally or parenterally, may be used for treating the inflammatory reaction associated with the late-phase response. Although their onset of action is slow (>4 hours), systemic corticosteroids may be used in the treatment of moderate to severe exacerbations because of their action in preventing the progression of the exacerbation, speeding recovery, and preventing early relapses.

Long-term Medications. The *long-term medications* are taken on a daily basis to achieve and maintain control of persistent asthma symptoms. They include inhaled corticosteroids, long-acting bronchodilators, cromolyn and nedocromil, leukotriene receptor antagonists, and theophylline.[19,21,31] The corticosteroids are considered the most effective anti-inflammatory agents for use in long-term treatment of asthma. Inhaled corticosteroids administered by MDI usually are preferred because of minimal systemic absorption and reduced disruption in hypothalamic-pituitary-adrenal function.

The long-acting β_2-agonists, available for administration by the inhaled or oral routes, act by relaxing bronchial smooth muscle. They are used as an adjunct to anti-inflammatory medications for providing long-term control of symptoms, especially nocturnal symptoms, and for preventing exercise-induced bronchospasm. The long-acting β_2-agonists have durations of action of at least 12 hours and should not be used to treat acute symptoms or exacerbations.[19]

The leukotriene receptor antagonists (monelukast and zafirlukast) block the action of the leukotrienes, which are arachidonic acid derivatives synthesized by a number of inflammatory cells in the airways, including eosinophils, mast cells, macrophages, and basophils.[19,31] Several of the leukotrienes exert many of the effects known to occur in asthma, including bronchoconstriction, increased bronchial reactivity, mucosal edema, and mucus hypersecretion. A particular advantage of the leukotriene receptor antagonists is that they are taken orally.

Theophylline, a phosphodiesterase inhibitor, is a bronchodilator that acts by relaxing bronchial smooth muscle. The sustained-release form of the drug is used as an adjuvant therapy, particularly to relieve nighttime symptoms.[19] It may be used as an alternative, but not preferred, medication in long-term preventative therapy when there are issues concerning adherence with regimens using inhaled medications or when cost is a factor. Because elimination of the drug varies widely among persons, blood levels are required to ensure that a therapeutic but not toxic dose is achieved.[17]

The anti-IgE monoclonal antibody omalizumab is the first biologic immunoregulatory agent available to treat asthma.[29] It binds to the portion of the IgE that recognizes its receptor on the surface of mast cells and basophils. Omalizumab, which is indicated for treatment of moderate and severe persistent asthma, is administered subcutaneously every 2 to 4 weeks, depending on the dose. The drug has been approved for adults and children 12 years of age and older.

Severe Asthma

Severe (or refractory) asthma represents a subgroup (probably <10%) of persons with asthma who have high medication requirements to maintain good symptom control, or who continue to have persistent symptoms despite high medication use.[32,33] The condition has been described as persistent asthma that required continuous high-dose inhaled or oral corticosteroids for more than 50% of the previous year and the need for additional daily treatment with controller medications, exhibited evidence of disease exacerbations or instability, and required hospitalizations or emergency room visits.[19,21,32,33] Persons with severe asthma are at increased risk for a fatal or near-fatal asthmatic attack. Underestimating the severity of the attack may be a contributing factor.[34] Deterioration often occurs rapidly during an acute attack, and underestimation of

its severity may lead to a life-threatening delay in seeking medical attention.

Little is known about the causes of severe asthma. Among the proposed risk factors are genetic predisposition, continued allergen or tobacco exposure, infection, intercurrent sinusitis or gastroesophageal reflux disease, and lack of compliance or adherence with treatment measures.[33] Because bronchial asthma likely involves multiple genes, mutations in genes regulating cytokines (e.g., IL-4), growth factors, or receptors for medications used in treatment of asthma (β_2-adrenergic agonist or glucocorticoid) could be involved. Environmental factors include both allergen and tobacco exposure, with the strongest reaction occurring in response to house dust mite antigens, cockroach allergen, and *Alternaria* exposure.

Bronchial Asthma in Children

Asthma is a common chronic illness in children. In the United States, asthma is the most common cause of childhood emergency department visits, hospitalizations, and missed school days.[35–38] Although childhood asthma may have its onset at any age, up to 80% of children who develop asthma are symptomatic before 5 years of age.[19] Asthma is more prevalent among black than white children.[36–39] Worldwide, childhood asthma appears to be increasing in prevalence.[35] It is particularly common in children living in suburban areas, as compared to rural areas of developing countries.

As with adults, asthma in children commonly is associated with an IgE-related reaction. It has been suggested that IgE directed against respiratory viruses in particular may be important in the pathogenesis of wheezing illnesses in infants (i.e., bronchiolitis), which often precede the onset of asthma.[37,38] Previous severe infections with the respiratory syncytial virus (RSV) are a risk factor in the development of asthma. Other contributing factors include exposure to environmental allergens such as pet dander, dust mite antigens, and cockroach allergens. Exposure to environmental tobacco smoke also contributes to asthma in children.[36–39]

The signs and symptoms of asthma in infants and small children vary with the stage and severity of an attack. Because airway patency decreases at night, many children have acute signs of asthma at this time. Often, previously well infants and children develop what may seem to be a cold with rhinorrhea, rapidly followed by irritability, nonproductive cough, wheezing, tachypnea, dyspnea with prolonged expiration, and use of accessory muscles of respiration. Cyanosis, hyperinflation of the chest, and tachycardia indicate increasing severity of the attack. Wheezing may be absent in children with extreme respiratory distress. The symptoms may progress rapidly and require a trip to the emergency department or hospitalization.

As with adults and older children, the Expert Panel of the NAEPP recommends a stepwise approach to diagnosing and managing childhood asthma.[19] Treatment involves not only pharmacologic agents but also recognition and modification of potential environmental triggers, such as tobacco smoke, and allergens, such as dust mites and pet dander. Inhaled corticosteroids should be used to control asthma symptoms and improve the child's quality of life but not to prevent more serious asthma or irreversible obstruction in later years.[19] The systemic side effects of inhaled corticosteroids are usually limited to children receiving very high doses and are similar to the side effects seen with systemic corticosteroids: adrenal suppression, growth suppression, decreased bone density, myopathy, and weight gain. Despite the low risk of side effects, growth velocity should be monitored in children and adolescents receiving long-term corticosteroid therapy.[19]Alternative or supplemental medications include long-acting β-agonists and leukotriene pathway inhibitors. Short-acting β-agonists may be used to relieve acute symptoms. Systemic corticosteroids may be required during episodes of severe disease.

Special delivery systems for administration of inhalation medications are available for infants and small children, including nebulizers with face masks and spacers or holding chambers for use with an MDI. For children younger than 2 years of age, nebulizer therapy usually is preferred. Children between 3 and 5 years of age may begin using an MDI with a spacer and holding chamber. The child's caregiver should be carefully instructed in the appropriate use of these devices. The Expert Panel recommends that adolescents (and younger children when appropriate) be directly involved in developing their asthma management plans.[19] Active participation in physical activities, exercise, and sports should be encouraged.

Chronic Obstructive Pulmonary Disease

Chronic obstructive pulmonary disease (COPD) denotes a group of respiratory disorders characterized by chronic and recurrent obstruction of airflow in the pulmonary airways.[15,16,40,41] The airflow obstruction is usually progressive, may be accompanied by airway hyperreactivity, and may be partially reversible. COPD remains a leading cause of morbidity and mortality worldwide. It is the fourth leading cause of death in the United States, and is projected to become the third leading cause of death worldwide.[41]

The most common cause of COPD is smoking, as evidenced by the fact that 85% to 90% of persons with COPD have a history of smoking.[15,16] Other predisposing factors include exposure to occupational dusts and chemicals, airway infections, and asthma or airway hyperresponsiveness.[41] Unfortunately, clinical findings are almost always absent during the early stages of COPD. By the time symptoms appear or are recognized, the disease is usually far advanced. For smokers with early signs of airway disease, there is hope that early recognition, combined with appropriate treatment and smoking cessation, may prevent or delay the usually relentless progression of the disease.

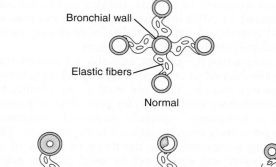
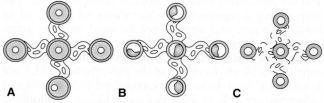

FIGURE 23-6. Mechanisms of airflow obstruction in chronic obstructive lung disease. (*Top*) Normal bronchial airway with elastic fibers that provide traction and hold the airway open. (*Bottom*) Obstruction of the airway caused by **(A)** inflammation and fibrosis of the bronchial wall, **(B)** hypersecretion of mucus, and **(C)** destruction of the elastic fibers that hold the airway open.

The term *chronic obstructive pulmonary disease* encompasses two types of obstructive airway disease: *emphysema*, with enlargement of air spaces and destruction of lung tissue, and *chronic obstructive bronchitis*, with increased mucus production, obstruction of small airways, and a chronic productive cough.[15,16] Persons with COPD often have overlapping features of both emphysema and chronic bronchitis.

The mechanisms involved in the pathogenesis of COPD usually are multiple and include inflammation and fibrosis of the bronchial wall, hypertrophy of the submucosal glands and hypersecretion of mucus, and loss of elastic lung fibers and alveolar tissue (Fig. 23-6). Inflammation and fibrosis of the bronchial wall, along with excess mucus secretion and destruction of elastic fibers, cause mismatching of ventilation and perfusion. Destruction of alveolar tissue decreases the surface area for gas exchange, and loss of elastic fibers, which normally provide traction and hold the airways open, impairs the expiratory flow rate, increases air trapping, and predisposes to airway collapse.

Emphysema

Emphysema is characterized by a loss of lung elasticity and abnormal enlargement of the air spaces distal to the terminal bronchioles, with destruction of the alveolar walls and capillary beds[16] (Fig. 23-7). Enlargement of the air spaces leads to hyperinflation of the lungs and produces an increase in total lung capacity (TLC). Two of the recognized causes of emphysema are smoking, which incites lung injury, and an inherited deficiency of α_1-antitrypsin, an antiprotease enzyme that protects the lung from injury. Genetic factors other than an inherited α_1-antitrypsin deficiency also may play a role in smokers who develop COPD at an early age.[41]

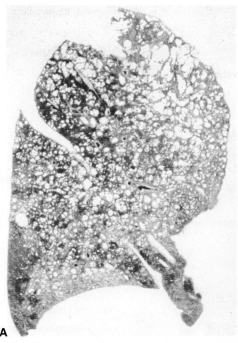

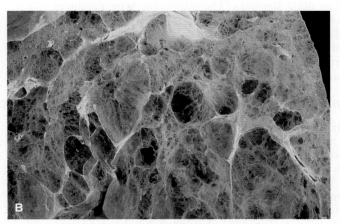

FIGURE 23-7. Panacinar emphysema. **(A)** A whole mount of the left lung from a patient with severe emphysema reveals widespread destruction of pulmonary parenchyma that in some areas leaves behind a lacy network of supporting tissue. **(B)** The lung from a patient with α_1-antitrypsin deficiency shows a panacinar pattern of emphysema. The loss of alveolar walls has resulted in markedly enlarged air spaces. (From Bearsley MB, Travis WD, Rubin E. The respiratory system. In: Rubin R, Strayer DS, eds. *Rubin's Pathology: Clinicopathologic Foundations of Medicine*. 6th ed. Philadelphia, PA: Wolters Kluwer Health | Lippincott Williams & Wilkins; 2012:569.)

Emphysema is thought to result from the breakdown of elastin and other alveolar wall components by enzymes, called *proteases*, which digest proteins. The proteases—particularly elastase, which is an enzyme that digests elastin—are released from polymorphonuclear leukocytes (i.e., neutrophils), alveolar macrophages, and other inflammatory cells.[16,17] Normally, the lung is protected by antiprotease enzymes, including α_1-antitrypsin. Cigarette smoke and other irritants stimulate the movement of inflammatory cells into the lungs, resulting in increased release of elastase and other proteases. In smokers in whom COPD develops, antiprotease production and release may be inadequate to neutralize the excess protease production such that the process of elastic tissue destruction goes unchecked (Fig. 23-8).

A hereditary deficiency in α_1-antitrypsin accounts for approximately 1% of all cases of COPD and is more common in young persons with emphysema.[40] The type and amount of α_1-antitrypsin that a person has are determined by a pair of codominant genes referred to as *protein inhibitor* (PI) genes. Homozygotes who carry two defective PI genes have only about 15% to 20% of the normal plasma concentration of α_1-antitrypsin.[16] Smoking and repeated respiratory tract infections, which also decrease α_1-antitrypsin levels, contribute to the risk for emphysema in persons with α_1-antitrypsin deficiency. Laboratory methods are available for measuring α_1-antitrypsin levels. Human α_1-antitrypsin is

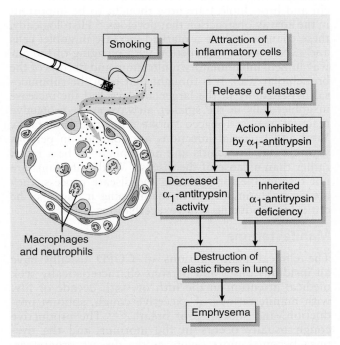

FIGURE 23-8. Protease (elastase)–antiprotease (antitrypsin) mechanisms of emphysema. The effects of smoking and an inherited α_1-antitrypsin deficiency on the destruction of elastic fibers in the lung and development of emphysema are shown.

available for replacement therapy in persons with a hereditary deficiency of the enzyme.

There are two commonly recognized types of emphysema: centriacinar or centrilobular, and panacinar (Fig. 23-9). The centriacinar type affects the bronchioles in the central part of the respiratory lobule, with initial preservation of the alveolar ducts and sacs.[16] It is the most common type of emphysema and is seen predominantly in male smokers. The panacinar type produces initial involvement of the peripheral alveoli and later extends to involve the more central bronchioles. This type of emphysema is more common in persons with α_1-antitrypsin deficiency. It also is found in smokers in association with centriacinar emphysema.

Chronic Bronchitis

Chronic bronchitis represents airway obstruction of the major and small airways.[15,16] The condition is seen most commonly in middle-aged men and is associated with chronic irritation from smoking and recurrent infections. A clinical diagnosis of chronic bronchitis requires a history of a chronic productive cough that has persisted for at least 3 consecutive months in at least 2 consecutive years.[44] Typically, the cough has been present for many years, with a gradual increase in acute exacerbations that produce frankly purulent sputum.

The earliest feature of chronic bronchitis is hypersecretion of mucus in the large airways, associated with hypertrophy of the submucosal glands in the trachea and bronchi.[15,16] Although mucus hypersecretion in the large airways is the cause of sputum overproduction, the accompanying changes in the small airways (small bronchi and bronchioles) are now thought to be important in the airway obstruction that develops.[15] Histologically, these changes include a marked increase in goblet cells and excess mucus production with plugging of the airway lumen, inflammatory infiltration, and fibrosis of the bronchiolar wall. It is thought that both the submucosal hypertrophy in the larger airways and the increase in goblet cells in the smaller airways are a protective reaction against tobacco smoke and other pollutants. Viral and bacterial infections are common in persons with chronic bronchitis and are thought to be a result rather than a cause of the disease. While infections are not responsible for initiating the disease process, they are probably important in maintaining it and may be critical in producing acute exacerbations.

Manifestations

The clinical manifestations of COPD usually have an insidious onset and persons characteristically seek medical attention in the fifth or sixth decade of life, with manifestations of excessive cough, sputum production, and shortness of breath.[10,44] The productive cough usually occurs in the morning and the dyspnea becomes more severe as the disease progresses. Frequent exacerbations of infection and respiratory insufficiency are common, causing absence from work and eventual disability. The late stages of COPD are characterized by recurrent respiratory infections and

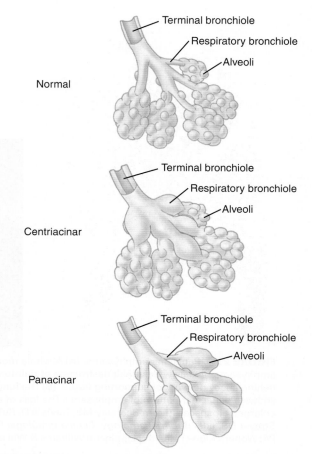

FIGURE 23-9. Centriacinar and panacinar emphysema. In centriacinar emphysema, the destruction is confined to the terminal (TB) and respiratory bronchioles (RB). In panacinar emphysema, the peripheral alveoli (A) are also involved. (Adapted from West JB. *Pulmonary Pathophysiology: The Essentials.* 7th ed. Philadelphia, PA: Wolters Kluwer Health | Lippincott Williams & Wilkins; 2008:56.)

chronic respiratory failure. Death usually occurs during an exacerbation of illness associated with infection and respiratory failure.

The mnemonics "pink puffer" and "blue bloater" have been used to differentiate the clinical manifestations of emphysema and chronic obstructive bronchitis.[15] Persons with predominant emphysema are classically referred to as *pink puffers,* a reference to the lack of cyanosis, the use of accessory muscles, and pursed-lip ("puffer") breathing. With loss of lung elasticity and hyperinflation of the lungs, the airways often collapse during expiration because pressure in surrounding lung tissues exceeds airway pressure. Air becomes trapped in the alveoli and lungs, producing an increase in the anteroposterior dimensions of the chest, the so-called *barrel chest* that is typical of persons with emphysema (Fig. 23-10). Such persons have a dramatic decrease in breath sounds throughout the chest. Because the diaphragm may be functioning near its maximum ability, the person is vulnerable to diaphragmatic fatigue and acute respiratory failure. Persons with a clinical syndrome of chronic bronchitis are classically

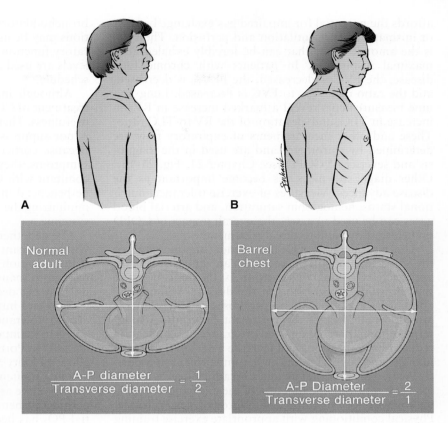

FIGURE 23-10. Characteristics of normal chest wall and chest wall in emphysema. The normal chest wall and its cross-section are illustrated on the left **(A)**. The barrel-shaped chest of emphysema and its cross-section are illustrated on the right **(B)**. (From Smeltzer SC, Bare BG. *Medical-Surgical Nursing.* 10th ed. Philadelphia, PA: Lippincott Williams & Wilkins; 2004:572.)

Normal adult

$$\frac{\text{A-P diameter}}{\text{Transverse diameter}} = \frac{1}{2}$$

Barrel chest

$$\frac{\text{A-P Diameter}}{\text{Transverse diameter}} = \frac{2}{1}$$

labeled *blue bloaters,* a reference to cyanosis and fluid retention associated with right-sided heart failure. In practice, differentiation between the two types of COPD is often difficult. This is because persons with COPD often have some degree of both emphysema and chronic bronchitis.

The manifestations of COPD are associated with episodes of moderate to severe respiratory impairment due to obstruction of airflow, which is greater on expiration than inspiration, resulting in increased work of breathing but decreased effectiveness. The development of exertional dyspnea, often described as increased effort to breathe, heaviness, air hunger, or gasping, can be insidious. Activities involving significant arm work, particularly above the shoulders, are usually difficult for persons with COPD. The breathing becomes increasingly more labored, even at rest; the expiratory phase of respiration is prolonged; and expiratory wheezes and crackles can be heard on auscultation. Persons with severe airflow obstruction may also exhibit use of the accessory muscles, often sitting in the characteristic "tripod" position in which the arms are braced to facilitate use of the sternocleidomastoid, scalene, and intercostal muscles. Pursed-lip breathing enhances airflow because it increases the resistance to the outflow of air and helps to prevent airway collapse by increasing airway pressure. Eventually, persons with COPD are unable to maintain normal blood gases by increasing their breathing effort. Hypoxemia, hypercapnia, and cyanosis develop, reflecting an imbalance between ventilation and perfusion.

Exacerbations, which are characterized by increased cough, sputum, dyspnea, and fatigue, are increasingly frequent as the disease progresses.[44,45] They are often difficult to distinguish from other causes of respiratory deterioration, such as pneumonia, congestive heart failure, pulmonary emboli, and pneumothorax with radiologic or laboratory tests. Persons with frequent exacerbations exhibit a faster decline in lung function and have a lower quality of life, an increased need for hospitalization, and a higher mortality rate.

Severe hypoxemia, in which arterial PO_2 levels fall below 55 mm Hg, causes reflex vasoconstriction of the pulmonary vessels and further impairment of gas exchange in the lung. It is more common in persons with the chronic bronchitis form of COPD. Hypoxemia also stimulates red blood cell production, causing polycythemia. The increase in pulmonary vasoconstriction and subsequent elevation in pulmonary artery pressure further increase the work of the right ventricle. As a result, persons with COPD may develop right-sided heart failure with peripheral edema (i.e., cor pulmonale). However, signs of overt right-sided heart failure are seen less frequently since the advent of supplemental oxygen therapy (to be discussed).

Diagnosis and Treatment

The diagnosis of COPD is based on a careful history and physical examination, pulmonary function studies, chest radiographs, and laboratory tests.[10,42,44] Airway obstruction prolongs the expiratory phase of respiration and affords the potential for impaired gas exchange because of mismatching of ventilation and perfusion. The FVC is the amount of air that can be forcibly exhaled after maximal inspiration. In patients with chronic lung disease, the FVC is decreased, the $FEV_{1.0}$ is decreased, and the ratio of $FEV_{1.0}$ to FVC is decreased. Lung volume measurements reveal a marked increase in RV, an increase in TLC, and elevation of the RV-to-TLC ratio. These and other measurements of expiratory flow are determined by spirometry and are used in the diagnosis and severity of COPD (see Chapter 21, Fig. 21-15). Other diagnostic measures become important as the disease advances. Measures of exercise tolerance, nutritional status, hemoglobin saturation, and arterial blood gases can be used to assess the overall impact of COPD on health status and to direct treatment.

The treatment of COPD depends on the stage of the disease and often requires an interdisciplinary approach.[10,44] Smoking cessation is the only measure that slows the progression of the disease. Maintaining and improving physical and psychosocial functioning is an important part of the treatment program. A long-term pulmonary rehabilitation program can significantly reduce hospitalizations and increase a person's ability to manage and cope with his or her impairment in a positive way. This program includes breathing exercises that focus on restoring the function of the diaphragm, reducing the work of breathing, and improving gas exchange. Physical conditioning with appropriate exercise training increases maximal oxygen consumption and reduces ventilatory effort and heart rate for a given workload. Work simplification and energy conservation strategies may be needed when impairment is severe.

Respiratory tract infections can prove life-threatening to persons with severe COPD. A person with COPD should avoid exposure to others with known respiratory tract infections and should avoid attending large gatherings during periods of the year when influenza or respiratory tract infections are prevalent. Immunization for influenza and pneumococcal infections decreases the likelihood of their occurrence. Although antibiotics are used to treat acute exacerbations of COPD due to bacterial infection, there is no evidence that the prophylactic use of antibiotics prevents acute exacerbations.

The pharmacologic treatment of COPD includes the use of bronchodilators, including inhaled adrenergic and anticholinergic agents.[10,44] Inhaled β_2-agonists have been the mainstay of treatment of COPD for many years. It has been suggested that long-acting inhaled β_2-agonists may be even more effective than the short-acting forms of the drug. The anticholinergic drugs, which are administered by inhalation, produce bronchodilation by blocking parasympathetic cholinergic receptors that produce contraction of bronchial smooth muscle. They also reduce the volume of sputum without altering its viscosity. Because these drugs have a slower onset and longer duration of action, they typically are used on a regular basis rather than as needed. Inhalers that combine an anticholinergic drug with a β_2-adrenergic agonist are available. Oral theophylline may be used in treatment of persons who fail to respond to inhaled

bronchodilators. The long-acting theophylline preparations may be used to reduce overnight declines in respiratory function. When theophylline is prescribed, blood levels are used as a guide in arriving at an effective dose schedule.

Although inhaled corticosteroids often are used in treatment of COPD, there is controversy regarding their usefulness. There is evidence that inflammation in COPD is not suppressed by inhaled or oral corticosteroids.[44] Because corticosteroids are useful in relieving asthma symptoms, they may benefit persons with asthma concomitant with COPD. Inhaled corticosteroids also may be beneficial in treating acute exacerbations of COPD, minimizing the undesirable effects that often accompany systemic use.

Oxygen therapy is prescribed for selected persons with significant hypoxemia (arterial $PO_2 < 55$ mm Hg). Administration of continuous low-flow (1 to 2 L/min) oxygen to maintain arterial PO_2 levels between 55 and 65 mm Hg decreases dyspnea and pulmonary hypertension and improves neuropsychological function and activity tolerance.[10,44] The overall goal of oxygen therapy is to maintain a hemoglobin oxygen saturation of at least 90%. Portable oxygen administration units, which allow mobility and the performance of activities of daily living, are often used in severe COPD. Because the ventilatory drive associated with hypoxic stimulation of the peripheral chemoreceptors does not occur until the arterial PO_2 has been reduced to about 60 mm Hg or less, increasing the arterial PO_2 above 60 mm Hg tends to depress the hypoxic stimulus for ventilation and often leads to hypoventilation and carbon dioxide retention.

Bronchiectasis

Bronchiectasis is characterized by a permanent dilation of bronchi caused by destruction of the bronchial muscle wall and elastic supporting tissue[16,46,47] (Fig. 23-11). It is not a primary disease but occurs secondary to a number of abnormalities that profoundly obstruct the airways or produce persistent infection, including atelectasis, obstruction of the smaller airways, diffuse bronchitis, and cystic fibrosis.[15] In the past, bronchiectasis often followed a necrotizing bacterial pneumonia that frequently complicated measles, pertussis (whooping cough), or influenza. Tuberculosis was also commonly associated with bronchiectasis. Thus, with the advent of antibiotics that more effectively treat respiratory infections such as tuberculosis, and with immunization against pertussis and measles, there has been a marked decrease in the prevalence of bronchiectasis.

Etiology and Pathogenesis

Two processes are critical to the pathogenesis of bronchiectasis: obstruction and chronic persistent infection.[15,16] Regardless of which may come first, both cause damage to the bronchial walls, leading to weakening and dilation. On gross examination, bronchial dilation is classified as saccular, cylindrical, or varicose.[16,47] Saccular bronchiectasis involves the proximal third to

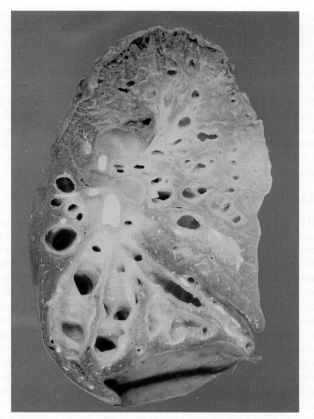

FIGURE 23-11. Bronchiectasis. The resected upper lobe shows widely dilated bronchi, with thickening of the bronchial walls and collapse and fibrosis of the pulmonary parenchyma. (From Bearsley MB, Travis WD, Rubin E. The respiratory system. In: Rubin R, Strayer DS, eds. *Rubin's Pathology: Clinicopathologic Foundations of Medicine.* 6th ed. Philadelphia, PA: Wolters Kluwer Health | Lippincott Williams & Wilkins; 2012:545.)

fourth generation of bronchi (see Chapter 21, Fig. 21-4). These bronchi become severely dilated and end blindly in dilated sacs, with collapse and fibrosis of more distal lung tissue. Cylindrical bronchiectasis involves uniform and moderate dilation of the sixth to eighth generations of airways. It is a milder form of disease than saccular bronchiectasis and leads to fewer symptoms. Varicose bronchiectasis involves the second through eighth branchings of bronchi and results in bronchi that resemble varicose veins. Bronchiolar obliteration is not as severe and symptoms are variable.

Bronchiectasis can present in either of two forms: a local obstructive process involving a lobe or segment of a lung or a diffuse process involving much of both lungs.[16] *Localized bronchiectasis* is most commonly caused by conditions such as tumors, foreign bodies, and mucus plugs that produce atelectasis and infection due to obstructed drainage of bronchial secretions. It can affect any area of the lung, the area being determined by the site of obstruction or infection. *Generalized bronchiectasis* usually is bilateral and most commonly affects the lower lobes. It is due largely to inherited impairments of host mechanisms or acquired disorders that permit introduction of infectious organisms

into the airways. They include cystic fibrosis, in which airway obstruction is caused by impairment of normal mucociliary function; congenital and acquired immunodeficiency states, which predispose to respiratory tract infections; lung infection (e.g., tuberculosis, fungal infections, lung abscess); and exposure to toxic gases that cause airway obstruction.

Manifestations

Bronchiectasis is usually manifested by a chronic productive cough, often with several hundred milliliters of foul-smelling, purulent sputum a day.[16] Hemoptysis is common. Dyspnea and wheezing occur in about 75% of patients.[6] Weight loss, anemia, and other systemic manifestations are common.[10] Clubbing of the fingers is infrequent in mild cases, but common in severe disease. Obstructive pulmonary dysfunction with hypoxemia is seen in moderate to severe cases. However, due to improved treatment with better antibiotics and physical therapy, outcome and life expectancy have improved considerably.

Diagnosis and Treatment

Diagnosis is based on history and imaging studies. The condition often is evident on chest radiographs. High-resolution CT scanning of the chest allows for definitive diagnosis. Accuracy of diagnosis is important because interventional bronchoscopy or surgery may be palliative or curative in some types of obstructive disease.

Treatment consists of early recognition and management of infections along with regular postural drainage and chest physical therapy. Persons with this disorder benefit from many of the rehabilitation and treatment measures used for chronic bronchitis and emphysema.

Cystic Fibrosis

Cystic fibrosis (CF), which is a major cause of severe chronic respiratory disease in children and young adults, is an inherited disorder involving fluid secretion by the exocrine glands in the epithelial lining of the respiratory, gastrointestinal, and reproductive tracts.[48–51] In addition to chronic respiratory disease, CF is manifested by pancreatic exocrine deficiency and elevation of sodium chloride in the sweat. Nasal polyps, sinus infections, pancreatitis, and cholelithiasis also are common. Excessive loss of sodium in the sweat predisposes young children to salt depletion episodes. Most males with CF have congenital bilateral absence of the vas deferens with azoospermia.

Cystic fibrosis is inherited as an autosomal recessive trait. Homozygotes have all or substantially all of the clinical symptoms of the disease, compared with heterozygotes, who are carriers of the disease but have no recognizable symptoms. Cystic fibrosis occurs most frequently in white populations of northern Europe, North America, and Australia/New Zealand.[51] Although it occurs less frequently among African, Hispanic, Middle Eastern, South Asian, and Eastern Asian populations, it may occur in these populations as well.

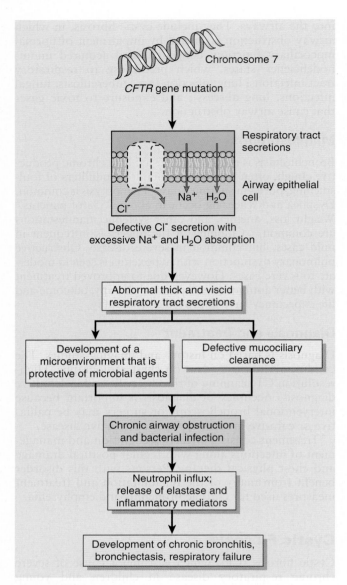

FIGURE 23-12. Pathogenesis of cystic fibrosis.

Etiology and Pathogenesis

Cystic fibrosis is caused by mutations in a single gene on the long arm of chromosome 7 that encodes for the cystic fibrosis transmembrane regulator (CFTR), which functions as a chloride channel in epithelial cell membranes.[49–51] Mutations in the *CFTR* gene render the epithelial membrane relatively impermeable to the chloride (Cl⁻) ion (Fig. 23-12).

The impact on impaired Cl⁻ transport is relatively tissue specific. In the sweat glands, the concentration of sodium (Na⁺) and Cl⁻ secreted into the lumen of the gland remain unaffected, whereas the reabsorption of Cl⁻ through the CFTR and accompanying reabsorption of Na⁺ in the ducts of the gland fail to occur. This defect accounts for the high concentration of NaCl in the sweat of persons with CF.[50,51] In the normal airway epithelium, Cl⁻ is secreted into airway lumen through the CFTR. As shown in Figure 23-12, in persons with CF, the transport

of Cl⁻ into airway lumen is impaired. This ultimately leads to a series of secondary events, including increased absorption of Na⁺ and water from the airways into the blood. This lowers the water content of the mucociliary blanket coating the respiratory epithelium, causing it to become more viscid. The resulting dehydration of the mucous layer leads to defective mucociliary function and accumulation of viscid secretions that obstruct the airways and predispose to recurrent pulmonary infections. Similar transport abnormalities and pathophysiologic events take place in the pancreatic and biliary ducts and in the vas deferens in males.

Manifestations

Respiratory manifestations of CF are caused by an accumulation of viscid mucus in the bronchi, impaired mucociliary clearance, and lung infections. Chronic bronchiolitis and bronchitis are the initial lung manifestations, but after months and years, structural changes in the bronchial wall lead to bronchiectasis. In addition to airway obstruction, the basic genetic defect that occurs with CF predisposes to chronic infection with a surprisingly limited number of organisms, the most common being *Pseudomonas aeruginosa, Burkholderia cepacia, Staphylococcus aureus,* and *Haemophilus influenzae.*[48–51] Soon after birth, initial infection with bacterial pathogens occurs and is associated with an excessive neutrophilic inflammatory response that appears to be independent of the infection itself. There is evidence that the airway secretions in persons with CF provide a favorable environment for harboring these organisms. *Pseudomonas aeruginosa,* in particular, has a propensity to undergo mucoid transformation in this environment. The complex polysaccharide produced by these organisms provides a hypoxic environment and generates a biofilm that protects *Pseudomonas* against antimicrobial agents. Pulmonary inflammation is another cause of decline in respiratory function in persons with CF and may precede the onset of chronic infection.

Exocrine pancreatic function is abnormal in more than 85% of affected children.[51] Steatorrhea, diarrhea, and abdominal pain are common. In the newborn, meconium ileus may cause intestinal obstruction, a fatal condition if left untreated. The degree of pancreatic involvement is highly variable. In some children, the defect is relatively mild, and in others, the involvement is severe and impairs intestinal absorption. In addition to exocrine pancreatic insufficiency, hyperglycemia may occur, especially after 10 years of age, when approximately 8% of persons with CF develop diabetes mellitus.[51]

Diagnosis and Treatment

Early diagnosis and treatment are important in delaying the onset and severity of chronic illness in children with CF. Diagnosis is based on the presence of respiratory and gastrointestinal manifestations typical of CF, a history of CF in a sibling, or a positive newborn screening test result. Confirmatory laboratory tests include the sweat test and DNA tests for *CFTR* gene mutations.[51] The *sweat test,* using pilocarpine iontophoresis to collect the sweat followed by chemical analysis of its chloride content, remains the standard approach to diagnosis. Newborns with CF have elevated blood levels of immunoreactive trypsinogen, presumably because of secretory obstruction in the pancreas. A variety of *newborn screening* tests are in place to identify infants with cystic fibrosis, most of which consist of a combination of immunoreactive trypsinogen and limited DNA analysis. These tests can be done on blood spots collected for routine newborn screening tests.

Treatment measures are directed toward early and aggressive measures to slow progression of secondary organ dysfunction and sequelae such as chronic lung infection and pancreatic insufficiency.[51] They include the use of antibiotics to prevent and manage infections, the use of chest physical therapy (chest percussion and postural drainage) and mucolytic agents to prevent airway obstruction, and nutritional therapy including pancreatic enzyme replacement. Routine laboratory evaluations are key to assessing pulmonary function and response to therapeutic interventions. These studies include radiologic examinations, pulmonary function testing, and microbiologic cultures of respiratory secretions.

Appropriate antibiotic therapy directed against bacterial pathogens isolated from the respiratory tract is an essential component in the management of CF lung disease. Antibiotics are initially used to prevent colonization with *P. aeruginosa*; they are used as maintenance therapy once the airways are colonized with *P. aeruginosa* and other organisms such as *S. aureus*; and they are administered as aggressive treatment during acute exacerbations of pulmonary symptoms caused by infections.[51] To avoid adverse effects and to obtain high airway concentrations, the inhalation route is often used as an option for home delivery of these agents, with other routes of delivery being used during periods of progressive symptoms.

The abnormal viscosity of airway secretions is attributed largely to the presence of polymorphonuclear white blood cells and their degradation products. A purified recombinant human deoxyribonuclease (rhDNase), an enzyme that breaks down these products, has been developed.[54] Clinical trials have shown that the drug, which is administered by inhalation, can decrease pulmonary symptoms and reduce the frequency of respiratory exacerbations. Although many persons benefit from the therapy, the drug is costly, and recommendations for its use are evolving.

Up to 90% of patients with CF have complete loss of exocrine pancreatic function and inadequate digestion of fats and proteins. They require supplemental vitamins and minerals and enteric-coated, pH-sensitive pancreatic enzyme supplements. At one time, a low-fat, high-protein, high-calorie diet was recommended. With the advent of improved pancreatic enzyme products, however, normal amounts of fat in the diet are usually tolerated and preferred.

Progress of the disease is variable. Improved medical management has led to longer survival.[49,51,52] Today, many people with the disease can expect to live into their 40s and beyond. Lung transplantation is being used as a treatment for persons with end-stage lung disease.

The last 10 years have seen promising results from research into the management of cystic fibrosis using small molecules called *cystic fibrosis transmembrane regulator protein (CFTR) modulators* designed to increase the time the CFTR channels in the cell surface remain open.[53]

SUMMARY CONCEPTS

- Obstructive airway disorders due to bronchial smooth muscle hyperreactivity or changes in bronchial wall structure, injury to the mucosal lining of the airways, or excess respiratory tract secretions are characterized by limitation in movement of atmospheric air into and out of the gas exchange portion of the lung.

- Bronchial asthma is a chronic disorder of the airways that causes reversible episodes of airway obstruction due to bronchial smooth muscle hyperreactivity and airway inflammation. Extrinsic (or atopic) asthma is a type I hypersensitivity reaction triggered by an allergen; whereas intrinsic asthma is triggered by respiratory tract infections, exercise, drugs and chemicals, airborne pollutants, and gastroesophageal reflux.

- An asthmatic episode is characterized by two types of responses—acute and late phase. The *acute-phase response* results in immediate bronchoconstriction on exposure to an inhaled antigen and usually subsides within 90 minutes. The *late-phase response* develops 4 to 8 hours after exposure to an asthmatic trigger; and involves inflammation and increased airway responsiveness that prolong the attack and cause a vicious cycle of exacerbations.

- Chronic obstructive pulmonary disease (COPD) encompasses two types of obstructive airway disease: *emphysema,* with enlargement of air spaces and destruction of lung tissue, and *chronic obstructive bronchitis,* with increased mucus production, obstruction of small airways, and a chronic productive cough. Persons with COPD often have overlapping features of both emphysema and chronic bronchitis, and both are manifested by eventual mismatching of ventilation and perfusion. As the conditions advance, signs of respiratory distress and impaired gas exchange become evident, with development of hypercapnia and hypoxemia.

- Bronchiectasis is an uncommon form of COPD that is characterized by an abnormal dilation of the large bronchi associated with infection and destruction of the bronchial walls.

(continued)

Interstitial Lung Diseases

The diffuse interstitial lung diseases, also called *diffuse parenchymal lung diseases*, are a diverse group of lung disorders that produce similar inflammatory and fibrotic changes in the interstitium or interalveolar septa of the lung. Because the interstitial lung diseases result in a stiff and noncompliant lung, they are commonly classified as *restrictive lung disorders*.

In contrast to the obstructive lung diseases, which primarily involve the airways of the lung, the interstitial lung disorders exert their effects on the collagen and elastic connective tissue found in the delicate interstitium of the alveolar walls.[10,15,54–56] Many of these diseases also involve the airways, arteries, and veins. The clinical hallmark of these widespread lung changes is diminished lung compliance, which presents as restrictive lung disease. The lungs are stiff and difficult to inflate. More pressure is needed to expand the lungs, which in turn necessitates more effort in breathing. Damage to alveolar epithelium and interstitial vasculature produces impaired gas exchange and hypoxemia. With progression, persons develop respiratory failure, often in association with pulmonary hypertension and cor pulmonale.

The interstitial lung diseases may be acute or insidious in onset; they may be rapidly progressive, slowly progressive, or static in their course. Over 100 distinct entities of interstitial lung diseases have been recognized including hypersensitivity pneumonitis (discussed in Chapter 16); lung diseases caused by medications (e.g., the cancer drug bleomycin and the antiarrhythmic drug amiodarone) and radiation therapy; the occupational lung diseases, including the pneumoconioses that are caused by the inhalation of inorganic dusts such as silica, coal dust, and asbestos; immunologic lung disorders, such as those that accompany rheumatoid arthritis and scleroderma; and granulomatous diseases such as sarcoidosis.[15,58] Examples of interstitial lung diseases and their causes are listed in Chart 23-1. The discussion in this chapter focuses on idiopathic pulmonary fibrosis and sarcoidosis, two of the most common interstitial lung diseases seen in the clinical setting.[55]

CHART 23-1 Causes of Interstitial Lung Disease*

Occupational and Environmental Inhalants
Pneumoconioses (coal miner's pneumoconiosis, silicosis, asbestosis)
Hypersensitivity pneumonitis (farmer's lung, bird breeder's lung)
Talcosis (talc inhalation in injection drug users)
Smoking related

Drugs and Therapeutic Agents
Cancer drugs (e.g., bleomycin, busulfan, cyclophosphamide, methotrexate)
Antiarrhythmic drugs (amiodarone)
Ionizing radiation (i.e., radiation therapy)

Granulomatous Disorders
Sarcoidosis

Immunologic Disorders
Systemic lupus erythematosus
Rheumatoid arthritis
Scleroderma

Unknown Causes
Idiopathic pulmonary fibrosis

*This list is not intended to be inclusive.

Pathogenesis

Current theory suggests that most interstitial lung diseases, regardless of their cause, have a common pathogenesis.[15] It is thought that these disorders are initiated by some type of injury to the alveolar epithelium, followed by an inflammatory process that involves the alveoli and interstitium of the lung. If the injury is mild and self-limited, resolution with restoration of normal lung structures follows. However, with persistence of the injurious agent, an accumulation of inflammatory and immune cells causes continued damage to lung tissue and replacement of normally functioning lung tissue with fibrous scar tissue. Alveolar macrophages secrete a host of fibrogenic factors, including fibroblast growth factor, transforming growth factor-β (TGF-β), and platelet-derived growth factor, which can attract fibroblasts as well as stimulate their proliferation. Alveolar cells also appear to play a role in the process. Destruction of type I alveolar cells is often accompanied by proliferation of type II alveolar cells (see Chapter 21). These cells secrete chemotactic factors that attract additional macrophages, growth factors, and cytokines such as TGF-β that contribute to fibrotic changes.

Clinical Features

In general, the interstitial lung diseases are characterized by clinical changes consistent with restrictive rather than obstructive changes in the lung. Persons with interstitial lung diseases have dyspnea, tachypnea, and eventual cyanosis, without evidence of wheezing or signs of airway obstruction. Usually, there is an insidious onset of breathlessness that initially occurs during exercise and may progress to the point at which the person is totally incapacitated. Typically, the person breathes with a tachypneic pattern of breathing, in which the respiratory rate is increased and the tidal volume is decreased. This pattern of breathing serves to maintain minute volume yet reduces the work of breathing because it takes less work to move air through the airways at an increased rate than it does to stretch a stiff lung to accommodate a larger tidal volume. A nonproductive cough may develop, particularly with continued exposure to the inhaled irritant. Clubbing of the fingers and toes may develop.

Lung volumes, including vital capacity and total lung capacity, are reduced in interstitial lung disease. In contrast to COPD, in which expiratory flow rates are reduced, the $FEV_{1.0}$ usually is preserved, even though the ratio of $FEV_{1.0}$ to FVC may increase. Although resting arterial blood gases usually are normal early in the course of the disease, arterial PO_2 levels may fall during exercise. In persons with advanced disease, hypoxemia often is present, even at rest. In the late stages of the disease, hypercapnia and respiratory acidosis develop. The impaired diffusion of gases is thought to be caused by alterations in the alveolar–capillary membrane as well as an increase in shunt resulting from unventilated regions of the lung.

The diagnosis of interstitial lung disease requires a careful personal and family history, with particular emphasis on exposure to environmental, occupational, and other injurious agents.[55,56] Chest radiographs may be used as an initial diagnostic method, and to follow the progress of the disease. A biopsy specimen for histologic study and culture may be obtained by surgical incision, bronchoscopy, or bronchoalveolar lavage, in which fluid is instilled into the alveoli through a bronchoscope and then removed by suction for laboratory study.

The treatment goals for persons with interstitial lung disease focus on identifying and removing the injurious agent, suppressing the inflammatory response (typically with corticosteroids), preventing progression of the disease, and providing supportive therapy for persons with advanced disease. Many of the supportive treatment measures, such as oxygen therapy and measures to prevent infection, are similar to those discussed for persons with COPD.

Idiopathic Pulmonary Fibrosis

The most common diagnosis among persons with interstitial lung disease is idiopathic pulmonary fibrosis. The disease is characterized by diffuse interstitial fibrosis, which in severe cases results in severe hypoxemia and cyanosis. As the name implies, the cause of the disorder is unknown. Men are affected more commonly than women and approximately two thirds

of persons are older than 60 years of age at the time of presentation.

A number of conditions and risk factors are associated with the disease.[15,56] Cigarette smoking increases the risk, as do certain occupations such as farming, hairdressing, stonecutting, and metal cutting. Although viruses have not been clearly implicated in the pathogenesis of idiopathic pulmonary fibrosis, several viral proteins and antibodies to viruses are associated with the disease. In addition, some people may have a genetic predisposition to the disease.

The disease is characterized by patchy interstitial fibrosis that causes collapse of alveolar walls and formation of cystic spaces lined by hyperplastic type II alveolar cells or bronchial epithelium. Secondary hypertensive changes due to intimal fibrosis and medial thickening of the pulmonary arteries are often present.

Idiopathopathic pulmonary fibrosis usually presents insidiously, with gradual onset of a nonproductive cough and progressive dyspnea. Cyanosis, cor pulmonale, and peripheral edema may present late in the disease. Diagnosis is confirmed by surgical biopsy. Unfortunately, the progress of the disease is relentless despite current methods of treatment. The mean survival after diagnosis is 3 to 5 years.

Sarcoidosis

Sarcoidosis is a multisystem disorder in which granulomas are found in many tissues and organs, particularly the lung.[15,16,57,58] The disorder predominantly affects adults younger than 40 years of age, although it can occur in older persons. The incidence is highest among North American blacks and northern European whites; and women are affected more frequently than men.

The cause of sarcoidosis remains unclear. It is thought that the disorder may result from exposure of genetically predisposed persons to specific environmental agents. Defective human leukocyte antigen (HLA) genes located in the major histocompatibility complex may be linked to disease susceptibility and prognosis. Multiple lines of evidence suggest that the inciting agent triggers an immune response that depends on host susceptibility.

The immune response is characterized by chronic inflammation, monocyte recruitment, and granuloma formation in which multinucleated giant cells are frequently seen. These granulomas do not show evidence of necrosis or caseation. The inflammation often involves the alveoli (alveolitis). It is composed largely of macrophages and lymphocytes, with the latter thought to be of particular importance in the pathogenesis of the disease.

Sarcoidosis has variable manifestations and an unpredictable course of progression in which any organ system can be affected. The three systems that most commonly manifest symptoms are the lungs, eyes, and skin. Persons with sarcoidosis frequently seek health care either as a result of abnormalities detected on an incidental chest film or because of insidious onset of respiratory symptoms (shortness of breath, nonproductive cough, chest pain) or constitutional signs and symptoms (e.g., fever, sweating, anorexia, weight loss, fatigue, myalgia). Eye involvement (anterior uveitis) and skin involvement (skin papules and plaques) are particularly common extrathoracic manifestations, but there may be cardiac, neuromuscular, hematologic, hepatic, endocrine, and lymph node findings.

Sarcoidosis is characterized by either progressive chronicity or periods of activity interspersed with remissions, sometimes permanent, that may be spontaneous or induced by corticosteroid therapy. Approximately 65% to 75% of persons recover with minimal clinical and radiographic abnormalities.[15] Other persons have persistent radiographic abnormalities and progression of their respiratory symptoms, with or without additional extrathoracic disease.

The diagnosis of sarcoidosis is based on history and physical examination, tests to exclude other diseases, chest radiography, and biopsy to obtain confirmation of noncaseating granulomas. A thorough ophthalmologic evaluation is recommended for most persons, even those without ocular symptoms.

Treatment is directed at interrupting the granulomatous inflammatory process that is characteristic of the disease and managing the associated complications. When treatment is indicated, corticosteroid drugs are used. These agents produce clearing of the lung, as seen on the chest radiograph, and improve pulmonary function, but it is not known whether they affect the long-term outcome of the disease.

SUMMARY CONCEPTS

■ The interstitial lung diseases are a diverse group of lung disorders that produce similar inflammatory and fibrotic changes in the interstitium or alveolar septa of the lung. As a result, the lungs become stiff and difficult to inflate, increasing the work of breathing and causing dyspnea and decreased exercise tolerance due to hypoxemia, without evidence of wheezing or signs of airway obstruction.

■ These diseases include drug- and radiation-induced lung disease, environmental and occupational lung diseases caused by inhalation of organic and inorganic dusts, immunologic lung disorders such as those that accompany scleroderma, idiopathic pulmonary fibrosis, and sarcoidosis.

■ The restrictive lung disorders reduce the diffusing capacity of the lung, producing various degrees of hypoxemia, dyspnea, tachypnea, and eventual cyanosis.

Disorders of the Pulmonary Circulation

As blood moves through the pulmonary capillaries, the oxygen content increases and the carbon dioxide decreases. These processes depend on the matching of ventilation (i.e., gas exchange) and perfusion (i.e., blood flow). This section discusses two major problems of the pulmonary circulation: pulmonary embolism and pulmonary hypertension. Pulmonary edema, another major problem of the pulmonary circulation, is discussed in Chapter 20.

Pulmonary Embolism

Pulmonary embolism develops when a blood-borne substance lodges in a branch of the pulmonary artery and obstructs blood flow.[15,16,59,61] The embolism may consist of a thrombus (Fig. 23-13), air that has accidentally been injected during intravenous infusion, fat that has been mobilized from the bone marrow after a fracture or from a traumatized fat depot, or amniotic fluid that has entered the maternal circulation during childbirth.

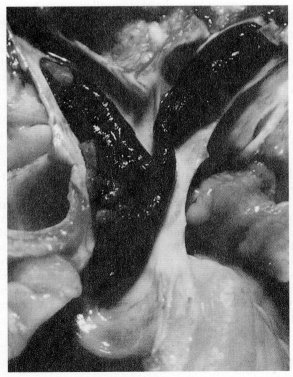

FIGURE 23-13. Pulmonary embolism. The main pulmonary artery and its bifurcation have been opened to reveal a large saddle embolus. (From McManus BM, Allard MF, Yanagawa R. Hemodynamic disorders. In: Rubin R, Strayer DS, eds. *Rubin's Pathology: Clinicopathologic Foundations of Medicine.* 6th ed. Philadelphia, PA: Wolters Kluwer Health | Lippincott Williams & Wilkins; 2012:275. Courtesy of Dr. Greg J. Davis.)

Pathogenesis

Athough pulmonary emboli can originate from a number of sources, most arise from deep vein thrombosis (DVT) in the large veins of the lower legs, typically originating in the popliteal vein or larger veins above it (see Chapter 18). The presence of thrombosis in the deep veins of the legs or pelvis often is unsuspected until embolism occurs. Among the physiologic factors that contribute to venous thrombosis are venous stasis, venous endothelial injury, and hypercoagulability states. Venous stasis and venous endothelial injury can result from prolonged bed rest (particularly with immobilization of the legs), severe trauma (including burns and fractures), surgery (particularly orthopedic surgery of the knee or hip), childbirth, myocardial infarction and congestive heart failure, and spinal cord injury. Hypercoagulability is related to various factors. Cancer cells can produce thrombin and synthesize procoagulation factors, increasing the risk for thromboembolism. Pregnancy, and hormone replacement therapy are thought to increase the resistance to endogenous anticoagulants and risk of pulmonary embolism. There is also increased risk for pulmonary embolism among users of oral contraceptives, particularly in women who smoke. The thrombophilias (e.g., antithrombin III deficiency, protein C and S deficiencies, factor V Leiden mutation) are a group of inherited disorders affecting coagulation that make an individual prone to the development of venous thromboemboli (see Chapter 12).

The pathophysiologic effects of thromboembolism depend largely on the size of the embolus and degree of pulmonary blood flow obstruction. Obstruction of pulmonary blood flow causes reflex bronchoconstriction in the affected area of the lung, ventilation without perfusion, impaired gas exchange, and loss of alveolar surfactant. Pulmonary hypertension and right heart strain may develop with large emboli or in those with poor cardiac reserve.

Although small areas of infarction may occur, pulmonary infarction is uncommon. This is because the lung is perfused not only by the pulmonary arteries but also by the bronchial arteries and air from the alveoli. If the bronchial circulation is normal and adequate ventilation is maintained, a decrease in pulmonary artery perfusion does not usually cause infarction.

Manifestations

The clinical manifestations of pulmonary embolism depend on the size and location of the obstruction. Small emboli that become lodged in the peripheral branches of the pulmonary artery are clinically silent and may go unrecognized, especially in the elderly and acutely ill. Persons with moderate-sized emboli often present with breathlessness accompanied by pleuritic pain, apprehension, slight fever, and cough productive of blood-streaked sputum. Tachycardia often occurs to compensate for decreased oxygenation, and the breathing pattern is rapid and shallow. Patients with massive emboli usually present with sudden collapse, crushing substernal chest pain, shock, and sometimes loss of consciousness. The pulse is rapid and weak, the blood pressure is low, the neck veins are distended, and the skin is cyanotic and diaphoretic. Massive pulmonary emboli often are fatal.

Diagnosis and Treatment

Diagnosis of pulmonary embolism is based on clinical signs and symptoms, blood gas determinations, D-dimer testing, lung perfusion scans, CT scans of the chest, and, in selected cases, pulmonary angiography.[59–61] Laboratory studies and radiologic films are useful in ruling out other conditions that might give rise to similar symptoms. Because emboli can cause an increase in pulmonary vascular resistance, the electrocardiogram (ECG) may be used to detect signs of right heart strain. There has been recent interest in combining several noninvasive methods (lower limb compression ultrasonography, D-dimer measurements, and clinical assessment measures) as a means of establishing a diagnosis of pulmonary embolism.

Because most pulmonary emboli originate from DVT, venous studies such as *lower limb compression ultrasonography, impedance plethysmography,* and *contrast venography* are often used as initial diagnostic procedures. Of these, lower limb compression ultrasonography has become an important noninvasive means for detecting DVT. *D-dimer testing* involves the measurement of plasma D-dimer, a degradation product of coagulation factors that have been activated as a result of a thromboembolic event. The *ventilation–perfusion scan* uses radiolabeled albumin, which is injected intravenously, and a radiolabeled gas, which is inhaled. A scintillation (gamma) camera is used to scan the various lung segments for blood flow and distribution of the radiolabeled gas. Ventilation–perfusion scans are useful only when their results are either normal or indicate a high probability of pulmonary embolism. *Helical (spiral) CT angiography* requires administration of an intravenous radiocontrast medium. It is sensitive for the detection of emboli in the proximal pulmonary arteries and provides another method of diagnosis. *Pulmonary angiography* involves the passage of a venous catheter through the right heart and into the pulmonary artery under fluoroscopy. Although it remains the most accurate method of diagnosis, it is an invasive procedure; therefore, its use is reserved for selected cases.

Treatment goals for pulmonary emboli include preventing DVT and the development of thromboemboli, protecting the lungs from exposure to thromboemboli when they occur, and in the case of large and life-threatening pulmonary emboli, sustaining life and restoring pulmonary blood flow.[60,61] Thrombolytic therapy using streptokinase, urokinase, or recombinant tissue plasminogen activator may be indicated in persons with life-threatening pulmonary emboli. Thrombolytic therapy is followed by anticoagulant therapy (e.g., heparin and then warfarin) to prevent clot reoccurrence but carries the risk of bleeding complications and is contraindicated in many post-surgical patients. Anticoagulation with unfractionated or low-molecular weight heparin is frequently employed to prevent additional clot burden when signs of right heart strain are absent. Surgical interruption of the vena cava or insertion of a filter to prevent emboli from traveling to the lung may be indicated in life-threatening situations or in cases where thrombolytic therapy or anticoagulation is contraindicated.

Venous thromboembolism is often clinically silent until it presents with significant morbidity and mortality. Thus, recognition of risk factors and appropriate preventative treatment are essential. Prophylactic measures include early ambulation for postoperative and postpartum patients and the use of graded compression elastic stockings and intermittent pneumatic compression (IPC) boots for bedridden patients. Intermittent pneumatic compression boots provide intermittent inflation of air-filled sleeves that prevent venous stasis. Some devices produce sequential gradient compression that moves blood upward in the leg. Anticoagulant therapy may be used to decrease the likelihood of deep vein thrombosis, thromboembolism, and fatal pulmonary embolism after major surgical procedures (see Chapter 12). Low–molecular-weight heparin, which can be administered subcutaneously, often is used. Warfarin, an oral anticoagulation drug, may be used for persons with a long-term risk for development of thromboemboli. Newer factor Xa inhibitors are gaining popularity as an alternative to warfarin due to their efficacy and fewer food and drug interactions.

Pulmonary Hypertension

The pulmonary circulation is normally a low-pressure system designed to accommodate varying amounts of blood delivered from the right heart. The main pulmonary artery and major branches are relatively thin-walled, compliant vessels. The distal pulmonary arterioles also are thin walled and have the capacity to dilate, collapse, or constrict depending on the presence of vasoactive substances released from the endothelial cells of the vessel, neurohumoral influences, flow velocity, oxygen tension, and alveolar ventilation.

Pulmonary hypertension is a disorder characterized by an abnormal elevation of pressure within the pulmonary circulation—namely, the pulmonary arterial system.[62,63] Once present, pulmonary hypertension is self-perpetuating. It introduces secondary structural abnormalities of pulmonary vessels including smooth muscle hypertrophy and proliferation of the vessel intima. Although pulmonary hypertension can develop as a primary disorder, most cases develop secondary to other conditions.

Secondary Pulmonary Hypertension

Secondary pulmonary hypertension refers to an increase in pulmonary pressures associated with other disease conditions, usually cardiac or pulmonary.[10,15,16] Often more than one disorder, such as COPD, heart failure, and sleep apnea, contributes. Secondary pulmonary hypertension may develop at any age. Mechanisms include: (1) elevation of pulmonary venous pressure, (2) increased pulmonary blood flow, (3) pulmonary vascular obstruction, and (4) hypoxemia.

Elevation of pulmonary venous pressure is common in conditions such as mitral valve disorders or left ventricular diastolic dysfunction. In each of these alterations, the elevated left atrial pressure is transmitted to the pulmonary circulation. Continued increases in left atrial pressure can lead to medial hypertrophy and intimal thickening of the small pulmonary arteries, causing sustained hypertension.

Increased pulmonary blood flow results from increased flow through left-to-right shunts in congenital heart diseases such as atrial or ventricular septal defects and patent ductus arteriosus. If the high-flow state is allowed to continue, morphologic changes occur in the pulmonary vessels, leading to sustained pulmonary hypertension. The pulmonary vascular changes that occur with congenital heart disorders are discussed in Chapter 19.

Obstruction of pulmonary blood flow is commonly due to pulmonary thromboemboli. Persons who are promptly treated for acute pulmonary thromboembolism with anticoagulants rarely develop pulmonary hypertension. However, in some persons chronic obstruction of the pulmonary vascular bed develops because of impaired resolution of the thromboemboli.

Continued exposure of the pulmonary vessels to hypoxemia is a common cause of pulmonary hypertension. Unlike blood vessels in the systemic circulation, most of which dilate in response to hypoxemia and hypercapnia, the pulmonary vessels constrict. The stimuli for constriction are thought to originate in the air spaces near the smaller branches of the pulmonary arteries. In regions of the lung that are poorly ventilated, the response is adaptive in that it diverts blood flow away from the poorly ventilated areas to those areas that are more adequately ventilated. This effect, however, becomes less beneficial as more and more areas of the lung become poorly ventilated. Pulmonary hypertension is a common problem resulting from hypoxemia that develops in persons with advanced COPD or interstitial lung disease.[62] It also may develop at high altitudes in persons with normal lung function. Persons who experience marked hypoxemia during sleep (such as those with sleep apnea) often experience marked elevations in pulmonary arterial pressure.

Secondary pulmonary hypertension is difficult to recognize in its early stages, when the signs and symptoms are primarily those of the underlying disease. Pulmonary hypertension may cause, or contribute to, dyspnea, present initially with exertion and later at rest. Fatigue and syncope on exertion also occur, presumably the result of reduced cardiac output and elevated pulmonary artery pressures.

Diagnosis is based on radiographic findings and echocardiography. Doppler ultrasonography is a reliable noninvasive method for estimating pulmonary artery systolic pressure. Treatment measures are directed toward the underlying disorder. Vasodilator therapy may be indicated.

Primary Pulmonary Arterial Hypertension

Primary pulmonary arterial hypertension (PAH) is persistent elevation in pulmonary artery pressure that occurs in the absence of identified cardiopulmonary or other secondary causes of pulmonary hypertension.[10,15,16,63–66]

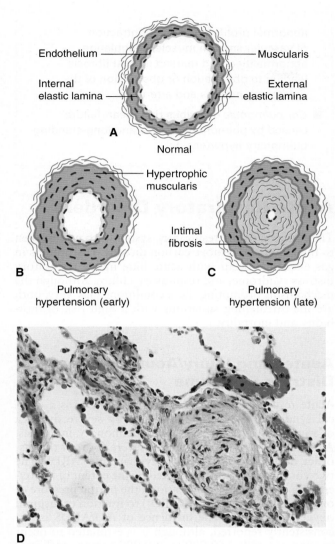

Endothelium

Muscularis

Internal elastic lamina

External elastic lamina

A

Normal

Hypertrophic muscularis

Intimal fibrosis

B

Pulmonary hypertension (early)

C

Pulmonary hypertension (late)

D

FIGURE 23-14. (A) Normal pulmonary artery. **(B)** Mild pulmonary hypertension with thickening of the media of the pulmonary artery. **(C)** Pulmonary artery with extensive intimal fibrosis and thickening of vascular smooth muscle. **(D)** Micrograph of a small pulmonary artery that is virtually occluded by concentrically thickened intimal fibrosis and thickening of the media due to pulmonary arterial hypertension. (From Bearsley MB, Travis WD, Rubin E. The respiratory system. In: Rubin R, Strayer DS, eds. *Rubin's Pathology: Clinicopathologic Foundations of Medicine*. 6th ed. Philadelphia, PA: Wolters Kluwer Health | Lippincott Williams & Wilkins; 2012:592.)

It is a rare and debilitating disorder characterized by abnormal proliferation and contraction of vascular smooth muscle, coagulation abnormalities, and marked intimal fibrosis leading to obliteration or obstruction of the pulmonary arteries and arterioles (Fig. 23-14). The resulting increase in pulmonary artery pressure results in progressive right heart failure, low cardiac output, and death if left untreated.

A familial form of PAH appears to be inherited as an autosomal dominant trait with a variable but low penetrance, with some individuals inheriting the trait without exhibiting the disease. A causal relationship has been established between several appetite-suppressant drugs, including fenfluramine, and the development of PAH. Although the drug has been removed from the world market, many were exposed before that time. Pulmonary arterial hypertension is also associated with human immunodeficiency virus (HIV) infection. The mechanism by which HIV infection produces PAH remains unknown, but treatment of HIV infection does not appear to affect the severity or natural history of the underlying pulmonary hypertension. Other conditions associated with PAH include portal hypertension and persistent pulmonary hypertension in the newborn.

Although the specific mechanisms responsible for the vascular changes that occur in PAH remain unknown, a number of mechanisms have been proposed[64] including diminished levels of nitric oxide and prostacyclin, two potent vasodilators. Nitric oxide is produced locally in the lungs, and prostacyclin is produced by the vascular endothelium. Moreover, increased levels of several growth factors, including endothelin-1, vascular endothelial growth factor, and platelet-derived growth factor, may contribute. Endothelin-1 is a peptide produced by the vascular endothelium that has potent vasoconstrictor and paracrine effects on vascular smooth muscle. Results of studies relating these mechanisms to the structure and function of the pulmonary arterial circulation have already been translated into targeted therapies for PAH.

Symptoms of PAH typically progress from shortness of breath and decreasing exercise tolerance to right heart failure, with marked peripheral edema and functional limitations. Other common symptoms include fatigue, angina, and syncope (fainting) or near-syncope. The diagnosis of primary pulmonary hypertension is based on an elevated pulmonary artery pressure and an absence of disorders that cause secondary pulmonary hypertension.

Treatment for primary pulmonary hypertension consists mainly of measures to improve right heart function as a means of reducing fatigue and peripheral edema. Supplemental oxygen may be used to increase exercise tolerance. The calcium channel blockers (nifedipine, diltiazem) may be effective early in the course of the disease but offer little in advanced stages.

More recent medications for treatment of primary pulmonary arterial hypertension include prostacyclin analogues, endothelin receptor antagonist, and phosphodiesterase type 5 inhibitors. Continuous long-term infusion of prostacyclin (e.g., epoprostenol), a potent pulmonary vasodilator, has been shown to provide symptomatic benefits and improved survival in selected patients.[63–66] Because of its short half-life (3 to 5 minutes), the drug must be administered by continuous intravenous infusion through an indwelling catheter with an automatic ambulatory pump. Properties of the drug other than its vasodilating effects include inhibition of platelet aggregation and beneficial vascular remodeling effects. Endothelin, which is a potent vasoconstrictor and stimulator of vascular smooth muscle proliferation, is believed to be important in the pathogenesis of primary pulmonary arterial hypertension. Oral endothelin antagonists (e.g., ambristan, bosentran) have proved to be effective in treating moderate to severe primary pulmonary hypertension and may become the treatment of choice for all stages of the disease.[66] Sildenafil (e.g., Revatio), a highly selective phosphodiesterase-5 inhibitor that acts in a manner similar to nitric oxide to produce vasodilation, is approved for use in pulmonary hypertension. Lung transplantation may be an alternative for persons who do not respond to other forms of treatment.

Cor Pulmonale

The term *cor pulmonale* refers to right heart failure resulting from primary lung disease or pulmonary hypertension. The increased pressures and work result in hypertrophy and eventual failure of the right ventricle. The manifestations of cor pulmonale include the signs and symptoms of the primary lung disease and the signs of right-sided heart failure (see Chapter 20). Signs of right-sided heart failure include venous congestion, peripheral edema, shortness of breath, and a productive cough, which becomes worse during periods of heart failure. Plethora (i.e., redness), cyanosis, and warm, moist skin may result from the compensatory polycythemia and desaturation of arterial blood that accompany chronic lung disease. Drowsiness and altered consciousness may occur as the result of carbon dioxide retention. Management of cor pulmonale focuses on the treatment of the lung disease and heart failure. Low-flow oxygen therapy may be used to reduce the pulmonary hypertension and polycythemia associated with severe hypoxemia caused by chronic lung disease.

> ### SUMMARY CONCEPTS
>
> ■ The pulmonary circulation is a low-pressure system that links the right heart and systemic venous system with the left heart and the systemic arterial system and functions as a conduit for exchange of the dissolved gases in the blood with the ventilated air in the alveoli.
>
> ■ Pulmonary embolism develops when a blood-borne substance lodges in a branch of the pulmonary artery and obstructs blood flow. The embolus can consist of a thrombus, air, fat, or amniotic fluid. The most common form is thromboemboli arising from the deep venous channels of the lower extremities.
>
> ■ Pulmonary hypertension represents an elevation in the pulmonary arterial pressure. It may arise as a secondary disorder associated with other disease conditions, usually cardiac or pulmonary, or as a primary disorder, characterized by

> abnormal proliferation and contraction of vascular smooth muscle, coagulation abnormalities, and marked intimal fibrosis leading to obliteration or obstruction of the pulmonary arteries and arterioles.
>
> ■ *Cor pulmonale* describes right heart failure caused by pulmonary disease and long-standing pulmonary hypertension.

Acute Respiratory Disorders

The function of the respiratory system is to add oxygen to the blood and remove carbon dioxide. Disruptions in gas exchange occur with acute lung injury respiratory distress syndrome, and respiratory failure. Although the mechanisms prompting these conditions may vary, both are life-threatening situations with a high risk of morbidity and mortality.

Acute Lung Injury/Acute Respiratory Distress Syndrome

Acute respiratory distress syndrome (ARDS) is a clinical syndrome that is characterized by severe dyspnea of rapid onset, hypoxemia, and pulmonary infiltrates. Acute lung injury (ALI) is a less-severe form of the disorder, but has the potential for evolving into ARDS. The two conditions are differentiated by the extent of hypoxemia as determined by the ratio of the partial pressure of oxygen in the arterial blood (PO_2) to fraction of inspired oxygen (FIO_2).[67–70] The incidence of ALI/ARDS is not consistently reported, although it is estimated to occur in approximately 150,000 to 200,000 persons each year in North America. Despite the most sophisticated interventions, the mortality rate varies from 35% to 60% and morbidity is extensive, including physical, cognitive, and emotional sequelae.[15,71]

Both ARDS and ALI can result from a number of conditions, including aspiration of gastric contents, major trauma (with or without fat emboli), sepsis secondary to pulmonary or nonpulmonary infections, acute pancreatitis, hematologic disorders, metabolic events, and reactions to drugs and toxins (Chart 23-2).

Etiology and Pathogenesis

Although a number of conditions may lead to ALI/ARDS, they all produce similar pathologic lung changes that include diffuse epithelial cell injury with increased permeability of the alveolar–capillary membrane (Fig. 23-15). The increased permeability permits fluid, plasma proteins, and blood cells to move out of the vascular compartment into the interstitium and alveoli of the lung.[15,69] Diffuse alveolar cell damage leads to accumulation of fluid, surfactant inactivation, and formation of a hyaline membrane that is fibrous and impervious to gas exchange.

CHART 23-2	Conditions in Which ARDS Can Develop*

Aspiration
Near-drowning
Aspiration of gastric contents

Drugs, Toxins, Therapeutic Agents
Free-base cocaine smoking
Heroin
Inhaled gases (e.g., smoke, ammonia)
Breathing high concentrations of oxygen
Radiation

Infections
Septicemia

Trauma and Shock
Burns
Fat embolism
Chest trauma

Disseminated Intravascular Coagulation

Multiple Blood Transfusions

*This list is not intended to be inclusive.

The pathogenesis of ALI/ARDS is unclear, although both local and systemic inflammatory responses occur. It is thought that dysregulated inflammation, accumulation of neutrophils, uncontrolled activation of coagulation pathways, and altered permeability of the endothelial and epithelial barriers all play a role.[67] Initially, a direct or indirect pulmonary insult is believed to promote the accumulation of neutrophils in the microcirculation. These neutrophils activate and migrate in large numbers across the alveolar epithelial surfaces, releasing proteases, cytokines, and reactive oxygen species that lead to increased permeability in the alveolar epithelial cells and damage to type I and type II alveolar cells. This in turn leads to pulmonary edema, hyaline membrane formation, and loss of surfactant that decrease pulmonary compliance and make air exchange difficult.

Clinical Features

Clinically, ALI/ARDS is marked by a rapid onset, usually within 12 to 18 hours of the initiating event, of respiratory distress, an increase in respiratory rate, and signs of respiratory failure. Chest radiography shows diffuse bilateral infiltrates of the lung tissue in the absence of cardiac dysfunction (non-cardiogenic pulmonary edema). Marked hypoxemia occurs that is refractory to treatment with supplemental oxygen therapy. Many persons with ARDS have a systemic response that results in multiple organ failure, particularly of the renal, gastrointestinal, cardiovascular, and central nervous systems.

The treatment goals in ARDS are to supply oxygen to vital organs and provide supportive care until the condition causing the pathologic process has been reversed and the lungs have had a chance to heal. Assisted ventilation using high concentrations of oxygen may be required to correct the hypoxemia. Positive end-expiratory pressure breathing, which increases the

As the disease progresses, the work of breathing becomes greatly increased as the lung stiffens and becomes more difficult to inflate. There is increased intrapulmonary shunting of blood, impaired gas exchange, and hypoxemia despite high supplemental oxygen therapy. Gas exchange is further compromised by alveolar collapse resulting from abnormalities in surfactant production. When injury to the alveolar epithelium is severe, disorganized epithelial repair may lead to fibrosis.

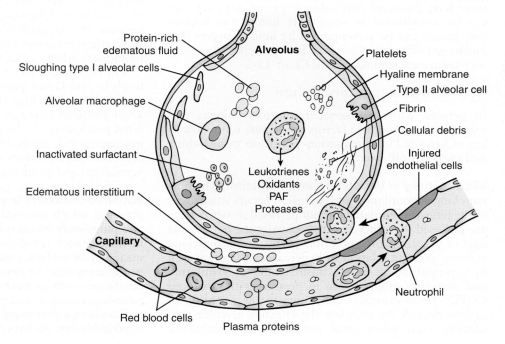

FIGURE 23-15. Mechanism of lung changes in acute respiratory distress syndrome. Injury and increased permeability of the alveolar capillary membrane allow fluid, protein, cellular debris, platelets, and blood cells to move out of the vascular compartment and enter the interstitium and alveoli. Activated neutrophils release a variety of products that damage the alveolar cells and lead to edema, surfactant inactivation, and formation of a hyaline membrane. PAF, platelet activating factor.

pressure in the airways during expiration, may be used to assist in reinflating the collapsed areas of the lung and to improve the matching of ventilation and perfusion. Smaller tidal volumes (6 mL/kg) based on ideal body weight have been shown to reduce barotrauma secondary to lower plateau pressures and optimal positive end expiratory pressure (PEEP) therapy prevents damage associated with the collapse and reinflation of alveoli.

Acute Respiratory Failure

Respiratory failure can be viewed as impaired gas exchange due to either pump (heart) or lung failure, or both.[3,72-74] It is not a specific disease, but can occur in the course of a number of conditions that impair ventilation, compromise the matching of ventilation and perfusion, or impair gas diffusion. Acute respiratory failure may occur in previously healthy persons as the result of acute disease or trauma involving the respiratory system, or it may develop in the course of a chronic neuromuscular or lung disease.

Respiratory failure is a condition in which the respiratory system fails in one or both of its gas exchange functions—oxygenation of mixed venous blood and removal of carbon dioxide. The function of the respiratory system can be said to consist of two aspects: (1) gas exchange (movement of gases across the alveolar–capillary membrane) and (2) ventilation (movement of gases into and out of the alveoli due to the action of the respiratory muscles, the respiratory center in the central nervous system [CNS], and the pathways that connect the centers in the CNS with the respiratory muscles). Thus, respiratory failure is commonly divided into two types: (1) hypoxemic respiratory failure due to failure of the gas exchange function of the lung and (2) hypercapnic/hypoxemic respiratory failure due to ventilatory failure.[3,70,71] The classification should not be viewed as rigid since lung disorders that cause impaired gas exchange can be complicated by ventilatory failure and ventilatory failure can be accompanied by lung disorders that impair gas diffusion. Causes of the two types of respiratory failure are summarized in Chart 23-3.

Hypoxemic Respiratory Failure

In persons with hypoxemic respiratory failure, two major pathophysiologic factors contribute to the lowering of arterial PO_2: ventilation–perfusion mismatching and impaired diffusion.

Mismatching of Ventilation and Perfusion. The mismatching of ventilation and perfusion occurs when areas of the lung are ventilated but not perfused or when areas are perfused but not ventilated. Usually the hypoxemia seen in situations of ventilation–perfusion mismatching is more severe in relation to hypercapnia than that seen in hypoventilation. Severe mismatching of ventilation and perfusion often is seen in persons with advanced COPD. These disorders contribute to the retention of carbon dioxide by reducing the effective alveolar ventilation, even when total ventilation is maintained.

CHART 23-3	**Causes of Respiratory Failure***

Hypoxemic Respiratory Failure
Chronic obstructive pulmonary disease
Restrictive lung disease
Severe pneumonia
Atelectasis
Impaired diffusion
    Pulmonary edema
    Acute lung injury/acute respiratory distress
      syndrome

Hypercapnic/Hypoxemic Respiratory Failure
Upper airway obstruction
    Infection (e.g., epiglottitis)
    Laryngospasm
    Tumors
Weakness or paralysis of respiratory muscles
    Brain injury
    Drug overdose
    Guillain-Barré syndrome
    Muscular dystrophy
    Spinal cord injury
Chest wall injury

*This list is not intended to be inclusive.

This occurs because a region of the lung is not perfused and gas exchange cannot take place or because an area of the lung is not being ventilated. Maintaining a high ventilation rate effectively prevents hypercapnia but also increases the work of breathing.

The hypoxemia associated with ventilation–perfusion disorders often is exaggerated by conditions such as hypoventilation and decreased cardiac output. For example, sedation can cause hypoventilation in persons with severe COPD, resulting in further impairment of ventilation. Likewise, a decrease in cardiac output because of myocardial infarction can exaggerate the ventilation–perfusion impairment in a person with mild pulmonary edema or COPD.

The beneficial effect of oxygen administration on PO_2 levels in ventilation–perfusion disorders depends on the degree of mismatching that is present. Because oxygen administration increases the diffusion gradient in ventilated portions of the lung, it usually is effective in raising arterial PO_2 levels. However, high-flow oxygen may decrease the respiratory drive, resulting in a decrease in ventilation and an increase in PCO_2.

Impaired Diffusion. Impaired diffusion describes a condition in which gas exchange between the alveolar air and pulmonary blood is impeded because of an increase in the distance for diffusion or a decrease in the permeability or surface area of the respiratory membranes to the movement of gases. It most commonly occurs in conditions such as interstitial lung disease, ALI/ARDS, pulmonary edema, and pneumonia.

Conditions that impair diffusion may produce severe hypoxemia but no hypercapnia because of the increase in ventilation and greater diffusion rate of carbon dioxide. Hypoxemia resulting from impaired diffusion can be partially or completely corrected by the administration of high concentrations of oxygen. In this case, the high concentration of oxygen serves to overcome the decrease in diffusion by establishing a larger alveolar-to-capillary diffusion gradient.

Hypercapnic/Hypoxemic Respiratory Failure

In the hypercapnic form of respiratory failure, patients are unable to maintain a level of alveolar ventilation sufficient to eliminate CO_2 and keep arterial O_2 levels within normal range. Because ventilation is determined by a sequence of events ranging from the generation of impulses in the CNS to movement of air through the conducting airways, there are several stages at which problems can adversely affect the total minute ventilation.

Hypoventilation or ventilatory failure occurs when the volume of "fresh" air moving into and out of the lung is significantly reduced. It is commonly caused by conditions outside the lung such as depression of the respiratory center (e.g., drug overdose, brain injury), diseases of the nerves supplying the respiratory muscles (e.g., Guillain-Barré syndrome, spinal cord injury), disorders of the respiratory muscles (e.g., muscular dystrophy), exacerbation of chronic lung disease (e.g., COPD), or thoracic cage disorders (e.g., severe scoliosis or crushed chest).

Hypoventilation has two important effects on arterial blood gases. First, it almost always causes an increase in PCO_2. The rise in PCO_2 is directly related to the level of ventilation; reducing the ventilation by one half causes a doubling of the PCO_2. Thus, the PCO_2 level is a good diagnostic measure for hypoventilation. Second, it may cause hypoxemia, although the hypoxemia that is caused by hypoventilation can be readily abolished by the administration of supplemental oxygen.

Clinical Features

Acute respiratory failure is usually manifested by varying degrees of hypoxemia and hypercapnia. There is no absolute definition of the levels of PO_2 and PCO_2 that indicate respiratory failure; however, it is conventionally defined as an arterial PO_2 of less than 60 mm Hg, an arterial PCO_2 of more than 45 mm Hg, or both when prior blood values have been normal.[71] Again, these cutoff values are not rigid, but serve as a general guide in combination with history and physical assessment data.

The signs and symptoms of acute respiratory failure are those of the underlying disease combined with those of hypoxemia and hypercapnia.[72,73] Hypoxemia is accompanied by increased respiratory drive and increased sympathetic tone. Potential signs include cyanosis, restlessness, confusion, anxiety, delirium, fatigue, tachypnea, hypertension, cardiac arrhythmias, and tremor. The initial cardiovascular effects are tachycardia with increased cardiac output and increased blood pressure. Serious cardiac arrhythmias may be triggered. The pulmonary vasculature constricts in response to low alveolar PO_2. If severe, the pulmonary vasoconstriction may result in acute right ventricular failure with

manifestations such as jugular vein distention and dependent edema. Profound acute hypoxemia can cause convulsions, retinal hemorrhages, and permanent brain damage. Hypotension and bradycardia often are preterminal events in persons with hypoxemic respiratory failure, indicating the failure of compensatory mechanisms.

Many of the adverse consequences of hypercapnia are the result of respiratory acidosis. Direct effects of acidosis include depression of cardiac contractility, decreased respiratory muscle contractility, and arterial vasodilation (see Chapter 8). Raised levels of PCO_2 greatly increase cerebral blood flow, which may result in headache, increased cerebrospinal fluid pressure, and sometimes papilledema (see Chapter 38, Fig. 38-9). The headache is due to dilation of the cerebral vessels. Additional indicators of hypercapnia are warm and flushed skin and hyperemic conjunctivae. Hypercapnia produces nervous system effects similar to those of an anesthetic—hence the term *carbon dioxide narcosis*. There is progressive somnolence, disorientation, and, if the condition is left untreated, coma. Mild to moderate increases in blood pressure are common. Air hunger and rapid breathing occur when alveolar PCO_2 levels rise to approximately 60 to 75 mm Hg; as PCO_2 levels reach 80 to 100 mm Hg, the person becomes lethargic and sometimes semicomatose.

The treatment of respiratory failure focuses on correcting the problem causing impaired gas exchange when possible and on relieving the hypoxemia and hypercapnia. A number of treatment modalities are available, including the establishment of an airway, use of bronchodilating drugs, and antibiotics for respiratory infections. Controlled oxygen therapy and mechanical ventilation are used in treating blood gas abnormalities associated with respiratory failure.[75]

When alveolar ventilation is inadequate to maintain PO_2 or PCO_2 levels because of respiratory or neurologic failure, mechanical ventilation may be lifesaving. Usually a nasotracheal, orotracheal, or tracheotomy tube is inserted into the trachea to provide the airway needed for mechanical ventilation. There has been recent interest in noninvasive forms of mechanical ventilation that use a face mask to deliver positive-pressure ventilation.[76]

SUMMARY CONCEPTS

■ The hallmark of acute lung injury and acute respiratory distress syndrome is a pronounced inflammatory response that affects the lung and may result in systemic organ failure. The acute inflammatory response results in damage and dysfunction of the alveolar–capillary membrane of the lung. Classically, there is interstitial edema of lung tissue, an increase in surface tension caused by inactivation of surfactant, collapse of alveolar structures, a stiff and noncompliant lung

(continued)

SUMMARY CONCEPTS (continued)

that is difficult to inflate, and impaired diffusion of the respiratory gases with severe hypoxia that is resistant to oxygen therapy.

■ Acute respiratory failure is a condition in which the lungs fail to oxygenate the blood adequately (hypoxemic respiratory failure) or prevent undue retention of carbon dioxide (hypercapnic/hypoxemic respiratory failure). The causes of respiratory failure are many. It may arise acutely in persons with previously healthy lungs, or it may be superimposed on chronic lung disease. Treatment of acute respiratory failure is directed toward treatment of the underlying disease, maintenance of adequate gas exchange and tissue oxygenation, and general supportive care. When alveolar ventilation is inadequate to maintain PO_2 or PCO_2 levels because of impaired respiratory function or neurologic failure, mechanical ventilation may be necessary.

REVIEW EXERCISES

1. A 30-year-old man is brought to the emergency department with a knife wound to the chest. On visual inspection, asymmetry of chest movement during inspiration, displacement of the trachea, and absence of breath sounds on the side of the wound are noted. His neck veins are distended, and his pulse is rapid and weak. A rapid diagnosis of tension pneumothorax is made.

   A. Explain the observed respiratory and cardiovascular function in terms of the impaired lung expansion and the air that has entered the chest as a result of the injury.
   B. What type of emergent treatment is necessary to save this man's life?

2. A 10-year-old boy who is having an acute asthmatic attack is brought to the emergency department by his parents. The boy is observed to be sitting up and struggling to breathe. His breathing is accompanied by use of the accessory muscles, a weak cough, and audible wheezing sounds. His pulse is rapid and weak and both heart and breath sounds are distant on auscultation. His parents relate that his asthma began to worsen after he developed a "cold," and now he doesn't even get relief from his "albuterol" inhaler.

   A. Explain the changes in physiologic function underlying this boy's signs and symptoms.
   B. What is the most probable reason for the progression of this boy's asthma in terms of the early- and late-phase responses?

   C. The boy is treated with a systemic corticosteroid and inhaled anticholinergic and β_2-adrenergic agonist and then transferred to the intensive care unit. Explain the action of each of these medications in terms of relieving this boy's symptoms.

3. A 62-year-old man with an 8-year history of chronic obstructive pulmonary disease (COPD) reports to his health care provider with complaints of increasing shortness of breath, ankle swelling, and a feeling of fullness in his upper abdomen. The expiratory phase of his respirations is prolonged, and expiratory wheezes and crackles are heard on auscultation. His blood pressure is 160/90 mm Hg, his red blood cell count is 6.0×10^6 μL (normal is 4.2 to 5.4×10^6 μL), his hematocrit is 65% (normal male value is 40% to 50%), his arterial PO_2 is 55 mm Hg, and his O_2 saturation, which is 85% while he is resting, drops to 55% during walking exercise.

   A. Explain the physiologic mechanisms responsible for his edema, hypertension, and elevated red blood cell count.
   B. His arterial PO_2 and O_2 saturation indicate that he is a candidate for continuous low-flow oxygen. Explain the benefits of this treatment in terms of his activity tolerance, blood pressure, and red blood cell count.
   C. Explain why the oxygen flow rate for persons with COPD is normally titrated to maintain the arterial PO_2 between 60 and 65 mm Hg.

4. An 18-year-old woman is admitted to the emergency department with a suspected drug overdose. Her respiratory rate is slow (4 to 6 breaths/min) and shallow. Arterial blood gases reveal a PCO_2 of 80 mm Hg and a PO_2 of 60 mm Hg.

   A. What is the cause of this woman's high PCO_2 and low PO_2?
   B. Hypoventilation almost always causes an increase in PCO_2. Explain.
   C. Even though her PO_2 increases to 90 mm Hg with institution of oxygen therapy, her PCO_2 remains elevated. Explain.

REFERENCES

1. Hall JE. *Guyton and Hall Textbook of Medical Physiology.* 12th ed. Philadelphia, PA: Elsevier Saunders; 2012:477–484, 515–523.
2. Koeppen BM, Stanton BA, eds. *Bern & Levy Physiology.* 6th ed. Philadelphia, PA: Mosby Elsevier; 2010:444–467.
3. West JB. *Pulmonary Pathophysiology: The Essentials.* 9th ed. Philadelphia, PA: Wolters Kluwer Health/Lippincott Williams & Wilkins; 2012:75.
4. Rajkumar A, Karmarkar A, Knotts J. Pulse oximetry: An overview. *J Perioper Pract.* 2006;6(10):502–504.
5. Chan ED, Chan MM, Chan MM. Pulse oximetry: understanding its basic principles facilitates appreciation of its limitations. *Respir Med.* 2013;107(6):789–799.

6. Weinberger SE, Schwartzstein RM, Weiss JW. Hypercapnia. *N Engl J Med.* 1989;321:1223–1230.
7. English JC, Leslie KO. Pathology of the pleura. *Clin Chest Med.* 2006;27:157–180.
8. Weldon E, Williams J. Pleural disease in the emergency room. *Emerg Med Clin North Am.* 2012;30:475–499.
9. Kass SM, Williams PM, Beamy BY. Pleurisy. *Am Fam Physician.* 2007;75:1357–1364.
10. Chestnut MS, Pendergast TJ, Tavan ET. Pulmonary disorders. In: Papadakis MA, McPhee SJ. *Current Medical Diagnosis & Treatment.* 52nd ed. New York, NY: McGraw-Hill Lange; 2013:242–343.
11. Light RW. Pleural effusions. *Med Clin North Am.* 2011;95: 1055–1070.
12. Romero S. Nontraumatic chylothorax. *Curr Opin Pulm Med.* 2000;6:287–291.
13. Haynes D, Baumann MH. Management of pneumothorax. *Semin Respir Crit Care Med.* 2010;31:769–780.
14. Baumann MH. Management of spontaneous pneumothorax. *Clin Chest Med.* 2006;27:369–381.
15. Husain AN. The lung. In: Kumar RS, Abbas AK, Fausto N, et al. *Robbins and Cotran Pathologic Basis of Disease.* 8th ed. Philadelphia, PA: Elsevier Saunders; 2010:677–737.
16. Bearsley MB, Travis WD, Rubin E. The respiratory system. In: Rubin R, Strayer DS, eds. *Rubin's Pathology: Clinicopathologic Foundations of Medicine.* 6th ed. Philadelphia, PA: Wolters Kluwer Health/Lippincott Williams & Wilkins; 2012:537–604.
17. Follenweider LM, Lambertino A. Epidemiology of asthma in the United States. *Nurs Clin North Am.* 2013;48:1–10.
18. American Lung Association. 2012. *Asthma in adults fact sheet* [Online]. Available at: http://www.lung.org/lung-disease/asthma/resources/facts-and-figures/asthma-in-adults.html. Accessed January 7, 2014.
19. National Asthma Education and Prevention Program. 2007. *EPR 3: Guidelines for the Diagnosis and Management of Asthma.* NIH Publication No. 12-5075, revised September 2012. Bethesda, MD: National Institutes of Health, National Heart, Lung, and Blood Institute. Available at: http://www.nhlbi.nih.gov/guidelines/asthma/asthma_qrg.pdf. Accessed October 12, 2013.
20. Martomez F, Vercelli D. Asthma. *Lancet.* 2013;383:1360–1372.
21. Murata A, Ling PM. Asthma diagnosis and management. *Emerg Med Clin North Am.* 2012;30:203–222.
22. Kileen K, Skora K. Pathophysiology, diagnosis, and clinical assessment of asthma in the adult. *Nurs Clin North Am.* 2013;48:13–23.
23. Weiler JM, Bonini S, Coifman R, et al. American Academy of Allergy, Asthma & Immunology Work Group Report: exercise-induced asthma. *J Allergy Clin Immunol.* 2007;119:1349–1358.
24. Young S, LeSouef PN, Geelhoed GC, et al. The influence of a family history of asthma and parental smoking on airway responsiveness in early infancy. *N Engl J Med.* 1991;324: 1168–1173.
25. Dykewicz MS. Occupational asthma: current concepts in pathogenesis, diagnosis, and management. *J Allergy Clin Immunol.* 2009;123:519–529.
26. Lenmenes L. Asthma in the workplace. *Nurs Clin North Am.* 2013;48:159–368.
27. Stevenson DD., Szczeklik F. Clinical and pathologic perspectives on aspirin sensitivity and asthma. *J Allergy Clin Immunol.* 2006; 118:773–786.
28. Tan KS, McFarlane LC, Lipworth BJ. Loss of normal cyclical B2 adrenoreceptor regulation and increased premenstrual responsiveness to adenosine monophosphate in stable female asthmatic patients. *Thorax.* 1997;52:608–611.
29. Haxhiu MA, Rust CF, Brooks C, et al. CNS determinants of sleep-related worsening of airway functions: implications for nocturnal asthma. *Respir Physiol Neurobiol.* 2006;151:1–30.

30. Sutherland ER. Nocturnal asthma. *J Allergy Clin Immunol.* 2005;116:1179–1186.
31. Fanta CH. Drug therapy in asthma. *N Engl J Med.* 2009;360(10): 1002–1014.
32. Wenzel S. Physiologic and pathologic abnormalities in severe asthma. *Clin Chest Med.* 2006;27:29–40.
33. Holgate ST, Polosa R. The mechanisms, diagnosis, and management of severe asthma in adults. *Lancet.* 2006;368: 780–793.
34. Magadle R, Berar-Yanay N, Weiner P. The risk of hospitalization and near-fatal and fatal asthma in relation to the perception of dyspnea. *Chest.* 2012;121:329–333.
35. U.S. National Library of Medicine. Asthma – children [Online]. Available at: http://www.ncbi.nlm.nih.gov/pubmedhealth/PMH0001985/. Accessed January 8, 2014.
36. Herzog R, Cunningham-Rundles S. Pediatric asthma: natural history, assessment and treatment. *Mt Sinai J Med.* 2011;78(5):645–660.
37. Kline-Krammes S, Robinson S. Childhood asthma: a Guide for Pediatric Medicine Providers. *Emerg Med Clin North Am.* 2013; 31:703–732.
38. Stewart LJ. Pediatric asthma. *Prim Care Clin Office Pract.* 2008;35:25–40.
39. Van Roeyen LS. Management of pediatric asthma at home and in school. *Nurs Clin North Am.* 2013;48:165–175.
40. Balkinssoon R, Lommatzsch S, Carolan B, et al. Chronic obstructive pulmonary disease: a concise review. *Med Clin North Am.* 2011;95:1125–1141.
41. Tam A. Pathologic mechanisms of chronic obstructive pulmonary disease. *Med Clin North Am.* 2012;96:681–698.
42. Rabe KF, Hurd S, Anzueto A, et al. Global strategy for diagnosis, management, and prevention of chronic obstructive lung disease: GOLD executive summary. *Am J Respir Crit Care Med.* 2007;176:532–555.
43. MacNee W. The pathogenesis of chronic obstructive pulmonary disease. *Clin Chest Med.* 2007;28:479–513.
44. Shapiro SD, Reilly JJ, Rennard SI. Chronic bronchitis and emphysema. In Mason JR, Broadus VC, Martin TR, et al., eds. *Mason, Murray, and Nadel's Textbook of Respiratory Medicine.* 5th ed. Philadelphia, PA: Elsevier Saunders; 2010:919–967.
45. McKay AJ, Hurst JR. COPD exacerbations: causes, prevention, and treatment. *Med Clin North Am.* 2010;96:789–809.
46. Barker AF. Bronchiectasis. *N Engl J Med.* 2002;346:1383–1393.
47. King PT. The pathophysiology of bronchiectasis. *Int J Chron Obstruct Pulmon Dis.* 2009;41:411–419.
48. Rowe SM, Miller S, Sorscher EJ. Cystic fibrosis. *N Engl J Med.* 2005;352:1992–2001.
49. Lobo J, Noone PG. Recent advances in cystic fibrosis. *Clin Chest Med.* 2012;33:307–328.
50. Strausbaugh SD, Davis PB. Cystic fibrosis: a review of epidemiology and pathobiology. *Clin Chest Med.* 2007;28:279–288.
51. Eagan M. Cystic fibrosis. In: Kliegman RM, Stanton BF, St. Geme JW, et al., eds. *Nelson Textbook of Pediatrics.* 19th ed. Philadelphia, PA: W.B. Saunders; 2011:1481–1497.
52. Flume PA, Van Devanter DR. State of progress in treating cystic fibrosis respiratory disease. *BMC Med.* 2012;10:88.
53. Derichs N. Targeting a genetic defect: cystic fibrosis transmembrane conductance regulator modulators in cystic fibrosis. *Eur Respir Rev.* 2012;22:58–65.
54. Selman M, Morrison LD, Noble PW, et al. Idiopathic interstitial pneumonias. In Mason RJ, Braddus VC, Martin TR, et al., eds. *Murray and Nadel's Textbook of Respiratory Medicine.* 5th ed. Philadelphia, PA: Elsevier Saunders; 2010:1356–1397.
55. Ryu JH, Daniels CE, Hartman T, et al. Diagnosis of interstitial lung diseases. *Mayo Clin Proc.* 2007;82(8):976–986.
56. Behr K. Approach to diagnosis of interstitial lung disease. *Clin Chest Med.* 2013;33:1–10.

57. Iannuzzi MC, Rybicki BA, Teirstein AS. Sarcoidosis. *N Engl J Med*. 2007;357(21):2153–2165.

58. Mihailovic-Vucinic V, Jovanovic D. Pulmonary sarcoidosis. *Clin Chest Med*. 2008;29:459–473.

59. Sadosty AT, Boie ET, Stead LG. Pulmonary embolism. *Emerg Med Clin North Am*. 2003;21:363–384.

60. Cardin T, Marinelli A. Pulmonary embolism. *Crit Care Nurs Q*. 2004;27:310–332.

61. Tapson VF. Acute pulmonary embolism. *N Engl J Med*. 2008;358:1037–1053.

62. Girgis RF, Mathai SC. Pulmonary hypertension associated with chronic respiratory disease. *Clin Chest Med*. 2007;28:219–232.

63. Farber HW, Lascalzo J. Pulmonary arterial hypertension. *N Engl J Med*. 2004;351:1655–1365.

64. Archer SL, Weir EK, Wilkins MR. The basic science of pulmonary arterial hypertension for the clinician. *Circulation*. 2010;121(18):2045–2066.

65. Stringham R, Shah N. Pulmonary arterial hypertension: an update on diagnosis and treatment. *Am Fam Physician*. 2010;82(4):370–377.

66. Rubin LJ, Badesch DB. Evaluation and management of the patient with pulmonary arterial hypertension. *Ann Intern Med*. 2005;143:282–292.

67. Mattihay MA, Ware LB, Zimmerman GA. The acute respiratory distress syndrome. *J Clin Invest*. 2012;122(8):2731–2740.

68. Bernard GRA, Artigas KL, Brigham J, et al. (Consensus Committee). The American-European Consensus Conference on ARDS: definitions, mechanisms, relevant outcomes, and clinical trial coordination. *Am J Respir Crit Care Med*. 1994;149:1807–1814.

69. Mendez JL, Hubmayr RD. New insights into the pathology of acute respiratory failure. *Curr Opin Crit Care*. 2005;11:29–36.

70. Saguil A, Fargo M. Acute respiratory distress syndrome: diagnosis and management. *Am Fam Physician*. 2012;84(4):352–358.

71. Rubenfeld GD, Caldwell E, Peabody E, et al. Incidence and outcomes of acute lung injury. *N Engl J Med*. 2005;353:1685–1693.

72. Roussos C, Koutsoukou A. Respiratory failure. *Eur Respir J Suppl*. 2003;47:1s–3s.

73. Chebbo A, Tfaili A, Jones SF. Hypoventilation syndromes. *Med Clin North Am*. 2010;95:1189–1202.

74. Markou NK, Myrianthefs PM, Baltopoulos GJ. Respiratory failure: an overview. *Crit Care Nurs Q*. 2004;27:353–379.

75. MacIntyre NR. Supporting oxygenation in acute respiratory failure. *Respir Care*. 2013;58(1):142–148.

76. Nava S, Hill N. Non-invasive ventilation in acute respiratory failure. *Lancet*. 2009;374:250–259.

Porth Essentials Resources

Explore these additional resources to enhance learning for this chapter:

- NCLEX-Style Questions and Other Resources on thePoint, http://thePoint.lww.com/PorthEssentials4e
- Study Guide for Essentials of Pathophysiology
- Concepts in Action Animations
- Adaptive Learning | Powered by PrepU, http://thepoint.lww.com/prepu

C h a p t e r 24

Structure and Function of the Kidney

It is no exaggeration to say that the composition of the blood is determined not so much by what the mouth takes in as by what the kidneys keep.
—Homer Smith, *From Fish to Philosopher*

The kidneys are remarkable organs. Each is smaller than a person's fist, but in a single day the two organs process approximately 1700 L of blood and combine their waste products into approximately 1.5 L of urine. As part of their function, the kidneys filter physiologically essential substances, such as sodium and potassium, from the blood and selectively reabsorb those substances that are needed to maintain the normal composition of internal body fluids. Substances that are not needed or are in excess of those needed pass into the urine. In addition to regulating the volume and composition of body fluids, the kidneys also perform endocrine functions. They release renin, an enzymatic hormone that participates in the regulation of blood pressure and maintenance of the circulating blood volume; they produce erythropoietin, a hormone that stimulates red blood cell production; and they convert vitamin D to its active form.

Functional Anatomy of the Kidney

The kidneys are paired, bean-shaped organs that lie outside the peritoneal cavity in the back of the upper abdomen, one on each side of the vertebral column at the level of the 12th

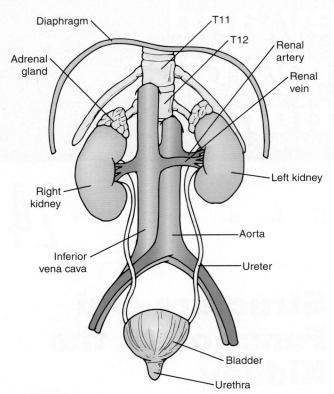

FIGURE 24-1. Kidneys, ureters, and bladder. (The right kidney is usually lower than the left.)

thoracic to 3rd lumbar vertebrae (Fig. 24-1). The right kidney normally is situated lower than the left, presumably because of the position of the liver. In the adult, each kidney is approximately 10 to 12 cm long, 5 to 6 cm wide, and 2.5 cm deep and weighs approximately 113 to 170 g. The medial border of the kidney is indented by a deep fissure called the *hilus*. It is here that blood vessels and nerves enter and leave the kidney. The ureters, which connect the kidneys with the bladder, also enter the kidney at the hilus.

Gross Structure

The kidney is composed of up to 18 lobes. Each lobular is in turn composed of nephrons, which are the functional units of the kidney. Two distinct regions can be identified on the bisected kidney—an outer cortex and an inner medulla (Fig. 24-2). The cortex has a reddish-brown granular appearance that is absent from the medulla. The medulla consists of light-colored, cone-shaped masses—the renal pyramids—that are divided by columns of the cortex that extend into the medulla. Each pyramid, topped by a region of cortex, forms a lobe of the kidney. The apices of the pyramids form the papillae (i.e., 8 to 18 per kidney, corresponding to the number of lobes), which are perforated by the openings of the collecting tubules. The renal pelvis is a wide, funnel-shaped structure at the upper end of the ureter. It is made up of the calyces or cuplike structures that drain the upper and lower halves of the kidney.

The kidney is sheathed in a fibrous external capsule and surrounded by a mass of fatty connective tissue, especially at its ends and borders. The adipose tissue protects the kidney from mechanical blows and assists, together with the attached blood vessels and fascia, in holding the kidney in place. Although the kidneys are relatively well protected, they may be bruised by blows to the loin or by compression between the lower ribs and the ileum. Because the kidneys are located outside the peritoneal cavity, injury and rupture do not produce the same threat of peritoneal involvement as that of other organs such as the liver or spleen.

Renal Blood Supply

Each kidney is supplied by a single renal artery that arises on either side of the aorta. As the renal artery approaches the kidney, it divides into segmental arteries that enter the hilus of the kidney. In the kidney, each segmental artery branches into several lobular arteries that

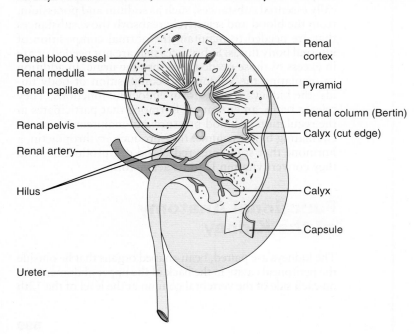

FIGURE 24-2. Internal structure of the kidney.

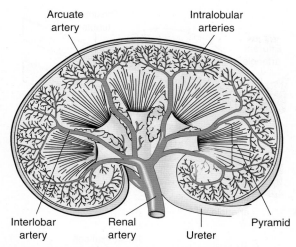

FIGURE 24-3. Simplified illustration of the arterial supply of the kidney. (From Cormack DH. *Ham's Histology.* 9th ed. Philadelphia, PA: J.B. Lippincott; 1987.)

supply the upper, middle, and lower parts of the kidney. The lobular arteries further subdivide to form the interlobular arteries at the level of the corticomedullary junction (Fig. 24-3). These arteries give off branches,

the arcuate arteries, which arch across the top of the pyramids. Small intralobular arteries radiate from the arcuate arteries to supply the cortex of the kidney. The afferent arterioles that supply the glomeruli arise from the intralobular arteries.

Although nearly all the blood that enters the kidney flows through the cortex, less than 10% passes into the medulla and only about 1% moves into the papillae. Under conditions of decreased perfusion or increased sympathetic nervous system stimulation, blood flow is redistributed away from the cortex toward the medulla. This redistribution of blood flow decreases glomerular filtration while maintaining the urine-concentrating ability of the kidneys, a factor that is important during conditions such as shock.

The Nephron

Each kidney is composed of more than 1 million tiny, closely packed functional units called *nephrons*, each of which is capable of producing urine (Fig. 24-4A). Each nephron consists of a glomerulus, where blood is filtered, and a system of tubular structures where water, electrolytes, and other substances needed to maintain the

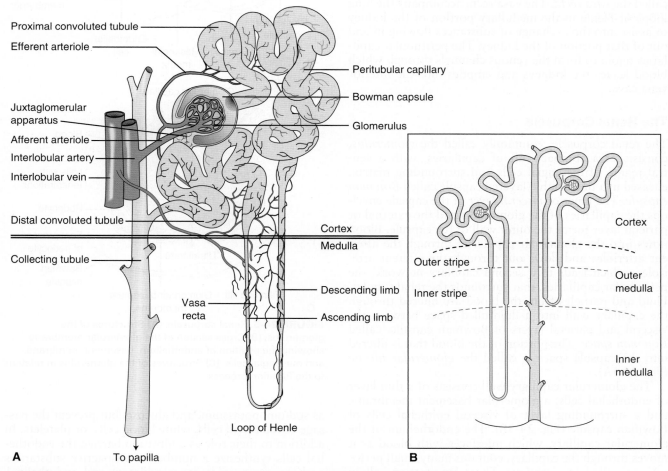

FIGURE 24-4. (A) Nephron showing the glomerular and tubular structures along with the blood supply. **(B)** Comparison of differences in location of tubular structures of the cortical and juxtamedullary nephrons.

constancy of the internal environment are reabsorbed into the bloodstream while other, unneeded materials are secreted into the tubular filtrate for elimination.

Nephrons can be roughly grouped into two categories. Approximately 85% of the nephrons originate in the superficial part of the cortex and are called *cortical nephrons* (Fig. 24-4B). They have short, thick loops of Henle that penetrate only a short distance into the medulla. The remaining 15% are called *juxtamedullary nephrons*. They originate deeper in the cortex and have longer and thinner loops of Henle that penetrate the entire length of the medulla. The juxtamedullary nephrons are largely concerned with urine concentration.

The nephrons are supplied by two capillary systems, the glomerulus and peritubular capillary network (see Fig. 24-4A). The *glomerulus* is a unique, high-pressure capillary filtration system located between two arterioles—the afferent and the efferent arterioles. The *peritubular capillaries* originate from the efferent arteriole. They are low-pressure vessels that are adapted for reabsorption rather than filtration. These capillaries surround all portions of the tubules, an arrangement that permits rapid movement of solutes and water between the fluid in the tubular lumen and the blood in the capillaries. In the deepest part of the renal cortex, the efferent arterioles continue as long, thin-walled looping vessels called the *vasa recta*. The vasa recta accompany the long loops of Henle in the medullary portion of the kidney to assist into the exchange of substances flowing in and out of that portion of the kidney. The peritubular capillaries rejoin to form the venous channels through which blood leaves the kidneys and empties into the inferior vena cava.

The Renal Corpuscle

The renal corpuscle, commonly called the *glomerulus*, consists of a compact tuft of capillaries, with a central region of mesangial cells and surrounding matrix, encased in a thin double-layered capsule called *Bowman capsule*. The inner or *visceral layer* of the capsule envelops the capillaries of the glomerulus and the external or parietal layer forms the outer wall of the capsule. Blood flows into the glomerular capillaries through the afferent arterioles and flows out through the efferent arterioles, which leads to a second capillary network, the peritubular capillaries, that surrounds the renal tubules. Fluid and particles from the blood are filtered through the capillary wall into a fluid-filled space between the visceral and parietal layers of Bowman capsule, called *Bowman space*. The portion of the blood that is filtered into the capsule space is called the *glomerular filtrate* (Fig. 24-5A).

The glomerular capillary wall consists of a thin layer of endothelial cells, a glomerular basement membrane, and a surrounding layer of visceral epithelial cells of Bowman capsule (Fig. 24-5B). The endothelium of the glomerular capillary, which interfaces with blood as it moves through the capillary, contains many small perforations, called *fenestrations*. These fenestrations allow for the free passage of water, and of small particles such

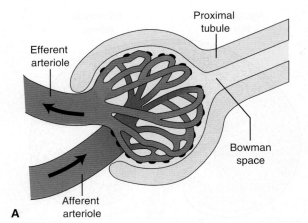

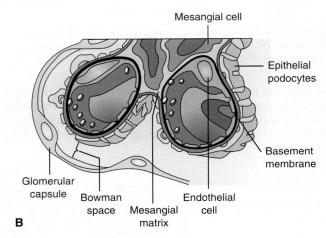

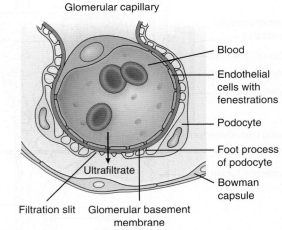

FIGURE 24-5. Renal corpuscle. **(A)** Structures of the glomerulus. **(B)** Cross-section of the glomerular membrane showing the position of endothelium, basement membrane, and mesangial cells. **(C)** Structures of the glomerulus in relation to the filtration process.

as sodium, potassium, and glucose, but prevent the passage of red blood cells, white blood cells, or platelets. In addition to their role as a filtration barrier, the endothelial cells synthesize a number of vasoactive substances such as nitric oxide (a vasodilator) and endothelin-1 (a vasoconstrictor) that control renal blood flow.

The glomerular basement membrane consists of a homogeneous acellular meshwork of collagen fibers, glycoproteins, and mucopolysaccharides (Fig. 24-5C). Because the endothelial and epithelial layers of the glomerular capillary have porous structures, the basement membrane determines the permeability of the capillary membrane. The spaces between the fibers that make up the basement membrane represent the pores of a filter and determine the size-dependent permeability barrier of the glomerulus. The size of the pores in the basement membrane normally prevents red blood cells and plasma proteins from passing into the filtrate. Alterations in the structure and function of the glomerular basement membrane are responsible for the leakage of proteins and blood cells into the filtrate that occurs in many forms of glomerular disease.

The visceral layer of the Bowman capsule is composed of epithelial cells that are highly modified to perform a filtering function. These large cells, called *podocytes,* have numerous finger-like processes that completely encircle the outer surface of the capillaries (see Fig. 24-5C). The elongated spaces between the interdigitating foot processes, called *filtration slits,* function as a size-selective filter that prevents proteins and macromolecules that have crossed the basement membrane from entering Bowman space.

Another important component of the glomerulus is the *mesangium.* In some areas, the capillary endothelium and the basement membrane do not completely surround each capillary tuft. Instead, the mesangial cells, which lie between the tufts, provide support for the glomerulus in these areas (Fig. 24-5B). The mesangial cells produce an intercellular substance similar to that of the basement membrane. This substance covers the endothelial cells where they are not covered by basement membrane. The mesangial cells also exhibit contractile properties and are thought to contribute to the regulation of blood flow through the glomerulus; possess phagocytic properties and remove macromolecular materials that enter the intercapillary spaces; and are capable of proliferation. Although the mesangial area is normally narrow and contains only a small number of cells, mesangial hyperplasia and increased mesangial matrix develop in many forms of glomerular disease.

Tubular Components of the Nephron

The nephron tubule is divided into several segments: the *proximal tubule,* which drains Bowman capsule; a thin looped structure, the *loop of Henle;* a distal coiled portion, the *distal convoluted tubule;* and the final segment, the *collecting tubule* (see Fig. 24-4A). The filtrate passes through each of these segments before reaching the pelvis of the kidney.

The proximal tubule is a highly coiled structure that lies in the cortex of the kidney and dips toward the renal pelvis to become the loop of Henle. The loop consists of a descending and ascending limb. The ascending loop of Henle returns to the region of the renal corpuscle, where it becomes much thicker, and is referred to as the *thick ascending limb.* Beyond the thick ascending limb of Henle is the distal convoluted tubule, which like the proximal tubule lies in the renal cortex. The distal convoluted tubule is divided into two segments: the *diluting segment* and the *late distal tubule.* The late distal tubule fuses with the collecting tubule The collecting tubule is divided into two segments: the *cortical tubule* and the *medullary collecting tubule.* The initial parts of 8 or 10 cortical collecting tubules join to form a single large tubule that moves down into the medulla to become the medullary collecting tubule.

Throughout its course, the tubule is composed of a single layer of epithelial cells resting on a basement membrane. The structure of the epithelial cells varies with tubular function. The cells of the proximal tubule have a fine, villous structure that increases the surface area for reabsorption; they also are rich in mitochondria, which support active transport processes. The epithelial layer thins in segments of the loop of Henle and has few mitochondria, indicating minimal metabolic activity and reabsorptive function.

SUMMARY CONCEPTS

■ The kidneys are paired, bean-shaped organs that lie outside the peritoneal cavity in the posterior abdomen, one on either side of the vertebral column. On longitudinal section, a kidney can be divided into an outer cortex and an inner medulla. The cortex and medulla are composed of nephrons, blood vessels, and nerves.

■ The nephrons, which are the functional units of the kidney, consist of a renal capsule (glomerulus and Bowman capsule) where blood is filtered, and tubular structures (proximal tubule, loop of Henle, distal tubule, and collecting tubule) where water, electrolytes, and soluble nutrients are reabsorbed into the blood and waste products are secreted from the blood into the tubular fluid.

■ The nephrons are supplied by two capillary systems, a glomerulus and peritubular capillary network. The glomerulus is a unique, high-pressure capillary filtration system located between two arterioles—the afferent and the efferent arterioles. The peritubular capillaries, which originate from the efferent arteriole and surround the tubules, are low-pressure vessels adapted for reabsorption rather than filtration.

Urine Formation

Urine formation involves the filtration of blood by the glomerulus to form an *ultrafiltrate of urine,* the selective reabsorption by the renal tubules of substances needed to maintain the constancy of the internal environment, and the secretion of unneeded and waste materials into the urine filtrate. The urine that is formed represents the sum of the three processes—glomerular filtration, tubular reabsorption, and tubular secretion.

Glomerular Filtration

Urine formation begins with the filtration of essentially protein-free plasma through the glomerular capillaries into the Bowman space. The movement of fluid through the glomerular capillaries is determined by the same factors (i.e., capillary filtration pressure, colloidal osmotic pressure, and capillary permeability) that affect fluid movement through other capillaries in the body. The glomerular filtrate has a chemical composition similar to plasma, but contains almost no proteins because large molecules do not readily pass through the openings in the glomerular capillary wall. Approximately 125 mL of filtrate is formed each minute. This is called the *glomerular filtration rate* (GFR). This rate can vary from a few milliliters per minute to as high as 200 mL/minute.

The location of the glomerulus between two arterioles allows for maintenance of a high-pressure filtration system. The capillary filtration pressure (approximately 60 mm Hg) in the glomerulus is approximately two to three times higher than that of other capillary beds in the body. The filtration pressure and the GFR are regulated by relaxation and constriction of the afferent and efferent arterioles. For example, relaxation of the afferent arteriole increases the filtration pressure and the GFR by increasing glomerular blood flow; whereas relaxation of the efferent arteriole decreases resistance to outflow of blood, decreasing the glomerular pressure and the GFR. The afferent and the efferent arterioles are innervated by the sympathetic nervous system and are sensitive to vasoactive hormones, such as angiotensin II. During periods of strong sympathetic stimulation, such as shock, constriction of the afferent arteriole causes a marked decrease in renal blood flow, and thus glomerular filtration pressure. Consequently, urine output can fall almost to zero.

Tubular Reabsorption and Secretion

From Bowman capsule, the glomerular filtrate moves into the tubular segments of the nephron. In its movement through the lumen of the tubular segments, the glomerular filtrate is changed considerably by the tubular transport of water and solutes. Tubular transport can result in reabsorption of substances from the tubular fluid into the peritubular capillaries or secretion of substances into the tubular fluid from the blood in the peritubular capillaries (Fig. 24-6).

The mechanisms of transport across the tubular cell membrane are similar to those of other cell membranes in the body and include active and passive transport mechanisms. Water and urea (a by-product of protein metabolism) are passively absorbed along concentration gradients. Sodium (Na+), other electrolytes, as well as urate (a metabolic end-product of purine metabolism), glucose, and amino acids, are reabsorbed using primary

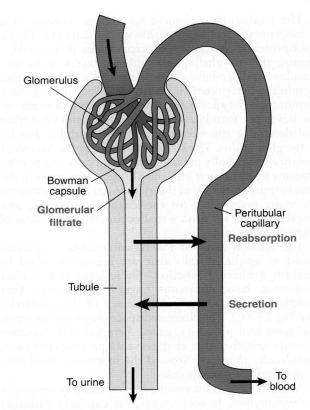

FIGURE 24-6. Reabsorption and secretion of substances between the renal tubules and the peritubular capillaries.

or secondary active transport mechanisms to move across the tubular membrane. Some substances, such excess K+ and urate, are secreted into the tubular fluids. Under normal conditions, approximately 1 mL of the 125 mL of glomerular filtrate that is formed each minute is excreted in the urine. The other 124 mL is reabsorbed in the tubules. This means that the average output of urine is approximately 60 mL/hour.

Renal tubular cells have two membrane surfaces through which substances must pass as they are reabsorbed from the tubular fluid. The outside membrane that lies adjacent to the interstitial fluid is called the *basolateral membrane,* and the side that is in contact with the tubular lumen and tubular filtrate is called the *luminal membrane.* In most cases, substances move from the tubular filtrate through the luminal membrane into the tubular cell along a concentration gradient, but they require facilitated transport or carrier systems to move across the basolateral membrane into the interstitial fluid, where they are absorbed into the peritubular capillaries.

The bulk of energy used by the kidney is for active sodium transport mechanisms that facilitate sodium reabsorption and cotransport of other electrolytes and substances such as glucose and amino acids. This is called *secondary active transport* or *cotransport* (Fig. 24-7). In secondary active transport, two or more substances interact with a specific membrane protein (a carrier protein) and are transported across the membrane. As one of the substances (in this case sodium) diffuses

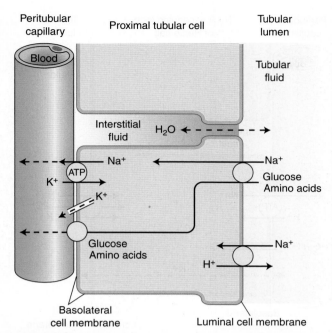

FIGURE 24-7. Mechanism for secondary active transport or cotransport of glucose and amino acids in the proximal tubule. The energy-dependent sodium–potassium pump on the basal lateral surface of the cell maintains a low intracellular gradient that facilitates the downhill movement of sodium and glucose or amino acids (cotransport) from the tubular lumen into the tubular cell and then into the peritubular capillary.

down its concentration gradient, the energy released is used to move another substance (for instance, glucose or an amino acid) against its concentration gradient. Thus, the secondary active transport of a substance such as glucose does not require energy directly from adenosine triphosphatase (ATPase), but depends on the energy-dependent Na^+/K^+-adenosine triphosphatase (ATPase) pump on the basolateral side of renal tubular cells. This pump maintains a low intracellular sodium

concentration that facilitates the downhill movement of sodium across the luminal membrane; it is this downhill diffusion of sodium to the interior of the cell that provides the energy for the simultaneous uphill transport of glucose across the luminal membrane. A few substances, such as hydrogen (H^+), are secreted into the tubule.

Proximal Tubule. Approximately 65% of all reabsorptive and secretory processes that occur in the tubular system take place in the proximal tubule. There is almost complete reabsorption of nutritionally important substances, such as glucose, amino acids, lactate, and water-soluble vitamins (Fig. 24-8). Electrolytes, such as Na^+, K^+, Cl^-, and bicarbonate (HCO_3^-), are 65% to 80% reabsorbed. As these solutes move into the tubular cells, their concentration in the tubular lumen decreases, providing a concentration gradient for the osmotic reabsorption of water and urea. The proximal tubule is highly permeable to water, and the osmotic movement of water occurs so rapidly that the concentration difference of solutes on either side of the membrane seldom is more than a few milliosmoles.

Many substances, such as glucose, are freely filtered in the glomerulus and reabsorbed by energy-dependent cotransport carrier mechanisms. The maximum amount of substance that these transport systems can reabsorb per unit time is called the *transport maximum*. The transport maximum is related to the number of carrier proteins that are available for transport and usually is sufficient to ensure that all of a filtered substance such as glucose can be reabsorbed rather than being eliminated in the urine. The plasma level at which the substance appears in the urine is called the *renal threshold*. Under some circumstances, the amount of substance filtered in the glomerulus exceeds the transport maximum. For example, when the blood glucose level is elevated in uncontrolled diabetes mellitus, the amount that is filtered in the glomerulus often exceeds the transport maximum (approximately 320 mg/minute), and glucose spills into the urine.

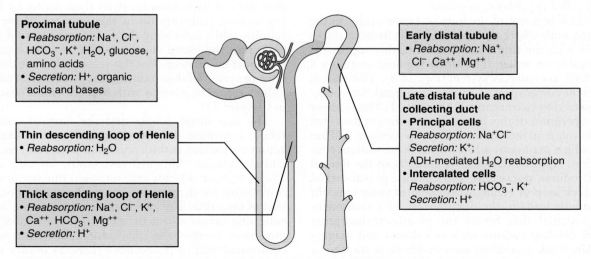

FIGURE 24-8. Sites of tubular water (H_2O), glucose, amino acids, Na^+ (sodium), Cl^- (chloride), HCO_3^- (bicarbonate), K^+ (potassium), Ca^{++} (calcium), and Mg^{++} (magnesium) reabsorption; and sites of organic acids and bases, H^+ (hydrogen), and K^+ secretion.

In addition to *reabsorbing* solutes and water, cells in the proximal tubule also *secrete* organic cations and anions into the urine filtrate (see Figs. 24-6 and 24-8). Many of these organic anions and cations are end products of metabolism (e.g., urate, oxalate) that circulate in the plasma. The proximal tubule also secretes exogenous organic compounds such as penicillin, aspirin, and morphine. Many of these compounds are bound to plasma proteins and not freely filtered in the glomerulus. Therefore, excretion by filtration alone eliminates only a small portion of these potentially toxic substances from the body.

Loop of Henle. The loop of Henle plays an important role in controlling the concentration of the urine. It does this by establishing a high concentration of osmotically active particles in the interstitium surrounding the medullary collecting tubules where the antidiuretic hormone exerts its effects.

The loop of Henle is divided into three segments: the thin descending segment, the thin ascending segment, and the thick ascending segment. Taken as a whole, the loop of Henle always reabsorbs more sodium and chloride than water. This is in contrast to the proximal tubule, which reabsorbs sodium and water in equal proportions. The thin descending limb is highly permeable to water and moderately permeable to urea, sodium, and other ions. As the urine filtrate moves down the descending limb, water moves out of the filtrate into the surrounding interstitium. Thus, the osmolality of the filtrate reaches its highest point at the elbow of the loop of Henle. In contrast to the descending limb, the ascending limb of the loop of Henle is impermeable to water. In this segment, solutes move out, but water cannot follow and remains in the filtrate. As a result, the tubular filtrate becomes more and more dilute, often reaching an osmolality of 100 mOsm/kg H_2O as it enters the distal convoluted tubule, compared with the 285 mOsm/kg H_2O in plasma. This allows for elimination of free water from the body. For this reason, the segment of the tubule is often called the *diluting segment*.

The thick segment of the loop of Henle begins in the ascending limb where the epithelial cells become thickened. As with the thin ascending limb, this segment is impermeable to water. The thick segment contains a $Na^+/K^+/2Cl^-$ cotransport system (Fig. 24-9). This system involves the cotransport of positively charged Na^+ and K^+ accompanied by two negatively charged Cl^-. The gradient for the operation of this cotransport system is provided by the basolateral membrane sodium–potassium ATPase pump, which maintains a low intracellular sodium concentration. Approximately 20% to 25% of the filtered load of sodium, potassium, and chloride is reabsorbed in the thick loop of Henle. Movement of these ions out of the tubule leads to the development of a transmembrane potential that favors the passive reabsorption of small divalent cations such as calcium and magnesium. The thick ascending loop of Henle is the site of the powerful "loop" diuretics (e.g., furosemide [Lasix]), which exert their action by inhibiting the $Na^+/K^+/2Cl^-$ cotransporters.

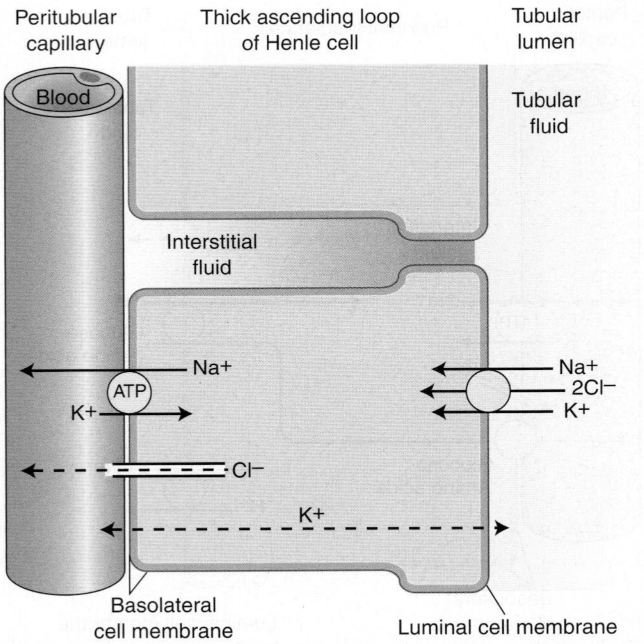

FIGURE 24-9. Sodium, chloride, and potassium reabsorption in the thick segment of the loop of Henle.

Distal and Collecting Tubules. Like the thick ascending loop of Henle, the distal convoluted tubule is relatively impermeable to water, and reabsorption of sodium chloride from this segment further dilutes the tubular fluid. Sodium reabsorption occurs through a Na^+/Cl^- cotransport mechanism. Approximately 5% of filtered sodium chloride is reabsorbed in this section of the tubule. Unlike the thick ascending loop of Henle, neither Ca^{++} nor Mg^{++} is passively absorbed in this segment of the tubule. Instead, Ca^{++} is actively reabsorbed in a process that is largely regulated by parathyroid hormone and possibly by vitamin D. The thiazide diuretics, which are widely used to treat disorders such as hypertension, exert their action by blocking sodium reabsorption in this segment of the renal tubules, while enhancing the active reabsorption of calcium into the blood via the calcium-sodium exchange transport mechanism. For this reason, thiazide diuretics have proved useful in reducing the incidence of calcium kidney stones in persons with hypercalciuria (discussed in Chapter 25).

The late distal tubule and the cortical collecting tubule constitute the site where aldosterone exerts its action on sodium reabsorption and potassium secretion and elimination. Although responsible for only 2% to 5% of sodium chloride reabsorption, this site is largely responsible for determining the final sodium concentration of the urine. The late distal tubule with the cortical collecting tubule also is the major site for regulation of potassium excretion by the kidney. When the body is confronted with a potassium excess, as occurs with a diet high in potassium content, the amount of potassium secreted into the urine filtrate at this site may exceed the amount filtered in the glomerulus.

The mechanism for sodium reabsorption and potassium secretion in this section of the nephron is distinct from other tubular segments. This tubular segment is composed of two types of cells, the intercalated cells and principal cells. The *intercalated cells* secrete hydrogen (H^+) ions and reabsorb bicarbonate (HCO_3^-) ions. Thus, they play a key role in acid–base regulation. H^+ secretion by the intercalated cells is mediated by the action of a hydrogen-ATPase transporter, in which H^+ are generated by the carbonic anhydrase-mediated reaction, in which water (H_2O) and carbon dioxide (CO_2) combine to form carbonic acid ($H_2CO_3^-$), which then dissociates to form H^+ and HCO_3^-. The H^+ ions are then secreted into the tubular fluid and the HCO_3^- become available for reabsorption.

The *principal cells* reabsorb sodium and water from the tubule lumen and secrete potassium into the lumen. Sodium reabsorption and potassium secretion depend on the activity of a sodium–potassium ATPase pump located on the basolateral membrane (Fig. 24-10). This pump maintains a low sodium concentration inside the cell by moving sodium down its concentration gradient into the cell through special sodium channels. The pump also establishes a high concentration of potassium within the cell, causing it to diffuse down its concentration gradient across the luminal membrane into the tubular fluid.

Regulation of Urine Concentration

The ability of the kidney to respond to changes in the osmolality of the extracellular fluids by producing either a concentrated or dilute urine depends on the establishment of a high concentration of osmotically active particles in the interstitium of the kidney medulla and the action of the antidiuretic hormone (ADH) in regulating the water permeability of the surrounding medullary collecting tubules (see Understanding How the Kidney Concentrates Urine).

In approximately one fifth of the juxtamedullary nephrons, the loops of Henle and vasa recta descend into the medullary portion of the kidney, forming a countercurrent system that controls water and solute movement so that water is kept out of the area surrounding the tubule and solutes are retained. The term *countercurrent* refers to a flow of fluids in opposite directions in adjacent structures. In this case, there is an exchange of solutes between the adjacent descending and ascending loops of Henle and between the ascending and descending sections of the vasa recta. Because of these exchange processes, a high concentration of osmotically active particles (approximately 1200 mOsm/kg H_2O) collects in the interstitium of the kidney medulla. The presence of these osmotically active particles in the interstitium surrounding the medullary collecting tubules facilitates the ADH-mediated reabsorption of water.

Antidiuretic hormone assists in the maintenance of the extracellular fluid volume by controlling the permeability of the medullary collecting tubules. Osmoreceptors in the hypothalamus sense an increase in osmolality of extracellular fluids and stimulate the release of ADH from the posterior pituitary gland. In exerting its effect, ADH, also known as *vasopressin,* binds to receptors on the basolateral side of the tubular cells. Binding of ADH to the vasopressin receptors causes water channels, known as *aquaporin-2 channels,* to move into the luminal side of the tubular cell membrane, producing a marked increase in water permeability. At the basolateral side of the membrane, water exits the tubular cell into the hyperosmotic interstitium of the medullary area, where it enters the peritubular capillaries for return to the vascular system. The aquaporin-2 channels are thought to have a critical role in inherited and acquired disorders of water reabsorption by the kidney, such as diabetes insipidus.

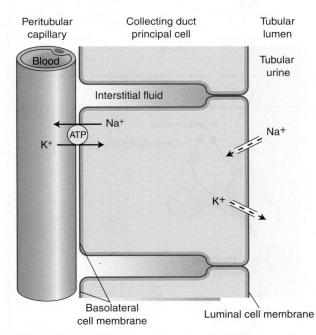

FIGURE 24-10. Mechanism of sodium reabsorption and potassium secretion by principal cells of the late distal and collecting tubules. Aldosterone exerts its action by increasing the activity of the Na$^+$/K$^+$-ATPase pump that transports sodium outward through the basolateral membrane of the cell and into the blood at the same time it pumps potassium into the cell. Aldosterone also increases the permeability of the luminal membrane for potassium.

Regulation of Renal Blood Flow and the GFR

In the adult, the kidneys are perfused with 1000 to 1300 mL of blood per minute, or 20% to 25% of the cardiac output. This large blood flow is mainly needed to ensure a sufficient GFR for the removal of waste products from the blood, rather than for the metabolic needs of the kidney. Feedback mechanisms, both intrarenal (e.g., autoregulation, local hormones) and extrarenal (e.g., sympathetic nervous system, blood-borne hormones), normally keep blood flow and the GFR constant despite changes in arterial blood pressure.

Neural and Humoral Control Mechanisms

The kidney is richly innervated by the sympathetic nervous system. Increased sympathetic activity causes

(*text continues on page 609*)

UNDERSTANDING ➜ How the Kidney

The osmolarity of body fluids relies heavily on the ability of the kidney to produce dilute or concentrated urine. Urine concentration depends on three factors: (1) the osmolarity of interstitial fluids in the urine-concentrating part of the kidney, (2) the antidiuretic hormone (ADH), and (3) the action of ADH on the cells in the collecting tubules of the kidney.

1

Osmolarity. In approximately one fifth of the juxtamedullary nephrons, the loops of Henle and special hairpin-shaped capillaries called the *vasa recta* descend into the medullary portion of the kidney to form a countercurrent system—a set of parallel passages in which the contents flow in opposite directions. The countercurrent design serves to increase the osmolarity in this part of the kidney by promoting the exchange of solutes between the adjacent descending and ascending loops of Henle and between the descending and ascending sections of the vasa recta. Because of these exchange processes, a high concentration of osmotically active particles (approximately 1200 mOsm/kg of H_2O) collects in the interstitium surrounding the collecting tubules where the ADH-mediated reabsorption of water takes place.

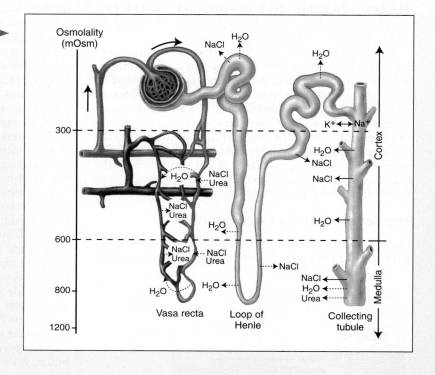

2

Antidiuretic Hormone. Antidiuretic hormone, which regulates the ability of the kidneys to concentrate urine, is synthesized by neurons in the hypothalamus and transported down their axons to the posterior pituitary gland and then released into the circulation. One of the main stimuli for synthesis and release of ADH is an increase in serum osmolarity. Antidiuretic hormone release is also controlled by cardiovascular reflexes that respond to changes in blood pressure or blood volume.

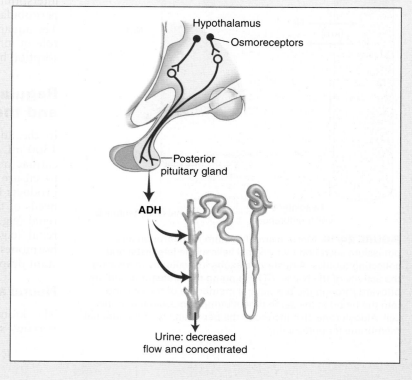

Concentrates Urine

3

Action of ADH. Antidiuretic hormone, also known as vasopressin, acts at the level of the collecting tubule to increase water absorption. It exerts its action by binding to vasopressin receptors on the basolateral membrane of the tubular cell. Binding of ADH to the vasopressin receptors causes water channels (*aquaporin-2 channels*) to move into the luminal side of the cell membrane, which is normally impermeable to water. Insertion of the channels allows water from the tubular fluids to move into the tubular cell and then out into the surrounding hyperosmotic interstitial fluid on the basolateral side of the cell. From there it moves into the peritubular capillaries for return to the circulatory system. Thus, when ADH is present, the water that moved from the blood into the urine filtrate in the glomeruli is returned to the circulatory system, and when ADH is absent, the water is excreted in the urine.

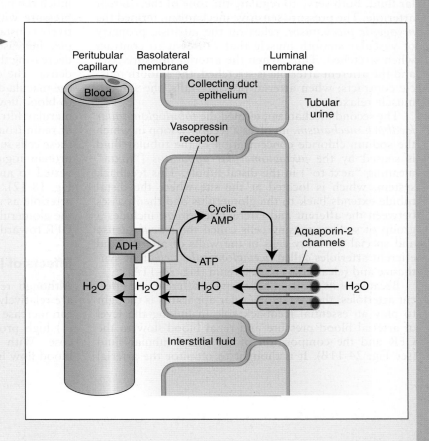

(*text continued from page 607*)

constriction of the afferent and efferent arterioles and thus a decrease in renal blood flow. Intense sympathetic stimulation such as occurs in shock and trauma can produce marked decreases in renal blood flow and GFR, even causing blood flow to cease altogether.

Several humoral substances, including angiotensin II, ADH, and the endothelins, produce vasoconstriction of renal vessels. The endothelins are a group of peptides released from damaged endothelial cells in the kidney and other tissues. Although not thought to be an important regulator of renal blood flow during everyday activities, endothelin I may play a role in the reduction of blood flow in conditions such as postischemic renal failure (see Chapter 26).

Other substances such as dopamine, nitric oxide, and prostaglandins (i.e., E_2 and I_2) produce vasodilation. Nitric oxide, a vasodilator produced by the vascular endothelium, appears to be important in preventing excessive vasoconstriction of renal blood vessels and allowing normal excretion of sodium and water. Prostaglandins are a group of mediators of cell function that are produced locally and exert their effects locally. Prostaglandins do not appear to play a major role in regulating renal blood flow and GFR under normal conditions, but may protect the kidneys against the vasoconstricting effects of sympathetic stimulation and angiotensin II. This effect is important because it prevents severe and potentially harmful vasoconstriction and ischemia during conditions such as hemorrhage and shock. Aspirin and other nonsteroidal anti-inflammatory drugs (NSAIDs) that inhibit prostaglandin synthesis may decrease renal blood flow and GFR under certain conditions.

Autoregulatory Mechanisms

The constancy of blood flow through body tissues is maintained by a process called *autoregulation*. In most tissues other than the kidneys, autoregulation functions to maintain blood flow at a level consistent with the metabolic needs of the tissues. In the kidney, autoregulation of blood flow also functions to maintain a relatively constant GFR and to allow for the precise regulation of solute and water excretion.

Two major systems are credited with maintaining the constancy of renal blood flow and GFR: one responds to changes in arterial pressure and the other to changes in the sodium chloride concentration in the distal tubular fluid. Both serve to regulate the tone of the afferent arteriole. The pressure sensitive mechanism, termed the *myogenic mechanism*, relies on the intrinsic property of vascular smooth muscle that causes it to contract when stretched. Thus, when the arterial pressure rises and the afferent arteriole is stretched, the smooth muscle contracts; when arterial pressure falls, the smooth muscle relaxes.

The second mechanism, termed the *tubuloglomerular feedback mechanism*, involves a feedback loop in which the sodium chloride concentration in the tubular fluid is sensed by the *juxtaglomerular apparatus* ("juxta" meaning "next to") in the distal tubule. This feedback system, which is located at the site where the distal tubule extends back to the glomerulus and then passes between the afferent and efferent arterioles, includes a group of sodium sensing cells called the *macula densa* and special secretory cells in the walls of afferent and efferent arterioles called *juxtaglomerular cells* that synthesize and release the enzyme renin (Fig. 24-11A).

Because of its location between the afferent and efferent arterioles, the juxtaglomerular apparatus is thought to play an essential feedback role in linking the level of arterial blood pressure and renal blood flow to the GFR and the composition of the distal tubular fluid (see Fig. 24-11B). It is thought to monitor the arterial blood pressure by sensing both the stretch of the afferent arteriole and the concentration of sodium chloride in the tubular filtrate as it passes through the macula densa. This information is then used in determining how much renin should be released to keep the arterial blood pressure within its normal range and maintain a relatively constant GFR. A decrease in the GFR, for example, increases sodium chloride reabsorption, thereby decreasing the delivery of sodium chloride to the macula densa. The decrease in delivery of sodium chloride to the macula densa has two effects: it decreases resistance to blood flow in the afferent arteriole, which raises glomerular filtration pressure; and it increases the release of renin from the juxtaglomerular cells. The renin from these cells functions as an enzyme to convert the plasma protein angiotensinogen to angiotensin I, which is converted to angiotensin II in the lungs (see Chapter 18, Fig. 18-12). Angiotensin II acts to constrict the efferent arteriole as a means of producing a further increase in the glomerular filtration pressure; thereby returning the GFR toward a more normal range.

Effects of Increased Protein and Glucose Load

Although renal blood flow and glomerular filtration are relatively stable under most conditions, two factors can increase renal blood flow and glomerular filtration: (1) high protein intake, (2) an increase in blood glucose. With ingestion of a high-protein meal, renal blood flow increases 20% to 30% within 1 to 2 hours.

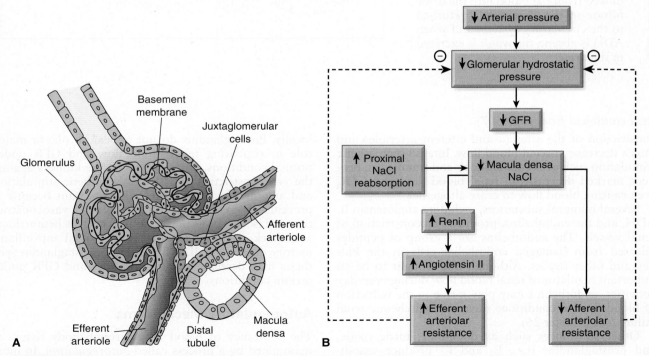

FIGURE 24-11. (A) Juxtaglomerular apparatus showing the close contact of the distal tubule with the afferent arteriole, the macula densa, and the juxtaglomerular cells. **(B)** Flow chart depicting the macula densa feedback mechanism for autoregulation of glomerular hydrostatic pressure and glomerular filtration rate (GFR) during changes in renal arterial pressure. (From Hall JE. *Guyton and Hall Textbook of Medical Physiology*. 12th ed. Philadelphia, PA: Saunders Elsevier; 2011:320.)

Although the exact mechanism for this increase is uncertain, it is thought to be related to the fact that amino acids and sodium are absorbed together in the proximal tubule via secondary active transport. As a result, delivery of sodium to the macula densa is decreased, which elicits an increase in renal blood flow through the juxtaglomerular apparatus feedback mechanism. The resultant increase in blood flow and GFR allows sodium excretion to be maintained at a near-normal level while increasing the excretion of the waste products of protein metabolism, such as urea. The same mechanism is thought to explain the large increases in renal blood flow and GFR that occur with high blood glucose levels in persons with uncontrolled diabetes mellitus.

SUMMARY CONCEPTS

■ Urine formation, which begins with the formation of a plasma ultrafiltrate from the glomerular capillaries into Bowman capsule, serves to regulate extracellular volume and concentration of electrolytes and other solutes.

■ Tubular mechanisms allow the kidneys to retain water, electrolytes, and nutrients that are essential and regulate their levels in the blood by altering the degree to which they are reabsorbed or secreted into the tubular fluid for elimination.

■ The kidney's ability to produce a dilute or concentrated urine as a means of controlling the osmolality of body fluids relies on the development of an osmotic gradient in the medullary interstitium of the thin loops of Henle and reabsorption of water from the collecting tubules under the influence of the antidiuretic hormone (ADH).

■ The *glomerular filtration rate* (GFR), which is the amount of filtrate that is formed each minute as blood moves through the glomeruli, is regulated by the arterial blood pressure and renal blood flow. Feedback mechanisms, both intrarenal (e.g., autoregulation, local hormones) and extrarenal (e.g., sympathetic nervous system, blood-borne hormones), normally keep blood flow and GFR constant despite changes in arterial blood pressure.

Elimination and Endocrine Functions of the Kidney

The kidneys play a critical role in maintaining the volume and composition of body fluids through the reabsoption of water and electrolytes, as well as in ridding the body of waste products. The kidneys also have endocrine functions that are important to the regulation of blood pressure, production of red blood cells, and absorption of calcium.

Elimination Functions of the Kidney

The functions of the kidney focus on elimination of water, excess electrolytes, metabolic acids, and waste products from the blood. As renal function declines, there is an increase in serum levels of substances such as urea, creatinine, phosphate, and potassium. The effect of renal failure on the concentration of serum electrolytes and metabolic end products is discussed in Chapter 26.

Sodium and Potassium Elimination

Elimination of sodium and potassium is regulated by the GFR and by humoral agents that control their reabsorption. Aldosterone, a hormone secreted by the adrenal gland, functions in the regulation of sodium and potassium elimination by the principal cells in the distal and collecting tubules.

Sodium reabsorption in the distal and collecting tubules is highly variable and depends on the presence of aldosterone. In the presence of aldosterone, which stimulates sodium absorption and simultaneous excretion of potassium into the tubular fluid, almost all the sodium in the distal tubular fluid is reabsorbed, and the urine essentially becomes sodium free. In the absence of aldosterone, virtually no sodium is reabsorbed from the distal tubule and excessive amounts of sodium are lost in the urine. The remarkable ability of the distal tubular and collecting duct cells to alter sodium reabsorption in relation to changes in aldosterone allows the kidneys to excrete urine with sodium levels that range from a few tenths of a gram to 40 g/day.

Atrial natriuretic peptide (ANP) is also believed to have an important role in salt and water excretion by the kidney. It is synthesized by muscle cells in the atria of the heart and released when the atria are stretched. Increased levels of this peptide directly inhibit the reabsorption of sodium and water in the renal tubules. Atrial natriuretic peptide also inhibits renin secretion and therefore angiotensin II formation, which in turn reduces reabsorption of sodium. This decreased sodium reabsorption increases urine output and helps return blood volume to normal. Atrial natriuretic peptide levels, which become elevated when the atria are stretched in congestive heart failure, help to decrease vascular volume by increasing urine output.

Like sodium, potassium is freely filtered in the glomerulus and reabsorbed in the proximal and distal tubule. Unlike sodium, however, potassium is both reabsorbed from and secreted into the tubular fluid. The amount of potassium that is delivered to the distal tubule each day is only about 70 mEq, yet the average person consumes that much or more in the diet. Therefore, the excess potassium that is not filtered in the glomerulus must be secreted into the tubular fluid so it can be eliminated in the urine. Potassium secretion occurs mainly in the distal and collecting tubules, with plasma potassium and aldosterone levels being the main physiological regulators of the secretory process. A rise in plasma potassium due to an increase in dietary intake increases potassium secretion and urinary excretion; correspondingly, a fall in plasma levels due to a decrease in dietary intake increases reabsorption and decreases urinary excretion. Aldosterone also exerts a strong influence on potassium secretion in the distal and collecting tubules. In the absence of aldosterone, as occurs in Addison disease, potassium secretion is markedly decreased, causing blood levels to increase (see Chapter 32).

Regulation of Body pH

The average North American diet results in the liberation of 40 to 80 mmol of H^+ each day. Neither blood buffer systems nor the respiratory control mechanisms for carbon dioxide elimination can eliminate H^+ from the body. This is accomplished by the kidneys. Virtually all the excess H^+ excreted in the urine are secreted into the tubular fluid by means of tubular secretory mechanisms.

The lowest tubular fluid pH that can be achieved without damaging the kidney structures is about 4.5. The ability of the kidneys to excrete large amounts of H^+ in the urine is accomplished by combining the excess ions with buffers in the urine. The three major urine buffers are HCO_3^-, phosphate (HPO_4^{2-}), and ammonia (NH_3). Bicarbonate ions, which are present in the urine filtrate, combine with H^+ that has been secreted into the tubular fluid, resulting in formation of carbon dioxide and water. The carbon dioxide is then absorbed into the tubular cells and bicarbonate is regenerated. The phosphate ion is a metabolic end product that is filtered into the tubular fluid; it combines with a secreted hydrogen ion and is not reabsorbed. Ammonia is synthesized in tubular cells by deamination of the amino acid glutamine; it diffuses into the tubular fluid and combines with the hydrogen ion. An important aspect of this buffer system is that the deamination process increases whenever the body's hydrogen ion concentration remains elevated for 1 to 2 days. These mechanisms for pH regulation are described more fully in Chapter 8.

Elimination of Organic Ions

The proximal tubule actively secretes large amounts of different organic anions. Exogenous anions (e.g., salicylates, penicillin) and those produced endogenously (e.g., bile acids, uric acid) are actively secreted into the tubular fluid. Most of the anions that are secreted use the same transport system, allowing the kidneys to rid the body of many different drugs and environmental agents. Because the same transport system is shared by different anions, there is competition for transport such that elevated levels of one substance tend to inhibit the secretion of other anions. The proximal tubules also possess an active transport system for organic cations that is analogous to that for organic anions.

Uric Acid Elimination

Uric acid is a product of purine metabolism (see Chapter 44). Excessively high blood levels (i.e., hyperuricemia) can cause gout, and excessive urine levels can cause kidney stones. Uric acid is freely filtered in the glomerulus and is reabsorbed and secreted into the proximal tubules, using the previously described anion transport system in the proximal tubule. Tubular reabsorption normally exceeds secretion, and the net effect is removal of uric acid from the filtrate. Although the rate of reabsorption exceeds secretion, the secretory process is homeostatically controlled to maintain a constant plasma level. Many persons with elevated uric acid levels secrete less uric acid than do persons with normal uric acid levels.

Uric acid uses the same transport systems as other anions, such as aspirin, sulfinpyrazone, and probenecid. Small doses of aspirin compete with uric acid for secretion into the tubular fluid and reduce uric acid secretion, and large doses compete with uric acid for reabsorption and increase uric acid excretion in the urine. Because of its effect on uric acid secretion, aspirin is not recommended for treatment of gouty arthritis. Thiazide and loop diuretics (i.e., furosemide and ethacrynic acid) also can cause hyperuricemia and gouty arthritis, presumably through a decrease in extracellular fluid volume and enhanced uric acid reabsorption.

Urea Elimination

Urea is an end product of protein metabolism. The normal adult produces 25 to 30 g of urea a day; the quantity rises when a high-protein diet is consumed, when there is excessive tissue breakdown, or in the presence of gastrointestinal bleeding. With gastrointestinal bleeding, blood proteins are broken down to form ammonia in the intestine. The ammonia is then absorbed into the portal circulation and converted to urea by the liver before being released into the bloodstream. The kidneys, in their role as regulators of blood urea nitrogen (BUN) levels, filter urea in the glomeruli and then reabsorb it in the tubules. This enables maintenance of a normal BUN level, which ranges from 8 to 25 mg/dL (2.9 to 8.9 mmol/L). During periods of dehydration, the blood volume and GFR drop, and BUN levels increase. The renal tubules are permeable to urea, which means that the longer the tubular fluid remains in the kidneys, the greater is the reabsorption of urea into the blood. Only small amounts of urea are reabsorbed into the blood when the GFR is high, but relatively large amounts of urea are returned to the blood when the GFR is reduced.

Drug Elimination

Many drugs are eliminated in the urine. These drugs are selectively filtered in the glomerulus and reabsorbed or secreted into the tubular fluid. Drugs that are not bound to plasma proteins are filtered in the glomerulus and therefore able to be eliminated by the kidneys. Many drugs are weak acids or weak bases and are present in the renal tubular fluid partly as ionized water-soluble and nonionized lipid-soluble molecules. The nonionized lipid soluble form of a drug diffuses more readily across the lipid bilayer of the tubular cell membrane and then back into the bloodstream, whereas the ionized water-soluble form remains in the urine filtrate. The ratio of ionized to nonionized drug depends on the pH of the urine. Aspirin, for example, is highly ionized in alkaline urine and in this form is rapidly excreted in the urine, and it is largely nonionized in acid urine and, as such, reabsorbed rather than excreted. Measures that alkalinize or acidify the urine may be used to increase elimination of drugs, particularly in situations of toxic overdose.

Endocrine Functions of the Kidney

In addition to their role in regulating fluid and electrolytes, the kidneys function as an endocrine organ in that they produce chemical mediators that travel through the blood to distant sites where they exert their actions. The kidneys participate in control of blood pressure through the renin-angiotensin-aldosterone mechanism, in calcium metabolism by activating vitamin D, and in regulating red blood cell production through the synthesis of erythropoietin.

The Renin-Angiotensin-Aldosterone Mechanism

The renin-angiotensin-aldosterone mechanism is important in short- and long-term regulation of blood pressure (see Chapter 18). Renin is an enzyme that is synthesized and stored in the juxtaglomerular cells of the kidney. This enzyme is thought to be released in response to a decrease in renal blood flow or a change in the composition of the distal tubular fluid, or as the result of sympathetic nervous system stimulation. Renin itself has no direct effect on blood pressure. Rather, it acts enzymatically to convert a circulating plasma protein called *angiotensinogen* to angiotensin I.

Angiotensin I, which has few vasoconstrictor properties, leaves the kidneys and enters the circulation; as it is circulated through the lungs, the *angiotensin-converting enzyme* catalyzes its conversion to angiotensin II. Angiotensin II is a potent vasoconstrictor, and it acts directly on the kidneys to decrease salt and water excretion. Both mechanisms have relatively short periods of action. Angiotensin II also stimulates the secretion of aldosterone by the adrenal gland, thereby exerting a more long-term effect on maintenance of blood pressure by increasing the reabsorption of sodium in the distal tubule. Renin also functions via angiotensin II to produce constriction of the efferent arteriole as a means of preventing a serious decrease in glomerular filtration pressure.

Erythropoietin

Erythropoietin is a polypeptide hormone that regulates the differentiation of red blood cells in the bone marrow (see Chapter 13). Between 89% and 95% of erythropoietin is formed in the kidneys. The synthesis of erythropoietin is stimulated by tissue hypoxia, which may be brought about by anemia, residence at high altitudes, or impaired oxygenation of tissues due to cardiac or pulmonary disease. Persons with chronic kidney disease often are anemic because of an inability of the kidneys to produce erythropoietin. This anemia usually is managed by the administration of a recombinant erythropoietin (epoetin alfa) produced through DNA technology to stimulate erythropoiesis.

Vitamin D

Activation of vitamin D occurs in the kidneys. Vitamin D increases calcium absorption from the gastrointestinal tract and helps to regulate calcium deposition in bone. It also has a weak stimulatory effect on renal calcium absorption. Although vitamin D is not synthesized and released from an endocrine gland, it is often considered as a hormone because of its pathway of molecular activation and mechanism of action.

Vitamin D exists in two forms: natural vitamin D (cholecalciferol), produced in the skin from ultraviolet irradiation, and synthetic vitamin D (ergocalciferol), derived from irradiation of ergosterol. The active form of vitamin D is 1,25-dihydroxycholecalciferol. Cholecalciferol and ergocalciferol must undergo chemical transformation to become active: first to 25-hydroxycholecalciferol in the liver and then to 1,25-dihydroxycholecalciferol in the kidneys. Persons with end-stage renal disease are unable to transform vitamin D to its active form and may require pharmacologic preparations of the active vitamin (calcitriol) for maintaining mineralization of their bones.

SUMMARY CONCEPTS

- The kidneys have multiple functions, including maintaining the volume and composition of body fluids through the regulation of electrolyte levels and excretion of various by-products of metabolism.

- Sodium and potassium levels are regulated by the GFR and by humoral agents such as aldosterone, which controls the final steps in regulating their absorption or elimination.

- The kidneys regulate the pH of body fluids by eliminating H^+ and conserving or generating bicarbonate ions.

- Various products of metabolism and exogenous organic anions, such as drugs, are bound to plasma proteins and are therefore unavailable for filtration in the glomerulus. Thus, secretion of substances into tubular fluid provides the route for elimination in the urine.

- The kidneys also function as endocrine organs. They participate in control of blood pressure by way of the renin-angiotensin-aldosterone mechanism, help regulate red blood cell production through the synthesis of erythropoietin, and aid in calcium metabolism through the conversion of vitamin D to its active form.

Tests of Renal Function

The function of the kidneys is to filter the blood, selectively reabsorb those substances that are needed to maintain the constancy of body fluid, and excrete metabolic wastes. Blood and urine tests can provide valuable information about the kidneys' ability to remove metabolic wastes and maintain the blood's normal electrolyte and pH composition. As renal function declines, there is an increase in serum levels of substances such as urea, creatinine, phosphate, and potassium. Radiologic tests, endoscopy, and renal biopsy afford means for viewing the gross and microscopic structures of the kidneys and urinary system.

Renal Clearance and Glomerular Filtration Rate

Both the renal clearance and GFR provide information about the kidneys' ability to filter and reabsorb and/or secrete substances into blood. Renal clearance measures the rate at which a substance is excreted into the urine and the GFR measures the volume of plasma that is filtered each minute.

In clinical practice, one way of estimating the clearance rate of endogenous creatinine is by collecting timed samples of blood and urine. *Creatinine* is a product of creatine metabolism in muscles; its formation and release are relatively constant and proportional to the amount of muscle mass present. Because creatinine is freely filtered in the glomeruli but is not reabsorbed from the tubules into the blood nor significantly secreted into the tubules from the blood, its blood and urine levels can be used to calculate the GFR.

Another serum protein, *cystatin C* can also be used as an estimate of GFR. It is produced by all body cells at a constant rate, is freely filtered at the glomerulus, and in several studies has shown a greater sensitivity in detecting a decrease in GFR than creatinine. Recent studies suggest that the use of a combined creatinine–cystatin C equation may provide a better estimate of GFR than either test used separately.

Blood Tests

Blood tests can provide valuable information about the kidneys' ability to remove metabolic wastes from the blood and maintain normal electrolyte and pH composition of the blood. Normal blood values are listed in Table 24-1. Serum levels of potassium, phosphate, BUN, and creatinine increase in renal failure while serum pH, calcium, and bicarbonate levels decrease.

Serum Creatinine

Serum creatinine levels reflect the GFR. Because these measurements are easily obtained and relatively inexpensive, they often are used as a screening measure of renal function. The normal creatinine value is approximately 0.7 mg/dL of blood for a woman with a small frame, approximately 1.0 mg/dL of blood for a normal adult man, and approximately 1.5 mg/dL of blood (60 to

TABLE 24-1	Normal Blood Chemistry Levels
Substance	**Normal Value***
Blood urea nitrogen	8.0–20.0 mg/dL (2.9–7.1 mmol/L)
Creatinine	0.6–1.2 mg/dL (50–100 mmol/L)
Sodium	135–145 mEq/L (135–145 mmol/L)
Chloride	98–106 mEq/L (98–106 mmol/L)
Potassium	3.5–5 mEq/L (3.5–5 mmol/L)
Carbon dioxide (CO_2 content)	24–29 mEq/L (24–29 mmol/L)
Calcium	8.5–10.5 mg/dL (2.1–2.6 mmol/L)
Phosphate	2.5–4.5 mg/dL (0.77–1.45 mmol/L)
Uric acid	
Male	2.4–7.4 mg/dL (140–440 μmol/L)
Female	1.4–5.8 mg/dL (80–350 μmol/L)
pH	7.35–7.45

*Values may vary among laboratories, depending on the method of analysis used.

130 mmol/L) for a muscular man. There is an age-related decline in creatinine clearance in many elderly persons because muscle mass and the GFR decline with age. A normal serum creatinine level usually indicates normal renal function. In addition to its use in calculating the GFR, the serum creatinine level is used in estimating the functional capacity of the kidneys (Fig. 24-12). If the value doubles, the GFR—and renal function—probably has fallen to one half of its normal state. A rise in the serum creatinine level to three times its normal value suggests that there is a 75% loss of renal function, and with creatinine values of 10 mg/dL or more, it can be assumed that approximately 90% of renal function has been lost.

Blood Urea Nitrogen

Urea is formed in the liver as a by-product of protein metabolism and is eliminated entirely by the kidneys. Therefore, the BUN is related to the GFR but, unlike creatinine, it also is influenced by protein intake, gastrointestinal bleeding, and hydration status. In gastrointestinal bleeding, the blood is broken down by the intestinal flora, and the nitrogenous waste is absorbed into the portal vein and transported to the liver, where it is converted to urea. During dehydration, elevated BUN levels result from increased concentration. Approximately two

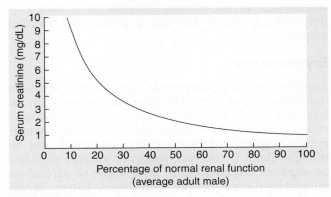

FIGURE 24-12. Relation between the percentage of renal function and serum creatinine levels.

thirds of renal function must be lost before a significant rise in the BUN level occurs.

The BUN is less specific for renal insufficiency than creatinine, but the *BUN–creatinine ratio* may provide useful diagnostic information. The ratio normally is approximately 10:1. Ratios greater than 15:1 represent prerenal conditions, such as congestive heart failure and upper gastrointestinal tract bleeding, that produce an increase in BUN but not in creatinine. A ratio of less than 10:1 occurs in persons with liver disease and in those who receive a low-protein diet or chronic dialysis because BUN is more readily dialyzable than creatinine.

Urine Tests

Urine is a clear, amber-colored fluid that is approximately 95% water and 5% dissolved solids. The kidneys normally produce approximately 1.5 L of urine each day. Normal urine contains metabolic wastes and few or no plasma proteins, blood cells, or glucose molecules. Urine tests can be performed on a single urine specimen or on a 24-hour urine specimen. First-voided morning specimens are useful for qualitative protein and specific gravity testing. A freshly voided specimen is most reliable. Urine specimens that have been left standing may contain lysed red blood cells, disintegrating *casts,* and rapidly multiplying bacteria. Table 24-2 describes urinalysis values for normal urine.

Casts are molds of the distal nephron lumen. A gel-like substance called *Tamm-Horsfall mucoprotein,* which is formed in the tubular epithelium, is the major protein constituent of urinary casts. Casts composed of this gel but devoid of cells are called *hyaline casts.* These casts develop when the protein concentration of the urine is high (as in nephrotic syndrome), urine osmolality is high, and urine pH is low. The inclusion of granules or cells in the matrix of the protein gel leads to the formation of various other types of casts.

Proteinuria

Proteinuria represents excessive protein excretion in the urine. Because of the glomerular capillary filtration barrier, less than 150 mg/L of protein is excreted in the urine over 24 hours in a healthy person. Urine tests for proteinuria are used to detect abnormal filtering of albumin in the glomeruli or defects in its reabsorption in the renal tubules. A protein reagent dipstick can be used as a rapid screening test for the presence of proteins in the urine. Once the presence of proteinuria has been detected, a 24-hour urine test is often used to quantify the amount of protein that is present.

Albumin, which is the smallest of the plasma proteins, is filtered more readily than globulins or other plasma proteins. Thus, *microalbuminuria* tends to occur long before clinical proteinuria becomes evident. A dipstick test for microalbuminuria is available for screening purposes. The microalbuminuria dipstick method, however, only indicates an increase in urinary albumin that is below the detectable range of the standard proteinuria test. It does not specify the amount of albumin that is present in the urine. Therefore, a 24-hour urine collection is the standard method for detecting microalbuminuria (an albumin excretion >30 mg/day is abnormal).

Specific Gravity and Osmolality

The *specific gravity* of urine is a measure of its concentration of solutes. Urine specific gravity provides a valuable index of the hydration status and functional ability of the kidneys. The usual range is from 1.010 to 1.025 with normal fluid intake. Healthy kidneys can produce concentrated urine with a specific gravity of 1.030 to 1.040 during periods of dehydration, and a dilute urine with a specific gravity that approaches 1.000 during periods of taking too much fluid. With diminished renal function, there is a loss of renal concentrating ability, and the urine specific gravity may fall to levels of 1.006 to 1.010. These low levels are particularly significant if they occur during periods that follow a decrease in water intake (e.g., during the first urine specimen on arising in the morning).

Urine osmolality, which depends on the number of particles of solute in a unit of solution, is a more exact measurement of urine concentration than specific gravity. More information concerning renal function can be obtained if the serum and urine osmolality tests are done at the same time. The normal ratio between urine and serum osmolality is 3:1. A high urine-to-serum ratio is seen in concentrated urine. With poor concentrating ability, the ratio is low.

TABLE 24-2 Normal Values for Routine Urinalysis

General Characteristics and Measurements	Chemical Determinations	Microscopic Examination of Sediment
Color: yellow-amber—indicates a high specific gravity and small output of urine Turbidity: clear to slightly hazy Specific gravity: 1.010–1.025 with a normal fluid intake pH: 4.6–8.0	Glucose: negative Ketones: negative Blood: negative Protein: negative Bilirubin: negative Urobilinogen: 0.5–4.0 mg/d Nitrate for bacteria: negative Leukocyte esterase: negative	Casts negative: occasional hyaline casts Red blood cells: negative or rare Crystals: negative (none) White blood cells: negative or rare Epithelial cells: few

From Fischbach FT, Dunning MB. *A Manual of Laboratory and Diagnostic Tests.* 8th ed. Philadelphia, PA: Wolters Kluwer Health | Lippincott Williams & Wilkins; 2014:203.

SUMMARY CONCEPTS

- The composition of urine and blood samples provides valuable information about kidney function.

- Blood tests that measure serum levels of pH, electrolytes, and by-products of metabolism provide information about renal function. Creatinine, a product of creatine metabolism in muscles, is freely filtered in the glomeruli and neither reabsorbed nor secreted into the tubules; therefore, serum creatinine levels are commonly used to estimate the GFR. Urea is formed in the liver as a by-product of protein metabolism and is eliminated entirely by the kidneys; thus, blood urea nitrogen (BUN) is related to the GFR but, unlike creatinine, is also influenced by protein intake, gastrointestinal bleeding, and hydration status.

- Urinalysis and urine specific gravity is used to assess the kidneys' ability to concentrate urine. Dipstick and 24-hour urine tests for proteinuria and microalbuminuria are used to detect abnormal filtering of albumin in the glomeruli.

REVIEW EXERCISES

1. A 32-year-old woman with diabetes is found to have a positive result on a urine dipstick test for microalbuminuria. A subsequent 24-hour urine specimen reveals an albumin excretion of 50 mg (an albumin excretion >30 mg/day is abnormal).

   A. Use the structures of the glomerulus in Figure 24-5 to provide a possible explanation for this finding. Why specifically test for the albumin rather than the globulins or other plasma proteins?

   B. Strict control of blood sugars and treatment of hypertension have been shown to decrease the progression of kidney disease in persons with diabetes. Explain the physiologic rationale for these two types of treatments.

2. A 10-year-old boy with enuresis (bed-wetting) was placed on an ADH nasal spray at bedtime as a means of treating the disorder.

   A. Explain the rationale for using ADH to treat bed-wetting.

3. A 54-year-old man, seen by his physician for an elevated blood pressure, was found to have a serum creatinine of 2.5 mg/dL. He complains that he has been urinating more frequently than usual. His first morning urine specimen reveals a dilute urine with a specific gravity of 1.010.

   A. Explain the elevation of serum creatinine in terms of a decrease in renal function.

   B. Explain the inability of persons with early renal failure to produce a concentrated urine as evidenced by the frequency of urination and the low specific gravity of his first morning urine specimen.

BIBLIOGRAPHY

Hall JE. *Guyton & Hall Textbook of Medical Physiology.* 12th ed. Philadelphia, PA: Elsevier Saunders; 2011:303–378.

Inker LA, Schmid CH, Tighiouart H, et al. Estimating glomerular filtration rate from serum creatinine and cystatin C. *N Engl J Med.* 2012;367(1):20–29.

National Kidney Foundation. Cystatin C: What's is its role in estimating GFR. 2008. www.kidney.org/professionals/tools/pdf/cystatinC.pdf. Accessed May 20013.

Nielson S, Kwon TH, Fenton RA, et al. Anatomy of the kidney. In: Taal MW, Chertow GM, Marsden PA, et al. *Brenner and Rector's The Kidney.* 9th ed. Philadelphia, PA: Elsevier Saunders; 2012:31–92.

Ross GI, Pawlina W. *Histology: A Text and Atlas.* 6th ed. Philadelphia, PA: Wolters Kluwer Health/Lippincott Williams & Wilkins; 2011:698–723.

Sherwood L. *Human Physiology: From Cells to Systems.* 8th ed. Belmont, CA: Brooks/Cole; 2013:505–547.

Simon J, Amode M, Poggio EG. Interpreting the estimated glomerular filtration rate in primary care: benefits and pitfalls. *Clev Clinic J Med.* 2011;78(3):189–195.

Smith H. *From Fish to Philosopher.* Boston, MA: Little, Brown; 1953:4.

Stanton BA, Koepen BM. Elements of renal function and solute and water transport along the nephron: Tubular function. In: Koeppen BM, Stanton BA, eds. *Berne & Levy Physiology.* 6th ed. Philadelphia, PA: Mosby Elsevier; 2010:557–618.

Stevens LA, Levey AS. Measurement of kidney function. *Med Clin North Am.* 2005;89:457–473.

Tanner GA. Kidney function. In: Rhoades RA, Bell DR, eds. *Medical Physiology.* 2nd ed. Philadelphia, PA: Wolters Kluwer Health/Lippincott Williams & Wilkins; 2013:399–406.

Porth Essentials Resources

Explore these additional resources to enhance learning for this chapter:

- NCLEX-Style Questions and Other Resources on the**Point**, http://thePoint.lww.com/PorthEssentials4e
- Study Guide for Essentials of Pathophysiology
- Concepts in Action Animations
- Adaptive Learning | Powered by PrepU, http://thepoint.lww.com/prepu

C h a p t e r 25

Disorders of Renal Function

The kidneys are subject to many of the same disease processes that affect other organs, including genetic and developmental defects, infections, immunologic disorders, and neoplasms. Although many disorders of renal function originate in the kidneys, others develop secondary to diseases such as systemic lupus erythematosus and diabetes mellitus. Some of these diseases are progressive, eventually leading to chronic kidney disease and the need for dialysis or transplantation. As a major cause of work loss, physicians' visits, and hospitalizations, kidney diseases remain among the most costly illnesses throughout the industrial world.

The content in this chapter focuses on congenital and hereditary disorders of the kidney, disorders of glomerular function, tubulointerstitial disorders, obstructive disorders, and malignant neoplasms. Acute renal injury and failure and chronic kidney disease are discussed in Chapter 26, and disorders that predominantly affect the lower urinary tract and bladder are discussed in Chapter 27.

Congenital and Hereditary Disorders of the Kidney

The kidneys begin to develop early in the fifth week of gestation and start to function approximately four weeks later.[1] Urine formation begins at about the ninth week of gestation, with the rate of urine production increasing throughout gestation to reach a volume of about 50 mL/hour at term.[2] The urine that is produced is excreted into the amniotic cavity and is the main constituent of amniotic fluid. In pregnancies that involve infants with nonfunctional kidneys or obstruction of urine outflow from the kidneys, the amount of amniotic fluid is small—a condition called *oligohydramnios*.[2,3]

Disorders of Kidney Development

About 10% of all people are born with potentially significant malformations of the urinary system.[4] These disorders sometimes result from hereditary influences, but most often are the result of an acquired defect that arises during embryonic development.

Agenesis, Hypoplasia, and Dysplasia

Defects in development of renal structures are frequently observed during the 1st year of life, when they collectively represent a significant cause of morbidity and mortality. Renal agenesis, hypogenesis, and dysplasia account for a significant portion of these defects.[3]

Renal Agenesis. The term *agenesis* refers to the complete failure of an organ to develop. Total agenesis of both kidneys is incompatible with extrauterine life. Infants are stillborn or die shortly after birth. Newborns with renal agenesis often have characteristic facial features, called *Potter syndrome*, that are caused by fetal compression due to a marked reduction in amniotic fluid levels.[1,2,4] The eyes are widely separated and have epicanthic folds, the ears are set low, the nose is broad and flat, and the chin is receding. The most life-threatening component of Potter syndrome is *pulmonary hypoplasia*, which is caused by inadequate stimulation from the amniotic fluid and by compression of the chest wall. Bilateral renal agenesis, which has an incidence of 1 in 3000 births with a male predominance, is usually suspected when maternal ultrasonography demonstrates oligohydramnios, nonvisualization of the bladder, and absent kidneys.[2]

Unilateral agenesis is more common than bilateral agenesis and is compatible with life if no other abnormality is present. The opposite kidney usually is enlarged as a result of compensatory hypertrophy. The disorder frequently goes undetected, unless discovered by chance observation on prenatal ultrasound.

Renal Hypoplasia. In *renal hypoplasia*, the kidneys are small in size and have less than the normal number of calyces and nephrons. Hypoplasia may affect one or both kidneys.[2–4] When unilateral, the condition is usually discovered during examination for another urinary tract problem or hypertension. When both kidneys are affected, there is progressive development of renal failure. A history of polyuria and polydipsia is common.

Renal Dysplasia. A developmental disorder, renal dysplasia, is characterized by maldifferentiated primitive structures, primarily of the renal tubules. The condition can affect all or only part of the kidney. If the entire kidney is affected with multiple cysts, the condition is referred to as a *multicystic dysplastic kidney disorder (MCDK)*.[2–4] Bilateral MCDKs cause oligohydramnios and Potter syndrome and are incompatible with life.

Multicystic dysplastic kidney disorder is generally unilateral.[2] In most children with MCDK, a palpable mass is discovered shortly after birth, although small multicystic kidneys may not be apparent until years later. Management is controversial, with complete cyst regression occurring in nearly half of children by age 7 years.[2] The risk of hypertension and Wilms tumors of the affected kidney is approximately 1 in 333.[2] Because of the risk of these neoplasms, annual follow-up with sonography and blood pressure measurement is usually recommended. The most important aspect of follow-up is to make certain that the unaffected kidney is functioning properly.

Alterations in Kidney Position and Form

During embryonic life, the kidneys can develop in an abnormal location, usually just above the pelvic rim or within the pelvis. Because of the abnormal position, kinking of the ureters and obstruction of urine flow may occur.

One of the most common alterations in kidney form is an abnormality called a *horseshoe kidney*. This abnormality occurs in approximately 1 in every 500 to 1000 persons.[4,5] In this disorder, the upper or lower poles of the two kidneys are fused, producing a horseshoe-shape structure that is continuous along the midline of the body anterior to the great vessels. Most horseshoe kidneys are fused at the lower poles (Fig. 25-1). The condition usually does not cause problems because its collecting system develops normally and the ureters enter the bladder.[1] If urinary flow is impeded, signs and symptoms and/or infection may appear.

Cystic Diseases of the Kidney

Renal cysts are epithelium-lined cavities filled with fluid or semisolid material. The cysts may be single or multiple, can vary in size from microscopic to several centimeters in diameter, and can be symptomatic or asymptomatic. Although they may arise as a developmental abnormality or be acquired later in life, most forms are hereditary.[4,5] The inherited cystic kidney diseases, which are single-gene disorders and are inherited as mendelian traits, include autosomal dominant polycystic kidney disease,

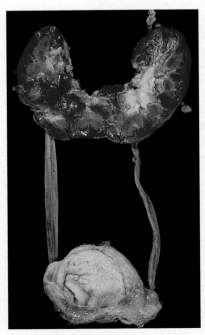

FIGURE 25-1. Horseshoe kidney. The kidneys are fused at the lower pole. (From Jennette JC. The kidney. In: Rubin R, Strayer DS, eds. *Rubin's Pathology: Clinicopathologic Foundations of Medicine*. 6th ed. Philadelphia, PA: Wolters Kluwer Health | Lippincott Williams & Wilkins; 2012:757.)

autosomal recessive polycystic kidney disease, and nephronophthisis and medullary cystic kidney diseases.

Autosomal Dominant Polycystic Kidney Disease

Autosomal dominant (adult) polycystic kidney disease (ADPKD) is the most common of all inherited kidney diseases, with 600,000 to 700,000 cases in the United States and about 12.5 million cases worldwide.[6] About 5000 to 6000 new cases are diagnosed in the United States each year, about 40% before the age of 45.[6] About 5% to 10% of these persons develop chronic kidney disease that requires dialysis or kidney transplant.[5]

The disorder is characterized by multiple expanding cysts of both kidneys that ultimately destroy the surrounding kidney structures and cause renal failure (Fig. 25-2A). There are two genetic forms of ADPKD: polycystin-1I which is caused by mutations in the *PKD1* gene and accounts for 85% of cases; and polycystin-2, which is caused by mutations in the *PKD2* gene and accounts for most of the remaining 15% of cases.[4–8] Although the two mutations produce almost identical renal and extrarenal disease, disease progression is typically more rapid in people with the *PKD1* gene.

Recent research suggests that the products of the polycystin genes are transmembrane proteins found on the primary cilia that line the apical surface of the tubular epithelial cells of the kidney. Because the cilia project out and above the tubular cell surface like antennas, they are currently thought to act as sensors of urinary flow and as signal transducers for tubular cell proliferation, differentiation, and apoptosis.[9] The polycystin genes also regulate vascular development in other organs such as the liver, brain, and pancreas, accounting for the extrarenal manifestations that often accompany the disorder.

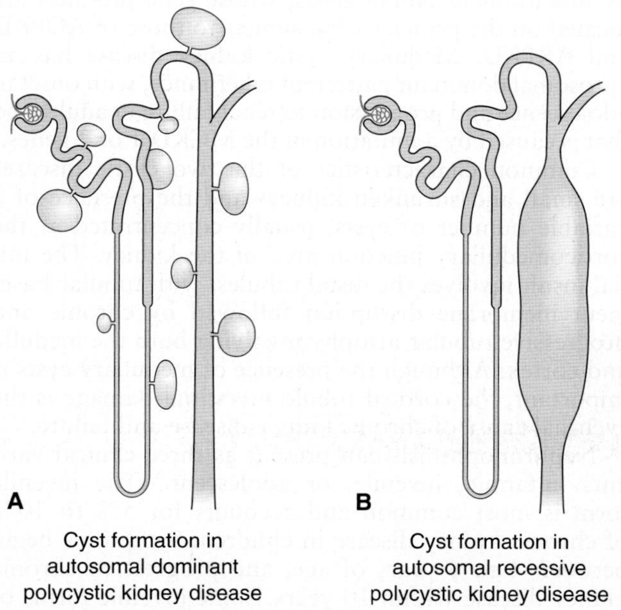

In ADPKD, cysts in the kidney increase in size over time, ultimately destroying normal renal tissue. The kidneys are usually enlarged and may achieve enormous sizes (Fig. 25-3). The external contours of the kidneys are distorted by numerous cysts, some as large as 5 cm in diameter, filled with straw-colored fluid.[5] Cysts also may be found in the liver and, less commonly, the pancreas and spleen. Hepatic cysts, which occur in one third of persons with ADPKD, are generally asymptomatic and liver function is normal.[5] Mitral valve prolapse and other valvular abnormalities are found in 20% to 25% of people, but most are asymptomatic. One of the most devastating extrarenal manifestations is a weakness in the walls of the cerebral arteries that can lead to aneurysm formation. It has been estimated that persons with ADPKD who have a family member with ADPKD and a history of intracranial aneurysm or cerebral hemorrhage have a 20% chance of developing an intracranial aneurysm.[6]

The manifestations of ADPKD include pain from the enlarging cysts that may reach debilitating levels, episodes of gross hematuria from bleeding into a cyst, infected cysts from ascending UTIs, and hypertension resulting from compression of intrarenal blood vessels with activation of the renin-angiotensin mechanism.[4,5] Renal colic caused by nephrolithiasis, or kidney stones, occurs in about 20% of persons with ADPKD.[6] The progress of the disease is slow, and chronic kidney disease is uncommon before 40 years of age.

Ultrasonography usually is the preferred technique for the diagnosis of ADPKD in symptomatic patients and for screening of asymptomatic family members. Computed tomography (CT) may be used for detection of small cysts. Genetic linkage studies are now available

A

Cyst formation in autosomal dominant polycystic kidney disease

B

Cyst formation in autosomal recessive polycystic kidney disease

FIGURE 25-2. Mechanism of cyst formation in polycystic kidney disease. **(A)** In autosomal dominant polycystic kidney disease, cystic outpouchings arise in every tubule segment and rapidly close off the nephron of origin. **(B)** In autosomal recessive polycystic kidney disease, cysts are derived from collecting tubules, which remain connected to the nephron of origin. (From Wilson PD. Polycystic kidney disease. *N Engl J Med.* 2004;350:155. Copyright © 2004. Massachusetts Medical Society.)

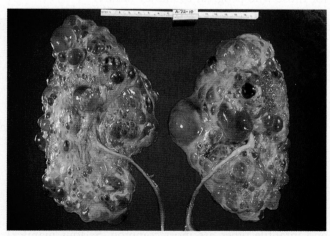

FIGURE 25-3. Gross pathology of polycystic kidneys. (From the Centers for Disease Control and Prevention Public Health Images Library. No. 861. Courtesy of Edwin P. Ewing, Jr).

for diagnosis of ADPKD, but are usually reserved for cases in which radiographic imaging is negative and the need for a definitive diagnosis is essential, such as when screening family members for potential kidney donation. Magnetic resonance angiography is recommended for persons who have a family history of cerebral aneurysm or stroke and for those with new-onset or severe headache.

The treatment of ADPKD is largely supportive and aimed at delaying progression of the disease. Control of hypertension and prevention of ascending UTIs are important. Pain is a common complaint of persons with ADPKD, and a systematic approach is needed to differentiate the etiology of the pain and define an approach for management.

Cyclic adenosine monophosphate (cAMP) has been shown to increase proliferation of epithelial cells in cyst walls and the rate of fluid secretion into cysts. One of the prime mediators of cell proliferation, acting through cAMP, is *arginine vasopressin* (AVP), also known as the *antidiuretic hormone*. In studies using genetically produced polycystic animals, the use of vasopressin V2 receptor inhibitors reduced cyst growth and preserved renal function. Because an increase in urine osmolality serves to increase vasopressin levels, it is often recommended that persons with ADPKD drink approximately 3000 L of water throughout the waking hours to reduce plasma AVP levels.[6,7] Normally cAMP is broken down by phosphodiesterases. Because caffeine raises cAMP levels by interfering with phosphodiesterase activity, it is also recommended that caffeinated beverages be avoided.[6,7]

In addition to increasing water intake to decrease vasopressin levels, the angiotensin-converting enzyme (ACE) inhibitors or angiotensin II receptor blockers (ARBs) may be used to interrupt the renin-angiotensin-aldosterone system as a means of reducing intraglomerular pressure and renal vasoconstriction. Although not approved by the Food and Drug Administration (FDA), there has been recent interest in the use of vasopressin receptor antagonists (vaptans) to decrease cyst development.[9] Dialysis and kidney transplantation are reserved for those who progress to kidney failure.

Autosomal Recessive Polycystic Kidney Disease

Autosomal recessive (childhood) polycystic kidney disease (ARPKD) is characterized by cystic dilation of the cortical and medullary collecting tubules[3–5] (see Fig. 25-2B). It is rare compared with ADPKD, occurring in 1 to 20,000 live births. Autosomal recessive (childhood) polycystic kidney disease is caused by mutations in the *PKHD1* gene. The gene product, fibrocystin, is found in the collecting ducts of the kidney, biliary ducts of the liver, and exocrine ducts of the pancreas, and appears to be involved in the regulation of cell proliferation and adhesion. Perinatal, neonatal, infantile, and juvenile subcategories have been defined, dependent on time of presentation. The perinatal and infantile types are most common. Serious manifestations are usually present at birth, with the infant progressing rapidly into renal failure.

The typical infant with ARPKD presents with bilateral flank masses, accompanied by severe renal failure, signs of impaired lung development, and variable degrees of liver fibrosis and portal hypertension. Potter facies and other defects associated with oligohydramnios may be present. Hypertension is usually noted within the first few weeks of life and is often severe. Approximately 75% of infants die during the perinatal period, often of pulmonary hypoplasia.[3] Children and juveniles who survive infancy develop a distinctive type of liver fibrosis. In older children, liver disease is the predominant clinical concern.

The treatment of ARPKD is largely supportive. Aggressive ventilatory support is often necessary in the neonatal period because of pulmonary hypoplasia and hypoventilation. Modern neonatal respiratory technology and renal replacement therapy (e.g., dialysis and kidney transplant) have increased the 10-year survival rate of children surviving beyond the 1st year of life. Morbidity and mortality in the older child is related to complications of kidney failure and liver disease.

Nephronophthisis and Medullary Cystic Kidney Disease

Nephronophthisis and adult-onset medullary cystic kidney disease both produce progressive medullary tubulointerstitial cystic disease, but vary in terms of genetic causes and patterns of inheritance.[4,5] Nephronophthisis has an autosomal recessive pattern of inheritance with onset in infancy, childhood, or adolescence. It is caused by mutations in NPHP genes, whose gene products are located on the primary cilia, similar to those of ADPKD and ARPKD. Medullary cystic kidney disease has an autosomal dominant pattern of inheritance, with onset in adolescence and progression to renal failure in adulthood that is caused by a mutation in the MCKD 1 or 2 genes.[4]

Common characteristics of the two cystic diseases are small and shrunken kidneys and the presence of a variable number of cysts, usually concentrated at the corticomedullary junction area of the kidney. The initial insult involves the distal tubules, with tubular basement membrane disruption followed by chronic and progressive tubular atrophy involving both the medulla and cortex. Although the presence of medullary cysts is important, the cortical tubulointerstitial damage is the eventual cause of chronic kidney disease and failure.[5]

Nephronophthisis can present as three clinical variants: infantile, juvenile, or adolescent.[4] The juvenile form is most common and accounts for 5% to 10% of chronic kidney disease in children. Symptoms begin between 4 to 6 years of age, and progress to chronic kidney disease within 10 years. Some juvenile forms of nephronophthisis have extrarenal complications, including ocular motor abnormalities, retinitis pigmentosa, liver fibrosis, and cerebellar abnormalities. The onset and progression of the adolescent form causes chronic kidney failure at 10 to 20 years of age, and the infantile form before 2 years of age.

Children with nephronophthisis and adults with medullary cystic kidney disease present first with polyuria, polydipsia, and enuresis (bed-wetting), which reflect impaired ability of the kidneys to concentrate urine. Other manifestations of the disorders include salt wasting, growth retardation, anemia, and progressive renal insufficiency.

Simple and Acquired Renal Cysts

Simple cysts are a common acquired disorder of the kidney. The cysts may be single or multiple, unilateral or bilateral, and they are commonly 1 to 5 cm in diameter, but may reach 10 cm or more. The cysts usually are confined to the cortex. In rare instances, massive cysts as large as 10 cm in diameter are encountered.[4,5] Most simple cysts do not produce signs or symptoms or compromise renal function. When symptomatic, they may cause flank pain, hematuria, infection, and hypertension related to ischemia-produced stimulation of the renin-angiotensin system. They are most common in persons older than 50 years. Although the cysts are benign, the main concern is to differentiate them from renal cell carcinoma. Ultrasound and CT scanning are the recommended procedures for evaluating these masses.[4,5]

An acquired form of renal cystic disease occurs in persons with chronic kidney disease who have undergone prolonged dialysis treatment.[4] Although the condition is largely asymptomatic, the cysts may bleed, causing hematuria. Tumors, usually adenomas but occasionally adenosarcomas, may develop in the walls of these cysts.

 SUMMARY CONCEPTS

■ Congenital abnormalities of the kidney include *agenesis* or failure of the kidneys to develop, which is incompatible with life if both kidneys are affected; *hypogenesis* or failure of the kidneys to develop to normal size, which usually causes no problems unless both kidneys are affected; and *renal dysplasia*, which is characterized by disorganized and maldifferentiated development of kidney tissue, usually accompanied by cyst formation. Other developmental kidney defects can result in kidneys that lie outside their normal position or are fused to form horseshoe-shaped kidneys.

■ Cystic diseases of the kidney are hereditary and nonhereditary disorders in which there is dilation of tubular structures with cyst formation.

■ There are two forms of polycystic kidney disease: *autosomal dominant* (ADPKD) and *autosomal recessive* (ARPKD). Autosomal dominant (adult) polycystic kidney disease results in the formation of numerous fluid-filled cysts in the tubular structures of both kidneys with the threat of progression to chronic kidney disease. ARPKD,

which is rare compared with ADPKD and usually presents as severe renal dysfunction during infancy, is characterized by cystic transformation of the collecting ducts.

■ Nephronophthisis and adult-onset medullary cystic kidney disease are characterized by the presence of similar progressive medullary cystic disease, but with different genetic causes and inheritance. *Nephronophthisis* is an autosomal recessive disorder, with onset in infancy, childhood, or adolescence; whereas *adult-onset medullary cystic disease* is an autosomal dominant disorder with onset in adolescence and renal failure in adulthood.

■ Simple cysts are an acquired disorder of the kidney. They may be single or multiple, unilateral or bilateral, and are commonly 1 to 5 cm in diameter. Although the cysts are benign, the main concern is to differentiate them from malignancies.

Disorders of Glomerular Function

Glomerular disorders are one of the most common forms of kidney disease. The glomeruli may be the major site of disease (primary glomerular disease) or part of a disease affecting other organs (secondary glomerular disease). Hereditary glomerular diseases such as Alport syndrome, although relatively rare, are an important category of glomerular disease because of their association with progressive loss of renal function and transmission to future generations.

Etiology and Pathogenesis of Glomerular Injury

Many of the clinical manifestations of glomerular disorders result from dysfunction of specific components of the glomeruli, which consist of a network of capillaries, lined with a fenestrated endothelium invested in two layers of epithelium (Fig. 25-4A). The visceral epithelium is incorporated into and becomes an intricate part of the capillary wall, separated from the endothelium by a basement membrane.[4,5] The parietal epithelium, which lines Bowman space within which urine collects, is attached to the basement membrane by long, footlike processes (*podocytes*) that encircle the outer surface of the capillaries. The glomerular capillary membrane is selectively permeable, allowing water and small particles (e.g., electrolytes and dissolved particles, such as glucose and amino acids) to leave the blood and enter the Bowman space while preventing larger particles (e.g., plasma proteins and blood cells) from leaving the blood.

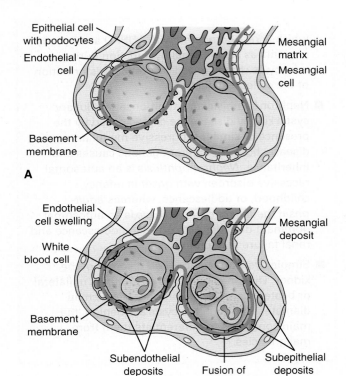

Epithelial cell with podocytes
Endothelial cell
Mesangial matrix
Mesangial cell
Basement membrane

A

Endothelial cell swelling
White blood cell
Mesangial deposit
Basement membrane
Subendothelial deposits
Fusion of epithelial cell podocytes
Subepithelial deposits

B

FIGURE 25-4. (A) Normal. **(B)** Localization of immune deposits (mesangial, subendothelial, subepithelial) and changes in glomerular architecture associated with injury.

The agents or events that trigger glomerular injury include infectious microorganisms, immunologic mechanisms, drugs, and environmental agents.[4,5,10–13] Most cases of primary and many cases of secondary glomerular disease probably have an immune origin. Although many glomerular diseases are driven by immunologic events, a variety of metabolic (e.g., diabetes), hemodynamic (e.g., hypertension), and toxic (e.g., drugs, chemicals) stresses can induce glomerular injury, either alone or in concert with immunologic mechanisms.

Two types of immune mechanisms have been implicated in the development of glomerular disease: (1) injury resulting from antibodies reacting with fixed glomerular antigens or antigens planted within the glomerulus and (2) injury resulting from circulating antigen–antibody complexes that become trapped in the glomerular membrane[4,5,12] (Fig. 25-5). Antigens responsible for development of the immune response may be of endogenous origin, such as autoantibodies to deoxyribonucleic acid (DNA) in systemic lupus erythematosus (SLE), or they may be of exogenous origin, such as streptococcal membrane antigens in poststreptococcal glomerulonephritis. Frequently, the source of the antigen is unknown.

Glomerular diseases have traditionally been named according to tissue appearance (i.e., proliferative, membranous, or sclerotic) rather than according to the underlying cause. Accordingly, the term *proliferative* is used to describe a hypercellular inflammatory process with proliferation of glomerular cells; *membranous,* an abnormal thickening of the glomerular basement membrane; and *sclerotic,* an increase in the amount of extracellular material in the mesangial, subendothelial, or subepithelial tissue of the glomerulus.[4,10] Glomerular changes can be *diffuse,* involving all glomeruli and all parts of the glomeruli; *focal,* in which only some glomeruli are affected and others are essentially normal; *segmental,* involving only a certain segment of each glomerulus; or *mesangial,* affecting only mesangial cells. Figure 25-4B illustrates the location of lesions associated with various types of glomerular disease.

Dependent upon the structures involved and the extent of their involvement, glomerular disorders can manifest with hematuria (red cells in the urine), proteinuria (protein in the urine), and the presence or absence of hypertension; azotemia (elevation of blood urea nitrogen); or renal insufficiency. The *nephritic syndrome* is due to glomerular disease that is usually of acute onset and is accompanied by grossly visible hematuria, mild to moderate proteinuria, and hypertension. The *nephrotic syndrome,* also due to glomerular disease, is characterized by heavy proteinuria, hypoalbuminemia, and severe edema.

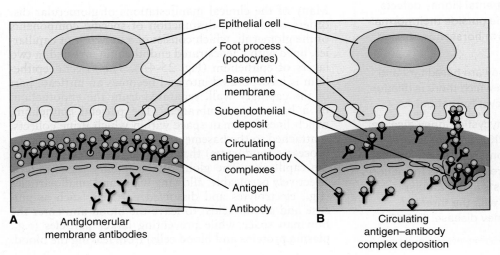

Epithelial cell
Foot process (podocytes)
Basement membrane
Subendothelial deposit
Circulating antigen–antibody complexes
Antigen
Antibody

A Antiglomerular membrane antibodies

B Circulating antigen–antibody complex deposition

FIGURE 25-5. Immune mechanisms of glomerular disease. **(A)** Antiglomerular membrane antibodies leave the circulation and interact with antigens that are present in the basement membrane of the glomerulus. **(B)** Antigen–antibody complexes circulating in the blood become trapped as they are filtered in the glomerulus.

Types of Glomerular Disease

The clinical manifestations of glomerular disorders generally fall into several categories: acute nephritic syndromes, rapidly progressive glomerulonephritis, nephrotic syndrome, IgA nephropathy, hereditary nephritis (e.g., Alport syndrome), and chronic glomerulonephritis.[4,5,10–13] The nephritic syndromes produce a proliferative inflammatory response, whereas the nephrotic syndrome produces increased permeability of the glomerulus. Because most glomerular disorders can produce mixed nephritic and nephrotic syndromes, a definitive diagnosis often requires renal biopsy.

Many cases of glomerular disease result in mild asymptomatic illness that is not recognized or is brought to the attention of a health care professional during routine screening or physical examination for another purpose. Disorders such as IgA nephropathy and Alport syndrome often present with asymptomatic hematuria and/or proteinuria.

Acute Nephritic Syndrome

Acute nephritic syndrome is an acute inflammatory process that occludes the glomerular capillary lumen and damages the capillary wall. It may occur as a renal-limited primary disorder, such as acute postinfectious glomerulonephritis, or as a secondary complicating disorder in systemic diseases, such as SLE. In its most dramatic form, acute nephritic syndrome is characterized by sudden onset of hematuria (either microscopic or grossly visible, with red cell casts), variable degrees of proteinuria, diminished glomerular filtration rate (GFR), oliguria, and signs of impaired renal function. Extracellular fluid accumulation, edema, and hypertension develop because of the decreased GFR and enhanced tubular reabsorption of salt and water.

Acute Postinfectious Glomerulonephritis. Acute postinfectious glomerulonephritis usually occurs after infection with certain strains of group A β-hemolytic streptococci and is caused by deposition of immune complexes.[4,5,10,14] It also may occur after infections by other organisms, including staphylococci and a number of viral agents, such as those responsible for mumps, measles, and chickenpox.[4] This type of glomerular disease is now rare in industrialized nations, but continues to be a common disorder in the underprivileged populations of the world.[5] Although the disease is seen primarily in children, persons of any age can be affected.

The acute phase of postinfectious glomerulonephritis is characterized by diffuse glomerular enlargement and hypercellularity. The hypercellularity is caused by infiltration of leukocytes, both neutrophils and monocytes; proliferation of endothelial and mesangial cells; and formation of electron-dense subepithelial deposits, often having the appearance of "humps" (see Fig. 25-4B). There is also swelling of the endothelial cells, and the combination of proliferation, swelling, and leukocyte infiltration obliterates the glomerular capillary lumens. On immunofluorescence microscopy there are granular deposits of immunoglobulin G (IgG) and

the complement component C3 in the mesangium and along the basement membrane (Fig. 25-6).

The classic case of poststreptococcal glomerulonephritis follows a streptococcal infection by approximately 7 to 12 days—the time needed for the development of antibodies. The primary infection usually involves the pharynx (pharyngitis), but can also result from a skin infection (impetigo). Oliguria, which develops as the GFR decreases, is one of the first symptoms. Proteinuria and hematuria follow because of increased glomerular capillary wall permeability. The red blood cells are degraded by materials in the urine, and cola-colored urine may be the first sign of the disorder. Sodium and water retention gives rise to edema (particularly of the face and hands) and hypertension. Important laboratory findings include an elevated antistreptococcal antibody (ASO) titer, a decline in serum concentrations of C3 and other components of the complement cascade, and cryoglobulins (i.e., large immune complexes) in the serum.

Treatment of acute poststreptococcal glomerulonephritis includes eliminating the streptococcal infection with antibiotics and providing supportive care. The disorder generally carries an excellent prognosis and rarely causes chronic kidney disease. In children, spontaneous resolution of the glomerular lesion and nephritic syndrome is usually the norm and occurs within 6 to 8 weeks. Adults tend to recover more slowly, often with some degree of persistent azotemia that may, in some cases, progress to chronic kidney disease.

Rapidly Progressive Glomerulonephritis

Rapidly progressive glomerulonephritis is a clinical syndrome characterized by signs of severe glomerular injury that does not have a specific cause. As its name indicates, this type of glomerulonephritis is rapidly progressive,

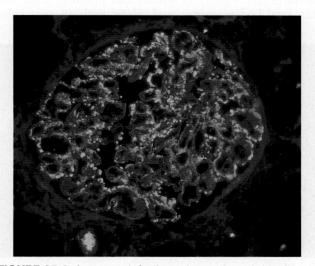

FIGURE 25-6. Acute postinfectious glomerulonephritis. An immunofluorescence micrograph demonstrates granular staining for complement C3 in capillary walls and the mesangium. (From Jennette JC. The kidney. In: Rubin R, Strayer DS, eds. *Rubin's Pathology: Clinicopathologic Foundations of Medicine.* 6th ed. Philadelphia, PA: Wolters Kluwer Health | Lippincott Williams & Wilkins; 2012:776.)

often within a matter of months. The disorder involves focal and segmental proliferation of glomerular cells and recruitment of monocytes and macrophages with the formation of crescent structures that obliterate the Bowman space.[5] Rapidly proliferative glomerulonephritis may be caused by a number of immunologic disorders, some systemic and others restricted to the kidney. Among the diseases associated with this form of glomerulonephritis are immune complex disorders such as SLE, and an aggressive form of glomerulonephritis called *Goodpasture syndrome.*

Goodpasture Syndrome. An uncommon and aggressive form of glomerulonephritis, Goodpasture syndrome is caused by antibodies to the glomerular basement membrane (GBM). The anti–glomerular membrane (anti-GBM) antibodies cross-react with the pulmonary alveolar basement membrane to produce the syndrome of pulmonary hemorrhage associated with renal failure. The pathologic hallmark of anti-GBM glomerulonephritis is diffuse linear staining of glomerular basement membranes for IgG (Fig. 25-7). The cause of the disorder is unknown, although influenza infection and exposure to hydrocarbon solvent (found in paints and dyes) have been implicated in some persons, as have various drugs and cancers. There is a high prevalence of certain human leukocyte antigen subtypes (e.g., HLA-DRB1) in those affected, suggesting a genetic predisposition.[4] Treatment includes plasmapheresis to remove circulating anti-GBM antibodies and immunosuppressive therapy (i.e., corticosteroids and cyclophosphamide) to inhibit antibody production.

Nephrotic Syndrome

The nephrotic syndrome is characterized by massive proteinuria (≥3.5 g/day in adults) and lipiduria (e.g., free fat, oval bodies, fatty casts), along with an associated

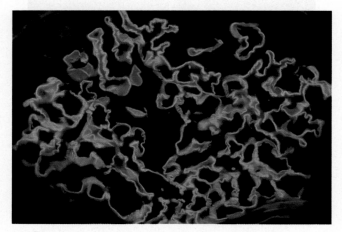

FIGURE 25-7. Anti–glomerular basement membrane glomerulonephritis. Linear immunofluorescence for IgG is seen along the glomerular basement membrane. (From Jennette JC. The kidney. In: Rubin R, Strayer DS, eds. *Rubin's Pathology: Clinicopathologic Foundations of Medicine.* 6th ed. Philadelphia, PA: Wolters Kluwer Health | Lippincott Williams & Wilkins; 2012:782.)

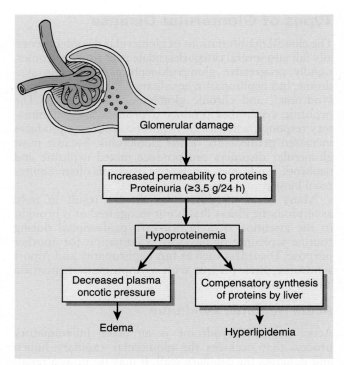

FIGURE 25-8. Pathophysiology of the nephrotic syndrome.

hypoalbuminemia (<3 g/dL), generalized edema, and hyperlipidemia.[4,5,10] The nephrotic syndrome is not a specific glomerular disease, but a constellation of clinical findings that result from an increase in glomerular permeability and loss of plasma proteins in the urine (Fig. 25-8).

The glomerular membrane acts as a size-specific barrier through which the glomerular filtrate must pass. An increase in permeability allows proteins to escape from the plasma into the glomerular filtrate, often leading to an excessive loss of albumin—the smallest and most abundant of the plasma proteins. Generalized edema, which is a hallmark of the nephrotic syndrome, results from a decrease in the plasma colloidal osmotic pressure due to the hypoalbuminemia that develops as albumin is lost from the vascular compartment (see Chapter 8). There is also salt and water retention, which aggravates the edema. Initially, the edema presents in dependent parts of the body such as the lower extremities, but becomes more generalized as the disease progresses (Fig. 25-9). Dyspnea due to pulmonary edema, pleural effusions, and diaphragmatic compromise due to ascites can develop in persons with nephrotic syndrome.

The hyperlipidemia that occurs in persons with nephrosis is characterized by elevated levels of triglycerides and low-density lipoproteins (LDLs). Levels of high-density lipoproteins (HDLs) usually are normal. It is thought that these abnormalities are related, at least in part, to increased synthesis of lipoproteins in the liver secondary to a compensatory increase in albumin production.[13] Because of the elevated LDL levels, persons with nephrotic syndrome are at increased risk for development of atherosclerosis.

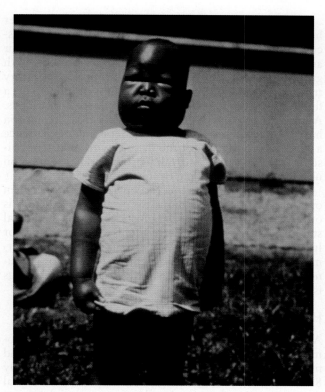

FIGURE 25-9. Photo of an African child with nephrosis associated with malaria. (From the Centers for Disease Control and Prevention Public Health Images Library. No. 3894. Courtesy of Myron Schultz.)

The largest proportion of protein lost in the urine is albumin, but globulins also may be lost. As a result, persons with nephrosis are often vulnerable to infections, particularly those caused by staphylococci and pneumococci.[4] This decreased resistance to infection probably is related to the loss of both immunoglobulins and low–molecular-weight complement components in the urine. Many binding proteins also are lost in the urine. Consequently, the plasma levels of many ions (iron, copper, zinc) and hormones (thyroid and sex hormones) may be low. Many drugs require protein binding for transport. Hypoalbuminemia reduces the number of available protein-binding sites, thereby producing a potential increase in the amount of free (active) drug that is available.

Persons with nephrotic syndrome are also at risk for thrombotic complications. These complications reflect a disruption in the function of the coagulation system brought about by a loss of coagulation and anticoagulation factors in the urine. Renal vein thrombosis, once thought to be a cause of the disorder, is more likely a consequence of the hypercoagulable state. Other thrombotic complications include deep vein thrombosis and pulmonary emboli.

The glomerular derangements that occur with nephrosis can develop as a primary disorder or secondary to changes caused by systemic diseases such as diabetes mellitus and SLE.[4,5] Among the primary glomerular lesions leading to nephrotic syndrome are minimal-change

disease (lipoid nephrosis), focal segmental glomerulosclerosis, and membranous glomerulonephritis. The relative frequency of these causes varies with age. In children younger than 15 years of age, nephrotic syndrome almost always is caused by primary idiopathic glomerular disease, whereas in adults it often is a secondary disorder.[4]

Minimal-Change Disease (Lipoid Nephrosis). Minimal-change disease is characterized by diffuse loss (through fusion) of the podocytes or foot processes of the visceral epithelial cells of the glomeruli. It is most commonly seen in children (peak incidence at 2 to 6 years of age),[5] but may occasionally occur in adults. Although the cause of minimal-change disease is unknown; children in whom the disease develops often have a history of recent upper respiratory infections or of receiving routine childhood immunizations.[4] Minimal-change disease does not usually progress to renal failure, but can cause significant complications, including predisposition to infection with gram-positive organisms, tendency toward thromboembolic events, hyperlipidemia, and protein malnutrition. The prognosis in children with the disorder is good; more than 90% respond to a short course of glucocorticoids. Adults also respond to corticosteroids, but the response is slower.[4]

Membranous Glomerulonephritis. Membranous glomerulonephritis is the most common cause of primary nephrosis in adults.[5,10,11] The disorder is caused by diffuse thickening of the glomerular basement membrane due to deposition of immune complexes. The disorder may be idiopathic or associated with a number of disorders, including autoimmune diseases such as SLE, infections such as chronic hepatitis B, metabolic disorders such as diabetes mellitus and thyroiditis, and use of certain drugs such as gold compounds, penicillamine, and captopril.[5]

The disorder usually begins with an insidious onset of the nephrotic syndrome with peripheral edema, hypoalbuminemia, and hyperlipidemia or, in a small percentage of patients, with nonnephrotic proteinuria. Hematuria and mild hypertension may be present. The progress of the disease is variable, with less than 40% eventually developing renal insufficiency. Spontaneous remissions and a relatively benign outcome occur more commonly in women and those with proteinuria in the nonnephrotic range. Treatment is controversial. Because of the variable course of the disease, the overall effectiveness of corticosteroids and other immunosuppressive therapy in controlling the progress of the disease has been difficult to evaluate.[5,10]

Focal Segmental Glomerulosclerosis. Focal segmental glomerulosclerosis (FSGS) is characterized by sclerosis (i.e., increased collagen deposition) in some but not all glomeruli. Moreover, in the affected glomeruli, only a portion of the glomerular tuft is involved.[4,5,10,11,15] Focal segmental glomerulosclerosis causes 30% of primary nephrotic syndrome in adults and 10% in children. It is more common in blacks than whites and is the leading cause of primary nephrotic syndrome in African Americans.[5]

Focal segmental glomerulosclerosis can be viewed as a heterogeneous group of glomerular diseases with different causes, pathologies, and outcomes. The disorder may be idiopathic (primary) or occur secondary to reduced oxygen in the blood (e.g., sickle cell disease and cyanotic congenital heart disease), human immunodeficiency virus (HIV) infection, or intravenous drug abuse.[4,5] It can also occur as a secondary event reflecting scarring from other glomerular disorders, such as IgA nephropathy. There is also evidence of a genetic basis for some cases of the disorder. Multiple factors probably lead to a common pathway of injury.

Clinical presentations and outcomes vary among the different patterns of injury. Most people with the disorder show persistent proteinuria and progressive decline in renal function. Many persons with the disorder progress to kidney failure within 5 to 20 years.[5] The disorder usually is treated with corticosteroids. Although kidney transplantation is the preferred treatment for end-stage kidney disease, focal segmental glomerulonephritis occurs in half of these people.

IgA Nephropathy

IgA nephropathy (i.e., Berger disease) is a primary glomerulonephritis characterized by the presence of glomerular IgA immune complex deposits. It can occur at any age, but most commonly has its onset in the second and third decades of life.[4,5,10,16,17] The disease occurs more commonly in men than women and is the most common cause of glomerular nephritis in Asians.

The disorder is characterized by the deposition of IgA-containing immune complexes in the mesangium of the glomerulus (Fig. 25-10). Once deposited in the kidney, the immune complexes are associated with glomerular inflammation. The cause of the disorder is unknown. Some people with the disorder have elevated serum IgA levels. Recent studies have focused on potential abnormalities of the IgA molecule as a factor in the pathogenesis of the disorder.[16]

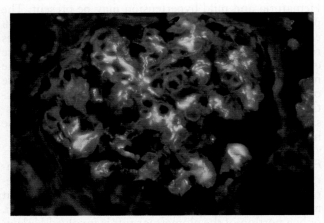

FIGURE 25-10. IgA nephropathy. An immunofluorescence micrograph shows deposits of IgA in the mesangial areas. (From Jennette JC. The kidney. In: Rubin R, Strayer D, eds. *Rubin's Pathology: Clinicopathologic Foundations of Medicine.* 6th ed. Philadelphia, PA: Wolters Kluwer Health | Lippincott Williams & Wilkins; 2012:781.)

Early in the disease, many people with the disorder have no obvious symptoms and the disorder is discovered during routine screening or examination for another condition. In others, the disorder presents with gross hematuria that is preceded by upper respiratory tract infection, gastrointestinal tract symptoms, or a flulike illness. The hematuria usually lasts 2 to 6 days. Approximately one half of those with gross hematuria have a single episode, whereas the remainder experience a gradual progression of the disease with recurrent episodes of hematuria and mild proteinuria. Progression usually is slow, extending over several decades.

Immunofluorescence microscopy, using a specimen obtained through renal biopsy, is essential for diagnosis of IgA nephropathy.[5] The diagnostic finding is mesangial staining for IgA that is more intense than staining for IgG or IgM. At present, there are no satisfactory treatment measures for IgA nephropathy. The role of immunosuppressive drugs such as steroids and cytotoxic drugs is not clear.

Hereditary Nephritis (Alport Syndrome)

Alport syndrome represents a hereditary defect of the glomerular basement membrane that results in hematuria and may progress to chronic renal failure.[4,5] Approximately 85% of cases are inherited as an X-linked autosomal dominant trait, whereas others have autosomal dominant and recessive patterns of inheritance.[5] In X-linked pedigrees, boys are usually affected more seriously than girls. Affected boys usually progress to renal failure as adults, but progression may occur during adolescence. Although many girls never have more than mild hematuria with or without mild proteinuria, some have more significant disease and may even progress to kidney failure.

Diagnosis of Alport syndrome is often made after examination of the urine of a child from a family with multiple cases of hereditary nephritis. Children may initially present with heavy microscopic hematuria (large amount of blood on dipstick), followed by the development of proteinuria. Many, but not all, persons with Alport syndrome have sensorineural deafness and various eye disorders, including lens dislocation, posterior cataracts, and corneal dystrophy. The hearing loss is bilateral and often is first detected during adolescence.

Chronic Glomerulonephritis

Chronic glomerulonephritis represents the chronic phase of a number of specific types of glomerulonephritis.[4,5] Some forms of acute glomerulonephritis (e.g., poststreptococcal glomerulonephritis) undergo complete resolution, whereas others progress at variable rates to chronic glomerulonephritis. Some persons who present with chronic glomerulonephritis have no history of glomerular disease. These cases may represent the end result of relatively asymptomatic forms of glomerulonephritis. Histologically, the condition is characterized by small kidneys with sclerosed glomeruli. In most cases, chronic glomerulonephritis develops insidiously and slowly progresses to chronic kidney disease over a period of years (see Chapter 26).

Glomerular Lesions Associated with Systemic Disease

Many systemic diseases (e.g., systemic lupus erythematosus, diabetes mellitus) are associated with glomerular injury. In some diseases the glomerular involvement may be the major clinical manifestation.

Systemic Lupus Erythematosus Glomerulonephritis. Renal involvement is one of the most common complications of SLE.[5,18] The pathogenesis of SLE (see Chapter 44) is uncertain, but appears to be related to dysregulated B-cell immunity with production of autoantibodies to a variety of nuclear, cytoplasmic, extracellular matrix, and cell membrane components. Most glomerular injury is triggered by the deposition of immune complexes within the glomerular wall. Immune complexes may derive from the circulation, develop locally, or both.

The clinical manifestations of SLE glomerulonephritis, commonly referred to as *lupus nephritis*, depend on the site of immune complex–mediated injury. Immune complexes confined to the mesangium cause less inflammation than subendothelial immune complexes, which have greater exposure to inflammatory cells and mediators in the blood and therefore are more likely to produce inflammation.[5,18] Immune complexes may also localize in the renal interstitium, walls of interstitial vessels, and basement membranes, causing the tubulointerstitial inflammation that occurs in persons with SLE.[5]

Because of the high risk for kidney disease, all persons with SLE should undergo routine urinalysis to monitor for the appearance of hematuria or proteinuria. If urinary abnormalities are noted, renal biopsy is often performed. Treatment depends on the extent of glomerular involvement. Oral corticosteroids and angiotensin-converting enzyme (ACE) inhibitors are the mainstays of treatment. Persons with more advanced disease may require treatment with immunosuppressive agents (e.g., intravenous cyclophosphamide or oral mycophenolate mofetil). Clinical trials using other immunosuppressant agents are ongoing.

Diabetic Glomerulosclerosis. Diabetic nephropathy is a major cause of chronic kidney disease and the most common cause of kidney failure treated by renal replacement therapy in the United States.[4,5,19,20] It occurs in both type 1 and type 2 diabetes mellitus.

The lesions of diabetic nephropathy most commonly involve the glomeruli and are associated with three glomerular syndromes: nonnephrotic proteinuria, nephrotic syndrome, and chronic renal failure. Widespread thickening of the glomerular capillary basement membrane occurs in almost all persons with diabetes and can occur without evidence of proteinuria. This is followed by a diffuse increase in mesangial matrix, with mild proliferation of mesangial cells. As the disease progresses, the mesangial cells impinge on the capillary lumen, reducing the surface area for glomerular filtration. In nodular glomerulosclerosis, also known as *Kimmelstiel-Wilson syndrome*, there is nodular deposition of hyaline in the mesangial portion of the glomerulus. As the sclerotic process progresses in the diffuse and nodular forms of glomerulosclerosis, there is complete obliteration of the glomerulus, with impairment of renal function.

Although the mechanisms of glomerular change in diabetes are uncertain, they are thought to represent enhanced or defective synthesis of the glomerular basement membrane and mesangial matrix with inappropriate incorporation of glucose into the noncellular components of these glomerular structures.[20] Alternatively, hemodynamic changes that occur secondary to elevated blood glucose levels may contribute to the initiation and progression of diabetic glomerulosclerosis.[4] It has been hypothesized that elevations in blood glucose produce an increase in GFR and glomerular pressure that leads to enlargement of glomerular capillary pores by a mechanism that is, at least partly, mediated by angiotensin II. This enlargement results in an increase in the protein content of the glomerular filtrate, which in turn requires increased endocytosis of the filtered proteins by tubular endothelial cells, a process that ultimately leads to nephron destruction and progressive deterioration of renal function.

The clinical manifestations of diabetic glomerulosclerosis are closely linked to those of diabetes. The increased GFR that occurs in persons with early alterations in renal function is associated with *microalbuminuria*, defined as urinary albumin excretion of 30 to 300 mg in 24 hours.[5] Microalbuminuria is an important predictor of future diabetic nephropathies.[4,19] In many cases, these early changes in glomerular function can be reversed by careful control of blood glucose levels (see Chapter 33). Inhibition of angiotensin by ACE inhibitors or ARBs has been shown to have a beneficial effect, possibly by reversing increased glomerular pressure. Hypertension and cigarette smoking have been implicated in the progression of diabetic nephropathy. Thus, control of blood pressure (to levels of 130/80 mm Hg or less) and smoking cessation are recommended as primary and secondary prevention strategies in persons with diabetes.

SUMMARY CONCEPTS

■ Glomerulonephritis represents a group of kidney diseases that result from inflammation and injury of the glomerulus. It may occur as a primary condition in which the glomerular abnormality is the only disease present, or as a secondary condition in which the glomerular abnormality results from another disease, such as diabetes mellitus or SLE. Most cases of primary and many cases of secondary glomerular disease probably have an immune origin.

(continued)

Tubular and Interstitial Disorders

Several disorders cause histologic and functional alterations that affect renal tubular structures, including the proximal and distal tubules. Most of these disorders also affect the interstitial tissue that surrounds the tubules. Although these disorders, sometimes referred to as *tubulointerstitial disorders*, may occur in the progression of diseases that primarily affect the glomerulus or as secondary manifestations of other diseases such as diabetes mellitus, they can also occur as a primary event. These diseases have diverse causes and different pathogenic mechanisms. They include acute tubular necrosis (discussed in Chapter 26), tubulointerstitial nephritis, acute and chronic pyelonephritis, reflux nephropathy, and nephropathy induced by drugs and toxins.

Tubulointerstitial Nephritis

Tubulointerstial nephritis represents acute or chronic inflammation of the renal tubules and surrounding interstitium. In chronic tubulointerstitial nephritis there is infiltration with mononuclear leukocytes, interstitial fibrosis, and widespread tubular atrophy.

The tubulointerstitial disorders are distinguished clinically from glomerular diseases by the absence, in the early stages, of such hallmarks of nephritis and nephrosis as hematuria and proteinuria, and by the presence of disorders in tubular function. These disorders, which are often subtle, include the inability to concentrate urine, as evidenced by polyuria and nocturia; interference with acidification of urine, resulting in metabolic acidosis; and diminished tubular reabsorption of sodium and other substances.[5] In their advanced forms, however, they are difficult to distinguish from other causes of renal insufficiency.

Pyelonephritis

Pyelonephritis is a renal disease affecting the tubules, interstitium, and pelvis of the kidney. Acute pyelonephritis is caused by bacterial infection; whereas chronic pyelonephritis is a more complex disorder involving not only bacterial infection but other factors such as reflux. Most infections of the kidney are ascending infections that occur secondary to infections of the lower urinary tract (discussed in Chapter 27).

Acute Pyelonephritis

Acute pyelonephritis is an acute suppurative inflammation of the kidney caused by bacterial infection.[4,5,21,22] *Escherichia coli* is the causative agent in about 80% of cases. Less common causative organisms include *Enterobacteriaceae*, *Pseudomonas* species, group B *Streptococcus*, *Staphylococcus*, and *enterococci*.[21] There are two forms of acute pyelonephritis: uncomplicated and complicated. Uncomplicated acute pyelonephritis most commonly occurs in healthy young women without structural or urinary tract obstructions or other contributing factors. Complicated acute pyelonephritis occurs in children or adults with structural or functional urinary tract abnormalities or predisposing medical conditions. Factors that contribute to the development of complicated acute pyelonephritis are outflow obstruction, catheterization and urinary instrumentation, vesicoureteral reflux, pregnancy, and neurogenic bladder.

There are two routes by which bacteria can gain access to the kidney: ascending infection from the lower urinary tract and through the bloodstream (hematogenous spread). Ascending infection from the lower urinary tract is the most important and common route by which bacteria reach the kidney. The hematogenous route results from seeding of the kidneys by bacteria from distant loci in the course of septicemia or infective endocarditis.[5] It is more likely to occur in debilitated, chronically ill persons and those receiving immunosuppressive therapy, and with nonenteric bacteria such as staphylococci and certain fungi.

Although outflow obstruction is an important predisposing factor in the pathogenesis of ascending infection, it is incompetence of the vesicoureteral orifice that allows bacteria to ascend the ureter into the renal pelvis.[4,5] The ureter normally inserts into the bladder at a steep angle and in its most distal portion courses parallel to the bladder wall, forming a mucosal flap[4] (Fig. 25-11A). The flap acts as a one-way valve: it is normally relaxed, allowing urine to flow into the bladder, but is compressed against the bladder wall during micturition, preventing urine from being forced into the ureter. In persons with vesicoureteral reflux, the ureter enters the bladder at an approximate right angle such that urine is forced into the ureter during micturition (Fig. 25-11B). It is seen most commonly in children with urinary tract infections

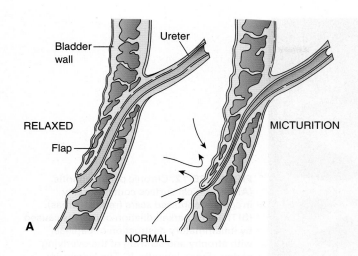

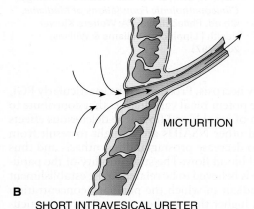

FIGURE 25-11. Anatomic features of the ureter and bladder and their relationship to vesicoureteral reflux. **(A)** In the normal bladder, the distal portion of the intravesical ureter courses between the mucosa and the muscularis of the bladder. A mucosal flap is thus formed. On micturition, the elevated intravesicular pressure compresses the flap against the bladder wall, thereby occluding the lumen. **(B)** Persons with a congenitally short intravesical ureter have no mucosal flap because the entry of the ureter into the bladder approaches at a right angle. Thus, micturition forces urine into the ureter. (Adapted from Jennette JC. The kidney. In: Rubin R., Strayer DS, eds. *Rubin's Pathology: Clinicopathologic Foundations of Medicine.* 6th ed. Philadelphia, PA: Wolters Kluwer Health | Lippincott Williams & Wilkins; 2012:795. Courtesy of Dmitri Karetnikov, artist.)

(UTIs) and is believed to result from congenital defects in length, diameter, muscle structure, or innervation of the submucosal segment of the ureter. Vesicoureteral reflux is discussed further in Chapter 27.

The onset of acute pyelonephritis is usually abrupt, with shaking chills, moderate to high fever, and a constant ache in the loin area of the back that is unilateral or bilateral.[5,21,22] Lower urinary tract symptoms, including dysuria, frequency, and urgency, also are common. There may be significant malaise, and the person usually looks and feels ill. Nausea and vomiting may occur along with abdominal pain. Palpation or percussion over the costovertebral angle on the affected side usually causes pain. Pyuria occurs but is not diagnostic because it also occurs in lower UTIs.

A second and infrequent form of acute pyelonephritis is characterized by ischemia and a condition known as *papillary necrosis*, the suppurative necrosis of one or several renal pyramids.[4,5] It occurs most commonly in persons with diabetes mellitus who develop acute pyelonephritis when there is significant urinary tract obstruction. The development of papillary necrosis is associated with a much poorer prognosis. There is often evidence of overwhelming sepsis with frequent development of kidney failure.

Acute pyelonephritis is treated with appropriate antimicrobial drugs. Unless obstruction or other complications occur, the symptoms usually disappear within several days. Treatment with an appropriate antimicrobial agent usually is continued for 10 to 14 days. Persons with complicated acute pyelonephritis and those who do not respond to outpatient treatment may require hospitalization.[22]

Chronic Pyelonephritis and Reflux Nephropathy

Chronic pyelonephritis represents a progressive process. There is scarring and deformation of the renal calyces and pelvis, along with atrophy and thinning of the overlying cortex[4,5] (Fig. 25-12). The disorder involves a recurrent or persistent bacterial infection superimposed on urinary tract obstruction, urine reflux, or both. Chronic obstructive pyelonephritis can be bilateral, caused by conditions that obstruct bladder outflow; or unilateral, such as occurs with ureteral obstruction. Reflux, which is the most common cause of chronic pyelonephritis, results from superimposition of infection on congenital vesicoureteral reflux or intrarenal reflux.

The symptoms of chronic pyelonephritis may be similar to those of acute pyelonephritis, or its onset may be insidious. Often there is a history of recurrent episodes of UTI or acute pyelonephritis. Loss of tubular function and the ability to concentrate urine give rise to polyuria and nocturia, and mild proteinuria is common. Severe hypertension often is a contributing factor in the progress of the disease. Chronic pyelonephritis is a significant cause of chronic kidney disease and renal failure.

Drug-Related Nephropathies

Drug-related nephropathies involve functional or structural changes in the kidneys that occur after exposure to a drug.[4,5,23–26] Because of their large blood flow and high filtration pressure, the kidneys are exposed to any substance that is in the blood. The kidneys also are active in the metabolic transformation of drugs and therefore are exposed to a number of toxic metabolites. Renal tubular cells, particularly proximal tubule cells, are vulnerable to the toxic effects of drugs because their role in concentrating and reabsorbing glomerular filtrate exposes them to high levels of circulating toxins. The tolerance to drugs varies with age and depends on renal function,

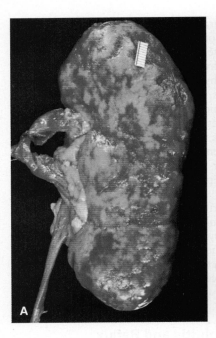
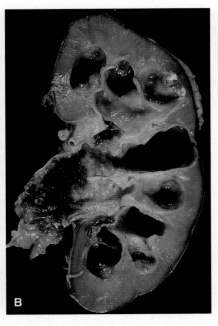

FIGURE 25-12. Chronic pyelonephritis. **(A)** The cortical surface contains many irregular depressed scars (reddish areas). **(B)** There is marked dilation of calyces caused by inflammatory destruction of papillae, with atrophy and scarring of the overlying cortex. (From Jennette JC. The kidney. In: Rubin R, Strayer DS, eds. *Rubin's Pathology: Clinicopathologic Foundations of Medicine.* 6th ed. Philadelphia, PA: Wolters Kluwer Health | Lippincott Williams & Wilkins; 2012:797.)

state of hydration, blood pressure, and the pH of the urine. Elderly persons are particularly susceptible to kidney damage caused by drugs and toxins. The dangers of nephrotoxicity are increased when two or more drugs capable of producing kidney damage are given at the same time.

Drugs and other toxic substances can damage the kidneys by causing a decrease in renal blood flow, directly damaging tubulointerstitial structures, producing hypersensitivity reactions, or obstructing urine flow. Some drugs, such as diuretics, high–molecular-weight radiocontrast media, the immunosuppressive drugs cyclosporine and tacrolimus, and the nonsteroidal anti-inflammatory drugs (NSAIDs), can cause acute kidney injury by decreasing renal blood flow (discussed in Chapter 26). Other drugs such as sulfonamides and vitamin C supplements can form crystals that cause kidney damage by obstructing urinary flow in the tubules.

Acute drug-related hypersensitivity reactions produce tubulointerstitial nephritis, with damage to the tubules and interstitium. This condition was observed initially in persons who were sensitive to the sulfonamide drugs; currently, it is observed most often with the use of methicillin and other synthetic antibiotics, and with the use of furosemide and the thiazide diuretics in persons sensitive to these drugs. The condition begins approximately 15 days (range, 2 to 40 days) after exposure to the drug.[4] At the onset, there is fever, eosinophilia, hematuria, mild proteinuria, and, in approximately one fourth of cases, a rash. In approximately 50% of cases, signs and symptoms of acute renal failure develop. Withdrawal of the drug commonly is followed by complete recovery, but there may be permanent damage, usually in older persons. Drug nephritis may not be recognized in its early stage because it is relatively uncommon.

Chronic analgesic nephritis, which is associated with analgesic abuse, causes tubulointerstitial nephritis with renal papillary necrosis. Prostaglandins (particularly PGI_2 and PGE_2) are potent renal vasodilators that contribute to the regulation of renal blood flow. The deleterious effects of aspirin and other NSAIDs are thought to result from their ability to decrease prostaglandin synthesis and thus decrease renal blood flow. The susceptibility of the papillae to damage is believed to be related to the establishment of a renal gradient in which the papillary concentration of the drug is higher than in the cortex. Persons particularly at risk are the elderly because of age-related changes in renal function, individuals who are dehydrated or have a decrease in blood volume, and those with preexisting kidney disease or renal insufficiency.

Chinese herbal drugs have also been implicated in drug-related kidney damage. Early recognition of the problem surfaced in the early 1990s with reports of an unusually rapid and progressive form of renal failure in women with a shared history of chronic ingestion of slimming herbs, such as ephedra (ma huang), from China as part of a weight loss program.[23] Growing evidence from both clinical and animal models suggests that this form of kidney damage is attributable, at least in part, to the presence of aristolochic acid in the slimming herb preparations.

Illicit drug use has also been implicated in a wide spectrum of kidney diseases.[26] For example, acute renal failure has been reported in persons presenting with acute cocaine intoxication. The cause is probably multifactorial and involves direct vasoconstriction, altered systemic hemodynamics, and myoglobin-induced renal failure. The chronic inhalation of solvents (e.g., glue, paint thinner), aerosols, gases, and nitrates has also been associated with a variety of toxic kidney effects, including acute and chronic renal failure. The tubular manifestations of solvent abuse probably result from the interference with intracellular metabolic processes involved in membrane transport.

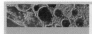

SUMMARY CONCEPTS

■ Tubulointerstitial diseases affect the tubules and the surrounding interstitium of the kidneys. These disorders include acute and chronic pyelonephritis and the effects of drugs and toxins. Pyelonephritis, or infection of the kidney and kidney pelvis, can occur as an acute or a chronic condition. Acute pyelonephritis typically is caused by ascending bladder infections or infections that come from the bloodstream; it usually is successfully treated with appropriate antimicrobial drugs. Chronic pyelonephritis is a progressive disease that produces scarring and deformation of the renal calyces and pelvis.

■ The susceptibility of the kidney to drug-induced damage reflects its significant exposure to medications and their metabolites. Some drugs, such as diuretics, high–molecular-weight radiocontrast media, the immunosuppressive drugs cyclosporine and tacrolimus, and the NSAIDs can cause acute prerenal failure by decreasing renal blood flow. Other drugs such as sulfonamides and vitamin C can form crystals that cause kidney damage by obstructing urinary flow in the tubules. Drugs can also directly damage tubulointerstitial structures, or provoke hypersensitivity reactions. Illicit drug use has also been implicated in a wide spectrum of kidney diseases.

Obstructive Disorders

Urinary obstruction can occur in persons of any age and can involve any level of the urinary tract, from the urethra to the renal pelvis[5,27] (Fig. 25-13). Obstruction may be sudden or insidious, partial or complete, and unilateral or bilateral. The conditions that cause urinary tract obstruction include congenital anomalies, urinary calculi (i.e., stones), pregnancy, benign prostatic hyperplasia, scar tissue resulting from infection and inflammation, tumors, and neurologic disorders such as spinal cord injury. The causes of urinary tract obstructions are summarized in Table 25-1.

Obstructive uropathy is usually classified according to site, degree, and duration of obstruction. Lower urinary tract obstructions are located below the ureterovesical junction and are bilateral in nature. Upper urinary tract obstructions are located above the ureterovesical junction and are usually unilateral. The condition causing the obstruction can cause complete or partial occlusion of urine outflow. When the obstruction is of short duration (i.e., less than a few days), it is said to be acute and is usually caused by conditions such as renal calculi.

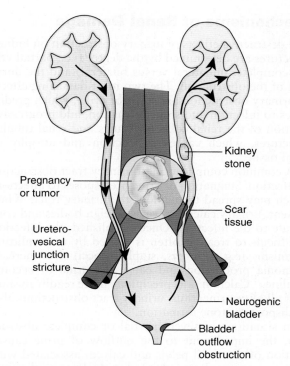

FIGURE 25-13. Locations and causes of urinary tract obstruction.

An obstruction that develops slowly and is longer lasting is said to be chronic and is usually caused by conditions such as congenital ureterovesical abnormalities. Bilateral acute urinary tract obstruction causes acute renal failure. Because many causes of acute obstruction are reversible, prompt recognition is important. When left untreated, an obstructed kidney undergoes atrophy, and in the case of bilateral obstruction, results in chronic kidney disease.

TABLE 25-1	Causes of Urinary Tract Obstruction
Level of Obstruction	**Cause**
Renal pelvis	Renal calculi
	Papillary necrosis
Ureter	Renal calculi
	Pregnancy
	Tumors that compress the ureter
	Ureteral stricture
	Congenital disorders of the uretero-vesical junction and ureteropelvic junction strictures
Bladder and urethra	Bladder cancer
	Neurogenic bladder
	Bladder stones
	Prostatic hyperplasia or cancer
	Urethral strictures
	Congenital urethral defects

Mechanisms of Renal Damage

The destructive effects of urinary obstruction on kidney structures are determined by the degree (i.e., partial versus complete, unilateral versus bilateral) and the duration of the obstruction. The two most damaging effects of urinary obstruction are stasis of urine, which predisposes to infection and stone formation, and progressive dilation of the renal collecting ducts and renal tubular structures, which causes destruction and atrophy of renal tissue.

A common complication of urinary tract obstruction is infection. Stagnation of urine predisposes to infection, which may spread throughout the urinary tract. When present, urinary calculi serve as foreign bodies and contribute to the infection. Once established, the infection is difficult to treat. It often is caused by urea-splitting organisms (e.g., *Proteus*, staphylococci) that increase ammonia production and cause the urine to become alkaline.[27] Calcium salts precipitate more readily in stagnant alkaline urine; thus, urinary tract obstructions also predispose to stone formation.

In situations of severe partial or complete obstruction, the impediment to the outflow of urine causes dilation of the renal pelvis and calyces associated with progressive atrophy of the kidney.[4,5] Even with complete obstruction, glomerular filtration continues for some time. Because of the continued filtration, the calyces and pelvis of the affected kidney become dilated, often markedly so. The high pressure in the renal pelvis is transmitted back through the collecting ducts of the kidney, compressing renal vasculature and causing renal atrophy. Initially, the functional alterations are largely tubular, manifested primarily by impaired urine-concentrating ability. Only later does the GFR begin to diminish.

Hydronephrosis

Hydronephrosis refers to urine-filled dilation of the renal pelvis and calyces associated with progressive atrophy of the kidney due to obstruction of urine outflow.[4,5,27] The degree of hydronephrosis depends on the duration, degree, and level of obstruction. In far-advanced cases, the kidney may be transformed into a thin-walled cystic structure with parenchymal atrophy, total obliteration of the pyramids, and thinning of the cortex (Fig. 25-14). The condition is usually unilateral; bilateral hydronephrosis occurs only when the obstruction is below the level of the ureterovesical junction. When the obstruction affects the outflow of urine from the distal ureter, the increased pressure dilates the ureter, a condition called *hydroureter*. Bilateral hydroureter may develop as a complication of bladder outflow obstruction due to prostatic hyperplasia (see Chapter 39).

Clinical Features

The manifestations of urinary obstruction depend on the site of obstruction, the cause, and the rapidity with which the condition developed. Most of the early symptoms are produced by the underlying pathologic process. Urinary tract obstruction encourages the growth

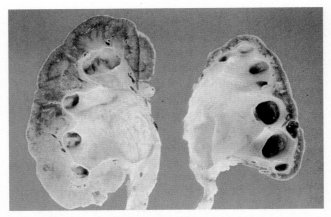

FIGURE 25-14. Hydronephrosis. Bilateral urinary tract obstruction has led to conspicuous dilation of the ureters, pelves, and calyces. The kidney on the right shows severe cortical atrophy. (From Jennette JC. The kidney. In: Rubin R, Strayer DS, eds. *Rubin's Pathology: Clinicopathologic Foundations of Medicine.* 6th ed. Philadelphia, PA: Wolters Kluwer Health | Lippincott Williams & Wilkins; 2012:801.)

of microorganisms and should be suspected in persons with recurrent urinary tract infections.

Complete or partial unilateral hydronephrosis may remain silent for long periods because the unaffected kidney can maintain adequate function. Obstruction may provoke pain due to distention of the collecting system and renal capsule. Whereas, acute supravesical obstruction, such as that due to a kidney stone lodged in the ureter, is associated with excruciating pain. More insidious causes of obstruction, such as narrowing of the ureteropelvic junction, may produce little pain but cause total destruction of the kidney.

Complete bilateral obstruction results in oliguria and anuria and renal failure. Acute bilateral obstruction may mimic prerenal failure. With partial bilateral obstruction, the earliest manifestation is an inability to concentrate urine, reflected by polyuria and nocturia. Hypertension is an occasional complication of urinary tract obstruction. It is more common in cases of unilateral obstruction in which renin secretion is enhanced, probably secondary to impaired renal blood flow. In these circumstances, removal of the obstruction often leads to a reduction in blood pressure. When hypertension accompanies bilateral obstruction, it is volume related. The relief of bilateral obstruction leads to a loss of volume and a decrease in blood pressure. In some cases, relieving the obstruction does not correct the hypertension.

Early diagnosis of urinary tract obstruction is important because the condition usually is treatable and a delay in therapy may result in permanent damage to the kidneys. Diagnostic methods vary with the symptoms. Ultrasonography has proved to be the single most useful noninvasive diagnostic modality for urinary obstruction. Radiologic methods, CT scans, and intravenous urography may also be used. Other diagnostic methods, such as urinalysis, are used to determine the extent of renal involvement and the presence of infection.

Treatment of urinary tract obstruction depends on the cause. Urinary stone removal may be necessary, or surgical treatment of structural defects may be indicated. Treatment of complicating urinary tract infections due to urinary stasis is also important.

Kidney Stones

The most common cause of upper urinary tract obstruction is urinary calculi. Although stones can form in any part of the urinary tract, most develop in the kidneys. Kidney stones, also known as *nephrolithiasis* or *renal calculi*, are the third most common disorder of the urinary tract, exceeded only by urinary tract infections and prostate disorders.[28]

Kidney stones are polycrystalline aggregates composed of materials that the kidneys normally excrete in the urine.[4,5,28–31] The etiology of urinary stone formation is complex. It is thought to encompass a number of factors, including increases in blood and urinary levels of stone-forming components and interactions among the components; anatomic changes in urinary tract structures; metabolic and endocrine influences; dietary and intestinal absorption factors; and urinary tract infections. Added to the mystery of stone formation is the fact that although both kidneys are exposed to the same urinary constituents, kidney stones tend to form in only one kidney.

Two factors implicated in kidney stone formation are a supersaturated urine and an environment that allows the stone to grow. The risk for stone formation is increased when the urine is supersaturated with stone components (e.g., calcium salts, uric acid, magnesium ammonium phosphate, and cystine). Supersaturation depends on urinary pH, solute concentration, ionic strength, and complexation. The greater the concentration of two ions, the more likely they are to precipitate. Complexation influences the availability of specific ions. For example, oxalate complexes with sodium and decreases the availability of free sodium ions to participate in stone formation.

In addition to supersaturated urine, kidney stone formation requires a nidus or nucleus that facilitates crystal aggregation. In supersaturated urine, stone formation begins with small clusters of crystals such as calcium oxalate. Most small clusters tend to disperse because the internal forces that hold them together are too weak to overcome the random tendency of ions to move apart. Larger ion clusters form nuclei and remain stable because the attraction forces balance surface losses. Once they are stable, nuclei can grow at levels of supersaturation below that needed for their creation. Organic materials, such as mucopolysaccharides derived from the epithelial cells that line the tubules, are also thought to act as nuclei for stone formation by lowering the level of supersaturation required for crystal aggregation.

The fact that many people experience supersaturation of their urine without developing kidney stones is believed to be due to the presence of natural stone inhibitors, including magnesium, citrate, and the Tamm-Horsfall mucoprotein. To date, the measurement and manipulation of stone inhibitors has not been part of clinical practice, with the exception of citrate.[28,29] Urine citrate reduces supersaturation by binding calcium and inhibiting nucleation and growth of calcium crystals. Citrate is a normal by-product of the citric acid cycle in renal cells. Metabolic stimuli that consume this product (as with metabolic acidosis due to fasting or hypokalemia) reduce the urinary concentration of citrate. Citrate supplementation (potassium citrate) may be used in the treatment of some forms of hypocitraturic kidney stones.

Types of Stones

There are four basic types of kidney stones: calcium (i.e., oxalate or phosphate), magnesium ammonium phosphate, uric acid, and cystine stones.[4,5,28–30] The causes and treatment measures for each of these types of renal stones are described in Table 25-2. Most kidney

---

TABLE 25-2 Composition, Contributing Factors, and Treatment of Kidney Stones

Type of Stone	Contributing Factors	Treatment
Calcium (oxalate and phosphate)	Hypercalcemia and hypercalciuria Immobilization	Treatment of underlying conditions Increased fluid intake Thiazide diuretics
	Hyperparathyroidism Vitamin D intoxication Diffuse bone disease Milk-alkali syndrome Renal tubular acidosis	
	Hyperoxaluria Intestinal bypass surgery	Dietary restriction of foods high in oxalate
Magnesium ammonium phosphate (struvite)	Urea-splitting urinary tract infections	Treatment of urinary tract infection Acidification of the urine Increased fluid intake
Uric acid (urate)	Formed in acid urine with pH of approximately 5.5	Increased fluid intake
	Gout High-purine diet	Allopurinol for hyperuricosuria Alkalinization of urine
Cystine	Cystinuria (inherited disorder of amino acid metabolism)	Increased fluid intake
		Alkalinization of urine

stones (70% to 80%) are calcium stones—calcium oxalate, calcium phosphate, or a combination of the two materials. Calcium stones usually are associated with increased concentrations of calcium in the blood and urine. Excessive bone resorption caused by immobility, bone disease, hyperparathyroidism, and renal tubular acidosis all are contributing conditions. High oxalate concentrations in the blood and urine predispose to formation of calcium oxalate stones.

Magnesium ammonium phosphate stones, also called *struvite stones,* form only in alkaline urine and in the presence of bacteria that possess an enzyme called *urease,* which splits the urea in the urine into ammonia and carbon dioxide. The ammonia that is formed takes up a hydrogen ion to become an ammonium ion, increasing the pH of the urine so that it becomes more alkaline. Because phosphate levels are increased in alkaline urine and because magnesium always is present in the urine, struvite stones form. These stones enlarge as the bacterial count grows, and they can increase in size until they fill an entire renal pelvis (Fig. 25-15). Because of their shape, they often are called *staghorn stones.* They almost always are associated with urinary tract infections and persistently alkaline urine. Because these stones act as a foreign body, treatment of the infection often is difficult. Struvite stones usually are too large to be passed and require lithotripsy or surgical removal.

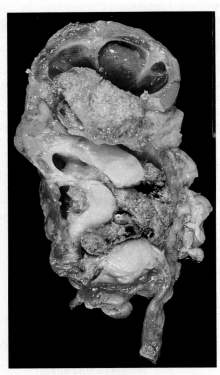

FIGURE 25-15. Staghorn stones. The kidney shows hydronephrosis and stones that are casts of the dilated calyces. (From Jennette JC. The kidney. In: Rubin R, Strayer DS, eds. *Rubin's Pathology: Clinicopathologic Foundations of Medicine,* 6th ed. Philadelphia, PA: Wolters Kluwer Health | Lippincott Williams & Wilkins; 2012:800.)

Uric acid stones develop in conditions of gout and high concentrations of uric acid in the urine. Hyperuricosuria also may contribute to calcium stone formation by acting as a nucleus for calcium oxalate stone formation. Unlike radiopaque calcium stones, uric acid stones are not visible on x-ray films. Uric acid stones form most readily in urine with a pH of 5.1 to 5.9. Thus, these stones can be treated by raising (alkalinizing) the urinary pH to 6.0 to 6.5 with potassium alkali salts.

Cystine stones account for less than 1% of kidney stones overall but represent a significant proportion of childhood calculi.[5] They are seen in cystinuria, which results from a genetic defect in renal transport of cystine. These stones resemble struvite stones except that infection is unlikely to be present.

Clinical Features

One of the major manifestations of kidney stones is pain. Depending on location, there are two types of pain associated with kidney stones: renal colic and noncolicky renal pain.[28] *Renal colic* is the term used to describe the colicky pain that accompanies stretching of the collecting system or ureter. The symptoms of renal colic are caused by stones 1 to 5 mm in diameter that can move into the ureter and obstruct flow. Classic ureteral colic is manifested by acute, intermittent, and excruciating pain in the flank and upper outer quadrant of the abdomen on the affected side. The pain may radiate to the lower abdominal quadrant, bladder area, perineum, or scrotum in the man. The skin may be cool and clammy, and nausea and vomiting are common. *Noncolicky pain* is caused by stones that produce distention of the renal calyces or renal pelvis. The pain usually is a dull, deep ache in the flank or back that can vary in intensity from mild to severe. The pain is often exaggerated by drinking large amounts of fluid.

The diagnosis of kidney stones is based on symptomatology and diagnostic tests, which include urinalysis, plain film radiography (X-ray), intravenous pyelography, and abdominal ultrasonography.[28,31] Urinalysis provides information related to hematuria, infection, presence of stone-forming crystals, and urine pH. Most stones are radiopaque and readily visible on a plain radiograph of the abdomen. The noncontrast spiral CT scan is the imaging modality of choice in persons with acute renal colic. Intravenous pyelography (IVP) uses an intravenously injected contrast medium that is filtered in the glomeruli to visualize the collecting system of the kidneys and ureters. Abdominal ultrasonography is highly sensitive to hydronephrosis, which may be a manifestation of ureteral obstruction. An imaging technique called *nuclear scintigraphy* uses bisphosphonate markers as a means of imaging stones. This method has been credited with identifying stones that are too small to be detected by other methods.

Treatment of acute renal colic usually is supportive. Pain relief may be needed during acute phases of obstruction, and antibiotic therapy may be necessary to treat urinary tract infections. Most stones that are less than 5 mm in diameter pass spontaneously. All urine should be strained during an attack in the hope of retrieving the stone for chemical analysis and determination of type. This information, along with a careful history and laboratory tests, provide the basis for long-term preventive measures.

A major goal of treatment in persons who have passed kidney stones or have had them removed is to prevent their recurrence. Prevention requires investigation into the cause of stone formation using urine tests, blood chemistries, and stone analysis. Underlying disease conditions, such as hyperparathyroidism, are treated. Adequate fluid intake reduces the concentration of stone-forming crystals in the urine and needs to be encouraged. Calcium supplementation with calcium salts such as calcium carbonate and calcium phosphate also may be used to bind oxalate in the intestine and decrease its absorption. Thiazide diuretics lower urinary calcium by increasing tubular reabsorption so that less remains in the urine. Drugs that bind calcium in the gut (e.g., cellulose phosphate) may be used to inhibit calcium absorption and urinary excretion.

Depending on the type of stone that is formed, dietary changes, medications, or both may be used to alter the concentration of stone-forming elements in the urine (Table 25-2). For example, persons who form calcium oxalate stones may need to decrease their intake of foods that are high in oxalate (e.g., spinach, Swiss chard, cocoa, chocolate, pecans, peanuts). Because of associated electrolyte disturbances and altered urine chemistry, obese persons are predisposed to hyperuricemia, gout, hypercitraturia, and uric acid stones.[31] Weight loss may improve or undermine management of these stones; however, it can be detrimental if associated with a high animal protein diet, laxative abuse, rapid loss of lean tissue, or poor hydration. High acid diets, such as the Atkins diet, increase the risk of uric acid stones.

Measures to change the pH of the urine also can influence kidney stone formation. In persons who lose the ability to acidify or lower the pH of their urine, there is an increase in the divalent and trivalent forms of urine phosphate that combine with calcium to form calcium phosphate stones. The formation of uric acid stones is increased in acid urine; stone formation can be reduced by raising the pH of urine to 6.0 to 6.5 with potassium alkali (e.g., potassium citrate) salts.

In some cases, stone removal may be necessary. Several methods are available for removing kidney stones: ureteroscopic removal, percutaneous removal, and extracorporeal lithotripsy.[28] All of these procedures eliminate the need for an open surgical procedure, which is another form of treatment. Open stone surgery may be required to remove large calculi or those that are resistant to other forms of removal. A nonsurgical treatment, called *extracorporeal shock-wave lithotripsy,* uses acoustic shock waves to fragment calculi into sandlike particles that are passed in the urine over the next few days. Because of the large amount of stone particles that are generated during the procedure, a ureteral stent (i.e., a tubelike device used to hold the ureter open) may be inserted to ensure adequate urine drainage.

SUMMARY CONCEPTS

■ Obstruction of urine flow can occur at any level of the urinary tract. Among the causes of urinary tract obstruction are developmental defects, pregnancy, infection and inflammation, kidney stones, neurologic defects, and prostatic hypertrophy.

■ Obstructive disorders produce stasis of urine, increase the risk for infection and calculi formation, and produce progressive dilation of the renal collecting ducts and renal tubular structures, which cause renal atrophy.

■ *Hydronephrosis* refers to urine-filled dilation of the renal pelvis and calyces associated with progressive atrophy of the kidney due to obstruction of urine outflow. Unilateral hydronephrosis may remain silent for long periods because the unaffected kidney can maintain adequate function. With partial bilateral obstruction, the earliest manifestation is an inability to concentrate urine, reflected by polyuria and nocturia. Complete bilateral obstruction results in oliguria, anuria, and renal failure.

■ Kidney stones are a major cause of upper urinary tract obstruction. The development of kidney stones is influenced by the concentration of stone components in the urine, the ability of the stone components to complex and form stones, and the presence of substances that inhibit stone formation.

■ There are four types of kidney stones: calcium (i.e., oxalate and phosphate) stones, which are associated with increased serum calcium levels; magnesium ammonium phosphate (i.e., struvite) stones, which are associated with urinary tract infections; uric acid stones, which are related to elevated uric acid levels; and cystine stones, which are seen in cystinuria. Treatment measures depend on stone type and include adequate fluid intake to prevent urine saturation, dietary modification to decrease intake of stone-forming constituents, treatment of urinary tract infections, measures to change urine pH, and the use of diuretics that decrease the calcium concentration of urine.

Malignant Tumors of the Kidney

There are two major groups of malignant tumors of the kidney: embryonic kidney tumors (i.e., Wilms tumor), which occur during childhood, and renal cell carcinoma, which occurs in adults.

 Wilms Tumor

Wilms tumor, also known as *nephroblastoma,* is one of the most common primary neoplasms of young children. It usually presents between 3 and 5 years of age and is the second most common malignant abdominal tumor in children.[4,32] It may occur in one or both kidneys. The incidence of bilateral Wilms tumor is 6% to 7%, with children having a horseshoe kidney being at twice the risk.

Histologically, the tumor is composed of elements that resemble normal fetal tissue: blastemic, stromal, and epithelial. An important feature of Wilms tumor is its association with other congenital anomalies, including aniridia (absence of the iris), hemihypertrophy (enlargement of one side of the face or body), and other congenital anomalies, usually of the genitourinary system. Several chromosomal abnormalities have been associated with Wilms tumor. One Wilms tumor gene, *WT1* located on chromosome 11, is a tumor-suppressor gene that regulates several other growth factor genes.[32]

Wilms tumor usually is a solitary mass that occurs in any part of the kidney. It usually is sharply demarcated, variably encapsulated, and grows to a large size, distorting kidney structure (Fig. 25-16). The tumors usually are staged using the National Wilms Tumor Study Group classification.[32] Stage I tumors are limited to the kidney and can be excised with the capsular surface intact. Stage II tumors extend into the renal capsule but can be excised. In stage III, extension of the tumor is confined to the abdomen, and in stage IV, hematogenous metastasis most commonly involves the lung.

The common presenting signs are a large asymptomatic abdominal mass and hypertension. The tumor is often discovered inadvertently, and it is not uncommon for the parent to discover it while bathing the child. Some children may present with abdominal pain, vomiting, or both. Microscopic and gross hematuria is present in 15% to 25% of children. CT scans are used to confirm the diagnosis.[32]

Treatment involves surgery, chemotherapy, and sometimes radiation therapy. Long-term survival rates have increased to more than 70% for all stages and to 91% to 96% for stages I through III.[32]

Renal Cell Carcinoma

Cancer of the kidney is the seventh leading malignancy among men and the twelfth among women, accounting for about 3% of all cancers.[33] Incidence peaks between 55 and 84 years of age.[34] Renal cell carcinoma

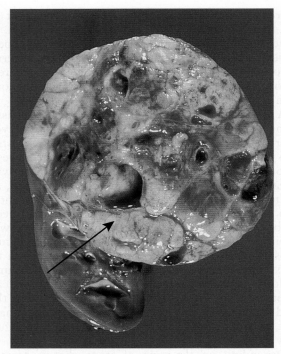

FIGURE 25-16. Wilms tumor. A cross-section of a pale tan neoplasm (*arrow*) attached to a residual portion of the kidney. (From Jennette JC. The kidney. In: Rubin R, Strayer DS, eds. *Rubin's Pathology: Clinicopathologic Foundations of Medicine.* 6th ed. Philadelphia, PA: Wolters Kluwer Health | Lippincott Williams & Wilkins; 2012:805.)

accounts for approximately 80% to 90% of all kidney cancers.[4,5,33–35] Most renal cell carcinomas are sporadic, but about 5% are inherited. Inherited tumors tend to be multifocal and bilateral, and appear at an earlier age than sporadic renal cell carcinomas.

A major advance in the understanding of renal cell carcinoma has been the realization that this neoplasm is not a single entity, but a collection of tumors that arise in different parts of the tubular or ductal epithelium. Clear cell carcinomas, so named because of their high cytoplasmic lipid content, accounts for 70% to 80% of all renal cell carcinomas.[5] They arise from proximal tubular epithelial cells and appear as solitary unilateral lesions located predominantly in the renal cortex (Fig. 25-17). Papillary carcinomas, which are characterized by a papillary growth pattern, account for another 10% to 15% of renal cancers.[5] Thought to arise from the proximal tubules, they can be multifocal and bilateral.

The cause of renal cell carcinoma remains elusive. Epidemiologic evidence suggests a correlation between heavy smoking and kidney cancer.[33,34] Obesity also is a risk factor, particularly in women. Additional risk factors include occupational exposure to petroleum products, heavy metals, and asbestos.[5] The risk for renal cell carcinoma also is increased in persons with acquired cystic kidney disease associated with chronic renal insufficiency.

Kidney cancer is largely a silent disorder during its early stages, and symptoms usually denote advanced

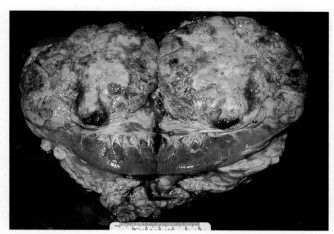

FIGURE 25-17. Gross pathology of a bisected kidney showing large renal cell carcinoma. Much of the kidney has been replaced by gray and yellow tumor tissue. A little remaining renal cortex and pericapsular fat are visible at the bottom of this surgical specimen. (From the Centers for Disease Control and Prevention Public Health Images Library. No. 863. Courtesy of Edwin P. Ewing, Jr.)

disease. Presenting features include hematuria, flank pain, and presence of a palpable flank mass. Gross or microscopic hematuria, which occurs in more than 50% of cases, is an important clinical clue.[4] It is, however, intermittent and may be microscopic; as a result, the tumor may reach considerable size before it is detected. One of the features of renal cell carcinoma is its ability to metastasize. In about 25% of new cases, there is radiologic evidence of metastasis, with the most common sites being lung and bone metastases.[35]

Ultrasonography and CT scanning are used to confirm the diagnosis. MRI may be used when involvement of the inferior vena cava is suspected. Surgery (radical nephrectomy with lymph node dissection) is the treatment of choice for all resectable tumors. Nephron-sparing surgery may be done when both kidneys are involved or when the contralateral kidney is threatened by an associated disease such as hypertension or diabetes mellitus. Single-agent and combination chemotherapy have been used with limited success. The 5-year survival rate is 90% if the tumor has not extended beyond the renal capsule, but drops to 30% if metastasis has occurred.[5]

SUMMARY CONCEPTS

■ There are two major groups of renal neoplasms: embryonic kidney tumors (i.e., Wilms tumor), which occur during childhood, and renal cell carcinoma, which occurs in adults.

■ Wilms tumor is one of the most common malignant tumors of children. The most common presenting signs are a large abdominal mass and hypertension. Treatment methods include surgery,

chemotherapy, and sometimes radiation therapy, with long-term survival rates of up to 96% with an aggressive plan of treatment.

■ Cancer of the kidney accounts for about 3% of all cancers, with renal cell carcinoma accounting for 80% to 90% of cases. The neoplasms are a collection of tumors from different parts of the nephron, each with different genetic profiles and histologic features that challenge both diagnostic and treatment methods. Many of these cancers are characterized by a lack of early warning signs, diverse clinical manifestations, and resistance to chemotherapy and radiation therapy.

REVIEW EXERCISES

1. A 6-year-old boy is diagnosed with acute glomerulonephritis that developed after a streptococcal throat infection. At this time, the following manifestations are noted: decrease in urine output, increasing lethargy, hyperventilation, and generalized edema. Trace amounts of protein are detected in his urine. Blood analysis reveals the following: pH = 7.35, HCO_3 = 18 mEq/L, hematocrit = 29%, Na = 132 mEq/L, K = 5.6 mEq/L, blood urea nitrogen (BUN) = 62 mg/dL, creatinine = 4.1 mg/dL, and albumin = 2 g/dL.

A. What is the probable cause of this boy's glomerular disease?
B. Use the laboratory values in the Appendix to interpret his laboratory test results. Which values are significant and why?
C. Is he progressing to uremia? How can you tell?

2. A 36-year-old man is admitted to the emergency department with a sudden onset of severe, intermittent, cramping pain that makes him feel nauseated. He describes the pain as originating in the left groin and radiating toward the flank. Microscopic examination of his urine reveals the presence of red blood cells. His temperature is normal, and he does not exhibit signs of sepsis.

A. What is the probable cause of this man's pain?
B. What diagnostic measure could be used to confirm the cause of his pain?
C. A plain-film radiograph reveals a 4- to 5-mm kidney stone in the left ureter. What are the chances that this man will pass the stone spontaneously?
D. What type of medications and other treatments should this man receive?
E. Once the stone has been passed, what type of measures can he use to prevent stone recurrence?

REFERENCES

1. Moore KL, Persaud TVN, Torchia MG. *The Developing Human: Clinically Oriented Embryology.* 9th ed. Philadelphia, PA: Elsevier Saunders; 2013:245–288.
2. Elder JS. Urologic disorders in infants and children. In: Kliegman RM, Statten BF, St. Gemell JW, et al., eds. *Kliegman & Nelson Textbook of Pediatrics.* 19th ed. Philadelphia, PA: Saunders Elsevier; 2011:1827–1829.
3. Sanna-Cherchi S, Caridi G, Weng PL. Genetic approaches to human renal agenesis/hypogenesis and dysplasia. *Pediatr Nephrol* 2007;22:1675–1684.
4. Jennette JC. The kidney. In: Rubin R, Strayer DS, eds. *Rubin's Pathology: Clinicopathologic Foundations of Medicine.* 6th ed. Philadelphia, PA: Wolters Kluwer Health/Lippincott Williams & Wilkins; 2012:753–807.
5. Alpers CE. The kidney. In: Kumar V, Abbas AK, Fautso N, et al. *Robbins and Cotran Pathologic Basis of Disease.* 8th ed. Philadelphia, PA: Saunders Elsevier; 2010:905–969.
6. Braun WE. Autosomal dominant polycystic kidney disease: emerging concepts of pathogenesis and new treatments. *Cleve Clin J Med.* 2009;76(2):97–104.
7. Wilson PD. Polycystic kidney disease. *N Engl J Med* 2004;350:151–164.
8. Gantham JJ. Autosomal dominant polycystic kidney disease. *N Engl J Med.* 2008;359(14):1477–1485.
9. Takier V, Caplan MJ. Polycystic kidney disease: Pathogenesis and potential treatment. *Biochim Biophys Acta.* 2011;1812(10):1337–1343.
10. Nachman PH, Jennette C, Falk FJ. Primary glomerular disease. In: Taal MW, Chertow GM, Marsten PA, et al. *Brenner and Rector's The Kidney.* Volume 2, 9th ed. Philadelphia, PA: Elsevier Saunders; 2012:1100–1191.
11. Thurman JM, Goldberg R. The glomerulopathies. In: Schrier RW, ed. *Renal and Electrolyte Disorders.* 7th ed. Philadelphia, PA: Wolters Kluwer Health/Lippincott Williams & Wilkins; 2010:559–607.
12. Chadban SJ, Atkins RC. Glomerulonephritis. *Lancet* 2005;365:1797–1806.
13. Beck LH, Salant DJ. Glomerular and tubulointerstitial diseases. *Prim Care Clin North Am.* 2008;35:265–296.
14. Rodriguez-Iturbe B, Musser JM. The current state of poststreptococcal glomerulonephritis. *J Am Soc Nephrol.* 2008;19:1855–1864.
15. D'Agati VD, Kaskel FJ, Falk RJ. Focal segmental glomerulonephritis. *N Engl J Med.* 2011;365(24):2398–2411.
16. Wyatt RJ, Julian BA. IgA nephropathy. *N Engl J Med.* 2013;368(25):2402–2414.
17. Baratt J, Feehally J. IgA nephropathy. *J Am Soc Nephrol* 2005;16:2088–2097.
18. Appel GB. New and future therapies for lupus nephritis. *Cleve Clin J Med.* 2012;79(2):134–140.
19. Ritz E. Clinical manifestations and natural history of diabetic kidney disease. *Med Clin North Am.* 2013;97:10–29.
20. Schena FP, Gesualdo L. Pathogenic mechanisms of diabetic nephropathy. *J Am Soc Nephrol.* 2005;16(Suppl 1):S30–S33.
21. Ramakrishnan K, Scheid D. Diagnosis and management of acute pyelonephritis in adults. *Am Fam Physician.* 2005;71:933–942.
22. Colgan R, Williams M, Johnson JR. Diagnosis and treatment of acute pyelonephritis in women. *Am Fam Physician.* 2011;84(5):519–526.
23. Kelley CJ, Neilson EC. Tubulointerstitial diseases. In: Taal MW, Chertow GM, Marsten PA, et al. *Brenner and Rector's the Kidney.* Volume 2, 9th ed. Philadelphia, PA: Elsevier Saunders; 2012:1332–1355.
24. Naughton C. Drug-induced nephrotoxicity. *Am Fam Physician.* 2008;78(6):743–750.
25. Taber SS, Mueller BA. Drug-associated renal dysfunction. *Crit Care Clin* 2006;22:357–374.
26. Blowey DL. Nephrotoxicity of over-the-counter analgesics, natural medicines, and illicit drugs. *Adolesc Med* 2005;16: 31–43.
27. Tanagho EA, Lue TF. Urinary obstruction and stasis. In: McAninch JW, Lue TF, eds. *Smith & Tanagho's General Urology.* 18th ed. New York, NY: McGraw-Hill Medical; 2013:170–181.
28. Stoller ML. Urinary stone disease. In: Tanagho EA, McAninch JW, eds. *Smith's General Urology.* 17th ed. New York, NY: McGraw-Hill Medical; 2008:256–290.
29. Miller NL, Evan AP, Lingeman JE. Pathogenesis of renal calculi. *Urol Clin North Am.* 2007;34:295–313.
30. Moe OW. Kidney stones: pathophysiology and medical management. *Lancet.* 2006;367:333–444.
31. Frassetto L, Kohlstadt I. Treatment and prevention of kidney stones: an update. *Am Fam Physician.* 2011;84:1234–1242.
32. Anderson PM, Dhamne CA, Huff V. Wilms tumor. In: Kliegman RM, Statten BF, St. Gemell JW, et al., eds. *Kliegman & Nelson Textbook of Pediatrics.* 19th ed. Philadelphia, PA: Saunders Elsevier; 2011:1757–1860.
33. Rini BI, Campbell SC, Escudler B. Renal cell cancer. *Lancet.* 2009;3669(28):1119–1132.
34. Cohen HT, McGovern FJ. Renal cell carcinoma. *N Engl J Med.* 2005;353:2477–2490.
35. Wood LS. Renal cell carcinoma, screening, diagnosis, and prognosis. *Clin J Oncol Nurs.* 2009;13(6 Suppl):3–7.

Porth Essentials Resources

Explore these additional resources to enhance learning for this chapter:

- NCLEX-Style Questions and Other Resources on the**Point**, http://thePoint.lww.com/PorthEssentials4e
- Study Guide for Essentials of Pathophysiology
- Adaptive Learning | Powered by PrepU, http://thepoint.lww.com/prepu

C h a p t e r **26**

Acute Kidney Injury and Chronic Kidney Disease

Renal failure is a condition in which the kidneys fail to remove metabolic end products from the blood and regulate the fluid, electrolyte, and pH balance of the extracellular fluids. The underlying cause may be renal disease, systemic disease, or urologic defects of nonrenal origin. Renal failure can occur as an acute or a chronic disorder. Acute kidney injury is abrupt in onset and often is reversible if recognized early and treated appropriately. In contrast, chronic kidney disease is the end result of irreparable damage to the kidneys. It develops slowly, usually over the course of a number of years and often requires dialysis therapy or transplantation.

Acute Kidney Injury

Acute kidney injury (AKI), formerly known as acute renal failure, represents an abrupt decline in kidney function, resulting in an inability to maintain fluid and electrolyte balance and excrete nitrogenous wastes.[1-7] Acute kidney injury is a common threat to seriously ill persons, in whom it is associated with a high rate of adverse outcomes, with mortality rates ranging between 25% and 80% depending on the cause and clinical status of the patient.[1] This high mortality rate probably reflects the facts that AKI is often seen in elderly persons and that it is frequently superimposed on other life-threatening conditions, such as trauma, shock, and sepsis.

Acute renal injury is commonly defined as an abrupt (within 48 hours) reduction in kidney function based on an increase in serum creatinine level, a reduction in urine output, and the need for dialysis, or a combination of these factors. The range of clinical manifestations can vary from mild to severe, based on the degree of rise in creatinine levels and decrease in urine output.

Types of Acute Kidney Injury

Acute kidney injury can be caused by several types of conditions, including a decrease in blood flow without

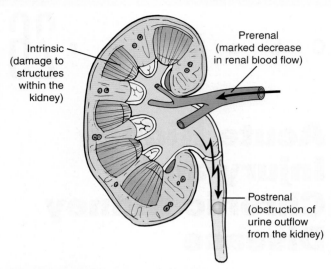

Intrinsic (damage to structures within the kidney)

Prerenal (marked decrease in renal blood flow)

Postrenal (obstruction of urine outflow from the kidney)

FIGURE 26-1. Types of acute kidney injury.

ischemic injury; ischemic, toxic, or obstructive tubular injury; and obstruction of urinary tract outflow. The causes of AKI commonly are categorized as prerenal, intrarenal, and postrenal[1-7] (Fig. 26-1). Collectively, prerenal and intrarenal causes account for 80% to 95% of AKI cases.[3] Causes of kidney injury within these categories are summarized in Chart 26-1.

CHART 26-1	**Causes of Acute Kidney Injury**

Prerenal

Hypovolemia
   Hemorrhage
   Dehydration
   Excessive loss of gastrointestinal tract fluids
   Excessive loss of fluid due to burn injury
Decreased vascular filling
   Anaphylactic shock
   Septic shock
Heart failure and cardiogenic shock
Decreased renal perfusion due to sepsis, vasoactive mediators, drugs, diagnostic agents

Intrarenal

Acute tubular necrosis
   Prolonged renal ischemia
   Exposure to nephrotoxic drugs, heavy metals, and organic solvents
   Intratubular obstruction resulting from hemoglobinuria, myoglobinuria, myeloma light chains, or uric acid casts
   Acute renal disease (acute glomerulonephritis, pyelonephritis)

Postrenal

Bilateral ureteral obstruction
Bladder outlet obstruction

Prerenal Injury

Prerenal kidney injury, the most common form of AKI, is characterized by a marked decrease in renal blood flow. It is reversible if the cause of the decreased renal blood flow can be identified and corrected before kidney damage occurs.

Normally, the kidneys receive 22% of the cardiac output.[8] This large blood supply is required to remove metabolic wastes and regulate body fluids and electrolytes. Fortunately, the normal kidney can tolerate relatively large reductions in blood flow before renal damage occurs. As renal blood flow falls, the glomerular filtration rate (GFR) decreases, the amount of sodium and other substances that are filtered by the glomeruli is reduced, and the blood flow needed for the energy-dependent mechanisms that reabsorb these substances is reduced (see Chapter 24). As the GFR and urine output approach zero, oxygen consumption by the kidney approximates that required to keep renal tubular cells alive. When blood flow falls below this level, which is about 25% of normal, ischemic changes occur.[9] Because of their high metabolic rate, the tubular epithelial cells are most vulnerable to ischemic injury. Improperly treated, prolonged renal hypoperfusion can lead to ischemic tubular necrosis with significant morbidity and mortality.

Causes of prerenal injury include profound depletion of vascular volume (e.g., hemorrhage, loss of extracellular fluid volume), impaired perfusion due to heart failure and cardiogenic shock, and decreased vascular filling because of increased vascular capacity (e.g., anaphylaxis or sepsis). Elderly persons are particularly at risk because of their predisposition to hypovolemia and their high prevalence of renal vascular disorders.

Some vasoactive mediators, drugs, and diagnostic agents stimulate intense intrarenal vasoconstriction and can induce glomerular hypoperfusion and prerenal injury. Examples include endotoxins, radiocontrast agents such as those used for cardiac catheterization, cyclosporine (an immunosuppressant drug that is used to prevent transplant rejection), amphotericin B (an antifungal agent), epinephrine, and high doses of dopamine.[3] Many of these agents also cause acute tubular necrosis (to be discussed).

In addition, several commonly used classes of drugs can impair renal adaptive mechanisms and can convert compensated renal hypoperfusion into prerenal injury. For example, angiotensin II is a potent renal vasoconstrictor that preferentially constricts the efferent arterioles of the kidney as a means of preserving the GFR in situations of arterial hypotension or volume depletion. The angiotensin converting enzyme (ACE) inhibitors and angiotensin receptor blockers (ARBs) reduce the effects of angiotensin II on renal blood flow. They also reduce intraglomerular pressure and may have a renal protective effect in persons with hypertension or type 2 diabetes. However, when combined with diuretics, they may cause prerenal injury in persons with decreased blood flow due to large-vessel or small-vessel kidney disease. Nonsteroidal anti-inflammatory drugs

(NSAIDs) can also reduce renal blood flow by inhibiting the synthesis of prostaglandins, which normally have a vasodilatory effect on renal blood vessels.

Prerenal injury is manifested by a sharp decrease in urine output and a disproportionate elevation of blood urea nitrogen (BUN) in relation to serum creatinine levels. The kidney normally responds to a decrease in the GFR with a decrease in urine output. Thus, an early sign of prerenal injury is a sharp decrease in urine output. A low fractional excretion of sodium (<1%) suggests that oliguria is due to decreased renal perfusion and that the nephrons are responding appropriately by decreasing the excretion of filtered sodium in an attempt to preserve vascular volume. Blood urea nitrogen levels also depend on the GFR. A low GFR allows more time for small particles such as urea to be reabsorbed into the blood. Creatinine, which is larger and nondiffusible, remains in the tubular fluid, and the total amount of creatinine that is filtered, although small, is excreted in the urine. Consequently, there also is a disproportionate elevation in the ratio of BUN to serum creatinine, from a normal value of 10:1 to a ratio greater than 20:1.[1]

Postrenal Injury

Postrenal injury results from obstruction of urine outflow from the kidneys. The obstruction can occur in the ureter (i.e., calculi and strictures), bladder (i.e., tumors or neurogenic bladder), or urethra (i.e., prostatic hyperplasia). Prostatic hyperplasia is the most common underlying problem. Because both ureters must be occluded to produce renal injury, obstruction of bladder outflow rarely causes AKI unless one of the kidneys already is damaged or a person has only one kidney. The treatment of acute postrenal injury consists of treating the underlying cause of obstruction so that urine flow can be reestablished before permanent nephron damage occurs.

Intrarenal Injury

Intrarenal injury results from conditions that damage structures within the kidney. The major causes of intrarenal injury are ischemia associated with prerenal injury, injury to the tubular structures of the nephron, and intratubular obstruction. Acute glomerulonephritis and acute pyelonephritis also are intrarenal causes of AKI. However, injury to the tubular structures of the nephron (acute tubular necrosis) is the most common cause and often is ischemic or toxic in origin.

Acute Tubular Necrosis. Acute tubular necrosis (ATN) is characterized by the destruction of tubular epithelial cells with acute suppression of renal function (Fig. 26-2). It can be caused by a number of conditions, including acute tubular damage due to ischemia, sepsis, nephrotoxic effects of drugs, tubular obstruction, and toxins from a massive infection.[3–5,10] Tubular epithelial cells are particularly sensitive to ischemia and toxins. The tubular injury that occurs in ATN frequently is reversible. The process depends on recovery of the injured cells, removal of the necrotic cells and intratubular casts, and

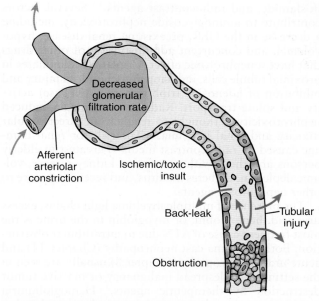

FIGURE 26-2. Pathogenesis of acute tubular necrosis (ATN). Sloughing and necrosis of tubular epithelial cells lead to obstruction and increased intraluminal pressure, which reduce glomerular filtration. Afferent arteriolar vasoconstriction caused in part by tubuloglomerular feedback mechanisms results in decreased glomerular capillary filtration pressure. Tubular injury and increased intraluminal pressure cause fluid to move from the tubular lumen into the interstitium (back-leak). (Modified from Jennette JC. The kidney. In: Rubin R, Strayer DS, eds. *Rubin's Pathology: Clinicopathologic Foundations of Medicine.* 6th ed. Philadelphia, PA: Wolters Kluwer Health | Lippincott Williams & Wilkins; 2012:792.)

regeneration of tubular cells to restore the normal continuity of the tubular epithelium.[5,10]

Acute tubular necrosis occurs most frequently in persons who have major surgery, severe hypovolemia, or overwhelming sepsis, trauma, or burns.[3] Sepsis produces ischemia by provoking a combination of systemic vasodilation and intrarenal hypoperfusion. In addition, sepsis results in the generation of toxins that sensitize renal tubular cells to the damaging effects of ischemia. ATN complicating trauma and burns frequently is multifactorial in origin, resulting from the combined effects of hypovolemia, myoglobinuria, and other toxins released from damaged tissue. In contrast to prerenal injury, the GFR does not improve with the restoration of renal blood flow in AKI caused by ischemic ATN.

Many drugs are nephrotoxic, causing tubular injury by inducing varying combinations of renal vasoconstriction, direct tubular damage, or intratubular obstruction. The kidney is particularly vulnerable to nephrotoxic injury because of its rich blood supply and ability to concentrate toxins to high levels in the medullary portion of the kidney. In addition, the kidney is an important site for metabolic processes that transform relatively harmless agents into toxic metabolites. Pharmacologic agents that are directly toxic to the renal tubule include antimicrobials such as aminoglycosides (e.g., gentamicin), cancer chemotherapeutic agents such as cisplatin and ifosfamide, and radiocontrast agents.[3,5] Several factors contribute to aminoglycoside nephrotoxicity, including a decrease in the GFR, preexisting renal disease, hypovolemia, and concurrent administration of other drugs that have a nephrotoxic effect. Cisplatin accumulates in proximal tubule cells, inducing mitochondrial injury and inhibition of adenosine triphosphatase (ATPase) activity and solute transport. Radiocontrast media–induced nephrotoxicity is thought to result from direct tubular toxicity and renal ischemia.[11] The risk for renal damage caused by radiocontrast media is greatest in elderly persons and those with preexisting kidney disease, volume depletion, diabetes mellitus, and recent exposure to other nephrotoxic agents.

The presence of multiple myeloma light chains, excess uric acid, hemoglobin, or myoglobin in the urine is the most frequent cause of ATN due to intratubular obstruction. Both myeloma cast nephropathy (Chapter 11) and acute urate nephropathy (Chapter 8) usually are seen in the setting of widespread malignancy or massive tumor destruction by therapeutic agents.[3] Hemoglobinuria results from blood transfusion reactions and other hemolytic crises. Skeletal and cardiac muscles contain myoglobin, which corresponds to hemoglobin in function, serving as an oxygen reservoir in the muscle fibers. Myoglobin normally is not found in the serum or urine. It has a low molecular weight; if it escapes into the circulation, it is rapidly filtered in the glomerulus. A life-threatening condition known as *rhabdomyolysis* occurs when increasing myoglobinuria levels cause myoglobin to precipitate in the renal tubules, leading to obstruction and damage to surrounding tubular cells. Myoglobinuria most commonly results from muscle trauma, but may result from extreme exertion, hyperthermia, sepsis, prolonged seizures, potassium or phosphate depletion, and alcoholism or drug abuse. Both myoglobin and hemoglobin discolor the urine, which may range from the color of tea to red, brown, or black.

Clinical Manifestations of Acute Tubular Necrosis. The clinical course of ATN, which is highly variable, is often divided into an initiation, maintenance and recovery phase. The onset or initiating phase, which lasts hours or days, is the time from the onset of the precipitating event (e.g., ischemic phase of prerenal failure or toxin exposure) until tubular injury occurs.

The maintenance phase can involve either an oliguric or nonoliguric phase. Nonoliguric ATN has a better outcome. Conversion from a nonoliguric to an oliguric state is characterized by a marked decrease in the GFR, accompanied by retention of metabolic wastes such creatinine, urea, and sulfate, which normally are cleared by the kidneys. The urine output usually is lowest at this point. Fluid retention gives rise to edema, water intoxication, and pulmonary congestion. If the period of oliguria is prolonged, hypertension develops and with it signs of uremia (accumulation of nitrogenous wastes in the blood). When untreated, the neurologic manifestations of uremia progress from neuromuscular irritability to seizures, somnolence, coma, and death.

The *recovery phase* is the period during which repair of renal tissue takes place. Its onset usually is heralded by a gradual increase in urine output and a fall in serum creatinine, indicating that the nephrons have recovered to the point at which urine excretion is possible. Diuresis often occurs before renal function has fully returned to normal. Consequently, BUN and serum creatinine, potassium, and phosphate levels may remain elevated or continue to rise even though urine output is increased. In some cases, the diuresis may result from impaired nephron function and may cause excessive loss of water and electrolytes. Eventually, renal tubular function is restored with improvement in concentrating ability. At about the same time, the creatinine and BUN begin to return to normal. In some cases, mild to moderate kidney damage persists.

Diagnosis and Treatment

Given the high morbidity and mortality rates associated with AKI, attention should be focused on prevention and early diagnosis. This includes assessment measures to identify persons at risk for development of AKI, including those with preexisting renal insufficiency and diabetes. These persons are particularly at risk for development of AKI due to nephrotoxic drugs (e.g., aminoglycosides and radiocontrast agents) or drugs such as the NSAIDs that alter intrarenal hemodynamics. Elderly persons are susceptible to all forms of AKI because of the effects of aging on renal reserve.

Careful observation of urine output is essential for persons at risk for development of AKI. Urine tests that measure urine osmolality, urinary sodium concentration, and fractional excretion of sodium help differentiate prerenal azotemia, in which the reabsorptive capacity of the tubular cells is maintained, from tubular necrosis, in which these functions are lost. One of the earliest manifestations of tubular damage is the inability to concentrate the urine. Further diagnostic information that can be obtained from the urinalysis includes evidence of proteinuria, hemoglobinuria, myoglobinuria, and casts or crystals in the urine. Blood tests for BUN and creatinine provide information regarding the ability to remove nitrogenous wastes from the blood.

A major concern in the treatment of AKI is identifying and correcting the cause (e.g., improving renal perfusion, discontinuing nephrotoxic drugs). Fluids are carefully regulated in an effort to maintain normal fluid volume and electrolyte concentrations. Adequate caloric intake is needed to prevent the breakdown of body proteins, which increases nitrogenous wastes.[5,8,10] Parenteral hyperalimentation may be used for this purpose. Because secondary infections are a major cause of death in persons with AKI, constant effort is needed to prevent and treat such infections.

Either hemodialysis (to be discussed) or continuous renal replacement therapy (CRRT) may be indicated when nitrogenous wastes and the water and electrolyte balance cannot be kept under control by other means.[5,10] Venovenous or arteriovenous CRRT has emerged as a method for treating AKI in patients too hemodynamically unstable to tolerate hemodialysis.[12] An associated advantage of CRRT is the ability to administer nutritional support. The disadvantages of CRRT are the need for prolonged anticoagulation therapy and continuous sophisticated monitoring.

SUMMARY CONCEPTS

■ Acute kidney injury (AKI) is an abrupt reduction in kidney function, as evidenced by an elevation in serum creatinine, reduction in urine output, the need for dialysis, or a combination of these factors.

■ Acute kidney injury can result from decreased blood flow to the kidney (prerenal injury), from conditions that interfere with the elimination of urine from the kidney (postrenal injury), or from disorders that disrupt the structures in the kidney (intrarenal injury).

■ Acute tubular necrosis (ATN), due to ischemia, sepsis, or nephrotoxic agents, is the most common cause of acute intrarenal injury. Acute tubular necrosis typically progresses through three phases: the initiation phase, during which tubular injury is induced; the maintenance phase, during which the GFR falls, nitrogenous wastes accumulate, and urine output decreases; and the recovery or reparative phase, during which the GFR, urine output, and blood levels of nitrogenous wastes return to normal.

■ Because of the high morbidity and mortality rates associated with AKI, identification of persons at risk is important to clinical decision making. Acute kidney injury often is reversible, making early identification and correction of the underlying cause (e.g., improving renal perfusion, discontinuing nephrotoxic drugs) important. Treatment includes the judicious administration of fluids and hemodialysis or continuous renal replacement therapy.

Chronic Kidney Disease

Chronic kidney disease (CKD) is a pathophysiologic process that results in the loss of nephrons and a decline in renal function as determined by a measured or estimated decrease in the GFR that has persisted for more than 3 months. Chronic kidney disease can result from a number of conditions including diabetes, hypertension, glomerulonephritis, systemic lupus erythematosus, and polycystic kidney disease.[13–16] The prevalence and incidence of the CKD continues to grow, reflecting the growing elderly population and the increasing number of people with diabetes and hypertension. In the United States alone, 26 million adults have CKD, and others are at increased risk.[17]

Regardless of cause, all forms of CKD are characterized by a reduction in the GFR, reflecting a corresponding reduction in the number of functioning nephrons (Fig. 26-3). The rate of nephron destruction differs from case to case, ranging from several months to many years. Typically, the signs and symptoms of CKD occur gradually and do not become evident until the disease is far advanced. This is because of the amazing compensatory ability of the kidneys. As kidney structures are destroyed, the remaining nephrons undergo structural and functional hypertrophy, each increasing its function as a means of compensating for those that have been lost. In the process, each of the remaining nephrons must filter more solute particles from the blood. It is only when the few remaining nephrons are destroyed that the manifestations of kidney failure become evident.

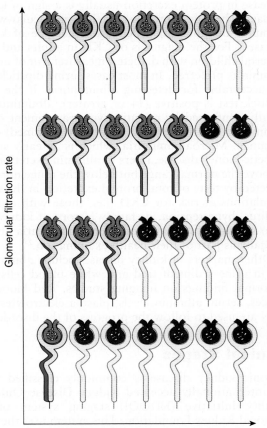

FIGURE 26-3. Relation of renal function and nephron mass. Each kidney contains about 1 million tiny nephrons. A proportional relation exists between the number of nephrons affected by a disease process and the resulting glomerular filtration rate.

Diagnostic Measures

The GFR is considered the best measure of overall function of the kidney. The normal GFR, which varies with age, sex, and body size, is approximately 120 to 130 mL/min/1.73 m² for normal young healthy adults.[18,19] A GFR below 60 mL/min/1.73 m² represents a loss of one half or more of the level of normal adult kidney function.

In clinical practice, GFR is usually estimated using the serum creatinine concentration (see Chapter 24). Although the GFR can be obtained from measurements of creatinine clearance using timed (e.g., 24-hour) urine collection methods, the levels gathered are reportedly no more reliable than the estimated levels obtained by using serum creatinine levels.[20] Because GFR varies with age, sex, ethnicity, and body size, the Modification of Diet in Renal Diseases (MDRD) equation that takes these factors into account is often used for estimating the GFR based on serum creatinine levels.[18] (GRR calculators are available online at http://www.kidney.org/professionals/kdoqi/gfr.cfm.)

Proteinuria serves as a key adjunctive tool for measuring nephron injury and repair. Urine normally contains small amounts of protein. However, a persistent increase in protein excretion usually is a sign of kidney damage. The type of protein (e.g., low–molecular-weight globulins or albumin) depends on the type of kidney disease.[21] For the diagnosis of CKD in adults and post-pubertal children with diabetes, measurement of urinary albumin is preferred. In most cases, urine dipstick tests are acceptable for detecting albuminuria. If the urine dipstick test is positive (1+ or greater), albuminuria is usually confirmed by quantitative measurement of the albumin-to-creatinine ratio in a spot (untimed) urine specimen. Microalbuminuria, which is an early sign of diabetic kidney disease, refers to albumin excretion that is above the normal range but below the range normally detected by tests of total protein excretion in the urine. Populations at risk for CKD (i.e., those with diabetes mellitus, hypertension, or family history of kidney disease) should be screened for microalbuminuria at least annually as part of their health examination.[21]

Other markers of kidney disease include abnormalities in urine sediment (red and white blood cells) and abnormal findings on imaging studies. Red blood cell indices, serum albumin levels, plasma electrolytes, and BUN are used to follow the progress of the disorder.

Clinical Stages

Chronic kidney disease is commonly classified using the internationally accepted Kidney Disease Outcome Quality Initiative (KDOQI) staging system of the National Kidney Foundation. This system uses the GFR to classify CKD into five stages, beginning with kidney damage accompanied by a normal or elevated GFR, progressing to CKD and, potentially, to kidney failure[18,19] (Table 26-1). Kidney damage that is present but undetected due to a normal or increased GFR is classified as stage 1. Individuals with a mild decrease in GFR

TABLE 26-1	Stages of Chronic Kidney Disease	
Stage	**Description**	**GFR (mL/min/1.73 m²)**
1	Kidney damage with normal or increased GFR	≥90
2	Kidney damage with mild decrease in GFR	60–89
3	Moderate decrease in GFR	30–59
4	Severe decrease in GFR	15–29
5	Kidney failure	<15 (or dialysis)

GFR, glomerular filtration rate.

Adapted from National Kidney Foundation. K/DOQI clinical practice guidelines for chronic kidney disease: Evaluation, classification, and stratification. 2002. Available at: http://www.kidney.org/professionals/KDOQI/guidelines_ckd/toc.htm. Reprinted with permission from National Kidney Foundation, Inc.

Chronic kidney disease is defined as either kidney damage or GFR <60 mL/min/1.73 m² for ≥3 months. Kidney damage is defined as pathologic abnormalities or markers of damage, including abnormalities in blood or urine tests or imaging studies.

of 60 to 89 mL/min/1.73 m² (corrected for body surface area) without kidney damage are classified as stage 2. Decreased GFR without recognized markers of kidney damage can occur in infants and older adults and is usually considered to be "normal for age." Other causes of chronically decreased GFR without kidney damage in adults include removal of one kidney, extracellular fluid volume depletion, and systemic illnesses associated with reduced kidney perfusion, such as heart failure and cirrhosis.[18] Even at this stage, there is often a characteristic loss of renal reserve.

Chronic kidney disease, or stage 3 or 4 kidney disease, is defined as either kidney damage or a GFR of 30 to 59 mL/min/1.73 m² for 3 months or longer.[18] Stage 5 CKD represents a GFR of less than 15 mL/min/1.73 m² that is accompanied by most of the signs and symptoms of uremia or a need for dialysis or transplantation.[18]

Clinical Manifestations

In its early stages, CKD is largely asymptomatic. When symptoms do appear, they develop slowly and are often nonspecific. Elevated levels of nitrogenous wastes in the blood, or *azotemia*, is often an early sign of kidney failure, occurring before other signs and symptoms become evident.[22] Urea is one of the first nitrogenous wastes to accumulate in the blood, and the BUN level becomes increasingly elevated as CKD progresses.

Uremia, which literally means "urine in the blood," is the term used to describe the clinical manifestations of kidney failure that are due to an accumulation of nitrogenous waste products in the blood. The uremic state is characterized by signs and symptoms of altered neuromuscular function (e.g., fatigue, peripheral neuropathy, restless leg syndrome, sleep disturbances, uremic encephalopathy); gastrointestinal disturbances such as anorexia and nausea; white blood cell and immune dysfunction; amenorrhea and sexual dysfunction; and dermatologic manifestations such as pruritus.[13,22-24] The onset of uremia in persons with CKD varies; some symptoms may be present to a lesser degree in persons with a GFR that is barely below 50% of normal. However, symptoms such as weakness and fatigue are often nonspecific and difficult to identify.

The manifestations of progressive CKD include disorders of fluid, electrolyte, and acid–base balance, cardiovascular function, anemia and blood coagulation, mineral metabolism, neuromuscular function, immunity, and drug elimination[13,22-24] (Fig. 26-4). The underlying mechanisms for many of these manifestations are often interrelated. The point at which these disorders make their appearance and the severity of the manifestations are determined largely by coexisting disease conditions and the extent to which kidney function has been reduced. Many of them make their appearance before the GFR has reached the kidney failure stage.

Fluid, Electrolyte, and Acid–Base Disorders

The kidneys function in the regulation of sodium and water balance, excrete potassium, and regulate the pH balance of blood. Thus, CKD can produce fluid, electrolyte, and acid–base imbalances.

Sodium and Water Balance. The kidneys function in the regulation of extracellular fluid volume. They do this by either eliminating or conserving sodium and water. Chronic kidney disease can produce dehydration or fluid overload, depending on the pathologic process of the kidney disease. In addition to volume regulation, the ability of the kidneys to concentrate the urine is diminished. An early symptom of kidney damage is *isosthenuria* or polyuria with urine that is almost isotonic with plasma and varies little from voiding to voiding.

As renal function declines further, the ability to regulate sodium excretion is reduced. The kidneys normally tolerate large variations in sodium intake while maintaining normal serum sodium levels. In CKD, they lose the ability to regulate sodium excretion.[13,24] There is impaired ability to adjust to a sudden reduction in sodium intake and poor tolerance of an acute sodium overload. Volume depletion with an accompanying decrease in the GFR can occur with a restricted sodium intake or excess sodium loss caused by diarrhea or vomiting. Salt wasting is a common problem in advanced kidney failure because of impaired tubular reabsorption of sodium. Increasing sodium intake in persons with kidney failure often improves the GFR and whatever renal function remains. In patients with associated hypertension, the possibility of increasing blood pressure or producing congestive heart failure often excludes supplemental sodium intake.

Potassium Balance. Approximately 90% of potassium excretion is through the kidneys. In CKD, potassium excretion by each nephron increases as the kidneys adapt to a decrease in the GFR. In addition, excretion in the gastrointestinal tract is increased. As a result, hyperkalemia usually does not develop until

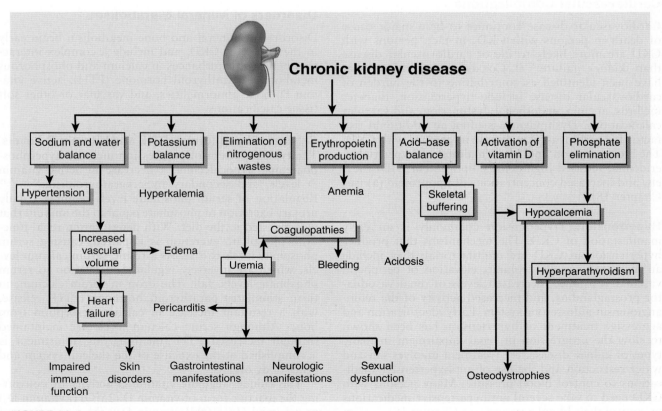

FIGURE 26-4. Mechanisms and manifestations of chronic kidney disease.

kidney function is severely compromised.[13,24] Because of this adaptive mechanism, it usually is not necessary to restrict potassium intake until the GFR has dropped below 5 to 10 mL/min/1.73 m^2.[13] In persons with kidney failure, hyperkalemia often results from failure to follow dietary potassium restrictions; constipation; acute acidosis that causes the release of intracellular potassium into the extracellular fluid; trauma or infection that causes release of potassium from body tissues; or exposure to medications that contain potassium, prevent its entry into cells, or block its secretion in distal nephrons.

Acid–base Balance.

The kidneys also regulate the pH of the blood by eliminating hydrogen ions produced in metabolic processes and regenerating bicarbonate.[13] This is achieved through hydrogen ion secretion, sodium and bicarbonate reabsorption, and the production of ammonia, which acts as a buffer for titratable acids (see Chapter 8). With a decline in kidney function, these mechanisms become impaired and metabolic acidosis may occur when the person is challenged with an excessive acid load or loses excessive alkali, as in diarrhea. The acidosis that occurs in persons with kidney failure seems to stabilize as the disease progresses, probably as a result of the tremendous buffering capacity of bone. However, this buffering action is thought to increase bone resorption and contribute to the skeletal disorders that occur in persons with CKD.

Cardiovascular Complications

Cardiovascular disease continues to be a major cause of death in persons with CKD. In fact, persons with CKD are more likely to die of cardiovascular disease than kidney failure.[22-24] Coexisting conditions that have been identified as contributing to the burden of cardiovascular disease include hypertension, diabetes mellitus, anemia, endothelial dysfunction, and vascular calcifications. Dyslipidemia is often an additional risk factor for cardiovascular disease in persons with CKD. The most common lipid abnormalities are hypertriglyceridemia, reduced high-density lipoprotein (HDL) levels, and increased concentrations of lipoprotein (a) (see Chapter 18).[25]

Hypertension.

Hypertension commonly is an early manifestation of CKD. The mechanisms that produce hypertension in CKD are multifactorial; they include an increased vascular volume, elevation of peripheral vascular resistance, decreased levels of renal vasodilator prostaglandins, and increased activity of the renin-angiotensin-aldosterone system. Early identification and aggressive treatment of hypertension has been shown to slow the progression of renal impairment in many types of kidney disease.[23,24] Treatment involves salt and water restriction and the use of antihypertensive medications to control blood pressure. Many persons with CKD need to take several antihypertensive medications to control their blood pressure (see Chapter 18).

Heart Disease.

The spectrum of heart diseases that occur with CKD include left ventricular hypertrophy, ischemic heart disease, and congestive heart failure.[23,26] People with CKD tend to have an increased prevalence of left ventricular dysfunction, with both depressed left ventricular ejection fraction, as in systolic dysfunction, and impaired ventricular filling, as in diastolic failure (see Chapter 19). Multiple factors lead to development of left ventricular dysfunction, including extracellular fluid overload, shunting of blood through an arteriovenous fistula for dialysis, and anemia. Anemia, in particular, has been correlated with the presence of left ventricular hypertrophy. These abnormalities, coupled with the hypertension that often is present, cause increased myocardial work and oxygen demand, with eventual development of heart failure.

Gastrointestinal Disorders

Most people with CKD have gastrointestinal symptoms. Anorexia, nausea, and vomiting are common in persons with uremia, along with a metallic taste in the mouth that further depresses the appetite.[13,24] Early-morning nausea is common. Ulceration and bleeding of the gastrointestinal mucosa may develop, and hiccups are common. A possible cause of nausea and vomiting is the decomposition of urea by intestinal flora, resulting in a high concentration of ammonia. Nausea and vomiting often improve with restriction of dietary protein and after initiation of dialysis, and disappear after kidney transplantation.

Disorders of Mineral Metabolism

Disorders of mineral and bone metabolism begin early in the course of CKD, and include a complex interaction between disturbances in calcium and phosphorous metabolism, parathyroid hormone (PTH), active vitamin D, bone abnormalities, and vascular or other soft tissue calcifications.

Calcium, Phosphorous, PTH, and Vitamin D Levels.

The typical pattern of progression includes hyperphosphatemia, hypocalcemia, a decrease in active vitamin D levels, and secondary hyperparathyroidism.[13,24,27-29] Regulation of serum phosphate levels requires a daily urinary excretion of phosphate equal to the amount that was ingested in the diet. With deteriorating renal function, phosphate excretion is impaired, causing serum phosphate levels to rise. As a result, serum calcium levels, which are inversely regulated in relation to serum phosphate levels, fall. The drop in serum calcium, in turn, stimulates parathyroid hormone (PTH) release, with a resultant increase in calcium resorption from bone. Although serum calcium levels are maintained through increased PTH function, this adjustment is accomplished at the expense of the skeletal system and other body organs.

The kidneys regulate vitamin D activity by converting the inactive form of vitamin D (25[OH] vitamin D$_3$) to calcitriol (1,25[OH] vitamin D$_3$), the active form of vitamin D.[30,31] Reduced levels of 1,25[OH] vitamin D_3 impair the absorption of calcium from the intestine. Calcitriol also has a direct suppressive effect on PTH production; therefore, reduced levels of calcitriol produce an increase in PTH levels. Most persons with CKD develop secondary hyperparathyroidism, the result of chronic stimulation of the parathyroid glands. Vitamin D also regulates osteoblast differentiation, thereby affecting bone replacement.

Metastatic Calcifications. When the calcium–phosphate product (serum calcium [mg/dL] × serum phosphate [mg/dL]) rises above 60 to 70, metastatic calcifications are commonly seen in arteries, visceral organs, and joints. Alkalemia, which often persists after hemodialysis and may even persist between dialysis treatments, may predispose to precipitation of calcium salts in soft tissues.[28]

Vascular calcifications may affect almost any of the medium-sized arteries, and has been seen in arteries of the forearm, wrist, eyes, feet, abdominal cavity, and brain.[13,28] They are seen more frequently in people older than 40 years of age and in persons on hemodialysis. *Visceral calcifications* may be found in the myocardium, lungs, and stomach.[13,28] In cardiac calcification, the deposits usually develop in the conduction system and may result in serious cardiac arrhythmias. When calcification occurs in the lungs, it causes a fibrotic response in the small arteries and alveolar septa, leading to restrictive and diffusion abnormalities. *Periarticular calcification* in the shoulders, wrists, phalangeal joints, hips, and ankles is common in people on dialysis.[13,28] The major symptom associated with these deposits is limitations in joint movement because of the deposits.

Bone Disease. A hallmark of CKD is renal osteodystrophy or bone disease, which is typically accompanied by reductions in bone mass, alterations in bone microstructure, bone pain, and skeletal fracture.[13,24,27–29] There are changes in bone turnover, mineralization, and bone volume, accompanied by bone pain and muscle weakness, risk of fractures, and other skeletal complications. Two major types of bone disease are commonly encountered in CKD: high-bone turnover due to enhanced bone resorption, and low-bone turnover due to impaired bone mineralization.[24,28] Mild forms of defective bone metabolism may be observed in early stages of CKD (stage 2), and they become more severe as kidney function deteriorates. All of the bone disorders can cause bone pain, proximal muscle weakness, and increased risk of fractures.

High-bone turnover osteodystrophy or *osteitis fibrosa,* the most common type of disease, is the result of secondary hyperparathyroidism and the osteoclast stimulation effects of PTH.[28] Because bone resorption and formation are coupled processes, osteoblast activity is also increased (see Chapter 42, Understanding Bone Remodeling). Although the osteoblasts produce excessive amounts of bone, mineralization fails to keep pace, and there is a decrease in bone density and formation of coarse fibrous bone.[13,28] Cortical bone is affected more severely than cancellous bone.

Low–bone-turnover osteodystrophy or lack of bone mineralization leads to rickets in children and osteomalacia in adults. *Osteomalacia* is characterized by a slow rate of bone formation and defects in bone mineralization, which may be caused by vitamin D deficiency, excess aluminum deposition, or metabolic acidosis.[13,28] Metabolic acidosis is thought to have a direct effect on both osteoblastic and osteoclastic activity, as well as on the mineralization process, by decreasing the availability of trivalent phosphate. Another type of low–bone-turnover osteodystrophy, *adynamic osteodystrophy,* which is almost as common as high–bone-turnover osteodystrophy and is especially common among persons with diabetes. It is characterized by a low number of osteoblasts, a normal or reduced number of osteoclasts, and reduced bone volume and mineralization that may result, in part, from excessive suppression of PTH production with calcitriol.

Early treatment of hyperphosphatemia and hypocalcemia is important to prevent or slow the development of skeletal complications.[28] Phosphate-binding antacids (aluminum salts, calcium carbonate, or calcium acetate) may be prescribed to decrease absorption of phosphate from the gastrointestinal tract. Aluminum-containing antacids can contribute to the development of osteodystrophy, whereas calcium-containing phosphate binders can lead to hypercalcemia, thus worsening soft tissue calcification, especially in persons receiving vitamin D therapy. Phosphate-binding agents that do not contain calcium or aluminum (e.g., sevelamer, lanthanum) are now available.[24] Pharmacologic forms of activated vitamin D often are used to increase serum calcium levels and, at least partially, reverse the secondary hyperparathyroidism and osteitis fibrosa that occur with CKD.[31,32] Secondary hyperparathyroidism may also be treated by activating the calcium-sensing receptor on the parathyroid gland (see Chapter 8). The calcimimetic agent cinacalcet, the first representative of a new class of drugs that act through the calcium-sensing receptor, has been approved for treatment of secondary hyperparathyroidism in CKD.[24]

Hematologic Complications

Anemia. Anemia tends to develop early in the course of CKD, often interfering with the quality of life.[32–34] The anemia of CKD is due to several factors, including chronic blood loss, hemolysis, bone marrow suppression due to retained uremic factors, and decreased red cell production due to impaired production of erythropoietin and iron deficiency. The kidneys are the primary site for the production of the hormone *erythropoietin,* which controls red blood cell production.[32–34] In renal failure, erythropoietin production usually is insufficient to stimulate adequate red blood cell production by the bone marrow. Among the causes of iron deficiency in persons with CKD are anorexia and dietary restrictions that limit intake, as well as the blood loss that occurs during dialysis.

When untreated, anemia causes or contributes to the weakness, fatigue, depression, insomnia, and decreased cognitive function that commonly accompany CKD. There also is an increasing concern regarding the physiologic effects of anemia on cardiovascular function.[32] The anemia of renal failure produces a decrease in blood viscosity and a compensatory increase in heart rate. The decreased blood viscosity also exacerbates peripheral vasodilation and contributes to decreased vascular resistance. Cardiac output increases in a compensatory fashion to maintain tissue perfusion. Anemia also limits myocardial oxygen supply, particularly in persons with coronary heart disease, predisposing to angina pectoris and other ischemic events.

A remarkable advance in the treatment of anemia in CKD was realized when recombinant human erythropoietin (rhEPO) became available. Because iron deficiency is common among persons with CKD, iron supplementation often is needed.[33] Iron can be given orally or intravenously. Intravenous iron is used for treatment of persons who are not able to maintain adequate iron status with oral iron. Although adverse reactions have been reported, intravenous preparations are generally safe and well tolerated.

Coagulation Disorders. The coagulation disorders of CKD are mainly caused by platelet dysfunction.[35] Platelet counts may be slightly decreased and the bleeding time is prolonged because of abnormal adhesiveness and aggregation. Clinically, persons with CKD can experience epistaxis (nosebleeds), menorrhagia (excessive menstrual bleeding), gastrointestinal bleeding, and bruising of the skin and subcutaneous tissues. Coagulative function improves with dialysis but does not completely normalize, suggesting that uremia contributes to the problem. Persons with CKD also have greater susceptibility to thrombotic disorders, particularly if their underlying disease was characterized by a nephrotic presentation.

Immunologic Disorders

All aspects of inflammation and immune function may be affected adversely by the high levels of urea and metabolic wastes seen in CKD. A decreased granulocyte count, defective phagocyte function, impaired acute inflammatory response, and impaired humoral and cell-mediated immunity are typical. These immunologic abnormalities decrease the efficiency of the immune response to infection, which is a common complication of CKD.[36] Skin and mucosal barriers to infection also may be defective. In persons who are maintained on dialysis, vascular access devices are common portals of entry for pathogens. Many persons with CKD fail to mount a fever with infection, making a diagnosis of infection more difficult. The delayed-type hypersensitivity response is also impaired. Although persons with CKD have normal humoral responses to vaccines, a more aggressive immunization program may be needed.

Neuromuscular Complications

Many persons with CKD have alterations in peripheral and central nervous system function.[13,37] Peripheral neuropathy, or involvement of the peripheral nerves, affects the lower limbs more frequently than the upper limbs. It is symmetric, affects both sensory and motor function, and is associated with atrophy and demyelination of nerve fibers, possibly due to uremic toxins. Restless leg syndrome is a manifestation of peripheral nerve involvement and can be seen in as many as two thirds of persons on dialysis. This syndrome is characterized by creeping, prickling, and itching sensations that typically are more intense at rest. Temporary relief is obtained by moving the legs. A burning sensation of the feet, which may be followed by muscle weakness and atrophy, is a manifestation of uremia.

The central nervous system disturbances in uremia are similar to those caused by other metabolic and toxic disorders. Sometimes referred to as *uremic encephalopathy,* the condition is poorly understood and may result, at least in part, from an excess of toxic organic acids that alter neural function. Electrolyte abnormalities, such as sodium shifts, also may contribute. The manifestations are more closely related to the progress of the uremic state than to the level of the metabolic end products. Reductions in alertness and awareness are the earliest and most significant indications of uremic encephalopathy. These often are followed by an inability to fix attention, loss of recent memory, and perceptual errors in identifying persons and objects. Delirium and coma occur late in the disease course; seizures are the preterminal event.

Disorders of motor function commonly accompany the neurologic manifestations of uremic encephalopathy. During the early stages, there often is difficulty in performing fine movements of the extremities; the gait becomes unsteady and clumsy with tremulousness of movement. Asterixis (dorsiflexion movements of the hands and feet) typically occurs as the disease progresses. It can be elicited by having the person hyperextend his or her arms at the elbow and wrist with the fingers spread apart. If asterixis is present, this position causes side-to-side flapping movements of the fingers.

Sexual Dysfunction

Alterations in sexual function and reproductive ability are common in CKD.[38] The cause probably is multifactorial and may result from high levels of uremic toxins, neuropathy, altered endocrine function, psychological factors, and medications (e.g., antihypertensive drugs).

Impotence occurs in as many as 56% of male patients on dialysis. Derangements of the pituitary and gonadal hormones, such as decreases in testosterone levels and increases in prolactin and luteinizing hormone levels, are common and cause erectile difficulties and decreased spermatocyte counts. Loss of libido may result from chronic anemia and decreased testosterone levels.

Impaired sexual function in women is manifested by abnormal levels of progesterone, luteinizing hormone, and prolactin. Hypofertility, menstrual abnormalities, decreased vaginal lubrication, and inability to achieve an orgasm have been described. Amenorrhea is common among women who are on dialysis therapy.

Skin Disorders

Skin disorders are common in persons with CKD.[13] The skin and mucous membranes often are dry, and subcutaneous bruising is common. Skin dryness is caused by a reduction in perspiration owing to the decreased size of sweat glands and the diminished activity of oil glands. Pruritus is common; it results from the high serum phosphate levels and the development of phosphate crystals that occur with hyperparathyroidism. Severe scratching and repeated needle sticks, especially with hemodialysis, break the skin integrity and increase the risk for infection. In the advanced stages of untreated kidney failure, urea crystals may precipitate on the skin as a result of the high urea concentration in body fluids. The fingernails may become thin and brittle, with a dark band just behind the leading edge of the nail followed by a white band. This appearance is known as *Terry nails*.

Treatment

Chronic kidney disease is treated by conservative management to prevent or slow the rate of nephron destruction and, when necessary, by renal replacement therapy with dialysis or transplantation.

Conservative Medical Management

Conservative treatment, which includes measures to retard deterioration of renal function and assist the body in managing the effects of impaired function, can often delay the progression of CKD.[13,39] Urinary tract infections should be treated promptly and medication nephrotoxic potential should be avoided. It should be noted that these strategies are complementary to the treatment of the original cause of the renal disorder, which is of the utmost importance and needs to be continually addressed.

Blood pressure control is important, as is control of blood glucose in persons with diabetes mellitus. In addition to reduction in cardiovascular risk, antihypertensive therapy in persons with CKD aims to slow the progression of nephron loss by lowering intraglomerular hypertension and hypertrophy.[18] Elevated blood pressure also increases proteinuria due to transmission of the elevated pressure to the glomeruli. This is the basis for the treatment guideline establishing 125/75 mm Hg as the target blood pressure for persons with CKD[18] (see Chapter 18). The angiotensin converting enzyme (ACE) and angiotensin receptor blockers (ARBx), which have a unique effect on the glomerular microcirculation (i.e., dilation of the efferent arteriole), are increasingly being used in the treatment of hypertension and proteinuria, particularly in persons with diabetes.[18]

It has also become apparent that smoking has a negative impact on kidney function, and it is one of the most remedial risk factors for CKD.[40] The mechanisms of smoking-induced renal damage appear to include both acute hemodynamic effects (i.e., increased blood pressure, intraglomerular pressure, and urinary albumin excretion) and chronic effects (endothelial cell dysfunction). Smoking is particularly nephrotoxic in elderly persons with hypertension and in those with diabetes. Importantly, the adverse effects of smoking appear to be independent of the underlying kidney disease.

Dietary Management

The goal of dietary management is to provide optimum nutrition while maintaining tolerable levels of metabolic wastes.[41,42] The specific diet prescription depends on the type and severity of renal disease and on the dialysis modality. Because of the severe restrictions placed on food and fluid intake, these diets may be complicated and unappetizing.

Dietary proteins may be restricted as a means of decreasing the progress of renal impairment in persons with advanced CKD. Proteins are broken down to form nitrogenous wastes, and reducing the amount of protein in the diet lowers the BUN and reduces symptoms. Moreover, a high-protein diet is high in phosphates and inorganic acids. Considerable controversy exists over the degree of restriction needed. If the diet is too low in protein, protein malnutrition can occur, with a loss of strength, muscle mass, and body weight. With protein restriction, adequate calories in the form of carbohydrates and fat are essential to meet energy needs. If sufficient calories are not available, the limited protein in the diet is metabolized for energy production, or body tissue itself is used, resulting in decreased strength and mass, as just noted.

Sodium and fluid restrictions depend on the kidneys' ability to excrete sodium and water and must be individually determined. Renal disease of glomerular origin is more likely to contribute to sodium retention, whereas disorders of tubular function tend to cause salt wasting. Fluid intake in excess of what the kidneys can excrete causes circulatory overload, edema, and water intoxication. Thirst is a common problem among patients on hemodialysis, often resulting in large weight gains between treatments. Inadequate intake, on the other hand, causes volume depletion and hypotension and can cause further decreases in the already compromised GFR. It is common practice to allow a daily fluid intake of 500 to 800 mL, which is equal to insensible water loss plus a quantity equal to the 24-hour urine output.

When the GFR falls to extremely low levels in CKD or during hemodialysis therapy, dietary restriction of potassium often becomes mandatory. Using salt substitutes that contain potassium or ingesting fruits, fruit juice, chocolate, potatoes, or other high-potassium foods can cause hyperkalemia.

Persons with CKD are usually encouraged to limit their dietary phosphorus as a means of preventing secondary hyperparathyroidism, renal osteodystrophy, and metastatic calcification. Unfortunately, many processed and convenience foods contain considerable amounts of added phosphorus. Common foods containing phosphorous are restructured meats (e.g., chicken nuggets, hot dogs), processed and spreadable cheeses, instant products (e.g., puddings, sauces), refrigerated bakery products, and beverages.[43] These phosphorus additives are highly absorbable. In a typical diet of grains, meats, and dairy products, only about 60% of phosphorus is absorbed, whereas phosphorus additives (e.g., polyphosphates, pyrophosphates) are almost 100% absorbed.[43] Identifying these newer phosphorus-containing foods is often challenging because manufacturers are no longer required to list the phosphorus content on food labels.

Medication Management

Chronic kidney disease and its treatment can interfere with the absorption, distribution, and elimination of drugs.[44] Many drugs are bound to plasma proteins, such as albumin for transport in the blood, with the unbound portion of the drug being free to act at the various receptor sites and metabolized. A decrease in plasma proteins, particularly albumin, that occurs in many persons with CKD results in less protein-bound drug and greater amounts of free drug.

In the process of metabolism, some drugs form intermediate metabolites that are toxic if not eliminated. Some pathways of drug metabolism, such as hydrolysis, are slowed with uremia. In persons with diabetes, for example, insulin requirements may be reduced as renal function deteriorates. Decreased elimination by the kidneys allows drugs or their metabolites to accumulate in the body and requires that drug dosages be adjusted accordingly. Some drugs contain unwanted nitrogen, sodium, potassium, and magnesium and must be avoided in patients with CKD. Penicillin, for example, contains potassium. Nitrofurantoin and ammonium chloride add to the body's nitrogen pool. Administration of large quantities of phosphate-binding antacids to control hyperphosphatemia and hypocalcemia in patients with CKD interferes with the absorption of some drugs. Because of problems with drug dosing and elimination, persons with CKD should be cautioned against the use of over-the-counter remedies.

Dialysis and Transplantation

Dialysis or renal replacement therapy is indicated when advanced uremia or serious electrolyte imbalances are present. The choice between dialysis and transplantation is dictated by age, related health problems, donor availability, and personal preference. Although transplantation often is the preferred treatment, dialysis plays a critical role as a treatment method for kidney failure. It is life sustaining for persons who are not candidates for transplantation or who are awaiting transplantation. There are two broad categories of dialysis: hemodialysis and peritoneal dialysis.

Hemodialysis. The basic principles of hemodialysis have remained unchanged over the years, although new technology has improved the efficiency and speed of dialysis.[45,46] A hemodialysis system, or artificial kidney, consists of three parts: a blood delivery system, a dialyzer, and a dialysis fluid delivery system. The dialyzer is usually a hollow cylinder composed of bundles of capillary tubes through which blood circulates, while the dialysate travels on the outside of the tubes. The walls of the capillary tubes in the dialysis chamber are made up of a semipermeable membrane material that allows all molecules except blood cells and plasma proteins to move freely in both directions—from the blood into the dialyzing solution and from the dialyzing solution into the blood. The direction of flow is determined by the concentration of the substances contained in the two solutions. The waste products and excess electrolytes in the blood normally diffuse into the dialyzing solution. If there is a need to replace or add substances, such as bicarbonate, to the blood, these can be added to the dialyzing solution (Fig. 26-5).

During dialysis, blood moves from an artery through the tubing and blood chamber in the dialysis machine and then back into the body through a vein. Access to the vascular system is accomplished through an external arteriovenous shunt (i.e., tubing implanted into an artery and a vein) or, more commonly, through an internal arteriovenous fistula (i.e., anastomosis of a vein to an artery, usually in the forearm). Heparin is used to prevent clotting during the dialysis treatment; it can be administered continuously or intermittently. Problems that may occur during dialysis, depending on the rates of blood flow and solute removal, include hypotension, nausea, vomiting, muscle cramps, headache, chest pain, and disequilibrium syndrome. Most persons are dialyzed three times each week for 3 to 4 hours. Many dialysis centers provide the option for patients to learn how to perform hemodialysis at home.

Peritoneal Dialysis. The same principles of diffusion, osmosis, and ultrafiltration that apply to hemodialysis apply to peritoneal dialysis, in which the thin serous membrane of the peritoneal cavity serves as the dialyzing membrane.[22,45] The procedure is facilitated by the surgical implantation of a silastic catheter into the peritoneal cavity at a point below the umbilicus. The catheter is tunneled through subcutaneous tissue and exits on the side of the abdomen (Fig. 26-6). The dialysis process involves instilling a sterile dialyzing solution (usually 1 to 3 L) through the catheter over a period of approximately 10 minutes. The solution then is allowed to remain, or *dwell*, in the peritoneal cavity for a prescribed amount of time, during which the metabolic end products and extracellular fluid diffuse into the dialysis solution. At the end of the dwell time, the dialysis fluid is drained out of the peritoneal cavity by gravity into a sterile bag. The osmotic effects of glucose in the dialysis solution account for water removal.

Peritoneal dialysis can be performed at home or in a dialysis center and can be carried out by continuous ambulatory peritoneal dialysis (CAPD), continuous

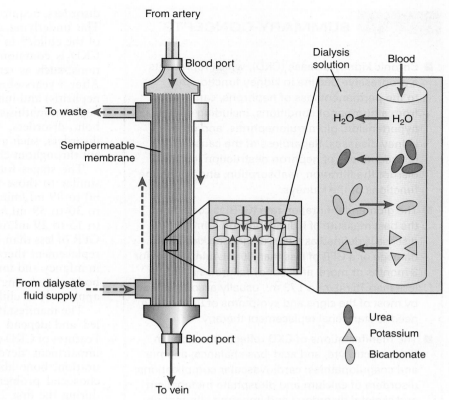

FIGURE 26-5. Schematic diagram of a hemodialysis system. The blood compartment and dialysis solution compartment are separated by a semipermeable membrane. This membrane is porous enough to allow all the constituents, except the plasma proteins and blood cells, to diffuse between the two compartments.

cyclic peritoneal dialysis (CCPD), or nocturnal intermittent peritoneal dialysis (NIPD)—all with variations in the number of exchanges and dwell times.[41] Individual preference, manual ability, lifestyle, knowledge of the procedure, and physiologic response to treatment are used to determine the type of dialysis that is used. The most common method is CAPD, a self-care procedure in which the person exchanges the dialysate four to six times a day. In CCPD, exchanges usually are performed at night, with the person connected to an automatic cycler. In the morning, with the last exchange remaining in the abdomen, the person is disconnected from the cycler and goes about his or her usual activities. In NIPD, the person is given approximately 10 hours of automatic cycling each night, with the abdomen left dry during the day.

Potential problems with peritoneal dialysis include infection, catheter malfunction, dehydration caused by excessive fluid removal, hyperglycemia, and hernia. The most serious complication is infection, which can occur at the catheter exit site, in the subcutaneous tunnel, or in the peritoneal cavity (i.e., peritonitis).

Transplantation. Greatly improved success rates have made kidney transplantation the treatment of choice for many patients with CKD. The availability of donor organs continues to limit the number of transplantations performed each year.[24] Donor organs are obtained from cadavers and living related donors (e.g., parent, sibling). Transplants from living unrelated donors (e.g., spouse) have been used in cases of suitable ABO

blood type and tissue compatibility. The success of transplantation depends primarily on the degree of histocompatibility, adequate organ preservation, and immunologic management. Maintenance immunosuppressive therapy plays an essential role in controlling T- and B-cell activation.

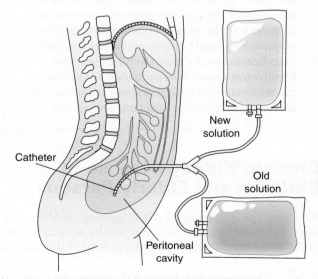

FIGURE 26-6. Peritoneal dialysis. A semipermeable membrane, richly supplied with small blood vessels, lines the peritoneal cavity. With dialysate dwelling in the peritoneal cavity, waste products diffuse from the network of blood vessels into the dialysate.

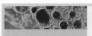

SUMMARY CONCEPTS

- Chronic kidney disease (CKD), which represents a progressive decline in kidney function due to the permanent loss of nephrons, can result from a number of conditions, including diabetes, hypertension, glomerulonephritis, and other kidney diseases. Regardless of the cause, the consequences of nephron destruction in CKD disrupt the filtration, reabsorption, and endocrine functions of the kidneys.

- The glomerular filtration rate (GFR) is considered the best measure of kidney function. Chronic disease is defined as either diagnosed kidney damage or a GFR of less than 60 mL/min/1.73 m² for 3 months or more, and kidney failure as a GFR of less than 15 mL/min/1.73 m², usually accompanied by most of the signs and symptoms of uremia or a need to start renal replacement therapy.

- The manifestations of CKD reflect alterations in fluid, electrolyte, and acid–base balance; anemia and coagulopathies; cardiovascular complications; disorders of calcium and phosphate metabolism and skeletal disorders; and impaired elimination of drugs that are excreted by the kidney. It also results in an accumulation of nitrogenous wastes and signs and symptoms of the uremic state, such as neuromuscular disorders, gastrointestinal disturbances, immune disorders, sexual dysfunction, and discomforting skin changes.

- Treatment measures for CKD can be divided into two types: conservative management and renal replacement therapy. The goals of conservative treatment are to prevent or retard deterioration in remaining renal function and assist the body in compensating for the existing impairment. Renal replacement therapy (dialysis or kidney transplantation) is indicated when advanced uremia and serious electrolyte problems are present.

Chronic Kidney Disease in Children and Elderly Persons

Although the spectrum of CKD among children and elderly persons is similar to that of adults, several unique issues affecting these groups warrant further discussion.

Chronic Kidney Disease in Children

Available data suggest that 1% to 2% of persons with CKD are in the pediatric age range.[47] The causes of CKD in children include congenital malformations, inherited disorders, acquired diseases, and metabolic syndromes. The underlying cause correlates closely with the age of the child.[48] In children younger than 5 years of age, CKD is commonly the result of congenital malformations, such as renal dysplasia or obstructive uropathy. After 5 years of age, acquired diseases (e.g., glomerulonephritis) and inherited disorders (e.g., familial juvenile nephronophthisis) predominate. CKD related to metabolic disorders, such as hyperoxaluria, and inherited disorders, such as polycystic kidney disease, may present throughout childhood.

The stages for progression of CKD in children are similar to those for adults: mild reduction of GFR to 60 to 89 mL/min/1.73 m²; moderate reduction of GFR to 30 to 59 mL/min/1.73 m²; severe reduction of GFR to 15 to 29 mL/min/1.73 m²; and kidney failure with a GFR of less than 15 mL/min/1.73 m², or a need for renal replacement therapy.[49] Because the GFR is much lower in infancy and undergoes gradual changes in relation to body size during the first 2 years of age, these values apply only to children older than 2 years of age.[49]

The manifestations of CKD in children are quite varied and depend on the underlying disease condition. Features of CKD during childhood include severe growth impairment, developmental delay, delay in sexual maturation, bone abnormalities, and development of psychosocial problems.[48,50] Critical growth periods occur during the first 2 years of life and during adolescence. Physical growth and cognitive development occur at a slower rate as consequences of CKD, especially among children with congenital kidney disease.[48] Puberty usually occurs at a later age in children with CKD, partly because of endocrine abnormalities. Renal osteodystrophies are more common and extensive in children than in adults. The most common condition seen in children is high–bone-turnover osteodystrophy caused by secondary hyperparathyroidism. Some hereditary renal diseases, such as medullary cystic disease, have patterns of skeletal involvement that further complicate the problems of renal osteodystrophy. Clinical manifestations of renal osteodystrophy include muscle weakness, bone pain, and fractures with minor trauma.[48,50,51] In growing children, rachitic bone changes, varus and valgus deformities of long bones, and slipped capital femoral epiphysis may be seen (see Chapter 43).

Factors related to impaired growth include deficient nutrition, anemia, renal osteodystrophy, chronic acidosis, and cases of nephrotic syndrome that require high-dose corticosteroid therapy. Nutrition is believed to be the most important determinant of growth during infancy. During childhood, growth hormone is important, and gonadotropic hormones become important during puberty. Parental heights provide a means of assessing growth potential (see Chapter 32). For many children, catch-up growth is important because a growth deficit frequently is established during the first months of life. Recombinant human growth hormone therapy has been used to improve growth in children with CKD.[48] Success of treatment depends on the level of bone maturation at the initiation of therapy.

All forms of renal replacement therapy can be safely and reliably used for children. Age is a defining factor in dialysis modality selection. The majority of North American children are treated with CCPD or NIPD, which leaves the child and family free of dialysis demands during waking hours, with the exchanges being performed automatically during sleep by the machine. Renal transplantation is considered the best alternative for children.[48] Early transplantation in young children is regarded as the best way to promote physical growth, improve cognitive function, and foster psychosocial development.[52] Immunosuppressive therapy in children is similar to that used in adults.[52] All immunosuppressive agents have side effects, including increased risk for infection. Corticosteroids, which have been the mainstay of chronic immunosuppressive therapy for decades, carry the risk for hypertension, orthopedic complications (especially aseptic necrosis), cataracts, and growth retardation.

 ## Chronic Kidney Disease in Elderly Persons

Chronic kidney disease is rather common among the elderly, who comprise the fastest growing subpopulation of the persons with CKD.[53] Aging is associated with structural and functional changes that predispose the aging kidney to insults that otherwise might not have serious consequences. With aging there is a decrease in renal mass and volume, a decrease in renal blood flow, decreased ability to concentrate the urine, and a decrease in the GFR.[54–56] These changes occur at varying stages of aging depending on predisposing genetic factors and exposure to risk factors such as cardiovascular disease and diabetes mellitus.

The reduction in GFR related to aging is not accompanied by a parallel rise in the serum creatinine level because the serum creatinine level, which results from muscle metabolism, is significantly reduced in elderly persons because of diminished muscle mass and other age-related changes. The KDOQI guidelines suggest that the same criteria for establishing the presence of CKD in younger adults (i.e., GFR < 60 mL/min/1.73 m^2) should be used for the elderly. Evaluation of elderly persons with a GFR of 60 to 89 mL/min/1.73 m^2 should include age-adjusted measurements of creatinine clearance, along with assessment of CKD risks, measurement of blood pressure, albumin-to-creatinine ratio in a "spot" urine specimen, and examination of the urine sediment for red and white blood cells.[18]

The prevalence of concurrent chronic disease affecting the cerebrovascular, cardiovascular, and skeletal systems is higher in this age group. As a result, the presenting symptoms of kidney disease in elderly persons may differ from those observed in younger adults. For example, congestive heart failure and hypertension may be the dominant clinical features indicating the onset of acute glomerulonephritis, whereas oliguria and discolored urine more often are the first signs in younger adults. In addition, the course of CKD may be more complicated in older patients with numerous chronic diseases, and its treatment more challenging.

Treatment of the elderly with CKD is usually based on the severity of kidney function impairment and stratification of risk for progression to renal failure and cardiovascular disease.[53,55,56] Persons with low risk may require only modification of dosages of medications excreted by the kidney, monitoring of blood pressure, avoidance of drugs and procedures that increase the risk of AKI, and lifestyle modification to reduce the risk of cardiovascular disease.

Elderly persons with more severe impairment of kidney function may require renal replacement therapy. Treatment options for CKD in elderly patients include hemodialysis, peritoneal dialysis, and transplantation, and acceptance of death from uremia. Neither hemodialysis nor peritoneal dialysis has proved to be superior in the elderly. The choice of therapy should be individualized, taking into account underlying medical and psychosocial factors. Most professional groups support renal transplantation for older people with end stage kidney disease.[53,57] In the past, reluctance to provide transplantation as an alternative may have been due, at least in part, to the scarcity of available organs and the view that younger persons are more likely to benefit for a longer time. The general reduction in T-lymphocyte function that occurs with aging has been suggested as a beneficial effect that increases transplant graft survival. With increasing experience, many transplantation centers have increased the age for acceptance on transplant waiting lists. When dialysis is not effective and transplantation is not an option, psychotherapy may help the person accept death from uremia.

 ## SUMMARY CONCEPTS

- Causes of CKD in infants and children include congenital malformations (e.g., renal dysplasia and obstructive uropathy), inherited disorders (e.g., polycystic kidney disease), acquired diseases (e.g., glomerulonephritis), and metabolic syndromes (e.g., hyperoxaluria). Problems associated with CKD in children include growth impairment, delay in sexual maturation, and more extensive bone abnormalities than in adults. Although all forms of renal replacement therapy can be safely and reliably used in children, CCPD, NIPD, and transplantation optimize growth and development.

- Normal aging is associated with a decline in the GFR, which makes elderly persons more susceptible to the detrimental effects of nephrotoxic drugs and other conditions that compromise renal function. Current guidelines for diagnosis of CKD and stratification of risk for progression to kidney failure are the same as for younger adults. Treatment options for chronic renal failure in elderly patients are also similar to those for younger adults.

REVIEW EXERCISES

1. A 55-year-old man with diabetes and coronary heart disease, who had undergone cardiac catheterization with the use of a radiocontrast agent 2 days ago, is admitted to the emergency department with a flulike syndrome including chills, nausea, vomiting, abdominal pain, fatigue, and pulmonary congestion. His serum creatinine is elevated, and he has protein in his urine. He is admitted to the intensive care unit with a tentative diagnosis of acute kidney injury due to radiocontrast nephropathy.

   A. Radiocontrast agents are thought to exert their effects through decreased renal perfusion and through direct toxic effects on renal tubular structures. Explain how each of these phenomena contributes to the development of acute kidney injury.

   B. Explain the elevated serum creatinine, proteinuria, and presence of pulmonary congestion.

2. A 35-year-old, 70-kg white man with diabetes mellitus is seen in the diabetic clinic for his 6-month check-up. His serum creatinine, which was slightly elevated at his last visit, is now 1.6 mg/dL.

   A. Use the following website to estimate his GFR: http://www.kidney.org/professionals/kdoqi/gfr_calculator.cfm

   B. Would he be classified as having chronic kidney disease? If so, what stage? What might be done to delay or prevent further deterioration of his kidney function?

3. Chronic kidney disease is accompanied by hyperphosphatemia, hypocalcemia, impaired activation of vitamin D, hyperparathyroidism, and skeletal complications.

   A. Explain the impaired activation of vitamin D and its consequences on calcium and phosphate homeostasis, parathyroid function, and mineralization of bone in persons with CKD.

   B. Explain the possible complications of the administration of activated forms of vitamin D on parathyroid function and calcium and phosphate homeostasis.

REFERENCES

1. Rahman M, Shad F, Smith MC. Acute renal injury: a guide to diagnosis and management. *Am Fam Physician.* 2012;86(7):631–639.
2. Kellum JA, Lameire N; for the KDIGO Guideline Work Group. Diagnosis, evaluation, and management of acute kidney injury: a KDIGO summary (Part 1). *Crit Care.* 2013;17:204, 1–15.
3. Martin RK. Acute kidney injury. *AACN Adv Crit Care.* 2010;21(6):350–356.
4. Belloma R, Kellum JA, Ranco C. Acute kidney injury. *Lancet.* 2012;380:756–766.
5. Khalil P, Murty P, Palevsky PM. The patient with acute renal injury. *Prim Care.* 2008;35:239–264.
6. Zarjou A, Agarwal A. Sepsis and acute kidney injury. *J Am Soc Nephrol.* 2011;22:999–1006.
7. Abuelo JG. Normotensive ischemic acute renal failure. *N Engl J Med.* 2007;357(8):797–805.
8. Hall JE. *Guyton and Hall Textbook of Medical Physiology.* 12th ed. Philadelphia, PA: Saunders Elsevier; 2011:399–410.
9. Jennette JC. The kidney. In: Rubin R, Strayer DS. eds. *Rubin's Pathology: Clinicopathologic Basis for Medical Practice.* 6th ed. Philadelphia, PA: Wolters Kluwer Health/Lippincott Williams & Wilkins; 2012:791–794.
10. Alpers CE. The kidney. In: Kumar V, Abbas AK, Fausto N, eds. *Robbins and Cotran Pathologic Basis of Disease.* 8th ed. Philadelphia, PA: Saunders Elsevier; 2010:935–938.
11. McCullough PA, Soman SS. Contrast-induced nephropathy. *Crit Care Clin.* 2005;21:261–280.
12. Tolwani A. Continuous renal-replacement therapy for acute kidney injury. *N Engl J Med.* 2012;367(26):2505–2514.
13. Chonchol M, Chan L. Chronic kidney disease: manifestations and pathogenesis. In: Schrier RW, ed. *Renal and Electrolyte Disorders.* 7th ed. Philadelphia, PA: Wolters Kluwer Health/Lippincott Williams & Wilkins; 2010:389–425.
14. Levey AS. Chronic kidney disease. *Lancet.* 2012;379:165–180.
15. Murphree DD, Thelen SM. Chronic kidney disease in primary care. *J Am Board Fam Med.* 2010;23(4):542–550.
16. Baumgarten M, Gehr T. Chronic kidney disease: detection and evaluation. *Am Fam Physician.* 2011;84(10):1138–1148.
17. National Kidney Foundation. Chronic kidney disease—a growing problems. 2013. Available at: http://www.kidney.org/news/factsheets/CKD-A-Growing problem. Accessed July 4, 2013.
18. National Kidney Foundation. KDOQI clinical practice guidelines for chronic kidney disease: evaluation, classification, and stratification. 2002. Available at: http://www.kidney.org/professionals/KDOQI/guidelines_ckd/toc.htm. Accessed July 30, 2013.
19. Levey AS, Eckardt KW, Tsukamato Y. Definition and classification of chronic kidney disease: a position statement from kidney disease: improving global outcomes (KDIGO). *Kidney Int.* 2005;67:2089–2100.
20. Stevens LA, Coresh J, Greene T, et al. Assessing kidney function: measured and estimated glomerular filtration rate. *N Engl J Med.* 2006;354:2473–2483.
21. Eknoyan G, Hostetter T, Barkis GL, et al. Proteinuria and other markers of chronic kidney disease: a position statement of the National Kidney Foundation (NKF) and the National Institute of Diabetes and Digestive and Kidney Diseases (NIDDK). *Am J Kidney Dis.* 2003;42:617–622.
22. Aimeras C, Argilés Á. The general picture of uremia. *Semin Dial.* 2009;22(4):329–333.
23. Thomas R, Kanso A, Sedor JR. Chronic kidney disease and its complications. *Prim Care.* 2008;35:329–344.
24. Watnick S, Dirkx T. Kidney disease. In: Papadakis MA, McPhee SJ, eds. *Current Medical Diagnosis and Treatment.* New York, NY: McGraw-Hill Lange; 2013:908–917.
25. Tsimihodimos V, Dounousi E, Siamopoulos KC. Dyslipidemia in chronic kidney disease: an approach to pathogenesis and treatment. *Am J Nephrol.* 2008;28:958–973.
26. Schiffrin EL, Lipman ML, Mann JFE. Chronic kidney disease: effects on cardiovascular function. *Circulation.* 2007;116:85–97.
27. Eknoyan G, Levin NW. Bone metabolism and disease in chronic kidney disease. *Am J Kidney Dis.* 2003;42(suppl 3):S1–S201.
28. National Kidney Foundation Inc. KDOQI clinical practice guideline for bone metabolism and disease in chronic kidney disease. *Am J Kidney Dis.* 2003;42(suppl 3):S1–S202.

29. Smith KR, Smelt SC. Consequences of chronic kidney disease: mineral and bone disorders: a progressive disease. *Nephrol Nurs J.* 2009;36(1):49–55.

30. Melamed ML, Thadharni RI. Vitamin D therapy in chronic kidney disease and end stage renal disease. *Clin J Am Soc Nephrol.* 2012;7:358–365.

31. Metamet ML, Thadham RI. Vitamin D therapy in chronic kidney disease and end stage kidney disease. *Clin J Am Soc Nephrol.* 2012;7:358–365.

32. Fishbone S, Nissenson AR. Anemia management in chronic kidney disease. *Kidney Int.* 2010;78(suppl 117):53–59.

33. National Kidney Foundation. KDOQI clinical practice guidelines and clinical practice recommendations for anemia in chronic kidney disease. 2007. Available at: http://www.kidney.org/professionals/KDOQI/guidelines_anemia/index.htm. Accessed July 27, 2013.

34. Pendse S, Singh AK. Complications of chronic renal kidney disease: anemia, mineral metabolism, and cardiovascular disease. *Med Clin North Am.* 2005;89:549–561.

35. Boccardo P, Remuzzi G, Galbusera M. Platelet dysfunction in renal failure. *Semin Thromb Hemost.* 2004;30:579–589.

36. Vaziri ND, Pahl MW, Crum A, et al. Effect of uremia on structure and function of the immune system. *J Ren Nutr.* 2012;22(1):149–156.

37. Brouns R, De Deyn PP. Neurological complications in renal failure: a review. *Clin Neurol Neurosurg.* 2004;107:1–16.

38. Anantharaman P, Schmidt RJ. Sexual function is chronic kidney disease. *Adv Chronic Kidney Dis.* 2007;14(2):119–125.

39. Jabor BL, Madias NE. Progression of chronic kidney disease: can it be prevented or arrested? *Am J Med.* 2005;118:1323–1330.

40. Orth SR. Effects of smoking on systemic and intrarenal hemodynamics: influence on renal function. *J Am Soc Nephrol.* 2004;15(suppl 1):S58–S63.

41. National Kidney Foundation. Clinical practice guidelines for nutrition in chronic renal failure. 2000. Available at: www.kidney.org/professionals/kdoqi/guidelines_updates/doqi_nut.html. Accessed January 19, 2007.

42. Fouque D, Pelletier S, Mafr D, et al. Nutrition and chronic kidney disease. *Kidney Int.* 2011;80:348–357.

43. Murphy-Gutekunst L. Hidden phosphorus in popular beverages. Parts I–IV. *J Ren Nutr.* 2005;15:e1–e6.

44. Quan DJ, Aweeks FT. Dosing of drugs in renal failure. In: Koda-Kimble MA, Young LY, Kradjan WA, et al., eds. *Applied Therapeutics: The Clinical Use of Drugs.* 8th ed. Philadelphia, PA: Lippincott Williams & Wilkins; 2005:34-1–34-26.

45. Flemming GF. Renal replacement therapy review. *Organogenesis.* 2011;7(1):2–12.

46. Himmelfarb J, Ikizer T. Hemodialysis. *N Engl J Med.* 2010;363(19):1833–1845.

47. Chan JCM, Williams DM, Roth KS. Kidney failure in infants and children. *Pediatr Rev.* 2002;23(2):47–60.

48. Sneedharan R, Avner ED. Chronic kidney disease. In: Kliegman RM, Stanton BF, Schor NF, et al., eds. *Nelson Textbook of Pediatrics.* 19th ed. Philadelphia, PA: Elsevier Saunders; 2011:1822.e1–1826.e1.

49. Hogg RJ, Furth S, Lemley KV, et al. National Kidney Foundation's Kidney Disease Outcomes Quality Initiative: clinical practice guidelines for chronic kidney disease in children and adolescents: evaluation, classification, and stratification. *Pediatrics.* 2003;111:1416–1423.

50. Greenbaum LA, Warady BA, Furth SL. Current advances in chronic kidney disease in children: growth, cardiovascular, and neurocognitive risk factors. *Semin Nephrol.* 2009;29(4):425–434.

51. Wesseling-Perry K. Bone disease in pediatric chronic kidney disease. *Pediatr Nephrol.* 2013;28:569–576.

52. Sarwl MM, Wong CJ. Renal transplantation. In: Kliegman RM, Stanton BF, Schor NF, et al., eds. *Nelson Textbook of Pediatrics.* 19th ed. Philadelphia, PA: Elsevier Saunders; 2011:1826.e1–1826.e8.

53. Dousdampanis P, Trigka K, Fourtounas C. Diagnosis and management of chronic kidney disease in the elderly: a field of ongoing debate. *Aging Dis.* 2012;3(5):160–172.

54. Abdelhafiz AH, Brown SHM, Bello A, et al. Chronic kidney disease in older people: physiology, pathology or both. *Nephron Clin Pract.* 2010;116:19–24.

55. Tedla FM, Friedman EA. The trend toward geriatric nephrology. *Prim Care.* 2008;35:515–530.

56. Ng BL, Anpalahan M. Management of chronic kidney disease in the elderly. *Intern Med J.* 2011:761–768.

57. Hansberry MR, Whittier WL, Krause MW. The elderly patient with chronic kidney disease. *Adv Chronic Kidney Dis.* 2005;12(1):71–77.

Porth Essentials Resources

Explore these additional resources to enhance learning for this chapter:

- NCLEX-Style Questions and Other Resources on thePoint, http://thePoint.lww.com/PorthEssentials4e
- Study Guide for Essentials of Pathophysiology
- Concepts in Action Animations
- Adaptive Learning | Powered by PrepU, http://thepoint.lww.com/prepu

Disorders of the Bladder and Lower Urinary Tract

Although the kidneys control the formation of urine, its storage and periodic elimination depend on the coordinated activity of the smooth and striated muscle of the two functional units of the lower urinary tract— the urinary bladder, which serves as reservoir for urine storage and the urethra and urethral sphincter, which function as an outlet for urine elimination. Alterations in the storage and expulsion functions of the lower urinary tract can result in urine retention, which has deleterious effects on ureteral and, ultimately, renal function; or incontinence, with its accompanying social and hygienic problems. The discussion in this chapter focuses on the control of urine elimination, disorders of lower urinary tract structures and function, lower urinary tract infections, and bladder cancer.

Control of Urine Elimination

The urinary bladder is a freely movable organ located retroperitoneally on the pelvic floor, just posterior to the pubic symphysis. It consists of two main components: the body in which urine collects, and the bladder neck, which is a funnel-shaped extension of the body that connects with the urethra.[1,2] In the male, the urethra continues anteriorly through the penis, with the prostate gland surrounding the neck of the bladder where it empties into the urethra. In the female, the bladder is located anterior to the vagina and uterus.

Urine passes from the kidneys to the bladder through the ureters. The interior of the bladder has openings for both the ureters and the urethra. The smooth triangular area that is bounded by these three openings is called the *trigone* (Fig. 27-1). There are no valves at the ureteral openings, but as the pressure of the urine in the bladder rises, the ends of the ureters are compressed against the bladder wall to prevent the backflow of urine.

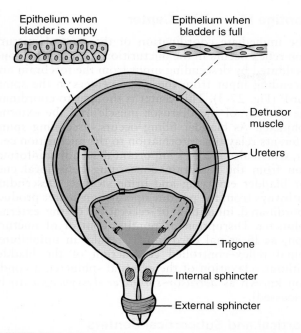

Epithelium when bladder is empty

Epithelium when bladder is full

Detrusor muscle

Ureters

Trigone

Internal sphincter

External sphincter

FIGURE 27-1. Diagram of the bladder, showing the detrusor muscle, ureters, trigone area, and urethral orifice. Note the folding of the epithelial (urothelial) cells when the bladder is empty and flattening of the cells when the bladder is full and the wall is stretched.

Bladder Structure

The bladder, also known as the *urinary vesicle,* is composed of four layers: an outer serosal layer covers the upper surface of the bladder and is continuous with the peritoneum; beneath it is an external network of smooth muscle fibers called the *detrusor muscle;* this is followed by a submucosal layer formed largely of connective and elastic tissue; and an innermost layer of transitional epithelium, often referred to as the *urothelium.*[1,3] Stretching of the bladder wall as a result of distention with urine is accomplished by flattening of its numerous mucosal folds and thick transitional epithelium (see Fig. 27-1).

The urothelium is essentially impermeable to urine solutes and water. The tonicity and composition of the urine often is quite different from that of the blood, and the urothelium acts as an effective barrier to prevent the passage of water and other urine elements between the bladder and the blood.[4] The surface of the urothelium is covered with a mucin layer that is thought to act as a nonspecific anti-adherence factor and as a defense mechanism against infection. The urothelium not only acts as barrier between the bladder contents and the underlying bladder tissues but also as a sensory organ by transmitting physical and chemical information to afferent sensory neurons in the underlying smooth muscle fibers.[4] It has been suggested that conditions such as overactive bladder and interstitial cystitis are associated with alterations in the function of this sensory system.

The detrusor muscle is the muscle of micturition or urination. When it contracts, urine is expelled from the bladder.[1,2] Muscles in the bladder neck, sometimes referred to as the *internal urethral sphincter,* are a continuation of the detrusor muscle. They run down obliquely behind the proximal urethra, forming the posterior urethra in males and the entire urethra in females. When the bladder is relaxed, these circular muscle fibers are closed and act as a sphincter. When the detrusor muscle contracts, the sphincter is pulled open as the shape of the bladder changes as urine is forced into the urethra.

Another muscle important to bladder function is the *external sphincter,* a circular muscle composed of striated skeletal muscle fibers that surrounds the urethra distal to the base of the bladder[1,2] (see Fig. 27-1). The external sphincter operates as a reserve mechanism to stop micturition when it is occurring and to maintain continence in the face of unusually high bladder pressure. The skeletal muscle of the pelvic floor also contributes to the support of the bladder and the maintenance of continence.

Neural Control of Bladder Function

To maintain continence, or retention of urine, the bladder must function as a low-pressure storage system, with the pressure in the bladder being lower than that in the urethra. To ensure that this condition is met, the increase in intravesical pressure that accompanies bladder filling is almost imperceptible.[5,6] Abnormal sustained elevations in intravesical pressures often are associated with vesicoureteral reflux (i.e., backflow of urine from the bladder into the ureter) and the development of ureteral dilation (see Chapter 25, Fig. 25-7). Although the pressure in the bladder is maintained at low levels, sphincter pressures remains high, preventing loss of urine as the bladder fills.

Micturition, or urination, involves the activity of both sensory and motor neurons. When the bladder is distended to 150 to 250 mL in the adult, the first sensation of fullness is transmitted to the spinal cord and then to the cerebral cortex, and at 350 to 450 mL there is a definite sense of bladder fullness.[5] During the act of micturition, the detrusor muscle of the bladder fundus and bladder neck contract down on the urine and the ureteral orifices are forced shut. The bladder neck is widened and shortened, and the external sphincter relaxes as urine moves out of the bladder. Descent of the diaphragm and contraction of the abdominal muscles raise intra-abdominal pressure and aid in the expulsion of urine from the bladder.

Normal bladder function requires coordinated interactions between the sensory and motor components of both the autonomic nervous system (ANS), which controls involuntary smooth muscle activity, and the somatic nervous system, which controls voluntary skeletal muscle activity.[5-7] The motor components of the neural reflex that causes bladder emptying is controlled by the parasympathetic division of the ANS, and the relaxation and storage functions of the bladder is controlled by the sympathetic division. The somatic nervous system innervates the skeletal muscles of the external sphincter and the pelvic floor muscles that together control the outflow of urine. These functions are controlled by three neurologic centers: the spinal cord reflex centers, the micturition center in the pons, and cortical and subcortical centers.[5-7]

Spinal Cord Centers

The centers for reflex control of bladder function are located in the sacral (S1 through S4) and thoracolumbar (T11 through L2) segments of the spinal cord (Fig. 27-2). The parasympathetic neurons for the detrusor muscle of the bladder are located in the sacral segments of the spinal cord; their axons travel to the bladder by way of the *pelvic nerve*. The lower motor neurons for the external sphincter also are located in the sacral segments of the spinal cord. These neurons receive their control from the motor cortex through the corticospinal tract and send impulses to the external sphincter through the *pudendal nerve*. The bladder neck and trigone area of the bladder, because of their different embryonic origins, receive sympathetic outflow from the thoracolumbar (T11 to L2) segments of the spinal cord. In the male, the seminal vesicles, ampulla, and vas deferens also receive sympathetic innervation from the thoracolumbar segments of the cord.

The afferent input from the bladder and urethra is carried to the central nervous system (CNS) by fibers that travel with the parasympathetic (pelvic), somatic (pudendal), and sympathetic (hypogastric) nerves. The pelvic nerve carries sensory fibers from the stretch receptors in the bladder wall, the pudendal nerve carries sensory fibers from the external sphincter and pelvic muscles, and the hypogastric nerve carries sensory fibers from the trigone area.

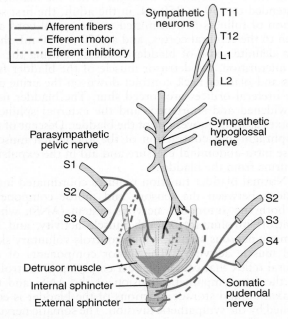

FIGURE 27-2. Nerve supply to the bladder and the urethra.

Pontine Micturition Center

The immediate coordination of the normal micturition reflex occurs in the micturition center in the pons, facilitated by descending input from the forebrain and ascending input from the reflex centers in the spinal cord[5] (Fig. 27-3). This center is thought to coordinate the activity of the detrusor muscle and the external sphincter. As bladder filling occurs, ascending spinal afferents relay this information to the micturition center, which also receives important descending information from the forebrain concerning behavioral cues for bladder emptying and urine storage. Descending pathways from the pontine micturition center produce coordinated inhibition or relaxation of the external sphincter. Disruption of pontine control of micturition, as in spinal cord injury, results in uninhibited spinal reflex–controlled contraction of the bladder without relaxation of the external sphincter, a condition known as *detrusor–sphincter dyssynergia* (to be discussed).

Cortical and Subcortical Centers

Cortical brain centers enable inhibition of the micturition center in the pons and conscious control of urination. Neural influences from the subcortical centers in the basal ganglia modulate the contractile response. They modify and delay the detrusor contractile response during filling and then modulate the expulsive activity of the bladder to facilitate complete emptying.

In infants and young children the pathways to the cortical and subcortical centers are not fully developed and micturition occurs whenever the bladder is sufficiently distended. At about age 2 1/2 years it begins to come under cortical control; in most children, complete control is achieved by 3 years of age.

Neuromediator Control of Bladder Function

The neuromediators for the ANS play a central role in micturition and maintenance of continence.[6,7] Parasympathetic innervation of the bladder is mediated by the neurotransmitter acetylcholine. Two types of cholinergic receptors, nicotinic and muscarinic, affect various aspects of micturition. *Nicotinic* (N) receptors are found in the synapses between the preganglionic and postganglionic neurons of the sympathetic and parasympathetic nervous systems, as well as motor endplates of the striated muscle fibers of the external sphincter and pelvic muscles. *Muscarinic* (M) receptors are found in the postganglionic parasympathetic endings of the detrusor muscle. Several subtypes of M receptors have been identified. Both M_2 and M_3 receptors appear to mediate detrusor muscle activity, with the M_3 subtype mediating direct activation of detrusor muscle contraction. The M_2 subtype appears to act indirectly by inhibiting sympathetically mediated detrusor muscle relaxation.[5-7] The identification of muscarinic receptor subtypes has facilitated the development of medications

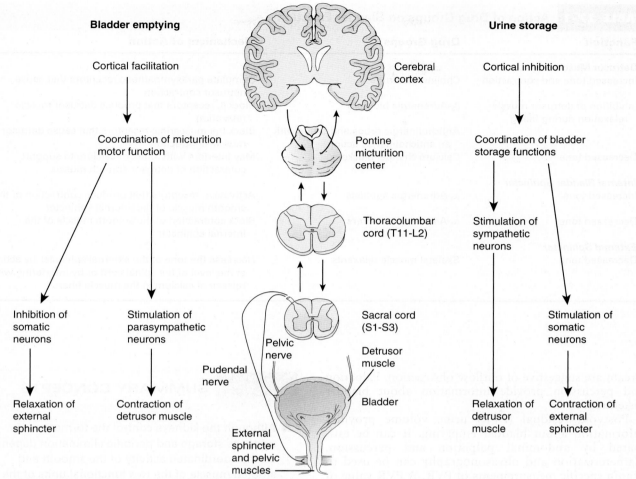

FIGURE 27-3. Pathways and central nervous system centers involved in the control of bladder emptying (*left*) and storage (*right*) functions. Efferent pathways for micturition (*left*) and urine storage (*right*) also are shown.

that selectively target bladder structures while minimizing undesired side effects.

Although sympathetic innervation is not essential to the act of micturition, it allows the bladder to store a large volume without the involuntary escape of urine—a mechanism that is consistent with the fight-or-flight function of the sympathetic nervous system. The bladder is supplied with α_1- and β_2-adrenergic receptors. The β_2-adrenergic receptors are found in the detrusor muscle. They produce relaxation of the detrusor muscle, increasing the bladder volume at which the micturition reflex is triggered. The α_1-adrenergic receptors are found in the trigone area, including the intramural ureteral musculature, bladder neck, and internal sphincter. The activation of α_1-adrenergic receptors produces contraction of these muscles. Sympathetic activity ceases when the micturition reflex is activated. During male ejaculation, which is mediated by the sympathetic nervous system, the musculature of the trigone area and that of the bladder neck and prostatic urethra contract

and prevent the backflow of seminal fluid into the bladder.

Because of their effects on bladder function, drugs that selectively activate or block ANS outflow or receptor activity can alter urine elimination. Table 27-1 describes the action of drug groups that impair bladder function or can be used in the treatment of micturition disorders. For example, many of the nonprescription cold preparations contain α-adrenergic agonists and antihistamine agents that have anticholinergic properties. These drugs can cause urinary retention. Many of the antidepressant and antipsychotic drugs also have anticholinergic actions that influence urination.

Evaluation of Bladder Function

Bladder function can be assessed by a number of methods.[8,9] Reports or observations of frequency, hesitancy, straining to urinate, and a weak or interrupted urine

TABLE 27-1	Action of Drug Groups on Bladder Function	
Function	**Drug Groups**	**Mechanism of Action**
Detrusor Muscle		
Increased tone and contraction	Cholinergic drugs	Stimulate parasympathetic receptors that cause detrusor contraction
Inhibition of detrusor muscle relaxation during filling	β_2-Adrenergic blockers	Block β_2 receptors that produce detrusor muscle relaxation
	Anticholinergic drugs and drugs with an anticholinergic action	Block the muscarinic receptors that cause detrusor muscle contraction
Decreased tone	Calcium channel blockers	May interfere with influx of calcium to support contraction of detrusor smooth muscle
Internal Bladder Sphincter		
Increased tone	α_1-Adrenergic agonists	Activate α_1 receptors that produce contraction of the smooth muscle of the internal sphincter
Decreased tone	α_1-Adrenergic blockers	Block contraction of the smooth muscle of the internal sphincter
External Sphincter		
Decreased tone	Skeletal muscle relaxants	Decrease the tone of the external sphincter by acting at the level of the spinal cord or by interfering with release of calcium in the muscle fibers

stream are suggestive of outflow obstruction. Palpation and percussion provide information about bladder distention.

Postvoid residual (PVR) urine volume provides information about bladder emptying. It can be estimated by abdominal palpation and percussion. Catheterization and ultrasonography can be used to obtain specific measurements of PVR. A PVR value of less than 50 mL is considered adequate bladder emptying, and more than 200 mL indicates inadequate bladder emptying.[8]

Pelvic examination is used in women to assess perineal skin condition, perivaginal muscle tone, genital atrophy, pelvic prolapse (e.g., cystocele, rectocele, uterine prolapse), pelvic mass, or other conditions that may impair bladder function (see Chapter 40). Bimanual examination (i.e., pelvic and abdominal palpation) can be used to assess PVR volume. Rectal examination is used to test for perineal sensation, sphincter tone, fecal impaction, and rectal mass. It is used to assess the contour of the prostate in men.

Urine tests provide information about kidney function and urinary tract infections. The presence of bacteriuria or pyuria suggests urinary tract infection and the possibility of urinary tract obstruction.[9] Blood tests (i.e., blood urea nitrogen and creatinine) provide information about renal function.

Bladder structures can be visualized indirectly by taking x-ray films of the abdomen and through excretory urography, which involves the use of a radiopaque dye, computed tomographic (CT) scanning, magnetic resonance imaging (MRI), or ultrasonography. Urodynamic studies are used to evaluate bladder function and voiding problems. Cystoscopy enables direct visualization of the urethra, bladder, and ureteral orifices.

 SUMMARY CONCEPTS

■ Although the kidneys control the formation of urine, its storage and periodic elimination depend on the coordinated activity of the smooth and striated muscle of the two functional units of the lower urinary tract—the urinary bladder, which serves as a storage reservoir; and the urethra and urethral sphincter, which function as an outlet for urine elimination.

■ The bladder is composed of four layers: an outer serosal layer, a smooth muscle layer called the *detrusor muscle*, a submucosal layer of connective and elastic tissue, and an inner epithelial layer. The detrusor muscle is the muscle of micturition or passage of urine. The inner epithelial layer prevents substances in the urine from moving into the bloodstream and its mucin layer acts as defense against infection.

■ Normal bladder function requires interaction between the sensory and motor components of both the autonomic nervous system (ANS), which controls the involuntary smooth muscle activity of the detrusor muscle, and the somatic nervous system, which controls voluntary skeletal muscle activity of the external sphincter. These functions are controlled by three ascending levels of nervous system control: the spinal cord reflex centers, the micturition center in the pons, and cortical and subcortical centers.

■ The sympathetic nervous system division of the ANS facilitates bladder filling by producing relaxation of the smooth muscle fibers of the detrusor muscle in the bladder wall and contraction of the internal sphincter. The parasympathetic nervous system facilitates bladder emptying by producing contraction of the detrusor muscle and relaxation of the internal sphincter.

■ The striated muscles in the external sphincter and pelvic floor, which are innervated by the somatic nervous system, provide for the voluntary control of urination and maintenance of continence.

Disorders of Lower Urinary Tract Structures and Function

Disorders of lower urinary tract structures and function include urinary obstruction with retention or stasis of urine, and urinary incontinence with involuntary loss of urine. Both types of disorders can have their origin in the structures of the lower urinary tract or in the neural mechanisms that control their function.

Lower Urinary Tract Obstruction and Stasis

In lower urinary tract obstruction and stasis, urine is produced normally by the kidneys but is retained in the bladder, a condition that predisposes to vesicoureteral reflux (VUR) and kidney damage. Obstructions can be classified according to their location (bladder neck, urethra, or external urethral meatus), cause (congenital or acquired), degree (partial or complete), and duration (acute or chronic).[10]

The common sites of congenital obstructions are the external meatus (i.e., meatal stenosis) in boys and just inside the external urinary meatus in girls. Another congenital cause of urinary stasis is the damage to sacral nerves that is seen in spina bifida and meningomyelocele (see Chapter 36). The acquired causes of lower urinary tract obstruction and stasis are numerous. In males, the most important cause of urinary obstruction is external compression of the urethra caused by enlargement of the prostate gland.[10,11] Gonorrhea and other sexually transmitted infections contribute to the incidence of infection-produced urethral strictures. Bladder tumors and secondary invasion of the bladder by tumors arising in structures that surround the bladder and urethra can compress the bladder neck or urethra and cause obstruction. Obstructive disorders in women include conditions related to relaxation of the pelvic support structures, such as cystocele and rectocele. Because of the proximity of the involved structures, severe constipation and fecal impaction can compress the urethra and produce urethral obstruction.

Compensatory and Decompensatory Changes

The body compensates for the obstruction of urine outflow with mechanisms designed to prevent urine retention. These mechanisms can be divided into two stages: a compensatory stage and a decompensatory stage.[10] The degree to which these changes occur and their effect on bladder structure and urinary function depend on the extent of the obstruction, the rapidity with which it occurs, and the presence of other contributing factors, such as neurologic impairment and infection.

During the early stage of obstruction, the bladder begins to hypertrophy and becomes hypersensitive to afferent stimuli arising from stretch receptors in the bladder wall. The ability to suppress urination is diminished, and the bladder contractions can become so strong that they virtually produce bladder spasms. There is urgency, sometimes to the point of incontinence, and frequency of urination during the day and at night.

With continuation and progression of the obstruction, there is further hypertrophy of the bladder muscle, and the pressure generated by detrusor contraction can increase from a normal 20 to 40 cm H_2O to 50 to 100 cm H_2O to overcome the resistance from the obstruction.[10] As the force needed to expel urine from the bladder increases, compensatory mechanisms may become ineffective, causing muscle fatigue before complete emptying can be accomplished. After a few minutes, voiding can again be initiated and completed, accounting for the frequency of urination.

Normally, the inner bladder surface forms smooth folds. With continued outflow obstruction, this smooth surface is replaced with coarsely woven structures (i.e., hypertrophied smooth muscle fibers) called *trabeculae*. Small pockets of mucosal tissue, called *cellulae*, commonly develop between the trabecular ridges. These pockets form diverticula when they extend between the actual fibers of the bladder muscle (Fig. 27-4). Because the diverticula have no muscle, they are unable to contract and expel their urine into the bladder, and secondary infections caused by stasis are common. Along with hypertrophy of the bladder wall, there is hypertrophy of the trigone area and the interureteric ridge, which is located between the two ureters. This causes backpressure on the ureters, the development of hydroureters, and, eventually, kidney damage. Stasis of urine also predisposes to urinary tract infections.

When compensatory mechanisms no longer are effective, signs of decompensation begin to appear. The period of detrusor muscle contraction becomes too short to expel the urine completely, and residual urine remains in the bladder. At this point, the symptoms of obstruction—frequency of urination, hesitancy, need to strain to initiate urination, a weak and small stream, and termination of the stream before the bladder is completely emptied—become pronounced. There may be signs of a complicating urinary tract infection such

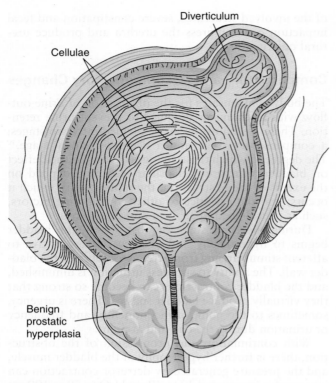

FIGURE 27-4. Destructive changes of the bladder wall with development of diverticulum caused by benign prostatic hyperplasia.

as burning on urination and cloudy urine. With progressive decompensation, the bladder may become severely overstretched, with a residual urine volume of 1000 to 3000 mL.[10] At this point, it loses its power of contraction and overflow incontinence occurs.

The immediate treatment of lower urinary tract obstruction and stasis is directed toward relief of bladder distention. This usually is accomplished through urinary catheterization. Long-term treatment is directed toward correcting the problem causing the obstruction.

Neurogenic Bladder Disorders

The urinary bladder is unique in that it is probably the only autonomically innervated visceral organ that is under CNS control. The neural control of bladder function can be interrupted at any level. It can be interrupted at the level of the peripheral nerves that innervate the bladder, the sacral cord reflex center, the ascending and descending tracts in the spinal cord, the pontine micturition center, or the cortical centers that are involved in voluntary control of micturition[7,11,12] (see Fig. 27-3).

Neurogenic disorders of bladder function commonly are manifested in one of two ways: bladder overactivity with a failure to relax and store urine; or areflexic bladder dysfunction, with a failure to contract and empty. Neurogenic detrusor overactivity usually results from neural lesions located above the level of the sacral micturition reflexes; in contrast, failure to contract (areflexic bladder dysfunction) results from lesions at the level of the sacral micturition center or the peripheral nerves that innervate the bladder. Less commonly, disorders of micturition occur when the neural control of external sphincter function is disrupted. Table 27-2 describes the characteristics of neurogenic bladder according to the level of the lesion.

Neurogenic Overactive Bladder: Failure to Store Urine

Neurogenic detrusor overactivity, or spastic bladder, is usually characterized by reflex bladder spasms and a decrease in bladder volume. It commonly is caused by conditions that produce partial or extensive neural damage above the level of the micturition reflex center

TABLE 27-2	**Types and Characteristics of Neurogenic Bladder**	
Level of Lesion	**Change in Bladder Function**	**Common Causes**
Sensory cortex, motor cortex, or corticospinal tract	Loss of ability to perceive bladder filling; low-volume, physiologically normal micturition that occurs suddenly and is difficult to inhibit	Stroke and advanced age
Basal ganglia or extrapyramidal tract	Detrusor contractions are elicited suddenly without warning and are difficult to control; bladder contraction is shorter than normal and does not produce full bladder emptying	Parkinson disease
Pontine micturition center or communicating tracts in the spinal cord	Storage reflexes are provoked during filling, and external sphincter responses are heightened; uninhibited bladder contractions occur at a lower volume than normal and do not continue until the bladder is emptied; antagonistic activity occurs between the detrusor muscle and the external sphincter	Spinal cord injury
Sacral cord or nerve roots	Areflexic bladder fills but does not contract; loss of external sphincter tone occurs when the lesion affects the α-adrenergic motor neurons or pudendal nerve	Injury to sacral cord or spinal roots
Pelvic nerve	Increased filling and impaired sphincter control cause increased intravesicular pressure	Radical pelvic surgery
Autonomic peripheral sensory pathways	Bladder overfilling occurs owing to a loss of ability to perceive bladder filling	Diabetic neuropathies, multiple sclerosis

in the sacral cord (see Fig. 27-3). As a result, bladder function is regulated by segmental reflexes, without control from higher brain centers. The degree of bladder spasticity and dysfunction depends on the level and extent of neural dysfunction. Usually, both the ANS neurons controlling bladder function and the somatic neurons controlling the function of the striated muscles in the external sphincter are affected. The most common causes of neurogenic detrusor overactivity are spinal cord lesions such as spinal cord injury, vascular lesions, tumors, or herniated intervertebral disk, and multiple sclerosis.

Bladder Dysfunction Caused by Spinal Cord Injury. Bladder dysfunction is a common problem in persons with spinal cord injury (see Chapter 36). The immediate and early effects of spinal cord injury on bladder function are quite different from those that follow recovery from the initial injury.[7,13] During the period immediately after spinal cord injury, a state of spinal shock develops in which all reflexes, including the micturition reflex, are depressed. During this stage, the bladder becomes atonic and cannot contract. Catheterization is necessary to prevent injury to urinary structures associated with overdistention of the bladder. Depression of reflexes lasts from a few weeks to 6 months (usually 2 to 3 months), after which the spinal reflexes return and become hyperactive.

After the acute stage of spinal cord injury, the micturition response changes to a segmental reflex. Because the sacral reflex arc remains intact, stimuli generated by bladder stretch receptors during filling produce frequent spontaneous contractions of the detrusor muscle. This creates a small, hyperactive bladder subject to high-pressure and short-duration uninhibited bladder contractions. Voiding is interrupted, involuntary, or incomplete. Dilation of the internal sphincter and spasticity of the external sphincter and perineal muscles occurs, producing resistance to bladder emptying. Overdistention of the bladder with hypertrophy of the trigone area develops, often leading to vesicoureteral reflux and risk for renal damage.

Overactive bladder due to spinal cord injuries at the cervical level is often accompanied by a condition known as *autonomic hyperreflexia* (see Chapter 36). Because the injury interrupts CNS control of sympathetic reflexes in the spinal cord, severe hypertension, bradycardia, and sweating can be triggered by even mild overdistention of the bladder or by insertion of a catheter.

Uninhibited Neurogenic Bladder. A mild form of reflex neurogenic bladder, sometimes called *uninhibited bladder*, can develop after a stroke, during the early stages of multiple sclerosis, or as a result of lesions located in the inhibitory centers of the cortex or associated structures.[13] With this type of disorder, sacral reflex motor function and sensation are retained, the urine stream is normal, and there is no residual urine. There usually is reduced awareness of bladder fullness and a low bladder capacity due to reduced inhibition by the pontine micturition center or cortical centers.

Detrusor–Sphincter Dyssynergia. Lesions that affect the micturition center in the pons or impair communication between the micturition center and spinal cord centers interrupt the coordinated activity of the detrusor muscle and the external sphincter.[13] This is called *detrusor–sphincter dyssynergia*. Instead of relaxing during micturition, the external sphincter becomes more constricted. This condition can lead to elevated intravesical pressures, vesicoureteral reflux, and kidney damage.

Neurogenic Areflexic Bladder: Failure to Empty Urine

Detrusor muscle areflexia, or flaccid neurogenic bladder, occurs when there is injury to nerves in the micturition center of the sacral cord, the cauda equina, or peripheral nerves that supply the bladder. Atony of the detrusor muscle and loss of the perception of bladder fullness permit overstretching of the detrusor muscle; which in turn, leads to weak and ineffective bladder contractions. External sphincter tone and perineal muscle tone are diminished. Voluntary urination does not occur, but fairly efficient emptying usually can be achieved by increasing the intra-abdominal pressure or applying manual suprapubic pressure. Among the causes of areflexic neurogenic bladder are trauma, tumors, and congenital anomalies (e.g., spina bifida, meningomyelocele).

Bladder Dysfunction Caused by Peripheral Neuropathies. Disorders of the peripheral (pelvic, pudendal, and hypogastric) nerves that supply the muscles of micturition can selectively interrupt sensory or motor pathways for the bladder or involve both pathways.

Bladder atony with dysfunction is a frequent complication of diabetes mellitus.[14,15] The disorder initially affects the sensory nerves of the bladder without involvement of the pudendal nerve. This leads to large residual volumes after micturition, sometimes complicated by infection. There frequently is a need for straining, accompanied by hesitation, weakness of the urinary stream, dribbling, and a sensation of incomplete bladder emptying.[15] The most common complications are vesicoureteral reflux and ascending urinary tract infection. Because persons with diabetes are already at risk for development of kidney disease, urinary stasis and reflux can have serious effects on renal function.

Nonrelaxing External Sphincter

Another condition that affects micturition and bladder function is the nonrelaxing external sphincter. This condition usually is related to a delay in maturation, developmental regression, psychomotor disorders, or locally irritative lesions. Inadequate relaxation of the external sphincter can also result from anxiety or depression. Any local irritation, including vaginitis or perineal irritation, can produce spasms of the sphincter through afferent sensory input from the pudendal nerve. In men, chronic prostatitis contributes to impaired relaxation of the external sphincter.

Treatment

The goals of treatment for neurogenic bladder disorders focus on preventing bladder overdistention, urinary tract infections, and potentially life-threatening kidney damage. The methods used in treatment are individualized based on the type of neurologic lesion that is involved; information obtained through the health history, including fluid intake; report or observation of voiding patterns; presence of other health problems; urodynamic studies when indicated; and the ability of the person to participate in the treatment. Treatment methods include catheterization, bladder training, pharmacologic manipulation of bladder function, and surgery.

Catheterization involves the insertion of a small-diameter latex or silicone tube into the bladder through the urethra. The catheter may be inserted on a one-time basis to relieve temporary bladder distention, left indwelling (i.e., retention catheter), or inserted intermittently. The methods used for bladder retraining depend on the type of lesion causing the disorder. Methods used to supplement bladder retraining include monitoring fluid intake to control urine volume and osmolality and prevent urinary tract infections, developing scheduled times for urination, and using body positions that facilitate micturition.

Pharmacologic manipulation includes the use of drugs to alter the contractile properties of the bladder, decrease the outflow resistance of the internal sphincter, and relax the external sphincter. Antimuscarinic drugs decrease detrusor muscle tone and increase bladder capacity in persons with spastic bladder dysfunction.[7] Cholinergic drugs that stimulate parasympathetic receptors provide increased bladder tone and may prove helpful in the symptomatic treatment of milder forms of flaccid neurogenic bladder. Muscle relaxants may be used to decrease the tone of the external sphincter. Intravesical injection of medications such as capsaicin and resiniferatoxin, which are specific C-fiber afferent neurotoxins, may be used to decrease bladder hyperactivity. Botulinum toxin type A injections may be used to produce paralysis of the striated muscles of the external sphincter in persons with neurogenic overactive bladder. The effects of the injection last about 6 months, after which the injection must be repeated.[12]

Among the surgical procedures used in the management of neurogenic bladder are sphincterectomy, reconstruction of the sphincter, and resection of the sacral reflex nerves that cause detrusor overactivity or the pudendal nerve that controls the external sphincter.[12] Extensive research is being conducted on methods of restoring voluntary control of the storage and evacuation functions of the bladder through the use of implanted electrodes.

Urinary Incontinence

Urinary incontinence represents the involuntary loss or leakage of urine. It can occur without the person's knowledge; at other times, the person may be aware of the condition but be unable to prevent it. A number of conditions can lead to incontinence, which is a common problem, particularly in older adults.[8,16–19]

Types and Causes of Incontinence

Urinary incontinence is commonly divided into three main types: stress incontinence, urge incontinence, and mixed incontinence, which is a combination of stress incontinence and urge incontinence. Other types of incontinence include overflow incontinence, which is a term used to describe leakage of urine associated with urinary retention, and nocturnal enuresis, which is the involuntary loss of urine during sleep. Post-micturition dribble and continuous urinary leakage are other forms of incontinence.[17-20]

Stress Incontinence. Stress incontinence represents the involuntary loss of urine that occurs when, in the absence of detrusor muscle action, the intravesical pressure exceeds the maximum urethral closure pressure.[21-24] Among the proposed causes of stress incontinence are changes in the anatomic relationship between the bladder and the urethra, so that increases in intra-abdominal pressure are unevenly distributed to the urethra.[8,19]

Stress incontinence, which is a common problem in women of all ages, occurs as the result of weakness or disruption of pelvic floor muscles leading to poor support of the vesicourethral sphincters. Except during the act of micturition, intraurethral pressure is normally greater than intravesical pressure. The pressure difference between the urethra and bladder is known as the *urethral closure pressure*. If intra-abdominal pressure increases as it does during actions such as coughing, laughing, or sneezing, and if this pressure is not equally transmitted to the urethra, then incontinence occurs. Diminution of muscle tone associated with normal aging, childbirth, or surgical procedures can cause weakness of the pelvic floor muscles and decrease the urethral closure pressure, resulting in stress incontinence by changing the relationship between the bladder base and the posterior urethral junction.

Another cause of stress incontinence is intrinsic urethral deficiency, which may result from congenital sphincter weakness, as occurs with meningomyelocele. It also may be acquired as a result of trauma, irradiation, or sacral cord lesions. Stress incontinence in men may result from trauma or surgery to the bladder outlet, as occurs with prostatectomy.[19,24] Neurologic dysfunction, as occurs with impaired sympathetic innervation of the bladder neck, impaired pelvic nerve innervation to the intrinsic sphincter, or impaired pudendal nerve innervation to the external sphincter, may also be a contributing factor.

Urge Incontinence. Urge incontinence is the involuntary loss of urine associated with a strong desire to void (urgency).[8,19] It is often associated with overactive bladder, which the International Continence Society defines as "urinary urgency, usually accompanied by frequency and nocturia, with or without urinary incontinence, in the absence of urinary tract infection or other obvious pathology."[25]

The symptoms of urge incontinence, which are caused by involuntary bladder contractions during filling, may occur alone or in any combination. They constitute overactive bladder when they occur in the absence of other pathologic processes.[8,19,26–28] Regardless of the primary cause of overactive bladder, two types of mechanisms are thought to contribute to its symptomatology: those involving CNS and neural control of bladder sensation and emptying (neurogenic) and those involving the smooth muscle of the bladder itself (myogenic).[8,26,27]

The *neurogenic* theory for overactive bladder proposes that the CNS functions as an on–off switching circuit for voluntary control of bladder function. Neurogenic causes of overactive bladder include stroke, Parkinson disease, and multiple sclerosis. Other neurogenic causes of overactive bladder include increased sensitization of the afferent nerves that sense bladder filling or increased excitability to efferent nerves that produce bladder emptying.

The *myogenic* causes of overactive bladder are thought to result from changes in the properties of the smooth muscle of the bladder itself. Bladder outlet obstruction can prompt such changes. It is hypothesized that the sustained increase in intravesical pressure that occurs with the outlet obstruction causes a partial destruction of the nerve endings that control bladder excitability.[7] This partial denervation produces hyperexcitability of the detrusor muscle, causing urgency and frequency of urination due to spontaneous bladder contractions. Disorders of detrusor muscle structure and excitability also can occur as the result of the aging process or disease conditions such as diabetes mellitus. Incomplete bladder emptying, a common accompaniment of overactive bladder, often exacerbates symptoms.

Overflow Incontinence. Overflow incontinence is an involuntary loss of urine that occurs when intravesical pressure exceeds the maximal urethral pressure because of bladder distention in the absence of detrusor activity.[8] It can occur with retention of urine owing to nervous system lesions or obstruction of the bladder neck or urethral stricture. Outflow obstruction may occur secondary to cystocele, uterine prolapse, or previous incontinence surgery in women. In men, one of the most common causes of obstructive incontinence is enlargement of the prostate gland. Person with this type of incontinence may experience dribbling, weak urinary stream, hesitancy, frequency, and nocturia.

Other Causes of Incontinence. Other causes of incontinence include decreased bladder compliance or distensibility. This abnormal bladder condition may result from radiation therapy, radical pelvic surgery, or interstitial cystitis. Many persons with this disorder have severe urgency related to bladder hypersensitivity that results in loss of bladder elasticity, such that any small increase in bladder volume or detrusor function causes a sharp rise in bladder pressure and severe urgency.

Incontinence may occur as a transient and correctable phenomenon, or it may not be totally correctable and may occur with various degrees of frequency. Incontinence may also present as nocturnal enuresis with involuntary loss of urine during sleep, as post-micturition dribble, or continuous urine leakage.[18] Among the transient causes of urinary incontinence are recurrent urinary tract infections; medications that alter bladder function or perception of bladder filling and the need to urinate; diuretics and conditions that increase bladder filling; restricted mobility; and a state of confusion. Night sedation may cause someone to sleep through the signal that normally would waken them so they could get up and empty their bladder and avoid wetting the bed. Incontinence also may be caused by factors outside the lower urinary tract, such as the inability to locate, reach, or receive assistance in reaching an appropriate place to void.

Diagnosis and Treatment

Urinary incontinence is not a single disease but a symptom with many possible causes. As a symptom, it requires full investigation to establish its cause.[20–24,27] This usually is accomplished through a careful history, physical examination, blood tests, and urinalysis. A voiding record (i.e., diary) may be used to determine the frequency, timing, and amount of voiding, as well as other factors associated with the incontinence. Because many drugs affect bladder function, a full drug history is essential. Estimation of the PVR volume is recommended for all persons with incontinence.

Treatment or management depends on the type of incontinence, accompanying health problems, and the person's age. It includes behavioral methods; exercises to strengthen the pelvic floor muscles; pharmacologic measures; surgical interventions; and, when urine flow cannot be controlled, noncatheter devices to obstruct urine flow or collect urine as it is passed.[28,29] Indwelling catheters, although a solution to the problem of urinary incontinence, usually are considered only after all other treatment methods have failed. In some types of incontinence, such as that associated with spinal cord injury or meningomyelocele, self-catheterization may provide the best means for controlling urine elimination (see Chapter 36).

Behavioral methods include fluid management, timed/prompted voiding, bladder retraining, and toileting assistance. Bladder retraining and biofeedback techniques seek to reestablish cortical control over bladder function by having the person ignore urgency and respond only to cortical signals during waking hours. Exercises of the pelvic muscles or Kegel exercises involve repetitive contraction and relaxation of the pelvic floor muscles and are an essential component of patient-dependent behavioral interventions.[19]

Pharmacologic treatment is aimed at using drugs to alter the physiologic mechanisms that contribute to the neurogenic or myogenic causes of incontinence (see Table 27-1).[19] They include the use of drugs that increase sphincter tone in stress incontinence, decrease hyperexcitability of the detrusor muscle in overactive bladder/urge incontinence, or relieve outflow obstruction in overflow incontinence.

Surgical intervention may be considered when other treatment methods have proved ineffective. The principal objective of surgical treatment of stress incontinence is to increase outlet resistance through restoration of the proper suspension and support of the vesicourethral segment of the urethra.[23] A minimally invasive procedure for the treatment of stress incontinence due to internal sphincter weakness is the periurethral injection of a bulking agent.[8,19] Surgically implanted artificial sphincters are available for use in treatment of incontinence due to severe sphincter damage.[8] Other procedures remove outflow obstruction to reduce overflow incontinence and detrusor muscle instability.

Special Needs of Elderly Persons

Urinary incontinence is a common problem in elderly persons, both male and female.[30-33] Incontinence increases social isolation, frequently leads to institutionalization, and predisposes to infections and skin breakdown. Many factors contribute to incontinence in elderly persons, including a reduction in bladder capacity and urethral closing pressure. Detrusor muscle function also tends to change with aging. There is often a reduction in the strength of bladder contraction and impairment in emptying that leads to larger PVR volumes. Detrusor overactivity is also common. It is characterized by symptoms of immediate urinary urgency and frequency and, in the case of involuntary urinary loss, urge incontinence. In men, benign prostatic hyperplasia may lead to outlet obstruction and overflow incontinence.[34] Men may also develop stress incontinence following radical prostatectomy for treatment of prostate cancer or transurethral resection for treatment of benign prostatic hyperplasia. In each of these cases, bladder pressure exceeds the closure pressure at the urethral outlet, leading to urine leakage.

Furthermore, advancing age often results in restricted mobility, comorbid illness, infection, and constipation or stool impaction, all of which can precipitate urinary incontinence. Many elderly persons have difficulty getting to the toilet in time. This can be caused by arthritis that makes walking or removing clothing difficult or by failing vision that makes trips to the bathroom precarious, especially in new and unfamiliar surroundings. Impaired thirst or limited access to fluids can lead to constipation, in which the impacted stool produces urethral obstruction, causing overflow incontinence.

Medications prescribed for other health problems may also contribute to incontinence. Potent, fast-acting diuretics are known for their ability to cause urge incontinence. Diuretics, particularly in elderly persons, increase the flow of urine and may contribute to incontinence, particularly in persons with diminished bladder

capacity and in those who have difficulty reaching the toilet in time. Drugs such as hypnotics, tranquilizers, and sedatives can interfere with the conscious inhibition of voiding, leading to urge incontinence.

Many nonurologic conditions predispose the elderly to urinary incontinence. The transient and often treatable causes of urinary incontinence may best be remembered with the acronym DIAPPERS, in which the D stands for dementia/dementias, I for infection (urinary or vaginal), A for atrophic vaginitis, P for pharmaceutical agents, P for psychological causes, E for endocrine conditions (diabetes), R for restricted mobility, and S for stool impaction.[32] These eight transient causes of incontinence should be identified and treated before other treatment options are considered.

As with urinary incontinence in younger persons, incontinence in elderly persons requires a thorough history and physical examination to determine the cause of the problem. A voiding history is important. A voiding diary provides a means for the person to provide objective information about the number of bathroom visits, the number of protective pads used, and even the volume of urine voided. A medication history is also important because, as just noted, medications can affect bladder function.

Treatment of incontinence in the elderly usually starts with conservation measures before considering the use of medications or surgery. Conservative treatment may involve changes in the physical environment so that the person can reach the bathroom more easily or remove clothing more quickly. Habit training with regularly scheduled toileting—usually every 2 to 4 hours—often is effective. The treatment plan may require dietary changes to prevent constipation or a plan to promote adequate fluid intake to ensure adequate bladder filling and prevent urinary stasis and symptomatic urinary tract infections.

SUMMARY CONCEPTS

■ Disorders of bladder structure and function include urinary obstruction with retention or stasis of urine, and urinary incontinence with involuntary loss of urine. Both types of disorders can have their origin in the structures of the lower urinary tract or in the neural mechanisms that control their function.

■ In lower urinary tract obstructive disorders, urine is produced normally by the kidneys but is retained in the bladder, a condition that predisposes to kidney damage. Obstructions can be classified according to their location (bladder neck, urethra, or external urethral meatus), cause (congenital or acquired), degree (partial or complete), and duration (acute or chronic).

■ Neurogenic disorders of the bladder commonly are manifested by a neurogenic overactive or spastic bladder dysfunction, in which there is failure to store urine, or an aflexic or flaccid bladder dysfunction, in which bladder emptying is impaired. Neurogenic overactive bladder dysfunction results from neural lesions above the level of the sacral cord that allow neurons in the micturition center to function reflexively without control from higher central nervous system centers; in contrast, areflexic bladder dysfunction results from neural disorders affecting the motor neurons in the sacral cord or peripheral nerves that control detrusor muscle contraction and bladder emptying.

■ Incontinence represents the involuntary loss of urine. Stress incontinence is caused by the decreased ability of the vesicourethral sphincter to prevent the escape of urine during activities, such as lifting and coughing, that raise bladder pressure above the external sphincter pressure. Urge or overactive bladder incontinence is caused by disorders that result in hyperactive bladder contractions. Overflow incontinence is caused by overfilling of the bladder with escape of urine.

Urinary Tract Infections

Urinary tract infections (UTIs) include several distinct entities—asymptomatic bacteriuria, symptomatic lower UTIs such as cystitis, and upper UTIs such as pyelonephritis. Because of their ability to cause renal damage, upper UTIs are considered more serious than lower UTIs. Acute pyelonephritis (discussed in Chapter 25) represents an infection of the renal parenchyma and renal pelvis. The discussion in this chapter focuses on lower urinary tract infections.

Etiologic Factors

Most uncomplicated lower UTIs are caused by *Escherichia coli*.[35-39] Other common uropathic pathogens include *Enterococcus faecalis*, *Staphylococcus saprophyticus*, *Klebsiella pneumoniae*, *Proteus mirabilis*, and *Pseudomonas* species. Most upper and lower UTIs are caused by bacteria that enter through the urethra. Although the distal portion of the urethra often contains pathogens, the urine formed in the kidneys and found in the bladder normally is sterile or free of bacteria. This is because of the *washout phenomenon*, in which urine from the bladder normally washes bacteria out of the urethra during urination.

There is an increased risk for UTIs in persons with urinary obstruction and reflux, in people with neurogenic disorders that impair bladder emptying, in women who are sexually active, in postmenopausal women, in men with diseases of the prostate, and in elderly persons. Instrumentation and urinary catheterization are the most common predisposing factors for nosocomial, or hospital-acquired, UTIs. Urinary tract infections occur more commonly in women with diabetes than in women without the disease. People with diabetes are also at increased risk for complications associated with UTIs, including pyelonephritis, and they are more susceptible to fungal infections (particularly *Candida* species) and infections with gram-negative pathogens other than *E. coli*, both of which are accompanied by increased severity and unusual manifestations.

Host–Agent Interactions

Because certain people tend to be predisposed to development of UTIs, considerable interest has been focused on host–pathogen interactions and factors that increase the risk for UTI.[35,36]

Host Defenses. In the development of a UTI, host defenses are matched against the virulence of the pathogen. The host defenses of the bladder have several components, including the washout phenomenon, in which bacteria are removed from the bladder and urethra during urination; the protective mucin layer that lines the bladder and protects against bacterial invasion; and local immune responses. Immune mechanisms, particularly secretory immunoglobulin (Ig) A, appear to provide an important antibacterial defense. Phagocytic blood cells further assist in the removal of bacteria from the urinary tract.

There has been a growing appreciation of the protective function of the bladder's mucin layer. It is thought that the epithelial cells that line the bladder produce protective substances that subsequently become incorporated into the mucin layer that adheres to the bladder wall. One theory proposes that the mucin layer acts by binding water, which then constitutes a protective barrier between the bacteria and the bladder epithelium. Elderly and postmenopausal women produce less mucin than younger women, suggesting that estrogen may play a role in mucin production in women.

Other important host factors include the normal flora of the periurethral area in women and prostate secretions in men. In women, the normal flora of the periurethral area, which consists of organisms such as *Lactobacillus*, provides a defense against the colonization of uropathic bacteria.[40] Alterations in the periurethral environment, such as occurs with a decrease in estrogen levels during menopause or the use of antibiotics, can alter the protective periurethral flora, allowing uropathogens to colonize and enter the urinary tract. In men, the prostatic fluid has antimicrobial properties that protect the urethra from colonization.

Pathogen Virulence. Pathogen virulence derives from its ability to gain access to and thrive in the environment of the urinary tract, to evade the destructive effects of the host's immune system, and to develop resistance to antimicrobial agents. Not all bacteria are capable of adhering to and infecting the urinary tract. Of the many strains of *E. coli*, only those with increased ability to adhere to the epithelial cells of the urinary tract are able to produce UTIs. These bacteria have fine protein filaments, called *pili* or *fimbriae*, that help them adhere to receptors on the lining of urinary tract structures.

Obstruction and Reflux

Obstruction and reflux are other factors that increase the risk for UTIs. Any microorganisms that enter the bladder normally are washed out during voiding. When outflow is obstructed, urine remains in the bladder and acts as a medium for microbial growth; the microorganisms in the contaminated urine can then ascend along the ureters to infect the kidneys. The presence of residual urine correlates closely with bacteriuria and with its recurrence after treatment. Another aspect of bladder outflow obstruction and bladder distention is increased intravesical pressure, which compresses blood vessels in the bladder wall, leading to a decrease in the mucosal defenses of the bladder.

In UTIs associated with stasis of urine flow, the obstruction may be anatomic or functional. Anatomic obstructions include urinary tract stones, prostatic hyperplasia, pregnancy, and malformations of the ureterovesical junction. Functional obstructions include neurogenic bladder, infrequent voiding, detrusor (bladder) muscle instability, and constipation.

A phenomenon called *urethrovesical reflux* occurs when urine from the urethra moves into the bladder. In women, urethrovesical reflux can occur during activities such as coughing or squatting, in which an increase in intra-abdominal pressure causes the urine to be squeezed into the urethra and then to flow back into the bladder as the pressure decreases.[40] This also can happen when voiding is abruptly interrupted. Because the urethral orifice frequently is contaminated with bacteria, the reflux mechanism may cause bacteria to be drawn back into the bladder. The *vesicoureteral reflux*, which occurs at the level of the bladder and ureter, allows urine and bacteria to ascend from the bladder to the kidney and is associated with pyelonephritis and infections of the upper urinary tract. (see Chapter 25, Fig. 25-11).

Catheter-Induced Infection

Urinary catheters are a source of urethral irritation and provide a means for entry of microorganisms into the urinary tract. Catheter-associated bacteriuria remains the most frequent cause of gram-negative septicemia in hospitalized patients. Studies have shown that bacteria adhere to the surface of the catheter and initiate the growth of a biofilm that then covers the surface of the catheter (see Chapter 14, Fig. 14-6).[41] The biofilm tends to protect the bacteria from the action of antibiotics and makes treatment difficult. A closed drainage system (i.e., closed to air and other sources of contamination) and careful attention to perineal hygiene (i.e., cleaning the area around the urethral meatus) help to prevent infections in persons who require an indwelling catheter. Careful hand-washing and early detection and treatment of UTIs also are essential.

Clinical Features

The manifestations of UTI depend on whether the infection involves the lower (bladder) or upper (kidney) urinary tract and whether the infection is acute or chronic. An acute episode of cystitis (bladder infection) is characterized by frequency of urination, lower abdominal or back discomfort, and burning and pain on urination (i.e., dysuria).[34,38] Occasionally, the urine is cloudy and foul smelling. In adults, fever and other signs of infection usually are absent. If there are no complications, the symptoms disappear within 48 hours of treatment. The symptoms of cystitis also may represent urethritis caused by *Chlamydia trachomatis*, *Neisseria gonorrhoeae*, or herpes simplex virus, or vaginitis attributable to *Trichomonas vaginalis* or *Candida* species (see Chapter 41).

Diagnosis and Treatment

The diagnosis of UTI usually is based on symptoms and on examination of the urine for the presence of microorganisms. When necessary, x-ray films, ultrasonography, and CT and renal scans are used to identify contributing factors, such as obstruction.

Urine tests are used to establish the presence of bacteria in the urine and a diagnosis of UTI. A commonly accepted criterion for diagnosis of a UTI is the presence of 100,000 colony-forming units (CFU) or more bacteria per milliliter (mL) of urine.[35] Colonization usually is defined as the multiplication of microorganisms in or on a host without apparent evidence of invasiveness or tissue injury. Pyuria (the presence of less than five to eight leukocytes per high-power field) indicates a host response to infection rather than asymptomatic bacterial colonization. A Gram stain may be done to determine the type (gram positive or gram negative) of organism that is present.

Chemical screening (urine dipstick) for markers of infection may provide useful information but is less sensitive than microscopic analysis.[35,36] These tests are relatively inexpensive, are easy to perform, and can be done in the clinic setting or even in the home. A urine culture may be done to confirm the presence of pathogenic bacteria in urine specimens, allow for their identification, and permit the determination of their sensitivity to specific antibiotics.

The treatment of UTI is based on the pathogen causing the infection and the presence of contributing host–agent factors. Other considerations include whether the infection is acute, recurrent, or chronic. Most acute lower UTIs, which occur mainly in women and are generally caused by *E. coli*, are treated successfully with a short course of antimicrobial therapy. Forcing fluids may relieve signs and symptoms, and this approach is used as an adjunct to antimicrobial treatment.

Recurrent lower UTIs are those that recur after treatment. They are due either to bacterial persistence or reinfection.[38] Bacterial persistence usually is curable by removal of the infectious source (e.g., urinary catheter or infected bladder stones). Reinfection is managed principally through education regarding pathogen transmission and prevention measures. Cranberry juice or blueberry juice has been suggested as a preventive measure for persons with frequent UTIs. Studies suggest that these juices reduce bacterial adherence to the epithelial lining of the urinary tract.[42] Because of their mechanism of action, these juices are used more appropriately in prevention rather than treatment of an established UTI.

Chronic UTIs are more difficult to treat. Because they often are associated with obstructive uropathy or reflux flow of urine, diagnostic tests usually are performed to detect such abnormalities. When possible, the condition causing the reflux flow or obstruction is corrected. Most persons with recurrent UTIs are treated with antimicrobial agents for longer periods of time in doses sufficient to maintain high urine levels of the drug, and they are examined for obstruction or other causes of infection. Men in particular should be investigated for obstructive disorders or a prostatic focus of infection.

Infections in Special Populations

Urinary tract infections affect persons of all ages. In infants, they occur more often in boys than in girls. After the first year of life UTIs occur more often in girls. Urinary tract infections are more common in women than men, specifically between 16 and 35 years of age, at which time women are 40 times more likely to develop a UTI than age-matched men.[35] This is because of the shorter length of the female urethra and because the vaginal vestibule can be easily contaminated with fecal flora. In men, the longer length of the urethra and the antibacterial properties of the prostatic fluid provide some protection from ascending UTIs until approximately 60 years of age.[43] After this age, prostatic hyperplasia becomes more common, and with it may come obstruction and increased risk for UTI (see Chapter 39).

Urinary Tract Infections in Non-pregnant Women

Approximately half of all adult women have at least one UTI during their lifetime.[37] The anterior urethra usually is colonized with bacteria; urethral massage or sexual intercourse can force these bacteria back into the bladder. Using a diaphragm and spermicide enhances the susceptibility to infection.[35,37] A nonpharmacologic approach to the treatment of frequent UTIs associated with sexual intercourse is to increase fluid intake before intercourse and to void soon after intercourse. This procedure uses the washout phenomenon to remove bacteria from the bladder.

 ## Urinary Tract Infections in Pregnant Women

Pregnant women are at increased risk for UTIs. Normal changes in the functioning of the urinary tract that occur during pregnancy predispose pregnant women to UTIs.[44-46] These changes involve the collecting system of the kidneys and include dilation of the renal calyces, pelves, and ureters that begins during the first trimester and becomes most pronounced during the third trimester. Dilation of the upper urinary system is accompanied by a reduction in the peristaltic activity of the ureters that is thought to result from the muscle-relaxing effects of progesterone-like hormones and mechanical obstruction from the enlarging uterus. In addition to the changes in the kidneys and ureters, the bladder becomes displaced from its pelvic position to a more abdominal position, producing further changes in ureteral position.

The complications of asymptomatic UTIs during pregnancy include persistent bacteriuria, acute and chronic pyelonephritis, and preterm delivery of infants with low birth weight. Evidence suggests that few women become bacteriuric during pregnancy. Rather, it appears that symptomatic UTIs during pregnancy reflect preexisting asymptomatic bacteriuria and that changes occurring during pregnancy simply permit the prior urinary colonization to progress to symptomatic infection and invasion of the kidneys. Because bacteriuria may occur as an asymptomatic condition in pregnant women, it is recommended that a urine culture be obtained at the time of their first prenatal visit.[45,46] A repeat culture should be obtained during the third trimester. Women with bacteriuria should be followed closely, and infections should be properly treated to prevent complications. The choice of antimicrobial agent should address the common infecting organisms and should be safe for both the mother and fetus.

 ## Urinary Tract Infections in Children

Acute urinary tract infection is considered to be the most common serious bacterial infection in childhood, affecting as many as 8% of girls and 2% of boys during the first 7 to 8 years of life.[47,48] In girls, the average age at first diagnosis is 5 years or younger, with peaks during infancy and toilet training.[49] In boys, most UTIs occur during the first year of life and are more common in uncircumcised than in circumcised boys.[49]

Vesicoureteral reflux (VUR), a common childhood disorder, is believed to predispose to UTI, with both VUR and UTI being associated with renal scarring and permanent kidney damage. Most UTIs that lead to scarring and diminished kidney growth occur in children younger than 4 years, especially infants younger than 1 year of age.[49] The incidence of renal scarring is greatest in children with gross VUR or obstruction, in children with recurrent UTIs, and in those with a delay in treatment.

Childhood UTIs usually are ascending, with inoculation of feces from the urethra and periurethral tissues into the bladder. The most common pathogen is *Escherichia coli*, followed by *Klebsiella* and *Proteus* species. In uncircumcised boys, the bacterial pathogens arise from the flora beneath the prepuce. In girls, UTIs often occur at the onset of toilet training because of urination dysfunction that occurs at that age.[49] The child is trying to retain urine to stay dry, yet the bladder may produce uninhibited contractions, forcing urine out. The result may be high-pressure, turbulent urine flow or incomplete bladder emptying, both of which predispose to bacteriuria. Similar problems can occur in school-age children who refuse to use the school bathroom.[49] Constipation may increase the risk of UTI recurrence in children with VUR by compressing the bladder and bladder neck, resulting in increased bladder storage pressure and incomplete bladder emptying.[50]

Unlike adults, children frequently do not present with the typical signs of a UTI.[47–51] Many neonates with UTIs have bacteremia and may show signs and symptoms of septicemia, including fever, hypothermia, apneic spells, poor skin perfusion, abdominal distention, diarrhea, vomiting, lethargy, and irritability. Older infants may present with feeding problems, failure to thrive, diarrhea, vomiting, fever, and foul-smelling urine. Toddlers often present with abdominal pain, vomiting, diarrhea, abnormal voiding patterns, foul-smelling urine, fever, and poor growth. In older children with lower UTIs, the classic features—enuresis, frequency, dysuria, and suprapubic discomfort—are more common. Fever is a common sign of UTI in children, and the possibility of UTI should be considered in any child with unexplained fever.

Diagnosis is based on a careful history of voiding patterns and symptomatology; physical examination to determine fever, hypertension, abdominal or suprapubic tenderness, and other manifestations of UTI; and urinalysis to determine bacteriuria, pyuria, proteinuria, and hematuria. A positive urine culture that is obtained correctly is essential for the diagnosis.[47–51] Additional diagnostic methods may be needed to determine the cause of the disorder. Children with a relatively uncomplicated first UTI may turn out to have significant reflux. Therefore, even a single documented UTI in a child requires careful diagnosis. Urinary symptoms in the absence of bacteriuria suggest vaginitis, urethritis, sexual molestation, the use of irritating bubble baths, pinworms, or viral cystitis. In adolescent girls, a history of dysuria, and vaginal discharge make vaginitis or vulvitis a consideration.[49]

The approach to treatment is based on the clinical severity of the infection, the site of infection (i.e., lower versus upper urinary tract), the risk for sepsis, and the presence of structural abnormalities. The immediate treatment of infants and young children is essential. Most infants with symptomatic UTIs and many children with clinical evidence of acute upper UTIs require hospitalization, rehydration, and intravenous antibiotic therapy.[50,51] Follow-up is essential for children with febrile UTIs to ensure resolution of the infection. Follow-up urine cultures often are done at the end of treatment. Imaging studies often are recommended for children after their first UTI to detect renal scarring, vesicoureteral reflux, or other abnormalities.

Urinary Tract Infections in the Elderly

Urinary tract infections are relatively common in elderly persons.[43,52,53] They are the second most common form of infection, after respiratory tract infections, among otherwise healthy community-dwelling elderly. They are particularly prevalent in elderly persons living in nursing homes or extended care facilities.[52]

Most of these infections follow invasion of the urinary tract by the ascending route. Several factors predispose elderly persons to UTIs, including underlying genitourinary abnormalities, immobility resulting in poor bladder emptying, diminished bactericidal properties of the urine, and constipation. Prostatic hyperplasia with bladder outflow obstruction is the most important contributing factor in older men, while alteration in the bacterial flora of the vagina is the most important contributing factor in older women. Added to these risks are other health problems that necessitate catheterization or instrumentation of the urinary tract.

Elderly persons with bacteriuria have varying symptoms, ranging from the absence of symptoms to the presence of typical UTI symptoms. Even when symptoms of lower UTIs are present, they may be difficult to interpret because elderly persons without UTIs commonly experience urgency, frequency, and incontinence. Alternatively, elderly persons may have vague symptoms such as anorexia, fatigue, weakness, or change in mental status. Even with more serious upper UTIs (e.g., pyelonephritis), the classic signs of infection such as fever, chills, flank pain, and tenderness may be altered or absent. Sometimes, no symptoms occur until the infection is far advanced.

Interstitial Cystitis/Painful Bladder Syndrome

Interstitial cystitis or painful bladder syndrome is a chronic, often debilitating, condition that is characterized by urinary frequency, urgency, and severe suprapubic pain.[54–56] Unlike bladder inflammation caused by a bacterial infection, the condition occurs in the absence of other pathology. Although previously reported to be a disorder of middle-aged women, it is now known that the condition affects both men and women of all ages.

Although the pathophysiology of interstitial cystitis/painful bladder syndrome is incompletely understood, it is thought to involve permeability changes of the urothelium, along with mast cell activation and neurogenic inflammation. Damage to the protective mucosal lining leads to impaired urothelial cell-barrier function, allowing urinary solutes to penetrate the epithelium and activate sensory nerve endings, leading to pain and inflammation.

At present there are no definitive diagnostic tests for interstitial cystitis/painful bladder syndrome. Diagnostic steps involve ruling out other diseases and overlapping syndromes. Although not universally accepted, the potassium sensitivity test is widely used to aid in the diagnosis. The test involves the instillation of a potassium chloride solution and sterile water directly into the bladder. Increased pain with instillation of the potassium solution is considered a positive test and indicates urothelium dysfunction.

There are a wide array of treatment options for interstitial cystitis/painful bladder syndrome.[55,56] Pentosan polysulfate sodium is the only FDA–approved oral therapy for the treatment of interstitial cystitis. The drug, which is an antidepressant, is thought to facilitate repair of the urothelium. Hydroxyzine (Vistaril), which is thought to control mast cell degranulation, and amitriptyline or nortriptyline, which inhibit neural activation, may also be used. Other nonspecific oral medications, such as analgesics, anti-inflammatory agents, and the urinary anesthetic phenazopyridine (Pyridium), can be used. Anticholinergic drugs are frequently used to control pain and frequency.

 SUMMARY CONCEPTS

- Urinary tract infections (UTIs) include several distinct entities, including asymptomatic bacteriuria, symptomatic lower UTIs such as cystitis, and upper UTIs such as pyelonephritis.

- UTIs involve host–agent interactions in which the defenses of the host compete with those of the infectious agent. *Host defenses* include the washout phenomenon in which the flow of urine washes bacteria out of the urethra, the bacteriostatic properties of the urine, the protective mucin layer that lines the bladder, and the antimicrobial properties of the normal periurethral flora in women and prostate secretions in men. Pathogen virulence derives from its ability to gain access to and thrive in the environment of the urinary tract, to evade the destructive effects of the host's immune system, and to develop resistance to antimicrobial agents.

- Most UTIs ascend from the urethra and bladder. A number of factors interact in determining the predisposition to development of ascending UTIs, including urinary tract obstruction, urine stasis and reflux, pregnancy-induced and aging changes in urinary tract function, and presence of urinary tract catheters.

- Interstitial cystitis or painful bladder syndrome is a chronic, often debilitating, condition that is characterized by urinary frequency, urgency, and severe suprapubic pain. Unlike bladder inflammation caused by a bacterial infection, the condition occurs in the absence of other pathology.

Cancer of the Bladder

Cancer of the bladder is the sixth most common malignancy in the United States, accounting for 7% of cancers in men and 3% of cancers in women.[57–60] For some as-yet unexplained reason, African Americans have only half the risk of white European Americans. Most cancer of the bladder occur in older persons and is rare in those under the age of 50 years.

Approximately 90% to 95% of bladder cancers are derived from the transitional epithelial (urothelial) cells that line the bladder.[57–60] These tumors can range from benign papillomas and low-grade papillary urothelial carcinomas to invasive urothelial cell carcinomas and highly malignant tumors.

Urothelial papillomas are rare benign tumors, of which there are two forms: exophytic papillomas and inverted papillomas.[59,60] *Exophytic papillomas* have fonts or finger-like papillae with a central core of loose fibrovascular tissue covered by epithelium. Although considered benign some exophytic papillomas may recur or progress to carcinoma, thus long-term follow-up is necessary after excision. *Inverted papillomas* are benign nodular lesions that are cured by excision.

Papillary urothelial neoplasms of low malignant potential share many histologic features with papillomas; however, they have a thicker urothelium and diffuse nuclear enlargement (Fig. 27-5). They may recur after excision and only rarely recur as higher grade tumors associated with invasion and progression.[59,60] Low-grade papillary urothelial carcinomas have fonts

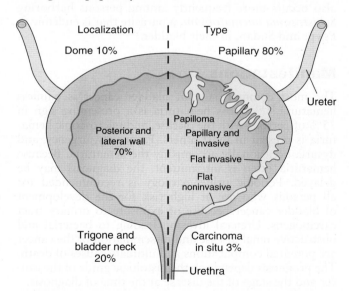

FIGURE 27-5. Urothelial neoplasms. Most tumors are located on the posterior and lateral walls; trigone and bladder neck are involved less commonly. Malignant tumors may be papillary or flat. Both flat and papillary tumors may be invasive or noninvasive. Benign transitional cell papillomas are rare. (Adapted from Damjanov I, McCure PA. The lower urinary tract and male reproductive system. In: Rubin R, Strayer DS, eds. *Rubin's Pathology: Clinicopathologic Foundations of Medicine.* 6th ed. Philadelphia, PA: Wolters Kluwer Health | Lippincott Williams & Wilkins; 2012:819.)

lined with neoplastic epithelium. Although these tumors may recur and rarely invade the underlying bladder wall, they are seldom life-threatening.[59,60]

High-grade carcinomas can be papillary or flat; they tend to cover larger areas of the mucosal surface and carry a high risk of invasion into the detrusor muscle and surrounding tissues, and when associated with invasion, a significant metastatic potential. Bladder cancers are commonly staged according to the TNM classification (see Chapter 7) of the World Health Organization (WHO) with stage T3 carcinomas invading perivesical tissues and T4 carcinomas spreading to adjacent organs and distant metastases.[59-61]

Etiology and Pathogenesis

Although the cause of bladder cancer is unknown, evidence suggests that its origin is related to local influences, such as carcinogens that are excreted in the urine and stored in the bladder.[57-62] Cigarette smoking is an important risk factor, with 30% to 50% of all bladder cancers among males who are current or past smokers. Other risk factors include the presence of arsenic in the drinking water and industrial exposure to the breakdown products of aromatic amines used in the dye industry and to chemicals used in the manufacture of rubber, textiles, paint, and petroleum products.[62] Both the heavy long-term use of cyclophosphamide, an immunosupressive agent, and prior exposure to bladder radiation, often administered for other pelvic malignancies, also increase the risk of bladder cancer. Bladder cancer also occurs more frequently among persons harboring *Schistosoma haematobium*, a parasite that is endemic in Egypt and Sudan, in their bladder.[59,61]

Manifestations

The most common sign of bladder cancer is painless hematuria.[58-61] Gross hematuria is a presenting sign in 75% of persons with the disease, and microscopic hematuria is present in most others. Frequency, urgency, and dysuria occasionally accompany the hematuria. Because hematuria often is intermittent, the diagnosis may be delayed. Periodic urine cytology is recommended for all persons who are at high risk for the development of bladder cancer because of exposure to urinary tract carcinogens. Ureteral invasion leading to bacterial and obstructive renal disease and dissemination of the cancer are potential complications and ultimate causes of death. The prognosis depends on the histologic grade of the cancer and the stage of the disease at the time of diagnosis.

Diagnosis and Treatment

Diagnostic methods include cytologic studies, excretory urography, cystoscopy, and biopsy. Ultrasonography, CT scans, and MRI are used as aids for staging the tumor. Cytologic studies performed on biopsy tissues or cells obtained from bladder washings may be used to detect the presence of malignant cells.[59]

The treatment of bladder cancer depends on the type and extent of the lesion and the health of the patient. Endoscopic resection usually is done for diagnostic purposes and may be used as a treatment for superficial lesions. For small papillary tumors that are not high grade, the initial diagnostic transurethral resection may be the only surgical procedure done. Segmental surgical resection may be used for removing a large single lesion. When the tumor is invasive, a cystectomy with resection of the pelvic lymph nodes frequently is the treatment of choice. Cystectomy requires urinary diversion, an alternative reservoir, usually created from the ileum (e.g., an ileal loop), that is designed to collect the urine. External-beam radiation therapy is an alternative to radical cystectomy in some patients with deeply infiltrating bladder cancer.[59]

Surgical treatment of superficial bladder cancer is often followed by intravesicular chemotherapy or immunotherapy, a procedure in which the therapeutic agent is directly instilled into the bladder. One of the agents used for this purpose is an attenuated strain of the tuberculosis bacillus, called *bacillus Calmette-Guérin* (BCG), which elicits an inflammatory response that destroys the tumor. Patients who are found to have regional invasion or distant metastasis are often treated with systemic chemotherapeutic agents. Therapy can be given before planned cystectomy (neoadjuvant) in an attempt to decrease recurrence or in some cases to allow for bladder preservation. Alternatively, adjuvant chemotherapy may administered after surgery to prevent tumor recurrence.

SUMMARY CONCEPTS

- Bladder cancers fall into two major groups: low-grade noninvasive tumors and high-grade invasive tumors that are associated with metastasis and a worse prognosis.

- Although the cause of cancer of the bladder is unknown, evidence suggests that carcinogens excreted in the urine may play a role. Cigarette smoking is an important risk factor. Other risk factors include the presence of arsenic in the drinking water and exposure to industrial chemicals.

- Microscopic and gross painless hematuria are the most frequent presenting signs of bladder cancer. The methods used in treatment of bladder cancer depend on the cytologic grade of the tumor and the lesion's degree of invasiveness.

- Treatment methods include surgical removal of the tumor, radiation therapy, and chemotherapy. In many cases, chemotherapeutic or immunotherapeutic agents can be instilled directly into the bladder, thereby avoiding the side effects of systemic therapy.

REVIEW EXERCISES

1. A 23-year-old man is recovering after the acute phase of a cervical (C6) spinal cord injury with complete loss of motor and sensory function below the level of injury. He is now experiencing spastic bladder contractions with involuntary and incomplete urination. Urodynamic studies reveal spastic contraction of the external sphincter with urine retention and high bladder pressures.

A. Explain the reason for the involuntary urination and incomplete emptying of the bladder despite high bladder pressures.

B. What are possible complications associated with overdistention and high pressure within the bladder?

2. A 66-year-old woman complains of leakage of urine during coughing, sneezing, laughing, or squatting down.

A. Explain the source of this woman's problem.

B. One of the recommended treatments for stress incontinence is the use of Kegel exercises, which focus on strengthening the muscles of the pelvic floor. Explain how these exercises contribute to the control of urine leakage in women with stress incontinence.

3. A 26-year-old woman makes an appointment with her health care provider, complaining of urinary frequency, urgency, and burning. She reports that her urine is cloudy and smells abnormal. A urine dipstick indicates the presence of infection, a urine sample is obtained for culture, and she is given a prescription for antibiotics.

A. What microorganism is most likely responsible for the infection?

B. What factors may have predisposed her to this disorder?

C. What could this woman do to prevent future infection?

REFERENCES

1. Tanagho EA, Lue TF. Anatomy of the genitourinary tract. In: McAninch JW, Lue TF, eds. *Smith and Tanagho's General Urology.* 18th ed. New York, NY: McGraw-Hill Medical; 2013:1–16.
2. Hall JE. *Guyton and Hall Textbook of Medical Physiology.* 12th ed. Philadelphia, PA: Saunders Elsevier; 2011:307–310.
3. Ross MH, Pawlina W. *Histology: A Text and Atlas.* 6th ed. Philadelphia, PA: Wolters Kluwer Health/Lippincott Williams & Wilkins; 2011:723–725.
4. Birder LA, Ruggieri M, Takeda M, et al. How does the urothelium affect bladder function in health and disease. *Neurourol Urodyn.* 2012;31(3):293–299.
5. Anderson K-E. Neurophysiology and pharmacology of the lower urinary tract. In: McAninch JW, Lue TF, eds. *Smith and Tanagho's General Urology.* 18th ed. New York, NY: McGraw-Hill Medical; 2013:429–441.
6. Clemens JQ. Basic bladder neurophysiology. *Urol Clin North Am.* 2010;37:487–494.
7. Lue TF, Tanagho EA. Neuropathic bladder disorders. In: McAninch JW, Lue TF, eds. *Smith and Tanagho's General Urology.* 18th ed. New York, NY: McGraw-Hill Medical; 2013:442–457.
8. Tanagho EA, Bella AJ, Lue TF. Urinary incontinence. In: McAninch JW, Lue, TF, eds. *Smith & Tanagho's General Urology.* 18th ed. New York, NY: McGraw-Hill Lange; 2013:489–497.
9. Porten SP, Greene KE. Urologic laboratory examination. In: McAninch JW, Lue TF, eds. *Smith & Tanagho's General Urology.* 18th ed. New York, NY: McGraw-Hill Lange; 2013:48–60.
10. Tanagho EA, Lue, TF. Urinary obstruction and stasis. In: McAninch JW, Lue TF, eds. *Smith and Tanagho's General Urology.* 18th ed. New York, NY: McGraw-Hill Lange; 2013:170–181.
11. Seliu BA, Subedi R. Urinary retention in adults: diagnosis and initial management. *Am Fam Physician.* 2008;77(5):643–650.
12. Dorsher PT, McIntosh PM. Neurogenic bladder. *Adv Urol.* 2012:1–16.
13. Jeong AJ, Cho CY, O S-J. Spinal cord injury and the neurogenic bladder. *Urol Clin North Am.* 2010;37:S37–S46.
14. Sasaki K, Yoshimura N, Chancellor MB. Implication of diabetes mellitus in urology. *Urol Clin North Am.* 2003;30:1–12.
15. Vinik AI, Maser RE, Mitchell BD, et al. Diabetic autonomic neuropathy. *Diabetes Care.* 2003;26:1553–1579.
16. Sampselle CM, Palmer MH, Boyington AR, et al. Prevention of urinary incontinence in adults. *Nurs Res.* 2004;53(6 suppl):S61–S67.
17. Lue FT. Urinary incontinence. In: McAninch JW, Lue TF, eds. *Smith and Tanagho's General Urology.* 18th ed. New York, NY: McGraw-Hill Lange; 2013:180–497.
18. Abrams P, Anderson KE, Birder L, et al. Fourth International Consultation on Incontinence Recommendations of the International Scientific Committee: evaluation and treatment of urinary incontinence, pelvic organ prolapse, and fecal incontinence. *Neurourol Urodyn.* 2010;29:213–240.
19. Fong E, Nitti VW. Urinary incontinence. *Prim Care.* 2010;37:599–612.
20. Khandelwal C, Disterler C. Diagnosis of urinary incontinence. *Am Fam Physician.* 2013;87(8):543–550.
21. Yoshimura N, Miyazato M. Neurophysiology and therapeutic receptor targets for stress urinary incontinence. *Int J Urol.* 2012;19:524–537.
22. Deng DY. Urinary incontinence in women. *Med Clin North Am.* 2011;95:101–109.
23. Smith PP, McCrery RJ, Appell RA. Current trends in the evaluation and management of female urinary incontinence. *Can Med Assoc J.* 2006;175:1233–1240.
24. Carpenter DA, Visovsky C. Stress urinary incontinence: a review of treatment options. *AORN J.* 2010;91(4):471–478.
25. Hayden RT, deRidder D, Freeman RM, et al. An International Urogynecological Association (IUGA) International Continence Society (ICS) joint report on the terminology for female pelvic floor dysfunction. *Neurourol Urodyn.* 2010;29:4–20.
26. Banackhar MA, Al-Shaiji TF, Hassouna MM. Pathophysiology of overactive bladder. *Int Urogynecol J.* 2012;23:975–982.
27. Chu FM, Dmochowski R. Pathology of overactive bladder. *Am J Med.* 2006;119(suppl 3A):3S–8S.
28. Nygaard I. Idiopathic urgency urinary incontinence. *N Engl J Med.* 2010;363(32):1156–1162.
29. Ouslander JG. Management of overactive bladder. *N Engl J Med.* 2004;350:786–799.
30. Gibbs CF, Johnson TM, Ouslander JG. Office management of geriatric urinary incontinence. *Am J Med.* 2007;120:213–220.

31. Goepel M, Kinschner-Hermanns R, Weiz-Barth A, et al. Urinary incontinence in the elderly. *Dtsch Arztebl Int.* 2010;107(30):531–536.

32. Griebling TL. Urinary incontinence in the elderly. *Clin Geriatr Med.* 2009;25:445–457.

33. Frank C. Office management of urinary incontinence among older patients. *Can Fam Physician.* 2010;56:1115–1120.

34. Madersbacher H, Madersbacher S. Men's bladder health: urinary incontinence in the elderly (Part I). *J Men' s Health Gender.* 2005;2(1):31–37.

35. Nguyen HT. Bacterial infections of the genitourinary tract. In: McAninch JW, Lue TF, eds. *Smith & Tanagho's General Urology.* 18th ed. New York, NY: McGraw-Hill Lange; 2013:197–222.

36. Niebubowicz GR, Mobley HLT. Host-pathogen interactions in urinary tract infections. *Nat Rev Urol.* 2010;7:430–436.

37. Hooton TM. Uncomplicated urinary tract infection. *N Engl J Infect.* 2012;366(11):1028–1037.

38. Litza JA, Brill JR. Urinary tract infection. *Prim Care.* 2010;37:491–507.

39. Drekonja DM, Johnson JR. Urinary tract infections. *Prim Care.* 2008;35:345–367.

40. Dielubaniza EJ, Schaeffer AJ. Urinary tract infections in women. *Med Clin North Am.* 2011;95:22–41.

41. Saint S, Chenoweth CE. Biofilms and catheter-associated urinary tract infections. *Infect Dis Clin North Am.* 2003;17:411–432.

42. Wang P. The effectiveness of cranberry products to reduce urinary tract infections in females: a literature review. *Urol Nurs.* 2012;33(1):38–45.

43. Nicole LE. Urinary tract infections in the elderly. *Clin Geriatr Med.* 2009;25:423–436.

44. Foster RT. Uncomplicated urinary tract infections in women. *Obstet Gynecol Clin North Am.* 2008;35:235–248.

45. Mittal P, Wing DA. Urinary tract infections in pregnancy. *Clin Perinatol.* 2005;32:749–764.

46. Macejko AM, Schaeffer AJ. Asymptomatic bacteriuria and symptomatic urinary tract infections during pregnancy. *Urol Clin North Am.* 2007;34:35–42.

47. White B. Diagnosis and treatment of urinary tract infections in children. *Am Fam Physician.* 2011;8(4):400–415.

48. Montini G, Tullus K, Hewitt I. Febrile urinary tract infections in children. *N Engl J Med.* 2011;365(3):239–250.

49. Elder JS. Urinary tract infections. In: Kliegman RM, Stanton BF, St. Geme JW, et al. *Nelson Textbook of Pediatrics.* 19th ed. New York, NY: Elsevier Saunders; 2011:1829–1834.

50. Bell LE, Mattoo TK. Update on childhood urinary tract infection and vesicoureteral reflux. *Semin Nephrol.* 2009;29:349–359.

51. Subcommittee on Urinary Tract Infections, Steering Committee on Quality Improvement and Management. Urinary tract infection: clinical practice guideline for the diagnosis and management of the initial UTI in febrile infants and children 2 to 24 years. *Pediatrics.* 2011;128(3):595–607.

52. Mathews SJ, Lancaster JW. Urinary tract infections in the elderly population. *Am J Geriatr Pharmacother.* 2011;9(5):286–309.

53. Genao L, Buhr GT. Urinary tract infections in older adults residing in long-term care facilities. *Ann Longterm Care.* 2012;20(4):33–38.

54. French LM, Bhambore N. Interstitial cystitis/painful bladder syndrome. *Am Fam Physician.* 2011;83(10):1175–1181.

55. Moutzouris D-A, Falagas ME. Interstitial cystitis: an unsolved enigma. *Clin J Am Soc Nephrol.* 2009;4:1844–1857.

56. Marinkovic SP, Moldwin R, Gillen LM, et al. The management of intersitial or painful bladder syndrome in women. *BMJ.* 2009;399:337–342.

57. Sharma S, Ksheersagar P, Sharma P. Diagnosis and treatment of bladder cancer. *Am Fam Physician.* 2009;80(7):717–723.

58. Konety BR, Carroll PR. Urothelial carcinoma: cancers of the bladder, ureter, and renal pelvis. In: McAninch JW, Lue TF, eds. *Smith & Tanagho's General Urology.* 18th ed. New York, NY: McGraw-Hill Lange; 2013:310–329.

59. Epstein JI. The lower urinary tract. In: Kumar V, Abbas AK, Fausto N, et al., eds. *Robbins and Cotran Pathologic Basis of Disease.* 8th ed. Philadelphia, PA: Saunders Elsevier; 2010:976–981.

60. Damjanov I, McCue PA. The lower urinary tract and male reproductive system. In: Rubin R, Strayer DS, eds. *Rubin's Pathology: Clinicopathologic Foundations of Medicine.* 6th ed. Philadelphia, PA: Wolters Kluwer Health/Lippincott Williams & Wilkins; 2012:819–823.

61. Jacobs BL, Lee CT, Montie JE. Bladder cancer in 2010. How far have we come? *CA Cancer J Clin.* 2010;20(10):244–272.

62. Letašiová S, Medvedd'ová A, Šovčíková A, et al. Bladder cancer, a review of environmental risk factors. *Environ Health* 2012;11(suppl 1):S11. Available online at http://www.ehjournal.net/content/11/S1/S11

Porth Essentials Resources

Explore these additional resources to enhance learning for this chapter:

- NCLEX-Style Questions and Other Resources on thePoint, http://thePoint.lww.com/PorthEssentials4e
- Study Guide for Essentials of Pathophysiology
- Adaptive Learning | Powered by PrepU, http://thepoint.lww.com/prepu

Chapter 28

Structure and Function of the Gastrointestinal System

The gastrointestinal (GI) tract is an amazing structure in which food is dismantled and its nutrients absorbed, wastes are collected and eliminated, and vitamins synthesized. The GI tract is also becoming increasingly recognized as an endocrine organ that produces and augments hormones that contribute to the regulation of appetite and food intake and function in the use and storage of nutrients.

As a matter of semantics, the GI tract also is referred to as the *digestive tract*, the *alimentary canal*, and, at times, the *gut*. The intestinal portion also may be called the *bowel*. For the purposes of this text, the liver and pancreas (discussed in Chapter 30), which produce secretions that aid in digestion, are considered *accessory organs*.

Organization and Function of the Gastrointestinal Tract

The major physiologic function of the GI tract is to provide the body with a continual supply of water and other nutrients. It carries out this function through processes involving motility, secretion, digestion, and absorption. In the digestive tract, as food moves slowly along its length it is systematically broken down into ions and molecules that can be absorbed into the blood and lymph. In the large intestine, unabsorbed wastes are collected for later elimination.

Structurally, the GI tract is a long, hollow tube, the lumen of which is an extension of the external environment (Fig. 28-1). Nutrients do not become part of the internal environment until they have passed through the intestinal wall and have entered the blood or lymph channels. For simplicity and understanding, the GI tract can be divided into three parts. The upper part—the mouth and pharynx, esophagus, and stomach—acts as an intake source and receptacle through which food passes and in which initial digestive processes take place. The middle portion—the duodenum, jejunum, and ileum of the small intestine—is where most digestive and absorptive processes occur. The lower segment—the cecum, colon, and rectum of the large intestine—serves as a storage channel for the efficient elimination of waste. The accessory organs, which include the salivary glands, liver, and pancreas, produce secretions that aid in digestion.

Upper Gastrointestinal Tract

The mouth forms the entryway into the GI tract for food; it contains the teeth, used in the mastication of food, and the tongue and other structures needed to direct food toward the pharynx and the esophagus. The mouth also serves as a receptacle for saliva produced by the salivary glands. Saliva moistens and lubricates food, so it is easier to swallow, and it contains enzymes (amylase and lipase) involved in the initial digestion of starches and lipids.

The esophagus is a straight, collapsible tube, about 25 cm (10 inches) in length, that lies behind the trachea and connects the pharynx with the stomach. The esophagus functions primarily as a conduit for the passage of food from the pharynx to the stomach. Its structure is uniquely designed for this purpose: the smooth muscle layers provide the peristaltic movements needed to move food along its length, and the mucosal and submucosal glands secrete mucus, which protects its surface and aids in lubricating food.

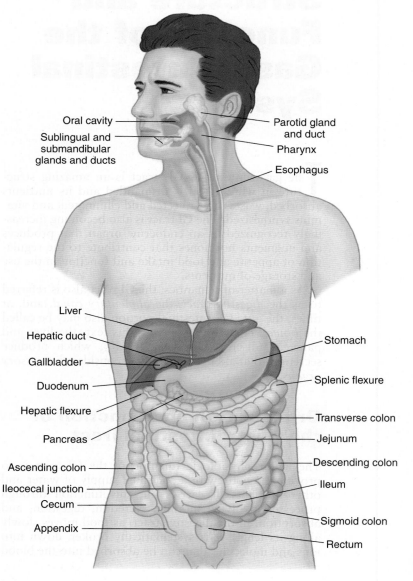

FIGURE 28-1. The gastrointestinal system.

There are sphincters at either end of the esophagus. The upper sphincter, the *pharyngoesophageal* sphincter, consists of a circular layer of striated muscle. It keeps air from entering the esophagus and stomach during breathing. The lower esophageal sphincter, also called the *gastroesophageal sphincter*, lies just above the area where the esophagus joins the stomach. The circular muscle in this area normally remains tonically contracted, creating a zone of high pressure that serves to prevent reflux of gastric contents into the esophagus. During swallowing, there is "receptive relaxation" of the lower esophageal sphincter that allows for easy propulsion of the esophageal contents into the stomach. The lower esophageal sphincter passes through an opening, or *hiatus*, in the diaphragm as it joins with the stomach, which is located in the abdomen. The portion of the diaphragm that surrounds the lower esophageal sphincter helps to maintain the zone of high pressure to support the function of the lower esophageal sphincter.

The stomach is a pouchlike structure that lies in the left side of the abdomen and serves as a food reservoir during the early stages of digestion. The esophagus opens into the stomach through an opening called the *cardiac orifice*, so named because of its proximity to the heart. The small part of the stomach that surrounds the cardiac orifice is called the *cardiac region*; the dome-shaped region that bulges above the cardiac region is called the *fundus;* the middle portion is called the *body;* and the funnel-shaped portion that connects with the small intestine is called the *pyloric region* (Fig. 28-2). The wider and more superior part of the pyloric region, the *antrum*, narrows to form the pyloric canal as it approaches the small intestine. At the end of the pyloric canal, the circular smooth muscle layer thickens to form the *pyloric sphincter*. This muscle serves as a valve that controls the rate of stomach emptying and prevents the regurgitation of intestinal contents back into the stomach.

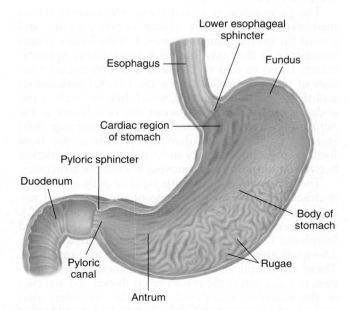

FIGURE 28-2. Structures of the stomach.

The inner surface of the empty stomach reveals a number of longitudinal folds or ridges called *rugae*. The rugae, which serve to accommodate expansion and filling of the stomach, almost disappear when the stomach is distended with food.

Small Intestine

The small intestine, which forms the middle portion of the GI tract, consists of three subdivisions: the duodenum, jejunum, and ileum (see Fig. 28-1). The duodenum, which is approximately 22 cm (10 inches) long, connects the stomach to the jejunum and contains the opening for the common bile duct and the main pancreatic duct. Bile, a fluid synthesized by the liver that breaks down lipids, and pancreatic juices, which facilitate digestion of lipids, carbohydrates, and proteins, enter the intestine through these ducts. It is in the jejunum and ileum, which together are approximately 7 m (23 ft) long and must be folded onto themselves to fit into the abdominal cavity, that food is digested and absorbed.

Lower Gastrointestinal Tract

The large intestine, which forms the lower GI tract, is approximately 1.5 m (5 ft) long. It is divided into the cecum, colon, rectum, and anal canal (see Fig. 28-1). The cecum is a blind pouch that projects down at the junction of the ileum and the colon. The ileocecal valve lies at the upper border of the cecum and prevents the return of feces from the cecum into the small intestine. The appendix arises from the cecum approximately 2.5 cm (1 inches) from the ileocecal valve. The colon is further divided into ascending, transverse, descending, and sigmoid portions. The ascending colon extends from the cecum to the undersurface of the liver, where it turns abruptly to form the right colic (hepatic) flexure. The transverse colon crosses the upper half of the abdominal cavity from right to left and then curves sharply downward beneath the lower end of the spleen, forming the left colic (splenic) flexure. The descending colon extends from the colic flexure to the rectum. The rectum extends from the sigmoid colon to the anus. The anal canal passes between the two medial borders of the levator ani muscles. Powerful sphincter muscles guard against fecal incontinence.

Gastrointestinal Wall Structure

Below the upper third of the esophagus, the GI tract is essentially a four-layered hollow tube of varying diameter, but similar structural organization. It consists of four distinct layers: the inner *mucosal layer*; the underlying *submucosal layer*, the *muscularis externa*, and the outer *serosal layer* (Fig. 28-3).

Mucosa

The *mucosa*, or inner mucosal layer, is made up of an epithelium lining; an underlying loose connective tissue, called the *lamina propriae*; and the muscularis

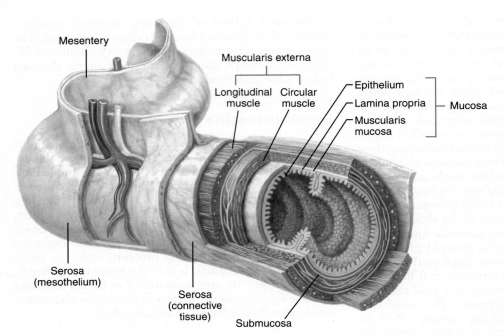

FIGURE 28-3. Transverse section of the gastrointestinal system.

mucosa, composed of smooth muscle cells that can contract and change the shape and surface area of the mucosal layer. The mucosal layer performs numerous functions in its role as an interface between the body and the external environment, including production of the mucus that protects and lubricates the inner lining of the GI tract lumen, secretion of the digestive enzymes and substances that break food down, absorption of the breakdown products of digestion, and maintenance of a barrier to prevent the entry of noxious substances and pathogenic organisms. Lymphatics within the mucosa serve as the body's first line of immune defense. The epithelial cells in the mucosal layer have a rapid turnover rate and are replaced every 4 to 5 days. Because of the regenerative capabilities of the mucosal layer, injury to this layer heals rapidly without leaving scar tissue.

Submucosa

The submucosal layer, or second layer, consists of dense connective tissue, aggregates of adipose tissue, and occasional glands. This layer contains the large blood vessels that send branches to the mucosa, muscular externa, and adventitia. It also contains the lymphatic vessels, as well as nerves that control motility and the secretory activity of glands in the mucosal layer.

Muscularis Externa

The *muscularis externa* consists of two concentric and relatively thick layers of smooth muscle: an inner layer made up of circularly arranged smooth muscle cells and an outer layer of longitudinally arranged smooth muscle. Located between the two muscle layers is a connective tissue layer that contains nerves that control smooth muscle movement, as well as blood and lymphatic vessels. Contraction of the smooth muscle in this

layer mixes and churns the GI contents and facilitates its movement along the GI tract.

Serosa and Adventitia

The serosa and adventitia constitute the outermost layer of the GI tract. The *serosa* is a serous membrane consisting of a layer of simple squamous epithelium, called the *mesothelium*, and a small amount of underlying connective tissue. It is equivalent to the visceral peritoneum and is continuous with the mesentery and omentum that enclose and support the abdominal viscera. Instead of the serosa, an *adventitia* consisting only of connective tissue is found where the wall of the GI tract is directly attached to the body wall.

The peritoneum is a continuous transparent serous membrane that lines the abdominopelvic cavity and invests the stomach and intestines. It is the largest serous membrane in the body, having a surface area approximately equal to that of the skin. The peritoneum consists of two continuous layers: the *visceral peritoneum* and the *parietal peritoneum*, which line the wall of the abdominopelvic cavity. Between the two layers is the *peritoneal cavity*, a potential space containing fluid secreted by the serous membranes. This serous fluid forms a moist and slippery surface that prevents friction between the continuously moving abdominal structures.

The *mesentery* is the double layer of peritoneum that encloses a portion or all of one of the abdominal viscera and attaches it to the abdominal wall (Fig. 28-4A). The mesentery contains the blood vessels, nerves, and lymphatic vessels that supply the intestinal wall (Fig. 28-4B). It also holds the organs in place and stores fat. There are dorsal as well as ventral mesenteries; however, in most places the mesentery is dorsal and attaches to the posterior abdominal wall. The mesentery that encloses the jejunum and ileum is gathered in folds that

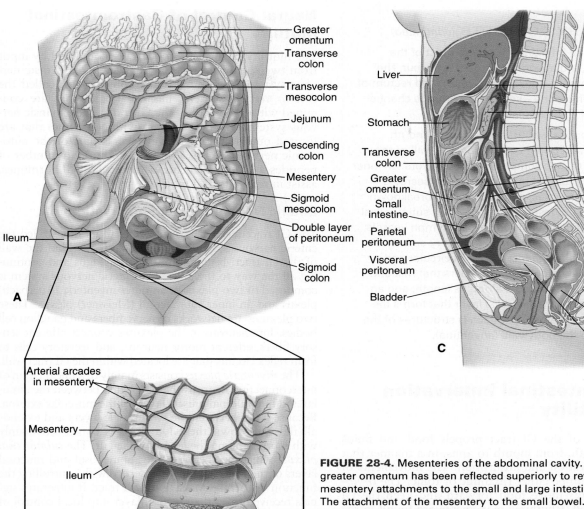

FIGURE 28-4. Mesenteries of the abdominal cavity. **(A)** The greater omentum has been reflected superiorly to reveal the mesentery attachments to the small and large intestines. **(B)** The attachment of the mesentery to the small bowel. The mesentery contains the blood vessels, nerves, and lymphatic vessels that supply the intestinal wall. **(C)** Sagittal section of the abdominopelvic cavity in a woman, showing the relationships of the peritoneal attachments and the greater and lesser omentums.

attach to the dorsal abdominal wall along a short line of insertion, giving a fan-shaped appearance, with the intestines at the edge.

An *omentum* is a double-layered extension or fold of peritoneum that passes from the stomach or proximal part of the duodenum to adjacent organs in the abdominal cavity or abdominal wall. The *greater omentum* extends from the stomach to cover the transverse colon and the folds of the intestine, whereas the *lesser omentum* extends between the transverse fissure of the liver and the lesser curvature of the stomach (see Fig. 28-4C). The greater omentum always contains some fat, which in obese persons can be a considerable amount. It has considerable mobility and moves around in the peritoneal cavity with the peristaltic movements of the intestines, and it cushions the abdominal organs against injury and provides insulation against the loss of body heat. It often forms adhesions (i.e., bands of fibrous scar tissue) adjacent to inflamed organs such as the appendix, walling off the infection and thereby preventing its spread.

SUMMARY CONCEPTS

■ The gastrointestinal (GI) tract is a long, hollow tube that is in contact with the external environment; food and fluids that enter the GI tract do not become part of the internal environment until they have been broken down and absorbed into the blood or lymph.

■ The digestive and absorptive functions of the GI tract are distributed among structures of the upper, middle, and lower parts of the tract. The upper part—the mouth, esophagus, and stomach—acts as an intake source and receptacle through which food passes and in which initial digestive processes take place. The middle portion—the duodenum, jejunum, and ileum

(continued)

SUMMARY CONCEPTS *(continued)*

of the small intestine—is where most of the digestive and absorptive processes occur. The lower segment—the cecum, colon, and rectum of the large intestine—serves as a storage channel for the efficient elimination of waste.

■ Throughout its length, except for the mouth, pharynx, and upper esophagus, the wall of the digestive tract is composed of four layers: an inner mucosal layer that produces mucus, secretes digestive enzymes, and absorbs the breakdown products of digestion; an underlying submucosal layer that contains blood vessels, lymph vessels, and nerves that control the secretory activity of the mucosal glands; a layer of circular and longitudinal smooth muscle fibers that mix and propel the gut contents along its length; and an outer *serosal* or *adventitial* layer that forms the peritoneum (serosa) or attaches structures of the GI tract to the body wall (adventitia).

Gastrointestinal Innervation and Motility

The motility of the GI tract propels food and fluids along its length, from mouth to anus, in a manner that facilitates digestion and absorption. The movements of the GI tract can be either rhythmic or tonic. The *rhythmic movements* move food forward and keep the GI contents mixed. Rhythmic movements are found in the esophagus, antrum of the stomach, and small intestine. The *tonic movements* consist of a constant level of contraction or tone without regular periods of relaxation. They are found in the lower esophagus, the upper region of the stomach, the ileocecal valve, and the internal anal sphincter.

All of the contractile tissue in the GI tract is smooth muscle, except for that in the mouth and pharynx, the upper third of the esophagus, and the external anal sphincter. Although the smooth muscle found in each region of the GI tract exhibits structural and functional differences, certain basic properties are common to all of the muscle cells. For example, all of the smooth muscle of the GI tract is unitary smooth muscle, in which the cells are electrically coupled by low-resistance pathways so that electrical signals initiating muscle contractions can move rapidly from one fiber to the next.

Like the self-excitable cardiac muscle cells in the heart, some smooth muscle cells throughout the GI tract function as pacemaker cells. These cells display rhythmic, spontaneous oscillations in membrane potentials, called *slow waves*, ranging in frequency from about 3 per minute in the stomach to 12 per minute in the duodenum. Slow waves are generated by a thin layer of interstitial cells located between the longitudinal and circular muscle layers.

Neural Control of Gastrointestinal Motility

The motility of the GI tract can be modulated by input from two sets of nerves, the intrinsic and extrinsic nervous systems. The intrinsic nervous system, called the *enteric nervous system*, has cell bodies that are contained within the wall of the GI tract. The extrinsic nervous system, which has nerves with cell bodies that are located outside the digestive tract, is part of the autonomic nervous system (ANS). In addition, a number of peptides, including neurotransmitters and GI hormones, assist in regulating GI motility.

Enteric Nervous System Innervation

The GI tract has a nervous system all its own called the enteric nervous system which lies entirely within the wall of the GI tract, beginning in the esophagus and continuing all the way to the anus. The enteric nervous system is composed of two plexuses: an outer myenteric (Auerbach) plexus and an inner submucosal (Meissner) plexus. These two plexuses are networks of nerve fibers and ganglion cell bodies. Interneurons in the plexuses connect afferent sensory fibers, efferent motor neurons, and secretory cells to form reflex circuits that are located within the GI tract wall.

The *myenteric plexus* consists mainly of a linear chain of interconnecting neurons that is located between the circular and longitudinal muscle layers of the muscular externa. Because it lies between the two muscle layers and extends all the way down the GI tract, it is concerned mainly with motility along the length of the gut. The *submucosal plexus*, which lies between the submucosal and mucosal layers of the wall, is mainly concerned with controlling the function of each segment of the GI tract. It integrates signals received from the mucosal layer into local control of motility, intestinal secretions, and absorption of nutrients.

The activity of the neurons in the myenteric and submucosal plexuses is regulated by local influences, input from the ANS, and interconnecting fibers that transmit information between the two plexuses. Mechanoreceptors monitor the stretch and distention of the GI tract wall, and chemoreceptors monitor the chemical composition (i.e., osmolarity, pH, and digestive products of protein and fat metabolism) of its contents. These receptors can communicate directly with ganglionic cells in the intramural plexuses or with visceral afferent fibers that influence ANS control of GI function.

Autonomic Innervation

The autonomic innervation of the GI system is mediated by both the sympathetic and parasympathetic nervous systems (see Chapter 34, Fig. 34-23). In general, stimulation of the parasympathetic nervous system causes a general increase in activity of the entire enteric nervous system, whereas sympathetic stimulation inhibits activity causing many effects.

Parasympathetic innervation to the stomach, small intestine, cecum, ascending colon, and transverse colon occurs through the vagus nerve. The remainder of the colon is innervated by parasympathetic fibers that exit the sacral segments of the spinal cord by way of the pelvic nerves. Preganglionic parasympathetic fibers can synapse with intramural plexus neurons, or they can act directly on intestinal smooth muscle. In addition, these same nerve bundles provide many afferent nerves whose receptors lie within the various tissues of the gut. Their nerves project to the spinal cord and brain to provide sensory input for integration. Most parasympathetic innervation is excitatory. Numerous vagovagal reflexes influence motility and secretions of the digestive tract.

Sympathetic innervation occurs through the thoracic chain of sympathetic ganglia and the celiac, superior mesenteric, and inferior mesenteric ganglia. The sympathetic nervous system exerts several effects on GI function. It controls the extent of mucus secretion by the mucosal glands, reduces motility by inhibiting the activity of intramural plexus neurons, enhances sphincter function, and increases the vascular smooth muscle tone of the blood vessels that supply the GI tract. Sympathetic stimulation suppresses the release of the excitatory neuromediators in the intramural plexuses, inhibiting GI motility.

Swallowing and Esophageal Motility

Chewing begins the digestive process—it breaks the food into particles of a size that can be swallowed, and lubricates it by mixing it with saliva. Although chewing usually is considered a voluntary act, it can be carried out involuntarily by a person who has lost the function of the cerebral cortex.

The swallowing reflex is a rigidly ordered sequence of events that results in the propulsion of food from the mouth to the stomach through the esophagus. Although swallowing is initiated as a voluntary activity, it becomes involuntary as food or fluid reaches the pharynx. Sensory impulses for the reflex begin at tactile receptors in the pharynx and esophagus and are integrated with the motor components of the response in an area of the reticular formation of the medulla and lower pons called the *swallowing center*. The motor impulses for the oral and pharyngeal phases of swallowing are carried in the trigeminal (V), glossopharyngeal (IX), vagus (X), and hypoglossal (XII) cranial nerves, and impulses for the esophageal phase are carried by the vagus nerve. Diseases that damage these brain centers or their cranial nerves disrupt the coordination of swallowing and predispose an individual to food and fluid lodging in the trachea and bronchi, leading to the risk of asphyxiation or aspiration pneumonia.

Swallowing consists of three phases: an oral, or voluntary, phase; a pharyngeal phase; and an esophageal phase. During the *oral phase*, the bolus of food is collected at the back of the mouth so the tongue can lift the food upward until it touches the posterior wall of the pharynx (Fig. 28-5A). At this point, the *pharyngeal*

(*text continues on page 684*)

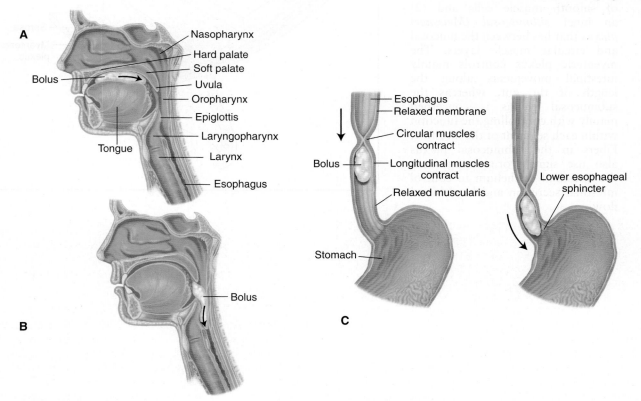

FIGURE 28-5. Steps in the swallowing reflex: **(A)** The *oral* or *voluntary phase* during which the bolus is collected at the back of the mouth so the tongue can lift the food upward and into the pharynx and the **(B)** *pharyngeal phase* during which food movement into the respiratory passages is prevented as the tongue is elevated and pressed against the soft palate closing the epiglottis, the upper esophageal sphincter relaxes, and the superior constrictor muscle contracts, forcing food into the esophagus; and **(C)** the *esophageal phase* during which peristalsis moves food through the esophagus and into the stomach.

UNDERSTANDING ➡ Intestinal Motility

Motility of the small intestine is organized to optimize the digestion and absorption of nutrients and the propulsion of undigested material toward the colon. Peristaltic movements mix the ingested foodstuffs with digestive enzymes and secretions and circulate the intestinal contents to facilitate contact with the intestinal mucosa. The regulation of motility results from an interplay of input from the (1) enteric and (2) autonomic nervous (ANS) systems and the intrinsic pacemaker activity of the (3) intestinal smooth muscle cells.

1

Enteric Nervous System Innervation. The gastrointestinal system has its own nervous system, called the *enteric nervous system.* The enteric nervous system is composed mainly of two plexuses: (1) the outer *myenteric (Auerbach) plexus* that is located between the longitudinal and circular layers of smooth muscle cells and (2) an inner *submucosal (Meissner) plexus* that lies between the mucosal and circular muscle layers. The myenteric plexus controls mainly intestinal movements along the length of the gut, whereas the submucosal plexus is concerned mainly with controlling the function within each segment of the intestine. Fibers in the submucosal plexus also use signals originating from the intestinal epithelium to control intestinal secretion and local blood flow.

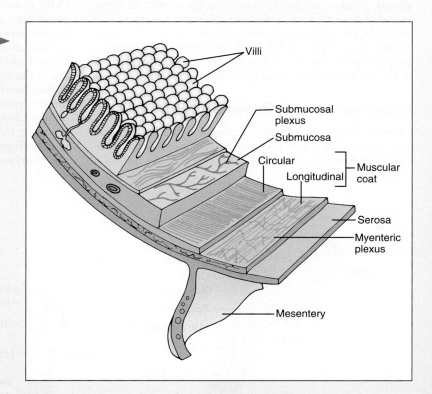

2

ANS Innervation. The intestine is also innervated by the parasympathetic and sympathetic branches of the ANS (see Chapter 35, Fig. 35-23). *Parasympathetic innervation* is supplied mainly by the vagus nerve with postganglionic neurons located primarily in the myenteric and submucosal plexuses. Stimulation of these parasympathetic nerves causes a general increase in both intestinal motility and secretory activity. *Sympathetic innervation* is supplied by nerves that run between the spinal cord and the prevertebral ganglia and between these ganglia and the intestine. Stimulation of the sympathetic nervous system is largely inhibitory, producing a decrease in intestinal motility and secretory activity.

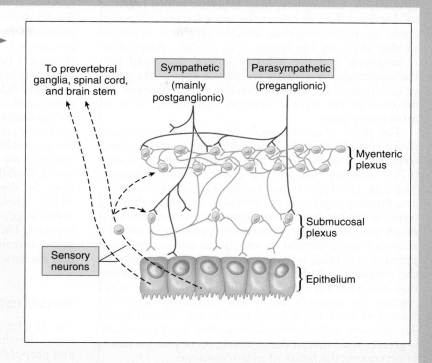

3

Intestinal Smooth Muscle. Intestinal smooth muscle has its own intrinsic slow-wave activity, which varies from about 12 waves minute in the duodenum to 8 or 9 waves per minute in the ileum. This slow-wave activity is thought to reside in a network of specialized pacemaker cells that are interposed between the smooth muscle cells. Slow waves are not action potentials and they do not directly induce muscle contraction; instead, they are rhythmic, wavelike fluctuations in the membrane potential that cyclically bring the membrane closer to threshold. If the peak voltage of the slow wave exceeds the cell's threshold potential, one or more action potentials may be triggered. Because action potentials occur at the peak of a slow wave, slow-wave frequency determines the rate of smooth muscle contractions. Stretching the intestinal smooth muscle and parasympathetic nervous system stimulation increase excitability of the smooth muscle cells, whereas sympathetic stimulation decreases excitability.

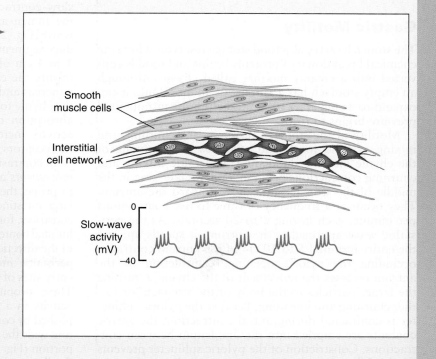

(*text continued from page 681*)

phase of swallowing is initiated. The soft palate is pulled upward, the palatopharyngeal folds are pulled together so that food does not enter the nasopharynx, the vocal cords are pulled together, and the epiglottis is moved so that it covers the larynx (Fig. 28-5B). Respiration is inhibited, and the bolus is moved backward into the esophagus by constrictive movements of the pharynx. Although the striated muscles of the pharynx are involved in the second stage of swallowing, it is an involuntary stage.

The third phase of swallowing is the *esophageal phase* (Fig. 29-5C). As food enters the esophagus and stretches its walls, local and central nervous system (CNS) reflexes that initiate peristalsis are triggered. There are two types of peristalsis—primary and secondary. Primary peristalsis is controlled by the swallowing center in the brain stem and begins when food enters the esophagus. Secondary peristalsis is partially mediated by smooth muscle fibers in the esophagus and occurs when primary peristalsis is inadequate to move food through the esophagus. Peristalsis begins at the site of distention and moves downward. Before the peristaltic wave reaches the stomach, the lower esophageal sphincter relaxes to allow the bolus of food to enter the stomach. The pressure in the lower esophageal sphincter normally is greater than that in the stomach, an important factor in preventing the reflux of gastric contents.

Gastric Motility

The stomach serves as a food storage reservoir where the chemical breakdown of proteins begins and food is converted into a creamy mixture called *chyme*. Although an empty stomach has a volume of about 50 mL, it can expand to as much as 1000 mL before the intraluminal pressure begins to rise.

Motility of the stomach results in the churning and mixing of solid foods and regulates the emptying of the chyme into the duodenum. Peristaltic mixing and churning contractions begin in a pacemaker area in the middle of the stomach and move toward the antrum. They occur at a frequency of three to five contractions per minute, each lasting 2 to 20 seconds. As the peristaltic wave approaches the antrum, it speeds up, and the entire terminal 5 to 10 cm of the antrum contracts, occluding the pyloric opening. Contraction of the antrum reverses the movement of the chyme, returning the larger particles to the body of the stomach for further churning and kneading. Because the pyloric sphincter is contracted during antral contraction, the gastric contents are emptied into the duodenum between contractions. Constriction of the pyloric sphincter prevents the backflow of gastric contents and allows them to flow into the duodenum at a rate commensurate with the ability of the duodenum to accept them. This is important because the regurgitation of bile salts and duodenal contents can damage the mucosal surface of the antrum and lead to gastric ulcers. Likewise, the duodenal mucosa can be damaged by the rapid influx of highly acid gastric contents.

The rate at which the stomach empties is regulated by neural and humoral signals from both the stomach and the duodenum. However, the duodenum provides by far the most potent of the signals, controlling the emptying of the chyme at a rate no greater than the rate at which the chyme can be digested and absorbed. Gastric emptying is slowed by hypertonic solutions in the duodenum, by duodenal pH below 3.5, and by the presence of fatty acids, amino acids, and peptides in the duodenum. The reflexes are transmitted directly from the duodenum to the stomach by the enteric nervous system and its connections with the sympathetic and parasympathetic nervous systems. Not only do nervous reflexes from the duodenum to the stomach inhibit gastric emptying, but hormones released from the duodenum and jejunum do so as well. These include cholecystokinin and glucose-dependent insulinotropic peptide (formerly known as *gastric inhibitory peptide*). The stimulus for releasing these inhibitory hormones is mainly fats entering the duodenum; other foods may decrease gastric emptying, but to a lesser degree.

Small Intestinal Motility

The rhythmic movements in the small intestine, like those elsewhere in the gastrointestinal tract, are mixing and propulsive. These movements involve segmentation and peristaltic contractions. With *segmentation waves*, slow contractions of the circular muscle layer occlude the lumen and drive the contents forward and backward (Fig. 28-6A). Most of the contractions that produce segmentation waves are local events involving only 1 to 4 cm of intestine at a time. They function mainly to mix the chyme with the digestive enzymes from the pancreas and to ensure adequate exposure of all parts of the chyme to the mucosal surface of the intestine, where absorption takes place. The frequency of segmenting activity increases after a meal, presumably stimulated by receptors in the stomach and intestine.

In contrast to the segmentation contractions, *peristaltic movements* are rhythmic propulsive movements designed to propel the chyme along the small intestine toward the large intestine. They occur when the smooth muscle layer constricts, forming a contractile band that forces the intraluminal contents forward. Normal peristalsis always moves in the direction from the mouth toward the anus. Regular peristaltic movements begin in the duodenum near the entry sites of the common duct and the main hepatic duct. These propulsive movements occur with synchronized activity in a section 10 to 20 cm long. They are accomplished by contraction of the proximal portion of the intestine with the sequential relaxation of its distal, or caudal, portion (Fig. 28-6B). After material has been propelled to the ileocecal junction by peristaltic movement, stretching of the distal ileum produces a local reflex that relaxes the sphincter and allows fluid to squirt into the cecum.

Motility disturbances of the small intestine are common, and auscultation of the abdomen for the presence of bowel sounds can be used to assess bowel activity. Inflammatory changes often increase motility. In many instances, it is not certain whether changes in motility

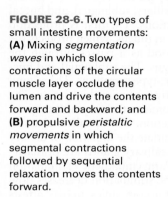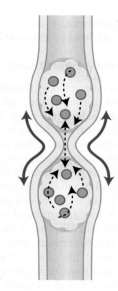

FIGURE 28-6. Two types of small intestine movements: **(A)** Mixing *segmentation waves* in which slow contractions of the circular muscle layer occlude the lumen and drive the contents forward and backward; and **(B)** propulsive *peristaltic movements* in which segmental contractions followed by sequential relaxation moves the contents forward.

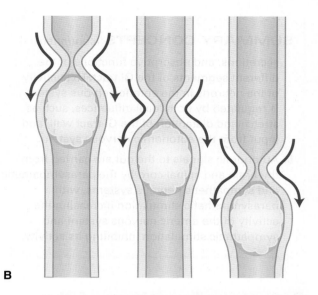

occur because of inflammation or are secondary to the effects of toxins or unabsorbed materials. Delayed passage of chyme in the small intestine also can be a problem. Transient interruption of intestinal motility often occurs after GI surgery. Intubation with suction often is required to remove the accumulating intestinal contents and gases until activity is resumed.

Colonic Motility and Defecation

The storage function of the colon dictates that movements in this section of the gut are different from those in the small intestine. Movements in the colon are of two types. First are the segmental mixing movements, called *haustrations*, so named because they occur within sacculations called *haustra*. These movements produce a local digging-type action, which ensures that all portions of the fecal mass are exposed to the intestinal surface. Second are the propulsive mass movements, in which a large segment of the colon (≥20 cm) contracts as a unit, moving the fecal contents forward as a unit. Mass movements last approximately 30 seconds, followed by a 2- to 3-minute period of relaxation, after which another contraction occurs. A series of mass movements lasts only for 10 to 30 minutes and may occur only several times a day. Defecation normally is initiated by the mass movements.

Defecation (discharge of feces from the rectum) is controlled by the action of two sphincters, the internal and external anal sphincters. The internal sphincter is a several-centimeters-long, circular thickening of smooth muscle that lies inside the anus. The external sphincter, which is composed of striated voluntary muscle, surrounds the internal sphincter. The external sphincter is controlled by nerve fibers in the pudendal nerve, which is part of the somatic nervous system and therefore under voluntary control. Defecation is controlled by defecation reflexes. One of these reflexes is the intrinsic myenteric reflex mediated by the local enteric nervous system. It is initiated by distention of the rectal wall, with initiation of reflex peristaltic waves that spread through the descending colon, sigmoid colon, and rectum.

A second defecation reflex, the parasympathetic reflex, is integrated at the level of the sacral cord. When the nerve endings in the rectum are stimulated, signals are transmitted first to the sacral cord and then reflexively back to the descending colon, sigmoid colon, rectum, and anus by the pelvic nerves. These impulses greatly increase peristaltic movements as well as relax the internal sphincter.

To prevent involuntary defecation from occurring, the external anal sphincter is under the conscious control of the cortex. As afferent impulses arrive at the sacral cord, signaling the presence of a distended rectum, messages are transmitted to the cortex. If defecation is inappropriate, the cortex initiates impulses that constrict the external sphincter and inhibit efferent parasympathetic activity. Normally, the afferent impulses in this reflex loop fatigue easily, and the urge to defecate soon ceases. At a more convenient time, contraction of the abdominal muscles compresses the contents in the large bowel, reinitiating afferent impulses to the cord.

(continued)

SUMMARY CONCEPTS (continued)

secretions, and absorptive functions of the different segments of the GI tract. The activity of the neurons in the enteric nervous system is regulated by both local influences, such as stretch and distention of the GI tract wall, and input from the autonomic nervous system.

■ Autonomic signals to the gut are carried from the brain and spinal cord by the parasympathetic and sympathetic nervous systems, with parasympathetic stimulation increasing the activity of the enteric nervous system and sympathetic stimulation inhibiting its activity.

Secretory Functions of the Gastrointestinal Tract

The GI tract produces a number of secretions, including mucus, hydrochloric acid, digestive enzymes, and hormones. Secretory activity, like motility, is influenced by local, humoral, and neural influences. Neural control of GI secretory activity is mediated through the ANS, with parasympathetic stimulation increasing secretory activity and sympathetic stimulation inhibiting secretory activity. Many local influences, including the pH and osmolarity of the GI contents, act as stimuli for neural and hormonal mechanisms.

Gastrointestinal Secretions

Throughout the GI tract, secretory glands serve two basic functions: production of mucus to lubricate and protect the mucosal layer of the GI tract wall and secretion of fluids and enzymes to aid in the digestion and absorption of nutrients. Each day, approximately 7000 mL of fluid is secreted into the GI tract (Table 28-1). Approximately 50 to 200 mL of this fluid leaves the body in the stool; the remainder is reabsorbed in the small and large intestines. These secretions are mainly water and have sodium and potassium concentrations similar to those of extracellular fluid. Because water and electrolytes for digestive tract secretions are derived from the extracellular fluid

TABLE 28-1	Secretions of the Gastrointestinal Tract
Secretions	**Amount Daily (mL)**
Salivary	1200
Gastric	2000
Pancreatic	1200
Biliary	700
Intestinal	2000
Total	7100

compartment, excessive secretion or impaired absorption can lead to extracellular fluid deficit.

Salivary Secretions

Saliva is secreted by the salivary glands. The salivary glands consist of the parotid, submaxillary, sublingual, and buccal glands. Saliva has three functions. The first is protection and lubrication. Saliva is rich in mucus, which protects the oral mucosa and coats the food as it passes through the mouth, pharynx, and esophagus. The sublingual and buccal glands produce only mucus-type secretions. The second function of saliva is its protective antimicrobial action. The saliva cleans the mouth and contains the enzyme lysozyme, which has an antibacterial action. Third, saliva contains ptyalin and amylase, which initiate the digestion of dietary starches. Secretions from the salivary glands are primarily regulated by the ANS. Parasympathetic stimulation increases flow and sympathetic stimulation decreases flow of saliva. The dry mouth that accompanies anxiety attests to the effects of sympathetic activity on salivary secretions.

Gastric Secretions

The otherwise smooth lining of the stomach is dotted with *gastric pits* that form the openings for two types of glands: pyloric and oxyntic or gastric glands (Fig. 28-7). The pyloric glands secrete gastrin and mucus for protection of the pyloric mucosa, and are located in the antral portion, or distal 20%, of the stomach. The oxyntic glands are located on the inside surfaces of the body and fundus of the stomach, which occupies about 80% of the stomach. They contain three types of cells: mucous neck cells, which secrete mainly mucus; peptic (chief cells), which secrete large quantities of pepsinogen; and parietal (oxyntic cells), which secrete HCl and intrinsic factor, which is needed for vitamin B_{12} absorption (Fig. 28-7). The pepsinogen that is secreted by the peptic cells is rapidly converted to pepsin (a protein-digesting enzyme) when exposed to the low pH of the gastric juices. A few stem cells are also found in the gastric pits. These cells are the parent cells for all new cells of the gastric mucosa.

The cellular mechanism for HCl secretion by the parietal cells in the stomach involves the hydrogen ion (H^+)/potassium ion (K^+)-adenosine triphosphatase (ATPase) transporter and chloride ion (Cl^-) channels located on their luminal membrane (Fig. 28-8). During the process of HCl secretion, carbon dioxide (CO_2) produced by aerobic metabolism combines with water (H_2O), catalyzed by the enzyme carbonic anhydrase, to form carbonic acid (H_2CO_3), which readily dissociates into H^+ and bicarbonate (HCO_3^-). The HCO_3^- moves out of the cell and into blood from the basolateral membrane. At the luminal side of the membrane, H^+ is secreted into the stomach by the H^+/K^+-ATPase transporter (also known as the *proton pump*). Chloride follows H^+ into the stomach by diffusing through Cl^- channels in the luminal membrane.

Three substances stimulate HCl secretion by the parietal cells: acetylcholine, gastrin, and histamine. Although each substance binds to different receptors on the parietal cell and has a different mechanism of action, they all serve to stimulate an increase in H^+ secretion through the H^+/K^+-ATPase transporter. Acetylcholine is released

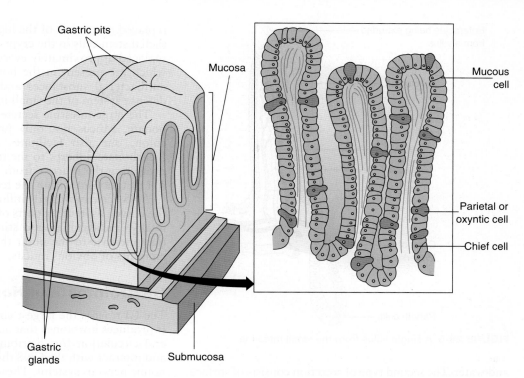

FIGURE 28-7. Gastric pit from body of the stomach.

from vagal nerves innervating the stomach and binds to acetylcholine receptors on the parietal cells. Gastrin is secreted by G cells in the antrum of the stomach and reaches the parietal cells through the circulation. It binds to as-yet uncharacterized receptors on the parietal cells. Histamine is released from special endocrine cells in the gastric mucosa and diffuses to nearby parietal cells, where it binds to histamine-2 (H_2) receptors.

One of the important characteristics of the gastric mucosa is resistance to the highly acid secretions that it produces. The mucosal surface is protected by prostaglandin E_2, which inhibits acid secretion and stimulates mucus production. Hence, it is an important factor in the maintenance of the gastric mucosal barrier. Aspirin and nonsteroidal anti-inflammatory drugs (NSAIDs) decrease prostaglandin synthesis, which can impair the integrity of the mucosal surface. Ethyl alcohol, or refluxed bile salts from the intestine, can also disrupt this barrier. When this occurs, hydrogen ions move into the tissue. Hydrogen ions accumulate in the mucosal cells, intracellular pH decreases, enzymatic reactions become impaired, and cellular structures are disrupted. The result is local ischemia, vascular stasis, hypoxia, and tissue necrosis.

Intestinal Secretions

The small intestine, which is where most of the digestion and absorption of food takes place, secretes digestive juices and receives secretions from the liver and pancreas (see Chapter 30). An extensive array of mucus-producing glands, called *Brunner glands*, is concentrated at the site where the contents from the stomach and secretions from the liver and pancreas enter the duodenum. These glands secrete large amounts of alkaline mucus that protect the duodenum from the acid content in the gastric chyme and from the action of the digestive enzymes.

In addition to mucus, the intestinal mucosa produces two other types of secretions. The first is an isotonic alkaline fluid (pH 6.5 to 7.5) secreted by specialized cells in the *crypts of Lieberkühn*, which are tubelike glands that dip down into the mucosal surface between the intestinal villi (Fig. 28-9). Unlike the gastric pits, the intestinal crypts do not secrete enzymes, but do secrete mucus, electrolytes,

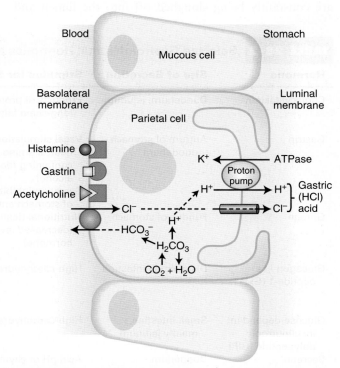

FIGURE 28-8. Mechanism of gastric acid secretion by the parietal cells in the stomach.

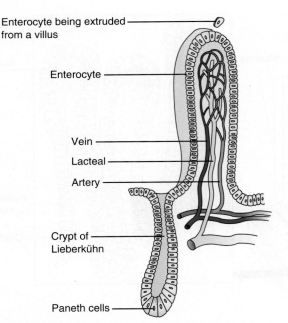

Enterocyte being extruded from a villus

Enterocyte

Vein

Lacteal

Artery

Crypt of Lieberkühn

Paneth cells

FIGURE 28-9. A single villus from the small intestine.

and water. The second type of secretion consists of surface enzymes that aid absorption. These enzymes include peptidases, which separate amino acids, and disaccharidases, which split sugars. Also present in intestinal secretions are mucins secreted by goblet cells. The mucins, which are glycoproteins high in carbohydrates, form a gel that serves to lubricate the mucosal surface and protect it from mechanical injury from solid food particles.

The crypts of Lieberkühn also function to replace epithelial cells. The epithelial cells lining the small intestine are constantly being sloughed off into the lumen and

replaced as a result of the high mitotic index of the epithelial stem cells in the crypts. The epithelium is entirely replaced approximately every 4 to 5 days. *Paneth cells*, which are present in the bottom of the crypts, secrete antibacterial substances and are involved in the host defense system of the small intestine.

The large intestine secretes mainly mucus and bicarbonate. Mucus not only protects the mucosa of the colon, but also facilitates compaction of the feces. Bicarbonate adheres to the mucus and acts as a buffer, protecting the mucosa from acid by-products of bacterial metabolism within the feces.

ANS activity strongly influences mucus production in the bowel, as in other parts of the digestive tract. During intense parasympathetic stimulation, mucus secretion may increase to the point that the stool contains large amounts of obvious mucus.

Gastrointestinal Hormones

The GI tract is the largest endocrine organ in the body. It produces hormones that act locally, pass into the general circulation for distribution to more distant sites, and interact with the CNS through the enteric and autonomic nervous systems. These hormones influence appetite, GI motility, enzyme activity, electrolyte levels, and the secretion and actions of hormones such as growth hormone, insulin, and glucagon. The actions of many of these hormones overlap: two or more GI hormones may affect the same process in the same direction, or they may inhibit each other. The GI tract hormones and their functions are summarized in Table 28-2.

The stomach is the source of two important GI hormones: gastrin and ghrelin. Gastrin is produced by G cells, located predominantly in the antrum of the

TABLE 28-2	Selected Gastrointestinal Hormones and Their Actions		
Hormone	**Site of Secretion**	**Stimulus for Secretion**	**Action**
Cholecystokinin	Duodenum, jejunum	Products of protein digestion and long-chain fatty acids	Stimulates contraction of gallbladder and secretion of pancreatic enzymes; slows gastric emptying; inhibits food intake
Gastrin	Antrum of stomach, duodenum	Vagal stimulation; epinephrine; neutral amino acids; calcium-containing foods such as milk; alcohol Secretion inhibited by acid content of stomach antrum (pH < 2.5)	Stimulates secretion of gastric acid and pepsinogen; increases gastric blood flow; stimulates gastric smooth muscle contractions; stimulates growth of gastric and intestinal mucosal cells
Ghrelin	Fundus of stomach	Nutritional (fasting) and hormonal (decreased levels of growth hormone)	Stimulates secretion of growth hormone; acts as an appetite-stimulating signal from stomach when an increase in metabolic efficiency is necessary
Glucagon-like peptide-1 (GLP-1)	Distal small intestine	High-carbohydrate meal	Augments insulin release; suppresses glucagon release; slows gastric emptying; decreases appetite and body weight
Glucose-dependent insulinotropic polypeptide (GIP)	Small intestine, mainly jejunum	High-carbohydrate meal	Augments insulin release
Secretin	Duodenum	Acid pH or chyme entering duodenum (pH < 3.0)	Stimulates secretion of bicarbonate-containing fluids by pancreas and liver

stomach. The primary function of *gastrin* is the stimulation of gastric acid secretion. Gastrin also has a trophic, or growth-producing, effect on the mucosa of the small intestine, colon, and acid-secreting area of the stomach. Removal of the tissue that produces gastrin results in atrophy of these structures. *Ghrelin* is a recently discovered peptide hormone produced by endocrine cells in the mucosal layer of the fundus of the stomach. It displays potent growth hormone–releasing activity and has a stimulatory effect on food intake and digestive function, while reducing energy expenditure. The isolation of this hormone has led to new insights into the gut–brain regulation of growth hormone secretion and energy balance.

The intestine is the source of secretin, cholecystokinin, and incretin hormones. *Secretin*, which is secreted by S cells in the mucosa of the duodenum and jejunum, inhibits gastric acid secretion. The entry of an acid chyme into the intestine stimulates the release of secretin, which inhibits the release of gastrin. Secretin also stimulates the pancreas to secrete large quantities of fluid with a high bicarbonate concentration and low chloride concentration. The primary function of *cholecystokinin* (CCK), secreted by I cells in the intestinal mucosa, is the stimulation of pancreatic enzyme secretion. It also potentiates the action of secretin, increasing the pancreatic bicarbonate response to low circulating levels of secretin; and regulates gallbladder contraction and gastric emptying. CCK has also been shown to inhibit food intake and to be an important mediator for appetite and amount of food consumed during a meal.

Several gut-derived hormones have been identified as having what is termed an *incretin* effect, meaning that they increase insulin release after an oral glucose load. This suggests that gut-derived factors can stimulate insulin secretion after a high-carbohydrate meal. The two hormones that account for about 90% of the incretin effect are glucagon-like peptide 1 (GLP-1), which is released from L cells in the distal small intestine, and glucose-dependent insulinotropic peptide (GIP), which is released by K cells in the upper small intestine (mainly the jejunum). Because increased levels of GLP-1 and GIP can lower blood glucose levels by augmenting insulin release in a glucose-dependent manner (i.e., at low blood glucose levels no further insulin is secreted, minimizing the risk of hypoglycemia), these hormones have been targeted as possible antidiabetic drugs. Moreover, GLP-1 can exert other metabolically beneficial effects, including suppression of glucagon release, slowing of gastric emptying, augmenting glucose clearance, and decreasing appetite and body weight.

SUMMARY CONCEPTS

- Secretory glands throughout the gastrointestinal tract serve two basic purposes: production of mucus to lubricate and protect its mucosal layer and secretion of fluids and enzymes to aid in the digestion and absorption of nutrients.

- The stomach, in addition to producing mucus, secretes hydrochloric acid (HCl); pepsinogen, which is converted to pepsin, which is important in protein metabolism; and intrinsic factor, which is involved in the absorption of vitamin B_{12}.

- The cells of the small intestine, where most digestion and absorption of foods take place, produces a watery alkaline fluid that aids in the digestive process and surface enzymes that aid in the digestion and absorption of carbohydrates and proteins. Digestive and absorptive processes in the small intestine are aided by bile from the liver and enzymes from the pancreas.

- In addition to secreting fluids containing digestive enzymes, the GI tract produces and secretes hormones that act locally, then pass into the general circulation for distribution to more distant sites. Among the hormones produced by the GI tract are gastrin, ghrelin, secretin, cholecystokinin, and incretin hormones (glucagon-like peptide-1 [GLP-1] and glucose-dependent insulinotropic polypeptide [GIP]). These hormones influence appetite, GI motility, enzyme activity, electrolyte levels, and the secretion and action of hormones such as growth hormone, insulin, and glucagon.

Digestion and Absorption in the Gastrointestinal Tract

Digestion involves the dismantling of foods into their constituent parts, a process that requires hydrolysis, enzyme cleavage, and fat emulsification. *Hydrolysis* is the breakdown of a compound that involves a chemical reaction with water. The importance of hydrolysis to digestion is evidenced by the amount of water (7 to 8 L) that is secreted into the GI tract daily. *Enzyme cleavage* requires the use of enzymes to cut substances into smaller components. *Emulsification* involves the breakdown of large globules of dietary fat into smaller particles.

Absorption is the process of moving nutrients and other materials from the external environment in the lumen of the GI tract into the blood or lymph of the internal environment. Absorption is accomplished by active transport and diffusion. A number of substances require a specific carrier or transport system. For example, vitamin B_{12} is not absorbed in the absence of intrinsic factor, which is secreted by the parietal cells of the stomach. Transport of amino acids and glucose occurs mainly in the presence of sodium. Water is absorbed passively along an osmotic gradient.

Small Intestinal Digestion and Absorption

Although some digestion of carbohydrates and proteins begins in the mouth and stomach respectively, digestion takes place mainly in the small intestine. The emulsification of fats to free fatty acids and monoglycerides takes place entirely in the small intestine. The liver, with its production of bile, and the pancreas, which supplies a number of digestive enzymes, play important roles in digestion.

The distinguishing characteristic of the small intestine is its large surface area, which in the adult is estimated to be approximately 250 m². Anatomic features that contribute to this enlarged surface area are the circular folds that extend into the lumen of the intestine and the villi, which are fingerlike projections of mucous membrane, numbering as many as 25,000, that line the entire small intestine (Fig. 28-10). Each villus is equipped with an artery, vein, and lymph vessel (i.e., lacteal), which bring blood to the surface of the intestine and transport the nutrients and other materials that have passed into the blood from the lumen of the intestine (see Fig. 28-9). Fats rely largely on the lymphatics for absorption. The villi are covered with cells called *enterocytes* that contribute to the absorptive and digestive functions of the small bowel, and goblet cells that provide mucus.

The enterocytes secrete enzymes that aid in the digestion of carbohydrates and proteins. These enzymes are called *brush border enzymes* because they adhere to the border of the microvilli that project from the surface of the enterocytes. In this way they have access to the carbohydrate and protein molecules as they come in contact with the absorptive surface of the intestine. This mechanism of secretion places the enzymes where they are needed and eliminates the need to produce enough enzymes to mix with the entire contents filling the lumen of the small bowel. The digested molecules diffuse through the membrane or are actively transported across the mucosal surface to enter the blood or, in the case of fatty acids, the lacteal. These molecules are then transported through the portal vein or lymphatics into the systemic circulation.

Carbohydrate Digestion and Absorption

Carbohydrates must be broken down into monosaccharides, or single sugars, before they can be absorbed from the small intestine. The average daily intake of carbohydrate in the American diet is approximately 350 to 400 g.

Digestion of starch begins in the mouth with the action of amylase. Pancreatic secretions also contain an amylase. Amylase breaks down starch into several disaccharides, including maltose, isomaltose, and α-dextrins. The brush border enzymes convert the disaccharides into monosaccharides that can be absorbed (Table 28-3). Sucrose yields glucose and fructose, lactose is converted to glucose and galactose, and maltose is converted to two glucose molecules. When the disaccharides are not broken down to monosaccharides, they cannot be absorbed but remain as osmotically active particles in the contents of the digestive system, causing diarrhea. For example, persons with a deficiency of lactase, the enzyme that breaks down lactose, experience diarrhea when they drink milk or eat dairy products.

Fructose is transported across the intestinal mucosa by facilitated diffusion, which does not require energy expenditure. Glucose and galactose move from the intestinal lumen into the intestinal cells by way of a sodium–glucose cotransporter (SGLT-1), against a chemical gradient. The energy for this step does not come directly from ATP, but from the sodium gradient created by the Na⁺/K⁺-ATPase pump located on the basolateral side of the membrane (Fig. 28-11). Glucose and galactose are transported from the cell into the blood across the basolateral membrane by facilitated diffusion using a glucose transporter-2 (GLUT-2) protein. Water absorption from the intestine is linked to absorption of osmotically active particles, such as glucose and sodium. It follows that an important consideration in facilitating the transport of water across the intestine (and decreasing diarrhea) after temporary disruption in bowel function is to include sodium and glucose in the fluids that are consumed.

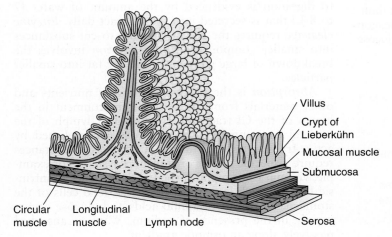

FIGURE 28-10. The mucous membrane of the small intestine. Note the numerous villi on a circular fold.

TABLE 28-3	Enzymes Used in Digestion of Carbohydrates	
Dietary Carbohydrates	**Enzyme**	**Monosaccharides Produced**
Lactose	Lactase	Glucose and galactose
Sucrose	Lactase	Fructose and glucose
Starch	Amylase	Maltose, maltotriose, and α-dextrins
Maltose and maltotriose	Maltase	Glucose and glucose
α-Dextrins	α-Dextrinase	Glucose and glucose

Protein Digestion and Absorption

Protein digestion begins in the stomach with the action of pepsin. Pepsinogen, the enzyme precursor of pepsin, is secreted by the chief cells in response to a meal and acid pH. Acid in the stomach is required for the conversion of pepsinogen to pepsin. Pepsin is inactivated when it enters the intestine by the alkaline pH.

Proteins are broken down further by pancreatic enzymes, such as trypsin, chymotrypsin, carboxypeptidase, and elastase. As with pepsin, the pancreatic enzymes are secreted as precursor molecules. Trypsinogen, which lacks enzymatic activity, is activated by an enzyme located on the brush border cells of the duodenal enterocytes. Activated trypsin activates additional trypsinogen molecules and other pancreatic precursor proteolytic enzymes. The amino acids are then liberated on the surface of the mucosal surface of the intestine by brush border enzymes that degrade proteins into peptides that are one, two, or three amino acids long.

As with glucose, many amino acids are transported across the mucosal membrane in a sodium-linked process that uses ATP as an energy source. Some amino acids are absorbed by facilitated diffusion processes that do not require sodium.

Fat Digestion and Absorption

The average adult eats approximately 60 to 100 g of fat daily, principally as triglycerides. The first step in digestion of lipids is to break the large globules of dietary fat into smaller particles so that water-soluble digestive enzymes can act on the surface molecules. This emulsification process begins in the stomach with agitation of the globules and continues in the duodenum under the influence of bile from the liver (Fig. 28-12). Emulsification greatly increases the number of triglyceride molecules exposed to pancreatic lipase, which splits triglycerides into free fatty acids and monoglycerides. Bile salts play an additional role by forming micelles that transport these

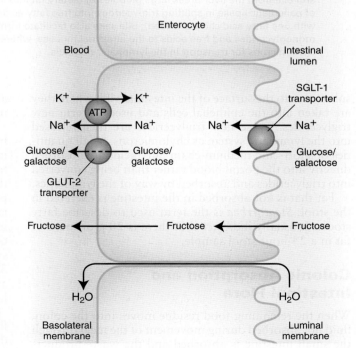

FIGURE 28-11. Intestinal transport of glucose, galactose, and fructose. Glucose and galactose are transported across the apical membrane by the sodium–glucose cotransporter (SGLT-1). Glucose moves out of the intestinal cell and into the blood using a glucose transporter-2 (GLUT-2) protein. Sodium is transported out of the cell by the Na^+/K^+-ATPase sodium pump. This creates the gradient needed to operate the transport system. Fructose is passively transported across the apical and basolateral membranes of the intestinal cell.

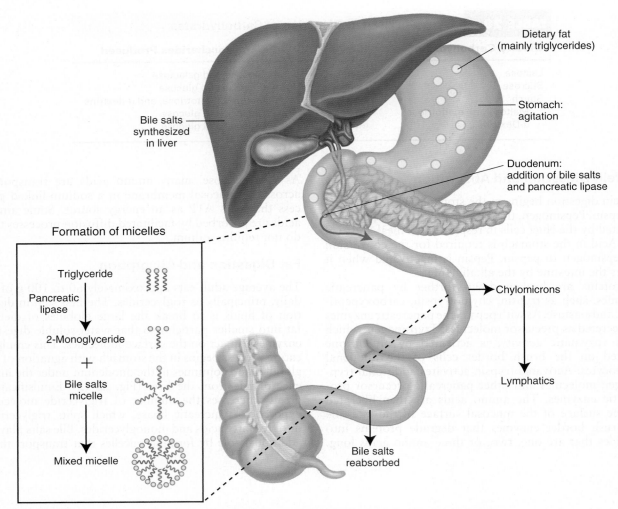

FIGURE 28-12. Mechanisms of dietary fat absorption. During digestion, agitation in the stomach and bile from the liver break large globules of dietary fat into small particles that facilitate the action of pancreatic lipase in splitting triglycerides into free fatty acids and monoglycerides (glycerol with one fatty acid chain attached). Bile salts also facilitate formation of micelles that transport the monoglycerides and free acids to the intestinal mucosa, where they are absorbed and converted to chylomicrons for transport in the lymphatic channels.

substances to the surface of the intestinal villi, where they are taken into the epithelial cells and used to form new triglycerides. These new triglycerides are then released into the lymphatic system as chylomicrons. Small quantities of short- and medium-chain fatty acids are absorbed directly into the portal blood rather than being converted into triglycerides and absorbed by way of the lymphatics.

Fat that is not absorbed in the intestine is excreted in the stool. *Steatorrhea* is the term used to describe fatty stools. It usually indicates that there is 20 g or more of fat in a 24-hour stool sample.

Colonic Absorption and Intestinal Flora

When the remaining food residue moves into the colon, fluid not absorbed during movement of the meal through the small intestine is absorbed and the waste products are stored in the large intestine until they can be conveniently eliminated.

While in the colon, food residues are acted upon by a large and diverse bacterial community called the intestinal flora. The stomach and small intestine contain only a few species of bacteria, probably because the composition of luminal contents (i.e., acids, bile, pancreatic secretions) kills most ingested microorganisms, and the propulsive movements of these organs impedes their colonization. The large intestine, on the other hand, contains a large and complex microbial ecosystem. It has been estimated that each individual has 300 to 500 different species of intestinal bacteria, with anaerobic bacteria outnumbering aerobic bacteria by a large percentage.

The major metabolic function of the intestinal flora is the fermentation of undigestible dietary residue including resistant starches, cellulose, pectins and other forms of dietary fibers, and unabsorbed sugars. Fermentation of these residues is a major source of energy for the microorganisms in the colon. The metabolic end point is the generation of short-chain fatty acids, which play a major role in intestinal epithelial cell growth and differentiation. Colonic microorganisms also play a role in vitamin synthesis and in absorption of calcium, magnesium, and iron. Vitamin K, for example, is synthesized by the intestinal flora. Lastly, the resident gut flora provides a crucial line of resistance to colonization by exogenous microbes, and therefore is highly protective against invasion of tissues by pathogens. The administration of broad-spectrum antibiotics can disrupt the microbial balance and allow overgrowth of species with potential pathogenicity, such as *Clostridium difficile* (see Chapter 29).

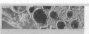

SUMMARY CONCEPTS

- Digestion is the process of dismantling foods into their constituent parts, and absorption is the process of moving nutrients and other materials from the GI tract into the internal environment.

- Carbohydrates must be broken down into monosaccharides before they can be absorbed, a process that involves both salivary and pancreatic amylase and the brush border enzymes of the small intestine.

- Digestion of proteins begins in the stomach with the action of pepsin and continues in the small intestine facilitated by the action of the proteolytic pancreatic enzymes, which split the protein molecules into dipeptides, tripeptides, or amino acids that are absorbed through the wall of the intestine.

- Fats are emulsified by bile into small droplets, which are broken down by pancreatic lipase into triglycerides containing medium- and long-chain fatty acids. Bile salts form micelles that transport these substances to the surface of intestinal villi, where they are absorbed by lymphatics.

- Fluid not absorbed during movement of a meal through the small intestine is absorbed in the colon, and food residues are fermented by the intestinal flora, resulting in short-chain fatty acids, which support epithelial cell proliferation and differentiation, and protects the colonized host against invasion by pathogenic organisms. Colonic microorganisms also play a role in vitamin synthesis and in absorption of calcium, magnesium, and iron and the synthesis of vitamins, including vitamin K.

Anorexia, Nausea, and Vomiting

Anorexia, nausea, and vomiting are physiologic responses common to many GI disorders. These responses are protective to the extent that they signal the presence of disease and, in the case of vomiting, remove noxious agents from the GI tract. They also can contribute to impaired intake or loss of fluids and nutrients.

Anorexia

Anorexia represents a loss of appetite. Several factors influence appetite. One is hunger, which is stimulated by contractions of the empty stomach. Appetite or the desire for food intake is regulated by the hypothalamus and other associated centers in the brain. Smell plays an important role, as evidenced by the fact that appetite can be stimulated or suppressed by the smell of food. Loss of appetite is associated with emotional factors, such as fear, depression, frustration, and anxiety. Many drugs and disease states cause anorexia. For example, in uremia the accumulation of nitrogenous wastes in the blood contributes to the development of anorexia. Anorexia often is a forerunner of nausea, and most conditions that cause nausea and vomiting also produce anorexia.

Nausea and Vomiting

Nausea is an ill-defined and unpleasant subjective sensation. It stimulates the vomiting center in the brain stem and often precedes or accompanies vomiting. Anorexia usually precedes nausea, and stimuli such as foods and drugs that cause anorexia in small doses usually produce nausea when given in larger doses. A common cause of nausea is distention of the duodenum or upper small intestinal tract. Nausea frequently is accompanied by autonomic nervous system manifestations such as watery salivation and vasoconstriction with pallor, sweating, and tachycardia. Nausea may function as an early warning signal of a pathologic process.

As a basic physiologic protective mechanism, vomiting limits the possibility of damage from ingested noxious agents by emptying the contents of the stomach and portions of the small intestine. Nausea and vomiting may also represent a total-body response to drug therapy, including overdose, cumulative effects, toxicity, and side effects.

The act of vomiting consists of taking a deep breath, closing the airways, and producing a strong, forceful contraction of the diaphragm and abdominal muscles along with relaxation of the gastroesophageal sphincter. Respiration ceases during the act of vomiting. Vomiting may be accompanied by dizziness, lightheadedness, a decrease in blood pressure, and bradycardia. *Retching* is the term used to describe the rhythmic spasmodic movements of the diaphragm, chest wall, and abdominal muscles without the expulsion of vomitus (dry heaves).

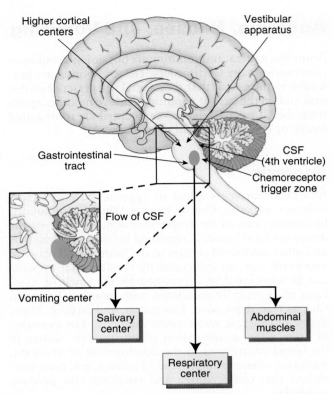

FIGURE 28-13. Physiologic events involved in vomiting. CSF, cerebrospinal fluid.

Several neurotransmitters and receptor subtypes are implicated as neuromediators in nausea and vomiting. Dopamine, serotonin, and opioid receptors are found in the GI tract and in the vomiting center and chemoreceptor trigger zone. Dopamine antagonists, such as prochlorperazine, depress vomiting caused by stimulation of the chemoreceptor trigger zone. Serotonin is believed to be involved in the nausea and emesis associated with cancer chemotherapy and radiation therapy. Serotonin (5-hydroxytryptamine [5HT]) antagonists (e.g., granisetron, ondansetron) are often effective in treating the nausea and vomiting associated with these stimuli. The recently developed neurokinin-1 (NK-1) receptor antagonists (e.g., aprepitant) may also be used for the treatment of acute and delayed chemotherapy-induced nausea and vomiting. These drugs act centrally to block the activation of the NK-1 receptors in the vomiting center. Motion sickness appears to be a CNS response to vestibular stimuli. Norepinephrine and acetylcholine receptors are located in the vestibular center. The acetylcholine receptors are thought to mediate the impulses responsible for exciting the vomiting center. Many of the motion sickness drugs (e.g., meclizine, dimenhydrinate, transdermal scopalamine) have a strong CNS anticholinergic effect and act on the receptors in the vomiting center and areas related to the vestibular system.

The act of vomiting is integrated in the vomiting center, which is located in the dorsal portion of the reticular formation of the medulla near the sensory nuclei of the vagus (Fig. 28-13). The vomiting center can be activated directly by irritants or indirectly following input from four different sources: (1) the GI tract and other abdominal organs; (2) higher central nervous system centers that respond to certain sights, sounds, or emotions that induce vomiting; (3) the vestibular apparatus, which is responsible for motion sickness; and (4) the chemoreceptor trigger zone, which is activated by chemical agents such as drugs and toxins. Hypoxia exerts a direct effect on the vomiting center, producing nausea and vomiting. This direct effect probably accounts for the vomiting that occurs during periods of decreased cardiac output, shock, environmental hypoxia, and brain ischemia caused by increased intracranial pressure. Inflammation of any of the intra-abdominal organs, including the liver, gallbladder, or urinary tract, can cause vomiting because of the stimulation of the visceral afferent pathways that communicate with the vomiting center. Distention or irritation of the GI tract also causes vomiting through the stimulation of visceral afferent neurons. The chemoreceptor trigger zone is located outside the blood–brain barrier in a small area between the medulla and the floor of the fourth ventricle, where it is exposed to both blood and cerebrospinal fluid. This region may be stimulated by drugs, chemotherapeutic agents, toxins, uremia, acidosis, and pregnancy.

SUMMARY CONCEPTS

- The signs and symptoms of many GI tract disorders are manifested by anorexia, nausea, and vomiting.

- Anorexia, or loss of appetite, may occur alone or may accompany nausea and vomiting.

- Nausea, which is an ill-defined, unpleasant sensation, signals the stimulation of the medullary vomiting center. It often precedes vomiting and frequently is accompanied by autonomic responses, such as salivation and vasoconstriction with pallor, sweating, and tachycardia.

- Vomiting, which is integrated by the vomiting center, involves the sudden and forceful oral expulsion of the gastric contents. The vomiting center can be activated directly by irritants or indirectly following input from the GI tract and other abdominal organs; higher central nervous system centers; the vestibular apparatus, which is responsible for motion sickness; or the chemoreceptor trigger zone, which is activated by chemical agents such as drugs and toxins.

REVIEW EXERCISES

1. Persons receiving chemotherapeutic agents, which interfere with the mitosis of cancer cells as well as the cells of other rapidly proliferating tissues in the body, often experience disorders such as ulcerations in the mucosal tissues of the mouth and other parts of the GI tract. These disorders are resolved once the chemotherapy treatment has been completed.

   A. Explain.

2. People with gastroesophageal reflux (movement of gastric contents into the esophagus) often complain of heartburn that becomes worse as the pressure in the stomach increases.

   A. Explain.
   B. Use information on hormonal control of gastric emptying to explain why eating a meal that is high in fat content often exaggerates the problem.

3. Infections of the GI tract, such as the "GI flu," often cause profound diarrhea.

   A. Describe the neural mechanisms involved in the increase in GI motility that produces the diarrhea.
   B. Explain the rationale for using a "drink" that contains both glucose and sodium to treat the fluid deficit that often occurs with diarrhea.

4. Explain the physiologic mechanisms associated with the occurrence of diarrhea in persons with:

   A. Lactase deficiency.
   B. Obstruction of bile flow into the intestine.
   C. Disruption of the normal intestinal flora due to antibiotic therapy.

5. Explain why anticholinergic drugs are often effective in treating the nausea and vomiting that accompany motion sickness but are relatively ineffective in treating the nausea and vomiting associated with chemotherapy agents used in the treatment of cancer.

BIBLIOGRAPHY

Becker DE. Nausea, vomiting, hiccups: a review of mechanisms and treatment. *Anesth Prog.* 2010;57:150–157.

Furness JB. The enteric nervous system and neurogastroenterology. *Nat Rev Gastroenterol Hepatol.* 2012;9(3):286–294.

Hall JE. *Guyton and Hall Textbook of Medical Physiology.* 12th ed. Philadelphia, PA: Elsevier Saunders; 2011:789–803.

Hargreaves R, Ferreira JC, Hughes D, et al. Development of aprepitant, the first neurokinin-1 receptor antagonist for prevention of chemotherapy-induced nausea and vomiting. *Ann N Y Acad Sci.* 2011;1222:40–48.

Hayes MR, DeJonghe BC, Kanosk SE. Role of glucagon-like perptide-1 receptor in control of energy balance. *Physiol Behav.* 2010;100(5):503–510.

Koeppen BM, Stanton BA, eds. *Berne and Levy Physiology.* 6th ed. Philadelphia, PA: Mosby; 2010:487–541.

Lindley C. Nausea and vomiting. In: Koda-Kimble MA, Young LY, Kradian WA, et al., eds. *Applied Therapeutics: The Clinical Use of Drugs.* 8th ed. Philadelphia, PA: Lippincott Williams & Wilkins; 2005:8-1–8-18.

Moore KL, Dalley AF, Agur AMR. *Clinically Oriented Anatomy.* 5th ed. Philadelphia, PA: Wolters Kluwer Health/Lippincott Williams & Wilkins; 2010:217–263.

O'Hara AM, Shanahan F. The gut flora as a forgotten organ. *EMBO Rep.* 2006;7:688–693.

Rhoades RA, Bell DR. *Medical Physiology: Principles for Clinical Medicine.* 4th ed. Philadelphia, PA: Wolters Kluwer Health/Lippincott Williams & Wilkins; 2013:471–535.

Ross MH, Pawlina W. *Histology: A Text and Atlas.* 6th ed. Philadelphia, PA: Wolters Kluwer Health/Lippincott Williams & Wilkins; 2011:568–625.

Sanders KM, Koh SD, Ward M. Interstitial cells of Cajal in the gastrointestinal tract. *Annu Rev Phys.* 2006;68:307–343.

Sherwood L. *Human Physiology: From Cells to Systems.* 8th ed. Belmont, CA: Brooks/Cole; 2013:581–634.

Porth Essentials Resources

Explore these additional resources to enhance learning for this chapter:

- NCLEX-Style Questions and Other Resources on the**Point**, http://thePoint.lww.com/PorthEssentials4e
- Study Guide for Essentials of Pathophysiology
- Concepts in Action Animations
- Adaptive Learning | Powered by PrepU, http://thepoint.lww.com/prepu

Disorders of Gastrointestinal Function

Gastrointestinal disorders are not cited as the leading cause of death in developed countries of the world, nor do they receive the same publicity as heart disease and cancer. However, digestive diseases rank high in the total economic burden of illness, resulting in considerable human suffering, personal expenditures for treatment, and lost working hours, as well as a drain on the nation's economy. In 2004 alone, digestive disorders accounted for an estimated 72 million ambulatory visits in the United States.[1] Visits were common for all age groups, with the highest rate among persons 65 years and older. Even more important is the fact that proper nutrition or a change in health practices could prevent or minimize many of these disorders.

Disruption in structure and function can occur at any level of the gastrointestinal tract, from the esophagus to the colon and rectum. This chapter is divided into three sections: (1) disorders of the esophagus, (2) disorders of the stomach, and (3) disorders of the small and large intestines. Disorders of the hepatobiliary system and exocrine pancreas are presented in Chapter 30.

Disorders of the Esophagus

The esophagus is a fixed muscular tube through which swallowed food and liquids pass as they move from the pharynx to the stomach. It lies posterior to the trachea and larynx and extends through the mediastinum, intersecting the diaphragm at the level of the T11 or T12 vertebra.[2] The wall of the esophagus is lined with a mucosal layer of abrasion-resistant nonkeratinized stratified epithelium; its submucosal layer contains mucus-secreting glands that produce a lubricating fluid that protects its mucosal surface and aids in the passage of food; and its muscularis layer provides the peristaltic movements needed to propel food along its length.

There are sphincters at either end of the esophagus: an upper esophageal, or pharyngoesophageal, sphincter that prevents reflux into the pharynx from the esophagus, and a lower esophageal, or gastroesophageal, sphincter that prevents reflux into the esophagus from the stomach.[3] The lower esophageal sphincter is a physiologic rather than a true anatomic sphincter. That is, it acts as a valve, but the only structural evidence of a sphincter is a slight thickening of the circular smooth muscle. The smooth muscle fibers in this portion of the esophagus normally remain tonically constricted except at times when a bolus of food is about to pass into the stomach or if a person is vomiting.[2] The lower esophageal sphincter passes through an opening, or *hiatus,* in the diaphragm as it joins with the stomach, which is located in the abdomen. The portion of the diaphragm that surrounds the lower esophageal sphincter helps to maintain the zone of high pressure needed to prevent reflux of stomach contents.

Disorders of Esophageal Structure and Function

The musculature of the pharyngeal wall and upper third of the esophagus is striated muscle, innervated by the glossopharyngeal and vagus nerves. The lower two thirds of the esophagus is smooth muscle, innervated by the vagus nerve. The act of swallowing depends on the coordinated action of the tongue, pharyngeal structures, and esophagus (see Chapter 28).

In general, swallowing can be divided into three stages (see Chapter 28, Fig. 28-6). The first, or voluntary, stage occurs in the mouth. Once the food has been chewed and well mixed with saliva, the bolus (food mass) is forced into the pharynx by the tongue. The second stage, the involuntary pharyngeal–esophageal phase, transports food through the pharynx and into the esophagus. The parasympathetic nervous system (primarily the vagus) controls this part of swallowing and promotes motility of the gastrointestinal tract from this point on. Once food reaches the distal end of the esophagus, it passes through the lower esophageal sphincter into the stomach (stage 3). The act of swallowing is complicated by the fact that the pharynx subserves respiration as well swallowing. Thus, it is important that breathing not be compromised because of swallowing.

Swallowing Disorders

Difficulty swallowing, often referred as *dysphagia,* can result from disorders that produce narrowing of the esophagus, lack of salivary secretion, weakness of the muscular structures that propel the food bolus, or disruption of the neural networks coordinating the swallowing mechanism. Lesions of the central nervous system (CNS), such as a stroke, often involve the cranial nerves that control swallowing. Cancer of the esophagus and strictures resulting from scarring can reduce the size of the esophageal lumen and make swallowing difficult. Scleroderma, an autoimmune disease that causes fibrous replacement of tissues in the muscularis layer of the gastrointestinal tract, is another important cause of dysphagia.[4,5] Persons with dysphagia usually complain of choking, coughing, or an abnormal sensation of food sticking in the back of the throat or upper chest when they swallow.

The term *achalasia* means "failure to relax" and in the context of esophageal function denotes an incomplete relaxation of the lower esophageal sphincter in relation to swallowing. In primary achalasia, the mesenteric ganglia that carry the vagal fibers for the lower esophagus are usually absent from the body of the esophagus. The condition usually becomes manifest in young adulthood, but may appear in infancy and childhood. Achalasia produces functional obstruction of the esophagus so that food has difficulty passing into the stomach and the esophagus above the lower esophageal sphincter becomes distended. Stasis of food may produce inflammation and ulceration proximal to the lower esophageal sphincter, and there is danger of aspiration of esophageal contents into the lungs when the person lies down. The most serious aspect of the condition is the potential for developing esophageal cancer.

Treatment of swallowing disorders depends on the cause and type of altered function that is present. Treatment often involves a multidisciplinary team of health professionals, including a speech therapist. Mechanical dilation or surgical procedures may be done to enlarge the lower esophageal sphincter in persons with esophageal strictures.

Esophageal Diverticula

A diverticulum of the esophagus is an outpouching of the esophageal wall caused by a weakness of the muscularis layer or motility problems (e.g., diffuse esophageal spasm, achalasia).[6,7] Esophageal diverticula tend to retain food. Complaints that the food stops before it reaches the stomach are common, as are reports of gurgling, belching, coughing, and foul-smelling breath. The trapped food may cause esophagitis and ulceration. Surgery is the optimal treatment for persons with severe symptoms or pulmonary complications.

Esophageal Lacerations

Longitudinal lacerations in the esophagus, also called *Mallory-Weiss syndrome,* represent nonpenetrating mucosal tears at the gastroesophageal junction.[6–8] They are most often encountered in persons with chronic alcoholism after a bout of severe retching or vomiting, but may also occur during acute illness with severe vomiting. The presumed pathogenesis is inadequate relaxation of the esophageal sphincter during vomiting, with stretching and tearing of the esophageal junction during propulsive expulsion of gastric contents. The tears, which range in length from millimeters to a few centimeters, usually cross the gastroesophageal junction and also may be located in the proximal gastric mucosa. Esophageal lacerations account for about 10% of all upper gastrointestinal bleeding, which often presents as hematemesis.[6] Most often bleeding is not severe and does not require surgical intervention. Healing is usually prompt, with minimal or no residual effects.

Hiatal Hernia

Hiatal hernia is characterized by a protrusion or herniation of the stomach through the esophageal hiatus of the diaphragm. There are two anatomic patterns of hiatal herniation: sliding (axial) and paraesophageal (nonaxial).[6] The sliding hiatal hernia is characterized by a bell-shaped protrusion of the stomach above the diaphragm (Fig. 29-1A). Small sliding hiatal hernias are common and considered to be of no significance in asymptomatic people. In paraesophageal hiatal hernias a separate portion of the stomach, usually along the fundus of the stomach, enters the thorax through a widened opening (Fig. 29-1B). The hernia progressively enlarges and increases in size. In extreme cases, most of the stomach herniates into the thorax. Large paraesophageal hernias may require surgical treatment.

Gastroesophageal Reflux

The term *reflux* refers to backward or return movement. In the context of gastroesophageal reflux, it refers to the backward movement of gastric contents into the esophagus, a condition that causes heartburn or pyrosis. Most people experience heartburn occasionally as a result of reflux. Such symptoms usually occur soon after eating, are short lived, and seldom cause more serious problems.

The lower esophageal sphincter regulates the flow of food from the esophagus into the stomach. Both internal and external mechanisms function in maintaining the antireflux function of the lower esophageal sphincter. The circular muscles of the distal esophagus constitute the internal mechanisms, and the portion of the diaphragm that surrounds the esophagus constitutes the external mechanism (Fig. 29-2). The oblique muscles of the stomach, located below the lower esophageal sphincter, form a flap that contributes to the antireflux function of the internal sphincter. Relaxation of the lower esophageal sphincter is a brain stem reflex that is mediated by the vagus nerve in response to a number of afferent stimuli. Transient relaxation with reflux is common after meals. Gastric distention and meals high in fat increase the frequency of relaxation. Normally, refluxed material is returned to the stomach by secondary peristaltic waves in the esophagus, with swallowed saliva neutralizing and washing away the refluxed acid.

Gastroesophageal Reflux Disease

The persistent reflux of gastric contents into the esophagus is referred to as *gastroesophageal reflux disease* (GERD).[8-10] It is thought to be associated with a weak or incompetent lower esophageal sphincter that allows reflux to occur, the irritant effects of the refluxate, and decreased clearance of the refluxed acid from the esophagus after it has occurred. In most cases, reflux occurs during transient relaxation of the esophagus. Delayed gastric emptying also may contribute to reflux by increasing gastric volume and pressure. Esophageal mucosal injury may occur and is related to the destructive nature of the refluxate and the amount of time it is in contact with mucosa. The mucosa is partially protected by mucin and alkaline secretions from the submucosal glands. Injury occurs when the reflux episodes are frequent and prolonged. Agents that decrease the tone of the lower esophageal

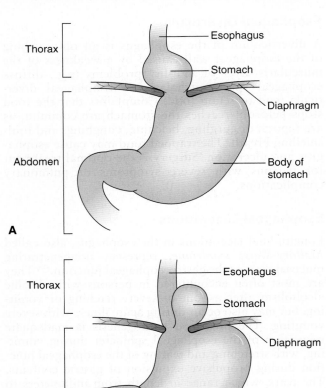

FIGURE 29-1. Hiatal hernia. **(A)** Sliding hiatal hernia. **(B)** Paraesophageal hiatal hernia.

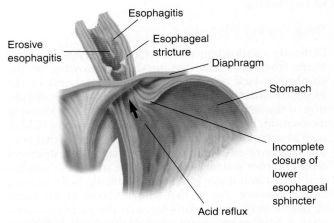

FIGURE 29-2. Gastroesophageal junction and site of gastroesophageal reflux. (From Anatomical Chart Company. *Atlas of Pathophysiology*. Springhouse, PA: Springhouse; 2004:171.)

6 weeks.[36] In most cases systemic manifestations are absent and the symptoms subside after the antibiotic has been discontinued. A more severe form of colitis, *pseudomembranous colitis,* is characterized by an adherent inflammatory membrane overlying the areas of mucosal injury. It is a life-threatening form of the disease. Persons with the disease are acutely ill, with lethargy, fever, tachycardia, abdominal pain and distention, and dehydration. The smooth muscle tone of the colon may be lost, resulting in toxic dilation of the colon. Prompt therapy is needed to prevent perforation of the bowel.

The diagnosis of *C. difficile* colitis requires a careful history, with particular emphasis on antibiotic use. Diagnostic findings include a history of antibiotic use and laboratory tests that confirm the presence of *C. difficile* toxins in the stool.[33,34] Patients with *C. difficile* infection should be put on contact precautions and placed in a single room with a bathroom or, if unavailable, with other infected patients.[35]

Treatment includes the immediate discontinuation of antibiotic therapy. Specific treatment aimed at eradicating *C. difficile* is used when symptoms are severe or persistent. Metronidazole is the drug of first choice, with vancomycin being reserved for persons who cannot tolerate metronidazole or do not respond to the drug. Both drugs are given orally.[33,34] Metronidazole is absorbed from the upper gastrointestinal tract and may cause side effects. Vancomycin is poorly absorbed, and its actions are limited to the gastrointestinal tract.

Escherichia coli O157:H7 Infection. Enterohemorrhagic *E. coli* O157:H7 has become recognized as an important cause of epidemic and sporadic colitis.[6] *E. coli* O157:H7 is a strain of *E. coli* found in the feces and contaminated milk of healthy dairy and beef cattle, but it also has been found in contaminated pork, poultry, and lamb. Infection usually is by food-borne transmission, often by ingesting undercooked ground beef. The organism also can be transferred to nonmeat products such as fruits and vegetables. Transmission has also been reported in persons swimming in a fecally contaminated lake as well as among visitors to farms and petting zoos who are in direct contact with animals. Person-to-person transmission may occur, particularly in nursing homes, day care settings, and hospitals. The very young and the very old are particularly at risk for the infection and its complications.

Although most strains of *E. coli* are harmless, *E. coli* O157:H7 produce *Shigella*-like toxins that attach to and damage the mucosal lining of the intestine, causing bloody diarrhea.[6,36,37] Subsequently, the *Shigella*-like toxins gain access to the circulatory system, where they damage the endothelium and initiate platelet activation. Two complications of the infection, hemolytic uremic syndrome and thrombotic thrombocytopenic purpura, reflect the effects of the *Shigella*-like toxins. The hemolytic uremic syndrome is characterized by hemolytic anemia, thrombocytopenia, and renal failure caused by platelet thrombi in the renal microvasculature. It occurs predominantly in infants and young children and is the most common cause of acute renal failure in children.

It has a mortality rate of 3% to 5%, and one third of the survivors are left with permanent disability. Thrombotic thrombocytopenic purpura is manifested by thrombocytopenia, renal failure, fever, and neurologic manifestations caused by microthrombi in the brain.

No specific therapy is available for *E. coli* O157:H7 infection. Treatment is largely symptomatic and directed toward treating the effects of complications. The use of antibiotics or antidiarrheal agents in the early stages of diarrhea has been shown to increase the risk of hemolytic uremic syndrome because the gut is exposed to a greater amount of toxins for a longer time. Because of the seriousness of the infection and its complications, education of the public about techniques for decreasing primary transmission of the infection from animal sources is important. Undercooked meats and unpasteurized milk are sources of transmission. Food handlers and consumers should be aware of the proper methods for handling uncooked meat to prevent cross-contamination of other foods. Particular attention should be paid to hygiene in day care centers and nursing homes, where the spread of infection to the very young and very old may result in severe complications.

Diverticular Disease

Diverticulosis is a disorder characterized by pseudodiverticula of the colonic mucosa and submucosa.[6,7,38–40] Although the disorder is prevalent in the developed countries of the world, it is almost nonexistent in many African nations and underdeveloped countries. This suggests that factors such as lack of fiber in the diet, a decrease in physical activity, and poor bowel habits (e.g., neglecting the urge to defecate), along with the effects of aging, contribute to the development of the disease.

True diverticula involve all layers of the intestinal wall. The abnormal structures in diverticulosis are instead pseudodiverticula, in which only the mucosa and submucosa are herniated through the muscle layers.[6,7] The diverticula are often multiple, ranging from a solitary herniation to several hundred (Fig. 29-8). They are most often located in the sigmoid colon, but more extensive areas may be involved in severe cases. Microscopically, colonic diverticula are small, flasklike outpouchings, usually 0.5 to 1.0 cm in diameter, that occur in a regular distribution alongside the teniae coli (Fig. 29-9).

Colonic diverticula result from the unique structure and elevated luminal pressures in the sigmoid colon.[6] In the colon, the longitudinal muscle does not form a continuous layer, as it does in the small bowel. Instead, there are three separate longitudinal bands of muscle called the *teniae coli.* In a manner similar to the small intestine, bands of circular muscle constrict the large intestine. As the circular muscle contracts at each of these points (approximately every 2.5 cm), the lumen of the bowel becomes constricted, so that it is almost occluded. The combined contraction of the circular muscle and the lack of a continuous longitudinal muscle

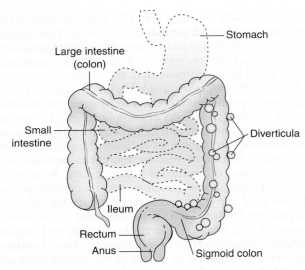

FIGURE 29-8. Location of diverticula in the sigmoid colon.

layer cause the intestine to bulge outward into pouches called *haustra*. Diverticula develop between the longitudinal muscle bands of the haustra, in the areas where blood vessels pierce the circular muscle layer to bring blood to the mucosal layer. An increase in intraluminal pressure in the haustra provides the force for creating these herniations.

Most people with diverticular disease remain asymptomatic.[38,39] The disease often is found when x-ray studies are done for other purposes. Ill-defined lower abdominal discomfort, a change in bowel habits (e.g., diarrhea, constipation), bloating, and flatulence are common. Diverticulitis is a complication of diverticulosis in which there is inflammation and gross or microscopic perforation of the diverticula.[40] One of the most common complaints of diverticulitis is pain in the lower

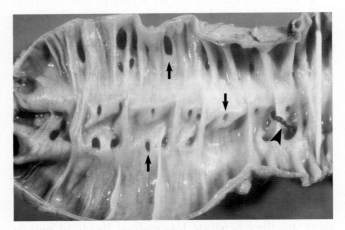

FIGURE 29-9. Diverticulosis of the colon. The colon was inflated with formalin. The mouths of numerous diverticula are seen between the taenia (*arrows*). There is a blood clot protruding from the mouth of one of the diverticula (*arrow*). (From Rubin R. The gastrointestinal tract. In: Rubin R, Strayer DS, eds. *Rubin's Pathophysiology: Clinicopathologic Foundations of Medicine.* 6th ed. Philadelphia, PA: Wolters Kluwer Health | Lippincott Williams & Wilkins; 2012:652.)

left quadrant, accompanied by nausea and vomiting, tenderness in the lower left quadrant, a slight fever, and an elevated white blood cell count. These symptoms usually last for several days, unless complications occur, and usually are caused by localized inflammation of the diverticula with perforation and development of a small, localized abscess. Complications include perforation with peritonitis, hemorrhage, and bowel obstruction. Fistulas can form, usually involving the bladder (i.e., vesicosigmoid fistula) but sometimes involving the skin, perianal area, or small bowel. Pneumaturia (i.e., air in the urine) is a sign of vesicosigmoid fistula.

The diagnosis of diverticular disease is based on history and presenting clinical manifestations.[39] The disease may be confirmed by CT scans or ultrasonographic studies. CT scans are the safest and most cost-effective method. Because of the risk of peritonitis, barium enema studies and endoscopy should be avoided in persons who are suspected of having acute diverticulitis. Flat abdominal radiographs may be used to detect complications associated with acute diverticulitis.

The usual treatment for diverticular disease is to prevent symptoms and complications. This includes increasing the bulk in the diet and bowel retraining so that the person has at least one bowel movement each day. The increased bulk promotes regular defecation and increases colonic contents and colon diameter, thereby decreasing intraluminal pressure. Acute diverticulitis is treated by withholding solid food and administering a broad-spectrum antibiotic. Hospitalization may be required for persons who show significant inflammation, are unable to tolerate oral fluids, or have significant comorbid conditions. Surgical treatment is reserved for complications.

Appendicitis

Acute appendicitis, or inflammation of the wall of the appendix, is extremely common. It is seen most frequently in the 20- to 30-year-old age group, but it can occur at any age.[6] The appendix becomes inflamed, swollen, and gangrenous, and it eventually perforates if not treated.[41] Although the cause of appendicitis is unknown, it is thought to be related to intraluminal obstruction with a fecalith (i.e., hard piece of stool) or to twisting.

Appendicitis usually has an abrupt onset, with pain referred to the epigastric or periumbilical area. This pain is caused by stretching of the appendix during the early inflammatory process. At approximately the same time that the pain appears, there are one or two episodes of nausea. Initially, the pain is vague, but over a period of 2 to 12 hours, it gradually increases and may become colicky. When the inflammatory process has extended to involve the serosal layer of the appendix and the peritoneum, the pain becomes localized to the lower right quadrant. There usually is an elevation in temperature and a white blood cell count greater than 10,000/mm^3, with 75% or more polymorphonuclear cells. Palpation of the abdomen usually reveals a deep tenderness in the lower right quadrant, which is confined to a small area approximately the size of the fingertip. It usually is located at approximately the site of the inflamed appendix. The person with appendicitis often is able to place his or her finger directly over the tender area. Rebound tenderness, which is pain that occurs when pressure is applied to the area and then released, and spasm of the overlying abdominal muscles are common.

Diagnosis is usually based on history and findings on physical examination. Ultrasonography or CT may be used to confirm the diagnosis.[41] Treatment consists of surgical removal of the appendix. Complications include peritonitis, localized periappendiceal abscess formation, and septicemia.

Disorders of Intestinal Motility

Intestinal motility, or the movement of contents through the gastrointestinal tract, is controlled by neurons located in the submucosal and myenteric plexuses of the gut (see Chapter 28). The axons from the cell bodies in the myenteric plexus innervate the circular and longitudinal smooth muscle layers of the gut. These neurons receive impulses from local receptors located in the mucosal and muscle layers of the gut and extrinsic input from the parasympathetic and sympathetic nervous systems. As a general rule, the parasympathetic nervous system tends to increase the motility of the bowel, whereas sympathetic stimulation tends to slow its activity.

The large intestine has sphincters at both ends: the ileocecal sphincter, which separates it from the small intestine; and the anal sphincter, which prevents the movement of feces to the outside of the body. About 1500 mL of fluid and undigested food normally pass through the ileocecal valve into the large intestine each day. Most of the water and electrolytes in the fluid are absorbed in the colon, usually leaving less than 100 mL to be excreted in the feces.[2] The large intestine can absorb a maximum of 5 to 8 L of fluid and electrolytes each day. When the total amount entering the large intestine through the ileocecal valve or by way of intestinal secretion exceeds this amount, the excess appears in the feces as diarrhea.

Diarrhea

The usual definition of *diarrhea* is excessively frequent passage of stools. Diarrhea can be acute or chronic and can be caused by infectious organisms, food intolerance, drugs, or intestinal disease. In developing countries, diarrhea is a common cause of mortality among children younger than 5 years of age, with an estimated 2 million deaths annually.[42] Even though diarrheal diseases are less prevalent in the United States than in other countries, they place a burden on the health care system.

Acute Diarrhea. Acute diarrhea is predominantly caused by infectious agents and follows a self-limited course of less than 2 weeks.[43] Acute diarrhea is commonly divided into noninflammatory (large-volume) and inflammatory (small-volume) diarrhea, based on the characteristics of the diarrheal stool. Enteric organisms cause diarrhea in several ways. Some organisms are noninvasive and do not cause inflammation, but secrete toxins that stimulate fluid secretion.[44,45] Others invade and destroy intestinal epithelial cells, thereby altering fluid transport so that secretory activity continues while absorption activity is halted.

Noninflammatory diarrhea is associated with large-volume watery and nonbloody stools, periumbilical cramps, bloating, and nausea or vomiting. It is commonly caused by toxin-producing bacteria (e.g., enterotoxigenic *E. coli*, *S. aureus*, *Vibrio cholerae*) or other agents (e.g., viruses, *Giardia*) that disrupt the normal absorption or secretory process in the small bowel. Prominent vomiting suggests viral enteritis or *S. aureus* food poisoning.[32] Although typically mild, diarrhea that originates in the small intestine can be voluminous and result in dehydration with hypokalemia and metabolic acidosis. Because tissue invasion and inflammation do not occur, leukocytes are not present in the feces.

Inflammatory diarrhea is usually characterized by the presence of fever and bloody diarrhea. It is caused by bacterial invasion of intestinal cells (e.g., *Shigella*, *Salmonella*, *Yersinia*, and *Campylobacter*) or the toxins associated with the previously described *C. difficile* or *E. coli* O157:H7 infection. Because infections associated with these organisms predominantly affect the colon, the diarrhea is small in volume (<1 L/day) and is associated with lower abdominal pain and the urgent desire to defecate. Infectious dysentery must be distinguished from acute ulcerative colitis, which may present with bloody diarrhea, fever, and abdominal pain. Diarrhea that persists for 14 days is usually not caused by bacterial pathogens (except for *C. difficile*), and the person should be evaluated for chronic diarrhea.

Chronic Diarrhea. Diarrhea is considered to be chronic when the symptoms persist for 3 to 4 weeks in children or adults and 4 weeks in infants. Chronic diarrhea is often associated with conditions such as irritable bowel and inflammatory bowel syndromes, malabsorption disorders, endocrine disorders (hyperthyroidism, diabetic autonomic neuropathy), or radiation colitis. There are four major causes of chronic diarrhea: presence of hyperosmotic luminal contents, increased intestinal secretory processes, inflammatory conditions, and infectious processes[8] (Chart 29-1). A condition called *factitious diarrhea* is caused by indiscriminate use of laxatives or excessive intake of laxative-type foods.

In *osmotic diarrhea*, water is pulled into the bowel by the hyperosmotic nature of its luminal contents. It occurs when osmotically active particles are not absorbed. In persons with lactase deficiency, the lactose in milk cannot be broken down and absorbed. Magnesium salts, which are contained in milk of magnesia and many antacids, are poorly absorbed and cause diarrhea when taken in sufficient quantities. Another cause of osmotic diarrhea is decreased transit time, which interferes with absorption.

CHART 29-1 **Chronic Diarrhea**

Hyperosmotic diarrhea
   Saline cathartics
   Lactase deficiency

Secretory diarrhea
   Acute infectious diarrhea
   Failure to absorb bile salts
   Fat malabsorption
   Chronic laxative abuse
   Carcinoid syndrome
   Zollinger-Ellison syndrome
   Fecal impaction

Inflammatory bowel disease
   Crohn disease
   Ulcerative colitis

Infectious disease
   Shigellosis
   Salmonellosis

Irritable bowel syndrome

Secretory diarrhea occurs when the secretory processes of the bowel are increased. Secretory diarrhea also occurs when excess bile acids remain in the intestinal contents as they enter the colon. This often occurs with disease processes of the ileum because bile salts are absorbed there. It also may occur with bacterial overgrowth in the small bowel, which interferes with bile absorption.

Inflammatory diarrhea commonly is associated with acute or chronic inflammation or intrinsic disease of the colon, such as ulcerative colitis or Crohn disease. Inflammatory diarrhea usually is evidenced by frequency and urgency and colicky abdominal pain. It commonly is accompanied by tenesmus (i.e., ineffectual and painful straining at stool), fecal soiling of clothing, and awakening during the night with the urge to defecate.

Chronic parasitic infections may cause chronic diarrhea through a number of mechanisms. Pathogens most commonly associated with chronic diarrhea include the protozoans *Entamoeba histolytica*, *Giardia*, and *Cyclospora*. Immunocompromised individuals are particularly susceptible to infectious organisms such as *Cryptosporidia*, cytomegalovirus (CMV), and *Mycobacterium avium-intracellulare* complex that can cause both acute and chronic diarrhea (see Chapter 16).

Diagnosis and Treatment. The diagnosis of diarrhea is based on complaints of frequent stools and a history of accompanying factors such as concurrent illnesses, medication use, and exposure to potential intestinal pathogens. Disorders such as Crohn disease and ulcerative colitis should be considered. If the onset of diarrhea is related to travel outside the United States, the possibility of traveler's diarrhea must be considered.

Although most acute forms of diarrhea are self-limited and require no treatment, diarrhea can be particularly serious in infants and small children, persons with other illnesses, and the elderly. Thus, the replacement of fluids and electrolytes is considered to be a primary therapeutic goal in the treatment of diarrhea. Oral replacement therapy (ORT) can be used in situations of uncomplicated diarrhea that can be treated at home. First applied to the treatment of diarrhea in developing countries, ORT can be regarded as a case of reverse technology, in which the protocols originally implemented in these countries have changed health care practices in industrialized countries as well.[42] Complete ORT solutions contain carbohydrate, sodium, potassium, chloride, and base to replace that lost in the diarrheal stool.[42,46] Commonly used beverages such as apple juice and cola drinks, which have increased osmolarity because of their high carbohydrate and low electrolyte content, are not recommended. The effectiveness of ORT is based on the coupled transport of sodium and glucose or other actively transported small organic molecules. ORT can be particularly effective in treating dehydration associated with diarrheal diseases in infants and small children. Children who are severely dehydrated with changes in vital signs or mental status require emergency intravenous fluid resuscitation. After initial treatment with intravenous fluids, these children can be given ORT.

Evidence suggests that feeding should be continued during diarrheal illness, particularly in children.[46] Starch and simple proteins are thought to provide co-transport molecules with little osmotic activity, increasing fluid and electrolyte uptake by intestinal cells. The luminal contents associated with early refeeding are also known to contain growth factor for enterocytes and help facilitate repair after injury. It is recommended that children who require rehydration therapy because of diarrhea be fed an age-appropriate diet. Although there is little agreement on which foods are best, fatty foods and foods high in simple sugars are best avoided. Almost all infants with acute gastroenteritis can tolerate breastfeeding. For formula-fed infants, diluted formula does not provide an advantage over full-strength formula.

Drugs used in the treatment of diarrhea include diphenoxylate (Lomotil) and loperamide (Imodium), which are opium-like drugs. These drugs decrease gastrointestinal motility and stimulate water and electrolyte absorption. Adsorbents, such as kaolin and pectin, adsorb irritants and toxins in the bowel. These ingredients are included in many over-the-counter antidiarrheal preparations because they adsorb toxins responsible for certain types of diarrhea. Antidiarrheal medications should not be used in persons with bloody diarrhea, high fever, or signs of toxicity because of the risk of worsening the disease. Antibiotics should be reserved for use in persons with identified enteric pathogens.

Constipation

Constipation can be defined as the infrequent or difficult passage of stools.[47–49] The difficulty with this definition arises from the many individual variations of function that are normal. What is considered normal for one person (e.g., two or three bowel movements per week) may be considered evidence of constipation by another.

Constipation can occur as a primary disorder of intestinal motility, as a side effect of drugs, as a problem associated with another disease condition, or as a symptom of obstructing lesions of the gastrointestinal tract. Some common causes of constipation are failure to respond to the urge to defecate, inadequate fiber in the diet, inadequate fluid intake, weakness of the abdominal muscles, inactivity and bed rest, pregnancy, and hemorrhoids.

The pathophysiology of constipation can be classified into three broad categories: normal-transit constipation, slow-transit constipation, and disorders of defecation. Normal-transit constipation (or functional constipation) is characterized by perceived difficulty in defecation and usually responds to increased fluid and fiber intake. Slow-transit constipation, which is characterized by infrequent bowel movements, is often caused by alterations in intestinal innervation. *Hirschsprung disease* is an extreme form of slow-transit constipation in which the ganglion cells in the distal bowel are absent because of a defect that occurred during embryonic development; the bowel narrows at the area that lacks ganglionic cells. Although most persons with this disorder present in infancy or early childhood, some with a relatively short segment of involved colon do not have symptoms until later in life. Defecatory disorders are most commonly due to dysfunction of the pelvic floor or anal sphincter.

Diseases associated with chronic constipation include neurologic diseases such as spinal cord injury, Parkinson disease, and multiple sclerosis; endocrine disorders such as hypothyroidism; and obstructive lesions in the gastrointestinal tract. Drugs such as narcotics, anticholinergic agents, calcium channel blockers, diuretics, calcium (antacids and supplements), iron supplements, and aluminum antacids tend to cause constipation. Elderly people with long-standing constipation may develop dilation of the rectum, colon, or both. This condition allows large amounts of stool to accumulate with little or no sensation. Constipation, in the context of a change in bowel habits, may be a sign of colorectal cancer.

Diagnosis of constipation usually is based on a history of infrequent stools, straining with defecation, the passing of hard and lumpy stools, or the sense of incomplete evacuation with defecation. Rectal examination is used to determine whether fecal impaction, anal stricture, or rectal masses are present. Constipation as a sign of another disease condition should be ruled out. Tests that measure colon transit time and defecatory function are reserved for refractory cases.

The treatment of constipation usually is directed toward relieving the cause. A conscious effort should be made to respond to the defecation urge. A time should be set aside after a meal, when mass movements in the colon are most likely to occur, for a bowel movement. Adequate fluid intake and bulk in the diet should be encouraged. Moderate exercise is essential, and persons on bed rest benefit from passive and active exercises. Laxatives and enemas should be used judiciously. They should not be used on a regular basis to treat simple constipation because they interfere with the defecation reflex and actually may damage the rectal mucosa.

Acute Intestinal Obstruction

Intestinal obstruction refers to impaired movement of intestinal contents in a cephalocaudal direction. The condition can be acute or chronic and may affect the small intestine or colon. In contrast to chronic obstructions, which often involve the colon and may last for weeks or months, acute obstructions usually present as severe disorders of the small intestine that are potentially lethal if not recognized early.[50,51] Acute intestinal obstruction can be mechanical or nonmechanical, resulting from paralytic obstruction of the ileus.

Mechanical obstruction can result from a number of conditions, intrinsic or extrinsic, that encroach on the patency of the bowel lumen (Fig. 29-10). Major inciting causes include an external hernia (i.e., inguinal, femoral, or umbilical) and postoperative adhesions.[52] Less common causes are strictures, tumors, foreign bodies, intussusception, and volvulus.[7] Intussusception involves the telescoping of bowel into the adjacent segment (Figs. 29-10A and 29-11). It is the most common cause of intestinal obstruction in children younger than 2 years of age. The most common form is intussusception of the terminal ileum into the right colon, but other areas of the bowel may be involved. In most cases, the cause of the disorder is unknown.[52] The condition can also occur in adults when an intraluminal mass or tumor acts as a traction force and pulls the segment along as it telescopes into the distal segment. Volvulus refers to a complete twisting of the bowel on an axis formed by its mesentery (see Fig. 29-10B). It can occur in any portion of the gastrointestinal tract, but most commonly involves the cecum, followed by the sigmoid colon. Mechanical bowel obstruction may be a simple obstruction, in which there is no alteration in blood flow, or a strangulated obstruction, in which there is impairment of blood flow and necrosis of bowel tissue.

Paralytic, or adynamic, obstruction of the ileus results from neurogenic or muscular impairment of peristalsis. Paralytic ileus is seen most commonly after abdominal surgery. It also accompanies inflammatory conditions of the abdomen, intestinal ischemia, pelvic fractures, and back injuries. It occurs early in the course of peritonitis and can result from chemical irritation caused by bile, bacterial toxins, electrolyte imbalances as in hypokalemia, and vascular insufficiency.

The major effects of intestinal obstruction are abdominal distention and loss of fluids and electrolytes[51] (Fig. 29-12). Distention is further aggravated by the accumulation of gases and fluid proximal to the site of obstruction. Approximately 70% to 80% of these gases are derived from swallowed air, and because this air is composed mainly of nitrogen, it is poorly absorbed from the intestinal lumen. As the process continues, the distention moves proximally (i.e., toward the mouth), involving additional segments of bowel. Either form of intestinal obstruction eventually may lead to strangulation (i.e., interruption of blood flow), gangrenous changes in the bowel wall, and, ultimately, perforation of the bowel. The increased pressure in the intestine tends to compromise mucosal blood flow, leading to

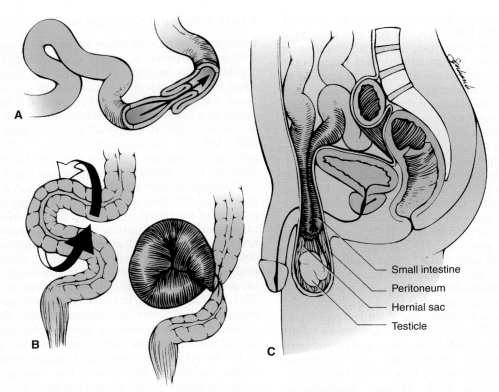

FIGURE 29-10. Three causes of intestinal obstruction. **(A)** Intussusception with invagination or shortening of the bowel caused by movement of one segment of the bowel into another. **(B)** Volvulus of the sigmoid colon; the twist is counterclockwise in most cases. Note the edematous section of bowel. **(C)** Hernia (inguinal). The sac of the hernia is a continuation of the peritoneum of the abdomen. The hernial contents are intestine, omentum, or other abdominal contents that pass through the hernial opening into the hernial sac. (From Smeltzer SC, Bare BG. *Brunner and Suddarth's Textbook of Medical–Surgical Nursing.* 10th ed. Philadelphia, PA: Lippincott Williams & Wilkins; 2004:1055.)

necrosis and movement of blood into the luminal fluids. This promotes rapid growth of bacteria, especially anaerobes that grow rapidly in this favorable environment and produce a lethal endotoxin.[54]

The manifestations of intestinal obstruction depend on the degree of obstruction and its duration. The major symptoms of acute intestinal obstruction are pain, absolute constipation, abdominal distention, and vomiting.[51] With mechanical obstruction, the pain is severe and colicky, in contrast with the continuous pain and silent abdomen of paralytic ileus. There also is borborygmus (i.e., rumbling sounds made by propulsion of gas in the intestine); audible, high-pitched peristalsis; and peristaltic rushes. Visible peristalsis may appear along the course of the distended intestine. Extreme restlessness and conscious awareness of intestinal movements are experienced along with weakness, perspiration, and anxiety. Should strangulation of the bowel occur, there is a change in symptoms. The character of the pain shifts from the intermittent colicky pain caused by the hyperperistaltic movements of the intestine to a severe and steady type of pain. Vomiting and fluid and electrolyte disorders occur with both types of obstruction.

Diagnosis of intestinal obstruction usually is based on history and physical findings. Plain film radiography of the abdomen may be used to detect the presence of a gas-filled bowel. CT scans and ultrasonography may also be used to detect the presence of mechanical obstruction.[51] Treatment depends on the cause and type of obstruction. Most cases of adynamic obstruction respond to decompression of the bowel through nasogastric suction and correction of fluid and electrolyte imbalances. Strangulation and complete bowel obstruction require surgical intervention.

Peritonitis

Peritonitis is an inflammatory response of the serous membrane that lines the abdominal cavity and covers the visceral organs.[6] It can be caused by bacterial invasion or chemical irritation. Most commonly, enteric bacteria enter the peritoneum because of a break in the wall of one of the abdominal organs. The most common causes of peritonitis are perforated peptic ulcer, ruptured appendix, perforated diverticulum, gangrenous bowel, pelvic inflammatory disease, and gangrenous gallbladder. Other causes are abdominal trauma and wounds.

The peritoneum has several characteristics that increase its vulnerability to or protect it from the effects

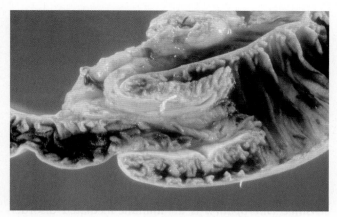

FIGURE 29-11. Intussusception. A cross-section through the area of the obstruction shows "telescoped" small intestine surround by dilated small intestine. (From Rubin R. The gastrointestinal tract. In: Rubin R, Strayer DS, eds. *Rubin's Pathophysiology: Clinicopathologic Foundations of Medicine.* 6th ed. Philadelphia, PA: Wolters Kluwer Health | Lippincott Williams & Wilkins; 2012:645.)

of peritonitis. One weakness of the peritoneal cavity is that it is a large, unbroken space that favors the dissemination of contaminants. For the same reason, it has a large surface that permits rapid absorption of bacterial toxins into the blood. The peritoneum is particularly well adapted for producing an inflammatory response as a means of controlling infection. It tends, for example, to exude a thick, sticky, and fibrinous substance that adheres to other structures, such as the mesentery and omentum, as a means of sealing off the perforation and localizing the process. Localization is enhanced by

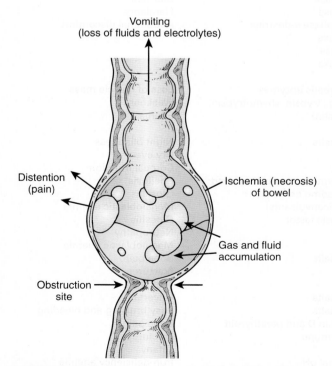

FIGURE 29-12. Pathophysiology of intestinal obstruction.

sympathetic stimulation that limits intestinal motility. Although the diminished or absent peristalsis that occurs tends to give rise to associated problems, it does inhibit the movement of contaminants throughout the peritoneal cavity.

The onset of peritonitis may be acute, as with a ruptured appendix, or it may have a more gradual onset, as occurs in pelvic inflammatory disease. Pain and tenderness are common symptoms. The pain usually is more intense over the inflamed area. The person with peritonitis usually lies still because any movement aggravates the pain. Breathing often is shallow to prevent movement of the abdominal muscles. The abdomen usually is rigid and sometimes described as boardlike because of reflex muscle guarding. Vomiting is also common. Fever, an elevated white blood cell count, tachycardia, and hypotension are common. Paralytic ileus occurs shortly after the onset of widespread peritonitis and is accompanied by abdominal distention. One of the most important manifestations of peritonitis is the translocation of extracellular fluid into the peritoneal cavity and into the bowel as a result of bowel obstruction. Nausea and vomiting cause further losses of fluid. The fluid loss may encourage development of hypovolemia and shock.

Treatment measures for peritonitis are directed toward preventing the extension of the inflammatory response, correcting the fluid and electrolyte imbalances that develop, and minimizing the effects of paralytic ileus and abdominal distention. Oral fluids are forbidden. Nasogastric suction, which entails the insertion of a tube placed through the nose into the stomach or intestine, is used to decompress the bowel and relieve the abdominal distention. Fluid and electrolyte replacement is essential. These fluids are prescribed on the basis of frequent blood chemistry determinations. Antibiotics are given to combat infection. Narcotics often are needed for pain relief. Surgical intervention may be needed to remove an acutely inflamed appendix or close the opening in a perforated peptic ulcer.

Disorders of Intestinal Absorption

Malabsorption is characterized by defective absorption of fats, carbohydrates, proteins, vitamins, minerals, and water from the intestine. It can selectively affect a single component, such as vitamin B_{12} or lactose, or its effects can extend to all the substances absorbed in a specific segment of the intestine.[6,7]

Malabsorption results from disturbances that impair one or more phases of nutrient absorption: intraluminal digestion, terminal digestion, transepithelial transport, and lymphatic transport. Intraluminal digestion involves the processing of proteins, carbohydrates, and fats into forms that are suitable for absorption. The most common causes are pancreatic insufficiency, hepatobiliary disease, and intraluminal bacterial growth. Terminal digestion involves the hydrolysis of carbohydrates and peptides, respectively, by brush border enzymes of the small intestine. Disorders of transepithelial transport are caused by mucosal lesions that impair uptake and transport of available intraluminal nutrients across the mucosal surface of the intestine. They include disorders such as celiac disease and Crohn disease. Disorders of lymphatic transport interfere with the transport of absorbed lipids. The process can be interrupted by congenital defects, neoplasms, trauma, and selected infectious diseases.

Malabsorption Syndrome

In many malabsorption disorders one or more of the intestinal absorptive processes predominate, but more than one usually contributes to the manifestations of the disorder. As a result, malabsorption syndromes resemble each other more than they differ. Weakness, muscle wasting, and weight loss occur despite normal or excessive caloric intake.

General symptoms include diarrhea (from nutrient malabsorption and intestinal secretion), flatulence, bloating, abdominal cramps, and weight loss. A hallmark of malabsorption is *steatorrhea,* characterized by fatty, bulky, yellow-gray, and foul-smelling stools. Along with loss of fat in the stools, there is failure to absorb the fat-soluble vitamins. This can lead to easy bruising and bleeding because of vitamin K deficiency, as well as bone pain and a predisposition to the development of fractures and tetany from vitamin D and calcium deficiency. In addition, there may be macrocytic anemia and peripheral neuropathy as a result of vitamin B_{12} deficiency. Table 29-2 describes the signs and symptoms of impaired absorption of dietary constituents.

Celiac Disease

Celiac disease, also known as *celiac sprue* and *gluten-sensitive enteropathy,* is an immune-mediated disorder triggered by ingestion of gluten-containing grains (wheat, barley, and rye).[53-56] Until recently, celiac disease was considered to be a rare malabsorption syndrome that manifested during early childhood, but today it is known

TABLE 29-2	**Sites of and Requirements for Absorption of Dietary Constituents and Manifestations of Malabsorption**		
Dietary Constituent	**Site of Absorption**	**Requirements**	**Manifestation**
Water and electrolytes	Mainly small bowel	Osmotic gradient	Diarrhea Dehydration Cramps
Fat	Upper jejunum	Pancreatic lipase Bile salts Functioning lymphatic channels	Weight loss Steatorrhea Fat-soluble vitamin deficiency
Carbohydrates			
Starch	Small intestine	Amylase Maltase Isomaltase α-dextrins	Diarrhea Flatulence Abdominal discomfort
Sucrose	Small intestine	Sucrase	
Lactose	Small intestine	Lactase	
Maltose	Small intestine	Maltase	
Fructose	Small intestine		
Protein	Small intestine	Pancreatic enzymes (e.g., trypsin, chymotrypsin, elastin)	Loss of muscle mass Weakness Edema
Vitamins			
A	Upper jejunum	Bile salts	Night blindness Dry eyes Corneal irritation
Folic acid	Duodenum and jejunum	Absorptive; may be impaired by some drugs (i.e., anticonvulsants)	Cheilosis Glossitis Megaloblastic anemia
B_{12}	Ileum	Intrinsic factor	Glossitis Neuropathy Megaloblastic anemia
D	Upper jejunum	Bile salts	Bone pain Fractures Tetany
E	Upper jejunum	Bile salts	Uncertain
K	Upper jejunum	Bile salts	Easy bruising and bleeding
Calcium	Duodenum	Vitamin D and parathyroid hormone	Bone pain Fractures Tetany
Iron	Duodenum and jejunum	Normal pH (hydrochloric acid secretion)	Iron-deficiency anemia Glossitis

to be one of the most common genetic diseases, with a mean prevalence of 1% in the general population. The disease is recognized not only in Europe and in countries populated by persons of European ancestry, but also in the Middle East, Asia, South America, and North Africa.

The disease results from an inappropriate T-cell–mediated immune response against the gliadin fraction of gluten contained in the diet. Almost all persons with the disorder share the major histocompatibility complex class II allele HLA-DQ2 or HLA-DQ8. Several non-HLA genes that may influence susceptibility to the disease have been identified, but their role has not been confirmed. Persons with the disease have increased levels of antibodies to a variety of antigens, including transglutaminase, endomysium, and gliadin. The resultant immune response produces an intense inflammatory reaction that results in loss of absorptive villi from the small intestine. When the resulting lesions are extensive, they may impair absorption of macronutrients (i.e., proteins, carbohydrates, fats) and micronutrients (i.e., vitamins and minerals). Small-bowel involvement is most prominent in the proximal part of the small intestine, where the exposure to gluten is greatest.

Populations at higher risk for celiac disease include persons with type 1 diabetes mellitus, those with other autoimmune endocrine disorders such as autoimmune thyroid disorders or Addison disease, first- and second-degree relatives of persons with celiac disease, and individuals with Turner syndrome. Various malignancies also appear to be a direct result of celiac disease, in that the increased incidence seen in persons with celiac disease returns to that of the general population after several years of a gluten-free diet. These malignancies include head and neck squamous cell carcinoma, small intestinal adenocarcinoma, and non-Hodgkin lymphoma.

The clinical manifestations of celiac disease vary greatly according to age group.[55,56] Infants and young children generally present with diarrhea, abdominal distention, failure to thrive, and, occasionally, severe malnutrition. Beyond infancy, the manifestations tend to be less dramatic. Older children may present with anemia, constitutional short stature, dental enamel defects, and constipation. Among adults, women constitute about 75% of newly diagnosed cases of celiac disease. The classic presentation in adults is diarrhea, which may be accompanied by abdominal pain or discomfort. It has been observed that fewer persons with celiac disease are presenting with the so-called "classic manifestations" of the disease. While diarrhea is still the most frequent mode of presentation, others include iron deficiency, osteoporosis, and recognition of mucosal changes in persons undergoing endoscopy for esophageal reflux or dyspepsia.[55] A prior diagnosis of irritable bowel syndrome is common.

Celiac disease is also becoming increasing recognized in the elderly population.[57] Rather than symptoms related to severe malabsorption, this age group often presents with anemia, accelerated osteoporosis, and osteomalacia. Although abdominal symptoms are still common in elderly persons, these individuals tend to present with milder symptoms such as abdominal bloating, flatulence, and abdominal discomfort, which make diagnosis difficult.

The diagnosis of celiac disease is based on clinical manifestations and confirmed by serologic tests and intestinal biopsy. Based on very high sensitivities, the best available tests are the immunoglobulin (Ig) A anti–human tissue transglutaminase (TTG) and IgA endomysial antibody (EMA) immunofluorescence tests.[56] Biopsies of the proximal small bowel are indicated in persons with a positive celiac disease antibody test. Usually, additional laboratory tests are done to determine if the disorder has resulted in nutritional disorders such as iron-deficiency anemia.

The primary treatment of celiac disease consists of removal of gluten and related proteins from the diet. Gluten is the primary protein in wheat, barley, and rye. Oat products, which are nontoxic, may be contaminated with wheat during processing. Many gluten-free types of bread, cereals, cookies, and other products are available.[56] Meats, vegetables, fruits, and dairy products are free of gluten as long as they are not contaminated during processing. Complete exclusion of dietary gluten generally results in rapid and complete healing of the intestinal mucosa.

Colorectal Neoplasms

Adenomatous Polyps

Adenomatous polyps (adenomas) are benign neoplasms that arise from the mucosal epithelium of the intestine.[6,7] They are composed of neoplastic cells that have proliferated in excess of those needed to replace the cells that normally are shed from the mucosal surface. The most common and clinically important neoplastic polyps are colonic adenomas that are precursors in the majority of colorectal adenocarcinomas.

Adenomas can range in size from a barely visible nodule to a large, sessile mass. They can be classified as tubular, villous, or tubulovillous adenomas. *Tubular adenomas,* which constitute approximately 65% of benign large bowel adenomas, typically are smooth-surfaced spheres, usually less than 2 cm in diameter, that are attached to the mucosal surface by a stalk.[7] Although most tubular adenomas display little epithelial dysplasia, approximately 20% show a range of dysplastic changes, from mild nuclear changes to frank invasive carcinoma. *Villous adenomas* constitute 10% of adenomas of the colon.[7] They typically are broad-based, elevated lesions with a shaggy, cauliflower-like surface and are found predominantly in the rectosigmoid colon. In contrast to tubular adenomas, villous adenomas are more likely to contain malignant cells. When invasive carcinoma develops, there is no stalk to isolate the tumor and invasion is directly into the wall of the colon. *Tubulovillous adenomas* manifest both tubular and villous architecture. They are intermediate between tubular and villous adenomas in terms of invasive carcinoma risk.

The pathogenesis of adenoma formation involves neoplastic alterations in the replication of the colonic crypt cells (Fig. 29-13). There may be diminished apoptosis (see Chapter 2), persistence of cell replication, and failure of cell maturation and differentiation of the cells that migrate to the surface of the crypts. Normally, DNA synthesis ceases as the cells reach the upper two

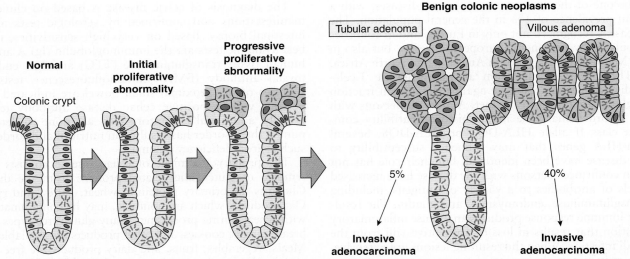

FIGURE 29-13. The histogenesis of adenomatous polyps of the colon. The initial proliferative abnormality of the colonic mucosa, the extension of the mitotic zone in the crypts, leads to accumulation of mucosal cells. The formation of adenomas may reflect epithelial–mesenchymal interactions. (From Rubin R. The gastrointestinal tract. In: Rubin R, Strayer DS, eds. *Rubin's Pathology: Clinicopathologic Foundations of Medicine.* 6th ed. Philadelphia, PA: Wolters Kluwer Health | Lippincott Williams & Wilkins; 2012:663.)

thirds of the crypts, after which they mature, migrate to the surface, and become senescent. They then become apoptotic and are shed from the surface.[7] Adenomas arise from a disruption in this sequence, such that the epithelial cells retain their proliferative ability throughout the entire length of the crypt. Aberrations in cell differentiation can lead to dysplasia and progress to the development of invasive adenocarcinoma.

Colorectal Cancer

Adenocarcinoma of the colon is the most common malignancy of the gastrointestinal tract and is the major cause of morbidity and mortality worldwide.[6,7,58–60] It affects approximately 150,000 Americans annually, approximately one third of whom die.[58] It affects approximately 250,000 persons annually in Europe and approximately 1 million persons worldwide.

Epidemiology. The incidence of colorectal cancer peaks at 60 to 70 years of age, and fewer than 20% of cases occur before age 50.[7] Its incidence is increased among persons with a family history of cancer, persons with Crohn disease or ulcerative colitis, and those with familial adenomatous polyposis of the colon. Persons with a familial risk—those who have two or more first- or second-degree relatives (or both) with colorectal cancer—make up approximately 20% of all persons with colorectal cancer.[61] Familial adenomatous polyposis is a rare autosomal dominant trait linked to a mutation in the long arm of chromosome 5. Persons with the disorder develop multiple adenomatous polyps of the colon at an early age.[7] Carcinoma of the colon is inevitable, often by 40 years of age, unless a total colectomy is performed.

Diet also is thought to play a role.[7] Attention has focused on dietary fat intake, refined sugar intake, fiber intake, and the adequacy of such protective micronutrients as vitamins A, C, and E in the diet. It has been hypothesized that a high level of fat in the diet increases the synthesis of bile acids in the liver, which may be converted to potential carcinogens by the bacterial flora in the colon. The proliferation of colonic bacteria is enhanced by a high dietary level of refined sugars. Dietary fiber is thought to increase stool bulk and thereby dilute and remove potential carcinogens. Refined diets often contain reduced amounts of vitamins A, C, and E, which may act as oxygen free radical scavengers.

In addition to dietary modification, pharmacologic chemoprevention has become an area of great interest. Several studies indicate that aspirin or other NSAIDs may protect against colorectal cancer.[62] An analysis of the incidence of colorectal cancer in the Nurses' Health Study showed a decreased incidence of colorectal cancer among women who took four to six aspirins per week. Although the mechanism of aspirin's action is unknown, it may be related to its effect on the synthesis of prostaglandins, one or more of which may be involved in signal systems that influence cell proliferation or tumor growth. Aspirin inhibits cyclooxygenase, the enzyme that catalyzes the conversion of arachidonic acid in cell membranes to prostaglandins. One form of cyclooxygenase, COX-2, promotes inflammation and cell proliferation, and colorectal cancers often overexpress this enzyme.

Clinical Manifestations. Cancer of the colon is usually present for a long period of time before it produces symptoms.[58,59] Bleeding is a highly significant early symptom and usually is the one that causes persons to seek medical care. Other symptoms include a change in bowel habits, diarrhea or constipation, and sometimes a sense of urgency or incomplete emptying of the bowel. Pain usually is a late symptom.

Diagnosis and Treatment. Cancer of the colon may be detected with a high degree of reliability with barium enema or colonoscopy. Colonoscopy permits biopsy for pathologic confirmation. CT scans, pelvic magnetic resonance imaging (MRI), and ultrasonography may be used to determine the extent of the lesions and whether metastasis has occurred.

The only recognized treatment for cancer of the colon and rectum is surgical removal.[65] Preoperative radiation therapy may be used and has in some cases demonstrated increased 5-year survival rates. Postoperative adjuvant chemotherapy may be used. Radiation therapy and chemotherapy are used as palliative treatment methods.

The prognosis for persons with colorectal cancer depends largely on the stage of the cancer. Colorectal cancer commonly is classified into four TNM (tumor, node, and metastasis) stages.[6,7] In this system, a stage I tumor is limited to invasion of the mucosal and submucosal layers of the colon and has a 5-year survival rate of 90% to 100%. Stage IV (metastatic) tumors penetrate the serosa or adjacent organs and have a much poorer prognosis.

Screening. The single most important prognostic indicator of colorectal cancer is the extent (stage) of the tumor at the time of diagnosis. The challenge, therefore, is to discover the tumors at their earliest stages. Among the methods used for early detection of colorectal cancers are the digital rectal examination and the fecal occult blood test, usually done during routine physical examinations; x-ray studies using barium (e.g., barium enema); and flexible sigmoidoscopy and colonoscopy.[58,59]

Almost all cancers of the colon and rectum bleed intermittently, although the amount of blood is small and usually not apparent in the stools. It therefore is feasible to screen for colorectal cancers using commercially prepared tests for occult blood in the stool. The sensitivity of fecal occult blood tests is improved by performing stool tests on three different occasions. Digital rectal examinations are most helpful in detecting neoplasms of the rectum. Rectal examination should be considered a routine part of a good physical examination. Flexible sigmoidoscopy involves examination of the rectum and sigmoid colon with a hollow, lighted tube that is inserted through the rectum. The procedure is performed without sedation and is well tolerated. Approximately 40% of cancers and polyps are out of the reach of the sigmoidoscope, emphasizing the need for fecal occult blood tests. Polyps can be removed or tissue can be obtained for biopsy during the procedure.

Colonoscopy provides a means for direct visualization of the rectum and colon. The colonoscope consists of a flexible, 4-cm–diameter glass fiber bundle that contains approximately 250,000 glass fibers and has a lens at either end to focus and magnify the image. Light from an external source is transmitted by the fiber-optic viewing bundle. Instruments are available that afford direct examination of the sigmoid colon or the entire colon. This method is used for screening persons at high risk for development of cancer of the colon (e.g., those with ulcerative colitis) and for those with symptoms. Colonoscopy also is useful for obtaining a biopsy and for removing polyps. Although this method is one of the most accurate for detecting early colorectal cancers, it is not suitable for mass screening because it is expensive and time consuming and must be done by a person who is highly trained in the use of the instrument.

It is recommended that persons at average risk for colonic adenomatous polyps or cancer should undergo colonoscopy every 10 years or alternative screening tests at periodically prescribed intervals beginning at age 50.[59] Persons who are members of high-risk groups, such as those with a family history of adenomatous polyps or disorders that predispose to colon cancer (e.g., ulcerative colitis), should undergo periodic surveillance more frequently.

SUMMARY CONCEPTS

■ Disorders of the small and large intestines include inflammatory bowel disease, infectious enterocolitis, diverticular disease, appendicitis, disorders of motility, peritonitis, alterations in intestinal absorption, and colorectal cancer.

■ The term inflammatory bowel disease is used to designate two inflammatory conditions: Crohn disease, which affects the small and large bowel, and ulcerative colitis, which affects the colon and rectum. Both are chronic diseases characterized by remissions and exacerbations of diarrhea, weight loss, fluid and electrolyte disorders, and systemic signs of inflammation.

■ Enterocolitis includes viral (e.g., rotavirus) and bacterial (e.g., *C. difficile* and *E. coli* O157:H7) infections.

■ Diverticular disease is a condition in which the mucosa and submucosa of the colon herniate through the muscularis layer, and diverticulitis, in which there is inflammation and gross or microscopic perforation of the diverticulum.

■ Diarrhea, constipation, and irritable bowel syndrome represent disorders of intestinal motility. *Diarrhea* or excessively frequent passage of stools can be caused by infectious organisms, food intolerance, drugs, or intestinal disease. *Constipation* or the infrequent passage of stools is commonly caused by failure to respond to the urge to defecate, inadequate fiber or fluid intake, weakness of the abdominal muscles, inactivity and bed rest, or pregnancy. *Irritable bowel syndrome* is characterized by a variable combination of chronic and recurrent intestinal symptoms, that are not related to a structural or biochemical abnormality.

(*continued*)

REVIEW EXERCISES

1. A 40-year-old man reports to his health care provider complaining of "heartburn" that occurs after eating and also wakens him at night. He is overweight, admits to enjoying fatty foods, and usually lies down on the sofa and watches TV after dinner. He also complains that lately he has been having a cough and some wheezing. A diagnosis of GERD was made.

   A. Explain the cause of heartburn and why it becomes worse after eating.
   B. Persons with GERD are advised to lose weight, avoid eating fatty foods, remain sitting after eating, and sleep with their head slightly elevated. Explain the possible relationship between these situations and the occurrence of reflux.
   C. Explain the possible relationship between GERD and the respiratory symptoms this man is having.

2. A 36-year-old woman who has been taking aspirin for back pain experiences a sudden episode of tachycardia and feeling faint, accompanied by the vomiting of a coffee-ground emesis and the passing of a tarry stool. She relates that she has not had any signs of a "stomach ulcer" such as pain or heartburn.

   A. Relate the mucosal protective effects of prostaglandins to the development of peptic ulcer associated with aspirin or NSAID use.
   B. Explain the apparent suddenness of the bleeding and the fact that the woman did not experience pain as a warning signal.
   C. Among the results of her initial laboratory tests is an elevated blood urea nitrogen (BUN) level. Explain the reason for the elevated BUN.

3. A 29-year-old woman has been diagnosed with Crohn disease. Her medical history reveals that she began having symptoms of the disease at 24 years of age and that her mother died of complications of the disease at 54 years of age. She complains of diarrhea and chronic cramping abdominal pain.

   A. Define the term *inflammatory bowel disease* and compare the pathophysiologic processes and manifestations of Crohn disease and ulcerative colitis.
   B. Describe the possible association between genetic and environmental factors in the pathogenesis of Crohn disease.
   C. Relate the use of the monoclonal antibody infliximab to the pathogenesis of the inflammatory lesions that occur in Crohn disease.

REFERENCES

1. Everhart JF. *The burden of digestive diseases in the United States.* 2009. National Institute of Diabetes and Digestive Diseases. NIH publication no. 09-6443. Available at: http://www2.niddk.nih.gov/AboutNIDDK/ReportsAndStrategicPlanning/BurdenOfDisease/DigestiveDiseases/. Accessed August 19, 2013.
2. Hall JE. *Guyton and Hall Textbook of Medical Physiology.* 12th ed. Philadelphia, PA: Saunders Elsevier; 2011:753–761, 789–805.
3. Epstein RK, Balaban DH. The esophagogastric junction. *N Engl J Med.* 1997;336(13):924–932.
4. Saud BM, Szyjkowski R. A diagnostic approach to dysphagia. *Gastroenterology* 2004;6:525–546.
5. Kuo P, Holloway RH, Nguyen NO. Current and future techniques in the evaluation of dysphagia. *J Gastroenterol Hepatol.* 2012;27(5):873–881.
6. Turner JR. The gastrointestinal tract. In: Kumar V, Abbas AK, Fausto N, et al., eds. *Robbins and Cotran Pathologic Basis of Disease.* 8th ed. Philadelphia, PA: Saunders Elsevier; 2010:763–831.
7. Rubin R. The gastrointestinal tract. In: Rubin R, Strayer DS, eds. *Rubin's Pathophysiology: Clinicopathologic Foundations of Medicine.* 5th ed. Philadelphia, PA: Wolters Kluwer Health/Lippincott Williams & Wilkins; 2012:605–675, 727–746.
8. McQuaid KR. Gastrointestinal disorders. In: Papadakis M, McPhee SJ, eds. *Current Medical Diagnosis and Treatment.* 52nd ed. New York, NY: McGraw-Hill Medical; 2013:564–661.
9. Richter JE. The many manifestations of gastrointestinal reflux disease: Presentation, evaluation, and treatment. *Gastroenterol Clin North Am.* 2007;37:577–599.
10. Rosemurgy AS, Donn N, Paul H, et al. Gastroesophageal reflux disease. *Surg Clin North Am.* 2011;91:1015–1029.
11. Spechler SJ. Barrett's esophagus. *N Engl J Med.* 2002;346:836–842.

12. Blanco FC, Davenport DP, Kane TD. Pediatric gastroesophageal reflux disease. *Surg Clin North Am.* 2012;92:541–558.

13. Hassall E. Decisions in diagnosis and managing chronic gastroesophageal reflux disease in children. *J Pediatr.* 2005;146:S3–S12.

14. Gold BD. Asthma and gastroesophageal reflux disease in children: exploring the relationship. *J Pediatr.* 2005;146:S13–S20.

15. Enzinger PC, Mayer RJ. Esophageal cancer. *N Engl J Med.* 2003;349:2241–2252.

16. Fromm D. Mechanisms involved in gastric mucosal resistance to injury. *Annu Rev Med.* 1987;38:119.

17. Wolfe MM, Lichtenstein DR, Singh G. Gastrointestinal toxicity of nonsteroidal anti-inflammatory drugs. *N Engl J Med.* 1999;340:1888–1899.

18. McColl KEL. *Helicobacter pylori* infections. *N Engl J Med.* 2010;362(17):1597–1604.

19. Vilaichone RK, Mahachai V, Graham DY. *Helicobacter pylori* diagnosis and management. *Gastroenterol Clin North Am.* 2006;35:229–247.

20. Saad RJ, Scheiman JM. Diagnosis and management of peptic ulcer disease. *Clin Fam Pract.* 2004;6:569–587.

21. Ramakrishnan K, Salinas RC. Peptic ulcer disease. *Am Fam Physician.* 2007;76:1005–1012.

22. Ali T, Harty RF. Stress-induced ulcer bleeding in critically ill patients. *Gastroenterol Clin North Am.* 2009;38:245–265.

23. Spirit MJ, Starily S. Update on stress ulcer prophylaxis in critically ill patients. *Crit Care Nurse.* 2006;26(1):18–29.

24. Layke JC, Lopez PP. Gastric cancer: diagnosis and treatment options. *Am Fam Physician.* 2004;69:1133–1146.

25. Videlock EJ, Chang L. Irritable bowel syndrome: Current approach to symptoms, evaluation, and treatment. *Gastroenterol Clin North Am.* 2007;36:665–685.

26. Abraham C, Choa JM. Inflammatory bowel disease. *N Engl J Med.* 2009;361(21):2066–2678.

27. Thoreson R, Cullen JJ. Pathophysiology of inflammatory bowel disease: an overview. *Surg Clin North Am.* 2007;87:575–585.

28. Wilkins T, Jarvis K, Jigneshkumar P. Diagnosis and management of Crohn's disease. *Am Fam Physician.* 2011;84(12):1365–1375.

29. Danese S, Fiocchi C. Ulcerative colitis. *N Engl J Med.* 2011;365(18):1713–1725.

30. Adams SM, Bornemann PH. Ulcerative colitis. *Am Fam Physician.* 2013;87(10):699–705.

31. Bass DM. Rotaviruses, caliciviruses, and astroviruses. In: Kliegman RM, Stanton BF, St. Gemelli JW, et al., eds. *Nelson Textbook of Pediatrics.* 19th ed. Philadelphia, PA: Elsevier Saunders; 2011:1134–1137.

32. DuPont H. Bacterial diarrhea. *N Engl J Med.* 2009;361(16):1560–1569.

33. Schroeder MS. *Clostridium difficile*–associated diarrhea. *Am Fam Physician.* 2005;71:921–928.

34. Kelly CP, LaMont JT. *Clostridia difficile*—More difficult than ever. *N Engl J Med.* 2008;350(18):1932–1940.

35. Gould CV, McDonald C. Bench-to-bedside review: *Clostridium difficile* colitis. *Morb Mortal Wkly Rep.* 2008;12(1):1–8.

36. Razzaq S. Hemolytic uremic syndrome. *Am Fam Physician.* 2006;74:991–996.

37. Moake JL. Thrombotic microangiopathies. *N Engl J Med.* 2002;347:589–600.

38. Weisman AV, Nguyen GC. Diverticular disease: epidemiology and management. *Can J Gastroenterol.* 2011;25(7):385–389.

39. Salzman H, Lillie D. Diverticular disease: diagnosis and treatment. *Am Fam Physician.* 2005;72:1229–1234.

40. Jacobs DO. Diverticulitis. *N Engl J Med.* 2007;357(20):2057–2066.

41. Paulson EK, Kalady MF, Pappas TN. Suspected appendicitis. *N Engl J Med.* 2003;348:236–242.

42. King CK, Glass R, Brewer JS, et al. Managing acute gastroenteritis among children: Oral rehydration, maintenance, and nutritional therapy. *MMWR Recomm Rep.* 2003;52(RR-16):1–16.

43. Deepak P, Ehrenpreis ED. Diarrhea. *Dis Mon.* 2011;57:490–510.

44. Field M, Rao MC, Chang EB. Intestinal electrolyte transport and diarrheal disease (part 2). *N Engl J Med.* 1989;321:879–883.

45. Field M. Intestinal ion transport and the pathophysiology of diarrhea. *J Clin Invest.* 2003;111:931–943.

46. Dennehy PH. Acute diarrheal disease in children: epidemiology, prevention, treatment. *Infect Dis Clin North Am.* 2005;19:585–602.

47. Wald A. Constipation in the primary care setting. *Am J Med.* 2006;119:736–739.

48. Hsieh C. Treatment of constipation in older adults. *Am Fam Physician.* 2005;72:2277–2285.

49. Lembo A, Camilleri M. Chronic constipation. *N Engl J Med.* 2003;349:1360–1368.

50. Ramano S, Bartone G, Romano L. Ischemia and infarction of the intestine related to obstruction. *Radiol Clin North Am.* 2008;46:925–942.

51. Jackson PG, Raiji M. Evaluation and management of intestinal obstruction. *Am Fam Physician.* 2011;83(2):159–165.

52. Wyllie R. Ileus, adhesions, intussusception, and closed-loop obstruction. In: Berman RE, Kliegman RM, Jenson HB, eds. *Nelson Textbook of Pediatrics.* 17th ed. Philadelphia, PA: Elsevier Saunders; 2004:1241–1243.

53. Evans KE, Sanders DS. Celiac disease. *Gastroenterol Clin North Am.* 2012;41:639–650.

54. Alaedini A, Green PHR. Narrative review: Celiac disease: Understanding a complex autoimmune disorder. *Ann Intern Med.* 2005;142:289–298.

55. Green PHR, Jabri B. Celiac disease. *Annu Rev Med.* 2006;57:207–221.

56. Niewinski MM. Advances in celiac disease and gluten-free diet. *J Am Diet Assoc.* 2008;108:661–672.

57. Rashtak S, Murray JA. Celiac disease in the elderly. *Gastroenterol Clin North Am.* 2009;38:433–446.

58. Cappell MS. Pathophysiology, clinical presentation, and management of colon cancer. *Gastroenterol Clin North Am.* 2007;37:1–24.

59. Cappell MS. The pathology, clinical presentation, and diagnosis of colon cancer and adenomatous polyps. *Med Clin North Am.* 2005;89:1–43.

60. Cornett PA, Dea TO. Cancer. In: Papadakis M, McPhee SJ, eds. *Current Medical Diagnosis and Treatment.* 52nd ed. New York, NY: McGraw-Hill Medical; 2013:1612–1629.

61. Guttmacher AE, de la Chapelle A. Hereditary colorectal cancer. *N Engl J Med.* 2003;348:919–932.

62. Chan AT, Ogino S, Fuchs CS. Aspirin and the risk of colorectal cancer in relation to the expression of COX-2. *N Engl J Med.* 2007;356:2131–2142.

Porth Essentials Resources

Explore these additional resources to enhance learning for this chapter:

- NCLEX-Style Questions and Other Resources on thePoint, http://thePoint.lww.com/PorthEssentials4e
- Study Guide for Essentials of Pathophysiology
- Concepts in Action Animations
- Adaptive Learning | Powered by PrepU, http://thepoint.lww.com/prepu

Disorders of Hepatobiliary and Exocrine Pancreas Function

The liver, the gallbladder, and the pancreas are classified as accessory organs of the gastrointestinal tract. The liver produces and the gallbladder stores and concentrates bile that is involved in the digestion of fats. The liver also plays an important role in the uptake, storage, and distribution of both nutrients and vitamins; it synthesizes most of the body's circulating plasma proteins; and it degrades and eliminates drugs and toxins. The exocrine pancreas secretes enzymes that are involved in the digestion of carbohydrates, lipids, and proteins,

This chapter is divided into two parts: the first focuses on functions and disorders of the liver, and the second on disorders of the gallbladder, biliary tract, and pancreas.

The Liver and Hepatobiliary System

The liver is the largest visceral organ in the body, weighing approximately 1.5 kg (3.3 lb) in the adult.[1,2] It is located immediately under the diaphragm in the upper right and partially in the upper left quadrants of the abdominal cavity, protected by the rib cage (Fig. 30-1). Anatomically, the liver is divided by deep grooves into two large lobes (the right and left lobes) and two smaller lobes (the caudate and quadrate lobes). Each lobe is divided into numerous lobules by small blood vessels and fibrous strands that form a supporting framework for them. The liver is enclosed in a capsule of fibrous connective tissue (*Glisson capsule*); a serous covering (visceral peritoneum) surrounds the capsule, except where the liver adheres to the diaphragm.

The liver is unique among the abdominal organs in having a dual blood supply consisting of a venous (portal) supply through the hepatic portal vein and an arterial

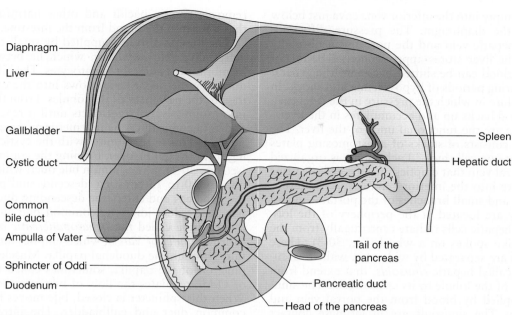

FIGURE 30-1. The liver and biliary system, including the gallbladder and bile ducts.

supply through the hepatic artery. Approximately 300 mL of blood per minute enters the liver through the hepatic artery; another 1050 mL/min enters by way of the valveless portal vein.[1] The venous blood delivered by the hepatic portal vein comes from the digestive tract and major abdominal organs, including the pancreas and spleen (Fig. 30-2). The portal blood supply carries nutrient and toxic materials absorbed in the intestine, blood cells and their breakdown products from the spleen, and insulin and glucagon from the pancreas. Although the blood from the portal vein is incompletely saturated with oxygen, it supplies approximately 60% to 70% of the oxygen needs of the liver. The venous outflow from the liver is carried by the valveless hepatic

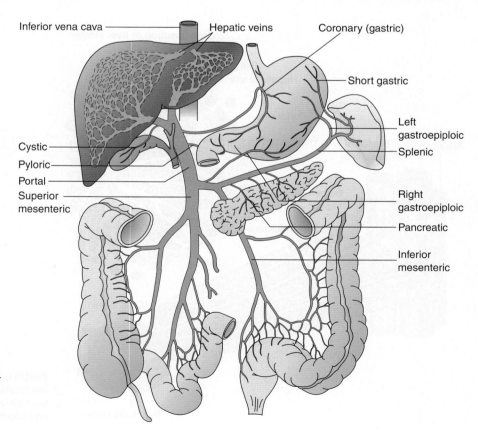

FIGURE 30-2. The portal circulation. Blood from the gastrointestinal tract, spleen, and pancreas travels to the liver through the portal vein before moving into the vena cava for return to the heart.

veins, which empty into the inferior vena cava just below the level of the diaphragm. The pressure difference between the hepatic vein and the portal vein normally is such that the liver stores approximately 450 mL of blood.[1] This blood can be shifted back into the general circulation during periods of hypovolemia and shock. In right heart failure in which the pressure in the vena cava increases, blood backs up and accumulates in the liver.

The *lobules* are the functional units of the liver. The classic lobule consists of stacks of anastomosing plates of hepatocytes one cell thick.[2] Each lobule is organized around a central vein that empties into the hepatic veins and from there into the inferior vena cava. The terminal bile ducts and small branches of the portal vein and hepatic artery are located at the periphery of the lobule. Plates of hepatic cells radiate centrifugally from the central vein like spokes on a wheel (Fig. 30-3). These hepatic plates are separated by wide, thin-walled vascular channels, called hepatic *sinusoids,* that extend from the periphery of the lobule to its central vein. The sinusoids are supplied by blood from the portal vein and hepatic artery. The sinusoids are in intimate contact with the hepatocytes and provide for the exchange of substances between the blood and liver cells.

The hepatic sinusoids are lined with two types of cells: the typical capillary endothelial cells and Kupffer cells. *Kupffer cells* (also called *reticuloendothelial cells*) are large resident macrophages that are capable of removing and phagocytizing old and defective blood cells, bacteria, and other foreign material from the portal blood as it flows through the sinusoid. This phagocytic action removes enteric bacilli and other harmful substances that filter into the blood from the intestine.

The lobules also are supplied by small tubular channels, called *bile canaliculi*, which lie between the cell membranes of adjacent hepatocytes. The bile that is produced by the hepatocytes flows into the canaliculi and then to the periphery of the lobules. From there it drains into progressively larger ducts until it reaches the right and left hepatic ducts, which merge as the common hepatic duct. This in turn unites with the cystic duct emerging from the gallbladder, forming the common bile duct (see Fig. 30-1). The common bile duct, which is approximately 10 to 15 cm long, descends and passes behind the pancreas and enters the descending duodenum. The pancreatic duct joins the common bile duct at a short dilated tube called the *hepatopancreatic ampulla* (also called *ampulla of Vater*), which empties into the duodenum through the duodenal papilla. Muscle tissue at the junction of the papilla, sometimes called the *sphincter of Oddi,* regulates the flow of bile into the duodenum. When this sphincter is closed, bile moves back into the common duct and gallbladder. The intrahepatic and extrahepatic bile ducts often are collectively referred to as the *hepatobiliary tree.*

Physiologic Functions of the Liver

The liver is one of the most versatile and active organs in the body, with a remarkable ability to regenerate after hepatic tissue loss. It produces bile, metabolizes

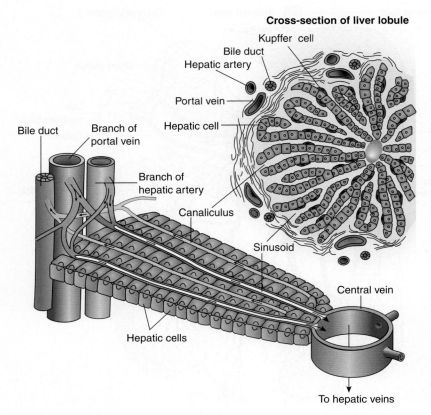

Cross-section of liver lobule

Kupffer cell

Bile duct

Hepatic artery

Portal vein

Hepatic cell

Bile duct

Branch of portal vein

Branch of hepatic artery

Canaliculus

Sinusoid

Central vein

Hepatic cells

To hepatic veins

FIGURE 30-3. A section of liver lobule showing the location of the hepatic veins, hepatic cells, liver sinusoids, and branches of the portal vein and hepatic artery.

TABLE 30-1　Functions of the Liver and Manifestations of Altered Function

Function	Manifestations of Altered Function
Production of bile salts	Malabsorption of fat and fat-soluble vitamins
Elimination of bilirubin	Elevation in serum bilirubin and jaundice
Metabolism of steroid hormones	
Sex hormones	Disturbances in gonadal function, including gynecomastia in the male
Glucocorticoids	Signs of increased cortisol levels (i.e., Cushing syndrome)
Aldosterone	Signs of hyperaldosteronism (e.g., sodium retention and hypokalemia)
Metabolism of drugs	Decreased drug metabolism
	Decreased plasma binding of drugs owing to a decrease in albumin production
Carbohydrate metabolism	Hypoglycemia may develop when glycogenolysis and gluconeogenesis are impaired
Stores glycogen and synthesizes glucose from amino acids, lactic acid, and glycerol	Abnormal glucose tolerance curve may occur because of impaired uptake and release of glucose by the liver
Fat metabolism	
Formation of lipoproteins	Impaired synthesis of lipoproteins
Conversion of carbohydrates and proteins to fat	
Synthesis, recycling, and elimination of cholesterol	Altered cholesterol levels
Formation of ketones from fatty acid	
Protein metabolism	
Deamination of proteins	
Formation of urea from ammonia	Elevated blood ammonia levels
Synthesis of plasma proteins	Decreased levels of plasma proteins, particularly albumin, which contributes to edema formation
Synthesis of clotting factors (fibrinogen, prothrombin, factors V, VII, IX, X)	Bleeding tendency
Storage of minerals and vitamins	Signs of deficiency of fat-soluble and other vitamins that are stored in the liver
Filtration of blood and removal of bacteria and particulate matter by Kupffer cells	Increased exposure of the body to colonic bacteria and other foreign matter

hormones and drugs, synthesizes plasma proteins and blood clotting factors, stores vitamins and minerals, maintains blood glucose levels, and regulates very–low-density lipoprotein (VLDL) levels. In its capacity for metabolizing drugs and hormones, the liver serves as an excretory organ. In this respect, the bile, which carries the end products of substances metabolized by the liver, is much like the urine, which carries the body wastes filtered by the kidneys. These functions, many of which are disrupted by the liver diseases discussed in this chapter, are summarized in Table 30-1.

Metabolic Functions

The liver is involved in many metabolic pathways including carbohydrate metabolism and maintenance of blood glucose, lipid metabolism, and protein synthesis and conversion of ammonia to urea. In addition to nutrients, several vitamins (e.g., A, D, K) are also taken up from the bloodstream and then stored or biochemically converted in the liver.

Carbohydrate Metabolism. The liver plays an essential role in carbohydrate metabolism and glucose homeostasis (Fig. 30-4A). It stores excess glucose as glycogen and synthesizes glucose from amino acids and other substrates as a means of maintaining blood glucose during periods of fasting or increased need. The liver also converts excess carbohydrates to triglycerides for storage in adipose tissue.

Pathways of Lipid Metabolism. Although most cells of the body metabolize fat, certain aspects of lipid metabolism occur mainly in the liver. These include the oxidation of free fatty acids to ketoacids; synthesis of cholesterol, phospholipids, and lipoproteins; and formation of triglycerides from carbohydrates and proteins (Fig. 30-4B). To derive energy from neutral fats (triglycerides), the molecule must first be split into glycerol and fatty acids, and then the fatty acids split into two-carbon acetyl-coenzyme A (acetyl-CoA units). Acetyl-CoA is readily channeled into the citric acid cycle to produce adenosine triphosphate ([ATP], see Chapter 1, Understanding Cell Metabolism). Because the liver cannot use all the acetyl-CoA that is formed, it converts the excess into acetoacetic acid, a highly soluble ketoacid that is released into the bloodstream and transported to other tissues, where it is used for energy. The acetyl-CoA derived from fat metabolism is also used to synthesize cholesterol and bile acids. Cholesterol has several fates in the liver. It can be esterified and stored, exported bound to VLDLs, or converted to bile acids.

Protein Synthesis and Conversion of Ammonia to Urea. In addition to its role in carbohydrate and lipid metabolism, the liver is also an important site for

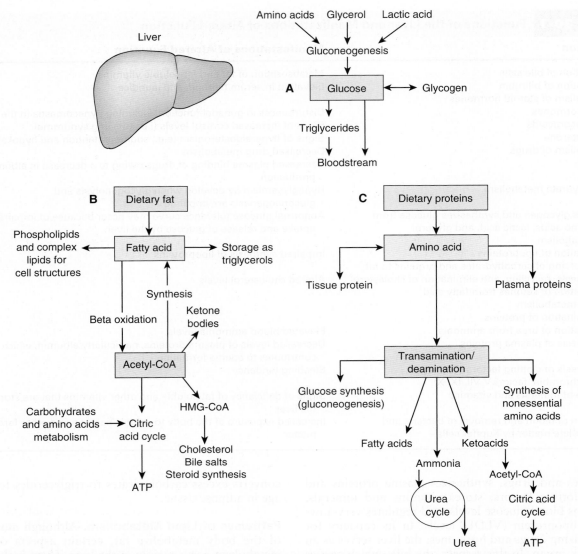

FIGURE 30-4. Hepatic pathways for **(A)** glucose metabolism, **(B)** lipid metabolism, and **(C)** protein metabolism and conversion of ammonia to urea. ATP, adenosine triphosphate; HMG-CoA, hydroxymethylglutaryl-CoA.

protein synthesis and degradation. It produces proteins for its own cellular needs, as well as secretory proteins (e.g., plasma proteins, fibrinogen, and coagulation factors) that are released into the circulation. One of the most important of these secretory proteins is albumin. Albumin contributes significantly to the plasma colloidal osmotic pressure (see Chapter 8) and to the binding and transport of numerous substances such as hormones, fatty acids, and bilirubin.

Proteins are made up of amino acids. Protein synthesis and degradation involves two major reactions: transamination and deamination[1] (Fig. 30-4C). In *transamination,* an amino group (NH_2) is transferred to an acceptor substance. The process is catalyzed by *aminotransferases,* enzymes that are found in high amounts in the liver. As a result of transamination, amino acids can participate in the intermediary metabolism of carbohydrates and lipids. During periods of fasting or starvation, amino acids are used for producing glucose

(i.e., gluconeogenesis). Most of the nonessential amino acids are synthesized in the liver by transamination.

Oxidative *deamination* involves the removal of the amino group and a hydrogen atom from an amino acid. This yields ammonia (NH_3). Because ammonia is very toxic to body tissues, particularly neurons, the ammonia that is released during the deamination process is rapidly removed from the blood by the liver and combined with carbon dioxide to form urea. Essentially all urea formed in the body is synthesized by the urea cycle in the liver and then excreted by the kidneys.

Although urea is mostly excreted by the kidneys, some diffuses into the intestine, where it is converted to ammonia by enteric bacteria. The intestinal production of ammonia also results from bacterial deamination of unabsorbed amino acids and proteins derived from the diet, exfoliated cells, or blood in the gastrointestinal tract. Ammonia produced in the intestine is absorbed into the portal circulation and transported to the liver, where it is converted to urea before being released into the systemic circulation. Intestinal production of ammonia is increased after ingestion of high-protein foods and gastrointestinal bleeding, a process that becomes impaired in persons with advanced liver disease.

Bile Formation and Flow

The secretion of bile is essential for digestion and absorption of dietary fats and fat-soluble vitamins from the intestine. The liver produces approximately 600 to 1200 mL of yellow-green bile daily.[1] Bile contains water, bile salts, bilirubin, cholesterol, and certain by-products of metabolism. Of these, only bile salts, which are formed from cholesterol, are important in digestion. The other components of bile depend on the secretion of sodium, chloride, bicarbonate, and potassium by the bile ducts.

Bile salts serve an important function in digestion; they aid in emulsifying dietary fats, and they are necessary for the formation of the micelles that transport fatty acids and fat-soluble vitamins to the surface of the intestinal mucosa for absorption. Approximately 94% of bile salts that enter the intestine are reabsorbed into the portal circulation by an active transport process that takes place in the distal ileum. From the portal circulation, the bile salts move into the liver cells and are recycled. Normally, bile salts travel this entire circuit approximately 18 times before being expelled in the feces.[1] The system for recirculation of bile is called the *enterohepatic circulation*.

Bilirubin Formation and Jaundice

Bilirubin is the substance that gives bile its color. It is formed from aging red blood cells. In the process of degradation, the hemoglobin from the red blood cell is broken down to form biliverdin, which is rapidly converted to free bilirubin (Fig. 30-5). Free bilirubin (unconjugated), which is insoluble in plasma, is transported in the blood attached to plasma albumin. As it passes through the liver, unconjugated bilirubin is absorbed through the hepatocytes' cell membrane and released from its albumin carrier molecule. Once inside the hepatocyte, unconjugated bilirubin combines with *glucuronic acid* (a molecule similar to glucose) to create a water-soluble form called *conjugated bilirubin*, which is secreted as a constituent of bile. In this form, it passes through the bile ducts into the small intestine. In the intestine, approximately one half of the bilirubin is converted into a highly soluble substance called *urobilinogen* by the intestinal flora. Urobilinogen is either absorbed into the portal circulation or excreted in the feces. Most of the urobilinogen that is absorbed is returned to the liver to be reexcreted into the bile. A small amount of urobilinogen, approximately 5%, is absorbed into the general circulation and then excreted by the kidneys.

Usually, only a small amount of bilirubin is found in the blood; the normal level of total serum bilirubin is 0.1 to 1.2 mg/dL (2 to 21 μmol/L).[3] Laboratory measurements of bilirubin usually determine the unconjugated and conjugated bilirubin as well as the total bilirubin. These are reported as the direct (conjugated) bilirubin and the indirect (unconjugated) bilirubin.

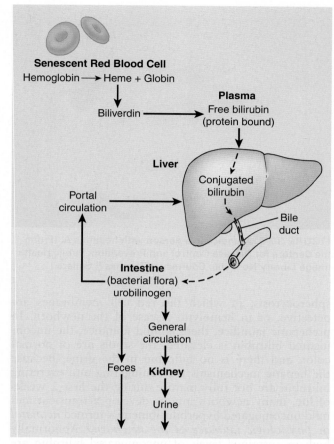

FIGURE 30-5. The process of bilirubin formation, circulation, and elimination.

Jaundice (i.e., icterus) is a yellowish discoloration of the skin and deep tissues resulting from abnormally high levels of bilirubin in the blood. Jaundice becomes evident when the serum bilirubin levels rise above 2 to 2.5 mg/dL (34.2 to 42.8 μmol/L).[3,4] Because normal skin has a yellow cast, the early signs of jaundice often are difficult to detect, especially in persons with dark skin. Bilirubin has a special affinity for elastic tissue. The sclera of the eye, which contains a high proportion of elastic fibers, usually is one of the first structures in which jaundice can be detected (Fig. 30-6).

The four major causes of jaundice are excessive destruction of red blood cells, impaired uptake of bilirubin by the liver cells, decreased conjugation of bilirubin, and obstruction of bile flow in the canaliculi of the hepatic lobules or in the intrahepatic or extrahepatic bile ducts. From an anatomic standpoint, jaundice can be categorized as prehepatic, intrahepatic, and posthepatic. Chart 30-1 lists the common causes of prehepatic, intrahepatic, and posthepatic jaundice.

The major cause of *prehepatic jaundice* is excessive hemolysis of red blood cells. Hemolytic jaundice occurs when red blood cells are destroyed at a rate in excess of the liver's ability to remove the bilirubin from the blood. It may follow a hemolytic blood transfusion reaction or may occur in diseases such as hereditary

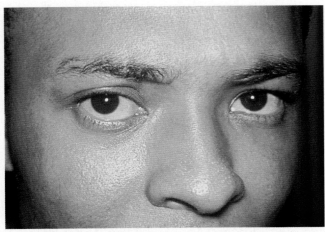

FIGURE 30-6. Jaundice in a person with hepatitis A. (From the Centers for Disease Control and Prevention. Public Health Image Library No. 2860. Courtesy of Thomas F. Sellers.)

spherocytosis, in which the red cell membranes are defective, or in hemolytic disease of the newborn. In prehepatic jaundice, there is mild jaundice, the unconjugated bilirubin is elevated, the stools are of normal color, and there is no bilirubin in the urine. Because the hepatic mechanisms for conjugating and excreting bilirubin are not fully mature during the first 2 weeks of life, many newborn infants develop a transient and mild unconjugated hyperbilirubinemia, termed *neonatal* or *physiologic jaundice of the newborn*.[3] Abnormally high or sustained levels of unconjugated bilirubin are

---

CHART 30-1 Causes of Jaundice

Prehepatic (Excessive Red Blood Cell Destruction)
Hemolytic blood transfusion reaction
Hereditary disorders of the red blood cell
Sickle cell disease
Thalassemia
Spherocytosis
Acquired hemolytic disorders
Hemolytic disease of the newborn
Autoimmune hemolytic anemias

Intrahepatic
Decreased bilirubin uptake by the liver
Decreased conjugation of bilirubin
Hepatocellular liver damage
Hepatitis
Cirrhosis
Cancer of the liver
Drug-induced cholestasis

Posthepatic (Obstruction of Bile Flow)
Structural disorders of the bile duct
Cholelithiasis
Congenital atresia of the extrahepatic bile ducts
Bile duct obstruction caused by tumors

---

abnormal, however, and require investigation and treatment (see Chapter 13).

Intrahepatic or *hepatocellular jaundice* is caused by disorders that directly affect the ability of the liver to remove bilirubin from the blood or conjugate it so it can be eliminated in the bile. Liver diseases such as hepatitis and cirrhosis are the most common causes of intrahepatic jaundice. Drugs such as the anesthetic agent halothane, oral contraceptives, estrogen, anabolic steroids, isoniazid, trimethoprim-sulfamethoxazole, amoxicillin-clavulanic acid, and chlorpromazine may also be implicated in this type of jaundice. Because intrahepatic jaundice usually interferes with all phases of bilirubin metabolism—uptake, conjugation, and excretion—both conjugated and unconjugated bilirubin are elevated, the urine often is dark because of bilirubin in the urine, and the serum alkaline phosphatase (ALP), an enzyme present in the bile duct epithelium and canalicular membrane of hepatocytes, is slightly elevated.

Posthepatic or *obstructive jaundice*, also called *cholestatic jaundice*, occurs when bile flow is obstructed between the liver and the intestine, with the obstruction located at any point between the junction of the right or left hepatic duct and the point where the common bile duct opens into the intestine. Among the causes are strictures of the bile duct, gallstones, and tumors of the bile duct or the pancreas. Conjugated bilirubin levels usually are elevated, the stools are clay colored because of the lack of bilirubin in the bile, the urine is dark, the levels of serum ALP are markedly elevated, and the aminotransferase levels are slightly increased. Blood levels of bile acids often are elevated in obstructive jaundice. As the bile acids accumulate in the blood, pruritus develops. A history of pruritus preceding jaundice is common in obstructive jaundice.

Cholestasis

Cholestasis represents a pathologic condition of impaired bile formation and bile flow, leading to accumulation of bile pigment in the parenchymal tissues of the liver. As a result, materials normally transferred to the bile, including bilirubin, cholesterol, and bile acids, accumulate in the blood.[3,4] The condition may be caused by intrinsic liver disease affecting the intrahepatic canaliculi and bile ducts, in which case it is referred to as intrahepatic cholestasis. Alternatively, it can by caused by obstruction of the large bile ducts, for example by strictures, gallstones, or neoplasms, a condition known as extrahepatic cholestasis. Genetic disorders involving the transport of bile into the canaliculi also can result in cholestasis.

The morphologic features of cholestasis depend on the underlying cause. Common to all types of obstructive and hepatocellular cholestasis is the accumulation of bile pigment in the liver. Elongated green-brown plugs of bile are visible in the dilated bile canaliculi. Rupture of the canaliculi leads to extravasation of bile and subsequent degenerative changes in the surrounding hepatocytes. Prolonged obstructive cholestasis leads not only to fatty changes in the hepatocytes but also to destruction of the supporting connective tissue.[3]

Unrelieved obstruction leads to biliary tract fibrosis and ultimately to end-stage biliary cirrhosis.

Pruritus is the most common presenting symptom in persons with cholestasis, probably related to an elevation in plasma bile acids. Skin xanthomas (focal accumulations of cholesterol) may occur as the result of hyperlipidemia and impaired excretion of cholesterol. A characteristic laboratory finding is elevated levels of serum ALP. Other manifestations of reduced bile flow relate to intestinal absorption, including nutritional deficiencies of the fat-soluble vitamins A, D, E, and K.

Tests of Hepatobiliary Function

The history and physical examination, in most instances, provide clues about liver function. Diagnostic tests help to evaluate liver function and the extent of liver damage. Laboratory tests commonly are used to assess liver function and confirm the diagnosis of liver disease.

Liver function tests, including serum levels of liver enzymes, are used to assess injury to liver cells, the liver's ability to synthesize proteins, and the excretory functions of the liver.[5,6] Elevated serum enzyme test results usually indicate liver injury earlier than other indicators of liver function. The key enzymes are alanine aminotransferase (ALT) and aspartate aminotransferase (AST), which are present in liver cells. ALT is liver specific, whereas AST is derived from organs other than the liver. In most cases of liver damage, there are parallel rises in ALT and AST. The most dramatic rise is seen in cases of acute hepatocellular injury, as occurs with viral hepatitis, autoimmune hepatitis, hypoxic or ischemic injury, acute toxic injury, or Reye syndrome. The liver's synthetic capacity is reflected in measures of serum protein levels (albumin) and prothrombin time (i.e., synthesis of coagulation factors). Deficiencies of fibrinogen and coagulation factors (II, VII, IX, and X) may occur.

Serum bilirubin, γ-glutamyltransferase (GGT), and ALP measure hepatic excretory function.[6] Alkaline phosphatase is present in the membranes between liver cells and the bile duct and is released by disorders affecting the bile duct. γ-glutamyltransferase, which is thought to function in the transport of amino acids and peptides into liver cells, is a sensitive indicator of hepatobiliary disease but not used much clinically as it has limited use in specific disease diagnosis.

Ultrasonography provides information about the size, composition, and blood flow of the liver. It is used predominately in detecting stones in the gallbladder or biliary tree. Computed tomography (CT) scanning and magnetic resonance imaging (MRI) provide information similar to that obtained by ultrasonography, but offer greater detail regarding composition, and blood and/or bile flow through the liver. Selective angiography of the celiac, superior mesenteric, or hepatic artery may be used to visualize the hepatic or portal circulation.

A liver biopsy affords a means of examining liver tissue without surgery. There are several methods for obtaining liver tissue: percutaneous liver biopsy, which uses a suction, cutting, or spring-loaded cutting needle; laparoscopic liver biopsy; and fine needle biopsy, which is performed under ultrasonographic or CT guidance.[7] The type of method used is based on the number of specimens needed and the amount of tissue required for evaluation. Laparoscopic liver biopsy provides the means for examining abdominal masses and staging liver cancers.

SUMMARY CONCEPTS

■ The liver, which is the largest and most versatile organ in the body, is located between the gastrointestinal tract and the systemic circulation. Venous blood from the intestine flows through the liver before it is returned to the heart, allowing nutrients to be removed for processing and storage, and bacteria and other foreign matter to be removed before the blood is returned to the systemic circulation.

■ The main functions of the liver include synthesis of plasma proteins, maintenance of blood glucose levels, regulation of circulating lipoprotein levels, and vitamin and mineral storage. The liver also plays an essential role in the metabolism and elimination of harmful toxins and drugs, conversion of ammonia to urea, and removal of bilirubin, a product of hemoglobin breakdown, from the blood.

■ Serum liver enzymes, especially alanine aminotransferase (ALT) and aspartate aminotransferase (AST), are used to assess injury to liver cells; plasma proteins (e.g., serum albumin) and blood clotting factors (prothrombin time) provide information related to the liver's synthetic capacity; and serum bilirubin, serum γ-glutamyltransferase (GGT), and alkaline phosphatase (ALP) are used as measures of hepatic excretory function.

Disorders of Hepatic and Biliary Function

The structures of the hepatobiliary system are subject to many of the same pathologic conditions that affect other body systems. This section focuses on alterations in liver function due to viral and autoimmune hepatitis; intrahepatic biliary disorders; drug- and alcohol-induced liver disease; nonalcoholic fatty liver disease; the hepatic syndromes of cirrhosis, portal hypertension, and liver failure; and cancer of the liver.

Hepatitis

Hepatitis refers to the acute or chronic inflammation of the liver. Although hepatitis viruses account for many cases of chronic hepatitis, there are many other causes including chronic alcoholism, drug toxicities, and auto-immune disorders. The discussion in this section focuses on viral and autoimmune hepatitis.

Viral Hepatitis

Viral hepatitis refers to hepatic infections due to a group of viruses known as *hepatotropic viruses* (hepatitis A [HAV], hepatitis B [HBV], hepatitis C [HCV], hepatitis D [HDV], and hepatitis E [HEV]) that have a particular affinity for the liver.[3,4] Although all of the hepatotropic viruses cause hepatitis, they differ in terms of their mode of transmission and incubation period; mechanism, degree, and chronicity of liver damage; and ability to evolve to a carrier state. Acute hepatitis may also occur in the course of other viral infections such as infectious mononucleosis, caused by the Epstein-Barr virus; and cytomegalovirus infection, particularly in newborn or immunosuppressed persons. These other forms of hepatitis must be distinguished from those caused by hepatotropic viruses.

Syndromes of Viral Hepatitis. The clinical course of viral hepatitis can involve a number of syndromes, including acute asymptomatic hepatitis with only serologic evidence of infection, acute symptomatic hepatitis, and chronic hepatitis, which can produce a carrier state. Fulminant hepatic failure, a syndrome of hepatic insufficiency with rapid progression to liver failure, occurs in a small percentage of persons with hepatitis B.[3]

The manifestations of *acute symptomatic viral hepatitis* can be divided into three phases: the prodromal or preicterus period, the icterus period, and the convalescent period. The onset of the *prodromal period* may vary from abrupt to insidious, with general malaise, myalgia, arthralgia, easy fatigability, and severe anorexia out of proportion to the degree of illness. Gastrointestinal symptoms such as nausea, vomiting, and diarrhea or constipation may occur. Abdominal pain is usually mild and felt on the right side. Chills and fever may mark an abrupt onset. In persons who smoke, there may be distaste for smoking that parallels the anorexia. Serum levels of AST and ALT show variable increases during the preicterus phase and precede a rise in bilirubin that accompanies the onset of the icterus or jaundice phase of infection. The *icterus phase*, if it occurs, usually follows the prodromal phase within 5 to 10 days. The prodromal symptoms may become worse with the onset of jaundice, followed by progressive clinical improvement. Severe pruritus and liver tenderness are common during the icterus period. The *convalescent phase* is characterized by an increased sense of well-being, return of appetite, and disappearance of jaundice. The acute illness usually subsides gradually over a 2- to 3-week period, with complete clinical recovery by approximately 9 weeks in hepatitis A and 16 weeks in uncomplicated hepatitis B.

Chronic hepatitis is defined as symptomatic, biochemical, or serological evidence of continuing or relapsing disease that has persisted for more than 6 months.[3] The clinical features of chronic hepatitis are extremely variable and not predictive of outcome. In many people the only manifestation is a persistent elevation of serum aminotransferases. If there are symptoms, the most frequently reported ones are fatigue, abdominal discomfort, and joint or muscle aches. However, even asymptomatic persons with normal serum aminotransferase levels are at risk for developing liver damage.

Infection with HBV/HDV, and HCV, can produce a *carrier state* in which the person does not have symptoms but harbors the virus and can therefore transmit the disease. There is no carrier state for HAV infection. There are two types of carriers: healthy carriers who have few or no ill effects, and those with chronic disease who may or may not have symptoms. Factors that increase the risk of becoming a carrier are age at time of infection and immune status. The carrier state for infections that occur early in life, as in infants of HBV-infected mothers, may be as high as 90% to 95%, compared with 1% to 10% of infected adults.[3]

Hepatitis A. Hepatitis A is usually a benign and self-limited disease caused by a small, nonenveloped, single-stranded ribonucleic acid (RNA) picornavirus. Lack of a lipid envelope confers resistance to lysis by bile acids in the intestine. Infection is contracted primarily by the fecal–oral route.[8]

Hepatitis A occurs throughout the world and is endemic in countries with poor sanitation. At special risk of infection are persons traveling abroad who have not been vaccinated or previously exposed to the virus. HAV has a brief incubation period, with an average of 25 to 30 days. The virus replicates in the liver, is excreted in the bile, and is shed in the stool. The fecal shedding of HAV occurs for 2 to 3 weeks before the development of symptoms and ends about 1 week after the onset of jaundice.[3] Because young children are asymptomatic, they play an important role in the spread of the disease. Oral behavior and lack of toilet training promote viral spread among children attending day care centers, who then carry the virus home to older siblings and parents. Infected workers in food industries may also be a source of spread. HAV usually is not transmitted by transfusion of blood or plasma derivatives, presumably because its short period of viremia usually coincides with clinical illness, so that the disease is apparent and blood donations are not accepted.

The onset of symptoms usually is abrupt and includes fever, malaise, nausea, anorexia, abdominal discomfort, dark urine, and jaundice. The likelihood of having symptoms is related to age. Children younger than 6 years often are asymptomatic. The illness in older children and adults usually is symptomatic and jaundice occurs in approximately 70% of cases.[9] Symptoms usually last approximately 2 months. HAV infection does not cause chronic hepatitis or induce a carrier state, and only rarely causes acute fulminant hepatitis.[3,8]

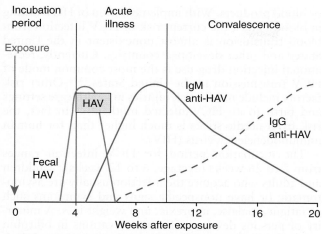

FIGURE 30-7. The sequence of fecal shedding of the hepatitis A virus (HAV), HAV viremia, and HAV antibody (IgM and IgG anti-HAV) changes in hepatitis A.

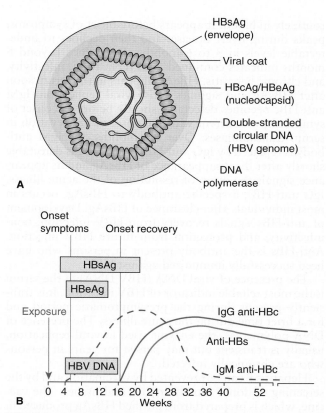

FIGURE 30-8. **(A)** The hepatitis B virus. **(B)** The sequence of hepatitis B virus (HBV) viral antigens (HBsAg, HBeAg), HBV DNA, and HBV antibody (IgM, IgG, anti-HBc, and anti-HBs) changes in acute resolving hepatitis B.

Antibodies to HAV (anti-HAV) appear early in the disease and tend to persist in the serum (Fig. 30-7). The immunoglobulin M (IgM) antibodies (see Chapter 15) usually appear during the first week of symptomatic disease and begin to decline in a few months.[3] Their presence coincides with a decline in fecal shedding of the virus. Peak levels of IgG antibodies occur after 1 month of illness and may persist for years; they provide long-term protective immunity against reinfection. The presence of IgM anti-HAV is indicative of acute hepatitis A, whereas IgG anti-HAV merely documents past infection.

A HAV vaccine is available for persons at high risk for HAV exposure.[9] These include international travelers to regions where sanitation is poor and endemic HAV infections are high, children living in communities with high rates of HAV infection, homosexually active men, and users of illicit drugs. A public health benefit also may be derived from vaccinating persons with increased potential for transmitting the disease (e.g., food handlers). The Centers for Disease Control and Prevention (CDC) has recently recommended vaccination of children in states, counties, and communities with high rates of infection.[9] Persons who have been exposed to HAV are advised to receive postexposure prophylaxis with a single dose of HAV vaccine or immune globulin (IgG) as soon as possible. The immune globulin is preferred for persons older than 40 years or younger than 1 year of age and for those who are immunocompromised or have chronic liver disease.

Hepatitis B. Hepatitis B is caused by a hepatotropic deoxyribonucleic acid (DNA)-containing *Hepadnavirus*. The complete hepatitis B virion, also called a *Dane particle*, consists of an outer envelope and an inner nucleocapsid that contains the viral DNA and viral polymerase that exhibits both DNA polymerase and reverse transcriptase activity (Fig. 30-8). HBV infection can produce acute hepatitis, chronic hepatitis, hepatocellular carcinoma, and fulminant hepatic failure. It also participates in the development of hepatitis D (delta hepatitis).[3,4,10] The virus usually is transmitted through inoculation

with infected blood or serum. However, the viral antigen can be found in most body secretions and can be spread by oral or sexual contact.

Hepatitis B has a longer incubation period and represents a more serious health problem than hepatitis A. More than 2 billion people—one third of the world's population—alive today have been infected with HBV, and of these more than 240 million remain infected.[3,11] The incidence of acute hepatitis B in the United States has dramatically declined since 1990, with the greatest declines in children and adolescents, coincident with HBV vaccination.

Worldwide, perinatal (vertical) transmission is the predominant mode of HBV transmission, whereas intravenous drug use and unprotected sexual intercourse are the main routes of transmission in low-prevalence areas such as the United States. Although the virus can be spread through transfusion or administration of blood products, routine screening methods have appreciably reduced transmission through this route.[12]

Three well-defined antigens are associated with the HBV virus: a core antigen, HBcAg; HBeAg, a precore protein; and a surface antigen, HBsAg. These HBV antigens evoke specific antibodies: anti-HBc, anti-HBe, and anti-HBs. The antigens and their antibodies serve as serologic markers for following the natural course of the disease[3,4] (see Fig. 30-8). HBsAg is the viral antigen measured most routinely in blood. It appears before onset of symptoms, peaks during overt disease, and then declines to undetectable levels in 3 to 6 months. Persistence beyond 6 months indicates continued viral replication, infectivity, and chronic hepatitis. HBeAg appears in the serum soon after HBsAg and signifies active viral replication. IgM anti-HBc becomes detectable shortly before the onset of symptoms, concurrent with the onset of an elevation in serum transaminases. Over the months, the IgM antibody is replaced by IgG anti-HBc. Anti-HBe is detectable shortly after the disappearance of HBeAg and its appearance signals the onset of resolution of the acute illness. IgG anti-HBs, a specific antibody to HBsAg, occurs in most individuals after clearance of HBsAg. Development of anti-HBs signals recovery from HBV infection, noninfectivity, and protection from future HBV infection. Anti-HBs is the antibody present in persons who have been successfully immunized against HBV.

The presence of viral DNA (HBV DNA) in the serum is the most reliable indicator of HBV infection. It is transiently present during the presymptomatic period and for a brief time during the acute illness. The presence of DNA polymerase, the enzyme used in viral replication, usually is transient but may persist for years in persons who are chronically infected.

Hepatitis B can be prevented by vaccination and by the screening of donor blood, organs, and tissues. The vaccine, which is prepared from purified HBsAg produced in yeast, induces a protective antibody response in 95% of vaccinated infants, children, and adolescents.[3] The CDC recommends vaccination of all children 0 to 18 years of age as a means of preventing HBV transmission.[12] The vaccine also is recommended for all unvaccinated adults who are at high risk for infection, international travelers to regions with high or intermediate levels of endemic HBV infection, persons with human immunodeficiency virus (HIV) infection, persons with chronic liver disease, injection drug users, and all other persons seeking protection.[12] It is also recommended that all pregnant women be routinely tested for HBsAg during an early prenatal visit and that infants born to HBsAg-positive mothers receive appropriate doses of hepatitis B immune globulin (HBIG) and hepatitis B vaccine.[9]

Hepatitis C. The hepatitis C virus, discovered in 1989, is a member of the *Flaviviridae* family. It is a small, enveloped, single-stranded RNA virus.[3,4] The virus is genetically unstable, giving rise to multiple genotypes and subtypes. This allows a divergent population of closely related variants to circulate in infected persons.[3] One of the HCV envelope proteins, the E2 protein, which is the target for anti-HCV antibodies, is the most variable region of the entire viral genome. It is likely that the wide diversity of genotypes contributes to the pathogenicity of the virus, allowing it to escape the actions of host immune mechanisms and antiviral medications, and to difficulties in developing a preventive vaccine.

Hepatitis C is the most common cause of chronic hepatitis, cirrhosis, and hepatocellular cancer in the world.[3,4,13,14] Before 1990, the main route of transmission of HCV was through contaminated blood transfusions

or blood products. With implementation of HCV testing in blood banks, the current risk of HCV infection from blood transfusion is almost nonexistent in the United States and other developed countries. Currently, recreational injection drug use is the most common mode of HCV transmission in the United States.[13,14] Other risk factors include needlestick injuries in health care settings and birth to an HCV-infected mother.[13,14] In fact, the risk from needle sticks is much higher than for human immunodeficiency virus (HIV).[3]

The incubation period for HCV infection ranges from 2 to 26 weeks (average, 6 to 12 weeks).[3] Children and adults who acquire the infection usually are asymptomatic or have nonspecific signs and symptoms such as fatigue, malaise, anorexia, and weight loss. A minority of persons develop sufficient elevations in bilirubin to produce overt jaundice or the development of dark urine. Only a few persons who are newly infected with HCV will clear the infection, with the majority going on to develop chronic hepatitis.[13–15] Factors associated with spontaneous clearing of HCV infection appear to include younger age, female sex, and certain histocompatibility genes. The most serious consequences of chronic HCV infection are progressive liver fibrosis leading to cirrhosis, and hepatocellular cancer.

Both HCV RNA and anti-HCV antibody tests are available for detecting the presence of HCV infection (Fig. 30-9). Unlike hepatitis A and B, antibodies to HCV are not protective, but they serve as markers for the disease. With anti-HCV antibody tests, infection often can be detected as early as 6 to 8 weeks after exposure, but false-negative results can occur in immunocompromised people and early in the course of the disease. Direct measurement of HCV RNA in the serum can detect the virus as early as 1 to 2 weeks after exposure with viral tests that use polymerase chain reaction (PCR) methods (see Chapter 14).

Hepatitis D and E. Hepatitis D virus, or the delta hepatitis agent, is a defective RNA virus that requires concomitant infection with HBV for its own replication.[16]

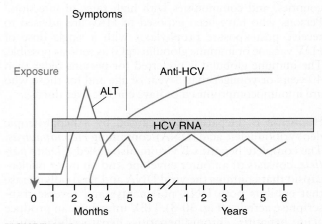

FIGURE 30-9. The sequence of serologic changes in chronic hepatitis C, with persistence of hepatitis C virus (HCV) RNA and exacerbations and remissions of clinical symptoms indicated by changes in serum alanine aminotransferase (ALT) levels.

Acute hepatitis D occurs in two forms: coinfection that occurs simultaneously with acute hepatitis B, and a superinfection in which hepatitis D is imposed on chronic hepatitis B.[3,16] The delta agent often increases the severity of HBV infection.

The routes of transmission of hepatitis D are similar to those for hepatitis B. In the United States, infection is restricted largely to persons at high risk for HBV infection, particularly injecting drug users. The greatest risk is in HBV carriers; these persons should be informed about the dangers of HDV superinfection. Hepatitis D is diagnosed by detection of antibody to HDV (anti-HDV) in the serum or HDV RNA in the serum. There is no specific treatment for hepatitis D. Because the infection is linked to hepatitis B, prevention of hepatitis D should begin with prevention of hepatitis B through vaccination.

The hepatitis E virus is an enveloped, single-stranded RNA virus. It is transmitted by the fecal–oral route and causes manifestations of acute hepatitis that are similar to hepatitis A. It does not cause chronic hepatitis or the carrier state.[3] A distinguishing feature of HEV infection is the high mortality rate (approximately 20%) among pregnant women, owing to the development of fulminant hepatitis. The infection occurs primarily in developing coutries of the world. The only reported cases in the United States have been in persons who have recently been in an endemic area.

Chronic Viral Hepatitis. Chronic hepatitis is defined as a chronic inflammatory reaction of the liver, or positive viral serologies of more than 6 months' duration. Chronic viral hepatitis is the principal cause of chronic liver disease, cirrhosis, and hepatocellular cancer in the world and now ranks as the chief reason for liver transplantation in adults.[17] Of the hepatotropic viruses, only three are known to cause chronic hepatitis—HBV/HDV and HCV. In both HBV and HCV, fibrosis and clinical manifestations of chronic disease result from host immune responses directed against viral antigens. In response to these viral antigens, the host immune system directs cytoxic T lymphocytes and cytokines to inhibit viral replication (Chapter 15), the effects of which induce inflammation and liver injury.

There are several treatment options for chronic viral hepatitis. Drugs used in the treatment of chronic hepatitis B include the recombinant human interferon-2α and peginterferon or nucleotide analog antiretroviral agent. Persons with active viral replication may be treated with recombinant human interferon-2α and peginterferon. Peginterferons were developed by adding a polyethylene glycol (PEG) moiety to an interferon molecule (PEG-IFN), resulting in a prolonged serum half-life and the ability to administer the compound once weekly. Nucleoside and nucleotide analogs (e.g., entecavir, tenofovir) have shown good efficacy and better tolerance and may be used instead of interferon for treatment of chronic HBV infection.[18] The current treatment for persons with chronic hepatitis C is a combination of peginterferon (alfa-2b or alfa-2a) plus ribavirin (a nucleoside analog), plus sofosbuvir (a polymerase inhibitor)

or sofosbuvir plus ribavirin.[19] Treatment for HCV is 70% to 80% effective, but is costly and has side effects. These side effects range from flulike symptoms, which are almost universal, to more serious and less common side effects, such as psychiatric symptoms (depression, anxiety), thyroid dysfunction, and bone marrow suppression. Although most persons with HCV infection are candidates for treatment, many have other health problems that are contraindications to therapy.

Liver transplantation is a treatment option for those with advanced decompensated cirrhosis from viral hepatitis. Liver transplantation, however, is not a cure for viral hepatitis, as it often reoccurs in the transplanted liver.

Autoimmune Hepatitis

Autoimmune hepatitis is a chronic and progressive form of hepatitis of unknown origin that is associated with high levels of serum immunoglobulins, including autoantibodies.[3,4,20] Although the disorder is usually seen in young women, it can occur in either sex at any age.

Clinical and laboratory observations have led to the hypothesis that autoimmune hepatitis is a multifactorial disorder, with genetic and environmental factors playing important roles. Most knowledge about the genetics of the disease has focused on the human leukocyte antigen (HLA) genes that reside in the major histocompatibility complex (MHC), located on the short arm of chromosome 6 (see Chapter 15). The environmental agents assumed to induce autoimmune hepatitis are viruses, immunizations, herbal products such as black cohash, and medications such as minocycline, methyldopa, atorvastatin, simvastatin, interferons, and nitrofurantoin.[3,20] Autoantibodies, in particular antinuclear antibody and anti–smooth muscle antibody, have been found in serum of those with autoimmune hepatitis, although the exact function of these antibodies in this condition is unknown.

Two distinct types of autoimmune hepatitis have been broadly identified based on the presence of circulating antibodies.[2,4,20] Type I autoimmune hepatitis, the most common form of the disease, is characterized by increased levels of anti–smooth muscle and antinuclear autoantibodies. Approximately 30% of cases occur in women younger than 40 years of age, a third of whom have other autoimmune diseases.[4] Type II autoimmune hepatitis, a rare disorder, occurs mainly in children 2 to 14 years of age and is characterized by the presence of antibody to liver and kidney microsomes and liver cytosol.[4] The disorder is often accompanied by other autoimmune disorders, especially type 1 diabetes mellitus and thyroiditis. The genetic component for this type of autoimmune hepatitis is less well defined than for type 1.

Clinical manifestations of the disorder cover a spectrum that extends from no apparent symptoms to the signs of liver failure. Physical examination may reveal no abnormalities, but may also reveal hepatomegaly, splenomegaly, jaundice, and signs and symptoms of chronic liver disease. In asymptomatic cases, the disorder may be discovered when abnormal serum enzyme levels are identified during performance of routine screening tests.

The differential diagnosis includes measures to exclude other causes of liver disease, including hepatitis B and C. A characteristic laboratory finding is that of a marked elevation in serum gamma globulins. A biopsy is used to confirm the diagnosis. Corticosteroid and immunosuppressant drugs are the treatment of choice. Although some persons remain in remission after drug treatment is withdrawn, most require long-term maintenance treatment. Liver transplantation may be required for persons who are refractory to or intolerant of immunosuppressive therapy and in whom end-stage liver disease develops.

Acute Fulminant Hepatitis

Acute fulminant hepatitis or hepatic failure is hepatic insufficiency that progresses from onset of hepatitis symptoms to hepatic encephalopathy within 2 to 3 weeks in persons who do not have chronic liver disease.[3] Viral hepatitis is responsible for about 10% of cases of fulminant hepatitis, with about 8% of those being caused by HBV and the rest by HAV.[3,21] Acetaminophen (Tylenol) toxicity (to be discussed) is the most common cause, accounting for at least 46% of cases in the United States.[21] Other causes include idiosyncratic drug reactions (now the second most common cause), poisonous mushrooms, fatty liver of pregnancy, and other disorders of fatty acid oxidation.

Acute fulminant liver failure often presents with gastrointestinal symptoms, signs of the systemic inflammatory response (see Chapter 20), and hemorrhagic phenomenon. Jaundice may be absent or minimal early, but laboratory tests show severe hepatocellular damage. The blood ammonia level is typically elevated and correlates with the development of encephalopathy and cerebral edema. Survival of more than a week may permit replication of residual hepatocytes.

The treatment for acute liver failure is directed toward correcting the underlying liver abnormality and providing supportive care. Liver transplantation is the only option for persons who do not succumb to secondary infections or other organ failure. The mortality rate of fulminant hepatitis is about 85% without transplant and about 35% with transplant.[3]

Intrahepatic Biliary Disorders

Intrahepatic biliary diseases disrupt the flow of bile through the liver, causing cholestasis and biliary cirrhosis. Among the causes of intrahepatic biliary disease are primary biliary cirrhosis and secondary biliary cirrhosis.

Primary Biliary Cirrhosis

Primary biliary cirrhosis is a chronic disease of the liver characterized by the autoimmune destruction of the medium-sized intrahepatic bile ducts with cholestasis and eventual development of cirrhosis and liver failure.[3,22] Cirrhosis develops only after many years; thus, the name *primary biliary cirrhosis* is somewhat misleading for persons diagnosed early in the precirrhotic stage.[3]

The disease is seen most commonly in women 40 to 60 years of age. Both the incidence and prevalence are increasing, and geographic clustering of the disease has been reported, suggesting genetic and environmental factors are important in its pathogenesis. Family members of persons with the disease have increased risk of developing the disease. The disease may be associated with other autoimmune disorders such as Sjögren syndrome (sicca complex of dry eyes and mouth), autoimmune thyroid disease, rheumatoid arthritis, Raynaud phenomenon, and celiac disease.

The disorder is characterized by an extremely insidious onset, and persons may be symptom-free for many years. Morphologically, there is progressive scarring and destruction of liver tissue. The liver becomes enlarged and takes on a green hue because of the accumulated bile. The earliest symptoms are unexplained pruritus (itching), weight loss, and fatigue, followed by dark urine and pale stools. Vitamin D malabsorption–related osteoporosis occurs in up to one third of persons with the disorder.[22] Jaundice is a late manifestation of the disorder, as are other signs of liver failure. Serum alkaline phosphatase (ALP) levels are elevated in persons with primary biliary cirrhosis.

Treatment for primary biliary cirrhosis is ursodeoxycholic acid (ursodiol), a drug that increases bile flow and decreases the toxicity of bile contents, and has been shown to decrease the rate of clinical deterioration. Cholestyramine, a bile acid–binding drug, or rifampicin can be beneficial for treatment of pruritus. Liver transplantation, however, remains the only treatment for advanced disease. Primary biliary cirrhosis does not recur after liver transplantation if appropriate immunosuppression is used.

Secondary Biliary Cirrhosis

Secondary biliary cirrhosis results from prolonged obstruction of the extrabiliary tree.[3] The most common cause is cholelithiasis (gallstones). Other causes of secondary biliary cirrhosis are malignant neoplasms of the biliary tree or head of the pancreas and strictures of the common duct caused by previous surgical procedures. Extrahepatic biliary cirrhosis may benefit from surgical procedures designed to relieve the obstruction.

Drug- and Alcohol-Induced Liver Disease

By virtue of its many enzyme systems that are involved in biochemical processes, the liver has an important role in the metabolism of many drugs and chemical substances. The liver is particularly important in the metabolism of lipid-soluble substances that cannot be directly excreted by the kidney.

Drug Metabolism

There are two major types of reactions involved in the hepatic detoxification and metabolism of drugs and other chemicals: phase 1 and phase 2 reactions.[23]

These reactions, often referred to as *biotransformations,* are important considerations in drug therapy.

Phase 1 reactions result in the chemical modification of reactive drug groups through oxidation, reduction, hydroxylation, or other chemical reactions. Many of these reactions involve drug-metabolizing enzymes that are located in the lipophilic endoplasmic reticulum membranes of liver cells. One of the enzymes involved is the product of a gene superfamily called *cytochrome P450* (abbreviated CYP or CYP P450). Multiple isoforms of the CYP enzyme have been identified and traced to the metabolism of specific drugs and to potential interactions among drugs. Of these isoforms, the CYP3A4 enzyme accounts for approximately 50% of the liver's drug-metabolizing activity.[23]

Many gene members of the *CYP* enzyme system can have their activity induced or suppressed as they undergo the task of metabolizing drugs. For example, drugs such as alcohol and barbiturates can induce certain members to increase enzyme production, accelerating drug metabolism and decreasing the pharmacologic action of the drug and of coadministered drugs that use the same member of the CYP system. In the case of drugs metabolically transformed to reactive intermediates, enzyme induction may exacerbate drug-mediated tissue toxicity. Certain drugs can also inhibit enzymes in the CYP system. For example, the antibiotic erythromycin and the antifungal agents fluconazole, itraconazole, and ketoconazole inhibit CYP3A4 enzyme activity, as does grapefruit juice, thereby decreasing the metabolism of drugs that use this enzyme system.[23]

Phase 2 reactions, which involve the conversion of lipid-soluble derivatives to water-soluble substances called *conjugates,* may follow phase 1 reactions or proceed independently. Conjugation, a process that couples the drug with an activated endogenous compound such as glutathione, renders the drug more water soluble so it can be excreted in the bile or urine. Although many water-soluble drugs and endogenous substances are excreted unchanged in the urine or bile, lipid-soluble substances tend to accumulate in the body unless they are converted to less active compounds or water-soluble metabolites. Because the endogenous substrates used in the conjugation process are obtained from the diet, nutrition plays a critical role in phase 2 reactions.

In addition to its role in metabolism of drugs and chemicals, the liver also is responsible for hormone inactivation or modification. Insulin and glucagon are inactivated by proteolysis or deamination. Thyroxine and triiodothyronine are metabolized by reactions involving deiodination. Steroid hormones such as the glucocorticoids are first inactivated by a phase 1 reaction and then conjugated by phase 2 reactions.

Drug-Induced Liver Disease

Many widely used therapeutic drugs, including over-the-counter medications and "natural" products, can cause hepatic injury.[23] Hepatotoxicity is the leading cause of acute liver failure in the United States. The drug most commonly involved is acetaminophen, with half the cases reported to be unintentional overdoses.[24] Unintentional overdoses may occur when people unknowingly take several over-the-counter preparations that contain acetaminophen (e.g., an acetaminophen-containing cold preparation and acetaminophen pain medication). Numerous host factors contribute to the susceptibility to drug-induced liver disease, including genetic predisposition, age, underlying chronic liver disease, diet and alcohol consumption, and the use of multiple interacting drugs.

Drugs and chemicals can exert their effects by causing hepatocyte injury and death or by cholestatic liver damage due to injury of biliary drainage structures. Drug reactions can be acute or chronic, and predictable based on the drug's chemical structure and metabolites or unpredictable (idiosyncratic) based on individual characteristics of the person receiving the drug.

Direct Predictable Injury. Some drugs are known to have toxic effects on the liver. Examples are acetaminophen, isoniazid, and phenytoin. Direct hepatic damage, which is often age and dose dependent, usually results from drug metabolism and the generation of toxic metabolites. Because of the greater activity of the drug-metabolizing enzymes in the central zones of the liver, these agents typically cause centrilobular necrosis. The injury is characterized by marked elevations in ALT and AST values with minimally elevated ALP. Bilirubin levels invariably are increased, and the prognosis often is worse when hepatocellular necrosis is accompanied by jaundice.

Idiosyncratic Reactions. In contrast to direct predictable drug reactions, idiosyncratic reactions are unpredictable, not related to dose, and sometimes accompanied by features suggesting an allergic reaction. Drugs are relatively small molecules and, therefore, unlikely to provoke an immune response. However, in the process of biotransformation, drugs may combine with enzymes, producing a compound large enough to serve as an antigen and induce the formation of antibodies or a direct cytotoxic T-cell response. In some cases, the reaction results directly from a metabolite that is produced only in certain persons based on a genetic predisposition. For example, certain people are capable of rapid acetylation of isoniazid, an antituberculosis drug.

Cholestatic Reactions. Cholestatic drug reactions result in decreased secretion of bile or obstruction of the biliary tree. Acute intrahepatic cholestasis is one of the most frequent types of idiosyncratic drug reactions. Among the drugs credited with causing cholestatic drug reactions are estradiol; chlorpromazine, an antipsychotic drug; and some of the antibiotics, including amoxicillin/clavulanic acid, erythromycin, and nafcillin. Typically, cholestatic drug reactions are characterized by an early onset of jaundice and pruritus, with little alteration in the person's general feeling of well-being. Most instances of acute drug-induced cholestasis subside once the drug is withdrawn.

Alcohol Metabolism

Alcohol is readily absorbed from the stomach and intestine. It is then distributed to all of the tissues and fluids in the body in direct proportion to the blood level. Most of the alcohol that a person drinks is metabolized by the liver. In the liver, alcohol metabolism proceeds simultaneously by two major pathways: the alcohol dehydrogenase (ADH) system and the microsomal ethanol-oxidizing system (MEOS).[25,26] Both pathways lead to the production of acetaldehyde which has many toxic effects and is responsible for some of the acute effects of alcohol.

Alcohol oxidation by ADH involves a reduction in the adenine dinucleotide (NAD–to–nicotinamide adenine dinucleotide [NADH]) ratio (see Chapter 1, Understanding Cell Metabolism), with a consequent decrease in NAD and increase in NADH. Since NAD is required for fatty acid oxidation, its deficiency is a main cause of the accumulation of fat in the liver of alcoholics. It also causes lactic acidosis in alcoholics.[25]

Metabolism of alcohol by the MEOS system involves the CYP drug-metabolizing enzymes, located in the smooth endoplasmic reticulum. One of these metabolizing enzymes also oxidizes a number of other compounds, including various drugs (e.g., acetaminophen, isoniazid), toxins (e.g., carbon tetrachloride, halothane), industrial solvents, and carcinogenic agents (e.g., aflatoxin, nitrosamines). Induction of this system by alcohol enhances the susceptibility of alcoholics to the hepatotoxic effects of these and other compounds metabolized by the same system.[25]

Alcohol-Induced Liver Disease

About 2 million people in the United States are suspected of having alcoholic liver disease, which causes 27,000 deaths each year.[3] Most of these deaths are attributable to liver failure, bleeding esophageal varices, or kidney failure. Because only approximately 10% to 15% of alcoholics develop cirrhosis, genetic and environmental factors are thought to contribute to alcoholic liver disease.[3]

The spectrum of alcoholic liver disease includes fatty liver disease, alcoholic hepatitis, and cirrhosis.[3,4] *Fatty liver disease* is characterized by the accumulation of fat in hepatocytes, a condition called *steatosis* (Fig. 30-10). As a consequence, the liver becomes yellow and enlarges. The pathogenesis of fatty liver is not completely understood and can depend on the amount of alcohol consumed, dietary fat content, body stores of fat, hormonal status, and other factors. There is evidence that ingestion of large amounts of alcohol can cause fatty liver changes even with an adequate diet. For example, young, nonalcoholic volunteers had fatty liver changes after 2 days of consuming an excess amount of alcohol, even though adequate carbohydrates, fats, and proteins were included in the diet. The fatty changes that occur with ingestion of alcohol usually do not produce symptoms and are reversible after the alcohol intake has been discontinued.

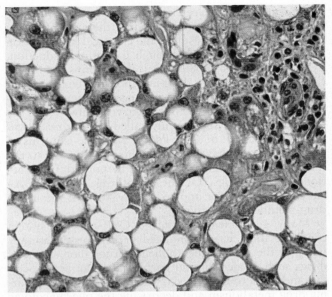

FIGURE 30-10. Alcoholic fatty liver. A photomicrograph shows the cytoplasm of almost all hepatocytes distended by fat that displaces the nucleus to the periphery. (From Herrine SK, Navarro VJ, Rubin R. The liver and biliary system. In: Rubin R, Strayer DS, eds. *Rubin's Pathology: Clinicopathologic Foundations of Medicine.* 6th ed. Philadelphia, PA: Wolters Kluwer Health | Lippincott Williams & Wilkins; 2012:708.)

Alcoholic hepatitis is characterized by inflammation and necrosis of liver cells caused by excessive alcohol intake.[3,4,27] The cardinal sign of alcoholic hepatitis is rapid onset of jaundice. Other manifestations include fever, hepatic tenderness, pain, anorexia, nausea, ascites, and liver failure. Persons with severe alcoholic hepatitis may have encephalopathy. The immediate prognosis correlates with severity of liver cell injury. In some cases, the disease progresses rapidly to liver failure and death. The mortality rate in the acute stage ranges from 10% to 50% depending on severity of inflammation.[4,28] In persons who survive and continue to drink, the acute phase often is followed by persistent alcoholic hepatitis with progression to cirrhosis in a matter of 1 to 2 years.

Alcoholic cirrhosis is the end result of repeated bouts of drinking-related hepatocyte injury and regeneration. The gross appearance of the early cirrhotic liver is one of fine, uniform nodules on its surface. The condition has traditionally been called *micronodular* or *Laennec cirrhosis*. Initially, the developing fibrous septa extend through the sinusoids from the central to the portal regions and the entrapped hepatocytes generate uniform micronodules. With more advanced cirrhosis, regenerative processes cause the nodules to become larger and more irregular in size and shape. As this occurs, the nodules cause the liver to become relobulized through the formation of new portal tracts and venous outflow channels. The nodules may compress the hepatic veins, curtailing blood flow out of the liver and producing portal hypertension, extrahepatic portosystemic shunts, and cholestasis.

Nonalcoholic Fatty Liver Disease

The term *nonalcoholic fatty liver disease* (NAFLD) is often used to describe fatty liver disease arising from causes other than alcohol.[29] The condition can range from simple steatosis (fatty infiltration of the liver) to nonalcoholic steatohepatitis (steatosis with inflammation and hepatocyte necrosis and cirrhosis). Although steatosis alone does not appear to be progressive, approximately 20% of persons with nonalcoholic steatohepatitis progress to cirrhosis over the course of a decade.[29] Obesity, type 2 diabetes, metabolic syndrome, and hyperlipidemia are coexisting conditions frequently associated with fatty liver disease (see Chapter 33). The condition is also associated with other nutritional abnormalities, surgical conditions, and drugs.

The pathogenesis of NAFLD is thought to involve both lipid accumulation within hepatocytes and formation of free radicals, in a manner similar to that which occurs with alcohol metabolism. The primary metabolic abnormalities leading to lipid accumulation are poorly understood but are thought to include alterations in the pathways for uptake, synthesis, degradation, or secretion of hepatic lipids resulting from insulin resistance. Obesity increases the synthesis and reduces the oxidation of free fatty acids. Type 2 diabetes or insulin resistance also increases adipose tissue lipolysis and the subsequent production of free fatty acids.[29] When the capacity of the liver to export triglyceride is exceeded, excess fatty acids contribute to the development of steatosis and fatty liver disease. Both ketones and free fatty acids are inducers of previously described CYP enzymes of the MEOS pathway, which results in free radical formation, including hydrogen peroxide and superoxide. Abnormal lipid peroxidation ensues, followed by direct hepatocyte injury, release of toxic by-products, inflammation, and fibrosis.

Nonalcoholic fatty liver disease is usually asymptomatic, although fatigue and discomfort in the right upper quadrant of the abdomen may be present. Mildly to moderately elevated serum levels of AST, ALT, or both are the most common and often the only abnormal laboratory findings. Other abnormalities, including hypoalbuminemia, a prolonged prothrombin time, and hyperbilirubinemia, may be present in persons with cirrhotic-stage liver disease. The diagnosis of NAFLD can be made clinically with plasma liver aminotransferase levels, ultrasonography, and exclusion of alcohol. Liver biopsy is not routinely used unless there is concern for nonalcoholic steatohepatitis or advanced fibrosis.

The aim of treatment is to slow progression of NAFLD and to prevent liver-related illness. Both weight loss and exercise improve insulin resistance and are recommended in conjunction with treatment of associated metabolic disturbances. Alcohol use should be avoided. Vitamin E replacement has recently been found to improve steatosis in those with aggressive steatosis who do not have diabetes or cirrhosis. Oxidative stress in the liver results from an imbalance between production of reactive oxygen species (free radicals) and decreased antioxidant defenses. Vitamin E is an antioxidant that prevents propagation of free radicals and thereby decreases liver inflammation caused by oxidative stress.[30] Disease progression is slow and the magnitude of disease-related morbidity and mortality is uncertain. Liver transplantation is an alternative for some persons with end-stage liver disease, but NAFLD may recur or develop after liver transplantation.[29]

Hepatic Syndromes

Like other organs, the liver responds to a variety of insults with similar cellular and tissue responses, including hepatocyte degeneration, necrosis and apoptosis, and fibrosis. Clinically, these changes can lead to one or more characteristic syndromes, including cirrhosis, portal hypertension, and liver failure.

Cirrhosis

Cirrhosis represents the end stage of chronic liver diseases in which much of the functional liver tissue has been replaced by fibrous tissue. Although cirrhosis usually is associated with alcoholism, it can develop in the course of other disorders, including viral hepatitis, nonalcoholic liver disease, and biliary disease.[31,32] Cirrhosis also accompanies metabolic disorders that cause the deposition of minerals in the liver. Two of these disorders are hemochromatosis (i.e., iron deposition) and Wilson disease (i.e., copper deposition).

Cirrhosis is characterized by diffuse fibrosis and conversion of normal liver architecture into nodules containing proliferating hepatocytes encircled by fibrosis. The formation of nodules, which vary in size from very small (<3 mm, micronodules) to large (several centimeters, macronodules), represents a balance between regenerative activity and constrictive scarring.[3,4] The fibrous tissue that replaces normally functioning liver tissue forms constrictive bands that disrupt flow in the vascular channels and biliary duct systems of the liver. The disruption of vascular channels predisposes to portal hypertension and its complications; obstruction of biliary channels and exposure to the destructive effects of bile stasis; and loss of liver cells, leading to liver failure.

The manifestations of cirrhosis are variable, ranging from asymptomatic hepatomegaly to hepatic failure (Fig. 30-11). Often there are no symptoms until the disease is far advanced.[31] The most common signs and symptoms of cirrhosis are weight loss (sometimes masked by ascites), cachexia, weakness, and anorexia. Diarrhea frequently is present, although some persons may complain of constipation. There may be abdominal pain because of liver enlargement or stretching of the liver's fibrous tissue capsule. This pain is located in the epigastric area or in the upper right quadrant and is described as dull, aching, and causing a sensation of fullness.

The late manifestations of cirrhosis are related to portal hypertension and liver cell failure. Splenomegaly, ascites, and portosystemic shunts (i.e., esophageal varices, gastric varices, and caput medusae) result from portal hypertension. Other complications include bleeding due

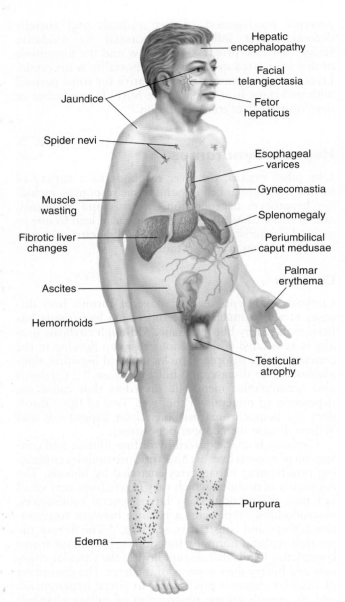

Hepatic encephalopathy

Facial telangiectasia

Fetor hepaticus

Jaundice

Spider nevi

Esophageal varices

Gynecomastia

Muscle wasting

Splenomegaly

Fibrotic liver changes

Periumbilical caput medusae

Palmar erythema

Ascites

Hemorrhoids

Testicular atrophy

Purpura

Edema

FIGURE 30-11. Clinical manifestations of cirrhosis.

obstructions.[3,4] *Prehepatic* causes of portal hypertension include obstructive thrombosis, narrowing of the portal vein before it enters the liver, and massive splenomegaly with increased splenic blood flow. The main *posthepatic* causes are right-sided heart failure and hepatic vein outflow obstruction. The dominant *intrahepatic* cause of portal hypertension is cirrhosis, in which bands of fibrous tissue and fibrous nodules distort the architecture of the liver and increase the resistance to blood flow.

The major clinical consequences of portal hypertension arise from the increased pressure and dilation of the venous channels behind the obstruction. In addition, collateral channels open that connect the portal circulation with the systemic venous circulation. The complications of the increased portal vein pressure and the opening of collateral channels are ascites, congestive splenomegaly, and the formation of portosystemic shunts with bleeding from esophageal varices (Fig. 30-12).

Ascites. Ascites occurs when the amount of fluid in the peritoneal cavity is increased. It is a late-stage manifestation of cirrhosis and portal hypertension.[3,4,34] Ascites usually becomes clinically evident when at least 500 mL of fluid has accumulated. However, the amount may be so great (frequently several liters) that it not only distends the abdomen, but also interferes with breathing. The fluid is generally serous, having less than 3 g of protein (largely albumin) and a concentration of solutes (glucose, sodium, and potassium) similar to that in the blood.

Although the mechanisms responsible for the development of ascites are not completely understood, several factors appear to contribute to fluid accumulation, including an increase in hydrostatic pressure due to portal hypertension, salt and water retention by the kidney, and decreased colloidal osmotic pressure due to impaired synthesis of albumin by the liver. Diminished blood volume (i.e., underfill theory) and excessive blood volume (i.e., overfill theory) have been used to explain the increased salt and water retention by the kidney. According to the underfill theory, a contraction in the effective blood volume causes the kidney to retain salt and water. The effective blood volume may be reduced because of loss of fluid into the peritoneal cavity or because of vasodilation caused by the presence of circulating vasodilating substances. The overfill theory proposes that the initial event in the development of ascites is renal retention of salt and water caused by disturbances in the liver itself. These disturbances include failure of the liver to metabolize aldosterone, causing an increase in salt and water retention by the kidney. Another likely contributing factor in the pathogenesis of ascites is a decreased colloidal osmotic pressure, which limits reabsorption of fluid from the peritoneal cavity (see Chapter 8).

Treatment of ascites usually focuses on dietary restriction of sodium and administration of diuretics.[34] Water intake also may need to be restricted. Because of the many limitations in sodium restriction, the use of diuretics has become the mainstay of treatment for ascites.

to decreased clotting factors, thrombocytopenia due to splenomegaly, gynecomastia, and a feminizing pattern of pubic hair distribution in men because of testicular atrophy, spider angiomas, palmar erythema, and hepatic encephalopathy.

Portal Hypertension

Portal hypertension is characterized by increased resistance to flow in the portal venous system and sustained increase in portal venous pressure.[3,4,33] Normally, venous blood returning to the heart from the abdominal organs collects in the portal vein and travels through the liver before entering the vena cava (see Fig. 30-2). Portal hypertension can be caused by a variety of conditions that increase resistance to hepatic blood flow, including prehepatic, posthepatic, and intrahepatic

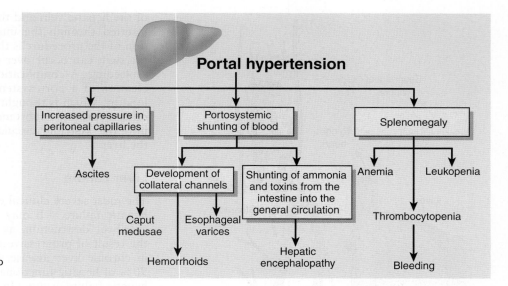

FIGURE 30-12. Mechanisms of disturbed liver function related to portal hypertension.

Two classes of diuretics are used: a diuretic that acts in the distal part of the nephron to inhibit aldosterone-dependent sodium reabsorption, and a loop diuretic such as furosemide (see Chapter 24). Oral potassium supplements often are given to prevent hypokalemia. Large-volume paracentesis (removal of 5 L or more of ascitic fluid) may be done in persons with massive ascites and pulmonary compromise.[34] Because the removal of fluid produces a decrease in vascular volume along with increased plasma renin activity and aldosterone-mediated sodium and water reabsorption by the kidneys, a volume expander such as albumin usually is administered to maintain the effective circulating volume. A transjugular intrahepatic portosystemic shunt may be inserted in persons with refractory ascites (to be discussed).[34]

Spontaneous bacterial peritonitis is a potential complication in persons with both cirrhosis and ascites. The infection is serious and carries a high mortality rate even when treated with antibiotics. Presumably, the peritoneal fluid is seeded with bacteria from the blood or lymph or from passage of bacteria through the bowel wall. Symptoms include fever and abdominal pain. Other symptoms include worsening of hepatic encephalopathy, diarrhea, hypothermia, and shock. It is diagnosed by a neutrophil count of 250/mm³ or higher and a protein concentration of 1 g/dL or less in the ascitic fluid.[34]

Splenomegaly. The spleen enlarges progressively in portal hypertension because of shunting of blood into the splenic vein.[3] The enlarged spleen often gives rise to sequestering of a significant number of blood elements and development of a syndrome known as *hypersplenism.* Hypersplenism is characterized by a decrease in the life span of all the formed elements of the blood and a subsequent decrease in their numbers, leading to anemia, thrombocytopenia, and leukopenia. The decreased life span of the blood elements is thought to result from an increased rate of removal because of the prolonged transit time through the enlarged spleen.

Portosystemic Shunts and Esophageal Varices. With the gradual obstruction of venous blood flow in the liver, the pressure in the portal vein increases, and large collateral channels develop between the portal and systemic veins that supply the lower rectum and esophagus and the umbilical veins of the falciform ligament that attaches to the anterior wall of the abdomen.[3,4] The collaterals between the inferior and internal iliac veins may give rise to hemorrhoids. In some persons, the fetal umbilical vein is not totally obliterated; it forms a channel on the anterior abdominal wall. Dilated veins around the umbilicus are called *caput medusae.* Portopulmonary shunts also may develop and cause blood to bypass the pulmonary capillaries, interfering with blood oxygenation and producing cyanosis.

Clinically, the most important collateral channels are those connecting the portal and coronary veins that lead to reversal of flow and formation of thin-walled varicosities in the submucosa of the esophagus and stomach[3,4,33,35] (Fig. 30-13). These thin-walled *varices* are subject to rupture, producing massive and sometimes fatal hemorrhage. Impaired hepatic synthesis of coagulation factors and decreased platelet levels (i.e., thrombocytopenia) due to splenomegaly may further complicate the control of esophageal bleeding.

Treatment of portal hypertension and esophageal varices is directed at prevention of initial hemorrhage, management of acute hemorrhage, and prevention of recurrent hemorrhage. Pharmacologic therapy is used to lower portal venous pressure and prevent initial hemorrhage. Nonselective β-adrenergic blocking drugs (propranolol, nadolol) commonly are used for this purpose.[33] These agents reduce portal venous pressure by decreasing splanchnic blood flow and thereby decreasing blood flow in collateral channels.

Several methods are used to control acute hemorrhage, including pharmacologic therapy, balloon tamponade, and emergent endoscopic therapy.[33,35] Pharmacologic methods include the administration of octreotide, a long-acting synthetic analog of somatostatin. Somatostatin,

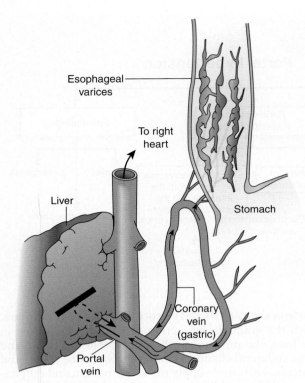

FIGURE 30-13. Obstruction of blood flow in the portal circulation, with portal hypertension and diversion of blood flow to other venous channels, including the gastric and esophageal veins.

which is normally produced by enteric cells in the gastrointestinal tract, by delta cells in the endocrine pancreas, and from the hypothalamus, reduces splanchnic and hepatic blood flow and portal pressures in persons with cirrhosis. The drug, which is given intravenously, provides control of variceal bleeding in up to 80% of cases.[35] Balloon tamponade provides compression of the varices and is accomplished through the insertion of a tube with inflatable gastric and esophageal balloons. After the tube has been inserted, the balloons are inflated; the esophageal balloon compresses the bleeding esophageal veins, and the gastric balloon helps to maintain the position of the tube. Emergent endoscopic procedures include sclerotherapy, in which the varices are injected with a sclerosing solution that obliterates the vessel lumen, and ligation, in which a band is inserted around the bleeding vessel.

Prevention of recurrent hemorrhage focuses on lowering portal venous pressure and diverting blood flow away from the easily ruptured collateral channels.[33] Two procedures may be used for this purpose: the surgical creation of a portosystemic shunt or a transjugular intrahepatic portosystemic shunt (TIPS). *Surgical portosystemic shunt* procedures involve the creation of an opening between the portal vein and a systemic vein. These shunts have a considerable complication rate, and TIPS has evolved as the preferred treatment for refractory portal hypertension. The TIPS procedure involves insertion of an expandable metal stent between a branch of the hepatic vein and the portal vein using a catheter inserted through the internal jugular vein. A limitation of the procedure is that stenosis and thrombosis of the stent can occur over time, with consequent risk of rebleeding. A complication that is associated with the creation of a portosystemic shunt is hepatic encephalopathy, which is thought to result when ammonia and other neurotoxic substances from the gut pass directly into the systemic circulation without going through the liver.

Liver Failure

The most severe clinical consequence of liver disease is hepatic failure.[3,4] It may result from sudden and massive liver destruction, as in fulminant hepatitis, or be the result of progressive damage to the liver, as occurs in chronic liver disease. Whatever the cause, 80% to 90% of hepatic functional capacity must be lost before hepatic failure occurs.[3] In many cases, the effects of progressive liver disease are hastened by disesase complications that results in gastrointestinal bleeding, systemic infection, electrolyte disturbances, or superimposed diseases such as heart failure.

Manifestations. The manifestations of liver failure reflect the various synthesis, storage, metabolic, and elimination functions of the liver (Fig. 30-14). *Fetor hepaticus* refers to a characteristic musty, sweetish odor of the breath in the person in advanced liver failure, resulting from the metabolic by-products of the intestinal bacteria.

Liver failure can cause *anemia, thrombocytopenia, coagulation defects,* and *leukopenia.* Anemia may be caused by blood loss, excessive red blood cell destruction, and impaired formation of red blood cells. A folic acid deficiency may lead to severe megaloblastic anemia. Changes in the lipid composition of the red blood cell membrane increase hemolysis. Because many clotting factors are synthesized by the liver, their decline in liver disease contributes to bleeding disorders. Malabsorption of the fat-soluble vitamin K contributes further to the impaired synthesis of these clotting factors. Thrombocytopenia often occurs as the result of splenomegaly. These factors increase the risk of easy bruising as well as abnormal menstrual bleeding and bleeding from the esophagus and other segments of the gastrointestinal tract.

Endocrine disorders, particularly disturbances in gonadal (sex hormone) function, are common accompaniments of cirrhosis and liver failure. Women may have menstrual irregularities (usually amenorrhea), loss of libido, and sterility. In men, testosterone levels usually fall, the testes atrophy, and loss of libido, impotence, and gynecomastia occur. A decrease in aldosterone metabolism may contribute to salt and water retention by the kidney, along with a lowering of serum potassium resulting from increased elimination of potassium.

Liver failure also brings on numerous *skin disorders.* These lesions, called variously *vascular spiders, telangiectases, spider angiomas,* and *spider nevi,* are seen most

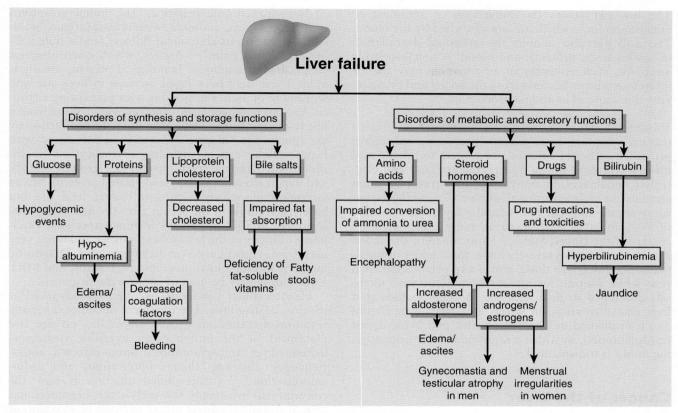

FIGURE 30-14. Alterations in liver function and manifestations of liver failure.

often in the upper half of the body. They consist of a central pulsating arteriole from which smaller vessels radiate. Palmar erythema is redness of the palms, probably caused by increased blood flow from higher cardiac output. Clubbing of the fingers may be seen in persons with cirrhosis. Jaundice usually is a late manifestation of liver failure.

The *hepatorenal syndrome* refers to a functional renal failure sometimes seen during the terminal stages of liver failure with ascites.[36] It is characterized by progressive azotemia, increased serum creatinine levels, and oliguria. Although the basic cause is unknown, a decrease in renal blood flow is believed to play a part. Ultimately, when renal failure is superimposed on liver failure, azotemia and elevated levels of blood ammonia occur; this condition is thought to contribute to hepatic encephalopathy and coma.

Hepatic encephalopathy refers to the totality of central nervous system manifestations of liver failure.[3,37] It is characterized by neural disturbances ranging from a lack of mental alertness to confusion, coma, and convulsions. A very early sign of hepatic encephalopathy is a flapping tremor called *asterixis*. Various degrees of memory loss may occur, coupled with personality changes such as euphoria, irritability, anxiety, and lack of concern about personal appearance and self. Speech may be impaired, and the person may be unable to perform certain purposeful movements. The encephalopathy may progress to decerebrate rigidity and then to a terminal deep coma.

Although the cause of hepatic encephalopathy is unknown, the accumulation of neurotoxins, which appear in the blood because the liver has lost its detoxifying capacity, is believed to be a factor. Hepatic encephalopathy develops in approximately 10% of persons with portosystemic shunts. One of the suspected neurotoxins is ammonia. A particularly important function of the liver is the conversion of ammonia, a by-product of protein and amino acid metabolism, to urea. The ammonium ion is produced in abundance in the intestinal tract, particularly in the colon, by the bacterial degradation of luminal proteins and amino acids. Normally, these ammonium ions diffuse into the portal blood and are transported to the liver, where they are converted to urea before entering the general circulation. When the blood from the intestine bypasses the liver or the liver is unable to convert ammonia to urea, ammonia moves directly into the general circulation and from there to the cerebral circulation. Hepatic encephalopathy may become worse after a large protein meal or gastrointestinal tract bleeding. Narcotics and tranquilizers are poorly metabolized by the liver, and administration of these drugs may contribute to central nervous system depression and precipitate hepatic encephalopathy.

Lactulose is a drug often used in hepatic encephalopathy. It is not absorbed from the small intestine but moves directly to the large intestine, where it is broken down by colonic bacteria to small organic acids that cause production of large, loose stools with a low pH.

The low pH favors the conversion of ammonia to ammonium ions, which are not absorbed by the blood. The acid pH also inhibits the intestinal degradation of amino acids, proteins, and blood. A nonabsorbable antibiotic, such as neomycin, or rifaximin may also be given to eradicate bacteria from the bowel and thus prevent this cause of ammonia production.[38]

Treatment. The treatment of liver failure is directed toward symptom management; preventing infections; providing sufficient calories and protein to rebuild and maintain protein stores; and correcting fluid and electrolyte imbalances. In many cases, liver transplantation remains the only effective treatment. Currently, 1-year survival rates approach 90%, and a 5-year survival rate of 70% to 80% is achieved at many transplantation centers in the United States.[39] Unfortunately, the shortage of donor organs severely limits the number of transplantations that are done, and many persons die each year while waiting for a transplant. Innovative methods developed to deal with the shortage include split liver transplantation, in which a cadaver liver is split and transplanted into two recipients, and living donor transplantation, in which a segment or lobe from a living donor is transplanted.[39]

Cancer of the Liver

Malignant tumors of the liver can be primary or metastatic. Although primary tumors of the liver are relatively rare in developed countries of the world, the liver shares with the lung the distinction of being the most common site of metastatic tumors.

Primary Liver Cancers

There are two major types of primary liver cancer: hepatocellular carcinoma, which arises from the liver cells, and cholangiocarcinoma, which is a primary cancer of bile duct cells.[3,4]

Hepatocellular Carcinoma. Hepatocellular carcinoma, the most common form of liver cancer, is the fifth most common cancer and third leading cause of cancer-related mortality worldwide.[40] In Europe, Australia, and the United States, the incidence is approximately 3 cases per 100,000. There has been an increased incidence, however, in developed countries as a consequence of chronic HCV infection.[40]

Among the factors identified as etiologic agents in liver cancer are chronic hepatitis B and C, chronic alcoholism, nonalcoholic fatty liver disease, and long-term exposure to environmental agents such as aflatoxin.[3,41] Aflatoxins, produced by food spoilage molds in certain areas endemic for hepatocellular carcinoma, are particularly potent carcinogenic agents.[3] They are activated by hepatocytes and their products incorporated into the host DNA with the potential for developing cancer-producing mutations.

The manifestations of hepatocellular cancer often are insidious in onset and masked by those related to cirrhosis or chronic hepatitis. The initial symptoms include weakness, anorexia, weight loss, fatigue, bloating, a sensation of abdominal fullness, and a dull, aching abdominal pain.[40,41] Ascites, which often obscures weight loss, is common. Jaundice, if present, usually is mild. There may be a rapid increase in liver size and worsening of ascites in persons with preexisting cirrhosis. Various paraneoplastic syndromes (e.g., disturbances due to ectopic hormone or growth factor production by the tumor (see Chapter 7) have been associated with hepatocellular cancer, including erythrocytosis (erythropoietin), hypoglycemia (insulin-like growth factor), and hypercalcemia (parathyroid-related protein). Serum α-fetoprotein, which is present during fetal life but barely detectable in the serum after the age of 2 years, is present in 50% of persons with hepatocellular carcinoma.[3] However, the test lacks specificity and is not very useful as a surveillance or diagnostic tool. Diagnostic methods include ultrasonography, CT scans, and MRI. Liver biopsy may be used to confirm the diagnosis.

Hepatocellular carcinoma is often far advanced at the time of diagnosis. The treatment of choice is hepatic resection if conditions permit. Depending on size and placement of the tumor, other available treatments include liver transplantation, tumor-directed radiofrequency ablation, chemoembolization, and radioembolization.[41,42] Image-guided ablation is now the conventional treatment for early-stage hepatocellular cancer. Ablation induces tumor necrosis by injection of chemicals (ethanol, acetic acid) or temperature modification (radiofrequency, microwave, laser, or cryoablation) into the tumor area. Sorefenib, a chemotherrapeutic agent that is taken orally, has recently been approved for the treatment of hepatocellular carcinoma.[41,42]

Cholangiocarcinoma. Cholangiocarcinoma is a malignancy of the biliary tree, arising from bile ducts within and outside the liver. It accounts for 7.6% of cancer deaths worldwide and 3% of cancer deaths in the United States.[3] The etiology, clinical features, and prognosis vary considerably with the part of the biliary tree that is the site of origin. Cholangiocarcinoma is not associated with the same risk factors as hepatocellular carcinoma. Instead, most of the risk factors revolve around long-standing inflammation and injury of the bile duct epithelium. Cholangiocarcinoma often presents with pain, weight loss, anorexia, and abdominal swelling or awareness of a mass in the right hypochondrium. Tumors affecting the central or distal bile ducts may present with jaundice.

Metastatic Tumors

Metastatic tumors of the liver are much more common than primary tumors.[3,4] Common sources include colorectal, breast, lung, and urogenital cancer. In addition, tumors of neuroendocrine origin spread to the liver. It often is difficult to distinguish primary from metastatic tumors with the use of CT scans, MRI, or ultrasonography. Usually the diagnosis is confirmed by biopsy.

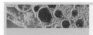
SUMMARY CONCEPTS

■ The liver is subject to most of the disease processes that affect other body structures, such as infections, autoimmune disorders, toxic injury, metabolic diseases, and neoplasms.

■ Hepatitis is characterized by inflammation of the liver. Viral hepatitis is caused by hepatitis viruses A, B, C, D, and E, which differ in terms of mode of transmission, incubation period, mechanism, degree and chronicity of liver damage, and ability to evolve to a carrier state. Autoimmune hepatitis involves the immune destruction of hepatocytes causing inflammation.

■ Intrahepatic biliary diseases disrupt the flow of bile through the liver, causing cholestasis and biliary cirrhosis. Causes of intrahepatic biliary diseases include primary biliary cirrhosis, primary sclerosing cholangitis, and secondary biliary cirrhosis.

■ The liver, which is the major drug-metabolizing and detoxifying organ in the body, is subject to potential damage from an enormous array of pharmaceutical and environmental chemicals. There are two types of drug reactions: predictable, based on the drug's chemical structure and metabolites, and idiosyncratic, based on individual characteristics of the person receiving the drug.

■ Cirrhosis represents the end stage of chronic liver disease in which much of the liver's functional tissue has been replaced by fibrous tissue that disrupts venous blood flow predisposing to portal hypertension and its complications, loss of liver cells, and eventual liver failure.

■ Portal hypertension is characterized by increased resistance to flow and increased pressure in the portal venous system, the pathologic consequences of which include ascites, the formation of collateral bypass channels (e.g., esophageal varices), and splenomegaly.

■ The manifestations of liver failure reflect the various functions of the liver, including hematologic disorders, disruption of endocrine function, skin disorders, hepatorenal syndrome, and hepatic encephalopathy.

■ There are two types of primary cancers of the liver. Hepatocellular cancer, the most common form, is derived from hepatocytes and their precursors and is associated with conditions such as chronic hepatitis B and C infection and alcoholic cirrhosis. Cholangiocarcinoma, or bile duct cancer, arises from the biliary epithelium, typically following long-standing inflammation of the bile ducts.

Disorders of the Hepatobiliary System and Exocrine Pancreas

The hepatobiliary system consists of the gallbladder; the left and right hepatic ducts, which come together to form the common hepatic duct; the cystic duct, which extends to the gallbladder; and the bile duct, which is formed by the union of the common hepatic duct and the cystic duct[2] (Fig. 30-15). The bile duct descends posteriorly to the first part of the duodenum, where it comes in contact with the main pancreatic duct. These ducts unite to form the hepatopancreatic ampulla. The circular muscle around the distal end of the bile duct is thickened to form the sphincter of the bile duct.

The pancreas lies transversely in the posterior part of the upper abdomen (see Fig. 30-1). The head of the pancreas is at the right of the abdomen; it rests against the curve of the duodenum in the area of the hepatopancreatic ampulla and its entrance into the duodenum. The body of the pancreas lies beneath the stomach, with the tail touching the spleen. The pancreas is virtually hidden because of its posterior position; unlike many other organs, it cannot be palpated. Because of the position of the pancreas and its large functional reserve, symptoms from conditions such as cancer of the pancreas do not usually appear until the disorder is far advanced.

Disorders of the Hepatobiliary System

The gallbladder is a distensible, pear-shaped muscular sac located on the ventral surface of the liver.[2] It has an outer serous peritoneal layer, a middle smooth muscle layer, and an inner mucosal layer that is continuous with the lining of the bile duct. The function of the gallbladder is to store and concentrate bile. In the gallbladder, water and electrolytes are absorbed from the bile, causing the concentration of bile salts and lecithin to increase, along with that of cholesterol; in this way, the solubility of cholesterol is maintained.

Entrance of food into the intestine causes the gallbladder to contract and the sphincter of the bile duct to relax, such that bile stored in the gallbladder moves into the duodenum. The stimulus for gallbladder contraction is primarily hormonal. Products of food digestion, particularly lipids, stimulate the release of a gastrointestinal hormone called *cholecystokinin* from the mucosa of the duodenum. Cholecystokinin provides a strong stimulus for gallbladder contraction. The role of other gastrointestinal hormones in bile release is less clearly understood.

Passage of bile into the intestine is regulated largely by the pressure in the common bile duct. Normally, the gallbladder regulates this pressure. It collects and stores bile as it relaxes and the pressure in the common bile duct decreases, and it empties bile into the intestine as the gallbladder contracts, producing an increase in common duct pressure. After gallbladder surgery, the

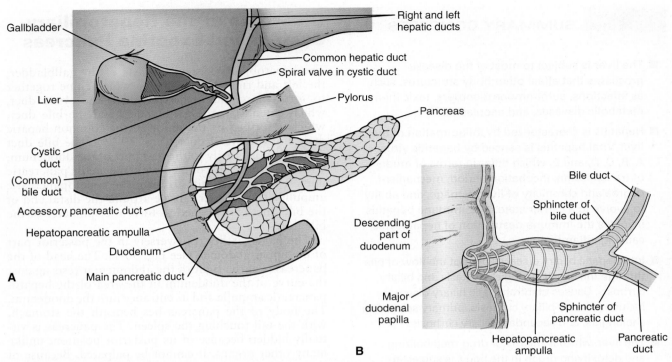

FIGURE 30-15. (A) Extrahepatic bile passages, gallbladder, and pancreatic ducts. **(B)** Entry of bile duct and pancreatic duct into the hepatopancreatic ampulla, which opens into the duodenum.

pressure in the common bile duct changes, causing it to dilate. The flow of bile then is regulated by the duct sphincters.

Common disorders of the biliary system are cholelithiasis (i.e., gallstones) and inflammation of the gallbladder (cholecystitis) or common bile duct (cholangitis). Cancer of the gallbladder is less common.

Cholelithiasis

Cholelithiasis is caused by precipitation of substances contained in bile, mainly cholesterol and bilirubin. Approximately 80% of gallstones are composed primarily of cholesterol; the other 20% are black or brown pigment stones consisting of calcium salts with bilirubin.[3] Pigment stones containing bilirubin are seen in persons with hemolytic disease (e.g., sickle cell disease) and hepatic cirrhosis. Many stones have a mixed composition. Figure 30-16 shows a gallbladder with numerous cholesterol gallstones.

Three factors contribute to the formation of gallstones: abnormalities in the composition of bile, stasis of bile, and inflammation of the gallbladder.[3,4] The formation of cholesterol stones is associated with obesity and occurs more frequently in women, especially women who have had multiple pregnancies or who are taking oral contraceptives. All of these factors cause the liver to excrete more cholesterol into the bile. Estrogen reduces the synthesis of bile acid in women. Gallbladder sludge (thickened gallbladder mucoprotein with tiny trapped cholesterol crystals) is thought to be a precursor of gallstones. Sludge frequently occurs with pregnancy,

starvation, and rapid weight loss. Drugs that lower serum cholesterol levels, such as clofibrate, also cause increased cholesterol excretion into the bile. Malabsorption disorders stemming from ileal disease or intestinal bypass surgery tend to interfere with the absorption of bile salts, which are needed to maintain the solubility of cholesterol. Inflammation of the gallbladder alters the absorptive characteristics of the mucosal layer, allowing excessive absorption of water and bile salts.

At least 10% of adults have gallstones.[3,4] There is an increased prevalence with age, and approximately twice as many white women as men have gallstones.[3] They are extremely common among Native Americans, which suggests that a genetic component may have a role in gallstone formation.

Many persons with gallstones have no symptoms. Gallstones cause symptoms when they obstruct bile flow.[43] Small stones (<8 mm in diameter) pass into the common duct, producing symptoms of indigestion and biliary colic. Larger stones are more likely to obstruct flow and cause jaundice. The pain of biliary colic is usually located in the upper right quadrant or epigastric area and may be referred to the upper back, right shoulder, or midscapular region. Typically the pain is abrupt in onset, increases steadily in intensity, persists for 2 to 8 hours, and is followed by soreness in the upper right quadrant.

Acute Cholecystitis

Acute cholecystitis is a diffuse inflammation of the gallbladder, usually secondary to obstruction of the gallbladder outlet. Most cases of acute cholecystitis

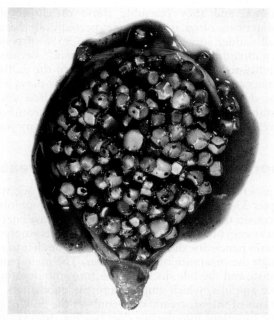

FIGURE 30-16. Cholesterol gallstones. The gallbladder has been opened to reveal numerous yellow cholesterol gallstones. (From Herrine SK, Navarro VJ, Rubin R. The liver and biliary system. In: Rubin R, Strayer DS, eds. *Rubin's Pathology: Clinicopathologic Foundations of Medicine.* 6th ed. Philadelphia, PA: Wolters Kluwer Health | Lippincott Williams & Wilkins; 2012:732.)

(85% to 90%) are associated with the presence of gallstones (calculous cholecystitis).[3,4,44,45] The remaining cases (acalculous cholecystitis) are associated with sepsis, severe trauma, or infection of the gallbladder. Acute acalculous cholecystitis, which involves ischemic rather than inflammatory changes associated with stones, can rapidly progress to gangrene and perforation.[44]

Acute *calculous* cholecystitis occurs when a stone becomes impacted in the cystic duct and inflammation develops behind the obstruction. It has been theorized that obstruction of the cystic duct leads to the release of mucosal phospholipase from the epithelium of the gallbladder. These lipases, in turn, lead to disruption of the normal glycoprotein mucous layer, exposing the mucosal epithelium to the destructive action of concentrated bile salts.[3,4] Acute *acalculous* cholecystitis is thought to result from ischemia. The cystic artery is an end artery with essentially no collateral circulation.[3] Contributing factors may include inflammation and edema of the gallbladder wall, stasis of bile, and conditions that lead to cystic duct obstruction in the absence of frank stone formation. Risk factors for acute acalculous cholecystitis include sepsis with hypotension and multisystem organ failure, immunosuppression, major trauma and burns, diabetes mellitus, and infections.[3,44]

Persons with acute cholecystitis usually experience an sudden onset of upper right quadrant or epigastric pain, frequently associated with mild fever, anorexia, nausea, vomiting.[43–45] Whereas in biliary colic the cystic duct obstruction is transient, in acute cholecystitis it is persistent. Persons with calculous cholecystitis usually, but

not always, have experienced previous episodes of biliary pain. The pain may appear with remarkable suddenness and constitute a surgical emergency. In the absence of medical attention, the attack usually subsides in 7 to 10 days and frequently within 24 hours. In persons who recover, recurrence is common. The onset of acalculous cholecystitis tends to be more insidious because the manifestations are obscured by the underlying conditions precipitating the attack. In the severely ill patient, early recognition is crucial because a delay in treatment can prove life-threatening. Persons with acute cholecystitis usually have an elevated white blood cell count and many have mild elevations in AST, ALT, ALP, and bilirubin.

Chronic Cholecystitis

Chronic cholecystitis results from repeated episodes of acute cholecystitis or chronic irritation of the gallbladder by stones.[3,4] It is characterized by varying degrees of chronic inflammation. Gallstones almost always are present. Cholelithiasis with chronic cholecystitis may be associated with acute exacerbations of gallbladder inflammation, common duct stones, pancreatitis, and, rarely, carcinoma of the gallbladder.

The manifestations of chronic cholecystitis are more vague than those of acute cholecystitis. There may be intolerance to fatty foods, belching, and other indications of discomfort. Often, there are episodes of colicky pain with obstruction of biliary flow caused by gallstones. The gallbladder, which in chronic cholecystitis usually contains stones, may be enlarged, shrunken, or of normal size.

Diagnosis and Treatment of Gallbladder Disease

The methods used to diagnose gallbladder disease include ultrasonography, cholescintigraphy (nuclear scanning), and CT scans.[43–45] Ultrasonography is widely used in diagnosing gallbladder disease and has largely replaced the oral cholecystogram in most medical centers. It can detect stones as small as 1 to 2 cm, and its overall accuracy in detecting gallbladder disease is high. In addition to stones, ultrasonography can detect wall thickening, which indicates inflammation. It also can rule out other causes of right upper quadrant pain such as tumors. Cholescintigraphy, also called a *gallbladder scan*, relies on the ability of the liver to extract a rapidly injected radionuclide, technetium-99m, bound to one of several iminodiacetic acids, that is excreted into the bile ducts. Serial scanning images are obtained within several minutes of the injection of the tracer and every 10 to 15 minutes during the next hour. The gallbladder scan is highly accurate in detecting acute cholecystitis. Although CT is not as accurate as ultrasonography in detecting gallstones, it can show thickening of the gallbladder wall or pericholecystic fluid associated with acute cholecystitis.

Gallbladder disease usually is treated by removing the gallbladder. The gallbladder stores and concentrates bile, and its removal usually does not interfere with digestion. Laparoscopic cholecystectomy has become the treatment of choice for symptomatic gallbladder disease.[45] The procedure involves insertion of a laparoscope through a small incision near the umbilicus, and surgical instruments are inserted through several stab wounds in the upper abdomen. Although the procedure requires more time than the older open surgical procedure, it usually requires only 1 night in the hospital. A major advantage of the procedure is that patients can return to work in 1 to 2 weeks, compared with 4 to 6 weeks after open cholecystectomy.

Choledocholithiasis and Cholangitis

Choledocholithiasis refers to stones in the common duct and *cholangitis* to inflammation of the common bile duct.[3,43] Common bile duct stones usually originate in the gallbladder, but can form spontaneously in the common duct.

The manifestations of choledocholithiasis are similar to those of gallstones and acute cholecystitis. There is a history of acute biliary colic and right upper abdominal pain, with chills, fever, and jaundice associated with episodes of abdominal pain. Bilirubinuria and an elevated serum bilirubin are present if the common duct is obstructed. Complications include acute suppurative cholangitis accompanied by pus in the common duct. It is characterized by the presence of an altered sensorium, lethargy, and septic shock.[3] Acute suppurative cholangitis represents an endoscopic or surgical emergency. Common duct stones also can obstruct the outflow of the pancreatic duct, causing secondary pancreatitis.

Ultrasonography, CT scans, and radionuclide imaging may be used to demonstrate dilation of bile ducts and impaired blood flow. Endoscopic ultrasonography and magnetic resonance cholangiography are used for detecting common duct stones. Both percutaneous transhepatic cholangiography (PTC) and endoscopic retrograde cholangiopancreatography (ERCP) provide a direct means for determining the cause, location, and extent of obstruction. Percutaneous transhepatic cholangiography involves the injection of dye directly into the biliary tree. It requires the insertion of a thin, flexible needle through a small incision in the skin with advancement into the biliary tree. Endoscopic retrograde cholangiopancreatography involves the passage of an endoscope into the duodenum and the passage of a catheter into the hepatopancreatic ampulla. Endoscopic retrograde cholangiopancreatography can be used to enlarge the opening of the sphincter of the bile duct, which may allow the lodged stone to pass, or an instrument may be inserted into the bile duct to remove the stone.

Common duct stones in persons with cholelithiasis usually are treated by stone extraction followed by laparoscopic cholecystectomy. Antibiotic therapy, with an agent that enters the bile, is used to treat suppurative cholangitis. Emergency decompression of the common duct, usually by ERCP, may be necessary for persons who are septic or fail to improve with antibiotic treatment.

Cancer of the Gallbladder

Cancer of the gallbladder is the fifth most common cancer of the gastrointestinal tract. It is slightly more common in women and occurs more often in the seventh decade of life. The onset of symptoms usually is insidious, and they resemble those of cholecystitis; the diagnosis often is made unexpectedly at the time of gallbladder surgery. About 80% to 85% of persons with gallbladder cancer have cholelithiasis.[46] Because of its ability to produce chronic irritation of the gallbladder mucosa, it is believed that cholelithiasis plays a role in the development of gallbladder cancer. It is seldom resectable at the time of diagnosis, and the mean 5-year survival rate has remained a dismal 1% for many years.[3]

Disorders of the Exocrine Pancreas

The pancreas is both an exocrine and endocrine organ (see Chapter 33). The exocrine pancreas is made up of lobules that consist of acinar cells, which secrete digestive enzymes into a system of microscopic ducts. These ducts empty into the main pancreatic duct, which extends from left to right through the substance of the pancreas. The main pancreatic duct and the bile duct unite to form the hepatopancreatic ampulla, which empties into the duodenum. The sphincter of the pancreatic duct controls the flow of pancreatic secretions into the bile duct (see Fig. 30-15).

The secretions of the pancreatic acinar cells contain proteolytic enzymes, including trypsin and several others, that break down dietary proteins. The pancreas also secretes pancreatic amylase, which breaks down starch, and lipases, which hydrolyze triglycerides into glycerol and fatty acids. The pancreatic enzymes are secreted in the inactive form and become activated in the intestine. This is important because the enzymes would digest the tissue of the pancreas itself if they were secreted in the active form. The acinar cells also secrete a trypsin inhibitor, which prevents trypsin activation. Because trypsin activates other proteolytic enzymes, the trypsin inhibitor prevents subsequent activation of the other enzymes.

Although the enzymes of the pancreatic secretions are secreted entirely by the acinar cells, the other two important ingredients—bicarbonate ions and water—are secreted entirely by the epithelial cells that line the ductules and ducts leading from the acinar cells. When the pancreas is stimulated to secrete copious amounts of digestive enzymes, the epithelial cells increase their production of bicarbonate that serves to neutralize the hydrochloric acid emptied into the stomach from the duodenum.[1]

Two types of pancreatic disease are discussed in this chapter: acute and chronic pancreatitis and cancer of the pancreas.

Acute Pancreatitis

Acute pancreatitis represents a reversible inflammatory process of the pancreatic acini brought about by premature activation of pancreatic enzymes.[47–51] Although the disease process may be limited to pancreatic tissue, it also can involve peripancreatic tissues or those of more distant organs.

The pathogenesis of acute pancreatitis involves the autodigestion of pancreatic tissue by inappropriately activated pancreatic enzymes. The process is thought to begin with the activation of trypsin. Once activated, trypsin can then activate a variety of digestive enzymes that cause pancreatic injury, resulting in an intense inflammatory response. The acute inflammatory response itself causes substantial tissue damage and may progress beyond the pancreas to produce a systemic inflammatory response syndrome and multiorgan failure (see Chapter 20). Although a number of factors are associated with the development of acute pancreatitis, in the United States alcohol abuse and gallstones account for 70% to 80% of all cases.[47-51] The precise mechanisms whereby alcohol exerts its action are largely unknown; however, alcohol is known to be a potent stimulator of pancreatic secretions, and it also is known to cause partial obstruction of the sphincter of the pancreatic duct. In the case of biliary tract obstruction due to gallstones, pancreatic duct obstruction or biliary reflux is believed to activate the enzymes in the pancreatic duct system. Acute pancreatitis also is associated with hyperlipidemia, hypercalcemia, infections (particularly viral), abdominal and surgical trauma, and drugs such as thiazide diuretics.

Clinical Manifestations. The manifestations of acute pancreatitis can range from mild with minimal organ dysfunction to severe and life-threatening. Overall, about 20% of persons with acute pancreatitis have a severe course, and 10% to 30% of those with severe pancreatitis die.[49,50] The diagnosis of acute pancreatits is made by the presence of 2 of the 3 following symptoms: (1) abdominal pain;which is usually severe, located in the epigastric or left upper quadarant and may radiate to the back, chest, or flank areas; (2) serum amylase or lipase greater than 3 times the upper limit of normal; and (3) classic signs on abdominal imaging. Serum lipase may remain elevated slightly longer than amylase. However, the level of elevation of the serum amylase or lipase does not correlate with the severity of the disorder. The white blood cell count may also be increased, and hyperglycemia and an elevated serum bilirubin level may be present. Abdominal ultrasonography is usually performed to assess for gallstones. Both CT scans and dynamic contrast-enhanced CT of the pancreas are used to detect necrosis and fluid accumulation.

Physical examination findings are variable and include fever, tachycardia, hypotension, severe abdominal tenderness, respiratory distress, and abdominal distention. Recognized markers of severe disease include laboratory values that measure the inflammatory response (e.g., C-reactive protein), scoring systems that assess inflammation or organ failure, and findings on imaging studies. Clinical findings such as thirst, poor urine output, progressive tachycardia, tachypnea, hypoxemia, agitation, confusion, a rising hematocrit level, and lack of improvement in symptoms within the first 48 hours are warning signs of impending severe disease. Complications include the systemic inflammatory response, acute respiratory distress syndrome, acute tubular necrosis, and organ failure. An important disturbance related to acute pancreatitis is the loss of a large volume of fluid into the retroperitoneal and peripancreatic spaces and the abdominal cavity. Signs of hypocalcemia may develop, probably as a result of the precipitation of serum calcium in the areas of fat necrosis.

Treatment. Determination of the cause is important in guiding the immediate management and preventing recurrence. Treatment measures depend on the severity of the disease. Persons who present with persistent or severe pain, vomiting, dehydration, or signs of impending severe acute pancreatitis require hospitalization. Treatment measures are directed at pain relief, "putting the pancreas to rest" by withholding oral foods and fluids, and restoration of lost plasma volume. Meperidine rather than morphine usually is given for pain relief because it causes fewer spasms of the sphincter of the pancreatic duct. Gastric suction is instituted to treat distention of the bowel and prevent further stimulation of the secretion of pancreatic enzymes. Intravenous fluids and electrolytes are administered to replace those lost from the circulation and to combat hypotension and shock. Intravenous colloid solutions are given to replace the fluid that has become sequestered in the abdomen and retroperitoneal space.

Complications. Sequelae in persons surviving an episode of severe acute pancreatitis include fluid collections and infection.[49] In 40% to 60% of persons with acute necrotizing pancreatitis, the necrotic debris becomes infected, usually by gram-negative organisms from the alimentary canal, further complicating the condition.[47] Fluid collections with a high level of pancreatic enzymes are usually associated with pancreatic duct disruptions and may eventually form pseudocysts (a collection of pancreatic fluid enclosed in a layer of inflammatory tissue). A pseudocyst most often is connected to a pancreatic duct, so that it continues to increase in mass. The symptoms depend on its location; for example, jaundice may occur when a cyst develops near the head of the pancreas, close to the common duct. Pseudocysts may resolve or, if they persist, may require surgical intervention.

Chronic Pancreatitis

Chronic pancreatitis is characterized by progressive and permanent destruction of the exocrine pancreas, fibrosis, and, in the later stages, destruction of the endocrine pancreas.[3,4,52,53] Most factors that cause acute pancreatitis can also cause chronic pancreatitis. However, the chief distinction between the two conditions is the irreversibility of pancreatic function that is characteristic of chronic pancreatitis. By far the most common cause of chronic pancreatitis is long-term alcohol abuse. Less common causes are long-standing obstruction of the pancreatic duct by pseudocysts, calculi, or neoplasms, autoimmune disorders, primary sclerosing cholangitis, inflammatory bowel disease, cystic fibrosis (discussed in Chapter 23), and hereditary pancreatitis, a rare autosomal dominant disorder.

Chronic pancreatitis is manifested by episodes that are similar, albeit of lesser severity, to those of acute pancreatitis. Patients have persistent, recurring episodes of epigastric and upper left quadrant pain; the attacks often are precipitated by alcohol abuse or overeating. Anorexia, nausea, vomiting, constipation, and flatulence are common. Eventually the disease progresses to the extent that endocrine and exocrine pancreatic functions become deficient. At this point, signs of diabetes mellitus and the malabsorption syndrome (e.g., weight loss, fatty stools [steatorrhea]) become apparent.

Treatment consists of measures to treat coexisting biliary tract disease. A low-fat diet usually is prescribed. The signs of malabsorption may be treated with pancreatic enzymes. When diabetes is present, it is treated with insulin. Alcohol is forbidden because it frequently precipitates attacks. Because of the frequent episodes of pain, narcotic addiction is a potential problem in persons with chronic pancreatitis. Surgical intervention sometimes is needed to relieve the pain and usually focuses on relieving any obstruction that may be present.

Cancer of the Pancreas

Pancreatic cancer is now the fourth leading cause of death from cancer in the United States, preceded only by lung, colon, and breast cancer.[47,48] Considered to be one of the most deadly malignancies, pancreatic cancer is associated with a 5-year survival rate of only 4% to 6%.[47,48,54,55] The incidence of pancreatic cancer seems to be increasing in all countries studied and has tripled in the United States over the past 50 years.[48]

The cause of pancreatic cancer is unknown. Age is a major risk factor. Pancreatic cancer rarely occurs in persons younger than 50 years of age, and the risk increases with age. The most significant and reproducible environmental risk factor is cigarette smoking, which doubles the risk.[47,48,54–56] Diabetes and chronic pancreatitis also are associated with pancreatic cancer, although neither the nature nor the sequence of the possible cause-and-effect relation has been established. There has been a recent focus on the molecular genetics of pancreatic cancer.

Clinical Manifestations. Almost all pancreatic cancers are adenocarcinomas of the ductal epithelium, and symptoms are primarily caused by mass effect rather than disruption of exocrine or endocrine function. The clinical manifestations depend on the size and location of the tumor as well as its metastasis.[54–56] Pain, jaundice, and weight loss constitute the classic presentation of the disease. The most common pain is a dull epigastric pain often accompanied by back pain, often worse in the supine position, and relieved by sitting forward. Patients may also present with diabetes or impaired glucose tolerance. Because of the proximity of the pancreas to the common duct and the hepatopancreatic ampulla, cancer of the head of the pancreas tends to obstruct bile flow. Jaundice frequently is the presenting symptom of a person with cancer of the head of the pancreas, and it usually is accompanied by complaints of pain and pruritus. Cancer of the body of the pancreas usually impinges on the celiac ganglion, causing pain. The pain usually worsens with ingestion of food or assumption of the supine position. Cancer of the tail of the pancreas usually has metastasized before symptoms appear.

Migratory thrombophlebitis (deep vein thrombosis) develops in about 10% of persons with pancreatic cancer, particularly when the tumor involves the body or tail of the pancreas. Thrombi develop in multiple veins, including the deep veins of the legs, the subclavian vein, the inferior and superior mesentery veins, and even the vena cava. It is not uncommon for the migratory thrombophlebitis to provide the first evidence of pancreatic cancer, although it may present in other cancers as well. The mechanism responsible for the hypercoagulable state is largely unclear, but may relate to activation of clotting factors by proteases released from the tumor cells.[48]

Diagnosis and Treatment. Patient history, physical examination, and elevated serum bilirubin and alkaline phosphate levels may suggest the presence of pancreatic cancer but are not diagnostic.[54–56] The serum cancer antigen (CA) 19–9, a Lewis blood group antigen, may help confirm the diagnosis in symptomatic patients and may help predict prognosis and recurrence after resection. However, CA 19–9 lacks the sensitivity and specificity to effectively screen asymptomatic patients.[56] Ultrasonography and CT scanning are the most frequently used diagnostic methods to confirm the disease. Intravenous and oral contrast–enhanced spiral CT is the preferred method for imaging the pancreas. Percutaneous fine needle aspiration cytology of the pancreas has been one of the major advances in the diagnosis of pancreatic cancer. Unfortunately, the smaller and more curable tumors are most likely to be missed by this procedure. Endoscopic retrograde cholangiopancreatography may be used for evaluation of persons with suspected pancreatic cancer and obstructive jaundice.

Most cancers of the pancreas have metastasized at the time of diagnosis. Surgical resection of the tumor is done when the tumor is localized or as a palliative measure. Radiation therapy may be useful when the disease is localized but not resectable. The use of irradiation and chemotherapy for pancreatic cancer continues to be investigated. Pain control is one of the most important aspects in the management of persons with end-stage pancreatic cancer.

SUMMARY CONCEPTS

■ The biliary tract, which consists of the bile ducts and gallbladder, serves as a passageway for the delivery of bile from the liver to the intestine.

■ The most common causes of biliary tract disease are cholelithiasis and cholecystitis. Three factors contribute to the development of cholelithiasis: abnormalities in the composition of bile, stasis of bile, and inflammation of the gallbladder. Cholelithiasis, in turn, predisposes to obstruction of bile flow, causing biliary colic and acute or chronic cholecystitis.

- The pancreas is an endocrine and exocrine organ. The exocrine function of the pancreas produces digestive enzymes that are secreted in an inactive form and transported to the small intestine through the main pancreatic duct, which empties into the hepatopancreatic ampulla and then into the duodenum through the sphincter of Oddi.

- Acute pancreatitis is an inflammatory condition of the pancreas due to inappropriate activation of pancreatic enzymes, with manifestations that can range from mild to severe and life-threatening.

- Chronic pancreatitis causes progressive destruction of the endocrine and exocrine pancreas. It is characterized by episodes of pain and epigastric distress that are similar to but less severe than those that occur with acute pancreatitis.

- Pancreatic cancer, the cause of which is unknown, is considered to be one of the most deadly malignancies.

REVIEW EXERCISES

1. A 24-year-old woman reports to her health care professional with complaints of a yellow discoloration of her skin, loss of appetite, and a feeling of upper gastric discomfort. She denies use of intravenous drugs and has not received blood products. She cannot recall eating uncooked shellfish or drinking water that might have been contaminated. She has a daughter who attends day care.

   A. What tests could be done to confirm a diagnosis of hepatitis A?
   B. What is the most common mode of transmission for hepatitis A? It is suggested that the source might be through the day care center that her daughter attends. Explain.
   C. What methods could be used to protect other family members from getting the disease?

2. A 56-year-old man with a history of heavy alcohol consumption and a previous diagnosis of alcoholic cirrhosis and portal hypertension is admitted to the emergency department with acute gastrointestinal bleeding due to a tentative diagnosis of bleeding esophageal varices and signs of circulatory shock.

   A. Relate the development of esophageal varices to portal hypertension in persons with cirrhosis of the liver.
   B. Many persons with esophageal varices have blood coagulation problems. Explain.
   C. What are the possible treatment measures for this man, both in terms of controlling the current bleeding episode and preventing further bleeding episodes?

3. A 40-year-old woman presents in the emergency department with a sudden episode of vomiting and severe right epigastric pain that developed after eating a fatty evening meal. Although there is no evidence of jaundice in her skin, the sclera of her eyes is noted to have a yellowish discoloration. Palpation reveals tenderness of the upper right quadrant with muscle splinting and rebound pain. Right upper quadrant abdominal ultrasonography confirms the presence of gallstones. The woman is treated conservatively with pain and antiemetic medications. She is subsequently scheduled for a laparoscopic cholecystectomy.

   A. Relate this woman's signs and symptoms to gallstones and their effect on gallbladder function.
   B. Explain the initial appearance of jaundice in the eyes as opposed to the skin. Which of the two laboratory tests for bilirubin would you expect to be elevated—direct (conjugated) or indirect (unconjugated or free)?
   C. What effect will removal of the gallbladder have on the woman's digestive system?

REFERENCES

1. Guyton A, Hall JE. *Textbook of Medical Physiology*. 12th ed. Philadelphia, PA: Elsevier Saunders; 2011:837–842.
2. Ross MH, Pawlina W. *Histology: A Test and Atlas*. 6th ed. Philadelphia, PA: Lippincott Williams & Wilkins; 2010:576–609.
3. Crawford JM, Liu C. Liver and biliary tract. In: Kumar V, Abbas AK, Fausto N, et al., eds. *Robbins and Cotran Pathologic Basis of Disease*. 8th ed. Philadelphia, PA: Saunders Elsevier; 2010:833–890.
4. Herrine S, Navarro V, Rubin R. The liver and biliary system. In: Rubin R, Strayer DS, eds. *Rubin's Pathophysiology: Clinicopathologic Foundations of Medicine*. 6th ed. Philadelphia, PA: Wolters Kluwer Health/Lippincott Williams & Wilkins; 2012:677–736.
5. Aragon G, Younoussi Z. When and how to evaluate mildy elevated serum enzymes in apparently healthy patients. *Cleve Clin J Med*. 2010;77(3):195–204.
6. Krier M, Ahmed A. The asymptomatic outpatient with abnormal liver function tests. *Clin Liver Dis*. 2009;13:167–177.
7. Rockey DC, Caldwell SH, Goodman ZD, et al. Liver biopsy. *Hepatology*. 2009;49:1017–1044.
8. Matheny SC, Kingery JE. Hepatitis A. *Am Fam Physician*. 2012;86:1027–1034.
9. Lavanchy D. Viral hepatitis: Global goals for vaccination. *J Clin Virol*. 2012;55(4):296–302.
10. Carey W, Anand B, Lauer G, et al. Viral hepatitis B and D. *First Consult*. 2012. Available at: https://www.clinicalkey.com. Accessed September 1, 2013.
11. World Health Organization. Hepatitis B. 2013. Available at: http://www.who.int/topics/hepatitis. Accessed August 28, 2013.
12. Centers for Disease Control and Prevention. Hepatitis B for health professionals. 2012. Available at: http://www.cdc.gov/hepatitis/HBV. Accessed August 28, 2013.
13. Hajarizadeh B, Grebely J, Dore GJ. Epidemiology and natural history of HCV infection. *Nat Rev Gastroenterol Hepatol*. 2013;10:553–562.

14. Centers for Disease Control and Prevention. Hepatitis C for health professionals. 2012. Available at: http://www.cdc.gov/hepatitis.HCV. Accessed August 28, 2013.

15. Blackard JT, Shata MT, Shira NJ, et al. Acute hepatitis C: a chronic problem. *Hepatology.* 2008;27(1):321–331.

16. Rizzetto M, Ciancio A. Epidemiology of hepatitis D. *Semin Liver Dis.* 2012;32:211–219.

17. Ghany MG, Strader DB, Thomas DL, et al. Diagnosis, management, and treatment of hepatitis C: an update. 2009 practice guideline by the American Association for the Study of Liver Diseases. *Hepatology.* 2009;49:1335–1374.

18. Lok A, McMahon B. Chronic hepatitis B: update 2009. 2009 practice guideline by the American Association for the Study of Liver Diseases. *Hepatology..* 2009;50:1–36.

19. American Association for Study of Liver Disease. Recommendations for Testing, Managing and Treating Hepatitis C. Available at: http://www.hcvguidelines.org/. Revised March 21, 2012. Accessed May 2, 2014.

20. Heneghan M, Yeoman AD, Verma S, et al. Autoimmune hepatitis. *Lancet.* 2013;382:1433–1444.

21. Stravitz RT, Kramer DJ. Acute liver failure. In: Boyer T, Manns M, Sayal A, eds. *Zakim and Boyer's Hepatology: A Textbook of Liver Disease.* 6th ed. Philadelphia, PA: Elsevier Saunders; 2012:327–251.

22. Selmi C, Bowlus CL, Gershwin ME, et al. Primary biliary cirrhosis. *Lancet.* 2011;377:1600–1609.

23. Correia MA. Drug biotransformation. In: Katzung BG, Masters SB, Trevor AJ, eds. *Basic and Clinical Pharmacology.* 12th ed. New York, NY: McGraw-Hill Medical; 2012:53–68.

24. Davern TJ. Drug induced liver disease. *Clin Liver Dis.* 2012;16:231–245.

25. Kumar V, Abbas AK, Fausto N, et al., eds. *Robbins and Cotran Pathologic Basis of Disease.* 8th ed. Philadelphia, PA: Saunders Elsevier; 2010:412–414.

26. Lieber CS. Metabolism of alcohol. *Clin Liver Dis.* 2005;9:1–35.

27. Lucey MR, Mthurin P, Morgan TP. Alcoholic hepatitis. *N Engl J Med.* 2009;360(26): 2758–2769.

28. O'Shea RS, Dasarathy S, McCullough A. AASLD practice guidelines for alcoholic liver disease. *Hepatology.* 2010;51:307–328.

29. Lomonaco R, Sunny N, Bril F, Cusi K. Nonalcoholic fatty liver disease: current issues and novel treatment approaches. *Drugs.* 2013;73:1–14.

30. Pacano T, Sanyal A. Vitamin E and nonalcoholic fatty liver disease. *Curr Opin Clin Nutr Metab Care.* 2012;15:641–648.

31. Starr SP, Raines D. Cirrhosis: diagnosis, management, and prevention. *Am Fam Physician.* 2011;84(12):1353–1359.

32. Lefton HB. Diagnosis and epidemiology of cirrhosis. *Med Clin North Am.* 2009;93:787–799.

33. Toubia N, Sanyal AJ. Portal hypertension and variceal hemorrhage. *Med Clin North Am.* 2008;92:351–374.

34. Runyon BA. Management of adult patients with ascites due to cirrhosis. *Hepatology.* 2013;57:1651–1653.

35. McQuaid KR. Esophageal varices. In: Papadakis MA, McPhee SJ, eds. *Current Medical Diagnosis and Treatment.* 52nd ed. New York, NY: McGraw-Hill Medical; 2013:601–604.

36. Arroyo V, Fernandez J. Management of hepatorenal syndrome in patients with cirrhosis. *Nat Rev Nephrol.* 2011;7:517–526.

37. Sundaram V. Hepatic encephalopathy: pathophysiology and emerging therapies. *Med Clin North Am.* 2009;93:819–836.

38. Rose CF. Ammonia lowering strategies for the treatment of hepatic encephalopathy. *Clin Pharmacol Ther.* 2012;92:321–331.

39. Merion RM. Current status and future of liver transplantation. *Semin Liver Dis.* 2010;30:411–421.

40. Parikh S, Hyman D. Hepatocellular cancer: a guide for the internist. *Am J Med.* 2007;120:194–202.

41. Forner A, Llovet JM, Bruix J. Hepatocellular carcinoma. *Lancet.* 2012;379:1245–1255.

42. Maluccio M, Covey A. Recent progress in understanding, diagnosing, and treating hepatocellular carcinoma. *CA Cancer J Clin.* 2012;62:394–399.

43. Vogt DP. Gallbladder disease. *Cleve Clin J Med.* 2002;69:977–984.

44. Strasberg SM. Acute calculous cholecystitis. *N Engl J Med.* 2008;358(26):2804–2811.

45. Bellows CF, Berger DH, Crass RA. Management of gallstones. *Am Fam Physician.* 2005;72:637–642.

46. Gourgiotis S, Kocher HM, Solaini L, et al. Gallbladder cancer. *Am J Surg.* 2008;196:252–264.

47. Hruban RH, Iacobuzio-Donahue C. The pancreas. In: Kumar V, Abbas AK, Fausto N, et al., eds. *Robbins and Cotran Pathologic Basis of Disease.* 8th ed. Philadelphia, PA: Saunders Elsevier; 2010:891–904.

48. Klimstra DS, Stelow EB. The pancreas. In: Rubin R, Strayer DS, eds. *Rubin's Pathophysiology: Clinicopathologic Foundations of Medicine.* 6th ed. Philadelphia, PA: Wolters Kluwer Health/Lippincott Williams & Wilkins; 2012:737–754.

49. Whitcomb DC. Acute pancreatitis. *N Engl J Med.* 2006;354:2142–2150.

50. Carroll JK, Herrick B, Gipson T, et al. Acute pancreatitis: diagnosis, prognosis, and treatment. *Am Fam Physician.* 2007;75:1513–1520.

51. Banks PA, Freeman ML; for the Practice Parameters Committee of the American College of Gastroenterologists. Practice guidelines for acute pancreatitis. *Am J Gastroenterol.* 2006;101: 2379–2400.

52. Nair RJ, Lawler L. Chronic pancreatitis. *Am Fam Physician.* 2007;76:1679–1688.

53. Forsmark CE. Management of chronic pancreatitis. *Gastroenterology.* 2013;144:1282–1291.

54. Wolfgang CL, Herman JM, Laheru DA, et al. Recent progress in pancreatic cancer. *CA Cancer J Clin.* 2013;63:318–348.

55. Vincent A, Herman J, Schulick R, et al. Pancreatic cancer. *Lancet.* 2011;607–620.

56. Kumar R, Herman JM, Wolfgang CL, Zeng L. Multidisciplinary management of pancreatic cancer. *Surg Oncol Clin North Am.* 2013;22:265–287.

Porth Essentials Resources

Explore these additional resources to enhance learning for this chapter:

- NCLEX-Style Questions and Other Resources on thePoint, http://thePoint.lww.com/PorthEssentials4e
- Study Guide for Essentials of Pathophysiology
- Concepts in Action Animations
- Adaptive Learning | Powered by PrepU, http://thepoint.lww.com/prepu

Chapter 31

Mechanisms of Endocrine Control

The endocrine system is involved in all of the integrative aspects of life, including growth, sex differentiation, metabolism, and adaptation to an ever-changing environment. This chapter focuses on general aspects of endocrine function, organization of the endocrine system, hormone receptors and hormone actions, and regulation of hormone levels.

The Endocrine System

The endocrine system uses chemical messengers called *hormones* as a means of controlling the flow of information between the different tissues and organs of the body. It does not act alone, however, but interacts with the nervous system to coordinate and integrate the activity of body cells. Each system can function alone or in concert with other systems as a single neuroendocrine system, performing the same general functions within the body of communication, integration, and control.

Although both the endocrine and nervous systems function in regulating body functions, the means and speed of control used by these two systems are different. The nervous system functions by means of neurotransmitter molecules transported by neurons over a short distance to muscles and glands that respond within milliseconds (see Chapter 34). The endocrine system, on the other hand, uses hormones released from glands into the blood and transported throughout the body to influence the activity of body tissues. Tissue and organ responses to endocrine hormones tend to take much longer than the response to neurotransmitters, but once initiated they tend to be much more prolonged than those induced by the nervous system.

The glands of the endocrine system are widely scattered throughout the body (Fig. 31-1). These glands include the pituitary, thyroid, parathyroid, and adrenal glands. In addition, several organs of the body contain discrete areas of endocrine tissue and produce hormones as well as exocrine products. Such organs, which include the pancreas and the gonads (testes and ovaries), are also major endocrine glands. The hypothalamus also falls into this category. In addition to its neural functions, it releases hormones that influence the secretion of hormones by other endocrine organs.

Besides the major endocrine glands, there are endocrine cells within organs whose primary function is not endocrine. These include cells within the heart that produce atrial natriuretic factor, cells within the kidney that produce erythropoietin, and numerous cell types within the gastrointestinal tract that produce hormones.

Hormones

The effects of hormones are many and varied. Their actions are involved in regulating water and electrolyte balance; responding to adverse conditions, such as infection, trauma, and stress; sequentially integrating the processes of growth and development; contributing to the processes of reproduction, including gamete (ovum and sperm) production, fertilization, and maintenance of a pregnancy; and digesting, using, and storing nutrients.

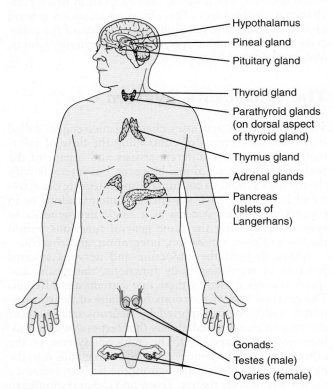

FIGURE 31-1. Location of endocrine glands.

- Hypothalamus
- Pineal gland
- Pituitary gland
- Thyroid gland
- Parathyroid glands (on dorsal aspect of thyroid gland)
- Thymus gland
- Adrenal glands
- Pancreas (Islets of Langerhans)
- Gonads:
- Testes (male)
- Ovaries (female)

A characteristic of endocrine hormones is that a single hormone can exert various effects in different tissues or, conversely, a single function can be regulated by several different hormones. For example, estradiol, which is produced by the ovary, can act on the ovarian follicles to promote their maturation, on the uterus to stimulate its growth and maintain the cyclic changes in the uterine mucosa, on the mammary gland to stimulate ductal growth, on the hypothalamic-pituitary system to regulate the secretion of gonadotropins and prolactin, on the bone to maintain skeletal integrity, and on general metabolic processes to affect adipose tissue distribution. Lipolysis, which is the release of free fatty acids from adipose tissue, is an example of a single function that is regulated by several hormones, including the catecholamines, insulin, and glucagon, and also by the cytokine tumor necrosis factor-α. Table 31-1 lists the major actions and sources of body hormones.

Although some hormones are released into the bloodstream and transported to distant target sites, where they exert their actions, other hormones and hormone-like substances never enter the bloodstream but instead act locally in the vicinity in which they are released (Fig. 31-2). When they act locally on cells other than those that produce the hormone, the action is called *paracrine*. The action of sex steroids on the ovary is a paracrine action. Hormones also can exert an *autocrine* action on the cells from which they were produced. For example, the release of insulin from pancreatic beta cells can inhibit its release from the same cells.

Structural Classification

Hormones, which have diverse chemical structures ranging from single amino acids to complex proteins and lipids, can be divided into three categories: (1) amines and amino acids; (2) peptides, polypeptides, proteins, and glycoproteins; and (3) steroids (Table 31-2).

The first category, the amines and amino acid hormones, includes norepinephrine and epinephrine, which are derived from a single amino acid (i.e., tyrosine), and the thyroid hormones, which are derived from two iodinated tyrosine amino acid residues. The second category, the peptide, polypeptide, protein, and glycoprotein hormones, can be as small as thyrotropin-releasing hormone (TRH), which contains 3 amino acids, and as large and complex as growth hormone (GH) and follicle-stimulating hormone (FSH), which have approximately 200 amino acids. Glycoproteins are large peptide hormones associated with a carbohydrate (e.g., FSH). The third category consists of the steroid hormones, such as the glucocorticoids, which are derivatives of cholesterol.

A group of compounds that have a hormone-like action are the eicosanoids, which are derived from polyunsaturated fatty acids in the cell membrane. Among these, *arachidonic acid* is the most important and abundant precursor of the various eicosanoids (see Chapter 3, Fig. 3-4). The most important of the eicosanoids are the prostaglandins, leukotrienes, and thromboxanes. These fatty acid derivatives are produced by most body cells, are rapidly cleared from the

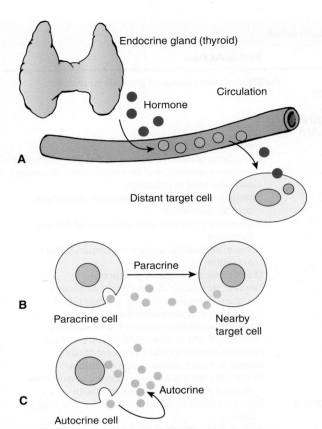

FIGURE 31-2. Examples of endocrine **(A)**, paracrine **(B)**, and autocrine **(C)** secretions.

circulation, and are thought to act mainly by paracrine and autocrine mechanisms. Eicosanoid synthesis often is stimulated in response to hormones, and they serve as mediators of hormone action.

An extension of the endocrine system is represented by numerous cell types with enzymes that modify inactive precursors or less active hormones into highly active hormones. An example is the conversion of the inactive circulating plasma protein *angiotensinogen* to highly active angiotensin II by the enzymatic action of renin, which is produced by the kidney, and angiotensin-converting enzyme, which is present in the lung (see Chapter 18, Fig. 18-13). Another example is the activation of vitamin D by two subsequent hydroxylation reactions in the liver and kidney to produce the highly bioactive form of vitamin D.

Hormone Synthesis

The mechanisms for hormone synthesis and release vary with hormone structure. Protein and polypeptide hormones are synthesized and stored in vesicles in the cytoplasm of the cell until secretion is required. Other hormones, such as the lipid-soluble steroid hormones, are released as they are synthesized.

Vesicle-Mediated Synthesis. The protein and polypeptide hormones comprise the most prominent class of hormones whose synthesis and release is vesicle mediated. These hormones are synthesized in the rough endoplasmic reticulum of the endocrine cell in a manner similar to the synthesis of other proteins (see Chapter 1). The appropriate amino acid sequence is dictated by messenger ribonucleic acids (mRNAs) from the nucleus. Usually, synthesis involves the production of a precursor hormone, which is modified by the addition of peptides or sugar units. These precursor hormones often contain extra peptide units that ensure proper folding of the molecule and insertion of essential linkages. If extra amino acids are present, as in insulin, the precursor hormone is called a *prohormone*.

After synthesis and sequestration in the endoplasmic reticulum, the protein and peptide hormones move into the Golgi complex, where they are packaged in vesicles. It is in the Golgi complex that prohormones are converted into hormones. Stimulation of the endocrine cell causes the vesicles to move to the cell membrane and release their hormones.

The vesicle-mediated pathway is also used for secretion of a number of nonpolypeptide hormones and neurotransmitters such as the catecholamines (epinephrine and norepinephrine). However, these small molecules do not pass through the full range of intracellular mechanisms seen in the synthesis and secretion of the larger protein and polypeptide hormones.

Non–Vesicle-Mediated Synthesis. Hormones synthesized by non–vesicle-mediated pathways include the glucocorticoids, androgens, estrogens, and mineralocorticoids—all steroids derived from cholesterol. These hormones are synthesized in the smooth endoplasmic reticulum, and steroid-secreting cells can be identified by their large amounts of smooth endoplasmic reticulum. Certain steroids serve as precursors for the production of other hormones. In the adrenal cortex, for example, progesterone and other steroid intermediates are enzymatically converted into aldosterone, cortisol, or androgens (see Chapter 32).

The release of hormones synthesized by non–vesicle-mediated pathways is not fully understood. Historically it was thought to occur by simple diffusion. In recent years, however, specific transporters have been implicated in directing some of these classes of hormones out of the cell. Whether all hormones produced by non–vesicle-mediated pathways depend on transporters for their secretion remains a subject for further investigation.

Hormone Transport and Clearance from the Blood

The signaling of the endocrine system relies on mechanisms that transport blood-borne chemical messengers to the site of action, and then clear them from the blood once their action is no longer needed.

Transport Mechanisms. Hormones that are released into the bloodstream circulate as either free or unbound molecules or as hormones attached to transport carriers (Fig. 31-3). Peptide hormones and protein hormones

TABLE 31-1 Major Action and Source of Selected Hormones

Source	Hormone	Major Action
Hypothalamus	Releasing and inhibiting hormones Corticotropin-releasing hormone (CRH) Thyrotropin-releasing hormone (TRH) Growth hormone–releasing hormone (GHRH) Gonadotropin-releasing hormone (GnRH) Somatostatin	Controls the release of pituitary hormones Inhibits GH and TSH
Anterior pituitary	Growth hormone (GH)	Stimulates growth of bone and muscle, promotes protein synthesis and fat metabolism, decreases carbohydrate metabolism
	Adrenocorticotropic hormone (ACTH)	Stimulates synthesis and secretion of adrenal cortical hormones
	Thyroid-stimulating hormone (TSH)	Stimulates synthesis and secretion of thyroid hormone
	Follicle-stimulating hormone (FSH)	Female: stimulates growth of ovarian follicle, ovulation Male: stimulates sperm production
	Luteinizing hormone (LH)	Female: stimulates development of corpus luteum, release of oocyte, production of estrogen and progesterone Male: stimulates secretion of testosterone, development of interstitial tissue of testes
	Prolactin	Prepares female breast for breast-feeding
Posterior pituitary	Antidiuretic hormone (ADH)	Increases water reabsorption by kidney
	Oxytocin	Stimulates contraction of pregnant uterus, milk ejection from breasts after childbirth
Adrenal cortex	Mineralocorticosteroids, mainly aldosterone	Increases sodium absorption, potassium loss by kidney
	Glucocorticoids, mainly cortisol	Affects metabolism of all nutrients; regulates blood glucose levels, affects growth, has anti-inflammatory action, and decreases effects of stress
	Adrenal androgens, mainly dehydroepiandrosterone (DHEA) and androstenedione	Have minimal intrinsic androgenic activity; they are converted to testosterone and dihydrotestosterone in the periphery
Adrenal medulla	Epinephrine Norepinephrine	Serve as neurotransmitters for the sympathetic nervous system
Thyroid (follicular cells)	Thyroid hormones: triiodothyronine (T_3), thyroxine (T_4)	Increase the metabolic rate; increase protein and bone turnover; increase responsiveness to catecholamines; necessary for fetal and infant growth and development
Thyroid C cells	Calcitonin	Lowers blood calcium and phosphate levels
Parathyroid glands	Parathyroid hormone (PTH)	Regulates serum calcium
Pancreatic islet cells	Insulin	Lowers blood glucose by facilitating glucose transport across cell membranes of muscle, liver, and adipose tissue
	Glucagon	Increases blood glucose concentration by stimulation of glycogenolysis and gluconeogenesis
	Somatostatin	Delays intestinal absorption of glucose
Kidney	1,25-Dihydroxyvitamin D	Stimulates calcium absorption from the intestine
Ovaries	Estrogen	Affects development of female sex organs and secondary sex characteristics
	Progesterone	Influences menstrual cycle; stimulates growth of uterine wall; maintains pregnancy
Testes	Androgens, mainly testosterone	Affect development of male sex organs and secondary sex characteristics; aid in sperm production

TABLE 31-2	Classes of Hormones Based on Structure	
Amines and Amino Acids	**Peptides, Polypeptides, and Proteins**	**Steroids**
Dopamine	Corticotropin-releasing hormone (CRH)	Aldosterone
Epinephrine	Growth hormone–releasing hormone (GHRH)	Glucocorticoids
Norepinephrine	Thyrotropin-releasing hormone (TRH)	Estrogens
Thyroid hormone	Adrenocorticotropic hormone (ACTH)	Testosterone
	Follicle-stimulating hormone (FSH)	Progesterone
	Luteinizing hormone (LH)	Androstenedione
	Thyroid-stimulating hormone (TSH)	1,25-Dihydroxyvitamin D
	Growth hormone (GH)	Dihydrotestosterone (DHT)
	Antidiuretic hormone (ADH)	Dehydroepiandrosterone (DHEA)
	Oxytocin	
	Insulin	
	Glucagon	
	Somatostatin	
	Calcitonin	
	Parathyroid hormone (PTH)	
	Prolactin	

are water soluble and usually circulate unbound in the blood. Steroid hormones and thyroid hormones are carried by specific carrier proteins synthesized in the liver. The extent of carrier binding influences the rate at which hormones leave the blood and enter the cells.

The half-life of a hormone—the time it takes for the body to reduce the concentration of the hormone by one half—is positively correlated with its percentage of protein binding. Thyroxine, which is more than 99% protein bound, has a half-life of 6 days. Aldosterone, which is only 15% bound, has a half-life of only 25 minutes.

Drugs that compete with a hormone for binding with transport carrier molecules increase hormone action by increasing the availability of the active unbound hormone. For example, aspirin competes with thyroid hormone for binding to transport proteins; when this drug is administered to persons with excessive levels of circulating thyroid hormone, such as during thyroid crisis, serious effects may occur due to the dissociation of free hormone from the binding proteins.

Inactivation and Elimination. Hormones secreted by endocrine cells must be inactivated continuously to prevent their accumulation. Intracellular and extracellular mechanisms participate in the termination of hormone function. Most peptide hormones and catecholamines are water soluble and circulate freely in the blood. They are usually degraded by enzymes in the blood or tissues and then excreted by the kidneys and liver. For example, the catecholamines are rapidly degraded by catechol O-methyl transferase (COMT) and monoamine oxidase (MAO). Because of their short half-life, their production is measured by some of their metabolites. In general, peptide hormones also have a short life span in the circulation. Their major mechanism of degradation is through binding to cell surface receptors, with subsequent uptake and degradation by peptide-splitting enzymes in the cell membrane or inside the cell.

Steroid hormones are bound to protein carriers for transport and are inactive in the bound state. Their activity depends on the availability of transport carriers. Unbound adrenal and gonadal steroid hormones are conjugated in the liver, which renders them inactive, and then excreted in the bile or urine. Thyroid hormones also are transported by carrier molecules. The free hormone is rendered inactive by the removal of amino acids (i.e., deamination) in the tissues, and the hormone is conjugated in the liver and eliminated in the bile.

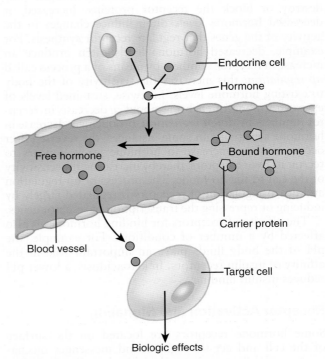

FIGURE 31-3. Relationship of free and carrier-bound hormones.

Receptor Control of Hormone Function

Hormones produce their effects through interaction with high-affinity receptors, which in turn are linked to one or more effector systems within the cell (see Understanding Hormone Receptors). These mechanisms involve many of the cell's metabolic activities, ranging from ion transport at the cell surface to stimulation of nuclear transcription of complex molecules. The rate at which hormones react depends on their mechanism of action. Thyroid hormone, which controls cell metabolism and synthesis of intracellular signaling molecules, requires days for its full effect to occur.

Control of Receptor Number and Affinity

Hormone receptors are complex molecular structures that are located either on the surface or inside target cells. The function of these receptors is to recognize a specific hormone and translate the hormonal signal into a cellular response. The structure of these receptors varies in a manner that allows target cells to respond to one hormone and not to others. For example, receptors in the thyroid are specific for thyroid-stimulating hormone, and receptors on the gonads respond to the gonadotropic hormones.

The response of a target cell to a hormone varies with the *number* of receptors present and with the *affinity* of these receptors for hormone binding. A variety of factors influence the number of receptors that are present on target cells and their affinity for hormone binding.

The number of hormone receptors on a cell may be altered for any of several reasons. Antibodies may destroy or block the receptor proteins. Increased or decreased hormone levels often induce changes in the activity of the genes that regulate receptor synthesis. For example, decreased hormone levels often produce an increase in receptor numbers by means of a process called *up-regulation;* this increases the sensitivity of the body to existing hormone levels. Likewise, sustained levels of excess hormone often bring about a decrease in receptor numbers by *down-regulation,* producing a decrease in hormone sensitivity. In some instances, the reverse effect occurs, and an increase in hormone levels appears to recruit its own receptors, thereby increasing the sensitivity of the cell to the hormone. The process of up-regulation and down-regulation of receptors is regulated largely by inducing or repressing the transcription of receptor genes.

The affinity of receptors for binding hormones is also affected by a number of conditions. For example, the pH of the body fluids plays an important role in the affinity of insulin receptors. In ketoacidosis, a lower pH reduces insulin binding.

Receptor Activation and Signaling

Some hormone receptors are located on the surface of the cell and act through second messenger mechanisms, and others are located within the cell, where they modulate the synthesis of enzymes, transport proteins, or structural proteins. The receptors for thyroid hormones, which are found in the nucleus, are thought to be directly involved in controlling the activity of genes located on one or more of the chromosomes in the nucleus. Chart 31-1 lists examples of hormones that act through the two types of receptors.

Cell Surface Receptors. Because of their low solubility in the lipid layer of cell membranes, peptide hormones and catecholamines cannot readily cross the cell membrane. Instead, these hormones interact with surface receptors in a manner that incites the generation of an intracellular signal or message. The intracellular signal system is termed the *second messenger,* and the hormone is considered to be the first messenger. For example, the first messenger glucagon binds to surface receptors on liver cells to incite glycogen breakdown by way of the second messenger system.

The most widely distributed second messenger is cyclic adenosine monophosphate (cAMP), which is formed from adenosine triphosphate (ATP) by the enzyme adenylate cyclase, a membrane-bound enzyme that is located on the inner aspect of the cell membrane (see Chapter 1, Fig. 1-9). Adenylate cyclase is functionally coupled to various cell surface receptors by the regulatory actions of G proteins. A second messenger similar to cAMP is cyclic guanosine monophosphate (cGMP), derived from guanosine triphosphate (GTP). As a result of binding to specific cell receptors, many peptide hormones incite a series of enzymatic reactions that produce an almost immediate increase in cAMP and target cell response. Some hormones act to decrease cAMP levels and have an opposite effect on cell responses.

In some cells, the binding of a hormone or neurotransmitter to a surface receptor acts directly, rather than through a second messenger, to open an ion channel in

CHART 31-1	Hormone–Receptor Interactions

Second Messenger Interactions

Glucagon
Insulin
Epinephrine
Parathyroid hormone (PTH)
Thyroid-stimulating hormone (TSH)
Adrenocorticotropic hormone (ACTH)
Follicle-stimulating hormone (FSH)
Luteinizing hormone (LH)
Antidiuretic hormone (ADH)
Secretin

Intracellular Interactions

Estrogens
Testosterone
Progesterone
Adrenal cortical hormones
Thyroid hormones
Vitamin D
Retinoids

the cell membrane. The influx of ions then serves as an intracellular signal to convey the hormone's message to the interior of the cell. In many instances, the activation of hormone receptors results in the opening of calcium channels, with the increasing intracellular concentration of calcium ions acting as the signal that elicits the cellular response.

Nuclear Receptors. A second type of receptor mechanism is involved in mediating the action of thyroid and steroid hormones, as well as vitamin D, retinoic acid, and other molecules. In contrast to peptide and catecholamine hormones, these hormones enter the cell and bind to receptors in the cell nucleus that are gene regulatory proteins. Many of these hormones and molecules bind to receptors in the cytoplasm, and the hormone–receptor complexes then travel to the nucleus. Nuclear receptors can also be activated by second messenger signaling pathways, thereby linking cell surface receptors to nuclear receptor activation pathways.

Several subfamilies of nuclear receptors are currently recognized on the basis of structural similarity. One subfamily consists of receptors for thyroid hormone and vitamin D. A second subfamily consists of glucocorticoid, progesterone, androgen, and estrogen receptors. Other subfamilies contain "orphan receptors" for which natural ligands have not as yet been identified.

Activated nuclear receptors act by binding to deoxyribonucleic acid (DNA) response elements in the promoter sites where gene transcription is initiated. These DNA-binding elements, which are termed *hormone response elements*, then activate or suppress intracellular mechanisms such as gene activity, with the subsequent production or inhibition of mRNA and protein synthesis. The importance of the nuclear effects of thyroid and steroid hormones is illustrated by the fact that each regulates protein synthesis. Proteins whose synthesis is regulated up or down by these hormones may be enzymes, structural proteins, receptor proteins, or transcriptional proteins that regulate the expression of other genes, or proteins that are exported from the cell.

Some nuclear receptors are regulated by intracellular metabolites rather than secreted signal molecules. The peroxisome proliferator-activated receptors (PPARs), for example, bind intracellular lipid metabolites and regulate the transcription of genes involved in lipid metabolism and adipose tissue metabolism. The thiazolidinedione medications, which are used in the treatment of type 2 diabetes mellitus, act at the level of nuclear PPAR-γ receptors to promote glucose uptake and utilization by adipose tissue cells (see Chapter 33).

Regulation of Hormone Levels

Hormone secretion varies widely over a 24-hour period. Some hormones, such as growth hormone (GH) and adrenocorticotropic hormone (ACTH), have diurnal fluctuations that vary with the sleep–wake cycle. Others, such as the female sex hormones, are secreted in a complicated

cyclic manner. The levels of hormones such as insulin and antidiuretic hormone (ADH) are regulated by feedback mechanisms that monitor substances such as glucose (insulin) and water (ADH) in the body. The levels of many of the hormones are regulated by feedback mechanisms that involve the hypothalamic-pituitary–target cell system.

Hypothalamic-Pituitary Regulation

The hypothalamus and pituitary gland, also known as the *hypophysis*, form a unit that exerts control over many functions of several endocrine glands as well as a wide range of other physiologic functions. These two structures are connected by blood flow in the hypophysial portal system, which begins in the hypothalamus and drains into the anterior pituitary gland, and by the nerve axons that connect the supraoptic and paraventricular nuclei of the hypothalamus with the posterior pituitary gland (Fig. 31-4).

Hypothalamic Hormones. The synthesis and release of anterior pituitary hormones are largely regulated by the action of releasing or inhibiting hormones from the hypothalamus, which is the coordinating center of the brain for endocrine, behavioral, and autonomic nervous system function. It is at the level of the hypothalamus that emotion, pain, body temperature, and other neural input are communicated to the endocrine system. The posterior pituitary hormones, ADH and oxytocin, are synthesized in the cell bodies of neurons in the hypothalamus that have axons that travel to the posterior pituitary.

The hypothalamic hormones that regulate the secretion of anterior pituitary hormones include GH-releasing hormone (GHRH), somatostatin, dopamine, TRH, corticotropin-releasing hormone (CRH), and gonadotropin-releasing hormone (GnRH). With the exception of GH and prolactin, most of the pituitary hormones are regulated by hypothalamic stimulatory hormones. GH secretion is stimulated by GHRH; thyroid-stimulating hormone (TSH) by TRH; adrenocorticotropic hormone (ACTH) by CRH; and luteinizing hormone (LH) and follicle-stimulating hormone (FSH) by GnRH. The secretion of prolactin, which is also produced by cells in the anterior pituitary gland, is inhibited by dopamine from the hypothalamus. Drugs that interfere with the synthesis or action of dopamine, such as some of the antipsychotic medications, increase prolactin secretion.

The activity of the hypothalamus is regulated by both hormonally mediated signals (e.g., negative feedback signals) and by neuronal input from a number of sources. Neuronal signals are mediated by neurotransmitters such as acetylcholine, dopamine, norepinephrine, serotonin, γ-aminobutyric acid (GABA), and opioids. Cytokines that are involved in immune and inflammatory responses, such as the interleukins, also are involved in the regulation of hypothalamic function (see Chapter 15). This is particularly true of the hormones involved in the hypothalamic-pituitary-adrenal axis. Thus, the hypothalamus can be viewed as a bridge by which signals from multiple systems are relayed to the pituitary gland.

(*text continues on page 761*)

UNDERSTANDING ➜ Hormone Receptors

Hormones bring about their effects on cell activity by binding to specific cell receptors. There are two general types of receptors: (1) cell surface receptors that exert their actions through cytoplasmic second messenger systems, and (2) intracellular nuclear receptors that modulate gene expression by binding to DNA or promoters of target genes.

1

Cell Surface Receptors. Water-soluble peptide hormones, such as parathyroid hormone and glucagon, which cannot penetrate the lipid layer of the cell plasma membrane, exert their effects through intracellular second messengers. They bind to a portion of a membrane receptor that protrudes through the surface of the cell. This produces a structural change in the receptor molecule itself, causing activation of a hormone-regulated signal system located on the inner aspect of the cell membrane. This system allows the cell to sense extracellular events and pass this information to the intracellular environment. There are several types of cell surface receptors, including G-protein–coupled receptors that mediate the actions of catecholamines, prostaglandins, thyroid-stimulating hormone, and others. Binding of the hormone to the receptor activates a G protein, which in turn acts on an effector (such as adenyl cyclase) to generate a second messenger (such as cyclic adenosine monophosphate, cAMP). The second messenger, in turn, activates other enzymes that participate in cellular secretion, gene activation, or other target cell responses.

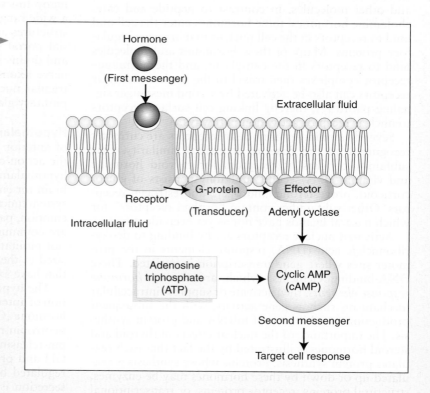

2 **Nuclear Receptors.** Steroid hormones, vitamin D, thyroid hormones, and other lipid-soluble hormones diffuse across the cell membrane into the cytoplasm of the target cell. Once inside, they bind to an intracellular receptor that is activated by the interaction. The activated hormone–receptor complex then moves to the nucleus, where the hormone binds to a hormone response element (HRE) in the promoters on a target gene or to another transcription factor. Attachment to the HRE results in transcription of a specific messenger RNA (mRNA). The mRNA then moves into the cytoplasm, where the "transcribed message" is translated and used by cytoplasmic ribosomes to produce new cellular proteins or changes in the production of existing proteins. These proteins promote a specific cellular response or, in some cases, the synthesis of a structural protein that is exported from the cell.

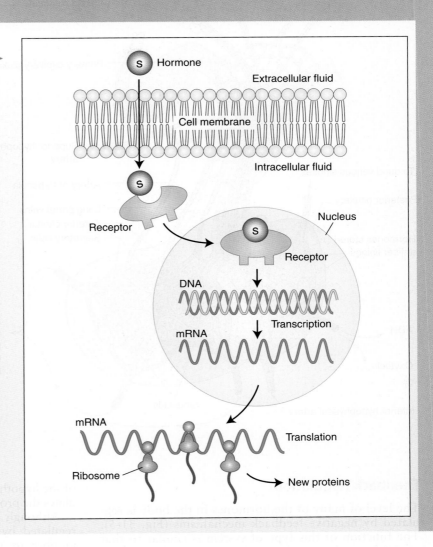

(text continued from page 759)

Pituitary Hormones. The pituitary is a pea-sized endocrine gland that is located at the base of the brain, where it lies in a saddle-shaped depression in the sphenoid bone called the *sella turcica*. The pituitary gland has two functional units: an anterior lobe, or *adenohypophysis*, and a posterior lobe, or *neurohypophysis*. Embryologically, the anterior lobe of the pituitary gland develops from glandular tissue and the posterior lobe from neural tissue.

The pituitary gland has been called the *master gland* because its hormones control the functions of many target glands and cells. The anterior pituitary gland contains five cell types: (1) thyrotrophs, which produce thyrotropin, also called *TSH*; (2) corticotrophs, which produce corticotropin, also called *ACTH*; (3) gonadotrophs, which produce the gonadotropins, LH, and FSH; (4) somatotrophs, which produce GH;

and (5) lactotrophs, which produce prolactin. The posterior pituitary gland stores and releases antidiuretic hormone (ADH) and oxytocin, which are synthesized in the hypothalamus. Hormones produced by the anterior pituitary control body growth and metabolism (GH), function of the thyroid gland (TSH), glucocorticoid hormone levels (ACTH), function of the gonads (FSH and LH), and breast growth and milk production (prolactin). Melanocyte-stimulating hormone (MSH), which is involved in the control of pigmentation of the skin, is produced by the pars intermedia (the region between the two lobes of the pituitary gland). The functions of many of these hormones are discussed in other parts of this book (e.g., thyroid hormone, GH, and the corticosteroids in Chapter 32; the sex hormones in Chapters 39 and 40; and ADH from the posterior pituitary in Chapter 8).

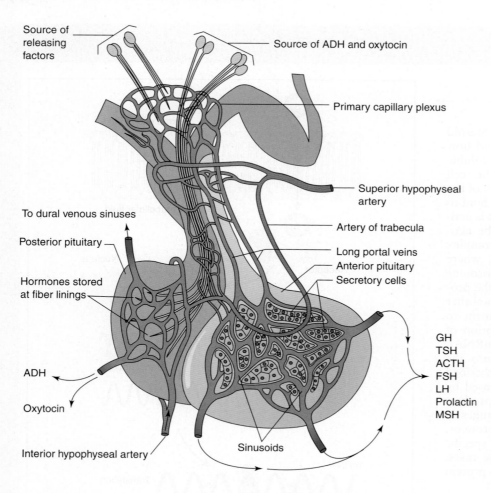

GH
TSH
ACTH
FSH
LH
Prolactin
MSH

FIGURE 31-4. The hypothalamus and the anterior and posterior pituitary. The hypothalamic releasing or inhibiting hormones are transported to the anterior pituitary through the portal vessels. Antidiuretic hormone and oxytocin are produced by nerve cells in the supraoptic and paraventricular nuclei of the hypothalamus and then transported through the nerve axon to the posterior pituitary, where they are released into the circulation. ADH, antidiuretic hormone; ACTH, adrenocorticotropic hormone; FSH, follicle stimulating hormone; GH, growth hormone; LH, luteinizing hormone; MSH, melanocyte stimulating hormone; TSH, thyroid stimulating hormone.

Feedback Regulation

The level of many of the hormones in the body is regulated by negative feedback mechanisms (Fig. 31-5). The function of this type of system is similar to that of the thermostat in a heating system. In the endocrine system, sensors detect a change in the hormone level and adjust hormone secretion so that blood levels are maintained within an appropriate range. When the sensors detect a decrease in blood levels, they initiate changes that cause an increase in hormone production; when blood levels rise above the set point of the system, the sensors cause hormone production and release to decrease. For example, an increase in thyroid hormone is detected by sensors in the hypothalamus or anterior pituitary gland, and this causes a reduction in the secretion of TSH, with a subsequent decrease in the output of thyroid hormone from the thyroid gland. The feedback loops for the hypothalamic-pituitary feedback mechanisms are illustrated in Figure 31-6.

Exogenous forms of hormones (given as drug preparations) can influence the normal feedback control of hormone production and release. One of the most common examples of this influence occurs with the administration of the corticosteroid hormones, which causes suppression of the hypothalamic-pituitary–target cell system that regulates the production of these hormones.

Although the blood levels of most hormones are regulated by negative feedback mechanisms, a small number are under positive feedback control, in which rising levels of a hormone cause another gland to release a hormone that is stimulating to the first. There must, however, be a mechanism for shutting off the release of the first hormone, or its production would continue unabated. An example of such a system is that of the female ovarian hormone estradiol. Increased estradiol production during the follicular stage of the menstrual cycle causes increased gonadotropin (FSH) production by the anterior pituitary gland. This stimulates further increases in estradiol levels until the demise of the follicle, which is the source of estradiol, results in a fall in gonadotropin levels.

In addition to positive and negative feedback mechanisms that monitor changes in hormone levels, some hormones are regulated by the level of the substance they regulate. For example, insulin levels normally are regulated in response to blood glucose levels, and those of aldosterone in response to blood levels of sodium and potassium. Other factors such as stress, environmental temperature, and nutritional status can alter feedback regulation of hormone levels.

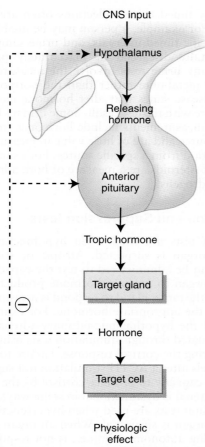

FIGURE 31-5. Hypothalamic-pituitary control of hormone levels. The *dashed line* represents feedback control. CNS, central nervous system.

Diagnostic Tests

Several techniques are available for assessing endocrine function and hormone levels. One technique measures the effect of a hormone on body function. Measurement of blood glucose, for example, is an indirect method of assessing insulin levels. However, insulin action (i.e., insulin activity) is also important in relation to glucose levels as hyperglycemia could occur if marked insulin resistance is present, despite the presence of a compensatory increase in insulin levels (i.e., hyperinsulinemia). This situation is common in type 2 diabetes (see Chapter 33). Thus, the most common method is to measure hormone levels directly.

Blood Tests

Hormones circulating in the plasma were first detected by bioassays using an intact animal or a portion of tissue from the animal. However, most bioassays lack the precision, sensitivity, and specificity to measure low concentrations of hormones in plasma, and they are inconvenient to perform.

Blood tests provide information about hormone levels at a specific time. For example, blood insulin levels can be measured along with blood glucose after administration of a challenge dose of glucose to measure the time course of change in blood insulin levels.

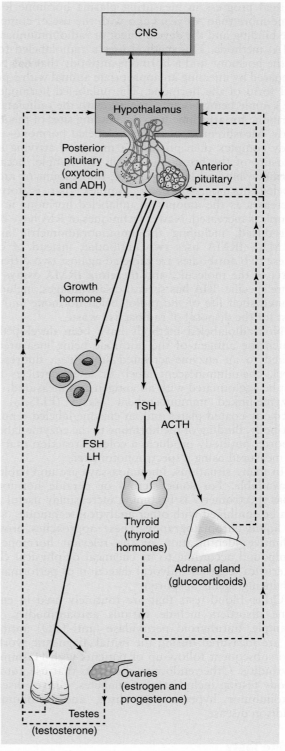

FIGURE 31-6. Control of hormone production by the hypothalamic-pituitary–target cell feedback mechanism. Hormone levels from the target glands regulate the release of hormones from the anterior pituitary through a negative feedback system. The *dashed line* represents feedback control. ADH, antidiuretic hormone; ACTH, adrenocorticotropic hormone; CNS, central nervous system; FSH, follicle stimulating hormone; LH, luteinizing hormone; TSH, thyroid stimulating hormone.

Real progress in measuring plasma hormone levels came more than 40 years ago with the use of competitive binding and the development of radioimmunoassay (RIA) methods. This method uses a radiolabeled form of the hormone and a hormone antibody that has been prepared by injecting an appropriate animal with a purified form of the hormone. The unlabeled hormone in the sample being tested competes with the radiolabeled hormone for attachment to the binding sites of the antibody. Measurement of the radiolabeled hormone–antibody complex then provides a means of arriving at a measure of the hormone level in the sample. Because hormone binding is competitive, the amount of radiolabeled hormone–antibody complex that is formed decreases as the amount of unlabeled hormone in the sample is increased. Newer techniques of RIA have been introduced, including the immunoradiometric assay (IRMA). IRMA uses two antibodies instead of one. These two antibodies are directed against two different parts of the molecule, and therefore IRMA assays are more specific. RIA has several disadvantages, including limited shelf life of the radiolabeled hormone and the cost for the disposal of radioactive waste.

Nonradiolabeled methods have been developed in which the antigen of the hormone being measured is linked to an enzyme-activated label (e.g., fluorescent label, chemiluminescent label) or latex particles that can be agglutinated with an antigen and measured. The enzyme-linked immunosorbent assays (ELISAs) use antibody-coated plates and an enzyme-labeled reporter antibody. Binding of the hormone to the enzyme-labeled reporter antibody produces a colored reaction that can be measured using a spectrophotometer.

In many situations, immunoassays are unreliable or unavailable. For some steroid or peptide hormones, mass spectrometry is becoming increasingly useful and can be combined with other analytical techniques, such as liquid chromatography. These approaches provide definitive identification of the relevant hormone or compound according to its chemical or physical characteristics (e.g., unequivocal detection of performance-enhancing agents in sports).

Other blood tests that are routinely used in endocrine disorders include various autoantibodies. For example, antithyroid peroxidase (anti-TPO) antibodies are measured during the initial diagnostic workup and subsequent follow-up of patients with Hashimoto thyroiditis. Other endocrine disorders that use autoantibody testing include type 1 diabetes, Graves disease, autoimmune hypoparathyroidism, and autoimmune Addison disease.

Urine Tests

Measurements of urinary hormone or hormone metabolites often are done on a 24-hour urine sample and provide a better measure of hormone levels during that period than hormones measured in an isolated blood sample. The advantages of a urine test include the relative ease of obtaining urine samples and the fact that blood sampling is not required. The disadvantage is that reliably timed urine collections often are difficult to obtain. For example, a person may be unable to urinate at specific timed intervals, and urine samples may be accidentally discarded or inaccurately preserved. Because many urine tests involve the measurement of a hormone metabolite rather than the hormone itself, drugs or disease states that alter hormone metabolism may interfere with the test result. Some urinary hormone metabolite measurements include hormones from more than one source and are of little value in measuring hormone secretion from a specific source. For example, urinary 17-ketosteroids are a measure of both adrenal and gonadal androgens.

Stimulation and Suppression Tests

Stimulation tests are used when hypofunction of an endocrine organ is suspected. Atropic or stimulating hormone can be administered to test the capacity of an endocrine organ to increase hormone production. The capacity of the target gland to respond is measured by an increase in the appropriate hormone. For example, the function of the hypothalamic-pituitary-adrenal system can be evaluated through stimulation tests using ACTH and measuring the cortisol response. Failure to increase cortisol levels after a ACTH stimulation test suggests an inadequate capacity to produce cortisol by the adrenals (i.e., the adrenal is dysfunctional in some way).

Suppression tests are used when hyperfunction of an endocrine organ is suspected. When an organ or tissue is functioning autonomously (i.e., is not responding to the normal negative feedback control mechanisms and continues to secrete excessive amounts of hormone), a suppression test may be useful to confirm the situation. For example, when a GH-secreting tumor is suspected, the GH response to a glucose load is measured as part of the diagnostic workup (see Chapter 32). Normally, a glucose load would suppress GH levels. However, in adults with GH-secreting tumors (a condition known as *acromegaly*), GH levels are not suppressed (and paradoxically increase in 50% of cases).

Genetic Tests

The diagnosis of genetic diseases using DNA analysis is rapidly becoming a routine part of endocrine practice. Completion of the human genome sequence has revealed the presence of about 30,000 genes. The considerable interest in the field of genomics (i.e., examination of the DNA) and transcriptomics (i.e., examination of the mRNA) has been complemented by advances in proteomics (i.e., examination of the proteome, which is all of the proteins expressed by a cell or tissue type). It is proposed that compared with the size of the genome, the proteome is far larger, with several hundred thousand to several million different protein forms possible. Analysis of the proteins produced by normal and abnormal endocrine cells, tissues, and organs will lead to a better understanding of the pathophysiologic processes of endocrine conditions. This may also lead to selective targeting for new drug development.

The cloning of many endocrine system genes has had an enormous impact on everyday clinical practice. For example, identification of a gene for a given disorder (e.g., the *RET* proto-oncogene in certain multiple endocrine neoplasia syndromes) means that faster diagnosis and more appropriate management for the affected individual can occur, but also that screening of family members for kindred harboring a known mutation can be undertaken.

Imaging Techniques

Imaging studies are important in the diagnosis and follow-up of endocrine disorders. Imaging modalities related to endocrinology can be divided into isotopic and nonisotopic types. Isotopic imaging includes radioactive scanning of the thyroid (e.g., using radioiodine) and parathyroids (e.g., using sestamibi). Nonisotopic imaging includes magnetic resonance imaging (MRI), which is the preferred choice for pituitary and hypothalamic imaging, and computed tomography (CT) scanning, which is preferred for adrenal lesions and abdominal endocrine lesions. Ultrasonographic scanning provides excellent and reproducible anatomic images for the thyroid, parathyroids, and neighboring structures. Thyroid ultrasonography is recommended for managing thyroid nodules and can aid in visualization of the nodule for biopsy (fine needle aspiration), which is necessary to help distinguish benign from malignant etiology. Selective venography is usually accompanied by venous sampling to determine hormonal output from a gland or organ (e.g., adrenal, pituitary, and kidney). Positron emission tomography (PET) scanning is being used more widely for evaluation of endocrine tumors. Dual electron x-ray absorptiometry (DEXA) is used routinely for the diagnosis and monitoring of osteoporosis and metabolic bone diseases.

SUMMARY CONCEPTS

■ The endocrine system acts as a communication system that uses hormones as chemical messengers. Hormones travel through the blood to distant target sites of action, or act locally as paracrine or autocrine messengers to incite more local effects.

■ Hormones exert their effects by interacting with high-affinity receptors, which in turn are linked to one or more effector systems in the cell. Some hormone receptors are located on the surface of the cell and act through second messenger mechanisms, and others are located in the cell, where they modulate the synthesis of enzymes, transport proteins, or structural proteins. Other hormones bind to nuclear receptors and act by directly regulating gene transcription.

■ Many of the endocrine glands are under the regulatory control of other parts of the endocrine and nervous systems. The hypothalamus and the pituitary gland form a complex integrative network that joins the nervous system and the endocrine system; this central network controls the output from many of the other glands in the body.

■ Many hormones are controlled by negative feedback loops that adjust their level and confer stability to the many functions of the endocrine system.

■ Endocrine function can be assessed directly by measuring blood hormone levels or indirectly by assessing the effects that a hormone has on the body (e.g., assessment of insulin function through blood glucose). Imaging techniques are increasingly used to visualize endocrine structures, and genetic techniques are used to determine the presence of genes that contribute to the development of endocrine disorders.

REVIEW EXERCISES

1. Vitamin D is often considered a hormone rather than a vitamin.

   A. Explain.

2. Thyroid hormones are transported in the serum bound to transport proteins such as thyroid-binding globulin and albumin.

   A. Explain why free thyroxine (T_4) levels are usually used to assess thyroid function rather than total T_4 levels.

3. People who are being treated with exogenous forms of corticosteroid hormones often experience diminished levels of ACTH and exogenously produced cortisol.

   A. Explain using information regarding the hypothalamic-pituitary feedback control of cortisol production by the adrenal cortex.

BIBLIOGRAPHY

Alberts B, Aranda A, Pascual A. Nuclear hormone receptors and gene expression. *Physiol Rev.* 2001;81(3):1239–1304.
Alberts B, Johnson A, Lewis V, et al. *Molecular Biology of the Cell.* 5th ed. New York, NY: Garland Science; 2008:889–903.

Gardner DG, Shoback D, eds. *Greenspan's Basic and Clinical Endocrinology*. 9th ed. New York, NY: Lange Medical Books/ McGraw-Hill; 2011.

White B. The endocrine system. In: Koeppen BM, Stanton BA. *Berne & Levy Physiology*. 6th ed. St. Louis, MO: Mosby Elsevier; 2010:653–663.

Griffin JE, Sergio RO. *Textbook of Endocrine Physiology*. 5th ed. New York, NY: Oxford University Press; 2005.

Hall JE. *Guyton & Hall Textbook of Medical Physiology*. 12th ed. Philadelphia, PA: Saunders Elsevier; 2011:881–893.

Holt RIG, Hanley NA. *Essential Endocrinology and Diabetes*. 5th ed. Malden, MA: Blackwell; 2013.

Jameson JL, ed. *Harrison's Endocrinology*. New York, NY: McGraw-Hill; 2013.

Kovacs WJ, Sergio RO. *Textbook of Endocrine Physiology*. 6th ed. New York, NY: Oxford University Press; 2011.

Rogers A, Thakler RV. Clinically relevant genetic advances in endocrinology. *Clin Med*. 2013;13:299–305.

Whiteheads S, Micelli J. *Clinical Endocrinology*. Banbury, UK: Scion Publishing; 2011.

Porth Essentials Resources

Explore these additional resources to enhance learning for this chapter:

- NCLEX-Style Questions and Other Resources on thePoint, http://thePoint.lww.com/PorthEssentials4e
- Study Guide for Essentials of Pathophysiology
- Concepts in Action Animations
- Adaptive Learning | Powered by PrepU, http://thepoint.lww.com/prepu

Disorders of Endocrine Control of Growth and Metabolism

The endocrine system, in concert with the nervous system, serves to regulate and integrate the functioning of the body's many cells and organ systems. Disorders of the endocrine system can affect many aspects of body functioning, including growth and development, energy metabolism, muscle and adipose tissue distribution, sexual development, fluid and electrolyte balance, and inflammatory and immune responses.

This chapter focuses on disorders of the anterior pituitary gland, growth and growth hormone, thyroid gland, and adrenocortical hormones. Disorders of the parathyroid hormone are discussed in Chapter 8, insulin in Chapter 33, and the male and female gonadal hormones in Chapters 39 and 40.

General Aspects of Altered Endocrine Function

Several processes can disturb the normal function of the endocrine system, including impaired or uncontrolled synthesis or release of hormones, altered interactions between hormones and their target tissues, or abnormal responses of the target tissues to their hormones. Diseases involving the endocrine system most commonly present with signs of hypofunction or hyperfunction.[1] The disorder can occur as a primary disorder of an endocrine organ or as a secondary or tertiary disorder involving hormones produced by the pituitary gland or hypothalamus.

Hypofunction and Hyperfunction

Hypofunction of an endocrine gland can occur for a variety of reasons. Congenital defects can result in the absence or impaired development of an endocrine gland or the absence of an enzyme needed for hormone synthesis. The gland may be destroyed by a disruption in blood flow, infection, inflammation, autoimmune responses, or neoplastic growth. There may be a decline in function with aging, or the gland may atrophy as the result of drug therapy or for unknown reasons. Some endocrine-deficient states are associated with receptor defects: hormone receptors may be absent, the receptor binding of hormones may be defective, or the cellular responsiveness to the hormone may be impaired. It is suspected that in some cases a gland may produce a biologically inactive hormone or that an active hormone may be destroyed by circulating antibodies before it can exert its action.

Hyperfunction usually is associated with excessive hormone production. This can result from excessive stimulation and hyperplasia of an endocrine gland or from a hormone-producing tumor. Hyperfunction symptoms may also be *paraneoplastic*, meaning they are caused by hormones secreted by tumors of nonendocrine tissue (see Chapter 7). In addition to excessive endogenous hormone production, syndromes of hormone excess may result from deliberate or inadvertent administration of exogenous hormones. For example, administration of glucocorticoid drugs to suppress the inflammatory response may lead to Cushing syndrome, or androgen excess with suppression of pituitary gonadotropins may occur in athletes who take androgens to improve their performance.

Primary, Secondary, and Tertiary Disorders

Endocrine disorders in general can be divided into primary, secondary, and tertiary disorders. *Primary* disorders originate in the target gland responsible for producing the hormone. In *secondary disorders* of endocrine function, the target gland is essentially normal, but its function is altered by defective levels of stimulating hormones or releasing hormones from the pituitary gland. For example, total thyroidectomy produces a primary deficiency of thyroid hormones. Removal or destruction of the pituitary gland eliminates thyroid-stimulating hormone stimulation of the thyroid and brings about a secondary deficiency. A *tertiary disorder* results from hypothalamic dysfunction (as may occur with craniopharyngiomas or cerebral irradiation); thus, both the pituitary and target glands are understimulated.

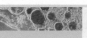

SUMMARY CONCEPTS

■ Disorders of the endocrine system, which provides the chemical messengers that serve to integrate the many functions of the body, can result from either a hypofunction or hyperfunction of an endocrine gland.

■ These disorders can occur as a primary defect in hormone production by a target gland that produces the hormone or as a secondary or tertiary disorder resulting from a defect in the hypothalamic-pituitary system that controls the target gland's function.

Anterior Pituitary and Growth Hormone Disorders

The pituitary gland, also known as the *hypophysis,* is a pea-sized gland located at the base of the brain, where it lies in a saddle-shaped depression in the sphenoid bone called the *sella turcica.* A short funnel-shaped stalk, the *infundibulum,* connects the pituitary gland with the hypothalamus. The pituitary gland has two components: a posterior lobe (neurohypophysis) or neural component, which stores and releases the oxytocin and the antidiuretic hormone (discussed in Chapter 8), and an anterior lobe (adenohypophysis) or glandular component (see Chapter 31, Fig. 31-3).

Control of Anterior Pituitary Function

The anterior lobe of the pituitary gland produces adrenocorticotropic hormone (ACTH), thyroid-stimulating hormone (TSH), growth hormone (GH), the gonadotropic hormones (follicle-stimulating hormone [FSH] and luteinizing hormone [LH]), and prolactin.[2,3] The release of these hormones is in turn under the control of hormones produced in the hypothalamus (see Chapter 31). All of the anterior pituitary hormones, except for GH, exert their primary effects by controlling the biosynthesis and secretion of hormones from other target endocrine glands. ACTH controls the release of cortisol from the adrenal gland, TSH controls the secretion of thyroid hormone from the thyroid gland, and LH and FSH control sex hormone production and fertility.

Clinical Manifestations of Hypothalamic-Pituitary Disorders

Diseases of the pituitary are uncommon but may present with a variety of manifestations including pituitary hormone hypersecretion, hyposecretion, and/or the localized mass effect that causes compression of the optic chiasm or basal portion of the brain. In adults, the most common cause of hypothalamic-pituitary dysfunction is a pituitary adenoma. In children, pituitary adenomas are uncommon; the most common cause of pituitary dysfunction is hypothalamic tumors, of which craniopharyngiomas (neoplasms arising from cells of an embryonic hypophysial structure) are the most common. These tumors usually manifest with signs of pituitary hyposecretion (e.g., short stature due to low GH levels and delayed puberty due to gonadotropin deficiency) prior to development of headache, visual loss, and other neurologic symptoms due to the mass effect of the expanding tumor.

Assessment of Hypothalamic-Pituitary Function

The precise assessment of hypothalamic-pituitary function has been made possible by radioimmunoassay of the anterior pituitary hormones and their specific target gland hormones. Magnetic resonance imaging (MRI) is used for imaging the hypothalamus and pituitary. It has largely replaced the use of computed tomography (CT) because it allows better visualization of normal structures and has better resolution in defining tumors.[2] When further information regarding pituitary function is required, combined hypothalamic-pituitary function tests (e.g., rapid ACTH stimulation test or GH suppression test) may be undertaken.[2]

Pituitary Adenomas and Hyperpituitarism

The most common cause of hyperpituitarism is a pituitary adenoma, or a benign tumor arising from the anterior pituitary.[2–5] Other, less common causes of hyperpituitarism are hyperplasia and carcinoma of the anterior pituitary, secretion of hormones by extrapituitary tumors, and certain hypothalamic lesions. Clinically diagnosed pituitary adenomas are responsible for about 10% of intracranial neoplasms. They are discovered incidentally in as many as 25% of routine autopsies and are increasingly being detected as incidental findings on MRI and CT scans of the head performed for other reasons.[6]

The usual pituitary adenoma is a well-circumscribed lesion that can range in size from small lesions that do not enlarge the gland (microadenomas, <1 cm) to large, expansive tumors (macroadenomas, >1 cm) that erode the sella turcica and impinge on surrounding cranial structures.[2,5] The adenomas can be divided into nonfunctional tumors and functional tumors that secrete pituitary hormones.

The signs and symptoms of pituitary adenomas include endocrine abnormalities related specifically to functional hormone-secreting adenomas and to the local mass effects of the expanding tumor. Lactotrophic adenomas are the most frequent type of hyperfunctioning pituitary adenoma, accounting for about 30% of all diagnosed cases.[2,4,5] Lactotrophic adenomas are usually small, benign tumors composed of prolactin-secreting cells. Hyperprolactinemia inhibits the pulsatile secretion of LH, which is essential for normal ovulation in women. Thus, the manifestations of hyperprolactinemia are most easily recognized in women of reproductive age and include amenorrhea (lack of menstruation), galactorrhea (spontaneous milk secretion unrelated to pregnancy), and infertility. In males, the symptoms of hyperprolactinemia are vague and may include erectile dysfunction and loss of libido.

Because of the close proximity of the sella turcica to the optic nerves and chiasm, expanding pituitary lesions often compress the decussating fibers of the optic chiasm, giving rise to visual field abnormalities.[2,5] Cranial nerve deficits, which are much less common, can result in blurred or double vision or, very rarely, paresthesia (abnormal nonpainful burning or prickling sensation) on one side of the face. As in the case of any expanding intracranial mass, pituitary adenomas may produce signs and symptoms of increased intracranial pressure, including headache, nausea, and vomiting. In some cases, pituitary adenomas may extend beyond the sella turcica into the base of the brain, producing seizures and obstructive hydrocephalus. On occasion, acute hemorrhage into an adenoma may occur, producing rapid enlargement of the pituitary. The condition, termed *pituitary apoplexy*, is accompanied by a combination of acute nerve palsies, severe headache, and systemic symptoms related to ACTH deficiency.

Hypopituitarism

Hypopituitarism is characterized by a decreased secretion of pituitary hormones that causes hypofunction of the secondary organs that depend on trophic stimuli from the pituitary.[1] It may selectively involve one subset of pituitary cells (e.g., somatotropes that produce growth hormone) or all of the pituitary cells, in which case it is referred to as *panhypopituitarism*. Typically, 70% to 90% of the anterior pituitary must be destroyed before hypopituitarism becomes clinically evident. The cause may be congenital, or result from a variety of acquired abnormalities that cause destruction of the anterior pituitary, or from a secondary phenomenon resulting from a deficiency of hypothalamic hormones that normally act on the pituitary. Space-occupying lesions cause hypopituitarism by destroying the pituitary gland or hypothalamic nuclei or by disrupting the hypothalamic-hypophysial portal system.

Anterior pituitary hormone loss is usually gradual, especially with progressive loss of pituitary reserve due to tumors or previous pituitary radiation therapy (which may take 10 to 20 years to produce hypopituitarism). The loss of pituitary function tends to follow a classic course beginning with the loss of GH, LH, and FSH secretion followed by deficiencies in TSH, then ACTH, and finally prolactin. Impairment of GH secretion causes decreased growth in children but may be clinically unapparent in adults. Hypogonadism, manifested by amenorrhea in women and decreased libido and erectile function in men, may precede the clinical appearance of other manifestations. The manifestations of hypothyroidism caused by TSH deficiency (e.g., cold intolerance, dry skin, mental dullness) are similar to those observed in primary thyroid failure but less severe. Adrenocorticotropic hormone deficiency is the most serious endocrine deficiency. It causes secondary adrenal insufficiency, leading to weakness, nausea, anorexia, fever, and postural hypotension.

Treatment of hypopituitarism includes treating any identified underlying cause. Hormone deficiencies require replacement therapy with appropriate hormones. Cortisol replacement is started when ACTH deficiency is present, thyroid replacement when TSH deficiency is detected, and sex hormone replacement when LH and FSH are deficient. Growth hormone replacement is indicated for pediatric GH deficiency and is being increasingly used to treat GH deficiency in adults.[2,7,8]

Growth and Growth Hormone Disorders

Several hormones are essential for normal body growth and maturation, including growth hormone, insulin, thyroid hormone, and androgens.[9] Insulin, for example, plays an essential role in growth processes, in addition to its actions on carbohydrate and fat metabolism. Children with diabetes, particularly those with poor control, often fail to grow normally even though GH levels are normal. When levels of thyroid hormone are lower than normal, bone growth and epiphyseal closure are delayed. Androgens such as testosterone and dihydrotestosterone exert anabolic growth effects through their actions on protein synthesis. Glucocorticoids at excessive levels inhibit growth, apparently because of their antagonistic effect on GH secretion.

Growth Hormone

Growth hormone, also called *somatotropin*, is a 191-amino-acid polypeptide hormone synthesized and secreted by special cells in the anterior pituitary called *somatotropes*.[2] For many years, it was thought that GH was produced primarily during periods of growth. However, this has proved to be incorrect because the rate of GH production in adults is almost as great as in children.

Growth hormone is necessary for growth and contributes to the regulation of metabolic functions (Fig. 32-1). All aspects of cartilage growth are stimulated by GH; one of the most striking effects of GH is on linear bone growth, resulting from its action on the epiphyseal growth plates of long bones. The width of bone also increases because of enhanced periosteal growth. Visceral and endocrine organs, skeletal and cardiac muscle, skin, and connective tissue all undergo increased growth in response to GH. In many instances, the increased growth of visceral and endocrine organs is accompanied by enhanced functional capacity. For example, increased growth of cardiac muscle is accompanied by an increase in cardiac output.

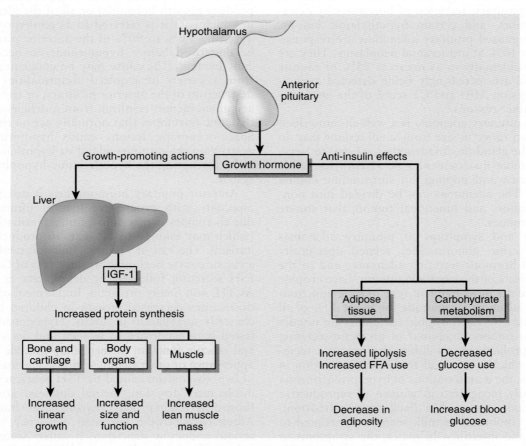

FIGURE 32-1. Growth-promoting and anti-insulin effects of growth hormone. FFA, free fatty acids; IGF-1, insulin-like growth factor-1.

In addition to its effects on growth, GH increases the rate of protein synthesis by all of the cells of the body, enhances fatty acid mobilization and increases the use of fatty acids for fuel, and maintains or increases blood glucose levels by decreasing the use of glucose for fuel. Growth hormone has an initial effect of increasing insulin levels. However, the predominant effect of prolonged GH excess is to increase blood glucose levels despite an insulin increase. This is because GH induces a resistance to insulin in the peripheral tissues, inhibiting the uptake of glucose by muscle and adipose tissues.[2]

Many of the effects of GH are mediated by *insulin-like growth factors* (IGFs), which are produced mainly by the liver.[9] Growth hormone cannot directly produce bone growth; instead, it acts indirectly by causing the liver to produce IGFs. These peptides act on cartilage and bone to promote their growth. Several IGFs have been identified; of these, IGF-1 (previously known as somatomedin C) appears to be the more important in terms of growth, and it is the one that usually is measured in laboratory tests. The IGFs have been sequenced and found to have structures that are similar to those of proinsulin. This undoubtedly explains the insulin-like activity of the IGFs and the weak action of insulin on growth. Insulin-like growth factor levels are themselves influenced by a family of at least six binding factors called *IGF-binding proteins* (IGFBPs).

Growth hormone is carried unbound in the plasma and has a half-life of approximately 20 to 50 minutes. The secretion of GH is regulated by two hypothalamic hormones: GH-releasing hormone (GHRH), which increases GH release, and somatostatin, which inhibits GH release. A third hormone, the recently identified *ghrelin*, also may be important (see Chapter 28). The hypothalamic influences of GHRH and somatostatin are tightly regulated by neural and metabolic influences. The secretion of GH fluctuates over a 24-hour period, with peak levels occurring 1 to 4 hours after onset of sleep. The nocturnal sleep bursts, which account for 70% of daily GH secretion, are greater in children than in adults.

Growth hormone secretion is stimulated by hypoglycemia, fasting, starvation, increased blood levels of amino acids (particularly arginine), and stress conditions such as excitement, emotional stress, heavy exercise, and trauma. Growth hormone is inhibited by increased glucose levels, free fatty acid release, cortisol, and obesity.

 Short Stature in Children

Short stature is a condition in which the attained height is well below the third percentile or linear growth is below normal for age and gender. Short stature, or growth retardation, has a variety of causes, including chromosomal abnormalities such as Turner syndrome (see Chapter 6), GH deficiency, hypothyroidism, and panhypopituitarism.[9] Other conditions known to cause short stature include protein-calorie malnutrition, chronic diseases such as chronic kidney disease and poorly controlled diabetes mellitus, malabsorption syndromes such as celiac disease, and certain therapies such as excessive glucocorticoid administration.

Emotional disturbances can lead to functional endocrine disorders, causing psychosocial dwarfism. The causes of short stature are summarized in Chart 32-1.

Accurate measurement of height is an extremely important part of the physical examination of children. Completion of the developmental history and growth charts is essential.[10,11] Growth curves and growth velocity studies also are needed. The Centers for Disease Control and Prevention (CDC) growth charts are available at http://www.cdc.gov/growthcharts. Diagnosis of short stature is not made on a single measurement, but is based on sequential height measurements and on velocity of growth and parental height.[9]

The diagnostic procedures for short stature include tests to exclude nonendocrine causes. If the cause is hormonal, extensive hormonal testing procedures are initiated. Usually, GH and IGF-1 levels are determined (IGFBP-3 levels also are useful). Tests can be performed using insulin (to induce hypoglycemia), GHRH, levodopa, and arginine, all of which stimulate GH secretion so that GH reserve can be evaluated.[9] Because administration of pharmacologic agents can result in false-negative responses, two or more tests usually are performed. If a prompt rise in GH is realized, the child is considered normal. Physiologic tests of GH reserve (e.g., GH response to exercise) also can be performed. Levels of IGF-1 usually reflect those of GH and may be used to indicate GH deficiency. Radiologic films are used to assess bone age, which most often is delayed. Magnetic resonance imaging of the hypothalamic-pituitary area is recommended if a

CHART 32-1   Causes of Short Stature

Variants of normal
Genetic or "familial" short stature
Constitutional growth delay
Low birth weight (e.g., intrauterine growth retardation)
Functional endocrine disorders (psychosocial dwarfism)
Growth hormone (GH) deficiency
  Primary GH deficiency (idiopathic GH deficiency, pituitary agenesis)
  Secondary GH deficiency (panhypopituitarism)
Biologically inactive GH production
Deficient IGF-1 production in response to normal or elevated GH (Laron-type dwarfism)
Hypothyroidism
Glucocorticoid excess
  Endogenous (Cushing syndrome)
  Exogenous (glucocorticoid drug treatment)
Abnormal mineral metabolism (e.g., pseudohypoparathyroidism)
Diabetes mellitus in poor control
Chronic illness and malnutrition (e.g., asthma, especially when treated with glucocorticoids; heart or renal disease)
Malabsorption syndrome (e.g., celiac sprue)
Chromosomal disorders (e.g., Turner syndrome)
Skeletal abnormalities (e.g., achondroplasia)

lesion is clinically suspected. After the cause of short stature has been determined, treatment can be initiated.

Idiopathic Short Stature. Idiopathic short stature, also referred to as normal-variant short stature, is short stature of undefined cause.[11–13] It has been defined as a condition in which the height of an individual is more than 2 standard deviations below the corresponding mean height for a given age, sex, and population group without evidence of systemic, endocrine, nutritional, or chromosomal abnormalities.[10] This definition includes children with familial short stature and constitutional delay in growth and puberty. Children with familial short stature tend to be well proportioned and to have a height close to the midparental height of their parents. The midparental height for boys can be calculated by adding 13 cm (5 inches) to the height of the mother, adding the father's height, and dividing the total by two. For girls, 13 cm (5 inches) is subtracted from the father's height, the result is added to the mother's height, and the total is divided by two.[9] Ninety-five percent of normal children are within 8 cm (i.e., ±2 standard deviations) of the midparental height.

Constitutional delay in growth and puberty describes children (particularly boys) who have moderately short stature, thin build, delayed skeletal and sexual maturation, and absence of other causes of decreased growth. *Catch-up growth* is a term used to describe an abnormally high growth rate that occurs as a child approaches normal height for age. It also occurs after the initiation of therapy for GH deficiency and hypothyroidism and the correction of chronic diseases.[9]

Psychosocial Dwarfism. Psychosocial dwarfism involves a functional hypopituitarism and is seen in some emotionally deprived children. These children usually present with poor growth, potbelly, and poor eating and drinking habits. Typically, there is a history of disturbed family relationships in which the child has been severely neglected or disciplined. Often, the neglect is confined to one child in the family. Growth hormone function usually returns to normal after the child is removed from the constraining environment. The prognosis depends on improvement in behavior and catch-up growth. Family therapy usually is indicated, and foster care may be necessary.

Growth Hormone and Insulin-Like Growth Factor Deficiencies in Children. There are several forms of GH deficiency that present in childhood. Children with idiopathic GH deficiency lack the hypothalamic GHRH but have adequate somatotropes, whereas children with pituitary tumors or agenesis of the pituitary lack somatotropes.

Congenital GH deficiency is associated with a shorter than normal birth length, followed by a decrease in growth rate that can be identified by careful measurement during the first year and that becomes obvious by 1 to 2 years of age. Children with classic GH deficiency have normal intelligence, short stature, obesity with immature facial features, and some delay in skeletal maturation (Fig. 32-2). Puberty often is delayed, and

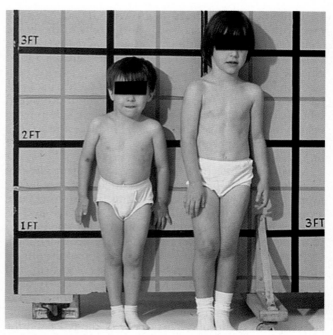

FIGURE 32-2. Child with growth hormone deficiency. A 5.5-year-old boy (*left*) with growth hormone deficiency was significantly shorter than his fraternal twin sister (*right*), with the discrepancy beginning early in childhood. Notice his chubby, immature appearance compared with his sister. (From Shulman D, Bercu B, volume eds. Atlas of Clinical Endocrinology, Volume IV: Neuroendocrinology and Pituitary Disease. Korenman S, series ed. Philadelphia, PA: Current Medicine; 2000. With kind permission of Springer Science + Business Media.)

males with the disorder have microphallus (abnormally small penis), especially if the condition is accompanied by gonadotropin-releasing hormone (GnRH) deficiency. In the neonate, GH deficiency can lead to hypoglycemia and seizures; if ACTH deficiency also is present, the hypoglycemia often is more severe. Acquired GH deficiency develops in later childhood. It may be caused by a hypothalamic-pituitary tumor, particularly if it is accompanied by other pituitary hormone deficiencies.

When short stature is caused by a GH deficiency, GH replacement therapy is the treatment of choice. Growth hormone is species specific, and only human GH is effective in humans. Human GH is now produced by recombinant deoxyribonucleic acid (DNA) technology, and is available in adequate supply. The hormone is administered daily by subcutaneous injection during the period of active growth and can be continued into adulthood.[9] Children with short stature due to Turner syndrome and chronic renal insufficiency also are treated with GH. Growth hormone therapy may also be considered for children with idiopathic short stature.[10]

In a rare condition called *Laron-type* dwarfism there is an extreme resistance to GH due to abnormalities in the growth hormone receptor.[9,14] Affected persons tend to be obese and have high levels of GH and low levels of IGF-1. The condition is seen predominantly in people of Mediterranean descent, especially Sephardic Jews.

The same pathology is responsible for dwarfism of the African pygmies. IGF-1 is now produced by recombinant DNA technology. Since GH produces its effects by promoting IGF-1 secretion, IGF-1 is an effective replacement therapy for Laron dwarfism, mimicking most of the effects ascribed to GH.[9]

Growth Hormone Deficiency in Adults

There are two categories of GH deficiency in adults: GH deficiency that was present in childhood, and GH deficiency that developed during adulthood, mainly as the result of hypopituitarism resulting from a pituitary tumor or its treatment.[15] Growth hormone levels also can decline with aging (described as the *somatopause*), and there has been interest in the effects of declining GH levels in the elderly.[16] Growth hormone replacement obviously is important in the growing child; however, the role in adults (especially for the somatopause) is being assessed.

The clinical features of adult GH deficiency include changes in body composition, such as a decrease in lean body mass and an increase in fat mass, hyperlipidemia, decreased bone mineral density, and reduced exercise capacity, and diminished sense of well-being. Growth hormone deficiency is associated with a cluster of cardiovascular risk factors including central adiposity (associated with increased visceral fat), insulin resistance, and dyslipidemia.[15] These features also are associated with the *metabolic syndrome* (see Chapter 33). In addition to these so-called traditional cardiovascular risk factors, nontraditional cardiovascular risk factors (e.g., C-reactive protein [CRP], which is a marker of the inflammatory pathway) are also elevated.[17]

Several recombinant human GH preparations have been approved for treatment of adults with diagnosed GH deficiency. The most common side effects of GH treatment in adults with hypopituitarism are peripheral edema, arthralgias and myalgias, carpal tunnel syndrome, paresthesias, and decreased glucose tolerance.[15] Side effects appear to be more common in people who are older, have greater weight, and are overtreated as determined by high serum IGF-1 levels during therapy.

Tall Stature and Growth Hormone Excess in Children

Just as there are children who are short for their age and gender, there also are children who are tall for their age and gender.[9,18] Normal variants of tall stature include genetic tall stature and constitutional tall stature. Children with exceptionally tall parents tend to be taller than children with shorter parents. The term *constitutional tall stature* is used to describe a child who is taller than his or her peers and is growing at a velocity that is within the normal range for bone age. Other causes of tall stature are genetic or chromosomal disorders such as Marfan syndrome or XYY syndrome (see Chapter 6). Endocrine causes of tall stature include sexual precocity because of early onset of estrogen and androgen secretion and excessive GH.

Exceptionally tall children (i.e., genetic tall stature and constitutional tall stature) can be treated with sex hormones—estrogens in girls and testosterone in boys—to effect early epiphyseal closure. Such treatment is undertaken only after full consideration of the risks involved. To be effective, such treatment must be instituted 3 to 4 years before expected epiphyseal fusion.[9,18]

Growth hormone excess occurring before puberty and the fusion of the epiphyses of the long bones results in *gigantism*[19] (Fig. 32-3). It usually develops when excessive secretion of GH by somatotrope adenomas leads to high levels of IGF-1, the mediator of excessive skeletal growth. Fortunately, the condition is rare because of early recognition and treatment of the adenoma.

Growth Hormone Excess in Adults

When GH excess occurs in adulthood or after the epiphyses of the long bones have fused, it causes a condition called *acromegaly* (from the Greek words *acros*, meaning "end portion," and *megalos*, meaning "large"),

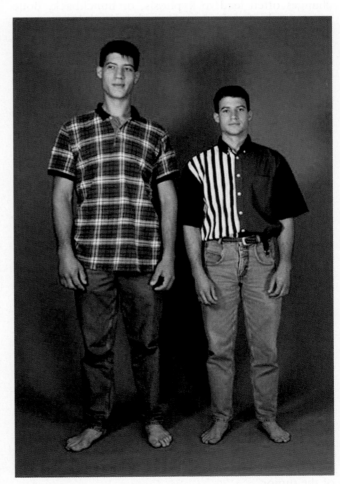

FIGURE 32-3. Primary gigantism. A 22-year-old man with gigantism due to excess growth hormone is shown to the left of his identical twin. (From Gagel RF, McCutcheon IE. Images in clinical medicine. *N Engl J Med.* 1999;340:524. Copyright © 2003. Massachusetts Medical Society.)

which represents an exaggerated growth of the ends of the extremities (fingers, hands, and toes). The annual incidence of acromegaly is 3 to 4 cases per 1 million people, with a mean age at the time of diagnosis of 40 to 45 years.[2,20,21]

The most common cause of acromegaly is GH-secreting adenomas, most of which are benign.[21] The disorder usually has an insidious onset, and symptoms often are present for a considerable period before a diagnosis is made. When the production of excessive GH occurs after the epiphyses of the long bones have closed, as in the adult, the person cannot grow taller, but the soft tissues continue to grow. Enlargement of the small bones of the hands and feet and of the membranous bones of the face and skull results in a pronounced enlargement of the hands and feet, a broad and bulbus nose, a protruding jaw, and a slanting forehead (Fig. 32-4). The teeth become splayed, causing a disturbed bite and difficulty in chewing. The cartilaginous structures in the larynx and respiratory tract also become enlarged, resulting in a deepening of the voice and tendency to develop bronchitis. Vertebral changes often lead to kyphosis, or hunchback. Bone overgrowth often leads to arthralgias and degenerative arthritis of the spine, hips, and knees. Virtually every organ of the body is increased in size. Enlargement of the heart and accelerated atherosclerosis may lead to an early death.

The metabolic effects of excess levels of GH include disorders of fat and carbohydrate metabolism. Growth hormone causes increased release of free fatty acids from adipose tissue, leading to increased concentration of free fatty acids in body fluids. In addition, GH exerts multiple effects on carbohydrate metabolism, including decreased glucose uptake by tissues such as skeletal muscle and adipose tissue, increased glucose production by the liver, and increased insulin secretion. Each of these changes results in GH-induced insulin resistance (see Chapter 33). Impaired glucose tolerance occurs in as many as 50% to 70% of persons with acromegaly; overt diabetes mellitus subsequently can result.

Other manifestations of acromegaly include excessive sweating with an unpleasant odor, oily skin, heat intolerance, moderate weight gain, muscle weakness and fatigue, menstrual irregularities, and decreased libido. Hypertension is relatively common. Sleep apnea syndrome is present in up to 90% of patients. The pathogenesis of the sleep apnea syndrome is obstructive in the majority of patients, due to increased pharyngeal soft tissue accumulation. Paresthesias may develop because of nerve entrapment and compression caused by excess soft tissue and accumulation of subcutaneous fluid (especially carpal tunnel syndrome). Headaches are frequent. Temporal hemianopia (loss of vision for one half of the visual field) may occur as a result of the optic chiasm being impinged by a suprasellar growth of the tumor.

The treatment goals for acromegaly focus on the correction of metabolic abnormalities and include normalization of the GH response to an oral glucose load; normalization of IGF-1 levels to age- and sex-matched control levels; removal or reduction of the tumor mass;

relieving the central mass effects; and improvement of adverse clinical features.[2] Pituitary tumors can be removed surgically using the transsphenoidal approach or, if that is not possible, a transfrontal craniotomy. Radiation therapy may be used, but remission (reduction in GH levels) may not occur for several years after therapy.

Somatostatin analogs (especially long-acting formulations of octreotide or lanreotide) produce feedback inhibition of GH and are effective in the medical management of acromegaly. Dopamine agonists also reduce GH levels and have been used with some success.[2] Growth hormone analogs (e.g., pegvisomant) antagonize the actions of GH by binding to GH receptors on the cell surfaces. These analogs produce symptom relief and normalize serum IGF-1 levels in most individuals with acromegaly.[2]

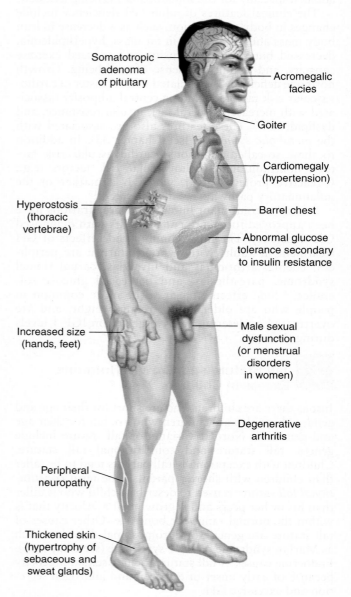

Somatotropic adenoma of pituitary

Acromegalic facies

Goiter

Cardiomegaly (hypertension)

Hyperostosis (thoracic vertebrae)

Barrel chest

Abnormal glucose tolerance secondary to insulin resistance

Increased size (hands, feet)

Male sexual dysfunction (or menstrual disorders in women)

Degenerative arthritis

Peripheral neuropathy

Thickened skin (hypertrophy of sebaceous and sweat glands)

FIGURE 32-4. Clinical manifestations of acromegaly.

Precocious Puberty

Precocious puberty is defined as early activation of the hypothalamic-pituitary-gonadal axis, resulting in the development of secondary sexual characteristics and fertility.[22,23] Classically, sexual development was considered precocious and warranting investigation when it occurred before 8 years of age for girls and before 9 years of age for boys. However, these criteria were revised based on an office pediatric study of more than 17,000 American girls.[24] Precocious puberty is now defined as the appearance of secondary sexual development before the age of 7 years in white girls and 6 years in African American girls.[23] In boys of both races, the lower age limit remains 9 years; however, it is recognized that puberty can develop earlier in boys with obesity (an increasingly common problem).[23] Precocious sexual development may be idiopathic or may be caused by gonadal, adrenal, or hypothalamic disorders. Benign and malignant tumors of the central nervous system (CNS) can cause precocious puberty. These tumors are thought to remove the inhibitory influences normally exerted on the hypothalamus during childhood. Central nervous system tumors are found more often in boys with precocious puberty than in girls. In girls, most cases are idiopathic.

Diagnosis of precocious puberty in girls is based on physical findings of early thelarche (i.e., beginning of breast development), adrenarche (i.e., beginning of augmented adrenal androgen production), and menarche (i.e., beginning of menstrual function) in girls. The most common sign in boys is early genital enlargement. Radiologic findings may indicate advanced bone age. Persons with precocious puberty usually are tall for their age as children but short as adults because of the early closure of the epiphyses. MRI or CT should be used to exclude intracranial lesions.

Depending on the cause of precocious puberty, the treatment may involve surgery, medication, or no treatment. The administration of a long-acting GnRH agonist results in a decrease in pituitary responsiveness to GnRH, leading to decreased secretion of gonadotropic hormones and sex steroids (i.e., due to down-regulation of GnRH receptors). Parents often need education, support, and anticipatory guidance in dealing with their feelings and the child's physical needs and in relating to a child who appears older than his or her years.

- or localized mass effects that cause compression of the optic chiasm or basal portion of the brain.
- Growth hormone, which is produced by somatotropes in the anterior pituitary, is necessary for linear bone growth in children, as well as affecting the rate at which cells transport amino acids across their cell membranes and the rate at which they utilize carbohydrates and fatty acids. The effects of GH on linear growth require insulin-like growth factors (IGFs), which are produced mainly by the liver.
- In children a GH (or IGF) deficiency interferes with linear bone growth, resulting in short stature or dwarfism, and an excess results in increased linear growth or gigantism. In adults, GH deficiency represents a deficiency carried over from childhood or one that develops during adulthood as the result of a pituitary tumor or its treatment; and a GH excess in adults results in acromegaly, which involves overgrowth of the cartilaginous parts of the skeleton, enlargement of the heart and other organs, and metabolic disturbances in fat and carbohydrate metabolism.
- Alterations in childhood growth include short or tall stature. Short stature can occur as a variant of normal growth, idiopathic short stature, or as the result of endocrine disorders, chronic illness, malnutrition, emotional disturbances, chromosomal disorders, or GH deficiency. Tall stature can occur as a variant of normal growth (i.e., genetic tall stature or constitutional tall stature) or as the result of a chromosomal abnormality or GH excess.
- Precocious puberty defines a condition of early activation of the hypothalamic-pituitary-gonadal axis (i.e., before 6 years of age in African American girls and 7 years of age in white girls, and before 9 years of age in boys of both races), resulting in the development of secondary sexual characteristics and fertility. It causes tall stature during childhood but results in short stature in adulthood because of the early closure of the epiphyses.

SUMMARY CONCEPTS

- With the exception of growth hormone (GH), the hypothalamus and anterior pituitary gland form a unit that controls the function of the thyroid gland, adrenal cortex, ovaries, and testes.
- Disorders of the anterior pituitary are uncommon but may present with a variety of manifestations including hormone hyper- or hyposecretion and/

Thyroid Hormone Disorders

The thyroid gland, which is the body's largest single organ specialized for hormone production, plays a major role in the processes of almost all body cells.

Structure and Function of the Thyroid Gland

The thyroid gland is a shield-shaped structure located immediately below the larynx in the anterior middle portion of the neck[25,26] (Fig. 32-5A). It is composed of

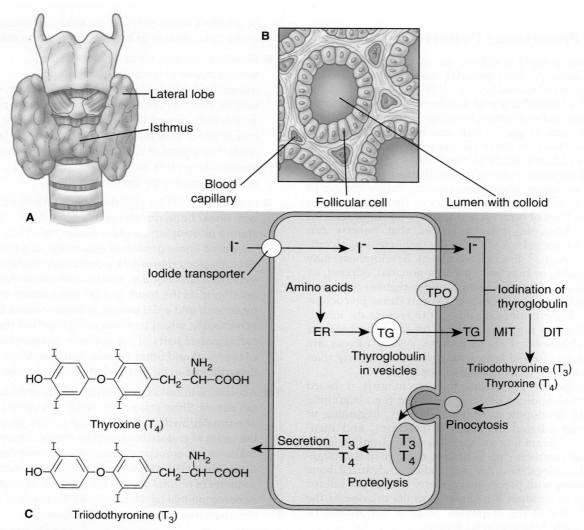

FIGURE 32-5. (A) The thyroid gland. **(B)** Microscopic structure of thyroid follicles. **(C)** Cellular mechanisms for transport of iodide (I⁻), oxidation of I⁻ by thyroperoxidase (TPO), coupling of oxidized I⁻ with thyroglobulin (TG) to form thyroid hormones, and movement of T_3 and T_4 into the follicular cell by pinocytosis and release into the blood. ER, endoplasmic reticulum; MIT, monoiodotyrosine; DIT, diiodotyrosine.

a large number of tiny, saclike structures called *follicles* (Fig. 32-5B). These are the functional units of the thyroid. Each follicle is formed by a single layer of epithelial (follicular) cells and is filled with a secretory substance called *colloid,* which consists largely of a glycoprotein–tyrosine complex called *thyroglobulin* that contains 140 tyrosine amino acids. In the process of thyroid hormone synthesis, iodide is attached to these tyrosine molecules. Both thyroglobulin and iodide are secreted into the colloid of the follicle by the follicular cells.

The thyroid is remarkably efficient in its use of iodide. A daily absorption of 150 to 200 μg of dietary iodide is sufficient to form normal quantities of thyroid hormone. In the process of removing it from the blood and storing it for future use, iodide (I⁻) is pumped into the follicular cells against a concentration gradient by an intrinsic membrane protein called the *Na⁺/I symporter* (NIS).[25] At the apical border, a second transport protein

called *pendrin* moves iodide into the colloid, where it is involved in hormone production. The NIS is stimulated by both TSH and the TSH receptor–stimulating antibody found in Graves' disease (to be discussed). Mutations in the pendrin gene (*PDS*) have been found in persons with goiter and congenital deafness (Pendred syndrome).

Synthesis of Thyroid Hormones

Once inside the follicle, most of the iodide is oxidized by the enzyme thyroid peroxidase (TPO) in a reaction that facilitates combination with a tyrosine molecule to form monoiodotyrosine (MIT), and a second iodide is then attached to make diiodotyrosine (DIT). Two diiodotyrosine molecules are coupled to form thyroxine (T_4), or a monoiodotyrosine and a diiodotyrosine are coupled to form triiodothyronine (T_3). Only T_4 (90%) and T_3 (10%) are released into the circulation (Fig. 32-5C).

There is evidence that T_3 is the active form of the hormone and that T_4 is converted to T_3 before it can act physiologically.

Thyroid hormones are bound to thyroxine-binding globulin (TBG) and other plasma proteins, mainly transthyretin and albumin, for transport in the blood. Only the free hormone enters cells and regulates the pituitary feedback mechanism. Protein-bound thyroid hormone forms a large reservoir that is slowly drawn on as free thyroid hormone is needed. More than 99% of T_4 and T_3 is carried in the bound form.[25,26] TBG carries approximately 75% of T_4 and T_3, transthyretin binds approximately 10% of circulating T_4 and lesser amounts of T_3, and albumin binds approximately 15% of circulating T_4 and T_3.

A number of conditions and pharmacologic agents can decrease the amount of binding protein in the plasma or influence hormone binding. Congenital TBG deficiency is an X-linked trait that occurs in 1 of every 5000 live births. Glucocorticoid medications and systemic disease conditions such as protein malnutrition, nephrotic syndrome, and cirrhosis decrease TBG concentrations. Medications such as phenytoin, salicylates, and diazepam can affect the binding of thyroid hormone to normal concentrations of binding proteins.

Regulation of Thyroid Hormone Secretion

The secretion of thyroid hormone is regulated by the hypothalamic-pituitary-thyroid feedback system (Fig. 32-6). In this system, thyrotropin-releasing hormone (TRH), which is produced by the hypothalamus, increases the release of TSH from the anterior pituitary gland. Thyroid stimulating hormone, in turn, binds to the TSH receptor on thyroid epithelial cells stimulating essentially every aspect of thyroid function, including promoting the release of thyroid hormones from the thyroid follicles into the bloodstream, and increasing the activity of the iodide pump and iodination of tyrosine to increase production of the thyroid hormones. Thyroid stimulating hormone also has a strong tropic effect, stimulating hypertrophy, hyperplasia, and survival of thyroid epithelial cells.

Increased levels of thyroid hormone act in the feedback inhibition of TRH or TSH. High levels of iodide (e.g., from iodide-containing cough syrup or kelp tablets) also cause a temporary decrease in thyroid activity that lasts for several weeks, probably through a direct inhibition of TSH on the thyroid. Cold exposure is one of the strongest stimuli for increased thyroid hormone production and probably is mediated through TRH from the hypothalamus. Various emotional reactions also can affect the output of TRH and TSH and therefore indirectly affect secretion of thyroid hormones.

Actions of Thyroid Hormone

Most of the major organs in the body are affected by altered levels of thyroid hormone. Thyroid hormone increases metabolism and protein synthesis; it is necessary for growth and development in children, including mental development and attainment of sexual maturity; and it affects the function of many other organ systems in the body. These actions are mainly mediated by T_3.

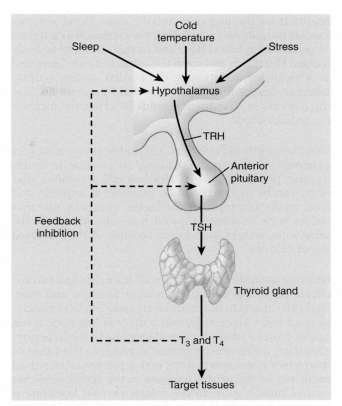

FIGURE 32-6. The hypothalamic-pituitary-thyroid feedback system, which regulates the body levels of thyroid hormone. TRH, thyrotropin-releasing hormone; TSH, thyroid-stimulating hormone.

In the cell, T_3 binds to a nuclear receptor, resulting in transcription of specific thyroid hormone response genes.[25,26]

Metabolic Rate. Thyroid hormone increases the metabolism of all body tissues except the retinas, spleen, testes, and lungs. The basal metabolic rate can increase to 60% to 100% above normal when large amounts of T_4 are present. As a result of this higher metabolism, the rate of glucose, fat, and protein use increases. Lipids are mobilized from adipose tissue, and the catabolism of cholesterol by the liver is increased. Blood levels of cholesterol are decreased in hyperthyroidism and increased in hypothyroidism. Muscle proteins are broken down and used as fuel, probably accounting for some of the muscle fatigue that occurs with hyperthyroidism. The absorption of glucose from the gastrointestinal tract is increased. Because vitamins are essential parts of metabolic enzymes and coenzymes, an increase in metabolic rate tends to accelerate the use of vitamins and cause vitamin deficiency.

Cardiorespiratory Function. Cardiovascular and respiratory functions are strongly affected by thyroid function. With an increase in metabolism, there is a rise in oxygen consumption and production of metabolic end products, with an accompanying increase in vasodilation. Blood flow to the skin, in particular, is augmented as a means of dissipating the body heat that results from the higher metabolic rate. Blood volume, cardiac output, and ventilation are increased as a means of maintaining blood flow and oxygen delivery to body tissues. Heart rate and cardiac contractility are increased as a means of maintaining the needed cardiac output, whereas there is little change in blood pressure because the increase in vasodilation tends to offset the increase in cardiac output.

Gastrointestinal Function. Thyroid hormone enhances gastrointestinal function, causing an increase in motility and production of gastrointestinal secretions that often results in diarrhea. An increase in appetite and food intake accompanies the higher metabolic rate that occurs with increased thyroid hormone levels. At the same time, weight loss occurs because of the increased use of calories.

Neuromuscular Effects. Thyroid hormone has marked effects on neural control of muscle function and tone. Slight elevations in hormone levels cause skeletal muscles to react more vigorously, and a drop in hormone levels causes muscles to react more sluggishly. In the hyperthyroid state, a fine muscle tremor is present. The cause of this tremor is unknown, but it may represent an increased sensitivity of the neural synapses in the spinal cord that control muscle tone. In the infant, thyroid hormone is necessary for normal brain development. The hormone enhances cerebration; in the hyperthyroid state, it causes extreme nervousness, anxiety, and difficulty in sleeping.

Evidence suggests a strong interaction between thyroid hormone and the sympathetic nervous system. Many of the signs and symptoms of hyperthyroidism suggest overactivity of the sympathetic division of the autonomic nervous system, such as tachycardia, palpitations, and sweating. Tremor, restlessness, anxiety, and diarrhea also may reflect autonomic nervous system imbalances. Drugs that block sympathetic activity have proved to be valuable adjuncts in the treatment of hyperthyroidism because of their ability to relieve some of these undesirable symptoms.

Tests of Thyroid Function

Various tests aid in the diagnosis of thyroid disorders.[25,27] Measures of T_3, T_4, and TSH have been made available through immunoassay methods. The free T_4 test measures the unbound portion of T_4 that is free to enter cells to produce its effects. TSH levels are used to differentiate between primary and secondary thyroid disorders. T_3, T_4, and free T_4 levels are low in primary hypothyroidism, and the TSH level is elevated. The assessment of thyroid autoantibodies (e.g., anti-TPO antibodies in Hashimoto thyroiditis) is important in the diagnostic workup and consequent follow-up of patients with thyroid disorders.

The radioiodine (^{123}I) uptake test measures the ability of the thyroid gland to remove and concentrate iodine from the blood. Thyroid scans (^{123}I, ^{99m}Tc-pertechnetate) can be used to detect thyroid nodules and determine the functional activity of the thyroid gland. Ultrasonography can be used to differentiate cystic from solid thyroid lesions, and CT and MRI scans are used to demonstrate tracheal compression or impingement on other neighboring structures. Fine needle aspiration biopsy of a thyroid nodule has proved to be the best method for differentiation of benign from malignant thyroid disease.

Thyroid Disorders

An alteration in thyroid function can present as a hypofunctional or a hyperfunctional state. The manifestations of these two altered states are summarized in Table 32-1. Disorders of the thyroid may be due to a

TABLE 32-1 Manifestations of Hypothyroid and Hyperthyroid States

Level of Organization	Hypothyroidism	Hyperthyroidism
Basal metabolic rate	Decreased	Increased
Sensitivity to catecholamines	Decreased	Increased
General features	Myxedematous features	Exophthalmos (in Graves' disease)
	Deep voice	Lid lag
	Impaired growth (child)	Accelerated growth (child)
Blood cholesterol levels	Increased	Decreased
General behavior	Mental retardation (infant)	Restlessness, irritability, anxiety
	Mental and physical sluggishness	Hyperkinesis
	Somnolence	Wakefulness
Cardiovascular function	Decreased cardiac output	Increased cardiac output
	Bradycardia	Tachycardia and palpitations
Gastrointestinal function	Constipation	Diarrhea
	Decreased appetite	Increased appetite
Respiratory function	Hypoventilation	Dyspnea
Muscle tone and reflexes	Decreased	Increased, with tremor and twitching
Temperature tolerance	Cold intolerance	Heat intolerance
Skin and hair	Decreased sweating	Increased sweating
	Coarse and dry skin and hair	Thin and silky skin and hair
Weight	Gain	Loss

congenital defect in thyroid development, or they may develop later in life, with a gradual or sudden onset.

Goiter is an increase in the size of the thyroid gland. It can occur in hypothyroid, euthyroid, and hyperthyroid states. Goiters may be toxic, producing signs of extreme hyperthyroidism or thyrotoxicosis, or they may be nontoxic. Goiters may be diffuse, involving the entire gland without evidence of nodularity, or they may contain nodules. Diffuse goiters usually become nodular.

Diffuse nontoxic and multinodular goiters are the result of compensatory hypertrophy and hyperplasia of follicular epithelium from some derangement that impairs thyroid hormone output. The degree of thyroid enlargement usually is proportional to the extent and duration of thyroid deficiency. Multinodular goiters produce the largest thyroid enlargements (Fig. 32-7). When sufficiently enlarged, they may compress the esophagus and trachea, causing difficulty in swallowing, a choking sensation, and inspiratory stridor. Such lesions also may compress the superior vena cava, producing distention of the veins of the neck and upper extremities, edema of the eyelids and conjunctiva, and syncope with coughing.

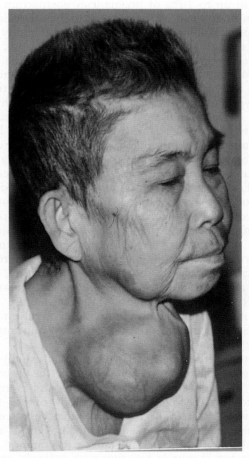

FIGURE 32-7. Nontoxic goiter in a middle aged woman. The thyroid has enlarged to produce a conspicuous neck mass. (From: Merino MJ, Quezado M. The endocrine system. In: Rubin R, Strayer DS, eds. *Rubin's Pathology: Clinicopathologic Foundations of Medicine*, 6th ed. Philadelphia, PA: Wolters Kluwer Health/Lippincott Williams & Wilkins; 2012:1047.)

Hypothyroidism

Hypothyroidism can occur as a congenital or an acquired defect. Congenital hypothyroidism develops prenatally and is present at birth. Acquired hypothyroidism develops later in life because of primary disease of the thyroid gland or secondary to disorders of hypothalamic or pituitary origin.

Congenital Hypothyroidism. Thyroid hormone is essential for normal growth and brain development, almost half of which occurs during the first 6 months of life.[25] Hypothyroidism in an infant may result from a congenital lack of the thyroid gland or from abnormal biosynthesis of thyroid hormone or deficient TSH secretion.[25] If untreated, congenital hypothyroidism causes mental retardation and impairs physical growth.

With congenital lack of the thyroid gland, the infant usually appears normal and functions normally at birth because of hormones supplied in utero by the mother. Prolongation of physiologic jaundice, caused by delayed maturation of the hepatic system for conjugating bilirubin, may be the first sign[26] (Fig. 32-8). There may be respiratory difficulties and a hoarse cry, due in part to the enlarged tongue; feeding difficulties, especially sluggishness, lack of interest, somnolence, and choking during nursing; an enlarged abdomen; and an umbilical hernia. The manifestations of untreated congenital

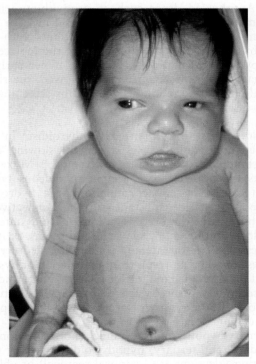

FIGURE 32-8. A 6-week-old female infant who presented with symptoms of jaundice, which was proven to be due to hypothyroidism. She was placed on supplemental thyroid hormonal therapy and appeared to be a normal healthy child at 1 year of age. (From the Centers for Disease Control and Prevention Public Health Images Library. No. 5604.)

hypothyroidism are referred to as *cretinism*. However, the term does not apply to the normally developing infant in whom replacement thyroid hormone therapy was instituted shortly after birth.

Long-term studies have shown that closely monitored T_4 supplementation begun in the first 6 weeks of life results in normal intelligence. Fortunately, developed countries throughout the world now routinely screen newborns for hypothyroidism, providing the means for early diagnosis and treatment. The screening test involves taking a drop of blood from the infant's heel and sending it to a central laboratory, where it is analyzed for T_4 or TSH.[25] Screening is done 24 to 48 hours after birth, usually in the hospital nursery.

Congenital hypothyroidism is treated by hormone replacement. Evidence indicates that it is important to normalize T_4 levels as rapidly as possible because a delay is accompanied by poorer psychomotor and mental development. Dosage levels are adjusted as the child grows.

Transient congenital hypothyroidism has been recognized more frequently since the introduction of neonatal screening. It is characterized by high TSH levels and low or normal thyroid hormone levels. The fetal and infant thyroids are sensitive to iodine excess. Iodine crosses the placenta and mammary glands and is readily absorbed by infant skin.[25] Transient hypothyroidism may be caused by maternal or infant exposure to substances such as povidone-iodine used as a disinfectant (i.e., vaginal douche or skin disinfectant in the nursery). Antithyroid drugs such as propylthiouracil and methimazole can cross the placenta and in large doses will impair fetal thyroid function. Infants with transient hypothyroidism usually can have the replacement therapy withdrawn at 6 to 12 months. When early and adequate treatment regimens are followed, the risk of mental retardation in infants detected by screening programs essentially is nonexistent.

Acquired Hypothyroidism. Hypothyroidism in older children and adults causes a general slowing down of metabolic processes and myxedema.[25] Myxedema implies the presence of a nonpitting mucous type of edema caused by an accumulation of a hydrophilic mucopolysaccharide substance in the connective tissues throughout the body. The hypothyroid state may be mild, with only a few signs and symptoms, or it may progress to a life-threatening condition called *myxedematous coma*. It can result from destruction or dysfunction of the thyroid gland (i.e., primary hypothyroidism), as a secondary disorder caused by impaired pituitary function, or as a tertiary disorder caused by a hypothalamic dysfunction.

Primary hypothyroidism is much more common than secondary (and tertiary) hypothyroidism. It may result from thyroidectomy (i.e., surgical removal) or ablation of the gland with radiation. Certain goitrogenic agents, such as lithium carbonate (used in the treatment of bipolar disorders), and the antithyroid drugs propylthiouracil and methimazole in continuous dosage can block hormone synthesis and produce hypothyroidism with goiter. Large amounts of iodine (i.e., ingestion of kelp

tablets or iodide-containing cough syrups, or administration of iodide-containing radiographic contrast media or the cardiac drug amiodarone, which contains 75 mg of iodine per 200-mg tablet) also can block thyroid hormone production and cause goiter, particularly in persons with autoimmune thyroid disease. Iodine deficiency, which can cause goiter and hypothyroidism, is rare in the United States because of the widespread use of iodized salt and other iodide sources.

The most common cause of hypothyroidism is *Hashimoto thyroiditis*, an autoimmune disorder in which the thyroid gland may be totally destroyed by an immunologic process.[28,29] It is the major cause of goiter and hypothyroidism in children and adults. Hashimoto thyroiditis is predominantly a disease of women, with a female-to-male ratio of 5:1. The course of the disease varies. At the onset, only a goiter may be present. In time, hypothyroidism usually becomes evident. Although the disorder usually causes hypothyroidism, a hyperthyroid state may develop midcourse in the disease. The transient hyperthyroid state is caused by leakage of preformed thyroid hormone from damaged cells of the thyroid gland. Subacute thyroiditis, which can occur in up to 10% of pregnancies postpartum (postpartum thyroiditis), also can result in hypothyroidism.

Hypothyroidism may affect almost all body functions (see Table 32-1).[25,29,30] The manifestations of the disorder are related largely to two factors: the hypometabolic state resulting from thyroid hormone deficiency, and myxedematous involvement of body tissues. The hypometabolic state associated with hypothyroidism is characterized by a gradual onset of weakness and fatigue, a tendency to gain weight despite a loss of appetite, and cold intolerance (Fig. 32-9). As the condition progresses, the skin becomes dry and rough and the hair becomes coarse and brittle. Reduced conversion of carotene to vitamin A and increased blood levels of carotene may give the skin a yellowish color. The face becomes puffy with edematous eyelids, and there is thinning of the outer third of the eyebrows. Fluid may collect in almost any serous cavity and in the middle ear, giving rise to conductive deafness. Gastrointestinal motility is decreased, producing constipation, flatulence, and abdominal distention. Delayed relaxation of deep tendon reflexes and bradycardia are sometimes noted. Central nervous system involvement is manifested in mental dullness, lethargy, and impaired memory.

Although the myxedematous fluid is usually most obvious in the face, it can collect in the interstitial spaces of almost any body structure and is responsible for many of the manifestations of the severe hypothyroid state. The tongue is often enlarged, and the voice becomes hoarse and husky. Carpal tunnel and other entrapment syndromes are common, as is impairment of muscle function with stiffness, cramps, and pain. Pericardial or pleural effusion may develop. Mucopolysaccharide deposits in the heart cause generalized cardiac dilation, bradycardia, and other signs of altered cardiac function.

Diagnosis of hypothyroidism is based on history, physical examination, and laboratory tests. A low

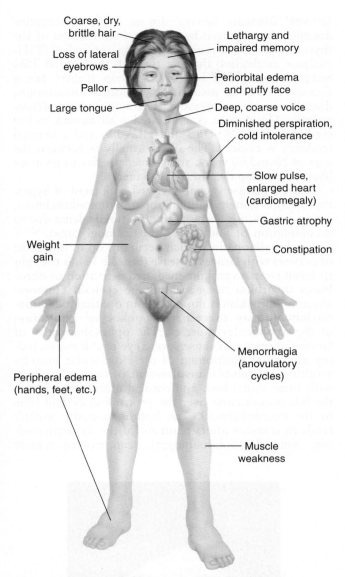

Coarse, dry, brittle hair

Loss of lateral eyebrows

Pallor

Large tongue

Weight gain

Peripheral edema (hands, feet, etc.)

Lethargy and impaired memory

Periorbital edema and puffy face

Deep, coarse voice

Diminished perspiration, cold intolerance

Slow pulse, enlarged heart (cardiomegaly)

Gastric atrophy

Constipation

Menorrhagia (anovulatory cycles)

Muscle weakness

FIGURE 32-9. Clinical manifestations of hypothyroidism.

cardiovascular collapse, hypoventilation, and severe metabolic disorders including hyponatremia, hypoglycemia, and lactic acidosis. The pathophysiology of myxedema coma involves three major aspects: (1) carbon dioxide retention and hypoxemia, (2) fluid and electrolyte imbalance, and (3) hypothermia.[31] It occurs most often in elderly women who have chronic hypothyroidism from a spectrum of causes. The fact that it occurs more frequently in winter months suggests that cold exposure may be a precipitating factor. The severely hypothyroid person is unable to metabolize sedatives, analgesics, and anesthetic drugs, and buildup of these agents may precipitate coma.

Treatment includes aggressive management of precipitating factors; supportive therapy such as management of cardiorespiratory status, hyponatremia, and hypoglycemia; and thyroid replacement therapy. If hypothermia is present (a low-reading thermometer should be used), active rewarming of the body is contraindicated because it may induce vasodilation and vascular collapse. Prevention is preferable to treatment and entails special attention to high-risk populations, such as women with a history of Hashimoto thyroiditis. These persons should be informed about the signs and symptoms of severe hypothyroidism and the need for early medical treatment.

Hyperthyroidism

Hyperthyroidism is the clinical syndrome that results when tissues are exposed to high levels of circulating thyroid hormone. In most instances, hyperthyroidism is due to hyperactivity of the thyroid gland.[25,32,33] The most common causes of hyperthyroidism are Graves' disease (to be discussed) and diffuse goiter. Other causes of hyperthyroidism are multinodular goiter, adenoma of the thyroid, and thyroiditis. Iodine-containing agents can induce hyperthyroidism as well as hypothyroidism. Thyroid crisis, or storm, is an acutely exaggerated manifestation of the thyrotoxic state.

Many of the manifestations of hyperthyroidism are related to the increase in oxygen consumption and use of metabolic fuels associated with the hypermetabolic state, as well as to the increase in sympathetic nervous system activity that occurs (see Table 32-1).[25,32,33] The fact that many of the signs and symptoms of hyperthyroidism resemble those of excessive sympathetic nervous system activity suggests that thyroid hormone may heighten the sensitivity of the body to the catecholamines or that it may act as a pseudocatecholamine. With the hypermetabolic state, there are frequent complaints of nervousness, irritability, and fatigability (Fig. 32-10). Weight loss is common despite a large appetite. Other manifestations include tachycardia, palpitations, shortness of breath, excessive sweating, muscle cramps, and heat intolerance. The person appears restless and has a fine muscle tremor. Even in persons without exophthalmos (i.e., bulging of the eyeballs seen in Graves' disease), there is an abnormal retraction of the eyelids and infrequent blinking such that they appear to be staring. The hair and skin usually are thin and have a silky appearance. About 15%

serum T_4 and elevated TSH levels are characteristic of primary hypothyroidism. The tests for antithyroid antibodies should be done when Hashimoto thyroiditis is suspected (anti-TPO antibody titer is the preferred test).

Hypothyroidism is treated by replacement therapy with synthetic preparations of T_3 or T_4. Most people are treated with T_4. Serum TSH levels are used to estimate the adequacy of T_4 replacement therapy. When the TSH level is normalized, the T_4 dosage is considered satisfactory (for primary hypothyroidism only). A "go low and go slow" approach should be considered in the treatment of elderly persons with hypothyroidism because of the risk of inducing acute coronary syndromes in susceptible individuals.

Myxedematous Coma. Myxedematous coma is a life-threatening, end-stage expression of hypothyroidism.[31] It is characterized by coma, hypothermia,

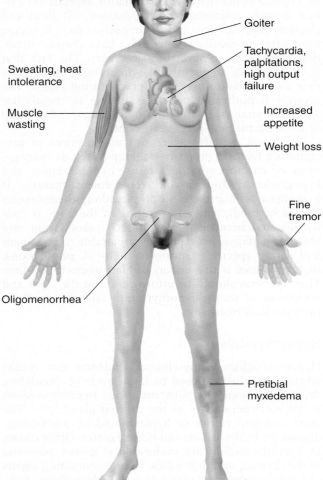

Fine hair

Exophthalmos

Nervousness
Restlessness
Emotional instability
Insomnia

Goiter

Tachycardia,
palpitations,
high output
failure

Sweating, heat
intolerance

Muscle
wasting

Increased
appetite

Weight loss

Fine
tremor

Oligomenorrhea

Pretibial
myxedema

FIGURE 32-10. Clinical manifestations of hyperthyroidism.

Graves' Disease. Graves' disease is an autoimmune disorder characterized by abnormal stimulation of the thyroid gland by thyroid-stimulating antibodies (TSH-receptor antibodies) that act through the normal TSH receptors. Identified by Irish surgeon Robert James Graves, it may be associated with other autoimmune disorders such as myasthenia gravis and pernicious anemia. The disease is associated with human leukocyte antigen (HLA)-DR3 and HLA-B8, and a familial tendency is evident. The onset usually is between the ages of 20 and 40 years, and women are five times more likely to develop the disease than men.

Graves' disease is characterized by a triad of hyperthyroidism, goiter, ophthalmopathy (exophthalmos), or less commonly, dermopathy (pretibial edema due to accumulation of fluid and glycosaminoglycans).[25,34–37] The ophthalmopathy, which occurs in up to one third of persons with Graves' disease (Fig. 32-11), is thought to result from a cytokine-mediated activation of fibroblasts in orbital tissue behind the eyeball. Humoral autoimmunity also is important; an ophthalmic immunoglobulin may exacerbate lymphocytic infiltration of the extraocular muscles. The ophthalmopathy of Graves' disease can cause severe eye problems, including abnormal positioning of the extraocular muscles resulting in diplopia; involvement of the optic nerve, with some visual loss; and corneal ulceration because the lids do not close over the protruding eyeball (due to the exophthalmos). The ophthalmopathy usually tends to stabilize after treatment of the hyperthyroidism. Since the ophthalmopathy can worsen acutely

of elderly individuals with new-onset atrial fibrillation have thyrotoxicosis.[32]

The treatment of hyperthyroidism is directed toward reducing the level of thyroid hormone. This can be accomplished with eradication of the thyroid gland with radioactive iodine, through surgical removal of part or all of the gland, or with the use of drugs that decrease thyroid function and thereby the effect of thyroid hormone on the peripheral tissues. Eradication of the thyroid with radioactive iodine is used more frequently than surgery. The β-adrenergic blocking drugs (e.g., propranolol, metoprolol, atenolol, nadolol) are administered to block the effects of the hyperthyroid state on sympathetic nervous system function. They are given in conjunction with antithyroid drugs (e.g., propylthiouracil and methimazole) that act by inhibiting the thyroid gland from using iodine in thyroid hormone synthesis and by blocking the conversion of T_4 to T_3 in the tissues (propylthiouracil only).

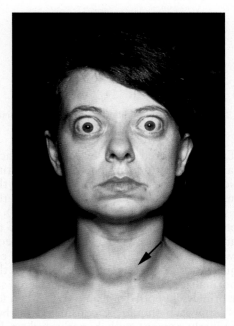

FIGURE 32-11. Graves' disease. A young woman with hyperthyroidism displays a mass in the neck and exophthalmos. (From: Merino MJ, Quezado M. The endocrine system. In: Rubin R, Strayer DS, eds. *Rubin's Pathology: Clinicopathologic Foundations of Medicine,* 6th ed. Philadelphia, PA: Wolters Kluwer Health | Lippincott Williams & Wilkins; 2012:1050. Courtesy of Novartis International AG.)

after radioiodine treatment, some physicians prescribe glucocorticoids for several weeks surrounding the radioiodine treatment if the person had signs of ophthalmopathy. Others do not use radioiodine therapy under these circumstances, but prefer antithyroid therapy with drugs (which may decrease the immune activation in the condition). Unfortunately, not all of the ocular changes are reversible with treatment. Ophthalmopathy also can be aggravated by smoking, which should be strongly discouraged.

Thyroid Storm. Thyroid storm, or crisis, is an extreme and life-threatening form of thyrotoxicosis, rarely seen today because of improved diagnosis and treatment methods.[25,38] When it does occur, it is seen most often in undiagnosed cases or in persons with hyperthyroidism who have not been adequately treated. It often is precipitated by stress such as an infection (usually respiratory), diabetic ketoacidosis, physical or emotional trauma, or manipulation of a hyperactive thyroid gland during thyroidectomy. Thyroid storm is manifested by a very high fever, extreme cardiovascular effects (i.e., tachycardia, congestive failure, and angina), and severe CNS effects (i.e., agitation, restlessness, and delirium). The mortality rate is high.

Thyroid storm requires rapid diagnosis and implementation of treatment. Peripheral cooling is initiated with cold packs and a cooling mattress. For cooling to be effective, the shivering response must be prevented. General supportive measures to replace fluids, glucose, and electrolytes are essential during the hypermetabolic state. A β-adrenergic blocking drug, such as propranolol, is used to block the undesirable effects of T_4 on cardiovascular function. Glucocorticoids are used to correct the relative adrenal insufficiency resulting from the stress imposed by the hyperthyroid state and to inhibit the peripheral conversion of T_4 to T_3. Propylthiouracil or methimazole may be given to block thyroid synthesis. Aspirin increases the level of free thyroid hormones by displacing the hormones from their protein carriers and should not be used during thyroid storm.

SUMMARY CONCEPTS

■ Thyroid hormones play a major role in the metabolic processes of almost all body cells and are necessary for normal physical and mental growth in infants and young children. Disorders of thyroid function can manifest as a hypothyroid or a hyperthyroid state.

■ Hypothyroidism can occur as a congenital or an acquired defect. Congenital hypothyroidism leads to mental retardation and impaired physical growth unless treatment is initiated during the first months of life. When hypothyroidism occurs in older children

or adults, it produces a hypometabolic state, an accumulation of a hydrophilic mucopolysaccharide substance (myxedema) in the connective tissues throughout the body, and an elevation in serum cholesterol. There is a gradual onset of weakness, a tendency to gain weight despite a loss of appetite, and cold intolerance. As the condition progresses, the skin becomes dry and rough, the hair becomes brittle, and the face becomes puffy with edematous eyelids.

■ Myxedematous coma, which is manifested by coma, hypothermia, severe fluid and electrolyte imbalances, and cardiovascular collapse, is a life-threatening, end-stage expression of hypothyroidism.

■ Hyperthyroidism has an effect opposite to that of hypothyroidism. It produces an increase in metabolic rate and oxygen consumption, increased use of metabolic fuels, and increased sympathetic nervous system responsiveness. Manifestations include nervousness, irritability, a fine muscle tremor, weight loss despite an increased appetite, excessive sweating, muscle cramps, and heat intolerance. Graves' disease is characterized by the triad of hyperthyroidism, goiter, and ophthalmopathy (exophthalmos or protruding eyeballs) or dermopathy (pretibial myxedema).

■ Thyroid storm or crisis, which is manifested by a very high fever, extreme cardiovascular effects (tachycardia, congestive failure, and angina), and severe central nervous system effects (agitation, restlessness, and delirium), is an extreme and life-threatening form of thyrotoxicosis.

Adrenal Cortical Hormone Disorders

The adrenal glands are small, bilateral structures that weigh approximately 5 g each and lie retroperitoneally at the apex of each kidney (Fig. 32-12A). The medulla or inner portion of the gland (which constitutes approximately 10% of each adrenal) secretes epinephrine and norepinephrine and is part of the sympathetic nervous system. The cortex forms the bulk of the adrenal gland (approximately 90%) and is responsible for secreting three types of hormones: glucocorticoids, mineralocorticoids, and adrenal androgens.[26,39] Because the sympathetic nervous system also secretes the neurotransmitters epinephrine and norepinephrine, adrenal medullary function is not essential for life, but adrenal cortical function is. If untreated, the total loss of adrenal cortical function is fatal in 4 to 14 days.

Adrenal Cortical Hormones

More than 30 hormones are produced by the adrenal cortex. Of these hormones, aldosterone is the principal mineralocorticoid, cortisol (hydrocortisone) is the major glucocorticoid, and androgens are the main sex hormones. All of the adrenal cortical hormones have a similar structure in that all are steroids and are synthesized from acetate and cholesterol. Each of the steps involved in the synthesis of the various hormones requires a specific enzyme (Fig. 32-12B). The secretion of both the glucocorticoids and adrenal androgens is controlled by ACTH secreted by the anterior pituitary gland.

Cortisol, aldosterone, and the adrenal androgens are secreted in an unbound state and bind to plasma proteins for transport in the circulatory system. Cortisol binds largely to corticosteroid-binding globulin and to a lesser extent to albumin. Aldosterone and androgens circulate mainly bound to albumin. It has been suggested that the pool of protein-bound hormones may extend the duration of their action by delaying metabolic clearance.

The main site for metabolism of the adrenal cortical hormones is the liver, where they undergo a number of metabolic conversions before being conjugated and made water soluble. They are then eliminated in either the urine or the bile.

Mineralocorticoid Hormones

The mineralocorticoids play an essential role in regulating potassium and sodium levels and water balance. They are produced in the zona glomerulosa or the outer layer of cells of the adrenal cortex. Aldosterone secretion is regulated by the renin-angiotensin mechanism and by blood levels of potassium. Increased levels of aldosterone promote sodium retention by the distal tubules of the kidney while increasing urinary losses of potassium. The influence of aldosterone on fluid and electrolyte balance is discussed in Chapter 8.

Glucocorticoid Hormones

The glucocorticoid hormones, mainly cortisol, are synthesized in the zona fasciculata and the zona reticularis of the adrenal cortex. The blood levels of these hormones are regulated by negative feedback mechanisms of the hypothalamic-pituitary-adrenal (HPA) system (Fig. 32-13). Just as other hormones from the hypothalamus control the release of their target pituitary hormones, corticotropin-releasing hormone (CRH) controls the release of ACTH. In turn, ACTH controls the release of cortisol. Levels of cortisol increase as ACTH levels rise and decrease as ACTH levels fall. There is considerable diurnal variation in ACTH levels, which reach their peak in the early morning (around 6 to 8 AM) and decline as the day progresses.[26] This appears to be due to rhythmic activity in the CNS, which causes bursts of CRH secretion and, in turn, ACTH secretion. This diurnal pattern is reversed in people who work during the night and sleep during the day. The rhythm also may be changed by physical and psychological stresses, endogenous depression, and liver disease or other conditions that affect cortisol metabolism. One of the earliest signs of Cushing syndrome, a disorder of glucocorticoid excess, is the loss of diurnal variation in CRH and ACTH secretion.[40,41]

The glucocorticoids perform a necessary function in response to stress and are essential for survival. When produced as part of the stress response, these hormones aid in regulating the metabolic functions of the body and in controlling the inflammatory response. The actions of cortisol are summarized in Table 32-2. Many of the anti-inflammatory actions attributed to cortisol result from the administration of pharmacologic levels of the hormone.

By far the best-known metabolic effect of cortisol and other glucocorticoids is their ability to stimulate gluconeogenesis (glucose production) by the liver. In the process, body proteins are broken down and their amino acids are mobilized and transported to the liver, where they are used in the production of glucose. In much the same manner that cortisol promotes amino acid mobilization from muscle, it promotes mobilization of fatty acids from adipose tissue. This increased mobilization of fats by cortisol converts cell metabolism from the use of glucose for energy to the use of

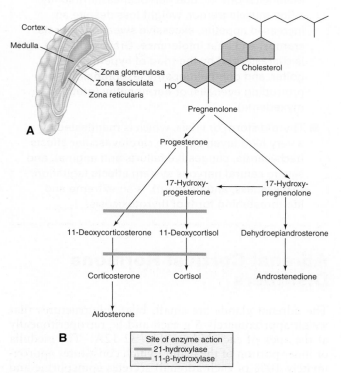

FIGURE 32-12. (A) The adrenal gland, showing the medulla and the three layers of the cortex. The outer layer of the cortex (zona glomerulosa) is primarily responsible for mineralocorticoid production, and the middle layer (zona fasciculata) and the inner layer (zona reticularis) produce the glucocorticoids and the adrenal androgens. **(B)** Predominant biosynthetic pathways of the adrenal cortex. Critical enzymes in the biosynthetic process include 11-β-hydroxylase and 21-hydroxylase. A deficiency in one of these enzymes blocks the synthesis of hormones dependent on that enzyme and routes the precursors into alternative pathways.

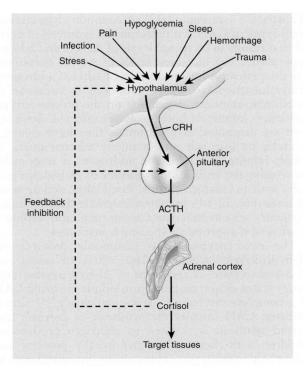

FIGURE 32-13. The hypothalamic-pituitary-adrenal (HPA) feedback system that regulates glucocorticoid (cortisol) levels. Cortisol release is regulated by adrenocorticotropic hormone (ACTH). Stress exerts its effects on cortisol release through the HPA system and corticotropin-releasing hormone (CRH), which controls the release of ACTH from the anterior pituitary gland. Increased cortisol levels incite a negative feedback inhibition of ACTH release.

TABLE 32-2	Actions of Cortisol
Major Influence	**Effect on Body**
Glucose metabolism	Stimulates gluconeogenesis
	Decreases glucose use by the tissues
Protein metabolism	Increases breakdown of proteins
	Increases plasma protein levels
Fat metabolism	Increases mobilization of fatty acids
	Increases use of fatty acids
Anti-inflammatory action (pharmacologic levels)	Stabilizes lysosomal membranes of the inflammatory cells, preventing the release of inflammatory mediators
	Decreases capillary permeability to prevent inflammatory edema
	Depresses phagocytosis by white blood cells to reduce the release of inflammatory mediators
	Suppresses the immune response
	Causes atrophy of lymphoid tissue
	Decreases eosinophils
	Decreases antibody formation
	Decreases the development of cell-mediated immunity
	Reduces fever
	Inhibits fibroblast activity
Psychic effect	May contribute to emotional instability
Permissive effect	Facilitates the response of the tissues to humoral and neural influences, such as those of the catecholamines, during trauma and extreme stress

fatty acids. As glucose production by the liver rises and peripheral glucose use falls, a moderate resistance to insulin develops. In persons with diabetes and those who are diabetes prone, this has the effect of raising the blood glucose level.

Cortisol also influences multiple aspects of immunologic function and inflammatory responsiveness. Large quantities of cortisol are required for an effective anti-inflammatory action. This is achieved by the administration of pharmacologic rather than physiologic doses of cortisol. The increased cortisol blocks inflammation at an early stage by decreasing capillary permeability and stabilizing the lysosomal membranes so that inflammatory mediators are not released. Cortisol suppresses the immune response by reducing humoral and cell-mediated immunity. During the healing phase, cortisol suppresses fibroblast activity and thereby lessens scar formation. Cortisol also inhibits prostaglandin synthesis, which may account in large part for its anti-inflammatory actions.

The glucocorticoid hormones also appear to be involved directly or indirectly in emotional behavior. Receptors for these hormones have been identified in brain tissue, which suggests that they play a role in the regulation of behavior. Persons treated with adrenal cortical hormones have been known to display behavior ranging from mildly aberrant to psychotic.

Adrenal Androgen Hormones

The adrenal androgens are synthesized primarily by the zona reticularis and the zona fasciculata of the adrenal cortex (see Fig. 32-12A). These sex hormones probably exert little effect on normal sexual function. There is evidence, however, that the adrenal androgens (the most important of which is dehydroepiandrosterone [DHEA] and its sulfate conjugate [DHEAS]) contribute to the pubertal growth of body hair, particularly pubic and axillary hair in women. They also may play a role in the steroid hormone economy of the pregnant woman and the fetal–placental unit. In women, DHEAS is increasingly being used in the treatment of both Addison disease (to be discussed) and those who have decreased levels of DHEAS. Because the testes produce these hormones, there is no rationale for using it in men. The levels of DHEAS decline to approximately one-sixth the levels of a 20-year-old by 60 years of age (the *adreno-pause*). The value of routine replacement of DHEAS in the adrenopause is largely unproven, but replacement may improve general well-being and sexuality and have other important effects in women.

Pharmacologic Suppression of Adrenal Function

A highly significant aspect of long-term therapy with pharmacologic preparations of the glucocorticoids is adrenal insufficiency upon withdrawal of the drugs. The deficiency results from suppression of the HPA system. Chronic suppression causes atrophy of the adrenal gland, and the abrupt withdrawal of drugs can cause acute adrenal insufficiency. Recovery to a state of normal adrenal function may be prolonged, requiring up to 12 months or more.

Tests of Adrenal Function

Several diagnostic tests can be used to evaluate adrenal cortical function and the HPA system.[17] Blood levels of cortisol, aldosterone, and ACTH can be measured using immunoassay methods. A 24-hour urine specimen measuring the excretion of various metabolic end products of the adrenal hormones provides information about alterations in the biosynthesis of the adrenal cortical hormones. The 24-hour urinary free cortisol, late-night (between 11 PM and midnight) serum or salivary cortisol levels, and the overnight 1-mg dexamethasone suppression test (see later) are excellent screening tests for Cushing syndrome.[39,40] Suppression and stimulation tests afford a means of assessing the state of the HPA feedback system. For example, a test dose of ACTH can be given to assess the response of the adrenal cortex to stimulation. Similarly, administration of dexamethasone, a synthetic glucocorticoid drug, provides a means of measuring negative feedback suppression of ACTH. The insulin-induced hypoglycemic test, which is the gold standard for assessing the function of the HPA axis, induces a central nervous system stress response, increases CRH release, and in this way increases ACTH and cortisol secretion. It therefore measures the integrity of the axis and its ability to respond to stress.

Adrenal Cortical Disorders

Disorders of the adrenal cortex include disorders of adrenocortical hormone insufficiency or excess. They can be congenital or acquired and can occur as the result of primary disorders of the adrenal cortex or secondary to altered ACTH secretion.

Congenital Adrenal Hyperplasia

Congenital adrenal hyperplasia (CAH), or the adrenogenital syndrome, describes a congenital disorder caused by an autosomal recessive trait in which there is a deficiency of any of the enzymes necessary for the synthesis

of cortisol[3,42] (see Fig. 32-12). A common characteristic of all types of CAH is a defect in the synthesis of cortisol that results in increased levels of ACTH and adrenal hyperplasia. The increased levels of ACTH overstimulate the pathways for production of adrenal androgens. Mineralocorticoids may be produced in excessive or insufficient amounts, depending on the precise enzyme deficiency. Infants of both sexes are affected. Boys seldom are diagnosed at birth unless they have enlarged genitalia or lose salt and manifest adrenal crisis. In female infants, an increase in androgens is responsible for creating the virilization syndrome of ambiguous genitalia with an enlarged clitoris, fused labia, and urogenital sinus (Fig. 32-14). In male and female children, other secondary sex characteristics are normal, and fertility is unaffected if appropriate therapy is instituted.

The two enzymes most commonly deficient are 21-hydroxylase (accounting for >90% of cases) and 11-β-hydroxylase. A spectrum of 21-hydroxylase deficiency states exists, ranging from simple virilizing CAH to a complete salt-losing enzyme deficiency.[42,43] Simple virilizing CAH impairs the synthesis of cortisol, and steroid synthesis is shunted to androgen production. Children with these deficiencies usually produce sufficient aldosterone or aldosterone intermediates to prevent signs and symptoms of mineralocorticoid deficiency. The salt-losing form is accompanied by deficient production of aldosterone and its intermediates. This results in fluid and electrolyte disorders after the 5th day of life (including hyponatremia, hyperkalemia, vomiting, dehydration, and shock). The 11-β-hydroxylase deficiency is rare and is manifested by a spectrum of severity. Affected children have excessive androgen production and impaired conversion of 11-deoxycorticosterone to corticosterone. The overproduction of 11-deoxycorticosterone, which has mineralocorticoid activity, is responsible for the hypertension that accompanies this deficiency.

Diagnosis of CAH depends on the precise biochemical evaluation of metabolites in the cortisol pathway

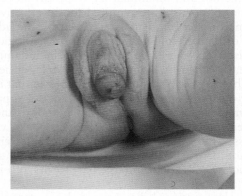

FIGURE 32-14. A female infant with congenital adrenal hyperplasia demonstrating virilization of the genitalia with hypertrophy of the clitoris and partial fusion of labioscrotal folds. (From Merino MJ, Quezado M. The endocrine system. In: Rubin R, Strayer DS, eds. *Rubin's Pathology: Clinicopathologic Foundations of Medicine.* 6th ed. Philadelphia, PA: Wolters Kluwer Health/Lippincott Williams & Wilkins; 2012:1067.)

and on clinical signs and symptoms. Genetic testing is also invaluable; however, correlation between the phenotype and genotype is not always straightforward.[42]

Medical treatment of CAH includes oral or parenteral glucocorticoid replacement. Fludrocortisone acetate, a mineralocorticoid, also may be given to children who are salt losers. Depending on the degree of virilization, reconstructive surgery during the first 2 years of life is indicated to reduce the size of the clitoris, separate the labia, and exteriorize the vagina. Advances in surgical techniques have led to earlier use of single-stage surgery—between 2 and 6 months of life in girls with 21-hydroxylase deficiency, a time when the tissues are maximally pliable and psychological trauma to the child is minimized.[21] Surgery has provided excellent results and does not usually impair sexual function.

Adrenal Cortical Insufficiency

There are two forms of adrenal insufficiency: primary and secondary[44-46] (Table 32-3). Primary adrenal insufficiency, or Addison disease, is caused by destruction of the adrenal gland. Secondary adrenal insufficiency results from a disorder of the HPA system.

Primary Adrenal Cortical Insufficiency. In 1855, Thomas Addison, an English physician, provided the first detailed clinical description of primary adrenal insufficiency, now called *Addison disease*.[46] The use of this term is reserved for primary adrenal insufficiency, in which adrenal cortical hormones are deficient and ACTH levels are elevated because of the lack of feedback inhibition.

Addison disease is a relatively rare disorder in which all the layers of the adrenal cortex are destroyed. Autoimmune destruction is the most common cause of Addison disease in the United States. Before 1950, tuberculosis was the major cause of Addison disease in the United States and Canada, and it continues to be a major cause of the disease in countries where the infection is more prevalent. Rare causes include metastatic carcinoma, fungal infection (particularly histoplasmosis), cytomegalovirus infection, amyloid disease, and hemochromatosis. Bilateral adrenal hemorrhage

may occur in persons taking anticoagulants, during open heart surgery, and during birth or major trauma. Adrenal insufficiency can be caused by acquired immunodeficiency syndrome (AIDS), in which the adrenal gland is destroyed by a variety of opportunistic infectious agents. Drugs (e.g., ketoconazole) that inhibit synthesis or cause excessive breakdown of glucocorticoids can also result in adrenal insufficiency.

Addison disease, like type 1 diabetes mellitus, is a chronic metabolic disorder that requires lifetime hormone replacement therapy. The adrenal cortex has a large reserve capacity, and the manifestations of adrenal insufficiency usually do not become apparent until approximately 90% of the gland has been destroyed.[4] These manifestations are related primarily to mineralocorticoid deficiency, glucocorticoid deficiency, and hyperpigmentation resulting from elevated ACTH levels. Although lack of the adrenal androgens (i.e., DHEAS) exerts few effects in men because the testes produce these hormones, women have sparse axillary and pubic hair.

Mineralocorticoid deficiency causes increased urinary losses of sodium, chloride, and water, along with decreased excretion of potassium (Fig. 32-15). The result is hyponatremia, loss of extracellular fluid, decreased cardiac output, and hyperkalemia. There may be an abnormal appetite for salt. Orthostatic hypotension is common. Dehydration, weakness, and fatigue are common early symptoms. If loss of sodium and water is extreme, cardiovascular collapse and shock ensue. Because of a lack of glucocorticoids, the person with Addison disease has poor tolerance to stress. This deficiency causes hypoglycemia, lethargy, weakness, fever, and gastrointestinal symptoms such as anorexia, nausea, vomiting, and weight loss.

Hyperpigmentation results from elevated levels of ACTH. The skin looks bronzed or suntanned in exposed and unexposed areas, and the normal creases and pressure points tend to become especially dark. The gums and oral mucous membranes may become bluish-black. The amino acid sequence of ACTH is strikingly similar to that of melanocyte-stimulating hormone; hyperpigmentation occurs in greater than 90% of persons with Addison disease and is helpful

TABLE 32-3   Clinical Findings of Adrenal Insufficiency

Finding	Primary	Secondary/Tertiary
Anorexia and weight loss	Yes (100%)	Yes (100%)
Fatigue and weakness	Yes (100%)	Yes (100%)
Gastrointestinal symptoms, nausea, diarrhea	Yes (50%)	Yes (50%)
Myalgia, arthralgia, abdominal pain	Yes (10%)	Yes (10%)
Orthostatic hypotension	Yes	Yes
Hyponatremia	Yes (85%–90%)	Yes (60%)
Hyperkalemia	Yes (60%–65%)	No
Hyperpigmentation	Yes (>90%)	No
Secondary deficiencies of testosterone, growth hormone, thyroxine, antidiuretic hormone	No	Yes
Associated autoimmune conditions	Yes	No

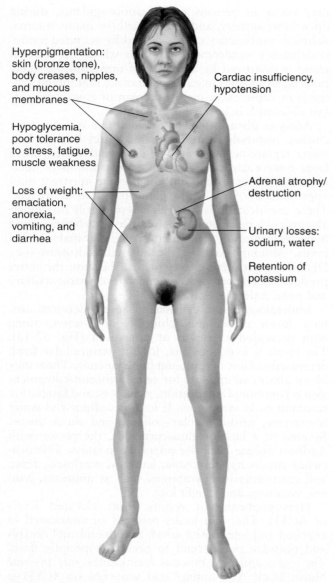

Hyperpigmentation: skin (bronze tone), body creases, nipples, and mucous membranes

Hypoglycemia, poor tolerance to stress, fatigue, muscle weakness

Loss of weight: emaciation, anorexia, vomiting, and diarrhea

Cardiac insufficiency, hypotension

Adrenal atrophy/destruction

Urinary losses: sodium, water

Retention of potassium

FIGURE 32-15. Clinical manifestations of primary (Addison disease) and secondary adrenal insufficiency.

in distinguishing the primary and secondary forms of adrenal insufficiency.

The daily regulation of the chronic phase of Addison disease usually is accomplished with oral replacement therapy, with higher doses being given during periods of stress. The pharmacologic agent that is used should have both glucocorticoid and mineralocorticoid activity. Mineralocorticoids are needed only in primary adrenal insufficiency. Hydrocortisone usually is the drug of choice. In mild cases, hydrocortisone alone may be adequate. Fludrocortisone (a mineralocorticoid) is used for persons who do not obtain a sufficient salt-retaining effect from hydrocortisone. DHEAS replacement also may be helpful in the female patient.[44] Because persons with the disorder are likely to have episodes of hyponatremia and hypoglycemia, they need to have a regular schedule for meals and exercise. Persons with Addison disease also have limited ability to respond to infections, trauma, and other stresses. Such situations require immediate medical attention and treatment. All persons with Addison disease should be advised to wear a medical alert bracelet or medal.

Secondary Adrenal Cortical Insufficiency. Secondary adrenal insufficiency can occur as the result of hypopituitarism or because the pituitary gland has been surgically removed. Tertiary adrenal insufficiency results from a hypothalamic defect. However, a far more common cause than either of these is the rapid withdrawal of glucocorticoids that have been administered therapeutically. These drugs suppress the HPA system, with resulting adrenal cortical atrophy and loss of cortisol production. This suppression continues long after drug therapy has been discontinued and can be critical during periods of stress or when surgery is performed.

Acute Adrenal Crisis. Acute adrenal crisis is a life-threatening situation.[44,45] If Addison disease is the underlying problem, exposure to even a minor illness or stress can precipitate nausea, vomiting, muscular weakness, hypotension, dehydration, and vascular collapse. The onset of adrenal crisis may be sudden, or it may progress over a period of several days. The symptoms may occur suddenly in children with salt-losing forms of CAH. Massive bilateral adrenal hemorrhage causes an acute fulminating form of adrenal insufficiency. Hemorrhage can be caused by meningococcal septicemia (i.e., Waterhouse-Friderichsen syndrome), adrenal trauma, anticoagulant therapy, adrenal vein thrombosis, or adrenal metastases.

Acute adrenal crisis is treated with extracellular fluid restoration and glucocorticosteroid replacement therapy. Extracellular fluid volume should be restored with several liters of 0.9% saline and 5% dextrose. Oral hydrocortisone replacement therapy can be resumed once the saline infusion has been discontinued and the person is taking food and fluids by mouth. Mineralocorticoid therapy is not required when large amounts of hydrocortisone are being given, but as the dose is reduced it usually is necessary to add fludrocortisone. Glucocorticoid and mineralocorticoid replacement therapy is monitored using heart rate and blood pressure measurements, serum electrolyte values, and titration of plasma renin activity into the upper-normal range. Since bacterial infection frequently precipitates acute adrenal crisis, broad-spectrum antibiotic therapy may be needed.

Glucocorticoid Hormone Excess

The term *Cushing syndrome* refers to the manifestations of hypercortisolism from any cause.[39,40,47] Three important forms of Cushing syndrome result from excess glucocorticoid production by the body. One is a pituitary form, which results from excessive production of ACTH by a tumor of the pituitary gland. This form of the disease was the one originally described by Cushing; therefore, it is called *Cushing disease*. The second form is the adrenal form, caused by a benign or malignant adrenal tumor. The third form is ectopic Cushing syndrome, caused by a nonpituitary ACTH-secreting tumor. Certain extrapituitary malignant tumors such as small cell carcinoma of the lung may secrete ACTH or, rarely, CRH and produce Cushing syndrome. Cushing syndrome also can result from long-term therapy with one of the potent pharmacologic preparations of glucocorticoids; this form is called *iatrogenic Cushing syndrome.*

The major manifestations of Cushing syndrome represent an exaggeration of the many actions of cortisol. Altered fat metabolism causes a peculiar deposition of fat characterized by a protruding abdomen; subclavicular fat pads or "buffalo hump" on the back; and a round, plethoric "moon face" (Fig. 32-16). There is muscle weakness, and the extremities are thin because of protein breakdown and muscle wasting. In advanced cases, the skin over the forearms and legs becomes thin, having the appearance of parchment. Purple striae, or stretch marks, from stretching of the catabolically weakened skin and subcutaneous tissues are distributed over the breast, thighs, and abdomen. Osteoporosis may develop because of destruction of bone proteins and alterations in calcium metabolism, resulting in back pain, compression fractures of the vertebrae, and rib fractures. As calcium is mobilized from bone, renal calculi may develop.

Derangements in glucose metabolism are found in approximately 75% of patients, with clinically overt diabetes mellitus occurring in approximately 20%. The glucocorticoids possess mineralocorticoid properties; this causes hypokalemia as a result of excessive potassium excretion and hypertension resulting from sodium retention. Inflammatory and immune responses are inhibited, resulting in increased susceptibility to infection. Cortisol increases gastric acid secretion, which may provoke gastric ulceration and bleeding. An accompanying increase in androgen levels causes hirsutism (facial hair), mild acne, and thinning of the hair, along with menstrual irregularities in women (Fig. 32-17). Excess levels of the glucocorticoids may give rise to extreme emotional lability, ranging from mild euphoria and absence of normal fatigue to grossly psychotic behavior.

Diagnosis of Cushing syndrome depends on the finding of cortisol hypersecretion.[39,40,47,48] The determination of 24-hour excretion of cortisol in urine provides a reliable and practical index of cortisol secretions. One of the prominent features of Cushing syndrome is loss of the diurnal pattern of cortisol secretion. This is why late-night (between 11 PM and midnight) serum or salivary cortisol levels can be inappropriately elevated, aiding in the diagnosis of Cushing syndrome. The overnight dexamethasone suppression test is also used as a screening tool for Cushing syndrome.

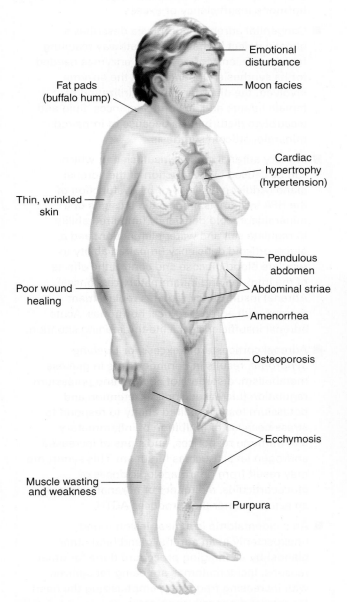

Emotional disturbance

Moon facies

Fat pads (buffalo hump)

Cardiac hypertrophy (hypertension)

Thin, wrinkled skin

Pendulous abdomen

Abdominal striae

Poor wound healing

Amenorrhea

Osteoporosis

Muscle wasting and weakness

Ecchymosis

Purpura

FIGURE 32-16. Clinical features of Cushing syndrome.

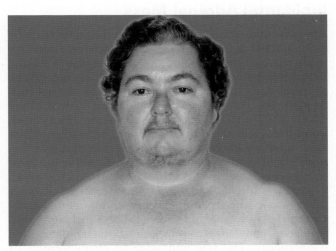

FIGURE 32-17. Cushing syndrome. A woman who suffered from a pituitary adenoma that produced adrenocorticotropic hormone exhibits a moon face, buffalo hump, increased facial hair, and thinning of scalp hair (From: Merino MJ, Quezado M. The endocrine system. In: Rubin R, Strayer DS, eds. *Rubin's Pathology: Clinicopathologic Foundations of Medicine.* 6th ed. Philadelphia, PA: Wolters Kluwer Health/Lippincott Williams & Wilkins; 2012:1073.)

Other tests include measurement of the plasma levels of ACTH.[39,40,47,48] Adrenocorticotropic hormone levels should be normal or elevated in ACTH-dependent Cushing syndrome (Cushing disease and ectopic ACTH), and low in non–ACTH-dependent Cushing syndrome (adrenal tumors). Various suppression or stimulation tests of the HPA system are performed to delineate the cause further. MRI or CT scans afford a means for locating adrenal or pituitary tumors.

Untreated, Cushing syndrome produces serious morbidity and even death. The choice of surgery, irradiation, or pharmacologic treatment is determined largely by the cause of the hypercortisolism. The goal of treatment for Cushing syndrome is to remove or correct the source of hypercortisolism without causing permanent pituitary or adrenal damage.[40,48] Transsphenoidal removal of a pituitary adenoma or a hemihypophysectomy is the preferred method of treatment for Cushing disease. This allows removal of only the tumor rather than the entire pituitary gland. After successful removal, the person must receive cortisol replacement therapy for 6 to 12 months or until adrenal function returns. Pituitary radiation therapy may also be used, but the full effects of treatment may not be realized for 3 to 12 months. Unilateral or bilateral adrenalectomy may be done in the case of adrenal adenoma. When possible, ectopic ACTH-producing tumors are removed. Pharmacologic agents that block steroid synthesis (i.e., mitotane, ketoconazole, and metyrapone) may be used to treat persons with ectopic tumors or adrenal carcinomas that cannot be resected.[39,40] Many of these patients also require *Pneumocystis jiroveci* (formerly known as *Pneumocystis carinii*) pneumonia prophylaxis because of the profound immunosuppression caused by the excessive glucocorticoid levels.

Incidental Adrenal Mass

An incidentaloma is a mass lesion found unexpectedly in an adrenal gland by an imaging procedure (done for other reasons), most commonly CT (but also MRI and ultrasonography).[49] It has been increasingly recognized since the early 1980s.[50] The prevalence of adrenal incidentalomas at autopsy is approximately 10 to 100 per 1000. In CT series, 0.6% to 4.4% are the usual figures published. Incidentalomas also can occur in other organs (e.g., pituitary, thyroid). The two most important questions are (1) is the mass malignant, and (2) is the mass hormonally active (i.e., is it functioning)?

Primary adrenal carcinoma is quite rare, but other cancers, particularly lung cancers, commonly metastasize to the adrenal gland (other cancers include breast, stomach, pancreas, colon, kidney, melanomas, and lymphomas). The size and imaging characteristics of the mass may help determine whether the tumor is benign or malignant. The risk of cancer is high in adrenal masses larger than 6 cm. Many experts recommend surgical removal of masses larger than 4 cm, particularly in younger patients.[49,50] Appropriate screening to exclude a hormonally active lesion includes tests to rule out pheochromocytoma, Cushing syndrome, and Conn syndrome (mineralocorticoid excess).

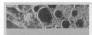

SUMMARY CONCEPTS

■ The adrenal cortex produces three types of hormones: mineralocorticoids, glucocorticoids, and adrenal androgens. The mineralocorticoids, along with the renin–angiotensin mechanism, aid in controlling body levels of sodium and potassium. The glucocorticoids have anti-inflammatory actions and aid in regulating glucose, protein, and fat metabolism during periods of stress. The adrenal androgens exert little effect on daily control of body function, but they probably contribute to the development of body hair in women. Disorders of the adrenal cortex include those that produce adrenocortical hormone insufficiency or excess.

■ Congenital adrenal hyperplasia describes a genetic defect in the cortisol pathway resulting from a deficiency of one of the enzymes needed for its synthesis. Depending on the enzyme involved, the disorder causes virilization of female infants and, in some instances, fluid and electrolyte disturbances because of impaired mineralocorticoid synthesis.

■ Primary adrenal cortical insufficiency, which can be caused by destruction of the adrenal gland (Addison disease) or by dysfunction of the HPA system, is manifested by signs of a mineralocorticoid deficiency (impaired ability to regulate salt and water elimination) and a glucocorticoid deficiency (impaired ability to regulate blood glucose and control the effects of the immune and inflammatory responses). Adrenal insufficiency requires replacement therapy with adrenal cortical hormones. Acute adrenal insufficiency is a life-threatening situation.

■ Adrenal corticosteroid excess, or *Cushing syndrome*, results in derangements in glucose metabolism, disorders of sodium and potassium regulation (increased sodium retention and potassium loss), impaired ability to respond to stress because of inhibition of inflammatory and immune responses, and signs of increased androgen levels such as hirsutism. This syndrome may result from pharmacologic doses of glucocorticoids, a pituitary or adrenal tumor, or an ectopic tumor that produces ACTH.

■ An incidentaloma is a mass lesion found unexpectedly in an adrenal gland (and other glands) by an imaging procedure done for other reasons. Incidentalomas are being recognized with increasing frequency, emphasizing the need for correct diagnosis and treatment.

REVIEW EXERCISES

1. A 59-year-old man was referred to a neurologist for evaluation of headaches. Subsequent MRI studies revealed a large suprasellar mass (2.5 × 2.4 cm), consistent with a pituitary tumor. His history is positive for hypertension and, on direct inquiry, he believes that his hands are slightly larger than previously, with increased sweating. Family history is negative, as are weight change, polyuria and polydipsia, visual disturbance, and erectile dysfunction. Subsequent laboratory findings reveal a baseline serum GH of 8.7 ng/mL (normal is 0 to 5 ng/mL), which is unsuppressed after oral glucose tolerance testing; glucose intolerance; and increased IGF-1 on two occasions (1044 and 1145 μg/L [upper limit of normal is 480 μg/L]). Other indices of pituitary function are within the normal range.

A. What diagnosis would this man's clinical features, MRI, and laboratory findings suggest?

B. What is the reason for asking the patient about weight change, polyuria and polydipsia, visual disturbance, and erectile dysfunction?

C. How would you explain his impaired glucose tolerance?

D. What are the possible local effects of a large pituitary tumor?

2. A 76-year-old woman presents with weight gain, subjective memory loss, dry skin, and cold intolerance. On examination she is found to have a multinodular goiter. Laboratory findings reveal a low serum T_4 and elevated TSH.

A. What diagnosis would this woman's history, physical, and laboratory tests suggest?

B. Explain the possible relationship between the diagnosis and her weight gain, dry skin, cold intolerance, and subjective memory loss.

C. What type of treatment would be indicated?

3. A 45-year-old woman presents with a history of progressive weakness, fatigue, weight loss, nausea, and increased skin pigmentation (especially of creases, pressure areas, and nipples). Her blood pressure is 120/78 mm Hg when supine and 105/52 mm Hg when standing. Laboratory findings reveal a serum sodium of 120 mEq/L (normal is 135 to 145 mEq/L), potassium level of 5.9 mEq/L (normal is 3.5 to 5 mEq/L), and low plasma cortisol and high ACTH levels.

A. What diagnosis would this woman's clinical features and laboratory findings suggest?

B. Would her diagnosis be classified as a primary or secondary endocrine disorder?

C. What is the significance of her darkened skin?

D. What type of treatment would be indicated?

REFERENCES

1. Webb P, Baxter JD. Introduction to endocrinology. In: Gardner DG, Shoback D, eds. *Basic and Clinical Endocrinology*. 9th ed. New York, NY: Lange Medical Books/McGraw-Hill Medical; 2011:1–26.
2. Aron DC, Findling JW, Tyrrell JB. Hypothalamus and pituitary gland. In: Gardner DG, Shoback D, eds. *Basic and Clinical Endocrinology*. 9th ed. New York, NY: Lange Medical Books/McGraw-Hill Medical; 2011:65–114.
3. Merino MJ, Quezado M, Rubin E, et al. The endocrine system. In: Rubin R, Strayer DS, eds. *Rubin's Pathology: Clinicopathologic Foundations of Medicine*. 5th ed. Philadelphia, PA: Wolters Kluwer Health/Lippincott Williams & Wilkins; 2008:933–955, 958–973.
4. Maitra A. The endocrine system. In: Kumar V, Abbas AK, Fausto N, et al., eds. *Robbins and Cotran Pathologic Basis of Disease*. 8th ed. Philadelphia, PA: Saunders Elsevier; 2010:1097–1129, 1148–1163.
5. Pickett CA. Diagnosis and management of pituitary tumors: recent advances. *Prim Care*. 2003;30:765–789.
6. Bevan J. Pituitary incidentalomas. *Clin Med*. 2013;13:296–298.
7. Toogood AA, Stewart PM. Hypopituitarism: clinical features, diagnosis, and management. *Endocrinol Metab Clin North Am*. 2008;37:235–261.
8. Molitch ME, Clemmons DR, Malzowski S, et al. Evaluation and treatment of adult growth hormone deficiency: an Endocrine Society clinical practice guideline. *J Clin Endocrinol Metab*. 2006;91:1621–1634.
9. Styne D. Growth. In: Gardner DG, Shoback D, eds. *Basic and Clinical Endocrinology*. 9th ed. New York, NY: Lange Medical Books/McGraw-Hill Medical; 2011:129–162.
10. Cohen P, Rogol AD, Deal CL, et al. Consensus statement of the diagnosis and treatment of children with idiopathic short stature: a summary of the Growth Hormone Research Society, the Lawson Wilkins Pediatric Endocrine Society, and the European Society of Paediatric Endocrinology Workshop. *J Clin Endocrinol Metab*. 2008;93(11):4210–4217.
11. Nwosu B, Lee MM. Evaluation of short and tall stature in children. *Am Fam Physician*. 2008;78(5):597–604.
12. Lee MM. Idiopathic short stature. *N Engl J Med*. 2006;354(24):2575–2582.
13. Guitosi-Kug RA, Cuttler L. Idiopathic short stature. *Endocrinol Metab Clin North Am*. 2005;34:565–580.
14. Laron Z. Laron syndrome (primary GH resistance): the personal experience 1958–2003. *J Clin Endocrinol Metab*. 2004;89:1031–1044.
15. Melmed S. Idiopathic adult growth hormone deficiency. *J Clin Endocrinol Metab*. 2013;98:2187–2197.
16. Nass R, Park J, Thorner MO. Growth hormone supplementation in the elderly. *Endocrinol Metab Clin North Am*. 2007;36:233–245.
17. Sesmilo G, Biller BM, Levadot J, et al. Effects of GH administration on inflammatory and other cardiovascular risk markers in men with GH deficiency. *Ann Intern Med*. 2000;133:111–122.
18. Root A. The tall, rapidly growing infant, child, and adolescent. *Curr Opin Endocrinol Diab*. 2001;8:6–16.
19. Hosana H, Cohen P. Hyperpituitarism, tall stature, and overgrowth syndromes. In: Kliegman RM, Stanton BF, St. Gemell JW, et al., eds. *Nelson Textbook of Pediatrics*. 19th ed. Philadelphia, PA: Saunders Elsevier; 2011:1886:e1–e6.
20. Melmed S. Acromegaly. *N Engl J Med*. 2006;355:2558–2573.
21. Ben-Shlomo A, Melmed S. Acromegaly. *Endocrinol Metab Clin North Am*. 2008;37:101–122.
22. Fuqua JS. Treatment and outcomes of precocious puberty. *J Clin Endocrinol Metab*. 2013;98:2198–2207.
23. Styne D. Puberty. In: Gardner DG, Shoback D, eds. *Basic and Clinical Endocrinology*. 8th ed. New York, NY: Lange Medical Books/McGraw-Hill Medical; 2007:611–640.

24. Kaplowitz PB, Oberfield SE. Reexamination of the age limit for defining when puberty is precocious in girls in the United States: implications for evaluation and treatment. *Pediatrics.* 1999;104:936–941.

25. Cooper DS, Greenspan FS, Ladenson PW. The thyroid gland. In: Gardner DG, Shoback D, eds. *Basic and Clinical Endocrinology.* 9th ed. New York, NY: Lange Medical Books/McGraw-Hill Medical; 2011:163–226.

26. Guyton AC, Hall JE. *Medical Physiology.* 12th ed. Philadelphia, PA: Elsevier Saunders; 2012:907–920.

27. Koulouri O, Gurnell M. Interpretation of thyroid function tests. *Clin Med.* 2013;13:282–286.

28. Pearce EN, Farwell AP, Braverman LE. Thyroiditis. *N Engl J Med.* 2003;348:2646–2655.

29. Devdhar M, Ousman YH, Burman KD. Hypothyroidism. *Endocrinol Metab Clin North Am.* 2007;36:595–615.

30. Fatourechl V. Subclinical hypothyroidism: an update for primary care physicians. *Mayo Clin Proc.* 2009;84(1):65–71.

31. Wartofsky L. Myxedema coma. *Endocrinol Metab Clin North Am.* 2006;35:687–698.

32. Cooper DS. Hyperthyroidism. *Lancet.* 2003;362:459–468.

33. Pearce EN, Hennessey JV, McDermott MT. New American Thyroid Association and American Association of Clinical Endocrinologists guidelines for thyrotoxicosis and other forms of hyperthyroidism: significant progress for the clinician and a guide to future research. *Thyroid.* 2011;21:573–576.

34. McKenna TJ. Graves' disease. *Lancet.* 2001;357:1793–1796.

35. Brent GA. Graves' disease. *N Engl J Med.* 2008;358(24):2594–2605.

36. Bartalena L, Tanda ML. Graves' ophthalmopathy. *N Engl J Med.* 2009;360(10):994–1001.

37. Bahn R. Pathophysiology of Graves' ophthalmopathy: the cycle of disease. *J Clin Endocrinol Metab.* 2003;88:1939–1946.

38. Matfin G. Endocrine and metabolic emergencies: thyroid storm. *Ther Adv Endocrinol Metab.* 2010;3:139–145.

39. Aron DC, Findling JW, Tyrrell JB, et al. Glucocorticoids and adrenal androgens. In: Gardner DG, Shoback D, eds. *Basic and Clinical Endocrinology.* 9th ed. New York, NY: Lange Medical Books/McGraw-Hill Medical; 2011:285–328.

40. Newell-Price J, Bertagna X, Grossman AB, et al. Cushing's syndrome. *Lancet.* 2006;367:1605–1617.

41. Pivonello R, Cristina M, DeMartino CM, et al. Cushing's syndrome. *Endocrinol Metab Clin North Am.* 2008;37:135–149.

42. White PC, Bachega T. Congenital adrenal hyperplasia. *Semin Reprod Med.* 2012;30:400.

43. Boos CJ, Rumsby G, Matfin G. Multiple tumors associated with late onset congenital hyperplasia due to aberrant splicing of adrenal 21-hydroxylase gene. *Endocr Pract.* 2002;8:470–473.

44. Arlt W, Allolio B. Adrenal insufficiency. *Lancet.* 2003;361:1881–1893.

45. Bouillon R. Acute adrenal insufficiency. *Endocrinol Metab Clin North Am.* 2006;35:767–775.

46. Bornstein SR. Predisposing factors for adrenal insufficiency. *N Engl J Med.* 2009;360(22):2328–2339.

47. Raff H, Findling JW. A physiological approach to the diagnosis of Cushing's syndrome. *Ann Intern Med.* 2003;138:980–991.

48. Nieman LK, Ilias I. Evaluation and treatment of Cushing's syndrome. *Am J Med.* 2005;118:1340–1346.

49. Gopan T, Remer E, Hamrahian AH. Evaluating and managing adrenal incidentalomas. *Cleve Clin J Med.* 2006;73:561–568.

50. Grumbach MM, Biller BMK, Braunstein GD, et al. Management of the clinically inapparent adrenal mass ("incidentaloma"). *Ann Intern Med.* 2003;138:424–429.

Porth Essentials Resources

Explore these additional resources to enhance learning for this chapter:
- NCLEX-Style Questions and Other Resources on **thePoint**, http://thePoint.lww.com/PorthEssentials4e
- Study Guide for Essentials of Pathophysiology
- Concepts in Action Animations
- Adaptive Learning | Powered by PrepU, http://thepoint.lww.com/prepu

C h a p t e r **33**

Diabetes Mellitus and the Metabolic Syndrome

Diabetes mellitus is an abnormality in blood glucose regulation and nutrient storage related to an absolute or relative deficiency of insulin and/or resistance to the actions of insulin. In the United States alone, diabetes mellitus affects 25.8 million people, or approximately 8.3% of the population.[1] Type 1 diabetes, which is caused by an absolute deficiency of insulin, accounts for 1 million of these people with the remainder having type 2 diabetes. In addition, another 79 million people have been categorized as having "prediabetes." Globally, the prevalence of prediabetes and type 2 diabetes is increasing at an alarming rate.

Hormonal Control of Nutrient Metabolism and Storage

Nutrient intake and storage in the form of adipose tissue, along with the action of insulin and other hormones, play an important role in the development of insulin resistance, the metabolic syndrome, and type 2 diabetes. This section provides a brief overview of nutrient (glucose, fat, protein) metabolism and storage and the hormones, including insulin, that are involved in the process. Overweight and obesity, as well as adipose tissue and its function in energy storage and as an endocrine organ, are discussed in Chapter 10.

Nutrient Metabolism and Storage

The body uses glucose, fatty acids, and other substrates as fuel to satisfy its energy needs. Although the respiratory and circulatory systems combine efforts to furnish the body with the oxygen needed for metabolic purposes, it is the liver, in concert with insulin and other hormones, that controls the storage and mobilization of the body's fuel supply.

Glucose Metabolism and Storage

Glucose, a six-carbon molecule, is an efficient fuel that, when metabolized in the presence of oxygen, breaks down to form carbon dioxide and water. Although many tissues and organ systems are able to use other forms of fuel, such as fatty acids and ketones, the brain and nervous system rely almost exclusively on glucose as a fuel source. Because the brain can neither synthesize nor store more than a few minutes' supply of glucose, normal cerebral function requires a continuous supply from the circulation. Severe and prolonged hypoglycemia can cause brain death, and even moderate hypoglycemia can result in substantial brain dysfunction.

Body tissues obtain glucose from the blood. Fasting blood glucose levels are tightly regulated between 70 and 99 mg/dL (4.0 and 5.5 mmol/L). After a meal, blood glucose levels rise, and insulin release from the beta cells in the pancreas enables its transport into body cells. Approximately two thirds of the glucose that is ingested with a meal is removed from the blood and stored in the liver or skeletal muscles as glycogen. When the liver and skeletal muscles become saturated with glycogen, any excess glucose is converted into fatty acids by the liver and then stored as triglycerides in the fat cells of adipose tissue.

When blood glucose levels fall below normal, as they do between meals, the liver converts stored glycogen back to glucose in a process called *glycogenolysis*. The glucose is then released in a homeostatic mechanism that maintains the blood glucose within its normal range. Although skeletal muscle has glycogen stores, it lacks the enzyme glucose-6-phosphatase that allows glucose to be broken down sufficiently to pass through the cell membrane and enter the bloodstream, limiting its usefulness to the muscle cell.

In addition to mobilizing its glycogen stores, the liver synthesizes glucose from amino acids, glycerol, and lactic acid in a process called *gluconeogenesis*. This glucose may be released directly into the circulation or stored as glycogen.

Fat Metabolism and Storage

Fat is the most efficient form of fuel storage, providing 9 kcal/g of stored energy, compared with the 4 kcal/g provided by carbohydrates and proteins. About 40% of the calories in the normal American diet are obtained from fats, which is about equal to the amount obtained from carbohydrates.[2] Fats are a major energy source for the body during rest as well as physical activity; in fact, the body's use of fats for energy is as important as its use of carbohydrates. In addition, dietary carbohydrates and proteins consumed in excess of body needs are converted to triglycerides for storage in adipose tissue.

A triglyceride contains three fatty acids linked by a glycerol molecule. The mobilization of fatty acids for use as an energy source is facilitated by the action of enzymes (lipases) that break triglycerides into their glycerol and fatty acid components. The glycerol molecule can enter the glycolytic pathway and be used along with glucose to produce energy, or it can be used to produce glucose. The fatty acids are transported to tissues where they are metabolized for energy. Almost all body cells, with the exception of the brain, nervous tissue, and red blood cells, can use fatty acids interchangeably with glucose for energy. Although many cells use fatty acids as a fuel source, fatty acids cannot be converted to the glucose needed by the brain for energy.

A large share of the initial degradation of fatty acids occurs in the liver, especially when excessive amounts of fatty acids are being used for energy. The liver uses only a small amount of the fatty acids for its own energy needs; it converts the rest into ketones and releases them into the blood. In situations that favor fat breakdown, such as fasting, large amounts of ketones are released into the bloodstream. Because ketones are organic acids, release of excessive amounts, as can occur in diabetes mellitus, can prompt ketoacidosis, an acute complication of diabetes.

Protein Metabolism and Storage

Proteins are essential for the formation of all body structures, including genes, enzymes, contractile structures in muscle, matrix of bone, and hemoglobin of red blood cells.[2] Amino acids are the building blocks of proteins. Unlike glucose and fatty acids, there is only a limited facility for the storage of excess amino acids in the body. Most of the stored amino acids are contained in body proteins. Amino acids in excess of those needed for protein synthesis are converted to fatty acids, ketones, or glucose and then stored or used as metabolic fuel. Because fatty acids cannot be converted to glucose, the body must break down proteins and use the amino acids as a major substrate for gluconeogenesis during periods when metabolic needs exceed food intake.

Glucose-Regulating Hormones

The hormonal control of blood glucose resides largely within the endocrine pancreas. The pancreas is made up of two major tissue types: the acini and the islets of Langerhans (Fig. 33-1). The acini secrete digestive juices into the duodenum, whereas the islets of Langerhans, which account for only about 1% to 2% of the volume of the pancreas, secrete hormones into the blood. Each islet is composed of beta cells that secrete insulin and amylin, alpha cells that secrete glucagon, and delta cells that secrete somatostatin. In addition, at least one other cell type, the F (or PP) cell, is present in small numbers in the islets and secretes a hormone of uncertain function called *pancreatic polypeptide*.[2,3] Blood glucose regulation is also influenced by several gut-derived hormones that increase insulin release after nutrient intake and by counterregulatory hormones that help to maintain blood glucose levels during periods of limited glucose intake or excessive glucose use.

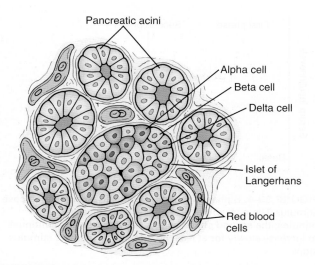

Pancreatic acini

Alpha cell

Beta cell

Delta cell

Islet of Langerhans

Red blood cells

FIGURE 33-1. Islet of Langerhans in the pancreas.

Insulin

Although several hormones are known to increase blood glucose levels, insulin is the only hormone known to have a direct effect in lowering blood glucose levels. The actions of insulin are threefold: (1) it promotes glucose uptake by target cells and provides for glucose storage as glycogen, (2) it prevents fat and glycogen breakdown, and (3) it inhibits gluconeogenesis and increases protein synthesis (Table 33-1).[2,3] Insulin acts to promote fat storage by increasing the transport of glucose into fat cells (Fig. 33-2). It also facilitates triglyceride synthesis from glucose in fat cells and inhibits the intracellular breakdown of stored triglycerides. Insulin also inhibits protein breakdown and increases protein synthesis by increasing the active transport of amino acids into body cells, and it inhibits gluconeogenesis, or the building of glucose from new sources, mainly amino acids. When sufficient glucose and insulin are present, protein breakdown is minimal because the body is able to use glucose and fatty acids as a fuel source. In children and adolescents, insulin is needed for normal growth and development.

The active form of insulin is composed of two polypeptide chains—an A chain and a B chain (Fig. 33-3). Active insulin is formed in the beta cells from a larger molecule called *proinsulin.* In converting proinsulin to insulin, enzymes in the beta cell cleave proinsulin at specific sites to form two separate substances: active insulin and a biologically inactive C-peptide (connecting peptide) chain that joined the A and B chains before they were separated. Active insulin and the inactive C-peptide chain are packaged into secretory granules and released simultaneously from the beta cell. The C-peptide chains can be measured clinically, and this measurement can be used to study beta cell function (i.e., persons with

	Insulin	Glucagon
Glucose		
Glucose transport	Increases glucose transport into skeletal muscle and adipose tissue	
Glycogen synthesis	Increases glycogen synthesis	Promotes glycogen breakdown
Gluconeogenesis	Decreases gluconeogenesis	Increases gluconeogenesis
Fats		
Fatty acid and triglyceride synthesis	Promotes fatty acid and triglyceride synthesis by the liver	
Fat storage in adipose tissue	Increases the transport of fatty acids into adipose cells	
	Increases conversion of fatty acids to triglycerides by increasing the availability of α-glycerol phosphate through increased transport of glucose in adipose cells	
	Maintains fat storage by inhibiting breakdown of stored triglycerides by adipose cell lipase	Activates adipose cell lipase, making increased amounts of fatty acids available to the body for use as energy
Proteins		
Amino acid transport	Increases active transport of amino acids into cells	Increases amino acid uptake by liver cells and their conversion to glucose by gluconeogenesis
Protein synthesis	Increases protein synthesis by increasing transcription of messenger RNA and accelerating protein synthesis by ribosomal RNA	
Protein breakdown	Decreases protein breakdown by enhancing the use of glucose and fatty acids as fuel	

TABLE 33-1 Actions of Insulin and Glucagon on Glucose, Fat, and Protein Metabolism

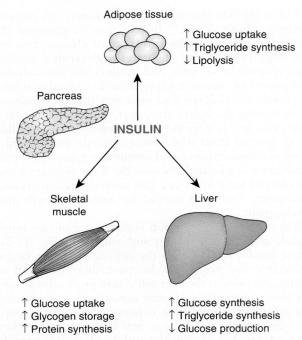

Adipose tissue

↑ Glucose uptake
↑ Triglyceride synthesis
↓ Lipolysis

Pancreas

INSULIN

Skeletal
muscle

Liver

↑ Glucose uptake
↑ Glycogen storage
↑ Protein synthesis

↑ Glucose synthesis
↑ Triglyceride synthesis
↓ Glucose production

FIGURE 33-2. Effects of insulin on glucose transport and storage.

type 2 diabetes with very little or no remaining beta cell function will have very low or nonexistent levels of C-peptide in their blood, and thus will likely need insulin replacement for treatment).

The release of insulin from the pancreatic beta cells is regulated by blood glucose levels, increasing as blood glucose levels rise and decreasing when blood glucose levels decline. Secretion of insulin occurs in a pulsatile fashion. After exposure to glucose, which is a nutrient secretagogue (a substance that prompts secretion of another substance), a first-phase release of stored

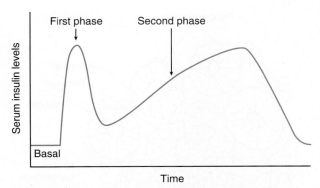

FIGURE 33-4. Biphasic insulin response to a constant glucose stimulus. The peak of the first phase in humans is 3 to 5 minutes; the second phase begins at 2 minutes and continues to increase slowly for at least 60 minutes or until the stimulus stops.

preformed insulin occurs, followed by a second-phase release of newly synthesized insulin (Fig. 33-4). Diabetes may result from dysregulation or deficiency in any of the steps involved in this process (e.g., impaired sensing of blood glucose levels and defects in insulin release or synthesis). Serum insulin levels begin to rise within minutes after a meal, reach a peak in approximately 3 to 5 minutes, and then return to baseline levels within 2 to 3 hours.

Insulin secreted by the beta cells enters the portal circulation and travels directly to the liver, where approximately 50% is used or degraded. Insulin, which is rapidly bound to peripheral tissues or destroyed by the liver or kidneys, has a half-life of approximately 5 to 10 minutes once it is released into the general circulation. To initiate its effects on target cells, insulin binds to a membrane receptor. The insulin receptor consists of four subunits—two larger α subunits that extend outside the cell membrane and are involved in insulin

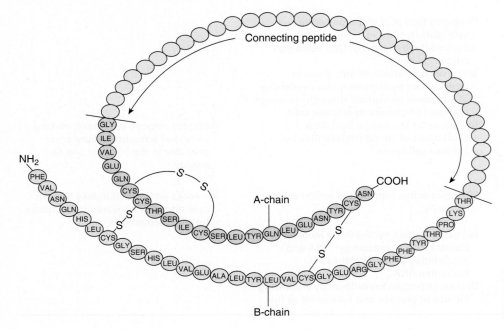

FIGURE 33-3. Structure of proinsulin. With removal of the connecting peptide (C peptide), proinsulin is converted to insulin.

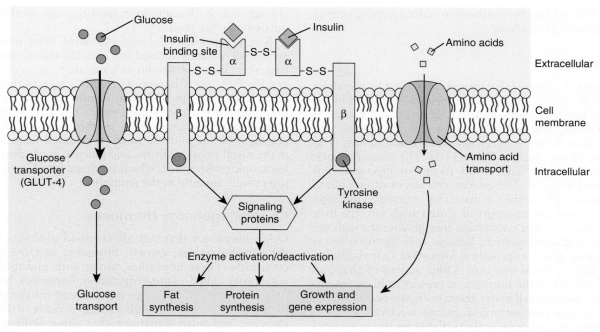

FIGURE 33-5. Insulin receptor. Insulin binds to the α subunits of the insulin receptor, which increases glucose and amino acid transport and causes autophosphorylation of the β subunit of the receptor, which induces tyrosine kinase activity. Tyrosine phosphorylation, in turn, activates a cascade of intracellular signaling proteins that mediate the effects of insulin on glucose, fat, and protein metabolism.

binding, and two smaller β subunits that are predominantly located inside the cell membrane and contain a kinase enzyme that becomes activated during insulin binding (Fig. 33-5). Activation of the kinase enzyme results in autophosphorylation of the β subunit itself. Phosphorylation of the β subunit in turn activates some enzymes and inactivates others; thereby, directing the desired intracellular effect of insulin on glucose, fat, and protein metabolism.

Because cell membranes are impermeable to glucose, they require a special carrier, called a *glucose transporter*, to move glucose from the blood into the cell. These transporters move glucose across the cell membrane at a faster rate than would occur by diffusion alone. Considerable research has revealed a family of glucose transporters termed *GLUT-1, GLUT-2,* and so forth.[4] GLUT-4 is the insulin-dependent glucose transporter for skeletal muscle and adipose tissue (Fig. 33-6). It is sequestered inside the membrane of these cells and thus is unable to function as a glucose transporter until a signal from insulin causes it to move from its inactive site into the cell membrane, where it facilitates glucose entry. GLUT-2 is the major transporter of glucose into beta cells and liver cells. It has a low affinity for glucose and acts as a transporter only when plasma glucose levels are relatively high, such as after a meal. GLUT-1 is present in all tissues. It does not require the actions of insulin and is important in tissues with a high demand for glucose such as the brain.

Another distinct group of glucose transporters have recently been identified. The sodium glucose cotransporters (SGLTs) are responsible for transporting glucose

from the lumen of the intestine across the brush border of the enterocytes and from the glomerular filtrate into the proximal tubules of the kidney. SGLT1 predominantly enables the small intestine to absorb glucose. In comparison, SGLT2 is mainly responsible for reabsorption of most (>90%) of the glucose filtered by the kidney. Pharmacologic inhibitors with varying specificities for these transporters (e.g., canagliflozin) can slow the rate of intestinal glucose absorption and increase the renal elimination of glucose into the urine. This new

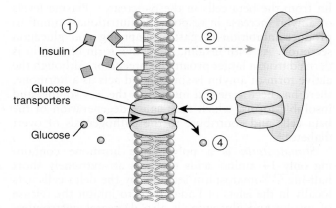

FIGURE 33-6. Insulin-dependent glucose transporter (GLUT-4). (*1*) Binding of insulin to insulin receptor on the surface of the cell membrane, (*2*) generation of intracellular signal, (*3*) insertion of GLUT-4 receptor from its inactive site into the cell membrane, and (*4*) transport of glucose across the cell membrane.

class of drugs has been shown to reduce hyperglycemia in patients with diabetes. [5]

Glucagon

Glucagon, a polypeptide molecule produced by the alpha cells of the islets of Langerhans, helps to maintain blood glucose between meals and during periods of fasting. [2,3] Like insulin, glucagon travels through the portal vein to the liver, where it exerts its main action, which is to increase blood glucose (Table 33-1). The most dramatic effect of glucagon is its ability to initiate glycogenolysis (the breakdown of glycogen) as a means of raising blood glucose, usually within a matter of minutes. Glucagon also increases the transport of amino acids into the liver and stimulates their conversion into glucose through the process of gluconeogenesis. Because liver glycogen stores are limited, gluconeogenesis is important in maintaining blood glucose levels over time. Other actions of glucagon occur only when the hormone is present in high concentrations, usually well above those normally present in the blood. At high concentrations, glucagon activates adipose cell lipase, making fatty acids available for use as energy. [2]

Glucagon secretion is regulated by blood glucose. A decrease in blood glucose concentration produces an immediate increase in glucagon secretion, and an increase produces a decrease in glucagon secretion. High concentrations of amino acids, as occur after a protein meal, also can stimulate glucagon secretion. In this way, glucagon increases the conversion of amino acids to glucose as a means of maintaining the body's glucose levels. Glucagon levels also increase during strenuous exercise as a means of preventing a decrease in blood glucose.

Amylin, Somatostatin, and Gut-Derived Hormones

Islet amyloid polypeptide, or *amylin,* was originally identified as a major constituent of pancreatic amyloid deposits in persons with type 2 diabetes and subsequently shown to be a polypeptide that is cosecreted with insulin from the beta cells in the pancreas. [3,5] Plasma levels of amylin increase in response to nutritional stimuli to produce inhibition of gastric emptying and glucagon secretion. As with insulin, the active form of amylin is derived from a larger proamylin precursor. Although the active form of amylin is soluble and acts as a hormone, there has been renewed interest in the less soluble and insoluble forms, which may cause degeneration of the beta cells and contribute to the pathogenesis of overt diabetes. [5]

Somatostatin is a polypeptide hormone containing only 14 amino acids that has an extremely short half-life. [2,3] Somatostatin secreted by the delta cells acts locally in the islets of Langerhans to inhibit the release of insulin and glucagon. It also decreases gastrointestinal activity after ingestion of food. Almost all factors related to ingestion of food stimulate somatostatin secretion. By decreasing gastrointestinal activity, somatostatin is thought to extend the time during which food is absorbed into the blood, and by inhibiting insulin and glucagon, it is thought to extend the use of absorbed nutrients by the tissues. [2]

Several *gut-derived hormones* have been identified as having what is termed an *incretin effect,* meaning that they increase insulin release after an oral nutrient load [2,3,6] (see Chapter 28). This suggests that gut-derived factors can stimulate insulin secretion after a predominantly carbohydrate meal. The two hormones that account for about 90% of the incretin effect are glucagon-like peptide-1, which is released from L cells in the distal small intestine, and glucose-dependent insulinotropic polypeptide, which is released by K cells more proximally (mainly in the jejunum).

Counterregulatory Hormones

Other hormones that can affect blood glucose include the catecholamines, growth hormone, and the glucocorticoids. These hormones, along with glucagon, are sometimes called *counterregulatory hormones* because they counteract the storage functions of insulin in regulating blood glucose levels during periods of fasting, exercise, and other situations that either limit glucose intake or deplete glucose stores.

Epinephrine. Epinephrine, a catecholamine, helps to maintain blood glucose levels during periods of stress. Epinephrine has the potent effect of stimulating glycogenolysis in the liver, thus causing large quantities of glucose to be released into the blood. It also inhibits insulin release from the beta cells and thereby decreases the movement of glucose into muscle cells, while at the same time increasing the breakdown of muscle glycogen stores. Although the glucose that is released from muscle glycogen cannot be released into the blood, the mobilization of these stores for muscle use conserves blood glucose for use by other tissues such as the brain and nervous system. Epinephrine also has a direct lipolytic effect on adipose cells, thereby increasing the mobilization of fatty acids for use as an energy source. The blood glucose–elevating effect of epinephrine is an important homeostatic mechanism during periods of hypoglycemia.

Growth Hormone. Growth hormone has many metabolic effects. It increases protein synthesis in all cells of the body, mobilizes fatty acids from adipose tissue, and antagonizes the effects of insulin. Growth hormone decreases cellular uptake and use of glucose, thereby increasing the level of blood glucose. The increased blood glucose level stimulates further insulin secretion by the beta cells. The secretion of growth hormone normally is inhibited by insulin and increased levels of blood glucose. During periods of fasting, when both blood glucose levels and insulin secretion fall, growth hormone levels increase. Exercise, such as running and cycling, and various stresses, including anesthesia, fever, and trauma, also increase growth hormone levels.

Chronic hypersecretion of growth hormone, such as occurs in acromegaly (see Chapter 32), can lead to glucose intolerance and the development of diabetes mellitus. In people who already have diabetes, moderate elevations in growth hormone levels that occur during periods of stress and periods of growth in children can produce the entire spectrum of metabolic abnormalities associated with poor regulation, despite optimized insulin treatment.

Glucocorticoid Hormones. The glucocorticoid hormones, which are synthesized in the adrenal cortex along with other corticosteroid hormones, are critical to survival during periods of fasting and starvation. They stimulate gluconeogenesis by the liver, sometimes producing a 6- to 10-fold increase in hepatic glucose production. These hormones also moderately decrease tissue use of glucose.

There are several steroid hormones with glucocorticoid activity; the most important of these is cortisol, which accounts for approximately 95% of all glucocorticoid activity (see Chapter 32). Almost any type of stress, whether physical or emotional, causes an immediate increase in adrenocorticotropic hormone (ACTH) secretion by the anterior pituitary gland, followed within minutes by greatly increased secretion of cortisol by the adrenal gland. Hypoglycemia is a potent stimulus for cortisol secretion. In predisposed persons, the prolonged elevation of glucocorticoid hormones can lead to hyperglycemia and the development of diabetes mellitus. In people with diabetes, even transient increases in cortisol can complicate control.

SUMMARY CONCEPTS

■ The body predominantly metabolizes glucose and fatty acids for energy. The brain depends exclusively on glucose for its energy. Body tissues obtain glucose from the blood. The liver stores excess glucose as glycogen and it uses gluconeogenesis to convert amino acids, lactate, and glycerol into glucose during fasting or when glucose intake does not keep pace with demand.

■ Blood glucose levels reflect the difference between the amount of glucose released into the circulation by the liver and the amount of glucose removed from the blood by body tissues. Fats, which serve as an efficient source of fuel for the body, are stored in adipose tissue as triglycerides, which consist of three fatty acids linked to a glycerol molecule. In situations that favor fat breakdown, such as fasting or diabetes mellitus, the triglycerides in adipose tissue are broken down and the fatty acids are used as fuel or transported to the liver, where they are converted to ketones.

■ Proteins, which are made up of amino acids, are essential for the formation of all body structures. Unlike glucose and fatty acids, there is only a limited facility for storage of excess amino

acids in the body. Because fatty acids cannot be converted to glucose, the body must break down proteins and use the amino acids for gluconeogenesis.

■ Energy metabolism is controlled by a number of hormones, including insulin, glucagon, epinephrine, growth hormone, and the glucocorticoids. Of these hormones, only insulin has the effect of lowering the blood glucose level. It does this by facilitating the transport of glucose into body cells and decreasing the liver's production and release of glucose into the bloodstream. Insulin also has the effect of decreasing lipolysis and the use of fats as a fuel source.

■ Other hormones—glucagon, epinephrine, growth hormone, and the glucocorticoids—maintain or increase blood glucose concentrations. Glucagon and epinephrine promote glycogenolysis, and glucagon and the glucocorticoids increase gluconeogenesis. Epinephrine and glucagon also increase the use of fat for energy by increasing the release of fatty acids from adipose tissue cells. Growth hormone decreases the peripheral utilization of glucose.

Diabetes Mellitus

The term *diabetes* is derived from a Greek word meaning "going through," and *mellitus* from the Latin word for "honey" or "sweet." Reports of the disorder can be traced back to the first century AD, when Aretaeus the Cappadocian described the disorder as a chronic affliction characterized by intense thirst and voluminous, honey-sweet urine: "the melting down of flesh into urine." It was the discovery of insulin by Banting and Best in 1922 that transformed the once-fatal disease into a manageable chronic health problem.[7]

Diabetes is a disorder of carbohydrate, protein, and fat metabolism resulting from a lack of insulin availability or a reduction in the biologic effects of insulin. It can represent an absolute insulin deficiency, impaired release of insulin by the pancreatic beta cells, inadequate or defective insulin receptors or postreceptor regulation, or the production of inactive insulin or insulin that is destroyed before it can carry out its action.

Classification and Etiology

Although diabetes mellitus clearly is a disorder of insulin availability, it is not a single disease. A revised classification system, which was developed in 1997 by the Expert Committee on the Diagnosis and Classification of Diabetes Mellitus, divides diabetes into four clinical classes[8] (Table 33-2). Included are the categories of type 1 diabetes (i.e., diabetes resulting from beta cell destruction and an absolute insulin deficiency); type 2 diabetes (i.e., diabetes due to insulin resistance and a relative insulin deficiency); gestational diabetes mellitus (i.e., glucose intolerance that develops during pregnancy that is not clearly overt diabetes [either type 1 or type 2]); and other specific types of diabetes, many of which occur secondary to other conditions (e.g., Cushing syndrome, acromegaly, and pancreatitis).

Categories of Risk for Diabetes

The revised classification system also includes a system for diagnosing diabetes according to stages of glucose intolerance.[8–11] The system relies on two tests: (1) a fasting plasma glucose (FPG) test, which measures plasma glucose levels after food has been withheld for at least 8 hours, and (2) an oral glucose tolerance test (OGTT), which measures the body's ability to remove glucose from the blood within 2 hours of consuming 75 g of glucose in 300 mL of water.

A FGP below 100 mg/dL or an OGTT less than 140 mg/dL is considered normal (Table 33-3). Persons whose glucose levels, although not meeting the criteria for diabetes, are too high to be considered normal are classified as having *impaired fasting plasma glucose* (IFG) and/or *impaired glucose tolerance* (IGT). Impaired fasting glucose is defined by an elevated FPG of 100 to 125 mg/dL and IGT as plasma glucose levels of 140 to 199 mg/dL with an OGTT (see Table 33-3).

Persons with IFG and/or IGT are often referred to as having *prediabetes*, meaning they are at relatively high risk for the future development of diabetes as well as cardiovascular disease.[10,11] Thus, calorie restriction and weight reduction (even 5% to 10%) are important in overweight people with prediabetes.

Person with a FPG greater than or equal to 126 mg/dL (7.0 mmol/L) or an OGTT 2-hour glucose level greater than or equal to 200 mg/dL (11.1 mmol/L) are considered to have provisional diabetes.[10,11] The criteria in Table 33-3 are used to confirm the diagnosis. Glycosylated hemoglobin (i.e., HbA$_{1c}$ [A1C]) is a widely used marker for chronic hyperglycemia, reflecting average blood glucose levels over a 2- to 3-month period of time (to be discussed). The A1C, which plays a critical role in the management of persons with diabetes, is now recommended for use in the diagnosis of diabetes, with a threshold of greater than 6.5%.[10,11] The test can also be used to identify persons at higher risk for developing diabetes (see Table 33-3).

Type 1 Diabetes Mellitus

Type 1 diabetes mellitus, which is characterized by destruction of the pancreatic beta cells and accounts for 5% to 10% of those with diabetes, is subdivided into type 1A immune-mediated diabetes and type 1B idiopathic (non–immune-related) diabetes.[10] In the United States and Europe, approximately 90% to 95% of people with type 1 diabetes mellitus have type 1A immune-mediated diabetes. The rate of beta cell destruction is

TABLE 33-2 Etiologic Classification of Diabetes Mellitus

Type	Subtypes	Etiology of Glucose Intolerance
I. Type 1*	Beta cell destruction usually leading to absolute insulin deficiency	
	A. Immune mediated	Autoimmune destruction of beta cells
	B. Idiopathic	Unknown
II. Type 2*	May range from predominantly insulin resistance with relative insulin deficiency to a predominantly secretory defect with insulin resistance	
III. Other specific types	A. Genetic defects in beta cell function (e.g., glucokinase)	Dysregulation insulin secretion due to a defect in glucokinase generation
	B. Genetic defects in insulin action (e.g., leprechaunism, Rabson-Mendenhall syndrome)	Pediatric syndromes that have mutations in insulin receptors
	C. Diseases of exocrine pancreas (e.g., pancreatitis, neoplasms, cystic fibrosis)	Loss or destruction of insulin-producing beta cells
	D. Endocrine disorders (e.g., acromegaly, Cushing syndrome)	Diabetogenic effects of excess hormone levels
IV. Gestational diabetes mellitus (GDM)	Any degree of glucose intolerance that develops during pregnancy that is not clearly diabetes (either type 1 or type 2)	Combination of insulin resistance and impaired insulin secretion

*Patients with any form of diabetes may require insulin treatment at some stage of the disease. Such use of insulin does not, in itself, classify the patient.

Adapted from The Expert Committee on the Diagnosis and Classification of Diabetes Mellitus. Report of the Expert Committee on the Diagnosis and Classification of Diabetes Mellitus. *Diabetes Care.* 2004;27:S5–S10. Reprinted with permission from the American Diabetes Association. Copyright © 2004 American Diabetes Association.

TABLE 33-3 Normal and Increased Fasting Plasma Glucose (FPG), Oral Glucose Tolerance Test (OGTT), and Hemoglobin A₁c (A1C) for Categories of Increased Risk for Diabetes and Criteria for Diagnosis of Diabetes

Test	Normoglycemia	Categories of Increased Risk for Diabetes*	Criteria for Diagnosis of Diabetes†
FPG‡	<100 mg/dL(5.6 mmol/L)	Impaired fasting glucose (IFG)100 mg/dL (5.6 mmol/L) to125 mg/dL (6.9 mmol/L)	≥126 mg/dL (7.0 mmol/L) or
2-h plasma glucose in 75-g OGTT	<140 mg/dL(7.8 mmol/L)	Impaired glucose tolerance (IGT)140 mg/dL (7.8 mmol/L) to199 mg/dL (11.0 mmol/L)	≥200 mg/dL (11.1 mmol/L) or
A1C§	3.9%–5.6%	5.7%–6.4%	≥6.5% or
Other			Classic symptoms of hyperglycemia or hyperglycemic crisis and a plasma glucose ≥200 mg/dL (11.1 mmol/L)

*For all three tests, risk is continuous below the lower limit of the range and becomes disproportionately greater at higher ends of the range.

†Diagnosis of diabetes can be based on criteria 1 (FP), 2 (OGTT), 3 (A1C), or 4 (Other). In the absence of unequivocal hyperglycemia, criteria for 1–3 should be confirmed by repeat testing.

‡Fasting is defined as no caloric intake for at least 8 hours.

§A1C should be performed using a method that is certified by the National Glycohemoglobin Standardization Program and standardized or traceable to the Diabetes Control and Complications Trial reference assay.

Developed from American Diabetes Association. Diagnosis and classification of diabetes mellitus—2010. *Diabetes Care*. 32(Suppl 1):S62–S69.

quite variable, being rapid in some individuals (mainly infants and children) and slow in others (mainly adults). Some individuals, particularly children and adolescents, may present with diabetic ketoacidosis (DKA) as the first manifestation of the disease (to be discussed). Others may have modest elevations in FPG that can rapidly change to severe hyperglycemia and DKA in the presence of stress and infection. Still others, particularly adults, may retain sufficient beta cell function to delay onset of clinical diabetes for many years.

The destruction of beta cells and absolute lack of insulin in people with type 1 diabetes mellitus mean that they are particularly prone to the development of DKA. One of the actions of insulin is the inhibition of *lipolysis* (i.e., fat breakdown) and release of free fatty acids (FFAs) from fat cells. In the absence of insulin, ketosis develops when these fatty acids are released from fat cells and converted to ketones in the liver. Because of the loss of insulin response, all people with type 1A diabetes require exogenous insulin replacement to reverse the catabolic state, control blood glucose levels, and prevent ketosis.

Type 1A Immune-Mediated Diabetes. Type 1A diabetes, commonly referred to as *type 1 diabetes*, is characterized by immune-mediated destruction of beta cells. This type of diabetes, formerly called *juvenile diabetes*, occurs more commonly in children and adolescents. In fact, three quarters of all cases of type 1 diabetes occur in individual younger than 18 years of age.[11]

Type 1A diabetes is an autoimmune disorder that is thought to result from a genetic predisposition (i.e., diabetogenic genes); an environmental triggering event, such as an infection; and a T-lymphocyte–mediated hypersensitivity reaction against some beta cell antigens. Much evidence has focused on the inherited major histocompatibility complex (MHC) genes on chromosome 6 that encode human leukocyte antigen (HLA)-DQ and HLA-DR, especially DR-3 and DR-4.[3] In addition to the MHC susceptibility genes on chromosome 6, an insulin gene regulating beta cell replication and function has been identified on chromosome 11.

Type 1A diabetes–associated autoantibodies may exist for years before the onset of hyperglycemia. There are two main types of autoantibodies: insulin autoantibodies (IAAs) and islet cell autoantibodies, including antibodies directed at other islet autoantigens, including glutamic acid decarboxylase (GAD) and the protein tyrosine phosphatase IA-2.[3,11] Testing for antibodies to GAD or IA-2 and for IAAs using sensitive assays can be used to identify new cases of type 1 diabetes when diagnostic confusion between type 1 and type 2 diabetes occurs or there is future risk of type 1 diabetes (e.g., in siblings of a person with type 1).[1] These persons also have increased predisposition to other autoimmune disorders such as Graves disease, rheumatoid arthritis, and Addison disease.

The fact that type 1 diabetes is thought to result from an interaction between genetic and environmental factors led to research into methods directed at prevention and early control of the disease. These methods include the identification of genetically susceptible persons and early intervention in newly diagnosed persons with type 1 diabetes. After the diagnosis of type 1 diabetes, there often is a short period of improved beta cell function, during which symptoms of diabetes disappear and insulin injections are reduced or not needed. This is sometimes called the *honeymoon period*. Immune interventions (immunomodulation) designed to interrupt the destruction of beta cells before development of type 1 diabetes are being investigated in various trials. Unfortunately, none of the interventions studied to date has shown real clinical utility.

Idiopathic Type 1B Diabetes. The term *idiopathic type 1B diabetes* is used to describe those cases of beta cell destruction in which no evidence of autoimmunity is present. Only a small number of people with type 1 diabetes fall into this category; most are of African or Asian descent. Type 1B diabetes is strongly inherited. People with the disorder have episodic DKA due to varying degrees of insulin deficiency with periods of absolute insulin deficiency that may come and go.

Type 2 Diabetes Mellitus and the Metabolic Syndrome

Type 2 diabetes mellitus, previously described as *non–insulin-dependent diabetes*, is a condition of hyperglycemia that accompanies a *relative* rather than an *absolute* insulin deficiency (although insulin therapy may be still be required for glycemic control).[3,10,11] It currently accounts for about 90% to 95% of the cases of diabetes. Most people with type 2 diabetes are overweight and older. Recently, however, type 2 diabetes has become a more common occurrence in obese children and adolescents.[12,13] Although type 1 diabetes remains the main form of diabetes in children worldwide, it seems likely that type 2 diabetes will become the predominant form within 10 years in some ethnic groups.[13]

Metabolic Abnormalities Involved in Type 2 Diabetes. The metabolic abnormalities involved in type 2 diabetes include (1) insulin resistance, (2) increased glucose production by the liver, and (3) impaired secretion of insulin by the pancreatic beta cells[14–16] (Fig. 33-7).

Insulin resistance, which can be defined as the failure of target tissues to respond to insulin, predates the development of hyperglycemia. That is, in the early stages of the evolution of type 2 diabetes, insulin resistance is usually accompanied by compensatory beta cell hyperfunction and hyperinsulinemia.

In skeletal muscle, insulin resistance prompts decreased uptake of glucose. Although muscle glucose uptake is slightly increased after a meal, the efficiency with which it is taken up (glucose clearance) is diminished, resulting in an increase in *postprandial* (following a meal) blood glucose levels.[16]

In contrast, in the liver, insulin resistance leads to impaired suppression of glucose production with an overproduction of glucose despite a fasting hyperinsulinemia. In fact, the excessive rate of hepatic glucose production is the primary determinant of elevated FPG in persons with type 2 diabetes.[15,16]

Several mechanisms can lead to impaired secretion of insulin by the pancreatic beta cells. These include an initial decrease in beta cell mass related to genetic or epigenetic factors, increased apoptosis or decreased regeneration of beta cells, or beta cell exhaustion due to long-standing insulin resistance.[15] According to one study, beta cell function was reduced by an average of 50% at the time of diagnosis in type 2 diabetes, and

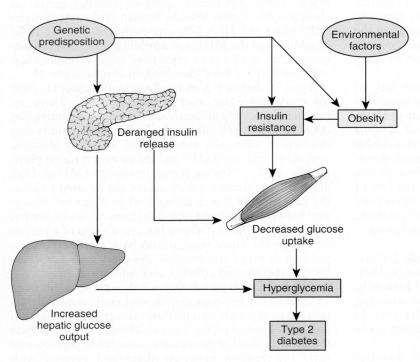

FIGURE 33-7. Pathogenesis of type 2 diabetes mellitus.

progressively decreased (by an average of approximately 4% per year), resulting in worsening hyperglycemia even when the degree of insulin resistance remained stable.[17]

Pathogenesis. The pathogenesis of type 2 diabetes involves genetic, epigenetic, behavioral, and environmentally mediated factors. A positive family history confers a twofold to fourfold increased risk for type 2 diabetes, and 15% to 25% of first-degree relatives of persons with type 2 diabetes develop impaired glucose tolerance or diabetes.[14] Despite the strong familial predisposition, the genetics of type 2 diabetes is poorly defined. This is probably because of the heterogeneous nature of the disorder as well as the difficulty in sorting out the contribution of acquired factors affecting insulin action and glycemic control.[15] However, so far more than 60 genetic loci associated with type 2 diabetes have been identified. Unfortunately, when all these loci are added together they still only account for approximately 10% of the apparent genetic causes (i.e., heritability) of type 2 diabetes. Regardless, most cases of type 2 diabetes develop in obese individuals who have a genetic predisposition to beta–cell dysfunction and failure.

Among the acquired factors that predispose to type 2 diabetes, obesity and physical inactivity are paramount.[14,15,18] As the body mass index (BMI) increases, the risk of developing diabetes increases, and approximately 90% of persons with type 2 diabetes are overweight. Obesity has profound effects on sensitivity of tissues to insulin, and as a consequence, on glucose homeostasis. Not only the absolute amount of body fat, but also its distribution has an effect on insulin resistance. People with upper body (or central) obesity who have increased stores of visceral (intra-abdominal) fat are at greater risk for developing type 2 diabetes and metabolic disturbances than persons with lower body (or peripheral) obesity (see Chapter 10). Waist circumference and waist–hip ratio, which are both surrogate measures of central obesity, have been shown to correlate well with insulin resistance. Thus, measures such as diet and exercise that reduce visceral adiposity are important in the management of type 2 diabetes. Other acquired factors include the patient's microbiome (i.e., the bacteria that live in or on us) related metabolic factors and inflammatory effects.

Role of Adipose Tissue in Type 2 Diabetes. Although many details of the relationship between adipose tissue, insulin resistance, and increased glucose production in obese people with type 2 diabetes remain to be elucidated, several pathways have been proposed. Primary among these is the role of an increased concentration of free fatty acids (FFAs).[15,19] Visceral obesity is accompanied by an increase in postprandial FFA concentrations and subsequent triglyceride storage, including in sites that do not normally store fat such as the liver, skeletal muscle, heart, and pancreatic beta cells.[20,21] This has several consequences. First, excessive and chronic elevation of FFAs can directly cause pancreatic beta cell dysfunction (lipotoxicity). Second, at the level of the peripheral tissues, FFAs inhibit glucose uptake and glycogen storage. Third, the accumulation of FFAs and triglycerides reduces hepatic insulin sensitivity, leading to increased hepatic glucose production and hyperglycemia, especially in the fasting state. In the liver, the uptake of FFAs from the portal blood can lead to hepatic triglyceride accumulation and nonalcoholic fatty liver disease (see Chapter 30).

In addition to the metabolic effects of visceral obesity, adipocytes are the source of a number of important factors (e.g., adiponectin, leptin, FFAs) involved in a wide range of other processes, including glucose and lipid metabolism, inflammation, and thrombosis.[15,20–23] In obesity and type 2 diabetes, there is a reduction in the production of some factors that are normally synthesized by adipocytes (i.e., adiponectin), whereas there is an accelerated release of other factors such as angiotensinogen, plasminogen activator inhibitor-1, leptin, and proinflammatory cytokines (e.g., tumor necrosis factor-α). Adiponectin, which is secreted by adipocytes and circulates in the blood, is the only known adipocyte-secreted factor that increases tissue sensitivity to insulin.[23] It has been shown that decreased levels of adiponectin coincide with insulin resistance in persons with obesity and type 2 diabetes. In skeletal muscle, adiponectin has been shown to decrease tissue triglyceride content by increasing the use of fatty acids as a fuel source. Adiponectin also appears to have antidiabetes, anti-inflammatory, and antiatherogenic effects.

Insulin Resistance and the Metabolic Syndrome. There is increasing evidence to suggest that when people with type 2 diabetes present predominantly with insulin resistance, the diabetes may represent only one aspect of a syndrome of metabolic disorders.[24] Hyperglycemia in these people is frequently associated with intra-abdominal obesity, high levels of plasma triglycerides and low levels of high-density lipoproteins (HDLs), hypertension, systemic inflammation (as detected by C-reactive protein [CRP] and other mediators), abnormal fibrinolysis, abnormal function of the vascular endothelium, and macrovascular disease (coronary artery, cerebrovascular, and peripheral arterial disease). This constellation of abnormalities often is referred to as the *insulin resistance syndrome, syndrome X,* or, the preferred term, *metabolic syndrome.*[21] In clinical practice, the definition of metabolic syndrome given in the Third Report of the National Cholesterol Education Program (NCEP III) is widely used[20] (Chart 33-1).

Other Specific Types of Diabetes

The category of other specific types of diabetes, formerly known as *secondary diabetes,* includes diabetes that is associated with certain other conditions and syndromes. Such diabetes can occur with pancreatic disease

---

---

or removal of pancreatic tissue and with other endocrine diseases, such as acromegaly, Cushing syndrome, or pheochromocytoma. Endocrine disorders that produce hyperglycemia do so by increasing the hepatic production of glucose or decreasing the cellular use of glucose.

Several specific types of diabetes are associated with single gene defects in beta cell function. These specific types of diabetes, which resemble type 2 diabetes but occur at an earlier age (usually before 25 years of age), were formerly referred to as *maturity-onset diabetes of the young* (MODY).[3] Cystic fibrosis–related diabetes (CFRD) is now recognized as the most common complication of cystic fibrosis. Glucose abnormalities are especially common in children younger than 10 years old. The pathophysiology of CFRD is poorly understood, but insulin deficiency is the major factor (possibly related to pancreatic scarring).[11]

Several diuretics—thiazide and loop diuretics—can elevate blood glucose. These diuretics increase potassium loss, which is thought to impair beta cell release of insulin. Other drugs and therapies known to cause hyperglycemia include diazoxide, glucocorticoids, oral contraceptives, antipsychotic agents, and total parenteral nutrition (i.e., hyperalimentation). Drug-related increases in blood glucose usually are reversed after the drug has been discontinued. A newly recognized form of diabetes, new-onset diabetes after transplant (NODAT), is a common complication after tissue or organ transplant and occurs in 15% to 30% of recipients. Several drugs are thought to be important in the pathophysiology of this condition including glucocorticoids (which can increase insulin resistance) and certain immunosuppressants such as cyclosporine (which are beta-cell toxic).[11] The advent of potent antiretroviral therapy (especially protease inhibitors) for the treatment of human immunodeficiency virus (HIV) infection has significantly improved survival in these conditions. However, these people are now developing metabolic derangements with features similar to those seen in the metabolic syndrome (see Chart 33-1).[25]

In addition, changes in fat distribution (peripheral lipoatrophy and visceral obesity), sometimes referred to as *lipodystrophy,* often occur (see Chapter 16). These people should be aggressively treated to prevent cardiovascular complications resulting from the abnormal risk factors.

Gestational Diabetes

Gestational diabetes mellitus (GDM) is defined as glucose intolerance that develops during pregnancy and is not clearly overt diabetes (either type 1 or type 2).[11] It occurs in 3% to 7% of pregnancies in the United States and is growing in prevalence.[26,27] The hyperglycemia varies in severity from glucose concentrations that would be diagnostic of diabetes apart from pregnancy to concentrations that are asymptomatic and only slightly above normal.[27] Factors that indicate a high risk for GDM include glycosuria, strong family history of type 2 diabetes, severe obesity, polycystic ovary disease, and prior history of GDM or delivery of a previous large-for-gestational-age infant.

All pregnant women should undergo risk assessment for diabetes during their first prenatal visit to determine the need for additional screening tests. Women who are younger than 25 years of age; were of normal body weight before pregnancy; have no family history of diabetes, prior history of GDM or large-for-gestational age infant, or presence of glycosuria; and are not members of a high-risk ethnic/racial group (e.g., Hispanic, Native American, Asian, African American) may not need to be screened.[11,26,27] Women at high risk for GDM should undergo glucose testing as soon as possible. An FPG greater than or equal to 126 mg/dL; or a casual plasma glucose greater than or equal to 200 mg/dL; or a A1C greater or equal to 6.5% meets the threshold for diagnosis of diabetes mellitus and should be confirmed on a subsequent day as soon as possible.[11] Women of average or low risk, including those not found to have diabetes early in pregnancy, should undergo GDM testing at 24 to 28 weeks of gestation using a 50-g OGTT. This screening test consists of 50 g of glucose given without regard to the last meal, followed in 1 hour by a venous blood sample for glucose concentration. If the plasma glucose level is greater than 140 mg/dL (7.8 mmol/L), a 100-g 3-hour OGTT is indicated to establish the diagnosis of GDM.[27] If the plasma glucose measured 3 hours after the test is greater or equal to 140 mg/dL (7.8 mmol/L), a diagnosis of GDM is made.[27]

Diagnosis and careful medical management are essential because women with GDM are at higher risk for complications of pregnancy, mortality, and fetal abnormalities.[3] Fetal abnormalities include macrosomia (i.e., large body size), hypoglycemia, hypocalcemia, polycythemia, and hyperbilirubinemia.

Treatment of GDM includes close observation of mother and fetus because even mild hyperglycemia has been shown to be detrimental to the fetus.[26,27] Maternal fasting and postprandial blood glucose levels should be measured regularly. The mother's diet should provide the necessary nutrients for maternal and fetal health, result in normoglycemia and proper weight gain, and prevent ketosis.[3] If dietary management alone does not achieve a capillary blood glucose of 90 to 99 mg/dL or a 2-hour postprandial blood glucose less than 120 mg/dL, the Fifth International Workshop on GDM recommends therapy with insulin.[28] More recently, several oral agents have also been used for the treatment of GDM, including glyburide and metformin. Self-monitoring of blood glucose levels is essential.

Approximately 50% of women with GDM will develop type 2 diabetes within 5 to 10 years.[26] Women in whom GDM is diagnosed should be followed after delivery to detect diabetes early in its course. These women should be evaluated during their first postpartum visit with a 2-hour OGTT with a 75-g glucose load.

Clinical Manifestations of Diabetes

Diabetes mellitus may have a rapid or an insidious onset. In type 1 diabetes, signs and symptoms often arise suddenly. Type 2 diabetes usually develops more insidiously; its presence may be detected during a routine medical examination or when a patient seeks medical care for other reasons.

The most commonly identified signs and symptoms of diabetes are often referred to as the *three polys:* (1) polyuria (i.e., excessive urination), (2) polydipsia (i.e., excessive thirst), and (3) polyphagia (i.e., excessive hunger). These three symptoms are closely related to the hyperglycemia and glycosuria of diabetes. Glucose is a small, osmotically active molecule. When blood glucose levels are sufficiently elevated, the amount of glucose filtered by the glomeruli of the kidney exceeds the amount that can be reabsorbed by the renal tubules; this results in glycosuria accompanied by large losses of water in the urine. Thirst results from the intracellular dehydration that occurs as blood glucose levels rise and water is pulled out of body cells, including those in the hypothalamic thirst center. This early symptom may be easily overlooked in people with type 2 diabetes, particularly in those who have had a gradual increase in blood glucose levels. Polyphagia usually is not present in people with type 2 diabetes. In type 1 diabetes, it probably results from cellular starvation and the depletion of cellular stores of carbohydrates, fats, and proteins.

Weight loss despite normal or increased appetite is a common occurrence in people with uncontrolled type 1 diabetes. The cause of weight loss is twofold. First, loss of body fluids results from osmotic diuresis. Vomiting may exaggerate the fluid loss in ketoacidosis. Second, body tissue is lost because the lack of insulin forces the body to use its fat stores and cellular proteins as sources of energy. In terms of weight loss, there often is a marked difference between type 2 diabetes and type 1 diabetes. Many people with uncomplicated type 2 diabetes often have problems with obesity.

Other signs and symptoms of hyperglycemia include recurrent blurred vision, fatigue, paresthesias, and skin infections. In type 2 diabetes, these often are the symptoms that prompt a person to seek medical treatment. Blurred vision develops as the lens and retina are exposed to hyperosmolar fluids. Lowered plasma volume produces weakness and fatigue. Paresthesias reflect a temporary dysfunction of the peripheral sensory nerves. Chronic skin infections can occur and are more common in people with type 2 diabetes. Hyperglycemia and glycosuria favor the growth of yeast organisms. Pruritus and vulvovaginitis due to *Candida* infections are common initial complaints in women with diabetes. Balanitis secondary to *Candida* infections can occur in men.

Diagnostic Tests

The diagnosis of diabetes mellitus is confirmed through the use of laboratory tests that measure blood glucose levels. Testing for diabetes should be considered in all individuals 45 years of age and older. Diabetes screening should be considered at a younger age in people who are obese, have a first-degree relative with diabetes, are members of a high-risk group, have delivered an infant weighing more than 9 pounds or been diagnosed with GDM, have hypertension or hyperlipidemia, or have met the criteria (IFG, IGT, elevated A1C) for increased risk of diabetes on previous testing.[28]

Blood Tests

Blood glucose measurements are used in both the diagnosis and management of diabetes. Diagnostic tests include the FPG, casual plasma glucose, the glucose tolerance test, and glycosylated hemoglobin (i.e., A1C).[10,11,28] Laboratory and capillary or finger-stick glucose tests are used for glucose management in people with diagnosed diabetes.

Fasting Plasma Glucose. The FPG represents plasma glucose levels after food has been withheld for at least 8 hours. Advantages of the FPG are convenience, patient acceptability, and cost. An FPG level below 100 mg/dL (5.6 mmol/L) is considered normal (see Table 33-3).

Casual Blood Glucose Test. A casual (or random) plasma glucose is one that is done without regard to the time of the last meal. A casual plasma glucose concentration that is unequivocally elevated ($\geq$200 mg/dL [11.1 mmol/L]) in the presence of classic symptoms of diabetes such as polydipsia, polyphagia, polyuria, and blurred vision is diagnostic of diabetes mellitus at any age.

Oral Glucose Tolerance Test. The OGTT is an important screening test for diabetes. The test measures the body's ability to store glucose by removing it from the blood. In men and women, the test measures the plasma glucose response to 75 g of concentrated glucose solution at selected intervals, usually 1 and 2 hours. In people with normal glucose tolerance, blood glucose levels return to normal within 2 to 3 hours after ingestion of a glucose load. Because people with diabetes lack the ability to respond to an increase in blood glucose by releasing adequate insulin to facilitate storage, their blood glucose levels rise above those observed in normal people and remain elevated for longer periods.

Capillary Blood Glucose Monitoring. Technological advances have provided the means for monitoring blood glucose levels by using a drop of capillary blood. This procedure has provided health professionals with a rapid and economical means for monitoring blood glucose and has given people with diabetes a way of maintaining near-normal blood glucose levels through self-monitoring of blood glucose. These methods use a drop of capillary blood obtained by pricking the finger or forearm with a special needle or small lancet. Small trigger devices make use of the lancet virtually painless. The drop of capillary blood is placed on or absorbed by a reagent strip, and glucose levels are determined electronically using a glucose meter.

Laboratory tests that use plasma for measurement of blood glucose give results that are 10% to 15% higher than the finger-stick method, which uses whole blood.[28] Many blood glucose monitors approved for home use and some test strips now calibrate blood glucose readings to plasma values. It is important that people with diabetes know whether their monitors or glucose strips provide whole-blood or plasma test results.

Continuous glucose monitoring (CGM) systems are becoming available to fine-tune glucose management. The various systems have small catheters implanted in the subcutaneous tissue to provide frequent samples. The variety and accuracy of these systems are continually improving. Finger-stick glucose monitoring remains the standard of care, but does not provide as much information regarding the glycemic profile as CGM (especially during the overnight period).

Glycosylated Hemoglobin. Glycosylated hemoglobin, hemoglobin A_{1C} (HbA_{1C}), and A1C are terms used to describe hemoglobin into which glucose has been incorporated. Hemoglobin normally does not contain glucose when it is released from the bone marrow. During its 120-day life span in the red blood cell, hemoglobin becomes glycosylated to form HbA1. The major form of HbA1 is HbA_{1C}, which makes up 2% to 6% of total hemoglobin.[3] Because glucose entry into red blood cells is not insulin dependent, the rate at which glucose becomes attached to the hemoglobin molecule depends on blood glucose levels. Glycosylation is essentially irreversible, and the level of A1C present in the blood provides an index of blood glucose levels over the previous 6 to 12 weeks. In uncontrolled diabetes or diabetes with hyperglycemia, there is an increase in the level of A1C. The American Diabetes Association (ADA) recommends initiating corrective measures for A1C levels greater than an individualized goal. For example, the presence of several factors including advanced age, history of severe hypoglycemic episodes, and presence of cardiovascular disease might suggest a glycemic goal of 7.5% to 8%, whereas the absence of these and other worrying factors may mean that a target goal of 6.5% or less is warranted as long as this can be achieved safely.[11]

The A1C may overestimate glycemic burden in certain individuals and ethnic groups (such as African Americans).[11] In addition, A1C can be misleading in persons with certain forms of anemia and hemoglobin disorders, and in pregnant women. For these populations, the diagnosis of diabetes must use glucose criteria exclusively. Also, the A1C may not be significantly elevated in rapidly evolving diabetes, such as the development of type 1 diabetes in children.

Urine Tests

The ease, accuracy, and convenience of self-administered blood glucose monitoring techniques have made urine testing for glucose obsolete for most people with diabetes. These tests only reflect urine glucose levels and are influenced by such factors as the renal threshold for glucose, fluid intake and urine concentration, urine testing methodologies, and some drugs. It is recommended that all people with diabetes self-monitor their blood glucose. Urine ketone determinations remain an important part of monitoring diabetic control, particularly in people with type 1 diabetes who are at risk for development of ketoacidosis, and in pregnant diabetic women to check the adequacy of nutrition and glycemic control.[28]

Diabetes Management

The desired outcome of glycemic control in both type 1 and type 2 diabetes is normalization of blood glucose as a means of preventing short- and long-term complications. Treatment plans involve dietary management (medical nutrition therapy), exercise, and antidiabetic agents. People with type 1 diabetes require insulin therapy from the time of diagnosis. Weight loss and dietary management may be sufficient to control blood glucose levels in people with type 2 diabetes. However, they require follow-up care because insulin secretion from the beta cells may decrease or insulin resistance may persist or worsen, in which case non-insulin agents are prescribed.

Among the methods used to achieve these treatment goals are education in self-management and problem solving. Individual treatment goals should take into account the person's age and other disease conditions, the person's capacity to understand and carry out the treatment regimen, and socioeconomic factors that might influence compliance with the treatment plan. Optimal control of both type 1 and type 2 diabetes is associated with prevention or delay of chronic diabetes complications.

Dietary Management

Dietary management usually is individualized to meet the specific needs of each person with diabetes.[11,29] Therapy goals include maintenance of near-normal blood glucose levels, achievement of optimal lipid levels, adequate calories to attain and maintain a reasonable weight, prevention and treatment of chronic diabetes complications, and improvement of overall health through optimal nutrition.

The diabetic diet has undergone marked changes over the years, particularly in the recommendations for distribution of calories among carbohydrates, proteins, and fats. There no longer is a generic diabetic or ADA diet, but rather an individualized dietary prescription based on metabolic parameters, medical history of factors such as renal impairment and gastrointestinal autonomic neuropathy, and treatment goals. For a person with type 1 diabetes, eating consistent amounts and types of food at specific and routine times is encouraged. Home blood glucose monitoring is used to fine-tune the plan. Most people with type 2 diabetes are overweight; thus nutrition therapy focuses on achieving glucose, lipid, and blood pressure goals, and weight loss if indicated. Mild to moderate weight loss (5% to 10% of total body weight) has been shown to improve diabetes control, even if desirable weight is not achieved.

Exercise

The benefits of exercise for anyone include increased cardiovascular fitness and psychological well-being. For many people with type 2 diabetes, the benefits of exercise include a decrease in body fat, better weight control, and improvement in insulin sensitivity.[11,30] Exercise is so important in diabetes management that an individualized program of regular exercise usually is considered an integral part of the therapeutic regimen for every diabetic. In general, sporadic exercise has only transient benefits; a regular program is necessary for cardiovascular conditioning and to maintain a muscle–fat ratio that enhances peripheral insulin receptivity.

In people with diabetes, the beneficial effects of exercise are accompanied by an increased risk of hypoglycemia. Although muscle uptake of glucose increases significantly, the ability to maintain blood glucose levels is hampered by failure to suppress the absorption of injected insulin and activate the counterregulatory mechanisms that maintain blood glucose. Not only is there an inability to suppress insulin levels, but insulin absorption may also increase. This increased absorption is more pronounced when insulin is injected into the subcutaneous tissue of the exercised muscle, but it occurs even when insulin is injected into other body areas. Even after exercise ceases, insulin's lowering effect on blood glucose continues. In some people with type 1 diabetes, the symptoms of hypoglycemia occur several hours after cessation of exercise, perhaps because subsequent insulin doses (in people using multiple daily insulin injections) are not adjusted to accommodate the exercise-induced decrease in blood glucose. The cause of hypoglycemia in people who do not administer a subsequent insulin dose is unclear. It may be related to the fact that the liver and skeletal muscles increase their uptake of glucose after exercise as a means of replenishing their glycogen stores, or that the liver and skeletal muscles are more sensitive to insulin during this time. People with diabetes should be aware that delayed hypoglycemia can occur after exercise and that they may need to alter their diabetes medication dose, their carbohydrate intake, or both.

Although of benefit to people with diabetes, exercise must be weighed on the risk–benefit scale. Before beginning an exercise program, persons with diabetes should undergo an appropriate evaluation for macrovascular and microvascular disease.[30] The goal of exercise is safe participation in activities consistent with an individual's lifestyle. As with nutrition guidelines, exercise recommendations need to be individualized. Considerations include the potential for hypoglycemia, hyperglycemia, ketosis, cardiovascular ischemia and arrhythmias (particularly silent ischemic heart disease), exacerbation of proliferative retinopathy, and lower extremity injury. For those with chronic diabetes, the complications of vigorous exercise can be harmful and cause eye hemorrhage and other problems.

Oral and Injectable Antidiabetic Agents

Historically, two categories of antidiabetic agents existed: insulin injections and oral medications. However, this classification has been set aside since the introduction of new injectable non-insulin antidiabetic agents. Because people with type 1 diabetes are deficient in insulin, they are in need of exogenous insulin replacement therapy from the start. People with type 2 diabetes can have increased hepatic glucose production, decreased peripheral utilization of glucose, decreased utilization of ingested carbohydrates, and, over time, impaired insulin secretion and excessive glucagon secretion from the pancreas (Fig. 33-8). The antidiabetic (non-insulin) agents used in the treatment of type 2 diabetes (insulin secretagogues, biguanides, α-glucosidase inhibitors, thiazolidinediones, SGLT2 inhibitors, and incretin-based agents) attack each one of these areas and sometimes all.[31,32] If good glycemic control cannot be achieved with one or a combination of non-insulin agents, insulin can be added or used by itself.

Insulin Secretagogues. The insulin secretagogues act at the level of the pancreatic beta cells to stimulate insulin secretion. There are two general classes of insulin secretagogues: (1) sulfonylureas and (2) meglitinides.[32] Both types require the presence of functioning beta cells, are used only in the treatment of type 2 diabetes, and have the potential for producing hypoglycemia.

The control of insulin release from the pancreatic beta cells by glucose or the sulfonylurea drugs requires the generation of adenosine triphosphate (ATP), closing of an ATP-gated potassium channel, and opening of a transmembrane calcium channel.[32] The sulfonylureas (e.g., glipizide, glyburide, glimepiride) act by binding to a high-affinity sulfonylurea receptor on the beta cell that is linked to an ATP-sensitive potassium channel (Fig. 33-9). Binding of a sulfonylurea closes the channel, resulting in a coupled reaction that leads to an influx of calcium ions and insulin secretion. Because the sulfonylureas increase insulin levels and the rate at which glucose is removed from the blood, it is important to recognize that they can cause hypoglycemic reactions. This problem is more common in elderly people with

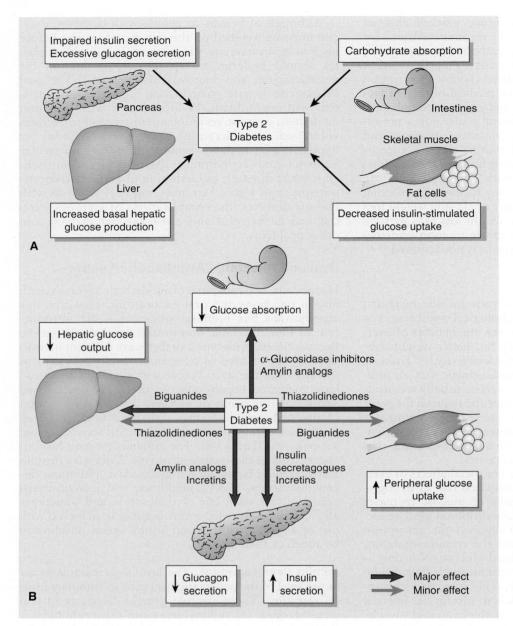

FIGURE 33-8. (A) Mechanisms of elevated blood glucose in type 2 diabetes mellitus. **(B)** Action sites of hypoglycemic agents and mechanisms of lowering blood glucose in type 2 diabetes. The incretins are the dipeptidyl peptidase-4 (DPP-4) inhibitors and glucagon-like peptide-1 (GLP-1) agonists.

impaired hepatic and renal function who are taking the longer-acting sulfonylureas.

The meglitinides (repaglinide) and related drugs (nateglinide) are shorter-acting insulin secretagogues (termed glinides) that target post-prandial glucose elevation. These agents, which are rapidly absorbed from the gastrointestinal tract, are taken shortly before meals. Both drugs can produce hypoglycemia; thus, proper timing of meals in relation to drug administration is essential.

Biguanides. Metformin, the only currently available biguanide, inhibits hepatic glucose production and increases the sensitivity of peripheral tissues to the actions of insulin. Secondary benefits of metformin therapy include weight loss and improved lipid profiles. This medication does not stimulate insulin secretion; therefore, it does not produce hypoglycemia. However,

it confers an increased risk for lactic acidosis, and is contraindicated in people with elevated serum creatinine levels, clinical and laboratory evidence of severe liver disease, or conditions associated with hypoxemia or dehydration.[32]

α-Glucosidase Inhibitors. The α-glucosidase inhibitors (acarbose, miglitol) block the action of intestinal brush border enzymes that break down complex carbohydrates.[32] By delaying the breakdown of complex carbohydrates, the α-glucosidase inhibitors delay the absorption of carbohydrates from the gut and blunt the postprandial increase in plasma glucose and insulin levels. Although not a problem with monotherapy or combination therapy with a biguanide, hypoglycemia may occur with concurrent sulfonylurea treatment. If hypoglycemia does occur, it should be treated with glucose (dextrose) and not

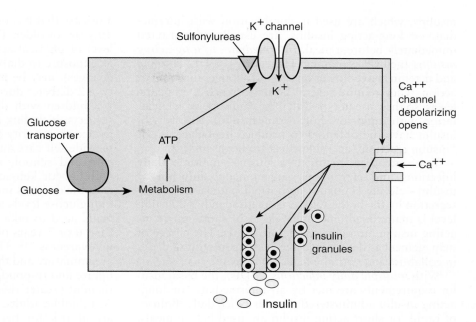

FIGURE 33-9. One model of control of release of insulin by the pancreatic beta cells and the action of the sulfonylurea agents. In the resting beta cell with low adenosine triphosphate (ATP) levels, potassium diffuses through the ATP-gated channels, maintaining the resting membrane potential. As blood glucose rises and is transported into the beta cell by the glucose transporter, ATP rises, causing the potassium channels to close and depolarization to occur. Depolarization results in opening of the voltage-gated calcium channels, which leads to insulin secretion. (Modified from Karam JH. Type II diabetes and syndrome X. *Endocrinol Metab Clin North Am.* 1992;21(2):329–350.)

sucrose (table sugar), whose breakdown may be blocked by the action of the α-glucosidase inhibitors.

Thiazolidinediones.

The thiazolidinediones (TZDs) or glitazones (e.g., pioglitazone, rosiglitazone) are the only class of drugs that directly target insulin resistance. They do this by increasing insulin sensitivity in the insulin-responsive tissues—liver, skeletal muscle, and fat—allowing the tissues to respond to endogenous insulin more efficiently without increased output from already dysfunctional beta cells.[3,32] Because of the previous problem with liver toxicity in this class of drugs, liver enzymes should be monitored before starting therapy according to guidelines. Both agents can cause fluid accumulation and are therefore contraindicated in patients with stage III and IV heart failure[33] (see Chapter 20, Table 20-1). Other potential adverse effects include an increased risk of bone fractures[34] and of bladder cancer.

Incretin-Based Agents.

Incretins are hormones released into the circulation by the gastrointestinal tract after a meal, especially one high in carbohydrates, that amplify the glucose-induced release of insulin (see Chapter 28).[3,6] The main incretins secreted are glucagon-like peptide 1 (GLP-1) and glucose-dependent insulinotropic polypeptide (GIP).[3,35,36] Both GLP-1 and GIP are rapidly degraded by the enzyme dipeptidyl peptidase-4 (DPP-4). DPP-4 enzyme inhibitors work by inhibiting the DPP-4 enzyme and increasing GLP-1 and GIP levels, which then increase insulin release. Glucagon-like peptide 1 also helps to suppress glucagon release.

Exenatide, a synthetic analog of GLP-1 that is resistant to DPP-4 degradation, is approved as an injectable adjunctive therapy for people with type 2 diabetes. The drug has been shown to have multiple actions such as potentiation of glucose-mediated insulin release, slowed gastric emptying, and a central loss of appetite. Although

exenatide was the first GLP-1 agonist to be developed and approved, other agents and formulations have also been approved.[36]

Many other novel classes of antidiabetes agents are also approved for type 2 diabetes including the SGLT2 inhibitor, canagliflozin. This agent, which works by inhibiting glucose reabsorption from the kidney, results in about 70 g (approximately 300 Kcal) glucose loss per day. The adverse effects are understandable, including polyuria due to osmotic diuresis and increased urinary tract infections and genitourinary *Candida* infections.

Insulin

Type 1 diabetes mellitus always requires treatment with insulin, and many people with type 2 diabetes eventually require insulin therapy. Insulin is destroyed in the gastrointestinal tract and must be administered by injection or inhalation. An inhaled form of insulin (Exubera) was on the market for a short time in the United States but was withdrawn for commercial reasons. Other inhaled insulin formulations are in clinical development.

Human insulin has become widely available, providing an alternative to forms of insulin obtained from bovine and porcine sources. Its manufacture uses recombinant deoxyribonucleic acid (DNA) technology. More recently, analogs to human insulin have become available that offer even better and more reproducible release characteristics.[37]

Four insulin types are classified by length and peaking of action: short acting, rapid acting, intermediate acting, and long acting.[32,37] *Short-acting insulin* (regular) is a soluble crystalline insulin whose effects begin within 30 minutes after subcutaneous injection and generally last for 5 to 8 hours. The *rapid-acting insulins* (lispro, aspart, glulisine) are produced by recombinant technology and have a more rapid onset, peak, and duration of action than short-acting regular insulin. The rapid-acting insulins, which are used in combination with intermediate or long-acting insulins, are usually administered immediately before a meal. *Intermediate- to long-acting insulins* (neutral protamine Hagedorn [NPH], glargine, and detemir) have slower onsets and a longer duration of action. They require several hours to reach therapeutic levels, so their use in type 1 diabetes requires supplementation with rapid- or short-acting insulin. All forms of insulin have the potential to produce hypoglycemia or "insulin reaction" as a side effect (to be discussed).

Two intensive treatment regimens—multiple daily injections and continuous subcutaneous infusion of insulin—closely simulate the normal pattern of insulin secretion by the body. With each method, a basal insulin level is maintained, and bolus doses of short- or rapid-acting insulin are delivered before meals. The choice of management is determined by the person with diabetes in collaboration with the health care team.

With *multiple daily injections* (MDIs), the basal insulin requirements are met by an intermediate- or long-acting insulin administered once or twice daily. Boluses of rapid- or short-acting insulin are used before meals. The development of convenient injection devices (e.g., pen injectors) has made it easier for people with diabetes to comply with algorithms for these insulins that are administered before meals.

The *continuous subcutaneous insulin infusion* (CSII) method uses an insulin pump. With this method, the basal insulin requirements are met by continuous infusion of subcutaneous insulin, the rate of which can be varied to accommodate diurnal variations.[38] The computer-operated pump then delivers one or more set basal amounts of insulin. In addition to the basal amount delivered by the pump, a bolus amount of insulin may be delivered when needed (e.g., before a meal) by pushing a button. Although the pump's safety has been proven, strict attention must be paid to signs of hyperglycemia. Self-monitoring of blood glucose levels is a necessity when using the CSII method of management. Hyperglycemia and ketotic episodes caused by pump failure, catheter clogging, and infections at the needle site also are possible complications. Candidate selection is crucial to the successful use of the insulin pump. Only people who are highly motivated to do frequent blood glucose tests and make daily insulin adjustments are candidates for this method of treatment.[38]

Pancreas or Islet Cell Transplantation

Pancreas or islet cell transplantation is not a lifesaving procedure. It does, however, afford the potential for significantly improving the quality of life. The most serious problems are the requirement for immunosuppression and the need for diagnosis and treatment of rejection. Investigators are looking for methods of transplanting islet cells and protecting the cells from destruction without the use of immunosuppressive drugs.[39]

Management of Diabetes in Children

Children with diabetes have traditionally been diagnosed with type 1 diabetes. However, health care providers are finding more children with type 2 diabetes, a disease that has usually been diagnosed in adults aged 40 years or older. The epidemics of obesity and the low level of physical activity among young people, as well as exposure to diabetes *in utero* (resulting in epigenetic changes), may be major contributors to the increase in type 2 diabetes during childhood and adolescence.

Children with diabetes differ from adults in many respects, including changes in insulin sensitivity related to sexual maturity and physical growth, their ability to provide self-care and their need for supervision in child care and school, and vulnerability to hypoglycemia and diabetic ketoacidosis.[11] While current standards of care for diabetes management reflect the need to maintain glucose levels as near normal as possible, glycemic goals need to take into account that children younger than 6 or 7 years of age have a form of "hypoglycemic unawareness."[11] Their counterregulatory mechanisms are immature and they lack the cognitive capacity to recognize and respond to hypoglycemic symptoms, placing them at greater risk for hypoglycemia and its sequelae. Also, unlike adults, young children under 5 years of age are at risk for permanent cognitive impairment after episodes of severe hypoglycemia.[11] Thus, the glycemic goals for children must consider the benefits of long-term health outcomes against the risks of hypoglycemia and the difficulties in achieving normoglycemia in children. Additional concerns include the effects of drugs developed and tested primarily for adults on growth and brain development in children.

Acute Complications

The three major acute complications of impaired blood glucose regulation are diabetic ketoacidosis (DKA), hyperglycemic hyperosmolar state (HHS), and hypoglycemia. All are life-threatening conditions that demand immediate recognition and treatment. The Somogyi effect and dawn phenomenon, which result from the mobilization of counterregulatory hormones, contribute to difficulties with diabetic control.

Diabetic Ketoacidosis

Diabetic ketoacidosis, characterized by hyperglycemia, ketosis, and metabolic acidosis, is an acute life-threatening complication of uncontrolled diabetes.[40–42] Diabetic ketoacidosis primarily affects persons with type 1 diabetes, but may also occur in persons with type 2 diabetes when severe stress such as sepsis or trauma is present. It may be an initial manifestation of previously undiagnosed type 1 diabetes or may result from increased insulin requirements in type 1 diabetes during stress situations, such as infection or trauma, that increase the release of stress hormones. For example, a mother may bring a child into the clinic or emergency department with reports of lethargy, vomiting, and abdominal pain, unaware that the child has diabetes. In clinical practice, ketoacidosis also occurs with the omission or inadequate use of insulin.

Ketoacidosis reflects the effect of insulin deficiency at multiple sites (Fig. 33-10). A lack of insulin results in the

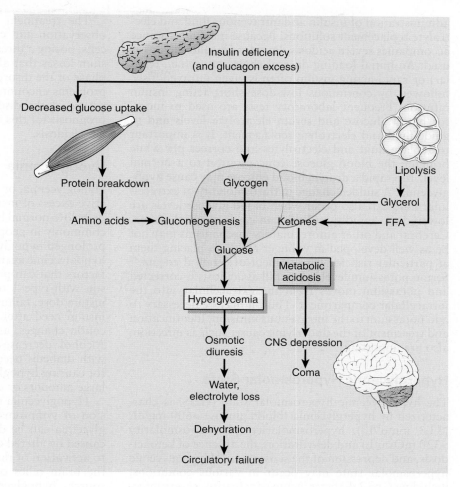

FIGURE 33-10. Mechanisms of diabetic ketoacidosis. Diabetic ketoacidosis is associated with very low insulin levels and extremely high levels of glucagon, catecholamines, and other counterregulatory hormones. Increased levels of glucagon and the catecholamines lead to mobilization of substrates for gluconeogenesis and ketogenesis by the liver. Gluconeogenesis in excess of that needed to supply glucose to the brain and other glucose-dependent tissues produces a rise in blood glucose levels. Mobilization of free fatty acids (FFAs) from triglyceride stores in adipose tissue leads to accelerated ketone production and ketosis. CNS, central nervous system.

rapid breakdown of energy stores from muscle and fat deposits, leading to increased movement of amino acids to the liver for conversion to glucose and of fatty acids for conversion to ketones. In the presence of ketosis, the levels of glucagon and counterregulatory hormones (i.e., glucocorticosteroids, epinephrine, and growth hormone) are consistently increased. Furthermore, in the absence of insulin, peripheral utilization of glucose and ketones is reduced. Metabolic acidosis is caused by the excess ketoacids that require buffering by bicarbonate ions; this leads to a marked decrease in serum bicarbonate levels.

The definitive diagnosis of DKA consists of *hyperglycemia* (blood glucose levels >250 mg/dL [13.8 mmol/L]), low serum bicarbonate, low arterial pH, and positive urine and serum ketones. It can be further subdivided into *mild DKA* (serum bicarbonate of 15 to 18 mEq/dL [15 to 18 mmol/L], pH 7.25 to 7.30); *moderate DKA* (serum bicarbonate 10 to <15 mEq/dL [10 to <15 mmol/L], pH 7.00 to 7.24); and *severe DKA* (serum bicarbonate <10 mEq/dL [<10 mmol/L], pH <7.00).[40,41] Hyperglycemia leads to osmotic diuresis, dehydration, and a critical loss of electrolytes. Hyperosmolality of extracellular fluids from hyperglycemia leads to a shift of water and potassium from the intracellular to the extracellular compartment. Extracellular sodium concentration frequently is low or normal despite enteric water losses because of an intracellular–extracellular fluid shift. This dilutional effect is referred to as *pseudohyponatremia*. Serum potassium levels may also be normal or elevated, despite total potassium depletion resulting from protracted polyuria and vomiting.

The development of DKA is commonly preceded by a day or more of polyuria, polydipsia, nausea, vomiting, and marked fatigue, with eventual stupor that can progress to coma. Abdominal pain and tenderness may be experienced without abdominal disease. The breath has a characteristic fruity smell because of the presence of volatile ketoacids. Hypotension and tachycardia may be present because of a decrease in blood volume. A number of the signs and symptoms that occur in DKA are related to compensatory mechanisms. The heart rate increases as the body compensates for a decrease in blood volume, and the rate and depth of respiration increase (i.e., Kussmaul respiration) as the body attempts to prevent further decreases in pH. Metabolic acidosis is discussed further in Chapter 8.

The goals in treating DKA are to improve circulatory volume and tissue perfusion, decrease blood glucose, and correct the acidosis and electrolyte imbalances. These objectives usually are accomplished through the administration of insulin and intravenous fluid and electrolyte replacement solutions. Because insulin resistance accompanies severe acidosis, low-dose insulin therapy is used. An initial loading dose of short-acting (i.e., regular) or rapid-acting insulin often is given intravenously, followed by continuous low-dose short-acting insulin infusion. Frequent laboratory tests are used to monitor blood glucose and serum electrolyte levels and to guide fluid and electrolyte replacement. It is important to replace fluid and electrolytes and correct pH while bringing the blood glucose concentration to a normal level. Too rapid a drop in blood glucose may cause hypoglycemia. A sudden change in the osmolality of extracellular fluid can also occur when blood glucose levels are lowered too rapidly, and this can cause cerebral edema. Cerebral and other autoregulatory mechanisms may not be as well developed in younger children, placing them at particular risk for development of cerebral edema.[42] Serum potassium levels often fall as acidosis is corrected and potassium moves from the extracellular into the intracellular compartment. Thus, it may be necessary to add potassium to the intravenous infusion. Identification and treatment of the underlying cause, such as infection, also are important.

Hyperglycemic Hyperosmolar State

The hyperglycemic hyperosmolar state (HHS) is characterized by hyperglycemia (blood glucose >600 mg/dL [33.3 mmol/L]), hyperosmolarity (plasma osmolarity >320 mOsm/L) and dehydration, the absence of ketoacidosis, and depression of the sensorium.[40] Hyperglycemic hyperosmolar state may occur in various conditions, including type 2 diabetes, acute pancreatitis, severe infection, myocardial infarction, and treatment with oral or parenteral nutrition solutions. It is seen most frequently in people with type 2 diabetes. A partial or relative insulin deficiency may initiate the syndrome by reducing glucose utilization while inducing a glucagon-stimulated increase in hepatic glucose output. With massive glycosuria, obligatory water loss occurs. If the person is unable to maintain adequate fluid intake because of associated acute or chronic illness or has excessive fluid loss, dehydration develops. As the plasma volume contracts, renal insufficiency develops and the resultant limitation of renal glucose losses leads to increasingly higher blood glucose levels and an increase in severity of the hyperosmolar state.

In hyperosmolar states, the increased serum osmolarity has the effect of pulling water out of body cells, including brain cells. The condition may be complicated by thromboembolic events arising because of the high serum osmolality. The most prominent manifestations are weakness, dehydration, polyuria, neurologic signs and symptoms, and excessive thirst. The neurologic signs include hemiparesis, Babinski reflex, aphasia, muscle fasciculations, hyperthermia, hemianopia, nystagmus, visual hallucinations, seizures, and coma. The onset of HHS often is insidious, and because it occurs most frequently in older people, it may be mistaken for a stroke.

The treatment of HHS requires judicious medical observation and care as water moves back into brain cells, posing a threat of cerebral edema. Extensive potassium losses that also have occurred during the diuretic phase of the disorder require correction. Because of the problems encountered in the treatment and the serious nature of the disease conditions that cause HHS, the prognosis for this disorder is less favorable than that for ketoacidosis.

Hypoglycemia

Hypoglycemia, or an insulin reaction, occurs from a relative excess of insulin in the blood and is characterized by below-normal blood glucose levels.[43,44] It occurs most commonly in people treated with insulin injections, but prolonged hypoglycemia also can result from some oral hypoglycemic agents (i.e., sulfonylurea). There are many factors that can precipitate an insulin reaction in a person with type 1 or type 2 diabetes, including error in insulin dose, failure to eat, increased exercise, decreased insulin need after removal of a stress situation, medication changes, and a change in insulin injection site. Alcohol decreases liver gluconeogenesis, and people with diabetes need to be cautioned about its potential for causing hypoglycemia, especially if it is consumed in large amounts or on an empty stomach.

Hypoglycemia usually has a rapid onset and progression of symptoms. The signs and symptoms of hypoglycemia can be divided into two categories: (1) those caused by altered cerebral function and (2) those related to activation of the autonomic nervous system. Because the brain relies on blood glucose as its main energy source, hypoglycemia produces behaviors related to altered cerebral function. Headache, difficulty in problem solving, disturbed or altered behavior, coma, and seizures may occur. At the onset of the hypoglycemic episode, activation of the parasympathetic nervous system often causes hunger. The initial parasympathetic response is followed by activation of the sympathetic nervous system; which causes anxiety, tachycardia, sweating, and a cool and clammy skin due to constriction of the skin vessels.

The signs and symptoms of hypoglycemia are highly variable, especially in children and the elderly, and not everyone manifests all or even most of the symptoms. Elderly people may not display the typical autonomic responses, but typically do display signs of altered cerebral function, including mental confusion. Also, some medications, such as β-adrenergic blocking drugs, interfere with the autonomic response normally seen in hypoglycemia. Some people develop hypoglycemic unawareness; that is, they do not report symptoms when their blood glucose concentrations are less than 50 to 60 mg/dL (2.8 to 3.3 mmol/L). This occurs most commonly in people who have a longer duration of diabetes and A1C levels within the normal range.[43]

The most effective treatment of an insulin reaction is the immediate administration of 15 g of glucose in a concentrated carbohydrate source. According to the so-called *rule of 15*, this 15 g of glucose can be repeated every 15 minutes for up to 3 doses. Monosaccharides such as glucose, which can be absorbed directly into the bloodstream, work best. Complex carbohydrates can be administered after the acute reaction has been controlled to sustain blood glucose levels. It is important not to overtreat hypoglycemia and cause rebound hyperglycemia. Alternative methods for increasing blood glucose may be required when the person having the reaction is unconscious or unable to swallow. Glucagon may be given intramuscularly or subcutaneously. Glucagon acts by hepatic glycogenolysis to raise blood glucose. Because the liver contains only a limited amount of glycogen (approximately 75 g), glucagon is ineffective in people whose glycogen stores have been depleted. In situations of severe or life-threatening hypoglycemia, it may be necessary to administer glucose (20 to 50 mL of a 50% solution) intravenously. If hypoglycemia occurs with α-glucosidase inhibitors, it should be treated with glucose (dextrose) and not sucrose (table sugar), whose breakdown may be blocked by the action of the α-glucosidase inhibitors.

The Somogyi Effect and Dawn Phenomenon

The *Somogyi effect* describes a cycle of insulin-induced posthypoglycemic episodes. In 1924, Joslin and associates noticed that hypoglycemia was associated with alternate episodes of hyperglycemia. It was not until 1959 that Somogyi presented the results of his 20 years of studies, which confirmed the observation that "hypoglycemia begets hyperglycemia."[45] In people with diabetes, insulin-induced hypoglycemia produces a compensatory increase in blood levels of catecholamines, glucagon, cortisol, and growth hormone. These counterregulatory hormones cause blood glucose to become elevated and produce some degree of insulin resistance. The cycle begins when the increase in blood glucose and insulin resistance is treated with larger insulin doses. The hypoglycemic episode often occurs during the night or at a time when it is not recognized, rendering the diagnosis of the phenomenon more difficult.

Research suggests that even mild insulin-associated hypoglycemia, which may be asymptomatic, can cause hyperglycemia in people with type 1 diabetes through the recruitment of counterregulatory mechanisms, although the insulin action does not wane. A waning of insulin's effects when it occurs (i.e., end of the duration of action) causes an exacerbation of the posthypoglycemic hyperglycemia that occurs and accelerates its development. These findings may explain the labile nature of the disease in some people with diabetes. Measures to prevent hypoglycemia and the subsequent activation of counterregulatory mechanisms include a redistribution of dietary carbohydrates and an alteration in insulin dose or time of administration.[46]

The *dawn phenomenon* is characterized by increased levels of fasting blood glucose, or insulin requirements, or both, between 5 AM and 9 AM without antecedent hypoglycemia. It occurs in people with type 1 or type 2 diabetes. It has been suggested that a change in the normal circadian rhythm for glucose tolerance, which usually is higher during the latter part of the morning, is altered in people with diabetes.[47] Growth hormone has been suggested as a possible factor. When the dawn phenomenon occurs alone, it may produce only mild hyperglycemia, but when it is combined with the Somogyi effect, it may produce profound hyperglycemia.

Chronic Complications

The chronic complications of diabetes include disorders of the microvasculature (i.e., neuropathies, nephropathies, and retinopathies), macrovascular complications (i.e., coronary artery, cerebrovascular, and peripheral arterial disease), and foot ulcers (Fig. 33-11). The level of chronic

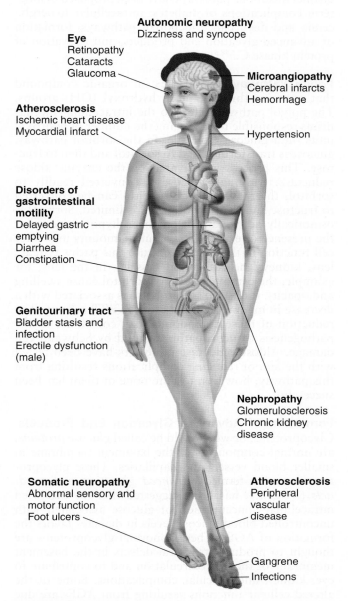

Autonomic neuropathy
Dizziness and syncope

Eye
Retinopathy
Cataracts
Glaucoma

Microangiopathy
Cerebral infarcts
Hemorrhage

Atherosclerosis
Ischemic heart disease
Myocardial infarct

Hypertension

Disorders of gastrointestinal motility
Delayed gastric emptying
Diarrhea
Constipation

Genitourinary tract
Bladder stasis and infection
Erectile dysfunction (male)

Nephropathy
Glomerulosclerosis
Chronic kidney disease

Somatic neuropathy
Abnormal sensory and motor function
Foot ulcers

Atherosclerosis
Peripheral vascular disease

Gangrene
Infections

FIGURE 33-11. Long-term complications of diabetes mellitus.

hyperglycemia is the best-established concomitant factor associated with diabetic complications.[48,49] The Diabetes Control and Complications Trial (DCCT) and its ongoing long-term observational study, the Epidemiology of Diabetes Interventions and Complications Study (EDIC) conducted in 1441 patients with type 1 diabetes, demonstrated that the incidence of retinopathy, nephropathy, and neuropathy can be reduced by intensive glycemic control.[49] Similar results have been demonstrated by the United Kingdom Prospective Diabetes Study (UKPDS) in 5000 patients with type 2 diabetes.[50]

Theories of Pathogenesis

The interest among researchers in explaining the causes and development of chronic lesions in a person with diabetes has led to a number of theories. At least three distinct metabolic pathways have been proposed in long-term complications of diabetes: intracellular hyperglycemia and disturbance in polyol pathways, formation of advanced glycation end products, and activation of protein kinase C.[3,48,51]

Polyol Pathway. A polyol is an organic compound that contains three or more hydroxyl (OH) groups. The polyol pathway refers to the intracellular mechanisms responsible for changing the number of hydroxyl units on a glucose molecule. In the sorbitol pathway, glucose is transformed first to sorbitol and then to fructose. This process is activated by the enzyme aldose reductase. Although glucose is converted readily to sorbitol, the rate at which sorbitol can be converted to fructose and then metabolized is limited. Sorbitol is osmotically active, and it has been hypothesized that the presence of excess intracellular amounts may alter cell function in the tissues that use this pathway (e.g., lens, kidneys, nerves, blood vessels). In the lens, for example, the osmotic effects of sorbitol cause swelling and opacity. Increased sorbitol also is associated with a decrease in myoinositol and reduced ATP activity. The reduction of these compounds may contribute to the pathogenesis of neuropathies caused by Schwann cell damage. Aldose reductase inhibitors have been tested with the aim of reducing complications resulting from this pathway; however, to date none of them has been successful.

Formation of Advanced Glycation End Products. Glycoproteins, or what could be called *glucose proteins*, are normal components of the basement membrane in smaller blood vessels and capillaries. These glycoproteins are also termed *advanced glycation end products* (AGEs). It has been suggested that the increased intracellular concentration of glucose associated with uncontrolled blood glucose levels in diabetes favors the formation of AGEs. These abnormal glycoproteins are thought to produce structural defects in the basement membrane of the microcirculation and to contribute to eye, kidney, and vascular complications. Some of the altered cellular functions resulting from AGEs are due to binding to specific receptors for AGEs (RAGEs).

Protein Kinase C. Diacylglycerol (DAG) and protein kinase C (PKC) are critical intracellular signaling molecules that can regulate many vascular functions, including permeability, vasodilator release, endothelial activation, and growth factor signaling. Levels of DAG and PKC are elevated in diabetes. Activation of PKC in blood vessels of the retina, kidney, and nerves can produce vascular damage. A PKC inhibitor was previously studied for the treatment of diabetic retinopathy and neuropathy, but showed variable results and is not marketed.[3]

Diabetic Neuropathies

Although the incidence of neuropathies is high among people with diabetes (approximately 50% compared with 2% in the general population and approximately 15% when age >40 years), it is difficult to document exactly how many people are affected by these disorders because of the diversity in clinical manifestations and because the condition often is far advanced before it is recognized. Results of the DCCT study showed that intensive diabetic therapy can reduce the incidence of clinical neuropathy by 60% compared with conventional therapy.[52]

Several types of pathologic changes have been observed in connection with diabetic neuropathies. These include thickening of the walls of the nutrient vessels that supply the nerve, leading to the assumption that vessel ischemia plays a major role in the development of these neural changes. Another finding is a segmental demyelinization process that affects the Schwann cell. This demyelinization process is accompanied by a slowing of nerve conduction.

Although there are several methods for classifying the diabetic peripheral neuropathies, a simplified system divides them into the somatic and autonomic nervous system neuropathies (Chart 33-2).

Somatic Neuropathy. A distal symmetric polyneuropathy, in which loss of function typically occurs in a stocking–glove pattern, is the most common form of peripheral neuropathy. Somatic sensory involvement usually occurs first, often is bilateral and symmetric, and is associated with diminished perception of vibration, pain, and temperature, particularly in the lower extremities.[53] In addition to the discomforts associated with the loss of sensory or motor function, lesions in the peripheral nervous system predispose a person with diabetes to other complications. The loss of feeling, touch, and position sense increases the risk of falling. Impairment of temperature and pain sensation increases the risk of serious burns and injuries to the feet. Denervation of the small muscles of the foot result in clawing of the toes and displacement of the submetatarsal fat pad anteriorly. These changes, together with joint and connective tissue changes, alter the biomechanics of the foot, increasing plantar pressure and predisposing to development of foot trauma and ulcers.[53]

Painful diabetic neuropathy involves the somatosensory neurons that carry pain impulses. This disorder, which causes hypersensitivity to light touch and

---

CHART 33-2	Classification of Diabetic Neuropathies

Somatic

Polyneuropathies (bilateral sensory)
   Paresthesias, including numbness and tingling
   Impaired pain, temperature, light touch, two-point
      discrimination, and vibratory sensation
   Decreased ankle and knee-jerk reflexes
Mononeuropathies
   Involvement of a mixed nerve trunk that includes
      loss of sensation, pain, and motor weakness
Amyotrophy
   Associated with muscle weakness, wasting, and
      severe pain of muscles in the pelvic girdle and
      thigh

Autonomic

Impaired vasomotor function
   Postural hypotension
Impaired gastrointestinal function
   Gastric atony
   Diarrhea, often postprandial and nocturnal
Impaired genitourinary function
   Paralytic bladder
   Incomplete voiding
   Erectile dysfunction
   Retrograde ejaculation
Cranial nerve involvement
   Extraocular nerve paralysis
   Impaired pupillary responses
   Impaired special senses

---

occasionally severe "burning pain," particularly at night, can become physically and emotionally disabling.[53]

Autonomic Neuropathy. The autonomic neuropathies involve disorders of sympathetic and parasympathetic nervous system function. There may be disorders of vasomotor function, decreased cardiac responses, inability to empty the bladder, gastrointestinal motility problems, and sexual dysfunction.[54] Defects in vasomotor reflexes can lead to dizziness and syncope due to postural hypotension when the person moves from the supine to the standing position (see Chapter 18). Incomplete emptying of the bladder predisposes to urinary stasis and bladder infection and increases the risk of renal complications.

Gastrointestinal motility disorders are common in persons with long-standing diabetes. The symptoms vary in severity and include gastroparesis, constipation, diarrhea, and fecal incontinence. Gastroparesis (delayed emptying of stomach) is commonly seen in persons with diabetes.[55] The disorder is characterized by complaints of epigastric discomfort, nausea, postprandial vomiting, bloating, and early satiety. Abnormal gastric emptying also jeopardizes the regulation of the blood glucose level. Diarrhea is another common symptom seen mostly in persons with poorly controlled type 1 diabetes and autonomic neuropathy.[56] The pathogenesis is thought to be multifactorial. Diabetic diarrhea is typically intermittent, watery, painless, and nocturnal and may be associated with fecal incontinence.

In the male, disruption of sensory and autonomic nervous system function may cause sexual dysfunction (see Chapter 39). Diabetes is the leading pathophysiological cause of erectile dysfunction (ED), and it occurs in both type 1 and type 2 diabetes. Of the 13 million men with diabetes in the United States, 30% to 60% have ED.[54]

Diabetic Nephropathies

Diabetic nephropathy, a term used to describe the combination of lesions that occur concurrently in the diabetic kidney, is the leading cause of chronic kidney disease (CKD) in persons starting renal replacement therapy (see Chapter 26).[57] Not all people with diabetes develop clinically significant nephropathy; for this reason, attention is focused on risk factors for the development of this complication. Among the suggested risk factors are genetic and familial predisposition, elevated blood pressure, poor glycemic control, smoking, hyperlipidemia, and increased albumin excretion.[11,58] Diabetic nephropathy occurs in family clusters, suggesting a familial predisposition, although this does not exclude the possibility of environmental factors shared by siblings. The risk for development of kidney disease is greater among Native Americans, Hispanic Americans (especially Mexican Americans), and African Americans.[11,58]

The most common kidney lesions in people with diabetes are those that affect the glomeruli. These include capillary basement membrane thickening, diffuse glomerular sclerosis, and nodular glomerulosclerosis, in which the development of nodular lesions in the glomerular capillaries causes impaired blood flow with progressive loss of kidney function and, eventually, renal failure (see Chapter 25). Nodular glomerulosclerosis is thought to occur only in people with diabetes. Changes in the basement membrane in diffuse nodular glomerulosclerosis allow plasma proteins to escape in the urine, causing albuminuria, hypoalbuminemia, edema, and other signs of impaired kidney function.

Kidney enlargement, nephron hypertrophy, and hyperfiltration are early accompaniments of diabetes, reflecting the increased work performed by the kidneys in reabsorbing excessive amounts of glucose. One of the first manifestations of diabetic nephropathy is an increase in urinary albumin excretion, which is defined as a urine protein loss greater or equal to 30 mg/day or an albumin-to-creatinine ratio (A/C ratio) greater or equal to 30 μg/mg (normal <30 μg/mg) from a spot urine collection.[58] It is recommended that the A/C ratio be the preferred screen for increased urinary albumin excretion. Both systolic and diastolic forms of hypertension accelerate the progression of diabetic nephropathy. Even moderate lowering of blood pressure can decrease the risk of CKD.[11] The estimated glomerular filtration rate (eGFR) should also be monitored on a regular basis.

Measures to prevent diabetic nephropathy or its progression in persons with diabetes include achievement of glycemic control, maintenance of blood pressure control (<140/80 mm Hg), prevention or reduction in the level of proteinuria (using angiotensin-converting enzyme inhibitors or angiotensin receptor blockers, or protein restriction in selected patients), treatment of hyperlipidemia, and smoking cessation in people who smoke.[11,57] Smoking increases the risk of CKD in both persons with and without diabetes. People with type 2 diabetes who smoke have a greater risk of increased urinary albumin excretion, and their rate of progression to CKD is approximately twice as rapid as in those who do not smoke.[11]

Diabetic Retinopathies

Diabetes is the leading cause of acquired blindness in the United States.[58,59] Although people with diabetes are at increased risk for development of cataracts and glaucoma, retinopathy is the most common pattern of eye disease. Diabetic retinopathy is estimated to be the most frequent cause of newly diagnosed blindness among Americans between the ages of 20 and 74 years.[59]

Diabetic retinopathy is characterized by abnormal retinal vascular permeability, microaneurysm formation, neovascularization and associated hemorrhage, scarring, diabetic macular edema, and retinal detachment[59] (see Chapter 38). Twenty years after the onset of diabetes, nearly all people with type 1 diabetes and more than 60% of people with type 2 diabetes have some degree of retinopathy. Pregnancy, puberty, and cataract surgery can accelerate these changes.[59] Risk factors associated with diabetic retinopathy are similar to those for other complications. Among the suggested risk factors associated with diabetic retinopathy are poor glycemic control, elevated blood pressure, dyslipidemia, and smoking. The strongest case for control of blood glucose comes from the DCCT/EDIC and UKPDS studies, which demonstrated a reduction in retinopathy with improved glucose control.[49,50]

Because of the risk of retinopathy, it is important that people with diabetes have regular dilated eye examinations. The recommendation for follow-up examinations is based on the type of examination that was done and the findings of that examination. People with persistently elevated glucose levels or proteinuria should be examined yearly.[59] Women who are planning a pregnancy should be counseled on the risk of development or progression of diabetic retinopathy. Women with diabetes who become pregnant should be followed closely throughout pregnancy. This does not apply to women in whom GDM develops because such women are not at risk for development of diabetic retinopathy.

People with macular edema, moderate to severe nonproliferative retinopathy, or any proliferative retinopathy should receive the care of an ophthalmologist who is knowledgeable and experienced in the management and treatment of diabetic retinopathy. Methods used in the treatment of diabetic retinopathy include the destruction and scarring of the proliferative lesions with laser photocoagulation. The use of antagonists to growth factors (e.g., vascular endothelial growth factor) administered by intra-vitreal injections also play an important role in the management of diabetic retinopathy, and are considered the gold-standard therapy in diabetic macular edema.

Macrovascular Complications

Diabetes mellitus is a major risk factor for atherosclerotic coronary artery disease, cerebrovascular disease, and peripheral vascular disease. The prevalence of these macrovascular complications is increased two- to fourfold in people with diabetes.

Multiple risk factors for macrovascular disease, including obesity, hypertension, hyperglycemia, hyperinsulinemia, hyperlipidemia, altered platelet function, endothelial dysfunction, systemic inflammation (as evidenced by increased CRP), and elevated fibrinogen levels, frequently are found in people with diabetes. There appear to be differences between type 1 and type 2 diabetes in terms of duration and development of macrovascular disease, with type 2 diabetics more commonly manifesting macrovascular disease at the time of diagnosis. This greater prevalence has been attributed to the associated cardiovascular risk factors that are part of the metabolic syndrome and which may have been present for many years before the diagnosis of type 2 diabetes.[19,20]

Aggressive management of cardiovascular risk factors should include smoking cessation, lifestyle changes including weight loss, and measures to control blood lipids, hypertension, and blood glucose, as appropriate.[19] Antiplatelet agents (aspirin or clopidogrel) may be prescribed to reduce the threat of blood clots. If treatment is warranted for peripheral arterial disease, the peroneal arteries between the knees and ankles commonly are involved in diabetes, making revascularization difficult.

Diabetic Foot Ulcers

Foot problems are common among people with diabetes and may become severe enough to cause ulceration, infection, and, eventually, the need for amputation.[60,61] Foot problems have been reported as the most common complication leading to hospitalization among people with diabetes. They represent the effects of neuropathy and vascular insufficiency. Approximately 60% to 70% of people with diabetic foot ulcers have neuropathy without vascular disease, 15% to 20% have vascular disease, and 15% to 20% have neuropathy and vascular disease.[60]

Distal symmetric neuropathy is a major risk factor for foot ulcers. People with sensory neuropathies have impaired pain sensation and often are unaware of the constant trauma to the feet caused by poorly fitting shoes, improper weight bearing, hard objects or pebbles in the shoes, or infections such as athlete's foot. Neuropathy may prevent people from detecting pain; they are unable to adjust their gait to avoid walking on an area of the foot where pressure is causing trauma and necrosis. Motor neuropathy with weakness of the intrinsic muscles of the foot may result in foot deformities, which lead to focal areas of high pressure. When the abnormal focus of pressure is coupled with loss of sensation, a foot ulcer can occur. Common sites of trauma are the back of the heel, the plantar metatarsal area, or the great toe, where weight is borne during walking (Fig. 33-12).

All persons with diabetes should receive a full foot examination at least once a year. This examination should include assessment of protective sensation, foot structure and biomechanics, vascular status, and skin integrity.[3,61] Evaluation should include a somatosensory test using the Semmes-Weinstein monofilament, a simple, inexpensive device for testing loss of protective sensation (Fig. 33-13). The monofilament is held in the hand or attached to a handle at one end. When the unattached or unsupported end of the monofilament is pressed against the skin until it buckles or bends slightly, it delivers 10 g of pressure at the point of contact.[61] The person tested reports when he or she is being touched by the monofilament. Usually four sites per foot are touched. An incorrect response at even one site indicates loss of protective sensation and increased risk of ulceration.

Because of the constant risk of foot problems, it is important that people with diabetes wear shoes that have been fitted correctly and inspect their feet daily, looking for blisters, open sores, and fungal infection (e.g., athlete's foot) between the toes. If their eyesight is poor, a family member should do this for them. In the event a lesion is detected, prompt medical attention is needed to prevent serious complications. Specially designed shoes have been demonstrated to be effective in preventing relapses in people with previous ulcerations.[61] Because cold produces vasoconstriction, appropriate foot coverings should be used to keep the feet warm and dry. Toenails should be cut straight across to prevent ingrown toenails. The toenails often are thickened and deformed, requiring the services of a podiatrist. Smoking should be

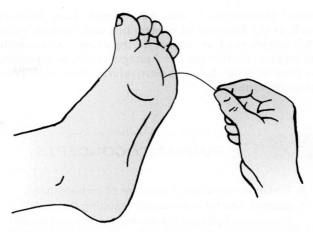

FIGURE 33-13. Use of a monofilament in testing for impaired sensation in the foot of a person with diabetes.

avoided because it causes vasoconstriction and contributes to vascular disease.

Cardiovascular risk factors should be addressed in patients with diabetic foot ulcers and peripheral arterial disease. Ulcers that are resistant to standard therapy may respond to application of growth factors. Growth factors provide a means by which cells communicate with each other and can have profound effects on cell proliferation, migration, and extracellular matrix synthesis. For example, becaplermin, a topical preparation of recombinant human platelet-derived growth factor, is used in the treatment of neuropathic lower extremity ulcers.

Infections

Although not specifically an acute or a chronic complication, infections are a common concern of people with diabetes. Certain types of infections occur with increased frequency in people with diabetes: soft tissue infections of the extremities, osteomyelitis, urinary tract infections and pyelonephritis, candidal infections of the skin and mucous surfaces, dental caries and periodontal disease, and tuberculosis.[62,63] Moreover, infections often are more serious in people with diabetes.

Suboptimal response to infection in a person with diabetes is caused by the presence of chronic complications, such as vascular disease and neuropathies, and by the presence of hyperglycemia and altered neutrophil function. Sensory deficits may cause a person with diabetes to ignore minor trauma and infection, and vascular disease may impair circulation and delivery of blood cells and other substances needed to produce an adequate inflammatory response and effect healing. Pyelonephritis and urinary tract infections are relatively common in persons with diabetes, and it has been suggested that these infections may bear some relation to the presence of a neurogenic bladder or nephrosclerotic changes in the kidneys. Hyperglycemia and glycosuria (including treatment with SGLT2 inhibitors) may influence the growth of microorganisms and increase the severity of the infection. Diabetes and elevated

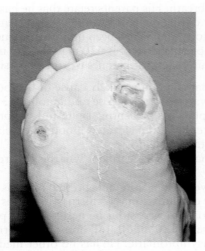

FIGURE 33-12. Neuropathic ulcers occur on pressure points in areas with diminished sensation in diabetic polyneuropathy. Pain is absent (and therefore the ulcer may go unnoticed). (From Bates BB. *A Guide to Physical Examination and History Taking*. 6th ed. Philadelphia, PA: J.B. Lippincott; 1995.)

blood glucose levels also may impair host defenses such as the function of neutrophils and immune cells. Polymorphonuclear leukocyte function, particularly adherence, chemotaxis, and phagocytosis, is depressed in persons with diabetes, particularly those with poor glycemic control.

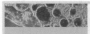

SUMMARY CONCEPTS

■ Diabetes mellitus is a disorder of carbohydrate, protein, and fat metabolism resulting from an imbalance between insulin availability and insulin need. In type 1 diabetes, there is destruction of beta cells and an absolute insulin deficiency. Type 2 diabetes is characterized by a lack of insulin availability or effectiveness. Diabetes can also occur secondary to some other condition that destroys beta cells (e.g., pancreatic disorders) or endocrine diseases that cause increased production of glucose by the liver and decreased use of glucose by the tissues (e.g., Cushing syndrome). Gestational diabetes develops during pregnancy.

■ The metabolic syndrome represents a constellation of metabolic abnormalities characterized by obesity, insulin resistance, high triglyceride levels and low HDL levels, hypertension, cardiovascular disease, and increased risk for development of type 2 diabetes.

■ The most commonly identified symptoms of type 1 diabetes are polyuria, polydipsia, polyphagia, and weight loss despite normal or increased appetite. Although persons with type 2 diabetes may present with one or more of these symptoms, they are often asymptomatic initially. The diagnosis of diabetes mellitus is based on clinical signs of the disease, fasting blood glucose levels, random plasma glucose measurements, and results of the glucose tolerance test. Glycosylation involves the irreversible attachment of glucose to the hemoglobin molecule; the measurement of glycosylated hemoglobin (A1C) provides an index of blood glucose levels over several months. Self-monitoring of capillary blood glucose provides a means of maintaining near-normal blood glucose levels through adjustment of insulin dosage.

■ Dietary management of diabetes focuses on maintaining a well-balanced diet, controlling calories to achieve and maintain an optimum weight, and regulating the distribution of carbohydrates, proteins, and fats.

■ Pharmacologic agents used in the management of diabetes include injectable insulin, injectable non-insulin agents including amylin and GLP-1 analogs, and oral diabetic drugs. Type 1 diabetes (and sometimes type 2 diabetes) requires treatment with injectable insulin. Oral antidiabetic drugs include the insulin secretagogues, biguanides, α-glucosidase inhibitors, thiazolidinediones, and incretin-based therapies. These drugs require a functioning pancreas and may be used in the treatment of type 2 diabetes.

■ The metabolic disturbances associated with diabetes affect almost every body system. The acute complications of diabetes include diabetic ketoacidosis, hyperglycemic hyperosmolar state, and hypoglycemia in people with insulin-treated diabetes. The chronic complications of diabetes affect the microvascular system (including the retina, kidneys, and peripheral nervous system) and the macrovascular system (coronary, cerebrovascular, and peripheral arteries). The diabetic foot is usually a combination of both microvascular and macrovascular dysfunction. Infection is also a frequent occurrence and is more likely to be severe in the diabetic patient.

REVIEW EXERCISES

1. A 6-year-old boy is admitted to the emergency department with nausea, vomiting, and abdominal pain. He is very lethargic; his skin is warm, dry, and flushed; his pulse is rapid; and he has a sweet smell to his breath. His parents relate that he has been very thirsty during the past several weeks, his appetite has been poor, and he has been urinating frequently. His initial plasma glucose is 420 mg/dL (23.1 mmol/L), and a urine test for ketones is strongly positive.

   A. What is the most likely cause of this boy's elevated blood glucose and ketonuria?
   B. Explain his presenting signs and symptoms in terms of the elevated blood glucose and metabolic acidosis.
   C. What type of treatment will this boy require?

2. A 53-year-old accountant presents for his routine yearly examination. His history indicates that on two prior occasions he had a fasting plasma glucose of 120 mg/dL (6.7 mmol/L). Currently he is asymptomatic. He has no other medical problems and does not use any medications. He neither smokes nor drinks alcohol. His father was diagnosed with type 2 diabetes at age 60 years. His physical examination reveals a blood pressure of 125/80 mm Hg,

BMI of 32 kg/m², and waist circumference of 45 inches (114 cm). Complete blood count (CBC), thyroid-stimulating hormone (TSH), and alanine aminotransferase (ALT) are within normal limits. The lipid panel shows that his HDL cholesterol (30 mg/dL [0.8 mmol/L]) and LDL cholesterol (136 mg/dL [3.5 mmol/L]) are within the normal range, and triglycerides are elevated (290 mg/dL [2.3 mmol/L]; normal is <165 mg/dL [1.9 mmol/L]).

A. What is this man's probable diagnosis?

B. Based on this man's blood glucose level and the ADA diabetes classification system, what glucose intolerance status would you place this man in? Does he need a 75-g OGTT for further assessment of his IFG?

C. His OGTT test result reveals a 2-hour glucose value of 175 mg/dL (9.6 mmol/L). What is the diagnosis? What type of treatment would be appropriate for this man?

REFERENCES

1. American Diabetes Association. *Diabetes statistics*. 2013. Available at: http://www.diabetes.org/diabetes-basics/diabetes-statistics/. Accessed September 10, 2013.
2. Hall JE. *Guyton and Hall's Medical Physiology*. 12th ed. Philadelphia, PA: Elsevier Saunders; 2011:939–954.
3. Masharani U, German MS. Pancreatic hormones and diabetes mellitus. In: Gardner DG, Shoback D, eds. *Greenspan's Basic and Clinical Endocrinology*. 9th ed. New York, NY: Lange Medical Books/McGraw-Hill; 2007:573–656.
4. Shepard PR, Kahn B. Glucose transporters and insulin action. *N Engl J Med*. 1999;341:248–256.
5. DeFronzo RA, Eldor R, Abdul-Ghani M. Pathophysiologic approach to therapy in patients with newly diagnosed type 2 diabetes. *Diabetes Care*. 2013;36(Suppl 2):S127–S138.
6. Drucker DJ. The biology of incretin hormones. *Cell Metab*. 2006;3:153–165.
7. Goldfine IR, Youngren JF. Contributions of the American Journal of Physiology to the discovery of insulin. *Am J Physiol*. 1998;274:E207–E209.
8. Expert Committee on the Diagnosis and Classification of Diabetes Mellitus. Report of the Expert Committee on the Diagnosis and Classification of Diabetes Mellitus. *Diabetes Care*. 1997;10:1183–1197.
9. Expert Committee on the Diagnosis and Classification of Diabetes Mellitus. Follow-up report on the diagnosis of diabetes mellitus. *Diabetes Care*. 2003;26(11):3160–3167.
10. American Diabetes Association. Diagnosis and classification of diabetes mellitus. *Diabetes Care*. 2013;36(Suppl 1):S62–S69.
11. American Diabetes Association. Standards of medical care in diabetes—2013. *Diabetes Care*. 2013;36(Suppl 1):S11–S61.
12. Jones KL. Role of obesity in complicating and confusing the diagnosis and treatment of diabetes in children. *Pediatrics*. 2008;121(2):361–368.
13. The International Diabetes Federation Consensus Workshop. Type 2 diabetes in the young: The evolving epidemic. *Diabetes Care*. 2004;27:1798–1811.
14. Nolan CJ, Damm P, Prentki M. Type 2 diabetes across the generations: from pathophysiology to prevention and management. *Lancet*. 2011;378:169–181.
15. Gerich JE. Contributions of insulin-resistance and insulin-secretory defects to the pathogenesis of type 2 diabetes. *Mayo Clin Proc*. 2003;78:447–456.
16. DeFronzo RA. Banting lecture. From the triumvirate to ominous octet: a new paradigm for the treatment of type 2 diabetes mellitus. *Diabetes*. 2009;32:1327–1334.
17. Matthews DR, Cull CA, Stratton IM, et al. for the United Kingdom Prospective Diabetes Study (UKPDS) Group. UKPDS 26: Sulfonylurea failure in non-insulin-dependent diabetic patients over six years. *Diabetes Med*. 1998;15:297–303.
18. Kahn SE, Hull RL, Utzschneider KM. Mechanisms linking obesity to insulin resistance and type 2 diabetes. *Nature*. 2006;444:840–846.
19. Matfin G. Developing therapies for the metabolic syndrome: Challenges. opportunities, and the unknown. *Ther Adv Endocrinol Metabol*. 2010;4(2):89–94.
20. Grundy SM, Panel Chair. Third Report of the National Cholesterol Education Program (NCEP) Expert Panel on Detection, Evaluation, and Treatment of High Blood Cholesterol in Adults (Adult Treatment Panel III). NIH publication no. 01–3670. Bethesda, MD: National Institutes of Health; 2001.
21. Guven S, El-Bershawi A, Sonnenberg GE, et al. Persistent elevation in plasma leptin level in ex-obese with normal body mass index: relation to body composition and insulin sensitivity. *Diabetes*. 1999;48:347–352.
22. Bays H, Mandarino L, DeFronzo RA. Role of adipocyte, free fatty acid, and ectopic fat in pathogenesis of type 2 diabetes: peroxisomal proliferator-activated receptor agonists provide a rationale therapeutic approach. *J Clin Endocrinol Metab*. 2004;89:463–478.
23. Kadowaki T, Yamauchi T, Kubota N, et al. Adiponectin and adiponectin receptors in insulin resistance, diabetes, and the metabolic syndrome. *J Clin Invest*. 2006;116:1784–1792.
24. Gallagher EJ, LeRoith D, Karnieli E. The metabolic syndrome—From insulin resistance to obesity and diabetes. *Endocrinol Metab Clin North Am*. 2008;37:559–579.
25. Kuritzkes DR, Currier J. Cardiovascular risk factors and antiretroviral therapy. *N Engl J Med*. 2003;348:679–680.
26. Landon MB, Gabbe SG. Gestational diabetes mellitus. *Obstet Gynecol*. 2011;118:1379–1393.
27. Metzger BE, Buchanan TA, Coustan DR, et al. Summary and recommendations of the Fifth International Workshop—Conference on Gestational Diabetes. *Diabetes Care*. 2007;30(Suppl 2):S251–S260.
28. American Diabetes Association. Guidelines and recommendations for laboratory analysis in the diagnosis and management of diabetes mellitus. *Diabetes Care*. 2011;34:e61–e99.
29. Bantle JP, Wylie-Rosett J, Albright AL, et al. Nutritional recommendations and interventions for diabetes—2006: a position statement of the American Diabetes Association. *Diabetes Care*. 2006;29:2140–2157.
30. American Diabetes Association. Physical activity/exercise and diabetes mellitus. *Diabetes Care*. 2004;27(Suppl 1):S55–S59.
31. Inzucchi SE, Bergenstal RM, Buse JB, et al.; for the American Diabetes Association, European Association for the Study of Diabetes. Management of hyperglycemia in type 2 diabetes: a patient-centered approach: Position statement of the American Diabetes Association (ADA) and the European Association for the Study of Diabetes (EASD). *Diabetes Care*. 2012;35:1364–1379.
32. Fonseca V. Diabetes mellitus in the next decade: novel pipeline medications to treat hyperglycemia. *Clin Ther*. 2013;35:714–72333.
33. Erdmann E, Wilcox RG. Weighing up cardiovascular benefits of thiazolidinedione therapy: the impact of increased risk of heart failure. *Eur Heart J*. 2008;29:12–20.
34. Meier BM, Kraenzlin ME, Meier CR. Risk of fractures with glitazones: a critical review of evidence to date. *Drug Saf*. 2009;32(7):539–547.

35. Zangeneh F, Kudva YC, Basu A. Insulin sensitizers. *Mayo Clin Proc.* 2003;78:471–479.

36. Davidson JA. Advances in therapy of type 2 diabetes: GLP-1 receptor agonists and DPP-4 inhibitors. *Cleve Clin J Med.* 2009;75(Suppl 5):S28–S38.

37. Hirsch I. Insulin analogs. *N Eng J Med.* 2005;352:174–183.

38. American Diabetes Association. Continuous subcutaneous insulin infusion. *Diabetes Care.* 2004;27(Suppl 1):S110.

39. American Diabetes Association. Pancreas transplantation for patients with type 1 diabetes. *Diabetes Care.* 2004;27(Suppl 1):S105.

40. American Diabetes Association. Hyperglycemic crises in patients with diabetes mellitus. *Diabetes Care.* 2004;27(Suppl 1):S94–S102.

41. Wilson JF. In the clinic. Diabetes ketoacidosis. *Ann Intern Med.* 2010;152(1):ITC1-1–ITC1-16.

42. American Diabetes Association. Diabetic ketoacidosis in infants, children and adolescents. *Diabetes Care.* 2006;29:1150–1159.

43. Mukherjee E, Carroll R, Matfin G. Endocrine and metabolic emergencies: hypoglycaemia. *Ther Adv Endocrinol Metab.* 2011;2:81–93.

44. Seaquist ER, Anderson J, Childs B, et al. Hypoglycemia and diabetes: a report of a workgroup of the American Diabetes Association and Endocrine Society. *Diabetes Care.* 2013;36:1384–1395.

45. Somogyi M. Exacerbation of diabetes in excess insulin action. *Am J Med.* 1959;26:169–191.

46. Bolli GB, Gotterman IS, Campbell PJ. Glucose counterregulation and waning of insulin in the Somogyi phenomenon (posthypoglycemic hyperglycemia). *N Engl J Med.* 1984;311:1214–1219.

47. Bolli GB, Gerich JE. The dawn phenomenon: a common occurrence in both non-insulin and insulin dependent diabetes mellitus. *N Engl J Med.* 1984;310:746–750.

48. Sheetz MJ, King GL. Molecular understanding of hyperglycemia's adverse effects for diabetic complications. *JAMA.* 2002;288:2579–2588.

49. The Diabetes Control and Complications Trial Research Group. The effect of intensified treatment of diabetes on the development and progression of long-term complications in insulin-dependent diabetes mellitus. *N Engl J Med.* 1993;329:955–977.

50. Stratton IM, Adler AI, Neil HA, et al. Association of glycaemia with macrovascular and microvascular complications in type 2 diabetes (UKPDS 35): prospective observational study. *BMJ.* 2000;321:405–412.

51. Maitra A. The endocrine system. In: Kumar V, Abbas AK, Fausto N, et al. *Robbins and Cotran Pathologic Basis of Diseases.* 8th ed. Philadelphia, PA: Elsevier Saunders; 2010:1130–1146.

52. Boulton AJM, Vinik AI, Arezzo JC, et al. Diabetic neuropathies. *Diabetes Care.* 2005;28:956–962.

53. Tesfaye S, Boulton AJM, Dickenson AH. Painful diabetic somatic neuropathies. *Diabetes Care.* 2013;36:2456–2465.

54. AACE Male Sexual Dysfunction Taskforce. AACE medical guidelines for clinical practice for the evaluation and treatment of male sexual dysfunction: a couple's problem—2003 update. *Endocr Pract.* 2003;9:77–95.

55. Camilleri M. Diabetic gastroparesis. *N Engl J Med.* 2007;356:820–829.

56. Shakil A, Church RJ, Rao SS. Gastrointestinal complications of diabetes. *Am Fam Physician.* 2008;77(12):1703–1704.

57. Gross JL, DeAzevedo MJ, Silveiro SP, et al. Diabetic nephropathy: diagnosis, prevention, and management. *Diabetes Care.* 2005;28:76–188.

58. American Diabetes Association. Diabetic retinopathy. *Diabetes Care.* 2004;27(Suppl 1):S84–S87.

59. Mohamed Q, Gillies MC, Wong TY. Management of diabetic retinopathy: A systematic review. *JAMA.* 2007;298(8):902–916.

60. Wukich DK, Armstrong DG, Attinger CE, et al. Inpatient management of diabetic foot disorders: a clinical guide. *Diabetes Care.* 2013;36(9):2862–2871.

61. American Diabetes Association. Preventative foot care in people with diabetes. *Diabetes Care.* 2004;27(Suppl 1):S63–S64.

62. Joshi N, Caputo GM, Weitekamp MR, et al. Infections in patients with diabetes mellitus. *N Engl J Med.* 1999;341:1906–1912.

63. Gupta S, Koirala J, Khardori R, et al. Infections in diabetes mellitus and hyperglycemia. *Infect Dis Clin North Am.* 2007;21:617–638.

Porth Essentials Resources

Explore these additional resources to enhance learning for this chapter:

- NCLEX-Style Questions and Other Resources on thePoint, http://thePoint.lww.com/PorthEssentials4e
- Study Guide for Essentials of Pathophysiology
- Concepts in Action Animations
- Adaptive Learning | Powered by PrepU, http://thepoint.lww.com/prepu

C h a p t e r *34*

Organization and Control of Neural Function

The nervous system, in coordination with the endocrine system, provides the means by which cell and tissue functions are integrated into an independent, living organism. It controls skeletal muscle movement and helps to regulate cardiac and visceral smooth muscle activity; it enables the reception, integration, and perception of sensory information; it provides the substratum necessary for intelligence, anticipation, and judgment; and it facilitates adjustment to an ever-changing external environment.

Nervous Tissue Cells

Anatomically, the nervous system can be divided into two basic components: the central and peripheral nervous systems. The *central nervous system* (CNS) consists of the brain and spinal cord, which are protected by the skull and vertebral column. The *peripheral nervous system* (PNS) includes the neurons outside the CNS (cranial nerves and their ganglia, and spinal nerves and their ganglia), which connect the brain and spinal cord with peripheral structures. Inherent in the basic design of the nervous system is the provision for the concentration of computational and control functions in the CNS, with the PNS relaying somatic and visceral sensory (afferent) input to the CNS for processing and transmitting efferent or motor output from the CNS to effector organs throughout the body (Fig. 34-1).

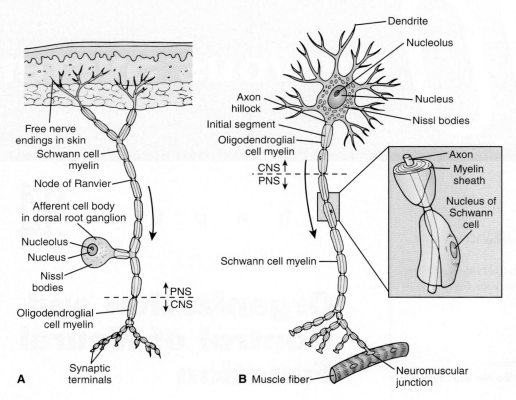

Free nerve endings in skin
Schwann cell myelin
Node of Ranvier
Afferent cell body in dorsal root ganglion
Nucleolus
Nucleus
Nissl bodies
Oligodendroglial cell myelin
↑PNS
↓CNS
Synaptic terminals
A

Dendrite
Nucleolus
Nucleus
Nissl bodies
Axon hillock
Initial segment
Oligodendroglial cell myelin
CNS↑
PNS↓
Schwann cell myelin
Axon
Myelin sheath
Nucleus of Schwann cell
B Muscle fiber
Neuromuscular junction

FIGURE 34-1. Afferent **(A)** and efferent neurons **(B)**, showing the soma or cell body, dendrites, and axon. *Arrows* indicate the direction for conduction of action potentials. CNS, central nervous system; PNS, peripheral nervous system.

Functionally, the nervous system is divided into two systems: the *somatic* and *autonomic* nervous systems. The somatic (Greek *soma,* "body") nervous system provides sensory and motor innervation for all parts of the CNS and PNS except viscera, smooth muscle, and glands. The autonomic nervous system (ANS) provides efferent innervation to smooth muscle in blood vessels and visceral structures, the conduction system of the heart, the sweat glands, and the exocrine glands of the gastrointestinal tract.

Nervous tissue consists of two principal types of cells—neurons and neuroglia or supporting cells. The neurons are the functional cells of the nervous system. They exhibit membrane excitability and conductivity and secrete neurotransmitters (signal-transmitting chemicals) and hormones, such as epinephrine and antidiuretic hormone (ADH). The neuroglial cells, such as the Schwann cells in the PNS and the oligodendrocytes in the CNS, protect the nervous system and provide metabolic support for the neurons.

Neurons

A typical neuron has three distinct parts: a cell body, dendrites, and an axon. The axonal and dendritic processes form the functional connections, or synapses, with other nerve cells, receptor cells, or effector cells. Afferent, or sensory, neurons of the PNS transmit information to the CNS (see Fig. 34-1A), whereas efferent, or motor, neurons carry information away from the CNS (see Fig. 34-1B). Interspersed between the afferent and

efferent neurons is a network of interconnecting neurons (also called *interneurons* or *internuncial* neurons) that modulate and control the body's response to changes in the internal and external environments.

The *cell body* of a neuron, also known as the *soma,* contains a large vesicular nucleus with one or more distinct nucleoli and a well-developed rough endoplasmic reticulum. A neuron's nucleus has the same deoxyribonucleic acid (DNA) and genetic information that is present in other cells of the body, and its nucleolus produces the ribonucleic acid (RNA) associated with protein synthesis. The cytoplasm contains large masses of ribosomes that are prominent in most neurons. These RNA masses, which are involved in protein synthesis, stain as dark Nissl bodies (see Fig. 34-1B). The Nissl bodies and free ribosomes extend into the dendrites, but not into the axon. The area of the cell body, called the *axon hillock,* is free of large cytoplasmic organelles and serves as a landmark to distinguish between axons and dendrites in microscopic preparations.

The *dendrites* (from the Greek *dendron,* "tree") are multiple, branched extensions of the nerve cell body; they conduct information toward the cell body and are the main source of information for the neuron. The dendrites and cell body are studded with synaptic terminals that communicate with axons and dendrites of other neurons (see Fig. 34-1A).

Axons are long efferent processes that project from the cell body and carry impulses away from the cell. Most neurons have only one axon; however, axons may exhibit multiple branching that results in many axonal terminals. The cytoplasm of the cell body extends to fill the dendrites and the axon. The proteins and other materials used by the axon are synthesized in the cell body and then flow down the axon through its cytoplasm.

The cell body of the neuron is equipped for a high level of metabolic activity. This is necessary because the cell body must synthesize the cytoplasmic and membrane constituents required to maintain the function of the axon and its terminals. Some of these axons extend for a distance of 1 to 1.5 m and have a volume that is 200 to 500 times greater than the cell body itself. Two axonal transport systems, one slow and one rapid, move molecules from the cell body through the cytoplasm of the axon to its terminals. Replacement proteins and nutrients slowly diffuse from the cell body, where they are transported down the axon, moving at the rate of approximately 1 mm/day. Other molecules, such as neurosecretory granules (e.g., neurotransmitters and neurohormones) or their precursors, are conveyed by a rapid, energy-dependent active transport system, moving at the rate of approximately 400 mm/day. For example, antidiuretic hormone (ADH) and oxytocin, which are synthesized by neurons in the hypothalamus, are carried by rapid axonal transport to the posterior pituitary, where the hormones are released into the bloodstream. A reverse (retrograde) axonal transport is responsible for moving molecules destined for degradation from the axon back to the cell body, where they are broken down.

Neuroglial Cells

The neuroglial, or supporting cells, which outnumber neurons 10 to 1, provide support and protection for neurons in both CNS and PNS. Although they do not participate directly in the short-term communication of information through the nervous system, the supporting cells segregate the neurons into isolated metabolic compartments, which are required for normal neural function.

The neuroglial cells in the PNS include the Schwann cells and satellite cells. The CNS has four types of glial cells: astrocytes, oligodendrocytes (oligodendroglia), microglia, and ependymal cells. Two of these cell types share a similar function: The Schwann cells of the PNS and the oligodendrocyte of the CNS wrap nerve axons in multiple layers, producing myelin sheaths that serve to increase the velocity of nerve impulse conduction in axons (see Fig. 34-1B, inset). Myelin has a high lipid content, which gives it a whitish color, and hence the name *white matter* is given to the masses of myelinated axons of the spinal cord and brain. Besides its role in increasing conduction velocity, the myelin sheath is essential for the survival of larger neuronal processes, perhaps by secreting neurotrophic compounds. In some pathologic conditions, such as multiple sclerosis in the CNS and Guillain-Barré syndrome involving the PNS, the myelin may degenerate or be destroyed, leaving a section of the axonal process without myelin while leaving the nearby Schwann or oligodendroglial cells intact. Unless remyelination takes place, the axon eventually dies.

Neuroglial Cells of the Peripheral Nervous System

The Schwann cells and satellite cells provide support and protection for the PNS. *Schwann cells* produce the myelin sheath that isolates nerve axons in the PNS from the surrounding extracellular compartment, ensuring rapid conduction of nerve impulses. They also aid in cleaning up PNS debris and guide the regrowth of PNS nerve fibers. During the process of myelination, the Schwann cell wraps around each nerve fiber several times in a "jelly roll" fashion (Fig. 34-2). Successive Schwann cells are separated by short extracellular fluid-filled gaps, called the *nodes of Ranvier*, where the myelin is missing and voltage-gated sodium channels are concentrated. The nodes of Ranvier increase the speed of nerve conduction by allowing the impulse to jump from node to node through the extracellular fluid in a process called *saltatory conduction*. In this way, the impulse can travel more rapidly than it could if it was required to move systematically along the entire nerve fiber. This increased conduction velocity greatly reduces reaction time, or time between the application of a stimulus and the subsequent motor response. The short reaction time is especially important in peripheral nerves with long distances for conduction between the CNS and distal effector organs.

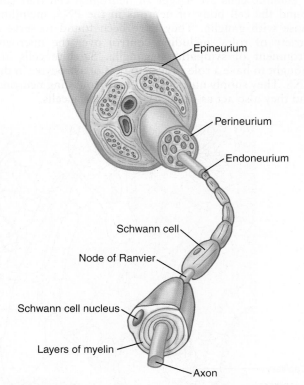

FIGURE 34-2. Section of a peripheral nerve containing both afferent (sensory) and efferent (motor) neurons. Schwann cells form a myelin sheath around the larger nerve fibers in the peripheral nervous system. Successive Schwann cells are separated by short extracellular fluid gaps called the *nodes of Ranvier*, where the myelin is missing and the voltage-gated sodium channels are concentrated.

Each of the Schwann cells along a peripheral nerve fiber is encased in a continuous tube of basement membrane, which in turn is surrounded by a multilayered sheath of loose connective tissue known as the *endoneurium* (see Fig. 34-2). The endoneurial sheath, which is essential to the regeneration of peripheral nerves, provides a collagenous tube through which a regenerating axon can again reach its former target. The endoneurial sheath does not penetrate the CNS. The absence of the endoneurial sheaths is thought to be a major factor in the limited axonal regeneration of CNS nerves compared with those of the PNS.

The endoneurial sheaths are bundled with blood vessels into small clusters of nerves called *fascicles*. In the nerve, fascicles consisting of bundles of nerve fibers are surrounded by another protective covering called the *perineurium*. Usually, several fascicles are further surrounded by the heavy, protective *epineurial sheath* of the peripheral nerve. The protective layers that surround the peripheral nerve processes are continuous with the connective tissue capsule of the sensory nerve endings and the connective tissue that surrounds the effector structures, such as the skeletal muscle cell. Centrally, the connective tissue layers continue along the dorsal and ventral roots of the nerve and fuse with the meninges that surround the spinal cord and brain.

Satellite cells are a type of neuroglial cell that surround the cell body of neurons in the PNS, including those with ganglia. They have been found to serve a variety of roles, including control over the microenvironment of sympathetic ganglia. Satellite cells are thought to have a role similar to that of astrocytes in the CNS. They supply nutrients to the surrounding neurons, and they also act as protective, cushioning cells.

Neuroglial Cells of the Central Nervous System

The neuroglial cells of the CNS consists of four types of cells: oligodendrocytes, astrocytes, microglia, and ependymal cells (Fig. 34-3). The *oligodendrocytes* form the myelin in the CNS. Instead of forming a myelin covering for a single axon, these cells reach out with several processes, each wrapping around and forming a multilayered myelin segment around several different axons. As within the PNS, the covering of axons in the CNS increases the velocity of nerve conduction.

Astrocytes are the largest and most numerous of neuroglia and are particularly prominent in the gray matter of the CNS. They form a network within the CNS and communicate with neurons to support and modulate their activities. Astrocytes have many processes, some stretching their processes from blood vessels to neurons and others filling most of the intercellular space within the CNS. It is now thought that astrocytes play an important role in the movement of metabolites and wastes to and from neurons and regulate ionic concentrations in the intercellular compartment. In addition, astrocytes take up neurotransmitters from synaptic zones after their release and thereby help regulate synaptic activity. They also have a role in maintaining the tight junctions of capillaries that form the blood-brain barrier. Astrocytes are also the principal cells responsible for repair and scar formation in the brain. They can fill their cytoplasm with microfibrils (i.e., fibrous astrocytes), and masses of these cells form the special type of scar tissue that develops in the CNS when tissue is destroyed, a process called *gliosis*.

A third type of neuroglia, the *microglia,* the microglial cells are the resident macrophages of the central nervous system. They are available for cleaning up debris after cellular damage, infection, or cell death. The fourth type

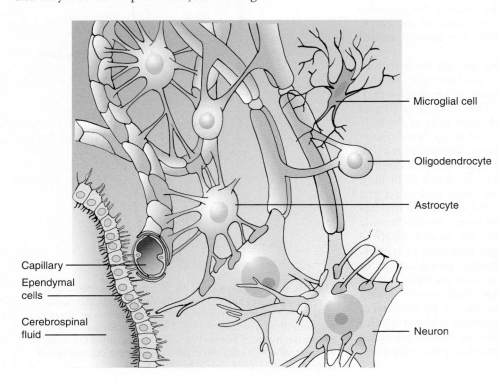

Microglial cell

Oligodendrocyte

Astrocyte

Capillary

Ependymal cells

Cerebrospinal fluid

Neuron

FIGURE 34-3. The supporting neuroglial cells of the central nervous system (CNS). Diagrammatic view of relationships between the glial elements (astrocyte, oligodendrocyte, microglial cell, and ependymal cells), capillaries, cerebrospinal fluid, and cell bodies of CNS neurons.

of cell, the *ependymal cell*, forms the lining of the neural tube cavity, the ventricular system. In some areas, these cells combine with a rich vascular network to form the *choroid plexus*, where production of the cerebrospinal fluid (CSF) takes place.

Metabolic Requirements of Nervous Tissue

Nervous tissue has a high rate of metabolism. Although the brain makes up only 2% of the body's weight, it receives approximately 15% of the resting cardiac output and consumes 20% of its oxygen. Despite its substantial metabolic requirements, the brain can neither store oxygen nor engage in anaerobic metabolism. An interruption in the blood or oxygen supply to the brain rapidly leads to clinically observable signs and symptoms. Without oxygen, brain cells continue to function for approximately 10 seconds. Unconsciousness occurs almost simultaneously with cardiac arrest, and the death of brain cells begins within 4 to 6 minutes. Interruption of blood flow also leads to the accumulation of metabolic by-products that are toxic to neural tissue.

Glucose is the major fuel source for the nervous system. Unlike muscle cells, neurons have no glycogen stores and must rely on glucose from the blood or the glycogen stores of supporting glial cells to meet their energy needs. Persons receiving insulin for diabetes may experience signs of neural dysfunction and unconsciousness (i.e., insulin reaction or shock) when blood glucose drops because of insulin excess (see Chapter 33).

SUMMARY CONCEPTS

■ Anatomically, the nervous system can be divided into two basic components: the *central nervous system* (CNS), consisting of the brain and spinal cord; and the *peripheral nervous system* (PNS), which relays *afferent* or sensory input to the CNS for processing and transmitting *efferent* or motor output from the CNS to effector organs throughout the body.

■ The nervous system contains two major types of cells: *neurons*, which are functioning cells of the nervous system, and neuroglial cells, which protect the nervous system and supply metabolic support.

■ Neurons (nerve cells), which are the functional components of the nervous system, are composed of three parts: a *cell body*, which controls cell activity; *dendrites*, which conduct information toward the cell body; and an *axon*, which carries impulses from the cell body.

■ The neuroglial cells that provide support and protection for the neurons consist of the Schwann and satellite cells of the PNS and the oligodendrocytes, astrocytes, microglial cells, and ependymal cells of the CNS. The Schwann cells of the PNS and the oligodendrocytes of the CNS form the myelin sheath that allows for rapid conduction of impulses.

■ The nervous system has a high level of metabolic activity, requiring a continuous supply of oxygen and glucose. Although the brain makes up only 2% of the body's weight, it receives approximately 15% of the resting cardiac output and consumes 20% of its oxygen.

Nerve Cell Communication

Neurons are characterized by their ability to communicate with other neurons and body cells through electrical impulses or action potentials, which are abrupt, pulsatile changes in the membrane potential that last a few ten thousandths to a few thousandths of a second. The frequency and pattern of action potentials constitute the code used by neurons to transfer information from one location to another.

Action Potentials

The cell membranes of excitable tissue, including those of nerve and muscle cells, contain ion channels that are responsible for generating action potentials (see Chapter 1, Understanding Membrane Potentials). These ion channels are guarded by voltage-dependent gates that open and close with changes in the membrane potential. Separate voltage-gated channels exist for the sodium, potassium, and calcium ions. Each type of ion channel has a characteristic membrane potential that opens and closes its channels. Also present are ligand-gated channels that respond to chemical messengers such as neurotransmitters, mechanically gated channels that respond to physical changes in the cell membrane, and light-gated channels that respond to fluctuations in light levels.

Action potentials can be divided into three phases: the resting or polarized state, depolarization, and repolarization (Fig. 34-4). The *resting membrane potential* (approximately –90 mV for large nerve fibers) is the undisturbed period of the action potential during which the nerve is not transmitting impulses. During this period, the membrane is said to be *"polarized"* because of the –90 mV negative membrane potential (i.e., positive on the outside and negative on the inside) that is present. The resting phase of the membrane potential continues until some event causes the membrane to increase its permeability to sodium. A *threshold potential*

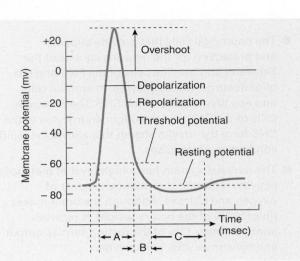

FIGURE 34-4. Time course of the action potential recorded at one point of an axon with one electrode inside and one outside the plasma membrane. The rising part of the action potential is called the *spike*. **(A)** The rising phase plus approximately the first half of the repolarization phase is the absolute refractory period. **(B)** The portion of the repolarization phase that extends from the threshold to the resting membrane potential represents the relative refractory period. **(C)** The remaining portion of the repolarization phase to the resting membrane potential is the negative afterpotential.

(approximately –60 mV in large nerve fibers) represents the membrane potential at which neurons or other excitable tissues are stimulated to fire. When the threshold potential is reached, the gatelike structures in the ion channels open. Below the threshold potential, these gates remain tightly closed. The gates function on an all-or-none basis, meaning they are either fully open or fully closed. Under ordinary circumstances, the threshold stimulus is sufficient to open many ion channels, triggering massive depolarization of the membrane (the action potential).

Depolarization is characterized by a rapid change in polarity of the resting membrane potential, which was negative on the inside and positive on the outside, to one that is positive on the inside and negative on the outside. During the depolarization phase, the membrane suddenly becomes permeable to sodium ions. The rapid inflow of sodium ions produces local electric currents that travel through the adjacent cell membrane, causing the sodium channels in this part of the membrane to open. In neurons, sodium ion gates remain open for approximately a quarter of a millisecond. During this phase of the action potential, the inner side of the membrane becomes positive (approximately +30 to +45 mV).

Repolarization is the phase during which the polarity of the resting membrane potential is reestablished. This is accomplished with closure of the sodium channels and opening of the potassium channels. The outflow of positively charged potassium ions across the cell membrane returns the resting membrane potential to negativity. The sodium/potassium–adenosine triphosphatase (Na^+/K^+-ATPase) pump gradually reestablishes the resting ionic concentrations on each side of the membrane. Membranes of excitable cells must be sufficiently repolarized before they can be re-excited. During repolarization, the membrane remains refractory (i.e., does not fire) until repolarization is approximately one-third complete. This period, which lasts approximately one half of a millisecond, is called the *absolute refractory period*. During one portion of the recovery period, the membrane can be excited, although only by a stronger-than-normal stimulus. This period is called the *relative refractory period*.

The excitability of neurons can be affected by conditions that alter the resting membrane potential, moving it either closer to or farther from the threshold potential. *Hypopolarization* increases the excitability of the postsynaptic neuron by bringing the membrane potential closer to the threshold potential so that a smaller subsequent stimulus is needed to cause the neuron to fire. *Hyperpolarization* brings the membrane potential further from the threshold and has the opposite, inhibitory effect, decreasing the likelihood that an action potential will be generated.

Synaptic Transmission

Neurons communicate with each other through structures known as *synapses*. There are two types of synapses in the nervous system: electrical and chemical. Electrical synapses permit the passage of current-carrying ions through small openings called *gap junctions* that penetrate the cell junction of adjoining cells. Although not important in synaptic transmission in the nervous system, gap junctions are important in cell-to-cell communication in smooth and cardiac muscle.

Chemical synapses, which are the more common type of synapse, involve special presynaptic and postsynaptic membrane structures, separated by a synaptic cleft. The presynaptic terminal secretes one and often several chemical transmitter molecules (e.g., neurotransmitters, neuromodulators). The secreted neurotransmitters diffuse into the synaptic cleft and bind to receptors on the postsynaptic membrane. In contrast to an electrical synapse, a chemical synapse permits only one-way communication. Chemical synapses are divided into two types: excitatory and inhibitory. In excitatory synapses, binding of the neurotransmitter to the receptor produces depolarization of the postsynaptic membrane; and in inhibitory synapses it reduces the postsynaptic neuron's ability to generate an action potential.

The process of neurotransmission involves the synthesis, storage, and release of a neurotransmitter; the reaction of the neurotransmitter with a receptor; and termination of the receptor action. Neurotransmitters are synthesized in the cytoplasm of the axon terminal. The synthesis of transmitters may require one or more enzyme-catalyzed steps (e.g., one for acetylcholine and three for norepinephrine). Each neuron generally produces only one type of neurotransmitter. After synthesis, the neurotransmitter molecules are stored in the axon terminal in tiny, membrane-bound sacs called *synaptic vesicles.*

These vesicles protect the neurotransmitters from enzyme destruction in the nerve terminal. There may be thousands of vesicles in a single terminal, each containing 10,000 to 100,000 transmitter molecules. Membrane depolarization due to arrival of an action potential causes the vesicles to move to the cell membrane and release their neurotransmitter molecules by fusion of the vesicular membrane with the outer cell membrane.

Once a neurotransmitter has exerted its effects on the postsynaptic membrane, its rapid removal is necessary to maintain precise control of neural transmission. A released transmitter can : (1) be broken down into inactive substances by enzymes, (2) be taken back up into the presynaptic neuron in a process called *reuptake*, or (3) diffuse away into the intercellular fluid until its concentration is too low to influence postsynaptic excitability. For example, acetylcholine is rapidly broken down by acetylcholinesterase into acetic acid and choline, with the choline being taken back into the presynaptic neuron for reuse in acetylcholine synthesis. The catecholamines are largely taken back into the neuron in an unchanged form for reuse. Catecholamines also can be degraded by enzymes, such as catechol-*O*-methyltransferase (COMT) in the synaptic space or monoamine oxidase (MAO) in the nerve terminals. Catechol-*O*-methyltransferase inhibitors and MAO inhibitors are used in the treatments of various conditions, such as Parkinson disease, major depression, and anxiety (see the Autonomic Neurotransmission section for detail).

Postsynaptic Potentials

A neuron's cell body and dendrites are covered by thousands of synapses, any or many of which can be active at any moment. Because of the interaction of this rich synaptic input, each neuron resembles a little computer, in which circuits of many neurons interact with one another. It is the complexity of these interactions and the subtle integrations involved in excitatory and inhibitory responses that give rise to the nervous system's intelligence.

Neurotransmitters exert their actions through specific proteins, called *receptors*, embedded in the postsynaptic membrane. These receptors are tailored precisely to match the size and shape of the transmitter. In each case, the interaction between a neurotransmitter and receptor causes the opening or closing of ion channels in the postsynaptic membrane, resulting in a transient, local change in the polarization of the postsynaptic membrane, called a *postsynaptic potential*. There are two types of postsynaptic potentials: excitatory and inhibitory. If opening of the ion channel results in a net gain of positive charge across the membrane, causing the potential to move close to zero, the membrane is said to be *depolarized*. This is called an *excitatory postsynaptic potential*, since it brings the resting potential closer to its firing threshold. If, on the other hand, opening of the ion channel results in a net gain of negative charge causing the potential to move further from zero, the membrane is said to be *hyperpolarized*. This is called an *inhibitory postsynaptic potential*, since it causes the resting membrane potential to move further from threshold.

Chemical Synaptic Transmission

The function of the nervous system relies on chemical substances that serve as synaptic messengers. These messengers include neurotransmitters, neuromodulators, and neurotrophic or nerve growth factors.

Neurotransmitters. Neurotransmitters are endogenous chemicals that facilitate the transmission of signals from one neuron to the next across synapses. There are many different ways to classify neurotransmitters, including by whether they produce excitatory or inhibitory effects on postsynaptic membranes and by their chemical structure.

A neurotransmitter is classified as *excitatory* if it activates a receptor; for example, glutamate, the most common excitatory neurotransmitter in the brain, increases the probability that the target cell will fire an action potential. A neurotransmitter is classified as *inhibitory* if it inhibits a receptor; gamma aminobutyric acid (GABA) is the brain's main inhibitory neurotransmitter. There are, however, other neurotransmitters for which both excitatory and inhibitory receptors exist; for example, acetylcholine is excitatory when it binds to a receptor at a myoneural junction, and it is inhibitory when it binds to a receptor at the sinoatrial node in the heart. Finally, some types of receptors activate complex metabolic pathways in the postsynaptic cell to produce effects that cannot appropriately be called either excitatory or inhibitory. Receptors are named according to the type of neurotransmitter with which they interact. For example, a *cholinergic receptor* is a receptor that binds acetylcholine.

In addition to function, neurotransmitters can be broadly categorized into three groups according to their chemical structure: (1) amino acids, (2) peptides, and (3) monoamines. Amino acids, such as glutamine, glycine, and GABA, serve as neurotransmitters at most CNS synapses. GABA mediates most synaptic inhibition in the CNS. Drugs such as the benzodiazepines (e.g., the tranquilizer diazepam) and the barbiturates exert their action by binding to their own distinct receptor on a GABA-operated ion channel. The drugs by themselves do not open the channel, but they change the effect that GABA has when it binds to the channel at the same time as the drug. *Peptides* are low–molecular-weight molecules that are made up of two or more amino acids. Neuropeptides are peptides used by neurons to communicate with each other. They include somatostatin, substance P, and opioid peptides such as endorphins and enkephalins, which are involved in pain sensation and perception (see Chapter 35). A *monoamine* is an amine molecule containing one amino group (–NH_2 group). All monoamines are derived from aromatic amino acids like phenylalanine, tyrosine, and tryptophan. Serotonin, dopamine, norepinephrine, and epinephrine are examples in this category.

Neuromodulators. Another class of messenger molecules, known as *neuromodulators*, also may be released from axon terminals. In contrast to neurotransmitters, neuromodulators do not directly activate ion-channel

(*text continues on page 829*)

UNDERSTANDING ➔ Synaptic Transmission

Neurons communicate with each other through chemical synapses and the use of neurotransmitters. Chemical synapses consist of a presynaptic neuron, a synaptic cleft, and a postsynaptic neuron. The communication process relies on (1) synthesis and release of the neurotransmitter from a presynaptic neuron, (2) binding of the neurotransmitter to receptors in the postsynaptic neuron, and (3) removal of the neurotransmitter from the receptor site.

1

Neurotransmitter Synthesis and Release. Neurotransmitters are synthesized in the presynaptic neuron, then stored in synaptic vesicles. Communication between the two neurons begins with a nerve impulse that stimulates the presynaptic neuron, followed by movement of the synaptic vesicles to the cell membrane and release of neurotransmitter into the synaptic cleft.

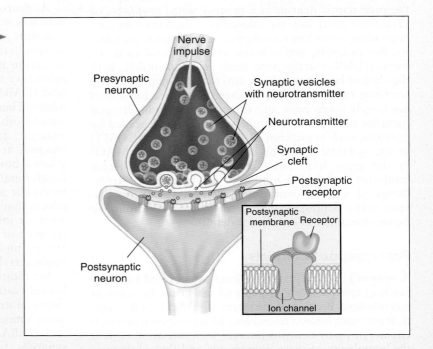

2

Receptor Binding. Once released from the presynaptic neuron, the neurotransmitter moves across the synaptic cleft and binds to receptors on the postsynaptic neuron. The action of a neurotransmitter is determined by the type of receptor (excitatory or inhibitory) to which it binds. Binding of a neurotransmitter to a receptor with an excitatory function often results in the opening of an ion channel, such as the sodium channel. Many presynaptic neurons also have receptors to which a neurotransmitter binds. The presynaptic receptors function in a negative feedback manner to inhibit further release of the neurotransmitter.

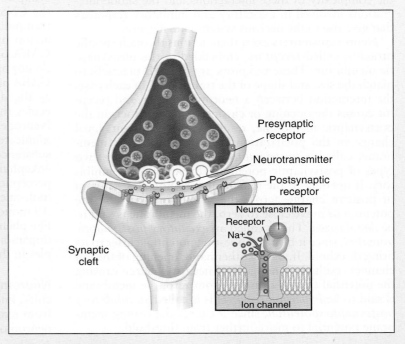

3

Neurotransmitter Removal.

Precise control of synaptic function relies on the rapid removal of the neurotransmitter from the receptor site. A released neurotransmitter can (1) be taken back up into the neuron through reuptake, (2) diffuse out of the synaptic cleft, or (3) be broken down by enzymes into inactive substances or metabolites. The action of norepinephrine is largely terminated by the reuptake process, in which the neurotransmitter is taken back into the neuron in an unchanged form and reused. It can also be broken down by enzymes in the synaptic cleft or in the nerve terminals. The neurotransmitter acetylcholine is rapidly broken down by the enzyme acetylcholinesterase.

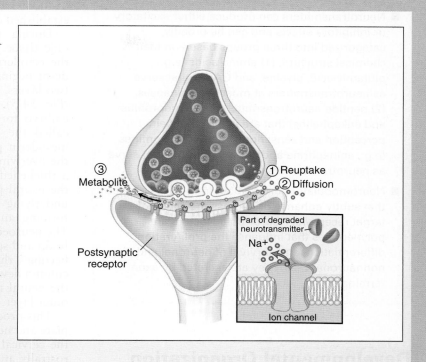

(text continued from page 827)

receptors, but bring about long-term changes that subtly enhance or depress the action of the receptors. Neuromodulators, such as dopamine, serotonin, acetylcholine, histamine, and others, may act at either presynaptic or postsynaptic sites. They may act on postsynaptic receptors to produce slower and longer-lasting changes in membrane excitability, by enhancing or decreasing the action of faster-acting neurotransmitter molecules. By combining with autoreceptors on its own presynaptic membrane, a transmitter can act as a neuromodulator by augmenting or inhibiting further nerve activity. In some nerves, such as the peripheral sympathetic nerves, a messenger molecule can have both transmitter and modulator functions. For example, norepinephrine can activate an α_1-adrenergic postsynaptic receptor to produce vasoconstriction or stimulate an α_2-adrenergic presynaptic receptor to inhibit further norepinephrine release.

Neurotrophic Factors. Neurotrophic factors, also known as *neurotrophins*, are a family of polypeptide growth factors that influence the proliferation, differentiation, and survival of neuronal and nonneuronal cells. Neurotrophins are secreted by axon terminals independent of action potentials. Examples include neuron-to-neuron trophic factors in the sequential synapses of CNS sensory neurons. Trophic factors from target cells that enter the axon and are necessary for the long-term survival of presynaptic neurons also have been demonstrated. Alterations in neurotrophin levels have been implicated in neurodegenerative disorders such as Alzheimer disease

and Huntington disease, as well as psychiatric disorders such as depression and substance abuse.

SUMMARY CONCEPTS

■ Neurons communicate with other neurons and body cells through electrical signals in their membrane called *action potentials*. Action potentials are divided into three parts: (1) the *resting membrane potential*, during which the membrane is polarized (positively charged on the outside of the membrane and negatively charged on the inside); (2) the *depolarization phase*, during which sodium channels open, allowing rapid inflow of the charged sodium ions that generate the electrical impulse; and (3) the *repolarization phase*, during which the outflow of potassium ions returns the membrane to its resting potential.

■ Neurotransmission or communication relies on chemical messengers or *neurotransmitters*, released from the presynaptic neuron, that cross the synaptic cleft and then interact with receptors on the postsynaptic neuron.

(continued)

Developmental Organization of the Nervous System

The organization of the nervous system can be understood in terms of its embryonic development, in which newer functions and greater complexity result from the modification and enlargement of earlier developed structures. Thus, the rostral or front end of the CNS, which is the last to develop, is more specialized in its functions than the caudal or tail end structures, namely the brain stem and spinal cord, which are the first to develop. The dominance of the rostral end of the CNS is reflected in what has been termed a hierarchy of control, with the forebrain having control over the brain stem and the brain stem having control over the spinal cord. In the developmental process, newer functions were added to the surface of earlier developed systems. As newer functions were added to the surface of earlier developed systems and became concentrated at the rostral end of the CNS, they also became more vulnerable to injury. Nothing exemplifies this principle better than the persistent vegetative state (discussed in Chapter 37) that occurs when severe brain injury causes irreversible damage to higher cortical centers, while lower brain stem centers such as those that control breathing remain functional.

Embryonic Development

The nervous system appears very early in embryonic development (22 to 23 days). This early development is essential because it influences the development and organization of many other body systems, including the axial skeleton, skeletal muscles, and sensory organs such as the eyes and ears. Throughout life, the organization of the nervous system retains many patterns that were established during embryonic life.

During the 2nd week of development, embryonic tissue consists of two layers, the endoderm and the ectoderm. At the beginning of week 3, the ectoderm begins to invaginate and migrates between the two layers, forming a third layer called the *mesoderm* (Fig. 34-5). Mesoderm along the entire midline of the embryo forms a specialized rod of embryonic tissue called the *notochord*. The notochord and adjacent mesoderm provide the necessary induction signal for the overlying neuroectoderm to differentiate and form a thickened structure called the *neural plate*. Within the neural plate a groove develops and sinks into the underlying mesoderm. Its walls fuse across the top, forming an ectodermal tube called the *neural tube*. The neuroectoderm of the neural plate gives rise to the brain and spinal cord of the CNS, while the notochord becomes the foundation around which the vertebral column develops. The surface ectoderm separates from the neural tube and fuses over the top to become the outer layer of skin.

This process involved in the formation of the neural plate and neural folds and closure of the folds begins at the cervical and high thoracic levels and zippers both rostrally and caudally. Complete closure occurs at the rostral-most end of the brain around day 25 and at about day 27 in the lumbosacral region. Most congenital defects, such as spina bifida, result from failure of fusion of one or more neural arches of the developing vertebral column during the fourth week of embryonic development.

As the neural tube closes, ectodermal cells called *neural crest cells* migrate away from the dorsal surface of the neural tube to become the progenitors or parent cells of the neurons and neuroglial cells of the PNS. Some of these cells gather into clusters to form the *dorsal root ganglia* at the sides of each spinal cord segment and the *cranial ganglia* that are present in most brain segments. Neurons of these ganglia become the afferent or sensory neurons of the PNS. Other neural crest cells become the pigment cells of the skin or contribute to the formation of many structures of the face, certain cells of the autonomic nervous system, and other structures.

During development, the more rostral (toward the head) portions of the embryonic neural tube—approximately 10 segments—undergo extensive modification and enlargement to form the brain (Fig. 34-6). In the early embryo, 3 swellings, or primary vesicles, develop, subdividing these 10 segments into the forebrain, containing the first 2 segments; the midbrain, which develops from segment 3; and the hindbrain, which develops from segments 4 to 10. In the prosencephalon or forebrain, two pairs of lateral outpouchings develop: the optic cup, which becomes the optic nerve and retina, and the telencephalic vesicles, which become the cerebral hemispheres. Within the prosencephalon, the hollow central canal expands to become enlarged

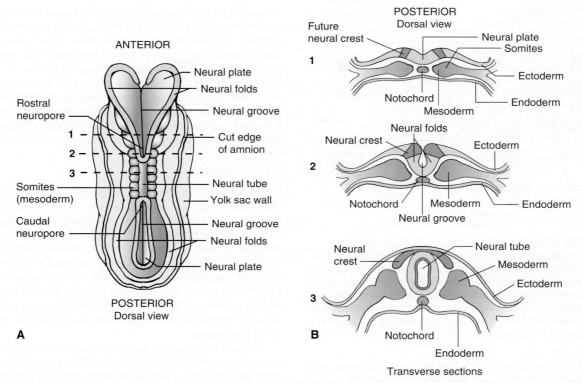

FIGURE 34-5. Folding of the neural tube. **(A)** Dorsal view of a six-somite embryo (22 to 23 days) showing the neural folds, neural groove, and fused neural tube. The anterior neuropore closes at about day 25 and the posterior neuropore at about day 27. **(B)** Three cross-sections taken at the levels indicated in A. The sections indicate where the neural tube is just beginning to form.

CSF-filled cavities, the first and second (lateral) ventricles. The remaining diencephalic portion of the neural tube develops into the thalamus and hypothalamus. The neurohypophysis (posterior pituitary) grows as a midline ventral outgrowth at the junctions of segments 1 and 2. A dorsal outgrowth, the pineal body, develops between segments 2 and 3.

Segmental Organization

Developmentally, the basic organizational pattern of the nervous system is that of a longitudinal series of segments, each repeating the same fundamental pattern that is retained in postnatal life. The CNS and its associated peripheral nerves consist of approximately 43 segments,

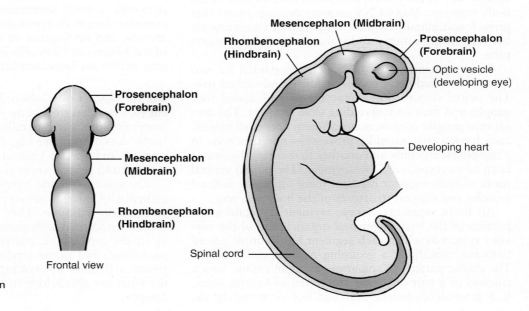

FIGURE 34-6. Frontal and lateral views of a 5-week-old embryo showing the brain vesicles and three embryonic divisions of the brain and brain stem.

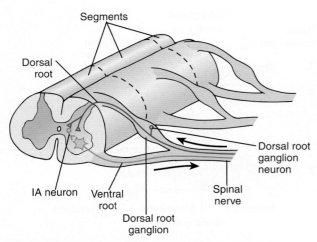

FIGURE 34-7. Three segments of the spinal cord showing dorsal roots entering the dorsal lateral surface of the cord and ventral roots exiting the ventral surface of the cord. The dorsal root ganglion contains dorsal root ganglion cells, whose axons bifurcate: one process enters the spinal cord in the dorsal root, and the other extends peripherally to supply the skin and muscle of the body. The ventral root is formed by axons from motor neurons in the spinal cord. IA, input association.

33 of which form the spinal cord and spinal nerves, and 10 of which form the brain and its cranial nerves.

The basic pattern of the CNS is that seen in the spinal cord—a central cavity surrounded by an inner core of gray matter and a superficial layer of white matter (Fig. 34-7). The brain retains this organization, but it also contains additional regions of gray matter that are not evident in the spinal cord. The gray matter is functionally divided into longitudinal columns of nerve cell bodies called the *cell columns*. The superficial white matter region contains the longitudinal tract systems of the CNS. The dorsal half or dorsal horn of the gray matter contains afferent neurons. The ventral portion, or *ventral horn*, contains efferent neurons that communicate by way of the ventral roots with effector cells of the body segment. Many CNS neurons develop axons that grow longitudinally as tract systems that communicate between neighboring and distal segments of the neural tube.

Each segment of the CNS is accompanied by two pairs of bundled nerve roots—a dorsal and ventral pair. The paired dorsal roots connect a pair of dorsal root ganglia and their corresponding CNS segment. The dorsal root ganglia contain many afferent nerve cell bodies, each having two axonlike processes—one that ends in a peripheral receptor and another that enters the dorsal horn of its respective CNS segment. The paired ventral roots of each segment contain fibers supplying skeletal muscles and visceral structures of the body segment.

All brain segments, except segment 2, retain some portion of the basic segmental organization of the nervous system in which each segment has multiple paired branches containing a grouping of component axons. The classic pattern of spinal nerve organization, which consists of a pair of dorsal and a pair of ventral roots, is a later development that has not occurred in the

cranial nerves. Consequently, the cranial nerves, which are arbitrarily numbered 1 through 12, retain the early pattern of development, with more than one cranial nerve branching from a single segment. The truly segmental nerve pattern of the cranial nerves is altered because all branches from segment 2 and most of the branches from segment 1 are missing. Cranial nerve 2, also called the *optic nerve*, is not a segmental nerve, but a brain tract connecting the retina (modified brain) with the first forebrain segment from which it developed.

Cell Columns

Anatomically, the body is organized into soma (e.g., skin, muscles, and skeletal structures of the body wall) and viscera (internal organs). The organizational structure of the nervous system can be best explained and simplified as a pattern in which functionally specific PNS and CNS afferent and efferent somatic and visceral neurons are repeated as parallel cell columns running lengthwise along the nervous system. In this organizational pattern, afferent neurons, dorsal horn cells, and ventral horn cells are organized as a bilateral series of 11 cell columns.

The cell columns on each side can be further grouped according to their location in the PNS: four in the dorsal root ganglia that contain sensory neurons, four in the dorsal horn that contain sensory *input association* (IA) interneurons, and three in the ventral horn that contain motor neurons (Fig. 34-8). The processes of sensory neurons that enter the dorsal horn communicate with IA neurons, which then distributes the afferent information to local reflex circuitry and to more rostral segments of the CNS. The ventral horns contain *output association* (OA) interneurons and lower motor neurons, which project to the effector muscles. The afferent and efferent cell columns of the PNS and CNS, their projections, and the type of information they transmit are summarized in Table 34-1.

Between the IA neurons and the OA neurons are networks of small interconnecting neurons arranged in complex circuits that provide the discreteness, appropriateness, and intelligence of responses to stimuli. Most of the billions of CNS cells in the spinal cord and brain gray matter are interconnecting neurons.

Dorsal Horn Cell Columns. Four columns of afferent (sensory) neurons in the dorsal root ganglia directly innervate four corresponding columns of IA neurons in the dorsal horn (see Fig. 34-8). These are the special somatic and special visceral afferents and the general somatic and general visceral afferents.

The special somatic afferent (SSA) neurons are concerned with internal sensory information such as joint and tendon sensation. They relay information to local reflexes concerned with posture and movement, as well as to the cerebellum, contributing to coordination of movement, and to the forebrain, contributing to experience. Afferents innervating the vestibular system of the inner ear also belong to the special somatic afferent category.

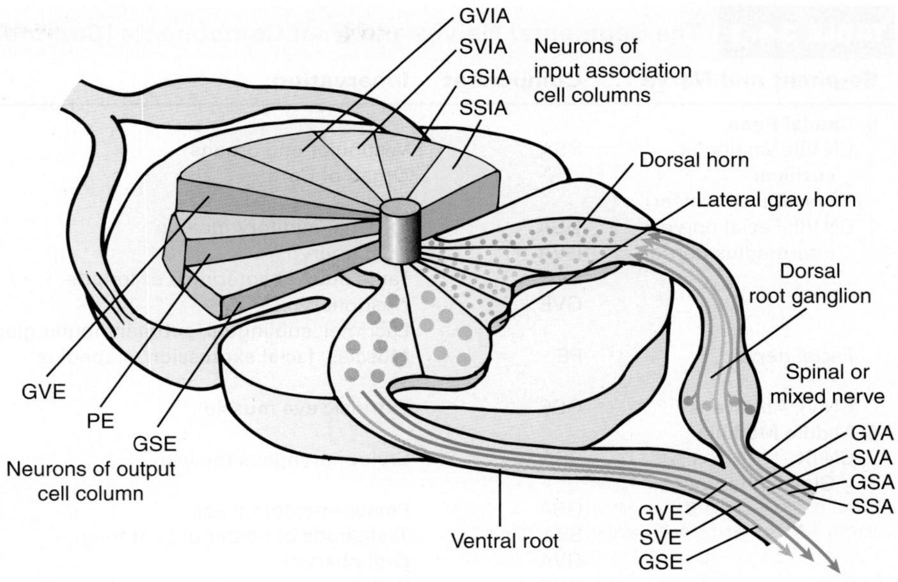

FIGURE 34-8. (A) Cell columns of the central nervous system. The cell columns in the dorsal horn contain input association (IA) neurons for the general visceral afferent (GVA), special visceral afferent (SVA), special sensory afferent (SSA), and general somatic afferent (GSA) neurons with cell bodies in the dorsal root ganglion. The cell columns in the ventral horn contain the general visceral efferent (GVE), pharyngeal efferent (PE), and general somite efferent (GSE) neurons and their output association (OA) neurons.

Special visceral afferent (SVA) neurons innervate specialized gut-related visceral receptors, such as the taste buds and receptors of the olfactory mucosa. They communicate with neurons involved in salivation, chewing, swallowing, and sensations of taste (i.e., gustation) and smell (i.e., olfaction).

General somatic afferent (GSA) neurons innervate the skin and other somatic structures, responding to stimuli such as those that produce pressure or pain. *General visceral afferent* (GVA) fibers innervate visceral structures such as the gastrointestinal tract, urinary bladder, and heart and great vessels; they communicate with neurons that send information to the forebrain regarding visceral sensations such as stomach fullness and bladder pressure.

Ventral Horn Cell Columns. The ventral horn contains three longitudinal cell columns: the general visceral efferent, general somatic efferent, and pharyngeal efferent (see Fig. 34-8). The efferent neurons for the ventral horn cell columns originate in brain centers (motor cortex and ANS centers) that control skeletal muscle and visceral function.

TABLE 34-1	The Segmental Nerves and Their Components			
Segment and Nerve	**Component**	**Innervation**		**Function**
1. Forebrain				
CN I: Olfactory	SVA	Receptors in olfactory mucosa		Reflexes, olfaction (smell)
2. CN II: Optic		Optic nerve and retina (part of brain system, not a peripheral nerve)		
3. Midbrain				
CN V: Trigeminal (V$_1$) ophthalmic division	SSA	Muscles of the upper face: forehead, upper lid		Facial expression, proprioception
	GSA	Skin, subcutaneous tissue; conjunctiva; frontal/ethmoid sinuses		Somesthesia Reflexes (blink)
CN III: Oculomotor	GVE	Iris sphincter Ciliary muscle		Pupillary constriction Accommodation
	GSE	Extrinsic eye muscles		Eye movement, lid movement
4. Pons				
CN V: Trigeminal (V$_2$) maxillary division	SSA	Muscles: facial expression		Proprioception Reflexes (sneeze), somesthesia
	GSA	Skin, oral mucosa, upper teeth, hard palate, maxillary sinus		
CN V: Trigeminal (V$_3$) mandibular division	SSA	Lower jaw, muscles: mastication		Proprioception, jaw jerk
	GSA	Skin, mucosa, teeth, anterior ⅔ of tongue		Reflexes, somesthesia
	PE	Muscles: mastication tensor tympani tensor veli palatini		Mastication: speech Protects ear from loud sounds Tenses soft palate
CN IV: Trochlear	GSE	Extrinsic eye muscle		Moves eye down and in

(Continued)

TABLE 34-1	The Segmental Nerves and Their Components (*Continued*)		
Segment and Nerve	**Component**	**Innervation**	**Function**
5. Caudal Pons			
CN VIII: Vestibular cochlear (vestibulocochlear)	SSA	Vestibular end organs	Reflexes, sense of head position
		Organ of Corti	Reflexes, hearing
CN VII: Facial nerve intermedius portion	GSA	External auditory meatus	Somesthesia
	GVA	Nasopharynx	Gag reflex: sensation
	SVA	Taste buds of anterior ⅔ of tongue	Reflexes: gustation (taste)
	GVE	Nasopharynx	Mucus secretion, reflexes
		Lacrimal, sublingual, submandibular glands	Lacrimation, salivation
Facial nerve	PE	Muscles: facial expression, stapedius	Facial expression
			Protects ear from loud sounds
CN VI: Abducens	GSE	Extrinsic eye muscle	Lateral eye deviation
6. Middle Medulla			
CN IX: Glossopharyngeal	SSA	Stylopharyngeus muscle	Proprioception
	GSA	Posterior external ear	Somesthesia
	SVA	Taste buds of posterior ⅓ of tongue	Gustation (taste)
	GVA	Oral pharynx	Gag reflex: sensation
	GVE	Parotid gland; pharyngeal mucosa	Salivary reflex: mucus secretion
	PE	Stylopharyngeus muscle	Assists swallowing
7, 8, 9, 10. Caudal Medulla			
CN X: Vagus	SSA	Muscles: pharynx, larynx	Proprioception
	GSA	Posterior external ear	Somesthesia
	SVA	Taste buds, pharynx, larynx	Reflexes, gustation
	GVA	Visceral organs (esophagus to midtransverse colon, liver, pancreas, heart, lungs)	Reflexes, sensation
	GVE	Visceral organs as above	Parasympathetic efferent
	PE	Muscles: pharynx, larynx	Swallowing, phonation, emesis
CN XII: Hypoglossal	GSE	Muscles of tongue	Tongue movement, reflexes
Spinal Segments			
C1–C4 Upper Cervical CN XI: accessory nerve	PE	Muscles: sternocleidomastoid, trapezius	Head, shoulder movement
Spinal nerves	SSA	Muscles of neck	Proprioception, DTRs
	GSA	Neck, back of head	Somesthesia
	GSE	Neck muscles	Head, shoulder movement
C5–C8 Lower Cervical	SSA	Upper limb muscles	Proprioception, DTRs
	GSA	Upper limbs	Reflexes, somesthesia
	GSE	Upper limb muscles	Movement, posture
T1–L2 Thoracic, Upper Lumbar	SSA	Muscles: trunk, abdominal wall	Proprioception
	GSA	Trunk, abdominal wall	Reflexes, somesthesia
	GVA	All of viscera	Reflexes and sensation
	GVE	All of viscera	Sympathetic reflexes, vasomotor control, sweating, piloerection
	GSE	Muscles: trunk, abdominal wall, back	Movement, posture, respiration
L2–S1 Lower Lumbar, Upper Sacral	SSA	Lower limb muscles	Proprioception, DTRs
	GSA	Lower trunk, limbs, back	Reflexes, somesthesia
	GSE	Muscles: trunk, lower limbs, back	Movement, posture
S2–S4 Lower Sacral	SSA	Muscles: pelvis, perineum	Proprioception
	GSA	Pelvis, genitalia	Reflexes, somesthesia
	GVA	Hindgut, bladder, uterus	Reflexes, sensation
	GVE	Hindgut, visceral organs	Visceral reflexes, defecation, urination, erection
S5–Co2 Lower Sacral, Coccygeal	SSA	Perineal muscles	Proprioception
	GSA	Lower sacrum, anus	Reflexes, somesthesia
	GSE	Perineal muscles	Reflexes, posture

Afferent (sensory) components: SSA, special somatic afferent; GSA, general somatic afferent; SVA, special visceral afferent; GVA, general visceral afferent.

Efferent (motor) components: GVE, general visceral efferent (autonomic nervous system); PE, pharyngeal efferent; GSE, general somatic efferent; DTRs, deep tendon reflexes.

The *general visceral efferent* (GVE) neurons are structurally and functionally divided between either the sympathetic or the parasympathetic nervous systems of the ANS (discussed later in this chapter). Their axons project through the segmental ventral roots to innervate smooth and cardiac muscle and glandular cells of the body, most of which are in the viscera.

The *general somatic efferent* (GSE) neurons supply skeletal muscles of the body and head, including those of the trunk, limbs, and tongue and the extrinsic eye muscles. Because they transmit the commands of the CNS to peripheral effectors, the skeletal muscles, they are considered the "final common pathway neurons" in the sequence leading to motor activity. They are often called *lower motor neurons* (LMNs) because they are under the control of *upper motor neurons* (UMNs) that have their origin in the CNS.

The *pharyngeal efferent* (PE) neurons innervate the muscles of mastication and facial expression, as well as the muscles of the pharynx and larynx. Pharyngeal efferent neurons also innervate the muscles responsible for moving the head.

Longitudinal Tracts

The gray matter of the cell columns in the CNS is surrounded by bundles of myelinated axons (i.e., white matter) and unmyelinated axons that travel longitudinally along the length of the neural axis. This white matter can be divided into three layers: inner, middle, and outer (Fig. 34-9). The inner layer contains short fibers that project for a maximum of approximately five segments before reentering the gray matter. The fibers of the middle layer project to six or more segments. The outer layer contains large-diameter axons that can travel the entire length of the nervous system (Table 34-2). *Suprasegmental* is a term that refers to higher levels of the CNS, such as the brain stem and cerebrum and structures above a given CNS segment. The middle and outer layer fibers have suprasegmental projections.

The longitudinal layers are arranged in bundles, or fiber tracts, that contain axons that have the same destination, origin, or function (Fig. 34-10). These longitudinal tracts are named systematically to reflect their origin and destination; the origin is named first, and the destination is named second. For example, the *spinothalamic tract* originates in the spinal cord and terminates in the

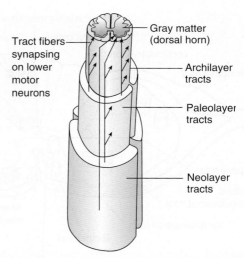

FIGURE 34-9. The three concentric subdivisions of the tract systems of the white matter of the spinal cord. Migration of neurons into the archilayer converts it into the reticular formation of the white matter.

thalamus and the *corticospinal tract* originates in the cerebral cortex and ends in the spinal cord.

The Inner Layer. The inner or archi layer of white matter contains the axons of neurons that connect neighboring segments of the nervous system. Axons of this layer permit the pool of motor neurons of several segments to work together as a functional unit. They also allow the afferent neurons of one segment to trigger reflexes that activate motor units in the same or a neighboring segment. The inner layer is the first of the longitudinal layers to become functional, and is the most primitive. Its circuitry may be limited to reflex movements, such as those of the fetus (i.e., quickening) that begin during the fifth month of intrauterine life.

The inner layer of the white matter differs from the other two layers in one important aspect. Many neurons in the embryonic gray matter migrate out into this layer, resulting in a rich mixture of neurons and local fibers called the *reticular formation*. The circuitry of most reflexes is contained in the reticular formation. In the brain stem, the reticular formation becomes quite large and acts in vital reflexes controlling respiration, cardiovascular function, swallowing, and vomiting. A functional system called the *reticular activating system* (RAS)

TABLE 34-2	Characteristics of the Concentric Subdivisions of the Longitudinal Tracts in the White Matter of the Central Nervous System		
Characteristics	**Archilayer Tracts**	**Paleolayer Tracts**	**Neolayer Tracts**
Segmental span	Intersegmental (<5 segments)	Suprasegmental (≥5 segments)	Suprasegmental
Number of synapses	Multisynaptic	Multisynaptic but fewer than archilayer tracts	Monosynaptic with target structures
Conduction velocity	Very slow	Fast	Fastest
Examples of functional systems	Flexor withdrawal reflex circuitry	Spinothalamic tracts	Corticospinal tracts

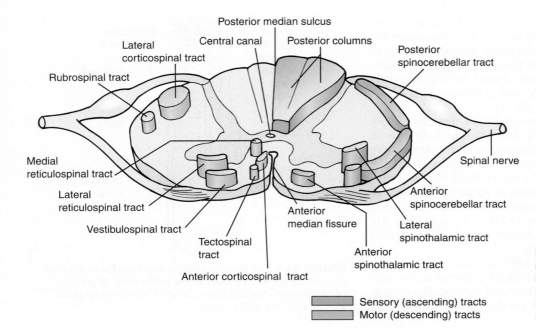

Posterior median sulcus

Central canal Posterior columns

Lateral
corticospinal tract

Rubrospinal tract

Posterior
spinocerebellar tract

Medial
reticulospinal tract

Spinal nerve

Lateral
reticulospinal tract

Anterior
spinocerebellar tract

Vestibulospinal tract

Anterior
median fissure

Lateral
spinothalamic tract

Tectospinal
tract

Anterior
spinothalamic tract

Anterior corticospinal tract

Sensory (ascending) tracts
Motor (descending) tracts

FIGURE 34-10. Transverse section of the spinal cord showing selected sensory and motor tracts. The tracts are bilateral but are indicated only on one half of the cord.

operates in the lateral portions of the reticular formation of the medulla, pons, and especially the midbrain.

The RAS has descending and ascending portions. The descending portion communicates with and serves to facilitate many cord-level reflexes. For example, it speeds reaction time and stabilizes postural reflexes. The ascending portion accelerates brain activity, particularly thalamic and cortical activity.

The Middle Layer. The middle or paleolayer layer of the white matter contains most of the major fiber tract systems required for sensation and movement. It contains the ascending spinoreticular and spinothalamic tracts. This layer consists of larger-diameter and longer suprasegmental fibers, which ascend to the brain stem and are largely functional at birth. It facilitates many primitive functions, such as the auditory startle reflex, which occurs in response to loud noises. This reflex consists of turning the head and body toward the sound, dilating the pupils of the eyes, catching of the breath, and quickening of the pulse.

The Outer Layer. The outer or neolayer layer of the tract systems develops after the other two layers. This pathway, which becomes functional at about 2 years of age, contains the pathways needed for bladder training. Myelination of these suprasegmental tracts, which include many pathways required for delicate and highly coordinated skills, is not complete until approximately the fifth year of life. This includes the development of tracts needed for fine manipulative skills, such as the finger–thumb coordination required for using tools and the toe movements needed for acrobatics. Being the last to be most developed and more superficial, the neolayer tracts are the most vulnerable to injury.

Collateral Communication Pathways. Axons in the inner and middle layer tracts characteristically possess many collateral branches that move into the gray cell columns or synapse with fibers of the reticular formation as the axon passes each succeeding CNS segment. Should a major axon be destroyed at some point along its course, these collaterals provide multisynaptic alternative pathways that bypass the local damage. Damage usually is followed by slow return of function, presumably through the collateral connections.

The outer layer tracts do not possess these collaterals but instead project mainly to the target neurons with which they communicate. When tracts in this layer are damaged, tracts in the middle and inner layers often remain functional, and rehabilitation methods can result in effective use of the older systems. Delicacy and refinement of motor movement may be lost, but basic function remains. For example, when the corticospinal system, an important outer layer system that permits the fine manipulative control required for writing, is damaged, the remaining middle systems, if intact, permit the grasping and holding of objects. The hand can still be used to perform its basic function, but the individual manipulation of the fingers is permanently lost.

SUMMARY CONCEPTS

■ The organization of the nervous system can be described in terms of its embryonic development, in which newer and more complex functions result from modification and enlargement of earlier developed structures. The dominance of the rostral end of the nervous system reflects a hierarchy of control, with the forebrain having control over the brain stem and the brain stem having control over the spinal cord.

- In terms of organization, the nervous system retains many early patterns of segmental development that were established during early embryonic life, with a longitudinal series of segments, each repeating the same fundamental pattern of a central cavity surrounded by an inner core of gray matter made up of nerve cells and a superficial layer of white matter containing axons of the longitudinal tract systems. Each of the body segments are connected to their corresponding central nervous system (CNS) segments by afferent sensory and efferent motor neurons of the peripheral nervous system (PNS).

- There are four types of afferent neurons that carry sensory information to the CNS through the dorsal root ganglia: *general somatic afferents* that carry sensory information from the skin and other somatic structures, *special somatic afferents* that are concerned with internal sensory information such as joint and tendon sensation, *general visceral afferents* that innervate visceral structures such as the gastrointestinal and genitourinary systems, and *special visceral afferents* that innervate gut-related visceral receptors such as taste buds and olfactory receptors.

- There are three types of efferent neurons in the ventral horn that synapse with lower motor neurons that exit the CNS in the ventral roots: general somatic efferent neurons that innervate skeletal muscles, general visceral efferent neurons that supply visceral structures innervated by the autonomic nervous system, and the pharyngeal efferent neurons that innervate pharyngeal muscles.

- Communication between longitudinal segments is provided by tracts that are arranged in three layers: an inner, a middle, and an outer layer. The *inner layer* of white matter contains the axons of neurons that connect neighboring segments of the nervous system. It contains a mixture of nerve cells and axons called the *reticular formation* and is the site of many important spinal cord and brain stem reflex circuits. The *middle layer* provides for longitudinal communication between the more distant segments of the nervous system; it contains most of the major fiber tract systems required for sensation and movement. The *outer layer* contains large-diameter axons that travel the entire length of the nervous system; it includes tracts needed for fine manipulative skills.

Spinal Cord and Brain

The central nervous system, which consists of the spinal cord and brain, gathers information about the environment from the peripheral nervous system, processes this information, perceives part of it, and organizes reflexes and other behavioral responses.

The Spinal Cord

In the adult, the spinal cord is found in the upper two thirds of the spinal canal of the vertebral column (Fig. 34-11A). It extends from the foramen magnum at the base of the skull to a cone-shaped termination, the conus medullaris, usually located at the level of the first or second lumbar vertebra (L1 or L2) in the adult. The dorsal and ventral roots of the more caudal portions of the cord elongate during development and angle downward from the cord, forming what is called the *cauda equina* (from the Latin for "horse's tail"). The filum terminale, which is composed of nonneural tissues and the pia mater, continues caudally and attaches to the second sacral vertebra (S2).

Cross-Sectional Anatomy of the Spinal Cord

The spinal cord is somewhat oval on transverse section, with the gray matter that forms the dorsal and ventral horns having the appearance of a butterfly or the letter "H" (see Fig. 34-11B). The central portion of the cord, which connects the dorsal and ventral horns, is called the *intermediate gray matter*. The intermediate gray matter surrounds the central canal. In the thoracic area, the small, slender projections that emerge from the intermediate gray matter are called the *intermediolateral columns* of the horns. These columns contain the visceral output association neurons and the efferent neurons of the sympathetic nervous system.

The gray matter is proportional to the amount of tissue innervated by a given segment of the cord (see Fig. 34-11B). Larger amounts of gray matter are present in the lower lumbar and upper sacral segments, which supply the lower extremities, and in the fifth cervical segment to the first thoracic segment, which supply the upper limbs. The white matter in the spinal cord also increases progressively toward the brain because ever more ascending fibers are added and the number of descending axons is greater.

The spinal cord and the dorsal and ventral roots are covered by a connective tissue sheath, the pia mater, which also contains the blood vessels that supply the white and gray matter of the cord (Fig. 34-12). On the lateral sides of the spinal cord, extensions of the pia mater, the denticulate ligaments, attach the sides of the spinal cord to the bony walls of the spinal canal. Thus, the cord is suspended by both the denticulate ligaments and the segmental nerves. A fat- and vessel-filled epidural space intervenes between the spinal dura mater and the inner wall of the spinal canal.

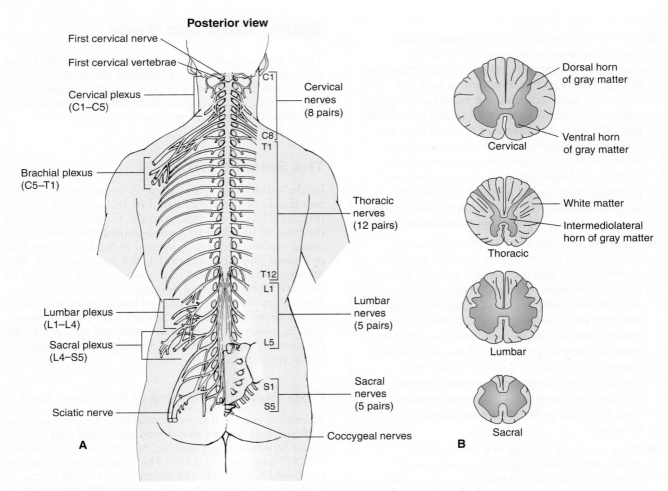

FIGURE 34-11. (A) Posterior view of the spinal cord, including portions of the major spinal nerves and some of the components of the major nerve plexuses. **(B)** Cross-sectional views of the spinal cord, showing regional variations in gray matter and increasing white matter as the cord ascends.

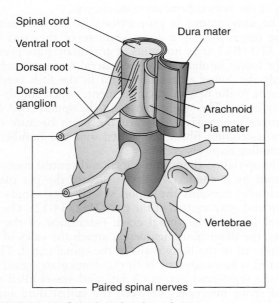

FIGURE 34-12. Spinal cord and meninges.

Protection of the Spinal Cord

The spinal cord, spinal nerves, and their supporting structures are protected by the bony structures of the vertebral column. The vertebral body is the anterior, more massive part of the bone that gives strength to the vertebral column and supports body weight. Each vertebral body has two pedicles that extend posteriorly and support the laterally oriented transverse processes of the laminae, which arch medially and fuse to continue as the spinal processes. The vertebral arch and posterior surface of the vertebral body form the wall of the vertebral foramen which is formed by the union of the vertebral arch with the vertebral body. The succession of vertebral foramina in the articulated spinal column forms the vertebral canal (spinal canal), which contains the spinal cord, meninges, fat, and spinal nerve roots. The spaces between the vertebral bodies are filled with fibrocartilaginous discs and stabilized with tough ligaments. A gap, the intervertebral foramen, occurs between each two succeeding pedicles, allowing for the exit of the segmental nerves and passage of blood vessels. Supporting structures of the spinal cord are discussed further in Chapter 36.

Early in fetal life, the spinal cord extends the entire length of the vertebral column and the spinal nerves exit through the intervertebral foramina (openings) near their level of origin. Because the vertebral column and spinal dura grow at a faster rate than the spinal cord, a disparity develops between each succeeding cord segment and the exit of its dorsal and ventral nerve roots through the corresponding intervertebral foramina. In the newborn, the cord terminates at the level of L2 or L3. In the adult, the cord usually terminates in the inferior border of L1, and the arachnoid mater and its enclosed subarachnoid space, which is filled with CSF, do not close down on the filum terminale until they reach the level of S2. This results in the formation of a pocket of CSF, the *dural cisterna spinalis*, which extends from approximately L2 to S2. Because this area contains an abundant supply of CSF and the spinal cord does not extend this far, the area often is used for sampling the CSF. A procedure called a *spinal tap*, or puncture, can be done by inserting a special needle into the dural sac at L3 or L4. The spinal roots, which are covered with pia mater, are in little danger of trauma from the needle used for this purpose.

Spinal Nerves

The peripheral nerves that carry information to and from the spinal cord are called *spinal nerves*. There are 31 left-right pairs of spinal nerves (8 cervical, 12 thoracic, 5 lumbar, 5 sacral, and 1 coccygeal); each pair is named for the segment of the spinal cord from which it exits. Because the first cervical spinal nerve exits the spinal cord just above the first cervical vertebra (C1), this nerve is given the number of the bony vertebra just below it (see Fig. 34-11A). However, the numbering is changed for all lower levels. An extra cervical nerve, the C8 nerve, exits above the T1 vertebra, and each of the subsequent nerves are numbered for the vertebra just above its point of exit.

Each spinal cord segment communicates with its corresponding body segment through the paired segmental spinal nerves. Each spinal nerve, accompanied by the blood vessels supplying the spinal cord, enters the spinal canal through an intervertebral foramen, where it divides into two branches, or roots. One branch enters the dorsolateral surface of the cord (i.e., dorsal root), carrying the axons of afferent neurons into the CNS. The other branch leaves the ventrolateral surface of the cord (i.e., ventral root), carrying the axons of efferent neurons into the periphery. These two branches or roots fuse at the intervertebral foramen, forming the mixed spinal nerve—"mixed" because it has both afferent and efferent axons.

After emerging from the vertebral column, the spinal nerve divides into two branches or *rami* (singular, *ramus*): a small dorsal primary ramus and a larger ventral primary ramus (Fig. 34-13). The thoracic and upper lumbar spinal nerves also lead to a third branch, the ramus communicans, which contains sympathetic axons supplying the blood vessels, the genitourinary system, and the gastrointestinal system. The dorsal ramus

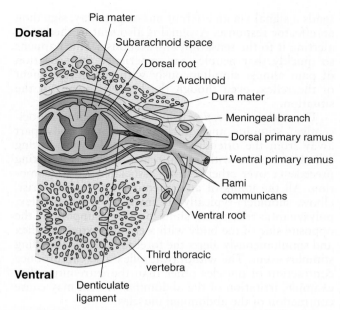

FIGURE 34-13. Cross-section of vertebral column at the level of the third thoracic vertebra, showing the meninges, the spinal cord, and the origin of a spinal nerve and its branches or rami.

contains sensory fibers from the skin and motor fibers to muscles of the back. The ventral primary ramus contains motor fibers that innervate the skeletal muscles of the anterior body wall and the legs and arms.

Spinal nerves do not go directly to skin and muscle fibers; instead, they form complicated nerve networks called *plexuses* (see Fig. 34-11A). A plexus is a site of intermixing nerve branches. Many spinal nerves enter a plexus and connect with other spinal nerves before exiting from the plexus. Nerves emerging from a plexus form progressively smaller branches that supply the skin and muscles of the various parts of the body. The PNS contains four major plexuses: the cervical, brachial, lumbar, and sacral plexuses.

Spinal Reflexes

A reflex is a highly predictable relationship between a stimulus and a motor response. A spinal reflex is a response mediated by cells in the spinal cord, bypassing any conscious effort from the brain. A reflex may involve neurons at a single spinal cord segment (i.e., segmental reflexes), several or many reflexes (i.e., segmental reflexes), or structures in the brain (i.e., suprasegmental reflexes).

A spinal reflex involves a sensory receptor, an afferent pathway, an integrating center in the spinal cord, an efferent pathway, and an effector muscle or gland. A classic example is the knee-jerk or patellar reflex, in which the leg jerks when the kneecap is briskly tapped with a reflex hammer. The reflex reaction is initiated by sensory receptors at the site of the stimulus, and relayed to the spinal cord via afferent sensory neurons. This happens in a fraction of a second, allowing people to jerk away before the brain is even aware of a problem. The integrating center in the spinal cord, in turn, sends a signal via an efferent motor pathway, signaling an effector response. A signal is also sent to the brain, alerting it to the sensation and response. This happens so quickly that people may experience the sensation of pain almost simultaneously with the development of the reflex, even though the brain is aware of the situation.

The *withdrawal reflex* is initiated by a painful (nociceptive) stimulus and quickly moves the body part away from the offending stimulus, usually by flexing a limb part. The withdrawal reflex is powerful, taking precedence over other reflexes associated with locomotion. All the joints of an extremity (e.g., finger, wrist, elbow, shoulder) typically are involved. This complex, polysynaptic reflex also shifts postural support to the opposite side of the body with a crossed extensor reflex and simultaneously alerts the forebrain to the offending stimulus event. The withdrawal reflex also can produce contraction of muscles other than the extremities. For example, irritation of the abdominal viscera may cause contraction of the abdominal muscles.

The Brain

The brain is divided into three regions, the hindbrain, the midbrain, and the forebrain (Fig. 34-14). The hindbrain includes the medulla oblongata, the pons, and its dorsal outgrowth, the cerebellum. Midbrain structures include two pairs of dorsal enlargements, the superior and inferior colliculi (not shown). The forebrain, which consists of two hemispheres covered by the cerebral cortex, contains central masses of gray matter, the basal ganglia (discussed in Chapter 36), and the rostral end of the neural tube, the diencephalon with its adult derivatives—the thalamus and hypothalamus. The olfactory and optic nerves are also considered part of the forebrain. In contrast, the motor and sensory nuclei of the 3rd to 12th cranial nerves are located in the midbrain and hindbrain.

An important concept is that the more rostral or recently developed parts of the neural tube gain dominance or control over regions and functions at lower levels. They do not replace the earlier developed circuitry but merely dominate it. After damage to the more vulnerable parts of the forebrain, as occurs with severe brain injury, a brain stem–controlled organism remains that is capable of breathing and may survive if the environmental temperature is regulated and nutrition and other aspects of care are provided. However, all aspects of intellectual function, experience, perception, and memory usually are permanently lost.

Hindbrain

During embryonic development, the hindbrain becomes subdivided into the cerebellum, the medulla oblongata—also referred to as the *medulla*—and the pons. The CSF-filled tube becomes the fourth ventricle, which is continuous with the cerebral aqueduct of the midbrain (see Fig. 34-14).

The cerebellum, the "little brain," is an important movement control center (see Chapter 36). It receives massive axonal inputs from the spinal cord and the pons. Neurons in the spinal cord provide information about the body's position in space, and those in the pons relay information from the cerebral cortex specifying the goals of the intended movements.

Brain Stem. The brain stem is the region of the brain that connects the cerebrum with the spinal cord. It consists of the midbrain, medulla oblongata, and the pons. In the brain stem, the reticular formation has been greatly expanded. Certain groups of neurons termed *vital centers* are located in the reticular formation of the pons and medulla. These centers include the respiratory, cardiovascular, and vasomotor centers. Still other centers in the brain stem are concerned with swallowing, intestinal movements, control of micturition, and a variety of more specific functions such as salivation and pupillary diameter.

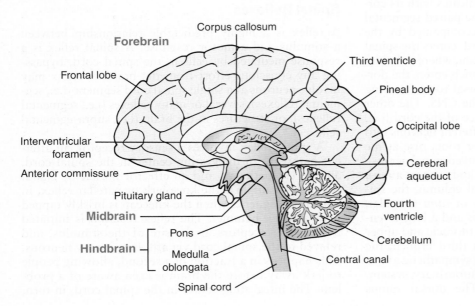

FIGURE 34-14. Midsagittal section showing structures of the hindbrain, midbrain, and forebrain.

The *medulla* represents the five caudal segments of the brain part of the neural tube; the cranial nerve branches entering and leaving it have functions similar to the spinal segmental nerves. Although the ventral horn areas in the medulla are quite small, the dorsal horn areas are enlarged, processing the large amount of information pouring through cranial nerves XII (hypoglossal), X (vagus), and IX (glossopharyngeal) (see Table 34-1).

The *pons*, which develops from the fifth neural tube segment, is located between the medulla and the midbrain. As the name implies (*pons*, Latin for "bridge"), the pons is composed chiefly of conduction fibers. The enlarged area on the ventral surface of the pons contains the pontine nuclei, which receive information from all parts of the cerebral cortex. The axons of these neurons form a massive bundle that enters the cerebellum. In the pons, the reticular formation is large and contains the circuitry for manipulating the jaws during chewing and speech. Cranial nerves VIII, VII, and VI have their origin in the pons (see Table 34-1).

Midbrain

The midbrain develops from the fourth segment of the neural tube, and its organization is similar to that of a spinal segment. Two prominent bundles of nerve fibers, the *cerebral peduncles*, pass along the ventral surface of the midbrain. These fibers include the corticospinal tracts and are the main motor pathways between the forebrain and the pons. On the dorsal surface, four "little hills," the *superior* and *inferior colliculi*, are areas of cortical formation. The inferior colliculus is involved in directional head turning and, to some extent, in experiencing the direction of sound sources. The superior colliculi are essential to the reflex mechanisms that coordinate eye movements when the visual environment is surveyed. Two cranial nerves, the oculomotor nerve

(CN III) and the trochlear nerve (CN IV), exit the midbrain (see Table 34-1).

Forebrain

The most rostral part of the brain, the forebrain consists of the diencephalon, or "between brain," and the telencephalon, or "end brain." The diencephalon forms the core of the forebrain, and the telencephalon forms the cerebral hemispheres.

Diencephalon. Three of the most forward brain segments form an enlarged dorsal horn and ventral horn with a narrow, CSF-filled central canal—the third ventricle—separating the two sides. This region is called the *diencephalon*. The dorsal horn part of the diencephalon is the thalamus and subthalamus, and the ventral horn part is the hypothalamus (Fig. 34-15). The optic nerve, or cranial nerve II, and retina are outgrowths of the diencephalon.

The thalamus consists of two large, egg-shaped masses, one on either side of the third ventricle. The thalamus is divided into several major parts, and each part is divided into distinct nuclei, which are the major relay stations for information going to and from the cerebral cortex. All sensory pathways have direct projections to thalamic nuclei, which convey the information to restricted areas of the sensory cortex. Coordination and integration of peripheral sensory stimuli occur in the thalamus, along with some crude interpretation of highly emotion-laden auditory experiences that not only occur but can be remembered. For example, a person can recover from a deep coma in which cerebral cortex activity was minimal and remember some of what was said at the bedside.

The thalamus also plays a role in relaying critical information regarding motor activities to and from

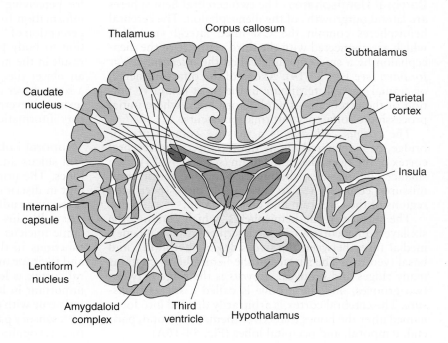

FIGURE 34-15. Frontal section of the brain passing through the third ventricle, showing the thalamus, subthalamus, hypothalamus, internal capsule, corpus callosum, basal ganglia (caudate nucleus, lentiform nucleus), amygdaloid complex, insula, and parietal cortex.

Thalamus

Corpus callosum

Subthalamus

Parietal cortex

Caudate nucleus

Insula

Internal capsule

Lentiform nucleus

Amygdaloid complex

Third ventricle

Hypothalamus

selected areas of the motor cortex. Two neuronal circuits are significant in this regard. One is the pathway from the cerebral cortex to the pons and cerebellum and then, by way of the thalamus, back to the motor cortex. The second is the feedback circuit that travels from the cortex to the basal ganglia, then to the thalamus, and from the thalamus back to the cortex. The subthalamus also contains movement control systems related to the basal ganglia.

Through its connections with the ascending reticular activating system, the thalamus processes neural influences that are basic to cortical excitatory rhythms (i.e., those recorded on the electroencephalogram), to essential sleep–wake cycles, and to the process of attending to stimuli. Besides their cortical connections, the thalamic nuclei have connections with each other and with neighboring nonthalamic brain structures such as the limbic system. Through their connections with the limbic system, some thalamic nuclei are involved in relating stimuli with the emotional responses they evoke.

The ventral horn portion of the diencephalon is the hypothalamus, which borders the third ventricle and includes a ventral extension, the posterior pituitary gland or neurohypophysis. The hypothalamus is the area of master-level integration of homeostatic control of the body's internal environment. Maintenance of blood gas concentration, water balance, food consumption, and major aspects of endocrine and ANS control require hypothalamic function.

The internal capsule is a broad band of projection fibers that lies between the thalamus medially and the basal ganglia laterally (see Fig. 34-15). It contains all of the fibers that connect the cerebral cortex with deeper structures, including the basal ganglia, thalamus, midbrain, pons, medulla, and spinal cord.

Cerebral Hemispheres. The two cerebral hemispheres are lateral outgrowths of the diencephalon. The cerebral hemispheres contain the CSF-filled lateral ventricles, which are connected with the third ventricle of the diencephalon by a small opening called the *interventricular foramen* (see Fig. 34-14). Axons of the olfactory nerve, or cranial nerve I, terminate in the most primitive portion of the cerebrum—the olfactory bulb, where initial processing of olfactory information occurs.

The *corpus callosum* is a massive commissure, or bridge, of myelinated axons that connects the cerebral cortex of the two sides of the brain (see Fig. 34-15). Two smaller commissures, the anterior and posterior commissures, connect the two sides of the more specialized regions of the cerebrum and diencephalon.

The surface of the hemispheres, which contains the six-layered neocortex, can be described as lateral (side), medial (area between the two sides of the brain), and basal (ventral). The surface of the hemispheres contains many ridges and grooves. A *gyrus* is the ridge between two grooves, and the groove is called a *sulcus* or *fissure*. The cerebral cortex is arbitrarily divided into lobes named after the bones that cover them: the frontal, parietal, temporal, and occipital lobes (Fig. 34-16A).

Frontal Lobe. The frontal lobe extends from the frontal pole to the central sulcus and is separated from the temporal lobe by the lateral sulcus. The frontal lobe can be subdivided rostrally into the frontal pole and laterally into the superior, middle, and inferior gyri, which continue on the undersurface over the eyes as the orbital cortex. These areas are associated with the medial thalamic nuclei, which also are related to the limbic system. In terms of function, the prefrontal cortex is thought to be involved in anticipation and prediction of consequences of behavior.

The precentral gyrus (area 4), next to the central sulcus, is the *primary motor cortex* (see Fig. 34-16B). This area of the cortex provides precise movement control for distal flexor muscles of the hands and feet and the phonation apparatus required for speech. Just rostral to the precentral gyrus is a region of the frontal cortex called the *premotor* or *motor association cortex*. This region (area 8 and rostral area 6) is involved in the planning of complex learned movement patterns. The primary motor cortex and the association motor cortex are connected with lateral thalamic nuclei, through which they receive feedback information from the basal ganglia and cerebellum. On the medial surface of the hemisphere, the premotor area includes a *supplementary motor cortex* involved in the control of bilateral movement patterns requiring great dexterity.

Parietal Lobe. The parietal lobe of the cerebrum lies behind the central sulcus and above the lateral sulcus. The strip of cortex bordering the central sulcus is called the *primary somatosensory cortex* (areas 1, 2, and 3) because it receives very discrete sensory information from the lateral nuclei of the thalamus. Just behind the primary sensory cortex is the *somatosensory association cortex* (areas 5 and 7), which is connected with the thalamic nuclei and the primary sensory cortex. This region is necessary for perceiving the meaningfulness of integrated sensory information from various sensory systems, especially the perception of "where" the stimulus is in space and in relation to body parts. Localized lesions of this region can result in the inability to recognize the meaningfulness of an object (i.e., agnosia). With the person's eyes closed, a screwdriver can be felt and described as to shape and texture. Nevertheless, the person cannot integrate the sensory information required to identify it as a screwdriver.

Temporal Lobe. The temporal lobe lies below the lateral sulcus and merges with the parietal and occipital lobes. The primary auditory cortex (area 41) is important in discrimination of sounds entering opposite ears. It receives auditory input projections by way of the inferior colliculus of the midbrain and a ventrolateral thalamic nucleus. The auditory association area (area 22) functions in the recognition of certain sound patterns and their meaning. The remaining portion of the temporal cortex is less defined functionally but apparently is important in long-term memory recall. This is particularly true with respect to perception and memory of complex sensory patterns, such as geometric figures and faces (i.e., recognition of "what" or "who" the stimulus is).

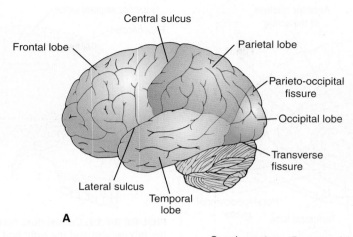

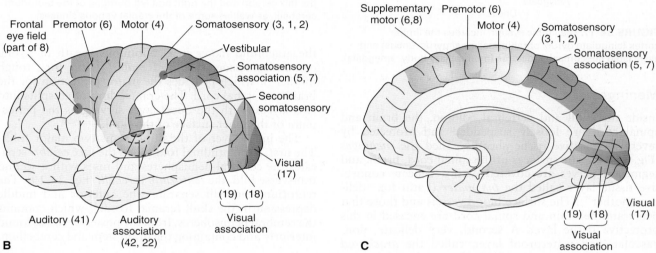

FIGURE 34-16. Cerebral hemispheres. **(A)** Lateral view of the cerebral hemispheres showing the frontal, parietal, occipital, and temporal lobes. **(B)** Left lateral view of the motor and sensory areas of the cerebral cortex. **(C)** Areas of the motor and sensory cortex in a brain that has been sectioned in the median plane.

Irritation or stimulation can result in vivid hallucinations of long-past events.

Occipital Lobe. The occipital lobe lies posterior to the temporal and parietal lobes. It contains the primary visual cortex (area 17), stimulation of which causes the experience of bright lights called phosphenes in the visual field. Just superior and inferior is the visual association cortex (areas 18 and 19), which is required for gnostic visual function, by which the meaningfulness of visual experience, including experiences of color, motion, depth perception, pattern, form, and location in space, occurs.

The neocortical areas of the parietal lobe, between the somatosensory and the visual cortices, have a function in relating the texture, or "feel," and location of an object with its visual image. Between the auditory and visual association areas, the *parieto-occipital region* is necessary for relating the meaningfulness of a sound and image to an object or person.

Limbic System. The medial aspect of the cerebrum is organized into concentric bands of cortex, the *limbic system* (from the Latin *limbus*, "border"), which surrounds the connection between the lateral and third ventricles. The innermost band just above and below the cut surface of the corpus callosum is folded out of sight but is a three-layered cortex ending as the hippocampus in the temporal lobe. Just outside the folded area is a band of transitional cortex, which includes the cingulate and the parahippocampal gyri (Fig. 34-17). The limbic lobe has reciprocal connections with the medial and the intralaminar nuclei of the thalamus, with the deep nuclei of the cerebrum, and with the hypothalamus. Overall, this region of the brain is involved in emotional experience and in the control of emotion-related behavior. Stimulation of specific areas in this system can lead to feelings of dread, high anxiety, or exquisite pleasure. It also can result in violent behaviors, including attack, defense, or explosive and emotional speech.

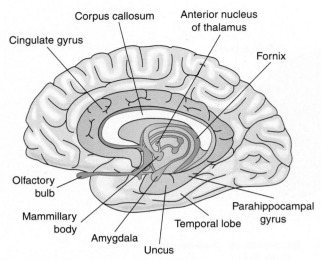

FIGURE 34-17. The limbic system includes the limbic cortex (cingulate gyrus, parahippocampal gyrus, uncus) and associated subcortical structures (mammillary body, amygdala).

Meninges

Inside the skull and vertebral column, the brain and spinal cord are loosely suspended and protected by several connective tissue sheaths called the *meninges* (Fig. 34-18). The surfaces of the spinal cord, brain, and segmental nerves are covered with a delicate connective tissue layer called the *pia mater* (Latin for "delicate mother"). The surface blood vessels and those that penetrate the brain and spinal cord are encased in this protective tissue layer. A second, very delicate, nonvascular, and waterproof layer, called the *arachnoid mater*, encloses the entire CNS. The arachnoid layer is named for its spider-web appearance. The CSF is contained in the subarachnoid space. Immediately outside

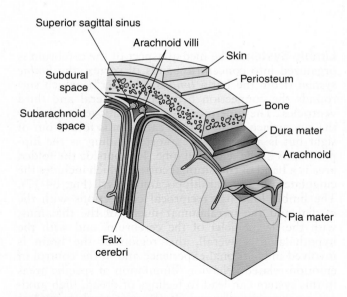

FIGURE 34-18. The cranial meninges. Arachnoid villi, shown within the superior sagittal sinus, are one site of cerebrospinal fluid absorption into the blood.

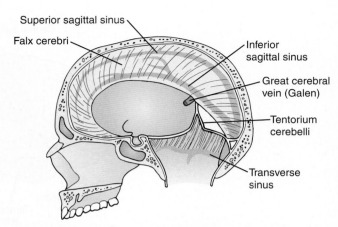

FIGURE 34-19. Cranial dura mater. The skull is open to show the falx cerebri and the right and left portions of the tentorium cerebelli, as well as some of the cranial venous sinuses.

the arachnoid mater is a continuous sheath of strong connective tissue, the *dura mater* (Latin for "tough mother"), which provides the major protection for the brain and spinal cord. The cranial dura often splits into two layers, with the outer layer serving as the periosteum of the inner surface of the skull.

The inner layer of the dura forms two major folds. The first, a longitudinal fold called the *falx cerebri* separates the cerebral hemispheres and fuses with a second transverse fold, the *tentorium cerebelli* (Fig. 34-19). The tentorium cerebelli separates the anterior and middle depression in the skull (cranial fossae), which contains the cerebral hemispheres, from the posterior fossa, found interiorly and containing the brain stem and cerebellum.

Ventricular System and Cerebrospinal Fluid

The ventricular system is a set of structures containing cerebrospinal fluid (CSF) in the brain (Fig. 34-20). The system comprises four ventricles: right and left lateral ventricles (the first and second ventricles), third ventricle, and fourth ventricle. Cerebrospinal fluid is a clear, colorless ultrafiltrate of blood plasma, composed of 99% water with other constituents, making it close to the composition of the brain extracellular fluid. The total volume of CSF is 135 to 150 mL. The daily production is about 500 to 600 mL/day, so the CSF turns over about 4 times per day.

The CSF provides a supporting and protective fluid in which the brain and spinal cord float, and it helps to maintain a constant ionic environment that serves as a medium for diffusion of nutrients, electrolytes, and metabolic end products into the extracellular fluid surrounding CNS neurons and glia. Filling the ventricles, the CSF supports the mass of the brain. Because it fills the subarachnoid space surrounding the CNS, a physical force delivered to either the skull or spine is to some extent diffused and cushioned.

The CSF is produced by tiny reddish masses of specialized capillaries from the pia mater, called the *choroid plexus*, which projects into the ventricles. Once produced, the CSF flows freely through the ventricles (Fig. 34-20B). Three openings, or foramina, allow the CSF to pass into

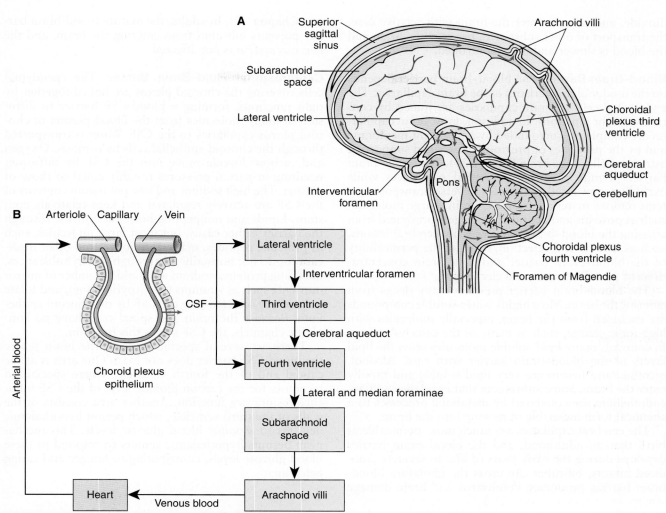

FIGURE 34-20. (A) The flow of cerebrospinal fluid (CSF) from the time of its formation from blood in the choroid plexuses until its return to the blood in the superior sagittal sinus. Plexuses in the lateral ventricles are not illustrated. **(B)** Cerebrospinal fluid is a blood filtrate produced by the choroid plexus epithelium that is found in each brain ventricle. The flow of CSF from the lateral ventricles flows through the interventricular foramen (Monro) into the third ventricle. From the third ventricle, CSF is conveyed to the fourth ventricle via the cerebral aqueduct (Sylvius). Three openings, a midline foramen of Magendie and two lateral foramina (Luschka), pass the CSF into the subarachnoid space, where it is returned to the venous circulation through the arachnoid villi.

the subarachnoid space. Two of these, the foramina of Luschka, are located at the lateral corners of the fourth ventricle. The third, the median foramen of Magendie, is in the midline at the caudal end of the fourth ventricle (see Fig. 34-20A). Approximately 30% of the CSF passes down into the subarachnoid space that surrounds the spinal cord, mainly on its dorsal surface, and moves back up to the cranial cavity along its ventral surface.

Reabsorption of CSF into the vascular system occurs along the sides of the superior sagittal sinus in the anterior and middle fossa. Here, the waterproof arachnoid mater has protuberances, the *arachnoid villi*, which penetrates the inner dura and venous walls of the superior sagittal sinus (see Fig. 34-20A). The arachnoid villi function as one-way valves, permitting CSF outflow into the blood but not allowing blood to pass into the arachnoid spaces.

Blood–Brain and Cerebrospinal Fluid–Brain Barriers

Maintenance of a chemically stable environment is essential to the function of the brain. In most regions of the body, extracellular fluid undergoes small fluctuations in pH and concentrations of hormones, amino acids, and potassium ions during routine daily activities such as eating and exercising. If the brain were to undergo these fluctuations, the result would be uncontrolled neural activity because some substances, such as amino acids, act as neurotransmitters, and ions such as potassium influence the threshold for neural firing. Two barriers, the blood–brain barrier and the CSF-brain barrier, provide the means for maintaining the stable chemical environment of the brain. Only water, carbon dioxide, and oxygen enter the brain with relative ease; the transport of other substances between the brain and the blood is slower and more controlled.

Blood–Brain Barrier. The blood–brain barrier depends on the unique characteristics of the brain capillaries. The endothelial cells of brain capillaries are joined by continuous tight junctions. In addition, most brain capillaries are completely surrounded by a basement membrane and by the processes of previously described supporting astrocyte cells of the brain (Fig. 34-21). The blood–brain barrier permits passage of essential substances while excluding unwanted materials. Reverse transport systems remove materials from the brain. Large molecules such as proteins and peptides are largely prevented from crossing the blood–brain barrier. Acute cerebral lesions, such as trauma and infection, increase the permeability of the blood–brain barrier and alter brain concentrations of proteins, water, and electrolytes.

The blood–brain barrier prevents many drugs from entering the brain. Most highly water-soluble compounds are excluded from the brain, especially molecules with high ionic charge, such as many of the catecholamines. In contrast, many lipid-soluble molecules cross the lipid layers of the blood–brain barrier with ease. Alcohol, nicotine, and heroin are very lipid soluble and rapidly enter the brain. Some substances that enter the capillary endothelium are converted by metabolic processes to a chemical form incapable of moving into the brain.

The cerebral capillaries are much more permeable at birth than in adulthood, and the blood–brain barrier develops during the early years of life. In severely jaundiced infants, bilirubin can cross the immature blood-brain barrier, producing kernicterus and brain damage (see Chapter 13). In adults, the mature blood-brain barrier prevents bilirubin from entering the brain, and the nervous system is not affected.

Cerebrospinal Fluid–Brain Barrier. The ependymal cells covering the choroid plexus are linked together by tight junctions, forming a blood-CSF barrier to diffusion of many molecules from the blood plasma of choroid plexus capillaries to the CSF. Water is transported through the choroid epithelial cells by osmosis. Oxygen and carbon dioxide move into the CSF by diffusion, resulting in partial pressures roughly equal to those of plasma. The high sodium and low potassium contents of the CSF are actively regulated and kept relatively constant. Lipids and nonpeptide hormones diffuse through the barrier rather easily, but most large molecules, such as proteins, peptides, many antibiotics, and other medications, do not normally get through. Many substances, including proteins, sodium ions, and a number of micronutrients such as vitamins C, B_6 (pyridoxine), and folate are actively secreted into the CSF by the choroid epithelium. Because the brain and spinal cord have no lymphatic channels, the CSF serves this function.

There are several specific areas of the brain where the blood-CSF barrier does not exist. One area is at the caudal end of the fourth ventricle, where specialized receptors for the carbon dioxide level of the CSF influence respiratory function. Another area consists of the walls of the third ventricle, which permit hypothalamic neurons to monitor blood glucose levels. This mechanism permits hypothalamic centers to respond to these blood glucose levels, contributing to hunger and eating behaviors.

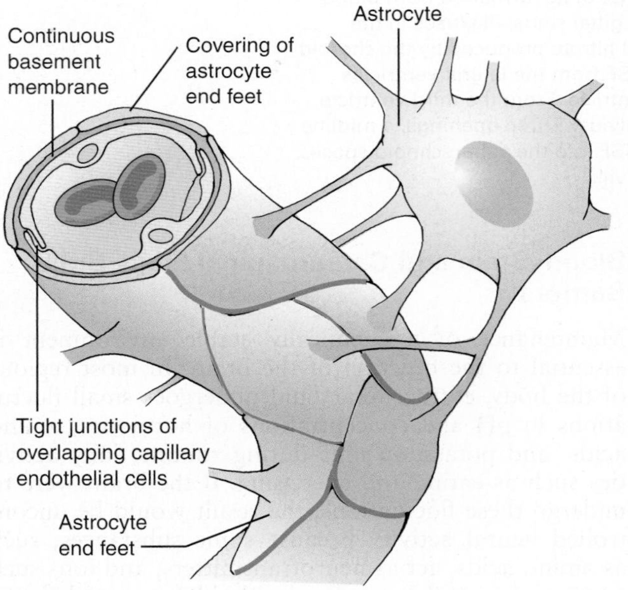

FIGURE 34-21. The three components of the blood-brain barrier: the astrocyte and astrocyte end feet that encircle the capillary, the capillary basement membrane, and the tight junctions that join the overlapping capillary endothelial cells.

Labels: Astrocyte; Continuous basement membrane; Covering of astrocyte end feet; Tight junctions of overlapping capillary endothelial cells; Astrocyte end feet

SUMMARY CONCEPTS

■ In the adult, the spinal cord is in the upper two thirds of the spinal canal of the vertebral column. On transverse section, the spinal cord has an oval shape, and the internal gray matter has the appearance of a butterfly or letter "H." The dorsal horns contain the input association (IA) neurons and receive afferent information from dorsal root and other connecting neurons. The ventral horns contain the output association neurons and lower motor neurons that leave the cord by the ventral roots.

■ There are 31 pairs of spinal nerves (8 cervical, 12 thoracic, 5 lumbar, 5 sacral, and 1 coccygeal), each communicating with its corresponding body segments. Each spinal nerve is formed by the combination of nerve fibers from the dorsal and ventral roots of the spinal cord. The dorsal roots carry afferent sensory axons entering the dorsal horn of the gray matter, while the ventral roots carry efferent axons from motor neurons located within the ventral horn of the gray matter. At its distal end, the ventral root joins with the dorsal root to form a mixed spinal nerve.

- The brain can be divided into three regions: the hindbrain, the midbrain, and the forebrain. The hindbrain, consisting of the medulla oblongata, pons, and cerebellum, contains the neuronal circuits for the eating, breathing, and locomotive functions required for survival and cranial nerves V through XII. The midbrain contains cranial nerves IV and III. The forebrain consists of the diencephalon, which forms the core of the forebrain; and the telencephalon, which forms the cerebral hemispheres.

- The diencephalon contains the thalamus and hypothalamus. All sensory pathways have direct projections to the thalamic nuclei, which convey the information to restricted parts of the sensory cortex. The hypothalamus functions in the homeostatic control of the internal environment.

- The cerebral hemispheres, which are the lateral outgrowths of the diencephalon, are divided into four lobes—the frontal, parietal, temporal, and occipital lobes. The premotor area and primary motor cortex are located in the frontal lobe; the primary sensory cortex and somatosensory association area are in the parietal cortex; the primary auditory cortex and the auditory association area are in the temporal lobe; and the primary visual cortex and association visual cortex are in the occipital lobe.

- The brain is enclosed and protected by connective tissue sheaths called the *meninges*, which consist of three layers: the dura mater, arachnoid mater, and pia mater. The CSF, in which the brain and spinal cord float, is secreted into the ventricles by the choroid plexus, circulates through the ventricular system, passes outside to surround the brain, and is reabsorbed into the venous system through the arachnoid villi. The blood-brain barrier and CSF-brain barrier protect the brain from substances in the blood that would disrupt brain function.

The Autonomic Nervous System

The autonomic nervous system (ANS), in contrast to the previously discussed somatic nervous system, provides a person with the ability to maintain internal physiologic homeostasis and perform the activities of daily living in an ever-changing physical environment. The term "autonomic" (self-governing) reflects the independent nature of this part of the nervous system or functioning largely below the level of consciousness. The ANS is involved in regulating, adjusting, and coordinating vital visceral functions such as heart rate and blood pressure. It is strongly affected by emotional influences and is involved in many of the expressive aspects of behavior, including blushing, pallor, palpitations, clammy hands, and dry mouth.

As with the somatic nervous system, the ANS is represented in both the CNS and the PNS. Traditionally, the ANS has been defined as a general efferent system innervating visceral organs. The efferent outflow from the ANS has two divisions: the sympathetic nervous system and the parasympathetic nervous system. The afferent input to the ANS is provided by visceral afferent neurons, usually not considered part of the ANS.

The functions of the sympathetic nervous system include maintaining body temperature, respiration, digestion, elimination, and adjusting blood flow and blood pressure to meet the changing needs of the body. The sympathoadrenal system also can discharge as a unit when there is a critical threat to the integrity of the individual—the so-called fight-or-flight response. During a stress situation, the heart rate accelerates, the blood pressure rises, blood flow shifts from the skin and gastrointestinal tract to the skeletal muscles and brain, blood sugar increases, the bronchioles and pupils dilate, the sphincters of the stomach and intestine and the internal sphincter of the urethra constrict, and the rate of secretion of exocrine glands that are involved in digestion diminishes. Emergency situations often require vasoconstriction and shunting of blood away from the skin and into the muscles and brain, a mechanism that, should a wound occur, would provide for a reduction in blood flow and preservation of vital functions needed for survival.

In contrast to the sympathetic nervous system, the functions of the parasympathetic nervous system are concerned with conservation of energy, resource replenishment and storage, and maintenance of organ function during periods of minimal activity. The parasympathetic nervous system slows heart rate, stimulates gastrointestinal function and related glandular secretion, promotes bowel and bladder elimination, and contracts the pupil, protecting the retina from excessive light during periods when visual function is not vital to survival.

The two divisions of the ANS usually are viewed as having opposite and antagonistic actions (i.e., if one activates, the other inhibits a function). Exceptions are functions, such as sweating and regulation of arteriolar blood vessel diameter, that are controlled by a single division of the ANS, in this case the sympathetic nervous system.

The sympathetic and parasympathetic nervous systems are continually active. The effect of this continual or basal (baseline) activity is referred to as *tone*. The tone of an effector organ or system can be increased or decreased and usually is regulated by a single division of the ANS. For example, vascular smooth muscle tone is controlled by the sympathetic nervous system. Increased sympathetic activity produces local vasoconstriction from increased vascular smooth muscle tone, and decreased activity results in vasodilatation caused by decreased tone. In structures such as the sinoatrial node and atrioventricular node of the heart, which are innervated by both divisions of the ANS, one division predominates in controlling tone. In this case, the tonically active parasympathetic nervous system exerts a constraining or braking effect on heart rate, and when parasympathetic outflow is withdrawn, similar to releasing a brake, the heart rate increases. The increase in heart rate that occurs with vagal withdrawal can be further augmented by sympathetic stimulation.

Autonomic Efferent Pathways

The outflow of both divisions of the ANS follows a two-neuron efferent pathway (Fig. 34-22). The cell body of the first motor neuron, called the *preganglionic neuron*, lies in the brain stem or the spinal cord. The second motor neuron, called the *postganglionic neuron*, synapses with a preganglionic neuron in an autonomic ganglion located in the PNS. The two divisions of the ANS differ in terms of location of preganglionic cell bodies, relative length of preganglionic fibers, general function, nature of peripheral responses, and preganglionic and postganglionic neurotransmitters and their postsynaptic receptors (Table 34-3).

Most visceral organs are innervated by both sympathetic and parasympathetic fibers. Exceptions include structures such as blood vessels and sweat glands that have input from only sympathetic division of the ANS. The fibers of the sympathetic nervous system are distributed to effectors throughout the body, and as a result, sympathetic actions tend to be more diffuse than those of the parasympathetic nervous system, in which there is a more localized distribution of fibers. The preganglionic fibers of the sympathetic nervous system may traverse a considerable distance and pass through several ganglia before synapsing with postganglionic neurons, and their terminals make contact with a large number of postganglionic fibers. In some ganglia, the ratio of preganglionic to postganglionic cells may be 1:20; because of this, the effects of sympathetic stimulation are diffuse. There is considerable overlap, and one ganglion cell may be supplied by several preganglionic fibers. In contrast to the sympathetic nervous system, the parasympathetic nervous system has its postganglionic neurons located very near or in the organ of innervation. Because the ratio of preganglionic to postganglionic communication often is 1:1, the effects of the parasympathetic nervous system are much more circumscribed.

Sympathetic Nervous System

The preganglionic neurons of the sympathetic nervous system are located primarily in the thoracic and upper lumbar segments (T1 to L2) of the spinal cord; thus, the

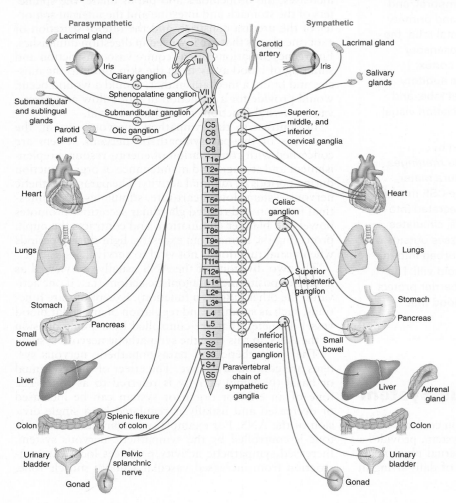

FIGURE 34-22. The autonomic nervous system with the parasympathetic division (craniosacral) indicated in red on the right and the sympathetic division (thoracolumbar) indicated in blue on the left. (Adapted from DeMyer W. *Neuroanatomy*, 2nd ed. Baltimore, MD: Williams & Wilkins; 1998.)

TABLE 34-3 Characteristics of the Sympathetic and Parasympathetic Nervous Systems

Characteristic	Sympathetic Outflow	Parasympathetic Outflow
Location of preganglionic cell bodies	T1–T12, L1 and L2	Cranial nerves: III, VII, IX, X; S2 to S4
Relative length of preganglionic fibers	Short—to paravertebral chain of ganglia or to aortic prevertebral of ganglia	Long—to ganglion cells near or in the innervated organ
General function	Catabolic—mobilizes resources in anticipation of challenge for survival (preparation for "fight-or-flight" response)	Anabolic—concerned with conservation, renewal, and storage of resources
Nature of peripheral response	Generalized	Localized
Neurotransmitter at ganglion	ACh	ACh
Receptor at ganglion	Nicotinic (N_N)	Nicotinic (N_N)
Transmitter of postganglionic neuron	NE (most synapses) * NE and Epi (secreted by adrenal gland)	ACh
Type of transmitter receptors at target synapse	Alpha (α) and Beta (β)	Muscarinic (M)
Target effectors	Smooth muscle, cardiac muscle, and secretory cells throughout body	Most viscera of the head and the thoracic, abdominal, and pelvic cavities

Ach, acetylcholine; NE, norepinephrine; Epi, epinephrine

*Postganglionic sympathetic nerve fibers to sweat glands, piloerector muscles, and a few blood vessels are cholinergic.

sympathetic nervous system often is referred to as the thoracolumbar division of the ANS. These preganglionic neurons have axons that are largely myelinated and relatively short. The postganglionic neurons of the sympathetic nervous system are located in the paravertebral ganglia of the sympathetic chain that lie on either side of the vertebral column, or in prevertebral sympathetic ganglia such as the celiac ganglia, the branches of which innervate the liver, stomach, and other visceral organs (Fig. 34-23). Besides postganglionic efferent neurons, the sympathetic ganglia contain interconnecting neurons similar to those associated with complex circuitry in the brain and spinal cord, many of which inhibit modulate preganglionic-to-postganglionic transmission.

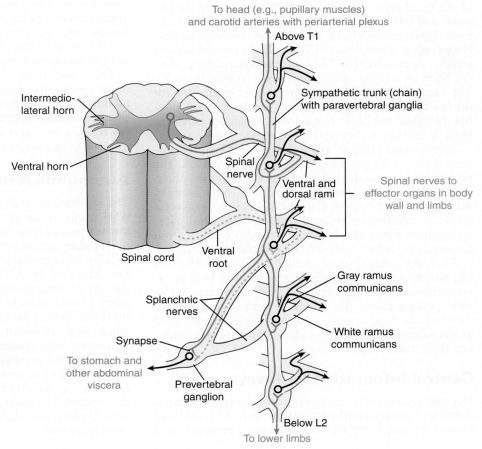

FIGURE 34-23. Sympathetic pathways. Sympathetic preganglionic fibers (*blue*) leave the spinal cord by way of the ventral root of the spinal nerves, enter the ventral primary rami, and pass through the white rami to the prevertebral or paravertebral ganglia of the sympathetic chain, where they synapse with postganglionic neurons (*black*). Other preganglionic neurons (*red dotted lines*) travel directly to their destination in the various effector organs.

The axons of the preganglionic neurons leave the spinal cord through the ventral root of the spinal nerves (T1 to L2), enter the ventral primary rami (i.e., nerve divisions) and leave the spinal nerve through white rami of the rami communicantes to reach the paravertebral ganglionic chain (see Fig. 34-23). In the sympathetic chain of ganglia, preganglionic fibers may synapse with neurons of the ganglion they enter, pass up or down the chain and synapse with one or more ganglia, or pass through the chain and move outward through a splanchnic nerve to terminate in one of the prevertebral ganglia (i.e., celiac, superior mesenteric, or inferior mesenteric) that are scattered along the dorsal aorta and its branches. The adrenal medulla, which is part of the sympathetic nervous system, contains postganglionic sympathetic neurons that secrete sympathetic neurotransmitters directly into the bloodstream.

Parasympathetic Nervous System

As is true in the sympathetic nervous system, efferent parasympathetic nerve signals are carried from the central nervous system to their targets by a two-neuron pathway. The preganglionic fibers of the parasympathetic nervous system, also referred to as the *craniosacral division* of the ANS, originate in some segments of the brain stem and sacral segments of the spinal cord (see Fig. 34-22). The central regions of origin are the midbrain, pons, medulla oblongata, and sacral part of the spinal cord. The outflow from the midbrain passes through the oculomotor nerve (cranial nerve III) to supply the pupillary sphincter muscle of each eye and the ciliary muscles that control lens thickness for accommodation. Caudal pontine outflow comes from branches of the facial nerve (cranial nerve VII) that supply the lacrimal and nasal glands. The medullary outflow develops from cranial nerves VII, IX, and X. Fibers in the glossopharyngeal nerve (cranial nerve IX) supply the parotid salivary glands. Approximately 75% of parasympathetic efferent fibers are carried in the vagus nerve (cranial nerve X). The vagus nerve provides parasympathetic innervation for the heart, trachea, lungs, esophagus, stomach, small intestine, proximal half of the colon, liver, gallbladder, pancreas, kidneys, and upper portions of the ureters.

Sacral preganglionic axons leave the S2 to S4 segmental nerves by gathering into the pelvic nerves. The pelvic nerves leave the sacral plexus on each side of the cord and distribute their peripheral fibers to the bladder, uterus, urethra, prostate, distal portion of the transverse colon, descending colon, and rectum. The sacral parasympathetic fibers also supply the venous outflow from the external genitalia to facilitate erectile function.

With the exception of cranial nerves III, VII, and IX, which synapse in discrete ganglia, the long parasympathetic preganglionic fibers pass uninterrupted to short postganglionic fibers located in the organ wall. In the walls of these organs, postganglionic neurons send axons to smooth muscle and glandular cells that modulate their functions.

Central Integrative Pathways

General visceral afferent fibers accompany the sympathetic and parasympathetic outflow into the spinal and cranial nerves, bringing chemoreceptor, pressure, and nociceptive (pain) information from organs of the viscera to the brain stem, thoracolumbar cord, and sacral cord. Local reflex circuits relating visceral afferent and autonomic efferent activity are integrated into a hierarchic control system in the spinal cord and brain stem. Progressively greater complexity in the responses and greater precision in their control occur at each higher level of the nervous system. Most visceral reflexes receive input from the lower motor neurons that innervate skeletal muscles as part of their response patterns.

For most autonomic-mediated functions, the hypothalamus serves as the major control center. The hypothalamus, which has connections with the cerebral cortex, the limbic system, and the pituitary gland, is in a prime position to receive, integrate, and transmit information to other areas of the nervous system. The neurons concerned with thermoregulation, thirst, and feeding behaviors are found in the hypothalamus. The hypothalamus also is the site for integrating neuroendocrine function. Hypothalamic releasing and inhibiting hormones control the secretion of the anterior pituitary hormones (see Chapter 31).

The organization of many life-support reflexes occurs in the reticular formation of the medulla and pons. These areas of reflex circuitry, often called *centers*, produce complex combinations of autonomic and somatic efferent functions required for the cough, sneeze, swallow, and vomit reflexes, as well as for the more purely autonomic control of the cardiovascular system. One of the striking features of ANS function is the rapidity and intensity with which it can change visceral function. Within 3 to 5 seconds, it can increase heart rate to approximately twice its resting level. Bronchial smooth muscle tone is largely controlled by parasympathetic fibers carried in the vagus nerve. These nerves produce mild to moderate constriction of the bronchioles.

Other important ANS reflexes are located at the level of the spinal cord. As with other spinal reflexes, these are modulated by input from higher centers. When there is loss of communication between the higher centers and the spinal reflexes, as occurs in spinal cord injury, these reflexes function in an unregulated manner (see Chapter 36).

Autonomic Neurotransmission

The generation and transmission of impulses in the ANS occur in the same manner as in the CNS. There are self-propagating action potentials with transmission of impulses across synapses and other tissue junctions by way of neurohumoral transmitters. The postganglionic fibers of the ANS form a diffuse neural plexus at the site of innervation. The membranes of the cells of many smooth muscle fibers are connected by gap junctions that permit rapid conduction of impulses through whole sheets of smooth muscle, often in repeating waves of contraction. Autonomic neurotransmitters released near a limited portion of these fibers provide a modulating function extending to a large number of effector cells, such as those of the muscle layers of the gut and of the bladder. The main neurotransmitters of the ANS are acetylcholine and the catecholamines, epinephrine and norepinephrine.

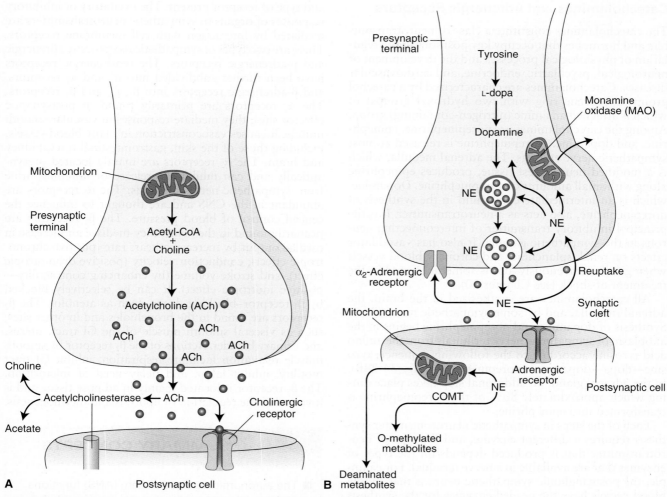

FIGURE 34-24. Schematic illustration of **(A)** parasympathetic cholinergic and **(B)** sympathetic noradrenergic neurotransmitter synthesis, release, receptor binding, neurotransmitter degradation, and metabolite transport back into the presynaptic neuron (acetylcholine) and reuptake (norepinephrine). COMT, catechol-*O*-methyltransferase; NE, norepinephrine; ChAT, Choline acetyltransferase.

Acetylcholine and Cholinergic Receptors

Acetylcholine (ACh) is the preganglionic neurotransmitter in autonomic ganglia of both the sympathetic and parasympathetic nerve fibers as well as the postganglionic neurotransmitter in parasympathetic nerve endings. It also is released at sympathetic nerve endings that innervate the sweat glands and cholinergic vasodilator fibers found in skeletal muscle. Acetylcholine is synthesized in cholinergic neurons from choline and acetyl coenzyme A (acetyl CoA) by a single step reaction catalyzed by the biosynthetic enzyme choline acetyltransferase (Fig. 34-24A). Once synthesized, ACh is transported from the cytoplasm into vesicles that are concentrated on the inner surface of the presynaptic neuron. Activation of the postsynaptic receptors occurs with action potential-mediated release of ACh from the presynaptic vesicles. Following dissociation from the postsynaptic receptors, ACh is rapidly hydrolyzed by the enzyme acetylcholinesterase (AChE) into acetate and choline in the synaptic cleft. The choline molecule is transported back into the nerve ending, where it is used again in the synthesis of ACh.

Cell membrane receptors that respond to acetylcholine are called *cholinergic receptors*. There are two types of cholinergic receptors: nicotinic and muscarinic. Nicotinic ACh receptors are of two types: muscle type receptor (N_M or N_1) and neuronal type receptor (N_N or N_2). N_M receptor is located in the neuromuscular junction, which causes the contraction of skeletal muscles by way of end-plate potential. N_N receptor causes depolarization in autonomic ganglia resulting in postganglionic impulse. Some skeletal muscle relaxants, such as succinylcholine and tubocurarine, can be used to induce muscle relaxation and short-term paralysis in anesthesia by blocking N_M receptors at the neuromuscular junction. Muscarinic acetylcholine receptors are present on the innervational targets of postganglionic fibers of the parasympathetic nervous system and the sweat glands, which are innervated by the sympathetic nervous system. The drug atropine is a competitive antagonist for the muscarinic acetylcholine receptor that prevents the action of acetylcholine at excitatory and inhibitory muscarinic receptor sites. Because it is a muscarinic-blocking drug, it exerts little effect at nicotinic receptor sites.

Catecholamines and Adrenergic Receptors

The catecholamines constitute a class of neurotransmitters and hormones that occupy key positions in the regulation of physiological processes and the development of neurological, psychiatric, endocrine, and cardiovascular diseases. Catecholamines are characterized by a catechol group (a benzene ring with two hydroxyl groups) to which is attached an amine (nitrogen-containing) group. Among the catecholamines are norepinephrine, epinephrine, and dopamine. Norepinephrine is released at most sympathetic nerve endings. The adrenal medulla, which is a modified neural crest tissue, produces epinephrine along with small amounts of norepinephrine. Dopamine, which is an intermediate compound in the synthesis of norepinephrine, also acts as a neurotransmitter. It is the principal inhibitory transmitter of interconnecting neurons in the sympathetic ganglia. It also has vasodilator effects on renal, splanchnic, and coronary blood vessels when given intravenously and is sometimes used in the treatment of shock (see Chapter 20).

All catecholamines are synthesized in the brain, the adrenal medulla, and by some sympathetic nerve fibers. Synthesis of dopamine and norepinephrine begins in the axoplasm of sympathetic nerve terminals from the amino acid tyrosine according to the following sequence: tyrosine→dopa→dopamine→norepinephrine (Fig. 34-24B). In the adrenal gland, an additional step takes place during which approximately 80% of the norepinephrine is transformed into epinephrine.

Each of the steps in sympathetic neurotransmitter synthesis requires a different enzyme, and the type of neurotransmitter that is produced depends on the types of enzymes that are available in a nerve terminal. For example, the postganglionic sympathetic neurons that supply blood vessels have the needed enzymes for the synthesis of norepinephrine, whereas those in the adrenal medulla have the enzymes needed to convert norepinephrine into epinephrine. As the catecholamines are synthesized, they are stored in vesicles. The final step of norepinephrine synthesis occurs in these vesicles. When an action potential reaches an axon terminal, the neurotransmitter molecules are released from the storage vesicles. The storage vesicles provide a means for concentrated storage of the catecholamines and protect them from the cytoplasmic enzymes that degrade the neurotransmitters.

In addition to neuronal synthesis, there is a second major mechanism for replenishment of norepinephrine in sympathetic nerve terminals. This mechanism consists of the active reuptake of the released neurotransmitter into the nerve terminal. Between 50% and 80% of the norepinephrine that is released during an action potential is removed from the synaptic area by an active reuptake process. This process terminates the action of the neurotransmitter and allows it to be reused by the neuron. The remainder of the released catecholamines diffuses into the surrounding tissue fluids or is degraded by two special enzymes: catechol-*O*-methyltransferase, which is diffusely present in all tissues, and monoamine oxidase (MAO), which is found in the nerve endings themselves. Catecholamines can cause excitation or inhibition of smooth muscle contraction, depending on the site, dose, and type of receptor present. The excitatory or inhibitory responses of organs to sympathetic neurotransmitters are mediated by interaction with cell membrane receptors. There are two types of sympathetic receptors: α-adrenergic and β-adrenergic receptors. The α-adrenergic receptors have been further subdivided into α_1 and α_2 receptors, and β-adrenergic receptors into β_1, β_2, and β_3 receptors. The α_1 receptors are primarily found in postsynaptic effector sites; they mediate responses in vascular smooth muscle. It causes vasoconstriction in many blood vessels, including those of the skin, gastrointestinal tract, kidney and brain. The α_2 receptors are mainly located presynaptically and can inhibit the release of norepinephrine from sympathetic nerve terminals. The α_2 receptors are abundant in the CNS and are thought to influence the central control of blood pressure. The β_1 receptors are primarily found in the heart; they mediate an increase in cardiac output by increasing heart rate (positive chronotropic effect), conduction velocity (positive dromotropic effect), and stroke volume (by enhancing contractility—positive inotropic effect). It can be selectively blocked by β_1-receptor–blocking drugs, such as atenolol. The β_2 receptors are found in the bronchioles and in other sites, such as visceral smooth muscle of the GI tract, uterus, and urinary bladder. Actions of the β_2 receptor by smooth muscle relaxation facilitate respiration, inhibit GI tract motility, inhibit labor, and delay need of micturition. The β_3 receptor is located mainly in adipose tissue and is involved in the regulation of lipolysis and thermogenesis.

SUMMARY CONCEPTS

■ The autonomic nervous system (ANS) functions at the subconscious level and is responsible for maintaining the visceral functions of the body. The two divisions of the ANS are the sympathetic and parasympathetic nervous systems. Although these divisions function in concert, they are generally viewed as having opposite and antagonistic actions. The sympathetic division maintains vital functions and responds when there is a critical threat to the integrity of the individual—the "fight-or-flight" response. The parasympathetic nervous system is concerned with conservation of energy, resource replenishment, and maintenance of organ function during periods of minimal activity.

■ The outflow of both divisions of the ANS consists of a two-neuron efferent pathway: a preganglionic and a postganglionic neuron. Acetylcholine is the neurotransmitter for the preganglionic neurons for both ANS divisions, as well as the postganglionic neurons of the parasympathetic nervous system. The catecholamines, including dopamine, norepinephrine, and epinephrine, are the neurotransmitters for most sympathetic postganglionic neurons.

REVIEW EXERCISES

1. An event such as cardiac arrest, which produces global ischemia of the brain, can result in a selective loss of recent memory and cognitive skills, while the more vegetative and life-sustaining functions such as breathing are preserved.

   A. Use principles related to the development of the nervous system and hierarchy of control to explain why.

2. Usually spinal cord injury or disease produces both sensory and motor deficits. An exception is infection by the poliomyelitis virus, which produces muscle weakness and paralysis without loss of sensation in the affected extremities.

   A. Explain using information on the cell column organization of the spinal cord.

3. The functions of the sympathetic nervous system are often described in relation to the "fight-or-flight" response. Using this description, explain the physiologic advantage for the following distribution of sympathetic nervous system receptors:

   A. The presence of β_2 receptors on the blood vessels that provide blood flow to the skeletal muscles during "fight or flight," and the presence of α_1 receptors on the resistance vessels that control blood pressure.

   B. The presence of acetylcholine receptors on the sweat glands that allow for evaporative loss of body heat during "fight or flight," and the presence of α_1 receptors that constrict the skin vessels that control blood flow to the skin.

   C. The presence of β_2 receptors that produce relaxation in the detrusor muscle of the bladder during "fight or flight," and the presence of α_1 receptors that produce contraction of the smooth muscle in the internal sphincter of the bladder.

BIBLIOGRAPHY

Alberts B, Johnson A, Lewis J, et al. *Molecular Biology of the Cell.* 5th ed. New York, NY: Garland Science; 2008:675–694, 1048–1050.

Brodal P. *The Central Nervous System: Structure and Function.* 4th ed. New York, NY: Oxford University Press; 2010.

Carlson BM. *Human Embryology and Developmental Biology.* 4th ed. St. Louis, MO: C. V. Mosby; 2008:65–81, 103–127, 233–275, 277–290.

Guyton AC, Hall JE. *Textbook of Medical Physiology.* 12th ed. Philadelphia, PA: Elsevier Saunders; 2010:555–619.

Haines DE, ed. *Fundamental Neuroscience.* 4th ed. New York, NY: Churchill Livingstone; 2012:115–121, 126–127, 146–148, 443–454.

Hanani M. Satellite glial cells in sympathetic and parasympathetic ganglia: in search of function. *Brain Res Rev.* 2010;64(2):304–327.

Jung C, Chylinski TM, Pimenta A, et al. Neurofilament transport is dependent on actin and myosin. *J Neurosci.* 2004;24:9486–9496.

Kandel ER, Schwartz JH, Jessell TM. *Principles of Neural Science.* 5th ed. New York, NY: McGraw-Hill; 2013.

Katzung B, Masters S, Trevor A. *Basic and Clinical Pharmacology.* 12th ed. New York, NY: Lange Basic Science; 2012.

Kierszenbaum AL. *Histology and Cell Biology: An Introduction to Pathology.* 3rd ed. St. Louis, MO: Elsevier Mosby; 2011: 221–250, 251–290.

Moore KL, Dalley AF, Agur AM. *Clinically Oriented Anatomy.* 6th ed. Philadelphia, PA: Wolters Kluwer Health/Lippincott Williams & Wilkins; 2010:878–888.

Moore KL, Persaud TVN. *The Developing Human: Clinically Oriented Embryology.* 8th ed. Philadelphia, PA: W.B. Saunders; 2013:389–427.

Purves D, Augustine GJ, Fitzpatrick D, et al. *Neuroscience.* 5th ed. Sunderland, MA: Sinauer Associates; 2011.

Ross MH, Pawlina W. *Histology: A Text and Atlas.* 6th ed. Philadelphia, PA: Wolters Kluwer Health/Lippincott Williams & Wilkins; 2010:318–363.

Sadler TW. *Langman's Medical Embryology.* 12th ed. Philadelphia, PA: Wolters Kluwer Health/Lippincott Williams & Wilkins; 2011:5–10, 67–72, 285–316.

Squire LR, Bloom FE, McConnell SK, et al. *Fundamental Neuroscience.* 4th ed. New York, NY: Academic Press; 2012:188–189, 391–416.

Takano T, Tian G, Peng W, et al. Astrocyte-mediated control of cerebral blood flow. *Nat Neurosci.* 2006;9:260–267.

Tortora GJ, Derrickson B. *Principles of Anatomy and Physiology.* 13th ed. Hoboken, NJ: John Wiley & Sons; 2011.

Porth Essentials Resources

Explore these additional resources to enhance learning for this chapter:

- NCLEX-Style Questions and Other Resources on the **Point**, http://thePoint.lww.com/PorthEssentials4e
- Study Guide for Essentials of Pathophysiology
- Concepts in Action Animations
- Adaptive Learning | Powered by PrepU, http://thepoint.lww.com/prepu

Somatosensory Function, Pain, and Headache

S ensory mechanisms provide individuals with a continuous stream of information about their bodies, the outside world, and the interactions between the two. The somatosensory component of the nervous system provides an awareness of pain, touch, temperature, and position, as compared to the specialized senses of sight and hearing (discussed in Chapter 38). Between 2 and 3 million nerve endings in the skin and deep body tissues provide a steady stream of encoded somatosensory information to the central nervous system. Only a small portion of this information reaches awareness; most of which provides input essential for the myriad of reflexes and automatic mechanisms that keep us functioning.

This chapter is organized into two distinct parts. The first part describes the organization and control of somatosensory function, and the second focuses on pain as a somatosensory modality.

Organization and Control of Somatosensory Function

The somatosensory system provides the central nervous system (CNS) with information related to deep and superficial body structures. It includes three types of neurons that vary in terms of distribution and type of sensation that is detected—general somatic, special somatic, and general visceral. *General somatic afferent neurons* have branches with widespread distribution throughout the body and with many distinct types of receptors that result in sensations such as pain, touch, and temperature. *Special somatic afferent neurons* have receptors located primarily in muscles, tendons, and joints. These receptors sense position and movement of the body. *General visceral afferent neurons* have receptors in various visceral structures that sense fullness and discomfort.

Somatosensory Systems

Sensory systems can be conceptualized as a series of first-order, second-order, and third-order neurons. *First-order neurons* transmit sensory information from the

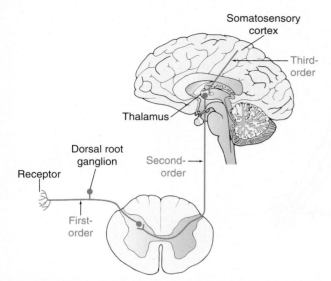

FIGURE 35-1. Arrangement of first-order, second-order, and third-order neurons of the somatosensory system.

periphery to the CNS. *Second-order neurons* communicate with various reflex networks and sensory pathways in the spinal cord and travel directly to the thalamus. *Third-order neurons* relay information from the thalamus to the cerebral cortex (Fig. 35-1).

This organizing framework corresponds with the three primary levels of neural integration in the somatosensory system: the sensory units, which contain the sensory receptors; the ascending pathways; and the central processing centers in the thalamus and cerebral cortex. Sensory information usually is relayed and processed in a cephalad (toward the head) direction by the three orders of neurons. Many interneurons process and modify the sensory information at the level of the second- and third-order neurons, and many more participate before coordinated and appropriate learned-movement responses occur. The number of participating neurons increases exponentially from the first-order through third-order levels.

The Sensory Unit

The somatosensory experience arises from information provided by a variety of receptors distributed throughout the body. These receptors monitor four major types or modalities of sensation: discriminative touch, which is required to identify the size and shape of objects and their movement across the skin; temperature sensation; sense of movement of the limbs and joints of the body; and nociception, or pain.

Each of these somatosensory modalities is mediated by a distinct system of receptors and pathways to the brain. However, all somatosensory information from the limbs and trunk shares a common class of first-order neurons called *dorsal root ganglion neurons*, and all somatosensory information from the face and cranial structures is transmitted by trigeminal sensory neurons, which function in the same manner as the dorsal root ganglion neurons. The cell body of the dorsal root

ganglion neuron, its peripheral branch (which innervates a small area of periphery), and its central axon (which projects to the CNS) form a sensory unit.

The fibers of different dorsal root ganglion neurons conduct impulses at varying rates, ranging from 0.5 to 120 m/second. This rate depends on the diameter of the nerve fiber. There are three types of nerve fibers that transmit somatosensory information: A, B, and C. Type A fibers, which are myelinated, have the fastest rate of conduction.[1,2] Type A fibers convey cutaneous pressure and touch sensation, cold sensation, mechanical pain, and heat pain. Type B fibers, which also are myelinated, transmit information from cutaneous and subcutaneous mechanoreceptors. The unmyelinated type C fibers have the smallest diameter and the slowest rate of conduction. They convey warm–hot sensation and mechanical and chemical as well as heat- and cold-induced pain sensation.

Dermatomal Pattern of Innervation

The somatosensory innervation of the body, including the head, retains a basic segmental pattern that was established during embryonic development. Thirty-three paired spinal (i.e., segmental) nerves provide sensory and motor innervation of the body wall, the limbs, and the viscera (see Chapter 34, Fig. 34-12). Sensory input to each spinal cord segment is provided by sensory neurons with cell bodies in the dorsal root ganglia. The head and face are innervated by the three branches of the trigeminal cranial nerve (CN V).

The region of the body wall that is supplied by a single pair of dorsal root ganglia is called a *dermatome*. These dorsal root ganglion–innervated strips occur in a regular sequence moving upward from the second coccygeal segment through the cervical segments, reflecting the basic segmental organization of the body and the nervous system (Fig. 35-2). Branches of the trigeminal nerve innervate the head, sending their axons to the equivalent nuclei in the brain stem. Neighboring dermatomes overlap one another sufficiently so that a loss of one dorsal root or root ganglion results in reduced but not total loss of sensory innervation of a dermatome (Fig. 35-3). Dermatome maps are helpful in interpreting the level and extent of sensory deficits that are the result of segmental nerve and spinal cord damage. For example, on the basis of the dermatomal map we can predict that sensory changes limited to the distal forearm and fourth and fifth fingers are the result of injury to the cervical (C) 8 and thoracic (T) 1 dorsal roots.

Spinal Circuitry and Ascending Neural Pathways

On entry into the spinal cord, the central axons of the somatosensory neurons branch extensively and project to neurons in the spinal cord gray matter. Some branches become involved in local spinal cord reflexes and directly initiate motor reflexes (e.g., flexor-withdrawal reflex). Two parallel pathways, the *discriminative pathway* and the *anterolateral pathway,* carry the information from the spinal cord to the thalamic level of sensation, each taking a different route through the CNS.[1,2] Having a

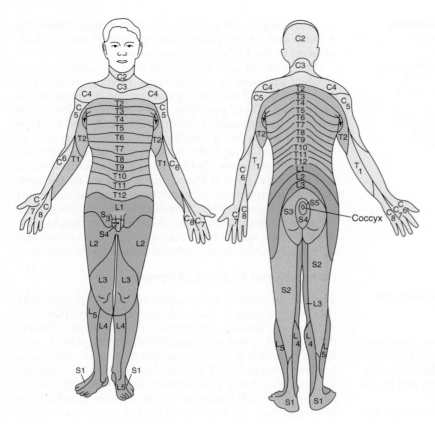

FIGURE 35-2. Cutaneous distribution of spinal nerves (dermatomes). (From Barr M. *The Human Nervous System.* New York, NY: Harper & Row; 1993.)

two-pathway system has several advantages. It adds richness to the sensory input by allowing sensory information to be handled in two different ways, and it ensures that if one pathway is damaged, the other still can provide input.

Discriminative Pathway. The *discriminative pathway* is used for the rapid transmission of sensory information, such as discriminative touch. It uses only three types of neurons to transmit information from a sensory receptor to the somatosensory cortex on the opposite side of the brain: (1) the dorsal root ganglion neurons,

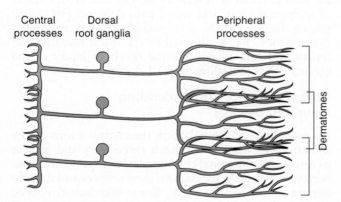

FIGURE 35-3. The dermatomes formed by the peripheral processes of adjacent spinal nerves overlap on the body surface. The central processes of these fibers also overlap in their spinal distribution.

which project their central axons to the dorsal horn in the spinal cord; (2) the dorsal column nuclei, which send their axons upward and across the midline of the medulla where they form a band of white matter called the *medial lemniscus* that passes upward to the thalamus; and (3) the thalamic neurons, which project to the primary sensory cortex (Fig. 35-4A). As the fibers in the medial lemniscus ascend through the brain stem, they are joined by sensory fibers from the trigeminal nerve that supplies the head and face. Sensory information arriving at the sensory cortex by this route can be discretely localized and discriminated in terms of intensity.

One of the distinct features of the discriminative pathway is that it relays precise information regarding spatial orientation. This is the only pathway taken by the sensations of muscle and joint movement, vibration, and delicate discriminative touch, which is required to correctly differentiate the location of touch on the skin at two neighboring points (i.e., two-point discrimination). One of the important functions of the discriminative pathway is to integrate the input from multiple receptors. The sense of shape and size of an object in the absence of visualization, called *stereognosis,* is based on precise afferent information from muscle, tendon, and joint receptors. For example, a screwdriver is perceived as being different from a knife in terms of its texture (tactile sensibility) and shape based on the relative position of the fingers as they move over the object. This complex interpretive perception requires that both the discriminative pathway and the somatosensory association area of the cerebral cortex are functioning properly. If the discriminative

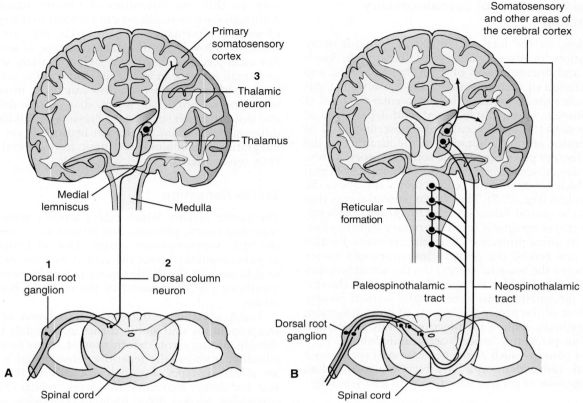

FIGURE 35-4. (A) Rapid-transmitting discriminative (dorsal column–medial lemniscal) pathway carrying axons mediating tactile sensation and proprioception. **(B)** Neospinothalamic and paleospinothalamic subdivisions of the anterolateral sensory pathway. The neurons of anterolateral pathways cross within the same segment as the cell body and ascend in the contralateral side of the spinal cord. The neospinothalamic tract travels mainly to thalamic nuclei that have third-order fibers projecting to the somatosensory cortex. The paleospinothalamic tract sends collaterals to the reticular formation and other structures, from which further fibers project to the thalamus.

pathway is functional but the association area has been damaged, the person can correctly describe the object but does not recognize it as a screwdriver. This deficit is called *astereognosis.*

Anterolateral Pathway. The anterolateral pathway (anterior and lateral spinothalamic tracts) consists of bilateral, multisynaptic, slow-conducting tracts (see Chapter 34, Fig. 34-11). These tracts provide for transmission of sensory information such as pain, thermal sensations, crude touch, and pressure that does not require discrete localization of signal source or fine discrimination of intensity. The fibers of the anterolateral pathway originate in the dorsal horns at the level of the segmental nerve, where the dorsal root ganglion neurons enter the spinal cord. These spinal neurons cross in the anterior commissure, within a few segments of origin, to the anterolateral column on the opposite side of the cord, and then ascend upward toward the brain. The anterolateral tract fibers synapse with several nuclei in the thalamus, but en route they give off numerous branches that travel to the reticular activating system of the brain stem. These projections provide the basis for increased wakefulness or awareness after

strong somatosensory stimulation and for the generalized startle reaction that occurs with sudden and intense stimuli. They also stimulate autonomic nervous system responses, such as a rise in heart rate and blood pressure, dilation of the pupils, and the pale, moist skin that results from constriction of the cutaneous blood vessels and activation of the sweat glands.

There are two subdivisions in the anterolateral pathway: the neospinothalamic and the paleospinothalamic tracts are important in pain perception[1] (see Fig. 35-4B). The *neospinothalamic tract* consists of a sequence of at least three neurons with long axons. It provides for relatively rapid transmission of sensory information to the thalamus. The *paleospinothalamic tract*, which is phylogenically older, consists of bilateral, multisynaptic, slow-conducting tracts that transmit sensory signals that do not require discrete localization or discrimination of fine gradations in intensity. This slower-conducting pathway also projects into the intralaminar nuclei of the thalamus, which have close connections with the limbic cortical systems. This circuitry gives touch its affective or emotional aspects, such as the particular unpleasantness of heavy pressure and the peculiar pleasantness of the tickling and gentle rubbing of the skin.

Central Processing of Somatosensory Information

Perception, or the final processing of somatosensory information, involves awareness of the stimuli, localization and discrimination of their characteristics, and interpretation of their meaning.[1,2] As sensory information reaches the thalamus, it begins to enter the level of consciousness, is roughly localized, and is perceived as a crude sense. The full localization, discrimination of the intensity, and interpretation of the meaning of the stimuli require processing by the somatosensory cortex.

The somatosensory cortex is located in the parietal lobe, which lies behind the central sulcus and above the lateral sulcus (Fig. 35-5). The strip of parietal cortex that borders the central sulcus is called the *primary somatosensory cortex* because it receives primary sensory information by direct projections from the thalamus. Parallel to and just behind the primary somatosensory cortex (i.e., toward the occipital cortex) lies the somatosensory association area, which is required to transform the raw sensory information into a meaningful learned perception. Most of the perceptive aspects of body sensation, or somesthesia, require the function of this association area. The perceptive aspect, or meaningfulness, of a stimulus pattern—such as the perception of sitting on a soft chair rather than on a hard bicycle seat—involves the integration of present sensation with past learning.

Somatosensory Modalities

Earlier, we noted that somatosensory experience can be divided into modalities, qualitative distinctions between the sensations of touch, temperature, position, and pain.[1,2] Somatosensory experience also involves quantitative discrimination; that is, the ability to distinguish between different intensities of sensory stimulation. Although sensory receptors can respond to many forms of sensory information at high levels, they are highly sensitive to low levels of a particular type of sensation. For example, a receptor may be particularly sensitive to a small increase in local skin temperature, yet stimulation with strong pressure also can result in receptor stimulation. Cool versus warm, sharp versus dull pain, and delicate touch versus deep pressure are all based on different populations of afferent neurons or on central integration of simultaneous input from several differently tuned afferents.

Tactile Sensation

The tactile system, which relays sensory information regarding touch, pressure, and vibration, is considered the basic somatosensory system. Loss of temperature or pain sensitivity leaves the person with no awareness of deficiency. If the tactile system is lost, however, total anesthesia (i.e., numbness) of the involved body part results.

Touch sensation results from stimulation of tactile receptors in the skin and in tissues immediately beneath the skin, pressure from deformation of deeper tissues, and vibration from rapidly repetitive sensory signals. There are at least six types of specialized tactile receptors in the skin and deeper structures: free nerve endings, Meissner corpuscles, Merkel disks, pacinian corpuscles, hair follicle end-organs, and Ruffini end-organs[1,2] (Fig. 35-6).

Free nerve endings are found in skin and many other tissues, including the cornea. They detect touch and pressure. *Meissner corpuscles* are elongated, encapsulated nerve endings present in nonhairy parts of the skin. They are particularly abundant in the fingertips, lips, and other areas where the sense of touch is highly developed. *Merkel disks* are dome-shaped receptors found in nonhairy and hairy parts of the skin. In contrast to Meissner corpuscles, which adapt within a fraction of a second, Merkel disks transmit an initial strong signal that diminishes in strength but is slow in adapting. They are responsible for giving steady-state signals that allow for continuous sense of touch against the skin.

Pacinian corpuscles are located immediately beneath the skin and deep in the fascial tissues. They are stimulated by rapid movements of the tissues and are important in detecting tissue vibration. The *hair follicle end-organs* consist of afferent unmyelinated fibers entwined around most of the length of the hair follicle. These receptors, which are rapidly adapting, detect movement on the surface of the body. *Ruffini end-organs* are found in the skin and deeper structures, including the joint capsules. These receptors, which have multibranched encapsulated endings, have very little adaptive capacity and are important for signaling continuous states of deformation, such as heavy and continuous touch and pressure.

Almost all the specialized touch receptors, with the exception of free nerve endings, transmit their signals through large myelinated nerve fibers (i.e., types $A\alpha$, $A\beta$) that have transmission velocities ranging from 25 to 70 m/second. Most free nerve endings transmit signals

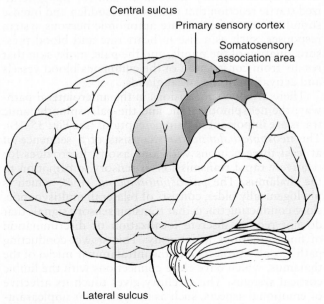

Central sulcus
Primary sensory cortex
Somatosensory association area
Lateral sulcus

FIGURE 35-5. Primary somatosensory cortex and somatosensory association area.

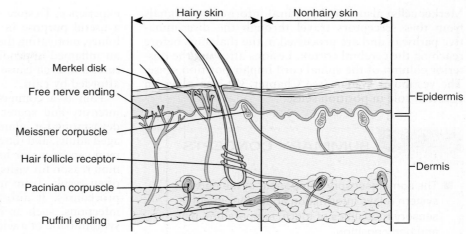

FIGURE 35-6. Somatic sensory receptors in the skin. Hairy skin and nonhairy skin have a variety of sensory receptors. (Adapted from Bear MF, Connors BW, Paradiso MA. *Neuroscience: Exploring the Brain*. Baltimore, MD: Lippincott-Raven; 1996:311.)

by way of small myelinated fibers (i.e., type Aδ) with conduction velocities of 10 to 30 m/second.

The sensory information for tactile sensation enters the spinal cord through the dorsal roots of the spinal nerves. All tactile sensation that requires rapid transmission is conducted through the discriminative pathway to the thalamus by way of the medial lemniscus. Tactile sensation also uses the more primitive and crude anterolateral pathway. Because of these multiple routes, total destruction of the anterolateral pathway seldom occurs. The only time this crude alternative system becomes essential is when the discriminative pathway is damaged. Then, despite projection of the anterolateral system information to the somatosensory cortex, only a poorly localized, high-threshold sense of touch remains. Such persons lose all sense of joint and muscle movement, body position, and two-point discrimination.

Thermal Sensation

Thermal sensation is discriminated by three types of receptors: cold, warmth, and pain. The cold and warmth receptors are located immediately under the skin at discrete but separate points, each serving an area of approximately 1 mm². Different gradations of heat and cold reception result from the relative degrees of stimulation of the different types of nerve endings. Warmth receptors respond proportionately to increases in skin temperature above resting values of 34°C and cold receptors to temperatures below 34°C.[2] The thermal pain receptors are stimulated only by extremes of temperature such as "freezing cold" (temperatures below 5°C) and "burning hot" (temperatures above 45°C) sensations.[2] Thermal receptors respond rapidly to sudden changes in temperature and then adapt over the next few minutes. They do not adapt completely, however, but continue to respond to steady states of temperature. For example, the sensation of heat one feels on entering a tub of hot water is the initial response to a change in temperature, followed by an adaptation in which one gets accustomed to the temperature change but still feels the heat because the receptors have not adapted completely.

Thermal afferents, with receptive thermal endings in the skin, send their central axons into the segmental dorsal horn of the spinal cord. On entering the dorsal horn, thermal signals are processed by second-order input association neurons. These association neurons activate projection neurons whose axons then cross to the opposite side of the cord and ascend in the multisynaptic, slow-conducting anterolateral system to the opposite side of the brain. Thalamic and cortical somatosensory regions for temperature are mixed with those for tactile sensibility.

Conduction of thermal information through peripheral nerves is quite slow compared with the rapid conduction of tactile sensation that travels through the discriminative system. If a person places a foot in a tub of hot water, the tactile sensation occurs well in advance of the burning sensation. The foot has been removed from the hot water by the local withdrawal reflex well before the excessive heat is perceived by the forebrain. Local anesthetic agents block the small-diameter afferents that carry thermal sensory information before they block the large-diameter axons that carry discriminative touch information.

Position Sense

Proprioception refers the sense or perception of limb and body movement and position without the use of vision. It is mediated by input from proprioceptive receptors (muscle spindle receptors and Golgi tendon organs) found primarily in muscles, tendons, and joint capsules (see Chapter 36). There are two submodalities of proprioception: the stationary or static component (limb position sense) and the dynamic aspects of position sense (kinesthesia). Both of these depend on constant transmission of information to the CNS regarding the degree of angulation of all joints and the rate of change in angulation. In addition, stretch-sensitive receptors in the skin (Ruffini end-organs, pacinian corpuscles, and Merkel cells) also signal postural information. Signals from these receptors are processed through the dorsal column–medial lemniscus pathway. In addition, stretch-sensitive receptors in the skin (Ruffini end-organs, pacinian corpuscles, and

Merkel cells) also signal postural information. Signals from these receptors travel through the discriminative pathway and are processed in the thalamus before reaching the cerebral cortex. Lesions affecting the posterior column of the spinal cord impair position sense. The vestibular system (see Chapter 38) also plays an essential role in position sense.

SUMMARY CONCEPTS

- The somatosensory component of the nervous system relays information about four major sensory modalities of touch, temperature, pain, and body position.

- Somatosensory information is sequentially transmitted over three types of neurons: *first-order neurons*, which transmit information from receptors in the sensory units of the system to dorsal horn neurons; *second-order association neurons* in the spinal cord, which communicate with various reflex circuits and transmit information to the thalamus, where it is roughly localized and perceived as a crude sense; and *third-order neurons*, which forward the information from the thalamus to the somatosensory cortex, where full localization, intensity discrimination, and interpretation occurs.

- The somatosensory system is organized segmentally into dermatomes, with each segment supplied by a single dorsal root ganglion that contains the neuronal cell bodies for the sensory units of the segment.

- There are two ascending pathways for transmission of somatosensory information: the discriminative and anteriolateral pathways. The discriminative pathway, which crosses at the medulla, uses only three neurons to rapidly transmit information such as position sense and discriminative touch from sensory receptors to somatosensory cortex. The anterolateral pathway, which crosses within the first few segments of entering the spinal cord, consists of bilateral, multisynaptic, slow-conducting tracts that transmit information such pain, thermal sensation, crude touch, and pressure.

Pain Sensation

Pain is an unpleasant sensory and emotional sensation associated with actual and potential tissue damage.[1-4] Unlike other somatic modalities, pain has an urgent and primitive quality, a quality responsible for the psychological, social, cultural, and cognitive aspects of the pain experience. Despite its unpleasantness, pain can serve a useful purpose in that it warns of impending tissue injury, motivating the person to seek relief. For example, an inflamed appendix could progress in severity, rupture, and even cause death were it not for the warning afforded by pain.

Pain is a common symptom that varies widely in intensity and spares no age group. It can be equally devastating for infants and children, young and middle-aged adults, and the elderly. Both acute pain and chronic pain can be major health problems. It is the most common reason for visits to health care facilities. Acute pain often results from injury, surgery, or invasive medical procedures. It also can be a presenting symptom of infections, such as otitis media. Chronic pain can be symptomatic of a wide range of health problems including arthritis, back injury, and cancer.

Pain Theories

Many theories, including the specific and pattern theories, have been offered to explain the physiologic basis for the pain experience. The *specificity theory* regards pain as a separate sensory modality evoked by the activity of specific receptors that transmit information by special nerve endings to pain centers or regions in the forebrain where pain is experienced.[5] *Pattern theory* proposes that pain receptors share endings or pathways with other sensory modalities, but that different patterns of activity (i.e., spatial or temporal) of the same neurons can be used to signal painful and nonpainful stimuli.[5] For example, light touch applied to the skin would produce the sensation of touch through low-frequency firing of the receptor; intense pressure would produce pain through high-frequency firing of the same receptor. Both of these theories focus on the neurophysiologic basis of pain, and aspects of both probably apply. Specific nociceptive afferents have been identified; however, almost all afferent stimuli, if driven at a very high frequency, can be experienced as painful.

Gate control theory, a modification of specificity theory proposed by Melzack and Wall in 1965, postulated that the presence of a neural gating mechanism at the segmental spinal cord level could block projection of pain information to the brain.[6] According to this theory, internuncial neurons involved in the gating mechanism are activated by large-diameter, faster-propagating fibers that carry tactile information capable of blocking the transmission of impulses from small-diameter myelinated and unmyelinated pain fibers. Pain therapists have long known that pain intensity can be temporarily modified by the stimulation of other sensory fibers. For example, repeated sweeping of a soft-bristled brush on the skin (i.e., brushing) over or near a painful area may result in pain reduction for several minutes to several hours.

Pain modulation is now known to be a much more complex phenomenon than that proposed by these theories. Tactile information is transmitted by small- and large-diameter fibers. Major interactions between sensory modalities, including the so-called gating phenomenon, occur at several levels of the CNS rostral to the input segment. Perhaps the most puzzling aspect of locally applied stimuli, such as brushing, that can block the experience of pain is the relatively long-lasting effect (minutes to hours) of such treatments. This prolonged effect has been difficult to explain on the basis of specificity theories, including the gate control theory. Other important factors include the effect of endogenous opioids and their receptors at the segmental and brain stem level, descending feedback modulation, altered sensitivity, learning, and culture.

More recently, Melzack has developed the *neuromatrix theory* to further address the brain's role in pain as well as the psychological and emotional dimensions of pain.[7] This theory proposes that the brain contains a widely distributed neural network, called the *body–self neuromatrix,* that has multiple somatosensory, limbic, and thalamocortical components. Genetic and sensory influences determine the architecture of each individual's neuromatrix, which integrates multiple sources of inputs. These include somatosensory inputs; other sensory inputs affecting interpretation of the situation; inputs from the brain addressing such things as attention, expectation, culture, and personality; various components of stress regulation systems; and other sources. The neuromatrix theory of pain, which places genetic and neuroendocrine mechanisms on a level equal to that of neural transmission, has important implications for research and therapy.[7]

Pain Mechanisms and Pathways

Pain can be either nociceptive or neuropathic in origin. The term *nociception*, which means "pain sense," comes from the Latin word *nocere*, "to injure." *Nociceptive pain* is initiated by nociceptors that are activated by injury to peripheral tissues. *Neuropathic pain,* on the other hand, arises from direct injury or dysfunction of the sensory axons of peripheral or central nerves.

Two aspects of pain affect an individual's response to a painful stimulus—pain threshold and tolerance. Although the terms often are used interchangeably, they have distinct meanings. *Pain threshold* is closely associated with the point at which a nociceptive stimulus is perceived as painful. *Pain tolerance* relates more to the total pain experience; it is defined as the maximum intensity or duration of pain that a person is willing to endure before the person wants something done about the pain. Psychological, familial, cultural, and environmental factors significantly influence the amount of pain a person is willing to tolerate. The threshold for pain is fairly uniform from one person to another, whereas pain tolerance is extremely variable.

The mechanisms of pain are many and complex. As with other forms of somatosensation, the pathways are composed of first-, second-, and third-order neurons[1,2] (Fig. 35-7). The first-order neurons and their receptive endings detect stimuli that threaten the integrity of innervated tissues. Second-order neurons are located in the spinal cord and process nociceptive information.

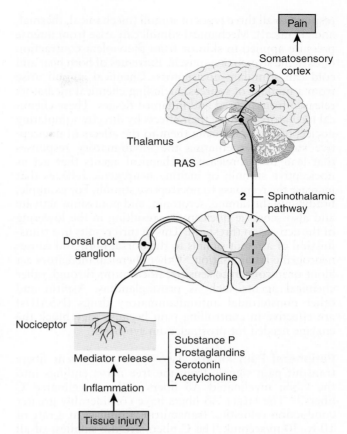

FIGURE 35-7. Mechanism of acute pain. Tissue injury leads to release of inflammatory mediators with subsequent nociceptor stimulation. Pain impulses are then transmitted to the dorsal horn of the spinal cord, where they make contact with second-order neurons that cross to the opposite side of the cord and ascend by the spinothalamic tract to the reticular activating system (RAS) and thalamus. The localization and meaning of pain occur at the level of the somatosensory cortex. 1, first-order sensory neurons; 2, second-order sensory neurons; 3, third-order sensory neurons.

Third-order neurons project pain information to the brain. The thalamus and somatosensory cortex integrate and modulate pain as well as the person's subjective reaction to the pain experience.

Pain Receptors and Primary Afferent Pathways

Nociceptors, or pain receptors, are activated by noxious insults to peripheral tissues. Structurally, they are free nerve endings of the peripheral pain fibers. These receptive endings translate noxious stimuli into signals that are transmitted by a dorsal root ganglion to the dorsal horn of the spinal cord.

Nociceptive Simulation. Unlike other sensory receptors, nociceptors respond to several forms of stimulation, including mechanical, thermal, and chemical. Some receptors respond to a single type of stimuli (mechanical or thermal) and others, called *polymodal receptors,* respond to all three types of stimuli (mechanical, thermal, and chemical). Mechanical stimuli can arise from intense pressure applied to skin or from the violent contraction or extreme stretch of a muscle. Extremes of both heat and cold can stimulate nociceptors. Chemical stimuli arise from a number of sources, including chemical mediators released from injured and inflamed tissues. These chemical mediators produce their effects by directly stimulating nociceptors or sensitizing them to the effects of nociceptive stimuli; perpetuating the inflammatory responses that lead to the release of chemical agents that act as nociceptive stimuli; or inciting neurogenic reflexes that increase the response to nociceptive stimuli. For example, bradykinin, histamine, serotonin, and potassium activate and also sensitize nociceptors, resulting in the lowering of the activation threshold. This in turn results in a transmission of afferent signals to the dorsal horn and causes neurogenic inflammation.[8] Other chemical mediators act alone or in concert to sensitize nociceptors through other chemical agents such as prostaglandins. Aspirin and other nonsteroidal anti-inflammatory drugs (NSAIDs) are effective in controlling pain because they block the enzyme needed for prostaglandin synthesis.

Peripheral Pain Fibers. Two types of afferent fibers transmit pain signals from the free nerve endings into the CNS: myelinated Aδ fibers and unmyelinated C fibers.[1,2] The larger Aδ fibers have considerably greater conduction velocities, transmitting impulses at a rate of 10 to 30 m/second. The C fibers are the smallest of all peripheral nerve fibers; they transmit impulses at the rate of 0.5 to 2.5 m/second. Pain conducted by Aδ fibers traditionally is called *fast pain* or first pain and typically is elicited by mechanical or thermal stimuli. C-fiber pain often is described as *slow-wave pain* or second pain because it is slower in onset and longer in duration, continuing to elicit pain for up to 80 hours.[9] It typically is incited by chemical stimuli or by persistent mechanical or thermal stimuli. The slow postexcitatory impulses generated in C fibers are now believed to be responsible for central sensitization to chronic pain.

Nociceptive stimulation that activates C fibers can cause a response known as *neurogenic inflammation* that produces vasodilation and an increased release of chemical mediators to which nociceptors respond. This inflammatory process results in vasodilation and the leakage of proteins and fluids into the extracellular space around the terminal end of the nociceptor. As a result, there is increased activity of immune cells, which further contributes to the inflammatory process.[8] This mechanism is thought to be mediated by a dorsal root neuron reflex that produces retrograde transport and release of chemical mediators, which in turn causes increasing inflammation of peripheral tissues. This reflex can set up a vicious cycle, which has implications for persistent pain and hyperalgesia (excessive sensitivity to pain), a condition in which the second-order neurons are overly sensitive to low levels of noxious stimulation.

The transmission of impulses between the peripheral nociceptive neurons and dorsal horn neurons in the spinal cord is mediated by neurotransmitters released from nerve endings of the nociceptive neurons.[10] Some of these neurotransmitters are amino acids (e.g., glutamate), others are amino acid derivatives (e.g., norepinephrine), and still others are low–molecular-weight peptides composed of two or more amino acids. The amino acid glutamate is a major excitatory neurotransmitter released from the central nerve endings of the nociceptive neurons. Substance P, a neuropeptide, also is released in the dorsal horn by C fibers in response to nociceptive stimulation. Substance P elicits slow excitatory potentials in dorsal horn neurons. Unlike glutamate, which confines its action to the immediate area of the synaptic terminal, some neuropeptides released in the dorsal horn can diffuse some distance because they are inactivated by reuptake mechanisms. This may help to explain the excitability and unlocalized nature of many persistently painful conditions. Neuropeptides such as substance P also appear to prolong and enhance the action of glutamate. If these neurotransmitters are released in large quantities or over extended periods, they can lead to secondary hyperalgesia.

Spinal Cord Circuitry and Ascending Pathways

On entering the spinal cord through the dorsal roots, the pain fibers bifurcate and ascend or descend one or two segments before synapsing with association neurons in the dorsal horn. From the dorsal horn, the axons of association projection neurons cross through the anterior commissure to the opposite side and then ascend upward in the previously described neospinothalamic and anterolateral pathways (Fig. 35-8).

The faster-conducting fibers in the neospinothalamic tract are associated mainly with the transmission of sharp–fast pain information to the thalamus. In the thalamus, synapses are made and the pathway continues to the contralateral parietal somatosensory area to provide the precise location of the pain. Typically, the pain is experienced as bright, sharp, or stabbing in nature.

The paleospinothalamic tract is a slower-conducting, multisynaptic tract concerned with the diffuse, dull, aching, and unpleasant sensations that commonly are associated with chronic and visceral pain. Fibers of this system also travel up the contralateral (i.e., opposite) anterolateral pathway to terminate in several thalamic regions, including the intralateral nuclei, which project to the limbic system. These projections are associated with the emotional or affective–motivational aspects of pain. Spinoreticular fibers from this pathway project bilaterally to the reticular formation of the brain stem. This component of the paleospinothalamic system facilitates avoidance reflexes at all levels. It also contributes to elevated levels of alertness and increased heart rate and blood pressure that can occur with pain.

Brain Centers and Pain Perception

Information from tissue injury is carried from the spinal cord to brain centers in the thalamus where the basic sensation of hurtfulness, or pain, occurs (see Fig. 35-8). In the neospinothalamic system, interconnections between the

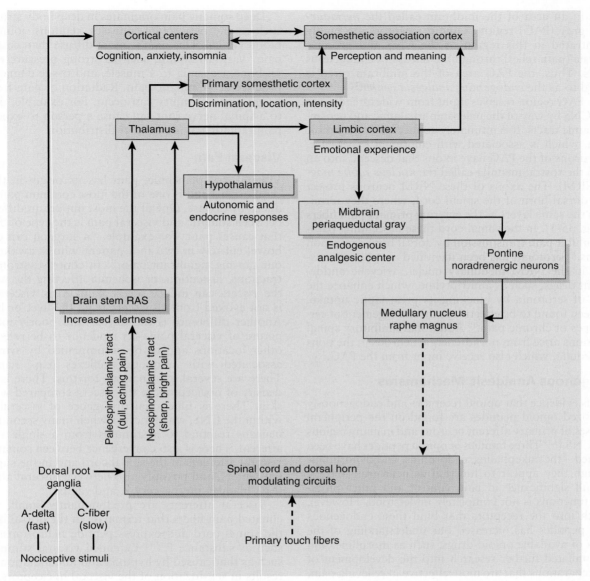

FIGURE 35-8. Primary pain pathways. The transmission of incoming nociceptive impulses is modulated by dorsal horn circuitry that receives input from primary touch receptors and from descending pathways that involve the limbic cortical systems (orbital frontal cortex, amygdala, and hypothalamus), the periaqueductal endogenous analgesic center in the midbrain, pontine noradrenergic neurons, and the nucleus raphe magnus (NRM) in the medulla. *Dashed lines* indicate inhibition or modulation of pain transmission by dorsal horn projection neurons. RAS, reticular activating system.

lateral thalamus and the somatosensory cortex are necessary to add precision, discrimination, and meaning to the pain sensation. The paleospinothalamic system projects diffusely from the intralaminar nuclei of the thalamus to large areas of the limbic cortex. These connections probably are associated with the hurtfulness and the mood-altering and attention-narrowing effect of pain.

Recent research has demonstrated cortical representation of fast–sharp and slow–chronic types of pain sensation. In healthy adults, nociceptive Aδ afferent stimulation is related to activation in the contralateral primary somatosensory cortex in the parietal lobe, whereas C afferent stimulation is related to activation of the secondary somatosensory cortices and the anterior cingulated cortex, which is part of the limbic system. With both afferents there is activation of the bilateral secondary somatosensory cortices in the posterior parietal lobes.[11]

Central Pathways for Pain Modulation

A major advance in understanding pain was the discovery of neuroanatomic pathways that arise in the midbrain and brain stem, descend to the spinal cord, and modulate ascending pain impulses. One such pathway begins in an area of the midbrain called the *periaque-ductal gray* (PAG) region. Opioid receptors are highly concentrated in this region of the CNS and produce analgesia (pain relief) through the release of endogenous opioids. Thus, the PAG area of the midbrain often is referred to as the *endogenous analgesia center*.[1]

The PAG region receives input from widespread areas of the CNS by way of the paleospinothalamic and neospinothalamic tracts. It is intimately connected to the limbic system, which is associated with emotional experience. The neurons of the PAG have axons that descend into an area in the rostral medulla called the *nucleus raphe magnus* (NRM). The axons of these NRM neurons project to the dorsal horn of the spinal cord, where they terminate in the same layers as the entering primary pain fibers (see Fig. 35-1). In the spinal cord these descending pathways inhibit pain transmission by dorsal horn projection neurons.[2] Serotonin has been identified as a neurotransmitter in the NRM medullary nuclei. Tricyclic antidepressant drugs, such as amitriptyline, which enhance the effects of serotonin by blocking its presynaptic uptake, have been found to be effective in the management of certain types of chronic pain.[12] Additional inhibitory spinal projections arise from noradrenergic neurons in the pons and medulla, which also receive input from the PAG.[2]

Endogenous Analgesic Mechanisms

There is evidence that opioid receptors and endogenously synthesized opioid peptides are found on the peripheral processes of primary afferent neurons and in many regions of the CNS.[13,14] Three families of opioid peptides have been identified—the enkephalins, endorphins, and dynorphins. Although they appear to function as neurotransmitters, their full significance in pain control and other physiologic functions is not completely understood. However, research into the receptors that bind these endogenous opioid peptides has increased our understanding of the actions of available opioid drugs, such as morphine, and has stimulated further research into the development of new preparations that are more effective in relieving pain, but with fewer side effects than existing drugs.[13,14]

Types of Pain

The most widely accepted classifications of pain are according to source or location (somatic or visceral), referral, and duration (acute or chronic). Classification based on associated medical diagnosis (e.g., surgery, trauma, cancer, sickle cell disease, fibromyalgia) is useful in planning appropriate interventions.

Cutaneous and Deep Somatic Pain

Cutaneous pain arises from superficial structures, such as the skin and subcutaneous tissues. It is a sharp pain with a burning quality and may be abrupt or slow in onset. It can be localized accurately and may be distributed along the dermatomes. Because there is an overlap of nerve fiber distribution between the dermatomes, the boundaries of pain frequently are not as clear-cut as dermatome diagrams indicate.

Deep somatic pain originates in deep body structures, such as the periosteum, muscles, tendons, joints, and blood vessels. This pain is more diffuse than cutaneous pain. Various stimuli, such as strong pressure exerted on bone, ischemia to a muscle, and tissue damage, can produce deep somatic pain. Radiation of pain from the original site of injury can occur. For example, damage to a spinal nerve root can cause a person to experience pain radiating along its fiber distribution.

Visceral Pain

Visceral, or splanchnic, pain has its origin in the visceral organs and is one of the most common pains produced by disease. One of the most important differences between somatic and visceral pain is the type of damage that causes pain. For example, "a surgeon can cut the bowel entirely in two in a patient who is awake without causing significant pain."[1] In contrast, strong contractions, distention, or ischemia affecting the walls of the viscera can induce severe pain. Also, visceral pain is not evoked from all viscera (e.g., the liver or lung).[14] Another difference is the diffuse and poorly localized nature of visceral pain—its tendency to be referred to other locations and to be accompanied by symptoms associated with autonomic reflexes (e.g., nausea).[15] There are several explanations for this. There is a low density of nociceptors in the viscera compared with the skin. There is functional divergence of visceral input within the CNS, which occurs when many second-order neurons respond to a stimulus from a single visceral afferent. There is also convergence between somatic and visceral afferents in the spinal cord and in the supraspinal centers, and possibly also between visceral afferents (e.g., bladder, uterus, cervix, and vagina).

Visceral afferents are predominantly small, unmyelinated pain fibers that terminate in the dorsal horn of the spinal cord and express peptide neurotransmitters such as substance P.[14,15] Extended visceral stimulation, such as that caused by hypoxia and inflammation, often results in sensitization of the visceral nociceptors. Once sensitized, these receptors begin to respond to otherwise innocuous stimuli (e.g., motility and secretory activity) that normally occur in the viscera. This sensitization may resolve more slowly than the initial injury, and thus visceral pain may persist longer than expected based on the initial injury.[14]

Referred Pain

Referred pain is pain that is perceived at a site different from its point of origin but innervated by the same spinal segment. It is hypothesized that visceral and somatic afferent neurons converge on the same dorsal horn projection neurons (Fig. 35-9). For this reason, it can be difficult for the brain to correctly identify the original source of pain. Pain that originates in the abdominal or thoracic viscera is diffuse and poorly localized and often perceived at a site far removed from the affected area. For example, the pain associated with myocardial infarction commonly is referred to the left arm, neck, and chest, which may delay diagnosis and treatment

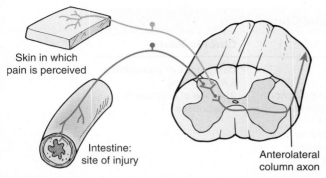

FIGURE 35-9. Convergence of cutaneous and visceral inputs onto the same second-order projection neuron in the dorsal horn of the spinal cord. Although virtually all visceral inputs converge with cutaneous inputs, most cutaneous inputs do not converge with other sensory inputs.

of a potentially life-threatening condition. Moreover, referred pain may arise alone or concurrent with pain located at the origin of the noxious stimuli.

Although the term *referred* usually is applied to pain that originates in the viscera and is experienced as if originating from the body wall, it also may be applied to pain that arises from somatic structures. For example, pain referred to the chest wall could be caused by nociceptive stimulation of the peripheral portion of the diaphragm, which receives somatosensory innervation from the intercostal nerves. An understanding of pain referral is of great value in diagnosing illness. The typical pattern of pain referral can be derived from understanding that the afferent neurons from visceral or deep somatic tissue enter the spinal cord at the same level as the afferent neurons from the cutaneous areas to which the pain is referred (Fig. 35-10).

The sites of referred pain are determined embryologically with the development of visceral and somatic structures that share the same site for entry of sensory information into the CNS and then move to more distant locations. For example, a person with peritonitis may complain of pain in the shoulder. Internally, there is inflammation of the peritoneum that lines the central part of the diaphragm. In the embryo, the diaphragm originates in the neck, and its central portion is innervated by the phrenic nerve, which enters the cord at the level of the third to fifth segments (C3 to C5). As the fetus develops, the diaphragm descends to its adult position between the thoracic and abdominal cavities while maintaining its embryonic pattern of innervation. Thus, fibers that enter the spinal cord at the C3 to C5 levels carry information from both the neck area and the diaphragm, and the diaphragmatic pain is interpreted by the forebrain as originating in the shoulder or neck area.

Although the visceral pleura, pericardium, and peritoneum are said to be relatively free of pain fibers, the parietal pleura, pericardium, and peritoneum do react to nociceptive stimuli. Visceral inflammation can involve parietal and somatic structures, and this may give rise to diffuse local or referred pain. For example, irritation of the parietal peritoneum resulting from appendicitis

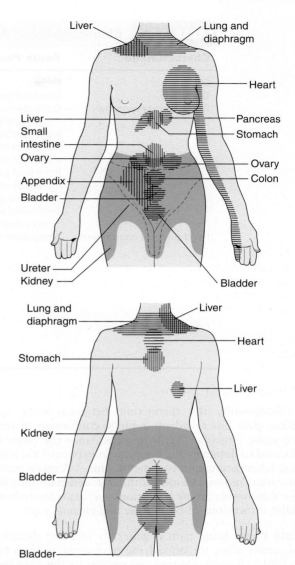

FIGURE 35-10. Areas of referred pain. (*Top*) Anterior view. (*Bottom*) Posterior view.

typically gives rise to pain directly over the inflamed area in the lower right quadrant, while producing referred pain in the umbilical area.

Muscle spasm, or *guarding,* occurs when somatic structures are involved. Guarding is a protective reflex rigidity; its purpose is to protect the affected body parts (e.g., an abscessed appendix or a sprained muscle). This protective guarding may cause blood vessel compression and give rise to the pain of muscle ischemia, causing local and referred pain.

Acute and Chronic Pain

It is common to classify pain according to its duration. Pain research of the last several decades has emphasized the importance of differentiating acute pain from chronic pain. The diagnosis and therapy for each is distinctive because they differ in cause, function, mechanisms, and psychological sequelae (Table 35-1).

TABLE 35-1	Characteristics of Acute and Chronic Pain	
Characteristic	**Acute Pain**	**Chronic Pain**
Onset	Recent	Continuous or intermittent
Duration	Short (<6 mo)	6 mo or more
Autonomic responses	Consistent with sympathetic fight-or-flight response	Absence of autonomic responses
	Increased heart rate	
	Increased stroke volume	
	Increased blood pressure	
	Increased pupillary dilation	
	Increased muscle tension	
	Decreased gut motility	
	Decreased salivary flow (dry mouth)	
Psychological component	Associated anxiety	Increased irritability
		Associated depression
		Somatic preoccupation
		Withdrawal from outside interests
		Decreased strength of relationships
Other types of response		Decreased sleep
		Decreased libido
		Appetite changes

Traditionally, the distinction between acute and chronic pain has relied on a single continuum of time with some interval (e.g., 6 months) since the onset of pain used to designate the onset of acute pain or the transition when acute pain became chronic.[16] A more recent conceptualization includes both time and pathophysiologic dimensions. Some conditions such as osteoarthritis exhibit dimensions of both acute and chronic pain.

Acute Pain. Acute pain is generally of short duration and remits when the underlying pathologic process has resolved.[17] Besides alerting the person to the existence of actual or impending tissue damage, acute pain typically prompts a search for professional help. The pain's location, radiation, intensity, and duration, as well as those factors that aggravate or relieve it, provide essential diagnostic clues.

Acute pain is elicited by surgery or trauma to body tissues and activation of nociceptive stimuli at the site of tissue damage.[16,18] This may induce an early wave of hyperexcitability of neurons within the CNS. The development of an inflammatory reaction to the tissue injury, with sensitization of peripheral receptors, often results in a second wave of longer-acting afferent input and a new increase in central hyperexcitability.[18,19] The resulting hyperalgesia can lead to increased postoperative and post-traumatic pain, usually about the second or third day, and in some cases an increased likelihood of developing chronic pain. A number of chronic pain syndromes, including whiplash injury and phantom pain, develop after trauma and surgery.[18]

Because acute pain is self-limited, in that it resolves as the injured tissues heal, long-term therapy usually is not needed. However, pain from acute illness, trauma, surgery, or medical procedures should be aggressively managed and preemptive analgesia provided before the pain becomes severe. The use of preemptive and multimodal therapy (two or more analgesics with differing analgesic mechanisms) not only allows the person to be more comfortable and active, but also helps to prevent peripheral sensitization of pain receptors and hyperexcitability of central pain centers.[19] Usually, less medication is needed when the drug is given before the pain becomes severe and the pain pathways become sensitized. Interventions that alleviate acute pain also relieve the anxiety and musculoskeletal spasms, as well increasing mobility and respiratory movements such as deep breathing and coughing.

Chronic Pain. Chronic pain is pain that persists longer than might be reasonably expected after an inciting event and is sustained by factors that are both pathologically and physically remote from the originating cause.[17,20,21] Chronic pain is highly variable. It may be unrelenting and extremely severe, as in metastatic bone pain. It can be relatively continuous with or without periods of escalation, as with some forms of back pain. Some conditions with recurring episodes of acute pain are particularly problematic because they have characteristics of both acute and chronic pain, as in sickle cell crisis or migraine headaches.

The biologic factors that contribute to chronic pain include peripheral mechanisms, peripheral–central mechanisms, and central mechanisms.[20] Peripheral mechanisms result from persistent stimulation of nociceptors, termed *peripheral sensitization.* Inflammatory mediators released from injured tissues increase the sensitivity of the C fibers and lead to increased duration of pain associated with chronic musculoskeletal, visceral, and vascular disorders. Peripheral–central mechanisms involve abnormal function of the peripheral and central portions of the somatosensory system.[21] They typically result from partial or complete loss of descending inhibitory pathways or spontaneous firing of regenerated nerve fibers. They include conditions such as causalgia, phantom limb pain, and postherpetic neuralgia. Central pain, which is associated with disease or injury of the CNS, is characterized by burning, aching, hyperalgesia, dysesthesia, and other abnormal sensations, and is experienced as superficial (skin) or deep (bone or muscle) pain. It is associated with conditions such as thalamic lesions, spinal cord injury, surgical interruption of pain pathways, and multiple sclerosis.

Unlike acute pain, chronic pain serves no useful purpose. It imposes physiologic, psychological, interpersonal, and economic stresses and may exhaust a person's resources. It is often associated with loss of appetite, sleep disturbances, and depression, which commonly is relieved once the pain is removed.

Chronic pain management is complex and treatment depends on the cause of the pain, the natural history of the underlying health problem, and the life expectancy of the individual.[20,21] If the organic illness causing the pain cannot be cured, then noncurative methods of pain control become the cornerstone of treatment. Chronic pain is best handled by a multidisciplinary team that includes specialists in areas such as anesthesiology, nursing, physical therapy, social services, and surgery.

Cancer is a common cause of chronic pain.[23–25] The goal of chronic cancer pain management should be pain alleviation and prevention. Preemptive therapy tends to reduce sensitization of pain pathways and provides for more effective pain control. Pharmacologic and nonpharmacologic interventions are the same as those used for other types of chronic pain. Depending on the form and stage of the cancer, other treatments such as palliative radiation, antineoplastic therapies, and palliative surgery may help to control the pain. In 1986, the World Health Organization (WHO) developed a three-step ladder that assists clinicians in choosing the appropriate analgesic medications.[26] Step 1 involves the use of nonopioid analgesics, and steps 2 and 3 involve the use of opioid analgesics.

Pain Management

Careful assessment of pain assists clinicians in diagnosing, managing, and relieving the patient's pain. As with other disease states, eliminating the cause of the pain is preferable to simply treating the symptom.

Assessment

Assessment includes such things as the nature, severity, location, and radiation of the pain. Reports of pain are almost entirely subjective. A careful history often provides information about the triggering factors (i.e., injury, infection, or disease) and the site of nociceptive stimuli (i.e., peripheral receptor or visceral organ).[21] A comprehensive pain history should include pain onset; description, localization, radiation, intensity, quality, and pattern of the pain; anything that relieves or exacerbates it; and the individual's personal reaction to the pain.

The single most reliable indicator of the existence and intensity of acute pain is probably the person's self-report.

Unlike many other bodily responses, such as temperature and blood pressure, the nature, severity, and distress of pain cannot be measured objectively. To overcome this problem, various methods have been developed for quantifying pain based on the person's report. They include numeric pain intensity, visual analog, and verbal descriptor scales. Most pain questionnaires assess a single aspect of pain such as pain intensity. For example, a *numeric pain intensity* scale would have patients select which number best represents the intensity of their pain, where 0 represents no pain and 10 represents the most intense pain imaginable. A *visual analog* scale also can be used; it is a straight line, often 10 cm in length, with a word description (e.g., "no pain" and "the most intense pain imaginable") at each of the ends of the line representing the continuum of pain intensity.

Nonpharmacologic Interventions

A number of nonpharmacologic methods of pain control are used in pain management. These include cognitive-behavioral interventions (e.g., relaxation, distraction, imagery, and biofeedback), physical agents (e.g., heat and cold), electroanalgesia (transcutaneous electrical nerve stimulation [TENS]), and acupuncture. Often these methods are used in addition to analgesics rather than as the sole form of pain management.

Pharmacologic Treatment

Pharmacologic treatment involves the use of drugs in the management of pain. It includes the use of nonnarcotic and narcotic analgesics, as well as adjuvant medications, such as antidepressants, anticonvulsants, and muscle relaxants. Topical medications (e.g., fentanyl patch) are a new aspect of pain management, whose full potential has yet to be determined.

An analgesic drug is a medication that acts on the nervous system to decrease or eliminate pain without inducing unconsciousness. Analgesic drugs do not cure the underlying cause of the pain, but their appropriate use makes the pain more tolerable and, in the case of acute pain, may prevent it from progressing to chronic pain. The ideal analgesic would be effective and nonaddictive and produce minimal adverse effects. Although long-term treatment with opioids can result in opioid tolerance (i.e., increasingly greater drug dosages being needed to achieve the same effect) and physical dependence, this should not be confused with addiction. Long-term drug-seeking behavior is rare in persons who are treated with opioids only during the time that they require pain relief. The unique needs and circumstances presented by each person in pain must be addressed to achieve satisfactory pain management.

Nonnarcotic Analgesics. Nonnarcotic oral analgesic medications include aspirin, other NSAIDs, and acetaminophen. Aspirin (acetylsalicylic acid) acts peripherally and centrally to block the transmission of pain impulses. It also has antipyretic and anti-inflammatory properties. The action of aspirin and other NSAIDs is through the inhibition of the cyclooxygenase (COX) enzymes, which mediate the biosynthesis of prostaglandins. Prostaglandins (particularly prostaglandin E_2) exert their effect through peripheral sensitization of nociceptors to chemical mediators such as bradykinin and histamine.[27] The NSAIDs also decrease the sensitivity of blood vessels to bradykinin and histamine, affect cytokine production by T lymphocytes, inhibit vasodilation, and decrease the release of inflammatory mediators from granulocytes and mast cells. Acetaminophen is an alternative to the NSAIDs. Although usually considered equivalent to aspirin as an analgesic and antipyretic agent, it lacks anti-inflammatory properties.

Opioid Analgesics. The term *opioid* or *narcotic* is used to refer to a group of medications, natural or synthetic, with morphinelike actions. The opioids (e.g., morphine, codeine, and many other semisynthetic congeners of morphine) exert their action through opioid receptors. There are three major categories of opioid receptors in the CNS, designated as mu (μ, for "morphine"), delta (δ), and kappa (κ).[27] Analgesia, as well as respiratory depression, miosis (constriction of the pupil), reduced gastrointestinal motility (causing constipation), feelings of well-being or euphoria, and physical dependence, principally result from morphine and morphinelike opioid analgesics that act at the mu receptors. Part of the pain-relieving properties of exogenous opioids such as morphine involve the release of endogenous opioids.[27]

Opioids are used in the management of acute and chronic pain. When given for temporary relief of severe pain, such as that occurring after surgery, there is much evidence that opioids given routinely before the pain starts or becomes extreme are far more effective than those administered in a sporadic manner. Persons who are treated in this manner usually require fewer doses and are able to resume regular activities sooner. Opioids also are used for persons with chronic pain such as that caused by cancer. Morphine remains the most useful strong opioid, and the WHO has recommended that oral morphine be part of the essential medication list and be made available throughout the world as the medication of choice for cancer pain.[24,27]

Adjuvant Analgesics. Adjuvant analgesics include medications such as tricyclic antidepressants, antiseizure medications, and neuroleptic anxiolytic agents.[28] Serotonin has been shown to play an important role in producing analgesia. In recent years the use of medications classified as serotonin norepinephrine reuptake inhibitors (SNRIs) have been shown to help with the treatment of chronic pain. The Food and Drug Administration (FDA) has approved two drugs in this class, duloxetine and milnacipran, for the treatment of chronic pain associated with fibromyalgia.[29] The use of these drugs has also shown potential benefit for the treatment of postherpetic neuralgia and painful diabetic neuropathy.[30] The tricyclic antidepressant medications that block the removal of serotonin from the synaptic cleft have been shown to produce pain relief in some

persons. These medications are particularly useful in some chronic painful conditions, such as postherpetic neuralgia. Antiseizure medications that suppress spontaneous neuronal firing are particularly useful in the management of pain that occurs after nerve injury (neuropathic pain), including diabetic neuropathy and chronic regional pain syndrome. Other agents, such as the corticosteroids, may be used to decrease inflammation and the nociceptive stimuli responsible for pain.

Surgical Interventions

If surgery removes the problem causing the pain, such as a tumor pressing on a nerve or an inflamed appendix, it can be curative. In other situations, surgery is used for symptom management rather than for cure. However, with rare exceptions, noninvasive analgesic approaches for pain relief should precede invasive surgical approaches.[16] Surgery for severe, intractable pain of peripheral or central origin has met with some success. It can be used to remove the cause or block the transmission of intractable pain from phantom limb pain, severe neuralgia, inoperable cancer of certain types, and other disorders.

SUMMARY CONCEPTS

■ Pain is both a protective and an unpleasant physically and emotionally disturbing sensation originating in pain receptors that respond to a number of stimuli that threaten tissue integrity. It is a symptom common to many illnesses and is a highly individualized experience that is shaped by a person's culture and previous life experiences.

■ Nociceptors, which are receptive nerve endings that respond to noxious or painful stimuli, transmit impulses to the dorsal horn neurons in the spinal cord using chemical neurotransmitters.

■ There are two pathways for pain transmission: The pathway for fast, sharply discriminated pain that moves directly from the receptor to the spinal cord and from the spinal cord to the thalamus using the neospinothalamic tract; and the pathway for slow, continuously conducted pain that is transmitted to the spinal cord and from the spinal cord to the thalamus using the more circuitous and slower-conducting paleospinothalamic tract.

■ The central processing of pain information includes transmission to the somatosensory cortex, where pain information is perceived and interpreted; the limbic system, where the emotional components of pain are experienced; and the brain stem centers, where autonomic nervous system responses are recruited.

■ Modulation of the pain experience occurs by way of the endogenous analgesic center in the midbrain, the pontine noradrenergic neurons, and the nucleus raphe magnus in the medulla, which sends inhibitory signals to dorsal horn neurons in the spinal cord or trigeminal nerve.

■ Pain can be classified according to location, referral, and duration as well as associated medical diagnoses. Pain can arise from stimulation of cutaneous, deep somatic, or visceral pain receptors. Referred pain is pain perceived at a site different from its origin. Acute pain is self-limiting pain that ends when the injured tissue heals. Chronic pain is pain that lasts much longer than the anticipated healing time for the underlying cause of the pain.

■ Treatment modalities for pain include the use of nonpharmacologic and pharmacologic agents either singly or in combination. Management of acute pain includes therapy directed at providing pain relief by interrupting the nociceptive stimulus. Chronic pain management is much more complex and is based on multiple considerations, including life expectancy.

Alterations in Pain Sensitivity and Special Types of Pain

Pain sensitivity and types of pain vary according to the body structures, the initiating event, and the duration of the pain. It also varies among persons and in the same person under different conditions.

Alterations in Pain Sensitivity

Sensitivity to and perception of pain varies among persons and in the same person under different conditions and in different parts of the body. Irritation, mild hypoxia, and mild compression of a peripheral nerve often result in hyperexcitability of the sensory nerve fibers or cell bodies. This is experienced as unpleasant hypersensitivity (i.e., *hyperesthesia*) or increased painfulness (i.e., *hyperalgesia*). Primary hyperalgesia describes pain sensitivity that occurs directly in damaged tissues. Secondary hyperalgesia occurs in the surrounding uninjured tissue. An example of primary hyperalgesia is the extreme sensitivity of sunburned skin, which results from sensitization of the skin pain endings by local products from the burn.

More severe pathologic processes can result in reduced or lost tactile (e.g., *hypoesthesia*, *anesthesia*), temperature (e.g., *hypothermia*, *athermia*), and pain sensation (i.e., *hypoalgesia*). *Analgesia*, in addition to meaning the relief of pain without loss of consciousness, is a pathology characterized by the absence of pain on noxious stimulation. The inability to sense pain may result in trauma, infection, and even loss of a body part or parts. It is thought to result from a peripheral nerve defect or a cortical defect, either of which disrupts the perception of pain. Whatever the cause, persons who lack the ability to perceive pain are at constant risk of tissue damage because pain cannot serve its protective function.

Allodynia (Greek *allo*, "other," and *odynia*, "painful") is the puzzling phenomenon of pain that follows a non-noxious stimulus to apparently normal skin.[2] Examples of such non-noxious stimuli are wind, touching sheets, and showering. The condition may arise when otherwise normal tissues are abnormally innervated or are referral sites. It can also result from increased responsiveness within the spinal cord (central sensitization) or a reduction in the threshold for nociceptor activation (peripheral sensitization). One type of allodynia involves *trigger points*, which are highly localized points on the skin or mucous membrane that can produce immediate intense pain at that site or elsewhere with light tactile stimulation.

Special Types of Pain

Neuropathic Pain

"Neuropathic pain refers to pain that originates from pathology of the nervous system."[31] When peripheral nerves are affected by injury or disease, it can lead to unusual and sometimes intractable sensory disturbances. The notable features that point to neuropathic processes as a cause of pain include widespread pain that is not otherwise explainable, evidence of sensory deficit (e.g., numbness, paresthesias), burning pain, pain that occurs with light stroking of the skin, and attacks of pain that occur without seeming provocation.[31] Depending on the cause, few or many axons could be damaged and the condition could be unilateral or bilateral.

Causes of neuropathic pain can be categorized according to the extent of peripheral nerve involvement. Conditions that can lead to pain by causing damage to peripheral nerves in a single area include nerve entrapment, nerve compression from a tumor mass, and various neuralgias (e.g., trigeminal, postherpetic, and post-traumatic). Conditions that can lead to pain by causing damage to peripheral nerves in a wide area include diabetes mellitus, long-term alcohol use, hypothyroidism, renal insufficiency, and drug treatment with neurotoxic agents.[32] Diabetes often causes a length-dependent neuropathy (meaning that the longest axons in a peripheral nerve are most vulnerable). Injury to a nerve also can lead to a multisymptom, multisystem syndrome, called *complex regional pain syndrome*. Nerve damage associated with amputation is believed to be a cause of phantom limb pain.

Neuropathic pain can vary with the extent and location of disease or injury. There may be allodynia or pain that is stabbing, jabbing, burning, or shooting.

The pain may be persistent or intermittent. The diagnosis depends on the mode of onset, the distribution of abnormal sensations, the quality of the pain, and other relevant medical conditions (e.g., diabetes, hypothyroidism, alcohol use, rash, or trauma). Injury to peripheral nerves sometimes results in pain that persists beyond the time required for the tissues to heal. Peripheral pathologic processes (e.g., neural degeneration, neuroma formation, and generation of abnormal spontaneous neural discharges from the injured sensory neuron) and neural plasticity (i.e., changes in CNS function) are the primary working hypotheses to explain persistent neuropathic pain.

Treatment methods include measures aimed at restoring or preventing further nerve damage (e.g., surgical resection of a tumor causing nerve compression, improving glycemic control for diabetic patients with painful neuropathies) and interventions for the palliation of pain. Although many adjuvant analgesics are used for neuropathic pain, pain control often is difficult. The initial approach in seeking adequate pain control is to try these drugs in sequence and then in combination. The adjuvant analgesics can be divided into three general classes according to the pain they are used to treat: burning, tingling, or aching pain; stabbing or shooting pain; and neurogenic pain. For pain that is burning, tingling, or aching, tricyclic antidepressants and the α_2-adrenergic agonist clonidine frequently are used. For the stabbing or shooting pain of neuralgias, antiseizure medications or baclofen, a drug used in the treatment of spasticity, may be used.[32] Nonpharmacologic therapies such as electrical stimulation of the peripheral or spinal nerves can be used for radiculopathies and neuralgias. As a last resort, neurolysis or neurosurgical blockade sometimes is used.

Neuralgia

Neuralgia is characterized by severe, brief, often repetitive attacks of lightninglike or throbbing pain. It occurs along the distribution of a spinal or cranial nerve and usually is precipitated by stimulation of the cutaneous region supplied by that nerve.

Trigeminal Neuralgia. Trigeminal neuralgia, or tic douloureux, is one of the most common and severe neuralgias. It is manifested by facial tics or spasms and characterized by paroxysmal attacks of stabbing pain that usually are limited to the unilateral sensory distribution of one or more branches of the trigeminal cranial nerve (CN V), most often the maxillary or mandibular divisions.[32,33] Although intermittent, the pain often is excruciating and may be triggered by light touch, movement, drafts, and eating. Considerable controversy remains regarding the pathophysiology of trigeminal neuralgia, but it is thought to be related to neurovascular compression. It also occurs secondary to major neurological diseases such as multiple sclerosis or tumor formation.[33]

Treatment of trigeminal neuralgia includes pharmacologic and surgical modalities. Other interventions include avoidance of precipitating factors (e.g., stimulation of trigger spots) and eye injury due to irritation; provision for adequate nutrition; and avoidance of social isolation. Carbamazepine, an antiseizure drug, is recognized as a first-line agent for treatment of trigeminal neuralgia. There is also some research showing the addition of lamotrigine, an anti-convulsant medication, to the treatment plan may be helpful.[33] Surgical release of vessels, dural structures, or scar tissue surrounding the semilunar ganglion or root in the middle cranial fossa often eliminates the symptoms. If not, percutaneous blocking or partial destruction of peripheral branches of the trigeminal nerve with heat, glycerol, or balloon compression may be used. Gamma knife radiosurgery, one of the newest techniques, involves imaging of the trigeminal nerve root entry zone, and radiation of the trigeminal nerve. There has also been recent interest in the use of botulinum toxin as a treatment modality.[33]

Postherpetic Neuralgia. Herpes zoster (also called *shingles*) is caused by the same herpes virus (varicella-zoster virus) that causes chickenpox and is thought to represent a localized recurrent infection by the varicella-zoster virus that has remained latent in the dorsal root ganglia since the initial attack of chickenpox[34] (see Chapter 46). Reactivation of viral replication is associated with a decline in cellular immunity, such as occurs with aging. Thus, the probability of developing herpes zoster increases strikingly with aging, and most cases occur in the elderly. Impaired cellular immunity also increases the risk.

During the acute stage of herpes zoster, the reactivated virus travels from the affected sensory ganglia and peripheral nerve to the skin of the corresponding dermatomes, causing a unilateral localized vesicular eruption and hyperpathia (i.e., abnormally exaggerated subjective response to pain).

Persons with postherpetic neuralgia may suffer from constant pain ("burning, aching, throbbing"), intermittent pain ("stabbing, shooting"), and stimulus-evoked pain (allodynia). Persons with allodynia often suffer from excruciating pain after the slightest touch to affected skin by such things as cold wind or clothing. These subtypes of pain may interfere with sleep and basic activities of living, causing chronic fatigue, depression, anorexia, weight loss, and social isolation.

Early treatment of shingles with antiviral drugs such as acyclovir or valacyclovir that inhibit herpes virus deoxyribonucleic acid (DNA) replication may reduce the severity of herpes zoster. Initially, postherpetic neuralgia can be treated with a topical anesthetic agent, lidocaine–prilocaine cream or 5% lidocaine gel. A tricyclic antidepressant medication, such as amitriptyline or desipramine, may be used for pain relief. Regional nerve blockade (i.e., stellate ganglion, epidural, local infiltration, or peripheral nerve block) has been used with limited success.

A live attenuated vaccine is now available for prevention of herpes zoster in adults 60 years of age and older. The vaccine is not indicated for treatment of herpes zoster or postherpetic neuralgia.[35]

Complex Regional Pain Syndrome

The complex regional pain syndrome (CRPS), formerly known as *reflex sympathetic dystrophy* (RSD), is a rare disorder of the extremities characterized by autonomic and vasomotor instability.[36–38] There are two forms of the CRPS: CRPS I (equivalent of RSD) and CRPS II, also known as *causalgia*. The International Association for the Study of Pain (IASP) lists the diagnostic criteria for CRPS I as the presence of an initiating traumatic event, continuing pain, allodynia (perception of pain from a nonpainful stimulus), or hyperalgesia disproportionate to the inciting event with evidence at some time of edema, changes in skin blood flow, or abnormal sensorimotor activity in the area of pain. The diagnosis is excluded by the existence of any condition that would otherwise account for the degree of pain and dysfunction.[39]

According to the IASP, CRPS II (i.e., causalgia) is diagnosed as the presence of continuing pain, allodynia, or hyperalgesia after a nerve injury, not necessarily limited to the distribution of the injured nerve, with evidence at some time of edema, changes in skin blood flow, or abnormal sensorimotor activity in the region of pain. The diagnosis is excluded by the existence of any condition that would otherwise account for the degree of pain and dysfunction. The primary difference between type I and type II is the identification of a definable nerve injury.

The hallmark of both types of CRPS is pain and mobility problems more severe than the injury warrants. Characteristically, the pain is severe and burning with or without deep aching. Usually, the pain can be elicited with the slightest movement or touch to the affected area, it increases with repetitive stimulation, and it lasts even after the stimulation has stopped. The pain can be exacerbated by emotional upsets or any increased peripheral sympathetic nerve stimulation. All the variations of CRPS include sympathetic components. These are characterized by vascular and trophic (e.g., dystrophic or atrophic) changes to the skin, soft tissue, and bone, and can include rubor or pallor, sweating or dryness, edema (often sharply demarcated), and, with time, patchy osteoporosis.

The pathophysiologic process of CRPS remains uncertain. Although abnormalities in sympathetic activity are observed, recent experimental data suggest that sensitization of small-diameter, polymodal C and Aδ fibers to noxious stimuli may be the basis for hyperalgia to heat and nociceptive stimuli.[38] There is also evidence that central mechanisms may play a role in sensitization of central neurons that occurs after intense peripheral mechanical stimuli or continuous activity in nociceptors. The sympathetic nervous system, either directly or indirectly through prostaglandin or α_1-adrenergic receptor activity, is considered to contribute to the excitation and sensitization of the nociceptive afferents. Other proposed mechanisms include neurogenic inflammation caused by the activation of neuromediators, such as substance P, calcitonin gene–related peptide, and histamine, which also mediates inflammation and vasodilation of

microvessels.[36] Recent research demonstrated the presence of autoantibodies against autonomic nervous system structures in patients with CRPS, especially CRPS II, suggesting that the disorder may result from dysfunction of the autonomic nervous system caused by an autoimmune attack.[39]

Early mobilization after injury or surgery reduces the likelihood of developing the syndrome.[38] In addition to addressing the underlying disorder, treatment is directed at restoration of function. Physical therapy is a cornerstone of therapy. Pain management involves the use of standard pharmacologic agents used in the management of neuropathic pain, namely, antidepressants (e.g., amitriptyline) and antiseizure drugs (e.g., gabapentin). Short-term corticosteroid (prednisone) treatment may be used in resistant cases. If this does not lead to improvement, treatment by sympathetic blockade may be used to provide pain relief and determine the extent to which the pain is sympathetically maintained. The latter mechanism, when present, might respond to the use of a α_1-adrenergic receptor antagonist (e.g., terazosin, phenoxybenzamine). Electrical neurostimulation of the spinal cord may also be considered. Neurostimulation not only may provide analgesia, but also may reduce the burning dysesthesia of which many patients complain. It may also improve circulation in the affected extremity by blocking the sympathetic efferent pathways.[38]

Phantom Limb Pain

Phantom limb pain, a type of neurologic pain, follows amputation of a limb or part of a limb.[40] Pain associated with the loss of a limb can fall into three categories: phantom limb pain, residual limb pain, and phantom limb sensations. It is estimated that up to 95% of all patients who have some form of limb loss will experience sensations in one of these categories.[40] The pain often begins as sensations of tingling, heat and cold, or heaviness, followed by burning, cramping, or shooting pain. It may disappear spontaneously or persist for many years and typically occurs within the first 6 months after the limb loss occurs.[40] One of the more troublesome aspects of phantom limb pain is that the person may experience painful sensations that were present before the amputation, such as that of a painful ulcer or bunion.

Several theories have been proposed as to the causes of phantom limb pain.[40] One theory is that the end of a regenerating nerve becomes trapped in the scar tissue of the amputation site. It is known that when a peripheral nerve is cut, the scar tissue that forms becomes a barrier to regenerating outgrowth of the axon, which often becomes trapped, forming a tangled growth (i.e., neuroma) of small-diameter axons, including nociceptive afferents and sympathetic efferents. It has been proposed that the afferents show increased sensitivity to innocuous mechanical stimuli and to sympathetic activity and circulating catecholamines. A related theory proposes that the source of phantom limb pain is in the spinal cord, suggesting that the pain is due to the spontaneous firing of spinal cord neurons that have lost their normal sensory input from the body. Another theory proposes that the phantom limb pain may be caused by changes in the flow of signals through somatosensory areas of the brain. Treatment of phantom limb pain has been accomplished by the use of sympathetic blocks, TENS of the large myelinated afferents innervating the area, hypnosis, and relaxation training.

SUMMARY CONCEPTS

- Pain may occur with or without an adequate stimulus, or it may be absent in the presence of an adequate stimulus—either of which describes a pain disorder. There may be *analgesia* (absence of pain), *hyperalgesia* (increased sensitivity to pain), *hypoalgesia* (a decreased sensitivity to painful stimuli), *hyperesthesia* (an abnormal increase in sensitivity to sensation), *hypoesthesia* (an abnormal decrease in sensitivity to sensations), or *allodynia* (pain produced by stimuli that do not normally cause pain).

- Neuropathic pain may be due to trauma or disease of neurons in a focal area or in a more global distribution (e.g., from endocrine disease or neurotoxic medications). *Neuralgia* is characterized by severe, brief, often repetitive attacks of lightninglike or throbbing pain that occurs along the distribution of a spinal or cranial nerve and usually is precipitated by stimulation of the cutaneous region supplied by that nerve. *Trigeminal neuralgia* is one of the most common and severe neuralgias. It is manifested by facial tics or spasms. *Postherpetic neuralgia* is a chronic pain that can occur after shingles, an infection of the dorsal root ganglia and corresponding areas of innervation by the varicella-zoster virus.

- Complex regional pain syndrome (CRPS) types I and II are pain syndromes characterized by severe pain or hyperalgesia, edema, changes in skin blood flow, and abnormal sensorimotor activity that typically follow an initiating traumatic event. The primary difference between CRPS I and II is the identification of a definable nerve injury, with type I occurring in the area of an initiating injury, and type II not necessarily limited to the distribution of the injured nerve.

- Phantom limb pain follows amputation of a limb or part of a limb. The pain sensations, which may disappear spontaneously or persist for many years, can be similar to those that were present before the amputation, as though the limb were still present.

Headache and Associated Pain

Although head and facial pain have characteristics that distinguish them from other pain disorders, they also share many of the same features.

Headache

Headache is a common health problem, with approximately 25% of adults reporting recurrent headaches and 4% reporting daily or nearly daily headaches.[41] Headache is caused by a number of conditions. Some headaches represent primary disorders and others occur secondary to other disease conditions in which head pain is a symptom. In 2004, the International Headache Society (IHS) published the second edition of *The International Classification of Headache Disorders* (ICHD-2). The classification system is divided into three sections: (1) primary headaches, (2) headaches secondary to other medical conditions, and (3) cranial neuralgias and facial pain.[42,43] The most common types of primary or chronic headaches are migraine headache, tension-type headache, cluster headache, and chronic daily headache.

Although most causes of secondary headache are benign, some are indications of serious disorders such as meningitis, brain tumor, or cerebral aneurysm. The sudden onset of a severe, intractable headache in an otherwise healthy person is more likely to be due to a serious intracranial disorder, as are headaches that disturb sleep, headaches prompted by exertion, and headaches accompanied by neurologic symptoms such as drowsiness, visual or limb disturbances, or altered mental status. Other indications of secondary headache disorder include a fundamental change or progression in headache pattern or a new headache in individuals younger than 5 or older than 50 years of age, or in individuals with cancer, immunosuppression, or pregnancy.[41]

The diagnosis and classification of headaches requires a comprehensive history and physical examination to exclude secondary causes. The history should include factors that precipitate headache, such as foods and food additives, missed meals, and association with the menstrual period. A careful medication history is essential because many medications can provoke or aggravate headaches. Alcohol also can cause or aggravate headache. A headache diary in which the person records his or her headaches and concurrent or antecedent events may be helpful in identifying factors that contribute to headache onset. Appropriate laboratory and imaging studies of the brain may be done to rule out secondary headaches.

Migraine Headache

Migraine headaches affect approximately 20 million persons in the United States. They occur in about 18% of women and 6% of men and result in considerable time lost from work and other activities.[44] Migraine headaches tend to run in families and are thought to be inherited as an autosomal dominant trait with incomplete penetrance.

There are two major types of migraine headache—migraine without aura and migraine with aura. *Migraine without aura*, which accounts for approximately 85% of migraines, is a pulsatile, throbbing, unilateral headache that typically lasts 1 to 2 days and is aggravated by routine physical activity. The headache is accompanied by nausea and vomiting, which often is disabling, and sensitivity to light and sound. Visual disturbances occur quite commonly and consist of visual hallucinations such as stars, sparks, and flashes of light.[43] *Migraine with aura* has similar symptoms, but is preceded by a sensory experience called an *aura*. It typically consists of visual symptoms, including flickering lights, spots, or loss of vision; sensory symptoms, including feeling of pins or needles, or numbness; and speech disturbances or other neurologic symptoms. These symptoms precede the headache, developing over a period of 5 to 20 minutes, and last from 5 minutes to 1 hour.[43] Although only a small percentage of persons with migraine experience an aura before an attack, many persons without aura have prodromal symptoms, such as fatigue and irritability, that precede the attack by hours or even days.

A retinal migraine is a rare form of migraine characterized by recurrent attacks of fully reversible scintillations (visual sensation of sparks or flashes of light), scotomata (visual blind spots), or blindness affecting one eye, followed within an hour by a headache. Migraines can also be chronic, occurring on 15 or more days per month for 3 months or more, in the absence of medication overuse. Migraine headache also can present as a mixed headache, including symptoms typically associated with tension-type or sinus headaches. These are called *transformed migraine* and are difficult to classify.

Migraine headaches occur in children as well as adults.[45,46] Before puberty, migraine headaches are equally distributed between the sexes. The essential diagnostic criterion for migraine in children is the presence of recurrent headaches separated by pain-free periods. Diagnosis is based on at least three of the following symptoms or associated findings: abdominal pain, nausea or vomiting, throbbing headache, unilateral location, associated aura (visual, sensory, motor), relief during sleep, and a positive family history.[46] Symptoms vary widely among children, from those that interrupt activities and cause the child to seek relief in a dark environment to those detectable only by direct questioning. A common feature of migraine in children is intense nausea and vomiting. The vomiting may be associated with abdominal pain and fever; thus, migraine may be confused with other conditions such as appendicitis. More than half of children with migraine undergo spontaneous prolonged remission after their 10th birthday. Because headaches in children can be a symptom of other, more serious disorders, including intracranial lesions, it is important that other causes of headache that require immediate treatment be ruled out.

The pathophysiologic mechanisms of the pain associated with migraine headaches remain poorly understood. Although many alternative theories exist, it is well established that during a migraine the trigeminal cranial nerve (CN V) becomes activated.[47] This may lead to the release of neuropeptides, causing painful neurogenic inflammation within the meningeal vasculature characterized by plasma protein extravasation, vasodilation, and mast cell degranulation. Another possible mechanism implicates neurogenic vasodilation of meningeal blood vessels as a key component of the inflammatory processes that occur during migraine. Supporting the neurogenic basis for migraine is the frequent presence of premonitory symptoms before the headache begins; the presence of focal neurologic disturbances, which cannot be explained in terms of cerebral blood flow; and the numerous accompanying symptoms, including those related to autonomic and somatic nervous system dysfunction.

Fluctuations in hormone levels, particularly in estrogen levels, are thought to play a role in the pattern of migraine attacks. For many women, migraine headaches coincide with their menstrual periods. Dietary substances, such as monosodium glutamate, aged cheese, and chocolate, also may precipitate migraine headaches. The actual triggers for migraine are the chemicals in the food, not allergens.

The treatment of migraine headaches includes preventive and abortive nonpharmacologic and pharmacologic treatment.[48] Nonpharmacologic treatment includes the avoidance of migraine triggers, such as foods, that precipitate an attack. Many persons with migraines benefit from maintaining regular eating and sleeping habits. Measures to control stress, which also can precipitate an attack, also are important. During an attack, many persons find it helpful to retire to a quiet, darkened room until symptoms subside.

Pharmacologic treatment involves both abortive therapy for acute attacks and preventive therapy. A wide range of medications is used to treat the acute symptoms of migraine headache. First-line agents include aspirin and other NSAIDs (e.g., naproxen sodium, ibuprofen), combinations of acetaminophen, acetylsalicylic acid, and caffeine; serotonin (5-HT$_1$) receptor agonists (e.g., sumatriptan); ergotamine derivatives (e.g., dihydroergotamine); and antiemetic medications (e.g., ondansetron, metoclopramide). Non-oral routes of administration may be preferred in individuals who develop severe pain rapidly or on awakening, or in those with severe nausea and vomiting. Both sumatriptan and dihydroergotamine have been approved for intranasal administration. For intractable migraine headache, dihydroergotamine may be administered parenterally with an antiemetic or opioid analgesic.[49] Frequent use of abortive headache medications may cause rebound headache. Because of the risk of coronary vasospasm, the 5-HT$_1$ receptor agonists should not be given to persons with coronary artery disease. Ergotamine preparations can cause uterine contractions and should not be given to pregnant women. They also can cause vasospasm and should be used with caution in persons with peripheral arterial disease.

Preventive pharmacologic treatment may be necessary if migraine headaches become disabling, if they occur more than two or three times a month, if abortive treatment is being used more than two times a week, or if the individual has hemiplegic migraine, migraine with prolonged aura, or migrainous infarction.[48] In most cases, preventative treatment must be taken daily for months to years. First-line agents include β-adrenergic blocking medications (e.g., propranolol, atenolol), antidepressants (amitriptyline), and antiseizure medications (e.g., divalproex, valproic acid). When a decision to discontinue preventive therapy is made, the medications should be gradually withdrawn.

Cluster Headache

Cluster headaches are relatively uncommon headaches that occur in about 1 in 1000 individuals, affecting men (80% to 85%) more frequently than women with the typical age of onset between 20 to 40 years of age.[50] These headaches tend to occur in clusters over weeks or months, followed by a long, headache-free remission period. Cluster headache is a type of primary neurovascular headache that typically includes severe, unrelenting, unilateral pain located, in order of decreasing frequency, in the orbital, retro-orbital, temporal, supraorbital, and infraorbital regions.[50-52] The pain is of rapid onset, builds to a peak in approximately 10 to 15 minutes, and lasts for 15 to 180 minutes. The pain behind the eye radiates to the ipsilateral trigeminal nerve (e.g., temple, cheek, gum). The headache frequently is associated with one or more symptoms such as restlessness or agitation, conjunctival redness, lacrimation, nasal congestion, rhinorrhea, forehead and facial sweating, miosis, ptosis, and eyelid edema. Because of their location and associated symptoms, cluster headaches are often mistaken for sinus infections or dental problems.

The underlying pathophysiologic mechanisms of cluster headaches are not completely known. It is thought that heredity, through an autosomal dominant gene, plays some role in the pathogenesis of the headaches. The most likely pathophysiologic mechanisms include the interplay of vascular, neurogenic, metabolic, and humoral factors. The regulating centers in the hypothalamus are thought to play a role because of circadian biologic changes and neuroendocrine disturbances (e.g., changes in cortisol, prolactin, and testosterone) that are observed both in active periods and during clinical remission.

Because of the relatively short duration and self-limited nature of cluster headache, oral preparations typically take too long to reach therapeutic levels. The most effective treatments are those that act quickly (e.g., oxygen inhalation and subcutaneous sumatriptan). Intranasal lidocaine also may be effective.[51,52] Oxygen inhalation may be indicated for home use. Prophylactic medications for cluster headaches include ergotamine derivatives, verapamil (a calcium channel blocker), corticosteroids, and valproic acid. Deep-brain surgical neurostimulation is an experimental approach beginning to show promise in the elimination of cluster headaches.[51]

Tension-Type Headache

The most common type of headache is tension-type headache. Unlike migraine and cluster headaches, tension-type headache usually is not sufficiently severe that it interferes with daily activities. Tension-type headaches frequently are described as dull, aching, diffuse, nondescript headaches, occurring in a hatband distribution around the head, and not associated with nausea or vomiting or worsened by activity. They can be infrequent, episodic, or chronic.

The exact mechanisms of tension-type headache are not known and the hypotheses of causation are contradictory. One popular theory is that it results from sustained tension of the muscles of the scalp and neck. Another theory suggests that migraine headache may be transformed gradually into chronic tension-type headache. Oromandibular dysfunction, psychogenic stress, anxiety, and depression may contribute, and overuse of analgesics or caffeine may also be involved.[53]

Tension-type headaches often are more responsive to nonpharmacologic techniques, such as biofeedback, massage, acupuncture, relaxation, imagery, and physical therapy, than other types of headache. For persons with poor posture, a combination of range-of-motion exercises, relaxation, and posture improvement may be helpful.

The medications of choice for acute treatment of tension-type headaches are analgesics, including acetylsalicylic acid, NSAIDs, and acetaminophen.[53] Persons with infrequent tension-type headache usually self-medicate using over-the-counter analgesics to treat the acute pain, and do not require prophylactic medication. These agents should be used cautiously because rebound headaches can develop when the medications are taken regularly. Other medications, including the entire range of migraine medications, may be tried in refractory cases.

Chronic Daily Headache

The term *chronic daily headache* (CDH) is used to refer to headaches that occur 15 days or more a month, including those due to medication overuse.[54,55] Little is known about the prevalence and incidence of CDH. Diagnostic criteria for CDH are not provided in the IHS Classification System. The cause of CDH is unknown, although there are several hypotheses. They include transformed migraine headache, evolved tension-type headache, new daily persistent headache, and posttraumatic headache. In many persons, CDH retains certain characteristics of migraine, whereas in others it resembles chronic tension-type headache. Chronic daily headache may be associated with chronic and episodic tension-type headache. New daily persistent headache may have a fairly rapid onset, with no history of migraine, tension-type headache, trauma, or psychological stress. Although overuse of symptomatic medications (e.g., analgesics, ergotamine) has been related to CDH, there is a group of patients in whom CDH is unrelated to excessive use of medications.

For patients with CDH, a combination of pharmacologic and behavioral interventions may be necessary. As with tension-type headaches, nonpharmacologic techniques, such as biofeedback, massage, acupuncture, relaxation, imagery, and physical therapy, may be helpful. Measures to reduce or eliminate medication and caffeine overuse may be helpful. If the patient is abusing medications, the overuse must be managed before prophylactic agents will be effective. Most of the medications used for prevention of CDH have not been examined in well-designed, double-blind studies.

Temporomandibular Joint Pain

A common cause of head pain is temporomandibular joint (TMJ) syndrome. It usually is caused by an imbalance in joint movement because of poor bite, bruxism (i.e., teeth grinding), or joint problems such as inflammation, trauma, and degenerative changes.[56] The pain almost always is referred and commonly presents as facial muscle pain, headache, neck ache, or earache. Referred pain is aggravated by jaw function. Headache associated with this syndrome is common in adults and children and can cause chronic pain problems.

Treatment of TMJ pain is aimed at correcting the problem, and in some cases this may be difficult. The initial therapy for TMJ pain should be directed toward relief of pain and improvement in function. Pain relief often can be achieved with use of the NSAIDs. Muscle relaxants may be used when muscle spasm is a problem. In some cases, the selected application of heat or cold, or both, may provide relief. Referral to a dentist who is associated with a team of therapists, such as a psychologist, physical therapist, or pain specialist, may be indicated.

SUMMARY CONCEPTS

- Headache is a common disorder that is caused by a number of conditions. Some headaches represent primary disorders and others occur secondary to another disease state in which head pain is a symptom.

- Primary headache disorders include migraine headache, tension-type headache, cluster headache, and chronic daily headache.

- Although most causes of secondary headache are benign, some are indications of serious disorders such as meningitis, brain tumor, or ruptured cerebral aneurysm.

- Temporomandibular joint (TMJ) syndrome is one of the major causes of headaches. It usually is caused by an imbalance in joint movement because of poor bite, teeth grinding, or joint problems such as inflammation, trauma, and degenerative changes.

Pain in Children and Older Adults

Pain frequently is under-recognized and undertreated in both children and the elderly. In addition to the concern about the effects of analgesia on respiratory status and the potential for addiction to opioids, another obstacle to adequate pain management in children and the elderly is the myth that patients in these age groups feel less pain than other patients, and even if they feel significant pain, they do not remember it. Moreover, it can be extremely difficult to accurately assess the location and intensity of pain in very young children, who are cognitively immature, or in cognitively impaired elderly. Research during the past few decades has added a great deal to the body of knowledge about pain in children and the elderly.

Pain in Children

Human responsiveness to painful stimuli begins in the neonatal period and continues through the life span. Although the specific and localized behavioral reactions are less marked in newborns, they clearly perceive and remember pain, as demonstrated by their integrated physiologic responses, including protective or withdrawal reflexes, to nociceptive stimuli.[57-59] For example, newborns in the neonatal intensive care unit (NICU) demonstrate protective withdrawal responses to a heel stick after repeated episodes. In fact, a newborn's pain may be accentuated because descending inhibitory pathways to the dorsal horn are not as well developed at birth.[58] Furthermore, the newborn's dorsal horn neurons have a wider receptive field and lower excitatory threshold than those of older children. The recognition that untreated pain can lead to serious consequences has resulted in a more liberal use of opioids for treatment of pain in the newborn, particularly in the NICU.[59]

As infants and children mature cognitively and developmentally, their responses to pain become more complex. Children do feel pain and have been shown to reliably and accurately report pain at as young as 3 years of age.[59] Like newborns, they also remember pain, as evidenced in studies of children with cancer, whose distress during painful procedures increases over time without intervention.

Pain Assessment

To manage pain adequately, ongoing assessment of the presence of pain and response to treatment is essential.[58,59] Behavior is a useful sign, but can be misleading. A toddler may scream during an ear examination because of fear rather than pain, and a child with inadequately relieved cancer pain may withdraw from his or her surroundings. Some physiologic measures, such as heart rate, are convenient to measure and respond rapidly to brief nociceptive stimuli, but they are nonspecific. Investigators have devised a range of behavioral distress scales for infants and young children, mostly emphasizing the child's facial expressions, crying, and bodily movements.

Children 3 to 7 years of age become more articulate in describing the intensity, location, and severity of the pain. There are self-report measures for children of this age, including scales with faces of actual children or cartoon faces. With children 8 years of age or older, numeric scales (i.e., 1 to 10) and word graphic scales (i.e., "none," "a little," "most I have ever experienced") can be used. Another supplementary strategy for assessing a child's pain is to use a body outline and ask the child to indicate "where it hurts."

Pain Management

The management of children's pain basically falls into two categories: pharmacologic and nonpharmacologic. In terms of pharmacologic interventions, many of the analgesics used in adults can be used safely and effectively in children and adolescents. However, it is critical when using specific medications to determine that the medication has been approved for use with children and that it is dosed appropriately according to the child's weight and level of physiologic development. Age-related differences in physiologic functioning, notably in neonates, will affect drug action. Neonates have decreased fat and muscle and increased water, which increases the duration of action for some water-soluble drugs; neonates also have decreased concentration of plasma proteins (albumin and α_1-glycoprotein), which increases the unbound concentration of protein-bound drugs.[58] Neonates and infants also have decreased levels of the hepatic enzymes needed for metabolism of many analgesics. The levels of these hepatic enzymes quickly increase to adult levels in the first few months of life. Drug clearance in the 2- to 6-year-old age group is actually higher than adult levels because of the larger hepatic mass relative to body weight.[58,60] The renal excretion of drugs depends on renal blood flow, glomerular filtration rate, and tubular secretion, all of which are decreased in neonates, particularly premature neonates. Renal function reaches adult levels by 1 year of age.[58,60]

The overriding principle in all pediatric pain management is to treat each child's pain on an individual basis and to match the analgesic agent with the cause and intensity of pain.[60] A second principle involves maintaining the balance between the level of side effects and pain relief such that pain relief is obtained with as little opioid and sedation as possible. One strategy toward this end is to time the administration of analgesia so that a steady blood level is achieved and, as much as possible, pain is prevented. This requires that the child receive analgesia on a regular dosing schedule, not "as needed." Also, most drugs are packaged primarily for adult use, and dose calculations and serial dilutions may predispose to medication errors. Common errors include milligram–microgram errors, decimal point errors, confusion between daily dose and fractional dose (e.g., 100 mg/kg/d divided by 6 hours versus 100 mg/kg per dose every 6 hours), and dilution errors.[60]

Nonpharmacologic strategies can be very effective in reducing the overall amount of pain and amount of analgesia used. In addition, some nonpharmacologic strategies can reduce anxiety and increase the child's level of self-control during pain. Pacifiers and sucrose are being used in the NICU. The effects of sucrose (sweet taste) are believed to be opioid mediated because its effects are reversed by naloxone (an opioid antagonist).[59]

Distraction helps children of any age divert their attention away from pain and onto other activities. Common attention diverters include bubbles, music, television, conversation, and games. Relaxation techniques and massage therapy are particularly useful in children with chronic pain. Other nonpharmacologic techniques can be taught to the child to provide psychological preparation for a painful procedure or surgery. These include positive self-talk, imagery, play therapy, modeling, and rehearsal. The nonpharmacologic interventions must be developmentally appropriate and, if possible, the child and parent should be taught these techniques when the child is not in pain (e.g., before surgery or a painful procedure) so that it is easier to practice the technique.

 Pain in Older Adults

Among adults, the prevalence of pain in the general population increases with age. Prevalence reports for persistent pain in older adults ranges from 25% to 80%, depending on whether the older adults are community dwelling or reside in a nursing home.[61] Among the common causes of pain in older adults are musculoskeletal disorders such as osteoarthritis and chronic low back pain; rheumatologic diseases such as rheumatoid arthritis and polymyalgia rheumatica; and neurologic conditions such as diabetic neuropathy, postherpetic neuralgia, and central post-stroke pain.

Unrelieved pain can have significant functional, cognitive, emotional, and societal effects in the elderly.[61,62] Decreased activity because of pain can lead to myofascial deconditioning and gait disturbances, which in turn can result in injuries from falls. Pain in the elderly has been associated with impaired appetite, increased sleep disturbances, and in some cases a decrease in cognitive function. These consequences can lead to less than optimal participation in rehabilitation efforts and decreased quality of life. Increased costs because of health care use have also been attributed to unrelieved pain in the elderly.

Pain Assessment

The assessment of pain in the elderly can range from relatively simple in a well-informed, alert, cognitively intact individual with pain from a single source and no comorbidities to extraordinarily difficult in a frail individual with severe dementia and many concurrent health problems.[61,63,64] When possible, a patient's report of pain is the gold standard, but behavioral signs of pain should be considered as well. Accurately diagnosing pain when the individual has many health problems or some decline in cognitive function can be particularly challenging. In recent years, there has been increased awareness of the need to address issues of pain in individuals with dementia. The Assessment for Discomfort in Dementia Protocol is one example of the efforts to improve assessment and pain management in these individuals. It includes behavioral criteria for assessing pain and recommended interventions for pain. Its use has been shown to improve pain management.[65]

Pain Management

When prescribing pharmacologic and nonpharmacologic methods of pain management for the older population, care must be taken to consider the cause of the pain, the person's health status, concurrent therapies, and mental status. In the older population, where the risk of adverse reaction to drugs is higher, the nonpharmacologic options are usually less costly and cause fewer side effects.

Common nonpharmacologic interventions include application of cold (which suppresses the release of products from tissue damage) and heat (which promotes the release of endogenous endorphins).[66] The role of mental focus and anxiety is important, and relaxation techniques, massage, and biofeedback may be useful. Physical therapy and occupational therapy bring a variety of modalities, including the use of braces or splints, changes in biomechanics, and exercise, all of which have been shown to promote pain relief.[65]

Although efficacy is important when considering the use of pharmacologic agents for pain relief in the elderly, safety must also be considered. The elderly may have physiologic changes that affect the pharmacokinetics of medications prescribed for pain management. These changes include decreased blood flow to organs, delayed gastric motility, reduced kidney function, and decreased albumin related to poor nutrition.[66] Also, the elderly often have coexisting health problems requiring medications. On average, a 70-year-old takes seven different medications.[66] The addition of analgesics to a complex medication regimen may cause drug interactions and complicate compliance; however, these considerations should not preclude the appropriate use of analgesic drugs to achieve pain relief. Non-opioids are generally the first line of therapy for mild to moderate pain, and acetaminophen is usually the first choice because it is relatively safe for older adults.[66] Opioids are used for more severe pain and for palliative care. As with younger persons, adjuvant analgesics are effectively used for treatment of pain in older adults. The use of some assessment tool to evaluate the level of pain and effectiveness of treatment is essential. Monitoring for side effects is also critical.

SUMMARY CONCEPTS

■ Children experience and remember pain, and even fairly young children are able to accurately and reliably report their pain. Recognition of this has changed the clinical practice of health professionals involved in the assessment of children's pain. Pharmacologic (including opioids) and nonpharmacologic pain management interventions have been shown to be effective in children. Nonpharmacologic techniques must be based on the developmental level of the child and should be taught to both children and parents.

■ Pain is a common symptom in the elderly. Assessment, diagnosis, and treatment of pain in the elderly can be complicated. The elderly may be reluctant or cognitively unable to report their pain. Diagnosis and treatment can be complicated by comorbidities and age-related changes in cognitive and physiologic function.

REVIEW EXERCISES

1. A 25-year-old man is admitted to the emergency department with acute abdominal pain that began in the epigastric area and has now shifted to the lower right quadrant of the abdomen. There is localized tenderness and guarding or spasm of the muscle over the area. His heart rate and blood pressure are elevated, and his skin is moist and cool from perspiring. He is given a tentative diagnosis of appendicitis and referred for surgical consultation.

   A. Describe the origin of the pain stimuli and the neural pathways involved in the pain that this man is experiencing.
   B. Explain the neural mechanisms involved in the spasm of the overlying abdominal muscles.
   C. What is the significance of his cool, moist skin and increased heart rate and blood pressure?

2. A 65-year-old woman with breast cancer is receiving hospice care in her home. She is currently receiving a long-acting opioid analgesic supplemented with a short-acting combination opioid and nonnarcotic medication for breakthrough pain.

   A. Explain the difference between the mechanisms and treatment of acute and chronic pain.
   B. Describe the action of opioid drugs in the treatment of pain.
   C. Define the term *tolerance* as it refers to the use of opioids for treatment of pain.

3. A 42-year-old woman presents with sudden, stabbing-type facial pain that arises near the right side of her mouth and then shoots toward the right ear, eye, and nostril. She is holding her hand to protect her face because the pain is "triggered by touch, movement, and drafts." Her initial diagnosis is trigeminal neuralgia.

   A. Explain the distribution and mechanisms of the pain, particularly the triggering of the pain by stimuli applied to the skin.
   B. What are possible treatment methods for this woman?

4. A 21-year-old woman presents to the student health center with complaints of a throbbing pain on the left side of her head, nausea and vomiting, and extreme sensitivity to light, noise, and head movement. She also tells you she had a similar headache 3 months ago that lasted for 2 days, and she thinks she is developing migraine headaches like her mother. She is concerned because she has been unable to attend classes and has exams next week.

A. Are this woman's history and symptoms consistent with migraine headaches? Explain.

B. Use the distribution of the trigeminal nerve and the concept of neurogenic inflammation to explain this woman's symptoms.

5. A 48-year-old man presents with complaints of severe pain in his right foot after a crush injury. He reports that although he had his ankle pinned surgically, it still causes severe pain now, almost 1 year after injury. He states that he cannot stand to have the sheets touch his foot, and even wearing shoes is painful. His physician has diagnosed chronic regional pain syndrome type I.

A. Differentiate chronic regional pain syndrome type I from type II.

B. Explain the proposed theories of why this pain syndrome develops.

REFERENCES

1. Guyton A, Hall JE. *Textbook of Medical Physiology*. 12th ed. Philadelphia, PA: Elsevier Saunders; 2011:543–592.
2. Kandel ER, Schwartz JH, Jessell TM, et al. *Principles of Neural Science*. 5th ed. New York, NY: McGraw-Hill; 2013:449–555.
3. Vanderah TW. Pathophysiology of pain. *Med Clin North Am*. 2007;91:1–12.
4. Polomano RC, Dunwoody CJ, Krenzischek DA, et al. Perspectives on pain management in the 21st century. *J Perianesth Nurs*. 2008;25(1A):S4–S14.
5. Bonica JJ. History of pain concepts and pain theory. *Mt Sinai J Med*. 1991;58:191–202.
6. Melzack R, Wall PD. Pain mechanisms: a new theory. *Science*. 1965;150:971–979.
7. Melzack R. Evolution of the matrix theory of pain. The Prithvi Raz Lecture. Presented at the third World Conference Institute of Pain, Barcelona 2004. *Pain Pract*. 2005;5(2):85–94.
8. Garland EL. Pain processing in the human nervous system: a selective review of nociceptive and biobehavioral pathways. *Prim Care*. 2012;39:561–571.
9. Grady K, Severn A, Eldridge P. *Key Topics in Pain Medicine*. 3rd ed. United Kingdom, UK: Informa Healthcare; 2007.
10. D'Mello R, Dickenson AH. Spinal cord mechanisms of pain. *Br J Anesth*. 2008;101(1):8–16.
11. Ploner M, Gross J, Timmerman L, et al. Cortical representation of first and second pain sensation in humans. *Proc Natl Acad Sci U S A* 2002;99:12444–12448.
12. Fields HL, Heinricher MM, Mason P. Neurotransmitters in nociceptive modulatory circuits. *Annu Rev Neurosci*. 1991;14:219–245.
13. Stein C. Opioid receptors on peripheral sensory neurons. In: Machelska H, Stein C, eds. *Immune Mechanisms of Pain and Analgesia*. New York, NY: Kluwer Academic/Plenum; 2003:69–76.
14. Banafscheh RA, Conzen P, Azad SC. Pharmacology of peripheral opioid receptors. *Curr Opin Anaesthesiol*. 2011;24(4):408–413.
15. Sengupta JN. Visceral pain: the neurophysiological mechanism. In: Canning BJ, Spina D, eds. *Handbook of Experimental Pharmacology*. Berlin, Germany: Springer-Verlag; 2009:31–73.
16. Fink WA. The pathophysiology of acute pain. *Emerg Med Clin North Am*. 2005;23:277–284.
17. Turk DD, Okifuji A. Pain terms and taxonomies of pain. In: Fishman SM, Ballantyne JC, Rathmell JP, eds. *Bonica's Management of Pain*. 4th ed. Philadelphia, PA: Wolters Kluwer Health/Lippincott Williams & Wilkins; 2010.
18. Peterson-Felix S, Curatolo M. Neuroplasticity—an important factor in acute and chronic pain. *Swiss Med Wkly*. 2002;132:273–278.
19. Polomano RC, Rathwell JP, Krenzischeck DA, et al. Emerging trends and new approaches to acute pain management. *J Perianesth Nurs*. 2008;25(1A):S45–S53.
20. Irving GA, Squire PL. Medical evaluation of the chronic pain patient. In: Fishman SM, Ballantyne JC, Rathmell JP, eds. *Bonica's Management of Pain*. 4th ed. Philadelphia, PA: Wolters Kluwer Health/Lippincott Williams & Wilkins; 2010.
21. Hainline B. Chronic pain: physiologic, diagnostic, and management considerations. *Psychiatr Clin North Am*. 2005;28:713–735.
22. Canavero S, Bonicalzi V. *Central Pain Syndrome: Pathophysiology, Diagnosis and Management*. New York, NY: Cambridge University Press; 2011.
23. Rustoen T, Gaardsrud T, Leegaard M, et al. Nursing pain management: a qualitative interview study of patients with pain, hospitalized for cancer treatment. *Pain Manag Nurs*. 2009;10(1):48–55.
24. De Pinto M, Dunbar PJ, Edwards WT. Pain management. *Anesthesiol Clin*. 2006;24:19–37.
25. DeSancire PL, Quest TE. Management of cancer-related pain. *Emerg Med Clin North Am*. 2009;27:179–194.
26. World Health Organization. *Cancer Pain Relief with Guide to Opioid Availability*. Geneva, Switzerland: World Health Organization; 1996.
27. Katzung BG, Masters SB, Trevor AJ. *Basic and Clinical Pharmacology*. 12th ed. New York, NY: Lange Basic Science/McGraw-Hill Medical; 2012.
28. Maizels M, McCarberg B. Antidepressant and antiepileptic drugs for chronic non-cancer pain. *Am Fam Physician*. 2005;71:483–490.
29. Hauser W, Wolfe F, Tolle T, et al. The role of antidepressants in the management of fibromyalgia syndrome: a systematic review and meta analysis. *CNS Drugs*. 2012;26:297–307.
30. Zin CS, Nissen LM, Smith MT, et al. An update on the pharmacological management of post-herpetic neuralgia and painful diabetic neuropathy. *CNS Drugs*. 2008;22:417–442.
31. Campbell JN, Meyer RA. Mechanisms of neuropathic pain. *Neuron*. 2006;52:77–92.
32. Rozen TD. Trigeminal neuralgia and glossopharyngeal neuralgia. *Neurol Clin*. 2004;22:185–206.
33. Cruccu G, Truini A. Refractory trigeminal neuralgia: non-surgical treatment options. *CNS Drugs*. 2012;21:91–96.
34. Schmader K. Herpes zoster and postherpetic neuralgia in older adults. *Clin Geriatr Med*. 2007;23:615–632.
35. Kimberlin DW, Whitley RJ. Varicella-zoster vaccine for the prevention of herpes zoster. *N Engl J Med*. 2007;356:1338–1343.
36. Pham T, Lafforgue P. Reflex sympathetic dystrophy syndrome and neuromediators. *Joint Bone Spine*. 2003;70:12–17.

37. Campell J, Basbaum A, Dray A, et al. *Emerging Strategies for the Treatment of Neuropathic Pain.* Seattle, WA: IASP Publications; 2006.
38. Watts D, Kremer MJ. Complex regional pain syndrome: a review of diagnostics, pathophysiologic mechanisms and treatment implications for certified nurse anesthetists. *AANA J.* 2011;79:505–510.
39. Blaes F, Schmitz K, Tschernatsch M. Autoimmune etiology of chronic regional pain syndrome. *Neurology.* 2004;63:1734–1736.
40. Hsu E, Cohen SP. Postamputation pain: epidemiology, mechanisms and treatment. *J Pain Res.* 2013;6:121–136.
41. Kaniecki R. Headache assessment and management. *JAMA.* 2003;289:1430–1433.
42. Headache Classification Subcommittee of the International Headache Committee. The International Classification of Headache Disorders. 3rd ed. *Cephalalgia.* 2013;33(9):629–808.
43. Hainer BL, Matheson EM. Approach to acute headache in adults. *Am Fam Physician.* 2013;87:683–687.
44. Mathew NT. Pathophysiology, epidemiology, and impact of migraine. *Clin Cornerstone.* 2001;4:1–17.
45. Lewis DJ. Headaches in children and adolescents. *Am Fam Physician.* 2002;65:625–632.
46. Hershey AD. In: Behrman RE, Kliegman RM, Stanton B, et al., eds. *Nelson Textbook of Pediatrics.* 19th ed. Philadelphia, PA: Saunders Elsevier; 2011:2039–2046.
47. Tepper SJ, Rapoport A, Sheftell F. The pathophysiology of migraine. *Neurologist.* 2001;7:279–786.
48. Snow V, Weiss K, Wall EM, et al. Pharmacologic management of acute attacks of migraine and prevention of migraine headache. *Ann Intern Med.* 2002;137:840–849.
49. Cady RJ, Shade CL, Cady RK. Advances in drug development for acute migraine. *Drugs.* 2012;72:2187–2205.
50. Weaver-Agostoni J. Cluster headache. *Am Fam Physician.* 2013;88:123–128.
51. May A. Cluster headache: pathogenesis, diagnosis, and management. *Lancet.* 2005;366:843–855.
52. Beck E, Sieber WJ, Trejo R. Management of cluster headache. *Am Fam Physician.* 2005;71:717–728.
53. Millea PJ, Brodie JJ. Tension-type headache. *Am Fam Physician.* 2002;66:797–804.
54. Biondi DM. Chronic daily headache. *Clin Fam Pract.* 2005;7:463–491.
55. Maizels M. The patient with daily headaches. *Am Fam Physician.* 2004;70:2299–2306, 2313–2314.
56. Lobbezoo F. Topical review: new insights into the pathology and diagnosis of disorders of the temporomandibular joint. *J Orofac Pain.* 2004;18:181–191.
57. Howard RF. Current status of pain management in children. *JAMA.* 2003;290:2464–2469.
58. Brislin RP, Rose JB. Pediatric acute pain management. *Anesthesiol Clin North America.* 2005;23:789–814.
59. Zeltzer LK, Krane EJ. Pediatric pain management. In: Behrman RE, Kliegman RM, Stanton B, et al., eds. *Nelson Textbook of Pediatrics.* 19th ed. Philadelphia, PA: Saunders Elsevier; 2011:360–375.
60. Berde CB, Sethna NF. Analgesics for the treatment of pain in children. *N Engl J Med.* 2002;347:1094–1103.
61. Bruckenthal P. Assessment of pain in the elderly adult. *Clin Geriatr Med.* 2008;24:213–236.
62. Deane G, Smith HS. Overview of pain management in older persons. *Clin Geriatr Med.* 2008;24:185–201.
63. Kovach CR, Weissman DE, Griffie J, et al. Assessment and treatment of discomfort for people with late-stage dementia. *J Pain Symptom Manage.* 1999;18:412–419.
64. Hutt E, Pepper GA, Vojir C, et al. Assessing the appropriateness of pain medication prescribing practices in nursing homes. *J Am Geriatr Soc.* 2006;54:231–239.
65. Barkin RL, Barkin SJ, Barkin DS. Perception, assessment, treatment, and management of pain in the elderly. *Clin Geriatr Med.* 2005;21:465–490.
66. Katzung BG. Special aspects of geriatric pharmacology. In: Katzung H, ed. *Basic and Clinical Pharmacology.* 12th ed. New York, NY: Lange Medical Books/McGraw-Hill Medical; 2012:1061–1080.

Porth Essentials Resources

Explore these additional resources to enhance learning for this chapter:

- NCLEX-Style Questions and Other Resources on **thePoint**, http://thePoint.lww.com/PorthEssentials4e
- Study Guide for Essentials of Pathophysiology
- Adaptive Learning | Powered by PrepU, http://thepoint.lww.com/prepu

C h a p t e r **36**

Disorders of Neuromuscular Function

Just as our perceptual skills reflect the ability of our sensory systems to detect, analyze, and estimate the significance of our physical environment, the ability to carry out these movements requires skeletal muscles that contract and neural pathways that plan, coordinate, and execute them in a manner that provides for smooth, purposeful, and coordinated movement. In some cases, purposeless and disruptive movements can be almost as disabling as relative or complete absence of movement. This chapter provides an introduction to the organization and control of motor function, followed by a discussion of disorders of motor function, including muscular dystrophy, and disorders of the neuromuscular junction, peripheral nerves, the basal ganglia and cerebellum, and upper motor neurons.

Organization and Control of Motor Function

Motor function, whether it involves walking, running, or precise finger movements, requires movement and maintenance of posture. Posture can be described as the relative position of the various parts of the body with respect to one another (limb extension, flexion) or to the environment (standing, supine).[1] Posture also can be described as the active muscular resistance to the displacement of the body by gravity or acceleration. The structures that control posture and movement are located throughout the neuromuscular system. The system consists of the motor unit (motor neuron and the muscle fibers it innervates); the spinal cord, which contains the basic reflex circuitry for posture and movement; and the descending pathways from brain stem circuits, the cerebellum, the basal ganglia, and the motor cortex.

Organization of Movement

As with other parts of the nervous system, the motor systems are organized in a functional hierarchy, each concerned with increased levels of complexity.[2] The lowest level of the hierarchy occurs at the spinal cord, which contains the basic reflex circuitry needed to coordinate the function of the motor units. Above the spinal cord is the brain stem, and above the brain stem are the cerebellum and basal ganglia, structures that modulate the actions of the brain stem systems. Overseeing these supraspinal structures are the motor centers in the cerebral cortex. The highest level of function, which occurs at the level of the frontal cortex, is concerned with the purpose and planning of motor movements. The efficiency of movement depends on input from sensory systems that operate in parallel with the motor systems.

The Spinal Cord

The spinal cord is the lowest level of motor hierarchical organization.[2] It contains the neuronal circuits that mediate a variety of reflexes and automatic rhythmic movements. Similar circuits governing reflex movements of the face and mouth are located in the brain stem. The simplest circuits are monosynaptic, containing only a primary motor neuron. However, most reflexes are polysynaptic, involving more than one interposed interneurons. Interneurons and motor neurons also receive input from axons descending from higher centers. These supraspinal signals can modify reflex responses to peripheral stimuli by facilitating or inhibiting different populations of interneurons. They also coordinate movements through these interneurons.

The Brain Stem

The next level of motor hierarchy is in the brain stem. The brain stem contains many groups of neurons that project from the spinal gray matter. These projections are grouped into two main systems—the medial and lateral brain stem systems—which receive input from the cerebral cortex and subcortical nuclei and project to the spinal cord.[2] The medial descending systems contribute to the control of posture by integrating visual, vestibular, and somatosensory information. The lateral descending systems control more distal limb muscles and are thus more concerned with goal-directed movements, especially of the arm and hand. Brain stem circuits also control movements of the eyes and head.

The Motor Cortex

The motor cortex represents the highest level of motor function. Precise, skillful, and intentional movements of the distal and especially flexor muscles of the limbs and speech apparatus are initiated and controlled by the primary, premotor, and supplementary motor cortices located in the posterior part of the frontal lobe[1,3] (Fig. 36-1). These motor areas receive information from the thalamus and somatosensory cortex and, indirectly, from the cerebellum and basal ganglia.

The primary motor cortex (Brodman area 4) is located on the medial surface of the brain, and adjacent portions of the central sulcus. It controls specific muscle

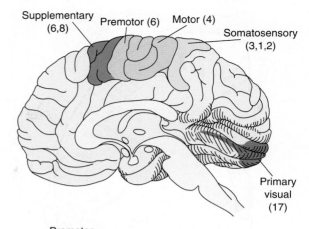

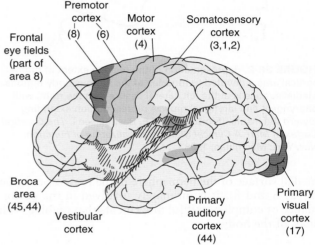

FIGURE 36-1. Primary motor cortex. (*Top*) The location of the primary, premotor, and supplementary cortex on the medial surface of the brain. (*Bottom*) The location of the primary and premotor cortex on the lateral surface of the brain.

movement sequences and is the first level of descending control for precise motor movements. The neurons in the primary motor cortex are arranged in a somatotopic array or distorted map of the body called the *motor homunculus*[4] (Fig. 36-2). The areas of the body that require the greatest dexterity have the largest cortical areas devoted to them. More than half of the primary motor cortex is concerned with controlling the muscles of the hands, of facial expression, and of speech.

The premotor cortex (areas 6 and 8), which is located just anterior to the primary motor cortex, sends some fibers into the corticospinal tract but mainly innervates the primary motor cortex. Nerve signals generated by the premotor cortex produce much more complex "patterns" of movement than the discrete patterns generated by the primary motor cortex. For example, the movement pattern to accomplish a particular objective, such as throwing a ball or picking up a fork, is programmed by the prefrontal association cortex and associated thalamic nuclei.

The supplementary motor cortex, which contains representations of all parts of the body, is located on the

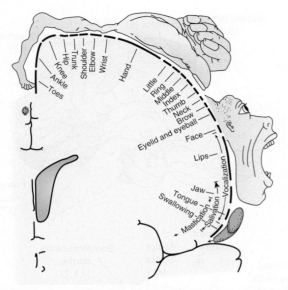

FIGURE 36-2. Representation of the relative extent of motor cortical area 4 devoted to muscles of the various body regions. Medial surface is at the left, lateral fissure is at the right, with pharyngeal and laryngeal muscle representation extending toward the insula. (From Penfield E, Rasmussen T. *The Cerebral Cortex in Man: A Clinical Study of Localization of Function.* New York: Macmillan; 1968.)

medial surface of the hemisphere in the premotor region (areas 6 and 8). It is intimately involved in the performance of complex, skillful movements that involve both sides of the body.

The Cerebellum and Basal Ganglia

In addition to the brain stem and cerebral cortex, the cerebellum and basal ganglia assist in the planning and execution of motor movements. They provide feedback circuits that regulate cortical and brain stem motor areas, and they receive indirect input from various areas of the motor cortex.[2] The cerebellum and basal ganglia do not send significant output directly to the spinal cord, but act on motor neurons in the brain stem.

Although the precise contributions of the cerebellum and basal ganglia are still unclear, both are necessary for smooth movement and posture. The basal ganglia provide the gracefulness of performance as well as the supportive posture for highly skilled movements. Cerebellar circuits are involved with the timing and coordination of movements that are in progress and with learning of motor skills. Damage to the cerebellum by vascular lesions of certain familial degenerative disorders produces cerebellar ataxia, a characteristic loss of coordination and accuracy of limb movement.

The Motor Unit

The motor neurons in the spinal cord represent the final pathway for integration of motor function.[2,3] Without the special neuronal circuits in the spinal cord, even the most complex motor control systems in the brain could not cause any purposeful muscle movement. Located in each segment of the anterior horn of the spinal cord are several thousand motor neurons called *lower motor neurons* (LMNs). Upper motor neurons (UMNs) control LMNs. They project from the motor strip in the cerebral cortex to the anterior horn of spinal cord and are fully contained in the central nervous system (CNS) (Fig. 36-3).

Motor neurons segregate into two major categories: *alpha* and *gamma.* The alpha motor neurons are large nerve fibers that innervate the extrafusal muscle fibers responsible for muscle contraction and force generation. The much-smaller gamma motor neurons innervate the intrafusal muscle fibers of the muscle spindles, which help control basic muscle tone (to be discussed under spinal reflexes). Each alpha motor neuron undergoes multiple branchings, making it possible for a single alpha motor neuron to innervate a few to thousands of muscle fibers. In general, large muscles—those containing hundreds or thousands of muscle fibers and providing gross motor movement—have large motor units. This contrasts sharply with those that control the hand, tongue, and eye movements, for which the motor units are small and permit very precise control.

The alpha motor neuron and the group of muscle fibers it innervates is called a *motor unit.* When an alpha motor neuron develops an action potential, all of the muscle fibers in the motor unit it innervates develop action potentials, causing them to contract simultaneously. Thus, a motor neuron and the muscle fibers it innervates function as a single unit—the basic unit of motor control.

Spinal Reflexes

The spinal cord contains neural reflexes or coordinated, involuntary motor responses that are initiated by a stimulus applied to peripheral receptors.[3,5] Some reflexes, such as the flexor-withdrawal reflex, initiate movements to avoid hazardous situations, whereas others, such as the stretch reflex or crossed-extensor reflex, serve to integrate motor movements so they function in a coordinated manner. The anatomic basis of a reflex consists of an afferent neuron that synapses either directly with an effector neuron that innervates a muscle or with an interneuron that synapses with an effector neuron. Reflexes are essentially "wired into" the CNS so that they are always ready to function. With training, most reflexes can be modified to become part of more complicated movements. A reflex may involve neurons in a single cord segment (i.e., segmental reflexes), several or many segments (i.e., intersegmental reflexes), or structures in the brain (i.e., suprasegmental reflexes).

In most cases, reflex activities go on without our conscious awareness. There is a significant amount of reflex circuitry in the spinal cord for the coordinated control of movements, particularly stereotyped movements concerned with locomotion. Many of these reflexes work equally well in decerebrate animals (those in which the brain has been destroyed) as long as the spinal cord is intact. Other spinal reflexes require the activity of the brain for their successful completion.

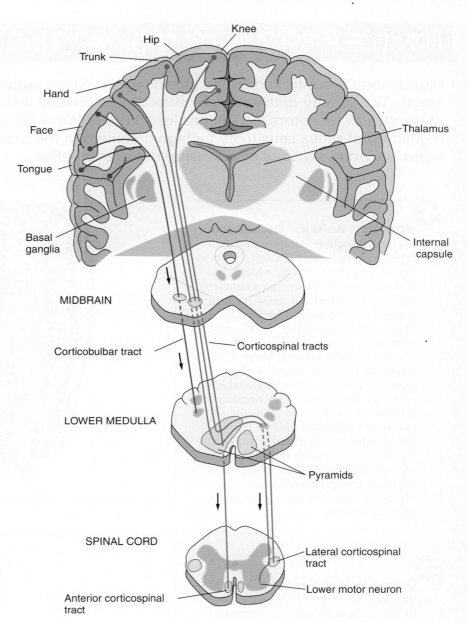

FIGURE 36-3. Upper motor neuron pathways: corticospinal (*red*) and corticobulbar tracts (*blue*). (Modified from Bickley LS. *Bates' Guide to Physical Examination and History Taking.* 8th ed. Philadelphia, PA: Lippincott Williams & Wilkins; 2003:543.)

If the skeletal muscles of the body are to perform normally, the brain must be continually informed of the current state of contraction, and the muscles must exhibit healthy tone (resistance to active and passive stretch at rest). The first requirement depends on the transmission of information regarding the sense of body position, movement, and muscle tone to the CNS. Information from sensory afferent neurons is relayed to the cerebellum and cerebral cortex and is experienced as *proprioception* or the sense of body movement and position, independent of vision. To provide this information, the muscles and their tendons are supplied with two types of receptors: muscle spindles and Golgi tendon organs. The *muscle spindles*, which are distributed throughout the belly of a muscle, relay information about muscle length and rate of stretch. The *Golgi tendon organs* are found in muscle tendons and transmit information

about muscle tension or force of contraction at the junction of the muscle and the tendon that attaches to bone.

Muscle Spindle and the Stretch Reflex. The muscle spindles consist of a group of specialized miniature skeletal muscle fibers called *intrafusal fibers* that are encased in a connective tissue capsule and attached to the extrafusal fibers of a skeletal muscle. In the center of the receptor area, a large sensory neuron spirals around the intrafusal fiber, forming the so-called *primary* or *annulospiral ending* (see Understanding the Stretch Reflex and Muscle Tone).

The intrafusal muscle fibers function as stretch receptors that increase their firing when the muscle is stretched and decrease their firing when the muscle is relaxed.[3] Axons of these spindle fiber neurons enter the spinal cord through several branches of the dorsal root. Some

(*text continues on page 886*)

UNDERSTANDING ➡ The Stretch Reflex

Muscle tone is controlled by the stretch reflex, which monitors changes in muscle length. The activity of the stretch reflex can be divided into three steps: (1) activation of the stretch receptors, (2) integration of the reflex in the spinal cord, and (3) regulation of reflex sensitivity by higher centers in the brain. Testing the (4) knee-jerk reflex provides a means of assessing the stretch reflex.

①

Stretch Reflex Receptors. Skeletal muscle is composed of two types of muscle fibers: a large number of extrafusal fibers, which control muscle movement, and a smaller number of intrafusal fibers, which control muscle tone. The intrafusal fibers are encapsulated in sheaths, forming a muscle spindle that runs parallel to the extrafusal fibers. Each intrafusal fiber is innervated by a large Ia sensory nerve fiber, which encircles the central noncontractile portion of the fiber to form the so-called *annulospiral ending*. Because the spindles are oriented parallel to the extrafusal muscle fibers, stretching of the extrafusal fibers also stretches the spindle fibers and stimulates the receptive endings of the Ia afferent neuron.

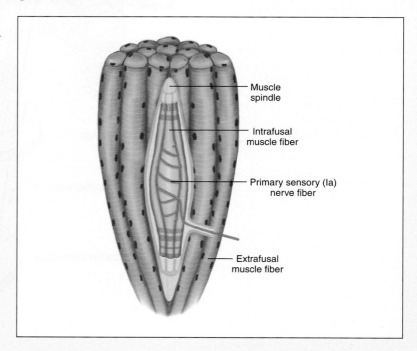

Muscle spindle

Intrafusal muscle fiber

Primary sensory (Ia) nerve fiber

Extrafusal muscle fiber

②

Spinal Reflex Centers. Afferent impulses from the Ia sensory fiber of the muscle spindle are transmitted to the spinal cord, where they synapse with α motor neurons of the stretched muscle to form a monosynaptic reflex arc. They are "monosynaptic" because only one synapse separates the primary sensory input from the motor neuron output. The reflex muscle contraction that follows resists further stretching of the muscle. As this spinal reflex activity is occurring, impulses providing information on muscle length are transmitted to higher centers in the brain. It is the coordinated activity of all the monosynaptic reflexes supplying the extrafusal fibers in a skeletal muscle that provides the muscle tone needed for organized movement.

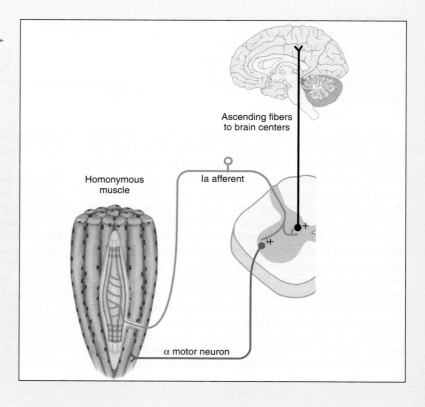

Homonymous muscle

Ascending fibers to brain centers

Ia afferent

α motor neuron

and Muscle Tone

3

Brain Center Connections. Although a spinal reflex can function independently, its sensitivity is adjusted by higher centers in the brain. Both types of muscle fibers are supplied with motor neurons—the extrafusal fibers with large alpha motor neurons, which produce muscle contraction; and the intrafusal fibers with smaller gamma motor neurons, which control the sensitivity of the stretch reflex. Descending fibers of motor pathways synapse with both alpha and gamma motor neurons, and the impulses are sent simultaneously to the large extrafusal fibers and to the intrafusal fibers to maintain muscle spindle tension (and sensitivity) during muscle contraction.

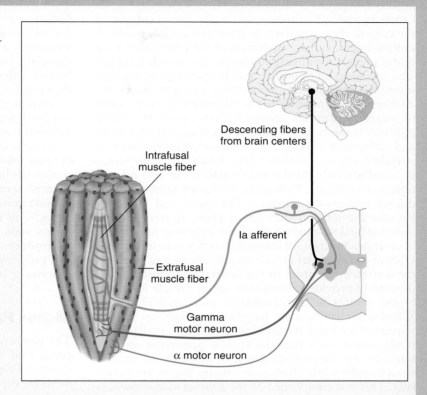

4

The Knee-Jerk Reflex. The knee-jerk reflex that occurs when the knee is tapped with a reflex hammer tests for the intactness of the stretch reflex arc in the quadriceps muscle. Stretching of the extrafusal fibers by tapping with a reflex hammer leads to lengthening of the intrafusal fibers and increased firing of the type Ia afferent neuron. Impulses from the Ia fiber enter the dorsal horn of the spinal cord and make monosynaptic contact with the anterior horn alpha motor neuron supplying the extrafusal fibers in the quadriceps muscle. The resultant reflex contraction (shortening) of the quadriceps muscle is responsible for the knee jerk. These muscle reflexes are called *deep tendon reflexes* (DTRs). They can be checked at the wrists, elbows, knees, and ankles as a means of assessing the components of the stretch reflex at different spinal cord segments.

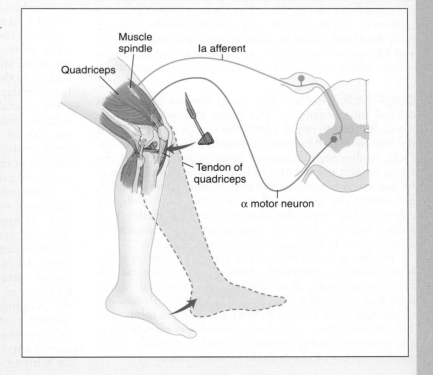

(text continued from page 883)

branches end in the segment of entry; others ascend to adjacent segments, influencing intersegmental reflex function; and still others ascend in the dorsal column of the cord to the brain stem. Segmental branches establish monosynaptic contact with each of the LMNs that have motor units in the muscle containing the spindle receptor. This produces an opposing muscle contraction. Another segmental branch of the same afferent neuron innervates an internuncial neuron that is inhibitory to motor units of antagonistic muscle groups. This disynaptic inhibitory pathway is the basis for the reciprocal activity of agonist and antagonist muscles (i.e., when an agonist muscle is stretched, the antagonists relax). Reciprocal innervation is useful not only for the stretch reflex, but also for voluntary movements. Relaxation of the antagonist muscle during movements enhances the speed and efficiency because the muscles that act as prime movers are not working against contraction of the opposing muscle.[1]

Another function of the stretch reflex is to inform the CNS of the status of muscle length. Ascending impulses from stretch receptors in the contracting muscle fibers ultimately provide information about muscle length to higher centers in the cerebellum and cerebral cortex. When a skeletal muscle lengthens or shortens against tension, a feedback mechanism needs to be available for readjustment such that the spindle apparatus remains sensitive to moment-to-moment changes in muscle stretch, even while changes in muscle length are occurring. This is accomplished by the *gamma motor neurons* that adjust spindle fiber length to match the length of the extrafusal muscle fiber. Descending fibers of motor pathways synapse with and simultaneously activate both the alpha motor neurons of the contracting muscle and gamma motor neurons so that the sensitivity of the spindle fibers is coordinated with muscle movement.

Golgi Tendon Reflex. The Golgi tendon organ helps control muscle tension. The major difference between the Golgi tendon organ versus the muscle spindle is that the muscle spindle monitors muscle length whereas the Golgi tendon organ monitors muscle tension.[3] When the Golgi tendon organs of a muscle tendon are stimulated by increased tension in the contracting muscle, signals are sent to the spinal cord to cause reflexive inhibitory effects in the respective muscle. Thus, this reflex provides a negative feedback mechanism that prevents the development of too much tension in the muscle.

Another possible function of the Golgi tendon reflex is to equalize contractile forces of separate muscle fibers by inhibiting those fibers that exert excessive tension and permitting those that exert too little tension to become more excited by withdrawing the inhibition. This spreads the muscle load over all the muscle fibers and prevents damage to isolated areas of a muscle where small numbers of fibers might be overloaded.

Central Control of the Spinal Reflexes. Normal muscle tone depends on stretch reflexes initiated by the muscle spindles, which monitor changes in muscle length; and the Golgi tendon organs, which monitor muscle tension. The neural circuits responsible for stretch reflexes provide higher centers of the nervous system with a mechanism for adjusting muscle tone. Disorders of muscle tone are frequently associated with lesions of the motor system, especially those that interfere with descending pathways. Stretch reflexes are hyperactive when lesions of the corticospinal tract (e.g., stroke or spinal cord injury) reduce or disrupt the inhibitory effect of the brain on the spinal cord, and they are hypoactive or absent in cases of peripheral nerve damage or anterior spinal cord injury.

Central control over the gamma motor neurons also permits increases or decreases in muscle tone in anticipation of changes in the muscle force. Through its coordinated control of the muscle's alpha and the spindle's gamma motor neurons, the CNS can suppress the stretch reflex. This occurs during centrally programmed movements, such as pitching a baseball, that require a muscle to produce a full range of unopposed motion. Without this programmed adjustability of the stretch reflex, any movement is immediately opposed and prevented.

Motor Pathways

The primary motor cortex (Brodman area 4) is structured into six well-defined layers. Those in layers I through IV project to the premotor and somatosensory areas on the same side of the brain, the opposite side of the brain, or to subcortical structures such as the thalamus and basal ganglia. Efferent motor neurons in layers V and VI descend to the brain stem and spinal cord. The axons of these UMNs project through the subcortical white matter and internal capsule to the deep surface of the brain stem, through the ventral bulge of the pons, and on to the ventral surface of the medulla, where they form a ridge or pyramid (see Fig. 36-3). The majority of corticospinal UMNs cross the midline in the pyramidal ridge to form the lateral corticospinal tract on the opposite side of the spinal cord. The remaining UMNs do not cross to the opposite side, but pass down the ventral column of the cord, mainly to cervical levels, where they cross and innervate contralateral LMNs.

Traditionally, motor tracts have been classified as belonging to one of two motor systems: the pyramidal and extrapyramidal systems. According to this classification system, the *pyramidal* system consists of the motor neurons that cross the midline in the pyramidal ridge. All other descending UMNs emanating from the motor cortex and basal ganglia are generally grouped together as the *extrapyramidal system*. Disorders of the pyramidal tracts (e.g., stroke) are characterized by spasticity and paralysis, whereas those affecting the extrapyramidal tracts (e.g., Parkinson disease) result in involuntary movements, muscle rigidity, and immobility without paralysis. As increased knowledge regarding motor pathways has emerged, it has become evident that the extrapyramidal and pyramidal systems are extensively interconnected and cooperate in the control of movement.[1]

Assessment of Motor Function

Disorders of the motor system produce signs and symptoms that can be used in localizing the disorder. These include changes in muscle characteristics (strength, bulk, and tone), spinal reflex activity, and motor coordination.[6] The distinction between LMNs and UMNs is important because each class of neurons produces distinctive symptoms.

Muscle Strength, Bulk, and Tone

Muscle Strength. Abnormalities in any part of the motor pathway can produce impaired strength or muscle weakness. *Paralysis* refers to loss of movement, and *paresis* to weakness or incomplete loss of strength. The pattern of weakness may be helpful in the localization of the lesion. *Monoparesis* or *monoplegia* results from the destruction of pyramidal UMN innervation of one limb; *hemiparesis* or *hemiplegia,* both limbs on one side; *diparesis* or *diplegia* or *paraparesis* or *paraplegia,* both upper or lower limbs; and *tetraparesis* or *tetraplegia,* also called *quadriparesis* or *quadriplegia,* all four limbs (Fig. 36-4).

Paresis or paralysis can be further designated as of UMN or LMN origin. UMN lesions of the motor cortex or corticospinal tract typically affect the flexors in the upper extremities more than the extensors, whereas in the lower extremities, the flexors are more affected. In LMN or peripheral nerve disorders, the weakness is predominantly in the distal limb, whereas in muscle disorders, such as muscular dystrophy, proximal limb function may be affected sooner than distal limb function.

Muscle Bulk. The size of muscle (whether muscles are normal sized, enlarged, or atrophied) also helps localize the lesion, and sometimes provides helpful hints to the pathologic process. Muscular atrophy, or loss of muscle bulk, usually results from LMN lesions as well as diseases of the muscles themselves. Hypertrophy refers to an increase in muscle bulk with a proportionate increase in strength. Pseudohypertrophy, as occurs with Duchenne muscular dystrophy, refers to an increase in bulk without an accompanying increase in strength.

Muscle Tone. Muscle tone is the normal state of muscle tension. It is assessed by palpating the muscle while at rest and during passive stretching. With the person at rest, the joints are put through the normal range of motion (flexion and extension) by the examiner. Disorders of skeletal muscle tone are characteristic of many nervous system lesions. Any interruption of the myotatic or stretch reflex circuitry by peripheral nerve injury, pathologic process of the neuromuscular junction, injury to the spinal cord, or damage to the corticospinal system can result in disturbances of muscle tone.

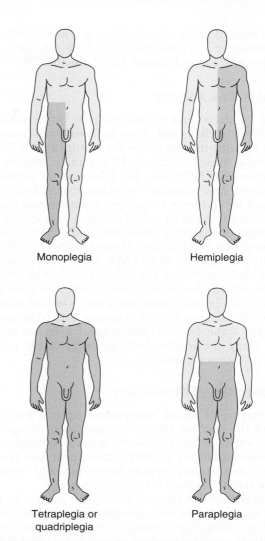

FIGURE 36-4. Areas of the body affected by monoplegia, hemiplegia, tetraplegia or quadriplegia, and paraplegia. The *shaded area* shows the extent of motor and sensory loss. (From Hickey JV. *The Clinical Practice of Neurological and Neurosurgical Nursing.* 3rd ed. Philadelphia, PA: J.B. Lippincott; 1997.)

Abnormalities of muscle tone may be described as hypotonia (less than normal), flaccidity (absent), or hypertonia, rigidity, spasticity, or tetany (all indicating higher-than-normal tone). Typically, UMN lesions produce increased tone, whereas LMN lesions produce decreased tone. Increased resistance that varies and commonly becomes worse at the extremes of the range of motion is called *spasticity.* Resistance that becomes worse throughout the range and in both directions is referred to as *lead-pipe rigidity.* Decreased resistance suggests disease of the LMNs or the acute stages of spinal cord injury. Marked floppiness indicates hypotonic or flaccid muscles.

Fasciculations. Fasciculations are visible squirming and twitching movements of muscle fibers that can be seen as flickers under the skin.[7] They are caused by spontaneous contractions of all the muscle fibers in a motor unit due to irritation and hyperexcitability of the cell body and its motor neuron, and suggest LMN disease.

Spinal Reflex Activity

Testing of deep tendon reflexes (see Understanding the Stretch Reflex and Muscle Tone) can provide important information about the status of the CNS in controlling muscle function. Hyperactive reflexes are suggestive of a UMN disorder. *Clonus* is the rhythmic contraction and alternate relaxation of a limb that is caused by suddenly stretching a muscle and gently maintaining it in the stretched position. It is seen in the hypertonia of spasticity associated with UMN lesions, such as spinal cord injury. *Hyporeflexia* or *areflexia* suggests the presence of an LMN lesion. The distribution of abnormality in the reflexes is also helpful in determining the location of the lesion. For example, hyperreflexia in both lower extremities would suggest a lesion in the spinal cord, whereas hyperreflexia on one side of the body would suggest a lesion in the UMN along the motor pathway (e.g., in the motor cortex or internal capsule).

Coordination of Movement

Coordination of muscle movement requires that four areas of the nervous system function in an integrated manner—the motor system for muscle strength, the cerebellar system for rhythmic movement and steady posture, the vestibular system for posture and balance, and the sensory system for position sense.

In cerebellar disease, one movement cannot be followed quickly by its opposite movement. Movements are slow, irregular, clumsy, unsteady, and inappropriately varying in their speed, force, and direction. *Dysdiadochokinesia* is the failure to accurately perform rapid alternating movements. *Ataxia* is a term used to describe a wide-based, unsteady gait. *Dysmetria* is a term used to describe inaccuracies of movements leading to a failure to reach a specified target. This can be tested by having the person touch the examiner's finger and then alternately touch his or her own finger. These movements are normally smooth and accurate. Asking the person to touch the examiner's finger with an outstretched arm and finger, first with the eyes open and then closed, provides a test for position sense. Repetitive and consistent deviation to one side (referred to as past pointing), which is worse with the eyes closed, suggests cerebellar or vestibular disease.

Chorea (abnormal writhing movements), *dystonia* (abnormal simultaneous contractions of agonist and antagonist muscles, leading to abnormal postures), *tremor* (rhythmic movements of a particular body part), *bradykinesia* (slowness of movements), and *myoclonus* (involuntary jerking movement) indicate abnormalities in the basal ganglia, although the exact localization may be difficult to determine.

SUMMARY CONCEPTS

■ Motor function, whether it involves walking, running, or precise finger movements, requires functioning neural pathways consisting of upper motor neurons (UMNs) that project from the motor cortex to the brain stem or spinal cord, where they innervate the lower motor neurons (LMNs) of the contracting muscles.

■ Proper control of muscle function requires not only excitation of the muscle by the LMNs located in the spinal cord, but also the function of reflex circuitry that monitors the functional status of the muscle fibers on a moment-by-moment basis. The muscle spindles of the stretch reflex function to monitor and correct for changes in muscle length when extrafusal fibers are either shortened (by contraction) or lengthened (by stretch).

■ Assessments of muscle strength and muscle bulk, muscle tone and motor reflexes, and patterns of motor movement and posture provide the means for determining the location of disorders of motor function. *Paresis* (weakness) and *paralysis* (loss of muscle movement) reflect a loss of muscle strength. UMN lesions tend to produce spastic paralysis, and LMN lesions flaccid paralysis. Changes in muscle bulk are characterized by a loss of muscle mass (atrophy) or an increase in muscle mass (hypertrophy). *Hypotonia* is a condition of less-than-normal muscle tone, and *hypertonia* or *spasticity* is a condition of excessive tone. Abnormal and uncoordinated movements and postures are suggestive of a cerebellar or basal ganglia pathologic process.

Disorders of the Motor Unit

Most of the diseases of the motor unit cause weakness and wasting of skeletal muscles. The distinguishing features of these diseases vary depending on which of the components of the motor unit is primarily affected—the cell body of the motor neuron, its axon, the neuromuscular junction, or the muscle fibers.[7-9] Disorders affecting the nerve cell body are often referred to as *LMN disorders*, those affecting the nerve axon as *peripheral neuropathies*, and primary disorders affecting the muscle fibers as *myopathies*.

Skeletal Muscle Disorders

Muscle Atrophy

Maintenance of muscle strength requires relatively frequent movements against resistance. Reduced use results in muscle atrophy, which is characterized by a reduction in the diameter of the muscle fibers because of a loss of protein filaments.[8] When a normally innervated muscle is not used for long periods, the muscle cells shrink in diameter, and although the muscle cells do not die, they lose much of their contractile proteins and become weakened. This is called *disuse atrophy*, and it occurs with conditions such as immobilization and chronic illness. The most extreme examples of muscle atrophy are found in persons with disorders that deprive muscles of their LMN innervation. This is called *denervation atrophy*.

Muscular Dystrophy

Muscular dystrophy is a term applied to a number of genetic disorders that produce progressive degeneration and necrosis of skeletal muscle fibers and eventual replacement with fat and connective tissue.[9–11] They are primary diseases of muscle tissue and probably do not involve the nervous system. As the muscle undergoes necrosis, fat and connective tissue replace the muscle fibers, which increases muscle size and results in muscle weakness. The increase in muscle size resulting from connective tissue infiltration is called *pseudohypertrophy*. Muscle weakness is insidious in onset but continually progressive, varying with the type of disorder.

The two most common forms of muscular dystrophy are Duchenne muscular dystrophy (DMD) and Becker muscular dystrophy (BMD), both of which are inherited as an X-linked recessive trait. Duchenne muscular dystrophy is the most common and severe form, with an incidence of 1 in every 3600 to 6000 live male births.[11] Despite the X-linked inheritance in DMD, about 30% of cases are due to new mutations and the mother is not a carrier.[10] Female carriers are usually asymptomatic. Affected girls are occasionally encountered, but usually have much milder symptoms than boys. Becker muscular dystrophy, which shares the same genetic locus as DMD, manifests later in childhood or adolescence and has a slower and less severe course of progression.

Both DMD and BMD are caused by mutations in the dystrophin gene, located on the short arm of the X chromosome. Dystrophin is a large protein that is expressed in a variety of tissues, including all types of muscle cells.[8–11] It attaches portions of the muscle sarcomere to the cell membrane, maintaining the structural integrity of skeletal and cardiac muscle cells. The role of dystrophin in transferring the force of contraction to the extracellular connective tissue matrix has been proposed as the basis for muscle cell degeneration that occurs with dystrophin defects or changes in other proteins that interact with dystrophin. The dystrophin gene is one of the largest in the human genome, spanning 2.3 million base pairs, a factor that is thought to make it particularly vulnerable to mutations. Muscle biopsy specimens from individuals with DMD show little or no dystrophin. In comparison, those with BMD, who also have mutations in the dystrophin gene, show diminished amounts of dystrophin, usually of an abnormal molecular weight, reflecting mutations that allow synthesis of an abnormal protein of smaller size.[8]

Clinical Course. Boys with DMD are usually asymptomatic at birth and during infancy.[8–11] Early gross movements such as rolling, sitting, and standing are usually achieved at the proper age. The postural muscles of the hips and shoulders are usually the first to be affected. Pseudohypertrophy of the calf muscle eventually develops (Fig. 36-5). Signs of muscle weakness usually become evident beginning at 2 to 3 years of age, when the child begins to fall frequently. Imbalances between agonist and antagonist muscles lead to abnormal postures and the development of contractures and joint immobility. Scoliosis (curvature of the spine) is common. Wheelchairs usually are needed at approximately 7 to 12 years of age.[10] Function of the distal muscles usually is preserved well enough that the child can continue to use eating utensils and a computer keyboard. The function of the extraocular muscles also is well preserved, as is the function of the muscles controlling urination and defecation. Incontinence is an uncommon and late event. Respiratory muscle involvement results in weak and ineffective cough, frequent respiratory infections, and decreasing respiratory reserve.

Cardiomyopathy is a common feature of the disease. The severity of cardiac involvement, however, does not necessarily correlate with skeletal muscle weakness. Some persons die early as the result of severe cardiomyopathy, whereas others maintain adequate cardiac function until the terminal stages of the disease. Death from respiratory and cardiac muscle involvement usually occurs in young adulthood.

Diagnosis and Treatment. Observation of the child's voluntary movement and a complete family history provide important diagnostic data for the disease. Serum levels of the enzyme creatine kinase (CK), which leaks out of damaged muscle fibers, suggests the presence of

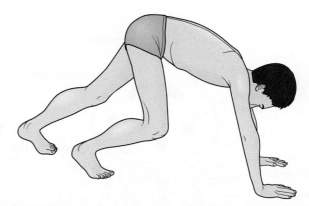

FIGURE 36-5. Pseudohypertrophy of the calves exercise for a child with proximal muscle weakness caused by Duchenne muscular dystrophy.

the disease.[10,11] A specific molecular genetic diagnosis is possible by demonstrating the defective dystrophin gene in a blood sample. Muscle biopsy, which shows a mixture of muscle cell degeneration and regeneration and reveals fat and scar tissue replacement, may be done to confirm the diagnosis. The same methods of genetic testing may be used on blood samples to establish carrier status in female relatives at risk, such as sisters and cousins. Prenatal diagnosis is possible as early as 12 weeks' gestation by sampling chorionic villi for DNA analysis[10] (see Chapter 6). Echocardiography, electrocardiography, and chest radiography are used to assess cardiac function.

Management of the disease is directed toward maintaining ambulation and preventing deformities. Passive stretching, correct or counterposturing, and splints help to prevent deformities. Precautions should be taken to avoid respiratory infections.

Glucocorticoids are the only medication currently available to slow the decline in muscle strength and function in DMD.[10,11] Steroids decrease inflammation, prevent fibrosis, and improve muscle regeneration.

Disorders of the Neuromuscular Junction

The neuromuscular junction serves as a synapse between a motor neuron and a skeletal muscle fiber.[3] It consists of the axon terminals of a motor neuron and a specialized region of the muscle membrane called the *endplate*. The transmission of impulses at the neuromuscular junction is mediated by the release of the neurotransmitter *acetylcholine* from the axon terminals. Acetylcholine binds to specific receptors in the endplate region of the muscle fiber surface to cause muscle contraction (Fig. 36-6A). Acetylcholine is active in the neuromuscular junction only for a brief period, during which an action potential is generated in the innervated muscle cell. Some of the transmitter diffuses out of the synapse, and the remaining transmitter is rapidly inactivated by an enzyme called *acetylcholinesterase*

(see Chapter 34, Fig. 34-25A). The rapid inactivation of acetylcholine allows repeated muscle contractions and gradations of contractile force.

Drug- and Toxin-Induced Disorders

A number of drugs and agents can alter neuromuscular function by changing the release, inactivation, or receptor binding of acetylcholine. Curare acts on the postjunctional membrane of the motor endplate to prevent the depolarizing effect of the neurotransmitter. Neuromuscular transmission is blocked by curare-type drugs during many types of surgical procedures to facilitate relaxation of involved musculature. Drugs such as physostigmine and neostigmine inhibit the action of acetylcholinesterase and allow acetylcholine released from the motor neuron to accumulate. These drugs are used in the treatment of myasthenia gravis.

Neurotoxins from the botulism organism (*Clostridium botulinum*) produce paralysis by blocking acetylcholine release.[3] Clostridia are anaerobic, gram-positive, spore-forming bacilli found worldwide in soils, marine and fresh water sediments, and the intestines of many animals. Classic food-borne botulism occurs through ingestion of soil-grown foods that are not properly cooked or preserved.[12] Canned vegetables, items preserved in garlic oil, and soups are usually the cause of sporadic outbreaks. Wound botulism occurs through colonization of wounds with *C. botulinum*.

Pharmacologic preparations of the botulinum toxin (botulinum type A toxin [Botox] and botulinum type B toxin [Myobloc]) have become available for use in treating eyelid and eye movement disorders such as blepharospasm and strabismus.[12,13] These agents also are used for treatment of spasmodic torticollis, spasmodic dysphonias (laryngeal dystonia), and other dystonias. The drug is injected into the target muscle using the electrical activity recorded from the tip of a special electromyographic injection needle to guide the injection. The treatment is not permanent and usually needs to be repeated approximately every 3 months.

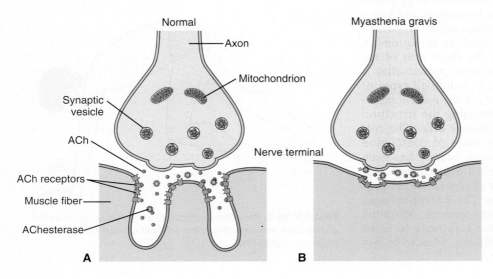

FIGURE 36-6. Neuromuscular junction. **(A)** Acetylcholine (ACh) released from the motor neurons in the myoneural junction crosses the synaptic space to reach receptors that are concentrated in the folds of the endplate of the muscle fiber. Once released, ACh is rapidly broken down by the enzyme acetylcholinesterase (AChesterase). **(B)** Decrease in ACh receptors in myasthenia gravis.

The aminoglycoside antibiotics (e.g., gentamicin) may produce a clinical disturbance similar to botulism by preventing the release of acetylcholine from nerve endings. The symptoms usually subside rapidly once the drug is eliminated from the body. These drugs are particularly dangerous in persons with preexisting disturbances of neuromuscular transmission, such as myasthenia gravis.

The organophosphates (e.g., malathion, parathion) that are used in some insecticides bind acetylcholinesterase to prevent the breakdown of acetylcholine. They produce excessive and prolonged acetylcholine action with a depolarization block of cholinergic receptors, including those of the neuromuscular junction.[12] The organophosphates are well absorbed from the skin, lungs, gut, and conjunctiva of the eye, making them particularly effective as insecticides but also potentially dangerous to humans. Malathion and certain other organophosphates are rapidly metabolized to inactive products in humans and are considered safe for sale to the general public. The sale of other insecticides, such as parathion, which is not effectively metabolized to inactive products, has been banned. Other organophosphate compounds (e.g., soman) were developed as "nerve gases"; if absorbed in high enough concentrations, they produce lethal effects through depolarization block and loss of respiratory muscle function.

Myasthenia Gravis

Myasthenia gravis is a disorder of the neuromuscular junction that affects impulse transmission between the motor neuron and the innervated muscle cell.[8,14-16] Women are affected nearly three times as often as men during early adulthood (age < 40 years), whereas the incidence is roughly equal during puberty and between ages 40 and 50. After 50 years of age, the incidence is higher in men. The Lambert-Eaton myasthenic syndrome is a special type of myasthenic syndrome that develops in association with neoplasms, particularly small cell carcinoma of the lung[8] (see Chapter 7).

Now recognized as an autoimmune disease, the disorder is caused by an antibody-mediated loss of acetylcholine receptors in the neuromuscular junction[8,14-16] (see Fig. 36-6B). Three mechanisms are thought to underlie the loss of functional acetylcholine receptors: (1) complement-mediated injury to the postsynaptic muscle membrane, (2) accelerated acetylcholine receptor degradation by receptor-specific antibodies, and (3) blockade of the receptors by antibodies attached to the acetylcholine-binding sites. Neonatal myasthenia gravis, caused by placental transfer of the acetylcholine receptor antibody, occurs in about 10% to 15% of infants born to mothers with the disease.[14,15] Spontaneous resolution of symptoms usually occurs within a few months of birth.

The trigger or inciting factor leading to the autoimmune derangement in myasthenia gravis remains unclear, but several lines of evidence implicate the thymus gland in the process. Approximately 75% of persons with myasthenia gravis also have thymic abnormalities, such as a thymoma (i.e., thymus tumor) or thymic hyperplasia (i.e., increased thymus weight from an increased number of thymus cells).[16]

Clinical Manifestations. In persons with myasthenia gravis who have a loss of functional acetylcholine receptors, each release of acetylcholine from the presynaptic membrane results in diminished motor response. This results in both muscle weakness and fatigability with sustained effort. Most commonly affected are the eye and periorbital muscles, with ptosis (drooping of eyelids) due to eyelid weakness or diplopia (double vision) due to weakness of the extraocular muscles as an initial symptom.[14-16] The disease may progress from ocular muscle weakness to generalized weakness, including respiratory muscle weakness. Chewing and swallowing may be difficult. Weakness in limb movement usually is more pronounced in the proximal rather than distal parts of the extremity, so that climbing stairs and lifting objects are difficult. As the disease progresses, the muscles of the lower face are affected, causing speech impairment. In most persons, symptoms are least evident when arising in the morning, but grow worse with effort and as the day proceeds.

Persons with myasthenia gravis may experience a sudden exacerbation of symptoms and weakness known as *myasthenic crisis*. Myasthenic crisis occurs when muscle weakness becomes severe enough to compromise ventilation to the extent that respiratory support and airway protection are needed. This usually occurs during a period of stress, such as infection, emotional upset, pregnancy, alcohol ingestion, cold exposure, or surgery. It also can result from inadequate or excessive doses of the anticholinesterase drugs used in treatment of the disorder.

Diagnosis and Treatment. The diagnosis of myasthenia gravis is based on history and physical examination and confirmed by the response to a short-acting anticholinesterase test. Edrophonium (Tensilon) commonly is used for the test.[14-16] The drug, which is administered intravenously, decreases the breakdown of acetylcholine in the neuromuscular junction. When weakness is caused by myasthenia gravis, a dramatic transitory improvement in muscle function occurs. Electrophysiologic studies can be done to demonstrate a decremental muscle response to repetitive motor nerve stimulation. An immunoassay test can be used to detect the presence of antiacetylcholine receptor antibodies circulating in the blood.

Treatment methods include the use of pharmacologic agents; immunosuppressive therapy, including corticosteroid drugs; management of myasthenic crisis; thymectomy; and plasmapheresis or intravenous immunoglobulin.[14-16] Medications that may exacerbate myasthenia gravis, such as the aminoglycoside antibiotics, should be avoided. Pharmacologic treatment with reversible anticholinesterase drugs (i.e., neostigmine, pyridostigmine) inhibits the breakdown of acetylcholine. Corticosteroid drugs, which suppress the immune response, are used in cases of a poor response to anticholinesterase drugs and thymectomy. Immunosuppressant drugs (e.g., azathioprine, cyclosporine) also may be used, often in combination with plasmapheresis.

Plasmapheresis removes antibodies from the circulation and provides short-term clinical improvement. It is used primarily to stabilize the condition of persons in myasthenic crisis or for short-term treatment in persons undergoing thymectomy. Intravenous immunoglobulin also produces improvement in persons with myasthenia gravis. Although the effect is temporary, it may last for weeks to months. Intravenous immunoglobulin therapy is very expensive, which limits its use.

Thymectomy, or surgical removal of the thymus, may be used as a treatment for myasthenia gravis. Because the mechanism whereby surgery exerts its effect is unknown, the treatment is controversial. Thymectomy may be performed in persons with thymoma, regardless of age, and in persons with generalized myasthenia gravis with onset before 50 years of age.[16]

Peripheral Nervous System Disorders

Peripheral nervous system (PNS) disorders involve neurons that are located outside the CNS. They include disorders of the motor and sensory branches of the somatic and visceral nervous systems and the peripheral branches of the autonomic nervous system (see Chapter 34). The result usually is muscle weakness, with or without atrophy, and sensory changes.

Unlike the nerves of the CNS, peripheral nerves are fairly strong and resilient. They contain a series of connective tissue sheaths: the outer *epineurium* that surrounds the medium-sized to large nerves, the *perineurium* that invests each bundle of nerve fibers; and the *endoneurium* that surrounds each nerve fiber (see Chapter 34, Fig. 34-2). Inside the endoneurium are the Schwann cells that produce the myelin sheath that surrounds the peripheral nerves. Each Schwann cell can myelinate only one segment of a single axon—the one that it covers—so that myelination of an entire axon requires the participation of a long line of these cells.

Peripheral Nerve Injury and Repair

There are two main types of peripheral nerve injury based on the target of the insult: segmental demyelination involving the Schwann cell and axonal degeneration involving the neuronal cell body or its axon.[8,17]

Segmental Demyelination. Segmental demyelination occurs when there is a disorder of the Schwann cell (as in hereditary motor and sensory neuropathies) or damage to the myelin sheath (e.g., Guillain-Barré syndrome) without a primary abnormality of the axon. It typically affects some Schwann cells while sparing others. The disintegrated myelin is engulfed initially by Schwann cells and then by macrophages. The denuded axon provides a stimulus for remyelination and the population of cells within the endoneurium has the capacity to replace the injured Schwann cells. These cells proliferate and encircle the axon, and in time remyelinate the denuded portion.

Axonal Degeneration. Axonal degeneration is caused by primary injury to a neuronal cell body or its axon. Damage to the axon may be due either to a focal event occurring at some point along the length of the nerve (e.g., trauma or ischemia) or to a more generalized abnormality affecting the neuronal cell body (neuropathy).

Damage to a peripheral nerve axon, whether by injury or neuropathy, results in degenerative changes, followed by breakdown of the myelin sheath and Schwann cells. In distal axonal degeneration, the proximal axon and neuronal cell body, which synthesizes the material required for nourishing and maintaining the axon, remain intact. In neuropathies and crushing injuries, in which the endoneurial tube remains intact, the outgrowing fiber grows down this tube to the structure that was originally innervated by the neuron (Fig. 36-7). However, it can take weeks or months for the regrowing fiber to reach its target organ and for communicative function to be reestablished. More time is required for the Schwann cells to form new myelin segments and for the axon to recover its original diameter and conduction velocity.

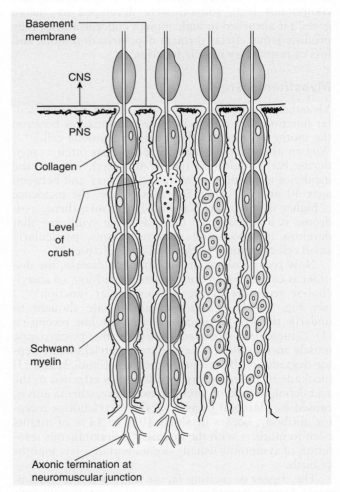

FIGURE 36-7. Sequential stages of efferent axon degeneration and regeneration within its endoneurial tube, after peripheral nerve crush injury. CNS, Central nervous system; PNS, Peripheral nervous system.

The successful regeneration of a nerve fiber in the PNS depends on many factors. If a nerve fiber is destroyed relatively close to the neuronal cell body, the chances are that the nerve cell will die; if it does, it will not be replaced. If a crushing type of injury has occurred, partial or often full recovery of function occurs. Cutting-type trauma to a nerve is an entirely different matter. Connective scar tissue forms rapidly at the wound site, and when it does, only the most rapidly regenerating axonal branches are able to get through to the intact distal endoneurial tubes. A number of scar-inhibiting agents have been used in an effort to reduce this hazard, but have met with only moderate success. In another attempt to improve nerve regeneration, various types of tubular implants have been used to fill longer gaps in the endoneurial tube.

Mononeuropathies

Mononeuropathies usually are caused by localized conditions such as trauma, compression, or infections that affect a single spinal nerve, plexus, or peripheral nerve trunk. Fractured bones may lacerate or compress nerves, excessively tight tourniquets may injure nerves directly or produce ischemic injury, and infections such as herpes zoster may affect a single segmental afferent nerve. Recovery of nerve function usually is complete after compression lesions and incomplete or faulty after nerve transection.

Carpal Tunnel Syndrome. Carpal tunnel syndrome is a relatively common entrapment mononeuropathy, caused by compression of the median nerve as it travels with the flexor tendons through a canal made by the carpal bones and transverse carpal ligament[18–20] (Fig. 36-8). It can be caused by a variety of conditions that produce a reduction in the capacity of the carpal tunnel (i.e., bony or ligamentous changes) or an increase in the volume of the tunnel contents (i.e., inflammation of the tendons, synovial swelling, or tumors). Carpal tunnel syndrome may be a feature of a number of systemic diseases, such as rheumatoid arthritis, hyperthyroidism, acromegaly, and diabetes mellitus. Most cases, however, are due to repetitive use of the wrist (i.e., flexion–extension movements and stress associated with pinching and gripping motions).

Carpal tunnel syndrome is characterized by pain, paresthesia (tingling), and numbness of the thumb and first, second, third, and half of the fourth digits of the hand; pain in the wrist and hand, which worsens at night; atrophy of the abductor pollicis muscle; and weakness in precision grip. All of these abnormalities may contribute to clumsiness of fine motor activity.

Diagnosis usually is based on sensory disturbances confined to median nerve distribution and a positive Tinel or Phalen sign.[18,20] The *Tinel sign* is the development of a tingling sensation radiating into the palm of the hand that is elicited by light percussion over the median nerve at the wrist. The *Phalen maneuver* is performed by having the person hold the wrist in complete flexion for approximately a minute; if numbness and

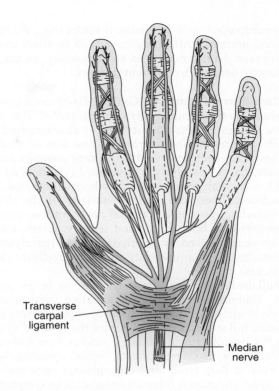

FIGURE 36-8. Carpal tunnel syndrome: compression of the median nerve by the transverse carpal ligament. (Courtesy of Carole Russell Hilmer, C.M.I.)

Labels: Transverse carpal ligament; Median nerve

paresthesia along the median nerve are reproduced or exaggerated, the test result is considered to be positive. Electromyography and nerve conduction studies often are done to confirm the diagnosis and exclude other causes of the disorder.

Treatment includes a variety of options including nonsteroidal anti-inflammatory agents, injection of corticosteroids, immobilization of the wrist with splints, rehabilitation modalities (e.g., ultrasound, stretching, and strengthening exercises), and surgery. Measures to decrease the causative repetitive movements should be initiated. Splints may be confined to nighttime use. When splinting is ineffective, corticosteroids may be injected into the carpal tunnel to reduce inflammation and swelling. Surgical intervention consists of operative division of the volar carpal ligaments as a means of relieving pressure on the median nerve.

Polyneuropathies

Polyneuropathies involve demyelination or axonal degeneration of multiple peripheral nerves that leads to symmetric sensory, motor, or mixed sensorimotor deficits. Typically, the longest axons are involved first, with symptoms beginning in the distal part of the extremities. If the autonomic nervous system is involved, there may be postural hypotension, constipation, and impotence. Polyneuropathies can result from immune mechanisms (e.g., Guillain-Barré syndrome), toxic agents (e.g., arsenic polyneuropathy, lead polyneuropathy, alcoholic polyneuropathy), and metabolic diseases (e.g., diabetes mellitus, uremia). Different causes tend to affect axons of different diameters and to affect sensory, motor, or autonomic neurons to different degrees.

Guillain-Barré Syndrome. Guillain-Barré syndrome is an acute life-threatening polyneuropathy.[21-24] The syndrome defines a clinical entity that is characterized by rapidly progressive limb weakness and loss of tendon reflexes. It has been described as the most common cause of acute, flaccid paralysis in developed countries of the world, now that poliomyelitis has been eliminated. As a syndrome, there are several subtypes of the disorder, including pure motor axonal degeneration, axonal degeneration of both motor and sensory nerves, and a variant characterized by ophthalmoplegia (paralysis of eye muscles), ataxia (unsteady gait), and areflexia (lack of reflexes).

Guillain-Barré syndrome is thought to be an acute onset immune-mediated demyelinating neuropathy. Approximately two thirds of patients report having had an acute, influenza-like illness before the onset of symptoms.[18] Controlled epidemiologic studies have linked it to infection with *Campylobacter jejuni*, cytomegalovirus, Epstein-Barr virus, and mycoplasma pneumoniae. A *C. jejuni* infection is often an antecedent to symptoms. In a few cases, the patient reports receiving a vaccination prior to onset of Guillain-Barré syndrome.

The disorder is characterized by progressive ascending muscle weakness of the limbs, producing a symmetric flaccid paralysis. Symptoms of paresthesia and numbness often accompany the loss of motor function. The rate of disease progression varies, and there may be disproportionate involvement of the upper or lower extremities. Paralysis may progress to involve the respiratory muscles. Autonomic nervous system involvement that causes postural hypotension, arrhythmias, facial flushing, abnormalities of sweating, and urinary retention is common. Pain is another common feature of Guillain-Barré syndrome. It is most common in the shoulder girdle, back, and posterior thighs and occurs with even the slightest of movements.

Guillain-Barré syndrome usually is a medical emergency. There may be a rapid development of respiratory failure and autonomic disturbances that threaten circulatory function. Treatment includes support of vital functions and prevention of complications such as skin breakdown and thrombophlebitis. Removing the circulating immune complexes via plasma exchange has been shown to decrease morbidity and shorten the course of the disease.[23,24] Treatment is most effective if initiated early in the course of the disease. High-dose intravenous immunoglobulin therapy also has proved effective. Approximately 85% of persons with the disease achieve a full and spontaneous recovery within 6 to 12 months.[21]

Back Pain and Spinal Nerve Root Disorders

The spinal cord and spinal nerve roots are located within the vertebral canal. The anterior portion of the spine consists of cylindrical vertebral bodies separated by intervertebral disks and held together by the anterior and posterior longitudinal ligaments (Fig. 36-9A). The posterior portion of the spine consists of the vertebral arches, each consisting of paired transverse processes, one posterior spinous process, and two superior articular facets. The functions of the posterior spine are to protect the spinal cord and nerves within the spinal canal and to stabilize the spine by providing sites for the attachment of muscles and ligaments.

Back pain is a common problem that affects an estimated two thirds of people at least once in their lifetime.[25] It can result from a number of causes, including problems involving the vertebrae and intervertebral joints or back muscles and ligaments, as well as disorders of the spinal nerve roots. Perhaps the most common causes are musculoligamentous injuries and age-related degenerative changes in the intervertebral disks and facet joints.[26] Other causes include spinal nerve root compression due to intervertebral disk herniation and narrowing of the central canal due to spinal stenosis.

Pain-sensitive structures in the spine include the periosteum of the vertebrae, dura, facet joints, annulus fibrosus of the intervertebral disk, and posterior longitudinal ligament. Pain sensation is conveyed through afferent fibers in the spinal nerves. Local pain is caused by stretching of pain-sensitive structures that compress or irritate sensory nerve endings. Pain referred to the back may arise from abdominal or pelvic structures. Pain associated with muscle spasm is usually dull, and often accompanied by abnormal posture and stiff paraspinal muscles.

Nerve root injury (radiculopathy) is a common cause of neck, arm, low back, and leg pain. The pain is typically sharp and radiates to the arm or leg within the territory of the spinal root. Disorders affecting the upper lumbar segments tend to be referred to the lumbar area, groin, or anterior thigh; and those affecting the lower lumbar and upper sacral segments, to the buttocks and posterior thighs.

Diagnosis and Treatment. Although back problems are commonly attributed to a herniated disk, most acute back disorders are caused by less-serious problems.[18,25-28] The diagnostic challenge is to identify those persons who require further evaluation for more serious problems such as malignancies, compression fractures, and vascular disorders. The diagnostic measures used in the evaluation of back pain include history and physical examination, including a thorough neurologic examination. Other diagnostic methods may include radiographs of the back and magnetic resonance imaging (MRI).

Treatment of back pain usually is conservative and consists of analgesic medications, muscle relaxants, and instruction in the correct mechanics for lifting and methods of protecting the back. Pain relief is usually provided using nonsteroidal anti-inflammatory drugs. Muscle relaxants may be used on a short-term basis. Bed rest, once the mainstay of conservative therapy, is now understood to be ineffective for acute back pain.

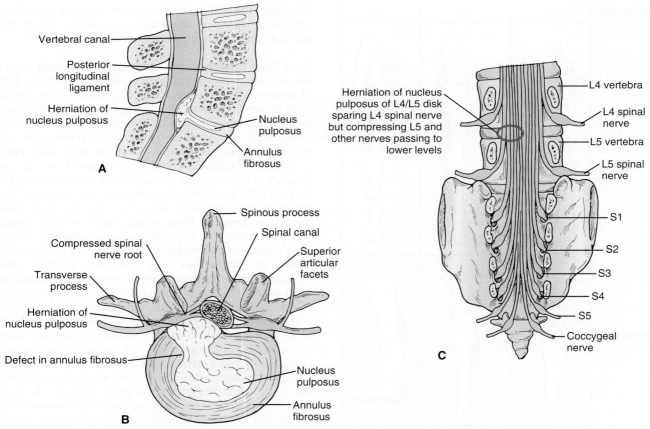

FIGURE 36-9. Herniated intervertebral disk. **(A)** Longitudinal section. **(B)** Cross-section. **(C)** Location of L4 to L5 and S1 to S5 spinal nerves, with site of L4/L5 herniation of nucleus pulposus indicated. (Modified from Moore KL, Dalley AF. *Clinically Oriented Anatomy.* 5th ed. Philadelphia, PA: Lippincott Williams & Wilkins; 2006:503.)

Conditioning exercises of the trunk muscles, particularly the back extensors, are often recommended.

Intervertebral Disk Disorders. The intervertebral disk is considered the most critical component of the load-bearing structures of the spinal column. It consists of a soft, gelatinous center called the *nucleus pulposus,* which is encircled by a strong ring of fibrocartilage called the *annulus fibrosus.*[29] The structural components of the disk make it capable of absorbing shock and changing shape while allowing movement. With dysfunction, the nucleus pulposus can be squeezed out of place and herniate through the annulus fibrosus, a condition referred to as a *herniated* or *slipped disk* (see Fig. 36-9B).

The intervertebral disk can become dysfunctional because of trauma, the effects of aging, or degenerative disorders of the spine. Protrusion of the nucleus pulposus usually occurs posteriorly and toward the intervertebral foramen and its contained spinal nerve root, where the annulus fibrosus is relatively thin and poorly supported by either the posterior or anterior ligaments[28,29] (see Fig. 36-9A). Trauma results from activities such as lifting while in the flexed position, slipping, falling on the buttocks or back, or suppressing a sneeze. With aging, the gelatinous center of the disk dries out and loses much of its elasticity.

The level at which a herniated disk occurs is important (see Fig. 36-9C). The cervical and lumbar regions are the most flexible areas of the spine and are most often involved in disk herniations. Usually, herniation occurs at the lower levels of the lumbar spine, where the mass being supported and the bending of the vertebral column are greatest. When the injury occurs in the lumbar area, only the nerve fibers of the cauda equina are involved. Because these elongated dorsal and ventral roots contain endoneurial tubes of connective tissue, regeneration of the nerve fibers is likely. However, months may be required for full recovery to occur because of the distance to the innervated muscle or skin of the lower limbs.

The signs and symptoms of a herniated disk are localized to the area of the body innervated by the spinal nerve roots and include both motor and sensory manifestations (Fig. 36-10). Pain is the first and most common symptom of a herniated disk. The nerve roots of L4, L5, S1, S2, and S3 give rise to a syndrome of back pain, sometimes referred to as *sciatica,* which spreads down the back of the leg and over the sole of the foot. The pain is usually intensified with coughing, sneezing, straining, stooping, standing, and the jarring motions that occur during walking or riding. Slight motor weakness may occur, although major weakness is rare.

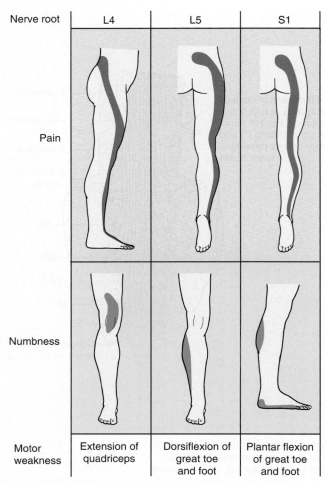

Nerve root	L4	L5	S1
Pain			
Numbness			
Motor weakness	Extension of quadriceps	Dorsiflexion of great toe and foot	Plantar flexion of great toe and foot

FIGURE 36-10. Dermatomes of the leg (L1 through S5) where pain and numbness would be experienced with spinal root irritation.

The most common sensory deficits from spinal nerve root compression are paresthesias and numbness, particularly of the leg and foot. Knee and ankle reflexes also may be diminished or absent.

A herniated disk must be differentiated from other causes of acute back pain. Diagnostic measures include history and physical examination. Neurologic assessment includes testing of muscle strength and reflexes. The straight-leg test is an important diagnostic maneuver. It is done with the person in the supine position and is performed by passively raising the person's leg. The test can also be done by slowly extending the knee while the person sits on a table, with both hip and knee flexed at 90 degrees. The maneuver is designed to apply traction along the nerve root, which exacerbates pain if the nerve root is acutely inflamed. Normally, it is possible to raise the leg approximately 90 degrees without causing discomfort of the hamstring muscles. The test result is positive if pain is produced when the leg is raised to 60 degrees or less. Other diagnostic methods include radiographs of the back, MRI, computed tomography (CT), and CT myelography.

Treatment usually is similar to that for back pain. Surgical treatment may be indicated when there is documentation of herniation by an imaging procedure, consistent pain, or consistent neurologic deficit that failed to respond to conservative therapy.

Back Pain Emergencies. Although acute back pain is usually a non–life-threatening condition, in 5% to 10% of persons it is a manifestation of a more serious pathologic process.[30] Vascular catastrophes (ruptured abdominal aortic aneurysms and dissecting aortic aneurysms), malignancy, spinal cord compression syndromes, and infectious processes may all present as acute back pain.

Clinical findings, commonly referred to as *red flags,* that indicate the possibility of more serious disease include gradual onset of pain; age younger than 20 years or older than 50 years; thoracic back pain; history of trauma, fever, chills, night sweats, immunosuppression, or malignancy; unintentional weight loss; recent procedure known to cause bacteremia; and history of intravenous drug use.[30] The gradual onset of pain may be indicative of malignancy or infection. Back pain that begins before 20 years of age suggests congenital or developmental disorders, and new-onset pain in persons 50 years of age or older is more likely to be a manifestation of serious conditions such as an aortic aneurysm, malignancy, or compression fracture. Pain that is aggravated by lying down is a red flag for malignancy or infection, and pain that improves with sitting or slight flexion of the spine suggests the presence of spinal stenosis. Persons with symptoms of large or rapidly evolving neurologic deficits require urgent evaluation for possible cauda equina syndrome, epidural abscess, or central disk herniation. Signs and symptoms that suggest possible cauda equina syndrome are low back pain associated with bilateral leg weakness (from multiple lumbar nerve root compressions), saddle area numbness, bowel and bladder incontinence, or impotence (indicating multiple sacral nerve compressions).[25,30] Reports of neurologic symptoms such as paresthesia, motor weakness, and gait abnormalities also require additional diagnostic tests to rule out spinal cord compression.

SUMMARY CONCEPTS

- *Muscular dystrophy* is a term used to describe a number of disorders, including Duchenne muscular dystrophy, that produce progressive deterioration of the skeletal muscles. *Myasthenia gravis* is a disorder of the neuromuscular junction resulting from a deficiency of functional acetylcholine receptors, which causes weakness of the skeletal muscles.

- Peripheral nerve disorders, which involve motor and sensory neurons outside the CNS, include the mononeuropathies, such as carpal tunnel syndrome, that involve a single peripheral nerve;

and the polyneuropathies, such as Guillain-Barré syndrome, which involve multiple peripheral nerves leading to symmetric sensory, motor, or mixed sensorimotor deficits.

■ Back pain and pain related to spinal nerve root irritation can be caused by a number of disorders including muscle and ligament strains, age-related degenerative spine disorders, disk herniation, and narrowing of the central vertebral canal due to spinal stenosis.

Disorders of the Cerebellum and Basal Ganglia

Aside from the areas in the cerebral cortex that stimulate muscle contraction, two other brain structures, the cerebellum and basal ganglia, are also essential for normal motor function. Neither one can control muscle function by itself. Instead, they always function in association with other components of motor control.

Disorders of the Cerebellum

The cerebellum has sometimes been referred to as the *silent area* of the brain because electrical stimulation does not produce any conscious sensation and rarely causes any motor movements.[3,31] However, removal or damage to the cerebellum causes movements to become highly abnormal. The cerebellum is especially vital during rapid muscular activities such as running, typing, and even talking. Loss of cerebellar function can result in total incoordination of these functions even though paralysis does not occur.

The functions of the cerebellum are integrated into many connected afferent and efferent pathways throughout the brain. An extensive and important afferent pathway is the *corticopontocerebellar* pathway, which originates in the cerebral motor and premotor cortices as well as the somatosensory cortex. Other important afferent pathways link the cerebellum to input from the basal ganglia, muscle and joint information from the stretch receptors, visual input from the eyes, and balance and equilibrium sensation from the vestibular system in the inner ear. There are three general efferent pathways leading out of the cerebellum: (1) the *vestibulocerebellar pathway* that functions in close association with the brain stem vestibular nuclei to maintain equilibrium and posture; (2) the *spinocerebellar pathway* that provides the circuitry for coordinating the movements of distal portions of the limbs, especially the hands and fingers; and (3) the *cerebrocerebellar pathway* that transmits output information in an upward direction to the cerebral cortex, functioning in a feedback manner with the motor and somatosensory systems to coordinate sequential body and limb movements.

The signs of cerebellar dysfunction include cerebellar ataxia and tremor. They result from defects in the smooth, continuously correcting functions of the cerebellum, and occur on the side of the cerebellar damage. Disorders of cerebellar function are typically caused by a congenital defect, cerebrovascular event, or growing tumor.

Cerebellar gait ataxia is characterized by wide-based staggering, lurching, and uncontrolled gait. Visual monitoring of movement cannot compensate for cerebellar defects, and these abnormalities occur whether the eyes are open or closed. Because ethanol specifically affects cerebellar function, persons who are inebriated often walk with a staggering and unsteady gait. Rapid alternating movements such as supination–pronation–supination of the hands are jerky and performed slowly. Reaching to touch a target breaks down into small sequential components, each going too far, followed by overcorrection. The finger moves jerkily toward the target, misses, corrects in the other direction, and misses again, until the target is finally reached. This is called *over- and underreaching* or *dysmetria*.

Cerebellar tremor is a rhythmic back-and-forth movement of a finger or toe that worsens as the target is approached. The tremor results from the inability of the damaged cerebellar system to maintain ongoing fixation of a body part and to make smooth, continuous corrections in the trajectory of the movement; overcorrection occurs, first in one direction and then the other. Often, the tremor of an arm or leg can be detected during the beginning of an intended movement. The common term for cerebellar tremor is *intention tremor*. Cerebellar function, as it relates to tremor, can be assessed by asking a person to touch one heel to the opposite knee, to gently move the toes along the back of the opposite shin, or to touch the nose with a finger.

The ability to fix the eyes on a target also can be affected. Constant conjugate readjustment of eye position, called *nystagmus*, results and makes reading extremely difficult, especially when the eyes are deviated toward the side of cerebellar damage. Cerebellar function also can affect the motor skills of chewing, swallowing, and speech. Normal speech requires smooth control of respiratory muscles and highly coordinated control of the laryngeal, lip, and tongue muscles. Cerebellar dysarthria is characterized by slow, slurred speech of continuously varying loudness. Rehabilitative efforts directed by speech therapists include learning to slow the rate of speech and to compensate as much as possible through the use of less-affected muscles.

Disorders of The Basal Ganglia

The basal ganglia are a group of deep, interrelated subcortical nuclei that play an essential role in control of movement. They function in the organization of inherited and highly learned and rather automatic movement programs, especially those affecting the trunk and proximal limbs. The basal ganglia are thought to be particularly important in starting, stopping, and monitoring movements executed by the cortex, especially those that are relatively slow and sustained, or stereotyped. They also help to regulate the intensity of these movements, and they act to inhibit antagonistic or unnecessary movements. The function of the basal ganglia is not limited to motor functions; they also are involved in cognitive and perceptual functions.

Functional Properties of The Basal Ganglia

The structural components of the basal ganglia include the caudate nucleus, putamen, and globus pallidus.[3,32] They are located lateral and caudal to the thalamus, occupying a large portion of the interior of both cerebral hemispheres. The caudate and putamen are collectively referred to as the *striatum*, and the putamen and globus pallidus form a wedge-shaped region called the *lentiform nucleus*. Two other structures, the *substantia nigra* of the midbrain and the *subthalamic nucleus* of the diencephalon, are considered part of the basal ganglia (Fig. 36-11). The dorsal part of the substantia nigra contains cells that synthesize dopamine and are rich in a black pigment called *melanin*. The high concentration of melanin gives the structure a black color, hence the name *substantia nigra*. The axons of the substantia nigra form the *nigrostriatal pathway,* which supplies dopamine to the striatum. The subthalamic nucleus lies just below the thalamus and above the anterior portion of the substantia nigra. The glutaminergic cells of this nucleus are the only excitatory projections to the basal ganglia.

The basal ganglia have input structures that receive afferent information from the cerebral cortex and thalamus, internal circuits that connect the various structures of the basal ganglia, and output structures that deliver information to other brain centers. The neostriatum represents the major input structure for the basal ganglia. Virtually all areas of the cortex and afferents from the thalamus project to the neostriatum. The output areas of the basal ganglia, including the lateral globus pallidus, have both ascending and descending components. The major ascending output is transmitted to thalamic nuclei, which process all incoming information that is transmitted to the cerebral cortex. Descending output is directed to the midbrain, brain stem, and spinal cord.

The output functions of the basal ganglia are mainly inhibitory. Looping circuits from specific cortical areas pass through the basal ganglia to modulate the excitability of specific thalamic nuclei and control the cortical activity involved in highly learned, automatic, and stereotyped motor functions. The most is known about the inhibitory basal ganglia loop that is involved in modulating cortical motor control. This loop regulates the release of stereotyped movement patterns that add efficiency and gracefulness to cortically controlled movements. These movements include inherited patterns that add precision, efficiency, and balance to motion, such as the swinging of the arms during walking and running and the highly learned automatic postural and follow-through movements of throwing a ball or swinging a bat.

The basal ganglia also have a cognitive function in that they monitor sensory information coming into the brain and apply it to information stored in memory as a means of planning and sequencing motor movements.[3] The cognitive control of motor activities determines, subconsciously and within seconds, which patterns of movement will be needed to achieve a goal. The caudate nucleus, which receives large amounts of input from the association areas of the brain, plays a major role in the cognitive control of motor activity.

Basal Ganglia–Associated Movement Disorders

Disorders of the basal ganglia comprise a complex group of motor disturbances characterized by tremor and other involuntary movements, changes in posture and muscle tone, and poverty and slowness of movement. They include tremors and tics, hypokinetic disorders, and hyperkinetic disorders[1] (Table 36-1).

Unlike disorders of the motor cortex and corticospinal (pyramidal) tract, lesions of the basal ganglia disrupt movement but do not cause paralysis. The various types of involuntary movements often occur in combination and appear to have a common underlying cause. Recent studies indicate that hypokinetic and hyperkinetic disorders can be explained as specific disturbances in the indirect and direct pathways that link the basal ganglia with the thalamocortical motor circuit.[32] Accordingly, overactivity of the indirect pathway relative to the direct pathway would result in hypokinetic disorders such as Parkinson disease, and underactivity of the indirect pathway would result in hyperkinetic disorders such as chorea and ballismus.

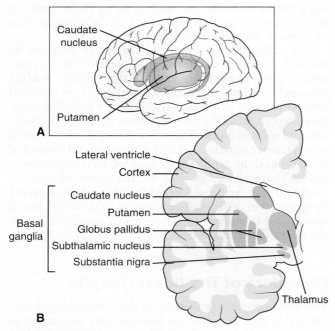

FIGURE 36-11. (A) Lateral view of the basal ganglia. **(B)** Coronal section showing the basal ganglia in relation to surrounding structures.

TABLE 36-1	Characteristics of Basal Ganglia–Associated Movement Disorders
Movement Disorder	**Characteristics**
Tremor	Involuntary, oscillating contractions of opposing muscle groups around a joint
	Usually fairly uniform in frequency and amplitude
	Can occur as resting tremors and postural tremors, which occur when the part is maintained in a stable position
Hypokinetic disorders	Slowness in initiating movement, and reduced range and force of the movement (bradykinesia)
Chorea	Irregular wriggling and writhing movements
	Accentuated by movement and by environmental stimulation; they often interfere with normal movement patterns
	May be grimacing movements of the face, raising the eyebrows, rolling of the eyes, and curling, protrusion, and withdrawal of the tongue
	In the limbs, the movements largely are distal; there may be piano playing–type movements with alternating extension and flexion of the fingers
Athetosis	Continuous, wormlike, twisting and turning motions of the joints of a limb or the body
Ballismus	Violent, sweeping, flinging motions, especially of the limbs on one side of the body (hemiballismus)
Dystonia	Abnormal maintenance of a posture resulting from a twisting, turning movement of the limbs, neck, or trunk
	Often the result of simultaneous contraction of agonist and antagonist muscles
	Can result in grotesque and twisted postures
Dyskinesias	Bizarre wriggling and writhing movements
	Frequently involve the face, mouth, jaw, and tongue, causing grimacing, pursing of the lips, or protrusion of the tongue
	Limbs affected less often
	Tardive dyskinesia is an untoward reaction that can develop with long-term use of some antipsychotic medications

Parkinson Disease

Parkinson disease is a progressive degenerative disorder of basal ganglia function that results in variable combinations of tremor, rigidity, and bradykinesia.[33,34] Parkinson disease is the second most common neurodegenerative disease after Alzheimer disease. It usually begins after 50 years of age, with the prevalence increasing to 4% to 5% in those older than 85 years of age.[33]

The clinical syndrome arising from the degenerative changes in basal ganglia function often is referred to as *parkinsonism*. Parkinson disease, the most common form of parkinsonism, is named after James Parkinson, a British physician who first described the disease in a paper he published in 1817 on the "shaking palsy."[35] In Parkinson disease, also known as *idiopathic parkinsonism*, dopamine depletion results from degeneration of the dopamine nigrostriatal system. Parkinsonism can also develop as a postencephalitic syndrome, as a side effect of therapy with antipsychotic drugs that block dopamine receptors, as a toxic reaction to a chemical agent, or as an outcome of severe carbon monoxide poisoning.[36] Drug-induced parkinsonism can follow the administration of antipsychotic drugs in high doses (e.g., phenothiazines, butyrophenones). These drugs block dopamine receptors and dopamine output by the cells of the substantia nigra. Symptoms of parkinsonism also may accompany conditions such as cerebral vascular disease, brain tumors, repeated head trauma, or degenerative neurologic diseases that structurally damage the nigrostriatal pathway.

The primary brain abnormality found in persons with Parkinson disease is degeneration of the nigrostriatal pathway, with subsequent reduction in striatal concentrations of dopamine. Other brain areas are affected to a lesser extent.[37,38] Although the cause of Parkinson disease is still unknown, it is widely believed that most cases are caused by an interaction of environmental and genetic factors. Over the past several decades, several pathologic processes (e.g., oxidative stress, apoptosis, and mitochondrial disorders) that might lead to degeneration have been identified.

There is increasing evidence that the development of Parkinson disease may be related to oxidative metabolites and the inability of neurons to render these products harmless. Of interest in terms of research was the development of Parkinson disease in several persons who had attempted to make a narcotic drug and instead synthesized a compound called *MPTP (1-methyl-phenyl-2,3,6-tetrahydropyridine)*.[37,38] This compound selectively destroys the dopaminergic neurons of the substantia nigra. This incident prompted investigations into the role of toxins that are produced by the body as a part of metabolic processes and those that enter the body from outside sources in the pathogenesis of Parkinson disease. One theory is that the auto-oxidation of catecholamines, such as dopamine, may injure neurons in the substantia nigra. MPTP is an inhibitor of the mitochondrial electron transport system that functions in the inactivation of these metabolites, suggesting that it may produce Parkinson disease in a manner similar to that of the naturally occurring disease.

The recent discovery of inherited forms of Parkinson disease suggests that genetic factors may also play a role in the pathogenesis of early-onset Parkinson disease.[37-39] The first genetic mutation associated with

Parkinson disease was found in the gene encoding α-*synuclein,* a member of a small family of proteins that are expressed preferentially in the substantia nigra.[37,38] Although mutations in this gene cause a very rare, autosomal dominant form of the disease, the mutation has received considerable attention because α-synuclein is one of the major components of the Lewy bodies that are found in the brain tissue of persons with Parkinson disease. Mutations in a second gene that encodes the protein *parkin* are associated with an autosomal recessive, early-onset form of Parkinson disease.[37] Numerous other genetic loci have been linked to Parkinson disease, but the genes remain to be mapped. Thus, the genetics of Parkinson disease are beginning to provide molecular clues that help explain the etiology, just as epidemiologic studies have delineated an array of environmental modulators of susceptibility, which can now be explored in the context of gene expression.[39]

Clinical Manifestations. The cardinal manifestations of Parkinson disease are tremor, rigidity, and bradykinesia or slowness of movement (Fig. 36-12).[33,34,40] Tremor is the most visible manifestation of the disorder. The tremor affects the distal segments of the limbs, mainly the hands and feet; head, neck, face, lips, and tongue; or jaw. It is characterized by rhythmic, alternating flexion and contraction movements (four to six beats per minute) that resemble the motion of rolling a pill between the thumb and forefinger. The tremor usually is unilateral, occurs when the limb is supported and at rest, and disappears with movement and sleep. The tremor eventually progresses to involve both sides of the body.

Rigidity is defined as resistance to movement of both flexors and extensors throughout the full range of motion. It is most evident during passive joint movement and involves jerky, cogwheel-type or ratchetlike movements that require considerable energy to perform. Flexion contractions may develop as a result of the rigidity. As with tremor, rigidity usually begins unilaterally but progresses to involve both sides of the body.

Bradykinesia is characterized by slowness in initiating and performing movements and difficulty with sudden, unexpected stopping of voluntary movements. Unconscious associative movements occur in a series of disconnected steps rather than in a smooth, coordinated manner. This is the most disabling of the symptoms of Parkinson disease. Persons with the disease have difficulty initiating walking and difficulty turning. While walking, they may freeze in place and feel as if their feet are glued to the floor, especially when moving through a doorway or preparing to turn. When they walk, they lean forward to maintain their center of gravity; take small, shuffling steps without swinging their arms; and have difficulty changing their stride.

Manifestations of advanced-stage parkinsonism include falls, fluctuations in motor function, neuropsychiatric disorders, and sleep disorders. Loss of postural reflexes predisposes to falling, often backward. Emotional and voluntary facial movements become limited and slow as the disease progresses, and facial expression becomes stiff and masklike. There is loss of the blinking reflex and a

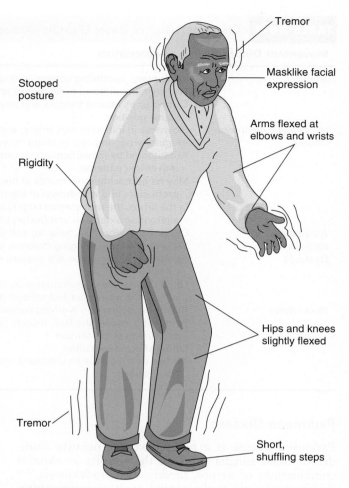

FIGURE 36-12. The clinical features of Parkinson disease. (From Timby BK, Smith NE. *Introductory Medical-Surgical Nursing.* 8th ed. Philadelphia, PA: Lippincott Williams & Wilkins; 2003:626.)

failure to express emotion. The tongue, palate, and throat muscles become rigid; the person may drool because of difficulty in moving the saliva to the back of the mouth and swallowing it. Speech becomes slow and monotonous, without modulation, and poorly articulated.

Because the basal ganglia also influence the autonomic nervous system, persons with Parkinson disease often have excessive and uncontrolled sweating, sebaceous gland secretion, and salivation. Autonomic symptoms, such as lacrimation, dysphagia, orthostatic hypotension, thermal regulation, constipation, impotence, and urinary incontinence, may be present, especially late in the disease.

Cognitive dysfunction may also be an important feature associated with Parkinson disease. It occurs in approximately 20% to 30% of persons with the disease and develops late in the course of the disease.[40] Deficits in executive functioning may be among the earliest signs of cognitive decline, as evidenced by difficulty in planning, starting, and carrying out tasks. Dementia, when it does occur, is usually a late manifestation of the disease, and the rate of decline is slow compared with Alzheimer disease.

Treatment. The approach to treatment of Parkinson disease must be highly individualized. It includes non-pharmacologic, pharmacologic, and, when indicated, surgical methods.[33,34,40] Nonpharmacologic interventions offer group support, education, daily exercise, and adequate nutrition. Botulinum toxin injections may be used in the treatment of dystonias such as eyelid spasm and limb dystonias that frequently are associated with Parkinson disease. Persons with parkinsonism other than idiopathic Parkinson disease usually do not respond significantly to medications developed for Parkinson disease.

Pharmacologic treatment usually is determined by the severity of symptoms. Antiparkinson drugs act by increasing the functional ability of the underactive dopaminergic system, or by reducing the excessive influence of excitatory cholinergic neurons. Drugs that improve the function of the dopaminergic system include those that increase dopamine levels (levodopa), stimulate dopamine receptors (dopamine receptor agonists), or retard the breakdown of dopamine (monoamine oxidase-B inhibitors).[40]

Levodopa, a dopamine agonist, is administered with carbidopa, which inhibits its peripheral metabolism, allowing therapeutic concentrations of the drug to enter the brain without disabling adverse effects. A later adverse effect of levodopa treatment is the so-called *on–off phenomenon,* in which frequent, abrupt, and unpredictable fluctuations in motor performance occur during the day. These fluctuations include "on" periods without dyskinesia, "on" periods with dyskinesia, and periods of bradykinesia (the "off" response). Some fluctuations reflect the timing of drug administration, in which case the "on" response coincides with peak drug levels and the "off" response with low drug levels.

Dopamine agonists such as pramipexole (Minaprex) and ropinirole (Requip) directly stimulate dopamine receptors. Rotigotine is a dopamine agonist that is supplied in a transdermal system. The dopamine agonists can be used as initial or adjunctive therapy in Parkinson disease and can be given in combination with carbidopa/levodopa. Rotigotine is only approved by the U.S. Food and Drug Administration (FDA) for initial treatment of Parkinson disease.

Amantidine, an antiviral agent, was found by chance to have antiparkinson properties. It is thought to augment release of dopamine from the remaining intact dopaminergic terminals in the nigrostriatal pathway of persons with Parkinson disease. It is used to treat persons with mild symptoms but no disability.

Several medications are used for adjuvant therapy as the initial therapy becomes less effective in controlling motor complications. As the therapy less effectively controls the symptoms, there is less "on time" (when the symptoms are controlled) and more "off time". Apomorphine is a dopamine agonist that can be given intravenously. It is often used as a rescue medication in patients experiencing sudden "off" periods or delayed "on" periods. Monamine oxidase-B inhibitors, such as selegiline and rasagiline, hinder the metabolic breakdown of dopamine. Selegiline and rasagiline may be used as adjunctive treatment to reduce mild on–off fluctuations in the responsiveness of persons who are receiving levodopa.

Because dopamine transmission is disrupted in Parkinson disease, there is a preponderance of cholinergic activity. Anticholinergic drugs (e.g., trihexyphenidyl, benztropine) are thought to restore a "balance" between reduced dopamine and uninhibited cholinergic neurons in the striatum. They are more useful in alleviating tremor and rigidity than bradykinesia. The anticholinergic drugs lessen the tremors and rigidity and afford some improvement of function. However, their potency seems to decrease over time, and increasing the dosage merely increases side effects such as blurred vision, dry mouth, bowel and bladder problems, cognitive dysfunction, and hallucinations.

Deep brain stimulation, which involves the surgical implantation of electrodes into the subthalamic nuclei or the pars interna of the globus pallidus, is an option for many persons who develop symptoms despite optimal medical therapy.[40,41] The electrodes are connected to a surgically implanted impulse generator that delivers electrical simulation to block the abnormal nerve activity that causes tremor and abnormal motor activity in Parkinson disease. The system allows the stimulation to be programmed to control the individual person's symptoms, and the stimulation parameters can be changed over time as the disease progresses. Deep brain stimulation is used for persons with Parkinson disease who respond to levodopa but experience side effects associated with it (e.g., motor fluctuation or dyskinesia). It is not a cure but serves to increase the duration of the "on" periods, allows for a reduction in medication dosages (in subthalamic nuclei stimulation), and improves function. Of note, other movement disorders can be treated by placing electrodes in different target sites (e.g., thalamus for tremor and globus pallidus internus for dystonia).

SUMMARY CONCEPTS

■ Both uncoordinated and abnormal muscle movements can result from disorders of the cerebellum and basal ganglia.

■ The functions of the cerebellum, which are especially vital during rapid muscular movements, use afferent input from various sources, including stretch receptors, proprioceptors, tactile receptors in the skin, visual input, and the vestibular system. Signs of cerebellar disorders include dystaxia, ataxia, tremor, and dysarthria.

■ The basal ganglia organize basic movement patterns into more complex patterns and release them when commanded by the motor cortex, contributing gracefulness to cortically initiated

(continued)

SUMMARY CONCEPTS (continued)

and controlled skilled movements. Disorders of the basal ganglia are characterized by involuntary movements, alterations in muscle tone, and disturbances in posture.

■ Parkinsonism is a disorder in which there is an imbalance between the dopaminergic inhibitory effects and excitatory cholinergic functions of the basal ganglia, and is manifested by resting tremor, increased muscle tonus and rigidity, slowness of movement (i.e., bradykinesia), gait disturbances, and impaired postural responses.

Upper Motor Neuron Disorders

Upper motor neuron disorders involve neurons that are fully contained within the CNS. They include the motor neurons arising in the motor areas of the cortex and their fibers as they project through the brain and descend in the spinal cord. Disorders that affect UMNs include multiple sclerosis and spinal cord injury. Stroke, which is a common cause of UMN damage, is discussed in Chapter 37. Amyotrophic lateral sclerosis is a mixed UMN and LMN disorder.

Amyotrophic Lateral Sclerosis

Amyotrophic lateral sclerosis (ALS), also known as *Lou Gehrig disease* after the famous New York Yankees baseball player, is a devastating neurologic disorder that selectively affects motor function. Amyotrophic lateral sclerosis has an annual incidence of about 2 cases per 100,000 population. It is primarily a disorder of middle to late adulthood, with men being affected more frequently than women. The disease typically follows a progressive course, with a mean survival period of 2 to 5 years from the onset of symptoms.

Amyotrophic lateral sclerosis is characterized by the loss of anterior LMNs in the spinal cord and motor nuclei of the brain stem and UMNs that originate in the motor cortex and descend via the pyramidal tract to synapse with the LMNs.[42–44] The death of LMNs leads to denervation, with subsequent muscle fiber atrophy and shinkage of skeletal muscles. It is this fiber atrophy, called *amyotrophy,* that appears in the name of the disease. The loss of nerve fibers in lateral columns of the white matter of the spinal cord, along with fibrillary gliosis, imparts a firmness or sclerosis to this CNS tissue; the term *lateral sclerosis* designates these changes. A remarkable feature of the disease is that the entire sensory system, the regulatory mechanisms of control and coordination of movement, and the intellect remain intact. The neurons for ocular motility and the parasympathetic neurons in the sacral spinal cord are also spared.

The pathogenesis of ALS is largely unknown, despite the identification of a number of genetic associations.[18,37,42,43,45]

Approximately 5% to 10% of cases are familial ALS, mostly with autosomal dominant inheritance. The rest are believed to be sporadic, with no family history of the disease. The gene for a subset of familial ALS has been mapped to the superoxide dismutase 1 (*SOD1*) gene on chromosome 21. SOD1 is a critical enzyme involved in protecting neurons from oxidative damage. Other suggested mechanisms of nerve injury are alterations in transport of molecules necessary for maintenance of the axon, neurofilament abnormalities, and glutamate-mediated excitotoxicity (see Chapter 37).

Manifestations of amyotrophic lateral sclerosis include those of both UMN and LMN dysfunction.[42–45] Muscle cramps involving the distal legs often are an early symptom. The most common clinical presentation is slowly progressive weakness and atrophy in distal muscles of one upper extremity. This is followed by regional spread of muscle weakness, reflecting involvement of neighboring areas of the spinal cord. Eventually, UMNs and LMNs involving multiple limbs and the head are affected. In the more advanced stages, muscles of the palate, pharynx, tongue, neck, and shoulders become involved, causing impairment of chewing, swallowing (dysphagia), and speech. Dysphagia with recurrent aspiration and weakness of the respiratory muscles produces the most significant acute complications of the disease. Death usually results from involvement of cranial nerves and respiratory musculature.

There are no specific tests for ALS. Diagnosis is based on a careful medical history, detailed physical and neurological examination, and electrophysiological studies.[43,44] Currently, there is no cure for ALS. The treatment of persons with ALS, which requires management of medical problems, severe disability, and psychosocial problems, is best provided by a multidisciplinary team.[42–44] Measures to assist persons with the disorder manage their symptoms (e.g., weakness and muscle spasms, dysphagia, communication difficulty, excessive salivation, and emotional lability), nutritional status, and respiratory muscle weakness increase survival time. An antiglutamate drug, riluzole, is the only drug approved for the treatment of ALS.[42] The drug is designed to decrease glutamate accumulation and slow the progression of the disease.

Multiple Sclerosis

Multiple sclerosis (MS) is an autoimmune demyelinating disorder characterized by inflammation and selective destruction of CNS myelin.[37,38,46–51] It affects approximately 350,000 persons in the United States and more than 1 million worldwide.[46] The age of onset is typically between 18 and 45 years.[46] Women are affected twice as frequently as men.

As with other autoimmune disorders, the pathogenesis appears to involve both genetic and environmental influences. The risk for developing MS is 15-fold higher when the disease is present in a first-degree relative, and is even greater in monozygotic twins.[37] People with the human leukocyte antigen (HLA)-DR2 haplotype (see

Chapter 15) are particularly susceptible. Alternatively, certain environmental factors such as residence in a northern latitude, particularly before age 15, may trigger disease in genetically susceptible persons. Recently, low vitamin D levels have been linked to MS. Because the penetrance of ultraviolet (UV) light declines rapidly with increased distance from the equator, it has been suggested that the quantities of UV light required for production of vitamin D may be insufficient, especially in winter.[46]

Pathophysiology

The pathophysiology of MS involves the demyelination of nerve fibers in the white matter of the brain, spinal cord, and optic nerve.[37,46–49] In the CNS, myelin is formed by the oligodendrocytes, chiefly those lying among the nerve fibers in the white matter. The properties of the myelin sheath—high electrical resistance and low capacitance—permit it to function as an electrical insulator. Demyelinated nerve fibers display a variety of conduction abnormalities, ranging from decreased conduction velocity to conduction blocks.

The lesions of MS consist of hard, sharp-edged, demyelinated or sclerotic patches that are macroscopically visible throughout the white matter of the CNS[37,38] (Fig. 36-13). These lesions, which represent the end result of acute myelin breakdown, are called *plaques*. The lesions have a predilection for the optic nerves, periventricular white matter, brain stem, cerebellum, and spinal cord white matter. Although the sequence of myelin breakdown is not well understood, it is known that the lesions contain small amounts of myelin basic proteins and increased amounts of proteolytic enzymes, macrophages, lymphocytes, and plasma cells. Acute, subacute, and chronic lesions often are seen at multiple sites throughout the CNS.

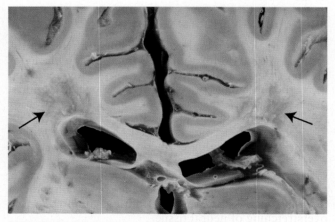

FIGURE 36-13. Multiple sclerosis. This fresh coronal section shows the darker hues of the somewhat irregular periventricular plaques (*arrows*) reflecting the loss of myelin, which imparts the normal glistening white appearance of white matter. (From Fuller GN, Goodman JC. In: Rubin E, Strayer DS, eds. *Rubin's Pathology: Clinicopathologic Foundations of Medicine.* 6th ed. Philadelphia, PA: Wolters Kluwer Health | Lippincott Williams & Wilkins; 2012:1336.)

Magnetic resonance imaging (MRI), which has had a major impact on the diagnosis and subsequent follow-up of MS, has shown that the lesions of MS may occur in two stages: a first stage that involves the sequential development of small inflammatory lesions, and a second stage during which the lesions extend and consolidate and when demyelination and gliosis (plaque formation) occur. It is not known whether the inflammatory process, present during the first stage, is directed against myelin or against the oligodendrocytes that produce myelin.

Clinical Manifestations

The interruption of neural conduction in the demyelinated nerves in MS is manifested by a variety of symptoms, depending on the location and extent of the lesion.[46,47,51] Areas commonly affected are the optic nerve (visual field), corticobulbar tracts (speech and swallowing), corticospinal tracts (muscle strength), cerebellar tracts (gait and coordination), spinocerebellar tracts (balance), medial longitudinal fasciculus (conjugate gaze function of the extraocular eye muscles), and posterior cell columns of the spinal cord (position and vibratory sensation). Typically, an otherwise healthy person presents with an acute or subacute episode of paresthesias, optic neuritis (i.e., visual clouding or loss of vision in part of the visual field with pain on movement of the globe), diplopia, or specific types of gaze paralysis.

Paresthesias are evidenced as numbness, tingling, burning sensations, or pressure on the face or involved extremities, with symptoms ranging from annoying to severe. The *Lhermitte sign* is an electric shock–like tingling down the back and onto the legs that is produced by flexion of the neck. Pain from spasticity also may be a factor that can be alleviated by appropriate stretching exercises. Other common symptoms are abnormal gait, bladder and sexual dysfunction, vertigo, nystagmus, fatigue, and speech disturbance. These symptoms usually last for several days to weeks, and then completely or partially resolve. After a period of normal or relatively normal function, new symptoms appear. Psychological manifestations, such as mood swings, may represent an emotional reaction to the nature of the disease or, more likely, involvement of the white matter of the cerebral cortex. Depression, euphoria, inattentiveness, apathy, forgetfulness, and loss of memory may occur.

Fatigue is one of the most common problems for persons with MS. Fatigue often is described as a generalized low-energy feeling not related to depression and different from weakness. Fatigue has a harmful impact on activities of daily living and sustained physical activity. Interventions such as spacing activities and setting priorities often are helpful.

The course of the disease may fall into one of four categories: relapsing-remitting, secondary progressive, primary progressive, or progressive relapsing.[46] The *relapsing-remitting* form of the disease is characterized by episodes of acute worsening with recovery and a stable course between relapses. *Secondary progressive disease* involves a gradual neurologic deterioration with or without superimposed acute relapses in a person with previous relapsing-remitting disease. *Primary progressive disease* is characterized by nearly continuous neurologic deterioration from onset of symptoms. The *progressive relapsing* category of disease involves gradual neurologic deterioration from the onset of symptoms but with subsequent superimposed relapses.

Diagnosis and Treatment

The diagnosis of MS is based on evidence of CNS lesions that are disseminated in time and space (i.e., occur in different parts of the CNS at least 3 months apart), with no explanation for the disease process.[46,47,51] MRI, which is a sensitive diagnostic tool that is an adjunct to clinical diagnosis, can detect lesions even when CT scans appear normal. A computer-assisted method of MRI can measure lesion size. Many new areas of myelin abnormality are asymptomatic. Serial MRI studies can be done to detect asymptomatic lesions, monitor the progress of existing lesions, and evaluate the effectiveness of treatment. Although MRI can be used to provide evidence of disseminated lesions in persons with the disease, normal findings do not exclude the diagnosis. Electrophysiologic evaluations (e.g., evoked potential studies) and CT scans may assist in the identification and documentation of lesions.

Most treatment measures for MS are directed at modifying the course and managing the primary symptoms of the disease.[46,47] The variability in symptoms, unpredictable course, and lack of specific diagnostic methods has made the evaluation and treatment of MS difficult. Persons who are minimally affected by the disorder require no specific treatment. The person should be encouraged to maintain as healthy a lifestyle as possible, including good nutrition and adequate rest and relaxation. Physical therapy may help maintain muscle tone. Every effort should be made to avoid excessive fatigue, physical deterioration, emotional stress, viral infections, and extremes of environmental temperature, which may precipitate an exacerbation of the disease.

The pharmacologic agents used in the treatment of MS fall into three categories: those used to (1) treat acute attacks or initial demyelinating episodes, (2) modify the course of the disease, and (3) treat symptoms of the disorder.[46] Corticosteroids are the mainstay of treatment for acute attacks of MS. These agents are thought to reduce the inflammation, improve nerve conduction, and exert important immunologic effects. Long-term administration does not, however, appear to alter the course of the disease and can have harmful side effects. Adrenocorticotropic hormone (ACTH) also may be used in the treatment of MS. Plasmapheresis has also proved beneficial in some cases.[46]

Disease-modifying agents include interferon-β and glatiramer acetate.[46,47,52] These agents have shown some benefit in reducing exacerbations in persons with relapsing-remitting MS. Interferon-β is a cytokine that acts as an immune enhancer. Two forms have been approved by the FDA for treatment of MS—interferon-β1a and interferon-β1b. Both are administered by injection, and both are usually well tolerated. Glatiramer acetate is a synthetic polypeptide that simulates parts of the myelin basic protein. Although the exact mechanism of action is unknown, the drug appears to block myelin-damaging T cells by acting as a myelin decoy. The drug is given daily by subcutaneous injection. Mitoxantrone, an anticancer drug, is recommended for persons with worsening forms of the disease. Because it is an anticancer drug, it is recommended that it only be administered by experienced health care professionals. Other promising therapies that focus on immune-mediated disease mechanisms are in development.

Among the medications used to manage the chronic problems associated with MS are dantrolene, baclofen, or diazepam for spasticity; cholinergic drugs for bladder problems; and antidepressant drugs for depression.

Vertebral and Spinal Cord Injury

Spinal cord injury (SCI) represents damage to the neural elements of the spinal cord. Spinal cord injury is primarily a disorder of young people, with nearly half of all injuries occurring in the 16- to 30-year-old age group.[53] The most common cause of SCI is motor vehicle accidents, followed by falls, violence (primarily gunshot wounds), and recreational sporting activities.[53] Life expectancy for persons with SCI continues to increase, but is somewhat below life expectancy for people without SCI.

Most SCIs involve damage to the vertebral column or supporting ligaments as well as the spinal cord. Because of extensive tract systems that connect sensory afferent neurons and LMNs with higher brain centers, SCIs commonly involve both sensory and motor function. Although the discussion in this section of the chapter focuses on traumatic SCI, much of the content is applicable to SCI caused by other disorders, such as congenital deformities (e.g., spina bifida), tumors, ischemia and infarction, and bone disease with pathologic fractures of the vertebrae.

Injury to the Vertebral Column

Injuries to the vertebral column include fractures, dislocations, and subluxations. A fracture can occur at any part of the bony vertebrae, causing fragmentation of the bone. It most often involves the pedicle, lamina, or processes (e.g., facets, see Fig. 36-9). Dislocation or subluxation (partial dislocation) injury causes the vertebral bodies to become displaced, with one overriding another and preventing correct alignment of the vertebral column. Damage to the ligaments or bony vertebrae may make the spine unstable. In an unstable spine, further unguarded movement of the spinal column can impinge on the spinal canal, causing compression or overstretching of neural tissue.

Most injuries result from some combination of compressive force or bending movements.[18] Flexion injuries occur when forward bending of the spinal column exceeds the limits of normal movement. Typical flexion injuries result, for example, when the head is struck from behind, as in a fall with the back of the head as the point of impact. Extension injuries occur with excessive forced bending (i.e., hyperextension) of the spine backward. A typical extension injury involves a fall in which the chin or face is the point of impact, causing hyperextension of the neck. Injuries of flexion and extension occur more commonly in the cervical spine (C4 to C6) than in any other area. Limitations imposed by the ribs, spinous processes, and joint capsules in the thoracic and lumbar spine make this area less flexible and less susceptible to flexion and extension injuries than the cervical spine.

A compression injury, causing the vertebral bones to shatter, squash, or even burst, occurs when there is spinal loading from a high-velocity blow to the top of the head or when landing forcefully on the feet or buttocks[18] (Fig. 36-14A). This typically occurs at the cervical level (e.g., diving injuries) or in the thoracolumbar area (e.g., falling from a distance and landing on the buttocks). Compression injuries may occur when the vertebrae are weakened by conditions such as osteoporosis and cancer with bone metastasis. Axial rotation injuries can produce highly unstable injuries. Maximal axial rotation occurs in the cervical region, especially between C1 and C2, and at the lumbosacral joint[18] (see Fig. 36-14B). Coupling of vertebral motions is common in injury when two or more individual motions occur (e.g., lateral bending and axial rotation).

Acute Spinal Cord Injury

Spinal cord injury involves damage to the neural elements of the spinal cord. The damage may result from direct trauma to the cord from penetrating wounds or indirect injury resulting from vertebral fractures, fracture-dislocations, or subluxations of the spine. The spinal cord may be contused, not only at the site of injury but also above and below the trauma site.[18] Traumatic injury may be complicated by the loss of blood flow to the cord, with resulting infarction.

Sudden, complete transection of the spinal cord results in complete loss of motor, sensory, reflex, and autonomic function below the level of injury. The immediate response to SCI is often referred to as *spinal shock*. It is characterized by flaccid paralysis with loss of tendon reflexes below the level of injury, absence of somatic and visceral sensations below the level of injury, and loss of bowel and bladder function. Loss of systemic sympathetic vasomotor tone may result in vasodilation, increased venous capacity, and hypotension. These manifestations occur regardless of whether the level of the lesion eventually will produce spastic (UMN) or flaccid (LMN) paralysis. The basic mechanisms accounting for transient spinal shock are unknown. Spinal shock may last for hours, days, or weeks. Usually, if reflex function returns by the time the person reaches the acute care setting, the neuromuscular changes are reversible. This type of reversible spinal shock may occur in football injuries, in which jarring of the spinal cord produces a concussionlike syndrome with loss of movement and reflexes, followed by full recovery within days. In persons in whom the loss of reflexes persists, hypotension and bradycardia may become a critical but manageable problem. In general, the higher the level of injury, the greater is the effect.

Pathophysiology. The pathophysiology of acute SCI can be divided into two types: primary and secondary.[18,54,55] The *primary neurologic injury* occurs at the time of injury and is irreversible. It is characterized by small hemorrhages in the gray matter of the cord, followed by edematous changes in the white matter that lead to necrosis of neural tissue. This type of injury results from the forces of compression, stretch, and

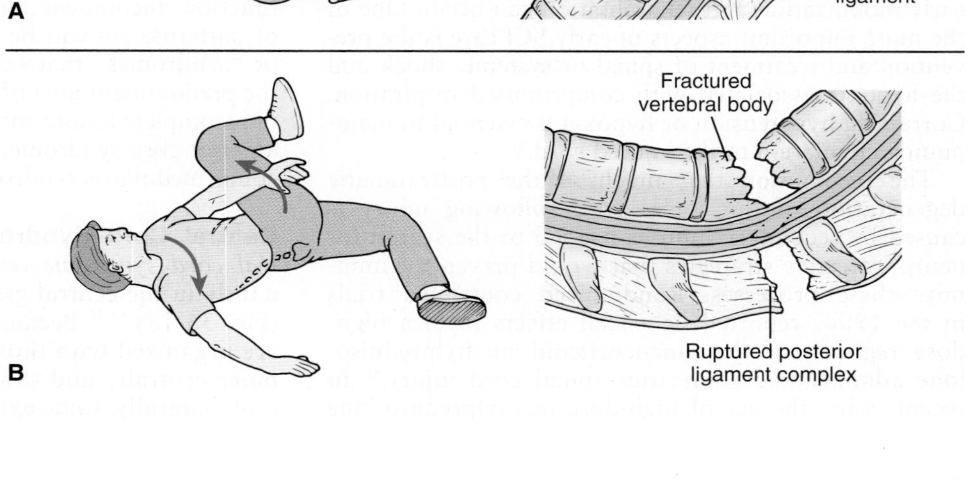

FIGURE 36-14. (A) Compression vertebral fracture secondary to axial loading as occurs when a person falls from a height and lands on the buttocks. **(B)** Rotational injury, in which there is concurrent fracture and tearing of the posterior ligamentous complex, is caused by extreme lateral flexion or twisting of the head or neck. (Modified from Hickey JV. *The Clinical Practice of Neurological and Neurosurgical Nursing.* 5th ed. Philadelphia, PA: Lippincott Williams & Wilkins; 2003:411–412.)

Force

A

Compression fracture of vertebral body

Stretched intraspinous ligament

Fractured vertebral body

Ruptured posterior ligament complex

B

shear associated with fracture or compression of the spinal vertebrae, dislocation of vertebrae (e.g., flexion, extension, subluxation) or contusions due to jarring of the cord in the spinal canal. Penetrating injuries produce lacerations and direct trauma to the cord and may occur with or without spinal column damage. Lacerations occur when there is cutting or tearing of the spinal cord, which injures nerve tissue and causes bleeding and edema.

Secondary injuries follow the primary injury and promote the spread of injury. Although there is considerable debate about the pathogenesis of secondary injuries, the tissue destruction that occurs ends in progressive neurologic damage. After SCI, several pathologic mechanisms come into play, including vascular damage, neuronal injury that leads to loss of reflexes below the level of injury, and release of vasoactive agents and cellular enzymes. Vascular lesions (i.e., vessel trauma and hemorrhage) can lead to ischemia, increased vascular permeability, and edema. Blood flow to the spinal cord may be further compromised by spinal shock that results from a loss of vasomotor tone and neural reflexes below the level of injury. The release of vasoactive substances (i.e., norepinephrine, serotonin, dopamine, and histamine) from the wound tissue causes vasospasm and impedes blood flow in the microcirculation, producing further necrosis of blood vessels and neurons. The release of proteolytic and lipolytic enzymes from injured cells causes delayed swelling, demyelination, and necrosis in the neural tissue in the spinal cord.

Management. The goal of management of acute SCI is to reduce the neurologic deficit and prevent any additional loss of neurologic function. The specific steps in resuscitation and initial evaluation can be carried out at the trauma site or in the emergency department, depending on the urgency of the situation.[18] Most traumatic injuries to the spinal column render it unstable, mandating immobilization measures such as collars and backboards and limiting the movement of persons at risk for or with known SCI. Every person with multiple trauma or head injury, including victims of traffic and sporting accidents, should be suspected of having sustained an acute SCI.

The goal of early surgical intervention for an unstable spine is to provide internal skeletal stabilization so that early mobilization and rehabilitation can occur. One of the more important aspects of early SCI care is the prevention and treatment of spinal or systemic shock and the hypoxia associated with compromised respiration. Correcting hypotension or hypoxia is essential to maintaining circulation to the injured cord.[18]

The recognition that much of the posttraumatic degeneration of the spinal cord following injury is caused by secondary injuries has led to the search for neuroprotective strategies that would prevent or minimize these processes. Randomized controlled trials in the 1990s reported beneficial effects from a high-dose regimen of the glucocorticoid methylprednisolone administered soon after spinal cord injury.[56] In recent years, the use of high-dose methylprednisolone

has become controversial, largely based on the risk of serious adverse effects (e.g., gastric bleeding, wound infection, venous thrombosis, and steroid myopathy) versus what is perceived to be a modest neurologic benefit.[57] Other neuroprotective agents, including monosialoganglioside sodium (GM-1 ganglioside), naloxone, and tirilazad, have been tested in multicenter clinical trials, but primary end points have not been achieved. Riluzole, a sodium-channel blocker, approved for treatment of ALS, has also shown some promise in preventing secondary injury by blocking sodium channels. Recent investigations are exploring the effects of early cooling strategies (i.e., mild and moderate hypothermia) on recovery outcomes in persons with spinal cord injury.[58]

Types and Classification of Spinal Cord Injury

Alterations in body function that result from SCI depend on the level of injury and the amount of cord involvement. *Tetraplegia*, sometimes referred to as *quadriplegia*, is the impairment or loss of motor or sensory function (or both) after damage to neural structures in the cervical segments of the spinal cord.[18,59] It results in impairment of function in the arms, trunk, legs, and pelvic organs (see Fig. 36-4). *Paraplegia* refers to impairment or loss of motor or sensory function (or both) from damage of neural elements in the spinal canal in the thoracic, lumbar, or sacral segments of the spinal cord.[18,59] With paraplegia, arm functioning is spared, but depending on the level of injury, functioning of the trunk, legs, and pelvic organs may be impaired. Paraplegia includes conus medullaris and cauda equina injuries (discussed later).

Further definitions of SCI describe the extent of neurologic damage as *complete* or *incomplete*[18,59] (Chart 36-1). Complete cord injuries can result from severance of the cord, disruption of nerve fibers although they remain intact, or interruption of blood supply to that segment, resulting in complete destruction of neural tissue and UMN or LMN paralysis. With complete injuries, no motor or sensory function is preserved in sacral segments S4 to S6. Incomplete SCI implies there is some residual motor or sensory function below the level of injury.

The prognosis for return of function is better in an incomplete injury because of preservation of axonal function. Incomplete injuries may manifest in a variety of patterns, but can be organized into certain patterns or "syndromes" that occur more frequently and reflect the predominant area of the cord that is involved. Types of incomplete lesions include the central cord syndrome, anterior cord syndrome, Brown-Séquard syndrome, and conus medullaris syndrome.

Central Cord Syndrome. A condition called *central cord syndrome* occurs when injury is predominantly in the central gray or white matter of the cord (Fig. 36-15).[18,59] Because the corticospinal tract fibers are organized with those controlling the arms located more centrally and those controlling the legs located more laterally, some external axonal transmission may

CHART 36-1   American Spinal Injury Association (ASIA) Impairment Scale

A = Complete: No motor or sensory function is preserved in sacral segments S4-S5.

B = Sensory Incomplete. Sensory but not motor function is preserved below the neurological level and includes the sacral segments S4-5 (light touch or pin prick at S4-S5 or deep anal pressure) AND no motor function is preserved more than three levels below the motor level on either side of the body.

C = Motor Incomplete. Motor function is preserved below the neurological level**, and more than half of key muscle functions below the neurological level of injury (NLI) have a muscle grade less than 3 (Grades 0–2).

D = Motor Incomplete. Motor function is preserved below the neurological level**, and *at least half* (half or more) of key muscle functions below the NLI have a muscle grade ≥3.

E = Normal. If sensation and motor function as tested with the ISNCSCI are graded as normal in all segments, and the patient had prior deficits, then the ASIA grade is E. Someone without an initial SCI does not receive an AIS grade.

****For an individual to receive a grade of C or D (i.e., motor incomplete status), they must have either (1) voluntary anal sphincter contraction or (2) sacral sensory sparing *with* sparing of motor function more than three levels below the motor level for that side of the body. The International Standards at this time allows even non-key muscle function more than 3 levels below the motor level to be used in determining motor incomplete status (AIS B versus C).

NOTE: When assessing the extent of motor sparing below the level for distinguishing between AIS B and C, the motor level on each side is used; whereas to differentiate between ASIA C and D (based on proportion of key muscle functions with strength grade 3 or greater) the neurological level of injury is used.

Muscle Function Grading: (0) = total paralysis; **(1)** = palpable or visible contraction; **(2)** = active movement, full range of motion (ROM) with gravity eliminated; **(3)** = active movement, full ROM against gravity; **(4)** = active movement, full ROM against gravity and moderate resistance in a muscle specific position; **(5)** = (normal) active movement, full ROM against gravity and full resistance in a functional muscle position expected from an otherwise unimpaired person; **(5*)** = (normal) active movement, full ROM against gravity and sufficient resistance to be considered normal if identified inhibiting factors (i.e., pain, disuse) were not present; **(NT)** = not testable (i.e., due to immobilization, severe pain such that the patient cannot be graded, amputation of limb, or contracture of >50% of the normal range of motion).

Sensory Grading : (0) = Absent; **(1)** = Altered, either decreased/impaired sensation or hypersensitivity; **(2)** = Normal; **(NT)** = Not testable.

Developed from the American Spinal Injury Association. International Standards for Neurological Classification of Spinal Cord Injury (ISNCSCI), revised 2013. Atlanta, GA; Reprinted 2013.

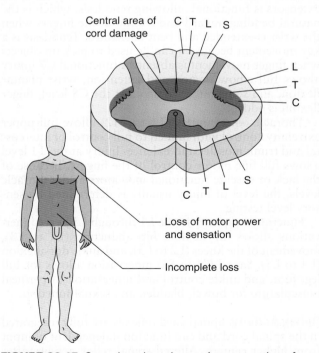

FIGURE 36-15. Central cord syndrome. A cross-section of the cord shows central damage and the associated motor and sensory loss. C, cervical; L, lumbar; S, sacral; T, thoracic.(From Kitt S, Kaiser J. *Emergency Nursing: A Physiological and Clinical Perspective*. Philadelphia, PA: W.B. Saunders; 1990.)

remain intact. Motor function of the upper extremities is affected, but the lower extremities may not be affected or may be affected to a lesser degree, with some sparing of sacral sensation. Bowel, bladder, and sexual functions usually are affected to various degrees, and this may parallel the degree of lower extremity involvement. This syndrome occurs almost exclusively in the cervical cord, rendering the lesion a UMN lesion with spastic paralysis. Central cord damage is more frequent in elderly persons with narrowing or stenotic changes in the spinal canal that are related to arthritis.

Anterior Cord Syndrome. Anterior cord syndrome usually is caused by damage from infarction of the anterior spinal artery, resulting in damage to the anterior two thirds of the cord[18,59] (Fig. 36-16). The deficits include loss of motor function provided by the corticospinal tracts and loss of pain and temperature sensations from damage to the lateral spinothalamic tracts. The posterior third of the cord is relatively unaffected, preserving the dorsal column axons that convey position, vibration, and touch sensations.

Brown-Séquard Syndrome. A condition called *Brown-Séquard syndrome* results from damage to a hemisection of the anterior and posterior cord[18,59] (Fig. 36-17). The effect is a loss of voluntary motor function from the

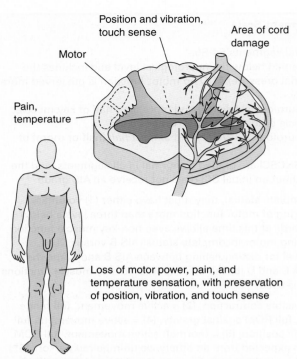

FIGURE 36-16. Anterior cord syndrome. Cord damage and associated motor and sensory loss are illustrated. (From Kitt S, Kaiser J. *Emergency Nursing: A Physiological and Clinical Perspective.* Philadelphia, PA: W.B. Saunders; 1990.)

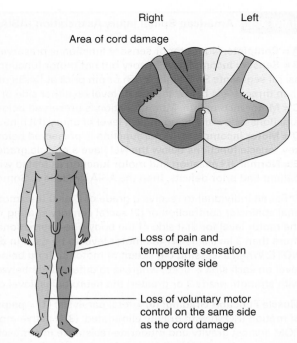

FIGURE 36-17. Brown-Séquard syndrome. Cord damage and associated motor and sensory loss are illustrated. (From Kitt S, Kaiser J. *Emergency Nursing: A Physiological and Clinical Perspective.* Philadelphia, PA: W.B. Saunders; 1990.)

corticospinal tract, proprioception loss from the ipsilateral side of the body, and contralateral loss of pain and temperature sensations from the lateral spinothalamic tracts for all levels below the lesion.

Conus Medullaris Syndrome. The conus medullaris syndrome involves damage to the conus medullaris or the sacral cord (i.e., conus) and lumbar nerve roots in the neural canal.[18,59] Functional deficits resulting from this type of injury usually result in flaccid bowel and bladder and altered sexual function. Sacral segments occasionally show preserved reflexes if only the conus is affected. Motor function in the legs and feet may be impaired without significant sensory impairment. Damage to the lumbosacral nerve roots in the spinal canal usually results in LMN and sensory neuron damage known as *cauda equina syndrome.* Functional deficits present as various patterns of asymmetric flaccid paralysis, sensory impairment, and pain.

Disruption of Somatosensory and Skeletal Muscle Function

Functional abilities after SCI are subject to various degrees of somatosensory and skeletal muscle function loss and altered reflex activity based on the level of cord injury and extent of cord damage (Table 36-2).

Motor and Somatosensory Function. Skeletal muscle function in cervical injuries ranges from complete dependence to independence with or without assistive devices in activities of mobility and self-care. The functional levels of cervical injury are related to C5, C6, C7, or

C8 innervation. At the C5 level, deltoid and biceps function is spared, allowing full head, neck, and diaphragm control with good shoulder strength and full elbow flexion. At the C6 level, wrist dorsiflexion by the wrist extensors is functional, allowing tenodesis, which is the natural bending inward and flexion of the fingers when the wrist is extended and bent backward. Tenodesis is a key movement because it can be used to pick up objects when finger movement is absent. A functional C7 injury allows full elbow flexion and extension, wrist plantar flexion, and some finger control. At the C8 level, finger flexion is added.

Thoracic cord injuries (T1 to T12) allow full upper extremity control with limited to full control of intercostal and trunk muscles and balance. Injury at the T1 level allows full fine motor control of the fingers. Because of the lack of specific functional indicators at the thoracic levels, the level of injury usually is determined by sensory level testing.

Functional capacity in the L1 through L5 nerve innervations allows hip flexion, hip abduction (L1 to L3), movement of the knees (L2 to L5), and ankle dorsiflexion (L4 to L5). Sacral (S1 to S5) innervation allows for full leg, foot, and ankle control and innervation of perineal musculature for bowel, bladder, and sexual function.

Reflex Activity. Spinal cord reflexes are fully integrated in the spinal cord and can function independent of input from higher centers. Altered spinal reflex activity after SCI is essentially determined by the level of injury and whether UMNs or LMNs are affected. With UMN injuries at T12 and above, the cord reflexes remain

TABLE 36-2   Functional Abilities by Level of Cord Injury

Injury Level	Segmental Sensorimotor Function	Dressing, Eating	Elimination	Mobility*
C1	Little or no sensation or control of head and neck; no diaphragm control; requires continuous ventilation	Dependent	Dependent	Limited. Voice-controlled or sip-n-puff electric wheelchair
C2–C3	Head and neck sensation; some neck control. Independent of mechanical ventilation for short periods.	Dependent	Dependent	Same as for C1
C4	Good head and neck sensation and motor control; some shoulder elevation; diaphragm movement	Dependent; may be able to eat with adaptive sling	Dependent	Limited to voice-, mouth-, head-, chin-, or shoulder-controlled electric wheelchair
C5	Full head and neck control; shoulder strength; elbow flexion	Independent with assistance	Maximal assistance	Electric or modified manual wheelchair, needs transfer assistance
C6	Fully innervated shoulder; wrist extension or dorsiflexion	Independent or with minimal assistance	Independent or with minimal assistance	Independent in transfers and wheelchair
C7–C8	Full elbow extension; wrist plantar flexion; some finger control	Independent	Independent	Independent; manual wheelchair
T1–T5	Full hand and finger control; use of intercostal and thoracic muscles	Independent	Independent	Independent; manual wheelchair
T6–T10	Abdominal muscle control, partial to good balance with trunk muscles	Independent	Independent	Independent; manual wheelchair
T11–L5	Hip flexors, hip abductors (L1–3); knee extension (L2–4); knee flexion and ankle dorsiflexion (L4–5)	Independent	Independent	Short distance to full ambulation with assistance
S1–S5	Full leg, foot, and ankle control; innervation of perineal muscles for bowel, bladder, and sexual function (S2–4)	Independent	Normal to impaired bowel and bladder function	Ambulate independently with or without assistance

*Assistance refers to adaptive equipment, setup, or physical assistance.

intact, whereas communication pathways with higher centers have been interrupted. This results in spasticity of involved skeletal muscle groups and of smooth and skeletal muscles that control bowel, bladder, and sexual function. In LMN injuries at T12 or below, the reflex circuitry itself has been damaged at the level of the spinal cord or spinal nerve, resulting in a decrease or absence of reflex function. The LMN injuries cause flaccid paralysis of involved skeletal muscle groups and the smooth and skeletal muscles that control bowel, bladder, and sexual function. However, injuries near the T12 level may result in mixed UMN and LMN deficits (e.g., spastic paralysis of the bowel and bladder with flaccid muscle tone).

After the period of spinal shock in a UMN injury, isolated spinal reflex activity and muscle tone that are not under the control of higher centers return. This may result in hypertonia and spasticity of skeletal muscles below the level of injury.[18] These spastic movements are involuntary instead of voluntary, a distinction that needs to be explained to persons with SCI and their families. The antigravity muscles, the flexors of the arms and extensors of the legs, are predominantly affected. Spastic movements are usually heightened initially after injury, reaching a peak and then becoming stable in approximately 1.5 to 2 years.[18]

The stimuli for reflex muscle spasm arise from somatic and visceral afferent pathways that enter the cord below the level of injury. The most common of these stimuli are muscle stretching, bladder infections or stones, fistulas, bowel distention or impaction, pressure areas or irritation of the skin, and infections. Because the stimuli that precipitate spasms vary from person to person, careful assessment is necessary to identify the factors that precipitate spasm in each person. Passive range-of-motion exercises to stretch the spastic muscles help to prevent spasm induced by muscle stretching, such as occurs with a change in body position.

Spasticity in itself is not detrimental and may even facilitate maintenance of muscle tone to prevent muscle wasting, improve venous return, and aid in mobility.

Spasms become detrimental when they impair safety; they also reduce the ability to make functional gains in mobility and activities of daily living. Spasms also may cause trauma to bones and tissues, leading to joint contractures and skin breakdown.

Respiratory Muscle Function. Ventilation requires movement of the expiratory and inspiratory muscles, all of which receive innervation from the spinal cord.[60,61] The main muscle of ventilation, the diaphragm, is innervated by segments C3 to C5 through the phrenic nerves. The intercostal muscles, which function in elevating the rib cage and are needed for coughing and deep breathing, are innervated by spinal segments T1 through T7. The major muscles of expiration are the abdominal muscles, which receive their innervation from levels T6 to T12.

Although the ability to inhale and exhale may be preserved at various levels of SCI, functional deficits in ventilation are most apparent in the quality of the breathing cycle and the ability to oxygenate tissues, eliminate carbon dioxide, and mobilize secretions. Cord injuries involving C1 to C3 result in a lack of respiratory effort, and affected patients require assisted ventilation. Although a C3 to C5 injury allows partial or full diaphragmatic function, ventilation is diminished because of the loss of intercostal muscle function, resulting in shallow breaths and a weak cough. Below the C5 level, as less intercostal and abdominal musculature is affected, the ability to take a deep breath and cough is less impaired. Maintenance therapy consists of muscle training to strengthen existing muscles for endurance and mobilization of secretions. The ability to speak is compromised with assisted ventilation, whether continuous or intermittent. Thus, ensuring adequate communication of needs is essential.

Disruption of Autonomic Nervous System Function

In addition to its effects on skeletal muscle function, SCI interrupts autonomic nervous system function below the site of injury.[62] This includes sympathetic outflow from the thoracic and upper lumbar cord and parasympathetic outflow from the sacral cord. Because of their sites of exit from the CNS, the cranial nerves, such as the vagus, are unaffected. Depending on the level of injury, the spinal reflexes that control autonomic nervous system function are largely isolated from the rest of the CNS. The regulation and integration of reflex function by centers in the brain and brain stem are lacking. This results in a situation in which the autonomic reflexes below the level of injury are uncontrolled, whereas those above the level of injury function in a relatively controlled manner.

Sympathetic nervous system regulation of circulatory function and body temperature (i.e., thermoregulation) presents some of the most severe problems in SCI. The higher the level of injury and the greater the surface area affected, the more profound are the effects on circulation and thermoregulation. Persons with injury at the T6 level or above experience problems in regulating vasomotor tone, whereas those with injuries below the T6 level usually have sufficient sympathetic function to maintain adequate vasomotor function. The level of injury and its corresponding problems may vary among persons, and some dysfunctional effects may be seen at levels below T6. With lower lumbar and sacral injuries, sympathetic function remains essentially unaltered.

Vasovagal Response. The vagus nerve (cranial nerve X), which is unaffected in SCI, normally exerts a continuous inhibitory effect on heart rate. Vagal stimulation that causes a marked bradycardia is called the *vasovagal response*. Visceral afferent input to the vagal centers in the brain stem of persons with tetraplegia or high-level paraplegia can produce marked bradycardia when unchecked by a dysfunctional sympathetic nervous system. Severe bradycardia and even asystole can result when the vasovagal response is elicited by deep endotracheal suctioning or rapid position change. Preventive measures, such as hyperoxygenation before, during, and after tracheal suctioning, are advised. Rapid position changes should also be avoided or anticipated, and anticholinergic drugs should be immediately available to counteract severe episodes of bradycardia.

Autonomic Dysreflexia. Autonomic dysreflexia represents an acute episode of exaggerated sympathetic reflex responses that occur in persons with injuries at T6 and above, in which CNS control of spinal reflexes is lost (Fig. 36-18). It does not occur until spinal shock has resolved and autonomic reflexes return, most often within the first 6 months after injury. It is most unpredictable during the first year after injury, but can occur throughout the person's lifetime.

Autonomic dysreflexia is characterized by vasospasm, hypertension ranging from mild (20 mm Hg above baseline) to severe (as high as 240/120 mm Hg, or higher), skin pallor, and gooseflesh associated with the piloerector response.[63] Because baroreceptor function and parasympathetic control of heart rate travel by way of the cranial nerves, these responses remain intact. Continued hypertension produces a baroreflex-mediated vagal slowing of the heart rate to bradycardic levels. There is an accompanying baroreflex-mediated vasodilation, with flushed skin and profuse sweating above the level of injury, headache ranging from dull to severe and pounding, nasal stuffiness, and feelings of anxiety. A person may experience one, several, or all of the symptoms with each episode.

The stimuli initiating the dysreflexic response include visceral distention, such as a full bladder or rectum; stimulation of pain receptors, as occurs with pressure ulcers, dressing changes, and diagnostic or operative procedures; and visceral contractions, such as ejaculation, bladder spasms, or uterine contractions. In many cases, the dysreflexic response results from a full bladder.

Autonomic dysreflexia is a clinical emergency, and without prompt and adequate treatment, convulsions, loss of consciousness, and even death can occur. The major components of treatment include monitoring blood pressure while removing or correcting the initiating

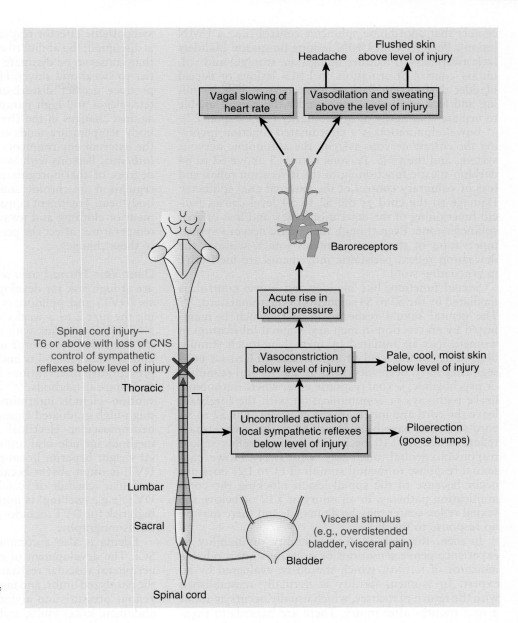

FIGURE 36-18. Mechanisms of autonomic dysreflexia.

cause or stimulus. The person should be placed in an upright position, and all support hose or binders should be removed to promote venous pooling of blood and reduce venous return, thereby decreasing blood pressure. If the stimuli have been removed or the stimuli cannot be identified and the upright position is established but the blood pressure remains elevated, drugs that block autonomic function are administered. Prevention of the type of stimuli that trigger the dysreflexic event is advocated.

Postural Hypotension. Postural, or orthostatic, hypotension usually occurs in persons with injuries at T4 to T6 and above and is related to the interruption of descending control of sympathetic outflow to blood vessels in the extremities and abdomen.[62] Pooling of blood, along with gravitational forces, impairs the return of venous blood to the heart, causing a decrease in cardiac

output along with a drop in arterial blood pressure when the person is placed in an upright position. The disorder is characterized by dizziness, pallor, excessive sweating above the level of the lesion, complaints of blurred vision, and possible fainting. Postural hypotension usually is prevented by slow changes in position and measures to promote venous return.

Disruption of Bladder, Bowel, and Sexual Function

Among the most devastating consequences of SCI are the loss of bladder, bowel, and sexual function.[18,64] Loss of bladder function results from disruption of neural pathways between the bladder and the reflex voiding center at the S2 to S4 level (i.e., a LMN lesion) or between the reflex voiding center and higher brain centers that coordinate sphincter control (i.e., a UMN lesion). Persons with UMN lesions or spastic bladders lack awareness of bladder filling (i.e., storage) and voluntary control of urination. In LMN lesions or flaccid bladder dysfunction, lack of awareness of bladder filling and lack of bladder tone render the person unable to urinate voluntarily or involuntarily (see Chapter 27).

Bowel elimination is a coordinated function involving the enteric nervous system, the autonomic nervous system, and the CNS. Persons with SCI above S2 to S4 develop spastic functioning of the defecation reflex and loss of voluntary control of the external anal sphincter. Damage to the cord at the S2 to S4 level causes flaccid functioning of the defecation reflex and loss of anal sphincter tone. Even though the enteric nervous system innervation of the bowel remains intact, without the defecation reflex, peristaltic movements are ineffective in evacuating stool.

Sexual function, like bladder and bowel control, is mediated by the S2 to S4 segments of the spinal cord.[18,65] The genital sexual response in SCI, which is manifested by an erection in men and vaginal lubrication in women, may be initiated by mental or touch stimuli, depending on the level of injury. The T11 to L2 cord segments have been identified as the mental-stimulus, or psychogenic, sexual response area, where autonomic nerve pathways in communication with the forebrain leave the cord and innervate the genitalia. The S2 to S4 cord segments have been identified as the sexual-touch reflex center. In T10 or higher injuries, reflex sexual response to genital touch may occur freely. However, a sexual response to mental stimuli (T11 to L2) does not occur because of the spinal lesion blocking the communication pathway. In an injury at T12 or below, the sexual reflex center may be damaged, and there may be no response to touch.

In men, the lack of erectile ability or inability to experience penile sensations or orgasm is not a reliable indicator of fertility, which should be evaluated by an expert. In women, fertility is normally reestablished with the return of menses, which usually occurs at about 3 to 5 months after injury. There are hazards to pregnancy, labor, and use of birth control devices relative to SCI that require the services of knowledgeable health care providers.

Disruption of Other Functions

Temperature Regulation. The central mechanisms for thermoregulation are located in the hypothalamus. In response to cold, the hypothalamus stimulates vasoconstrictor responses in peripheral blood vessels, particularly those of the skin. This results in decreased loss of body heat. Heat production results from increased metabolism, voluntary activity, or shivering. To reduce heat, hypothalamus-stimulated mechanisms produce vasodilation of skin blood vessels to dissipate heat, and sweating to increase evaporative heat losses.

After SCI, the communication between the thermoregulatory centers in the hypothalamus and the sympathetic effector responses below the level of injury is disrupted; the ability to control blood vessel responses that conserve or dissipate heat is lost, as are the abilities to sweat and shiver. Higher levels of injury tend to produce greater disturbances in thermoregulation. In tetraplegia and high paraplegia, there are few defenses against changes in the environmental temperature, and body temperature tends to assume the temperature of the external environment, a condition known as *poikilothermy*. Persons with lower-level injuries have various degrees of thermoregulation. Disturbances in thermoregulation are chronic and may cause continual loss of body heat. Treatment consists of education in the adjustment of clothing and awareness of how environmental temperatures affect the person's ability to accommodate to these changes.

Deep Vein Thrombosis and Edema. Persons with SCI are at high risk for development of deep vein thrombosis (DVT) and pulmonary embolism, particularly during the first 2 to 3 weeks after injury.[60,66] The high risk for DVT in patients with acute SCI is due to immobility, decreased vasomotor tone below the level of injury, and hypercoagulability and stasis of blood flow. Current preventative interventions include mechanical and pharmacological methods.[18,60] Mechanical methods of prevention include intermittent pneumatic compression, thigh-high graduated elastic compression stockings, and neuromuscular electrical stimulation. Pharmacologic methods include oral anticoagulants and low–molecular-weight heparin. Local pain, a common symptom of DVT, is often absent because of sensory deficits. Thus, a regular schedule of visual inspection for local signs of DVT (e.g., swelling) is important. Testing of persons at high risk for DVT includes plethysmography and duplex ultrasonography.

Edema is also a common problem in persons with SCI. The development of edema is related to decreased peripheral vascular resistance, decreased muscle tone in the paralyzed limbs, and immobility that causes increased venous pressure and abnormal pooling of blood in the abdomen, lower limbs, and upper extremities. Edema in the dependent body parts usually is relieved by positioning to minimize gravitational forces or by using compression devices (e.g., support stockings, binders) that encourage venous return.

Skin Integrity. The entire surface of the skin is innervated by cranial or spinal nerves organized into dermatomes that show cutaneous distribution. The CNS and autonomic nervous system also play a vital role in skin function. The sympathetic nervous system, through control of vasomotor and sweat gland activity, influences the health of the skin by providing adequate circulation, excretion of body fluids, and temperature regulation. The lack of sensory warning mechanisms and voluntary motor ability below the level of injury, coupled with circulatory changes, place the spinal cord–injured person at major risk for disruption of skin integrity (see Chapter 46). Significant factors associated with disruption of skin integrity are pressure, shearing forces, and localized trauma and irritation. Relieving pressure, allowing adequate circulation to the skin, and skin inspection are primary ways of maintaining skin integrity. Of all the complications after SCI, skin breakdown is the most preventable.

Future Directions in Repair of the Injured Spinal Cord

There is a continued effort to determine new and innovative strategies for repairing the injured spinal cord.[7,67–71] At present, these strategies focus on promoting the regrowth of interrupted nerve fiber tracts, using nerve growth–stimulating factors or molecules that suppress inhibitors of neuronal extension; bridging spinal cord lesions with scaffolds that are impregnated with nerve growth factors, which promote axon growth and reduce the barriers caused by scar tissue; repairing damaged myelin and restoring nerve fiber conductivity in the lesion area; and enhancing CNS plasticity by promoting compensatory growth of spared, intact nerve fibers above and below the level of injury. Stem cell transplantation offers a promising therapeutic strategy for spinal cord injury repair.[68] Although these strategies may not allow for complete repair of the spinal cord or to recreate what was present before the injury, even small successes may be useful for someone with SCI.

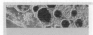

SUMMARY CONCEPTS

- Upper motor neuron (UMN) lesions are those involving neurons completely contained in the central nervous system (CNS).

- Amyotrophic lateral sclerosis is a progressive and devastating neurologic disorder that selectively affects motor function. It affects lower motor neurons (LMNs) in the spinal cord as well as UMNs in the brain stem and cerebral cortex.

- Multiple sclerosis is a slowly progressive demyelinating disease of the CNS that is characterized by exacerbations and remissions of paresthesias, optic neuritis, and motor weakness.

- Spinal cord injury (SCI) is a disabling neurologic condition of UMNs in the spinal cord that produces various degrees of sensorimotor loss and altered reflex activity based on the level of injury and extent of cord damage. Depending on the level of injury, SCI is associated with ventilation and communication problems; autonomic nervous system dysfunction that predisposes to the vasovagal response, autonomic hyperreflexia, impaired body temperature regulation, and postural hypotension; impaired muscle pump and venous innervation leading to edema of dependent areas of the body and risk for deep vein thrombosis; altered sensorimotor integrity that contributes to uncontrolled muscle spasms, altered pain responses, and threats to skin integrity; alterations in bowel and bladder elimination; and impaired sexual function.

REVIEW EXERCISES

1. A 32-year-old woman presents with complaints of "drooping eyelids," difficulty chewing and swallowing, and weakness of her arms and legs that is less severe in the morning but becomes worse as the day progresses. She complains that climbing stairs and lifting objects are becoming increasingly difficult. Clinical examination confirms weakness of the eyelid and jaw muscles. She is told that she may have myasthenia gravis and is scheduled for testing using the short-acting acetylcholinesterase inhibitor edrophonium (Tensilon).

   A. Explain the pathogenesis of this woman's symptoms as it relates to myasthenia gravis.
   B. Explain how information from the administration of the acetylcholinesterase inhibitor edrophonium can be used to assist in the diagnosis of the disorder.

2. A 20-year-old man suffered spinal cord injury at the C2 to C3 level as the result of a motorcycle accident.

   A. Explain the effects of this man's injury on ventilation and communication; sensorimotor function; autonomic nervous system function; bowel, bladder, and sexual function; and temperature regulation.
   B. Autonomic dysreflexia, which is a threat to persons with spinal cord injuries at T6 or above, is manifested by hypertension, often to extreme levels, and bradycardia; constriction of skin vessels below the level of injury; and severe headache and nasal stuffiness. Explain the origin of the elevated blood pressure and bradycardia. The condition does not occur until spinal shock has resolved, and usually occurs only in persons with injuries at T6 and above. Explain.

REFERENCES

1. Macpherson JM, Horak FB. Posture. In: Kandel ER, Schwartz JH, Jessell TM, et al., eds. *Principles of Neural Science.* 5th ed. New York: McGraw-Hill; 2013:935–959.
2. Wolpert DM, Pearson KG, Ghea CPJ. The organization and planning of movement. In: Kandel ER, Schwartz JH, Jessell TM, eds. *Principles of Neural Science.* 5th ed. New York: McGraw-Hill; 2013:744–767.
3. Hall JE. *Guyton and Hall Textbook of Medical Physiology.* 12th ed. Philadelphia, PA: Elsevier Saunders; 2010:85–91, 655–666, 673–684, 685–692, 698–713.
4. Penfield W, Rasmussen T. *The Cerebral Cortex of Man.* New York: Macmillan; 1950.
5. Pearson K, Gordon J. Spinal reflexes. In: Kandel ER, Schwartz JH, Jessell TM, eds. *Principles of Neural Science.* 5th ed. New York: McGraw-Hill.
6. Bickley LS, Szilagyi PG. *Bates' Guide to Physical Examination and History Taking.* 8th ed. Philadelphia, PA: Lippincott Williams & Wilkins; 2003:571–592.
7. Enocke RM, Pearson KG. The motor unit and muscle action. In: Kandel ER, Schwartz JH, Jessell TM, eds. *Principles of Neural Science.* 5th ed. New York: McGraw-Hill; 2013:768–769.
8. Anthony DP, Frosch MP, DeGirolami U. Peripheral nerve and skeletal muscle. In: Kumar V, Abbas AK, Fausto N, eds. *Robbins and Cotran Pathologic Basis of Disease.* 8th ed. Philadelphia, PA: Elsevier Saunders; 2010:1257–1277.
9. Kenyon LC. Skeletal muscle. In: Rubin R, Strayer DS, eds. *Rubin's Pathology: Clinicopathologic Foundations of Medicine.* 6th ed. Philadelphia, PA: Wolters Kluwer Health | Lippincott Williams & Wilkins; 2012:1273–1294.
10. Sarnat HB. Muscular dystrophies. In: Kliegman RM, Stanton BM, St. Geme JW, et al., eds. *Nelson Textbook of Pediatrics.* 17th ed. Philadelphia, PA: Elsevier Saunders; 2011:2118–2129.
11. Busby K, Finkel R, Birnkrant DJ, et al. Diagnosis and management of Duchenne muscular dystrophy, part 1; diagnosis, and pharmacological and psychosocial management. *Lancet Neurol.* 2010;9(1):77–93.
12. Katzung BG, Masters SB, Trevor AJ. *Basic and Clinical Pharmacology.* 12th ed. New York: Lange Medical Books/McGraw-Hill; 2012:465–482, 1006–1008.
13. Horowitz BZ. Botulinum toxin. *Crit Care Clin.* 2005;21:825–839.
14. Meriggioli MN, Sanders DB. Autoimmune myasthenia gravis: emerging clinical and biologic heterogeneity. *Lancet Neurol.* 2009;8:475–490.
15. Silvestri NJ, Wolfe GI. Myasthenia gravis. *Semin Neurol.* 2012;32(3):215–226.
16. Drachman DB. Myasthenia gravis and other diseases of the neuromuscular junction. In: Hauser SL, Josephson SA, eds. *Harrison's Neurology in Clinical Medicine.* 2nd ed. New York: McGraw-Hill; 2010:559–567.
17. Fuller GN, Goodman JC, Gouldin TW. The nervous system. In: Rubin R, Strayer DS, eds. *Rubin's Pathology: Clinicopathologic Foundations of Medicine.* 6th ed. Philadelphia, PA: Wolters Kluwer Health/Lippincott Williams & Wilkins; 2012:1295–1392.
18. Hickey JV. *Neurological and Neurosurgical Nursing.* 6th ed. Philadelphia, PA: Wolters Kluwer Health/Lippincott Williams & Wilkins; 2009:410–453, 460–485, 702–703, 704–708, 716–719.
19. Edward K, Cestia W. Carpal tunnel syndrome. *Am Fam Physician.* 2011;83:952–958.
20. Bickel KD. Carpal tunnel syndrome. *J Hand Surg Am.* 2010;35A:147–152.
21. Hauser SL, Asbury AK. Guillain-Barré syndrome and other immune-mediated neuropathies. In: Hauser SL, Josephson SA, eds. *Harrison's Neurology in Clinical Medicine.* 2nd ed. New York: McGraw-Hill; 2010:554–558.
22. Doom PA. Clinical features, pathogenesis, and treatment of Guillain-Barré syndrome. *Lancet Neurol.* 2008;7:939–950.
23. Yuki N, Hartlung H-P. Guillain-Barré syndrome. *N Engl J Med.* 2013;366(24):2294–2304.
24. Walling AD, Dickson G. Guillain-Barré syndrome. *Am Fam Physician.* 2013;87(3):191–197.
25. Casazza B. Diagnosis and treatment of low back pain. *Am Fam Physician.* 2012;85(4):343–350.
26. Devereaux M. Low back pain. *Med Clin North Am.* 2009;93:477–501.
27. Salzberg L. The physiology of low back pain. *Prim Care.* 2012;38:487–498.
28. Karppinen J, Shen FH, Luk KD, et al. Management of degenerative disk disease and chronic low back pain. *Orthop Clin North Am.* 2011;42:513–528.
29. Moore KL, Dalley AF, Agur AM. *Clinically Oriented Anatomy.* 6th ed. Philadelphia, PA: Wolters Kluwer Health/Lippincott Williams & Wilkins; 2010:495–507.
30. Cornwell BN. The emergency department evaluation, management, and treatment of low back pain. *Emerg Med Clin North Am.* 2010;28:811–839.
31. Lisberger SC, Thach WT. The cerebellum. In: Kandel ER, Schwartz JH, Jessell TM, et al., eds. *Principles of Neural Science.* 5th ed. New York. McGraw-Hill; 2013:960–981.
32. Wickmann T, DeLong MR. The basal ganglia. In: Kandel ER, Schwartz JH, Jessell TM, eds. *Principles of Neural Science.* 5th ed. New York: McGraw-Hill; 2013:963–998.
33. Gazewood JD, Richards DR, Clerbak K. Parkinson disease: an update. *Am Fam Physician.* 2013;87(4):267–273.
34. Samil A, Nutt JG, Ransom BR. Parkinson's disease. *Lancet.* 2004;363:1783–1793.
35. Parkinson J. *An Essay on the Shaking Palsy.* London, England: Sherwood, Nelley & Jones; 1817.
36. Fernandez HH. Updates in the medical management of Parkinson disease. *Cleve Clin J Med.* 2012;79(1):29–35.
37. Frosch MP, Anthony DC, De Girolami U. The central nervous system. In: Kumar V, Abbas AK, Fausto N, et al., eds. *Robbins and Cotran Pathologic Basis of Disease.* 8th ed. Philadelphia, PA: Elsevier Saunders; 2010:1309–1325.
38. Trojanowski JQ, Kenyon L. The nervous system. In: Rubin R, Strayer DS, eds. *Rubin's Pathology: Clinicopathologic Foundations of Medicine.* 6th ed. Philadelphia, PA: Wolters Kluwer Health/Lippincott Williams & Wilkins; 2010:1211–1213, 1221–1224.
39. Klein C, Schlossmacher MG. Parkinson disease, 10 years after its genetic revolution: multiple clues to a complex disorder. *Neurology.* 2007;69:2093–2104.
40. DeLong M, Juncos JL. Parkinson's disease and other movement disorders. In: Hauser SL, Josephson SA, eds. *Harrison's Neurology in Clinical Medicine.* 2nd ed. New York: McGraw-Hill; 2010:320–336.
41. Okun MS. Deep-brain stimulation for Parkinson's disease. *N Engl J Med* 2012;367:1529–1538.
42. Kierman MC, Vucic S, Cheah BC, et al. Amyotrophic lateral sclerosis. *Lancet* 2013;377:942–955.
43. Clarke K, Levine T. Clinical recognition and management of amyotrophic lateral sclerosis: the nurse's role. *J Neurosci Nurs* 2011;43:205–214.
44. Radunović A, Mitsumoto H, Leigh PN. Clinical care of patients with amyotrophic lateral sclerosis. *Lancet Neurol.* 2007;6:913–925.
45. Brown RH Jr. Amyotrophic lateral sclerosis and other motor neuron diseases, In: Hauser SL, Josephson SA, eds. *Harrison's Neurology in Clinical Medicine.* 2nd ed. New York: McGraw-Hill; 2010:559–567.
46. Hauser SL, Goodin DS. Multiple sclerosis and other demyelinating diseases. In: Hauser SL, Josephson SA, eds.

Harrison's Neurology in Clinical Medicine. 2nd ed. New York: McGraw-Hill; 2010:435–450.

47. Courtney AM, Treadaway K, Remington G, et al. Multiple sclerosis. *Med Clin North Am.* 2009;93:451–476.

48. Peterson JW, Trapp BD. Neuropathology of multiple sclerosis. *Neurol Clin.* 2005;23:107–129.

49. Nylander A, Hafler DA. Multiple sclerosis. *J Clin Invest.* 2012;122(4):1180–1186.

50. Frohman EM, Racke MK, Raine CS. Mulltiple sclerosis—the plaque and its pathogenesis. *N Engl J Med.* 2006;345(9):942–955.

51. Lubin DD. Clinical features and diagnosis of multiple sclerosis. *Neurol Clin.* 2005;23:1–15.

52. Kita M. FDA-approved preventative therapies for MS; first-line agents. *Neurol Clin.* 2011;29:401–409.

53. NSCISC National Spinal Cord Injury Statistical Center. *Spinal cord injury: Facts and figures at a glance.* Birmingham, AL: University of Alabama; 2013. [Online] Available at: https://www.nscisc.uab.edu/PublicDocuments/fact_figures_docs/Facts%202013.pdf. Accessed September 19, 2013.

54. McDonald JW. Spinal cord injury. *Lancet.* 2002;359:417–425.

55. Wilson JR, Fehlings MG. Emerging approaches to the surgical management of acute traumatic spinal cord injury. *Neurotherapeutics.* 2011;8:187–194.

56. Gupta R, Bathen ME, Smith JS, et al. Advances in the management of spinal cord injury. *J Am Acad Orthop Surg.* 2010;18(4):210–222.

57. Branco F, Cardenas DD, Svircev JN. Spinal cord injury: a comprehensive review. *Phys Med Rehabil Clin N Am.* 2007;18:651–679.

58. Dietrich WD. Therapeutic hypothermia in spinal cord injury. *Crit Care Med.* 2009;37(7):S238–S243.

59. Kirshblum SC, Burns SP, Biering-Sorensen F. International standards for neurological classification of spinal cord injury (revised 2011). *J Spinal Cord Med.* 2011;34(6):535–547.

60. Lo V, Esquenazi A, Han MK, et al. Critical care management of patients with acute spinal cord injury. *J Neurosurg Sci.* 2013;57(4):281–292.

61. Zimmer MB, Nantwi K, Goshgarian HG. Effect of spinal cord injury on the respiratory system: basic research and current clinical treatment options. *J Spinal Cord Med.* 2007;30:319–330.

62. Garstang SV, Miller-Smith SA. Autonomic nervous system dysfunction after spinal cord injury. *Phys Med Rehabil Clin N Am.* 2007:18, 275–296.

63. Krassioukov A, Warburton DER, Tessel R, et al. A systematic review of the management of autonomic dysreflexia following spinal cord injury. *Arch Phys Med Rehabil.* 2009;90(4):682–695.

64. Cruz CD, Cruz F. Spinal cord injury and bladder dysfunction: new ideas about an old problem. *Scientific World Journal.* 2011;11:214–234.

65. Riccardi R, Szabo CM, Poullos AY. Sexuality and spinal cord injury. *Nurs Clin North Am.* 2007;42:677–684.

66. Tessell RW, Hsieh TJ, Aubut JAL, et al. Venous thromboembolism following spinal cord injury. *Arch Phys Med Rehabil.* 2009;90(2):232–245.

67. Tohda C, Kuboyama T. Current and future therapeutic strategies for functional repair of spinal cord injury. *Pharmacol Ther.* ;2011;132(1):57–71.

68. Mothe A, Tator CH. Advances in stem cell therapy for spinal cord injury. *J Clin Invest.* 2012;122(11):3823–3834.

69. Wilson J, Forgione N, Fehlings MG. Emerging therapies for acute traumatic spinal cord injury. *CMAJ.* 2013;185(6):485–492.

70. Varma AK, Das A, Wallace G IV, et al. Spinal cord injury: a review of current therapy, future treatments, and basic science frontiers. *Neurochem Res.* 2013;38:895–905.

71. Bracken MB. Steroids for acute spinal cord injury. *Cochrane Database Syst Rev* 2012;1:CD001046.

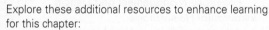

Porth Essentials Resources

Explore these additional resources to enhance learning for this chapter:

- NCLEX-Style Questions and Other Resources on thePoint, http://thePoint.lww.com/PorthEssentials4e
- Study Guide for Essentials of Pathophysiology
- Adaptive Learning | Powered by PrepU, http://thepoint.lww.com/prepu

(continued on page 917)

Chapter 37

Disorders of Brain Function

Anatomically and functionally, the brain is the most complex structure in the body. It controls our ability to think, our awareness of things around us, and our interactions with the outside world. Signals to and from various parts of the body are controlled by very specific areas in the brain. Therefore, the brain is much more vulnerable to lesions that in other organs might produce no significant effects. For example, an isolated renal infarct would not be expected to have a significant effect on kidney function, whereas an infarct of comparable size in a specific area of the brain could produce complete paralysis on one side of the body. Alterations in brain function can result from injury, cerebrovascular disease, infection, tumors, disruptions in electrical activity (seizures), or impairment of memory (impaired cognition or dementia).

Brain Injury

The brain is protected from external forces by the rigid confines of the skull and the cushioning afforded by the cerebrospinal fluid (CSF). The metabolic stability required by its electrically active cells is maintained by a number of regulatory mechanisms, including the blood–brain barrier and autoregulatory mechanisms that ensure adequate blood supply.

Mechanisms of Brain Injury

Injury to brain tissue can result from a number of conditions, including trauma, infections, tumors, and degenerative processes. Brain damage resulting from these disorders involves several common pathways, including hypoxia and ischemia, the effects of excitatory amino acid injury, and cerebral edema. In many cases the mechanisms are interrelated.

Hypoxic and Ischemic Injury

The brain relies on the ability of the cerebral circulation to deliver sufficient oxygen for its energy needs. Although the brain makes up only 2% of the body

Neurocognitive Disorders
  Alzheimer Disease
    Pathology
    Manifestations
    Diagnosis and Treatment

Other Types of Dementia
  Vascular Dementia
  Frontotemporal Dementia
  Wernicke-Korsakoff Syndrome
  Huntington Disease

weight, it receives one sixth of the resting cardiac output and accounts for 20% of the body's oxygen consumption.[2] By definition, *hypoxia* denotes a deprivation of oxygen with maintained blood flow, whereas *ischemia* represents a situation of greatly reduced or interrupted blood flow. The cellular effects of hypoxia and ischemia are quite different, and the brain tends to have different sensitivities to the two conditions. Hypoxia interferes with the delivery of oxygen, whereas ischemia interferes with the delivery of oxygen and glucose as well as the removal of metabolic wastes.

Hypoxia usually is seen in conditions such as exposure to reduced atmospheric pressure, carbon monoxide poisoning, severe anemia, and failure of the lungs to oxygenate the blood. Contrary to popular belief, hypoxia is fairly well tolerated, particularly in situations of chronic hypoxia. Neurons are capable of substantial anaerobic metabolism and are fairly tolerant of pure hypoxia, in which case it produces listlessness, drowsiness, and impaired problem solving. Unconsciousness and convulsions may occur when hypoxia is sudden and severe. However, the effects of severe hypoxia on brain function seldom are seen because the condition rapidly leads to cardiac arrest and ischemia.

Ischemia is seen in conditions of low blood flow. Cerebral ischemia can be focal, as in a stroke due to cerebral artery occlusion, or global, as in cardiac arrest.[3] Cerebral artery occlusion leads to focal ischemia, and if sustained, to infarction (death) of brain tissue in the distribution of the affected vessel. The location of the infarct and extent of tissue damage that results is determined by modifying variables, of which collateral blood flow is the most important. The collateral circulation may even provide sufficient blood flow to the borders of the focal ischemic region to maintain a low level of metabolic activity, thereby preserving tissue integrity.

Within the brain, certain regions and cell populations are more susceptible than others to ischemic injury[4] (Fig. 37-1). Areas of the brain located at the border zones between the overlapping territories supplied by the major cerebral arteries, sometimes called the *watershed areas,* are extremely vulnerable to ischemia. During events such as severe hypotension, these distal territories undergo a profound lowering of blood flow, predisposing to ischemia and infarction of brain tissues. As a consequence, areas of the cortex that are supplied by the major cerebral arteries usually regain function on recovery of adequate blood flow, whereas infarctions may occur in the watershed strips, resulting in focal neurologic deficits. *Laminar necrosis* refers to short, creeping segments of necrosis that occur within and parallel to the cerebral cortex, in areas supplied by the penetrating arteries

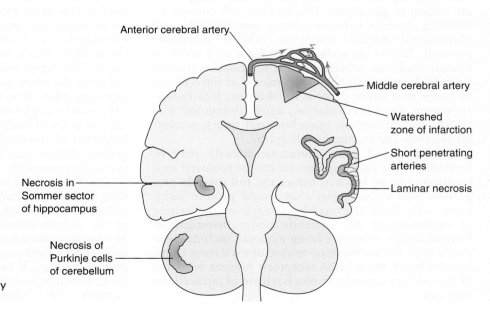

FIGURE 37-1. Consequences of global ischemia. A global insult induces lesions that reflect the vascular architecture (watershed infarcts, laminar necrosis) and the sensitivity of individual neuronal systems (pyramidal cells of the Sommer section, Purkinje cells). (From Trojanowsi JQ, Kenyon L. The central nervous system. In: Rubin R, Strayer DS, eds. *Rubin's Pathology: Clinicopathologic Foundations of Medicine,* 5th ed. Philadelphia, PA: Wolters Kluwer Health | Lippincott Williams & Wilkins; 2008:1191. Courtesy of Dmitri Karetnikov, artist.)

Anterior cerebral artery

Middle cerebral artery

Watershed zone of infarction

Short penetrating arteries

Laminar necrosis

Necrosis in Sommer sector of hippocampus

Necrosis of Purkinje cells of cerebellum

(see Fig. 37-1). The gray matter of the cerebral cortex receives its major blood supply through short penetrating arteries that emerge at right angles from larger vessels and then form a cascade as they repeatedly branch, forming a rich capillary network. An abrupt loss of arterial blood pressure markedly diminishes flow through these capillary channels.

Global ischemia occurs when blood flow is inadequate to meet the metabolic needs of the entire brain.[3] The result is a spectrum of neurologic disorders reflecting diffuse brain dysfunction. Unconsciousness occurs within seconds of severe global ischemia, such as that resulting from cardiac arrest. If the cerebral circulation is restored immediately, consciousness is regained quickly. The unique vulnerability of the brain is attributed to its limited tolerance of ischemia and its response to reperfusion. The metabolic depletion of energy associated with ischemia can result in an inappropriate release of excitatory amino acid neurotransmitters, disrupted calcium homeostasis, free radical formation, mitochondrial injury, and activation of cell-death pathways.[1,4] Although the threshold for ischemic neuronal injury is unknown, there is a period during which neurons can survive if blood flow is reestablished. Unfortunately, brain injury may be irreversible if the duration of ischemia is such that the threshold of injury has been reached.

Excitatory Amino Acid Injury

In many neurologic disorders, injury to neurons may be caused by inappropriate release of excitatory amino acid neurotransmitters such as glutamate.[1,3,5,6] The neurologic conditions involved in excitotoxic injury range from acute events such as stroke, hypoglycemic injury, and trauma to chronic degenerative disorders such as Huntington disease and possibly Alzheimer dementia.

During prolonged ischemia, metabolic depletion of adenosine triphosphate (ATP) results in the inappropriate release of glutamate. This initiates cell damage by allowing excessive influx of calcium ions (Ca^{++}) through glutamate–N-methyl-D-aspartate (NMDA) glutamate channels. Excess intracellular Ca^{++} leads to a series of calcium-mediated processes called the *calcium cascade* (Fig. 37-2), which results in the release of intracellular enzymes that cause protein breakdown, free radical formation, lipid peroxidation, deoxyribonucleic acid (DNA) fragmentation, mitochondrial injury, nuclear breakdown, and eventually cell death.

The effects of acute glutamate toxicity may be reversible if the excess glutamate can be removed or if its effects can be blocked before the full cascade progresses. Various strategies that would protect viable brain cells from irreversible damage in the setting of excitotoxicity are currently under investigation. Pharmacologic strategies being explored include those that inhibit the synthesis or release of excitatory transmitters; block the NMDA receptors; prevent initiation of the calcium cascade; or block release of intracellular enzymes.

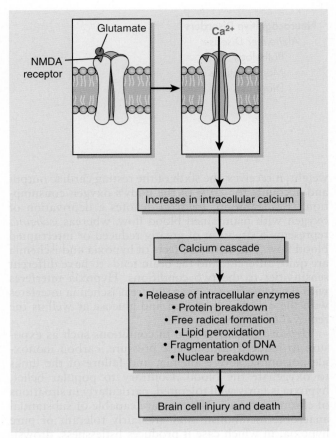

FIGURE 37-2. The role of the glutamate–N-methyl-D-aspartate (NMDA) receptor in brain cell injury. DNA, deoxyribonucleic acid.

Cerebral Edema

Cerebral edema, or brain swelling, is an increase in tissue volume secondary to abnormal fluid accumulation. There are two types of brain edema: vasogenic and cytotoxic.[1,7]

Vasogenic edema occurs with conditions that impair the function of the blood–brain barrier and allow transfer of water and proteins from the vascular into the interstitial space. It occurs in conditions such as hemorrhage, brain injury, and infectious processes (e.g., meningitis). Vasogenic edema occurs primarily in the white matter of the brain, possibly because the white matter is more compliant than the gray matter. Vasogenic edema can result in displacement of a cerebral hemisphere and various types of brain herniation. The functional manifestations of vasogenic edema include focal neurologic deficits, disturbances in consciousness, and severe intracranial hypertension.

Cytotoxic edema involves an increase in intracellular fluid. It can result from hypoosmotic states such as water intoxication or severe ischemia that impair the function of the sodium–potassium membrane pump. Ischemia also results in the inadequate removal of anaerobic metabolic end products such as lactic acid, producing extracellular acidosis. If blood flow is reduced to low levels for extended periods or to extremely low levels for a few minutes, cellular edema can cause the cell membrane to rupture, allowing the escape of intracellular contents into the surrounding extracellular fluid. This leads to damage of neighboring cells. Major changes in cerebral function, such as stupor and coma, occur with cytotoxic edema. The edema associated with ischemia may be severe enough to produce cerebral infarction with necrosis of brain tissue.

Increased Intracranial Pressure, Herniation, and Hydrocephalus

Intracranial pressure is, literally, the pressure inside the cranium. Its increase can cause herniations or hydrocephalus. Neurons can be injured when excessive pressure is exerted upon brain tissue, whether that pressure builds up gradually, such as from increasing CSF levels, or occurs suddenly, as from trauma.

The cranial cavity contains blood (approximately 10%), brain tissue (approximately 80%), and CSF (approximately 10%) in the rigid confines of a nonexpandable skull.[7,8] Each of these three intracranial volumes contributes to the intracranial pressure, which normally is maintained within a range of 0 to 15 mm Hg when measured in the lateral ventricles. Increased intracranial pressure (ICP) is a common pathway for brain injury from different types of insults and agents.

The volumes of each of three intracranial components can vary slightly without causing marked changes in ICP. This is because small increases in the volume of one component can be compensated for by a decrease in the volume of one or both of the other two components. This association is called the *Monro-Kellie hypothesis*.[4,7,8] Reciprocal compensation occurs among the three intracranial compartments. Of the three intracranial compartments, the CSF and blood volume are best able to compensate for changes in ICP, with the tissue volume being relatively restricted in its ability to change.

Initial increases in ICP are buffered by a translocation of CSF to the spinal subarachnoid space and increased reabsorption of CSF. The compensatory ability of the blood compartment is limited by the small amount of blood that is in the cerebral circulation, most of which is contained in the low-pressure venous system. As the volume-buffering capacity of this compartment becomes exhausted, venous pressure increases, and cerebral blood volume and ICP rise. Also, cerebral blood flow is highly controlled by autoregulatory mechanisms, which affect its compensatory capacity. For example, conditions such as ischemia and an elevated partial pressure of carbon dioxide (PCO_2) in the blood produce a compensatory vasodilation of the cerebral blood vessels. A decrease in PCO_2 has the opposite effect. For this reason, hyperventilation, which results in a decrease in PCO_2 levels, is sometimes used in the treatment of ICP.

The impact of increases in blood, brain tissue, or CSF volumes on ICP varies among individuals and depends on the amount of increase, effectiveness of compensatory mechanisms, and compliance or "distensibility" of brain tissue.[7] An increase in intracranial volume will have little or no effect on ICP as long as the compliance is high. Factors that influence compliance include the amount of volume increase, the time frame for accommodation, and the size of the intracranial compartments. For example, small volume increments over long periods of time can be better accommodated than a comparable increase introduced over a short period of time.

The cerebral perfusion pressure (CPP), which represents the difference between the mean arterial blood pressure (MABP) and the ICP (CPP = MABP − ICP), is the pressure perfusing the brain.[7,8] CPP (normally 70 to 100 mm Hg) is determined by the pressure gradient between the internal carotid artery and the subarachnoid veins. The MABP and ICP are monitored frequently in persons with brain conditions that increase ICP and impair brain perfusion. When the pressure in the cranial cavity approaches or exceeds the MABP, tissue perfusion becomes inadequate, cellular hypoxia results, and neuronal death may occur. The highly specialized cortical neurons are the most sensitive to oxygen deficit; a decrease in the level of consciousness is one of the earliest and most reliable signs of increased ICP. Continued cellular hypoxia leads to general neurologic deterioration, with the level of consciousness deteriorating from alertness to confusion, lethargy, obtundation, stupor, and coma.

Brain Herniation

The brain is protected by the nonexpandable skull and two supporting septa, the falx cerebri and the tentorium cerebelli, which divide the intracranial cavity into compartments that normally protect against excessive movement (Fig. 37-3A).[1,4,7] The *falx cerebri* is a sickle-shaped septum that divides the supratentorial space into right and left hemispheres. The *tentorium cerebelli* (so named because it is shaped like a tent) is a double fold of dura mater that forms a sloping partition between the cerebrum and cerebellum. In the center of the tentorium is a large semicircular opening called the *incisura* or *tentorial notch* (Fig. 37-3B). The brain stem, blood vessels (anterior cerebral, internal carotid, posterior communicating, and posterior and superior cerebellar arteries), and oculomotor nerve (cranial nerve [CN] III) pass through the inciscura.

Brain herniation represents a displacement of brain tissue under the falx cerebri or through the tentorial notch of the tentorium cerebelli. It occurs when an elevated ICP in one brain compartment causes displacement of the cerebral tissue toward an area of lower pressure. The different types of herniation syndromes are based on the area of the brain that has herniated and the structure under which it has been pushed. They commonly are divided into two broad categories, *supratentorial* and *infratentorial*, based on whether they are located above or below the tentorium.

Supratentorial Herniation. Progressive supratentorial lesions develop sequential signs and symptoms of ocular, motor, and respiratory function. This pattern follows the predictable continuum of rostal-to-caudal (head to tail) failure that proceeds from the diencephalon to the midbrain (ocular), followed by pons (motor),

(*text continues on page 921*)

UNDERSTANDING → Intracranial Pressure

The intracranial pressure (ICP) is the pressure within the intracranial cavity. It is determined by (1) the pressure-volume relationships among the brain tissue, cerebrospinal fluid (CSF), and blood in the intracranial cavity; (2) the Monro-Kellie hypothesis, which relates to reciprocal changes among the intracranial volumes; and (3) the compliance of the brain and its ability to buffer changes in intracranial volume.

1

Intracranial Volumes and Pressure. The ICP represents the pressure exerted by the essentially incompressible tissue and fluid volumes of the three compartments contained within the rigid confines of the skull—the brain tissue and interstitial fluid (80%), the blood (10%), and the CSF (10%).

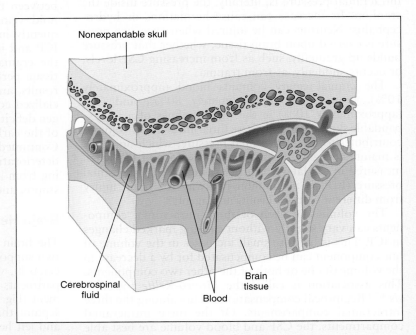

Nonexpandable skull

Cerebrospinal fluid

Blood

Brain tissue

2

Monro-Kellie Hypothesis. Normally, a reciprocal relationship exists among the three intracranial volumes such that the ICP is maintained within normal limits. Because these volumes are practically incompressible, a change in one component must be balanced by an almost equal and opposite effect in one or both of the remaining components. This is known as the *Monro-Kellie hypothesis.* Of the three intracranial volumes, the fluid in the CSF compartment is the most easily displaced. The CSF (**A**) can be displaced from the ventricles and cerebral subarachnoid space to the spinal subarachnoid space, and it can also undergo increased absorption or decreased production. Because most of the blood in the cranial cavity is contained in the low-pressure venous system, venous compression (**B**) serves as a means of displacing blood volume.

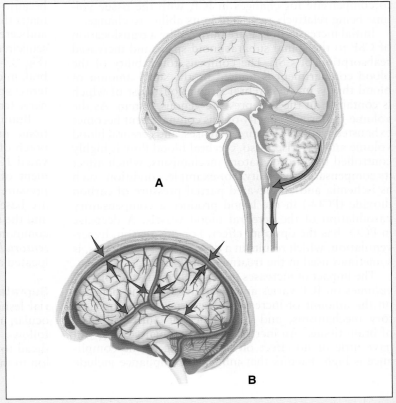

A

B

③ **Compliance and the Volume-Pressure Curve.** Compliance, which refers to the ease with which a substance can be compressed or deformed, is a measure of the brain's ability to maintain its ICP during changes in intracranial volume. Compliance (C) represents the ratio of change (Δ) in volume (V) to change in pressure (P): C = ΔV/ΔP.

The dynamic effects of changes in intracranial volume and compliance on ICP can be illustrated on a graph with the volume represented on the horizontal axis and ICP on the vertical axis. The shape of the curve demonstrates the effect on ICP of adding volume to the intracranial cavity. From points A to B, the compensatory mechanisms are adequate, compliance is high, and the ICP remains relatively constant as volume is added to the intracranial cavity. At point B, the ICP is relatively normal, but the compensatory mechanisms have reached their limits, compliance is decreased, and ICP begins to rise with each change in volume. From points C to D, the compensatory mechanisms have been exceeded and ICP rises significantly with each increase in volume as compliance is lost.

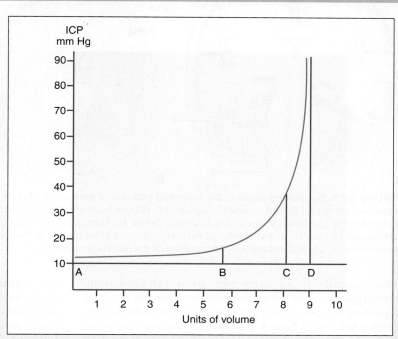

(From Hickey JV. *Neurological and Neurosurgical Nursing.* 5th ed. Philadelphia, PA: Lippincott Williams & Wilkins; 2003:286.)

(text continued from page 919)

and eventually medullary (respiratory) function. The pattern of deterioration is fairly predictable unless vascular or obstructive complications occur and exaggerate the condition. Pupillary reactions to light is upper brain stem function (oculomotor nerve [CNIII]) and are especially useful when assessing the unconscious patient.

There are two major types of supratentorial herniation: cingulate and transtentorial.[1,4,7] A *cingulate herniation* (see Fig. 37-3C [1]), which poses the less serious threat in terms of clinical outcomes, involves displacement of the cingulate gyrus and hemisphere beneath the sharp edges of the falx cerebri to the opposite side of the brain.[7] This displacement can compress local blood supply and cerebral tissue, causing edema and ischemia, which further increase the degree of ICP elevation. There may also be compression of branches of the anterior cerebral artery with unilateral or bilateral leg weakness.

Transtentorial herniations result in two distinct syndromes: a central syndrome and an uncal syndrome, which is the most common herniation syndrome.[7] Clinically, they display distinct patterns early in their course, but both merge in a similar pattern once they begin to involve structures at the level of the midbrain and below. *Central transtentorial herniations* (see Fig. 37-3C [2]) involve the downward displacement of the cerebral hemispheres, basal ganglia, diencephalon, and midbrain through the tentorial incisura. Bilateral small, reactive pupils and drowsiness are heralding signs. The *uncal herniation syndrome* occurs when an expanding lesion pushes the medial aspect of the temporal lobe, which contains the uncus and hippocampal gyrus, through the incisura of the tentorium (see Fig 37-3C [3]). As a result, the diencephalon and midbrain are compressed and displaced laterally to the opposite side of the tentorium. The oculomotor nerve (CN III) and the posterior cerebral artery are frequently compressed. The oculomotor nerve controls pupillary constriction; entrapment of this nerve results in ipsilateral pupillary dilation,

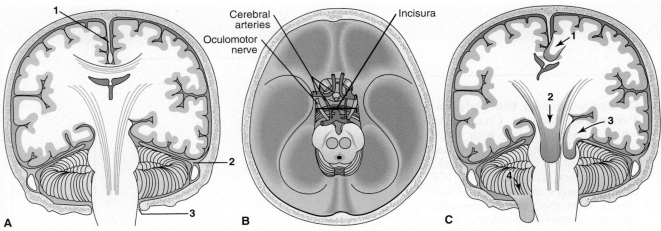

FIGURE 37-3. Supporting septa of the brain and patterns of herniation. **(A)** The falx cerebri [*1*], tentorium cerebelli [*2*], and foramen magnum [*3*]. **(B)** The location of the incisura or tentorial notch in relation to the cerebral arteries and oculomotor nerve. **(C)** Herniation of the cingulate gyrus under the falx cerebri [*1*], central or transtentorial herniation [*2*], uncal herniation of the temporal lobe into the tentorial notch [*3*], and infratentorial herniation of the cerebellar tonsils [*4*].

which usually is an early sign of uncal herniation. Consciousness may be unimpaired because the reticular activating system, which is responsible for wakefulness, has not yet been affected. As uncal herniations progress, there are changes in motor strength and coordination of voluntary movements because of compression of the descending motor pathways. It is not unusual for initial changes in motor function to occur ipsilateral to the side of the brain damage because of compression of the contralateral cerebral peduncles. Changes in consciousness and coma may follow due to compression of the midbrain against the opposite tentorial edge. Decerebrate posturing (Fig. 37-4B) may develop, followed by dilated, fixed pupils; flaccidity; and respiratory arrest.

Infratentorial Herniation. Infratentorial compartment lesions contributing to herniation are much less frequent than those of the supratentorial region.[7] The infratentorial compartment contains both the brain stem and cerebellum. Herniation may occur superiorly (upward) through the tentorial incisura or inferiorly (downward) through the foramen magnum. Upward displacement of the brain stem and cerebellum through the tentorium results maximum pressure on the midbrain. The most prominent signs of upward herniation include: immediate onset of deep coma; small equal, fixed pupils; and abnormal respirations (slow rate with intermittent sighs or ataxia) and other vital signs. Downward herniation involves displacement of the midbrain through the tentorial notch or the cerebellar tonsils through the foramen magnum (Fig. 37-3C [*4*]). It often progresses rapidly and can cause death because it is likely to involve the lower brain stem centers that control vital cardiopulmonary functions.

Hydrocephalus

Hydrocephalus represents a progressive enlargement of the ventricular system due to an abnormal increase in CSF volume (see Chapter 34, Fig. 34-21). It can result because of overproduction of CSF, impaired

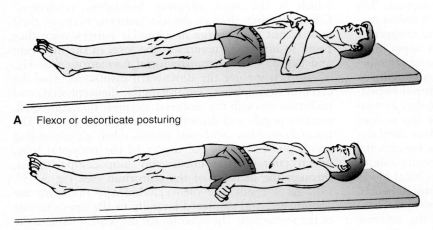

A Flexor or decorticate posturing

B Extensor or decerebrate posturing

FIGURE 37-4. Abnormal posturing. **(A)** Decorticate rigidity. In decorticate rigidity, the upper arms are held at the sides, with elbows, wrists, and fingers flexed. The legs are extended and internally rotated. The feet are plantar flexed. **(B)** Decerebrate rigidity. In decerebrate rigidity, the jaws are clenched and neck extended. The arms are adducted and stiffly extended at the elbows with the forearms pronated, wrists and fingers flexed. (From Fuller J, Schaller-Ayers J. *Health Assessment: A Nursing Approach.* 2nd ed. Philadelphia, PA: J.B. Lippincott; 1994.)

reabsorption of CSF, or obstruction of CSF flow in the ventricular system.

Pathophysiology. There are two types of hydrocephalus: communicating and noncommunicating.[4,7] *Communicating hydrocephalus* is caused by impaired reabsorption of CSF from the arachnoid villi into the venous system. Decreased absorption can result from a block in the CSF pathway to the arachnoid villi or a failure of the villi to transfer the CSF to the venous system. It can occur if too few villi are formed, if postinfective (meningitis) scarring occludes them, or if the villi become obstructed with fragments of blood or infectious debris. Adenomas of the choroid plexus can cause an overproduction of CSF. This form of hydrocephalus is much less common than that resulting from decreased absorption of CSF.

Noncommunicating or obstructive hydrocephalus occurs when obstruction in the ventricular system prevents the CSF from reaching the arachnoid villi. Cerebrospinal fluid flow can be obstructed due to congenital malformations, tumors encroaching on the ventricular system, or inflammation or hemorrhage. Similar pathologic patterns occur with noncommunicating and communicating types of hydrocephalus. The cerebral hemispheres become enlarged, and the ventricular system beyond the point of obstruction becomes dilated[4] (Fig. 37-5). The sulci on the surface of the brain become effaced and shallow, and the white matter reduced in volume.

Clinical Manifestations. In adults and children in whom the cranial sutures have fused, head enlargement does not occur.[4] Acute-onset hydrocephalus usually is marked by symptoms of increased ICP, including headache, vomiting, and papilledema or deviation in eye movements due to pressure on the cranial nerves.[7] If the obstruction is not relieved, progression to herniation ensues.

Signs and symptoms of hydrocephalus vary greatly, depending on age and rapidity of onset. When hydrocephalus develops in utero or before the cranial sutures of the skull have fused in infancy, the ventricles expand beyond the point of obstruction, the cranial sutures separate, the head expands, and there is bulging of the fontanels. Because the skull is able to expand, signs of increased ICP may be absent, and intelligence spared. However, seizures are not uncommon, and in severe cases, optic nerve atrophy leads to blindness. Weakness and uncoordinated movement are common. Surgical placement of a shunt allows for diversion of excess CSF fluid, preventing extreme enlargement of the head and neurologic deficits.

Diagnosis and Treatment. The most common diagnostic studies are computed tomographic (CT) and magnetic resonance imaging (MRI). The usual treatment is a ventricular shunting procedure, which provides an alternative route for return of CSF to the circulation.[7]

Normal Pressure Hydrocephalus. An important type of communicating hydrocephalus that is seen in older adults is called *normal-pressure hydrocephalus*.[4,7] In normal-pressure hydrocephalus, there is ventricular enlargement with compression of cerebral tissue, but a normal CSF pressure. The signs and symptoms of normal-pressure hydrocephalus, which include memory changes, disturbances in gait, and urinary incontinence, usually have an insidious onset. The changes occur so slowly that they can be easily overlooked by the patient or his or her family or they may be attributed to the aging process.[7] The accepted treatment for normal-pressure hydrocephalus is a ventricular shunt.

Traumatic Brain Injury

The term "head injury" is used to describe all structural damage to the head, including injury to the skull, brain, or both. The leading causes of head injury are motor vehicle accidents, bicycle crashes, battlefield trauma, sports injuries, falls, and assaults.[9,10] Head injury with concussion is becoming increasingly recognized as a significant medical problem with significant morbidity and sometimes devastating complications.[9] High-profile cases involving athletes and large numbers of returning armed services personnel with battlefield injuries have brought concussions to the forefront of concern for school athletic personnel and health care professionals.

The physical forces associated with head injury may result in skull fractures, brain injury, and vascular damage, all three of which can coexist.[1,4] Skull fractures are frequently accompanied by intracranial lesions, and the presence of skull fracture greatly increases the risk of an underlying subdural and/or epidural hemorrhage.

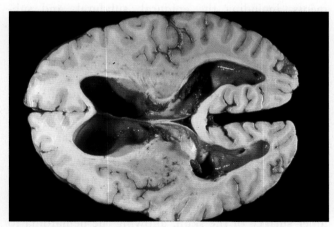

FIGURE 37-5. Hydrocephalus. Horizonatal section of the brain from a patient who died of a brain tumor that obstructed the aqueduct of Sylvius shows marked dilation of the lateral ventricles. (From Fuller GN, Goodman JC. Central nervous system. In: Rubin R, Strayer DS, eds. *Rubin's Pathology: Clinicopathologic Foundations of Medicine.* 6th ed. Philadelphia, PA: Wolters Kluwer Health | Lippincott Williams & Wilkins; 2012:1302.)

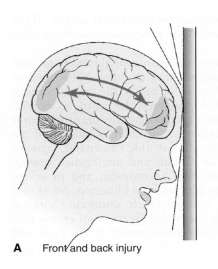

A Front and back injury

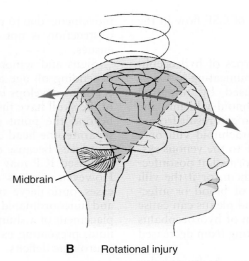

Midbrain

B Rotational injury

FIGURE 37-6. Mechanism of brain injury **(A)** acceleration–deceleration and **(B)** acceleration–decelerations with rotational motion of the cerebral hemispheres around the fixed-in-place brainstem that affects neurons in reticular activating system (RAS), which extends through the central core of the brainstem. (Adapted from Hickey JV. *The Clinical Practice of Neurological and Neurosurgical Nursing.* 6th ed. Philadelphia, PA: Wolters Kluwer Health | Lippincott Williams & Wilkins; 2009:372.)

Because the brain floats freely in the CSF within the rigid confines of the skull, blunt force to the head causes the brain to accelerate within the skull, and then decelerate abruptly upon hitting the inner skull surfaces.[7,10–12] As the brain strikes the rough surface of the cranial vault, brain tissue, blood vessels, nerve tracts, and other structures are bruised and torn, resulting in contusions and hematomas (Fig. 37-6). A special type of acceleration-deceleration motion is angular rotation.[7,12] It involves the rotational motion of the cerebral hemispheres in the anterior-posterior plane around the fixed-in-place brain stem, causing disruption of electrical and subcellular activities of neurons in the reticular activating system (RAS), which extends through the central core of the brain stem (Fig. 37-6).

There are two main stages in the development of brain damage after brain injury: primary and secondary. Primary injuries, which represent the immediate response to the initial injury, include focal lesions (contusions and hemorrhage) and diffuse injuries (concussion and diffuse axonal injuries).[1,4] Secondary injures involve complicating processes resulting from the initial injury, including brain swelling, and infection.[7,9–12] Ischemia is considered the most common cause of secondary brain injury. It can result from the hypoxia and hypotension that occur during the resuscitation process or from the impairment of regulatory mechanisms that control cerebrovascular responses that maintain blood flow and oxygen supply.

Contusions

Contusions represent a bruising on the brain surface or a lacerations or tearing of brain tissue.[1,4] Contusions can result from direct force, a depressed skull fracture, or a closed acceleration-deceleration injury. Closed injury contusions are often distributed along the rough, irregular inner surface of the brain and are more likely to occur in the frontal or temporal lobes,

resulting in cognitive and motor deficits. The clinical effects of a contusion depend on its size and related cerebral edema. Small, unilateral, frontal lesions may be asymptomatic; whereas larger lesions may result in neurological defects. They can cause secondary mass effects from edema resulting in an increased ICF, and possible herniation syndromes. Persons suffering from cerebral contusions are usually managed medically with emphasis toward prevention of secondary injuries.

Hematomas

Hematomas result from vascular injury and bleeding. Depending on the anatomic position of the ruptured vessel, bleeding can occur in any of several compartments, including the epidural, subdural, and subarachnoid spaces, or into the brain itself (intracerebral hematoma).

Epidural Hematoma. An epidural hematoma is one that develops between the inner side of the skull and the dura[1,4,7] (Fig. 37-7). It usually results from a tear in an artery, most often the middle meningeal, usually in association with a head injury in which the skull is fractured.[1,5,17] Because bleeding is arterial in origin, rapid expansion of the hematoma compresses the brain. Epidural hematoma is more common in a young person because the dura is less firmly attached to the skull surface than in an older person; as a consequence, the dura can be easily separated from the inner surface of the skull, allowing the hematoma to grow.

Typically, a person with an epidural hematoma presents with a history of head injury and a brief period of unconsciousness followed by a lucid period in which consciousness is regained. There is then a rapid progression to unconsciousness. The lucid interval does not always occur, but when it does, it is of great diagnostic value. With rapidly developing unconsciousness,

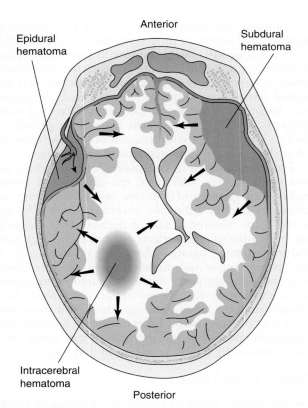

FIGURE 37-7. Location of epidural, subdural, and intracerebral hematomas.

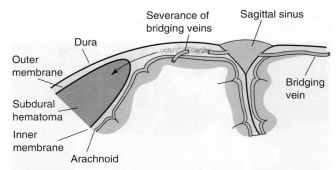

FIGURE 37-8. Mechanism of bleeding in subdural hematoma. (From Trojanowski JQ. The central nervous system. In: Rubin E, Gorstein F, Rubin R, et al; eds. *Rubin's Pathology: Clinicopathologic Foundations of Medicine.* 4th ed. Philadelphia, PA: Lippincott Williams & Wilkins; 2005:1430. Courtesy of Dmitri Karetnikov, artist.)

there are focal symptoms related to the area of the brain involved. These symptoms can include ipsilateral pupil dilation and contralateral (opposite side) hemiparesis from uncal herniation. If the hematoma is not removed, the condition progresses, with increased ICP, tentorial herniation, and death. The prognosis is excellent, however, if the hematoma is removed before loss of consciousness occurs.

Subdural Hematoma. A subdural hematoma develops in the area between the dura and the arachnoid (subdural space) and usually is the result of a tear in the small bridging veins that connect veins on the surface of the cortex to dural sinuses. The bridging veins pass from the pial vessels through the CSF-filled subarachnoid space, penetrate the arachnoid and the dura, and empty into the intradural sinuses.[1,4,7] These veins are readily snapped in head injury when the brain moves suddenly in relation to the cranium (Fig. 37-8). Bleeding can occur between the dura and arachnoid (i.e., subdural hematoma) or into the CSF-filled subarachnoid space (i.e., subarachnoid hematoma).

The venous source of bleeding in a subdural hematoma develops more slowly than the arterial bleeding in an epidural hematoma. Subdural hematomas are classified as acute, subacute, or chronic. This classification system is based on the approximate time before the appearance of symptoms. Symptoms of acute hematoma are seen within 24 hours of the injury, whereas subacute hematoma does not produce symptoms until 2 to 10 days

after injury. Symptoms of chronic subdural hematoma may not arise until several weeks after the injury.

Acute subdural hematomas progress rapidly and have a high mortality rate because of the severe secondary injuries related to edema and increased ICP. The high mortality rate has been associated with uncontrolled ICP increase, loss of consciousness, decerebrate posturing (see Fig. 37-4B), and delay in surgical removal of the hematoma. The clinical picture is similar to that of epidural hematoma, except that there usually is no lucid interval. By contrast, in subacute subdural hematoma, there may be a period of improvement in the level of consciousness and neurologic symptoms, only to be followed by deterioration if the hematoma is not removed.

Symptoms of chronic subdural hematoma develop weeks after a head injury, so much later that the person may not remember having had a head injury. Chronic subdural hematoma is more common in older persons because brain atrophy causes the brain to shrink away from the dura and stretch fragile bridging veins. When these veins rupture, there is slow seepage of blood into the subdural space. Fibroblastic activity causes the hematoma to become encapsulated. The sanguinous (blood fluid) in this encapsulated mass, with its high concentration of osmotically-active particles, draws fluid from the surrounding subarachnoid space, causing the hematoma to expand and exert pressure on the surrounding brain tissue. In some instances, the clinical picture is less defined, with the most prominent symptom being a decreasing level of consciousness, as manifested by drowsiness, confusion, headache, and apathy

Traumatic Intracerebral Hematomas. Traumatic intracerebral hematomas may be single or multiple. They can occur in any lobe of the brain but are most common in the frontal or temporal lobes, related to the bony prominences on the inner skull surface (Fig. 37-9). They may occur in association with the severe motion that the brain undergoes during head injury, or a contusion can coalesce into a hematoma. Intracerebral hematomas occur more frequently in older persons and alcoholics, whose cerebral vessels are more friable.

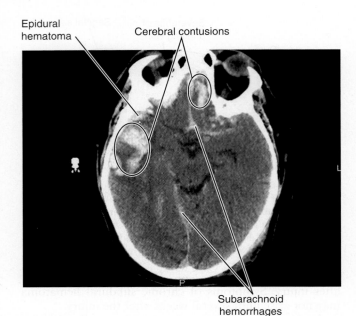

Epidural hematoma

Cerebral contusions

Subarachnoid hemorrhages

FIGURE 37-9. Computed tomography scan of brain in traumatic brain injury, showing hemorrhagic cerebral contusions in right temporal and bifrontal lobes, subarachnoid hemorrhages, and epidural hematoma.

The signs and symptoms produced by an intracerebral hematoma depend on its size and location in the brain. Signs of increased ICP can be manifested if the hematoma is large and encroaching on vital structures. A hematoma in the temporal lobe can be dangerous because of the potential for lateral herniation.

Concussions

A cerebral concussion can be defined as a transient neurogenic dysfunction caused by mechanical force to the brain.[7,10–12] Acceleration–deceleration is the mechanism of injury, usually due to a nonpenetrating force such as a sudden blow to the head. There may be a momentary loss of consciousness without demonstrable symptoms, except for residual amnesia. Microscopic changes can often be detected in neurons and neuroglia within hours of injury, but brain imaging is usually negative. Although recovery usually takes place within 24 hours, mild symptoms, such as headache, irritability, insomnia, and poor concentration and memory, may persist for months. This is known as the *postconcussion syndrome*. The amnesia or memory loss usually includes an interval of time preceding the injury (retrograde amnesia) and following the injury (anterograde amnesia). The duration of retrograde amnesia correlates with the severity of the brain injury.

Traditionally, the diagnosis and management of concussion has relied heavily on the person's self-reporting of symptoms. Because symptom resolution often precedes cognitive recovery and because many persons don't report symptoms in an effort to return to their normal activities, additional neurophysiologic testing and monitoring can be useful. Neurophysiologic tests commonly evaluate decision-making ability, reaction time, attention, memory, and cognitive processing speed in an objective fashion. CT or MRI imaging is usually reserved for cases in which intracranial bleeding is suspected. Treatment, which is largely supportive, includes both physical and mental rest. Once symptoms have resolved, the person may begin shortened work days with decreased work demands. Students may benefit from short periods of reading and studying with frequent breaks. Athletes are advised to follow a slow stepwise return to play.

The complications of concussion, although rare, are potentially serious. Currently, the clinical and neuropathic consequences of repeated mild head injury are known as *chronic traumatic encephalopathy*. The disorders often manifests years or decades after the inciting head injuries with effects on behavior, cognition, and movement. Cognitive changes may occur early in the disease course and include loss of executive function and poor memory. A widely feared complication of concussion is the *second-impact syndrome*. It is thought to occur when someone who is still recovering from a recent concussion suffers a second head trauma. Significant morbidity and even death can result from edema caused by cerebral congestion that occurs.

Diffuse Axonal Injury

Diffuse axonal injury is caused by shearing of fragile axons by acceleration-deceleration forces at the time of trauma.[1,4,7] The difference in acceleration–deceleration gradient on certain areas of the brain, permits generation of rotational forces that cause axonal shearing injury. It is characterized by distinct and microscopic findings, including axonal swelling, that are widely distributed in the cerebral hemispheric white matter, corpus callosum, and upper brain stem.

Diffuse axonal injury is characterized clinically by functional cerebral impairment, which may range from confusion to coma and death. The clinical diagnosis of diffuse axonal injury is based on immediate onset of unconsciousness in a person with significant cerebral trauma and no intracranial lesion noted on CT scan. Current treatment modalities focus on supportive care, especially for the unconscious person. Studies indicate that axonal injury evolves over a period of hours or days, suggesting that there may be an opportunity to arrest its progression and preserve axonal integrity.

Manifestations of Diffuse Brain Injury

Diffuse (global) brain injury, whether due to head trauma or other pathologic processes, is manifested by alterations in sensory, motor, and cognitive function and by changes in the level of consciousness. In contrast to a localized injury, which causes focal neurologic deficits without altered consciousness, global injury nearly always results in altered levels of consciousness, ranging from inattention to stupor or coma. Severe injury that seriously compromises brain function may result in brain death.

TABLE 37-1	Key Signs in Rostral-to-Caudal Progression of Brain Lesions
Level of Brain Injury	**Key Clinical Signs**
Diencephalon	Impaired consciousness; small, reactive pupils; intact oculocephalic reflex; decorticate posturing; Cheyne-Stokes respirations
Midbrain	Coma; fixed, midsize pupils; impaired oculocephalic reflex; neurogenic hyperventilation; decerebrate posturing
Pons	Coma; fixed, irregular pupils; dysconjugate gaze; impaired cold caloric stimulation; loss of corneal reflex; hemiparesis/quadriparesis; decerebrate posturing; apneustic respirations
Medulla	Coma; fixed pupils; flaccidity; loss of gag and cough reflexes; ataxic/apneic respirations

The cerebral hemispheres are the most susceptible to damage, and the most frequent sign of brain dysfunction is an altered level of consciousness and change in behavior. As the brain structures in the diencephalon, midbrain, pons, and medulla are sequentially affected, additional signs related to pupillary and eye movement reflexes, motor function, and respiration become evident (Table 37-1). Hemodynamic and respiratory instability are the last signs to occur because their regulatory centers are located low in the medulla.

In progressive brain deterioration, the person's neurologic capabilities appear to deteriorate in stepwise fashion. Similarly, as neurologic function returns, there usually is a stepwise progression to higher levels of consciousness. Deterioration of brain function from supratentorial lesions tends to follow a stepwise rostral-to-caudal progression, which is observed as the brain initially compensates for injury and subsequently decompensates with loss of autoregulation and cerebral perfusion. Infratentorial (brain stem) lesions may lead to an early, sometimes abrupt disturbance in consciousness without any orderly rostral to caudal progression of neurologic signs.

Consciousness

Consciousness is the state of awareness of self and the environment and of being able to become oriented to new stimuli.[13–15] Its two major components are content and arousal. Content represents the sum of all the functions of the cerebral cortex, including both cognition and affective responses. Arousal and wakefulness require the concurrent functioning of both cerebral hemispheres and an intact RAS in the brain stem.

The RAS is a diffuse, primitive system of interlacing nerve cells and fibers in the brain stem that receives input from multiple sensory pathways (Fig. 37-10). Anatomically, the RAS constitutes the central core of the brain stem, extending from the medulla through the pons to the midbrain, which is continuous caudally with the spinal cord and rostrally with the subthalamus, hypothalamus, and thalamus. Fibers from the reticular formation also project to the autonomic nervous system and motor systems. The hypothalamus plays a predominant role in maintaining homeostasis through

integration of somatic, visceral, and endocrine functions. Inputs from the reticular formation, vestibulospinal projections, and other motor systems are integrated to provide a continuously adapting background of muscle tone and posture to facilitate voluntary motor actions. Reticular formation neurons that function in regulation of cardiovascular, respiratory, and other visceral functions are intermingled with those that maintain other reticular formation functions.

The pathways for the ascending RAS travel from the medulla through the midbrain, such that lesions of the brain stem can interrupt RAS activity, leading to altered levels of consciousness and coma. Any deficit in level of consciousness, from mild confusion to stupor or coma, indicates injury to either the RAS or to both cerebral hemispheres concurrently. For example, consciousness may decline owing to severe systemic metabolic derangements that affect both hemispheres, or from head trauma causing shear injuries to white matter of both the RAS and the cerebral hemispheres. Brain injuries that affect a

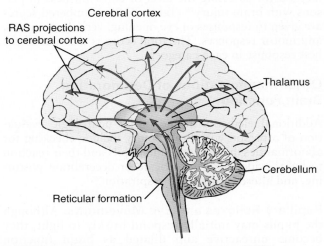

FIGURE 37-10. The reticular activating system (RAS). Ascending sensory tracts send axon collateral fibers to the reticular formation. These give rise to fibers synapsing in the nonspecific nuclei of the thalamus. From there, the nonspecific thalamic projections influence widespread areas of the cerebral cortex and limbic system.

TABLE 37-2 Descending Levels of Consciousness and Their Characteristics

Level of Consciousness	Characteristics
Confusion	Disturbance of consciousness characterized by impaired ability to think clearly and to perceive, respond to, and remember current stimuli; also, disorientation
Delirium	State of disturbed consciousness with motor restlessness, transient hallucinations, disorientation, and sometimes delusions
Obtundation	Disorder of decreased alertness with associated psychomotor retardation
Stupor	A state in which the person is not unconscious but exhibits little or no spontaneous activity
Coma	A state of being unarousable and unresponsive to external stimuli or internal needs; often determined by the Glasgow Coma Scale

Data from Bates D. The management of medical coma. *J Neurol Neurosurg Psychiatry.* 1993;56:590.

hemisphere unilaterally and also spare the RAS, such as cerebral infarction, usually do not impair consciousness.

Levels of Consciousness. Levels of consciousness reflect awareness and response to the environment. A fully conscious person is totally aware of his or her surroundings and able to react to stimuli in the environment.[14,15] Levels of consciousness exist on a continuum that includes consciousness, confusion, delirium, obtundation, stupor, and coma[4] (Table 37-2).

The earliest signs of diminution in level of consciousness are inattention, mild confusion, disorientation, and blunted responsiveness. With further deterioration, the delirious person becomes markedly inattentive and variably lethargic or agitated. The person may progress to become obtunded and may respond only to vigorous or noxious stimuli.

Because of its simplicity of application, the Glasgow Coma Scale has gained almost universal acceptance as a method for assessing the level of consciousness in persons with brain injury[16] (Table 37-3). Numbered scores are given to responses of eye opening, verbal utterances, and motor responses. The total score is the sum of the best response in each category.

Other Manifestations of Deteriorating Brain Function

Additional elements in the initial neurologic evaluation of a person with brain injury include checking for abnormalities in the size of the pupils and their reaction to light, evidence of decorticate or decerebrate posturing, and altered patterns of respiration.[4,7]

Pupillary Reflexes and Eye Movements. Although the pupils may initially respond briskly to light, they become unreactive and dilated as brain function deteriorates. A bilateral loss of the pupillary light response is indicative of lesions of the brain stem. A unilateral loss of the pupillary light response may be due to a lesion of the optic or oculomotor pathways. The oculocephalic reflex (doll's-head eye movement)

can be used to determine whether the brain stem centers for eye movement are intact (Fig. 37-11). If the oculocephalic reflex is inconclusive, and if there are no contraindications, the oculovestibular test (i.e., cold caloric test, in which cold water is instilled into the ear canal) may be used to elicit nystagmus (see Chapter 38).

Decorticate and Decerebrate Posturing. With the early onset of unconsciousness, there is some combative and purposeful movement in response to pain. As coma progresses, noxious stimuli can initiate rigidity and abnormal postures if the motor tracts are interrupted at specific levels. These abnormal postures are classified as decorticate and decerebrate.[7] Both are poor prognostic signs.

TABLE 37-3 The Glasgow Coma Scale

Test	Score*
Eye Opening (E)	
Spontaneous	4
To call	3
To pain	2
None	1
Motor Response (M)	
Obeys commands	6
Localizes pain	5
Normal flexion (withdrawal)	4
Abnormal flexion (decorticate)	3
Extension (decerebrate)	2
None (flaccid)	1
Verbal Response (V)	
Oriented	5
Confused conversation	4
Inappropriate words	3
Incomprehensible sounds	2
None	1

*GCS Score = E + M + V. Best possible score = 15; worst possible score = 3.

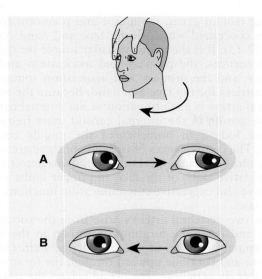

FIGURE 37-11. The *doll's-head eye response* demonstrates the always-present vestibular static reflexes without forebrain interference or suppression. Severe damage to the forebrain or to the brain stem rostral to the pons often results in loss of rostral control of these static vestibular reflexes. If the person's head is moved from side to side or up and down, the eyes will move in conjugate gaze to the opposite side **(A)**, much like those of a doll with counterweighted eyes. If the doll's-head phenomenon is observed, brain stem function at the level of the pons is considered intact (in a comatose person). In the unconscious person without intact brain stem function and vestibular static reflexes, the eyes stay in midposition (fixed) or turn in the same direction **(B)** as the head is turned.

Decorticate (flexion) posturing is characterized by the arms being held tightly to the sides, with flexion of the arms, wrists, and fingers; and extension and internal rotation of the legs with plantar flexion of the feet (see Fig. 37-4A). Decorticate posturing results from lesions of the cerebral hemisphere or internal capsule.

Decerebrate (extensor) posturing results from increased muscle excitability (see Fig. 37-4B). It is characterized by rigidity of the arms with the wrists and fingers flexed and turned away from the body and with stiffly extended legs and plantar flexion of the feet. This response occurs with rostral-to-caudal deterioration, when lesions of the diencephalon extend to involve the midbrain and upper brain stem.

Respiratory Responses. Early respiratory changes include yawning and sighing, with progression to Cheyne-Stokes breathing, in which there is waxing and waning of respirations with variable periods of apnea. When the progression of injury continues to the midbrain, respirations change to neurogenic hyperventilation, in which the frequency of respirations may exceed 40 breaths per minute because of uninhibited stimulation of inspiratory and expiratory centers. With medullary involvement, respirations become ataxic (i.e., totally uncoordinated and irregular). Apnea may occur because of a lack of responsiveness to carbon dioxide stimulation. Complete ventilatory assistance is often required at this point.

SUMMARY CONCEPTS

■ Many of the agents that cause brain damage do so through common and often interrelated pathways, including hypoxia or ischemia, accumulation of excitatory amino-acid neurotransmitters, and cerebral edema.

■ Deprivation of oxygen (i.e., hypoxia) or blood flow (i.e., ischemia) can have deleterious effects on the brain structures. Ischemia can be focal, as in stroke, or global as occurs during cardiac arrest when blood flow is inadequate to meet the metabolic needs of the entire brain.

■ *Excitotoxicity* is a final common pathway for neuronal cell injury and death. It is associated with excessive activity of excitatory amino-acid neurotransmitters, particularly glutamate.

■ Cerebral edema represents an increase in brain volume secondary to abnormal fluid accumulation. Vasogenic edema occurs when integrity of the blood–brain is disrupted allowing intravasular fluid to move into the extracellular fluid surround brain cells; whereas, cytotoxic edema involves swelling of brain cells due to the movement of the extracellular fluid into the brain cells.

■ The intracranial pressure (ICP) is the pressure exerted by the essentially incompressible tissue and fluid volumes of the three compartments contained within the rigid confines of the skull— brain tissue, blood, and cerebral spinal fluid (CSF). Excessive ICP can obstruct cerebral blood flow, destroy brain cells, displace brain tissue as in herniation, and otherwise damage delicate brain structures.

■ Hydrocephalus represents enlargement of the CSF compartment owing to an abnormal CSF volume. It can result from impaired reabsorption from the arachnoid villi into the venous system (communicating hydrocephalus) or from obstruction of the ventricular system (noncommunicating hydrocephalus), which prevents the CSF from reaching the arachnoid villi.

■ The term traumatic brain injury refers to injuries to the skull, brain, or both. The brain injuries can be primary, because of direct impact, or secondary, resulting from complicating processes that were initiated at the time of injury. They can be focal, as occurs with contusions and hematoma formation; or diffuse, as in concussion or diffuse axonal injury.

(continued)

Cerebrovascular Disease

Cerebrovascular disease encompasses a number of disorders involving vessels in the cerebral circulation. As elsewhere in the circulation, cerebrovascular disorders can involve vessel occlusion or rupture that leads to either focal or localized brain damage or to global hypoxia-ischemia that causes widespread brain injury.

The Cerebral Circulation

The blood flow to the brain is supplied by the two internal carotid arteries anteriorly and the vertebral arteries posteriorly[17] (Fig. 37-12A). The internal carotid artery, a terminal branch of the common carotid artery, branches into several arteries—the ophthalmic, posterior communicating, anterior choroidal, anterior cerebral, and middle cerebral arteries. Most of the arterial blood in the internal carotid arteries is distributed through the anterior and middle cerebral arteries (see Fig. 37-12B). The anterior cerebral arteries supply the medial surface of the frontal and parietal lobes and the anterior half of the thalamus, the corpus striatum, part of the corpus callosum, and the anterior limb of the internal capsule. The genu and posterior limb of the internal capsule and medial globus pallidus are fed by the anterior choroidal branch of the internal carotid artery.

The middle cerebral artery passes laterally, supplying the lateral basal ganglia and the insula, and then emerges on the lateral cortical surface, supplying the inferior frontal gyrus, the motor and premotor frontal cortex concerned with delicate face and hand control (Fig. 37-13). It is the major vascular source for the language cortices, the primary and association auditory cortices, and the primary and association somatosensory cortices for the face and hand. Because the middle cerebral artery is a continuation of the internal carotid, emboli arising in the internal carotid most frequently become lodged in branches of the middle cerebral artery. The consequences of ischemia of these areas may be the most devastating, resulting in damage to the fine manipulative skills of the face and upper limbs and to receptive and expressive communication functions (e.g., aphasia).

The two vertebral arteries arise from the subclavian artery and enter the foramina (opening) in the transverse spinal processes at the level of the sixth cervical vertebra and continue upward through the foramina of the upper six vertebrae. They wind behind the atlas and enter the skull through the foramen magnum and unite to form the basilar artery, which then diverges to terminate in the posterior cerebral arteries. Branches of the basilar and vertebral arteries supply the medulla, pons, cerebellum, midbrain, and caudal part of the diencephalon. The posterior cerebral arteries supply the remaining occipital and inferior regions of the temporal lobes and the thalamus.

The distal branches of the internal carotid and vertebral arteries communicate at the base of the brain through the circle of Willis; this anastomosis of arteries can provide continued circulation if blood flow through one of the main vessels is disrupted (see Fig. 37-12B). For instance, occlusion of one middle cerebral artery may have limited consequences if the anterior and posterior communicating arteries are patent, allowing collateral flow from the ipsilateral posterior cerebral and opposite carotid arteries. There are many normal variants across individuals in the completeness of the circle of Willis, such that collateral supply may be limited. Without collateral input, disruption of blood flow in a cerebral artery results in ischemic neural damage as metabolic needs of electrically active cells exceed nutrient supply.

The cerebral circulation is drained by two sets of veins that empty into the dural venous sinuses: the deep (great) cerebral venous system and the superficial venous system. In contrast to the superficial cerebral veins that travel through the pia mater on the surface of the cerebral cortex, the deep venous system is well protected. These vessels are directly connected to the sagittal sinuses in the falx cerebri by bridging veins. They travel through the CSF-filled subarachnoid space and penetrate the arachnoid and then the dura to reach the dural venous sinuses. This system of sinuses returns blood to the heart primarily through the internal jugular veins. The intracranial veins do not have valves. The direction of flow depends on gravity and pressures in the venous sinuses as compared with those of the extracranial veins. Increases in intrathoracic pressure, as can occur with coughing or performance of the Valsalva maneuver (i.e., exhaling against a closed glottis), produce a rise in

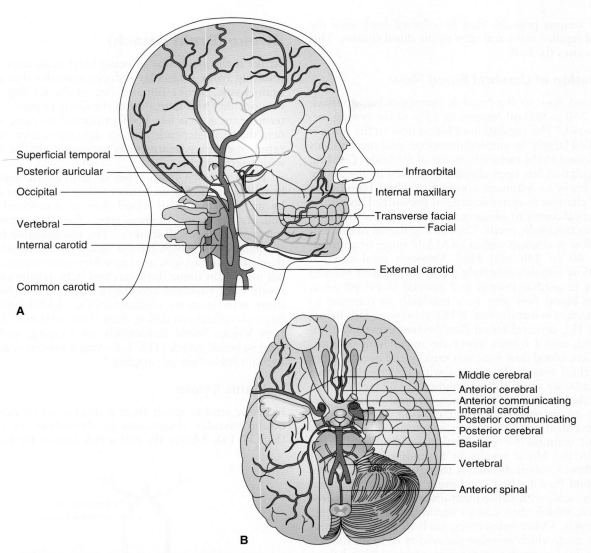

FIGURE 37-12. Cerebral circulation. **(A)** The internal carotid artery ascends to the base of the brain. The right vertebral artery is also shown as it ascends through the transverse foramina of the cervical vertebrae. **(B)** The cerebral arterial circle (circle of Willis).

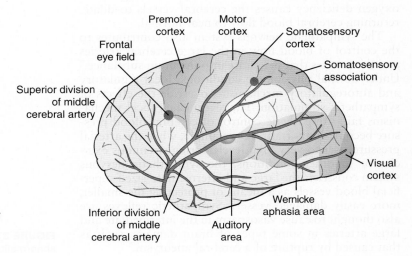

FIGURE 37-13. Lateral view of the cerebral hemisphere, showing areas of the cortex supplied by the superior and inferior divisions of the middle cerebral artery.

central venous pressure that is reflected back into the internal jugular veins and then to the dural sinuses. This briefly raises the ICP.

Regulation of Cerebral Blood Flow

The blood flow to the brain is maintained at approximately 750 to 900 mL/minute or 15% of the resting cardiac output.[2] The regulation of blood flow to the brain is controlled largely by autoregulatory or local mechanisms that respond to the metabolic needs of the brain. Cerebral autoregulation has been classically defined as the ability of the brain to maintain constant cerebral blood flow despite changes in systemic arterial pressure. This allows the cerebral cortex to adjust cerebral blood flow locally to satisfy its metabolic needs. The autoregulation of cerebral blood flow is efficient within an MABP range of approximately 60 to 140 mm Hg.[2] Although total cerebral blood flow remains relatively stable throughout marked changes in cardiac output and arterial blood pressure, regional blood flow may vary markedly in response to local changes in metabolism. If blood pressure falls below 60 mm Hg, cerebral blood flow becomes severely compromised, and if it rises above the upper limit of autoregulation, blood flow increases rapidly and overstretches the cerebral vessels. In persons with hypertension, this autoregulatory range shifts to higher MABP levels.

Metabolic factors affecting cerebral blood flow include an increase in carbon dioxide and hydrogen ion concentrations. Increased carbon dioxide provides a potent stimulus for vasodilation—a doubling of the PCO_2 in the blood results in a doubling of cerebral blood flow. Carbon dioxide is thought to increase cerebral blood flow by first combining with water to form carbonic acid, with subsequent dissociation into hydrogen ions, which then causes vasodilation of the cerebral vessels. Other substances, such as lactic acid and pyruvic acid, which increase the acidity of brain tissues, will produce a similar increase in cerebral blood flow. Oxygen deficiency also influences cerebral blood flow. Except during periods of intense brain activity, the rate of oxygen utilization by the brain remains within a narrow range. If blood flow to the brain becomes insufficient to supply this needed amount of oxygen, the oxygen deficiency causes the cerebral vessels to dilate, returning cerebral blood flow to near normal.

The sympathetic nervous system also contributes to the control of blood flow in the large cerebral arteries and the arteries that penetrate into the brain substance.[2] Under normal physiologic conditions, local regulatory and autoregulatory mechanisms override the effects of sympathetic stimulation. However, when local mechanisms fail, sympathetic control of cerebral blood pressure becomes important. For example, when the arterial pressure rises to very high levels during strenuous exercise or in other conditions, the sympathetic nervous system constricts the large and intermediate-sized superficial blood vessels as a means of protecting the smaller, more easily damaged vessels. Sympathetic reflexes are also thought to cause vasospasm in the intermediate and large arteries in some types of brain damage, such as that caused by rupture of a cerebral aneurysm.

Stroke (Brain Attack)

Stroke is the syndrome of acute focal neurologic deficit resulting from a vascular induced disorder that injures brain tissue. Stroke remains one of the leading causes of morbidity and mortality in the United States.[18,19] The term *brain attack* has been promoted to raise awareness that time-dependent tissue damage occurs and that rapid emergency treatment is necessary, similar to that with heart attack.

There are two main types of strokes: ischemic and hemorrhagic. Ischemic strokes reflect infarctions caused by an interruption of blood flow in a cerebral vessel and are the most common type of stroke, accounting for about 87% of all strokes.[7] The less common hemorrhagic strokes, which have a much higher fatality rate than ischemic strokes, are caused by spontaneous bleeding into brain tissue. Intracerebral hemorrhage can also result from ruptured cerebral aneurysms and bleeding from arteriovenous malformations. Additionally, the latest classifications define silent CNS infarction as ischemic lesions found incidentally on imaging, and transient ischemic attack (TIA) reflecting transient symptoms without infarction on imaging.[20]

Ischemic Stroke

Ischemic strokes result from a diverse set of causes of cerebrovascular obstruction by thrombosis or emboli (Fig. 37-14). Among the major risk factors for ischemic

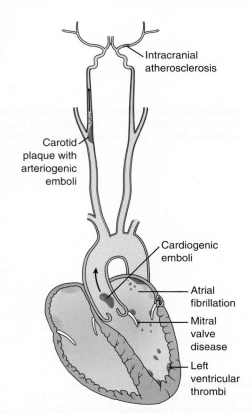

FIGURE 37-14. The most frequent sites of arterial and cardiac abnormalities causing ischemic stroke.

TABLE 37-4	Modifiable and Unmodifiable Risk Factors for Stroke
Modifiable Factors	**Unmodifiable Factors**

• Hypertension
• Hyperlipidemia
• Smoking
• Diabetes
• Heart disease
    Atrial fibrillation
    Wall motion defects
• Carotid artery disease
• Coagulation disorders
• Obesity/inactivity
• Heavy alcohol use
• Cocaine use
	• Age
	• Gender
	• Race
	• Heredity

stroke are family history of ischemic stroke, hypertension, cigarette smoking, overweight and obesity, high blood cholesterol and other lipids, diabetes mellitus, disorders of cardiac rhythm (e.g., atrial fibrillation), and chronic kidney disease[21] (Table 37-4). The incidence of stroke increases with age, and varies by sex and ethnicity. Men have higher rates in the younger age groups, though women catch up after menopause and live longer, resulting in higher rates of death among women. African Americans have almost twice the risk of first-ever strokes as whites. Blood pressure is a powerful determinant of stroke risk. Individuals with a blood pressure less than 120/80 mm Hg have about half the lifetime risk of stroke compared with persons with hypertension. Heart disease, particularly atrial fibrillation and other conditions that predispose to clot formation on the wall of the heart or valve leaflets, or to paradoxical embolism through right-to-left shunting, predisposes to cardioembolic stroke. Polycythemia, sickle cell disease (during sickle cell crisis), and blood disorders predispose to clot formation in the cerebral vessels.

Other, less well-documented risk factors include obesity, physical inactivity, alcohol and drug abuse, hypercoagulability disorders, hormone replacement therapy, and oral contraceptive use. Clinical trial data indicate that estrogen plus progestin, as well as estrogen alone, increase stroke risk in postmenopausal, generally healthy women, and provide no protection for women with established heart disease. Although extensively used in the past, the use of hormone therapy is no longer recommended (see Chapter 40). Heavy alcohol consumption can lead to hypertension, hypercoagulability of blood, reduction of cerebral blood flow, and greater likelihood of atrial fibrillation. Cocaine use causes both ischemic and hemorrhagic strokes by inducing vasospasm, enhanced platelet activity, and increased blood pressure, heart rate, body temperature, and metabolic rate.[22]

Classification. Various methods have been used to classify ischemic cerebrovascular disease. A common classification system identifies the five main mechanisms of stroke as stroke subtypes and their frequency: 20% large artery atherosclerotic disease (both thrombosis and arterial emboli); 25% small vessel or penetrating artery disease (so-called lacunar stroke); 20% cardiogenic embolism; 30% cryptogenic stroke (undetermined cause); and 5% other causes (i.e., migraine, vessel dissection, coagulopathy).[7]

Ischemic Penumbra in Evolving Stroke. During the evolution of a stroke, there usually is a central core of dead or dying cells, surrounded by an ischemic band or area of minimally perfused cells called the *penumbra* ("halo"). Brain cells of the penumbra receive marginal blood flow, and their metabolic activities are impaired. Although the area undergoes an "electrical failure," the structural integrity of the brain cells is maintained.[4,23] Reversal of the penumbral injury depends on the successful and timely return of adequate circulation, the volume of toxic products released by the neighboring dying cells, the degree of cerebral edema, and alterations in local blood flow. If the toxic products result in additional death of cells in the penumbra, the core of dead or dying tissue enlarges, and the volume of surrounding ischemic tissue increases.

Transient Ischemic Attacks. Transient ischemic attacks (TIAs) are brief episodes of neurologic dysfunction resulting from focal cerebral ischemia not associated with infarction.[18,24–26] A TIA or "ministroke" is equivalent to "brain angina" and reflects a temporary disturbance in cerebral blood flow, which reverses before infarction occurs, analogous to angina in relation to heart attack. The traditional definition of TIAs as a neurologic deficit resolving within 24 hours was developed before the mechanisms of ischemic cell damage and the penumbra were known and before the newer, more advanced methods of neuroimaging became available. A more accurate definition now is a transient deficit without time limits, best described as a zone of penumbra without central infarction.[20] The causes of TIAs are the same as those of ischemic stroke and include atherosclerotic disease of cerebral vessels and emboli. Transient ischemic attacks are important because they may provide warning of impending stroke. In fact, the risk for stroke is 15% in the 3 months following a TIA.[20] Diagnosis of TIA before a stroke may permit surgical or medical intervention that prevents an eventual stroke and associated neurologic deficits.

Large Vessel (Thrombotic) Stroke. Thrombi are the most common cause of ischemic strokes, usually occurring in atherosclerotic blood vessels.[1,4] In the cerebral circulation, atherosclerotic plaques are most commonly found at arterial bifurcations of large arteries. Common sites of plaque formation include the origins of the internal carotid and vertebral arteries, and junctions of the basilar and vertebral arteries. Cerebral infarction can result from an acute local thrombosis and occlusion at the site of chronic atherosclerosis, with or without embolization of the plaque material distally, or from critical perfusion failure distal to a stenosis (watershed). These infarcts often affect the cortex, causing aphasia or hemineglect, visual field defects, or transient monocular blindness (amaurosis fugax). In most cases of stroke, a single cerebral artery and its territories are affected. Usually, thrombotic strokes are seen in older persons and frequently are accompanied by evidence of atherosclerotic heart or peripheral arterial disease. The thrombotic stroke is not associated with activity and may occur in a person at rest.

Small Vessel Stroke (Lacunar Infarct). Lacunar infarcts are small (<15 mm wide) infarcts located in the deep, noncortical parts of the brain or in the brain stem.[1] They are found in the territory of single, deep, penetrating arteries supplying the internal capsule, basal ganglia, or brain stem. They result from occlusion of the smaller penetrating branches of large cerebral arteries, commonly the middle cerebral and posterior cerebral arteries. The infarcted tissue eventually scars to leave small, rounded cavities, or *lacunae* ("lakes"). They are thought to result from arteriosclerosis, commonly in the settings of chronic hypertension or diabetes. Because of their size and location, lacunar infarcts usually do not cause cortical deficits such as aphasia or apraxia. Instead, they produce classic recognizable "lacunar syndromes" such as pure motor hemiplegia, pure sensory hemiplegia, and dysarthria with clumsy hand syndrome. Because CT scans are not sensitive enough to detect these tiny infarcts, diagnosis used to depend on clinical features alone. The use of MRI has allowed frequent visualization of small vessel infarcts and is obligatory to confirm such a lesion.

Embolic Stroke. An embolic stroke is caused by a moving blood clot that travels from its origin to the brain. It usually affects the larger proximal cerebral vessels, with emboli often lodging at bifurcations. The most frequent site of embolic strokes is the middle cerebral artery, reflecting the large territory of this vessel and its position at the terminus of the carotid artery. Although most cerebral emboli originate from a thrombus in the left heart, they also may originate in an atherosclerotic plaque in the carotid arteries. The embolus travels quickly to the brain and becomes lodged in a smaller artery through which it cannot pass. Embolic stroke usually has a sudden onset with immediate maximum deficit.

Various cardiac conditions predispose to formation of emboli that produce embolic stroke, including rheumatic heart disease, atrial fibrillation, recent myocardial infarction, ventricular aneurysm, and bacterial endocarditis. More recently, the use of transesophageal echocardiography, which better images the interatrial septum, has implicated a patent foramen ovale as a source for paradoxical venous emboli to the arterial system. Advances in the diagnosis and treatment of heart disease can be expected to favorably alter the incidence of embolic stroke.

Hemorrhagic Stroke

The most frequently fatal stroke is caused by the spontaneous rupture of an intracerebral vessel.[27,28] With rupture of a blood vessel, hemorrhage into the brain tissue occurs, resulting in a focal hematoma and sometimes intraventricular hemorrhage, edema, compression of the brain contents, or spasm of the adjacent blood vessels. The most common predisposing factors are advancing age and hypertension. Other causes of hemorrhage are aneurysm, trauma, erosion of the vessels by tumors, arteriovenous malformations, blood coagulation disorders, vasculitis, and drugs. A cerebral hemorrhage occurs suddenly, usually when the person is active. Vomiting commonly occurs at the onset, and headache is common. Focal symptoms depend on which vessel is involved. In the most common situation, hemorrhage into the basal ganglia results in contralateral hemiplegia, with initial flaccidity progressing to spasticity. The hemorrhage and resultant edema exert great pressure on the brain substance, and the clinical course progresses rapidly to coma and frequently to death.

Treatment of hemorrhagic stroke focuses on intensive management of the increased arterial and intracranial pressures, and prevention of hematoma expansion. Initial promising results with use of recombinant factor VII to limit hematoma expansion were deflated by the occurrence of thromboembolic complications.[28] In patients with anticoagulant-associated hemorrhages, use of prothrombin complex concentrate has been more successful than vitamin K administration.[29]

Acute Stroke Management

The specific manifestations of stroke or TIA are determined by the cerebral artery that is affected, by the area of brain tissue that is supplied by that vessel, and by the adequacy of the collateral circulation.[7,18] Symptoms of stroke/TIA always are sudden in onset and focal, and usually are one-sided. The most common symptom is weakness of the face and arm, and sometimes also of the leg. Other frequent stroke symptoms are unilateral numbness, vision loss in one eye (amaurosis fugax) or to one side (hemianopia), language disturbance (aphasia), slurred speech (dysarthria), and sudden, unexplained imbalance or ataxia. In the event of TIA, symptoms rapidly resolve spontaneously, usually within minutes, although the underlying mechanisms are the same as for stroke.

Stroke signs depend on the specific vascular territory compromised (Table 37-5). As a generalization, carotid ischemia causes monocular visual loss or aphasia (dominant hemisphere) or hemineglect (nondominant hemisphere), contralateral sensory or motor loss, or other discrete cortical signs such as apraxia and agnosia. Vertebrobasilar ischemia induces ataxia, diplopia, hemianopia, vertigo, cranial nerve deficits, contralateral hemiplegia, sensory deficits (either contralateral or crossed, i.e., contralateral body and ipsilateral face), and arousal defects. Discrete subsets of these vascular syndromes usually occur, depending on which branches of the involved artery are blocked.

Diagnosis. Accurate diagnosis of acute stroke, based on a complete history and thorough physical and neurologic examination, is designed to determine the presence of

TABLE 37-5	Signs and Symptoms of Stroke by Involved Cerebral Artery	
Cerebral Artery	**Brain Area Involved**	**Signs and Symptoms***
Anterior cerebral	Infarction of the medial aspect of one frontal lobe if lesion is distal to communicating artery; bilateral frontal infarction if flow in other anterior cerebral artery is inadequate	Paralysis of contralateral foot or leg; impaired gait; paresis of contralateral arm; contralateral sensory loss over toes, foot, and leg; problems making decisions or performing acts voluntarily; lack of spontaneity, easily distracted; slowness of thought; aphasia depends on the hemisphere involved; urinary incontinence; cognitive and affective disorders
Middle cerebral	Massive infarction of most of lateral hemisphere and deeper structures of the frontal, parietal, and temporal lobes; internal capsule; basal ganglia	Contralateral hemiplegia (face and arm); contralateral sensory impairment; aphasia; homonymous hemianopia; altered consciousness (confusion to coma); inability to turn eyes toward paralyzed side; denial of paralyzed side or limb (hemiattention); possible acalculia, alexia, finger agnosia, and left–right confusion; vasomotor paresis and instability
Posterior cerebral	Occipital lobe; anterior and medial portion of temporal lobe	Homonymous hemianopia and other visual defects such as color blindness, loss of central vision, and visual hallucinations; memory deficits, perseveration (repeated performance of same verbal or motor response)
	Thalamus involvement	Loss of all sensory modalities; spontaneous pain; intentional tremor; mild hemiparesis; aphasia
Basilar and vertebral	Cerebral peduncle involvement	Oculomotor nerve palsy with contralateral hemiplegia
	Cerebellum and brain stem	Visual disturbance such as diplopia, dystaxia, vertigo, dysphagia, dysphonia

*Depend on hemisphere involved and adequacy of collaterals.

hemorrhage or ischemia, identify the stroke or TIA mechanism (i.e., large-vessel or small-vessel, atherothrombotic, cardioembolic, hemorrhagic, cryptogenic, or other), characterize the severity of clinical deficits, and unmask the presence of risk factors.[31–34] A careful history, including documentation of previous TIAs, the time of onset and pattern and rapidity of system progression, the specific focal symptoms (to determine the likely vascular territory), and any coexisting diseases, can help to determine the type of stroke that is involved.

Computed tomographic scans and magnetic resonance imaging have become essential brain imaging tools in diagnosing stroke, differentiating cerebral hemorrhage from ischemia, and excluding intracranial lesions that mimic stroke clinically. CT scans are a necessary screening tool in the acute setting for rapid identification of hemorrhage, but are insensitive to ischemia within 24 hours and to any brain stem or small infarcts. MRI is superior for imaging ischemic lesions in all territories and differentiating other nonstroke pathologic processes (e.g., tumors, contusion, infection). Newer MRI techniques such as perfusion- and diffusion-weighted imaging (DWI) can reveal cerebral ischemia immediately after onset and identify areas of potentially reversible damage (i.e., penumbra).

Vascular imaging is accomplished with CT angiography (CTA), magnetic resonance angiography (MRA), catheter-based "conventional" arteriography, and ultrasonography. All except ultrasonography can demonstrate the site of vascular abnormality (intracranial and extracranial) and afford visualization of most intracranial vascular areas. MRA is noninvasive and most widely available, but less sensitive and specific than CTA or catheter

angiography. CT angiography is exquisitely detailed for a noninvasive technique, but is limited in availability and requires iodinated contrast, which is nephrotoxic. Catheter angiography remains the gold standard in sensitivity and allows visualization of dynamic patterns of collateral flow, but is invasive and requires significant contrast doses. CT angiography and magnetic resonance angiography have largely replaced angiography as a screening tool for vascular lesions. Ultrasonographic techniques allow quick bedside assessment of the carotid bifurcation (duplex ultrasonography) or of flow velocities in the cerebral circulation (transcranial Doppler).

Treatment. Treatment of acute ischemic stroke has changed markedly since the early 1990s, with an emphasis on salvaging brain tissue, preventing secondary stroke, and minimizing long-term disability. The care of patients with stroke has shifted away from the "nearest hospital" to stroke centers that have been certified by some external agency, most commonly the state or Joint Commission.[33] Certification establishes that a hospital can manage stroke patients with appropriate care throughout the continuum—from emergency treatments, through the inpatient stay, and into the rehabilitation phase. With this advancement, the medical and lay communities acknowledge that care of the patient with stroke requires specialized personnel and resources to minimize stroke's devastating effects, as stroke is the leading cause of adult disability in the United States.

Stroke care begins with emergency treatments aimed at reversing the evolving ischemic brain injury. The realization that there is a window of opportunity during which ischemic but viable brain tissue can be salvaged has led to the use of reperfusion techniques and neuro-protective strategies in the early treatment of ischemic stroke.[18,30–33] Although the results of emergent treatment of hemorrhagic stroke have been less dramatic, continued efforts to reduce disability have been promising.

Reperfusion techniques include thrombolytic therapy (administered either intravenously or intra-arterially), catheter-directed mechanical clot disruption, and augmentation of cerebral perfusion pressure during acute stroke.[34] The first and only agent approved by the U.S. Food and Drug Administration (FDA) for treatment of acute ischemic stroke is tissue plasminogen activator (tPA). A subcommittee of the Stroke Council of the American Heart Association has developed guidelines for the use of tPA for acute stroke.[20] These guidelines recommend that in persons with suspected stroke, the diagnosis of hemorrhagic stroke be excluded through the use of CT scanning before administration of I.V. thrombolytic therapy, which must be administered within 3 hours of onset of symptoms, or 4.5 hours in some cases.[34] The major risk of treatment with thrombolytic agents is intracranial hemorrhage of the infarcted brain. A number of conditions, including therapeutic levels of oral anticoagulant medications, a history of gastrointestinal or urinary tract bleeding in the previous 21 days, prior stroke or head injury within 3 months, major surgery within the past 14 days, and a blood pressure greater than 185/110 mm Hg, are considered contraindications to intravenous thrombolytic therapy.[33]

Emerging experimental treatments for ischemic stroke are being increasingly used as alternative methods of reperfusion beyond intravenous thrombolysis. New catheter-based methods allow recanalization of a directly visualized cerebral clot with intra-arterial techniques, often beyond the 4.5-hour window. Patient candidates for invasive reperfusion strategies are generally identified using newer perfusion imaging techniques such as CT or MR perfusion in order to detect a region of reversible injury (ischemic penumbra) and to exclude completed infarcts. Once a penumbra is found, the interventional specialist might mechanically disrupt the clot, extract the clot (thrombectomy), or deliver the thrombolytic drug intra-arterially at the clot surface, or urgently stent intracranial vessels to restore flow and rescue the penumbra. Additional methods (drugs, ultrasound, hypothermia) aimed at either extending that therapeutic window until revascularization occurs or improving recanalization rates are under active investigation.[36] These methods require an experienced interventional angiography team, neurocritical care services, and extensive institutional infrastructure, and thus remain limited to tertiary care centers.

Poststroke Management and Deficits

Poststroke treatment is aimed at preventing recurrent stroke and medical complications while promoting the fullest possible recovery of function.[37] The risk of stroke recurrence is highest in the first week after a stroke or TIA, so the early implementation of antiplatelet agents in most cases, or warfarin (an anticoagulant) in cardioembolic stroke, is imperative. Long-term stroke recurrence is most effectively prevented with aggressive reduction of risk factors, primarily hypertension, diabetes, smoking, and hyperlipidemia. In cases of carotid territory stroke with carotid stenosis, revascularization with surgery or stenting should be considered. Early hospital care also requires careful prevention of aspiration, deep vein thrombosis, and falls. Recovery is maximized with early and aggressive rehabilitation efforts that include all members of the rehabilitation team—physician, nurse, speech therapist, physical therapist, and occupational therapist—and the family.

Poststroke Motor Deficits. Poststroke motor deficits are most common, followed by deficits of language, sensation, and cognition. After a stroke affecting the corticospinal tract such as the motor cortex, posterior limb of the internal capsule, basis pontis, or medullary pyramids, there is profound weakness on the contralateral side (hemiparesis; see Chapter 36, Fig. 36-4). Involvement at the level of the motor cortex is most often in the territory of the middle cerebral artery, usually with a sparing of the leg, which is supplied by the anterior cerebral artery. Subcortical lesions of the corticospinal tracts cause equal weakness of the face, arm, and leg. Within 6 to 8 weeks, the initial weakness and flaccidity are replaced by hyperreflexia and spasticity.

Spasticity involves an increase in the tone of affected muscles and usually an element of weakness. The flexor muscles usually are more strongly affected in the upper extremities and the extensor muscles more strongly affected in the lower extremities. There is a tendency toward foot drop; outward rotation and circumduction of the leg with gait; flexion at the wrist, elbow, and fingers; lower facial paresis; slurred speech; an upgoing toe to plantar stimulation (Babinski sign); and dependent edema in the affected extremities. A slight corticospinal lesion may be indicated only by clumsiness in carrying out fine coordinated movements rather than obvious weakness. Passive range-of-motion exercises help to maintain joint function and to prevent edema, shoulder subluxation (i.e., incomplete dislocation), and muscle atrophy, and may help to reestablish motor patterns. If no voluntary movement or movement on command appears within a few months, significant function usually will not return to that extremity.

Poststroke Dysarthria and Aphasia. Two key aspects of verbal communication are speech and language. Speech involves the mechanical act of articulating verbal sounds, the "motor act" of verbal expression, whereas language involves the written or spoken use of symbolic formulations, such as words or numbers.[7] *Dysarthria* is a disorder of speech, which manifests as the imperfect articulation of speech sounds or changes in voice pitch or quality. It results from a stroke affecting the muscles of the pharynx, palate, tongue, lips, or mouth and does not relate to the content of speech. A person with dysarthria may demonstrate slurred speech while still retaining language ability, or may have a concurrent language problem as well. *Aphasia* is a general term that encompasses varying degrees of inability to comprehend, integrate, and express language. Aphasia may be localized to the dominant cerebral cortex or thalamus—on the left side in 95% of people who are right handed and 70% of people who are left handed. In children, language dominance can readily shift to the unaffected hemisphere, resulting in more transient language deficits after stroke. A stroke in the territory of the middle cerebral artery is the most common aphasia-producing stroke.

Aphasia can be categorized as receptive or expressive, or as fluent or nonfluent. Receptive or fluent speech requires little or no effort, is intelligible, and is of increased quantity. The term *fluent* refers only to the ease and rate of verbal output, and does not relate to the content of speech or the ability of the person to comprehend what is being said. Verbal utterances are often paraphasic, meaning that letters, syllables, or whole words are substituted for the target words. There are three categories of fluent aphasia: Wernicke, anomic, and conduction aphasia. *Wernicke aphasia* is characterized by an inability to comprehend the speech of others or to comprehend written material. Lesions of the posterior superior temporal or lower parietal lobe (areas 22 and 39) are associated with receptive or *fluent aphasia*. *Anomic aphasia* is speech that is nearly normal except for difficulty with finding singular words. Conduction aphasia is manifest as impaired repetition and speech riddled with letter substitutions, despite good comprehension and fluency. *Conduction aphasia* (i.e., disconnection syndrome) results from destruction of the fiber system under the insula that connects the Wernicke and Broca areas.

Expressive or *nonfluent aphasia* is characterized by an inability to easily communicate spontaneously or translate thoughts or ideas into meaningful speech or writing. Speech production is limited, effortful, and halting and often may be poorly articulated because of a concurrent dysarthria. The person may be able, with difficulty, to utter or write two or three words, especially those with an emotional overlay. Comprehension is normal, and the person seems to be fully aware of his or her deficits but is unable to correct them. This often leads to frustration, anger, and depression. Expressive, nonfluent aphasia is associated with lesions of the Broca area at the dominant inferior frontal lobe cortex (areas 44 and 45).

Poststroke Cognitive and Other Deficits. Stroke can also cause cognitive, sensory, visual, and behavioral deficits. One distinct cognitive syndrome is that of hemineglect or hemi-inattention. Usually caused by strokes affecting the nondominant (right) hemisphere, hemineglect is the inability to attend to and react to stimuli coming from the contralateral (left) side of space. Affected persons may not visually track, orient, or reach to the neglected side. They may neglect to use the limbs on that side, despite normal motor function, and may not shave, wash, or comb that side. Such persons are unaware of this deficit, which is another form of their neglect (*anosognosia*). Other cognitive deficits include impaired ability to carry out previously learned motor activities despite normal sensory and motor function (*apraxia*), impaired recognition with normal sensory function (*agnosia*), memory loss, behavioral syndromes, and depression. Sensory deficits affect the body contralateral to the lesion and can manifest as numbness, tingling paresthesias, or distorted sensations such as dysesthesia and neuropathic pain. Visual disturbances from stroke are diverse, but most common are hemianopia from a lesion of the optic radiations between the lateral geniculate body and the temporal or occipital lobes, and monocular blindness from occlusion of the ipsilateral central retinal artery, a branch of the internal carotid artery.

Intracranial Hemorrhage

Intracranial hemorrhages can occur at any site within the brain. They usually result from rupture of small atherosclerotic vessels, as in hemorrhagic stroke; rupture of an aneurysm; or arteriovenous malformations.

Aneurysmal Subarachnoid Hemorrhage

An aneurysm is a bulge at the site of a localized weakness in the muscular wall of an arterial vessel. Most cerebral aneurysms are small saccular aneurysms called *berry aneurysms*. They usually occur in the anterior circulation and are found at bifurcations and other junctions of vessels such as those in the circle of Willis (Fig. 37-15). They are thought to arise from a congenital defect in the media of the involved vessels. Their incidence is higher in persons with certain disorders, including polycystic kidney disease, fibromuscular dysplasia, coarctation of the aorta, and arteriovenous malformations of the brain.[1,4] Other causes of cerebral aneurysms are atherosclerosis, hypertension, and bacterial infections.

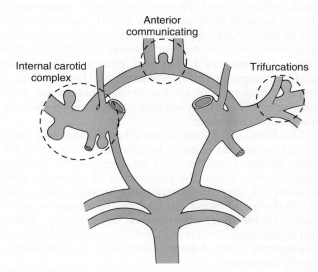

FIGURE 37-15. Common sites of berry aneurysms.

Aneurysmal subarachnoid hemorrhage represents bleeding into the subarachnoid space caused by a ruptured cerebral aneurysm. Bleeding into the subarachnoid space can extend well beyond the site of origin, flooding the basal cistern, ventricles, and spinal subarachnoid space. The incidence of rupture increases with age, occurring most commonly between 40 and 60 years of age.[43] The probability of rupture increases with the size of the aneurysm; aneurysms larger than 10 mm in diameter have a 50% chance of bleeding at some point during the course of a year.[1] Of the various factors that may predispose to aneurysmal subarachnoid hemorrhage, cigarette smoking, hypertension, and excessive alcohol intake appear to constitute the greatest threat.[38] Rupture may occur at any time, but often occurs with acute increases in ICP, such as with straining at stool. The mortality rate for subarachnoid hemorrhage is high (33% to 50%), with the majority of deaths occurring within the first few days of hemorrhage.[38]

The signs and symptoms of cerebral aneurysms can be divided into two phases: those presenting before rupture and those presenting after rupture. Most small aneurysms are asymptomatic; intact aneurysms frequently are found at autopsy as an incidental finding. Large aneurysms may cause chronic headache, neurologic deficits, or both.[38,39] Persons with subarachnoid hemorrhage often have a history of atypical headaches occurring days to weeks before the onset of hemorrhage, suggesting the presence of a small leak. These headaches are characterized by sudden onset and often are accompanied by nausea, vomiting, and dizziness. Persons with these symptoms may be mistakenly diagnosed as having tension or migraine headaches.

The onset of subarachnoid aneurysmal rupture often is heralded by a sudden and severe headache, described as "the worst headache of my life."[38] If the bleeding is severe, the headache may be accompanied by collapse and loss of consciousness. Vomiting may accompany the presenting symptoms. Other manifestations include signs of meningeal irritation such as nuchal rigidity (neck stiffness) and photophobia (light intolerance); cranial nerve deficits, especially CN II, and sometimes CN III and CN IV (diplopia and blurred vision); stroke syndromes (focal motor and sensory deficits); cerebral edema and increased ICP; and pituitary dysfunction (diabetes insipidus and hyponatremia). Hypertension, a frequent finding, and cardiac arrhythmias result from massive release of catecholamines triggered by the subarachnoid hemorrhage.

The diagnosis of subarachnoid hemorrhage and intracranial aneurysms is made by clinical presentation, CT scan, lumbar puncture, and angiography.[38,39] Lumbar puncture may reveal the presence of blood in the CSF, whereas CT may demonstrate the location and extent of subarachnoid blood. To identify the aneurysm at the source of bleeding, conventional angiography, MRA, and helical (spiral) CTA are used. Conventional catheter angiography is the definitive diagnostic tool for detecting the aneurysm.

The course of treatment after aneurysm rupture depends on the extent of neurologic deficit. The best outcomes are achieved when the aneurysm can be secured early and prevention of complications initiated.[39] Persons with mild to no neurologic deficits may undergo cerebral arteriography and early aneurysm obliteration with surgery or endovascular coiling, usually within 24 to 72 hours. Surgery involves craniotomy and inserting a specially designed silver clip that is tightened around the neck of the aneurysm. This procedure offers protection from rebleeding and may permit removal of the hematoma. The use of endovascular techniques such as balloon embolization and platinum coil electrothrombosis is an alternative to surgery, particularly in posterior circulation aneurysms or poor surgical candidates. Early outcomes and fewer complications are better with coiling, while long-term rebleeding rates are reduced with surgery.[39] Some persons with subarachnoid hemorrhage are managed medically for 10 days or more in an attempt to improve their clinical status before surgery or coiling.

The complications of aneurysmal rupture include rebleeding, vasospasm with cerebral ischemia, hydrocephalus, hypothalamic dysfunction, and seizure activity. Rebleeding and vasospasm are the most serious and most difficult to treat. Rebleeding, which usually occurs on the first day after the initial rupture, results in further and usually catastrophic neurologic deficits.

Cerebral vasospasm is a dreaded complication of aneurysmal rupture. The condition is difficult to treat and is associated with a high incidence of morbidity and mortality. Usually, the condition develops within 3 to 10 days (peak, 7 days) after aneurysm rupture and involves a focal narrowing of the cerebral artery or arteries that can be visualized on arteriography or by transcranial Doppler. The neurologic status gradually deteriorates as blood supply to the brain in the region of the spasm is decreased; this usually can be differentiated from the rapid deterioration seen in rebleeding. Vasospasm is treated by attempting to maintain adequate cerebral perfusion pressure through the use of vasoactive drugs or administration of large amounts of intravenous fluids to increase intravascular volume and produce hemodilution. There is risk for rebleeding from this therapy. Early surgery may provide some protection from vasospasm. Endovascular techniques, including balloon dilation, have been developed to treat spasmodic arterial segments mechanically. Nimodipine, a drug that blocks calcium channels and selectively acts on cerebral blood vessels, may be used to prevent or treat vasospasm.

Another complication of aneurysm rupture is the development of hydrocephalus. It is caused by plugging of the arachnoid villi with products from lysis of blood in the subarachnoid space. Hydrocephalus is diagnosed by serial CT scans showing increasing size of the ventricles and by the clinical signs of increased ICP. Hydrocephalus may respond to osmotic diuretics, but if neurologic deterioration is significant, surgical placement of a shunt is indicated.

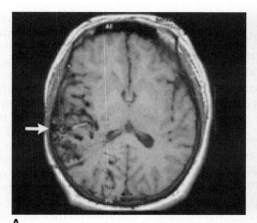
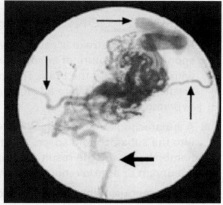

FIGURE 37-16. (A) Computed tomography scan of an arteriovenous malformation in the right parietal region of the brain (*arrow*). **(B)** Angiographic study of the internal carotid artery delineating the malformation in the middle cerebral artery distribution (*large arrow*), with draining veins (*small arrows*) to the superior sagittal sinus. (From Vermillion JM, Harris FS. Hemispheric arteriovenous malformation. *N Engl J Med* 2004;350[17]:e15. Copyright © 2004. Massachusetts Medical Society.)

A   **B**

Arteriovenous Malformations

Arteriovenous malformations are a complex tangle of abnormal arteries and veins linked by one or more fistulas[40,41] (Fig. 37-16). These vascular networks lack a capillary bed, and the small arteries have a deficient muscularis layer. Arteriovenous malformations are thought to arise from failure in development of the capillary network in the embryonic brain. As the child's brain grows, the malformation acquires additional arterial contributions that enlarge to form a tangled collection of thin-walled vessels that shunt blood directly from the arterial to the venous circulation. Arteriovenous malformations typically present before 40 years of age and affect men and women equally. Rupture of vessels in the malformation causing hemorrhagic stroke accounts for approximately 2% of all strokes.[40]

The hemodynamic effects of arteriovenous malformations are twofold. First, blood is shunted from the high-pressure arterial system to the low-pressure venous system without the buffering advantage of the capillary network. The draining venous channels are exposed to high levels of pressure, predisposing them to rupture and hemorrhage. Second, the elevated arterial and venous pressures divert blood away from the surrounding tissue, impairing tissue perfusion. Clinically, this is evidenced by slowly progressive neurologic deficits. The major clinical manifestations of arteriovenous malformations are intracerebral and subarachnoid hemorrhage, seizures, headache, and progressive neurologic deficits. Headaches often are severe, and persons with the disorder may describe them as throbbing and synchronous with their heartbeat. Other, focal symptoms depend on the location of the lesion and include visual symptoms (i.e., diplopia and hemianopia), hemiparesis, mental deterioration, and speech deficits.

Definitive diagnosis often is obtained through cerebral angiography. Treatment methods include surgical excision, endovascular occlusion, and radiation therapy.[40] Because of the nature of the malformation, each of these methods is accompanied by some risk for complications. If the arteriovenous malformation is accessible, surgical excision usually is the treatment of choice. Endovascular treatment involves the insertion of microcatheters into the cerebral circulation for delivery of embolic materials (e.g., microballoons, sclerosing agents, microcoils, or quick-drying glue) into the arteriovenous malformation vessels.[41] Radiation therapy (also known as *radiosurgery*) may involve the use of a gamma knife, proton beam, or linear accelerator.

SUMMARY CONCEPTS

■ Cerebrovascular disorders produce focal neurologic deficits caused by a disturbance in cerebral blood flow due to a thrombus or embolus (ischemic stroke), intracerebral hemorrhage due to spontaneous rupture of small fragile intracerebral vessels (hemorrhagic stroke), or subarachnoid hemorrhage due to a ruptured aneurysm or arteriovenous malformation.

■ During the evolution of an ischemic stroke, there usually is a central core of dead or dying cells surrounded by an ischemic band of minimally perfused cells called a *penumbra*. Whether the cells of the penumbra continue to survive depends on the successful and timely return of adequate circulation.

■ Transient ischemic attacks (TIAs), which are brief episodes of neurologic dysfunction resulting from focal cerebral ischemia, are a warning sign of an impending stroke.

■ The acute manifestations of stroke can include motor, sensory, language, speech, and cognitive disorders, depending on the location of the blood vessel that is involved.

(continued)

Infections

Infections of the brain may be classified according to the structure involved—meninges (meningitis) or parenchymal brain tissue (encephalitis). They also may be classified by the type of invading organism: bacterial, viral, or other. In general, pathogens enter the CNS from the bloodstream or by direct invasion through a skull fracture, or, rarely, by contamination during surgery or lumbar puncture. Local extension from an adjacent structure (e.g., infected sinus, tooth, middle ear) may also occur.

Meningitis

Meningitis is an inflammation of the pia mater, the arachnoid, and the CSF-filled subarachnoid space. Inflammation spreads rapidly because of CSF circulation around the brain and spinal cord. The inflammation usually is caused by an infection, but chemical meningitis can occur. There are two types of acute infectious meningitis: acute purulent meningitis (usually bacterial) and acute lymphocytic (usually viral) meningitis.[1] Factors responsible for the severity of meningitis include virulence of the pathogen, host factors, brain edema, and the presence of permanent neurologic sequelae.

Acute Bacterial Meningitis

Acute bacterial meningitis, which has a high potential for morbidity and mortality, is an inflammatory process of the leptomeninges and CSF within the subarachnoid space.[1,4,42,43] Most cases of bacterial meningitis are caused by *Streptococcus pneumoniae* (pneumococcus) or *Neisseria meningitidis* (meningococcus), except in neonates, who are more commonly infected by group B streptococci. The development of effective vaccines against *Haemophilus influenzae* and *S. pneumoniae* has resulted in a profound decline in bacterial meningitis among children in the United States.[44] Among adults, however, the incidence of meningitis has not changed. Epidemics of meningococcal meningitis occur in settings such as colleges and the military, where young people reside in close contact with each other. Other pathogens in adults are gram-negative bacilli and *Listeria monocytogenes*. The very young and the very old are at highest risk for pneumococcal meningitis. Risk factors associated with contracting meningitis include head trauma with basilar skull fractures, otitis media, sinusitis or mastoiditis, neurosurgery, dermal sinus tracts, systemic sepsis, or immunocompromise.

In the pathophysiologic process of bacterial meningitis, the microorganisms replicate and undergo lysis in the CSF, releasing endotoxins and cell wall fragments that cause inflammation, characterized by a cloudy, purulent exudate (Fig. 37-17). Thrombophlebitis of the bridging veins and dural sinuses or obliteration of arterioles by inflammation may develop, causing vascular congestion and infarction in the surrounding tissues. Ultimately, the meninges thicken and adhesions form. These adhesions may impinge on the cranial nerves, giving rise to cranial nerve palsies, or may impair the outflow of CSF, causing hydrocephalus.

The most common symptoms of acute bacterial meningitis are sudden onset of headache, fever, and stiffness of the neck (nuchal rigidity), sometimes accompanied

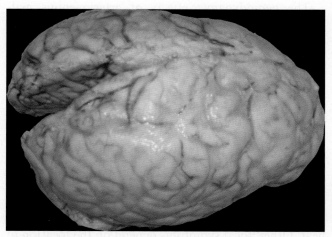

FIGURE 37-17. Purlent meningitis. A creamy exudate opacifies the leptomeninges in bacterial bacterial meningitis. The superficial veins are engorged and may develop thrombosis and the arteries on the surface of the brain may also develop thrombosis leading to infarcts. (From Fuller GN, Bouldin TW. The nervous system. In: Rubin R, Strayer DS, eds. *Rubin's Pathology: Clinicopathologic Foundations of Medicine*. 6th ed. Philadelphia, PA: Wolters Kluwer Health | Lippincott Williams & Wilkins; 2012:1318.)

by nausea, vomiting, photophobia, and altered mental status.[42,44] Other signs include seizures, cranial nerve palsies, and focal cerebral signs. Meningococcal meningitis is characterized by a petechial (petite hemorrhagic spots) rash with palpable purpura (bleeding into the skin) in most people. These petechiae vary in size from pinhead to large ecchymoses or even areas of skin gangrene, often associated with rapid onset of hypotension, acute adrenal hemorrhage (Waterhouse-Friderichsen syndrome), and multiple organ failure. Persons infected with *H. influenzae* or *S. pneumoniae* may present with difficulty in arousal and seizures, whereas those with *N. meningitidis* infection may present with delirium or coma. Cranial nerve damage (especially CN VIII, with resulting deafness) and hydrocephalus may occur as complications of pyogenic meningitis.

Diagnosis of bacterial meningitis is based on the history and physical examination, along with laboratory data. A stiff neck is an early sign of meningeal irritation. Moving the neck forward, either actively or passively, is difficult. Two assessment techniques can help determine whether meningeal irritation is present.[7] The *Kernig sign* is resistance to extension of the knee while the person is lying with the hip flexed at a right angle. The *Brudzinski sign* is elicited when flexion of the neck induces flexion of the hip and knee. These postures reflect resistance to the painful stretching of the inflamed meninges from the lumbar level to the head. Lumbar puncture findings, which are necessary for accurate diagnosis, include a cloudy and purulent CSF under increased pressure. Bacteria can be seen on smears and can easily be cultured with appropriate media. Occasionally, previous antibiotic use limits culture sensitivities, in which case latex agglutination or polymerase chain reaction (PCR) testing for *N. meningitidis*, *H. influenzae*, and *Listeria* species can be used. Because complications associated with lumbar puncture include life-threatening cerebral herniation, at-risk patients (i.e., those who are immunocompromised, had a seizure within a week, have papilledema, or have specific neurologic abnormalities) should have a CT scan before undergoing the procedure.

Treatment includes urgent administration of antimicrobial therapy while diagnostic testing ensues. Delay in initiation of antimicrobial therapy, most frequently because of performance of medical imaging before performance of lumbar puncture or transfer to another medical facility, can result in poor outcomes.[43,44] Because of the emergence of penicillin- and cephalosporin-resistant strains of *S. pneumoniae*, a combination of antimicrobial agents is usually used. Effective antimicrobial treatment produces rapid lysis of the pathogen, which produces inflammatory mediators that have the potential for exacerbating the abnormalities of the blood–brain barrier. To suppress this pathologic inflammation, adjunctive corticosteroid therapy is increasingly administered with or just before the first dose of antibiotics in patients of all ages.[43,44]

Persons who have been exposed to someone with meningococcal meningitis should be treated prophylactically with antibiotics. A quadrivalent polysaccharide–protein conjugate vaccine is now available to protect against meningococcal meningitis. The vaccine is recommended for adolescents aged 11 to 18 years, first-year college students living in dormitories, military recruits, and microbiologists with occupational exposure. The vaccine is also recommended for persons aged ≥ 9 months who travel to or reside in regions in which meningococcal disease is endemic and for all persons aged ≥ 2 months with conditions such as complement component deficiencies or anatomic or functional asplenia. The vaccine dosing schedule varies by age at time of previous vaccination.[45]

Viral Meningitis

Viral meningitis can be caused by many different viruses, most often enteroviruses, including coxsackievirus, poliovirus, and echovirus. Others include Epstein-Barr virus, mumps virus, herpes simplex virus (HSV), and West Nile virus. Often the virus cannot be identified.

Viral meningitis manifests in much the same way as bacterial meningitis, but the course is less severe and the CSF findings are markedly different. There are lymphocytes in the CSF rather than polymorphonuclear cells, the protein content is only moderately elevated, and the sugar content usually is normal. The acute viral meningitides are self-limited and usually require only symptomatic treatment, except for herpes simplex virus (HSV) type 2, which responds to intravenous acyclovir.

Encephalitis

Encephalitis represents a generalized infection of the parenchyma of the brain or spinal cord.[1,4,7,46] It usually is caused by a virus, but it also may be caused by bacteria, fungi, and other organisms. The nervous system is subject to invasion by many viruses, such as arbovirus, poliovirus, and rabies virus. The mode of transmission may be the bite of a mosquito (arbovirus), a rabid animal (rabies virus), or ingestion (poliovirus). Common causes of encephalitis in the United States are herpes simplex virus (HSV) and West Nile virus. Lessfrequent causes of encephalitis are toxic substances such as ingested lead and vaccines for measles and mumps. Encephalitis caused by human immunodeficiency virus (HIV) infection is discussed in Chapter 16.

The pathologic picture of encephalitis includes local necrotizing hemorrhage, which ultimately becomes generalized, with prominent edema. There is progressive degeneration of nerve cell bodies. The histologic picture, although rather general, may demonstrate some specific characteristics. For example, the poliovirus selectively destroys the cells of the anterior horn of the spinal cord.

Like meningitis, encephalitis is characterized by fever, headache, and nuchal rigidity, but more often patients also experience neurologic disturbances, such as lethargy, disorientation, seizures, focal paralysis, delirium, and coma. Diagnosis of encephalitis is made by clinical history and presenting symptoms, in addition to traditional CSF studies.

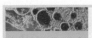

SUMMARY CONCEPTS

- Infections of the CNS may be classified according to the structures involved (the meninges [meningitis] or brain parenchyma [encephalitis]) and the type of organism causing the infection (bacteria or virus). The damage caused by infection may predispose to hydrocephalus, seizures, or other neurologic defects.

- Except in neonates, most cases of bacterial meningitis are pneumococcal or meningococcal. The most common symptoms are sudden onset of headache, fever, and stiffness of the neck (nuchal rigidity).

- Viral meningitis manifests in much the same way as bacterial meningitis, but the course is less severe and symptoms resolve spontaneously.

- Encephalitis is usually a viral infection of the brain. In addition to fever, headache, and nuchal rigidity, patients often experience neurologic disturbances.

Brain Tumors

Primary brain tumors account for 2% of all cancers in the United States.[4,47] Metastasis to the brain from other sites is more common. Central nervous system tumors are the second most common malignancy in children and adolescents, with the incidence rate being highest in infants and children 5 years of age or younger.[48]

The etiology of brain tumors is largely unknown. Several CNS tumors are associated with rare genetic conditions, most commonly the autosomal dominant disorder neurofibromatosis 1 (see Chapter 6). Although a large number of studies have examined the relationship between environmental and occupational factors, only high-dose radiation is a proven risk factor.[49,50] Irradiation given to treat intracranial and extracranial cancers, including prophylactic irradiation for leukemia, increases the incidence of brain tumors.

Types of Tumors

The term *brain tumor* refers to a collection of intracranial neoplasms, each with its own histology, site of origin, treatment, and prognosis.[1,4] For most neoplasms, the term *malignant* is used to describe the tumor's lack of cell differentiation, its invasive nature, and its ability to metastasize. However, the terms *benign* and *malignant* do not apply to brain tumors in the same sense as they do to tumors in other parts of the body. In the brain, even a well-differentiated and histologically benign tumor may grow and cause death because of its location. Also, tumors in the brain are rarely benign because surgery rarely cures. Most histologically benign tumors infiltrate the normal brain tissue, preventing total resection and allowing for tumor recurrence. Furthermore, brain tumors seldom metastasize, except within the CNS itself.

Brain tumors can be divided into three basic types: primary intracranial tumors of neuroepithelial tissue (e.g., neuroglia, neurons), primary intracranial tumors that originate in the cranial cavity but are not derived from the brain tissue itself (e.g., meninges, primary CNS lymphoma, pituitary gland tumors [discussed in Chapter 32]), and metastatic tumors.[1,4,50] Collectively, neurogliomas of astrocytic origin are the most common type of primary brain tumor in adults, and medulloblastomas the most common type in children. Whatever the type, brain tumors commonly present with symptoms related to a disruption in neuronal activity (seizures), signs of increased ICP (progressive headache, nausea and vomiting, drowsiness, visual abnormalities), focal motor or sensory deficits, and cognitive dysfunction.[7,50]

Neuroglial Tumors

Neuroglial tumors, which are the most common form of primary brain tumors, derive from astrocytes, oligodendrocytes, and ependymal cells.[1,4,51] Gliomas are divided into four grades: grades I and II are low-grade tumors, whereas grade III and IV are high-grade tumors.

Astrocytomas. There are two types of astrocyte tumors: infiltrating and noninfiltrating astrocytomas. Infiltrating astrocytomas account for 80% of adult primary brain tumors.[1] They occur most commonly in the fourth through the sixth decade. Although they usually are found in the cerebral hemispheres, they also can occur in the cerebellum, brain stem, or spinal cord. The most common presenting signs and symptoms are seizures, headaches, and focal neurologic deficits related to the location of the tumor. Infiltrating astrocytomas are characterized by a spectrum of histologic differentiation that includes diffuse astrocytomas (grade II); anaplastic astrocytomas (grade III); and the least differentiated and most aggressive, glioblastomas (grade IV).[1]

The grade I designation is reserved for the noninfiltrating pilocytic astrocytomas, which are distinguished from other astrocytomas by their cellular appearance and their benign behavior. Typically, they occur in children and young adults and usually are located in the cerebellum, but they also can be found in the floor and walls of the third ventricle, in the optic chiasm and nerves, and occasionally in the cerebral hemispheres. These tumors grow slowly and, in the cerebellum particularly, may be treated by resection.

Oligodendrogliomas. Oligodendrogliomas are tumors of the oligodendrocytes or their precursors.[1] They represent approximately 5% to 15% of neuroglial tumors and are most common in the fourth and fifth decades of life. The tumors are found mostly in the cerebral hemispheres, with a predilection for white matter. The prognosis of persons with oligodendrogliomas is less predictable than for persons with infiltrating astrocytomas.

It depends on the histologic grade of the tumor, its location, and, more recently, recognition of molecular features that can be linked to chemosensitivity.[50] Due to their delicate vasculature, the oligodendroglial tumors are prone to spontaneous hemorrhage.

Ependymomas. Ependymomas are derived from the single layer of epithelium that lines the ventricles and spinal canal. Although they can occur at any age, they are most likely to occur in the first two decades of life and most frequently affect the fourth ventricle; they constitute 5% to 10% of brain tumors in this age group.[1] In adults, the spinal cord is the most common location. The clinical features depend on the location of the neoplasm. Intracranial tumors are often associated with hydrocephalus and evidence of increased ICP.

Medulloblastomas

Tumors of neuronal origin (e.g., medulloblastomas) usually occur during infancy and childhood.[48] This is in accord with the principle that a cell must be capable of replication to undergo neoplastic transformation. Medulloblastoma is thought to originate from a primitive cell type in the cerebellum arising from one of two cerebellar germinal zones: the ventricular zone that forms the outermost boundary, or the external germinal layer that lines the outside of the cerebellum.

Medulloblastomas have a bimodal distribution, peaking at 3 or 4 years of age and then again at 8 or 9 years of age.[48] Children usually present with signs and symptoms of increased ICP (i.e., headache, nausea, vomiting, mental status changes, hypertension) and cerebellar dysfunction (i.e., ataxia, balance problems, movement disorders). The tumor is highly malignant, and the prognosis for untreated children is dismal. However, the tumor is highly radiosensitive; with total excision and irradiation, the 5-year survival rate is as high as 75%.

Meningiomas

Meningiomas develop from the meningothelial cells of the arachnoid and are outside the brain. They usually have their onset in the middle or later years of life and constitute approximately 20% of primary brain tumors in this age group.[1] Meningiomas are slow-growing, well-circumscribed, and often highly vascular tumors. They usually are benign, and complete removal is possible if the tumor does not involve vital structures.

Primary Central Nervous System Lymphomas

Primary CNS lymphomas have increased in incidence by a factor of 10 in the past several decades.[1,4] These deep, periventricular, and diffuse tumors are especially common in immunocompromised persons, including those with acquired immunodeficiency syndrome (AIDS) and immunosuppression after transplantation.

Most primary brain lymphomas are of B-cell origin. Primary lymphomas of the CNS are highly aggressive, and recurrence is common despite treatment. Behavioral and cognitive changes, which are the most common presenting symptoms, occur in about 65% of patients; hemiparesis, aphasia, and visual field deficits in about 50%; and seizures in 15% to 20%.

Metastatic Tumors

Metastatic tumors, mostly carcinomas, affect approximately 20% to 40% of persons with cancer.[50] The five most common sites for metastasis are the lung, breast, skin (melanoma), kidney, and gastrointestinal tract.[1,52,53] Within the brain there is regional selectivity for growth metastasis from the different primary types of cancer: melanoma is more typically found in the frontal and temporal lobes, breast cancer in the cerebellum and basal ganglia, and non–small cell lung cancer in the occipital lobe. Thus, it appears that tumor-specific interactions with brain tissue mediate the establishment and proliferation of brain metastasis. Recent investigations have begun to elucidate the mechanisms of such molecular mechanisms. For women with breast cancer, hormone receptor and human epidermal growth factor receptor-2 status is predictive of brain metastasis risk.[50]

Clinically evident brain metastases present with signs of increased ICP, mental status changes, seizures, and focal neurologic deficits. Management of persons with CNS metastasis consists of symptomatic and definitive therapies. The mainstays of symptomatic control are corticosteroids for tumor-related edema, antiepileptic drugs for seizure control, and multidisciplinary interventions aimed at minimizing neurologic disability.[50–52]

Manifestations

The clinical manifestations of brain tumors depend on the size and location of the tumor. General signs and symptoms include headache, nausea, vomiting, mental changes, papilledema, visual disturbances (e.g., diplopia), alterations in sensory and motor function, and seizures.[7,47] Because the volume of the intracranial cavity is fixed, brain tumors cause a generalized increase in ICP when they reach sufficient size or produce edema. Cerebral edema usually is of the vasogenic type, which develops around the tumors and is characterized by an increased extracellular fluid volume. The edema is thought to result from increased permeability of tumor capillary endothelial cells. Tumors can also obstruct the flow of CSF in the ventricular cavities and produce hydrocephalic dilation of the proximal ventricles and atrophy of the cerebral hemispheres. With very slow-growing tumors, complete compensation of ventricular volumes can occur, but with rapidly growing tumors, increased ICP is an early sign.

The brain itself is insensitive to pain. The headache that accompanies brain tumors results from compression or distortion of pain-sensitive dural or vascular structures. It may be felt on the same side of the head as the tumor, but more commonly is diffuse. In the early stages, the headache is mild and occurs in the morning on awakening and improves with head elevation. The headache becomes more constant as the tumor enlarges and often is worsened by coughing, bending, or sudden movements of the head.

Vomiting occurs with or without nausea, may be projectile, and is a common symptom of increased ICP and brain stem compression. Direct stimulation of the vomiting center, which is located in the medulla, may contribute to the vomiting that occurs with brain tumors. The vomiting is often associated with headache. Papilledema (edema of the optic disk) results from increased ICP and obstruction of the CSF pathways. It is associated with decreased visual acuity, diplopia, and deficits in the visual fields. Visual defects associated with papilledema often are the reason that persons with a brain tumor seek medical care.

Personality and mental changes such as depression are common with brain tumors. Persons with brain tumors often are irritable initially and later become quiet and apathetic. They may become forgetful, seem preoccupied, and appear to be psychologically depressed. Because of the mental changes, a psychiatric consultation may be sought before a diagnosis of brain tumor is made.

Focal signs and symptoms are determined by the location of the tumor. Tumors arising in the frontal lobe may grow to a large size, increase the ICP, and cause signs of generalized brain dysfunction before focal signs are recognized. Tumors that impinge on the visual system cause visual loss or visual field defects long before generalized signs develop. Certain areas of the brain have a relatively low threshold for seizure activity. Temporal lobe tumors often produce seizures as their first symptom. Hallucinations of smell or hearing and déjà vu phenomena are common focal manifestations of temporal lobe tumors. Brain stem tumors commonly produce upper and lower motor neuron signs, such as weakness of facial muscles and ocular palsies that occur with or without involvement of sensory or long motor tracts. Cerebellar tumors often cause ataxia of gait.

Diagnosis and Treatment

The diagnosis of brain tumors relies mainly on MRI.[7,47,50] Gadolinium-enhanced MRI is the test of choice for identifying and localizing the presence and extent of tumor involvement. Computed tomographic scans may fail to reveal certain mass lesions such as low-grade tumors or posterior fossa masses. Diagnostic maneuvers that suggest a possible tumor and indicate the need for MRI include physical and neurologic examinations, visual field and funduscopic examination, and sometimes electroencephalography (EEG). Approximately 75% of persons with a brain tumor have an abnormal EEG, which can indicate an underlying structural lesion warranting MRI. Cerebral angiography can be used to visualize the tumor's vascular supply, information that is important when planning surgery. MRI may be supplemented with positron emission tomography to better characterize the metabolic properties of the tumor, which is useful in planning treatment.[54] Magnetic resonance angiography and CT angiography can be used to distinguish vascular masses from tumors.

The three general methods for treatment of brain tumors are surgery, irradiation, and chemotherapy.

Surgery is part of the initial management of virtually all brain tumors; it establishes the diagnosis and achieves tumor removal in many cases. However, the degree of removal may be limited by the location of the tumor and its invasiveness. Stereotactic surgery uses three-dimensional coordinates and CT and MRI to precisely localize a brain lesion. Ultrasonographic technology has been used for localizing and removing tumors. The ultrasonic aspirator, which combines a vibrating head with suction, permits atraumatic removal of tumors from cranial nerves and important cortical areas. An important adjunct to some types of surgery is intraoperative monitoring of evoked potentials. For example, evoked potentials can be used to monitor auditory, visual, speech, or motor responses during surgery done under local anesthesia.

Most malignant brain tumors respond to external irradiation. Irradiation can increase longevity and sometimes can allay symptoms when tumors recur. The treatment dose depends on the tumor's histologic type, radioresponsiveness, and anatomic site and on the level of tolerance of the surrounding tissue. A newer technique called *gamma knife* combines stereotactic localization of the tumor with radiosurgery, allowing delivery of high-dose radiation to deep tumors while sparing the surrounding brain tissue. Radiation therapy is avoided in children younger than 2 years of age because of the long-term effects, which include developmental delay, panhypopituitarism, and secondary tumors.

The use of chemotherapy for brain tumors is somewhat limited by the blood–brain barrier. Chemotherapeutic agents can be administered intravenously, intra-arterially, intrathecally (i.e., into the spinal canal), as wafers impregnated with a drug and implanted into the tumor at the time of surgery.

SUMMARY CONCEPTS

- Brain tumors can be divided into primary intracranial tumors of neuroepithelial tissue (e.g., neuroglia, neurons), primary intracranial tumors that originate in the skull cavity but are not derived from the brain tissue itself (e.g., meninges, primary CNS lymphoma, pituitary gland tumors), and metastatic tumors.

- The clinical manifestations of brain tumor depend on the size and location of the tumor. Focal disturbances result from brain compression, tumor infiltration, disturbances in blood flow, and cerebral edema. General signs and symptoms include headache, nausea, vomiting, mental changes, papilledema, visual disturbances, alterations in motor and sensory function, and seizures.

- The three general methods for treatment of brain tumors are surgery, irradiation, and chemotherapy.

Seizure Disorders

A *seizure* represents an abrupt and transient occurrence of signs and/or symptoms resulting from an abnormal, excessive discharge from an aggregate of neurons in the brain.[7,54-57] Manifestations of a seizure, which vary according to site of discharge, can include sensory, motor, autonomic, or psychic phenomena. A *convulsion* refers specifically to a motor seizure involving the entire body. Seizure activity is the most common disorder encountered in pediatric neurology, and among adults its incidence is exceeded only by cerebrovascular disorders.[57] In most persons, the first seizure episode occurs before 20 years of age.[58] After 20 years of age, a seizure is caused most often by a structural change, trauma, tumor, or stroke.

Clinically, seizures may be categorized as provoked (secondary or acute symptomatic) or unprovoked (primary or idiopathic).[7,55] *Provoked seizures* may occur during almost all serious illnesses or injuries affecting the brain, including metabolic derangements, infections, tumors, drug abuse, vascular lesions, and brain injury. *Unprovoked seizures* are those for which no identifiable cause can be determined, and are thought to be genetic. Most unprovoked seizures occur in the setting of an epileptic syndrome. Persons with this type of seizure usually require chronic administration of antiepileptic medications to limit seizure recurrences. *Epilepsy* is characterized by recurrent seizures that are not provoked by other illnesses or circumstances.[55-60]

Many theories have been proposed to explain the cause of the abnormal brain electrical activity that occurs with seizures. Seizures may be caused by alterations in permeability or distribution of ions across neuronal cell membranes. Another cause may be decreased inhibition of excitability of neurons. Neurotransmitter imbalances such as an acetylcholine excess or γ-aminobutyric acid (GABA, an inhibitory neurotransmitter) deficiency have also been proposed as causes. Certain epilepsy syndromes have been linked to specific genetic mutations in ion channels.

Provoked Seizures

Provoked seizures include febrile seizures, seizures precipitated by systemic metabolic conditions, and those that follow a primary insult to the CNS. Transient systemic metabolic disturbances may precipitate seizures. Examples include electrolyte imbalances, hypoglycemia, hypoxia, hypocalcemia, uremia, alkalosis, and rapid withdrawal of sedative drugs. Specific CNS injuries such as toxemia of pregnancy, water intoxication, meningitis, trauma, cerebral hemorrhage and stroke, and brain tumors may precipitate a seizure. In most cases of provoked seizures, treatment of the immediate underlying cause often results in their resolution.

Febrile Seizures

One form of provoked seizures is febrile seizures that occur in children, between the ages of 6 and 60 months, with a temperature of 100.4°F (38°C) or higher that is not the result of a CNS infection or metabolic disorder. The fact that febrile seizures occur in this age group suggest that factors related to specific stages of brain development contribute to their occurrence.[59] A simple febrile seizure is a primary generalized seizure associated with fever that lasts for a maximum of 15 minutes and does not recur within a 24-hour period. Between 2% and 5% of neurologically healthy infants experience one simple seizure without any long-term ill effects.[59] Complex febrile seizures are more prolonged (>15 minutes), are focal, and/or recur within 24 hours. Febrile status epilepticus is a febrile seizure lasting longer than 30 minutes. Whether prolonged febrile seizures lead to epilepsy is still uncertain.[59] Children who present with complex febrile seizures or status epilepticus require a detailed history and thorough general and neurological examination.

Unprovoked (Epileptic) Seizures

The International League Against Epilepsy (ILAE) Commission on Classification and Terminology determines seizure type by clinical symptoms and EEG activity.[60] It divides epileptic seizures into two broad categories: focal and generalized. *Focal seizures* are those in which the seizure begins in a specific or focal area of one cerebral hemisphere. *Generalized seizures* are those which begin simultaneously in both hemispheres. The system also has a category of unknown origin, such as epileptic spasms (Chart 37-1).

Focal Seizures

Focal seizures, which are the most common type of seizures among newly diagnosed cases of epilepsy, can be viewed as those with neural networks limited to one

---

CHART 37-1 Classification of Epileptic Seizures

Generalized Seizures
Tonic–clonic (in any combination)[a]
Absence
  Typical
  Atypical
    Absence with special features
  Myoclonic
    Myoclonic atonic
    Myoclonic tonic
Clonic
Tonic
Atonic
Focal Seizures
Unknown
  Epileptic spasms

Adapted from Berg AT, Berkovic SF, Brodie MJ, et al. Revised terminology and concepts for organization of seizures and epilepsy: Report of ILAE Committee on Classification and Terminology, 2005–2009. *Epilepsia.* 2010;51(4):678.

hemisphere or the other. They may originate in subcortical structures, and may be discretely localized or widely distributed. For each seizure type, the site of onset is consistent from one seizure to another, with preferential propagation patterns that can involve the contralateral hemisphere.[60] Focal seizures are described according to their manifestations; that is, they may occur without or with impairment of consciousness or awareness.

Focal Seizures Without Impairment of Consciousness or Awareness.
This type of seizure usually involves one hemisphere and is not accompanied by loss of consciousness or awareness. The observed clinical signs and symptoms depend on the area of the brain where the abnormal electrical activity is taking place. There may be involuntary motor movements; somatosensory disturbances, such as tingling and crawling sensations; or special sensory disturbances, such as visual, auditory, gustatory, or olfactory phenomena. When abnormal cortical discharge stimulates the autonomic nervous system, flushing, tachycardia, diaphoresis, hypotension or hypertension, or pupillary changes may be evident.[60]

This type of focal seizure may be preceded by an *aura*, a term that has traditionally been used to describe the stereotyped warning sign of an impending seizure activity described by the affected person. The aura actually represents a simple partial seizure, affecting only a small area of electrical activity. A history of an aura is clinically useful to identify the seizure as focal and not generalized in onset. However, absence of an aura does not reliably exclude a focal onset because many focal seizures generalize too rapidly to generate an aura.

Focal Seizures with Impairment of Consciousness.
These types of seizures, which arise from the temporal lobe, involve impairment of consciousness.[60] The seizure begins in a localized area of the brain but may progress rapidly to involve both hemispheres. These seizures, sometimes referred to as *psychomotor seizures*, are often accompanied by automatisms or repetitive non-purposeful activities such as lip smacking, grimacing, patting, or rubbing clothing. Confusion during the postictal period (after a seizure) is common. Hallucinations and illusional experiences such as déja vu (a sense of unfamiliarity with a known environment) have been reported. There may be overwhelming fear, uncontrolled forced thinking or a flood of ideas, and a feeling of detachment and depersonalization. A person with this type of seizure disorder may be misdiagnosed as having a psychiatric disorder.

Generalized Seizures

Generalized-onset seizures are the most common type in young children. The seizures are classified as primary or generalized when clinical signs, symptoms, and supporting EEG changes indicate involvement of both hemispheres at onset. The clinical symptoms include unconsciousness and involve varying bilateral degrees of symmetric motor responses without evidence of localization to one hemisphere. These seizures are divided into six broad categories: tonic–clonic, absence seizures (typical, atypical, myoclonic absence, absence of eyelid myoclonia), myoclonic seizures (myoclonic, myoclonic atonic, myotonic clonic), clonic seizures, tonic seizures, and atonic seizures (Chart 37-1).[60]

Tonic-Clonic Seizures.
Tonic-clonic seizures, formerly called *grand mal seizures,* are the most common major motor seizures.[60] Frequently, a person has a vague warning (probably a simple focal seizure) and experiences a sharp tonic contraction of the muscles with extension of the extremities and immediate loss of consciousness. Incontinence of bladder and bowel is common. Cyanosis may occur from contraction of airway and respiratory muscles. The tonic phase is followed by the clonic phase, which involves rhythmic bilateral contraction and relaxation of the extremities. At the end of the clonic phase, the person remains unconscious until the RAS begins to function again. This is called the *postictal phase.* The tonic-clonic phases last approximately 60 to 90 seconds.

Absence Seizures.
Absence seizures are generalized, nonconvulsive epileptic events and are expressed mainly as disturbances in consciousness.[60] Formerly referred to as *petit mal seizures,* absence seizures typically occur only in children and cease in adulthood or evolve to generalized motor seizures. Children may present with a history of school failure that predates the first evidence of seizure episodes. Although typical absence seizures have been characterized by a blank stare, motionlessness, and unresponsiveness, motion occurs in many cases of absence seizures. This motion takes the form of automatisms such as lip smacking, mild clonic motion (usually in the eyelids), increased or decreased postural tone, and autonomic phenomena. There often is a brief loss of contact with the environment. The seizure usually lasts only a few seconds, and then the child is immediately able to resume normal activity. The manifestations often are so subtle that they may pass unnoticed.

Atypical absence seizures are similar to typical absence seizures except for greater alterations in muscle tone and less-abrupt onset and cessation. In practice, it is difficult to distinguish typical from atypical absence seizures without the benefit of supporting EEG findings. However, it is important to distinguish between complex focal and absence seizures because the drugs of choice for treatment are different. Medications that are effective for focal seizures may increase the frequency of absence seizures.

Myoclonic Seizures.
Myoclonic seizures involve brief involuntary muscle contractions induced by stimuli of cerebral origin. A myoclonic seizure involves bilateral jerking of muscles, generalized or confined to the face, trunk, or one or more extremities. Tonic seizures are characterized by a rigid, violent contraction of the muscles, fixing the limbs in a strained position. Clonic seizures consist of repeated contractions and relaxations of the major muscle groups.

Tonic Seizures.
Similar to the tonic phase of tonic–clonic seizures, tonic seizures are characterized by contraction of the voluntary muscles so that the body stiffens with

legs and arms extended. If the person is standing, they may fall to the ground.

Clonic Seizures. Clonic seizures, which are similar to those seen during the clonic phase of a tonic-clonic seizure, are characterized by repetitive rhythmic muscular contractions that are bilateral and symmetric, and are accompanied by hyperventilation.

Atonic Seizures. In atonic seizures, there is a sudden, split-second loss of muscle tone leading to slackening of the jaw, drooping of the limbs, and falling to the ground. These seizures also are known as "drop attacks."

Diagnosis and Treatment

The diagnosis of seizure disorders is based on a thorough history and neurologic examination, including a full description of the seizure.[7,56,60,61] The physical examination and laboratory studies help exclude any metabolic disorder (e.g., hyponatremia) that could precipitate seizures. Magnetic resonance imaging scans are used to identify structural defects such as temporal lobe sclerosis or underlying congenital malformations causing the seizure. One of the most useful diagnostic tests is the EEG, which is used to record changes in the brain's electrical activity. It is used to support the clinical diagnosis of epilepsy, to provide a guide for prognosis, and to assist in classifying the seizure disorder.

The first rules of treatment are to protect the person from injury during a seizure, preserve brain function by aborting or preventing seizure activity, and treat any underlying disease. People with epilepsy should be advised to avoid situations that could be dangerous or life-threatening if seizures occur. The management of seizure disorders focuses on treatment of the underlying conditions that cause or contribute to the seizures, avoidance of precipitating factors, suppression of recurrent seizures by prophylactic therapy with antiepileptic medications, surgery or neurostimulation, and addressing psychological and social issues.[7,56,60]

Antiepileptic Drug Therapy

Antiepileptic drug therapy is the mainstay of treatment for most persons with epilepsy. It is individualized for each patient based on the different types and causes of seizures as well as medication efficacy and side effects.

Antiepileptic drugs act mainly by suppressing repetitive firing of isolated neurons that act as epileptogenic foci for seizure activity or by inhibiting the transmission of electrical impulses involved in seizure activity.[62] Because of their selective mechanisms of action, different drugs are used to treat the different types of seizures. For example, ethosuximide, which suppresses the brain wave activity associated with lapses of consciousness, is used in the treatment of absence seizures, but is not effective for tonic-clonic seizures that progress from focal seizures.

More than 20 drugs are available for the treatment of epilepsy.[64] This group includes 12 new antiepileptic drugs that have been approved for use in the United States in the past several decades.[63] The goal of pharmacologic treatment is to bring the seizures under control with the least possible disruption in lifestyle and minimum of side effects from the medication. Whenever possible, a single drug should be used. Monotherapy eliminates drug interactions and additive side effects. Determining the proper dose of the anticonvulsant drug is often a long and tedious process, which can be very frustrating for the person with epilepsy.[64] Blood tests are often used to determine that the blood concentration is within the therapeutic range. Consistency in taking the medication is essential. Antiepileptic drug use never should be discontinued abruptly. Special consideration is needed when a person taking an antiepileptic medication becomes ill and must take additional medications. Some drugs act synergistically, and others interfere with the actions of other medications. This situation needs to be carefully monitored to avoid overmedication or interference with successful seizure control.

Women of child-bearing age require special consideration concerning fertility, contraception, and pregnancy. Many of the drugs interact with oral contraceptives; some affect hormone function or decrease fertility. All such women should be advised to take folic acid supplementation. For women with epilepsy who become pregnant, antiseizure drugs increase the risk for congenital abnormalities and other perinatal complications. Carbamazepine, phenytoin, phenobarbital, primidone, and valproic acid can interfere with vitamin D metabolism and predispose to osteoporosis.

Surgical and Neurostimulation Therapy

Surgical treatment may be an option for persons with epilepsy who are refractory to drug treatment.[7,60] With the use of modern neuroimaging and surgical techniques, a single epileptogenic lesion can often be identified and removed without leaving a neurologic deficit. The most common surgery consists of removal of the amygdala and an anterior part of the hippocampus and entorhinal cortex, as well as a small part of the temporal pole, leaving the lateral temporal neocortex intact. Another surgical procedure involves partial removal of the corpus callosum to prevent spread of a unilateral seizure to a generalized seizure.

Neurostimulation, with the development of a variety of different devices and targets of stimulation, is a rapidly evolving field in the treatment of epilepsy.[65] Methods of external (noninvasive) trigeminal stimulation have been developed and are currently being evaluated. These methods seem promising not only as therapy, but also as a useful predictor of success with other forms of stimulation therapy. A subcutaneous implantable device is also being evaluated.

Generalized Convulsive Status Epilepticus

Seizures that do not stop spontaneously or occur in succession without recovery are called *status epilepticus*.

There are as many types of status epilepticus as there are types of seizures. Tonic–clonic status epilepticus is a medical emergency and, if not promptly treated, may lead to respiratory failure and death. The disorder occurs most frequently in the young and old. Morbidity and mortality rates are highest in elderly persons and persons with acute symptomatic seizures, such as those related to anoxia or cerebral infarction.[65] If status epilepticus is caused by neurologic or systemic disease, the cause needs to be identified and treated immediately because the seizures probably will not respond until the underlying cause has been corrected.

Treatment consists of appropriate life support measures. Medications are given to control seizure activity. Intravenously administered diazepam or lorazepam is considered first-line therapy for the condition. The prognosis is related to the underlying cause as well as the duration of the seizures themselves.

SUMMARY CONCEPTS

- Seizures are paroxysmal motor, sensory, or cognitive manifestations of abnormal spontaneous electrical discharges from neural networks in the brain, thought to result directly or indirectly from changes in excitability of single neurons or groups of neurons. The site of seizure generation and the extent to which the abnormal neural activity is conducted to other areas of the brain determine the type and manifestations of the seizure activity.

- Focal seizures originate in a small group of neurons in one hemisphere with secondary spread of seizure activity to other parts of the brain. Seizure activity may involve impairment of consciousness, involuntary motor movements, somatosensory disturbances, special sensory sensations, flushing, tachycardia, diaphoresis, hypotension or hypertension, or pupillary changes due to stimulation of the autonomic nervous system.

- Generalized seizures show simultaneous disruption of electrical activity in both hemispheres from the onset. They include unconsciousness and varying bilateral degrees of symmetric motor responses with evidence of localization to one hemisphere. *Absence seizures* are generalized nonconvulsive seizure events that are expressed mainly by brief periods of unconsciousness. *Tonic–clonic seizures* involve unconsciousness along with both tonic and clonic muscle contractions.

Neurocognitive Disorders

Neurocognitive disorders involve changes in spectrum of memory and cognitive functions. *Memory* is the process by which information is encoded, stored, and later retrieved, while cognition is the process by which information is reduced, elaborated, transformed, and used.

Cognition involves the perception of sensory input and the ability to learn and manipulate new information, recognize familiar objects and recall past experiences, solve problems, think abstractly, and make judgments.

Dementia or nonnormative cognitive decline can be caused by any disorder that permanently damages large association areas of the cerebral hemispheres or subcortical areas subserving memory and cognition.[66,67] It is a common and disabling disorder in the elderly and, because of the rapidly increasing elderly population, is a growing public health problem. The disorder is characterized by impairment of short- and long-term memory, deficits in abstract thinking, impaired judgment and other higher cortical functions, abnormalities of speech, and personality changes. These changes eventually become severe enough that they interfere with day-to-day functioning. Common causes of dementia are Alzheimer disease, vascular dementia, frontotemporal dementia, Wernicke-Korsakoff syndrome, and Huntington chorea.

The diagnosis of dementia is based on assessment of the presenting problem; history about the person that is provided by an informant (someone who has known the person, usually a family member); complete physical and neurologic examination; evaluation of cognitive, behavioral, and functional status; and laboratory and imaging studies. Depression is the most common treatable illness that may masquerade as dementia, and it must be excluded when a diagnosis of dementia is considered. This is important because cognitive functioning usually returns to baseline levels after depression is treated. Screening evaluations for subdural hematoma, cerebral infarcts, cerebral tumors, and normal-pressure hydrocephalus are also recommended. These and other reversible forms of dementia that should be ruled out can be remembered by the mnemonic DEMENTIA: *D*rugs (drugs with anticholinergic activity), *E*motional (depression), *M*etabolic (hypothyroidism), *E*yes and ears (declining vision and hearing), *N*ormal-pressure hydrocephalus, *T*umor or other space-occupying lesions, *I*nfection (human immunodeficiency virus infection or syphilis), *A*nemia (vitamin B_{12} or folate deficiency).[67]

Alzheimer Disease

Dementia of the Alzheimer type is the most common type of dementia.[68–70] The disorder affects more than 5.2 million Americans, and is the sixth leading cause of death.[70] The risk for development of Alzheimer disease (AD) increases with age, starting at a level of 4% of persons under age 65 years, 13% of persons 65 to 74 years, 44% of persons 75 to 84 years, and 38% of persons age 85 years or older.[69]

Pathology

Alzheimer disease most often presents with a subtle onset of memory loss followed by slowly progressive dementia that has a course of several years. Evidence from familial forms of AD indicates that the accumulation of a peptide (amyloid beta or Aβ) in the brain initiates a chain of events that result in the morphologic changes of AD and dementia. This peptide is derived from a larger membrane-spanning protein known as *amyloid precursor protein* (APP), which can be processed in either of two ways. It can be cleaved by the enzymes, α-secretase and γ-secretase, in a proteolytic pathway that prevents the formation of Aβ, or it can be cleaved by β-secretase and γ-secretase in a pathway that generates Aβ.[1]

Diagnostic imaging of the brain reveals diffuse atrophy of the cerebral cortex with enlargement of the ventricles (Fig. 37-18). The major microscopic features of Alzheimer disease include *neuritic (senile) plaques*, patches or flat areas composed of clusters of degenerating nerve terminals arranged around a central amyloid core. In the cytoplasm of abnormal neurons are *neurofibrillary tangles*, which consist of fibrous proteins that are wound around each other in a helical fashion. These tangles are resistant to chemical or enzymatic breakdown, and they persist in brain tissue long after the neuron in which they arose has died and disappeared. Smaller cerebral vessels also exhibit amyloid angiopathy, in which there is deposition of Aβ in vessel walls.

Some plaques and tangles can be found in the brains of older persons who do not show cognitive impairment. The number and distribution of the plaques and tangles appear to contribute to the intellectual deterioration that occurs with Alzheimer disease. In persons with the disease, the plaques and tangles are found throughout the neocortex and in the hippocampus and amygdala, with relative sparing of the primary sensory cortex.[1] Hippocampal function in particular may be compromised by the pathologic changes. The hippocampus is crucial to information processing, acquisition of new memories, and retrieval of old memories.

Neurochemically, AD has been associated with a decrease in the level of choline acetyltransferase activity in the cortex and hippocampus. This enzyme is required for the synthesis of acetylcholine, a neurotransmitter that is associated with memory. The reduction in choline acetyltransferase is quantitatively related to the numbers of neuritic plaques and severity of dementia.

It is likely that AD is caused by several factors that interact differently in different persons. Progress in the genetics of inherited early-onset AD shows that mutations in at least three genes—the *APP* gene on chromosome 21; presenilin-1 (*PS1*), a gene on chromosome 14; and presenilin-2 (*PS2*), a gene on chromosome 1—can cause AD in certain families.[1,4] The *APP* gene is associated with an autosomal dominant form of early-onset AD and can be tested clinically. Virtually all persons with Down syndrome (trisomy 21) exhibit the pathologic features of AD as they age. Presenilin-1 and presenilin-2, both intracellular proteins, are components of γ-secretase and possibly part of a multiprotein complex containing the proteolytic site for breakdown of Aβ.

A fourth gene, the apolipoprotein E (ApoE) gene, has been found to increase the risk of AD and lowers the age of onset of the disease.[4,68] The gene, which is found on chromosome 19, has three common alleles—E2, E3, or E4. Each person inherits one copy of the gene from each parent. An increased risk of late-onset and sporadic AD is associated with inheritance of the E4 gene, particularly if it is inherited from both parents. Conversely, the E2 gene may confer some protection. The age of onset in late-onset AD also correlates with the gene, with E4/E4

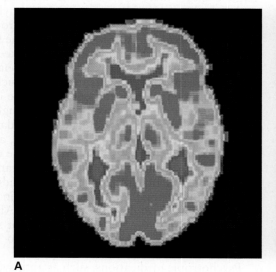 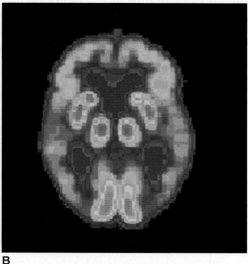

A   B

FIGURE 37-18. Functional imaging of the brain with positron emission tomography (PET). Perfusion and metabolism in a normal brain **(A)** and hypoperfusion and hypometabolism due to brain atrophy in a brain with Alzheimer disease **(B)** (From Alzheimer's Disease: Unraveling the Mystery Images. National Institutes of Health, National Institute of Aging.)

inheritance exhibiting the earliest age (younger than 70 years). The APoE genotype is not, however, an absolute determinant of who will develop AD. Just how these different APo alleles influence the risk of AD continues to remain poorly understood.

Manifestations

Alzheimer-type dementia follows an insidious and progressive course. The hallmark symptoms are loss of short-term memory and denial of such memory loss, with eventual disorientation, impaired abstract thinking, apraxias, and changes in personality and affect.[70] Various stages of the disease have been recognized; all are characterized by progressive degenerative changes. The initial changes are often subtle, characterized by a short-term memory loss that often is difficult to differentiate from the normal memory loss that often occurs in the elderly, and usually is reported by caregivers and denied by the person. Although most elderly persons have trouble retrieving from memory incidental information and proper names, persons with AD randomly forget important and unimportant details. They forget where things are placed, get lost easily, and have trouble remembering appointments and performing novel tasks. Mild changes in personality, such as lack of spontaneity, social withdrawal, and loss of a previous sense of humor, occur during this stage.

As the disease progresses, the person with AD enters the moderate stage. This stage may last several years and is marked by a more global impairment of cognitive functioning. During this stage, there are changes in higher cortical functioning needed for language, spatial relationships, and problem solving. Depression may occur in persons who are aware of their deficits. There is extreme confusion, disorientation, lack of insight, and inability to carry out the activities of daily living. Personal hygiene is neglected, and language becomes impaired because of difficulty in remembering and retrieving words. Behavioral changes can include agitation, sleep problems, restlessness and wandering, aggression, and suspiciousness. Some persons may become hostile and abusive toward family members. Persons who enter this stage become unable to live alone and should be assisted in making decisions about supervised placement with family members or friends or in a community-based facility.

Severe AD is the last stage of the disease. It is characterized by a loss of ability to respond to the environment. Individuals in this stage require total care and spend most of their time bedridden. Death can occur as a result of complications related to chronic debilitation.

Diagnosis and Treatment

Alzheimer disease is essentially a diagnosis of exclusion. There are no peripheral biochemical markers or tests for the disease. The diagnosis can be confirmed only by microscopic examination of tissue obtained from a cerebral biopsy or at autopsy. The diagnosis is based on clinical findings.

A diagnosis of Alzheimer disease requires the presence of dementia established by clinical examination and documented by results of a Mini-Mental State Examination, Blessed Dementia Test, or similar mental status test; no disturbance in consciousness; onset between 40 and 90 years of age, most often after 65 years of age; and absence of systemic or brain disorders that could account for the memory or cognitive deficits. Brain imaging, CT scan, or MRI is done to exclude other brain disease. Metabolic screening should be done for known reversible causes of dementia such as vitamin B_{12} deficiency, thyroid dysfunction, and electrolyte imbalance.

There is no curative treatment for Alzheimer disease.[70] Drugs are used primarily to slow the progression and to control depression, agitation, or sleep disorders. Two major goals of care are maintaining the person's socialization and providing support for the family. Self-help groups that provide support for family and friends have become available, with support from the AD and Related Disorders Association. Day care and respite centers are available in many areas to provide relief for caregivers and appropriate stimulation for the patient.

Although there is no current drug therapy that is curative for Alzheimer disease, cholinesterase inhibitors have been shown to be effective in slowing the progression of the disease by potentiating the action of available acetylcholine.[71,72] These drugs (e.g., donepezil, rivastigmine, galantamine) inhibit acetylcholinesterase, preventing the metabolism of endogenous acetylcholine, and are used in the early stages of the disease for mild cognitive impairment. Again, such therapy does not halt the disease but can slow its progression. Memantine, an N-methyl-D-aspartate antagonist, has been approved by the FDA for treatment of moderate to severe AD.[72] This medication may act by interfering with the glutamatergic excitotoxicity caused by the ischemia (discussed under mechanisms of brain injury) and amyloid deposits associated with the disease, or it may provide symptomatic improvement through effects on the function of hippocampal neurons. This medication, like the cholinesterase inhibitors, modestly delays functional loss.

Other treatments for Alzheimer disease include agents that are thought to have a neuroprotective effect.[70] Aβ seems to exert its neurotoxic effects through a variety of secondary mechanisms, including oxidative injury and lipid peroxidation of cell membranes, and inflammation. Several strategies have involved the use of anti-inflammatory agents and antioxidants (vitamins E and C). Several, but not all, epidemiologic studies provide evidence supporting the concept that vitamin E and vitamin C have a role in delaying the onset of AD. In some, but not all, trials, *G. biloba* had small but statistically significant effects compared with placebo in persons with Alzheimer disease.

Psychotropic medications, such as antipsychotics and mood stabilizers, may be used to assist in the behavioral management of the disease. Interventions also include environmental adjustments, behavioral intervention, and education and support for caregivers.

Other Types of Dementia

Cerebrovascular injury, brain tissue atrophy, alcoholism, and genetic disorders can also result in dementia.

Vascular Dementia

Vascular dementia is caused by brain injury resulting from ischemic or hemorrhagic damage. Vascular dementia is the second most common cause of cognitive impairment in the elderly. The incidence is closely associated with hypertension, but also with arrhythmias, stroke, peripheral vascular disease, lipid abnormalities, and diabetes mellitus.[73–75] The usual onset is between the ages of 55 and 70 years, and more men are affected than women.

The vessel disorders associated with vascular dementia include atherosclerosis, small vessel disease, cerebral amyloid angiopathy, brain infarcts, and cerebral hemorrhage. In addition to the impact of cerebral vascular lesions on dementia, the association between Alzheimer disease and vascular dementia points to a possible pathogenic link between AD and blood vessel causes of dementia.

Slowness in psychomotor functioning is a main clinical feature of this dementia, and symptoms of depression are present in up to 60% of patients with this disease.[4] The onset may be gradual or abrupt, the course usually is a stepwise progression, and there are focal neurologic symptoms related to local areas of infarction.

Frontotemporal Dementia

Frontotemporal dementia (FTD) refers to a group of disorders associated with atrophy of the frontal and anterior temporal lobes of the brain.[76,77] Originally known as *Pick disease,* FTD now refers to a syndrome that includes primary progressive aphasia, corticobasal degeneration, progressive supranuclear palsy, and semantic dementias. The disease often begins between 45 and 64 years of age, and is one of the most common forms of dementia in persons younger than 65 years.

The pathophysiology of FTD is not well understood. The disease is characterized by extensive atrophy of the frontotemporal regions, with the involved cortex being severely depleted of neurons. Most recently, mutations of the prograndin gene on chromosome 17 have been associated with intranuclear inclusions found in the brain tissue of persons with the disorder. Prograndin is a growth factor with multiple functions, including neuronal survival. Other than mutations linked to chromosome 17, several other chromosomes have been implicated in FTD, including mutations in chromosomes 3 and 9.

There are two distinct clinical presentations of FTD: behavior and language. The former is more common, with behavioral presentations of disinhibited and impulsive actions or apathy, with inappropriate social behavior. Unlike Alzheimer disease, which usually begins with memory difficulties, FTD begins with very disruptive behaviors that can be quite extreme, and can be misdiagnosed as schizophrenia or psychotic depression. The second type of FTD behavior involves disturbances in understanding or expressing language.

Diagnosis of FTD is based on evidence of cognitive impairment and exclusion of other illnesses that cause cognitive and behavioral deficits. Neuroimaging can be helpful in distinguishing FTD from other types of cognitive disorders. Typically, structural imaging shows anterior temporal and frontal lobe atrophy.

There is no specific cure for FTD. Treatment is focused on symptom management and support for patients, families, and caregivers. Current research focuses on molecular biology to better understand the underlying disease and the potential for identification of novel treatments, particularly disease-modifying treatments.

Wernicke-Korsakoff Syndrome

Wernicke-Korsakoff syndrome most commonly results from chronic alcoholism. Wernicke disease is characterized by acute weakness and paralysis of the extraocular muscles, nystagmus, ataxia, and confusion.[4] The affected person also may have signs of peripheral neuropathy. The person has an unsteady gait and complains of diplopia. There may be signs attributable to alcohol withdrawal such as delirium, confusion, and hallucinations. This disorder is caused by a deficiency of thiamine (vitamin B_{12}), which directly interferes with production of glucose, the brain's main nutrient. Many of the symptoms are reversed when nutrition is improved with supplemental thiamine.

The Korsakoff component of the syndrome involves the chronic phase with severe impairment of recent memory. There often is difficulty in dealing with abstractions, and the person's capacity to learn is defective. Confabulation (i.e., recitation of imaginary experiences to fill in gaps in memory) probably is the most distinctive feature of the disease. Polyneuritis also is common. Unlike Wernicke disease, Korsakoff psychosis does not improve significantly with treatment.

Huntington Disease

Huntington disease (HD) is a hereditary disorder characterized by chronic progressive chorea, psychological changes, and dementia.[1,4,78–81] Although the disease is inherited as an autosomal dominant disorder, the age of onset most commonly is in the fourth and fifth decades. By the time the disease has been diagnosed, the person often has passed the gene on to his or her children. Approximately 10% of HD cases are juvenile onset.[80] Children with the disease rarely live to adulthood.

Huntington disease is caused by a polyglutamine trinucleotide repeat expansion in the HD gene. The HD gene, located on chromosome 4, encodes a protein known as *huntingtin.*[1,78–80] Normal HD genes contain 6 to 35 copies of the trinucleotide repeat; an expansion of repeats beyond this level is associated with disease. There is an inverse relationship between repeat number and age of onset, such that longer repeats are associated with earlier onset. Repeat expansions occur during spermatogenesis, so that paternal transmission is associated with early onset in the next generation. Although the biologic function of normal huntingtin remains unknown, there is little evidence to suggest that the disease is caused by an insufficiency related to the mutated gene. Rather, the expansion of the polyglutamine region of the HD gene seems to bestow a toxic gain of function on the protein.[1]

Huntington disease produces localized death of brain cells. The first and most severely affected neurons are those of the basal ganglia that modulate motor output. These neurons normally function to dampen motor activity; thus, their degeneration in HD results in increased motor output, often manifested as choreiform movements. Although chorea is the prototypical movement disorder, the full spectrum of motor impairment in HD includes eye movement disorders, myoclonus, ataxia, dysarthria and dysphagia, and spasticity. Depression and personality changes are the most common early psychological manifestations; memory loss often is accompanied by impulsive behavior, moodiness, antisocial behavior, and a tendency toward emotional outbursts. Persons with HD universally go through cognitive decline, mental slowing, and impaired problem-solving abilities, and eventually become demented. Cognitive decline also heralds the juvenile onset of HD.

There is no cure for Huntington disease. The treatment is largely symptomatic. Drugs may be used to treat the dyskinesias and behavioral disturbances. Genetic testing can predict whether a person will develop the disease.

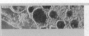

SUMMARY CONCEPTS

■ Cognition refers to all the processes by which sensory input is transformed, reduced, elaborated, stored, recovered, and used.

■ Dementia represents a syndrome of deterioration in cognitive function severe enough to interfere with occupational or social performance. The most common cause of dementia is Alzheimer disease, an insidious and progressive disorder that begins with memory impairment and terminates in an inability to recognize family or friends and the loss of control over bodily functions.

■ Other forms of dementia include vascular dementia due brain injury resulting from ischemic or hemorrhagic damage; frontotemporal dementia with atrophy of the frontal and temporal lobes; Wernicke-Korsakoff syndrome most often resulting from chronic alcoholism; and Huntington disease, a hereditary disorder characterized by chronic and progressive chorea, psychological changes, and dementia.

REVIEW EXERCISES

1. A 20-year-old man who was an unbelted driver involved in a motor vehicle accident presents in coma.

   A. What are the clinical signs of coma?
   B. What areas of the brain are involved in coma?
   C. Which complications of traumatic head injury might lead to coma?
   D. What are the key treatment options to manage elevated intracranial pressure?

2. A 65-year-old woman presents with a 1-hour history of right-sided weakness and aphasia. An immediate CT scan of the brain is negative.

   A. Where in the brain is the pathology?
   B. What are the indications to administer intravenous tissue plasminogen activator?
   C. What are the possible causes of stroke, and what diagnostic tests would reveal the cause?

3. A child is taken to the emergency department with lethargy, fever, and a stiff neck on examination.

   A. What findings on initial lumbar puncture indicate bacterial versus viral meningitis?
   B. In the case of bacterial meningitis, what are the most likely organisms, and which antibiotics should be started?

4. A 60-year-old man develops involuntary shaking of his right arm that spreads to the face, after which he collapses with whole-body shaking and loss of consciousness. After 1 minute, the shaking stops and he is confused and disoriented.

   A. What type of seizure is suggested by the clinical manifestations?
   B. Assuming this is his first seizure, what diagnostic tests should be performed to identify a cause for the seizure?
   C. If he has a long history of similar recurrent seizures, what treatments should be instituted? What treatments should be considered if he has failed multiple adequate trials of anticonvulsant medications?

REFERENCES

1. Frosch MP, Anthony D, DeGirofami U. The central nervous system. In: Kumar V, Abbas AK, Fausto N, eds. *Robbins and Cotran Pathologic Basis of Disease*. 8th ed. Philadelphia, PA: Elsevier Saunders; 2010:1279–1344.
2. Hall JE. *Guyton & Hall Textbook of Medical Physiology*. 12th ed. Philadelphia, PA: Saunders Elsevier; 2011:742–750.
3. Harukuni I, Bhardwaj A. Mechanisms of brain injury after global cerebral ischemia. *Neurol Clin*. 2006;24:1–21.

4. Fuller GN, Goodman JC, Bouldin TW, et al. The nervous system. In: Rubin R, Strayer DE, eds. *Rubin's Pathology: Clinicopathologic Foundations of Medicine.* 5th ed. Philadelphia, PA: Wolters Kluwer Health/Lippincott Williams & Wilkins; 2012:1295–1392.

5. Arundine M, Tymianski M. Molecular mechanisms of glutamate-dependent neurogeneration in ischemia and traumatic brain injury. *Cell Mol Life Sci.* 2004;61:657–668.

6. Kalia LW, Kalia SK, Salter MW. NMDA receptors in clinical neurology: excitatory times ahead. *Lancet Neurol.* 2008;7:742–755.

7. Hickey JV. *The Clinical Practice of Neurological and Neurosurgical Nursing.* 6th ed. Philadelphia, PA: Lippincott, Williams & Wilkins; 2009:117–120, 270–307, 370–409, 496–520, 588–619, 646–664.

8. Noble KA. Traumatic brain injury and increased intracranial pressure. *J Perianesth Nurs.* 2010;25(4):242–250.

9. Ropper AH. Coma. In: Hauser SL, ed. *Harrison's Neurology in Clinical Medicine.* New York, NY: McGraw-Hill; 2010:130–139.

10. Biennow K. The neuropathology and neurobiology of traumatic brain injury. *Neuron.* 2012;76(Dec 6):886–899.

11. Almasi SJ, Wilson JJ. An update on the diagnosis and management of concussion. *WMJ.* 2012;111(1):21–27.

12. Ropper AH, Gorson KC. Concussion. *N Engl J Med.* 2007;356(2):166–172.

13. Goldfine AM, Schiff ND. Consciousness: its neurobiology and the major classes of impairment. *Neurol Clin.* 2011;29(4):723–737.

14. Posner JB, Stupor CB, Schiff ND, et al. *Plum and Posner's Diagnosis of Stupor and Coma.* New York, NY: Oxford University Press; 2007.

15. Ingersoll GL, Leyden DB. The glasgow coma scale for patients with head injuries. *Crit Care Nurs.* 1987;7(5):26–32.

16. Teasdale GM. Revisiting the glasgow coma scale and coma score. *Intensive Care Med.* 2000;26:153–154.

17. Moore KL, Dalley AF, Agur AMP. *Clinically Oriented Anatomy.* 6th ed. Philadelphia, PA: Wolters Kluwer Health/Lippincott Williams & Wilkins; 2010:882–886.

18. Smith WS, English JD, Johnston SC. Cerebrovascular disease. In Hauser SL, ed. *Harrison's Neurology in Clinical Medicine.* New York, NY: McGraw-Hill; 2010:246–281.

19. American Stroke Association. Heart disease and stroke statistics—2012 update. *Circulation.* 2012;125:e2–e225.

20. Sacco RL, Kasner SE, Broderick JP, et al. An updated definition of stroke for the 21st century: a statement for healthcare professionals from the American Heart Association/American Stroke Association. *Stroke.* 2013;44:2064–2089.

21. Goldstein LB, Bushnell CD, Adams RJ. Guidelines for primary prevention of stroke: a guideline for healthcare professionals from the American Heart Association/American Stroke Association. *Stroke.* 2011;42:517–584.

22. Treadwell SD, Robinson TG. Cocaine use and stroke. *Postgrad Med.* 2007;83:389–394.

23. Paciaroni M, Caso V, Agnelli G. The concept of ischemic penumbra in acute stroke and therapeutic opportunities. *Eur Neurol.* 2009;61:321–330.

24. Siket MS, Edlow JA. Transient ischemic attack. *Emerg Med Clin North Am.* 2012;30(3):745–770.

25. Manglia A, Navi BB, Layton K. Transient global ishemia and risk of stroke. *Stroke.* 2013;44:2064–2089.

26. Easton JD, Chair. Definition and evaluation of transient ischemic attack: a scientific statement from the American Heart Association/American Stroke Council; Council on Cardiovascular Surgery and Anesthesia; Council on Cardiovascular Radiology and Intervention; Council on Cardiovascular Nursing; and the Interdisciplinary Council on Peripheral Vascular Disease. *Stroke.* 2009;40:2276–2293.

27. Aguilar MI, Freeman VVD. Spontaneous intracerebral hemorrhage. *Semin Neurol.* 2010;30(5):555–564.

28. Morgenstern LB, Hemphill Claude H III, Anderson C, et al. Guidelines for management of spontaneous intracerebral hemorrhage in adults: A guideline for Healthcare Professionals from the American Heart Association/American Stroke Association/American Stroke Association. *Stroke.* 2010;41:2108–2129.

29. Mayer SA, Brun NC, Bergtrup MS, et al. Recombinant activated factor VII for acute intracerebral hemorrhage. *N Engl J Med.* 2005;352(8):777–785.

30. Leissinger CA, Blatt PM, Hoots K, et al. Role of prothrombin complex concentrates in reversing anticoagulation: a review of the literature. *Am J Hematol.* 2008;83(2):137–143.

31. Jauch EC, Saver JL, Adams HP, et al. Guidelines for early management of patients with acute ischemic stroke: a guideline for healthcare professionals from the American Heart Association/American Stroke Association. *Stroke.* 2013;44:870–947.

32. Caulfield AF, Wijman CAC. Management of acute ischemic stroke. *Neurol Clin.* 2008;26:345–371.

33. van der Worp HB, van Gijn J. Acute ischemic stroke. *N Engl J Med.* 2007;357(6):572–579.

34. Gorelick AR, Gorelick P, Sloan EP. Emergency department evaluation and management of stroke: acute assessment, stroke teams and care pathways. *Neurol Clin.* 2008;26:923–942.

35. Lansberg MG, O'Connell MJ, Khartri P, et al. Antithrombotic and thrombolytic therapy for ischemic stroke. *Chest.* 2012;141 (2 Suppl):e601S–e636S.

36. del Zoppo GJ, Saver JL, Jauch EC, et al. Expansion of the time window for acute ischemic stroke: a science advisory from the American Heart Association/American Stroke Association. *Stroke.* 2009;40:2945–2948.

37. Demchuk AM, Gupta AM, Pooja RK. Emerging therapies. *Continuum.* 2008;14(6):80–97.

38. Duncan PW, Zorowitz R, Bates B, et al. Management of adult stroke rehabilitation care: a clinical practice guideline. *Stroke.* 2005;36:e100–e143.

39. Suarez JI, Tarr RW, Selman WR. Aneurysmal subarachnoid hemorrhage. *N Engl J Med.* 2006;354:387–396.

40. Connelly ES, Rabinstein AA, Carbuapoma JR, et al. Guidelines for the management of aneurysmal subarachnoid hemorrhage: a statement for healthcare professionals from the American Heart Association/American Stroke Association. *Stroke.* 2012;43:1711–1737.

41. Friedlander RM. Arteriovenous malformations of the brain. *N Engl J Med.* 2007;356:2704–2712.

42. Ogilvy CS. Chair, Special Writing Group of the Stroke Council, American Heart Association. Recommendations for management of intracranial arteriovenous malformations. *Stroke.* 2001;32:1458–1471.

43. Roos KL, Tyler KL. Meningitis, encephalitis, brain abscesses, and empyema. In Hauser SL, ed. *Harrison's Neurology in Clinical Medicine.* 2nd ed. New York, NY: McGraw-Hill; 2010:451–483.

44. Bamberger DM. Diagnosis, initial management, and prevention of meningitis. *Am Fam Physician.* 2010;82(2):1491–1498.

45. Honda H, Warren DK. Central nervous system infections: meningitis and brain abscesses. *Infect Dis Clin North Am.* 2009;23:609–623.

46. Centers for Disease Control and Prevention. Prevention and control of meningococcal disease: Recommendations of the Advisory Committee on Immunization Practices (AICP). *MMWR.* 2013;62(2):1–30.

47. Kelly D. An encephalitis primer. *Adv Exp Med Biol.* 2013;764:133–140.

48. Huffner A. Overview of primary brain tumors. *Hematol Oncol Clin North Am.* 2012;26:715–732.

49. Kuttesch JF Jr, Rush SZ, Ater JL. Brain tumors in childhood. In: Kliegman RM, Stanton BF, St. Geme JW, et al., eds. *Nelson Textbook of Pediatrics*. 19th ed. Philadelphia, PA: Saunders Elsevier; 2011:1747e1–1753.e1.

50. Ostrom QT, Barnabulz-Sloan JS. Current state of our knowledge on brain tumor epidemiology. *Curr Neurol Neurosci Rep*. 2011;11:329–335.

51. Sagar SM, Isrel MA. Primary and metastatic tumors of the nervous system. In: Hauser SL, ed. *Harrison's Neurology in Clinical Practice*. 2nd ed. New York, NY: McGraw-Hill; 2010:408–422.

52. Wen PY, Kesari S. Malignant gliomas in adults. *N Engl J Med*. 2008;359(5):492–507.

53. Nguyen TD, DeAngelis LM. Brain metastases. *Neurol Clin*. 2007;25:1173–1192.

54. Nguyen TD, Abrey LS. Brain metastasis: old problems, new strategies. *Hematol Oncol Clin North Am* 2007;21:369–387.

55. Lowenstein DH. Seizures and epilepsy. In: Hauser SL, ed. *Harrison's Neurology in Clinical Practice*. 2nd ed. New York, NY: McGraw-Hill; 2010:222–245.

56. National Library Medicine & National Institutes of Health. Epilepsy 2013. MedlinePlus. Available at: http://www.ninds.nih.gov/disorders/epilepsy/detail_epilepsy.htm. Accessed June 13, 2013.

57. Mikati MA. Seizures in childhood. In Kleigman RM, Stanton BF, St. Geme JW, et al., eds. *Nelson Textbook of Pediatrics*. 19th ed. Philadelphia, PA: Elsevier Saunders; 2011:2013e1–2039.e1.

58. French JA, Pedley TA. Initial management of epilepsy. *N Engl J Med*. 2008;359(2):166–176.

59. Schachter SC. Seizure disorders. *Med Clin North Am*. 2009;93: 343–351.

60. Dube C, Brewster AL, Baram TZ. Febrile seizures: mechanisms and relationship to epilepsy. *Brain Dev*. 2009;31(5):366–371.

61. Berg A, Berkovic S, Brodie MJ, et al. Revised terminology and concepts for organization of seizures and epilepsies: Report of the ILAE Commission on Classification and Terminology, 2005–2009. *Epilepsia*. 2010;51(4):676–685.

62. Wilden JA, Cohen-Gadol A. Evaluation of first nonfebrile seizure. *Am Fam Physician*. 2012;86(4):334–340.

63. Porter RJ, Meldrum MB. Antiseizure drugs. In Katzung BG, ed. *Basic and Clinical Pharmacology*. 12th ed. New York, NY: McGraw-Hill Medical; 2012:403–427.

64. Privitera M. Current challenges in the management of epilepsy. *Am J Manag Care*. 2011;17(7S):195–203.

65. Asconapé JJ. Epilepsy: new drug targets and neurostimulators. *Neurol Clin*. 2013;31:785–798.

66. Khaled KJA, Hirsch LJ. Updates in the management of seizures and status epilepticus in critically ill patients. *Neurol Clin*. 2008;26:385–408.

67. Peterson RC. Mild cognitive impairment. *N Engl J Med*. 2011;364:2227–2234.

68. Josshi S, Morley JE. Cognitive impairment. *Med Clin North Am*. 2006;90:769–787.

69. Bird TD, Miller BL. Alzheimer's disease and other dementias. In Hauser SL, ed., *Harrison's Neurology in Clinical Medicine*. 2nd ed. New York, NY: McGraw-Hill; 2010:298–319.

70. Alzheimer's Association. *2013 Alzheimer's disease: Facts and Figures* 2013:1–71. Available at: http://www.alz.org/professionals_and_researchers. Accessed June 12, 2013.

71. Querfurth HW, LaFerla FM. Alzheimer disease. *N Engl J Med*. 2010;362:329–344.

72. Mongialache F, Solomon A, Mecocci P, et al. Alzheimer's disease: clinical trials and drug development. *Lancet Neurol*. 2010;9: 202–216.

73. Katzung BG. Special aspects of geriatric pharmacology. In: Katzung BG, ed. *Basic and Clinical Pharmacology*. 12th ed. New York, NY, McGraw-Hill Medical; 2012:403–427, 1054–1055.

74. Kotczyn AD, Vakhopova V, Grinberg LT. Vascular dementia. *J Neurol Sci* 2012;322:2–10.

75. Gorelick PB, Scuteri A, Black SE, et al. Vascular contributions to cognitive impairment and dementia: a statement for healthcare professionals from American Heart Association/American Stroke Association. *Stroke*. 2011;42:2672–2713.

76. Thai DR, Grinberg LT, Atterns J. Vascular dementia: different forms of vessel disorders contribute to development of dementia in elderly brains. *Exp Gerontol*. 2012;47:816–824.

77. Cardarelli R, Kertesz A, Knebl JA. Frontotemporal dementia: a review for primary care physicians. *Am Fam Physician*. 2010;82(11):1372–1377.

78. Arvanitakis Z. Update on frontotemporal dementia. *Neurologist*. 2010;16(1):16–22.

79. Sturrock A, Leavitt BR. The clinical and genetic features of Huntington's disease. *J Geriatr Psychiatry*. 2013;23(4):243–259.

80. Huntington's Disease Society of America. *A juvenile HD handbook*. [Online]. Available at: http://www.hdsa.org/images/content/1/1/11702.pdf. Accessed November 7, 2013.

81. Cardosa F. Huntington disease and other choreas. *Neurol Clin*. 2009;27:719–736.

Porth Essentials Resources

Explore these additional resources to enhance learning for this chapter:

- NCLEX-Style Questions and Other Resources on thePoint, http://thePoint.lww.com/PorthEssentials4e
- Study Guide for Essentials of Pathophysiology
- Concepts in Action Animations
- Adaptive Learning | Powered by PrepU, http://thepoint.lww.com/prepu

C h a p t e r **38**

Disorders of Special Sensory Function: Vision, Hearing, and Vestibular Function

The special senses allow us to view and hear what is going on around us, to maintain our balance, and to communicate effectively with others. This chapter focuses on the eye and disorders of vision; the ear and disorders of hearing; and the vestibular system and disorders of equilibrium and balance.

The Eye and Disorders of Vision

There are 286 million people worldwide who are visually impaired—38 million are blind and 248 million have partial vision loss that cannot be corrected.[1] Disorders of vision can result from a number of conditions including those that affect the lens (cataract), retina (retinopathy and macular degeneration), and intraocular pressure (glaucoma) (Fig. 38-1).

General Structure of the Eye

The optic globe, commonly called the *eyeball,* is a remarkably mobile, nearly spherical structure contained in a pyramid-shaped cavity of the skull called the *orbit.* The eyeball is composed of three layers: an outer layer, which includes the white, opaque sclera and the transparent cornea; a middle vascular layer called the *uvea,* which includes the choroid, ciliary body, and iris; and an inner neural layer, which includes an outer pigment epithelium and an inner neural retina (Fig. 38-2).[2] Exposed surfaces of the eyes are protected by the eyelids, which are mucous membrane–lined skin flaps that provide a means for shutting out most light. Tears bathe the anterior surface of the eye, keeping the conjunctiva and corneal epithelium moist and washing away foreign material.

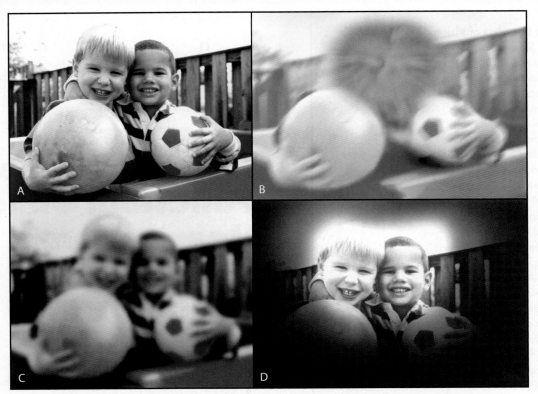

FIGURE 38-1. A scene as it might be viewed by a person with **(A)** normal vision, **(B)** age-related macular degeneration, **(C)** cataract, and **(D)** glaucoma. (Courtesy of the National Eye Institute, National Institutes of Health.)

Disorders of the Conjunctiva and Cornea

The conjunctiva is a thin layer of mucous membrane that lines the anterior surface of both eyelids as the palpebral conjunctiva and folds back over the anterior surface of the optic globe as the ocular or bulbar conjunctiva (see Fig. 38-2). The bulbar conjunctiva covers the sclera or white portion of the eyeball, but not the cornea. The conjunctiva provides a barrier against foreign objects and produces lubricating mucus that bathes the eye and keeps it moist.

The cornea functions as a protective membrane and transparent window through which light passes as it

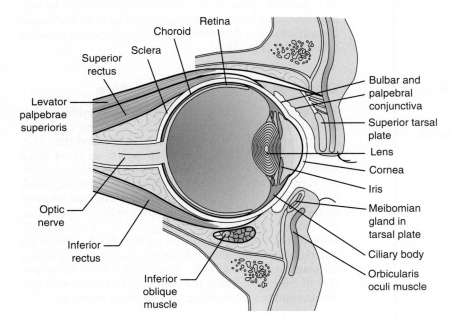

FIGURE 38-2. The eye and its appendages: lateral view.

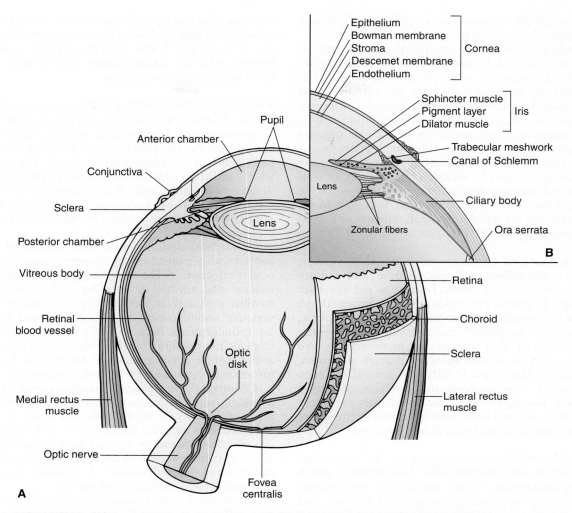

FIGURE 38-3. (A) Transverse section of the eyeball. **(B)** Enlargement of the anterior and posterior chambers of the eye, showing the layers of the cornea, the structures of the iris, the aqueous drainage system (trabecular meshwork, canal of Schlemm), and the ciliary process and ciliary muscle.

moves toward the retina (Fig. 38-3A). The cornea also contributes to the refraction (i.e., bending) of light rays and focusing of vision.

Although transparent, the cornea consists of three cellular layers: an extremely thin outer epithelial layer, which is continuous with the bulbar conjunctiva; a middle layer called the *substantia propria;* and an inner endothelial layer, which lies next to the aqueous humor of the anterior chamber.[2] The substantia propria is composed of regularly arranged collagen bundles embedded in a mucopolysaccharide matrix. This organization of the collagen fibers, which makes the substantia propria transparent, is necessary for light transmission. Hydration within a limited range is necessary to maintain the spacing of the collagen fibers and transparency. The three layers of the cornea are separated by two important basement membranes: Bowman and Descemet membranes (Fig. 38-3B). *Bowman membrane,* which lies between the corneal epithelium and the underlying corneal stroma, acts as a barrier to infection. It does not regenerate; if damaged, an opaque scar forms that can impair vision. *Descemet*

membrane, which lies between the corneal endothelium and stroma, has a feltlike appearance and consists of interwoven fibers and pores. Unlike Bowman membrane, it regenerates readily after injury.

The cornea is avascular and obtains its nutrient and oxygen supply by diffusion from the blood vessels of the adjacent sclera, the aqueous humor at its deep surface, and tears that bathe its surface. The corneal epithelium is heavily innervated by sensory neurons. Epithelial damage causes discomfort that ranges from a foreign body sensation and burning of the eyes to severe, incapacitating pain. Reflex lacrimation is also common.

Conjunctivitis

Conjunctivitis, or inflammation of the conjunctiva (i.e., red eye), is one of the most common eye disorders.[3–5] Most cases are due to viral or bacterial infections. Other causes include allergens, chemical agents, and physical irritants. The mode of transmission of infectious conjunctivitis is usually direct contact by way of the fingers, towels, etc., to the opposite eye or other persons. It may also be through contaminated eye drops.

Depending on the cause, conjunctivitis can vary in severity from a mild hyperemia (redness) with tearing to severe conjunctivitis with purulent drainage. The conjunctiva is extremely sensitive to irritation and inflammation. Symptoms of conjunctivitis include a foreign body sensation, a scratching or burning sensation, itching, and photophobia or light sensitivity. Severe pain suggests corneal rather than conjunctival disease. A discharge, or exudate, may be present. It is usually watery when the conjunctivitis is caused by allergy, a foreign body, or viral infection, and mucopurulent (mucus mixed with pus) in the presence of bacterial or fungal infection. Infectious forms of conjunctivitis are usually bilateral, whereas unilateral disease suggests sources of irritation such as foreign bodies.

The diagnosis of conjunctivitis is based on history, physical examination, and microscopic and culture studies to identify the cause. Because a red eye may be the sign of several eye conditions, it is important to differentiate between redness caused by conjunctivitis, which affects peripheral conjunctival blood vessels (Fig. 38-4), and that caused by more serious eye disorders, such as corneal lesions and acute glaucoma, which affects blood vessels radiating around the edge of the cornea. Conjunctivitis also produces only mild discomfort compared with the moderate to severe discomfort associated with corneal lesions or the severe and deep pain associated with acute glaucoma.

Viral Conjunctivitis. Adenoviruses are the most common causes of viral conjunctivitis.[3] The infection, which is highly contagious, causes generalized conjunctival hyperemia, copious tearing, and minimal exudate, and is often accompanied by pharyngitis, fever, and malaise. Viral conjunctivitis usually spreads through direct contact with contaminated fingers, swimming pool water, or personal items. Children are affected more often than adults. The disease usually lasts for at least 2 weeks and may be complicated by visual symptoms due to epithelial and subepithelial corneal involvement. There is no specific treatment for this type of viral conjunctivitis. Preventive measures include hygienic measures and avoiding shared use of eyedroppers, eye makeup, goggles, and towels. Persons who use contact lenses should wear wearing them until the infection clears.

Bacterial Conjunctivitis. Common agents of bacterial conjunctivitis are staphylococci, streptococci (particularly *S. pneumoniae*), *Haemophilus* species, *Pseudomonas*, and *Moraxella*. The infection usually is characterized by large amounts of yellow-green drainage. The eyelids are sticky, and there may be excoriation of the lid margins. Treatment measures include local application of antimicrobial agents. The disorder usually is self-limited, lasting approximately 10 to 14 days if untreated and 1 to 3 days if properly treated.[3]

Gonorrheal conjunctivitis, usually acquired through contact with genital secretions, is a severe, sight-threatening ocular infection.[3-5] The symptoms, include conjunctival redness and edema; lid swelling and tenderness; and swollen preauricular lymph nodes. Treatment includes systemic antimicrobial drugs supplemented with ocular antimicrobials. Because of the increasing prevalence of penicillin-resistant *N. gonorrhoeae*, the choice of an antimicrobial agent should be determined by current information regarding antimicrobial sensitivity.

Chlamydial, or *inclusion*, *conjunctivitis*, is usually a benign, suppurative conjunctivitis transmitted by the types of *Chlamydia trachomatis* (serotypes D through K) that causes venereal infections[3-6] (see Chapter 41). It is commonly spread by contact with genital secretions and occurs in newborns of mothers with *C. trachomatis* infections of the birth canal.[3-6] It is usually treated with appropriate oral antimicrobial agents.

Trachoma, a more serious form of infection, is caused by a different strain of *C. trachomatis* (serotypes A, B, and C).[6] This form of chlamydial infection affects the conjunctiva and causes ulceration and scarring of the cornea. It is the leading cause of preventable blindness in the world, and is seen mostly in developing countries.[3,6] It is transmitted by direct human contact, contaminated objects (fomites), and flies.

Allergic Conjunctivitis. Allergic conjunctivitis encompasses a spectrum of conjunctival conditions usually characterized by itching.[3-5,7] The most common of these is seasonal allergic rhinoconjunctivitis, or hay fever. Seasonal allergic conjunctivitis is an immunoglobulin E (IgE)-mediated hypersensitivity reaction precipitated by small air-borne allergens such as pollens.[7] It typically causes bilateral tearing, itching, and redness of the eyes.

The treatment of seasonal allergic rhinoconjunctivitis includes allergen avoidance and the use of cold compresses and eye washes with tear substitute. Allergic conjunctivitis also has been successfully treated with topical mast cell stabilizers, histamine type 1 (H_1) receptor antagonists, and topical nonsteroidal anti-inflammatory drugs.[7] Systemic antihistamines may be useful in prolonged allergic conjunctivitis. In severe cases, a short course of topical corticosteroids may be required to afford symptomatic relief.

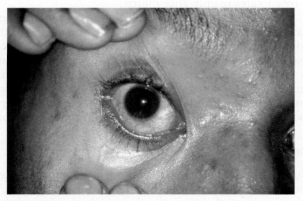

FIGURE 38-4. Gonococcal conjunctivitis of right eye. Note injection (redness) of the peripheral conjunctival blood vessels. (From the Centers for Disease Control and Prevention Public Health Images Library. No. 6784.)

Corneal Trauma

The integrity of the epithelium and endothelium is necessary to maintain hydration of the cornea within a limited range.[8] The integrity of the endothelium is more important than the epithelium, and damage to the endothelial cells is far more serious, causing edema of the cornea and loss of transparency. With corneal edema, the cornea appears dull, uneven, and hazy; visual acuity decreases; and iridescent vision (i.e., rainbows around lights) occurs.

Trauma that causes abrasions of the cornea can be extremely painful, but if minor, the abrasions usually heal in a few days. The epithelial layer can regenerate, and small defects heal without scarring. If the stroma is damaged, healing occurs more slowly, and the danger of infection is increased. Injuries to the Bowman membrane and the stromal layer heal with scar formation that impairs the transmission of light.

Keratitis

Keratitis, or inflammation of the cornea, can be caused by infections, misuse of contact lenses, hypersensitivity reactions, ischemia, trauma, defects in tearing, and interruption in sensory innervation, as occurs with local anesthesia. Scar tissue formation due to keratitis is the leading cause of blindness and impaired vision throughout the world. Most of this vision loss is preventable if the condition is diagnosed early and appropriate treatment is begun.

Keratitis can be infectious or noninfectious and nonulcerative or ulcerative.[8,9] In *nonulcerative* keratitis, all the layers of the epithelium may be affected, but the epithelium remains intact. There are a number of causes of epithelial keratitis, including epidemic keratoconjunctivitis caused by adenoviruses 8 and 19 and ultraviolet (UV) light exposure. Most cases of UV keratitis occur in welders with inadequate eye protection, but may also occur with tanning booth and other UV lamp exposure, and from sun reflecting off snow.[10]

Ulcerative keratitis is an inflammatory process in which parts of the corneal epithelium, stroma, or both are destroyed. Causes of ulcerative keratitis include infectious agents (e.g., *S. aureus, S. pneumoniae, C. trachomatis*), exposure trauma, and use of extended-wear contact lenses (i.e., *Pseudomonas* and *Acanthamoeba* keratitis). Bacterial keratitis is aggressive and demands immediate care. *Mooren ulcer* is a chronic, indolent, but painful ulcerative keratitis that occurs in the absence of infection. It is usually seen in older persons and may affect both eyes. Although the cause is unknown, an autoimmune origin is suspected.

Herpes Simplex Keratitis. Herpes simplex virus (HSV) keratitis, which usually is unilateral, is an important cause of ocular morbidity.[11,12] With the exception of neonatal infections, which are usually due to HSV type 2 (genital herpes) acquired during the birth process, most cases of herpes keratitis are caused by HSV type 1 (labial [lip] herpes). The disease can occur as either a primary or recurrent infection. Primary epithelial infections are the optical counterpart of labial herpes with similar immunologic and pathologic features as well as a similar time course (see Chapter 46).

The first manifestations of recurrent herpes keratitis are irritation, photophobia, and tearing. Some reduction in vision may occur when the lesion affects the central part of the cornea. Because corneal anesthesia occurs early in the disease, the symptoms may be minimal. A history of fever blisters or other herpetic infection is often noted, but corneal lesions may be the only sign of recurrent herpes infection. Typically, the corneal lesions involve the epithelium and heal without scarring. Lesions that involve the stromal layer of the cornea produce increasingly severe corneal opacities.

Any person with herpes simplex keratitis and an acute red eye should be referred urgently to an ophthalmologist. The treatment of HSV keratitis includes the use of topical antiviral agents to promote healing.[8] Oral antiviral agents (e.g., acyclovir) may be helpful for treatment of severe keratitis and as prophylaxis against recurrence, particularly in persons with compromised immune function. Although corticosteroids may control the damaging inflammatory responses, they do so at the expense of facilitating viral replication. With a few exceptions, their use is contraindicated.[11]

Varicella Zoster Ophthalmicus. Herpes zoster or *shingles* is a relatively common infection due to the herpesvirus that causes varicella (chickenpox).[8,12] Herpes ophthalmicus, which represents 10% to 25% of all cases of herpes zoster, occurs when reactivation of the latent virus occurs in the ganglia of the ophthalmic division of the trigeminal nerve.[12] Immunocompromised persons, particularly those with human immunodeficiency virus (HIV) infection, are at higher risk for developing herpes zoster ophthalmicus than those with a normally functioning immune system.

Herpes zoster ophthalmicus usually presents with malaise, fever, headache, and burning and itching of the periorbital area. These symptoms commonly precede the ocular eruption by a day or two. The rash, which is initially vesicular, becomes pustular and then crusting (see Chapter 46). Involvement of the tip of the nose and lid margins indicates a high likelihood of ocular involvement. Ocular signs include conjunctivitis, keratitis, and anterior uveitis, often with elevated intraocular pressure. Persons with corneal disease present with varying degrees of decreased vision, pain, and sensitivity to light.

Treatment includes the use of oral and intravenous antiviral drugs. Initiation of treatment within the first 72 hours after the appearance of the rash reduces the incidence of ocular complications but not the postherpetic neuralgia[8] (see Chapter 35). Many cases of herpes zoster and herpes zoster ophthalmicus can now be prevented with the herpes zoster vaccine.

Acanthamoeba Keratitis. *Acanthamoeba* is a free-living cyst-forming protozoan that thrives in polluted water containing bacteria and organic material.[8,13,14] *Acanthamoeba* keratitis is a rare but sight-threatening complication that typically occurs in people who wear soft contact lens, particularly overnight or without proper disinfection.[14] It also may occur in non–contact lens wearers after exposure to contaminated water or soil.

Acanthamoeba keratitis is characterized by severe pain, redness of the eye, and photophobia. Diagnosis is confirmed by scrapings and culture with specially prepared medium. In the early stages of infection, epithelial debridement may be beneficial. Treatment includes intensive use of topical antimicrobials. However, the organism may encyst within the corneal stroma, making treatment more difficult. Keratoplasty may be necessary in advanced disease to arrest the progression of the infection.

Disorders of the Lens

The lens is a remarkable structure, which like that in a camera, functions to bring images into focus on the retina. The lens is an avascular, transparent, biconvex structure, the posterior side of which is more convex than the anterior side.[2,15,16] It is positioned just posterior to the iris and is held in place by suspensory ligaments known as the *zonules*, which are composed of numerous fibrils that arise from the ciliary body (see Fig. 38-3B). The pull of the zonular fibers and lens capsule is normally under tension, causing the lens to have a flattened shape for distant vision. Relaxation of the fibers allows the lens to assume a more spherical shape for near vision. There are no pain fibers, blood vessels, or nerves in the lens.

The lens has three principal components: the lens capsule, a subcapsular epithelium, and lens fibers. The lens capsule is a transparent elastic structure that envelops the entire lens. The subcapsular epithelium is a cuboidal layer of cells that is present on the anterior surface of the lens. The lens fibers, which constitute the bulk of the lens, continue to produce new fibers throughout life, with the older fibers being compressed into the central nucleus of the lens. This causes the lens to gradually become larger and less elastic with age.

Refraction refers to deflection or bending of light as it passes from one transparent medium to another of different density. When parallel light rays pass through the center of a lens, their direction is not changed; however, the divergent rays passing peripherally through a lens are bent (Fig. 38-5A). The refractive power of a lens is usually described as the distance (in meters) from its surface to the point at which the rays come into focus on the retina (i.e., focal length). Usually, this is reported as the reciprocal of this distance (i.e., diopters).[16] For example, a lens that brings an object into focus at 0.5 m has a refractive power of 2 diopters (1.0/0.5 = 2.0). The closer the object, the more divergent the peripheral rays, and the stronger and more precise the focusing system must be.

In the eye, the major refraction of light begins at the convex corneal surface. Further refraction occurs as light moves from the posterior corneal surface to the aqueous humor, from the aqueous humor to the anterior lens surface, from the anterior lens surface to the posterior lens surface, and from the posterior lens surface to the vitreous humor.

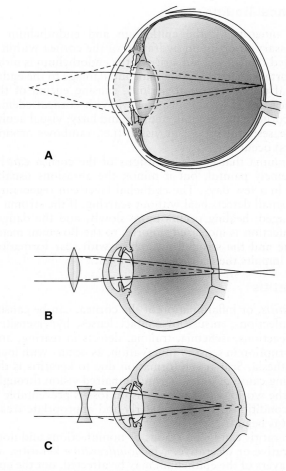

FIGURE 38-5. (A) Accommodation. The *solid lines* represent rays of light from a distant object, and the *dotted lines* represent rays from a near object. The lens is flatter for the former and more convex for the latter. In each case, the rays of light are brought to a focus on the retina. **(B)** Hyperopia corrected by a biconvex lens, shown by the *dotted lines*. **(C)** Myopia corrected by a biconcave lens, shown by the *dotted lines*.

Disorders of Refraction

A perfectly shaped eyeball and cornea result in optimal visual acuity, producing a sharp image in focus at all points on the surface of the retina. Unfortunately, individual differences in eyeball length result in inappropriate focal image formation. If the anterior-posterior dimension of the eyeball is too short, the point of focus will fall behind the retina. This is called *hyperopia*, or *farsightedness*[16] (see Fig. 38-5B). In such cases, the accommodative changes of the lens (to be discussed) can bring distant images into focus, but near images become blurred. If the anterior-posterior dimension of the eyeball is too long, the focus point falls in front of the retina. This condition is called *myopia*, or *nearsightedness*[16] (see Fig. 38-5C). Persons with myopia can see close objects without a problem because accommodative changes in their lens bring near objects into focus, but distant objects are blurred. A refractive defect of the corneal surface, or *astigmatism*, is usually the result of an asymmetric bowing of the cornea, but it also can result from defects in the cornea, lens, or retina.

Both hyperopia and myopia, as well as astigmatism, can be corrected with the appropriate lens. Refractive corneal surgeries such as laser in situ keratomileusis (LASIK), photorefractive keratectomy, and radial keratotomy can be performed to correct the corneal curvature in persons with myopia.[17]

Disorders of Accommodation

The ability of the eye to adjust its focus from far to near objects by changing the shape of its lens is called *accommodation*. Accommodation is associated with convergence of the eyes (focusing the vision on a near point), pupillary constriction, and thickening of the lens through contraction of the ciliary muscle of the eye.[16] Contraction of muscle fibers in the ciliary body is controlled mainly by parasympathetic stimulation of the oculomotor nerve (CN III). Paralysis of the ciliary muscle resulting in pupillary dilation, with loss of accommodation, is called *cycloplegia*. Pharmacologic cycloplegia through the use of a topical anticholinergic agent is sometimes used to aid in refractive examination of the eye, particularly in small children.

The term *presbyopia* refers to a decrease in accommodation that occurs because of aging.[16] The normal proliferative process in the lens nucleus that occurs throughout life causes the lens to thicken and its capsule to become less elastic, so that the range of focus or accommodation is diminished. As a result, the person begins to notice the inability to read small print or discriminate close objects. This is usually worse in dim light, on arising in the morning, or when the person is fatigued.

Cataracts

A cataract is a lens opacity that interferes with the transmission of light to the retina. Aging is the most common cause of cataracts, and most people over age 60 have some degree of lens opacity. Although aging is the most important cause of cataracts, other factors such as heredity, environmental influences, systemic diseases (e.g., diabetes mellitus), drugs, and trauma may be involved.[15,18] Long-term exposure to sunlight (ultraviolet radiation) has been associated with increased risk of cataract formation. Corticosteroids have been implicated as causative agents in cataract formation. Both systemic and inhaled corticosteroids have been cited as risk factors.[19]

Clinical Manifestations. The manifestations of cataracts depend on the extent of opacity and whether the defect is bilateral or unilateral. Cataracts are usually bilateral (with the exception of traumatic or congenital cataracts). Age-related cataracts, which are typically the result of opacification of the lens nucleus (nuclear sclerosis), are characterized by increasingly blurred vision and visual distortion.[15,20] Dilation of the pupil in dim light improves vision. In addition to decreased visual acuity, cataracts tend to cause light entering the eye to be scattered, thereby producing glare or the abnormal presence of light in the visual field (see Fig. 38-1C).

Diagnosis and Treatment. Diagnosis of cataracts is based on ophthalmoscopic examination and the degree of visual impairment on the Snellen vision test. On ophthalmoscopic examination, a cataract may appear as a gross opacity filling the pupillary aperture, or as an opacity silhouetted against the red background of the fundus. Other tests that determine the potential ability to see well after surgery, such as electrophysiologic testing in which the response to visual stimuli is measured electronically, may be done.

There is no effective medical treatment for cataract. Although strong bifocal lenses, magnification, appropriate lighting, and visual aids may help, surgery is the only treatment for cataract.[15,20] It is commonly performed on an outpatient basis with the use of local anesthesia. The cataract lens is typically fragmented into fine pieces, which then are aspirated from the eye, and an intraocular lens implanted. Monofocal intraocular lenses that correct for distance vision are available. Although eyeglasses may still be needed for near vision, the recent introduction of multifocal intraocular lenses has reduced the need for both distance and near vision corrective eyeglasses.

Childhood Cataract. Childhood cataracts can be divided into two groups: congenital (infantile) cataracts, which are present at birth or appear shortly thereafter, and acquired cataracts, which occur later and are usually related to a specific cause.[15,21] About one third of childhood cataracts are hereditary; another third are secondary to metabolic or infectious processes or associated with a variety of syndromes; and the final third results from undetermined causes. The development of congenital or infantile cataracts depend on the total dose of the agent and the stage of development at the time of exposure. It is during the last trimester of fetal life, genetically or environmentally influenced malformation of the superficial lens fibers can occur. Congenital lens opacities may occur in children of diabetic mothers. The presence of bilateral cataracts is often inherited and associated with other disease conditions, so genetic testing is required.

Most congenital cataracts are not progressive and are not dense enough to cause significant visual impairment.[15] However, cataracts that are dense, central, and larger than 2 mm in diameter require surgical management on an urgent basis. If not treated within the first 2 months of life, visual deprivation produces irreversible loss of vision[15,21] (i.e., ambylopia, to be discussed).

Disorders of The Retina

The retina is the most complex structure of the eye. It receives visual images produced by the optical system of the eye and converts the light energy into an electrical signal that is transmitted by way of the optic nerve to the visual cortex, where the image is perceived.[16,22,23] Disorders of the retina and its function include disorders of the retinal vessels such as retinopathies that cause

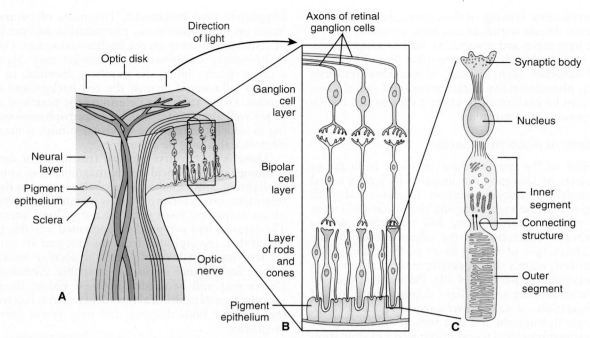

FIGURE 38-6. Organization of the retina. **(A)** Organization of the retina showing the inner neural layer and the outer pigment epithelium. **(B)** The three layers of the neural retina: a posterior layer of photoreceptors (rods and cones), a middle layer of bipolar cells, and an inner layer of ganglionic cells. **(C)** Photoreceptor structure: a retinal rod, showing its component parts and distribution of organelles.

hemorrhage and the development of opacities; separation of the pigment and sensory layers of the retina (i.e., retinal detachment); and macular degeneration. Because the retina has no pain fibers, most diseases of the retina do not cause pain, nor do they produce redness of the eye.

The retina is composed of two layers: an outer pigment (melanin-containing) epithelium and an inner neural layer[16,22] (Fig. 38-6A). The outer surface of the pigmented layer, a single-cell–thick lining, abuts the choroid and extends anteriorly to cover the ciliary body and the posterior side of the iris. Its pigmented epithelial cells, like those of the choroid, absorb light and prevent it from scattering. The pigment layer also stores large quantities of vitamin A, which is an important precursor of the photosensitive visual pigments.

The inner light-sensitive neural retina covers the inner aspect of the eyeball.[16,22] The neural retina is composed of three layers of neurons: a posterior layer of photoreceptors (rods and cones), a middle layer of bipolar cells, and an inner layer of ganglion cells that communicate with the photoreceptors (see Fig. 38-6B). Light must pass through the transparent inner layers of the sensory retina before it reaches the photoreceptors. Impulses produced in response to light spread from the photoreceptors to the bipolar neurons and other interneurons and then to the ganglionic cells, where action potentials are generated. The interneurons, which have cell bodies in the bipolar layer, play an important role in modulating retinal function. The optic disk, where the optic nerve exits the eye, is the weak part of the eye because it is not reinforced by the sclera. It also forms the blind

spot because it is not backed by photoreceptors, and light focused on it cannot be seen. People do not notice the blind spot because of a sophisticated visual function called "filling in," which the brain uses to deal with missing visual input.

Two types of photoreceptors are present in the retina: rods capable of black–white discrimination and cones capable of color discrimination.[16,22,24] Rod-based vision is particularly sensitive to detecting light, especially moving light stimuli, at the expense of clear pattern discrimination. Rod vision is particularly adapted for night and low-level illumination. Cone receptors, which are selectively sensitive to different wavelengths of light, provide the basis for color vision. Three types of cones, or cone-color systems, respond to the blue, green, and red portions of the visible electromagnetic spectrum. Cones do not have the dark adaptation capability of rods. Consequently, the dark-adapted eye is a rod receptor eye with only black–gray–white experience (scotopic or night vision). The light-adapted eye (*photopic vision*) adds the capacity for color discrimination.

Both rods and cones contain chemicals that change configuration on exposure to light and, in the process, generate electric signals that lead to the action potentials generated by the ganglionic cells. The light-sensitive chemical in rods is called *rhodopsin*, and the light-sensitive chemicals in cones are called *cone* or *color pigments*. Both types of photoreceptors are thin, elongated, mitochondria-filled cells with a single, highly modified cilium (Fig. 38-6C). The cilium has a short base, or inner segment, and a highly modified outer segment. The cell membrane of the outer segment is tightly folded to form membranous disks (rods) or conical shapes (cones) containing visual pigment. These disks are continuously synthesized at the base of the outer segment and shed at the distal end. Discarded membranes are phagocytized by the retinal pigment cells. If this phagocytosis is disrupted, as in a condition called *retinitis pigmentosa*, the sensory retina degenerates.

An area near the center of the retina, called the *macula lutea* (i.e., "yellow spot"), is especially adapted for acute and detailed vision.[16] This area is composed entirely of cones. In the central portion of the macula, the *fovea centralis* (foveola), the blood vessels and innermost layers are displaced to one side instead of resting on top of the cones. This allows light to pass unimpeded to the cones without passing through several layers of the retina. Many of these cones are connected one to one with ganglionic cells, an arrangement that favors high acuity.

Retinal Blood Supply

The blood supply for the retina is derived from two sources: the choriocapillaris (i.e., the capillary layer of the choroid) and branches of the central retinal artery (Fig. 38-7A). Oxygen and other nutrients are supplied by diffusion from blood vessels in the choroid. Because the choriocapillaris provides the only blood supply for the fovea centralis, detachment of this part of the sensory retina from the pigment epithelium causes irreparable loss of vision. The central artery, which is a branch of the ophthalmic artery, supplies the rest of the retina. Retinal veins follow a distribution parallel to the arterial branches and carry venous blood to the central vein of the retina, which exits the back of the eye through the optic disk.

Funduscopic examination of the eye with an ophthalmoscope provides the means for examining the retinal blood vessels and other aspects of the retina (Fig. 38-7B). Because the retina is an embryonic outgrowth of the brain and the blood vessels are to a considerable extent representative of brain blood vessels, the ophthalmoscopic examination of the fundus of the eye permits the study and diagnosis of metabolic and vascular diseases of the brain as well as pathologic processes that are specific to the retina.

Retinopathies

Retinopathies, which involve the small blood vessels of the retina, are characterized by changes in vessel structure and the development of microaneurysms, neovascularization, hemorrhage, and retinal opacities.[24,25] *Microaneurysms* are outpouchings of the retinal vasculature. On ophthalmoscopic examination, they appear as minute, unchanging red dots associated with blood vessels. Microaneurysms tend to leak plasma, resulting in localized edema that gives the retina a hazy appearance. They may also bleed, but areas of hemorrhage and edema tend to clear spontaneously. However, they reduce visual acuity if they encroach on the macula and cause degeneration before they are absorbed. *Neovascularization* involves the formation of new blood vessels. They can develop from the choriocapillaris, extending between the pigment and the sensory layers of the retina; or from the retinal veins, extending between the sensory retina and the vitreous cavity and sometimes into the vitreous. These new blood vessels are fragile, leak protein, and are likely to bleed. Although

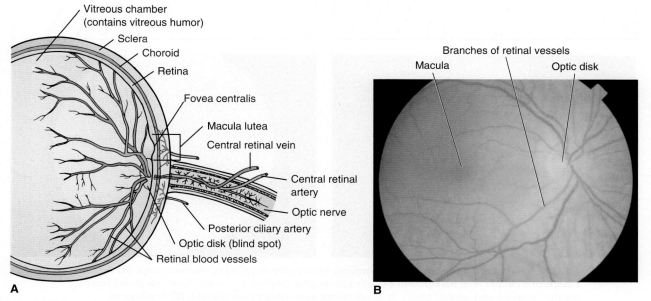

A   **B**

FIGURE 38-7. (A) Retinal circulation showing the distribution of the central retinal and posterior ciliary arteries and the central retinal vein. **(B)** Funduscopic image of the normal retina (From Moore KL, Daley AF, Agur AMR. *Clinically Oriented Anatomy.* 6th ed. Philadelphia, PA: Wolters Kluwer Health | Lippincott Williams & Wilkins; 2010:897.)

the cause of neovascularization is uncertain, research links the process with a vascular endothelial growth factor (VEGF) produced by the lining of blood vessels.[25–27] Hypoxia is a key regulator of VEGF-induced retinal neovascularization. It is likely that other growth factors and signaling systems are also involved.

Opacities represent a loss of retinal transparency due to hemorrhages, exudates, cotton-wool spots, edema, and tissue proliferation. The development of exudates often results in the destruction of the underlying retinal pigment and choroid layer. *Cotton-wool patches* are retinal opacities with hazy, irregular outlines. They occur in the nerve fiber layer of the retina and are associated with retinal trauma, severe anemia, papilledema, and diabetic retinopathy.

Diabetic Retinopathy. Diabetic retinopathy is one of the leading causes of blindness in the Western world, particularly among individuals of working age.[6,25–28] Chronic hyperglycemia, hypertension, hypercholesteremia, and smoking are all risk factors for the development and progression of the disorder. People with type 1 (insulin-dependent) diabetes do not usually develop the disorder until at least 3 to 5 years after the onset of the disease, whereas those with type 2 diabetes may have retinopathy as a presenting symptom at the time of diagnosis.[25]

Diabetic retinopathy can be divided into two types: nonproliferative (or background) and proliferative.[6,25] *Nonproliferative* retinopathy is confined to the retina. It involves engorgement of the retinal veins, thickening of the capillary endothelial basement membrane, and development of capillary microaneurysms (Fig. 38-8A,B). Small intraretinal hemorrhages may develop and microinfarcts may cause cotton-wool spots and leakage of exudates. The most common cause of decreased vision in persons with background retinopathy is macular edema. The edema is caused primarily by the breakdown of the blood-retina barrier at the level of the capillary endothelium, allowing leakage of fluid and plasma constituents into the surrounding retina.

Proliferative diabetic retinopathy represents a more severe retinal change than background retinopathy (Fig. 38-8C,D). It is characterized by formation of new fragile blood vessels (i.e., neovascularization) at the optic disk and elsewhere in the retina, which is often the

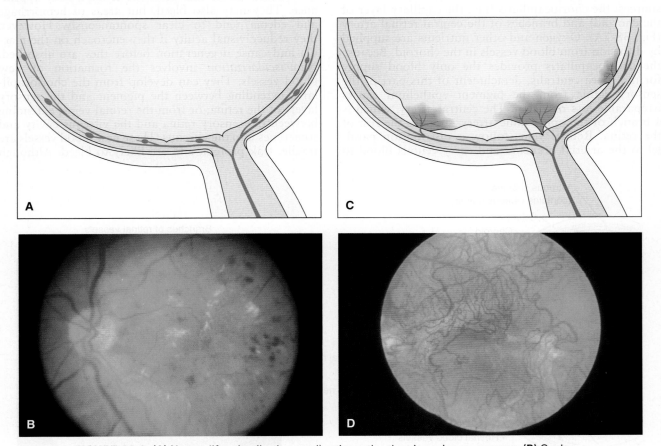

FIGURE 38-8. (A) Nonproliferative (background) retinopathy showing microaneurysms. **(B)** Ocular fundus of a patient with background diabetic retinopathy. Several yellowish "hard" exudates (which are rich in lipids) and several relatively small retinal hemorrhages are present. **(C)** Proliferative retinopathy. **(D)** Ocular fundus in a patient with proliferative retinopathy. A vascular frond (branching pattern of preretinal neovascularization) has extended anterior to the retina. (B and D from Klintworth GK. The eye. In: Rubin R, Strayer DS, eds. *Rubin's Pathology: Clinicopathologic Foundations of Medicine.* 6th ed. Philadelphia, PA: Wolters Kluwer Health | Lippincott Williams & Wilkins; 2012:1403.)

first detectable sign of diabetic retinopathy. These vessels grow in front of the retina along the posterior surface of the vitreous or into the vitreous. They threaten vision in two ways. First, they often leak blood into the vitreous cavity and decrease visual acuity. Second, they attach firmly to the retinal surface and the posterior surface of the vitreous chamber, such that normal movement of the vitreous humor may exert a pull on the retina, causing retinal detachment and progressive blindness.

Current guidelines recommend that persons with diabetes have yearly eye examinations.[27] Persons with any level of macular edema, severe nonproliferative diabetic retinopathy, or any proliferative retinopathy require the prompt care of an ophthalmologist experienced in the management and treatment of diabetic retinopathy. Women with preexisting diabetes who plan to become pregnant or are pregnant should have a comprehensive eye examination and be counseled about the risk for initiation or progression of diabetic retinopathy.

Preventing diabetic retinopathy from developing or progressing is considered the best approach to preserving vision. Growing evidence suggests that careful control of blood glucose levels in persons with diabetes mellitus may retard the onset and progression of retinopathy. There also is a need for intensive management of hypertension and hyperlipidemia, both of which have been shown to increase the risk of diabetic retinopathy in persons with diabetes.[28]

Treatment strategies for diabetic retinopathy include laser photocoagulation applied directly to leaking microaneurysms and grid photocoagulation with a checkerboard pattern of laser burns applied to diffuse areas of leakage and thickening. Because laser photocoagulation destroys the proliferating vessels and the ischemic retina, it reduces the stimulus for further neovascularization. Intravitreal injections of anti-VEGF agents are also being used to reduce active neovascularization and vitreous hemorrhage.[28] Vitrectomy may be used for removing vitreous hemorrhage and severing vitreoretinal membranes that develop.

Hypertensive Retinopathy. As with other blood vessels in the body, the retinal vessels undergo changes in response to chronically elevated blood pressure. In the initial, vasoconstrictor stage, there is vasospasm and an increase in retinal arterial tone because of local autoregulatory mechanisms. On ophthalmoscopy, this stage is represented by a general narrowing of the retinal arterioles. Persistently elevated blood pressure results in the compensatory thickening of arteriolar walls, which effectively reduces capillary perfusion pressure.[29] With severe uncontrolled hypertension, there is disruption of the blood-retina barrier, necrosis of smooth muscle and endothelial cells, exudation of blood and lipids, and retinal ischemia. These changes are manifested in the retina by microaneurysms, intraretinal hemorrhages, hard exudates, and cotton-wool patches. Swelling of the optic disk may occur at this stage and usually indicates severely elevated blood pressure (malignant hypertension). Elderly persons often have more rigid vessels that are unable to respond to the same degree as those in younger individuals.

Retinal Detachment

Retinal detachment involves the separation of the neurosensory retina from the pigment epithelium. The disorder, which is one of most time-critical events seen in an emergency department, occurs when traction on the inner sensory layer or a tear in this layer allows fluid, usually vitreous, to accumulate between the two layers of the retina.[6,23,30] There are three types of retinal detachments: exudative, traction, and rhegmatogenous.

Exudative Detachment. Exudative (or serous) retinal detachment results from the accumulation of serous or hemorrhagic fluid in the subretinal space due to severe hypertension, inflammation, or neoplastic effusions. It usually resolves with successful treatment of the underlying disease and without visual impairment.

Traction Retinal Detachment. *Traction retinal deattachment* occurs with mechanical forces on the retina, usually mediated by fibrotic tissue, resulting from previous hemorrhage (e.g., from diabetic retinopathy), injury, infection, or inflammation. Intraocular surgery such as cataract extraction may produce traction on the peripheral retina that causes eventual detachment months or even years after surgery. Correction of traction retinal detachment requires disengaging scar tissue from the retinal surface, and vision outcomes are often poor.

Rhegmatogenous Detachment. Rhegmatogenous detachment, the most common type of retinal detachment, is a full thickness break ("rhegma") in the sensory retina, with the passage of liquefied vitreous through the break into the subretinal space. Although typically an acute event, detachment is a consequence of lifelong liquefaction of the vitreous humor, and is highly age-dependent with 27% of patients in their seventies and 63% in their eighties.[30] As the collagenous and mucopolysaccharide matrix of the vitreous humor begins to liquefy and shrink, it pulls away from the retinal surface. Rhegmatogenous detachment occurs when the liquid vitreous enters the subretinal space through a retinal tear (Fig. 38-9). Detachment of the neural retina from the retinal pigment layer separates the visual receptors from their major blood supply, the choroid. If retinal detachment continues for some time, permanent destruction and blindness of that part of the retina occur. Persons with high grades of myopia or nearsightedness may have abnormalities in the peripheral retina that predispose to sudden detachment. In moderate to severe myopia, the anteroposterior length of the eye is increased, and the retina tends to be thinner and more prone to formation of a hole or tear.[30] As a result, there is greater vitreoretinal traction, and posterior vitreous detachment may occur at a younger age than in persons without myopia.

Clinical Manifestations. The primary symptom of retinal detachment is painless changes in vision. Commonly, flashing lights or sparks, followed by small floaters or spots in the field of vision, are early symptoms. As detachment progresses, the person

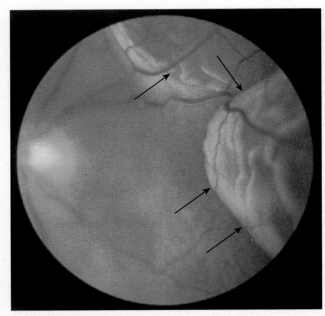

FIGURE 38-9. Ophthalmoscopic view of retinal detachment (arrows, wrinkles in detached retina). (From Moore KL, Daley AF, Agur AMR. *Clinically Oriented Anatomy.* 6th ed. Philadelphia, PA: Wolters Kluwer Health | Lippincott Williams & Wilkins; 2010:910).

perceives a shadow or dark curtain progressing across the visual field. Large peripheral detachments may occur without involvement of the macula, so that visual acuity remains unaffected.

Diagnosis and Treatment. Diagnosis of retinal detachment is based on a history of visual disturbances (e.g., presence of floaters, luminous rays, or light flashes) and the ophthalmoscopic appearance of the retina. The direct (handheld) ophthalmoscope is useful in detecting an altered red reflex sometimes associated with retinal detachment. However, because the view is narrow, a negative examination with direct ophthalmoscopy cannot exclude the diagnosis of retinal detachment. Ophthalmologists and optometrists use

indirect examination techniques that greatly enhance visualization of the peripheral retina.[30]

Because there is a variable interval between a retinal break and retinal detachment, treatment methods focus on early detection and prevention of further vitreous detachment and retinal tear formation. Symptomatic retinal breaks are usually treated with laser or cryotherapy to seal the retinal tears so that the vitreous humor can no longer leak into the subretinal space.[30] The primary treatment of traction retinal detachment is vitreoretinal surgery.[23,30]

Macular Degeneration

Macular degeneration is characterized by degenerative changes in the central portion of the retina (the macula) that result primarily in loss of central vision (see Figure 38-1B). Age-related macular degeneration (AMD) is the most common cause of reduced vision in the elderly.[23,25,31–33] The causes are poorly understood. In addition to older age, identifiable risk factors include cigarette smoking, obesity, and low dietary intake of lutein, omega 3 fatty acids, zinc, and vitamins A, C, and E.[32] Increasing evidence suggests that genetic factors may also play a role.

Age-related macular degeneration is commonly classified simply as "early" or "late." Late AMD is further subdivided into geographic atrophy ("dry") and neovascular ("wet"). Although both late forms are progressive and usually bilateral, they differ in manifestations, prognosis, and management.

Geographic Atrophic Degeneration. Geographic atrophic degeneration is characterized by gradually progressive visual loss of moderate severity due to atrophy and degeneration of the outer retina and retinal pigment epithelium. Because it does not involve leakage of blood or serum, it is commonly referred to as dry macular degeneration. The level of associated visual impairment is variable and may be minimal, and the atrophic changes may stabilize or progress slowly (Fig. 38-10A). However, people with this form of AMD need to be followed closely because the neovascular form may

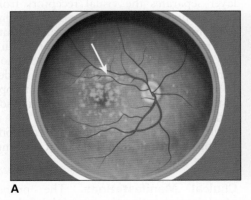

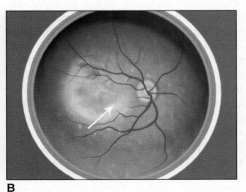

A   **B**

FIGURE 38-10. Funduscopic view of age-related macular degeneration (AMD). **(A)** Intermediate AMD with pale yellow spots or drusen scattered throughout the retina. **(B)** Advanced AMD with formation of scar tissue representing death of the underlying retinal tissue and loss of all visual function in the corresponding macular area. (Courtesy of the National Eye Institute, National Institutes of Health.)

develop suddenly at any time. Careful monitoring for metamorphopsia, or distorted vision of straight lines, can aid in the early detection of retinal damage.

Neovascular Degeneration.
The neovascular form of AMD is characterized by the formation of a choroidal neovascular membrane. These new blood vessels have weaker walls than normal and are prone to leakage; thus, this form is commonly referred to as "wet." The leakage of serous or hemorrhagic fluid into the subretinal space causes separation of the pigmented epithelium from the neurosensory retina. Over time, the subretinal hemorrhages organize to form scar tissue, causing death of the underlying retinal tissue and loss of all visual function in the corresponding macular area (see Fig. 38-10B). Although some subretinal neovascular membranes may regress spontaneously, the natural course is toward irreversible loss of central vision.

Diagnosis and Treatment.
The early stages of subretinal neovascularization may be difficult to detect with an ophthalmoscope. Therefore, there is a need to be alert for recent or sudden changes in central vision, blurred vision, or scotomata (visual field areas in which vision is depressed or absent). Persons with late-stage disease often find it difficult to see at long distances (e.g., in driving), do close work (e.g., reading), see faces clearly, or distinguish colors. However, they may not be severely incapacitated because the peripheral retinal function usually remains intact.

Effective therapies for neovascular macular degeneration include thermal laser photocoagulation, photodynamic therapy, and intravitreal injections of VEGF inhibitors.[23,31-33] Conventional retinal laser photocoagulation can achieve direct destruction of a choroidal neovascular membrane. Photodynamic laser therapy involves the intravenous injection of a dye that is subsequently activated by retinal laser irradiation to produce selective vascular damage. Recognition of the key role that VEGF plays in choroidal neovascularization pathogenesis led to development of VEGF inhibitors, a class of drugs that has now become the preferred treatment for neovascular macular degeneration. These drugs are given by intravitreal injection.

In addition to currently used and forthcoming treatments, there is interest in the so-called preventative category of treatments.[21,31-33] Tobacco smoking is consistently identified as a preventable age-related macular degeneration risk; thus, its elimination should be one of the first therapeutic recommendations. Preventative recommendations also include dietary supplementation containing high-dose antioxidants and minerals (vitamins E and C, zinc, and β-carotene) for persons at risk for developing macular degeneration and for slowing the progression of age-related macular degeneration in persons with the disease.[30] However, more experimental data and randomized clinical trials are needed to support their therapeutic value, the most effective composition in terms of single- or multiple-supplement combinations, and dosing of the particular supplements.

Disorders of Intraocular Pressure

The intraocular pressure reflects that of the aqueous humor that fills the anterior and posterior chambers of the eye. The aqueous humor is produced by the ciliary body and passes from the posterior chamber through the pupil into the anterior chamber[6,25,34,35] (Fig. 38-11A). Aqueous humor leaves through the trabecular meshwork at the iridocorneal angle between the anterior iris and the cornea. It then drains into the canal of Schlemm, a thin-walled vein that extends circumferentially around the iris, for return to the venous circulation. Intraocular pressure results from a balance of several factors, including the rate of aqueous humor production by the ciliary body, the resistance to flow between the iris and ciliary body, and its rate of removal by the drainage system (trabecular meshwork and canal of Schlemm). Normally, the rate of aqueous humor secretion is equal to the rate of outflow, and the intraocular pressure is maintained within a normal range of 10 to 21 mm Hg.[34]

Glaucoma is a chronic, pressure-induced degenerative neuropathy that produces changes in the optic nerve and visual field loss (see Fig. 38-1D). Glaucoma is commonly classified as open-angle or angle-closure glaucoma depending on the appearance of the iridocorneal angle, and according to whether it is a primary or secondary disorder.[6,25,34,35]

Open-Angle Glaucoma

Open-angle glaucoma, which is the most common form of glaucoma, results from an abnormality of the trabecular meshwork that controls the flow of aqueous humor into the canal of Schlemm without obstruction at the iridocorneal angle[34-36] (see Fig. 38-11B). Open-angle glaucoma is usually asymptomatic and chronic, causing progressive damage to the optic nerve and vision loss unless it is appropriately treated. Elevated intraocular pressure is a primary factor; however, some eyes tolerate elevated intraocular pressure without developing disk or visual field changes, whereas others develop glaucomatous changes with consistently normal intraocular pressures (normal-tension glaucoma).

Clinical Manifestations.
Because open-angle glaucoma is usually asymptomatic, it is often suspected when abnormal intraocular pressure measurements or optic disk abnormalities are found during a routine eye examination. The normal optic disk has a central depression called the *optic nerve cup* (Fig. 38-12). In glaucoma, the neuroretinal rim of the optic nerve becomes progressively thinner, thereby enlarging the optic nerve cup, a phenomenon referred to as *optic nerve cupping*. Its cause is loss of retinal ganglionic cell axons, along with supporting glia and vasculature.[6] Because changes in the optic cup precede visual field loss, regular ophthalmoscopic examinations are important to detect damage to retinal ganglion axons before visual field loss occurs.

Diagnosis and Treatment.
Diagnostic methods include applanation tonometry (measurement of intraocular

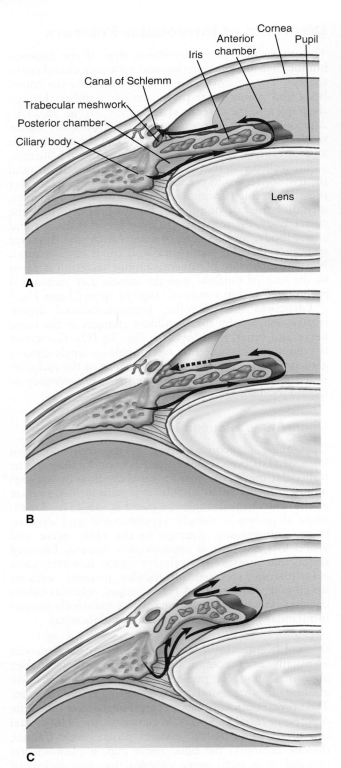

A

B

C

FIGURE 38-11. (A) Normally, aqueous humor, which is secreted in the posterior chamber, gains access to the anterior chamber by flowing through the pupil. In the angle of the anterior chamber, it passes through the canal of Schlemm into the venous system. **(B)** In open-angle glaucoma, the outflow of aqueous humor is obstructed at the trabecular meshwork. **(C)** In angle-closure glaucoma, the aqueous humor encounters resistance to flow through the pupil. Increased pressure in the posterior chamber produces a forward bowing of the peripheral iris, so that the iris blocks the trabecular meshwork.

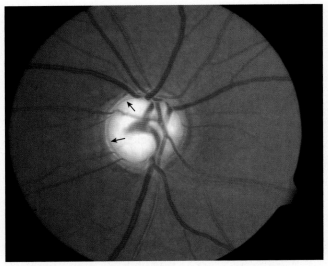

FIGURE 38-12. Optic nerve head in glaucoma. The anterior part of the optic nerve is decompressed ("optic cupping" arrows), and the blood vessels crossing the margin of the optic nerve head are displaced to the nasal side. The fundus appears dark because the eye of an African-American patient contains numerous pigmented melanocytes in the choroid. (From Klintworth GK. The eye. In: Rubin R, Strayer DS, eds. *Pathology; Clinicopathologic Foundations of Medicine.* 6th ed. Philadelphia, PA: Wolters Kluwer Health | Lippincott Williams & Wilkins; 2012:1410).

pressure), opthalmoscopic visualization of the optic nerve, and visual field testing.

The elevation in intraocular pressure in persons with open-angle glaucoma is usually treated pharmacologically or, in cases where pharmacologic treatment fails, by increasing aqueous outflow through a surgically created pathway. Drugs used in the long-term management of glaucoma fall into five classes: β-adrenergic antagonists, prostaglandin analogs, α-adrenergic agonists, carbonic anhydrase inhibitors, and cholinergic agonists.[34,37] Most glaucoma drugs are applied topically as eye drops. Topical β-adrenergic antagonists, which are thought to lower intraocular pressure by decreasing aqueous humor production, are usually the drugs of first choice. Prostaglandin analogs, which increase the outflow of aqueous humor through the iris root and ciliary body, are highly effective first-line or adjuvant agents.[34] The α-adrenergic agonists cause an early decrease in production of aqueous humor by constricting the vessels supplying the ciliary body. Carbonic anhydrase inhibitors reduce the secretion of aqueous humor. Cholinergic drugs, which exert their effects by increasing the effects of acetylcholine (a postganglionic neurotransmitter for the parasympathetic nervous system), increase aqueous outflow through contraction of the ciliary muscle and pupillary constriction.

When a reduction in intraocular pressure cannot be maintained through pharmacologic methods, laser or surgical trabeculoplasty may become necessary.[34] With laser trabeculoplasty, the microburns created by the laser treatment scar rather than penetrate the trabecular meshwork, a process thought to enlarge the outflow channels by increasing the tension exerted on the trabecular meshwork. Cryotherapy, diathermy, and high-frequency ultrasound may be used in some cases to destroy the ciliary epithelium and reduce aqueous humor production.

Angle-Closure Glaucoma

Angle-closure glaucoma results from occlusion of the iridocorneal angle itself, impairing access to the drainage aqueous humor (see Fig. 38-11C). An acute attack is often precipitated by pupillary dilation, which causes the iris to thicken, thus blocking the circulation between the posterior and anterior chambers.[6,25,34,35] Angle-closure glaucoma usually occurs as the result of an inherited anatomic defect that causes a shallow anterior chamber. It is more commonly seen in people of Asian or Inuit (Eskimo) descent and in people with hyperopia. This defect becomes exaggerated in older adults as the peripheral iris is anteriorly displaced by the increase in lens thickness that occurs with aging.

Clinical Manifestations. Manifestations of acute angle-closure glaucoma are related to sudden, intermittent increases in intraocular pressure. These occur after prolonged periods in the dark, emotional upset, and other conditions that cause extensive and prolonged dilation of the pupil. Administration of pharmacologic agents, such as atropine, that cause pupillary dilation (mydriasis) also can precipitate an acute episode. Attacks of increased intraocular pressure are manifested by ocular pain and blurred or iridescent vision caused by corneal edema. The pupil may be enlarged and fixed. Symptoms are often spontaneously relieved by sleep and conditions that promote pupillary constriction. With repeated or prolonged attacks, the eye becomes reddened, and edema of the cornea may develop, giving the cornea a hazy appearance. A unilateral, often excruciating, headache is common. Nausea and vomiting may occur, causing the headache to be confused with migraine.

Subacute angle-closure glaucoma is characterized by short episodes of elevated intraocular pressure that subside spontaneously. There are recurrent short episodes of unilateral pain, conjunctival redness, and blurring of vision associated with halos around lights. Attacks often occur in the evenings and resolve overnight.[34] Examination between attacks may show only a narrow anterior chamber angle. Although the episodes resolve spontaneously, there is accumulated damage to the anterior chamber angle. Subacute angle closure may also progress to acute angle closure.

Diagnosis and Treatment. Acute angle-closure glaucoma is an ophthalmic emergency that must be differentiated from conjunctivitis, uveitis, or corneal disorders. Treatment is initially directed at reducing the intraocular pressure, usually with pharmacologic agents. Once the intraocular pressure is under control, a laser peripheral iridotomy may be performed to create a permanent opening between the anterior and posterior chambers, allowing the aqueous humor to bypass the pupillary block. The anatomic abnormalities responsible for angle-closure glaucoma are usually bilateral, and prophylactic surgery is often performed on the other eye.

 ## Congenital and Infantile Glaucoma

Infantile (congenital) glaucoma is defined as glaucoma that begins within the first 3 years of life.[34,38] It can occur as a primary or secondary condition. Primary infantile glaucoma is caused by an isolated anomaly in development of the anterior chamber. In secondary glaucoma, other ocular defects or systemic disorders are present.

The clinical manifestations of infantile glaucoma include excessive lacrimation (tearing), conjunctival injection (redness of the eye), photophobia (sensitivity to light), and blepharospasm (eyelid squeezing). Affected infants tend to be fussy, have poor eating habits, and rub their eyes frequently. Because the sclera and cornea are more elastic in early childhood than later in life, chronic elevation of the intraocular pressure causes enlargement of the entire optic globe, including the cornea, and development of what is termed *buphthalmos* ("ox eye"). Diffuse edema of the cornea usually occurs, giving the eye a grayish-white appearance. Children with unilateral glaucoma generally present earlier because differences in the corneal size between the two eyes can be noticed. When both eyes are affected, the parents may not recognize the increased corneal size. Early surgical treatment is necessary to prevent blindness. Many children require several surgeries, as well as long-term medical therapy to maintain a lowering of their intraocular pressure.

Disorders of Neural Pathways and Cortical Centers

Full visual function requires the normally developed brain-related functions of photoreception and the pupillary reflex. These functions depend on the integrity of all visual pathways, including retinal circuitry and the pathway from the optic nerve to the visual cortex and other visual regions of the brain and brain stem.[16,24]

Visual information is carried to the brain by axons of the retinal ganglion cells, which form the optic nerve. The two optic nerves meet and fuse in the optic chiasm, beyond which they are continued as the optic tracts (Fig. 38-13). In the optic chiasm, axons from the nasal retina of each eye cross to the opposite side and join with the axons of the temporal retina of the contralateral eye to form the optic tracts.

Fibers of the optic tracts synapse in the lateral geniculate nucleus (LGN) of the thalamus. Axons from neurons in the LGN form the optic radiations that travel to the primary visual cortex in the occipital lobe. The pattern of information transmission established in the optic tract is retained in the optic radiations. For example, the axons from the right visual field, represented by the nasal retina of the right eye and the temporal retina of the left eye, are united at the chiasm. They continue through the left optic tract and left optic radiation to the left visual cortex (area 17), which is located in the occipital lobe of the brain (Fig. 38-14). Immediately surrounding the visual cortex are the visual association cortices (areas 18 and 19), which function in adding meaningfulness to the visual experience.

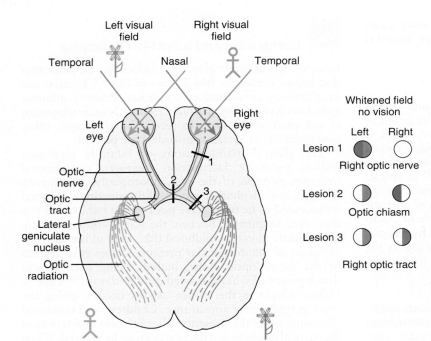

FIGURE 38-13. Diagram of optic pathways. The *red lines* indicate the right visual field and the *blue lines* the left visual field. Note the crossing of fibers from the medial half of each retina at the optic chiasm. Lesion 1 (right optic nerve) produces unilateral blindness. Lesion 2 (optic chiasm) may involve only those fibers that originate in the nasal half of each retina and cross to the opposite side in the optic chiasm; visual loss involves the temporal half of each field (bi-temporal hemianopia). Lesion 3 (right optic tract) interrupts fibers (and vision) originating on the same side of both eyes (homonymous), with loss of vision from half of each field (hemianopia).

The visual field refers to the area that is visible during fixation of vision in one direction[16,22,24] (see Fig. 38-13). As with a camera, the simple lens system of the eye inverts the image of the external world on each retina. In addition, the right and left sides of the visual field also are reversed. Most of the visual field is binocular, with both eyes focusing on one object and then fusing two images into one. The right binocular visual field (the nasal half of the right eye and the temporal half of the left eye) is seen by the left retinal halves of each eye. Likewise, the left binocular field is seen by the right retinal halves of each eye. This binocular field is subdivided into central and peripheral portions. Central portions of the retina provide high visual acuity and correspond to the field focused on the central fovea. The peripheral and surrounding portion provides the capacity to detect objects, particularly moving objects. Beyond the visual field shared by both eyes, the left lateral periphery of the visual field is seen exclusively by the left nasal retina, and the right peripheral field by the right nasal retina.

Disorders of the Optic Pathways

Among the disorders that can interrupt the visual pathway are trauma, tumors, and vascular lesions. Trauma and tumors can produce direct injury or impinge on the optic pathways. Vascular insufficiency in any one of the arterial systems of the retina or visual pathways can seriously affect vision. For example, normal visual function depends on the adequacy of blood flow in the ophthalmic artery and its branches—the central retinal artery; the anterior and middle cerebral arteries, which supply the intracranial optic nerve, chiasm, and optic tracts; and the posterior cerebral artery, which supplies the LGN, optic radiation, and visual cortex. The adequacy of posterior cerebral artery function depends on that of the vertebral and basilar arteries that supply the brain stem.

Visual Field Defects

Visual field defects result from damage to the visual pathways or the visual cortex (see Fig. 38-13). The testing of the visual fields of each eye and of the two eyes together is useful in localizing lesions affecting the system. Perimetry or visual field testing, in which the visual field of each eye is measured and plotted in an arc, is used to identify defects and determine the location of lesions.

Blindness in one eye is called *anopia*. If half of the visual field for one eye is lost, the defect is called *hemianopia*; if a quarter of the field is lost, it is called *quadrantanopia*. Loss of the temporal or peripheral visual fields on both sides results in a narrow binocular field, commonly called *tunnel vision*. The loss of different

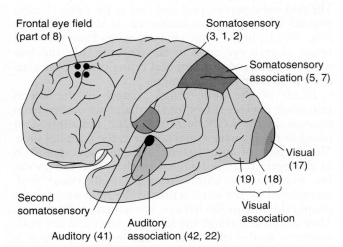

FIGURE 38-14. Lateral view of the cortex illustrating the location of the visual, visual association, auditory, and auditory association areas.

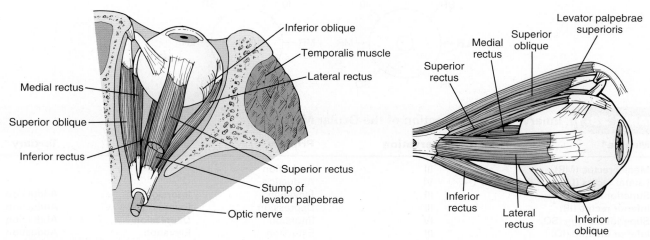

FIGURE 38-15. Extraocular muscles of the right eye.

half-fields in the two eyes is called a *heteronymous loss,* and the abnormality is called *heteronymous hemianopia.* Destruction of one or both lateral halves of the chiasm is common with multiple aneurysms of the circle of Willis (see Chapter 37). In this condition, the function of one or both temporal retinas is lost, and the nasal fields of one or both eyes are lost. The loss of the temporal fields (nasal retina) of both eyes is called *bitemporal heteronymous anopia.* With both eyes open, the person with bilateral defects still has the full binocular visual field.

Loss of the optic tract, LGN, full optic radiation, or complete visual cortex on one side results in loss of the corresponding visual half-fields in each eye. *Homonymous* means "the same" for both eyes. In left-side lesions, the right visual field is lost for each eye and is called *complete right homonymous hemianopia.* Partial injury to the left optic tract, LGN, or optic radiation can result in the loss of a quarter of the visual field in both eyes. This is called *homonymous quadrantanopia,* and depending on the lesion it can involve the upper (superior) or lower (inferior) fields. The LGN, optic radiation, and visual cortex all receive their major blood supply from the posterior cerebral artery; unilateral occlusion of this artery results in complete loss of the opposite field (i.e., homonymous hemianopia). Bilateral occlusion of these arteries results in total cortical blindness.

The Extraocular Eye Muscles and Disorders of Eye Movement

For complete function of the eyes, it is necessary that the two eyes point toward the same fixation point and that the retinal and central nervous system (CNS) visual acuity mechanisms are functional. Despite slight variations in the view of the external world for each eye, it is important that these two images become fused, which is a forebrain function. Binocular fusion is controlled by ocular reflex mechanisms that adjust the orientation of each eye to produce a single image. If these reflexes fail, *diplopia* or double vision occurs.

Binocular vision depends on three pairs of extraocular muscles—the medial and lateral recti, the superior and inferior recti, and the superior and inferior obliques[16] (Fig. 38-15). Each of the three sets of muscles in each eye is reciprocally innervated so that one muscle relaxes when the other contracts. Reciprocal contraction of the medial and lateral recti moves the eye from side to side (adduction and abduction); the superior and inferior recti move the eye up and down (elevation and depression). The oblique muscles rotate (intorsion and extorsion) the eye around its optic axis. A seventh muscle, the levator palpebrae superioris, elevates the upper eye lid.

The extraocular muscles are innervated by three cranial nerves. The trochlear nerve (CN IV) innervates the superior oblique, the abducens nerve (CN VI) innervates the lateral rectus, and the oculomotor nerve (CN III) innervates the remaining four muscles. Table 38-1 describes the function and innervation of the extraocular muscles.

Normal vision depends on the coordinated action of the entire visual system and a number of central control systems. It is through these mechanisms that an object is simultaneously imaged on the fovea of both eyes and perceived as a single image. Strabismus and amblyopia are two disorders that affect this highly integrated system.

 Strabismus

Strabismus, or squint, refers to any abnormality of eye coordination or alignment that results in loss of binocular vision. Strabismus affects approximately 4% of children younger than 6 years of age.[39–41] Because 30% to 50% of these children sustain permanent secondary loss of vision, or amblyopia (to be discussed), early diagnosis and treatment are essential.

Strabismus may be divided into two forms: paralytic, in which there is weakness or paralysis of one or more of the extraocular muscles; and nonparalytic, in which there is no primary muscle impairment. In terms of

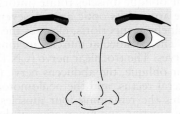

TABLE 38-1 Innervation and Function of the Ocular Muscles

Muscle*	CN Innervation	Primary	Secondary	Tertiary
Medial rectus (MR)	III	Adduction		
Lateral rectus (LR)	VI	Abduction		
Superior rectus (SR)	III	Elevation	Intorsion	Adduction
Inferior rectus (IR)	III	Depression	Extorsion	Adduction
Superior oblique (SO)	IV	Intorsion	Depression	Abduction
Inferior oblique (IO)	III	Extorsion	Elevation	Abduction

*In the schema of the functional roles of the six extraocular muscles, the major directional force applied by each muscle is indicated on the top. These muscles are arranged in functionally opposing pairs per eye and in parallel opposing pairs for conjugate movements of the two eyes. CN, cranial nerve.

standard terminology, the disorders of eye movement are described according to the direction of movement. *Esotropia* refers to medial deviation, *exotropia* to lateral deviation, *hypertropia* to upward deviation, *hypotropia* to downward deviation, and *cyclotropia* to torsional deviation (Fig. 38-16).

Nonparalytic Strabismus. Nonparalytic esotropia is the most common type of strabismus. The individual ocular muscles have no obvious defect and the amount of deviation is constant or relatively constant in the various directions of gaze. With persistent deviation, secondary abnormalities may develop because of

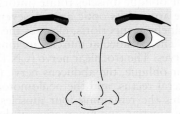

A Primary position: right esotropia

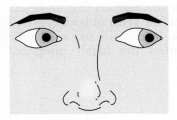

B Left gaze: no deviation

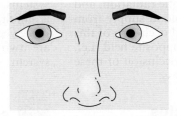

C Right gaze: left esotropia

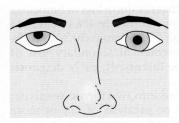

D Right hypertropia

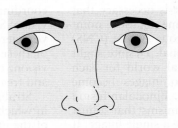

E Right exotropia

FIGURE 38-16. (A–C) Paralytic strabismus associated with paralysis of the right lateral rectus muscle: **(A)** primary position of the eyes (looking straight ahead); **(B)** left gaze with no deviation; **(C)** right gaze with left esotropia. **(D)** Primary position of the eyes with weakness of the right inferior rectus and right hypertropia. **(E)** Primary position of the eyes with weakness of the right medial rectus and right exotropia.

overactivity or underactivity of the extraocular muscles in some fields of gaze.

The disorder may be nonaccommodative, accommodative, or a combination of the two. Infantile esotropia is the most common cause of nonaccommodative strabismus. It occurs in the first 6 months of life, with large-angle deviations, in otherwise developmentally and neurologically normal infants. Eye movements are full, and the child often uses each eye independently to alter fixation (cross-fixation). The cause of the disorder is unclear. Research suggests that idiopathic strabismus may have a genetic basis, since siblings often present with similar disorders. Accommodative strabismus is caused by disorders such as uncorrected hyperopia of a significant degree, in which the esotropia occurs with accommodation that is undertaken to focus clearly. Onset of this type of esotropia characteristically occurs between 18 months and 4 years of age because accommodation is not well developed until that time. The disorder most often is monocular but may be alternating.

Paralytic Strabismus. Paralytic strabismus results from paresis (i.e., weakness) or plegia (i.e., paralysis) of one or more of the extraocular muscles. When the normal eye fixates, the affected eye is in the position of primary deviation. In the case of esotropia, there is weakness of one of the lateral rectus muscles. When the affected eye fixates, the unaffected eye is in a position of secondary deviation.[39]

Paralytic strabismus is uncommon in children but accounts for nearly all cases of adult strabismus; it can be caused by infiltrative processes (e.g., Graves disease; see Chapter 32), myasthenia gravis, stroke, and direct optical trauma.[38] In infants, paralytic strabismus can be caused by birth injuries affecting the extraocular muscles or the cranial nerves supplying these muscles. In general, binocular vision can be maintained when paralytic strabismus is corrected.

Treatment. Treatment of strabismus is directed toward the development of normal visual acuity, correction of the deviation, and superimposition of the retinal images to provide binocular vision. Early and adequate treatment is crucial because a delay in or lack of treatment can lead to amblyopia and permanent loss of vision.

Treatment includes both surgical and nonsurgical methods. Infantile esotropia is usually treated surgically by weakening the medial rectus muscle on each eye while the infant is under general anesthesia. Recurrences are common with infantile esotropia, and multiple surgeries are often required.

Nonsurgical treatment includes glasses, occlusive patching, and eye exercises (i.e., pleoptics). Glasses are often used in the treatment of accommodative esotropia that occurs with hypermetropia. Because accommodation is linked with convergence, focusing drives the eyes inward, producing esotropia. In infants and toddlers, intermittent exotropia is commonly treated with patching for 1 to 2 hours daily for several months. The use of over-minus glasses stimulates accommodative convergences, which contracts the exotropic drift. Vision therapy involves

exercises to stimulate convergence and techniques to train the visual system to recognize the suppressed images. Surgical treatment of intermittent exotropia is indicted when conservative methods fail to correct the deviation. Early treatment of children with intermittent exotropia is not as crucial as it is for those with constant deviations because stereopsis can still develop.

A relatively new form of treatment involves the injection of botulinum toxin type A (Botox) into the extraocular muscle to produce paralysis of that extraocular muscle.[39] Paralysis of the muscle shifts the eye into the field of action of the antagonist muscle. During the time the eye is deviated, the paralyzed muscle is stretched, whereas the antagonistic muscle is contracted. Usually two or more injections of the drug are necessary to obtain a lasting effect.

 ## Amblyopia

Amblyopia, sometimes called *lazy eye,* describes a decrease in visual acuity resulting from abnormal visual development in infancy or early childhood.[42–44] It is the most common cause of monocular visual impairment, affecting 1% to 4% of the population. With early detection and treatment, most cases of amblyopia are reversible and the most severe forms of the condition can be prevented.

Normal development of the thalamic and cortical circuitry necessary for binocular visual perception requires simultaneous binocular use of each fovea during a critical period early in life (0 to 5 years). Amblyopia can result from visual deprivation (e.g., cataracts, ptosis) or abnormal binocular interactions (e.g., strabismus, anisometropia) during visual immaturity. In infants with unilateral cataracts that are dense, central, and larger than 2 mm in diameter, this period is before 2 months of age.[15,21] In conditions causing abnormal binocular interactions, one image is suppressed to provide clearer vision. In esotropia, vision of the deviated eye is suppressed to prevent diplopia. A similar situation exists in anisometropia, in which the refractive indexes of the two eyes are different. Although the eyes are correctly aligned, they are unable to focus together, and the image of one eye is suppressed.

The reversibility of amblyopia depends on the maturity of the visual system at the time of onset and the duration of the abnormal experience. Occasionally in strabismus, some persons alternate eye fixation and do not experience significant amblyopia or diplopia. With late adolescent or adult onset, this habit pattern must be unlearned after correction. Amblyopia is remarkably responsive to treatment if the treatment is initiated early in life; thus, all infants and young children should be evaluated for visual conditions that could lead to amblyopia.

The American Academy of Pediatrics in association with the American Association of Certified Orthoptists, American Association of Pediatric Ophthalmology and Strabismus, and American Academy of Ophthalmology recommends that all newborn infants be examined in the nursery for structural abnormalities and have a red reflex test performed to check for abnormalities in the back of the eye (posterior segment) and opacities in the visual axis, such as cataracts or corneal opacity.[45] Visual examinations should then be performed during all well-child visits. These should include age-appropriate evaluation of visual acuity, ocular alignment, and ocular media clarity (cataracts, tumors).

The treatment of children at risk for development of amblyopia must be instituted well before the age of 6 years to avoid the suppression phenomenon. Surgery for congenital cataracts and ptosis should be done early. Severe refractive errors should be corrected. In children with strabismus, the alternate blocking of the vision in one eye and then the other with a patch forces the child to use both eyes for form discrimination. The duration of occlusion of vision in the good eye must be short (2 to 4 hours per day) and closely monitored, or deprivation amblyopia can develop in the good eye as well.

SUMMARY CONCEPTS

- The eyeball, or optic globe, which is a complex sensory organ that provides the sense of vision, is protected posteriorly by the bony structures of the orbital cavity and anteriorly by the eyelids. The eyeball is composed of three layers: an outer layer, which includes the white, opaque sclera and the transparent cornea; a middle vascular layer called the *uvea*, which includes the choroid, ciliary body, and iris; and an inner neural layer, which includes an outer pigment epithelium and the inner, light-sensitive retina, which is connected to the optic nerve.

- A conjunctiva lines the inner surface of the eyelids and covers the eyeball to the junction of the cornea and sclera. Conjunctivitis, also called *red eye* or *pink eye,* may result from bacterial or viral infection, allergic reactions, or the injurious effects of chemical agents, physical agents, or radiant energy.

- Keratitis, or inflammation of the cornea, can be caused by infections, hypersensitivity reactions, ischemia, defects in tearing, or trauma. Trauma or disease that involves the stromal layer of the cornea heals with scar formation and permanent opacification. These opacities interfere with the transmission of light and may impair vision.

- The lens is a biconvex, transparent, flexible structure that can change shape to allow precise focusing of light on the retina. Refraction refers to the ability of the lens to bend light rays in order to focus an object on the retina. In *hyperopia,* or farsightedness, the image falls behind the retina, and in *myopia,* or nearsightedness, it falls in front of the retina. Accommodation is the process by which a clear image is maintained as the gaze is shifted from a far object to a near object. *Presbyopia* is a change in the lens that occurs because of aging such that the lens becomes thicker and less able to change shape and accommodate for near vision. A cataract is characterized by increased lens opacity.

- The retina covers the inner aspect of the posterior two thirds of the eyeball and is continuous with the optic nerve. It contains the photoreceptors for vision: the rods, for black and white discrimination, and the cones, for color vision. The *retinopathies* are visual disorders involving the small blood vessels of the retina, which can result from a number of local and systemic disorders, including diabetes mellitus and hypertension. *Retinal detachment* involves separation of the sensory receptors from their blood supply; it causes blindness unless reattachment is accomplished promptly. *Macular degeneration,* which is a leading cause of blindness in the elderly, is characterized by loss of central vision resulting from destructive changes in the central fovea.

- Glaucoma is a chronic, degenerative visual field loss usually associated with an increase in intraocular pressure due to impaired outflow of aqueous humor from the anterior chamber of the eye. Glaucoma is commonly classified as *open-angle glaucoma,* in which impaired outflow of aqueous humor is due to dysfunction of the drainage system, and *angle-closure glaucoma,* in which occlusion of the anterior chamber angle impairs access to the drainage system.

- Eye movement, which is controlled by the extraocular muscles, provides for alignment of the eyes and binocular vision. *Strabismus,* which involves abnormalities in coordination of eye movements, can be caused by weakness or paralysis of the extraocular muscles (paralytic strabismus), inappropriate length or insertion of the extraocular muscles (nonparalytic strabismus), or accommodation disorders. The neural pathways for vision develop during infancy. *Amblyopia* is a condition of diminished vision that results from inadequately developed CNS circuitry due to visual deprivation or abnormal binocular interactions during the period of visual immaturity.

The Ear and Disorders of Auditory Function

The ears are paired organs consisting of an external and middle ear, which function in capturing, transmitting, and amplifying sound; and an inner ear, which contains the receptive organs that are stimulated by sound waves (i.e., hearing) or head position and movement (i.e., balance).

Disorders of the External Ear

The external ear is a funnel-shaped structure that conducts sound waves to the tympanic membrane. It consists of the auricle, the external acoustic meatus (ear canal), and the lateral surface of the tympanic membrane[2,46] (Fig. 38-17). Modified sebaceous glands in the auditory canal secrete a waxlike substance called *cerumen* or *earwax* that has certain antimicrobial properties and is thought to serve a protective function.

The tympanic membrane or eardrum is a thin, transparent membrane, approximately 1 cm in diameter, which separates the external ear from the middle ear. It is covered with thin skin externally and the mucous membrane of the middle ear internally. The tympanic membrane is attached in a manner that allows it to vibrate freely when audible sound waves enter the external auditory canal. Movements of the membrane are transmitted through the middle ear to the inner ear.

Impacted Cerumen

Although the ear normally is self-cleaning, the cerumen can accumulate in the narrow ear canal, causing reversible hearing loss.[47] Impacted cerumen usually produces no symptoms unless it hardens and touches the tympanic membrane, or the canal becomes irritated by a buildup of hardened cerumen, causing pain, itching, and a sensation of fullness. As the canal becomes completely occluded, there may be a feeling of fullness, a conductive hearing loss, and tinnitus (i.e., ringing in the ears).

In most cases, cerumen can be removed by gentle irrigation using a bulb syringe and warm tap water. Alternatively, health care professionals may remove cerumen using an otoscope for guidance along with a wire loop or plastic cerumen curette. A ceruminolytic agent is usually reserved for impacted or hardened cerumen that occurs without ear discharge, pain, rash, or irritation.

Otitis Externa

Otitis externa is an inflammation of the external ear that can vary in severity from mild dermatitis to severe cellulitis.[46,48] It can be caused by infectious agents, irritation (e.g., wearing hearing aids or earphones), or allergic reactions. Predisposing factors include frequent exposure to moisture in the ear canal (i.e., swimmer's ear), trauma to the canal caused by cleaning or scratching, and allergies or skin conditions such as psoriasis. It commonly occurs in the summer and is manifested by itching, redness, tenderness, and narrowing of the ear canal because of swelling. Inflammation of the auricle or ear canal makes movement of the ear painful. There may be watery or purulent drainage and intermittent hearing loss.

Treatment usually includes the use of ear drops containing an appropriate antimicrobial or antifungal agent in combination with a corticosteroid to reduce inflammation.[48] Persons with acute otitis externa (AOE) should preferably abstain from water sports, protect the

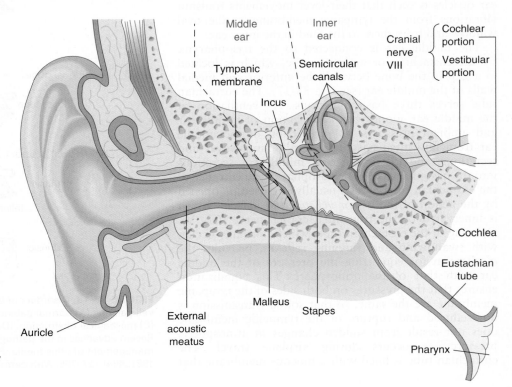

FIGURE 38-17. External, middle, and internal subdivisions of the ear.

ear if showering, and limit insertion of hearing aids or ear phones until pain or discharge subside.

Persistent external otitis in diabetic or immunocompromised persons may evolve into osteomyelitis of the skull base, often called *malignant external otitis*.[48] Usually caused by *Pseudomonas aeruginosa*, it begins in the floor of the ear canal, and may extend to the middle fossa floor, and even to the contralateral skull base. Persons with the disorder usually present with complaints of severe pain, foul-smelling ear discharge, fever, granulation tissue in the ear canal, possibly vertigo (dizziness), and in advanced cases, cranial nerve palsies. Diagnosis is confirmed by demonstration of osseous involvement on CT and radionuclide imaging.

Disorders of the Middle Ear and Eustachian Tube

The middle ear, or tympanic cavity, is a small, air-filled, mucosa-lined cavity in the petrous portion of the temporal bone[2,46] (see Fig. 38-17). It is bounded anteriorly by the tympanic membrane, and spanned by three tiny bones, the *auditory ossicles*, which are connected by two synovial joints and are covered with the epithelial lining of the cavity. There are two openings in the medial wall of the middle ear—the oval (vestibular) window and the round (cochlear) window—that communicate with the inner ear.

The three auditory ossicles (the malleus, the incus, and the stapes) connect the tympanic membrane with the oval window.[2,46] The *malleus* ("hammer") has its handle firmly fixed to the upper portion of the tympanic membrane. The head of the malleus articulates with the *incus* ("anvil"), which links the malleus to the *stapes* ("stirrup"), whose footplate fits into the oval window. Arrangement of the ear ossicles is such that their lever movements transmit vibrations from the tympanic membrane to the oval window and from there to the fluid in the inner ear.

The middle ear is connected to the nasopharynx by the eustachian or auditory tube, which is located in a gap in the bone between the anterior and medial walls of the middle ear (see Fig. 38-17). The eustachian tube serves three basic functions: (1) ventilation of the middle ear, along with equalization of middle ear and ambient pressures; (2) protection of the middle ear from unwanted nasopharyngeal sound waves and secretions; and (3) drainage of middle ear secretions into the nasopharynx.[49] The nasopharyngeal entrance to the eustachian tube, which usually is closed, is opened by the action of the *tensor veli palatini muscle*, which is innervated by the trigeminal cranial nerve (CN V). Opening of the eustachian tube, which normally occurs with swallowing and yawning reflexes, provides the mechanism for equalizing the pressure of the middle ear with that of the atmosphere. This equalization ensures that the pressures on both sides of the tympanic membrane are the same, so that sound transmission is not reduced and rupture of the tympanic membrane does not result from sudden changes in atmospheric pressure, as occurs during airplane travel. The eustachian tube is lined with a mucous membrane that

is continuous posteriorly with the tympanic cavity and anteriorly with that of the nasopharynx. Infections from the nasopharynx can travel from the nasopharynx along the mucous membrane of the eustachian tube to the middle ear, causing acute otitis media. Toward the nasopharynx, the eustachian tube becomes lined by columnar epithelium with mucus-secreting cells. Hypertrophy of these mucus-secreting cells is thought to contribute to the mucoid secretions that develop during certain types of otitis media.

Eustachian Tube Disorders

Abnormalities in eustachian tube function are important factors in the pathogenesis of middle ear infections. There are two important types of eustachian tube dysfunction: abnormal patency and obstruction (Fig. 38-18). The *abnormally patent tube* either does not close or does not close completely. In infants and children with an abnormally patent tube, air and secretions often are pumped into the eustachian tube during crying and nose blowing.

Obstruction can be functional or mechanical. *Functional obstruction* results from the persistent collapse of the eustachian tube due to a lack of tubal stiffness or poor function of the tensor veli palatini muscle that controls the opening of the eustachian tube (see Fig. 38-18B). It is common in infants and young children because the amount and stiffness of the cartilage supporting the eustachian tube are less than in older children and adults. Changes in the structure

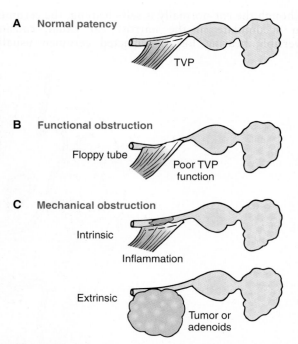

FIGURE 38-18. Disorders of the eustachian tube. TVP, tensor veli palatini: **(A)** normal patency, **(B)** functional obstruction, **(C)** mechanical obstruction. (Developed from Bluestone CD. Recent advances in the pathogenesis, diagnosis, and management of otitis media. *Pediatr Clin North Am.* 1981;28(4):727–755. With permission from Elsevier Science.)

of the craniofacial base also render the tensor muscle less efficient for opening the eustachian tube in this age group. In addition, craniofacial disorders, such as a cleft palate, alter the attachment of the tensor muscle, producing functional obstruction of the eustachian tube.

Mechanical obstruction results from internal obstruction or external compression of the eustachian tube (see Fig. 38-18C). Ethnic differences in the structure of the palate may increase the likelihood of obstruction. The most common internal obstruction is caused by swelling and secretions resulting from allergy and viral respiratory infections. With obstruction, air in the middle ear is absorbed, causing a negative pressure and the transudation of serous capillary fluid into the middle ear.

Otitis Media

Otitis media (OM) refers to inflammation of the middle ear without reference to etiology or pathogenesis (Fig. 38-19A). Inflammation of the middle ear may present as acute otitis media or otitis media with effusion.[50–52] Acute otitis media (AOM) refers to the rapid onset of signs and symptoms of a middle ear infection. Otitis media with effusion (OME) refers to inflammation of the middle ear with the presence of fluid in the middle ear without signs and symptoms of an acute ear infection.[53] It is important to differentiate OME from AOM to avoid unnecessary use of antimicrobial agents.

Risk Factors. Otitis media may occur in any age group, but is seen most frequently in infants and young children between the ages of 3 months and 3 years, with the peak incidence between 6 and 11 months.[51] There is a second peak incidence at about 5 years of age that is believed to be associated with entrance into school.[50] Risk factors include premature birth, male gender, ethnicity (Native American, Inuit), family history of recurrent OM, presence of siblings in the household, genetic syndromes, and low socioeconomic status.[51] It is more frequent in children with orofacial abnormalities such as cleft lip and palate.

The most important factor that contributes to OM is believed to be a dysfunction of the eustachian tube that allows reflux of fluid and bacteria into the middle ear from the nasopharynx. There are two reasons for the increased risk of OM in infants and young children: the eustachian tube is shorter, more horizontal, and wider in this age group than in older children and adults; and infection can spread more easily through the eustachian canal of infants who spend most of their day in the supine position.[51] Bottle-fed infants have a higher incidence of OM than breast-fed infants, probably because they are held in a more horizontal position during feeding, and swallowing while in the horizontal position facilitates the reflux of milk into the middle ear. Breast-feeding also provides for the transfer of protective maternal antibodies to the infant.

Measures to reduce the risk for development of OM during the first 6 months of life include breast-feeding, avoidance or elimination of bottle propping, and reduction or elimination of pacifier use.[51] Other ways

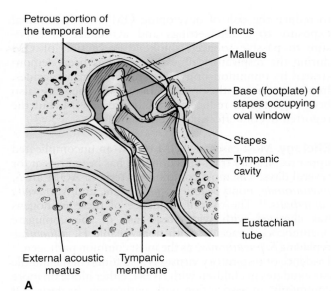

A

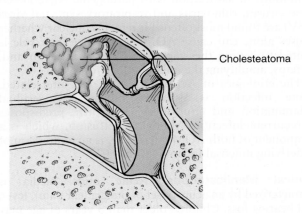

B

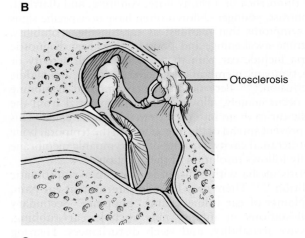

C

FIGURE 38-19. Disorders of the middle ear. **(A)** Otitis media. Otitis involves inflammation of the tympanic cavity. Infection often enters through the eustachian tube. **(B)** Cholesteatoma, a cystlike mass of the middle ear that often extends to involve the temporal bone. **(C)** Otosclerosis involving formation of new, spongy bone around the stapes and oval window.

to reduce the risk of developing OM include minimal exposure to group settings and avoidance of exposure to passive tobacco smoke.[51] Prevention of OM during the respiratory illness season has been demonstrated by immunoprophylaxis with influenza vaccines. Immunization with pneumococcal vaccine has also been reported to reduce the incidence of OM, but the reported overall effect has been small.[51,52]

Etiology. Most cases of AOM follow an uncomplicated upper respiratory tract infection that has been present for several days. The most common bacteria in AOM are *S. pneumoniae*, nontypeable *H. influenzae*, and *Moraxella catarrhalis*.[51] The overall incidence of these pathogens has changed with widespread use of the conjugate pneumococcal vaccine, with nontypeable *H. influenzae* replacing *S. pneumoniae* as the most common pathogen.[51] Evidence of respiratory viruses is also found in the middle ear exudates in children with AOM, either alone or, more commonly, in association with pathogenic bacteria. Of these viruses, rhinovirus and respiratory syncytial virus (RSV) are found most often.[51] It remains unclear whether viruses alone can cause AOM or whether their role is limited to setting the stage for bacterial invasion and, perhaps, amplifying the inflammatory response.

The etiologies of AOM and OME are interrelated. Acute infection is usually followed by residual inflammation and effusion that, in turn, predisposes to recurrent infection. Middle ear effusion, which is a component of both AOM and OME, is an expression of underlying mucosal inflammation.

Clinical Manifestations. Acute otitis media is characterized by an acute onset of otalgia (ear pain), fever, and hearing loss. Children older than 3 years of age may have rhinorrhea or a runny nose, vomiting, and diarrhea. In contrast, younger children often have nonspecific signs and symptoms that manifest as ear tugging, irritability, nighttime awakening, and poor feeding. Key diagnostic criteria include ear pain that interferes with activity or sleep, tympanic membrane erythema (redness), and middle ear effusion.[50–52] Perforation of the tympanic membrane may occur acutely, allowing purulent material from the middle ear to drain into the external auditory canal. This may prevent spread of the infection into the temporal bone or intracranial cavity. Healing of the tympanic membrane usually follows resolution of the infection.

Otitis media with effusion is often an asymptomatic condition.[51,53] There may be mild intermittent ear pain, complaints of ear fullness, and "popping." Secondary manifestations in infants may include ear rubbing, excessive irritability, and sleep disturbances. Hearing loss, even when not suggested by the child, is evidenced by a seeming lack of attentiveness, behavioral changes, and failure to respond to conversation-level speech. There may be problems related to school performance, balance problems and unexplained clumsiness, or delayed speech and language development.[52] The duration of the effusion may range from less than 3 weeks to more than 3 months. Many cases of OME resolve spontaneously, but 30% to 40% of children have recurrent OME, and 5% to 10% of episodes last 1 year or longer.[52]

Diagnosis. The diagnosis of OM is based on recent and usually acute onset of symptoms, presence of middle ear effusion, and signs and symptoms of middle ear inflammation, including erythema or redness with mild bulging of the tympanic membrane and otalgia or ear pain. Younger, nonverbal children with OM may present with holding, tugging, or rubbing of the ear. Nonspecific symptoms may include excessive crying, fever, or changes in sleep or behavior patterns.[54] Other evidence of infection includes mild bulging of the tympanic membrane, onset of ear pain of less than 48 hours, or intense redness of the tympanic membrane.

Both AOM without otorrhea (drainage from the ear) and OME are accompanied by otoscopic signs of middle ear effusion—namely, the presence of at least two of three tympanic membrane abnormalities: white, yellow, amber, or occasionally blue discoloration; opacification other than scarring; and decreased or absent motility. With OME the tympanic membrane is often cloudy with distinct impairment of mobility, and an air–fluid level or bubble may be visible in the middle ear. The overall importance of distinguishing normal ear status from AOM versus OME is avoidance of unnecessary use of antibiotics along with the potential of adverse effects and antimicrobial resistance.

The diagnosis of AOM can also be confirmed using tympanometry or acoustic reflectometry. A *tympanogram* is obtained by using a small probe that is placed snugly into the external ear canal. A sound stimulus generator then transmits acoustic energy into the canal, while a vacuum pump introduces positive and negative pressures into the ear canal. A microphone in the instrument detects returning sound energy. The tympanogram provides a determination of the degree of negative pressure present in the middle ear. It detects disease when present but is less reliable when disease is absent. *Acoustic reflectometry* detects reflected sound waves from the middle ear and provides information on whether an effusion is absent or present. Increased reflected sound correlates with an increased likelihood of effusion. This technique is most useful in children older than 3 months, and its success depends on user technique.

Tympanocentesis (puncture of the tympanic membrane with a needle) may be done to relieve pain from an effusion or to obtain a specimen of middle ear fluid for culture and sensitivity testing. In instances where the tympanic membrane has perforated with resultant drainage into the external ear, a specimen can be obtained and microbiologic studies can be done to identify the organism.

Treatment. The treatment of AOM focuses on symptom control and management of the underlying pathologic process. A number of options for pain management are available, including the local application of heat and use of analgesic drugs such as acetaminophen and ibuprofen.[51] Myringotomy (incision in the tympanic membrane) can be used for relief of pressure in the child with severe pain, providing almost immediate relief.

The extensive use of antimicrobial agents contributes to the development of bacterial resistance. Observation without antimicrobial agents is an option in a child with uncomplicated AOM. This approach involves joint decision making between the clinician and parents, a system for close follow-up, and beginning antibiotics if symptoms worsen or there is no improvement within 48 to 72 hours.[52]

Most cases of OME resolve spontaneously within a 3-week to 3-month period. The management options for this duration include observation only, antimicrobial therapy, or combination antimicrobial and corticosteroid therapy.[52,54] A hearing evaluation is recommended when OME persists for 3 months or longer or at any time that language delay, learning problems, or a significant hearing loss is suspected. Children with recurrent OM should be evaluated to rule out any anatomic variations (e.g., enlarged adenoids), allergies, and immunologic abnormalities. Referral to an otolaryngologist is indicated if the effusion persists for 4 months or longer.

Surgical treatment (e.g., tympanostomy tubes, adenoidectomy) may be indicated for OME if the effusion has persisted for 4 months or longer and is accompanied by persistent hearing loss and other manifestations; if recurrent or persistent effusion occurs in children at risk regardless of hearing status; or if there is structural damage to the tympanic membrane or middle ear.[54] Tympanostomy tube insertion is the preferred initial procedure and does not typically include the removal of adenoids unless the child has additional indications, such as postnasal obstruction from enlarged adenoids. Adenoidectomy plus myringotomy (without tube insertion) has been shown to have comparable efficacy in children 4 years of age or older but is more invasive, with additional surgical and anesthetic risks.[54]

Complications of Otitis Media. The complications of OM include hearing loss and extratemporal complications, including those affecting the middle ear, mastoid, adjacent structures of the temporal bone, and intracranial structures.

Hearing loss, which is a common complication of OM, usually is conductive and temporary based on the duration of the effusion. Hearing loss that is associated with fluid collection usually resolves when the effusion clears. Permanent hearing loss may occur as the result of damage to the tympanic membrane or other middle ear structures. Cases of sensorineural hearing loss are rare.

The mastoid antrum and air cells constitute a portion of the temporal bone and may become inflamed as an extension of acute or chronic OM.[51] The disorder causes necrosis of the mastoid process and destruction of the bony intercellular matrix, which are visible by radiologic examination. Mastoid tenderness and drainage of exudate through a perforated tympanic membrane can occur. Chronic mastoiditis can develop as the result of chronic middle ear infection. The usefulness of antimicrobial agents for this condition is limited. Mastoid or middle ear surgery, along with other medical treatment, may be indicated.

Cholesteatomas are cystlike lesions of the middle ear, usually associated with chronic otitis media (see Fig. 38-19B). Measuring 1 to 4 cm in diameter, they are lined with keratinizing squamous epithelium or mucus-secreting epithelium and filled with amorphous debris (derived largely from desquamated epithelium).[51] Although precise mechanisms involved in their development are unclear, it is proposed that chronic inflammation and perforation of the eardrum with ingrowth of squamous epithelium or metaplasia of the secretory epithelium of the middle ear are contributing factors. These lesions can erode the ossicles, the labyrinth, the adjacent mastoid bone, and the surrounding soft tissues. Although often thought of as a complication of otitis media, a cholesteatoma may also occur as a congenital condition. Symptoms commonly include painless drainage from the ear and hearing loss. Treatment involves microsurgical techniques to remove the cholesteatomatous material.

Intracranial complications are uncommon since the advent of antimicrobial therapy. Although rare, these complications can develop when the infection spreads through vascular channels, by direct extension, or through preformed pathways such as the round window.[48] These complications are seen more often with chronic suppurative OM and mastoiditis. They include otogenic meningitis, brain abscess, lateral sinus thrombophlebitis or thrombosis, labyrinthitis, and facial nerve paralysis. Any child who develops persistent headache, tinnitus, stiff neck, or visual or other neurologic symptoms should be investigated for possible intracranial complications.

Otosclerosis

Otosclerosis refers to the formation of new spongy bone around the stapes and oval window, which results in progressive deafness[55,56] (see Fig. 38-19C). In most cases, the condition is familial and follows an autosomal dominant pattern with variable penetrance. Otosclerosis may begin at any time in life but usually does not appear until after puberty, most frequently between the ages of 20 and 30 years. The disease process accelerates during pregnancy.

Otosclerosis begins with resorption of bone in one or more foci. During active bone resorption, the bone structure appears spongy and softer than normal (i.e., otospongiosis). The resorbed bone is replaced by an overgrowth of new, hard, sclerotic bone. The process is slowly progressive, involving more areas of the temporal bone, especially in front of and posterior to the stapes footplate. As it invades the footplate, the pathologic bone increasingly immobilizes the stapes, reducing the transmission of sound. Pressure of otosclerotic bone on middle ear structures or the vestibulocochlear nerve (CN VIII) may contribute to the development of sensorineural hearing loss, tinnitus, and vertigo (to be discussed).

The symptoms of otosclerosis involve an insidious conductive hearing loss. Initially, the affected person is unable to hear a whisper or someone speaking at a distance. In the earliest stages, the bone conduction by which the person's own voice is heard remains relatively unaffected. At this point, the person's own voice sounds unusually loud, and the sound of chewing becomes intensified. Because of bone conduction, most of these persons can hear fairly well on the telephone, which provides an amplified signal.

The treatment of otosclerosis can be medical or surgical. A carefully selected, well-fitting hearing aid may allow a person with conductive deafness to lead a normal life. Sodium fluoride has been used with some success in the medical treatment of otospongiosis.[55] Because much of the conductive hearing loss associated with otosclerosis is caused by stapedial fixation, surgical treatment involves stapedectomy with stapedial reconstruction using the patient's own stapes or a stapedial prosthesis.

Disorders of Inner Ear and Central Auditory Pathways

Located in the bony wall of the petrous part of the temporal bone, the inner ear contains a bony labyrinth (meaning 'maze'), or system of intercommunicating channels and the receptors for hearing and position sense.[2,57,22,46] A thin-walled, membranous labyrinth floats inside the outer bony wall, or the bony labyrinth (see Fig. 38-17). Two separate fluids are found in the inner ear: the perilymph or periotic fluid, which separates the bony labyrinth from the membranous labyrinth, and the endolymph or otic fluid, which fills the membranous labyrinth. Localized dilatations of the labyrinth develop into three main sensory areas: the semicircular canals, the vestibule, and the cochlea (see Fig. 38-17). The receptors in the cochlea are sensitive to sound, and those in the semicircular canals and vestibule are sensitive to changes in head position and maintenance of balance.

The cochlea is a shell-shaped part of the bony labyrinth that consists of three parallel compartments: the scala media or middle compartment of the cochlear canal, the scala vestibuli, and the scala tympani (Fig. 38-20). The scala media is an endolymph-containing space that is continuous with the lumen of the saccule and contains the spiral organ of Corti, the receptor organs for hearing. The scala vestibuli and scala tympani are perilymph spaces that communicate with each other at the apex of the cochlea through a small channel called the *helicotrema*. The scala vestibuli begins at the oval window, and the scala tympani ends at the round window.

The organ of Corti is composed of supporting cells; a flexible, fibrous "floor" called the basilar membrane; and several long rows of cochlear hair cells. Sound waves, delivered to the oval window by the stapes footplate, are transmitted to the perilymph and vibrate the basilar membrane. Transduction of sound stimuli occurs when the cilia of the cochlear hair cells are bent by this sound-induced movement.

Afferent fibers from the organ of Corti have their cell bodies in the spiral ganglion of the cochlear nerve. Auditory information travels along the vestibulocochlear nerve (CN VIII) and then to the cochlear nuclei in the caudal pons and midbrain to the thalamus. On the way many secondary nerve fibers pass to the opposite side of the brain. From the thalamus, the auditory pathway passes to the primary auditory cortex (area 41) and the auditory association cortex (areas 42 and 22) where the meaningfulness of sound is perceived (see Fig. 38-14). Because some of the fibers from each ear cross, each auditory cortex receives impulses from both ears.

Tinnitus

Tinnitus is the perception of abnormal ear or head noises not produced by an external stimulus.[58–60] Although it often is described as "ringing of the ears," it may also assume a hissing, roaring, buzzing, or humming sound. Tinnitus may be constant, intermittent, and unilateral or bilateral. The condition affects both sexes equally, is most prevalent between 40 and 70 years of age, and occasionally affects children.

Although tinnitus is a subjective experience, for clinical purposes it is subdivided into objective and subjective tinnitus. *Objective tinnitus* refers to those rare cases in which the sound is detected or potentially detectable by another observer. Typical causes of objective tinnitus include vascular abnormalities or neuromuscular disorders. For example, in some vascular disorders, sounds generated by turbulent blood flow (e.g., arterial bruits or venous hums) are conducted to the auditory system. Vascular disorders typically produce a pulsatile form of tinnitus. *Subjective tinnitus* refers to noise perception when there is no sound stimulation of the cochlea. A number of causes and conditions have been associated with subjective

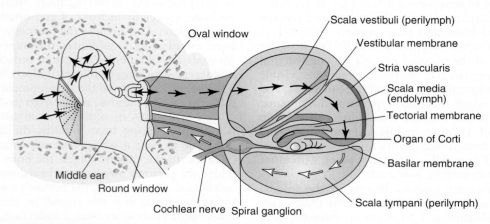

FIGURE 38-20. Path taken by sound waves reaching the inner ear.

tinnitus. Intermittent periods of mild, high-pitched tinnitus lasting for several minutes are common in normal-hearing persons. Impacted cerumen is a benign cause of tinnitus, which resolves after the earwax is removed. Medications such as aspirin and stimulants such as nicotine and caffeine can cause transient tinnitus. Conditions associated with more persistent tinnitus include noise-induced hearing loss, presbycusis (sensorineural hearing loss that occurs with aging), hypertension, atherosclerosis, head injury, and cochlear or labyrinthine infection or inflammation. The physiologic mechanism underlying subjective tinnitus is largely unknown. It seems likely that there are several mechanisms, including abnormal firing of auditory receptors, dysfunction of cochlear neurotransmitter function or ionic balance, and alterations in central processing of the signal.

Treatment measures for tinnitus are designed to reduce the symptoms, rather than effect a cure.[58,59] They include elimination of drugs or other substances, such as caffeine, some cheeses, red wine, and foods containing monosodium glutamate, that are suspected of causing tinnitus. Tinnitus retraining therapy, which includes directive counseling and extended use of low-noise generators to facilitate auditory adaptation to the tinnitus, has met with considerable success.

Central Auditory Pathway Disorders

The auditory pathways in the brain involve communication between the two sides of the brain at many levels. As a result, strokes, tumors, abscesses, and other focal abnormalities seldom produce more than a mild reduction in auditory acuity on the side opposite the lesion. For intelligibility of auditory language, lateral dominance becomes important. On the dominant side, usually the left side, the more medial and dorsal portion of the auditory association cortex is of crucial importance. This area is called the *Wernicke area*, and damage to it is associated with auditory receptive aphasia. Persons with damage to this area of the brain can speak intelligibly and read normally but are unable to understand the meaning of major aspects of audible speech.

Irritative foci that affect the auditory radiation or the primary auditory cortex can produce roaring or clicking sounds, which appear to come from the auditory environment of the opposite side (i.e., auditory hallucinations). Focal seizures that originate in or near the auditory cortex often are immediately preceded by the perception of ringing or other sounds preceded by a prodrome (i.e., aura). Damage to the auditory association cortex, especially if bilateral, results in deficiencies of sound recognition and memory. If the damage is in the dominant hemisphere, speech recognition can be affected (i.e., sensory or receptive aphasia).

Hearing Loss

Nearly 36 million Americans have some degree of hearing loss.[61] It affects persons of all age groups. Two to 3 out of every 1000 children in the United States are born deaf or hard of hearing.[61] Approximately 30% of adults between the ages of 65 and 74 years and approximately 47% of those age 75 and older have hearing loss.[61]

The level of hearing is measured in decibels (dB), where 0 dB is the threshold for perception of sound at a given frequency in persons with normal hearing. A 10-fold increase in sound pressure level from 0 dB is measured as 20 dB. Hearing loss is classified as mild (26 to 40 dB), moderate (41 to 55 dB), severe (71 to 90 dB), or profound (91 dB or greater).[61–63] "Hard of hearing" is defined as hearing loss between 20 and 25 dB in adults and greater than 15 dB in children. Profound deafness is defined as hearing loss greater than 90 dB in adults[62] or 70 dB in children.[64]

There are many causes of hearing loss or deafness. Most fit into the categories of conductive, sensorineural, or mixed deficiencies that involve a combination of conductive and sensorineural function deficiencies of the same ear.[63] Chart 38-1 summarizes common causes of hearing loss. Hearing loss may be genetic or acquired, sudden or progressive, unilateral or bilateral, partial or complete, reversible or irreversible.

CHART 38-1   Common Causes of Conductive and Sensorineural Hearing Loss

Conductive Hearing Loss
- External ear conditions
  - Impacted earwax or foreign body
  - Otitis externa
- Middle ear conditions
  - Trauma
  - Otitis media (acute and with effusion)
  - Otosclerosis
  - Tumors

Sensorineural Hearing Loss
- Trauma
  - Head injury
  - Noise
- Central nervous system infections (e.g., meningitis)
- Degenerative conditions
  - Presbycusis
- Vascular
  - Atherosclerosis
  - Sudden deafness
- Ototoxic drugs (e.g., aminoglycosides, salicylates, loop diuretics)
- Tumors
  - Vestibular schwannoma (acoustic neuroma)
  - Meningioma
  - Metastatic tumors
- Idiopathic
  - Ménière disease

Mixed Conductive and Sensorineural Hearing Loss
- Middle ear conditions
  - Barotrauma
  - Cholesteatoma
  - Otosclerosis
- Temporal bone fractures

Conductive Hearing Loss

Conductive hearing loss occurs when auditory stimuli are not adequately transmitted through the auditory canal, tympanic membrane, middle ear, or ossicle chain to the inner ear. Temporary hearing loss can occur as the result of impacted cerumen in the outer ear or fluid in the middle ear. Foreign bodies, including pieces of cotton and insects, may impair hearing. More permanent causes of hearing loss are thickening or damage of the tympanic membrane or involvement of the bony structures (ossicles and oval window) of the middle ear caused by otosclerosis or Paget disease.

Sensorineural Hearing Loss

Sensorineural, or perceptive, hearing loss occurs with disorders that affect the inner ear, auditory nerve, or auditory pathways of the brain.[62,63] With this type of deafness, sound waves are conducted to the inner ear, but abnormalities of the cochlear apparatus or auditory nerve decrease or distort the transfer of information to the brain. Abnormal function resulting from damage or malformation of the central auditory pathways and circuitry is included in this category.

Sensorineural hearing loss can vary with respect to onset and severity, and can affect one or both ears. It may have a genetic cause or result from an infection, other illness, trauma, or exposure to loud noise. Hearing loss that has its onset before speech-language acquisition is typically defined as prelingual, and that known to have developed after speech development as postlingual.

Genetic hearing loss may result from mutation in a single gene (monogenetic) or from a combination of mutations in different genes and environmental factors (multifactorial). Genetic forms of hearing loss also can be classified as being part of a syndrome in which other abnormalities are present, or as nonsyndromic, in which deafness is the only abnormality.

Environmentally induced deafness can occur through direct exposure to excessively intense sound, as in the workplace or at a concert. Sustained or repeated exposure to noise pollution at sound intensities greater than 100 to 120 dB can cause corresponding mechanical damage to the organ of Corti. Severe damage can result in permanent sensorineural deafness to the affected sound frequencies.

A number of infections can cause sensorineural hearing loss. Deafness or some degree of hearing impairment is the most common serious complication of bacterial meningitis in infants and children. The mechanism causing hearing impairment is thought to be a suppurative labyrinthitis or neuritis resulting in the loss of hair cells and damage to the auditory nerve. Sudden sensorineural hearing loss represents an abrupt loss of hearing that occurs instantaneously or on awakening. It is most commonly caused by viral infections or circulatory disorders.

Among the neoplasms that impair hearing are *acoustic neuromas*. Acoustic neuromas are benign Schwann cell tumors affecting CN VIII. These tumors usually are unilateral and cause hearing loss by compressing the cochlear nerve or interfering with blood supply to the nerve and cochlea. Other neoplasms that can affect hearing include meningiomas and metastatic brain tumors. The temporal bone is a common site of metastases.

Drugs that damage inner ear structures are labeled *ototoxic.*[65] Vestibular symptoms of ototoxicity include light-headedness, giddiness, and dizziness; if toxicity is severe, cochlear symptoms consisting of tinnitus or hearing loss occur. Hearing loss is sensorineural and may be bilateral or unilateral, or they may be transient, as often is the case with salicylate toxicity, or they may be permanent. Several classes of drugs have been identified as having ototoxic potential, including the aminoglycoside antimicrobials and some other basic antimicrobials, antimalarial drugs, some chemotherapeutic drugs, loop diuretics, and salicylates (aspirin). The risk of ototoxicity depends on the total dose of the drug and its concentration in the bloodstream. It is increased in persons with impaired kidney functioning and in those previously or currently treated with another potentially ototoxic drug.

Diagnosis and Treatment of Hearing Loss

Diagnosis of hearing loss is aided by careful history of associated otologic factors such as otalgia, otorrhea, tinnitus, and self-described hearing difficulties; physical examination to detect the presence of conditions such as otorrhea, impacted cerumen, or injury to the tympanic membrane; and hearing tests. Testing for hearing loss involves a number of methods, including a person's reported ability to hear an observer's voice, use of a tuning fork to test air and bone conduction, audioscopes, and auditory brain stem evoked responses (ABRs).[62]

Tuning forks are used to differentiate conductive and sensorineural hearing loss. Audioscopes can be used to assess a person's ability to hear pure tones at 1000 to 2000 Hz (usual speech frequencies). The ABR uses electroencephalographic (EEG) electrodes and high-gain amplifiers to produce a record of brain wave activity elicited during repeated acoustic stimulations of either or both ears. It involves subjecting the ear to loud clicks and using a computer to analyze nerve impulses as they are processed in the midbrain. Imaging studies such as computed tomography (CT) scans and magnetic resonance imaging (MRI) can be done to determine the site of a lesion and the extent of damage.[66]

Untreated hearing loss can have many consequences. Social isolation and depressive disorders are common in the hearing-impaired. Hearing-impaired people may avoid social situations where background noise makes conversation difficult to hear. Safety issues, both in and out of the home, may become significant. Treatment measures for hearing loss range from simple removal of impacted cerumen in the external auditory canal to surgical procedures, such as those used to reconstruct the tympanic membrane.

Hearing aids remain the mainstay of treatment for many persons with conductive and sensorineural hearing loss. With the advent of microcircuitry, hearing aids are now being designed with computer chips that allow multiple programs to be placed in a single hearing aid. The various programs allow the user to select a specific setting for different listening situations. The development of microcircuitry has also made it possible for hearing aids to be miniaturized to the point that, in many cases, they can be placed deep in the ear where they take advantage of the normal shape of the external ear and ear canal. Although modern hearing aids have improved greatly, they cannot replicate the person's ability to hear both soft and loud noises. They also fail consistently to filter out distorted or background noise.[57]

Surgically implantable cochlear prostheses for the profoundly deaf have been developed and are available for use in adults and children.[67] These prostheses are inserted into the cochlea and work by providing direct stimulation to the auditory nerve. For the implant to work, the auditory nerve must be functional. Although early implants used a single electrode, current implants use multielectrode placement, enhancing speech perception. Much of the progress in implant performance has been achieved through improvements in the speech processors that convert sound into electrical stimuli. Advances in the development of the multichannel implant have improved performance such that cochlear implants have been established as an effective option for adults and children with profound hearing impairment.[67,68]

 ## Hearing Loss in Infants and Children

Even mild or unilateral hearing loss can have a detrimental effect on the language development and hearing-associated learning of the young child.[69,70] In the United States, the average incidence of hearing loss is 1.1 per 1000 infants.[70] The cause of hearing impairment in children depends on whether the hearing loss is conductive or sensorineural. Most conductive hearing loss is caused by middle ear infections. Causes of sensorineural hearing impairment include genetic, infectious, traumatic, and ototoxic factors.

Genetic causes are probably responsible for as much as 50% of sensorineural hearing loss in children. The most common infectious cause of congenital sensorineural hearing loss is cytomegalovirus (CMV), which infects 1 out of every 100 newborns in the United States each year; of these, about 1200 to 2000 have sensorineural hearing loss.[70] Of particular concern is the fact that congenital CMV infection can cause both symptomatic and asymptomatic hearing loss in the newborn. Some children with congenital CMV infection, who were asymptomatic as newborns, have suddenly lost residual hearing at 4 to 5 years of age. Postnatal causes of sensorineural hearing loss include β-hemolytic streptococcal sepsis in the newborn, and although less frequent with the routine administration of the conjugate pneumococcal vaccine, *S. pneumoniae* bacterial meningitis is the most frequent cause after the neonatal period. Other causes of sensorineural hearing loss are toxins and trauma.

Hearing impairment can have a major impact on the development of a child; therefore, early identification through screening programs is strongly advocated.[70–72] The currently recommended screening techniques are either the transient evoked otoacoustic emissions (OAE) or the ABR.[70] Both methodologies are noninvasive, relatively quick (<5 minutes), and easy to perform. The

OAE measures sound waves generated in the inner ear (cochlea) in response to clicks or tone bursts emitted and recorded by a minute microphone placed in the external ear canals of the infant. The ABR uses three electrodes pasted to the infant's scalp to measure the EEG waves generated by clicks. Because many children become hearing impaired after the neonatal period and are not identified by neonatal screening programs, it is recommended that all infants with risk factors for delayed onset of progressive hearing loss receive ongoing audiologic and medical monitoring for 3 years and at appropriate intervals thereafter.[72]

Once hearing loss has been identified, a full developmental and speech and language evaluation is needed. Parental involvement and counseling are essential. Children with sensorineural hearing loss should be evaluated for possible hearing aid use by a pediatric audiologist. Hearing aids may be fitted for infants as young as 2 months of age.[70] Infants and young children with profound congenital or prelingual deafness have benefited from multichannel cochlear implants.[70] Because of the increased risk of pneumococcal meningitis, children who receive implants should receive age-appropriate immunization against pneumococcal disease.

 ## Hearing Loss in the Elderly

The term *presbycusis* is used to describe degenerative hearing loss that occurs with advancing age.[73,74] The degenerative changes that impair hearing may begin in the fifth decade of life and may not be clinically apparent until later. The hearing loss is typically gradual, bilateral, and characterized by high-frequency hearing loss. It is further characterized by reduced hearing sensitivity and speech understanding in noisy environments, slowed central processing of acoustic information, and impaired localization of sound sources. The disorder first reduces the ability to understand speech and, later, the ability to detect, identify, and localize sounds. The most common complaint of persons with presbycusis is not that they cannot hear, but rather that they cannot understand what is being said. High-frequency warning sounds, such as beepers, turn signals, and escaping steam, are not heard and localized, with potentially dangerous results.

Given the high prevalence of hearing loss in people of retirement age and its adverse effects on well-being, screening for hearing loss should be performed at annual health care visits. Clinical measures for hearing loss such as whispered voice tests and finger friction tests are reportedly imprecise and are not reliable methods for screening. Screening audiometry administered by someone trained in its use is a practical and cost-effective method for detecting significant hearing loss.

The majority of hearing loss in the elderly is sensorineural. In mild to severe loss, the most effective treatment is hearing amplification with hearing aids, lip reading, and assistive listening devices (e.g., hearing aids with the telephone, captioning on televised programs, flashing alarms). Cochlear implants are indicated at any age for people with bilateral hearing losses not materially helped by hearing aids.

SUMMARY CONCEPTS

- The outer ear collects sound vibrations and channels them to the tympanic membrane, which separates the outer ear from the middle ear. The middle ear is an air-filled cavity in the temporal bone that amplifies the sound waves and transmits them to the fluid-filled inner ear.

- The middle ear is connected to the nasopharynx by the eustachian tube, which opens briefly during swallowing to allow for equalization of air pressures on either side of the tympanic membrane. The eustachian tube is lined with a mucous membrane that is continuous with the nasopharynx, allowing infections from the nasopharynx to travel along the eustachian tube to the middle ear.

- Otitis media (OM) refers to inflammation of the middle ear. It can represent an acute otitis media (AOM) that has an abrupt onset and is usually related to bacterial infection, or otitis media with effusion (OME) that is associated with fluid in the middle ear without the manifestations of infection and which does not usually require treatment with antimicrobial agents.

- The inner ear houses two separate sensory systems: the auditory and vestibular systems. The auditory system contains the *cochlea* whose receptors convert sound waves to nerve impulses that are transmitted via the cochlear nerve to the auditory cortex.

- Hearing is a special sensory function that incorporates the sound-transmitting properties of the external ear canal, the eardrum that separates the external and middle ear, the bony ossicles of the middle ear, the sensory receptors of the cochlea in the inner ear, the neural pathways of the vestibulocochlear or auditory nerve, and the primary auditory and auditory association cortices.

- Hearing loss or deafness can be caused by conductive disorders, in which auditory stimuli are not transmitted through the structures of the outer and middle ears to the sensory receptors in the inner ear; by sensorineural disorders that affect the inner ear, auditory nerve, or auditory pathways; or by a combination of conductive and sensorineural disorders.

The Vestibular System and Disorders of Equilibrium

The vestibular apparatus, which is part of the inner ear, serves to maintain a sense of equilibrium and orientation in space. The equilibrium sense, which is also dependent on vision and input from stretch receptors in muscles and tendons, serves to maintain and assist recovery of a stable body and head position through control of postural reflexes, and to maintain a stable visual field despite marked changes in head position.

The Vestibular System

The structures of vestibular system, collectively referred to as the *vestibular apparatus,* are located in the bony labyrinth of the inner ear next to and continuous with the cochlea of the auditory system. Like the cochlea, the vestibular apparatus consists of two fluid-filled compartments—an outer bony labyrinth that is filled with perilymph and an inner membranous labyrinth that is filled with endolymph.[2,16,22] The bony membranous labyrinth is divided into three semicircular ducts and two large chambers known as the *utricle and saccule* (Fig. 38-21A). The semicircular ducts sense angular and rotary movements of the head, and the utricle and saccule sense forward and backward movement of the head.

The three semicircular ducts (anterior, posterior, and lateral) are arranged at right angles to each other and represent all three planes of space. Each of these ducts has an enlarged swelling at one end called an *ampulla.* The ampulla of each of the semicircular ducts contains a ridge that is covered by a sensory epithelium with tufts of hair cells that are covered by a flexible gelatinous cap called the *cupula* (see Fig. 38-21B). The ampulla of the three semicircular ductls, the lateral, anterior, and posterior ducts, are oriented in one of three planes of space. The lateral (horizontal) ducts are in the same plane, whereas the anterior (superior) duct of one side is parallel with the posterior (inferior) duct on the other side, and the two function as a pair. Thus, regardless of which plane one moves in, there will be receptors to detect movement. Impulses from the semicircular ducts are particularly important in reflex movement of the eyes. During head rotation the eyes slowly drift in the opposite direction and then jump rapidly back toward the direction of rotation to establish a new fixation point.

Located on the inside surface of each utricle and saccule is a small sensory area about 2 mm in diameter called the *macula* that responds to our sense of static equilibrium (see Fig. 38-21C). Each macula is a flat epithelial patch containing supporting cells and sensory hair cells, which synapse with sensory endings of the vestibular nerve. These hair cells are embedded in a gelatinous mass, the *otolithic membrane,* which is studded with tiny stones (calcium carbonate crystals) called *otoliths.* Although they are small, the density of the otoliths increases the membrane's weight and its resistance to change in

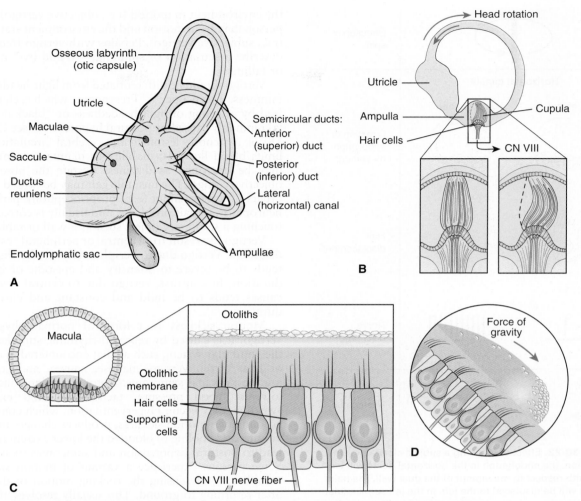

FIGURE 38-21. Vestibular labyrinth. **(A)** Osseous and membranous vestibular labyrinth of the middle ear showing the utricle and saccule with their maculae and three semicircular ducts and their ampullae. **(B)** Diagram of the crista ampullaris within the semicircular duct and location of the cupula and movement of the hair cells with head movement. **(C)** Relationship of the otoliths to the sensory hair cells, which synapse with the sensory endings of the vestibular nerve (CN VIII) in the maculae of the utricle and saccule. **(D)** Movement of the otoliths and bending of the macular hair cells when the head is tilted due to the forces of gravity.

motion. When the head is tilted, the gelatinous mass shifts its position because of the pull of the gravitational field, bending the cilia of the macular hair cells (see Fig. 38-21D). In a condition called *benign paroxysmal positional vertigo* (sensation of whirling or spinning motion), the otoliths become dislodged from their gelatinous base, causing a vertigo that is precipitated by changes in the recumbent head position (to be discussed).

The response to body imbalance, such as stumbling, must be fast and reflexive. Hence, information from the vestibular system goes directly to vestibular nuclei in the brain stem or to the cerebellum. The vestibular nuclei, which form the main integrative center for balance, also receive input from visual and somatic receptors, particularly from stretch receptors in the neck muscles that report the angle or inclination of the head. The vestibular nuclei integrate this information and then send impulses to the brain stem centers that control the extraocular eye movements and reflex movements of the neck, limb,

and trunk muscles. These reflex movements include the *vestibulo-ocular reflexes* that keep the eyes still as the head moves and the *vestibulospinal reflexes* that allow the body to maintain or regain balance. Neurons of the vestibular nuclei also project to the thalamus and cortex, providing the basis for the subjective experiences of position in space and of rotation. Moreover, connections with the chemoreceptor trigger zone of the brain stem stimulate the vomiting center, accounting for the nausea and vomiting that often are associated with motion sickness and vestibular disorders.

Nystagmus

The term *nystagmus* refers to the involuntary eye movements that preserve eye fixation on stable objects in the visual field during angular and rotational movements of the head.[16] As the body rotates, the vestibulo-ocular reflexes cause a slow compensatory

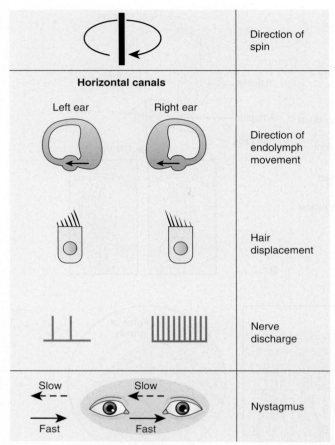

Horizontal canals

	Direction of spin
	Direction of endolymph movement
	Hair displacement
	Nerve discharge
	Nystagmus

Left ear — Right ear

Slow — Slow

Fast — Fast

FIGURE 38-22. Effect of spinning a subject clockwise. On acceleration, the endolymph in the horizontal ducts will lag behind with respect to movement of the duct wall. The hairs of cristae will be displaced to the left. In the left semicircular duct, hair displacement is away from the kinocilium, leading to decreased nerve discharges below the resting level. On the right, hair displacement is toward the kinocilium, leading to an increase in nerve discharge above the resting level. (From Sekurt FE. *Basic Physiology for the Health Professions.* 2nd ed. Boston, MA: Little, Brown; 1982:140.)

drifting of eye movement in the opposite direction, thus stabilizing the binocular fixation point. This pattern of slow–fast–slow movements is *nystagmus* (Fig. 38-22). Clinically, the direction of nystagmus is named for the fast phase of nystagmus.

Spontaneous nystagmus that occurs without head movement or visual stimuli is always pathologic. It seems to appear more readily and more severely with fatigue and to some extent can be influenced by psychological factors. Nystagmus due to a CNS pathologic process, in contrast to vestibular end-organ or vestibulocochlear nerve sources, seldom is accompanied by vertigo. If present, the vertigo is mild. Nystagmus eye movements can be tested by caloric stimulation or rotation (to be discussed).

Vertigo

Disorders of vestibular function are characterized by a condition called *vertigo,* in which an illusion of motion occurs. With vertigo, the person may be stationary and

the environment in motion (i.e., objective vertigo) or the person may be in motion and the environment stationary (i.e., subjective vertigo). Persons with vertigo frequently describe a sensation of spinning, "to-and-fro" motion, or falling.

Vertigo should be differentiated from light-headedness, faintness, or syncope.[74–77] Presyncope, which is characterized by a feeling of light-headedness or "blacking out," is commonly caused by postural hypotension (see Chapter 18) or a stenotic lesion in the cerebral circulation that limits blood flow. An inability to maintain normal gait may be described as dizziness despite the absence of objective vertigo. The unstable gait may be caused by disorders of sensory input (e.g., proprioception), peripheral neuropathy, or gait problems, and usually is corrected by touching a stationary object such as a wall or table.

Vertigo can result from central or peripheral vestibular disorders. Vertigo due to peripheral vestibular disorders tends to be severe in intensity and episodic or brief in duration. In contrast, vertigo due to central vestibular causes tends to be mild and constant and chronic in duration.

Motion sickness is a form of normal physiologic vertigo. It is caused by repeated rhythmic stimulation of the vestibular system, such as that encountered in car, air, or boat travel. Vertigo, malaise, nausea, and vomiting are the principal symptoms. Autonomic signs, including lowered blood pressure, tachycardia, and excessive sweating, may occur. Hyperventilation, which commonly accompanies motion sickness, produces changes in blood volume and pooling of blood in the lower extremities that lead to postural hypotension and sometimes to syncope. Some persons experience a variant of motion sickness, complaining of sensing the rocking motion of the boat after returning to ground. This usually resolves after the vestibular system becomes accustomed to the stationary influence of being back on land.

Disorders of Peripheral Vestibular Function

Disorders of peripheral vestibular function occur when signals from the vestibular apparatus are distorted, as in benign paroxysmal positional vertigo, or are unbalanced by unilateral involvement of one of the vestibular organs, as in Ménière disease. The inner ear is vulnerable to injury caused by fracture of the petrous portion of the temporal bones; by infection of nearby structures, including the middle ear and meninges; and by blood-borne toxins and infections. Damage to the vestibular system can occur as an adverse effect of certain drugs or from allergic reactions to foods. The aminoglycosides (e.g., streptomycin, gentamicin) have a specific toxic affinity for the vestibular portion of the inner ear. Alcohol can cause transient episodes of vertigo. The cause of peripheral vertigo remains unknown in approximately half of the cases.

Severe irritation or damage of the vestibular end-organs or nerves results in severe balance disorders reflected by instability of posture, ataxia, and falling accompanied by vertigo. Adaptation usually occurs within a few days, after which the person is usually able to walk and even drive a car. Such a person relies heavily on visual and proprioceptive input from muscle and joint sensors, and has severe orientation difficulty in the dark, particularly when traversing uneven terrain.

Benign Paroxysmal Positional Vertigo

Benign paroxysmal positional vertigo (BPPV) is the most common cause of pathologic vertigo and usually develops after the fourth decade of life. It is characterized by brief periods of vertigo, usually lasting less than 1 minute, that are precipitated by a change in head position.[77,78] The most prominent symptom of BPPV is vertigo that occurs in bed when the person rolls into a lateral position. It also commonly occurs when the person is getting in and out of bed, bending over and straightening up, or extending the head to look up.

Benign paroxysmal positional vertigo is thought to result from damage to the delicate sensory organs of the inner ear, the semicircular ducts, and otoliths (see Fig. 38-21). In persons with BPPV, the calcium carbonate particles (otoliths) from the utricle become dislodged and become free-floating debris within the endolymph of a semicircular duct, most commonly the posterior duct, which is the most dependent part of the inner ear. Movement of the free-floating debris causes this portion of the vestibular apparatus to become more sensitive, such that any movement of the head in the plane parallel to the posterior duct may cause vertigo and nystagmus. There usually is a several-second delay between head movement and onset of vertigo, representing the time it takes to generate the exaggerated endolymph activity. Symptoms usually subside with continued movement, probably because the movement causes the debris to be redistributed throughout the endolymph system and away from the posterior semicircular duct.

Diagnosis is based on tests that involve the use of a change in head position to elicit vertigo and nystagmus. BPPV often is successfully treated with drug therapy to control vertigo-induced nausea. Nondrug therapies using habituation exercises and otolith repositioning are successful in many people. Otolith repositioning involves a series of maneuvers in which the head is moved to different positions in an effort to reposition the free-floating debris in the endolymph of the semicircular ducts.

Acute Vestibular Neuronitis

Acute vestibular neuronitis represents an inflammation of the vestibular nerve and is characterized by an acute onset (usually hours) of vertigo, nausea, and vomiting lasting several days and not associated with auditory or other neurologic manifestations. Most persons experience gradual improvement over 1 to 2 weeks, but some develop recurrent episodes.[79] A large percentage report an upper respiratory tract illness 1 to 2 weeks before onset of symptoms, suggesting a viral origin. The condition also can occur in persons with herpes zoster oticus. In some persons, attacks of acute vestibulopathy recur over months or years. There is no way to determine whether a person who experiences a first attack will have repeated attacks.

Ménière Disease

Ménière disease is a disorder of the inner ear due to distention of the endolymphatic compartment of the inner ear, causing a triad of hearing loss, vertigo, and tinnitus.[80–82] A number of mechanisms have been postulated, including an increased production of endolymph, decreased production of perilymph accompanied by a compensatory increase in volume of the endolymphatic sac, and decreased absorption of endolymph caused by malfunction of the endolymphatic sac or blockage of endolymphatic pathways.

A number of conditions, such as trauma, infection (e.g., syphilis), and immunologic, endocrine (i.e., adrenal-pituitary insufficiency and hypothyroidism), and vascular disorders have been proposed as possible causes of Ménière disease. The most common form of the disease is an idiopathic form thought to be caused by a single viral injury to the fluid transport system of the inner ear. One area of investigation has been the relation between autoimmune disorders and Ménière disease.

Ménière disease is characterized by fluctuating episodes of tinnitus, feelings of ear fullness, and violent rotary vertigo that often renders the person unable to sit or walk. There is a need to lie quietly with the head fixed in a comfortable position, avoiding all head movements that aggravate the vertigo. Symptoms referable to the autonomic nervous system, including pallor, sweating, nausea, and vomiting, usually are present. The more severe the attack, the more prominent are the autonomic manifestations. Fluctuating hearing loss occurs with a return to normal after the episode subsides. Initially the symptoms tend to be unilateral, resulting in rotary nystagmus caused by an imbalance in vestibular control of eye movements. Because initial involvement usually is unilateral and the sense of hearing is bilateral, many persons with the disorder are not aware of the full extent of their hearing loss. However, as the disease progresses, the hearing loss stops fluctuating and progressively worsens, with both ears tending to be affected so that the prime disability becomes one of deafness. The episodes of vertigo diminish and then disappear, although the person may be unsteady, especially in the dark.

Methods used in the diagnosis of Ménière disease include audiograms, vestibular testing by electronystagmography, and petrous pyramid radiographs. The administration of hyperosmolar substances, such as glycerin and urea, often produces acute temporary hearing improvement in persons with Ménière disease and sometimes is used as a diagnostic measure of endolymphatic hydrops. The diuretic furosemide also may be used for this purpose.

The management of Ménière disease focuses on attempts to reduce the distention of the endolymphatic space, and can be medical or surgical. Pharmacologic management consists of suppressant drugs (e.g., prochlorperazine, promethazine, diazepam), which act centrally to decrease the activity of the vestibular system. Diuretics are used to reduce endolymph fluid volume. A low-sodium diet is recommended in addition to these medications. The steroid hormone prednisone may be used to maintain satisfactory hearing and resolve dizziness. Intratympanic gentamicin therapy has been used for ablation of the vestibular system.[81] This treatment is mainly effective in controlling vertigo and does not alter the underlying pathologic process. Surgical methods include the creation of an endolymphatic shunt in which excess endolymph from the inner ear is diverted into the subarachnoid space or the mastoid (endolymphatic sac surgery), and vestibular nerve section. Advances in vestibular nerve section have facilitated the monitoring of CN VII and CN VIII potentials as a means of preventing hearing damage.

Disorders of Central Vestibular Function

Abnormal nystagmus and vertigo can occur as a result of CNS lesions involving the cerebellum and lower brain stem. Central causes of vertigo include brain stem ischemia, tumors, and the demyelinating effects of multiple sclerosis. When brain stem ischemia is the cause of vertigo, it usually is associated with other brain stem signs, such as diplopia, ataxia, dysarthria, or facial weakness. Compression of the vestibular nuclei by cerebellar tumors invading the fourth ventricle results in progressively severe signs and symptoms. In addition to abnormal nystagmus and vertigo, vomiting and a broad-based and dystaxic gait become progressively more evident.

In contrast to peripherally generated nystagmus, CNS-derived nystagmus is relatively constant rather than episodic; can occur in any direction rather than being primarily horizontal or rotatory; often changes direction through time; cannot be suppressed by visual fixation; and does result in rapid diminution or "fatigue," as with peripheral abnormalities.

Tests of Vestibular Function

Diagnosis of vestibular disorders is based on a description of the symptoms, a history of trauma or exposure to agents that are destructive to vestibular structures, and physical examination. Tests of eye movements (i.e., nystagmus) and muscle control of balance and equilibrium often are used.

Electronystagmography (ENG) is a precise and objective diagnostic method of evaluating nystagmic eye movements. Electrodes are placed lateral to the outer canthus of each eye and above and below each eye, and a ground electrode is placed on the forehead. With ENG, the velocity, frequency, and amplitude of spontaneous or induced nystagmus and the changes in these measurements brought by a loss of fixation, with the eyes open or closed, can be quantified. *Caloric testing* involves elevating the head 30 degrees and irrigating each external auditory canal separately with 30 to 50 mL of ice water. The resulting changes in temperature, which are conducted through the petrous portion of the temporal bone, set up convection currents that mimic

the effects of angular acceleration. In an unconscious person with a functional brain stem and intact vestibulo-ocular reflexes, the eyes exhibit a jerk nystagmus lasting 2 to 3 minutes, with the slow component toward the irrigated ear followed by rapid movement away from the ear. With impairment of brain stem function, the response becomes perverted and eventually disappears. An advantage of the caloric stimulation method is the ability to test the vestibular apparatus on one side at a time. The test is never done on a person who does not have an intact eardrum or those who have blood or fluid collected behind the eardrum.

Rotational testing involves the use of a motor-driven revolving chair or platform. Unlike caloric testing, rotational testing depends only on the inner ear and is unrelated to conditions of the external ear or temporal bone. Motor-driven chairs or platforms can be precisely controlled, and multiple graded stimuli can be delivered in a relatively short period. Testing usually is performed in the dark without visual influence and with selected light stimuli. Eye movements are usually monitored using ENG. A major disadvantage of the method is that both ears are tested simultaneously.

The *Romberg test* is used to demonstrate disorders of static vestibular function. It is done be having a person stand with his or her feet together and arms extended forward so that the degree of sway and arm stability can be observed. The person then is asked to close his or her eyes. Deficiency in vestibular static input is indicated by greatly increased sway and a tendency for the arms to drift toward the side of deficiency. If vestibular input is severely deficient, the subject falls toward the deficient side.

Treatment of Vestibular Disorders

Depending on the cause, vertigo may be treated pharmacologically. There are two types of drugs used in the treatment of vertigo. First are the drugs used to suppress the illusion of motion. These include drugs such as antihistamines (e.g., meclizine, cyclizine, dimenhydrinate, and promethazine) and anticholinergic drugs (e.g., scopolamine, atropine) that suppress the vestibular system. The second type includes drugs used to relieve the nausea and vomiting that commonly accompany the condition. Antidopaminergic drugs (e.g., phenothiazines) and benzodiazepines commonly are used for this purpose.

Vestibular rehabilitation, a relatively new treatment modality for peripheral vestibular disorders, has met with considerable success.[83] It commonly is done by physical therapists and uses a home exercise program that incorporates habituation exercises, balance retraining exercises, and a general conditioning program. The habituation exercises take advantage of physiologic fatigue of the neurovegetative response to repetitive movement or positional stimulation and are done to decrease motion-provoked vertigo, light-headedness, and unsteadiness. The exercises are selected to provoke the vestibular symptoms. The person moves quickly into the position that causes symptoms, holds the position until the symptoms subside, relaxes, and then repeats the exercise for a prescribed number of times. The exercises usually are repeated twice daily.

The habituation effect is characterized by decreased sensitivity and duration of symptoms. It may occur in as little as 2 weeks or take as long as 6 months. Balance retraining exercises consist of activities directed toward improving individual components of balance that may be abnormal. General conditioning exercises, a vital part of the rehabilitation process, are individualized to the person's preferences and lifestyle.

SUMMARY CONCEPTS

■ Receptors for the vestibular system that respond to changes in rotational and linear acceleration of the head are located in the fluid-filled semicircular ducts of the inner ear.

■ The vestibular system has extensive interconnections with neural pathways controlling vision, hearing, balance, and autonomic nervous system function. Signals from the vestibular system initiate head and eye movements to stabilize the visual field and make adjustments in the posture muscles that maintain balance.

■ Disorders of vestibular function can result from repeated stimulation of the vestibular system such as during car, air, and boat travel (motion sickness); acute infection of the vestibular pathways (acute vestibular neuritis); dislodgement of otoliths that participate in the receptor function of the vestibular system (benign paroxysmal positional vertigo); or distention of the endolymphatic compartment of the inner ear (Ménière disease).

REVIEW EXERCISES

1. The mother of a 3-year-old boy notices that his left eye is red and watering when she picks him up from day care. He keeps rubbing his eye as though it itches. The next morning, she notices that both eyes are red, swollen, and watering. Being concerned, she takes him to the pediatrician in the morning and is told that he has "conjunctivitis." She is told that the infection should go away by itself.

    A. What part of the eye is involved?
    B. What type of conjunctivitis do you think this child has (bacterial, viral, or allergic)?
    C. Why didn't the pediatrician order an antimicrobial drug?
    D. Is the condition contagious? What measures should she take to prevent its spread?

2. During a routine eye examination to get new glasses because she had been having difficulty with her distant vision, a 75-year-old woman is told that she is developing cataracts.

    A. What types of visual changes occur as the result of a cataract?
    B. What can the woman do to prevent the cataracts from getting worse?
    C. What treatment may she eventually need?

3. A 50-year-old woman is told by her eye doctor that her intraocular pressure is slightly elevated and that although there is no evidence of damage to her eyes at this time, she is at risk for developing glaucoma and should have regular eye examinations.

    A. Describe the physiologic mechanisms involved in the regulation of intraocular pressure.
    B. Differentiate between open-angle and angle-closure glaucoma in terms of their pathology, manifestations, and treatment.
    C. See Figure 38-12 to relate the "optic disk cupping" that occurs with glaucoma to the visual field loss that occurs with the disorder.

4. The parents of a newborn infant have been told that their son has congenital cataracts and will require cataract surgery to prevent losing his sight.

    A. Explain why the infant is at risk for losing his sight if the cataracts are not removed.
    B. When should this procedure be done to prevent loss of vision?

5. A mother notices that her 13-month-old child is fussy and tugging at his ear and refuses to eat his breakfast. When she takes his temperature, it is 100°F. Although the child attends day care, his mother has kept him home and made an appointment with the child's pediatrician. In the physician's office, his temperature is 100.2°F, he is somewhat irritable, and he has a clear nasal drainage. His left tympanic membrane shows normal landmarks and motility on pneumatic otoscopy. His right tympanic membrane is erythematous and there is decreased motility on pneumatic otoscopy.

    A. What risk factors are present that predispose this child to the development of acute otitis media?
    B. Are his signs and symptoms typical of otitis media in a child of this age?
    C. What are the most likely pathogens? What treatment would be indicated?
    D. Later in the week, the mother notices that the child does not seem to hear as well as he did before developing the infection. Is this a common occurrence, and should the mother be concerned about transient hearing loss in a child of this age?

6. A granddaughter is worried that her grandfather is "losing his hearing." Lately, he has been staying away from social gatherings that he always enjoyed, saying everybody mumbles. He is defiant in maintaining that there is nothing wrong with his hearing. However, he does complain that his ears have been ringing a lot lately.

   A. What are common manifestations of hearing loss in the elderly?
   B. What type of evaluation would be appropriate for determining if this man has a hearing loss, and the extent of his hearing loss?
   C. What are some things the granddaughter might do so that her grandfather could hear her better when she is talking to him?

7. A 70-year-old man complains that he gets this terrible feeling "like the room is moving around" and becomes nauseated when he rolls over in bed or bends over suddenly. It usually goes away once he has been up for a while. He has been told that his symptoms are consistent with benign paroxysmal positional vertigo.

   A. What is the pathophysiology associated with this man's vertigo?
   B. Why do the symptoms subside once he has been up for a while?
   C. What methods are available for treatment of the disorder?

REFERENCES

1. Lighthouse International. About us [Online]. Available: http://www.lighthouse.org/research/statistics-on-vision-impairment/prevalence-of-vision-impairment/. Accessed August 7, 2013.
2. Ross MH, Pawlina W. *Histology: A Text and Atlas.* 5th ed. Philadelphia, PA: Wolters Kluwer Health/Lippincott Williams & Wilkins; 2011:896–919.
3. Nijm LM, Garcio FJ, Schwab IR. Conjunctiva and tears. In: Riordan-Eva P, Cunningham ET Jr., eds., *Vaughan & Asbury's General Ophthalmology.* 18th ed. New York: Lange Medical Books/McGraw-Hill; 2011:98–125.
4. Pasternak A, Irish B. Ophthalmologic infections in primary care. *Clin Fam Pract.* 2004;6(1):19–33.
5. Cronau H, Kankanala RR, Mauger T. Diagnosis and management of red eye in primary care. *Am Fam Physician.* 2010;81(2):137–144.
6. Rubin E, Strayer DS, eds. *Rubin's Pathology: Clinicopathologic Foundations of Medicine.* 6th ed. Philadelphia, PA: Wolters Kluwer Health/Lippincott Williams & Wilkins; 2012:180–182, 1393–1414.
7. Ono SJ, Abelson MB. Allergic conjunctivitis: Update on pathophysiology and prospects for future treatment. *J Allergy Clin Immunol.* 2006;115(1):118–122.
8. Biswell R. Cornea. In: Riordan-Eva P, Cunningham ET, eds., *Vaughan & Ashbury's General Ophthalmology.* 18th ed. New York: Lange Medical Books/McGraw-Hill; 2011:120–144.
9. DelMonte DW, Kim T. Anatomy and physiology of the cornea. *J Cataract Refract Surg.* 2011;37:588–598.
10. Dargin JM, Lowenstein RA. The painful eye. *Emerg Med Clin North Am.* 2008;26:199–216.
11. Pepose JS, Keadle TL, Morrison LA. Ocular herpes simplex: changing epidemiology, emerging disease patterns, and potential of vaccine prevention and therapy. *Am J Ophthalmol.* 2006;141:547–557.
12. Shaikh S, Ta C. Evaluation and management of herpes zoster ophthalmicus. *Am Fam Physician.* 2002;66:1723–1732.
13. Dart JKG, Saw VPL, Kilvington S. Acanthamoeba keratitis: diagnosis and treatment update 2009. *Am J Ophthalmol.* 2009;148(4):487–499.
14. Stapleton F, Carnt N. Contact lens-related microbial keratitis: how have epidemiology and genetics helped us with pathogenesis and prophylaxis. *Eye (Lond).* 2012;26:185–193.
15. Harper RA, Shock JP. Lens. In: Riordan-Eva P, Cunningham ET, eds. *Vaughan & Asbury's General Ophthalmology.* 18th ed. New York: McGraw-Hill Medical; 2011:174–182.
16. Hall JE. *Guyton & Hall Textbook of Medical Physiology.* 12th ed. Philadelphia, PA: Elsevier Saunders; 2011:557–631, 633–644.
17. Packer M, Fine H, Hoffman RS. Refractive lens surgery. *Ophthalmol Clin North Am.* 2006;19:77–88.
18. Abraham AG, Condon NG, Gower EW. The new epidemiology of cataract. *Ophthalmol Clin North Am.* 2006;19:415–425.
19. James ER. The etiology of steroid cataracts. *J Ocul Pharmacol Ther.* 2007;23(5):403–420.
20. Asbell PA, Dualan I, Mindel J, et al. Age-related cataract. *Lancet.* 2005;365:599–609.
21. Chan WH, Susmito B-J A, Lloyd LC. Congenital and infantile cataract: aetiology and management. *Eur J Pediatr.* 2012; 171:625–630.
22. Kandel ER, Schwartz JH, Jessell TM, et al. *Principles of Neural Science.* 5th ed. New York: McGraw-Hill; 2013:577–601, 639–653, 654–711, 917–935.
23. Fletcher EC, Chong GV, Augsburger JJ, et al. Retina. In: Riordan-Eva P, Cunningham ET, eds. *Vaughan & Asbury's General Ophthalmology.* 18th ed. New York: McGraw-Hill Medical; 2011:271–313.
24. Riordan-Eva P, Hoyt WF. Neuro-ophthalmology. In: Riordan-Eva P, Cunningham ET, eds. *Vaughan & Asbury's General Ophthalmology.* 18th ed. New York: McGraw-Hill Medical; 2011:190–221.
25. In: Kumar V, Abbas AK, Fausto N, eds. *Robbins and Cotran Pathologic Basis of Disease,* 8th ed. Philadelphia, PA: Elsevier Saunders; 2010:1345–1368.
26. Antonetti DA, Klein R, Gardner TW. Diabetic retinopathy. *N Engl J Med.* 2012;366(13):1227–1239.
27. Cheung N, Mitchel P, Wong TW. Diabetic retinopathy. *Lancet.* 2010;276:124–136.
28. Simó R, Hernández C. Advances in medical treatment of diabetic retinopathy. *Diabetes Care.* 2009;32(8):1556–1562.
29. Wong TY, Mitchell P. Hypertensive retinopathy. *N Engl J Med.* 2004;351(22):2310–2317.
30. D'Amico DJ. Primary retinal detachment. *N Engl J Med.* 2008;359(22):2346–2354.
31. Michenbaum JW. Geriatric vision loss due to cataracts, macular degeneration, and glaucoma. *Mt Sinai J Med.* 2012;79:276–294.
32. Lim L, Mitchell P, Sheldon JM, et al. Age-related macular degeneration. *Lancet.* 2012;379:1728–1738.
33. Kaufman SR. Developments in age-related macular degeneration: diagnosis and treatment. *Geriatrics.* 2009;64(2):16–19.
34. Salmon JF. Glaucoma. In: Riordan-Eva P, Cunningham ET Jr, eds. *Vaughan & Asbury's General Ophthalmology.* 18th ed. New York: McGraw-Hill Medical; 2011:222–237.
35. Quigley HA. Glaucoma. *Lancet.* 2012;377:1367–1377.
36. Kwon YH, Fingert JH, Kuehn MH, et al. Primary open-angle glaucoma. *N Engl J Med.* 2009;360(11):1113–1124.
37. Singh A. Medical therapy of glaucoma. *Ophthalmol Clin North Am.* 2005;18:397–408.

38. Kipp MA. Childhood glaucoma. *Pediatr Clin North Am.* 2003; 50:89–104.

39. Motley WW, Asbury T. Strabismus. In: Riordan-Eva P, Cunningham ET Jr., eds. *Vaughan & Asbury's General Ophthalmology.* 18th ed. New York: McGraw-Hill Medical; 2011:238–258.

40. Donahue SP. Pediatric strabismus. *N Engl J Med.* 2007;356(10):1040–1047.

41. Olitsky SE, Hug D, Plummer LS, et al. Disorders of eye movement and alignment. In: Kliegman RM, Stanton BF, St. Geme J, et al., eds. *Nelson Textbook of Pediatrics.* 19th ed. Philadelphia, PA: Elsevier Saunders; 2011:2157.e1–2162.e1.

42. Bradfield YS. Amblyopia. *Am Fam Physician.* 2013;87(5):348–352.

43. Gunton KB. Advances in amblyopia: what have we learned from PEDIG trials. *Pediatrics.* 2013;131:540–547.

44. Wu C, Hunter DG. Amblyopia: diagnostic and therapeutic options. *Am J Ophthalmol.* 2006;141(1):175–184.

45. American Academy of Pediatrics Committee on Practice and Ambulatory Medicine, Section of Ophthalmology. Eye examination in infants, children, and young adults by pediatrician. *Pediatrics.* 2003;111(4):902–907.

46. Moore KL, Dallen AF, Agur AMR. *Clinically Oriented Anatomy.* 5th ed. Philadelphia, PA: Wolters Kluwer Health/Lippincott Williams & Wilkins; 2010:966–980.

47. McCarter DF, Pollart SM. Cerumen impaction. *Am Fam Physician.* 2007;75(10):1523–1530.

48. Lustig LR, Schindler J. Ear, nose & throat. In: Papadakis MA, McPhee SJ, eds. *Current Medical Diagnosis and Treatment.* 52nd ed. New York: McGraw-Hill Medical; 2013:198–213.

49. Danner CJ. Eustachian tube function and the middle ear. *Otolaryngol Clin North Am.* 2006;39:1221–1235.

50. Lee H, Kim J, Nguyen V. Ear infections. *Prim Care.* 2013;40:671–686.

51. Kerschner JE. Otitis media. In: Kliegman RM, Stanton BF, St. Geme J, et al., eds. *Nelson Textbook of Pediatrics.* 19th ed. Philadelphia, PA: Elsevier Saunders; 2011:2198.

52. Pichichero MF. Otitis media. *Pediatr Clin North Am.* 2013;69:391–407.

53. American Academy of Pediatrics and American Academy of Family Physicians. Otitis media with effusion. *Pediatrics.* 2004;113:1412–1429.

54. Lieberthal AS, Carroll AE, Chonmatree T, et al. Clinical practice guidelines: the diagnosis and management of acute otitis media. *Pediatrics.* 2013;131(3):e963–e991.

55. Ealy M, Smith RJH. Otosclerosis. *Adv Otorhinolaryngol.* 2011;70:122–129.

56. Siddig MA. Otosclerosis: a review of aetiology, management and outcomes. *Br J Hosp Med (Lond).* 2006;67(9):472–476.

57. Palmer CV, Ortmann A. Hearing loss and hearing aids. *Neurol Clin.* 2005;23:901–918.

58. Lockwood AH. Tinnitus. *Neurol Clin.* 2005;23:893–900.

59. Holmes S, Padgham ND. "Ringing in the ears" Narrative review of tinnitus and its impact. *Biol Res Nurs.* 2011;13(1):97–108.

60. Møller AR. Pathophysiology of tinnitus. *Otolaryngol Clin North Am.* 2003;36:246–266.

61. National Institute on Deafness and Other Communication Disorders. *Quick statistics about hearing disorders, ear infections, and deafness.* Dec 2010. Available at: http://www.nidcd.nih.gov/health/statistics/pages/hearing.aspx. Accessed August 24, 2013.

62. Issacson B. Hearing loss. *Med Clin North Am.* 2010;94:973–988.

63. Kozak AT. Hearing loss. *Otolaryngol Clin North Am.* 2009;42:79–85.

64. Willems PJ. Genetic causes of hearing loss. *N Engl J Med.* 2000;342:1101–1109.

65. Love SR, VandeWaa E, DeRulter M, et al. Ototoxicity and vestibulotoxicity. *Clin Rev.* 2013;April:32–40.

66. Isaacson JE, Vora NM. Differential diagnosis and treatment of hearing loss. *Am Fam Physician.* 2003;68(5):1125–1132.

67. National Institute of Deafness and Other Communicative Disorders. *Cochlear implants.* Available at: http://www.nidcd.nih.gov/health/hearing/pages/coch.aspx. Accessed August 24, 2013.

68. Papsin BC, Gordon KA. Cochlear implants for children with severe-to-profound hearing loss. *N Engl J Med.* 2007;357(23):2380–2387.

69. Katbamna B, Patel DR. Hearing impairment in children. *Pediatr Clin North Am.* 2008;55:1175–1188.

70. Haddad J. Hearing loss. In: Kliegman RM, Stanton BF, St. Geme J, et al., eds. *Nelson Textbook of Pediatrics.* 19th ed. Philadelphia, PA: Elsevier Saunders; 2011:2188.e1–2196.e1.

71. Wrightson AS. Universal newborn hearing screening. *Am Fam Physician.* 2007;75(9):1349–1352.

72. Harbor ADB, Bower C. Hearing assessment in children: recommendations beyond neonatal screening. *Pediatrics.* 2009;124:1252–1263.

73. Gates GA, Mills JH. Presbycusis. *Lancet.* 2005;366:1111–1119.

74. Bance M. Hearing and aging. *Can Med Assoc J.* 2007;176(7):925–927.

75. Chawla N, Olshaker JS. Diagnosis and management of dizziness and vertigo. *Med Clin North Am.* 2006;90:291–304.

76. Post RE, Dickerson LM. Dizziness: a diagnostic approach. *Am Fam Physician.* 2010;82(4):363–368.

77. Kerber KA. Vertigo and dizziness in the emergency room. *Emerg Med Clin North Am.* 2009;27(1):1–13.

78. Fifa TD. Benign paroxysmal positional vertigo. *Semin Neurol.* 2009;29:500–508.

79. Baloh RW. Vestibular neuritis. *N Engl J Med.* 2003;348(11):1027–1032.

80. Berlinge MT. Meniere's disease: new concepts, new treatments. *Minn Med.* 2011;94(11):33–36.

81. Rauch SD. Clinical hints and precipitating factors in patients suffering from Meniere's disease. *Otolaryngol Clin North Am.* 2010;43:1011–1017.

82. Agrawal Y, Minor LB. Physiologic effects on the vestibular system in Meniere's disease. *Otolaryngol Clin North Am.* 2010;43:985–993.

83. Hall C. The role of vestibular rehabilitation in the balance disorder patient. *Otolaryngol Clin North Am.* 2009;42:161–169.

Porth Essentials Resources

Explore these additional resources to enhance learning for this chapter:

- NCLEX-Style Questions and Other Resources on **the**Point, http://thePoint.lww.com/PorthEssentials4e
- Study Guide for Essentials of Pathophysiology
- Concepts in Action Animations
- Adaptive Learning | Powered by PrepU, http://thepoint.lww.com/prepu

C h a p t e r **39**

Disorders of the Male Genitourinary System

The male genitourinary system is subject to a number of structural and functional disorders, all of which can affect urine elimination, sexual function, and fertility. This chapter is divided into three parts: (1) the physiologic basis of male reproductive function, including hormone production, spermatogenesis, and neural control of sexual function; (2) disorders of the male genitourinary structures, including the penis, scrotum and testes, and prostate gland; and (3) disorders of childhood and changes that occur as a result of the aging process.

Physiologic Basis of Male Reproductive Function

The male genitourinary system is composed of the paired gonads, or testes; genital ducts; accessory genital organs; and penis (Fig. 39-1). The testes function in the production of androgens or male sex hormones and spermatozoa; the ductile system aids in the storage and transport of spermatozoa; and the accessory genital organs produce the fluid constituents of semen. The penis functions in both urine elimination and sexual function.

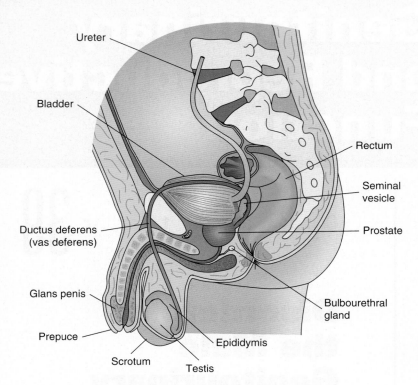

FIGURE 39-1. Structures of the male reproductive system, including the testes, scrotum, and excretory ducts.

Testicular Function

The two primary functions of the testes or male gonads are *steroidogenesis*, or synthesis of androgens or male sex hormones, and *spermatogenesis*, or sperm production.[1-3] The testes are paired ovoid organs that lie within the scrotum, which hangs outside the abdominal cavity. The testes are surrounded by two tunics. The outer tunic is the two-layered tunica vaginalis derived from the peritoneum. The inner tunic is the *tunica albuginea*, the dense connective tissue capsule of the testes (Fig. 39-2).

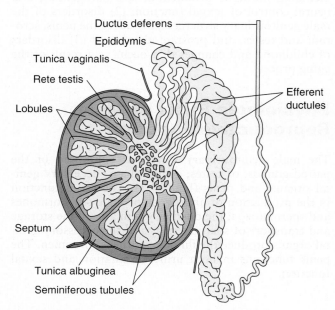

FIGURE 39-2. The parts of the testes and epididymis.

Septal extensions of the tunica albuginea divide the testes into 200 to 300 wedge-shaped compartments or lobules. Each lobule contains one to four tightly coiled *seminiferous tubules*, in which sperm are produced, and a connective tissue stroma, in which the androgen-producing *Leydig* or *interstitial cells* are located.

Hormone Production

The testes produce several male sex hormones, including *testosterone, dihydrotestosterone,* and *androstenedione*.[1-3] Testosterone, which is the most abundant of these hormones, is considered the main testicular hormone. The adrenal cortex also produces androgens, albeit in much smaller quantities (<5% of the total male androgens) than the testes. Larger amounts of testosterone are formed from dihydrotestosterone and androstenedione in other tissues of the body, especially the liver.[1] In addition to testosterone, small amounts of estrogens are formed in the male. Some of this estrogen, thought to be formed from testosterone, plays an important role in spermatogenesis.

Testosterone is metabolized in the liver and excreted by the kidneys. In the bloodstream, testosterone exists in an unbound (free) or a bound form. The bound form is attached to plasma proteins, including albumin and the sex hormone–binding protein produced by the liver. Only approximately 3% of circulating testosterone is unbound and therefore able to enter the cell and exert its metabolic effects.[1] Much of the testosterone that becomes fixed to the tissues is converted to dihydrotestosterone, especially in certain target tissues such as the prostate gland. Some of the actions of testosterone depend on this conversion, whereas others do not.

Testosterone exerts a number of biologic effects in the male (Chart 39-1). In the male embryo, it is essential for appropriate differentiation of the internal and external genitalia, and in the fetus it is necessary for descent of the testes. Testosterone is essential to the development of primary and secondary male sex characteristics during puberty and for the maintenance of these characteristics during adult life. It causes growth of pubic, chest, and facial hair; it produces changes in the larynx that result in the male bass voice; and it increases the thickness of the skin and the activity of the sebaceous glands, predisposing to acne.

Most of the actions of testosterone and other androgens result from increased protein synthesis in target tissues. Androgens function as anabolic agents in males and females to promote metabolism and musculoskeletal growth. They greatly affect the development of muscle mass during puberty, with boys averaging approximately 50% more of an increase in muscle mass than girls.[1]

Spermatogenesis

Spermatogenesis, which occurs in the seminiferous tubules of the testes, is the sequence of events that leads to the formation of male germ cells or spermatozoa. The process begins shortly before puberty and continues throughout a man's life.

The seminiferous tubules are composed of two types of cells: Sertoli cells and spermatogenic cells[1-3] (Fig. 39-3A). Sertoli cells are tall columnar cells with extensive cytoplasmic processes that surround the spermatogenic cells and form tight junctions with other Sertoli cells. Also known as *supporting* or *sustentacular cells*, Sertoli cells provide structural organization for the tubules; they supply both physical and nutritional support for the developing germ cells; and their tight junctions prevent the passage of proteins from the interstitial space into the lumen of the seminiferous tubules, thus forming a blood-testis barrier.[2,3] In addition, these cells have been shown to be responsible for the movement of spermatozoa

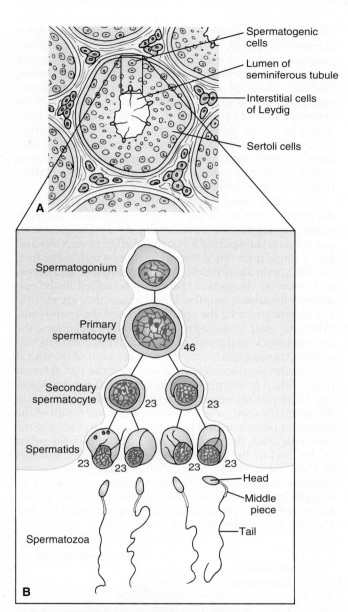

FIGURE 39-3. (A) Cross-section of seminiferous tubule and **(B)** stages of development of spermatozoa. (46, 23 = number of chromosomes.)

from the base of the tubule toward the lumen and for the release of mature sperm into the lumen. They also phagocytose damaged germ cells and residual bodies formed during the last stage of spermatogenesis. Finally, in response to follicle-stimulating hormone (FSH) or testosterone, the Sertoli cells secrete androgen-binding protein. This substance, which has a high affinity for androgens, provides high concentrations of testosterone to the developing germ cells during spermatogenesis.

Spermatogenic cells, the source of spermatozoa, are organized in poorly defined layers of progressive development between adjacent Sertoli cells. Both spermatogenesis and oogenesis, its counterpart in the female, involve a unique kind of nuclear division in which the chromosome number is reduced from 46 to 23 (see Chapter 5).

The process of spermatogenesis begins with the spermatogonial phase, during which the spermatogonia undergo mitotic division to form more spermatogonia as well as primary spermatocytes (Fig. 39-3B). During the next phase of spermatogenesis, the primary spermatocyte undergoes meiotic division during which its 46 chromosomes (23 pairs) are divided so that 23 chromosomes go to one secondary spermatocyte and the other 23 to another secondary spermatocyte. During the final stage of spermatogenesis, the secondary spermatocytes divide to form spermatids, which develop into mature spermatozoa or sperm cells.

After their development in the seminiferous tubules, the spermatozoa move into a highly convoluted network of ducts called the *rete testis* (see Fig. 39-2). The spermatozoa are then transported through the efferent ductules and into a single duct called the *epididymis*, which is the final site for sperm maturation.[1,2] The epididymis also serves as a reservoir for sperm. Sperm can be stored in the epididymis for several months. If held longer they are eventually phagocytized by the epithelial cells of the epididymis. When the male is sexually stimulated and ejaculates, the smooth muscle in the wall of the epididymis contracts vigorously, moving sperm into the next segment of the ductal system, the *ductus deferens*, also called the *vas deferens* (Fig. 39-4). The ductus deferens ascends along the posterior border of the testes and then enters the abdomen in the spermatic cord, which serves as a conduit for all of the structures passing to and from the testes. After leaving the spermatic cord, the ductus deferens descends in the pelvis to the level of the bladder, where its distal end enlarges to form the *ampulla*. Surgical disconnection of the vas deferens in the scrotal area (i.e., vasectomy) serves as an effective method of male contraception. Because sperm are stored in the ampulla, men can remain fertile for 4 to 5 weeks after performance of a vasectomy.

Semen Production

The accessory genital glands include the paired seminal vesicles and bulbourethral glands and the single prostate gland (see Fig. 39-1).[1,2] These glands secrete fluids that form the bulk of the ejaculatory fluid or semen.

The seminal vesicles, which lie on the posterior wall of the bladder, consist of highly tortuous tubes that secrete fluid for the semen. Each of the paired seminal vesicles is lined with secretory epithelium containing an abundance of fructose, prostaglandins, and several other proteins. The fructose secreted by the seminal vesicles provides the energy for sperm motility. The prostaglandins are thought to assist in fertilization by making the cervical mucus more receptive to sperm and by causing reverse peristaltic contractions in the uterus and fallopian tubes to move the sperm toward the ovaries. A short excretory duct from the each seminal vesicle combines with the ampulla of the ductus deferens to form the ejaculatory duct, which enters the posterior part of the prostate and continues through until it ends in the prostatic portion of the urethra. Contraction of the smooth muscle coat of the seminal vesicles during ejaculation discharges their secretion into the ejaculatory ducts and helps to flush sperm out of the urethra.

The prostate, which is the largest of the accessory glands, is located in the pelvis, inferior to the bladder, where it surrounds the prostatic portion of the urethra. The prostate gland secretes a thin, milky, alkaline fluid containing citric acid, calcium, acid phosphate, a clotting enzyme, and a profibrinolysin.[2] During ejaculation, the capsule of the prostate contracts, and the added fluid increases the bulk of the semen. Both vaginal secretions and the fluid from the vas deferens are strongly acidic. Because sperm mobilization occurs at a pH of 6.0 to 6.5, the alkaline nature of the prostatic secretions is essential for successful fertilization of the ovum.

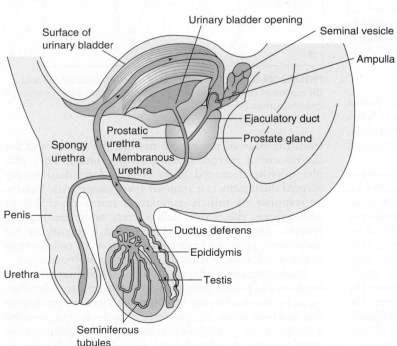

Surface of urinary bladder
Urinary bladder opening
Seminal vesicle
Ampulla
Ejaculatory duct
Prostate gland
Prostatic urethra
Membranous urethra
Spongy urethra
Penis
Urethra
Ductus deferens
Epididymis
Testis
Seminiferous tubules

FIGURE 39-4. The excretory ducts of the male reproductive system and the path that sperm follows as it leaves the testis and travels to the urethra.

The bulbourethral glands are peanut-sized glands located on either side of the membranous urethra (see Fig. 39-1). A duct of each gland joins the initial portion of the penile urethra. The glands, which structurally resemble mucus-secreting glands, produce a clear mucus-like secretion.[2] Sexual stimulation causes release of the secretion, which constitutes the major portion of the pre-seminal fluid and serves to lubricate the penile urethra.

Hypothalamic/Pituitary Control of Testicular Function

The hypothalamus and the anterior pituitary gland play an essential role in promoting spermatogenesis in the testes and maintaining the endocrine function of the testes by means of the gonadotropic hormones (i.e., anterior pituitary hormones that promote the function and growth of the testes in the male).[1,3] The synthesis and release of the gonadotropic hormones from the pituitary gland are regulated by gonadotropin-releasing hormone (GnRH), which is synthesized by the hypothalamus and secreted into the hypothalamohypophysial portal circulation (Fig. 39-5).

Two gonadotropic hormones are secreted by the pituitary gland: FSH and luteinizing hormone (LH). In the male, LH also is called *interstitial cell–stimulating hormone*. The production of testosterone by the interstitial cells of Leydig is regulated by LH. Follicle-stimulating hormone binds selectively to Sertoli cells surrounding the seminiferous tubules, where it functions in the initiation of spermatogenesis. Under the influence of FSH, Sertoli cells produce androgen-binding protein, plasminogen activator, and inhibin. Androgen-binding protein binds testosterone and serves as a carrier and storage site for testosterone in Sertoli cells. Although FSH is necessary for the initiation of spermatogenesis, full maturation of the spermatozoa requires testosterone. Androgen-binding protein also serves as a carrier of testosterone from the testes to the epididymis. Plasminogen activator, which converts plasminogen to plasmin, functions in the final detachment of mature spermatozoa from Sertoli cells.

Circulating levels of the gonadotropic hormones are regulated in a negative feedback manner by testosterone.[1,3] High levels of testosterone suppress LH secretion through a direct action on the pituitary and an inhibitory effect on the hypothalamus. Follicle-stimulating hormone is thought to be inhibited by a substance called *inhibin*, produced by Sertoli cells. Although two forms of inhibin have been identified, only inhibin B has been found in males.[3] Inhibin suppresses FSH release from the pituitary gland without effecting LH release. The pituitary gonadotropic hormones and Sertoli cells in the testes form a classic negative feedback loop in which FSH stimulates inhibin secretion and increased inhibin levels suppress FSH release from the hypothalamus. Unlike the cyclic hormonal pattern in the woman, in the man, FSH, LH, and testosterone secretion and spermatogenesis occur at relatively unchanging rates during adulthood.

Sexual Function

The penis is the male external genital organ through which the urethra passes. It functions both as a sexual organ and as an organ of urine elimination. Anatomically, the external penis consists of a shaft that ends in a tip called the *glans* (see Fig. 39-1). The loose skin of the shaft folds to cover the glans, forming what is called the *prepuce*, or *foreskin*. It is the foreskin that is removed during circumcision. The glans of the penis contains many sensory nerves, making this the most sensitive portion of the penile shaft. The shaft of the penis is composed of three masses of erectile tissue held together by fibrous strands and covered with a thin layer of skin (Fig. 39-6B). The two dorsal masses of tissue are called the *corpora cavernosa* and the third ventral mass, in which the spongy part of the urethra is enclosed, is called the *corpus spongiosum*.[2] The corpora cavernosa and corpus spongiosum are cavernous sinuses that normally are relatively empty but become engorged with blood during penile erection.

The physiology of the male sex act involves a complex interaction between autonomic nervous system–mediated spinal cord reflexes, higher neural centers, and the vascular system[1,2] (Fig. 39-6A). It involves erection, emission, ejaculation, and detumescence. *Erection* involves increased flow of blood into the corpora cavernosa and penile rigidity, *emission* is the contraction of the vas deferens and ampulla with expulsion of sperm into the internal urethra, and *ejaculation* is the

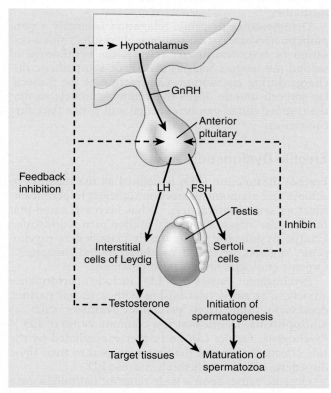

FIGURE 39-5. Hypothalamic-pituitary feedback control of spermatogenesis and testosterone levels in the male. The *dashed line* represents negative feedback. FSH, follicle-stimulating hormone; GnRH, gonadotropin-releasing hormone; LH, luteinizing hormone.

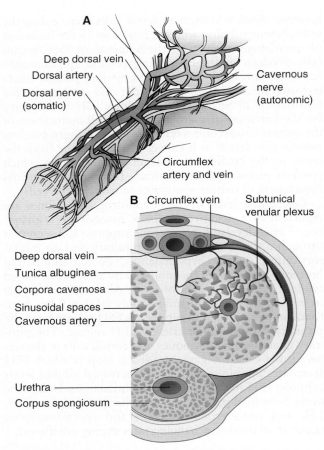

FIGURE 39-6. Anatomy and mechanism of penile erection. **(A)** Innervation and arterial and venous blood supply to penis. **(B)** Cross-section of penis, showing the corpus spongiosum and the sinusoidal system of the corpora cavernosa.

expulsion of semen from the urethra. *Detumescence*, or penile relaxation, results from outflow of blood from the corpora cavernosa.

Neural Control of Male Sexual Function

The penis is innervated by both the autonomic and somatic nervous systems. In the pelvis, the sympathetic and parasympathetic components of the autonomic nervous system merge to form what are called the *cavernous nerves*.[4] Erection is under the control of the parasympathetic nervous system, and ejaculation and detumescence are under the control of the sympathetic nervous system. Somatic innervation, which occurs through the pudendal nerve, is responsible for penile sensation and contraction and relaxation of the extracorporeal striated bulbocavernosus and ischiocavernous muscles.

Erection is a neurovascular process involving the autonomic nervous system, neurotransmitters and endothelial relaxing factors, the vascular smooth muscle of the arteries and veins supplying the penile tissue, and the trabecular smooth muscle of the sinusoids of the corpora cavernosa.[4] It involves increased flow of blood into the corpora cavernosa due to relaxation of the trabecular smooth muscle that surrounds the sinusoidal spaces and compression of the veins controlling outflow of blood

from the venous plexus. Erection is mediated by parasympathetic impulses that pass from the sacral segments of the spinal cord through the pelvic nerves to the penis. Parasympathetic stimulation results in release of nitric oxide, a nonadrenergic–noncholinergic neurotransmitter, which causes relaxation of the trabecular smooth muscle of the corpora cavernosa. This relaxation permits the inflow of blood into the sinuses of the cavernosa at pressures approaching those of the arterial blood pressure. Because the erectile tissues of the cavernosa are surrounded by a nonelastic fibrous covering, high pressure in the sinusoids causes ballooning of the erectile tissue to such an extent that the penis becomes hard and elongated. At the same time, contraction of the somatic-innervated ischiocavernous muscles forcefully compresses the blood-filled corpora cavernosa, producing a further increase in intercavernous pressures. During this phase of erection, inflow and outflow of blood cease.

Parasympathetic innervation must be intact and nitric oxide synthesis must be active for erection to occur. Nitric oxide activates guanyl cyclase, an enzyme that increases the concentration of cyclic guanosine monophosphate (cGMP), which in turn causes smooth muscle relaxation. Other smooth muscle relaxants (e.g., prostaglandin E_1 analogs and α-adrenergic antagonists), if present in high enough concentrations, can independently cause sufficient cavernosal relaxation to result in erection.[4] Many of the drugs that have been developed to treat erectile dysfunction act at the levels of these mediators.[5,6]

Detumescence or penile relaxation is largely a sympathetic nervous system response. It results from a cessation of neurotransmitter release, the breakdown of second messengers such as cGMP, or sympathetic discharge during ejaculation. Contraction of the trabecular smooth muscle opens the venous channels so that the trapped blood can be expelled and penile flaccidity can return.

Erectile Dysfunction

Erectile dysfunction (ED) is defined as the inability to achieve and maintain an erection sufficient to permit satisfactory sexual intercourse.[7] It has been estimated that the disorder affects about 150 million men worldwide.[6] Erectile dysfunction is commonly classified as psychogenic, organic, or mixed psychogenic and organic.[5,6,8] Organic etiologies are the most common.

Psychogenic causes of ED include performance anxiety, a strained relationship with a sexual partner, depression, and overt psychotic disorders such as schizophrenia. Depression is a common cause of ED.[5,8] Psychogenic factors can be further exacerbated by the side effects of many of the therapies used to treat these disorders, which can themselves cause ED.

Organic causes span a wide range of pathologic processes. They include neurogenic, hormonal, vascular, drug-induced, and penile-related etiologies. Neurogenic disorders such as Parkinson disease, stroke, and cerebral trauma often contribute to ED by decreasing libido or preventing the initiation of erection. In spinal cord injury, the extent of neural impairment depends on the level, location, and extent of the lesion. Somatosensory innervation of the genitalia is essential to the reflex mechanisms involved in erection; this becomes important with aging and conditions such as diabetes that impair peripheral nerve function. Extensive pelvis surgery, especially radical prostatectomy (even so-called "nerve-sparing" procedures), are common causes of erectile dysfunction (ED) due to both direct and indirect nerve damage.

Hormonal causes of ED include a decrease in androgen levels because of both primary and secondary hypogonadism. Androgen levels may be decreased because of aging (andropause). Hyperprolactinemia from any cause interferes with both reproduction and erectile function. This is because prolactin acts centrally to inhibit the release of the hypothalamic GnRH that controls the release of the pituitary gonadotropic hormones, LH and FSH. Elevated prolactin levels may also interfere with normal functioning at the level of the gonad.

Common risk factors for generalized penile arterial insufficiency include hypertension, hyperlipidemia, cigarette smoking, diabetes mellitus, and pelvic irradiation.[8] In hypertension, erectile function is impaired not so much by the increased blood pressure as by the associated stenotic arterial lesions. Focal stenosis of the common penile artery most often occurs in men who sustained blunt pelvic or perineal trauma (e.g., from bicycling accidents). Failure of the veins to close completely during an erection (veno-occlusive dysfunction) may occur in men with large venous channels that drain the corpora cavernosa. Other disorders that impair venous occlusion are degenerative changes involving the tunica albuginea, as in Peyronie disease.

Many drugs are reported to cause ED, including antidepressant, antipsychotic, antiandrogen, and antihypertensive medications.[5,6,8] Cigarette smoking can induce vasoconstriction and penile venous leakage because of its effects on cavernous smooth muscle and can double the risk of erectile dysfunction.[8] Alcohol in small amounts may increase libido and improve erection; however, in large amounts it can cause central sedation, decreased libido, and transient ED.

Aging is known to increase the risk of ED.[9] After 50 years of age, the overall prevalence of ED is reported to be greater than 50%.[10] Many of the pathologic processes that contribute to ED are more common in older men, including diabetes, hyperlipidemia, vascular disease, and the long-term effects of cigarette smoking. Age-related declines in testosterone may also play a role (andropause). Psychosocial problems such as depression, esteem issues, partner relationships, history of substance abuse, and anxiety and fear of performance failure also may contribute to ED in older men.[10]

A diagnosis of ED requires careful history (medical, sexual, and psychosocial), physical examination, and laboratory tests aimed at determining what other tests are needed to rule out organic causes of the disorder. Because many medications, including prescribed, over-the-counter, and illicit drugs, can cause ED, a careful drug history is indicated.

Erectile dysfunction is now recognized as a marker for cardiovascular disease, and is now considered a component of the metabolic syndrome (a collection of cardiovascular risk factors; see Chapter 33).[5,6,11,12] The presence of ED can be an early warning sign of underlying vascular disease (coronary, cerebrovascular, and peripheral) which can be asymptomatic especially in patients with type 2 diabetes. It has been proposed that men with smaller penile arteries (diameter 1–2 mm) suffer obstruction from artherosclerotic plaque burden earlier than those with larger coronary (3–4 mm), carotid (5–7 mm), or ileofemoral (6–8 mm) arteries, hence ED may be symptomatic before a coronary event. In addition, the association between ED and the metabolic syndrome may be related to the underlying endothelial dysfunction seen in both conditions (see Chapter 18). Men with ED should be evaluated for coexisting vascular disease and cardiovascular risk factors should be modified or treated (e.g., smoking, diabetes, hypertension, and hyperlipidemia).[5,6,11]

Treatment methods include psychosexual counseling, androgen replacement therapy (when androgen deficiency is confirmed), oral and intracavernous drug therapy, vacuum constriction devices, and surgical treatment (prosthesis and vascular surgery).[5,6,8] Among the commonly prescribed drugs used for the treatment of ED are the selective inhibitors of phosphodiesterase type 5 (PDE-5), the enzyme that inactivates cGMP (sildenafil, vardenafil, and tadalafil). These drugs act by facilitating corporeal smooth muscle relaxation in response to sexual stimulation. The concomitant use of PDE-5 inhibitors and nitrates (used, for example, in ischemic heart disease) is absolutely contraindicated because of the risk of profound hypotension.[11] The PDE-5 inhibitors are taken orally. Alprostadil, a prostaglandin E_1 analog, acts by producing relaxation of cavernous smooth muscle. It is either injected directly into the cavernosa (with diffusion into the opposite cavernosa) or placed in the urethra as a minisuppository. Phentolamine (α_2-adrenergic receptor antagonist) and papaverine (smooth muscle relaxant) are also administered by intracavernous injection.

SUMMARY CONCEPTS

- The male genitourinary system, which consists of the genital ducts, accessory genital organs, and penis, functions in both urine elimination and reproduction. The testes or male gonads function in both production of male germ cells (spermatogenesis) and the secretion of the male sex hormone, testosterone.

- Testosterone is essential for differentiation of the internal and external genitalia in the male embryo, descent of the testes in the fetus, development of primary and secondary male sex characteristics during puberty, and maintenance of these characteristics during adult life.

(continued)

■ The function of the male reproductive system is under the negative feedback control of the hypothalamus and the anterior pituitary gonadotropic hormones—FSH and LH. Spermatogenesis is initiated by FSH, and the production of testosterone is regulated by LH.

■ The male sex act involves erection, emission, ejaculation, and detumescence. The physiology of these functions involves a complex interaction between autonomic-mediated spinal cord reflexes, higher neural centers, and the vascular system. Erection is mediated by the parasympathetic nervous system and emission and ejaculation by the sympathetic nervous system.

■ Erection is a neurovascular process involving the autonomic nervous system, the somatic nervous system by way of the pudendal nerve, the vascular system, and the sinusoidal spaces of the corpora cavernosa. Erectile dysfunction is defined as the inability to achieve and maintain an erection sufficient to permit satisfactory sexual intercourse. It can be due to psychogenic factors, organic disorders, or mixed psychogenic and organic conditions. Erectile dysfunction is now recognized as a marker for cardiovascular disease and men with the disorder should be evaluated for coexisting vascular disease.

Disorders of the Penis, the Scrotum and Testes, and the Prostate

The male genitourinary system is subject to structural defects, inflammation and infection, and neoplasms, all of which can affect urine elimination, sexual function, and fertility.

Disorders of the Penis

Disorders of the penis include congenital defects (discussed in the section on disorders of childhood), acute and chronic inflammatory conditions, Peyronie disease, priapism, and neoplasms.

Inflammation and Infection

The term *balanitis* refers to local inflammation of the glans penis and *balanoposthitis* to inflammation of the glans penis and overlying prepuce.[13–15] The condition may result from trauma, irritation, or infection caused by a wide array of organisms. Among the most common infectious agents are *Candida albicans*, anaerobic bacteria, and pyogenic bacteria. A significant number of inflammatory conditions are caused by sexually transmitted infections (see Chapter 41). Balanitis due to *C. albicans* infection may be a presenting feature or result from poorly controlled diabetes mellitus.

Acute superficial balanoposthitis is characterized by erythema of the glans and prepuce. An exudate in the form of malodorous discharge may be present. It usually is encountered in males with phimosis (a tight foreskin) or a large, redundant prepuce that interferes with cleanliness and predisposes to bacterial growth in the accumulated secretions and smegma (i.e., debris from the desquamated epithelia). Extension of the erythema and edema may lead to extensive scarring and a condition called *phimosis*, in which the prepuce cannot be retracted easily over the glans prepuce. When the stenotic prepuce is forcibly retracted over the glans prepuce, the circulation can be compromised causing congestion, swelling, and pain, a condition known as *paraphimosis*.

Balanitis xerotica obliterans is a chronic, sclerosing, atrophic process of the glans penis that occurs in uncircumcised men. It is clinically and histologically similar to the lichen sclerosus that is seen in women[15] (see Chapter 40). Typically, the lesions consist of grayish-white plaques on the surface of the glans penis and the prepuce. The foreskin is thickened and fibrous and is not retractable. Although balanitis xerotica obliterans was once considered a benign condition, it is now recognized as a precancerous state.[16] Treatment measures include circumcision and topical or intralesional injections of corticosteroids.[13]

Peyronie Disease

Peyronie disease involves a localized and progressive fibrosis of unknown origin that affects the tunica albuginea (i.e., the tough, fibrous sheath that surrounds the corpora cavernosa) of the penis. It is named after Francois de la Peyronie, who in 1743 described a patient who had "rosary beads of scar tissue to cause upward curvature of the penis during erection."[17,18] The disorder is characterized initially by an inflammatory process that results in dense fibrous plaque formation. The plaque usually is on the dorsal midline of the shaft, causing upward bowing of the shaft during erection (Fig. 39-7). Some men may develop scarring on both the dorsal and ventral aspects of the shaft, causing the penis to be straight but shortened or have a lateral bend. The fibrous tissue prevents lengthening of the involved area during erection, making intercourse difficult and painful. The disease usually occurs in middle-aged or elderly men.

The manifestations of Peyronie disease include painful erection, bent erection, and the presence of a hard mass at the site of fibrosis. Approximately two thirds of men complain of pain as a symptom. The pain is thought to be generated by inflammation of the adjacent fascial tissue and usually disappears as the inflammation resolves.

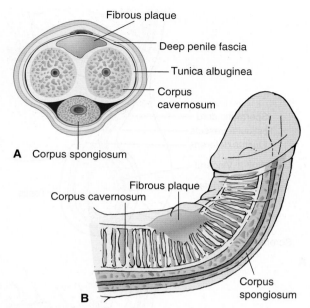

FIGURE 39-7. Peyronie disease. **(A)** Penile cross-section showing plaque between the corpora. **(B)** Penile curvature.

During the 1st year or so after formation of the plaque, while the scar tissue is undergoing the process of remodeling, penile distortion may increase, remain static, or resolve and disappear completely. In some cases, the scar tissue may progress to calcification and formation of bonelike tissue.

Diagnosis is based on history and physical examination. Ultrasonography may be used to diagnose the disorder. Although surgical intervention can be used to correct the disorder, it often is delayed because in many cases the disorder is self-limiting. Less invasive treatments include the administration of oral agents with antioxidant properties (e.g., vitamin E, colchicine); pentoxifylline, a drug that is thought to reduce blood viscosity, allowing it to flow more easily through partially obstructed areas; and intralesional treatments, including corticosteroids.

Priapism

Priapism is an involuntary, prolonged (>4 hours), abnormal and painful erection that continues beyond, or is unrelated to, sexual stimulation.[19,20] Priapism is a true urologic emergency because the prolonged erection can result in ischemia and fibrosis of the erectile tissue with significant risk of subsequent impotence. Priapism can occur at any age, in the newborn as well as other age groups. Sickle cell disease or neoplasms are the most common cause in boys between 5 and 10 years of age.[21]

Priapism is caused by impaired blood flow in the corpora cavernosa of the penis. Priapism is classified as primary (idiopathic) or secondary to a disease or drug effect. Secondary causes include hematologic conditions (e.g., leukemia, sickle cell disease, polycythemia), neurologic conditions (e.g., stroke, spinal cord injury), and renal failure. Between 6% and 42% of males with sickle cell

disease are affected at some stage by priapism.[21] The relative deoxygenation and stasis of cavernosal blood during erection is thought to increase sickling. Various medications, such as erectile dysfunction drugs, antihypertensive drugs, anticoagulant drugs, antidepressant agents, alcohol, and marijuana, can contribute to the development of priapism. Currently, intracavernous injection therapy for erectile dysfunction is one of the more common causes of priapism.

The diagnosis of priapism usually is based on clinical findings. Color Doppler studies of penile blood flow, penile ultrasonography, and computed tomography (CT) scans may be used to determine intrapelvic pathology. Initial treatment measures include analgesics, sedation, and hydration. Urinary retention may necessitate catheterization. Local measures include ice packs and cold saline enemas, aspiration and irrigation of the corpus cavernosum with plain or heparinized saline, or instillation of α-adrenergic drugs. If less aggressive treatment does not produce detumescence, a temporary surgical shunt may be established between the corpus cavernosum and the corpus spongiosum.

The prognosis for whether fibrosis or erectile failure will occur is determined by the severity and duration of blood stasis. Persistent stasis priapism is known to result in impaired erectile function and tissue fibrosis unless resolved within 24 to 48 hours of onset.[20]

Neoplasms of the Penis

Although relatively rare (<1% of male genital tumors) in developed countries of the world, cancer of the penis may account for 10% to 20% of all genital malignancies in areas such as Africa and South America.[22] When it is diagnosed early, penile cancer is highly curable. The greatest hindrance to early diagnosis is a delay in seeking medical attention.

The cause of penile cancer is unknown.[16,22,23] Several risk factors have been proposed, including poor genital hygiene, human papillomavirus (HPV) infection, ultraviolet radiation exposure, increasing age, and immunodeficiency states. Circumcision confers protection, and hence cancer of the penis is extremely rare in men circumcised at birth.[14,15] It is thought that circumcision is associated with better genital hygiene, which, in turn, reduces exposure to carcinogens that may accumulate in smegma and decreases the likelihood of potentially oncogenic strains of HPV. Ultraviolet radiation is thought to have a carcinogenic effect on the penis.[23] Men who were treated for psoriasis with ultraviolet A radiation (i.e., PUVA) have had a reported increased incidence of genital squamous cell carcinomas. Because of this observation, it is suggested that men should shield their genital area when using tanning salons. Immunodeficiency states (e.g., acquired immunodeficiency syndrome [AIDS]) also may play a role in the pathogenesis of penile cancer.[16,23] Dermatologic lesions with precancerous potential include balanitis xerotica obliterans (discussed under penile inflammatory conditions) and giant condylomata acuminata.[22] Giant condylomata acuminata, or genital warts, are cauliflower-like lesions arising on the prepuce or glans as a result of HPV infection (see Chapter 41).

Most penile cancers are of squamous epithelial cell origin and include carcinoma in situ, which is restricted to the epithelium and does not infiltrate the underlying dermis, and invasive carcinomas.[14–16] In situ carcinomas of the penis are include *Bowen disease* and *erythroplasia of Queyrat*.[15] Bowen disease appears as a sharply demarcated, erythematous or grayish-white plaque on the shaft of the penis. Erythroplasia of Queyrat manifests as single or multiple shiny red, sometimes velvety plaques on the glans or foreskin. In approximately 10% of men, these lesions may transform into infiltrating squamous cell cancer.[14,15]

Invasive squamous cell carcinoma of the penis usually begins as a small lump or ulcer on the glans or inner surface of the prepuce. The lesions are usually slow growing and have often been present for a year or more before being brought to medical attention. The lesions are usually nonpainful until they undergo secondary ulceration and infection.[14–16,22] If phimosis is present, there may be painful swelling, purulent drainage, or difficulty urinating. Metastasis to the inguinal lymph node is characteristic of early-stage disease, but widespread dissemination is uncommon until the lesion is far advanced.

Diagnosis usually is based on physical examination and biopsy results. Computed tomography scans, penile ultrasonographic studies, and magnetic resonance imaging (MRI) may be used in the diagnostic workup. Treatment options vary according to stage, size, location, and invasiveness of the tumor. Carcinoma in situ may be treated conservatively with fluorouracil cream application or laser treatment.[22] Conservative treatment requires frequent follow-up examinations. Surgery remains the mainstay of treatment for invasive carcinoma.

Disorders of the Scrotum and Testes

The testes, or male gonads, are two egg-shaped structures located outside the abdominal cavity in the scrotum. Embryologically, they develop in the abdominal cavity and then descend through the inguinal canal into a pouch of peritoneum (which becomes the tunica vaginalis) in the scrotum during the seventh to ninth months of fetal life.[23] As they descend, the testes pull their arteries, veins, lymphatics, nerves, and conducting excretory ducts with them. These structures are encased by the cremaster muscle and layers of fascia that constitute the spermatic cord (Fig. 39-8A). The descent of the testes is thought to be mediated by testosterone, which is active during this stage of fetal development.

After descent of the testes, the inguinal canal closes almost completely. Failure of this canal to close predisposes to the development of an inguinal hernia later in life (Fig. 39-8B). An inguinal hernia or "rupture" is a protrusion of the parietal peritoneum and part of the intestine through an abnormal opening from the abdominal cavity. A loop of small bowel may become incarcerated in an inguinal hernia (strangulated hernia), in which case the lumen of the bowel may become obstructed and its vascular supply compromised.

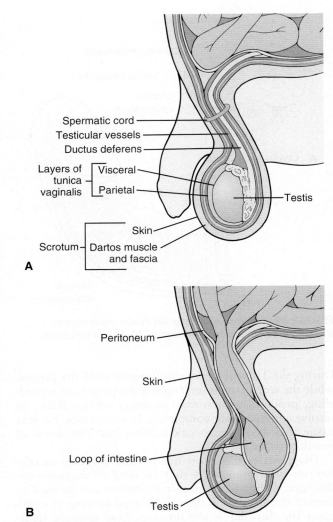

FIGURE 39-8. (A) Anterior view of the spermatic cord and inguinal canal and coverings of the spermatic cord and testes. **(B)** Indirect inguinal hernia. (Adapted from Moore KL, Agur AM. *Essentials of Clinical Anatomy.* 2nd ed. Philadelphia, PA: Lippincott Williams & Wilkins; 2002:130, 138.)

The testes and epididymis are completely surrounded by the tunica vaginalis, a serous pouch derived from the peritoneum during fetal descent of the testes into the scrotum. The tunica vaginalis has an outer parietal layer and a deeper visceral layer that adheres to the dense fibrous covering of the testes, the tunica albuginea. The tunica albuginea protects the testes and gives them their ovoid shape. A space exists between these two layers that typically contains a few milliliters of clear fluid. The cremaster muscles, which are bands of skeletal muscle arising from the internal oblique muscles of the trunk, elevate the testes. The testes receive their arterial blood supply from the long testicular arteries, which branch from the aorta. The testicular veins, which drain the testes, arise from a venous network called the *pampiniform plexus* that surrounds the spermatic artery. The testes are innervated by fibers from both divisions of the autonomic nervous system. Associated sensory nerves transmit pain impulses, resulting in excruciating pain, especially when the testes are hit forcibly.

The scrotum, which houses the testes, is made up of a thin outer layer of darkly pigmented skin that is continuous with the outer skin of the groin. Under the outer skin lies the closely related dartos fascia, a fat-free fascial layer with smooth muscle fibers (i.e., dartos muscle) that is responsible for the wrinkled appearance of the scrotum. This layer contains a septum that separates the two testes. Because the dartos muscle attaches to the skin, its contraction causes the scrotum to wrinkle when cold, reducing the surface area of the scrotum and assisting the cremaster muscles in holding the testes closer to the body.

The location of the testes in the scrotum is important for sperm production, which is optimal at 2°C to 3°C below body temperature (35°C to 37.4°C). Two mechanisms maintain the temperature of the testes at a level consistent with sperm production. One is the pampiniform plexus of testicular veins that surround the testicular artery. This plexus absorbs heat from the arterial blood, cooling it as it enters the testes. The other is the dartos and cremaster muscles, which respond to decreases in testicular temperature by moving the testes closer to the body. Prolonged exposure to elevated temperatures, as a result of prolonged fever or the dysfunction of thermoregulatory mechanisms, can impair spermatogenesis. Some tight-fitting undergarments hold the testes against the body and are thought to contribute to a decrease in sperm counts and infertility by interfering with the thermoregulatory function of the scrotum.

Disorders of the Testicular Tunica

Disorders of the testicular tunica represent scrotal swelling or enlargement due to an accumulation of fluid (hydrocele), blood (hematocele), or sperm (spermatocele) between the layers of the tunica vaginalis, or to dilation of the testicular veins (varicocele) (Fig. 39-9).

Hydrocele. A hydrocele forms when excess fluid collects between the layers of the tunica vaginalis[15,23] (Fig. 39-9B). It may be unilateral or bilateral and can develop as a primary congenital defect or as a secondary condition. Acute hydrocele may develop after local injury, epididymitis or orchitis, gonorrhea, lymph obstruction, or germ cell testicular tumor, or as a side effect of radiation therapy. Chronic hydrocele is more common. Fluid collects about the testis, and the mass grows gradually. Its cause is unknown, and it usually develops in men older than 40 years.

Most cases of hydrocele in male infants and children are caused by a patent processus vaginalis, which is continuous with the peritoneal cavity. There usually are reports that the mass increases in size during the day and decreases at night if the hydrocele communicates with the peritoneal cavity. In many cases hydrocele is associated with an indirect inguinal hernia.[24] Most hydroceles of infancy close spontaneously; therefore, they are not repaired before 1 year of age. If the hydrocele persists beyond 2 years of age, surgical treatment usually is indicated.

Hydroceles are palpated as cystic masses that may attain massive proportions. If there is enough fluid, the mass may be mistaken for a solid tumor. Transillumination of the scrotum (i.e., shining a light through the scrotum to visualize its internal structures) or ultrasonography can help to determine whether the mass is solid or cystic and whether the testicle is normal. A dense hydrocele that does not illuminate should be differentiated from a testicular tumor. If a hydrocele develops in a young man without apparent cause, careful evaluation is needed to exclude cancer or infection.

In an adult male, a hydrocele is a relatively benign condition. The condition often is asymptomatic, and no treatment is necessary. When symptoms do occur, the feeling may be that of heaviness in the scrotum or pain in the lower back. In cases of secondary hydrocele, the primary condition is treated. If the hydrocele is painful or cosmetically undesirable, surgical correction is indicated.

Hematocele. A hematocele is an accumulation of blood in the tunica vaginalis, which causes the scrotal skin to become dark red or purple.[15] It may develop as a result of an abdominal surgical procedure, scrotal trauma, a bleeding disorder, or a testicular tumor.

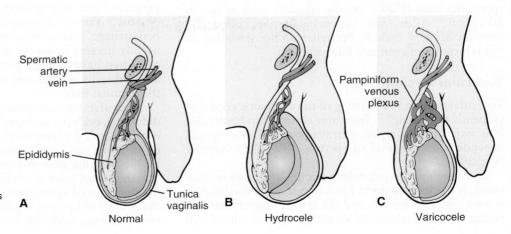

FIGURE 39-9. (A) Normal testis and appendages, **(B)** hydrocele, and **(C)** varicocele.

Spermatic artery
vein
Epididymis
Tunica vaginalis
A Normal

B Hydrocele

Pampiniform venous plexus

C Varicocele

Spermatocele. A spermatocele is a painless, sperm-containing cyst that forms at the end of the epididymis.[15] It is located above and posterior to the testis, is attached to the epididymis, and is separate from the testes. Spermatoceles may be solitary or multiple and usually are less than 1 cm in diameter. They are freely movable and should transilluminate. Spermatoceles rarely cause problems, but a large one may become painful and require excision.

Varicocele. A varicocele is characterized by varicosities of the pampiniform plexus, a network of veins supplying the testes[25] (Fig. 39-9C). The left side is more commonly affected because the left internal spermatic vein inserts into the left renal vein at a right angle, whereas the right spermatic vein has a more oblique insertion into the inferior vena cava. In the standing male, this particular anatomy may cause higher pressures to be transmitted to the left scrotal veins and result in retrograde reflux into veins of the pampiniform plexus. If the condition persists, there may be damage to the elastic fibers and hypertrophy of the vein walls, as occurs in formation of varicose veins in the leg. Sperm concentration and motility are decreased in men with varicoceles.

Varicoceles rarely are found before puberty, and the incidence is highest in males between 15 and 35 years of age. Symptoms of varicocele include an abnormal feeling of heaviness in the left scrotum, although many are asymptomatic. Usually, a varicocele is readily diagnosed on physical examination with the man in the standing and recumbent positions. Typically, the varicocele disappears in the lying position because of venous decompression into the renal vein. Scrotal palpation of a varicocele has been compared to feeling a "bag of worms." Additional diagnostic methods include ultrasonography, radioisotope scanning, and spermatic venography.

Treatment options for varicocele include surgical ligation or sclerosis using a percutaneous transvenous catheter under fluoroscopic guidance. It has been suggested that men with abnormalities in their semen and a varicocele show some degree of improvement in fertility after obliteration of the dilated veins.[25] However, the effectiveness of varicocele treatment in men from subfertile couples is still debated, especially when other assisted reproductive techniques (e.g., intracytoplasmic sperm injection [ICSI]) may be effective with as few as 20 sperm.[25] Aside from improving fertility, other reasons for surgery include the relief of the sensation of "heaviness" and cosmetic improvement.

Testicular Torsion

Testicular torsion is a twisting of the spermatic cord that suspends the testis.[26,27] Testicular torsion can be divided into two distinct types, extravaginal or intravaginal, depending on the level of spermatic cord involvement (Fig. 39-10).

Extravaginal torsion, which occurs in fetuses or neonates, is the less common form of testicular torsion.[28] It occurs when the testicle and the fascial tunicae that surround it rotate around the spermatic cord at a level well

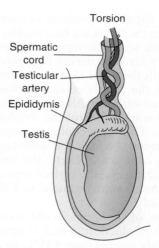

FIGURE 39-10. Testicular torsion with twisting of the spermatic cord that suspends the testis and the spermatic vessels that supply the testis with blood.

above the tunica vaginalis. The torsion probably occurs during fetal or neonatal descent of the testes before the tunica adheres to the scrotal wall. When the torsion occurs in utero, the baby is born with a large firm, non-tender testis. Usually the ipsilateral testis is ecchymotic. In these cases the torsed testis is rarely viable because of the time that has elapsed. In other cases the initial examination is normal, and acute scrotal swelling is recognized subsequently. In these cases, the torsed testis may occasionally be saved. The use of surgical treatment (orchiopexy [in which the testes is attached to the scrotum] and orchiectomy [removal of the testis]) is controversial. There are multiple animal studies indicating that failure to remove the torsed testis may produce an autoimmune response that affects the normal testis.[28]

Intravaginal torsion involves twisting of the spermatic cord within the tunica vaginalis. It is a true surgical emergency, and early recognition and treatment are necessary if the testicle is to be saved.[26–28] Intravaginal testicular torsion can occur at any age, but is more common during adolescence. Torsion usually occurs in the absence of any precipitating event and is thought to be due to abnormal fixation of the testis within the tunica vaginalis, allowing the testis to twist, especially during periods of testicular growth such as puberty. The torsion obstructs venous drainage, with resultant edema and hemorrhage, and subsequent arterial obstruction. Males usually present in severe distress within hours of onset and often have nausea, vomiting, and tachycardia. The affected testis is large and tender, with pain radiating to the inguinal area.

Testicular torsion must be differentiated from epididymitis, orchitis, and trauma to the testis. On physical examination, the testicle often is high in the scrotum and in an abnormal orientation. These changes are caused by the twisting and shortening of the spermatic cord. The degree of scrotal swelling and redness depends on the duration of symptoms. The cremasteric reflex, normally elicited by stroking the medial aspect of the thigh and observing testicular retraction, frequently is absent.

Color Doppler ultrasonography is increasingly used in the evaluation of suspected testicular torsion.

Treatment includes surgical detorsion and orchiectomy. Orchiectomy is carried out when the testis is deemed nonviable after surgical detorsion. Testicular salvage rates are directly related to the duration of torsion. Because the opposite testicle usually is affected by the same abnormal attachments, prophylactic fixation of that testis often is performed.

Epididymitis

Epididymitis is an inflammation of the epididymis, the elongated cordlike structure that is located along the posterior border of the testis and functions in the transport and storage of sperm[29,30] (see Fig. 39-4). The cause of epididymitis varies with age. Most cases of epididymitis in men younger than 35 years are due to sexually transmitted infections such as *Chlamydia trachomatis* and *Neisseria gonorrhoeae*. In men older than 35, epididymitis is generally caused by infection with common urinary tract pathogens, such as *Escherichia coli* and *Pseudomonas*. In prepubertal children, the disorder usually is associated with congenital urinary tract abnormalities and infection with gram-negative rods.

Infections may reach the epididymis through the vas deferens, in which case the pressure associated with voiding or physical strain may force pathogen-containing urine from the urethra or prostate up the ejaculatory duct and through the vas deferens into the epididymis. Infections may also reach the epididymis through the lymphatics of the spermatic cord. Risk factors for epididymitis in all men include sexual activity, heavy physical exertion, and bicycle or motorcycle riding. Recent urinary tract surgery or instrumentation and anatomic abnormalities such as prostatic obstruction are risk factors in older men.

Epididymitis is characterized by unilateral pain and swelling, accompanied by erythema and edema of the overlying scrotal skin that develops over a period of 24 to 48 hours. Initially, the swelling and induration are limited to the epididymis. The distinction between the testis and epididymis becomes less evident as the inflammation progresses, and the testis and epididymis become one mass. There may be tenderness over the groin (spermatic cord) or in the lower abdomen. Symptoms of lower urinary tract infection, such as fever, frequency, urgency, and dysuria, may be present. Whether urethral discharge is present depends on the organism causing the infection; it usually accompanies gonorrheal infections, is common in chlamydial infections, and is less common in infections caused by gram-negative organisms.

Laboratory findings usually reveal an elevated white blood cell count. Urinalysis and urine culture are important in the diagnosis of epididymitis, with bacteriuria and pyuria suggestive of the disorder; however, the urinalysis may be normal. If the diagnosis remains uncertain, color Doppler ultrasonography may be useful, revealing increased blood flow to the affected testis.

Treatment of epididymitis includes bed rest, scrotal elevation and support, analgesics, nonsteroidal anti-inflammatory agents, and antibiotics. Bed rest with scrotal support improves lymphatic drainage.[29,30] The choice of antibiotics is determined by age, physical findings, urinalysis, Gram stain results, cultures, and sexual history. Sexual activity or physical strain may exacerbate the infection and worsen the symptoms, and should be avoided. If a sexually transmitted disease is suspected, it is important to ensure that the sexual partner receives treatment.

Orchitis

Orchitis is an infection of the testes. It can be precipitated by a primary infection in the genitourinary tract, or the infection can be spread to the testes through the epididymis, bloodstream, or lymphatics.[29] It can develop as a complication of a systemic infection, such as parotitis (i.e., mumps), scarlet fever, or pneumonia. Probably the best known of these complications is orchitis caused by the mumps virus.[31]

Mumps orchitis is now rarely seen in children younger than 10, but is the most common complication of mumps infection in the postpubertal male, occurring in approximately 20% to 30% of adolescent boys and young men with mumps. Although the incidence of mumps orchitis has dramatically declined since the introduction of childhood vaccination programs, a sharp increase in mumps and mumps orchitis has recently been reported in both the United States[32] and the United Kingdom.[31] It is also important to note that mumps remains epidemic in many countries throughout the world, and the mumps vaccine is only used in 57% of the World Health Organization member-countries.[31]

The onset of mumps orchitis is sudden; it usually occurs approximately 3 to 4 days after the onset of the parotitis and is characterized by fever, painful enlargement of the testes, and small hemorrhages into the tunica albuginea. Unlike epididymitis, the urinary symptoms are absent. The symptoms usually run their course in 7 to 10 days. The residual effects seen after the acute phase of the infection include hyalinization of the seminiferous tubules and atrophy of the testes (seen in half of affected men). Spermatogenesis is irreversibly impaired in approximately 30% of testes damaged by mumps orchitis. If both testes are involved (which occurs in 10% to 30% of cases), permanent sterility can result, but is rare.[31] Androgenic hormone function is usually maintained in these cases.

Neoplasms of the Scrotum and Testes

Tumors can develop in the scrotum or the testes. Benign scrotal tumors are common and often do not require treatment. Carcinoma of the scrotum is rare and usually is associated with exposure to carcinogenic agents. Almost all solid tumors of the testes are malignant.

Scrotal Cancer. Cancer of the scrotum was the first cancer directly linked to a specific occupation when, in the 1800s, it was associated with chimney sweeps.[33]

Studies have linked this cancer to exposure to tar, soot, and oils. Most squamous cell cancers of the scrotum are linked to poor hygiene and chronic inflammation. Exposure to PUVA or HPV also has been associated with the disease. The mean age of presentation with the disease is 60 years, often preceded by 20 to 30 years of chronic irritation.

In the early stages, cancer of the scrotum may appear as a small tumor or wartlike growth that eventually ulcerates. The thin scrotal wall lacks the tissue reactivity needed to block the malignant process; more than one half of the cases seen involve metastasis to the lymph nodes. Because this tumor does not respond well to chemotherapy or irradiation, the treatment includes wide local excision of the tumor with inguinal and femoral node dissection.[34] Prognosis correlates with lymph node involvement.

Testicular Cancer. Testicular cancer accounts for 1% to 2% of all neoplasms in men.[35] Although relatively rare, it is the most common cause of cancer in 20- to 35-year-old males.[35] In the past, testicular cancer was a leading cause of death among men entering their most productive years. Since the late 1970s, however, advances in therapy have transformed an almost invariably fatal disease into one that is highly curable.

Although the cause of testicular cancer is unknown, several predisposing influences may be important: cryptorchidism, genetic factors, and disorders of testicular development.[14,15,35] The strongest association has been with cryptorchid or undescended testis. Genetic predisposition also appears to be important. Family clustering of the disorder has been described, although a well-defined pattern of inheritance has not been established. Men with disorders of testicular development, including those with Klinefelter syndrome and testicular feminization, also have a higher risk.

The majority of testicular tumors are of germ cell origin.[14,15] Germ cell tumors can be classified as seminomas and nonseminomas. *Seminomas* account for approximately 50% of germ cell tumors and are most frequent in the fourth decade of life.[14,15] Seminomas tend to retain the phenotypic features of spermatogonia and are the type of germ cell tumor most likely to produce a uniform population of cells. The *nonseminoma* tumors include embryonal carcinoma, teratoma, choriocarcinoma, and yolk cell carcinoma derivatives. They usually contain more than one cell type and are less differentiated than seminomas. *Embryonal carcinomas* are the least differentiated of the tumors, with the capacity to differentiate into other nonseminomatous cell types. They occur most commonly in the 20- to 30-year-old age group. *Choriocarcinoma* is a rare and highly malignant form of testicular cancer that is identical to tumors that arise in placental tissue. *Yolk sac tumors* mimic the embryonic yolk sac histologically. They are the most common type of testicular tumors in infants and children up to 3 years of age, and in this age group have a very good prognosis. Teratomas are composed of somatic cell types from two or more germline layers (ectoderm, mesoderm, or endoderm). They constitute less than 3% of germ cell tumors and can occur at any age from infancy to old age.

They usually behave as benign tumors in children, but contain minute foci of cancer cells in adults.

Often the first sign of testicular cancer is a slight enlargement of the testicle that may be accompanied by some degree of discomfort. This may be an ache in the abdomen or groin or a sensation of dragging or heaviness in the scrotum. Frank pain may be experienced in the later stages, when the tumor is growing rapidly and hemorrhaging occurs. Testicular cancer can spread when the tumor may be barely palpable. Approximately 10% of men present with symptoms related to metastatic disease.[35] Signs of metastatic spread include swelling of the lower extremities, back pain, neck mass, cough, hemoptysis, or dizziness. Gynecomastia (breast enlargement) may result from human chorionic gonadotropin (hCG)-producing tumors and occurs in about 5% of men with germ cell tumors. Although routine screening and monthly self-examination in young men has been recommended, studies have not shown that they improve outcomes.[35] However, men with suggestive signs and symptoms should be carefully evaluated to avoid delayed diagnosis or misdiagnosis.

The diagnosis of testicular cancer requires a thorough urologic history and physical examination. A painless testicular mass may be cancer. Conditions that produce an intrascrotal mass similar to testicular cancer include epididymitis, orchitis, hydrocele, or hematocele. The examination for masses should include palpation of the testes and surrounding structures, transillumination of the scrotum, and abdominal palpation. Testicular ultrasonography can be used to differentiate testicular masses. CT scans and MRI are used in assessing metastatic spread.

Tumor markers that measure protein antigens produced by malignant cells may provide information about the existence of a tumor and the type of tumor present. Three tumor markers are of importance in the diagnosis and management of testicular cancer: α-fetoprotein (AFP), β-hCG, and lactic acid dehydrogenase (LDH).[14,35] α-Fetoprotein is normally present in fetal serum in high levels, but should be present in only trace amounts beyond the age of 1 year. β-Human chorionic gonadotropin is a hormone produced by the placenta in pregnant women, and should not be present in significant levels in the normal male. Elevated serum LDH levels, a cellular enzyme found in muscle, liver, kidneys, and brain, has been shown to correlate with the mass of tumor cells. Lactic acid dehydrogenase is often elevated in widespread, metastatic testicular cancer.

The basic treatment of all testicular cancers includes orchiectomy, which is done at the time of diagnostic exploration. Depending on the histologic characteristics of the tumor and the clinical stage of disease, radiation or chemotherapy may be used after orchiectomy. Rigorous follow-up in all men with testicular cancer is necessary to detect recurrences, most of which occur within 2 years of the end of treatment.[35,36] Testicular cancer is a disease in which even recurrence is highly treatable. With appropriate treatment, the prognosis for men with testicular cancer is excellent. Even patients with more advanced disease have excellent chances for long-term survival.

Disorders of the Prostate

The prostate gland is a walnut-sized fibromuscular and glandular organ that encircles the urethra just inferior to the bladder (see Fig. 39-1). The segment of urethra that travels through the prostate gland is called the *prostatic urethra*. The prostatic urethra is lined by a thin layer of smooth muscle that is continuous with the bladder wall. This smooth muscle represents the true involuntary sphincter of the male posterior urethra. Because the prostate surrounds the urethra, it can produce urinary obstruction when it becomes enlarged.

The prostate gland is made up of many secretory glands arranged in three concentric areas surrounding the prostatic urethra, into which they open. The component glands of the prostate include the (1) small mucosal glands associated with the urethral mucosa, (2) intermediate submucosal glands that lie peripheral to the mucosal glands, and (3) large main prostatic glands that are situated toward the outside of the gland.

Prostatitis

Prostatitis refers to a variety of inflammatory disorders of the prostate gland, some bacterial and some not. It may occur spontaneously, as a result of catheterization or instrumentation, or secondary to other diseases of the male genitourinary system. As an outcome of two consensus conferences, the National Institutes of Health has established a classification system with four categories of prostatitis syndromes: acute bacterial prostatitis, chronic bacterial prostatitis, chronic prostatitis/pelvic pain syndrome, and asymptomatic inflammatory prostatitis.[37] Men with *asymptomatic inflammatory prostatitis* have no subjective symptoms and are detected incidentally on biopsy or examination of prostatic fluid.

Acute Bacterial Prostatitis. Acute bacterial prostatitis often is considered a subtype of urinary tract infection.[38,39] The most likely etiology of acute bacterial prostatitis is an ascending urethral infection or reflux of infected urine into the prostatic ducts. *E. coli*, other gram-negative rods, and enterococci, organisms known to cause urethritis, are the most common infectious agents. Risk of infection is increased in persons with impaired host defenses (e.g., due to diabetes or human immunodeficiency [HIV] infection), recent catheterization or instrumentation of the urinary tract, or urethral strictures.

The manifestations of acute bacterial prostatitis include fever and chills, malaise, myalgia, arthralgia, frequent and urgent urination, dysuria, and urethral discharge. Dull, aching pain often is present in the perineum, rectum, or sacrococcygeal region. The urine may be cloudy and malodorous because of urinary tract infection. Rectal examination reveals a swollen, tender, warm prostate with scattered soft areas. Prostatic massage produces a thick discharge with white blood cells that grows large numbers of pathogens on culture.

Acute prostatitis usually responds to appropriate antimicrobial therapy chosen in accordance with the sensitivity of the causative agents in the urethral discharge. Depending on the urine culture results, antibiotic therapy usually is continued for at least 4 to 6 weeks. Because acute prostatitis often is associated with anatomic abnormalities, a thorough urologic examination usually is performed after treatment is completed.

A persistent fever indicates the need for further investigation for an additional site of infection or a prostatic abscess. Computed tomography scans and transrectal ultrasonography of the prostate are useful in the diagnosis of prostatic abscesses. Prostatic abscesses, which are relatively uncommon since the advent of effective antibiotic therapy, are found more commonly in men with diabetes mellitus.

Chronic Bacterial Prostatitis. In contrast to acute bacterial prostatitis, chronic bacterial prostatitis is a subtle disorder that is difficult to treat. Men with the disorder typically present with recurrent urinary tract infections with persistence of the same strain of pathogenic bacteria in the prostatic fluid and urine.[39–41] Organisms responsible for chronic bacterial prostatitis usually are the gram-negative enterobacteria (*E. coli*, *Proteus*, or *Klebsiella*) or *Pseudomonas*.

The symptoms are variable and include frequent and urgent urination, dysuria, perineal discomfort, and low back pain. Occasionally, myalgia and arthralgia accompany the other symptoms. Secondary epididymitis sometimes is associated with the disorder. Most men are afebrile but have a history of recurrent or relapsing urinary tract infections. Others may be asymptomatic and the diagnosis made after investigation of bacteriuria.

The most accurate method of establishing a diagnosis is by urine cultures. Even after an accurate diagnosis has been established, treatment of chronic prostatitis often is difficult and frustrating.[39–41] Long-term therapy with an appropriate oral antimicrobial agent is the mainstay of treatment. Selection of an appropriate agent is important since antimicrobial drugs penetrate poorly into the chronically inflamed prostate.

Chronic Prostatitis/Chronic Pelvic Pain Syndrome. Chronic prostatitis/pelvic pain syndrome is both the most common and least understood of the prostatitis syndromes.[42] The category is divided into two types, inflammatory and noninflammatory, based on the presence of leukocytes in the prostatic fluid. The inflammatory type was previously referred to as *nonbacterial prostatitis*, and the noninflammatory type as *prostatodynia*.

A large group of men with prostatitis have pain along the penis, testicles, and scrotum; painful ejaculation; low back pain; rectal pain radiating to the inner thighs; urinary symptoms; decreased libido; and impotence, but they have no bacteria in the urinary system. Men with nonbacterial prostatitis often have inflammation of the prostate with an elevated leukocyte count and abnormal inflammatory cells in their prostatic secretions. The cause of the disorder is unknown, and efforts to prove the presence of unusual pathogens (e.g., mycoplasmas, *Chlamydia*, trichomonads, viruses) have been largely unsuccessful. It also is thought that nonbacterial prostatitis may be an autoimmune disorder.

Men with noninflammatory prostatitis have symptoms resembling those of nonbacterial prostatitis but have negative urine culture results and no evidence of prostatic inflammation (i.e., normal leukocyte count). The cause of noninflammatory prostatitis is unknown, but because of the absence of inflammation, the search for the cause of symptoms has been directed toward extraprostatic sources. In some cases, there is an apparent functional obstruction of the bladder neck near the external urethral sphincter; during voiding, this results in higher-than-normal pressures in the prostatic urethra that cause intraprostatic urine reflux and chemical irritation of the prostate by urine. In other cases, there is an apparent myalgia (i.e., muscle pain) associated with prolonged tension of the pelvic floor muscles. Emotional stress also may play a role.

Treatment methods for chronic prostatitis/pelvic pain syndrome are highly variable and require further study. Antibiotic therapy is used when an occult infection is suspected. Treatment often is directed toward symptom control. In men with irritative urination symptoms, α-adrenergic blocking agents and/or 5α-reductase inhibitors (such as finasteride) may be beneficial. Noncentered treatment methods such as physical therapy, myofascial trigger point release therapy, and relaxation techniques may provide some symptom relief.[43]

Benign Prostatic Hyperplasia

Benign prostatic hyperplasia (BPH), also called nodular hyperplasia of the prostate, is a common age-related, nonmalignant enlargement of the prostate gland[14,15,44–46] (Fig. 39-11). It has been reported that more than 50% of men older than 60 years of age have BPH.[44] The disorder is seen most frequently in Europe and the United States, and is seen least commonly in Asia.[15] The prevalence of the disorder in the United States is higher among blacks than among whites.

Pathogenesis. The pathogenesis of BPH is not completely understood, but appears to involve an imbalance between cell proliferation and cell death that results in an overgrowth of the mucosal glands of the prostate. There is an increased number of epithelial cells and stromal components of the periurethral area of the prostate, but no clear evidence of increased epithelial cell proliferation. Instead, it has been proposed that the cause of the hyperplastic process is decreased cell death, resulting in an accumulation of senescent cells.[14] The main androgen in the prostate is dihydrotestosterone (DHT), which is formed in the prostate from the conversion of testosterone by the enzyme 5α-reductase. It is thought that DHT-induced growth factors increase the proliferation of prostatic stromal cells and decrease the death of the epithelial cells. The discovery that DHT is the active factor in BPH provides the rationale for the use of 5α-reductase inhibitors in the treatment of the disorder.

Benign prostatic hyperplasia is characterized by the formation of large, discrete lesions in the periurethral region

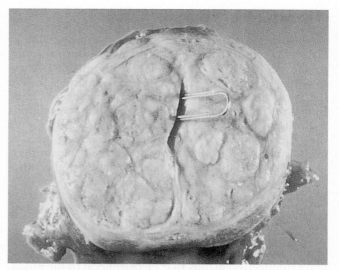

FIGURE 39-11. Nodular hyperplasia of the prostate. Cut surface of a prostate enlarged by nodular hyperplasia shows numerous, well-circumscribed nodules of prostatic tissue. The prostatic urethra (*paper clip*) has been compressed to a narrow slit. (From Damjanov I, McCue PA. The lower urinary tract and male reproductive system. In: Rubin R, Strayer DS, eds. *Rubin's Pathology: Clinicopathologic Foundations of Medicine.* 6th ed. Philadelphia, PA: Wolters Kluwer Health | Lippincott Williams & Wilkins; 2012:841.)

of the prostate rather than the peripheral zones, which commonly are affected by prostate cancer (Fig. 39-12). The anatomic location of the prostate at the bladder neck contributes to the obstructive properties of BPH and development of lower urinary tract symptoms. There are two distinct components of the obstruction: static and dynamic.[44,45] The static component of BPH is related to an increase in prostatic size and gives rise to symptoms such as a weak urinary stream, postvoid dribbling, frequency of urination, and nocturia. The dynamic component of BPH is related to prostatic smooth muscle tone, which is mediated by α₁-adrenergic receptors. The recognition of the role of α₁-adrenergic receptors on neuromuscular function in the prostate is the basis for use of α₁-adrenergic receptor blockers in treating BPH. A third component, detrusor instability and impaired bladder contractility, may contribute to the symptoms of BPH independent of the outlet obstruction created by an enlarged prostate (see Chapter 27). It has been suggested that some of the symptoms of BPH might be related to a decompensating or aging bladder rather than being primarily related to outflow obstruction. An example is the involuntary contraction that results in urgency and an attempt to void that occurs because of small bladder volume.[45]

Clinical Course. The clinical significance of BPH resides in its tendency to compress the urethra and cause partial or complete obstruction of urinary outflow. As the obstruction increases, acute retention of urine may occur with overdistention of the bladder. The residual urine in the bladder causes increased frequency of urination and a constant desire to empty the bladder, which becomes worse at night. With marked bladder

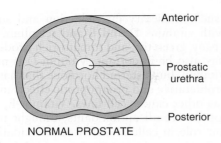

NORMAL PROSTATE

Anterior

Prostatic
urethra

Posterior

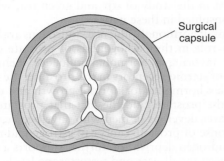

Surgical
capsule

NODULAR PROSTATIC
HYPERPLASIA

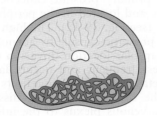

CARCINOMA
OF PROSTATE

FIGURE 39-12. Normal prostate, nodular benign prostatic hyperplasia, and cancer of the prostate. In prostatic hyperplasia, which involves predominantly the periurethral part of the gland, the nodules compress and distort the urethra. The expansion of the central prostatic glands leads to compression of the peripheral parts and fibrosis, resulting in the formation of the so-called surgical capsule. Prostatic cancer usually arises from the peripheral glands and compression of the urethra is a late clinical event. (From Damjanov I, McCue PA. The lower urinary tract and male reproductive system. In: Rubin R, Strayer DS, eds. *Rubin's Pathology: Clinicopathologic Foundations of Medicine.* 6th ed. Philadelphia, PA: Wolters Kluwer Health | Lippincott Williams & Wilkins; 2012:840.)

distention, overflow incontinence may occur with the slightest increase in intra-abdominal pressure. The resulting obstruction to urinary flow can give rise to urinary tract infection, destructive changes of the bladder wall, hydroureter, and hydronephrosis. Hypertrophy and changes in bladder wall structure develop in stages. Initially, the hypertrophied fibers form trabeculations and then herniations, or sacculations; finally, diverticula develop as the herniations extend through the bladder wall (see Chapter 27, Fig. 27-4). Because urine seldom is completely emptied from them, these diverticula are readily infected. Back-pressure on the ureters and

collecting system of the kidneys promotes hydroureter, hydronephrosis, and danger of eventual renal failure.

Current practice suggests that the single most important factor in the evaluation and treatment of BPH is the man's own experiences related to the disorder. The American Urological Association Symptom Index consists of seven questions about symptoms regarding incomplete emptying, frequency, intermittency, urgency, weak stream, straining, and nocturia.[46]

The diagnosis of BPH is based on history, physical examination, digital rectal examination, urinalysis, blood tests for serum creatinine and prostate-specific antigen (PSA), and urine flow rate. The digital rectal examination is used to examine the external surface and size of the prostate. An enlarged prostate found during a digital rectal examination does not always correlate with the degree of urinary obstruction. Some men can have greatly enlarged prostate glands with no urinary obstruction, but others may have severe symptoms without a palpable enlargement of the prostate. Urinalysis is done to detect bacteria, white blood cells, or microscopic hematuria in the presence of infection and inflammation. The serum creatinine test is used as an estimate of the glomerular filtration rate and renal function. The PSA test is used to screen for prostate cancer. These evaluation measures, along with the symptom index, are used to describe the extent of obstruction, determine if other diagnostic tests are needed, and establish the need for treatment.

Treatment of BPH is determined by the degree of symptoms that the condition produces and complications due to obstruction. When a man develops mild symptoms related to BPH, a "watchful waiting" stance often is taken.[44–46] The condition does not always run a predictable course; it may remain stable or even improve. Until the 1980s, surgery was the mainstay of treatment to alleviate urinary obstruction due to BPH. Currently, there is an emphasis on less invasive methods of treatment, including use of pharmacologic agents. However, when more severe signs of obstruction develop, surgical treatment is indicated to provide comfort and avoid serious kidney damage.

Pharmacologic management includes the use of 5α-reductase inhibitors, α₁-adrenergic blocking drugs, or a combination of the two drugs.[44,45] The 5α-reductase inhibitors such as finasteride reduce prostate size by blocking the effect of androgens on the prostate. Finasteride causes atrophy of the prostate glandular epithelial cells, which results in a 20% to 30% reduction in volume. The onset is slow (3 to 6 months), but long-lasting. The presence of α-adrenergic receptors in prostatic smooth muscle has prompted the use of α₁-adrenergic blocking drugs (e.g., prazosin, terazosin) to relieve prostatic obstruction and increase urine flow.

Herbal therapies have been used for many years by men for the treatment of BPH and lower urinary tract symptoms.[44–46] Several studies have looked at the effects of these agents, including the extract of the saw palmetto berry. Improvements in peak urine flow rates and nocturia can occur compared with placebo, but the durability of these effects is unproven. The long-term toxicity and mechanism of action of these agents remain unclear. Standardization of these products is also worrisome (as with all herbal therapies).

The surgical removal of an enlarged prostate can be accomplished by the transurethral, suprapubic, or perineal approach.[44–46] Currently, transurethral prostatectomy (TURP) is the most commonly used technique. With this approach, an instrument is introduced through the urethra, and prostate tissue is removed using a resectoscope and electrocautery. Late complications of TURP include sexual dysfunction, incontinence, and bladder neck constriction. Many new and experimental techniques have also been used to treat BPH including transurethral incision of the prostate, laser surgery, transurethral vaporization, transurethral microwave therapy, and transurethral needle ablation. For men who have heart or lung disease or a condition that precludes major surgery, a stent may be used to widen and maintain the patency of the urethra. A stent is a device made of tubular mesh that is inserted under local or regional anesthesia. Within several months, the lining of the urethra grows to cover the inside of the stent.

Cancer of the Prostate

Globally, prostate cancer is the second most frequently diagnosed cancer in men. An estimated 900,000 new cases were projected to occur in 2008. Nearly three quarters of these cases were expected to be diagnosed in developed countries, with the highest rates being recorded in the United States (233,000 cases in 2014).[47] The increase in diagnosed cases is thought to reflect earlier diagnosis because of widespread use of PSA testing since the early 1990s. African American men have the highest reported incidence rate for prostate cancer at all ages, and the cancer also tends to be diagnosed at a later stage.[47,48] Asians and Native American men have the lowest rate. Prostate cancer also is a disease of aging. The incidence increases rapidly after 50 years of age; more than 85% of all prostate cancers are diagnosed in men older than 65 years of age.[48]

Etiology and Pathogenesis. The precise cause of prostate cancer is unclear. As with other cancers, it appears that the development of prostate cancer is a multistep process involving genes that control cell differentiation and growth. The incidence of prostate cancer appears to be higher in relatives of men with prostate cancer. It has been estimated that men who have an affected first-degree relative (e.g., father, brother) and an affected second-degree relative (e.g., grandfather, uncle) have an eightfold increase in risk.[14,15,49] It has been suggested that dietary patterns, including increased dietary fats, may alter the production of sex hormones and growth factors and increase the risk of prostate cancer. Supporting the role of dietary fats as a risk factor for prostate cancer has been the observation that the diet of Japanese men, who have a low rate of prostate cancer, is much lower in fat content than that of U.S. men, who have a much higher incidence.

Several factors appear to be protective against the development of prostate cancer. These include dietary factors such as dietary fat reduction and supplementation with vitamins D and E and selenium.[50] Dietary intake of soy, green tea, and tomato-rich products (lycopene) may also be important. Vitamin D is not technically a vitamin, but a steroid hormone that has a variety of antiproliferative and proapoptotic effects in prostatic as well as other cancer cell lines. Vitamin E, selenium, and lycopene are all antioxidants, thought to play an important role in cellular defenses to oxidative stress. The low incidence of prostate cancer in Asia has led to an interest in the study of soy and green tea, which are highly consumed in these nations.

In terms of hormonal influence, androgens are believed to play a role in the pathogenesis of prostate cancer.[14] Evidence favoring a hormonal influence includes the presence of steroid receptors in the prostate, the requirement of sex hormones for normal growth and development of the prostate, and the fact that prostate cancer almost never develops in men who have been castrated. The response of prostate cancer to estrogen administration or androgen deprivation further supports a correlation between the disease and testosterone levels.[14]

Clinical Features. Prostatic adenocarcinomas, which account for most primary prostate cancers, are commonly multicentric and located in the peripheral zones of the prostate[14,15] (see Fig. 39-12). The high frequency of invasion of the prostatic capsule by adenocarcinoma relates to its subcapsular location. Invasion of the urinary bladder is less frequent and occurs later in the clinical course. Metastasis to the lung reflects lymphatic spread through the thoracic duct and dissemination from the prostatic venous plexus to the inferior vena cava. Bony metastases, particularly to the vertebral column, ribs, and pelvis, produce pain that often presents as a first sign of the disease.

Most men with early-stage prostate cancer are asymptomatic.[51] The presence of symptoms often suggests locally advanced or metastatic disease. Depending on the size and location in the prostate of the cancer at the time of diagnosis, there may be changes associated with the voiding pattern similar to those found in BPH. These include urgency, frequency, nocturia, hesitancy, dysuria, hematuria, or blood in the ejaculate.[44] On digital rectal examination, the prostate can be nodular and fixed. Bone metastasis often is characterized by low back pain. Pathologic fractures can occur at the site of metastasis. Men with metastatic disease may experience weight loss, anemia, or shortness of breath.

Screening. Whether screening for prostate cancer results in a decrease in prostate cancer deaths is a subject of much debate.[52,53] The screening tests currently available are digital rectal examination, PSA testing, and transrectal ultrasonography. Depending on the population studied, detection using digital rectal examination varies from 1.5% to 7%, with most cancers being far advanced when they are detected.[53] Prostate-specific antigen is a glycoprotein secreted into the cytoplasm of benign and malignant prostatic cells that is not found in other normal tissues or tumors. However, a positive

PSA test indicates only the possible presence of prostate cancer. It also can be positive in cases of BPH and prostatitis. Thus, the test can result in a large number of men undergoing biopsy and being treated unnecessarily. Transrectal ultrasonography is not used for first-line detection because of its expense, but may benefit men who are at high risk for development of prostate cancer.

The U.S. Preventative Services Task Force (USPSTF) recommends against prostate-specific antigen (PSA)-based screening for prostate cancer.[52] The American Cancer Society advocates that men aged 50 at average risk who are interested in PSA screening should discuss it with their health care provider.[52,53] Before screening, they should understand the benefits and limitations of screening.

Diagnosis. The diagnosis of prostate cancer is based on history and physical examination and confirmed through biopsy methods.[44,51] Transrectal ultrasonography is used to guide a biopsy needle and document the exact location of the sampled tissue. It also is used for providing staging information. Newly developed small probes for transrectal MRI have been shown to be effective in detecting the presence of cancer in the prostate. Radiologic examination of the bones of the skull, ribs, spine, and pelvis can be used to reveal metastases, although radionuclide bone scans are more sensitive.

Prostatic cancer, like other forms of cancer, is graded and staged[14,15] (see Chapter 7). Prostate-specific antigen levels are important in the staging and management of prostate cancer. In untreated cases, the level of PSA correlates with the volume and stage of disease. A rising PSA after treatment is consistent with progressive disease, whether it is locally recurring or metastatic. Measurement of PSA is used to detect recurrence after total prostatectomy. Because the prostate is the source of PSA, levels should drop to zero after surgery; a rising PSA indicates recurring disease.

Treatment. Cancer of the prostate is treated by surgery, radiation therapy, and hormonal manipulations.[44,51] Chemotherapy has shown limited effectiveness in the treatment of prostate cancer. Treatment decisions are based on tumor grade and stage and on the age and health of the man. Expectant therapy (watchful waiting) may be used if the tumor is not producing symptoms, is expected to grow slowly, and is small and contained in one area of the prostate. This approach is particularly suited for men who are elderly or have other health problems.

Radical prostatectomy involves complete removal of the seminal vesicles, prostate, and ampullae of the vas deferens. Refinements in surgical techniques ("nerve-sparing" prostatectomy) have allowed maintenance of continence in most men and erectile function in selected cases. Radiation therapy can be delivered by a variety of techniques, including external-beam radiation therapy and transperineal implantation of radioisotopes (brachytherapy).

Metastatic disease often is treated with androgen deprivation therapy. Androgen deprivation may be induced at several levels along the hypothalamic-pituitary-gonadal axis using a variety of methods or agents.[44,51] Orchiectomy or surgical removal of the testes eliminates the source of testosterone. The use of luteinizing hormone–releasing hormone (LHRH) agonists (e.g., leuprolide, goserelin), which act at the hypothalamic-pituitary level to achieve androgen deprivation without orchiectomy or administration of diethylstilbestrol (a synthetic estrogenic compound), currently is the most common method of reducing testosterone levels. Although testosterone is the main circulating androgen, the adrenal gland also secretes androgens. Inhibitors of adrenal androgen synthesis (i.e., ketoconazole and aminoglutethimide) block the synthesis of adrenal androgens. Complete androgen blockade can be achieved by combining an antiandrogen with use of an LHRH agonist or orchiectomy. The nonsteroidal antiandrogens (e.g., flutamide, bicalutamide) block the uptake and actions of androgens in the prostate cells. Abiraterone blocks the synthesis of androgens in the tumor as well as in the testes and adrenal glands. Patients treated with abiraterone are at risk for adrenal insufficiency and require concurrent steroid replacement therapy.

SUMMARY CONCEPTS

■ Disorders of the male reproductive system include those that affect the penis, the scrotum and testes, and the prostate gland.

■ Disorders of the penis include balanitis, an acute or chronic inflammation of the glans penis; and balanoposthitis, an inflammation of the glans and prepuce. Peyronie disease is characterized by the growth of a band of fibrous tissue on top of the penile shaft. Priapism is an abnormal, painful, sustained erection that can lead to ischemic damage of penile structures. It can occur at any age and is one of the possible complications of sickle cell disease.

■ Disorders of the scrotum and testes include collection of fluid (hydrocele), blood (hematocele), or sperm (spermatocele) in the tunica vaginalis; varicosities of the veins in the pampiniform venous plexus (varicocele); and twisting of the spermatic cord with a resulting compromise of the blood supply to the testis (testicular torsion). Inflammatory conditions can involve the scrotal sac, epididymis, or testes.

■ Tumors can arise in the scrotum or the testes. Scrotal cancers usually are associated with exposure to petroleum products such as tar, pitch, and soot. Testicular cancer is the most common cancer in 20- to 35-year-old males. With current treatment methods, a large percentage of men with these tumors can be cured.

(continued)

SUMMARY CONCEPTS *(continued)*

■ The prostate gland is a firm walnut-sized structure that surrounds the urethra. Inflammation of the prostate occurs as an acute or a chronic process. Benign prostatic hyperplasia (BPH) is an age-related enlargement of the prostate gland which compresses the urethra and produces symptoms of dysuria, increased frequency of urination, and marked bladder distention with overflow incontinence or difficulty urinating. Prostate cancer begins in the peripheral zones of the prostate gland and usually is asymptomatic until the disease is far advanced and the tumor has eroded the outer prostatic capsule and spread to adjacent pelvic tissues or metastasized.

Disorders in Childhood and Aging

Disorders of Childhood

Disorders of the male reproductive system that present in childhood include hypospadias, epispadias, phimosis and paraphimosis, and cryptorchidism.

Hypospadias and Epispadias

Hypospadias and epispadias are congenital disorders of the penis resulting from embryologic defects in the development of the urethral groove and penile urethra (Fig. 39-13). In hypospadias, which affects approximately 1 in 250 male infants, the termination of the urethra is on the ventral surface of the penis (the surface in contact with the scrotum).[54–57] The testes are undescended (cryptorchidism) in 8% to 10% of boys born with hypospadias and chordee (i.e., ventral bowing of the penis), and inguinal hernia also may accompany the disorder.[54] In the newborn with severe hypospadias and cryptorchidism, the differential diagnosis should consider ambiguous genitalia and masculinization that is seen in female infants with congenital adrenal hyperplasia[58] (see Chapter 32). Because many chromosomal aberrations result in ambiguity of the external genitalia, chromosomal studies often are recommended for male infants with hypospadias and cryptorchidism.[57]

Surgery is the treatment of choice for hypospadias.[57] Circumcision is avoided because the foreskin is used for surgical repair. Factors that influence the timing of surgical repair include anesthetic risk, penile size, and the psychological effects of the surgery on the child. In mild cases, the surgery is done for cosmetic reasons only. In more severe cases, surgical repair becomes essential for normal sexual functioning and to prevent the psychological effects of having malformed genitalia. When indicated, surgical repair is usually done between the ages of 6 and 12 months.[54–57]

Epispadias, in which the opening of the urethra is on the dorsal surface of the penis, is a less common defect, and is often associated with exstrophy of the bladder, a condition in which the abdominal wall fails to cover the bladder. The treatment depends on the extent of the developmental defect.

Phimosis and Paraphimosis

Embryologically, the foreskin begins to develop during the 8th week of gestation as a fold of skin at the distal edge of the penis that eventually grows forward over the base of the glans. By the 16th week of gestation, the prepuce and the glans are adherent. Only a small percentage of newborns have a fully retractable foreskin.[55] With growth, a space develops between the glans and foreskin, and by 3 years of age, approximately 90% of male children have retractable foreskins.

Phimosis refers to a tightening of the prepuce or penile foreskin that prevents its retraction over the glans.[58] In *paraphimosis*, the foreskin is so tight and constricted that it cannot cover the glans, a condition that can constrict the blood supply to the glans resulting in ischemia and necrosis.

Because the foreskin of many boys cannot be fully retracted in early childhood, it is important that the area be cleaned thoroughly. There is no need to retract the foreskin forcibly because this could lead to infection, scarring, or *paraphimosis*. As the child grows, the foreskin becomes retractable, and the glans and foreskin should be cleaned routinely. If symptomatic phimosis occurs after childhood, it can cause difficulty with voiding or sexual activity. Circumcision is then the treatment of choice.

Cryptorchidism

Cryptorchidism, or undescended testes, occurs when one or both of the testicles fail to move down into the scrotal sac.[59,60] The condition is bilateral in 10% to

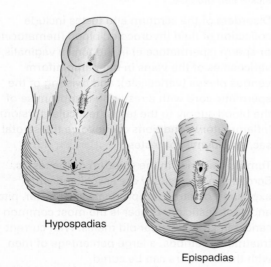

Hypospadias

Epispadias

FIGURE 39-13. Hypospadias and epispadias.

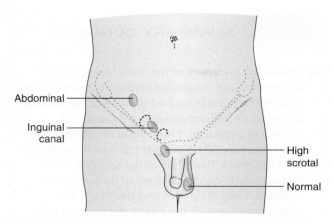

Abdominal

Inguinal canal

High scrotal

Normal

FIGURE 39-14. Possible locations of undescended testicles.

20% of cases. The testes develop intra-abdominally in the fetus and usually descend into the scrotum through the inguinal canal during the seventh to ninth months of gestation. The undescended testes may remain in the lower abdomen or at a point of descent in the inguinal canal (Fig. 39-14).

The incidence of cryptorchidism is directly related to birth weight and gestational age; infants who are born prematurely or are small for gestational age have the highest incidence of the disorder. The cause of cryptorchidism in full-term infants is poorly understood. Most cases are idiopathic, but some may result from genetic or hormonal factors.

The major manifestation of cryptorchidism is the absence of one or both of the testes in the scrotum. The testis either is not palpable or can be felt external to the inguinal ring. Spontaneous descent often occurs during the first 3 months of life, and by 6 months of age the incidence decreases to 0.8%.[54] Spontaneous descent rarely occurs after 4 months of age.

In children with cryptorchidism, histologic abnormalities of the testes reflect intrinsic defects in the testicle or adverse effects of the extrascrotal environment. The undescended testicle is normal at birth, but pathologic changes can be demonstrated at 6 to 12 months.[54] There is a delay in germ cell development, changes in the spermatic tubules, and reduced number of Leydig cells. These changes are progressive if the testes remain undescended. When the disorder is unilateral, it also may produce morphologic changes in the contralateral descended testis.

The consequences of cryptorchidism include infertility, testicular torsion, malignancy, and the possible psychological effects of an empty scrotum.[54,59,60] Indirect inguinal hernias usually accompany the undescended testes but rarely are symptomatic. Recognition of the condition and early treatment are important steps in preventing adverse consequences. The risk of malignancy in the undescended testis is 4 to 10 times higher than in the general population.[54] The increased risk of testicular cancer is not significantly affected by orchiopexy, hormonal therapy, or late spontaneous descent after the age of 2 years. However, orchiopexy does allow for earlier

detection of a testicular malignancy by positioning the testis in a more easily palpable location.

As a group, men with unilateral or bilateral cryptorchidism usually have decreased sperm counts, poorer-quality sperm, and lower fertility rates than do men whose testicles descend normally. The likelihood of decreased fertility increases when the condition is bilateral. Early orchiopexy appears to provide some protection of fertility.[60]

Diagnosis is based on careful examination of the genitalia in male infants. Undescended testes due to cryptorchidism should be differentiated from retractable testes that retract into the inguinal canal in response to an exaggerated cremaster muscle reflex. Retractable testes usually are palpable at birth but later become nonpalpable. They can be brought down with careful palpation in a warm room. Retractable testes usually assume a scrotal position during puberty. They have none of the complications associated with cryptorchidism.[54] Because imaging has not proven to be 100% reliable, laparoscopy has become standard practice for localization of nonpalpable testes.

The treatment goals for the child with cryptorchidism include measures to enhance future fertility potential, placement of the gonad in a favorable place for cancer detection, and improved cosmetic appearance. Surgical treatment is the cornerstone of therapy. Current information suggests that placement of the testes in the scrotum should be accomplished by 1 year of age to maximize the potential for fertility. Although hormonal treatment has been used in Europe, randomized clinical trials have not shown it to be effective in stimulating testicular descent.[54]

Treatment of men with undescended testis should include lifelong follow-up, considering the sequelae of testicular cancer and infertility. Parents need to be aware of the potential issues of infertility and increased risk of testicular cancer. On reaching puberty, boys should be instructed in the necessity of testicular self-examination.

Changes Related to Aging

Like other body systems, the male reproductive system undergoes degenerative changes as a result of the aging process; it becomes less efficient with age. The declining physiologic efficiency of male reproductive function occurs gradually and involves the endocrine, circulatory, and neuromuscular systems.[61] Compared with the marked physiologic change in aging women, the changes in the aging man are more gradual and less drastic. Gonadal and reproductive failures usually are not related directly to age because a man remains fertile into advanced age; 80- and 90-year-old men have been known to father children.

As the man ages, his reproductive system becomes measurably different in structure and function from that of the younger man. Male sex hormone levels, particularly testosterone, decrease with age, with the decline starting later on average than in women.

The term *andropause* has been used to describe an ill-defined collection of symptoms in aging men, typically those older than 50 years, who may have a low androgen level.[61]

The sex hormones play a part in the structure and function of the reproductive system and other body systems from conception to old age; they affect protein synthesis, salt and water balance, bone growth, and cardiovascular function. Decreasing levels of testosterone affect sexual energy, muscle strength, and the genital tissues. The testes become smaller and lose their firmness. The seminiferous tubules, which produce spermatozoa, thicken and begin a degenerative process that finally inhibits sperm production, resulting in a decrease of viable spermatozoa. The prostate gland enlarges, and its contractions become weaker. The force of ejaculation also decreases because of a reduction in the volume and viscosity of the seminal fluid. The seminal vesicles change little from childhood to puberty. The pubertal increases in the fluid capacity of the gland remain throughout adulthood and decline after the age of 60 years. After age 60 years, the walls of the seminal vesicles thin, the epithelium decreases, and the muscle layer is replaced by connective tissue. Age-related changes in the penis consist of fibrotic changes in the trabeculae in the corpus spongiosum, with progressive sclerotic changes in arteries and veins. Sclerotic changes also follow in the corpora cavernosa, with the condition becoming generalized in 55- to 60-year-old men.

Erectile dysfunction in the elderly man often is directly related to the man's general physical condition, including the presence of age-related diseases. Various cardiovascular, respiratory, hormonal, neurologic, and hematologic disorders can be responsible for secondary ED. For example, vascular disease affects male potency because it may impair blood flow to the pudendal arteries or their tributaries, resulting in loss of blood volume with subsequent poor distention of the vascular spaces of erectile tissue. Other diseases affecting potency include hypertension, diabetes, cardiac disease, and malignancies of the reproductive organs. In addition, certain medications can have an effect on sexual function.

Testosterone and other synthetic androgens may be used in older men with low androgen levels to improve muscle strength and vigor.[62] Preliminary studies of androgen replacement in aging men with low androgen levels show an increase in lean body mass and a decrease in bone turnover. Before testosterone replacement therapy is initiated, all men should be screened for prostate cancer and other androgen-related diseases. Testosterone is available in an injectable form that is administered every 2 to 4 weeks (a formulation taken every 10 to 12 weeks is also available outside the United States), as a buccal tablet, or as a transdermal patch, gel, or solution (administered via the axilla). Side effects of replacement therapy may include acne, gynecomastia, and reduced high-density lipoprotein levels. It also may contribute to a worsening of sleep apnea in men who are troubled by this problem.

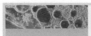

SUMMARY CONCEPTS

■ Childhood disorders of the male reproductive system include congenital disorders in which the urethral opening is located on the ventral surface of the penis (hypospadias) or on the dorsal surface (epispadias). Phimosis is the condition in which the foreskin is too tight to permit retraction over the glans. Disorders of the scrotum and testes include cryptorchidism or undescended testicles. Early diagnosis and treatment are important to reduce the risk of malignancy and infertility.

■ Like other body systems, the male reproductive system undergoes changes as a result of the aging process. The changes occur gradually and involve changes in endocrine, circulatory, and neuromuscular function. Testosterone levels decrease, the size and firmness of the testes decrease, sperm production declines, and the prostate gland enlarges. There often is a decrease in erectile function related to diseases that accompany the aging process.

REVIEW EXERCISES

1. A 64-year-old man presents to his family physician with erectile dysfunction. He is on multiple medications for "his heart disease." An initial physical examination is unremarkable.

   A. What additional information should be obtained?
   B. Given his medical history, what are possible factors contributing to his problem?

2. A 23-year-old man presents in the emergency department in severe distress. His left testicle is large and tender and he has pain radiating to the inguinal area.

   A. What would be a tentative diagnosis for this man?
   B. Why would this problem necessitate immediate diagnosis and surgical intervention?

3. A 72-year-old man had a radical prostatectomy for localized prostate cancer. After surgery his PSA level was undetectable. He presents 5 years later having been "lost to follow-up." He complains of pain in his hip and lower back. His PSA level is now markedly elevated.

   A. What initial investigations are warranted?
   B. What therapies are available for this complication?

REFERENCES

1. Hall JE. *Guyton and Hall Textbook of Medical Physiology*. 12th ed. Philadelphia, PA: Elsevier Saunders; 2011:973–986.
2. Ross MH, Pawlina W. *Histology: A Text and Atlas*. 5th ed. Philadelphia, PA: Wolters Kluwer Health/Lippincott Williams & Wilkins; 2007:728–771.
3. Braunstein GD. Testes. In: Gardner DG, Shoback D, eds. *Greenspan's Basic and Clinical Endocrinology*. 9th ed. New York. NY: McGraw-Hill; 2011:395–422.
4. Lue TF. Male sexual function. In: McAninch JW, Lue TF, eds. *Smith and Tanagho's General Urology*. 18th ed. New York, NY: McGraw-Hill; 2013:596–616.
5. Matfin G. Erectile dysfunction as a component of the metabolic syndrome. *Curr Diab Rep*. 2005;5:64–69.
6. Matfin G. Sexual dysfunction and cardiovascular disease—links and solutions. In: Fonseca V, ed. *Cardiovascular Endocrinology— Shared Pathways and Clinical Crossroads*. Totowa, NJ: Humana Press; 2009:119–215.
7. NIH Consensus Development Panel on Impotence. NIH Consensus Conference: impotence. *JAMA*. 1993;270:83–90.
8. AACE Male Sexual Dysfunction Taskforce. AACE medical guidelines for clinical practice for the evaluation and treatment of male sexual dysfunction: a couple's problem—2003 update. *Endocr Pract*. 2003;9:77–95.
9. Bacon CG, Mittleman MA, Kawachi I, et al. Sexual function in men older than 50 years of age: results from the Health Professionals Follow-Up Study. *Ann Intern Med*. 2003;139:161–168.
10. Feldman HA, Goldstein J, Hatzichristou DG, et al. Impotence and its medical and psychosocial effects: results of the Massachusetts Male Aging Study. *J Urol*. 1994;151:54–61.
11. Grant P, Jackson G, Baig I, Quin J. Erectile dysfunction in general medicine. *Clin Med*. 2013;13(2):136–140.
12. Minor MM, Kuritzky L. Erectile dysfunction: a sentinel marker for cardiovascular disease in primary care. *Cleve Clin J Med*. 2007;74(Suppl 2):530–537.
13. Edwards S. Balanitis and balanoposthitis: a review. *Genitourin Med*. 1996;72:155–159.
14. Epstein JI. The male genital tract. In: Kumar V, Abbas AK, Fausto N, et al. *Robbins and Cotran Pathologic Basis of Medicine*. 8th ed. Philadelphia, PA: Saunders Elsevier; 2010:982–1002.
15. Damajanov I. The lower urinary tract and male reproductive system. In: Rubin R, Strayer DS, eds. *Rubin's Pathology: Clinicopathologic Foundations of Medicine*. 5th ed. Philadelphia, PA: Wolters Kluwer Health/Lippincott Williams & Wilkins; 2008:758–779.
16. Micali G, Nasca MR, Innocenzi D. Penile cancer. *J Am Acad Dermatol*. 2006;54:369–391.
17. Chaudary M, Sheikh N, Asterling S, et al. Peyronie's disease with erectile dysfunction: modeling over inflatable penile prosthesis. *Urology*. 2005;65:760–764.
18. Taylor FL, Levine LA. Peyronie's disease. *Urol Clin North Am*. 2007;34:517–534.
19. Burnett AL, Bivalacqua TJ. Priapism: current principles and practice. *Urol Clin North Am*. 2007;34:631–642.
20. American Urological Association. *Guidelines on the Management of Priapism*. 2003. Available at: http://www.auanet.org. Accessed September 4, 2013.
21. Broderick GA. Priapism and sickle-cell anemia: diagnosis and nonsurgical therapy. *J Sex Med*. 2012;9(1):88–103.
22. Presti JC. Genital tumors. In: McAninch JW, Lue TF, eds. *Smith and Tanagho's General Urology*. 18th ed. New York, NY: McGraw-Hill; 2013:380–392.
23. Moore KL, Dalley AF, Agur AMR. *Clinically Oriented Anatomy*. 7th ed. Philadelphia, PA: Wolters Kluwer Health/Lippincott Williams & Wilkins; 2014:376–381.
24. Kapur P, Caty MG, Glick PL. Pediatric hernias and hydroceles. *Ped Clin North Am*. 1998;45:773–789.
25. Biyani CS, Cartledge J, Janetschek G. Varicocele. *Clin Evid*. 2006;15:339–340.
26. Lavallee ME, Cash J. Testicular torsion. *Curr Sports Med Rep*. 2005;4(2):102–104.
27. Sessions AE, Rabinowitz R, Hulbert WC, et al. Testicular torsion: direction, degree, duration, and disinformation. *J Urol*. 2003;169:663–665.
28. Leslie JA, Cain MP. Pediatric urologic emergencies and urgencies. *Ped Clin North Am*. 2006; 53:513–527.
29. Tojian TH, Lishnak TS, Heiman D. Epididymitis and orchitis: an overview. *Am Fam Physician*. 2009;79(7):583–587.
30. Tracy CR, Steers WD, Constabile R. Diagnosis and management of epididymitis. *Urol Clin North Am*. 2008;35:101–108.
31. Masarani M, Wazait H, Dinneen M. Mumps orchitis. *J R Soc Med*. 2006;99:573–575.
32. Centers for Disease Control and Prevention. *Prevention of Specific Infectious Disease: Mumps*. August 1, 2013. Available at: http://wwwn.cdc.gov/travel/yellowbook/ch4/mumps.aspx. Accessed September 4, 2013.
33. Mebcow MM. Percivall Pott (1713–1788): 200th anniversary of first report of occupation-induced cancer of the scrotum in chimney sweepers (1745). *Urology*. 1975;6:745.
34. Lowe FC. Squamous cell carcinoma of the scrotum. *Urol Clin North Am*. 1992;19:297–405.
35. Shaw J. Diagnosis and treatment of testicular cancer. *Am Fam Physician*. 2008;77(4):469–476.
36. Vaughn DJ, Gignac GA, Meadows AT. Long-term medical care of testicular cancer survivors. *Ann Intern Med*. 2002;136: 463–470.
37. Krieger JN, Nyberg L, Nickel JC. NIH consensus definition and classification of prostatitis. *JAMA*. 1999;282:721–725.
38. Brede CM, Shoskes DA. The etiology and management of acute prostatitis. *Nat Rev Urol*. 2011;8:207–212.
39. Ngugen HJ. Bacterial infections of the genitourinary system. In: McAninch JW, Lue TF, eds. *Smith and Tanagho's General Urology*. 18th ed. New York, NY: McGraw-Hill; 2013:197–222.
40. Benway BM, Moon TD. Bacterial prostatitis. *Urol Clin North Am*. 2008;35:23–32.
41. Erickson BA, Jang TL, Ching L, et al. Chronic prostatitis. *Clin Evid*. 2006;15:331–333.
42. Pontari MA. Chronic prostatitis/chronic pelvic pain syndrome. *Urol Clin North Am*. 2008;33:81–89.
43. Collins MM, MacDonald R, Wilt TJ. Diagnosis and treatment of chronic abacterial prostatitis: a systemic review. *Ann Intern Med*. 2000;133:367–381.
44. Cooperberg MR, Presti JC Jr, Shinahara K, Carroll PR. Neoplasms of the prostate gland. In: McAninch JW, Lue TF, eds. *Smith and Tanagho's General Urology*. 18th ed. New York, NY: McGraw-Hill; 2013:350–379.
45. Edwards JL. Diagnosis and management of benign prostatic hyperplasia. *Am Fam Physician*. 2008;77(10):1403–1413.
46. The American Urological Association. *Guideline on Management of Prostatic Hyperplasia (BPH)*. 2010. Available at: http://www.auanet.org/content/guidelines-and-quality-care/clinical-guidelines.cfm?sub=bph. Accessed September 4, 2013.
47. American Cancer Society. *Cancer Facts & Figures 2014*. 2014. Available at: http://www.cancer.org. Accessed May 18, 2014.
48. Crawford ED. Understanding the epidemiology, natural history, and key pathways involved in prostate cancer. *Urology*. 2009;73(Suppl 5A):4–10.
49. Nelson WG, De Manzo AM, Isaacs WB. Prostate cancer. *N Engl J Med*. 2003;349:366–381.
50. Fleshner N, Ziotta AR. Prostate cancer prevention: past, present, and future. *Cancer*. 2007;110(9):1889–1899.

51. Cornett P, Dea TO. Cancer. In: McPhee SJ, Papadakis MA, eds. *Current Medical Diagnosis and Treatment.* 52nd ed. New York, NY: McGraw-Hill; 2013:1593–1663.

52. U.S. Preventive Services Task Force. Screening for prostate cancer: U.S. Preventative Services Task Force recommendations statement. *Ann Intern Med.* 2012;157(2):120–134.

53. American Cancer Society. *Prostate Cancer: Early Detection.* 2013. Available at: http://www.cancer.org. Accessed September 4, 2013.

54. Elder J. Anomalies of the penis and urethra, and disorders and anomalies of the scrotal contents. In: Behrman R, Kliegman RM, Jenson HB, et al., eds. *Nelson Textbook of Pediatrics.* 19th ed. Philadelphia, PA: Elsevier Saunders; 2007:1852–1858, 1858–1864.

55. Moore KL, Persaud TVN, Torchia MG. *The Developing Human: Clinically Oriented Embryology.* 9th ed. Philadelphia, PA: W.B. Saunders; 2013:245–288.

56. Hughes IA, Houk C, Ahmed SF, et al. Consensus statement on management of intersex disorders. *Arch Dis Child.* 2006;91:554–563.

57. Shukla AR, Patel RP. Hypospadias. *Urol Clin N Am.* 2004;31:445–460.

58. Docimo SG, Silver RI, Cromie W. The undescended testicle: diagnosis and management. *Am Fam Physician.* 2000;62:2037–2048.

59. Leung AKC, Robson WLM. Current status of cryptorchidism. *Adv Pediatr.* 2004;51:351–377.

60. Kolon TF, Patel RP, Huff DS. Cryptorchidism: diagnosis, treatment, and long-term prognosis. *Urol Clin North Am.* 2004;31:469–480.

61. Basaria S. Aging and endocrinology reproductive aging in men. *Endocrinol Metab Clin North Am.* 2013;42:255–270.

62. Matsumoto AM. Aging and endocrinology testosterone administration in older men. *Endocrinol Metab Clin North Am.* 2013;42:271–286.

Porth Essentials Resources

Explore these additional resources to enhance learning for this chapter:

- NCLEX-Style Questions and Other Resources on the Point, http://thePoint.lww.com/PorthEssentials4e
- Study Guide for Essentials of Pathophysiology
- Adaptive Learning | Powered by PrepU, http://thepoint.lww.com/prepu

Disorders of the Female Genitourinary System

Disorders of the female reproductive system have widespread effects on physical and psychological function, including general health status, sexuality, and reproductive potential. This chapter provides a review of the structure and function of the female reproductive system and a discussion of disorders of the external and internal female reproductive organs, menstrual disorders, and disorders of the breast.

Structure and Function of the Female Reproductive System

The female reproductive system consists of the external and internal genital structures.[1,2] The external structures, or genitalia, are situated in the anterior part of the perineum, and the internal structures (vagina, uterus, fallopian tubes, and ovaries) are located in the pelvic cavity (Fig. 40-1).

External Genitalia

The external genitalia, which are collectively referred to as the *vulva*, include the mons pubis, labia majora, labia minora, clitoris, and perineal body (Fig. 40-2). Because of their location, the urethra and anus usually are considered in a discussion of the external genitalia.

The *mons pubis* is a rounded, skin-covered fat pad located anterior to the symphysis pubis. Running posteriorly from the mons pubis are two elongated, hair-covered, fatty folds, the *labia majora*. The labia majora enclose the *labia minora*, which may be smaller than the *labia majora* and are composed of skin, fat, and some erectile tissue. The *clitoris* is located below the clitoral hood, which is formed by the joining of the two labia minora to form the *prepuce*. The clitoris is an erectile organ, rich in vascular and nervous supply. Analogous to the male penis, it is a highly sensitive organ that becomes engorged during sexual stimulation.

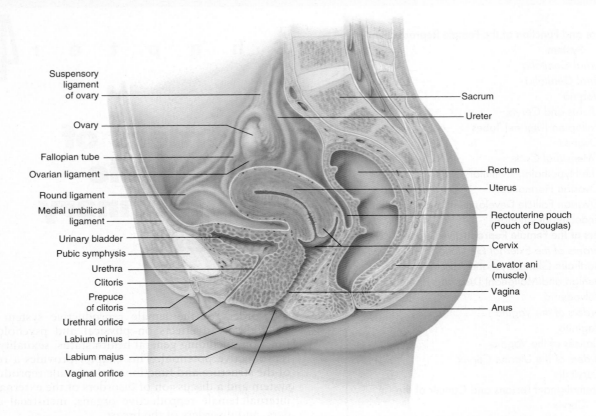

FIGURE 40-1. Female reproductive system as seen in sagittal section. (Adapted from Anatomical Chart Company. *Atlas of Human Anatomy.* Springhouse, PA: Springhouse; 2001:253.)

The area between the labia minora is called the *vestibule*. Located in the vestibule are the urethral and vaginal openings. The urethra is located posterior to the clitoris and usually is closer to the vaginal opening than to the clitoris. The vaginal orifice, commonly known as the *introitus*, is the opening between the external and internal genitalia. The ducts of the lesser vestibular (Skene) and greater vestibular (Bartholin) glands also open into the vestibule. Secretions from the Bartholin glands are responsible for sexually stimulated vaginal lubrication (see Fig. 40-2).

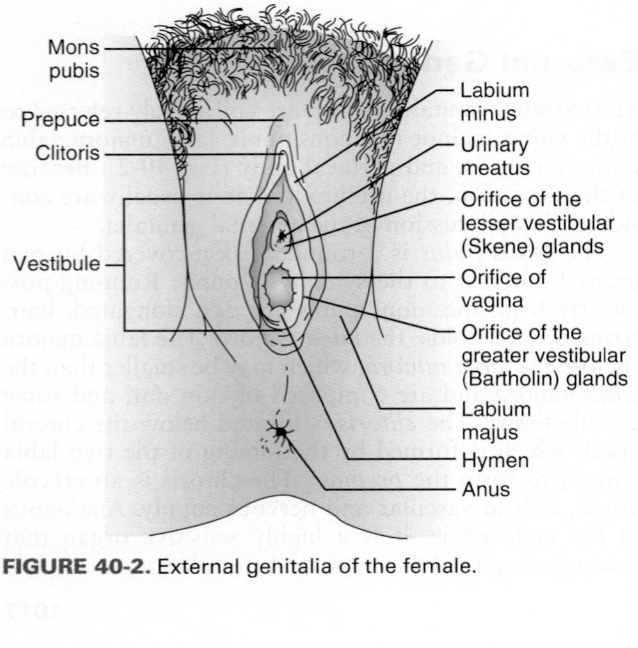

Internal Genitalia

The female internal genital organs include the vagina, uterus and cervix, and the paired fallopian tubes and ovaries.

Vagina

The vagina is a fibromuscular tube that connects the external and internal genitalia. It is located behind the urinary bladder and urethra and anterior to the rectum (Fig. 40-3). The uterine cervix projects into the vagina at its upper end, forming recesses called *fornices*. The vagina functions as a route for discharge of menses and other secretions, as well as an organ of sexual fulfillment and reproduction.

Uterus and Cervix

The uterus is a thick-walled muscular organ. This pear-shaped, hollow structure is located between the bladder and the rectum. The uterus can be divided into three parts: the upper portion above the insertion of the fallopian tubes, called the *fundus*; the central tapering

FIGURE 40-2. External genitalia of the female.

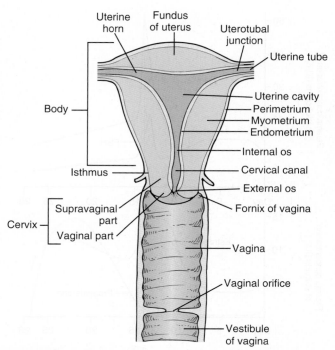

FIGURE 40-3. Median section of the vagina and uterus. (From Moore KL, Agur AMR. *Essential Clinical Anatomy*. 2nd ed. Philadelphia, PA: Lippincott Williams & Wilkins; 2002:238.)

portion, called the body; and the inferior constricted part, called the *cervix*[1,2] (see Fig. 40-3). The uterus is supported on both sides by four sets of ligaments: the *broad ligaments*, which run laterally from the body of the uterus to the pelvic side walls; the *round ligaments*, which run from the fundus laterally into each labium

majus; the *uterosacral ligaments*, which run from the uterocervical junction to the sacrum; and the *cardinal* or *transverse cervical* ligaments, which are attached to the side of the uterus (Fig. 40-4).

The wall of the uterus is composed of three layers: the perimetrium, the myometrium, and the endometrium.[2] The *perimetrium*, or outer serosal layer, is derived from the abdominal peritoneum. This outer layer merges with the peritoneum that covers the broad ligaments. Anteriorly, the perimetrium is reflected over the bladder wall, forming the *vesicouterine pouch*; posteriorly, it extends to form the *rectouterine pouch* (see Fig. 40-1). Because of the proximity of the perimetrium to the urinary bladder, a bladder infection often causes uterine symptoms, particularly during pregnancy.

The *myometrium*, or middle muscle layer of smooth muscle fibers, forms the major portion of the uterine wall. It is continuous with the muscle layer of the uterine tubes and the vagina. The smooth muscle also extends into the ligaments connected to the uterus. The inner fibers of the myometrium run in various directions, giving it an interwoven appearance. Contractions of these muscle fibers help to expel menstrual flow and the products of conception during miscarriage or childbirth.

The *endometrium*, or inner mucosal layer of the uterus, is continuous with the epithelial lining of the uterine tubes and vagina. It is actively involved in the menstrual cycle, differing in structure with each stage of the cycle (to be discussed). If conception occurs, the products of conception are implanted in this layer; if conception does not occur, the inner surface of this layer is shed through menstruation.

The round cervix forms the neck of the uterus. The opening, or os, of the cervix forms a pathway between the vagina and the uterus. The vaginal opening is called

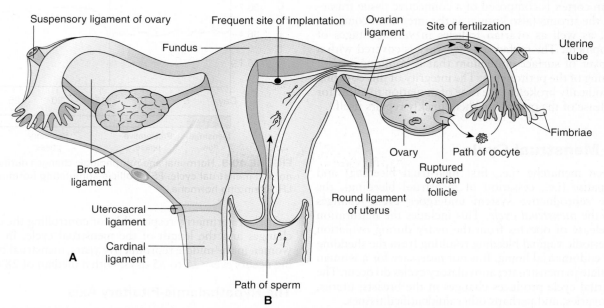

FIGURE 40-4. Schematic drawing of female reproductive organs, showing **(A)** suspensory ligament of the ovary and the broad, uterosacral, and cardinal ligaments on the left, and **(B)** the path of the oocyte as it moves from the ovary into the fallopian (uterine) tube; the path of sperm is also shown, as is the usual site of fertilization.

the *external os*, and the uterine opening, the *internal os*. The space between these two openings, which is called the *endocervical (cervical) canal*, provides a route for menstrual discharge and entry of sperm. Secretions from the columnar epithelium of the endocervix protect the uterus from infection, alter receptivity to sperm, and form a mucoid "plug" during pregnancy.

Fallopian (Uterine) Tubes

The *fallopian*, or *uterine*, tubes are slender cylindrical structures attached bilaterally to the uterus and supported by the upper folds of the broad ligament.[1,2] They are formed by smooth muscle and lined with a ciliated, mucus-producing epithelial layer. The end of the fallopian tube nearest the ovary forms a funnel-like opening with fringed, fingerlike projections, called *fimbriae*, that pick up the oocyte (egg cell) after its release into the peritoneal cavity following ovulation (see Fig. 40-4). The beating of the cilia, along with contractile movements of the smooth muscle, propel the nonmobile oocyte toward the uterus. Besides providing a passageway for ova and sperm, the fallopian tubes permit drainage of tubal secretions into the uterus.

Ovaries

The ovaries are almond-shaped organs located on either side of the uterus below the ends of the two fallopian tubes.[2] The ovaries are attached to the posterior surface of the broad ligament and to the uterus by the ovarian ligament (see Fig. 40-4). Structurally, the mature ovary is divided into a highly vascular inner medulla and an outer cortex. The medulla or medullary region is located in the central part of the ovary. It contains loose connective tissue, blood vessels, lymphatic vessels, and nerves. The ovarian cortex is composed of a connective tissue framework, the stroma (also known as the interstitial compartment), as well as ovarian follicles in various stages of development. The surface of the ovary is covered with a thin layer of surface epithelium that is continuous with the lining of the peritoneum. The integrity of this covering is periodically broken at the time of ovulation to allow for the release of the ovum, but then quickly repairs itself.

The Menstrual Cycle

Between menarche (i.e., first menstrual bleeding) and menopause (i.e., cessation of menstrual bleeding), the female reproductive system undergoes cyclic changes called the *menstrual cycle*. This includes the maturation and release of oocytes from the ovary during ovulation and periodic vaginal bleeding resulting from the shedding of the endometrial lining. It is not necessary for a woman to ovulate to menstruate; anovulatory cycles do occur. The menstrual cycle produces changes in the breasts, uterus, skin, ovaries, and perhaps other unidentified tissues.

The menstrual cycle is regulated by a complex interaction between the hypothalamic-pituitary axis, the ovaries, and the uterus[3,4] (Fig. 40-5). Although each part of the reproductive system is essential to normal function, the

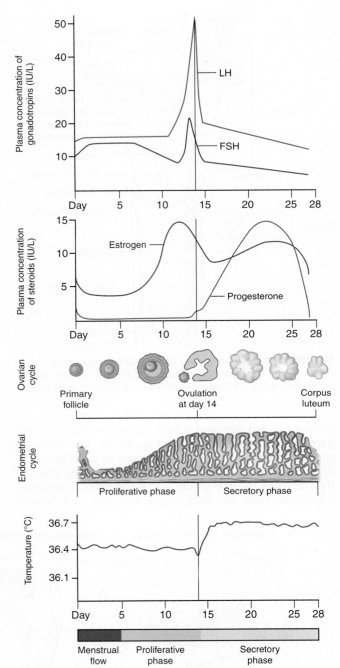

FIGURE 40-5. Hormonal and morphologic changes during the normal menstrual cycle. FSH, follicle-stimulating hormone; LH, luteinizing hormone.

ovaries are primarily responsible for controlling the cyclic changes and the length of the menstrual cycle. In most women in the middle reproductive years, menstrual bleeding occurs every 25 to 35 days, with a median of 28 days.

The Hypothalamic-Pituitary Axis

The ovaries perform two interrelated functions—steroidogenesis, or production of the female sex hormones, and gametogenesis, or production of ova. Both of these functions are regulated by follicle-stimulating hormone

(FSH) and luteinizing hormone (LH) from the anterior pituitary gland[3,4] (Fig. 40-6). Because these hormones promote the growth of cells in the ovaries and testes as a means of stimulating the production of sex hormones, they are called the *gonadotropic hormones*. The secretion of LH and FSH is stimulated by gonadotropin-releasing hormone (GnRH) from the hypothalamus. These gonadotropins then trigger the ovary to release an oocyte that is capable of being fertilized. Concurrently, the ovary secretes hormones that act on the endometrial lining of the uterus to prepare for implantation. In addition, the ovarian hormones provide feedback to the hypothalamus and pituitary regarding the secretion of gonadotropins during the menstrual cycle.

In addition to LH and FSH, the anterior pituitary secretes a third reproductive hormone called *prolactin*. The primary function of prolactin is the stimulation of lactation in the postpartum period. During pregnancy, prolactin, along with other hormones such as estrogen, progesterone, insulin, and cortisol, contributes to breast development in preparation for lactation. Although prolactin does not appear to play a physiologic role in ovarian function, hyperprolactinemia can lead to hypogonadism. This may include an initial shortening of the luteal phase with subsequent absence of menstruation, scanty menstruation, infrequent menstruation (periods more that 35 days apart), and infertility. The hypothalamic control of prolactin secretion is primarily inhibitory, and dopamine is the most important inhibitory factor. Hyperprolactinemia may occur as an adverse effect of drug treatment using phenothiazine derivatives (i.e., antipsychotic drugs that block dopamine receptors).

Ovarian Hormones

The ovaries produce estrogens, progesterone, and androgens (e.g., testosterone). In the ovary, the main source of hormone production are the maturing follicles, including the theca cells and granulosa cells (Fig. 40-7A), and the corpus luteum, the cell mass remaining in the ovary after the oocyte has been released (Fig. 40-7B). The theca cells produce androgens, the granulosa cells produce estrogen, and the corpus luteum produces progesterone. The other stromal cells that contribute to the production of androgens can be divided into two populations: the secondary interstitial cells (derived from the theca) and the cells of the hilum, the bridge of tissue through which blood vessels and nerves enter and exit the ovary (see Fig. 40-7B). These cells are the major ones involved in androgen production during menopause.[3,4]

Estrogens. Estrogens are a family of structurally related female sex hormones synthesized and secreted by cells in the ovaries and, in small amounts, by cells in the adrenal cortex.[3–5] Androgens can be converted to estrogens peripherally, especially in adipose tissue. Three estrogens occur naturally in humans: estrone, estradiol, and estriol. Of these, estradiol is the most biologically potent and the most abundantly secreted product of the ovary. Estrogens are transported in the blood bound to specific plasma globulins, inactivated and conjugated in the liver, and then excreted in the bile.

Estrogens are necessary for normal female development.[3–5] They stimulate the development of the vagina, uterus, and uterine tubes in the embryo. They also stimulate the stromal development and ductal growth of the breasts at puberty, are responsible for the accelerated pubertal skeletal growth phase and for closure of the epiphyses of the long bones, contribute to the growth of axillary and pubic hair, and alter the distribution of body fat to produce the typical female body contours. In concert with other hormones, estrogens provide for the reproductive processes of ovulation, implantation of the products of conception, pregnancy, parturition, and lactation by stimulating the development and maintaining the growth of the reproductive organs.

Estrogens also have a number of other important metabolic effects. They are responsible for maintaining the normal structure of skin and blood vessels in women. Estrogens decrease the rate of bone resorption by antagonizing the effects of calcitonin on bone; for this reason, osteoporosis is a common problem in estrogen-deficient postmenopausal women (see Chapter 44). In the liver, estrogens increase the synthesis of transport proteins for thyroxine, estrogen, testosterone, and other hormones. Estrogens also affect the composition of the plasma

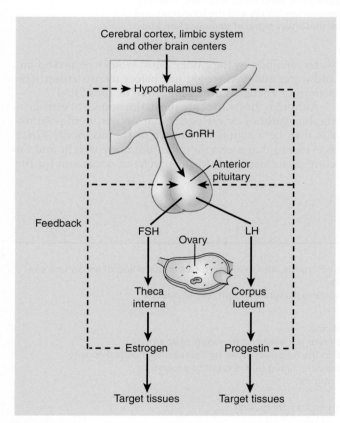

FIGURE 40-6. Hypothalamic-pituitary feedback control of estrogen and progesterone levels in the female. The *dashed line* represents negative feedback. FSH, follicle-stimulating hormone; GnRH, gonadotropin-releasing hormone; LH, luteinizing hormone.

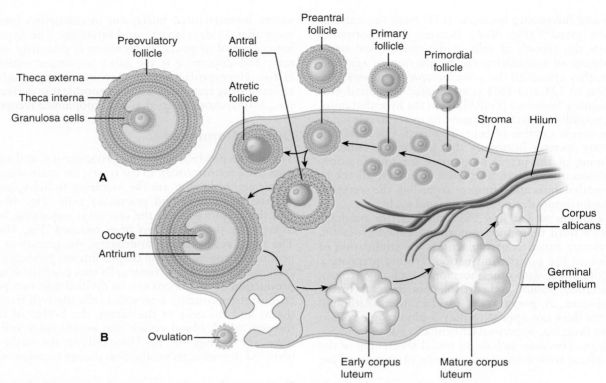

FIGURE 40-7. (A) Cross-section of preovulatory follicle. **(B)** Schematic diagram of an ovary, showing the sequence of events in the origin, growth, and rupture of an ovarian follicle and the formation and retrogression of a corpus luteum. The atretic follicles are those that show signs of degeneration and death.

lipoproteins. They produce an increase in high-density lipoproteins (HDLs), a slight reduction in low-density lipoproteins (LDLs), and a reduction in cholesterol levels. Estrogens also increase plasma triglyceride levels, and they enhance the coagulability of blood by increasing the circulating levels of plasminogen and factors II, VII, IX, and X. Estrogens, which have a chemical structure similar to adrenal cortical hormones, can also cause sodium and

water retention by the kidney. Most women retain sodium and water and gain weight just before menstruation. The actions of estrogens are summarized in Table 40-1.

Although the ovaries are the major source of estrogen, the biosynthesis of estrogens that occurs in adipose tissue may be a significant source of the hormone. There is evidence that a certain minimum body weight and fat content are necessary for menarche to occur and for the

TABLE 40-1	**Actions of Estrogens**
General Function	**Specific Actions**
Growth and development	
Reproductive organs	Stimulate development of vagina, uterus, and fallopian tubes in utero and of secondary sex characteristics during puberty
Skeleton	Accelerate growth of long bones and closure of epiphyses at puberty
Reproductive processes	
Ovulation	Promote growth of ovarian follicles
Fertilization	Alter the cervical secretions to favor survival and transport of sperm
	Promote motility of sperm within the fallopian tubes by decreasing mucus viscosity
Implantation	Promote development of endometrial lining in the event of pregnancy
Vagina	Proliferate and cornify vaginal mucosa
Cervix	Increase mucus consistency
Breasts	Stimulate stromal development and ductal growth
General metabolic effects	
Bone resorption	Decrease rate of bone resorption
Plasma proteins	Increase production of thyroid and other binding globulins
Lipoproteins	Increase high-density and slightly decrease low-density lipoproteins

menstrual cycle to be maintained.[4] This is supported by the observation of amenorrhea in women with anorexia nervosa, chronic disease, and malnutrition and in those who are elite athletes. In these women, gonadotropin and estradiol secretion, including LH release and responsiveness to the hypothalamic GnRH, can revert to prepubertal levels. With resumption of weight gain and attainment of sufficient body mass, the normal hormonal pattern usually is reinstated. Obesity or significant weight gain also is associated with disruption of the menstrual cycle, including oligomenorrhea or amenorrhea and infertility, although the mechanism is not well understood.

Progesterone. Although the word *progesterone* literally means a substance that maintains pregnancy, progesterone is secreted as part of the normal menstrual cycle.[3,4] The corpus luteum of the ovary secretes large amounts of progesterone after ovulation, and the adrenal cortex secretes small amounts. The hormone circulates in the blood attached to a specific plasma protein. It is metabolized in the liver and conjugated for excretion in the bile.

The local effects of progesterone on reproductive organs include the glandular development of the lobular and alveolar tissue of the breasts and the cyclic glandular development of the endometrium. Progesterone also can compete with aldosterone at the level of the renal tubule, causing a decrease in sodium reabsorption, with a resultant increase in secretion of aldosterone by the adrenal cortex (as occurs in pregnancy). Although the mechanism is uncertain, progesterone increases basal body temperature and is responsible for the increase in body temperature that occurs with ovulation. Smooth muscle relaxation under the influence of progesterone plays an important role in maintaining pregnancy by decreasing uterine contractions and is responsible for many of the common discomforts of pregnancy, such as edema, nausea, constipation, flatulence, and headaches. The increased progesterone present during pregnancy and the luteal phase of the menstrual cycle enhances the ventilatory response to carbon dioxide, leading to a measurable decrease in arterial and alveolar carbon dioxide (PCO_2) levels.

Androgens. Ovarian cells also secrete androgens. In the female, androgens contribute to normal hair growth at puberty and may have other important metabolic effects. Androgen production takes place in the stroma that surrounds the follicles.[4] During the reproductive years, the ovaries are directly responsible for one third of testosterone production. The remaining two thirds comes from the periphery and adrenal precursors— mainly androstenedione, which is produced in equal proportions by the adrenal gland and ovary. The adrenal gland may directly secrete testosterone, but its main contribution is derived from precursor hormones.

Ovarian Follicle Development and Ovulation

Unlike the male gonads, which produce sperm throughout a man's reproductive life, the female gonads contain a fixed number of ova at birth (1 to 2 million at birth—no further oocytes are produced). The process of oogenesis (generation of ova by mitotic division) begins during the 6th week of fetal life and proceeds to the development of the primary oocytes, which become surrounded by a single layer of granulosa cells.[2–4] The primary oocytes with their surrounding granulosa cells are referred to as *primordial follicles*. Throughout childhood, the granulosa cells provide nourishment for the ovum and secrete an inhibiting factor that keeps it suspended in a primordial state.

Beginning at puberty, a cyclic rise in the anterior pituitary hormones FSH and LH stimulates the development of several mature (graafian) follicles. Follicles at all stages of development can be found in both ovaries, except in menopausal women (see Fig. 40-7). Most follicles exist as primary follicles, each of which consists of a round oocyte surrounded by a single layer of flattened epithelial cells called *granulosa cells*. The primary follicles constitute an inactive pool of follicles from which all the ovulating follicles develop. Under the influence of endocrine stimulation, 6 to 12 primary follicles develop into secondary follicles during every ovulatory cycle. During the development of the secondary follicle, the primary oocyte increases in size, and the granulosa cells proliferate to form a multilayered wall around it. During this time, a membrane called the *zona pellucida* develops and surrounds the oocyte and small pockets of fluid begin to appear between the granulosa cells.

As the follicles mature, FSH stimulates the development of the cell layers. Cells from the surrounding stromal tissue align themselves to form a sheath of connective tissue cells, known as the *theca folliculi*. The cells of the theca folliculi become differentiated into two layers: an inner layer of highly vascularized androgen-producing cells, called the *theca interna*, and an outer layer of connective tissue, called the *theca externa*. As the follicle enlarges, a single large cavity, or *antrum*, is formed, and a portion of the granulosa cells and the oocyte are displaced to one side of the follicle by the fluid that accumulates. The secondary oocyte remains surrounded by a crown of granulosa cells, the *corona radiata*. As the follicle matures, ovarian estrogen is produced by the granulosa cells.

Selection of a dominant follicle occurs with the conversion to an estrogen microenvironment. The lesser follicles, although continuing to produce some estrogen, degenerate or become atretic. The dominant preovulatory follicle accumulates a greater mass of granulosa cells, and the theca becomes richly vascular, giving the follicle a hyperemic appearance. High levels of estrogen exert a negative feedback effect on FSH, inhibiting the development of multiple follicles and causing an increase in LH levels. This represents the follicular stage of the menstrual cycle. As estrogen suppresses FSH, the actions of LH predominate, and the mature follicle (measuring approximately 20 mm) bursts; the oocyte, along with the corona radiata, is ejected from the follicle. The ovum normally is then picked up and transported through the fallopian tube toward the uterus.

After ovulation, the follicle collapses, and the luteal stage of the menstrual cycle begins. The granulosa cells are invaded by blood vessels and yellow lipochrome-bearing cells from the theca layer. A rapid accumulation of blood and fluid forms a mass called the *corpus luteum*. Leakage of this blood onto the peritoneal surface that surrounds the ovary is thought to contribute to the *mittelschmerz* ("middle [or intermenstrual] pain") of ovulation. During the luteal stage, progesterone is secreted from the corpus luteum. If fertilization does not take place, the corpus luteum atrophies and is replaced by white scar tissue called the *corpus albicans*; the hormonal support of the endometrium is withdrawn and menstruation occurs. In the event of fertilization, the multiplying cells produce a hormone called *human chorionic gonadotropin*. This hormone prevents luteal regression. As a result the corpus luteum remains functional for 3 months, producing hormonal support for pregnancy until the placenta is fully functional.

Endometrial Changes

The endometrium consists of two distinct layers, or zones, that are responsive to hormonal stimulation: a basal layer and a functional layer. The *basal layer* lies adjacent to the myometrium and is not sloughed during menstruation.[2–4] The *functional layer* rises from the basal layer and undergoes proliferative changes and menstrual sloughing. It can be subdivided into two components: a thin, superficial, compact layer, and a deeper spongiosa layer that makes up most of the secretory and fully developed endometrium.

The endometrial cycle can be divided into three phases: proliferative, secretory, and menstrual (see Fig. 40-5). The proliferative, or preovulatory, phase is the period during which the glands and stroma of the superficial layer grow rapidly under the influence of estrogen. The secretory, or postovulatory, phase is the period during which progesterone produces glandular dilatation and active mucus secretion and the endometrium becomes highly vascular and edematous. The menstrual phase is the period during which the superficial layer degenerates and sloughs off.

SUMMARY CONCEPTS

- The female reproductive system, which consists of the external and internal genitalia, has both sexual and reproductive functions. The external genitalia (labia majora, labia minora, clitoris, and vestibular glands) surround the openings of the urethra and vagina. The internal genitalia of the female reproductive system are specialized to participate in sexual intercourse (the vagina), produce and maintain the female egg cells (the ovaries), transport these cells to the site of fertilization (the fallopian tubes), provide a favorable environment for development of offspring (the uterus), and produce the female sex hormones (the ovaries).

- The uterus is a thick-walled muscular organ, the wall of which is composed of an outer perimetrium, a middle myometrium, and an inner endometrium. The paired gonads, or ovaries, have the dual function of steroidogenesis, or production of the female sex hormones, and gametogenesis, or production of female germ cells (oocytes).

- Between menarche and menopause, the female reproductive system undergoes cyclic changes called the *menstrual cycle*. These changes involve complex interactions among four organs: the hypothalamus, which produces gonadotropin-releasing hormone (GnRH); the anterior pituitary gland, which synthesizes and releases the follicle stimulating hormone (FSH), the luteinizing hormone (LH), and prolactin; the ovaries, which synthesize and release estrogens, progesterone, and androgens; and the endometrium, which undergoes proliferative changes and sloughing.

- Although each component of the system is essential for normal functioning, the ovarian hormones are largely responsible for controlling the cyclic changes and length of the menstrual cycle. Estrogens are necessary for normal female physical maturation, for growth of ovarian follicles, for generation of a climate that is favorable to fertilization and implantation of the ovum, and for promoting the development of the endometrium in the event of pregnancy. The functions of progesterone include the glandular development of the lobular and alveolar tissue of the breasts, as well as maintenance of pregnancy.

Disorders of the Female Reproductive Organs

Disorders of the female reproductive system have widespread effects on physical, psychological, sexual, and reproductive function. Since the reproductive organs are located close to other pelvic structures, particularly those of the urinary system, disorders of the reproductive system may affect urinary function. This section of the chapter focuses on infections and benign and malignant disorders of the external and internal genitalia.

Disorders of the External Genitalia

The external genitalia, which are covered with stratified squamous epithelium, are subject to dermatologic conditions that affect skin elsewhere in the body. The discussion in this section of the chapter focuses on

Bartholin gland cysts and benign and malignant disorders of the vulva.

Bartholin Gland Cyst and Abscess

A Bartholin gland cyst is a fluid-filled sac located near the vaginal introitus that results from obstruction of the main duct of the gland (see Fig. 40-2).[6–8] It may become large, up to 3 to 5 cm in diameter, and produce pain and local discomfort. Infection of a Bartholin cyst produces acute inflammation within the gland and may result in an abscess. Acute symptoms are usually the result of infection and include pain, tenderness, and dyspareunia.

The treatment of symptomatic Bartholin gland cysts consists of the administration of appropriate antibiotics, local application of moist heat, and incision and drainage. Cysts that frequently are abscessed or are large enough to cause blockage of the introitus may require surgical intervention (i.e., marsupialization, a procedure that involves removal of a wedge of vulvar skin and the cyst wall).[8] Because the Bartholin glands usually shrink during menopause, a vulvar growth in postmenopausal women should be evaluated for malignancy.

Benign and Malignant Disorders of the Vulva

Disorders of the vulva often present as white lesions of the vulvar skin and mucosa that may produce pruritus (itching) and scaling. Although commonly referred to as *leukoplakia* because of their plaquelike appearance, these lesions can represent a number of disorders including inflammatory dermatoses (e.g., psoriasis or chronic dermatitis, discussed in Chapter 46), non-neoplastic epithelial disorders, and premalignant and malignant lesions of the vulva.[6]

Non-neoplastic Epithelial Disorders. The term *non-neoplastic epithelial disorders* refers to nonmalignant atrophic and hyperplastic changes of the vulvar skin and mucosa.[6,7,9] Depending on clinical and histologic characteristics, the lesions can be further categorized as lichen sclerosus, lichen planus, and squamous cell hyperplasia (also known as *lichen simplex chronicus*).

Lichen sclerosus is an inflammatory disease of the vulva characterized by plaquelike areas that may progress to parchment-thin epithelium with focal areas of ecchymosis and superficial ulcerations secondary to scratching. Atrophy and contracture of the vulvar tissues with eventual stenosis of the introitus are common when this condition becomes chronic. Itching is common and dyspareunia (painful intercourse) is frequent. The condition develops insidiously and is progressive.

Lichen planus, while similar to lichen sclerosus, is an intensely inflammatory autoimmune disorder. Although the symptoms and sequelae are similar to lichen sclerosus, lichen planus may also involve the mucosal and keratinized skin of the oral, anal, and vulvovaginal mucosa. Erosive lichen planus is characterized erythematous erosions surrounded by white lacey edges called *Wickam's striae*. Unlike lichen sclerosus, which is usually limited to the vulva, up to 70% of women with erosive lichen planus have vaginal involvement.[9]

Squamous cell hyperplasia, or *lichen simplex chronicus*, which usually presents as thickened, gray-white plaques with an irregular surface, is a nonspecific condition resulting from rubbing or scratching the skin to relieve pruritus. Presumed to be a response of the genital skin to some type of irritant, this diagnosis is used only when human papillomavirus (HPV) infection (see Chapter 41), fungal infections, or other known causative conditions have been excluded. Pruritus is the most common presenting complaint. Scaling is generally present, and excoriations due to recent scratching can often be seen. There is generally no increased predisposition to cancer, but similar lesions are often present at the margins of established cancer of the vulva.

Current treatment for lichen sclerosus, lichen planus, and squamous cell hyperplasia includes the use of topical corticosteroids. Lichen sclerosus frequently recurs, and lifetime maintenance therapy may be required. Hyperplastic areas that occur in the field of lichen sclerosus may be sites of malignant change and warrant close follow-up and possible biopsy.

Premalignant and Malignant Neoplasms. Carcinoma of the vulva is a relatively rare cancer that accounts for approximately 3% to 5% of all cancers of the female reproductive system in the United States, occurring most often in women 60 years of age or older.[6,10,11] Approximately 85% to 95% of vulvar malignancies are squamous cell carcinomas.[11] Less common forms of vulvar cancer include malignant melanomas, adenocarcinoma, basal cell carcinoma, and metastatic cancers from various other sites.

In terms of etiology, pathogenesis, and clinical presentation, vulvar carcinoma can be divided into two general groups: (1) basaloid and warty carcinomas, related to infection with oncogenic strains of HPV (about 30% of cases), and (2) keratinizing squamous cell carcinoma, not related to the human papillomavirus (HPV) infection (about 70% of cases).[6,7] Invasive basaloid and warty-type carcinomas develop from a precancerous in situ lesion called *vulvar intraepithelial neoplasia* (VIN). This type of lesion occurs in reproductive-age women, and risk factors are similar to those for cancer in situ of the cervix.[6] Spontaneous resolution of VIN lesions has occurred. The risk of progression to invasive cancer increases in older women and in women with suppressed immune function. The second form of vulvar cancer, which is seen more often in older women, is generally preceded by vulvar non-neoplastic disorders such as chronic vulvar irritation or lichen sclerosus. The etiology of this group of vulvar cancers is unclear, but they are not typically associated with HPV. Neoplastic changes may arise from lichen sclerosus lesions or hyperplasia, leading directly to invasion, or through an intermediate step involving cellular atypia.[6]

Approximately 50% of women with vulvar cancer present with pruritus and a visible lesion.[11] The lesion may appear as an inconspicuous thickening of the skin, a small raised area or lump, or an ulceration that fails to heal. It may be single or multiple and vary in color from white to velvety red or black. The lesions may resemble eczema or dermatitis and may produce few symptoms other than pruritus, local discomfort, and exudation. The lesion may become secondarily infected, causing pain and discomfort. The malignant lesion gradually spreads superficially or as a deep furrow involving all of one labial side. Because there are many lymph channels around the vulva, the cancer metastasizes freely to the regional lymph nodes, including those of the inguinal and femoral chains.

Early diagnosis is important in the treatment of vulvar carcinoma. Because malignant lesions can vary in appearance and commonly are mistaken for other conditions, biopsy and treatment often are delayed. Any vulvar lesion that is increasing in size or has an unusual wartlike appearance should be biopsied. Treatment is primarily wide surgical excision of the lesion for noninvasive cancer and radical excision or vulvectomy with node resection for invasive cancer.

Vulvodynia

Vulvodynia is a syndrome of unexplained vulvar pain, previously referred to as *vulvar pain syndrome* or *burning vulva syndrome*.[12,13] The terminology and diagnostic criteria used for this chronic disorder remain in flux, but the most recent classification system of the International Society for the Study of Vulvovaginal Disorders (ISSVD) defines it as a condition characterized by a sensation of burning, stinging, irritation, soreness or rawness in the absence of relevant visible findings or a specific, clinically identifiable neurological disorder.[12,14] Vulvodynia is further classified as localized or generalized, and as to whether it is provoked, unprovoked, or of mixed origin.

Localized vulvodynia or *vestibulodynia*, formerly referred to as *vulvar vestibulitis syndrome*, is characterized by pain at onset of intercourse, localized point tenderness near the vaginal opening, and sensitivity to tampon placement, tight-fitting pants, bicycling, or prolonged sitting. It is the leading cause of dyspareunia in women younger than 50 years of age. The pain can be primary (present from first contact) or secondary (developing after a period of comfortable sexual relations). The etiology is unknown, but the problem may evolve from chronic vulvar inflammation or trauma. Nerve fibers that supply the vestibular epithelium may become highly sensitized, causing neurons in the dorsal horn of the spinal cord to respond abnormally, thus transforming the sensation of touch in the vestibule into pain.

Generalized vulvodynia, formerly called *vulvar dysesthesia* or *essential vulvodynia*, involves severe, constant, widespread burning the vulvar area that interferes with daily activities. No abnormalities are found on examination, but there is diffuse and variable hypersensitivity and altered sensation to light touch. The quality of this unprovoked pain shares many of the features of other neuropathic pain disorders, particularly complex regional pain syndrome (see Chapter 35) or pudendal neuralgia. Although the cause of the neuropathic pain is unknown, it has been suggested that it may result from myofascial restrictions affecting the sacral and pelvic floor nerves.[12,13]

There are many proposed triggers for vulvodynia, including chronic recurrent vaginal infections; chemical irritation or drug effects, especially prolonged use of topical steroid creams; the irritating effects of elevated urinary levels of calcium oxalate; and immunoglobulin A deficiency or other disorders of immune regulation. Often it is multifactorial in origin.

Careful history taking and physical assessment are essential for differential diagnosis and treatment. *Vulvodynia* is a diagnosis of exclusion after ruling out infections, such as candidiasis and genital herpes; inflammatory conditions, such as squamous cell hyperplasia and lichen sclerosus; vulvar cancer; or neurologic disorders, such as herpes neuralgia or spinal nerve compression, as causes for the pain.

Treatment of vulvodynia is aimed at symptom relief, is frequently long term, and often needs to be managed from a multidimensional, chronic pain perspective.[12,13] Local measures include avoidance of harsh soaps and perfumed products, use of sitz baths, and application of topical anesthetic agents (i.e., lidocaine gel). Because dermatologic conditions such as atopic dermatitis and candidiasis are responsible for many of the symptoms of vulvodynia, some health care providers recommend treatment with antihistamines and oral antifungal medications, as well as avoiding contact with potential irritants.[14] Biofeedback and physical therapy may be used to reverse the changes in pelvic floor musculature and help women control the muscles, regaining strength and improving relaxation.[14] Oral medications, including tricyclic antidepressants and other antidepressants, are often used to treat the neuropathic pain associated with vulvodynia. Botulism toxin A injections block the cholinergic innervation of the target tissues and have been shown to be effective in some women with vulvodynia.[14] Another treatment option for women with severe discomfort is surgical excision of the vestibule. It is commonly the last option and should be reserved for women with long-standing severe symptoms after all other management has yielded unsatisfactory results.[14]

Disorders of the Vagina

The normal vaginal ecology depends on the delicate balance of hormones and bacterial flora. Normal estrogen levels maintain a thick, protective squamous epithelium that contains glycogen. Döderlein bacilli, part of the normal vaginal flora, metabolize glycogen, and in the process produce the lactic acid that normally maintains the vaginal pH of 3.8 to 4.5.[15] Disruptions in these normal environmental conditions predispose to infection.

Vaginitis

Vaginitis represents an inflammation of the vagina that is characterized by vaginal discharge and burning, itching, redness, and swelling of vaginal tissues.[15,16] Pain often occurs with urination and sexual intercourse. Vaginitis may be caused by chemical irritants, foreign bodies, or infectious agents. The causes of vaginitis differ in various age groups. In premenarchal girls, most vaginal infections have nonspecific causes, such as poor hygiene, intestinal parasites, or the presence of foreign bodies. *Candida albicans, Trichomonas vaginalis*, and bacterial vaginosis are the most common causes of vaginitis in the childbearing years, and some organisms can be transmitted sexually[15,16] (see Chapter 41).

The decrease in estrogen levels that occurs during perimenopause and post menopause can lead to an atrophic form of vaginitis. Estrogen deficiency results in a lack of regenerative growth of the vaginal epithelium and changes in the vaginal pH and flora, rendering these tissues more susceptible to infection and irritation. Döderlein bacilli disappear, and the vaginal secretions become less acidic. The symptoms of atrophic vaginitis include itching, burning, and dyspareunia. These symptoms usually can be reversed by local application of estrogen.

Every woman normally experiences vaginal discharge during the menstrual cycle, but it should not cause burning or itching or have an unpleasant odor. These symptoms suggest inflammation or infection. Because these symptoms are common to the different types of vaginitis, precise identification of the organism is essential for proper treatment. A careful history should include information about systemic disease conditions, the use of drugs such as antibiotics that foster the growth of yeast, dietary habits, stress, and other factors that alter the resistance of vaginal tissue to infections. A physical examination usually is done to evaluate the nature of the discharge and its effects on the genital structures. Microscopic examination of a saline wet-mount smear is the primary means of identifying the organism responsible for the infection.[15] Culture methods and deoxyribonucleic acid (DNA) probe tests may be needed when the organism is not apparent on a wet-mount preparation.

Cancer of the Vagina

Primary cancers of the vagina are extremely rare, accounting for approximately 1% to 2% of all cancers of the female reproductive system.[6,7,11] Like vulvar carcinoma, cancer of the vagina is largely a disease of older women, with a peak incidence between 60 and 70 years of age.[7] Vaginal cancers may also result from local extension of cervical cancer, from exposure to sexually transmitted HPV, or rarely from local irritation such as occurs with prolonged use of a pessary. Smoking and human immunodeficiency virus (HIV) infection also increase the risk of vaginal cancer.

Approximately 70% of vaginal cancers are squamous cell carcinomas, with other less common types being adenocarcinomas (15%), malignant melanomas (9%), and sarcomas (up to 4%).[17] Squamous cell carcinomas begin in the epithelium and progress over many years from precancerous lesions called *vaginal intraepithelial neoplasia* (VAIN). Not infrequently, squamous cell carcinoma develops some years after cervical or vulvar carcinoma, a sequence that supports the carcinogenic effect in the lower genital tract related to HPV infection.

The most common symptom of vaginal carcinoma is abnormal bleeding. Other signs or symptoms include an abnormal vaginal discharge, a palpable mass, or dyspareunia. Most women with preinvasive vaginal carcinoma are asymptomatic, with the cancer being discovered during a routine pelvic examination. The anatomic proximity of the vagina to other pelvic structures (urethra, bladder, and rectum) permits early spread to these areas. Pelvic pain, dysuria, and constipation are associated symptoms.

Since most preinvasive and early invasive cancers are silent, the routine use of vaginal cytology (Papanicolaou [Pap] smear) is the most effective method of detection. Diagnosis requires biopsy of suspect lesions or areas. Because vaginal cancer is rare, there is not standard treatment.[11] Both radiation and surgical methods are used, with the treatment plan being determined by the cancer type, stage of the disease (i.e., size, location, and spread), and the woman's age.[11]

Disorders of the Uterine Cervix

The cervix is composed of two types of epithelial tissue: stratified squamous and columnar epithelium. The exocervix, or visible portion, is covered with stratified squamous epithelium, which also lines the vagina. The endocervix, which is the canal that leads to the endometrial cavity, is lined with columnar epithelium that contains large, branched mucus-secreting glands. The amount and properties of the mucus secreted by the gland cells vary during the menstrual cycle. Blockage of the mucosal glands results in trapping of mucus in the deeper glands, leading to the formation of dilated cysts in the cervix called *nabothian cysts*. These are benign cysts that require no treatment unless they become so numerous that they cause cervical enlargement.

The junction of the squamous epithelium of the exocervix and mucus-secreting columnar epithelium of the endocervix (i.e., squamocolumnar junction) appears at various locations on the cervix at different points in a woman's life (Fig. 40-8). During childhood, the squamocolumnar junction is located just inside the external os. High levels of hormones which occur during puberty, first

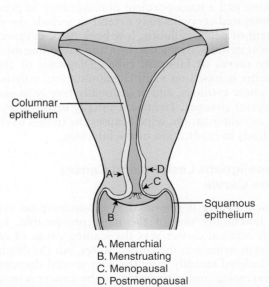

A. Menarchial
B. Menstruating
C. Menopausal
D. Postmenopausal

FIGURE 40-8. Location of the squamocolumnar junction (transformation zone) in menarchial, menstruating, menopausal, and postmenopausal women.

pregnancy and prolonged oral contraceptive use cause the squamocolumnar junction to "roll out" or evert from its original position inside the external os to a position of enlarged cervical surface. Exposure of the columnar cells to low pH vaginal secretions, irritants, and a changing hormonal environment lead to a gradual transformation from columnar to squamous epithelium—a process called *metaplasia* (see Chapter 2). The area of dynamic change where metaplasia takes place is called the *transformation zone*.[6,7] The transformation zone is a critical area for the development of cervical cancer.

Cervicitis

Cervicitis is an acute or chronic inflammation of the cervix. Acute cervicitis may result from the direct infection of the cervix or it may occur secondary to a vaginal or uterine infection. It may be caused by a variety of infective agents, particularly endogenous vaginal aerobes and anaerobes, *Streptococcus*, *Staphlococcus*, and *Enterococcus*.[7] Other specific organisms include *C. albicans* and herpes simplex virus. Some agents are sexually transmitted, whereas others may be introduced by foreign objects such as tampons or pessaries.[7]

With acute cervicitis, the cervix becomes reddened and edematous. Irritation from the infection results in copious mucopurulent drainage. Depending on the causative agent, acute cervicitis is treated with appropriate antibiotic therapy.[7]

Chronic cervicitis represents a low-grade inflammatory process. It is seen most commonly in parous women and may be sequelae to minute lacerations that occur during childbirth, instrumentation, or other trauma. The organisms usually are nonspecific—often staphylococcal, streptococcal, or coliform bacilli. The symptoms of chronic cervicitis are well defined. The cervix may be ulcerated or normal in appearance; it may contain nabothian cysts; the cervical os may be distorted by old lacerations or everted to expose areas of columnar epithelium; and a mucopurulent drainage may be present.

Untreated cervicitis may extend to include the development of pelvic cellulitis, low back pain, dyspareunia, cervical stenosis, dysmenorrhea, and ascending infection of the uterus or fallopian tubes. Diagnosis of chronic cervicitis is based on vaginal examination, colposcopy, Pap smear cytology, and occasionally biopsy to exclude malignant changes. Treatment usually involves cryosurgery or cauterization, which causes the tissues to slough and leads to eradication of the infection.

Premalignant Lesions and Cancer of the Cervix

Cervical cancer is one of the best-understood cancers and potentially one of the most preventable. In the 1950s cervical cancer was the leading cause of cancer deaths in women in the United States, but the death rate has declined steadily over the past several decades due to prevention and early detection by cancer screening.[6] Worldwide, however, cervical cancer remains the second most common cancer in women.[7]

Pathogenesis and Risk Factors. The pathogenesis of cervical cancer has been linked to HPV infection by a series of epidemiologic, pathologic, and molecular genetic studies. Of the approximate 100 types of HPV, about 40 affect the anogenital tract. About 15 of these types are associated with cancer and are known as high-risk groups, with subtypes 16 and 18 being the most important in terms of cervical cancer pathology (see Chapter 41).[6] HPV 16 accounts for almost 60% of cervical cancer cases, and HPV 18 for another 10%.[7] By contrast, low-risk types 6 and 11 are associated with genital warts (condylomata acuminata).

Most cervical cancers begin their development in the squamous columnar cells of the transformation zone. The metaplastic cells within this zone represent the newest and least mature cells in the cervix. HPV infects immature basal cells of the squamous epithelium, but not mature superficial cells that cover the exocervix, vagina, or vulva, explaining the vulnerability of cells in the transformation zone to malignant transformation. Even though HPV has been firmly established as a causative factor in cervical cancer, the evidence does not implicate HPV as the only risk factor. Most HPV infections are transient, indicating the host's defense system is able to eradicate the virus before it can cause neoplastic changes in cervical cells. Other factors such as cigarette smoking, dietary and nutritional factors, early age of first sexual intercourse, family history of cervical cancer, immunodeficiency (e.g., HIV infection), multiparity, and hormonal and other factors may play a role in determining whether a woman with HPV infection develops cervical cancer.[6,18]

Two types of HPV vaccines are currently available to prevent HPV infection: a quadrivalent vaccine (Gardasil) to prevent infection by HPV subtypes 16, 18, 6, and 11,[19] and a bivalent vaccine (Cervarix) to prevent infection by subtypes 16 and 18.[20] The quadrivalent vaccine has been approved for females and males between the ages of 9 and 26 years, optimally before initiation of sexual activity. Human papillomavirus subtypes 6 and 11 cause the majority of venereal warts, while types 16 and 18 are responsible for over 80% of all cervical cancers. Because the bivalent vaccine does not protect again HPV subtypes 6 and 11, which are responsible for the majority of condyloma acuminiata (genital warts), it is approved for females between the ages of 9 and 26 years, but not for males.

Premalignant and Malignant Lesions. One of the most important advances in the early diagnosis and treatment of cancer of the cervix was made possible by the observation that this cancer arises from precancerous lesions that begin with the development of atypical cervical cells. There are variations in cell size and shape and changes in the nuclear and cytoplasmic parts of the cell, commonly referred to as *dysplasia* (see Chapter 7). These precancerous changes represent a continuum of morphologic changes with indistinct boundaries that may gradually progress to cancer in situ and then to invasive cancer, or they may spontaneously regress.

The classification of cervical precancerous lesions has changed over time, and terms from different classification systems are currently used interchangeably.[6,7] Precancerous cell epithelial lesions are often described as either atypical squamous cells (ASCs), low-grade intraepithelial lesions (LSILs), or high-grade intraepithelial lesions (HSILs), and cancerous lesions are termed invasive squamous carcinoma. Atypical squamous cells can be further divided into "ASC of underdetermined significance" (ASC-US) and "ASC, cannot exclude HSIL." Precancerous glandular lesions are classified in a similar manner as atypical glandular cells (AGC). Cancerous glandular lesions are classified as adenocarcinoma.[6,11,22]

The atypical cellular changes that precede frank neoplastic changes consistent with cancer of the cervix can be recognized by a number of direct and microscopic techniques, including the cytology (Pap smear), colposcopy, and cervicography. The appropriate use of Pap smear cytology in cervical screening programs has been controversial. The American Cancer Society (ACS), the American College of Obstetricians and Gynecologists (ACOG), and the U.S. Preventative Services Task Force (USPSTF) have developed evidence-based guidelines for cancer screening.[21–23] The ACOG guidelines recommend that screening begin at age 21 regardless of sexual history and be done every 3 years between the ages of 21 and 29 years. For women ages 30 to 65 the preferred approach is to be screened every 5 years with the combination HPV and Pap smear cytology. Women who prefer may continue to be screened every 3 years with Pap smear cytology. It is recommended that women discontinue screening after the age of 65 if they have had negative cytology results in the previous 10 years. Women who have had a total hysterectomy (removal of the uterus and cervix) for noncancerous reasons should discontinue cytology and HPV testing. For women who have had a total hysterectomy because of a cancer diagnosis, cytology and HPV testing may still be warranted. Women who have had a supra-cervical hysterectomy (the uterus is removed, but the cervix remains) should continue cytology and HPV testing as recommended by cervical cancer screening guidelines.

Diagnosis and Treatment. In its early stages, cervical cancer often manifests as a poorly defined lesion of the endocervix. Frequently, women with cervical cancer present with abnormal vaginal bleeding, spotting, and discharge. Although bleeding may assume any course, it is reported most frequently after intercourse. Women with more advanced disease may present with pelvic or back pain that may radiate down the leg, hematuria, fistulas (rectovaginal or vesicovaginal), or evidence of metastatic disease to supraclavicular or inguinal lymph node areas.

Diagnosis of cervical cancer requires pathologic confirmation. Pap smear cytology results demonstrating squamous intraepithelial lesions often require further evaluation by colposcopy, during which a biopsy sample may be obtained from suspect areas and examined microscopically.[7,24] Diagnostic endocervical currettage may also be done to determine the extent of endocervical involvement.[7]

Early treatment of cervical cancer involves removal of the lesion by one of various techniques. Biopsy or local destruction of the affected cervical tissue may be therapeutic in and of itself. Electrocautery, cryosurgery, or carbon dioxide laser therapy may be used to treat moderate to severe dysplasia that is limited to the exocervix (i.e., squamocolumnar junction clearly visible). Therapeutic conization becomes necessary if the lesion extends into the endocervical canal and can be done surgically or with a large loop electrocautery procedure (LEEP) in the physician's office.[18]

Depending on the stage of involvement of the cervix, invasive cancer is treated with surgery, radiation therapy, chemoradiation, or chemotherapy.[18] External-beam irradiation and intracavitary irradiation or *brachytherapy* (i.e., insertion of radioactive materials into the body) can be used in the treatment of cervical cancer. Intracavitary radiation provides direct access to the central lesion and increases the tolerance of the cervix and surrounding tissues, permitting curative levels of radiation to be used. External-beam radiation eliminates metastatic disease in pelvic lymph nodes and other structures, as well as shrinking the cervical lesion to optimize the effects of intracavitary radiation. Surgery can include extended hysterectomy (i.e., removal of the uterus, fallopian tubes, ovaries, and upper portion of the vagina) without pelvic lymph node dissection, and radical hysterectomy with pelvic lymph node dissection. The choice of treatment is influenced by the stage of the disease as well as the woman's age and health.

Disorders of the Uterus

The uterus is subject to a number of disorders, the most common being infectious processes, endocrine imbalances, neoplasms, and defects in uterine support.

Infectious Disorders of the Uterus and Pelvic Structures

The uterus and pelvic structures are subject to infections by a number of agents, including the sexually transmitted organisms *N. gonorrhoeae* and *C. trachomatis*, as well as endogenous microorganisms such as anaerobes, *Haemophilus influenzae*, enteric gram-negative rods, and streptococci. Tuberculosis salpingitis is rare in the United States but more common in developing countries.

Endometritis. The endometrium and myometrium are relatively resistant to infections, primarily because the endocervix normally forms a barrier to ascending infections. Acute endometritis is uncommon and usually occurs after the cervical barrier is compromised by abortion, delivery, or instrumentation.[6,7] Curettage (scraping of the uterine cavity) is diagnostic and often curative because it removes the necrotic tissue that has served as a site for microbial growth.

Chronic inflammation of the endometrium is associated with intrauterine devices (IUDs), pelvic inflammatory disease, and retained products of conception after delivery or abortion. The presence of plasma cells (which are not present in the normal endometrium) is required for diagnosis. The clinical picture is variable, but often includes abnormal vaginal bleeding, mild to severe uterine tenderness, fever, malaise, and foul-smelling discharge. Treatment involves oral or intravenous antibiotic therapy, depending on the severity of the condition.

Pelvic Inflammatory Disease. Pelvic inflammatory disease (PID) is a polymicrobial infection of the upper reproductive tract (uterus, fallopian tubes, or ovaries) associated with sexually transmitted and endogenous organisms.[25–27] The organisms ascend through the endocervical canal to the endometrial cavity, and then to the fallopian tubes and ovaries (Fig. 40-9). The endocervical canal is slightly dilated during menstruation, allowing bacteria to gain entrance to the uterus and other pelvic structures. After entering the upper reproductive tract, the organisms multiply rapidly in the favorable environment of the sloughing endometrium and ascend to the fallopian tube.

Factors that predispose women to the development of PID include an age younger than 25 years; young age at first intercourse (<15 years); use of nonbarrier contraception, especially IUD or oral contraception; history of new, multiple, or symptomatic sex partners; and previous history of PID or sexually transmitted infection. [25]

The symptoms of PID include lower abdominal pain, which may start just after a menstrual period; dyspareunia; back pain; purulent cervical discharge; and the presence of lower abdominal tenderness and exquisitely painful cervix on bimanual pelvic examination. New-onset breakthrough bleeding in women who are on oral contraceptives or medroxyprogesterone contraceptive injection (Depo-Provera) has been associated with PID. Fever (>101°F), increased erythrocyte sedimentation rate, and an elevated white blood cell count (>10,000 cells/mL) commonly are seen, even though the woman may not appear acutely ill. Elevated C-reactive protein (CRP) levels equate with inflammation and can be used as another diagnostic tool. Laparoscopy, which allows for direct visualization of the ovaries, fallopian tubes, and uterus, is one of the most specific procedures for diagnosing PID, but is costly and carries the inherent risks of surgery and anesthesia.[27] Minimal criteria for a presumptive diagnosis of PID require only the presence of lower abdominal pain, adnexal (area adjoining the uterus, fallopian tubes, and ovaries) tenderness, and cervical motion tenderness on bimanual examination with no other apparent cause.

Treatment may involve hospitalization with intravenous administration of antibiotics. If the condition is diagnosed early, outpatient antibiotic therapy may be sufficient. Treatment is aimed at preventing complications, which can include pelvic adhesions, infertility, ectopic pregnancy, chronic abdominal pain, and tubo-ovarian abscesses.

Endometriosis

Endometriosis is the condition in which functional endometrial tissue is found in ectopic sites outside the uterus.[28–30] The site may be the ovaries, posterior broad ligaments, uterosacral ligaments, rectouterine pouch, pelvis, vagina, vulva, perineum, or intestines (Fig. 40-10).

The cause of endometriosis is largely unknown. There appears to have been an increase in its incidence in developed Western countries during the past four

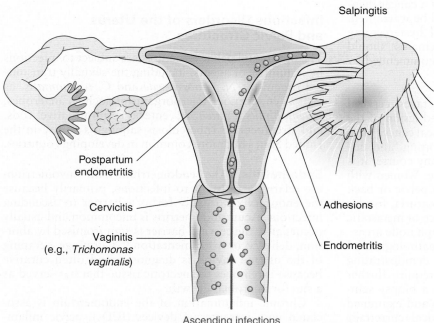

Salpingitis

Postpartum endometritis

Cervicitis

Vaginitis (e.g., *Trichomonas vaginalis*)

Adhesions

Endometritis

Ascending infections (e.g., *Gonococcus, Staphylococcus*, anaerobes, *Streptococcus, Chlamydia*)

FIGURE 40-9. Pelvic inflammatory disease. Microbial agents enter through the vagina and ascend to involve the uterus, fallopian tubes, and pelvic structures.

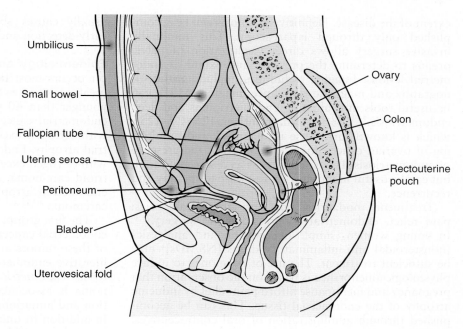

Umbilicus

Small bowel

Fallopian tube

Uterine serosa

Peritoneum

Bladder

Uterovesical fold

Ovary

Colon

Rectouterine pouch

FIGURE 40-10. Common locations of endometriosis in the pelvis and abdomen.

to five decades. Approximately 5% to 10% of reproductive-age women have some degree of endometriosis.[28,30] Risk factors may include early menarche and late menopause; short menstrual cycles (<28 days), longer duration (>5 days) or heavier flow cycles; increased menstrual pain; and other first-degree relatives with the condition.

Several theories attempt to explain the origin of the dispersed endometrial lesions that occur in women with endometriosis.[6,7,28] One theory, the *regurgitation/implantation theory*, suggests that menstrual blood containing fragments of endometrium is forced upward through the fallopian tubes into the peritoneal cavity. Retrograde menstruation is not an uncommon phenomenon, and it is unknown why endometrial cells implant and grow in some women but not in others. A second theory, the *vascular* or *lymphatic theory*, suggests that the endometrial tissue may metastasize through the lymphatics or vascular system. Another theory, the *metaplastic theory*, proposes that dormant, immature cellular elements, spread over a wide area during embryonic development, persist into adult life and then differentiate into endometrial tissue. Genetic and immune factors also have been studied as contributing factors to the development of endometriosis.

Endometriosis usually becomes apparent in the reproductive years when the lesions are stimulated by ovarian hormones in the same way as normal endometrium, becoming proliferative, then secretory, and finally undergoing menstrual breakdown. Bleeding into the surrounding structures can cause pain and the development of significant pelvic adhesions. Symptoms tend to be more severe premenstrually, subsiding after cessation of menstruation. Pelvic pain is the most common presenting symptom; other symptoms include back pain, dyspareunia, and pain on defecation and micturition. Endometriosis is associated with infertility because of adhesions that distort the pelvic anatomy and cause impaired ovum release and transport.

The gross pathologic changes that occur in endometriosis differ with location and duration. In the ovary, the endometrial tissue may form cysts (i.e., endometriomas filled with old blood that resembles chocolate syrup [chocolate cysts]).[6] Rupture of these cysts can cause peritonitis and adhesions. Elsewhere in the pelvis, the tissue may take the form of small hemorrhagic lesions that may be black, bluish, red, clear, or opaque (Fig. 40-11). Some may be surrounded by scar tissue.

Endometriosis may be difficult to diagnose because its symptoms mimic those of other pelvic disorders and the severity of the symptoms does not always reflect the

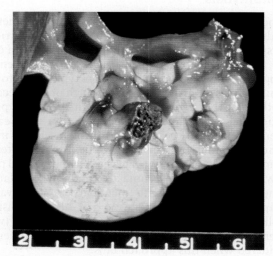

FIGURE 40-11. Endometriosis. Implants of endometrium on the ovary appear as red-blue nodules. (From Mutter GL, Prat J, Schwartz DA. The female reproductive system, the peritoneum and pregnancy. In: Rubin R, Strayer DS, eds. *Rubin's Pathology: Clinicopathologic Foundations of Medicine*. 6th ed. Philadelphia, PA: Wolters Kluwer Health | Lippincott Williams & Wilkins; 2012:903.)

extent of the disease. Definitive diagnosis can be accomplished only through laparoscopy. This minimally invasive surgery allows direct visualization of pelvic organs to determine the presence and extent of endometrial lesions. Imaging techniques, including ultrasonography and magnetic resonance imaging (MRI), can be useful tools in evaluating endometriomas and deep endometriosis.[29,30] Serum cancer antigen 125 (CA-125), which is known for its use in diagnosis and monitoring of ovarian cancer, may be elevated in the presence of endometriosis. It has limitations as a screening tool, but can be useful in monitoring response to therapy and recurrence.

Treatment modalities fall into three categories: pain relief, endometrial suppression, and surgery.[29,30] In young women, simple observation and analgesics (nonsteroidal anti-inflammatory drugs [NSAIDs]) may be sufficient treatment. The use of hormones to induce physiologic amenorrhea is based on the observation that pregnancy and menopause afford pain relief by inducing atrophy of the endometrial tissue. This can be accomplished through administration of oral contraceptives, continuous progestogen therapy, androgenic agents (danazol), or long-acting GnRH analogs that inhibit the pituitary gonadotropins and suppress ovulation.

Surgery may offer more definitive therapy for women with large or symptomatic endometriomas (endometrial cysts) that do not respond to medical therapy because of the concentration of endometriosis within the cyst.[29,30] Laproscopic surgical options include the use of cautery, laser ablation, or excision techniques. Definitive surgical treatment involves total hysterectomy and bilateral salpingo-oophorectomy (removal of the uterus, ovaries, and fallopian tubes) when the symptoms are unbearable or the woman's childbearing is completed.

Adenomyosis

Adenomyosis is the condition in which endometrial glands and stroma are found within the myometrium, interspersed between the smooth muscle fibers.[6,7] In contrast to endometriosis, which usually is a problem in young, infertile women, adenomyosis typically is found in multiparous women in their late fourth or fifth decade. It is thought that events associated with repeated pregnancies, deliveries, and uterine involution may cause the endometrium to be displaced throughout the myometrium. Adenomyosis frequently coexists with uterine myomas or endometrial hyperplasia. Heavy, painful periods with clots and dyspareunia are common complaints. Adenomyosis resolves with menopause. Conservative therapy using oral contraceptives or GnRH agonists is usually the first choice of treatment. Hysterectomy (with preservation of the ovaries in premenopausal women) is considered when this approach fails.

Endometrial Cancer

Endometrial cancer is the most frequent invasive cancer of the female reproductive tract and accounts for 7% of all invasive cancers in women.[6,7] It is typically a disease of postmenopausal women. Because endometrial cancer usually causes abnormal (postmenopausal) bleeding, early detection and cures are possible.

Epidemiology and Pathogenesis. Endometrial cancer occurs most frequently in postmenopausal women (peak age of 55 to 65 years) and is uncommon in women younger than 40 years of age.[6] Two groups in which endometrial cancers arise are perimenopausal women with estrogen excess and older women with endometrial atrophy. Endometrial cancers that arise in women with estrogen excess are described as type I or endometrioid carcinoma, and those that arise in women with endometrial atrophy as type II or serous or clear-cell carcinoma.[6,7,31–34]

The first group, or type I, is the most common type of endometrial cancer, accounting for 80% of cases. Most of these tumors are well differentiated and mimic proliferative endometrial glands, and as such are referred to as *endometrioid carcinoma*. Endometrioid carcinoma is associated with prolonged estrogen stimulation and mutations in PTEN, a tumor-suppressor gene. In addition to unopposed estrogen therapy, other risks for endometrioid carcinoma are obesity, diabetes, nulliparity (having borne no children), early menarche, and late menopause. Many of these risk factors are the same as those for endometrial hyperplasia. Obesity predisposes to insulin resistance, ovarian androgen excess, anovulation, and chronic progesterone deficiency. These hormonal changes stimulate endometrial cell proliferation, inhibit apoptosis, and promote angiogenesis. Progesterone counteracts the effects of estrogen. Pregnancy, with intense placental production of progestins, protects against endometrial cancer. Thus, multiparity protects against endometrial cancer, whereas nulliparity increases risk, especially when infertility is also present. Diabetes mellitus, hypertension, and polycystic ovary syndrome are conditions that also alter estrogen metabolism and elevate estrogen levels.

Type II endometrial cancers occur in a small subset of women who do not exhibit increased estrogen levels. These women usually acquire the disease at an older age and in a setting of endometrial atrophy rather than hyperplasia. This type of endometrial cancer usually is associated with a poorer prognosis than type I carcinomas.[7]

Clinical Features. The major symptom of endometrial hyperplasia or overt endometrial cancer is abnormal, painless bleeding. Abnormal bleeding is an early warning sign of endometrial cancer in up to 90% of women, and because endometrial cancer tends to be slow growing in its early stages, the chances of cure are good if prompt medical care is sought.[31] In menstruating women, this takes the form of bleeding between periods or excessive, prolonged menstrual flow. In postmenopausal women, any bleeding is abnormal and warrants investigation. Later signs of uterine cancer may include cramping, pelvic discomfort, postcoital bleeding, lower abdominal discomfort, and enlarged lymph nodes.

Although Pap smear cytology can identify a small percentage of endometrial cancers, it is not a good screening tool for the tumor. Endometrial biopsy is far more accurate. Direct visualization of the endometrium with hysteroscopy and dilatation of the cervix and curettage of the uterine cavity (D&C) is the definitive procedure for diagnosis because it provides a more thorough evaluation. Transvaginal ultrasonography may be used to determine the endometrial thickness as an indicator of hypertrophy and possible neoplastic change.

The prognosis for endometrial cancer depends on the clinical stage of the disease when it is diagnosed and its histologic grade and type. Surgery and radiation therapy are the most successful methods of treatment for endometrial cancer. With early diagnosis and treatment, the 5-year survival rate is approximately 80% to 85%.[6]

Uterine Leiomyomas

Uterine leiomyomas (commonly called *fibroids*) are benign neoplasms of smooth muscle origin.[6,7,35] They are the most common female reproductive tumor. Leiomyomas usually develop in the corpus of the uterus as intramural, subserosal, or submucosal growths (Fig. 40-12). Intramural fibroids are embedded in the myometrium. They are the most common type of fibroid and present as a symmetric enlargement of the nonpregnant uterus. Subserosal tumors are located beneath the perimetrium of the uterus. These tumors are recognized as irregular projections on the uterine surface; they may become pedunculated, displacing or impinging on other genitourinary structures and causing hydroureter or bladder problems. Submucosal fibroids displace endometrial tissue and are more likely to cause bleeding, necrosis, and infection than either of the other types.

Leiomyomas are asymptomatic approximately half of the time and may be discovered during routine pelvic examination, or they may cause menorrhagia (excessive menstrual bleeding), anemia, urinary frequency, rectal pressure/constipation, abdominal distention, and infrequently pain. Their rate of growth is variable, but they may increase in size during pregnancy or with exogenous estrogen stimulation (i.e., oral contraceptives or menopausal estrogen replacement therapy). Interference with pregnancy is rare unless the tumor is submucosal and interferes with implantation or obstructs the cervical outlet. These tumors may outgrow their blood supply, become infarcted, and undergo degenerative changes.

Most leiomyomas regress with menopause, but if bleeding, pressure on the bladder, pain, or other problems persist, hysterectomy may be indicated. Myomectomy (removal of just the tumors) can be done to preserve the uterus for future childbearing. Following myomectomy, cesarean section may be recommended for childbirth. Hypothalamic GnRH agonists may be used to suppress leiomyoma growth before surgery. Uterine artery embolization, which shrinks the fibroids by blocking the blood supply to the uterus, is a minimally invasive procedure for management of heavy bleeding and other symptoms. Uterine artery embolization is only used in women who have completed childbearing as there may not be enough circulation to the uterus to support a pregnancy.[35]

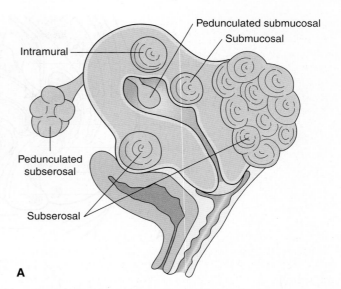

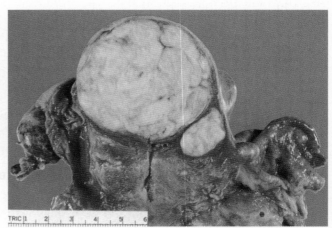

FIGURE 40-12. (A) Submucosal, intramural, and subserosal leiomyomas. **(B)** A bisected uterus displays a prominent, sharply circumscribed, fleshy tumor. (From Mutter GL, Pratt J, Schwartz DA. The female reproductive system, the peritoneum and pregnancy. In: Rubin R, Strayer DS, eds. *Rubin's Pathology: Clinicopathologic Foundations of Medicine.* 6th ed. Philadelphia, PA: Wolters Kluwer Health | Lippincott Williams & Wilkins; 2012:883.)

Disorders of Uterine Support

The uterus and the pelvic structures are maintained in proper position by the uterosacral ligaments, round ligaments, broad ligament, and cardinal ligaments.[1] The two cardinal ligaments maintain the cervix in its normal position (see Fig. 40-4A). The uterosacral ligaments hold the uterus in a forward position, and the broad ligaments suspend the uterus, fallopian tubes, and ovaries in the pelvis. The vagina is encased in the semirigid structure of the strong supporting fascia (Fig. 40-13A). The muscular floor of the pelvis is a strong, slinglike structure that supports the uterus, vagina, urinary bladder, and rectum (Fig. 40-14).

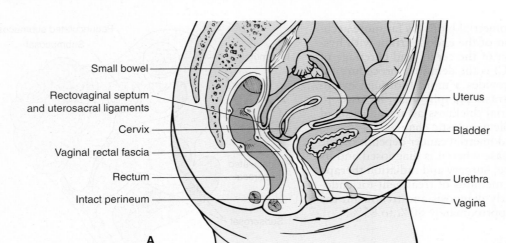

FIGURE 40-13. (A) Normal support of the uterus and vagina, **(B)** cystocele, **(C)** rectocele, and **(D)** uterine prolapse.

In the female anatomy, nature is faced with the problems of supporting the pelvic viscera against the force of gravity and the increases in intra-abdominal pressure associated with coughing, sneezing, defecation, and laughing, while at the same time allowing for urination, defecation, and normal reproductive tract function, especially the delivery of an infant.

Relaxation of the pelvic outlet usually comes about because of overstretching of the perineal supporting tissues during pregnancy and childbirth or years of prolonged straining with hard stools. Although the tissues are stretched only during these times, there may be no difficulty until later in life, such as in the fifth or sixth decade, when further loss of elasticity and muscle tone occurs. Even in a woman who has not borne children, the combination of aging and postmenopausal changes may give rise to problems related to relaxation of the pelvic support structures. The three most common conditions associated with this relaxation are cystocele, rectocele, and uterine prolapse.[36] These may occur separately or together.

Cystocele is a herniation of the bladder into the vagina. It occurs when the normal muscle support for the bladder is weakened, and the bladder sags below the uterus. This causes the anterior vaginal wall to stretch and bulge downward, allowing the bladder to herniate into the vagina due to the force of gravity and pressures from coughing, lifting, or straining at stool (see Fig. 40-13B). The symptoms of cystocele include an annoying bearing-down sensation, difficulty

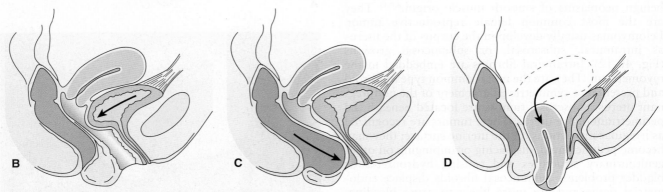

FIGURE 40-14. Muscles of the pelvic floor (female perineum).

in emptying the bladder, frequency and urgency of urination, and cystitis. Stress incontinence may occur at times of increased abdominal pressure, such as during squatting, straining, coughing, sneezing, laughing, or lifting (see Chapter 27).

Rectocele is the herniation of the rectum into the vagina. It occurs when the posterior vaginal wall and underlying rectum bulge forward, ultimately protruding through the introitus as the pelvic floor and perineal muscles are weakened. The symptoms include discomfort because of the protrusion of the rectum and difficulty in defecation (see Fig. 40-13C). Digital pressure (i.e., splinting) on the bulging posterior wall of the vagina may become necessary for defecation. The area between the uterosacral ligaments just posterior to the cervix may weaken and form a hernial sac into which the small bowel protrudes when the woman is standing. This defect, called an *enterocele*, may extend into the rectovaginal septum. It may be congenital or acquired through birth trauma. Enterocele can be asymptomatic or cause a dull, dragging sensation and occasionally low backache.

Uterine prolapse is the bulging of the uterus into the vagina that occurs when the primary supportive ligaments (i.e., cardinal ligaments) are stretched[1] (see Fig. 40-13D). Prolapse is ranked as first, second, or third degree, depending on how far the uterus protrudes through the introitus. First-degree prolapse shows some descent, but the cervix has not reached the introitus. In second-degree prolapse, the cervix or part of the uterus has passed through the introitus. The entire uterus protrudes through the vaginal opening in third-degree prolapse (i.e., procidentia). The symptoms associated with uterine prolapse result from irritation of the exposed mucous membranes of the cervix and vagina and the discomfort of the protruding mass.

Most of the disorders of pelvic relaxation may require surgical correction. These are elective surgeries and usually are deferred until after the childbearing years. The symptoms associated with the disorders often are not severe enough to warrant surgical correction. In other cases, the stress of surgery is contraindicated because of other physical disorders; this is particularly true of older women, in whom many of these disorders occur. Kegel exercises, which strengthen the pubococcygeus muscle, may be helpful in cases of mild cystocele or rectocele or after surgical repair to help maintain the improved function. In women with uterine prolapse, a pessary may be inserted to hold the uterus in place and may stave off surgical intervention in women who want to have children or in older women for whom the surgery may pose a significant health risk.

Disorders of the Ovaries

Disorders of the ovaries frequently cause menstrual and fertility problems. Benign conditions can present as primary lesions of the ovarian structures or as secondary disorders related to hypothalamic, pituitary, or adrenal dysfunction.

Cystic Lesions of the Ovaries

Cysts are the most common cause of enlarged ovaries.[7] Many are benign. A follicular cyst is one that results from occlusion of the duct of the follicle. Each month, several follicles begin to develop and are blighted at various stages of development. These follicles form cavities that fill with fluid, producing a cyst. The dominant follicle normally ruptures to release the egg (i.e., ovulation) but occasionally persists and continues growing. Likewise, a luteal cyst is a persistent cystic enlargement of the corpus luteum that is formed after ovulation and does not regress in the absence of pregnancy. Functional cysts are asymptomatic unless there is substantial enlargement or bleeding into the cyst. This can cause considerable discomfort or a dull, aching sensation on the affected side. However, these cysts usually regress spontaneously. Occasionally, a cyst may become twisted or may rupture into the intra-abdominal cavity (Fig. 40-15).

Polycystic Ovary Syndrome

Polycystic ovary syndrome (PCOS) is a common endocrine disorder affecting 5% to 10% of women of reproductive age, and is a frequent source of chronic anovulation. The disorder is characterized by varying degrees of menstrual irregularity, signs of hyperandrogenism (acne and hirsutism or male-pattern hair loss), infertility, and hyperinsulinemia or insulin resistance.[4,37-40] A substantial number of women who are diagnosed with PCOS are obese, and most have polycystic ovaries.

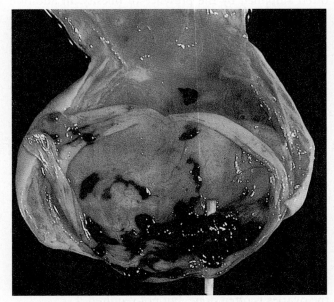

FIGURE 40-15. Follicular cyst of the ovary. The rupture of this thin-walled follicular cyst (dowel stick) led to intra-abdominal hemorrhage. (From Mutter GL, Pratt J, Schwartz DA. The female reproductive system, the peritoneum and pregnancy. In: Rubin R, Strayer DS, eds. *Rubin's Pathology: Clinicopathologic Foundations of Medicine.* 6th ed. Philadelphia, PA: Wolters Kluwer Health | Lippincott Williams & Wilkins; 2012:886).

Chronic anovulation, causing amenorrhea or irregular menses, is now thought to be the underlying cause of the bilaterally enlarged "polycystic" ovaries. Hence, the polycystic ovary is a sign of the disease, not the cause of the disease. There is increasing evidence that the disorder may begin before adolescence and that many of the manifestations of PCOS begin to make their appearance at that time. Because many of the symptoms common to PCOS, such as hirsutism, acne, and obesity, can be detrimental to a teenage girl's health and self-esteem, early detection and treatment of PCOS in adolescents are essential.[40]

The underlying etiology of the disorder is unknown, although most women have altered gonadotropin levels.[4,40] This is manifested by increased release of LH in relation to FSH release, with a resultant increase in production of androstenedione and testosterone by the theca cells of the ovary. Androstenedione, in turn, is converted to estrone within adipocytes. Although estrone is a weak estrogen, it stimulates LH release and suppresses FSH release. The resultant decrease in FSH levels allows for new follicular development, but full maturation is not attained and ovulation does not occur. The elevated LH levels result in increased androgen production, which in turn, prevents normal follicular development and contributes to a vicious cycle of anovulation and multiple cyst formation. Increased androgen levels also lead to the development of acne and hirsutism.

The typical woman with PCOS has hyperinsulinemia and many of the signs of the metabolic syndrome (see Chapter 33).[4] It has been shown that the cause of hyperinsulinemia is insulin resistance. The frequency and degree of hyperinsulinemia in women with PCOS is often amplified by the presence of obesity. In addition to its clinical manifestations, long-term health problems linked to PCOS include cardiovascular disease and type 2 diabetes. Classic lipid abnormalities include elevated triglyceride levels, low HDL levels, and elevated LDL levels. Hypertension is also common in women with PCOS. There is also concern that women with PCOS who are anovulatory do not produce progesterone. This, in turn, may subject the endometrium to an unopposed estrogen environment, which is a significant risk factor for development of endometrial cancer.[4,40]

The diagnosis of PCOS can be suspected from the clinical presentation. Although there is no consensus as to which tests should be used, laboratory evaluation to exclude hyperprolactinemia, late-onset adrenal hyperplasia, and androgen-secreting tumors of the ovary and adrenal gland are commonly done. Because of the high risk of insulin resistance, a fasting blood glucose, 2-hour oral glucose tolerance test, and insulin levels may be done to evaluate for hyperinsulinemia. Confirmation with ultrasonography or laparoscopic visualization of the ovaries is often done, but not required.[38]

The overall goal of treatment of PCOS should be directed toward symptom relief, prevention of potential malignant endometrial sequelae, and reduction in risk for development of diabetes and cardiovascular disease. The preferred and most effective treatment for PCOS is lifestyle modification. Weight loss may be beneficial in restoring normal ovulation when obesity is present. Combined oral contraceptive agents ameliorate menstrual irregularities and improve hirsutism and acne. The addition of spironolactone, a mineralocorticoid antagonist that inhibits the production of androgens by the adrenal gland, may be beneficial to women with severe hirsutism.[4]

Insulin-sensitizing agents (e.g., metformin) alone or with ovulation-inducing medications are emerging as an important component of PCOS treatment.[40] In addition to expected improvements in insulin sensitivity and glucose metabolism, they have been associated with reductions in androgen and LH levels and are highly effective in restoring normal menstrual regularity and ovulatory cycles.

Ovarian Cancer

Ovarian cancer is the second most frequent gynecologic malignancy after endometrial cancer in the United States, and it carries the highest mortality rate of all genital cancers combined.[6] The incidence of ovarian cancer and mortality rate increases with age, with most cases occurring in women older than 50 years of age.[41]

Malignant ovarian tumors are categorized according to cell type of origin—epithelial cell tumors, germ cell tumors, and gonadal stromal cell tumors (see Fig. 40-16). Approximately 90% of ovarian cancers are of epithelial cell origin.[6,7] These tumors tend to occur in older women, are usually discovered late in the disease, and have a high mortality rate. The nonepithelial ovarian cancers, which include germ cell tumors and stromal cell tumors, tend to occur in a younger population of women. They typically present with earlier signs of disease and excellent survival potential when detected early.

The most significant risk factor for ovarian cancer appears to be ovulatory age—the length of time during a woman's life when her ovarian cycle is not suppressed by pregnancy, lactation, or oral contraceptive use.[41–43] The incidence of ovarian cancer is much lower in countries where women bear numerous children. Epithelial cancer of the ovaries derives from malignant transformation of the epithelium of the ovarian surface. When these epithelial cells are situated over developing follicles, they undergo metaplastic transformation whenever ovulation occurs. It follows that repeated stimulation of the epithelium of the ovarian surface, which occurs with uninterrupted ovulation, may predispose the epithelium to malignant transformation. Family history also is a significant risk factor for ovarian cancer. The breast cancer susceptibility genes, *BRCA1* and *BRCA2* mutations, which are tumor-suppressor genes, increase the susceptibility to ovarian cancer[6,7,41–43] (see Chapter 7). The estimated lifetime risk of ovarian cancer in women bearing the BRCA1 and BRCA2 mutations is 23% to 54%. A high-fat Western diet and use of powders containing talc in the genital area are other factors that have been linked to the development of ovarian cancer.

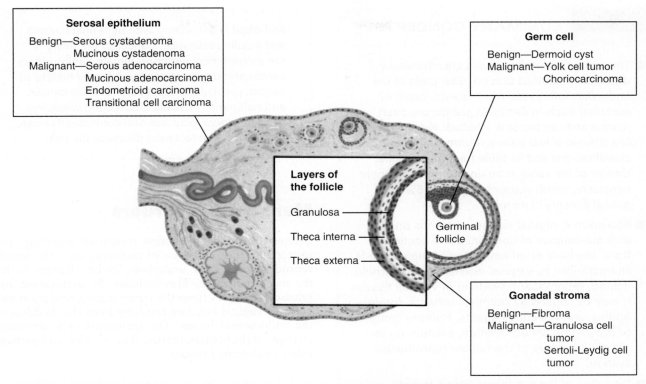

Serosal epithelium

Benign—Serous cystadenoma
        Mucinous cystadenoma
Malignant—Serous adenocarcinoma
        Mucinous adenocarcinoma
        Endometrioid carcinoma
        Transitional cell carcinoma

Germ cell

Benign—Dermoid cyst
Malignant—Yolk cell tumor
        Choriocarcinoma

**Layers of
the follicle**

Granulosa

Theca interna

Theca externa

Germinal
follicle

Gonadal stroma

Benign—Fibroma
Malignant—Granulosa cell
        tumor
        Sertoli-Leydig cell
        tumor

FIGURE 40-16. Classification of ovarian neoplasms based on cell type. (From Mutter GL, Pratt J, Schwartz DA. The female reproductive system, the peritoneum and pregnancy. In: Rubin R, Strayer DS, eds. *Rubin's Pathology: Clinicopathologic Foundations of Medicine.* 6th ed. Philadelphia, PA: Wolters Kluwer Health | Lippincott Williams & Wilkins; 2012:888.)

Clinical Features. Until recently it was believed that most cancers of the ovary produce no symptoms. Several studies have now established that symptoms are often present and reported by women before diagnosis, but are nonspecific and therefore difficult to interpret. Symptoms that are believed to have a strong correlation to ovarian cancer include increased abdominal size, epigastric distress, early satiety, or bloating as the result of increased pressure from ascites (i.e., fluid in the peritoneal cavity) or involvement of the omentum. Occasionally, women with early-onset disease present with abdominal or pelvic pain, due to ovarian torsion, although most women with early-stage disease are asymptomatic. Because the gastrointestinal manifestations can occur for a variety of reasons, many women self-treat with antacids and other remedies for a time before seeking treatment, and health care providers may dismiss the woman's complaints as being caused by other conditions, further delaying diagnosis and treatment. Recent onset (<12 months) and frequent occurrence (>12 times per month) of these symptoms should increase the index of suspicion for ovarian cancer and suggest the need for further evaluation.[44] It is not fully understood why the initial symptoms of ovarian cancer are manifested as gastrointestinal disturbances. It is thought that biochemical changes in peritoneal fluids may irritate the bowel or that pain originating in the ovary may be referred to the abdomen and be interpreted as a gastrointestinal disturbance.

At present, no good screening tests or other early methods of detection exist for ovarian cancer.[41,42] The serum tumor marker CA-125 is a cell surface antigen that can be used in monitoring therapy and recurrences when preoperative levels have been elevated. Despite its role in diagnostic evaluation and follow-up, CA-125 is not cancer or tissue specific for ovarian cancer. Levels also are elevated in the presence of endometriosis, uterine fibroids, pregnancy, liver disease, and other benign conditions and with cancers of the endometrium, cervix, fallopian tube, and pancreas. Transvaginal ultrasonography (TVS) has been used to evaluate ovarian masses for malignant potential. Although TVS has demonstrated high sensitivity and specificity as a screening tool, cost precludes its use as a universal screening method.

When ovarian cancer is suspected, surgical evaluation is required for diagnosis, complete and accurate staging, and cytoreduction and debulking procedures to reduce the size of the tumor. The most common surgery involves removal of the uterus, fallopian tubes, ovaries, and omentum. Recommendations regarding treatment beyond surgery and prognosis depend on the stage of the disease. Women with early-stage disease usually do not require adjuvant treatment; women with intermediate disease or advanced disease can often benefit from chemotherapy using a combination of a platinum compound (cisplatin or carboplatin) and a taxane (paclitaxel or docetaxel). When this combination therapy fails, salvage chemotherapy with newer drugs may prolong survival.

SUMMARY CONCEPTS

- The female external genitalia are affected by disorders that affect skin on other parts of the body. *Bartholin cysts,* which are the result of occluded ducts in Bartholin glands, are often painful and can become infected. *Vulvodynia* is a chronic vulvar pain syndrome with several classifications and variable treatment results. *Cancer of the vulva,* is an uncommon malignant neoplasm, which accounts for 3% to 5% of all genital cancers in women.

- The normal vaginal ecology depends on a delicate balance of hormones and bacterial flora. *Vaginitis* or inflammation of the vagina is characterized by vaginal discharge and burning, itching, redness, and swelling of vaginal tissues. It may be caused by chemical irritants, foreign bodies, and infectious agents. Primary *cancers of the vagina* is uncommon, accounting for 1% of all cancers of the female reproductive system.

- Disorders of the cervix and uterus include inflammatory conditions such as cervicitis and endometritis. *Endometriosis* is a condition in which functional endometrial tissue is found in ectopic sites outside the uterus. *Cervical cancer* is caused by HPV and arises from precursor lesions that can be detected on Pap smear cytology, and if detected early, is the most easily cured of all the cancers of the female reproductive system. *Endometrial cancer* is the most common cancer of the female pelvis. *Leiomyomas* are benign neoplasms of the uterine wall.

- *Pelvic inflammatory disease* (PID) is an inflammation of the upper reproductive tract that involves the uterus (endometritis), fallopian tubes (salpingitis), or ovaries (oophoritis).

- Disorders of uterine support result from weakness and relaxation of the pelvic floor muscles. *Cystocele* and *rectocele* involve herniation of the bladder or rectum into the vagina. *Uterine prolapse* occurs when the uterus bulges into the vagina.

- Disorders of the ovaries include cystic disorders, polycystic ovary syndrome (PCOS), and cancer of the ovary. *Functional cysts* usually are asymptomatic unless there is substantial enlargement or bleeding into the cyst or the cyst becomes twisted or ruptures. *Polycystic ovary syndrome* is a disorder characterized by various degrees of hirsutism, obesity, and infertility,

and often is associated with hyperinsulinemia and insulin resistance. *Cancer of the ovary* is the second most common female genitourinary cancer and the most deadly. A family history of cancer, particularly breast and ovarian cancer, and nulliparity increase the risk of developing ovarian cancer, whereas oral contraceptive use, pregnancy, and lactation decrease the risk.

Menstrual Disorders

Between menarche (i.e., first menstrual bleeding) and menopause (i.e., cessation of menstruation), the female reproductive system undergoes cyclic changes called the *menstrual cycle.* This includes the maturation and release of oocytes from the ovary during ovulation and periodic vaginal bleeding resulting from the shedding of the endometrial lining. The menstrual cycle produces changes in the breasts, uterus, skin, ovaries, and perhaps other unidentified tissues.

Dysfunctional Menstrual Cycles

Dysfunctional menstrual cycles may take many forms, including dysfunctional bleeding, and *amenorrhea* (absence of menstruation) is failure to menstruate, *hypomenorrhea* (scanty menstruation), *oligomenorrhea* (infrequent menstruation, periods more than 35 days apart), *polymenorrhea* (frequent menstruation, periods <21 days apart), *menorrhagia* (excessive menstruation), or *metrorrhagia* (bleeding between periods).[45] *Menometrorrhagia* is heavy bleeding during and between menstrual periods.

Although unexplained bleeding can occur because of pregnancy, spontaneous abortion, neoplasms, or other reasons, the frequent cause in the nonpregnant woman is a condition commonly called *dysfunctional bleeding.* Dysfunctional bleeding is related to alterations in the hormones that support normal cyclic endometrial changes. Estrogen deprivation causes retrogression of a previously built-up endometrium and bleeding. Such bleeding often is irregular in amount and duration, with the flow varying with the time and degree of estrogen stimulation and with the degree of estrogen withdrawal.[45] A lack of progesterone can cause abnormal menstrual bleeding. In its absence, estrogen induces development of a much thicker endometrial layer with a richer blood supply.

Periodic bleeding episodes alternating with amenorrhea are caused by variations in the number of functioning ovarian follicles present. When too many follicles are present and active, high levels of estrogen develop, causing the endometrium to proliferate for weeks or even months. In time, either of two events occurs that lead to an estrogen deficiency and bleeding: several follicles may simultaneously degenerate, or the needs of an enlarged endometrial tissue mass may exceed the capabilities of the functioning follicles. Estrogen and progesterone deficiencies are associated with the absence of ovulation, hence the term *anovulatory bleeding*. Because the vasoconstriction and myometrial contractions that normally accompany menstruation are caused by progesterone, anovulatory bleeding seldom is accompanied by cramps, and the flow frequently is heavy. Anovulatory cycles are common among adolescents during the first several years after menarche, when ovarian function is becoming established, and among perimenopausal women, whose ovarian function is beginning to decline.

Dysfunctional bleeding can originate as a primary disorder of the ovaries or uterus or as a secondary defect in ovarian function related to hypothalamic-pituitary stimulation. The latter can be initiated by emotional stress, marked variation in weight (i.e., sudden gain or loss), or nonspecific endocrine or metabolic disturbances. Nonhormonal causes of irregular menstrual bleeding include endometrial polyps, submucosal myoma (i.e., fibroid), bleeding disorder (e.g., von Willebrand disease, platelet dysfunction), endometrial dysplasia, and cancer.

The treatment of dysfunctional bleeding depends on what is identified as the probable cause. The minimum evaluation should include a detailed history with emphasis on bleeding pattern and a physical examination. A pregnancy test is important to rule out any complications of pregnancy. Endocrine studies (e.g., FSH/LH ratio, prolactin, androgen levels), ultrasonography of the endometrium, and endometrial biopsy may be needed for diagnosis. Nonhormonal causes generally require surgical intervention. Dilatation of cervix and scraping of the endometrium (D&C) can be therapeutic as well as diagnostic. Endometrial ablation (destruction of the basal layer of the endometrium from which the monthly buildup generates) has become a primary treatment method for abnormal uterine bleeding.[11] Various ablation devices are available; some use heat while others use cryotherapy. If nonhormonal problems have been excluded and alterations in hormone levels are the primary cause, treatment may include the use of oral contraceptives, cyclic progesterone therapy, or long-acting progesterone injections or implants.

Amenorrhea

There are two types of amenorrhea: primary and secondary. Primary amenorrhea is the failure to menstruate by 15 years of age, or by 13 years of age if failure to menstruate is accompanied by absence of secondary sex characteristics.[46] Secondary amenorrhea is the cessation of menses for at least 6 months in a woman who has established normal menstrual cycles. Primary amenorrhea usually is caused by gonadal dysgenesis, congenital müllerian agenesis, testicular feminization, or a hypothalamic-pituitary-ovarian axis disorder. Causes of secondary amenorrhea include ovarian, pituitary, or hypothalamic dysfunction; intrauterine adhesions; infections (e.g., tuberculosis, syphilis); pituitary

tumors; anorexia nervosa; or strenuous physical exercise, which can alter the critical body fat–to–muscle ratio needed for menses to occur.[46]

Diagnostic evaluation resembles that for dysfunctional uterine bleeding, with the possible addition of a computed tomographic scan or MRI to exclude a pituitary tumor. Treatment is based on correcting the underlying cause and inducing menstruation with cyclic progesterone or combined estrogen–progesterone regimens.

Dysmenorrhea

Dysmenorrhea is pain or discomfort with menstruation. Although not usually a serious medical problem, it causes some degree of monthly disability for a significant number of women. There are two forms of dysmenorrhea: primary and secondary. Primary dysmenorrhea is caused by the effects of excess prostaglandin production in the endometrium.[47] Prostaglandins are potent smooth muscle stimulants that cause intense uterine contractions. Prostaglandin production in the uterus normally increases under the influence of progesterone, reaching a peak at or soon after the onset of menstruation. With onset of menstruation, formed prostaglandins are released from the shedding endometrium. Prostaglandins also cause contraction of smooth muscle elsewhere in the body. Severe dysmenorrhea may be associated with systemic symptoms such as headache, nausea, vomiting, and diarrhea. The pain of primary dysmenorrhea is often diffusely located in the lower abdomen or suprapubic area, radiating to the lower back. The pain is often described as cramping and spasmodic, or similar to labor pains. Secondary dysmenorrhea is menstrual pain caused by structural abnormalities or disease processes such as endometriosis, uterine fibroids, adenomyosis, pelvic adhesions, IUDs, or PID. In women with secondary dysmenorrhea, the pain often lasts longer than the menstrual period; it may begin before menstrual bleeding begins; and it may become worse during menstruation.

Treatment for primary dysmenorrhea is directed at symptom control.[47] Women with primary dysmenorrhea generally experience dramatic pain relief with the nonsteroidal anti-inflammatory drugs (e.g., ibuprofen, naproxen, mefenamic acid), which are prostaglandin synthetase inhibitors. Ovulation suppression and symptomatic relief of dysmenorrhea can be instituted simultaneously with the use of hormonal contraceptives. Relief of secondary dysmenorrhea depends on identifying the cause of the problem. Medical or surgical intervention may be needed to eliminate the problem.

Premenstrual Syndrome Disorders

Premenstrual syndrome disorders are a group of physical, emotional, and behavioral changes that occur in a regular, cyclic relationship to the luteal phase of the menstrual cycle and that interfere with some aspect of a woman's life.[48–51] The severity of this cyclic symptom complex can vary from *premenstrual molimina* on the mild end; through *premenstrual syndrome* (PMS), which is characterized by mild to moderate physical and psychological symptoms preceding menstruation and relieved by onset of the menses; to *premenstrual dysphoric disorder* (PMDD), which is the most severe form of premenstrual distress and generally is associated with mood disorders.

Up to 80% of women in the United States experience some emotional or physical symptoms during the luteal phase of their menstrual cycle, without experiencing a substantial impact on their daily functioning. The PMS disorder, which results in moderate disruptions in a woman's life, occurs in 20% to 30% of premenstrual women and another 3% to 8% suffer from the extreme or severe symptoms of PMDD.[50] The incidence of PMS and PMDD seems to increase with age. It is less common in women in their teens and twenties, and most women seeking help for the problem are in their mid-thirties. The disorder is not culturally distinct; it affects both Westerners and non-Westerners.

Physical symptoms of PMS include painful and swollen breasts, bloating, abdominal pain, headache, and backache. Psychologically, there may be depression, anxiety, irritability, and behavioral changes. In some cases, there are puzzling alterations in motor function, such as clumsiness and altered handwriting. Women with PMS may report one or several symptoms, with symptoms varying from woman to woman and from month to month in the same woman. The disorder can significantly affect a woman's ability to perform at normal levels. Family responsibilities and relationships may suffer and she may lose time from or function ineffectively at work.

Although the causes of PMS and PMDD are poorly documented, they probably are multifactorial. Like dysmenorrhea, it is only recently that PMS has been recognized as a bona fide disorder rather than merely a psychosomatic illness. Because there appear to be no measurable differences in hormone levels between women with and without PMS, it is presumed that normal cyclic variation in the hormones is the trigger for symptoms in vulnerable or predisposed women. Currently, data suggest a relationship between normal gonadal fluctuations and central neurotransmitter activity, particularly serotonin. It is unclear whether decreased levels of serotonin are present during the luteal phase and only susceptible women respond with varying degrees of premenstrual symptoms, or if women with PMDD have a neurotransmitter abnormality.[48]

Diagnosis of PMS and PMDD focuses on documentation of the relationship of a woman's symptoms to the luteal phase of the menstrual cycle. A complete history and physical examination are necessary to exclude other physical causes of the symptoms. Depending on the symptom pattern, blood studies, including thyroid hormones, glucose, and prolactin assays, may be done. Psychosocial evaluation is helpful to exclude emotional illness that is merely exacerbated premenstrually.

Management of PMS/PMDD has been largely symptomatic and includes education and support directed toward lifestyle changes for women with mild symptoms.[48–51] An integrated program of personal assessment by diary, regular exercise, avoidance of caffeine, and a diet low in simple sugars and high in lean proteins is often beneficial. In addition to lifestyle changes. In addition to lifestyle changes, pharmacologic treatment includes the use of diuretics to reduce fluid retention, nonsteroidal anti-inflammatory agents for pain, and anxiolytic drugs to treat mood changes. Because symptoms are associated with ovulatory cycles, suppressing ovulation may be beneficial for some women with PMS and can be accomplished using hormonal contraceptives, danazol (a synthetic androgen), or GnRH agonists.[48] Hormonal contraceptives can be used for women who also require contraception. However, some women find their symptoms worsen when taking contraceptives. The pharmacologic treatment of PMDD differs from that of PMS. Ovulation suppression does not seem to help women with PMDD. Although many medications have been studied, only three antidepressants (fluoxetine, sertraline, and paroxetine controlled release) and an oral contraceptive that contains drospirenone (a spironolactone derivative) have been approved for treatment of the emotional and physical symptoms of PMDD.[48]

Menopause and Aging Changes

Menopause is the cessation of menstrual cycles. Like menarche, it is more of a process than a single event.[52,53] Most women stop menstruating between 48 and 55 years of age. *Perimenopause* (the years immediately surrounding menopause) precedes menopause by approximately 4 years and is characterized by menstrual irregularity and other menopausal symptoms. *Climacteric* refers to the entire transition to the nonreproductive period of life. Premature ovarian failure describes the approximately 1% of women who experience menopause before the age of 40 years. A woman who has not menstruated for a full year or has an FSH level greater than 30 mIU/mL is considered menopausal.

Menopause results from the gradual cessation of ovarian function and the resultant diminished levels of estrogen. Although estrogens derived from the adrenal cortex continue to circulate in a woman's body, they are insufficient to maintain the secondary sexual characteristics in the same manner as ovarian estrogens. As a result, breast tissue, body hair, skin elasticity, and subcutaneous fat decrease; the ovaries and uterus diminish in size; and the cervix and vagina become pale and friable. Problems that can arise as a result of this urogenital atrophy include vaginal dryness, urinary stress incontinence, urgency, nocturia, vaginitis, and urinary tract infection.[52,53] The woman may find intercourse painful and traumatic, although some type of vaginal lubrication may be helpful.

Systemically, a woman may experience significant vasomotor instability secondary to the decrease in estrogens and the relative increase in other hormones, including FSH, LH, GnRH, dehydroepiandrosterone, and androstenedione. This instability may give rise to "hot flashes," palpitations, dizziness, and headaches as the blood vessels dilate. Despite the association with these biochemical changes, the underlying cause of hot flashes is unknown. Tremendous variation exists in the onset, frequency, severity, and length of time that women experience hot flashes. When they occur at night and are accompanied by significant perspiration, they are referred to as *night sweats*. Insomnia as well as frequent awakening because of vasomotor symptoms can lead to sleep deprivation. A woman may experience irritability, anxiety, and depression as a result of these uncontrollable and unpredictable events.

Consequences of long-term estrogen deprivation include osteoporosis due to an imbalance in bone remodeling (see Chapter 44), and an increased risk for cardiovascular disease, which is the leading cause of death for women after menopause. With perimenopause, changes occur in the cardiovascular lipid profile: total cholesterol increases, HDL cholesterol decreases, and LDL cholesterol increases.

Menopausal hormonal therapy has come under scrutiny with the publication of the Women's Health Initiative.[54,55] Since the publication of these trials, there has been great interest in developing alternative doses, delivery systems, and medications for hormone therapy. Many products are now available, including transdermal delivery systems and lower-dose traditional hormone therapy. Vaginal estrogen preparations are available to treat symptoms related to vaginal atrophy. Selective estrogen receptor modulators (SERMs) may be used in place of estrogen to alleviate vulvovaginal atrophy and prevent osteoporosis.

SUMMARY CONCEPTS

- Dysfunctional menstrual cycles, including amenorrhea (absence of menstruation), hypomenorrhea (scanty menstruation), oligomenorrhea (infrequent menstruation), and polymenorrhea (excessive menstruation) are most often due to a lack of ovulation and disturbances in the pattern of ovarian hormone secretion

- Dysmenorrhea, or pain or discomfort during menses, can occur as a primary disorder due to intense uterine contractions caused by excess prostaglandin secretion or as a secondary disorder due to structural abnormalities or disease processes such as endometriosis, pelvic adhesions, or pelvic inflammatory disease.

- The terms *premenstrual syndrome* and *premenstrual dysphoric disorder* represent an array of predictable physical, cognitive, affective, and behavioral symptoms that occur during the luteal phase of the menstrual cycle and that are resolved by menstruation or within a few days of onset. Although the etiology of these disorders is currently unknown, it is probably the result of an interaction between the sex hormones and central neurotransmitters, particularly serotonin.

- Menopause is the cessation of ovarian function and menstrual cycles. It is accompanied by a decline in secondary sexual characteristics, vasomotor instability, and long-term consequences, including increased risk of osteoporosis and heart disease.

Disorders of the Breast

Although anatomically separate, the breasts are functionally related to the female reproductive system in that they respond to the cyclic changes in sex hormones and produce milk for infant nourishment. The breasts are composed of specialized epithelium and stroma that may give rise to both benign and malignant lesions.

Breast Structures

The breasts, or mammary glands, are located between the third and seventh ribs of the anterior chest wall and are supported by the pectoral muscles and superficial fascia. They are specialized glandular structures that have an abundant shared nervous, vascular, and lymphatic supply[1,2] (Fig. 40-17). Structurally the breast consists of fat, fibrous connective tissue, and glandular tissue. The superficial fibrous connective tissue is attached to the skin, a fact that is important in the visual observation of skin movement over the breast during breast self-examination. A nipple is located near the tip of the breast at about the level of the fourth intercostal space and is surrounded by an area of pigmented skin called the *areola* (Fig. 40-18). The areola contains sebaceous glands and modified sweat glands (glands of Montgomery). These glands have a structure intermediate between sweat glands and true mammary glands, and produce small elevations at the surface of the areola.

The breast mass is supported by the fascia of the pectoralis major and minor muscles and by the fibrous connective tissue of the breast. Fibrous tissue ligaments, called *Cooper ligaments*, extend from the outer boundaries of the breast to the nipple area in a radial manner, like the spokes on a wheel (see Fig. 40-17). These ligaments further support the breast and form septa that divide the breast into 15 to 20 lobes. Each lobe consists of grapelike clusters of glands (alveolar glands) and a duct (lactiferous duct) that lead to the nipple and opens to the outside (see Fig. 40-18). Two epithelial cell types line the

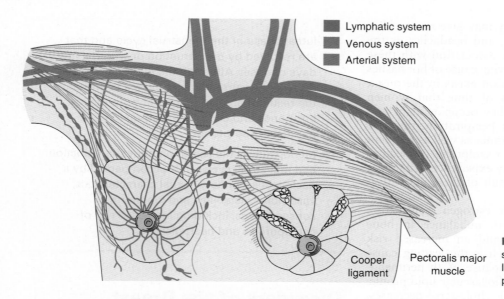

Lymphatic system
Venous system
Arterial system

FIGURE 40-17. The breasts, showing the shared vascular and lymphatic supply as well as the pectoral muscles.

Cooper ligament

Pectoralis major muscle

ducts and alveolar glands of the lobules—myoepithelial and luminal epithelial cells. Contractile epithelial cells, which lie between the surface epithelium and the basement membrane, provide structural support for the lobules, and assist in milk ejection during lactation. The luminal epithelial cells, which are the only cells capable of producing milk, overlie the myoepithelial cells.

The structure of the breast changes with the menstrual cycle and pregnancy. Estrogen stimulates the growth of the ductal system, whereas progesterone stimulates the growth and development of the ductile and glandular secretory epithelium. Early in the menstrual cycle, the ducts appear as cords with little or no lumen. Under estrogen stimulation, at the time of ovulation, the secretory cells increase in size, lumina appear in the ducts as small amounts of secretions accumulate, and fluid collects in the connective tissue. This causes a feeling of breast fullness and discomfort. During pregnancy, placental estrogen and progesterone produce further changes in the mammary glands. Beginning at about the

5th week of pregnancy, the anterior pituitary releases increasing amounts of the hormone *prolactin*. The alveolar glands are lined with secretory cells capable of producing milk under the influence of prolactin. However, milk production does not occur until after birth. This is because placental hormones inhibit milk production. Following childbirth and expulsion of the placenta, the maternal concentration of placental hormones declines rapidly and the action of prolactin is no longer inhibited.

Benign Disorders

Breast disease may be described as benign or cancerous.[56–58] Benign breast conditions are nonmalignant conditions of the breast. They include inflammatory disorders and benign epithelial disorders. Some benign disorders may increase the risk of malignant disease and others may present with signs that resemble malignant disease.

Inflammatory Disorders

Inflammatory diseases of the breast are uncommon, accounting for less than 1% of breast disorders. They include mastitis, mammary duct ectasia, and fat necrosis.

Mastitis. Mastitis is inflammation of the breast.[57,58] It most frequently occurs during lactation but may also result from other disorders. In the lactating woman, inflammation results from an ascending infection that travels from the nipple to the ductal structures. The most common organisms isolated are *Staphylococcus aureus* and *Streptococcus*.[57] The offending organisms often originate from the suckling infant's nasopharynx or the mother's hands. During the early weeks of nursing, the breast is particularly vulnerable to bacterial invasion because of minor cracks and fissures that occur with vigorous suckling. Infection and inflammation cause obstruction of the ductal system. The breast area becomes hard, inflamed, and tender if not treated early. Without treatment, the area becomes walled off and may abscess, requiring incision and drainage. It is

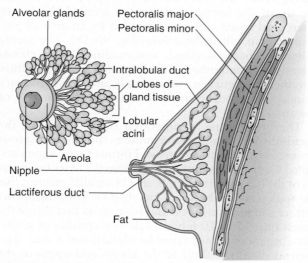

Alveolar glands

Pectoralis major
Pectoralis minor

Intralobular duct
Lobes of gland tissue

Lobular acini

Areola

Nipple

Lactiferous duct

Fat

FIGURE 40-18. The breast, showing the glandular tissue and ducts of the mammary glands.

advisable for the mother to continue breast-feeding during antibiotic therapy to prevent this.

Mastitis is not confined to the postpartum period; it can occur as a result of hormonal fluctuations, tumors, trauma, or skin infection. Cyclic inflammation of the breast occurs most frequently in adolescents, who commonly have fluctuating hormone levels. Tumors may cause mastitis secondary to skin involvement or lymphatic obstruction. Local trauma or infection may develop into mastitis because of ductal blockage of trapped blood, cellular debris, or the extension of superficial inflammation. The treatment for mastitis symptoms may include application of heat or cold, excision, aspiration, mild analgesics, antibiotics, and a supportive brassiere or breast binder.

Mammary Duct Ectasia. Mammary duct ectasia refers to the presence of dilated breast ducts containing a thick pasty material, with accompanying periductal inflammation and fibrosis.[57] The dilated ducts may rupture, resulting in grayish-green nipple discharge. Palpation of the breast increases the discharge. The disorder is usually unilateral, occurring after menopause, most often in elderly multiparous women. Women typically present with a poorly defined perialveolar mass that is often associated with thick, white nipple secretions and sometimes with nipple retraction. Pain and erythema are uncommon. Duct ectasia may be difficult to distinguish clinically from carcinoma and may require biopsy.

Fat Necrosis. Fat necrosis is a distinct clinical and histologic entity, resulting in either a localized or diffuse mass lesion of the breast. The majority of women have a history of trauma, surgery, or radiation therapy.[57,58] Initially the lesion consists of necrotic adipocytes and hemorrhage, after which the inflammatory cells phagocytize the lipid debris. Macrophages may produce a granulomatous inflammatory response. Fibroblast proliferation and collagen deposition during healing may lead to scar tissue (fibrosis). As a result, an irregular fixed hard mass may form that clinically resembles breast cancer. Unlike a malignant mass, however, fat necrosis is typically very tender and has a specific mammographic appearance.

Benign Epithelial Disorders

A wide variety of benign alterations in ducts and lobules are observed in the breast. Most are detected by mammography or as incidental findings on surgical specimens. These lesions have been divided into three groups according to the subsequent risk of developing carcinoma: nonproliferative (fibrocystic) changes, proliferative breast disease without atypia, and proliferative breast disease with atypia.[57]

Nonproliferative (Fibrocystic) Breast Changes. Formerly called *fibrocystic disease*, fibrocystic changes are the most frequent lesions of the breast. They encompass a wide variety of lesions and breast changes. Microscopically, fibrocystic changes refer to a constellation of morphologic changes manifested by (1) cystic dilation of terminal ducts, (2) relative increase in fibrous tissue, and (3) variable proliferation of terminal duct epithelial elements.[57] They are most common in women 30 to 50 years of age and are rare in postmenopausal women not receiving hormone therapy.[56,57]

Fibrocystic changes usually present as nodular (i.e., "shotty"), granular breast masses that are more prominent and painful during the luteal or progesterone-dominant portion of the menstrual cycle. Discomfort ranges from heaviness to exquisite tenderness, depending on the degree of vascular engorgement and cystic distention.

Although fibrocystic changes have been thought to increase the risk of breast cancer, only certain variants in which proliferation of the epithelial components is demonstrated represent a true risk. Fibrocystic changes with giant cysts and proliferative epithelial lesions with atypia are more common in women who are at increased risk for development of breast cancer. The nonproliferative form of fibrocystic changes that does not carry an increased risk for development of cancer is more common.

Diagnosis of fibrocystic changes is made by physical examination, mammography, ultrasonography, and biopsy (i.e., aspiration or tissue sample). Mammography may be helpful in establishing the diagnosis, but increased breast tissue density in women with fibrocystic changes may make an abnormal or cancerous mass difficult to discern among the other structures. Ultrasonography is useful in differentiating a cystic from a solid mass. Because a mass caused by fibrocystic changes may be indistinguishable from carcinoma on the basis of clinical findings, suspect lesions should undergo biopsy. Any discrete mass or lump on the breast should be viewed as possible carcinoma, and cancer should be excluded before instituting the conservative measures used to treat fibrocystic changes.

Treatment for fibrocystic changes is usually symptomatic. Mild analgesics (e.g., aspirin, acetaminophen, or NSAIDs), vitamin E, and local application of heat or cold may be used for pain relief. Prominent or persistent cysts may be aspirated and any fluid obtained sent to the laboratory for cytologic analysis. Women should be encouraged to wear a good supporting brassiere, and are advised to avoid foods that contain xanthines (e.g., coffee, cola, chocolate, and tea) in their daily diets, particularly premenstrually.

Proliferative Lesions without Atypia. Proliferative lesions without atypia, which are commonly detected as mammographic densities or calcifications, include epithelial hyperplasia, sclerosing adenosis, and intraductal papillomas.[57] These lesions are characterized by proliferation of ductile or lobular epithelial cells and/or are stromal without the cytologic or structural changes suggestive of carcinoma in situ. If there is increased fibrosis within the lobule with distortion and compression of the epithelium, the lesion is termed *sclerosing adenosis*. Papillomas are intraductal growths composed of multiple fibrovascular cores, each having a connective tissue axis lined with epithelial cells.[57] Solitary *intraductal papillomas* are found in the major lactiferous ducts of women, typically between the ages of 30 and 50 years. The papillomas, which can range in size from 2 mm to 5 cm, often present with serous or serosanguineous drainage.

Proliferative Lesions with Atypia. Proliferative disease with atypia includes atypical ductile hyperplasia and atypical lobular hyperplasia.[57] The hyperplasia is accompanied by replacement of the normal epithelial cells lining the ducts or lobules with atypical cells resembling those of carcinoma in situ. The basement membrane remains intact and, therefore, the cells cannot metastasize.

There are two types of atypical hyperplasia: lobular and ductile.[57] Atypical ductile hyperplasia is recognized by its histologic resemblance to ductile carcinoma in situ (DCIS). Atypical lobular hyperplasia is defined by proliferation of cells identical to those of lobular carcinoma in situ (LCIS), but the cells do not fill or distend more than 50% of the acini within the lobule. Management of LCIS consists of excisional biopsy. Women with DCIS are at increased risk for developing invasive cancer or recurrence of the DCIS lesion. For this reason, DCIS is evaluated with core-needle biopsy (to be discussed) followed by surgical biopsy or excision. Women with both types of lesions require careful follow-up to prevent and detect the presence of invasive cancer.

Breast Cancer

Cancer of the breast is the most common female cancer. Although the breast cancer mortality rate has shown a slight decline, it is second only to lung cancer as a cause of cancer-related deaths in women. The decline in the breast cancer mortality is due to a number of factors, especially improvements in screening and treatment.

Risk factors for breast cancer include increasing age, personal or family history of breast cancer (i.e., at highest risk are those with multiple affected first-order relatives), history of benign breast disease (i.e., primary "atypical" hyperplasia), and hormonal influences that promote breast maturation and may increase the chance of cell mutation (i.e., early menarche, late menopause, and no term pregnancies or first child after 30 years of age). Modifiable risk factors include obesity (particularly after menopause), physical inactivity, caffeine, moderate to heavy consumption of alcohol, cigarette smoking, and long-term use of postmenopausal hormone therapy (especially combined estrogen and progestin).[57] Most women with breast cancer have no identifiable risk factors.

Approximately 12% of all breast cancers are hereditary. The probability of a hereditary etiology increases with multiple affected first-degree relatives, with women who are affected before 50 years of age, and those who have multiple cancers.[57] Mutations in two breast cancer susceptibility genes—BRCA1 on chromosome 17 and BRCA2 on chromosome 13—may account for most inherited forms of breast cancer (see Chapter 7). BRCA1 is known to be involved in tumor suppression. A woman with known mutations in BRCA1 has a lifetime risk of approximately 57% for breast cancer and approximately 40% for ovarian cancer. BRCA2 is another susceptibility gene that elevates lifetime breast cancer risk to 49% and ovarian cancer risk to 18%.[59,60] Breast cancer risk reduction options

available to known carriers of BRCA1 and BRCA2 mutations include surveillance and surgery. Breast evaluation using MRI, digital mammography, and breast ultrasound give the best sensitivity for detecting breast cancer. Prophylactic surgery, in the form of bilateral mastectomy, bilateral oophorectomy, or both, has been shown to decrease the risk of developing cancer. These controversial surgeries can have physical and psychological side effects that warrant careful consideration before proceeding.

Detection

Cancer of the breast may manifest clinically as a mass, a puckering, nipple retraction, or unusual discharge. Many cancers are found by women themselves—sometimes when only a thickening or subtle change in breast contour is noticed. The variety of symptoms and potential for self-discovery underscore the need for all women to have an awareness of what their normal breast appearance and texture are like.

Mammography is the only effective screening technique for the early detection of clinically inapparent breast lesions. A generally slow-growing form of cancer, breast cancer may have been present for 2 to 9 years before it reaches 1 cm, the smallest mass normally detected by palpation. Mammography can disclose lesions as small as 1 mm and the clustering of calcifications that may warrant biopsy to exclude cancer.

In 2003, the American Cancer Society dropped its recommendation that all women perform regular, systematic breast self-examination (BSE). Research has indicated that most women who discover their own cancer do so at times other than scheduled BSE. The American Cancer Society screening guidelines now place primary emphasis for breast cancer diagnosis on clinical breast examination (CBE) by a trained health professional and mammography, while encouraging women in the area of self-awarenenss.[21] Between the ages of 20 and 39 years, average risk women should undergo CBE every 3 years, and after age 40 years CBE should take place annually, ideally prior to the woman's annual mammogram.[21] There is no specific upper age at which mammogram should be discontinued. Instead it is suggested that decision to stop mammogram screening should be individualized based on the potential risks and benefits. As long as the woman is in good health and would be a candidate for cancer treatment, it is recommended that she continue to be screened with mammography.[21]

Diagnosis and Classification

Procedures used in the diagnosis of breast cancer include physical examination, mammography, ultrasonography, percutaneous needle aspiration, stereotactic needle biopsy (i.e., core biopsy), and excisional biopsy. Figure 40-19 illustrates the appearance of breast cancer on mammography. Breast cancer often manifests as a solitary, painless, firm, fixed lesion with poorly defined borders. It can be found anywhere in the breast but is most common in the upper outer quadrant. Because of the variability in presentation, any suspect change in breast tissue warrants further investigation. The diagnostic

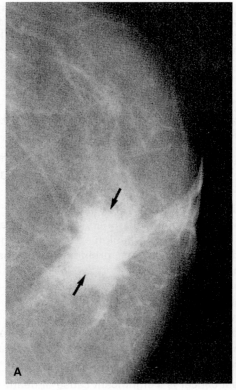
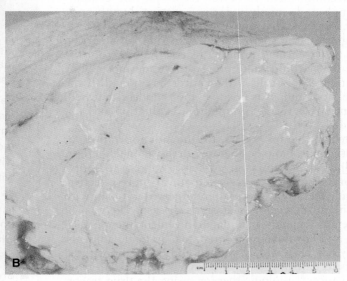

FIGURE 40-19. Carcinoma of the breast. **(A)** Mammogram. An irregularly shaped, dense mass (*arrows*) is seen in this otherwise fatty breast. **(B)** Mastectomy specimen. The irregular white, firm mass in the center is surrounded by fatty tissue. (From Thor AD, Osunkoya AO. The breast. In: Rubin R, Strayer DS, eds. *Rubin's Pathology: Clinicopathologic Foundations of Medicine.* 5th ed. Philadelphia, PA: Wolters Kluwer Health | Lippincott Williams & Wilkins; 2008:851.)

use of mammography enables additional definition of the clinically suspect area (e.g., appearance, character, calcification). Placement of a wire marker under radiographic guidance can ensure accurate surgical biopsy of nonpalpable suspect areas. Ultrasonography is useful as a diagnostic adjunct to differentiate cystic from solid tissue in women with nonspecific thickening.

Fine needle aspiration is a simple in-office procedure that can be performed repeatedly in multiple sites and with minimal discomfort. It can be accomplished by stabilizing a palpable mass between two fingers or in conjunction with handheld sonography to define cystic masses or fibrocystic changes and to provide specimens for cytologic examination. Fine needle aspiration can identify the presence of malignant cells, but it cannot differentiate in situ from infiltrating cancers. Stereotactic needle biopsy is an outpatient procedure done with the guidance of a mammography machine. After the lesion is localized radiologically, a large-bore needle is mechanically thrust quickly into the area, removing a core of tissue. Cells are available for histologic evaluation with 96% accuracy in detecting cancer. This procedure is less costly than excisional biopsy. Excisional biopsy to remove the entire lump provides the only definitive diagnosis of breast cancer, and often is therapeutic without additional surgery. Magnetic resonance imaging, positron emission tomography (PET), and computer-based or digital mammography are available as additional diagnostic modalities for breast cancer,

and may be recommended to supplement conventional mammography in women with radiographically dense breasts or a strong family history of cancer, or who are known carriers of *BRCA1* or *BRCA2*.[58]

Tumors are classified histologically according to tissue characteristics and staged clinically according to tumor size, nodal involvement, and presence of metastasis. It is recommended that estrogen and progesterone receptor analysis be performed on surgical specimens. Information about the presence or absence of estrogen and progesterone receptors can be used in predicting tumor responsiveness to hormonal manipulation. High levels of both receptors improve the prognosis and increase the likelihood of remission.

Treatment

The treatment methods for breast cancer include surgery, chemotherapy, radiation therapy, and hormonal manipulation. Radical mastectomy (i.e., removal of the entire breast, underlying muscles, and all axillary nodes) rarely is used today as a primary surgical therapy unless breast cancer is advanced at the time of diagnosis.[61,62] Modified surgical techniques (i.e., mastectomy plus axillary dissection or lumpectomy for breast conservation) accompanied by chemotherapy or radiation therapy have achieved outcomes comparable with those obtained with radical surgical methods and constitute the preferred treatment methods.

The prognosis for women with breast cancer is related more to the extent of nodal involvement than to the extent of breast involvement. Greater nodal involvement requires more aggressive postsurgical treatment, and many cancer specialists believe that a diagnosis of breast cancer is not complete until dissection and testing of the axillary lymph nodes have been accomplished. A newer technique for evaluating lymph node involvement is a sentinel lymph node biopsy. A radioactive substance or dye is injected into the region of the tumor. In theory, the dye is carried to the first (sentinel) node to receive lymph from the tumor. This would therefore be the node most likely to contain cancer cells if the cancer has spread. If the sentinel node biopsy is positive, more nodes are tested. If it is negative, further lymph node evaluation may not be needed.

Systemic therapy refers to the administration of chemotherapy, biologic therapy, or hormonal therapy. Neoadjuvant therapy is given before surgery to shrink the tumor and make surgical removal more effective. Adjuvant therapy is given after surgery to women with and without detectable metastatic disease. The goal of this therapy depends on nodal involvement, menopausal status, and hormone receptor status. Systemic adjuvant therapy has been widely studied and has demonstrated benefits in reducing rates of recurrence and death from breast cancer.[61] Biologic therapy, using the drug trastuzumab (Herceptin), is used to stop the growth of breast tumors that express the HER2/neu receptor on their cell surface. The HER2/neu receptor binds an epidermal growth factor that contributes to cancer cell growth.[63] Trastuzumab is a recombinant DNA-derived monoclonal antibody that binds to the HER2/neu receptor, thereby inhibiting proliferation of tumor cells that overexpress the receptor gene.[63]

Hormone therapy is used to block the effects of estrogen on the growth of breast cancer cells. Tamoxifen is a nonsteroidal antiestrogen that binds to estrogen receptors and blocks the effects of estrogens on the growth of malignant cells in the breast. Studies have shown decreased cancer recurrence, decreased mortality rates, and increased 5-year survival rates in women with estrogen receptor–positive tissue samples who have been treated with the drug. Aromatase inhibitors block the enzyme that converts androstenedione and testosterone to estrogen in the peripheral tissues. This reduces the circulating estrogen levels in postmenopausal women and is becoming the most effective adjuvant therapy for women with early-stage breast cancer.[64] Autologous bone marrow transplantation and peripheral stem cell transplantation are experimental therapies that may be used for treatment of advanced disease or in women at increased risk for recurrence.

Paget Disease

Paget disease accounts for 1% of all breast cancers.[57,58] The disease presents as an eczematoid lesion of the nipple and areola. Paget disease usually is associated with an infiltrating, intraductal carcinoma. When the lesion is limited to the nipple only, the rate of axillary metastasis is approximately 5%. Complete examination is required and includes a mammogram and biopsy. Treatment depends on the extent of spread.

SUMMARY CONCEPTS

- The breast contains alveolar glands and ducts that are lined with epithelial tissue that may give rise to benign and malignant lesions.

- Benign conditions include inflammatory disorders (mastitis, mammary duct dysplasia, and fat necrosis) and benign epithelial lesions (nonproliferative lesions, proliferative lesions without atypia, and proliferative lesions with atypia). Some benign conditions, such as proliferative lesions, may predispose to malignant disease, and others, such as fibrocystic changes and fat necrosis, may present with a mass and signs that resemble malignant disease.

- Breast cancer is a significant cause of death for women. Some inherited breast cancers are associated with mutations in breast cancer genes *BRCA1* and *BRCA2*. The combination of clinical breast exam and mammography afford women the best opportunity for detection of breast cancer which allows for earlier treatment and improved outcomes. The choice of treatment, which includes surgical resection, radiation, and chemotherapy, depends on the stage of the disease.

REVIEW EXERCISES

1. Most oral contraceptive agents use low doses of estrogen and progestin to prevent conception.

   A. Use Figures 40-5 and 40-6 to explain how these oral agents prevent ovulation and pregnancy.

2. A 32-year-old woman has been told that the report of her annual Pap test revealed the presence of mild cervical dysplasia.

   A. What questions should this woman ask to become informed about the significance of these findings?
   B. Cervical cancer is often referred to as a sexually transmitted disease. Explain.
   C. What type of follow-up care would be indicated?

3. A 30-year-old woman consults her gynecologist because of amenorrhea and inability to become pregnant. Physical examination reveals an obese woman with hirsutism. The physician tells her that she might have a condition known as *polycystic ovary syndrome* and that further laboratory tests are indicated.

A. Among tests ordered were a fasting blood glucose and serum LH, FSH, and dehydroepiandrosterone levels. What information can these tests provide that would help in establishing a diagnosis of polycystic ovary syndrome?

B. What is the probable cause of this woman's amenorrhea, hirsutism, and failure to become pregnant?

C. What type of treatment might be used to help this woman become pregnant?

4. A 45-year-old woman makes an appointment to see her physician because of a painless lump in her breast that she has discovered.

A. What tests should be done to confirm the presence or absence of breast cancer?

B. During the removal of breast cancer, a sentinel node biopsy is often done to determine whether the cancer has spread to the lymph nodes. Explain how this procedure is done and its value in determining lymph node spread.

C. After surgical removal of breast cancer, tamoxifen may be used as an adjuvant systemic therapy for women without detectable metastatic disease. The presence or absence of estrogen receptors in the cytoplasm of tumor cells is important in determining the selection of an agent for use in adjuvant therapy. Explain.

REFERENCES

1. Moore KL, Aqur AM, Dalley AF. *Clinically Oriented Anatomy.* 7th ed. Philadelphia, PA: Wolters Kluwer Health/Lippincott Williams & Wilkins; 2014: 98–108, 382–417.

2. Ross MH, Pawlina W. *Histology: A Text and Atlas.* 6th ed. Philadelphia, PA: Wolters Kluwer Health/Lippincott Williams & Wilkins; 2011:830–894.

3. Hall JE. *Guyton & Hall Textbook of Medical Physiology.* 12th ed. Philadelphia, PA: Elsevier Saunders; 2010:987–1005.

4. Rosen MP, Cedars MI. Female reproductive endocrinology and infertility. In: Gardner DG, Shoback D, eds. *Greenspan's Basic & Clinical Endocrinology.* 9th ed. New York, NY: Lange Medical Books/McGraw-Hill Medical; 2011:423–475.

5. Gruber CJ, Tschugguel W, Huber J. Production and actions of estrogens. *N Engl J Med.* 2002;346:340–350.

6. Ellenson LH, Pirog EC. The female genital tract. In: Kumar V, Abbas AK, Fausto N, et al., eds. *Robbins and Cotran Pathologic Basis of Disease.* 8th ed. Philadelphia, PA: Saunders Elsevier; 2010:1005–1063.

7. Mutter GL, Prat J, Schwartz DA. The female reproductive system. In: Rubin R, Strayer DA, eds. *Rubin's Pathology: Clinicopathologic Foundation of Medicine.* 6th ed. Philadelphia, PA: Wolters Kluwer Health/Lippincott Williams & Wilkins; 2012:847–923.

8. Kushnir VA, Mosquera C. Novel technique for management of Bartholin gland cysts and abscesses. *J Emerg Med.* 2009;36(4):388–390.

9. Burrows L, Goldstein G, Mowad G, et al. Vulvar dermatoses as a cause of dyspareunia. In: Goldstein A, Pukall C, Goldstein I, eds. *Female Sexual Pain Disorders.* 1st ed. Hoboken, NJ: Wiley-Blackwell; 2009:49–57, 112–116.

10. Ellas JC, Berek JS. Vulvar cancer: staging, treatment, and prognosis. May 8, 2013. Available at: http://www.uptodate.com/contents/vulvar-cancer-staging-treatment-and-prognosis. Accessed July, 10, 2013.

11. Carter JS, Downs LS. Vulvar and vaginal cancer. *Obstet Gynecol Clin North Am.* 2012;213–231.

12. Andrews JC. Vulvodynia interventions—systematic review and evidence grading. *Obstet Gynecol Surv.* 2011;66(5):299–315.

13. Groysman V. Vulvodynia: new concepts and review of the literature. *Dermatol Clin.* 2010;28:681–696.

14. Cox KJ, Neville CE. Assessment and management options for women with vulvodynia. *J Midwifery Womens Health.* 2012; 57(3):231–240.

15. Sobel J. Approach to women with symptoms of vaginitis. May 16, 2013. Available at: http://www.uptodate.com/contents/approach-to-women-with-symptoms-of-vaginitis. Accessed July 10, 2013.

16. Hainer BL, Gibson MV. Vaginitis: diagnosis and treatment. *Am Fam Physician.* 2011;83(7):807–815.

17. American Cancer Society. *Detailed Guide: Vaginal Cancer.* 2013. Available at: http://www.cancer.org/cancer/vaginalcancer/detailedguide/. Accessed July 10, 2013.

18. American Cancer Society. *Detailed Guide: Cervical Cancer.* 2013. Available at: http://www.cancer.org/cancer/cervicalcancer/detailedguide/. Accessed July 10, 2013.

19. Centers for Disease Control and Prevention Advisory Committee on Immunization Practices (ACIP). Recommendations on the use of quadrivalent human papillomavirus vaccine in males. *Morb Mortal Wkly Rep.* 2011;60(50):1705–1708.

20. Centers for Disease Control and Prevention. FDA licensure of bivalent human papillomavirus vaccine (HPV$_2$ Cerarix) for use in females and Updated Vaccination Recommendations from Advisory Committee on Immunization Practices (ACIP). *MMWR Morb Mortal Wkly Rep.* 2010;59(20):626–629.

21. Smith RA, Brooks D, Cokkindes V, et al. Cancer screening in the United States, 2013. *CA Cancer J Clin.* 2013;63:87–105.

22. U.S. Preventive Services Task Force. Screening for cervical cancer. 2012. Available at: http://www.uspreventiveservicestaskforce.org/uspstf/uspscerv.htm. Accessed July 23, 2013.

23. American College of Obstetricians and Gynecologists. *Screening for Cervical Cancer.* ACOG Practice Bulletin No. 131. Available at: http://www.acog.org. 2012. Accessed July 16, 2013.

24. Massad LS, et al. 2012 updated consensus guidelines for the management of abnormal cervical cancer screening tests and cancer precursors. *J Low Genit Tract Dis.* 2013;17(5):S1–S27.

25. Gradison M. Pelvic inflammatory disease. *Am Fam Physician.* 2012;85(8):791–796.

26. Lareau SM, Beigi RH. Pelvic inflammatory disease and tubo-ovarian abscess. *Infect Dis Clin North Am.* 2008;22:693–708.

27. Workowski KA, Berman S, Centers for Disease Control and Prevention (CDC). Sexually transmitted diseases treatment guidelines. *Morb Mortal Wkly Rep.* 2010;59(RR12):1–110.

28. Bulun SE. Endometriosis. *N Engl J Med.* 2009;360(3):268–279.

29. Schrager S, Fallerone J, Edgoose J. Evaluation and treatment of endometriosis. *Am Fam Physician.* 2013;87(2):1007–1113.

30. Falcone T, Lebovic DI. Clinical management of endometriosis. *Obstet Gynecol.* 2011;118:691–705.

31. Bakkum-Gamez J, Gonzalez-Bosquet J, Laack NN, et al. Current issues in the management of endometrial cancer. *Mayo Clin Proc.* 2008;83(1):97–112.

32. Wright JD, Mendel NIB, Schauli J, et al. Contemporary management of endometrial cancer. *Lancet.* 2012;379:1352–1360.

33. Buchanan EM, Weinstein LC, Hillson C. Endometrial cancer. *Am Fam Physician.* 2009;80(10):1075–1989.

34. DiCristofano A, Ellenson LH. Endometrial carcinoma. *Annu Rev Pathol Mech Dis.* 2007;2:57–85.

35. Evans P, Brunsell S. Uterine fibroid tumors: diagnosis and treatment. *Am Fam Physician.* 2007;75:1503–1508.

36. Lentz GM. Anatomic defects of the abdominal wall and pelvic floor. In: Lentz GM, Lobo RA, Gershenson DM, et al., eds. *Comprehensive Gynecology.* 6th ed. Philadelphia, PA: Elsevier Mosby; 2012:453.e3–477.e3.

37. Azziz R. Diagnostic criteria for polycystic ovary syndrome: a reappraisal. *Fertil Steril.* 2005;83:1343–1346.

38. Goodarzi MO, Dumesic DA, Chazenbath G, et al. (2013). Polycystic ovary syndrome: etiology, pathogenesis and diagnosis. *Nat Rev Endocrinol.* 7:219–231.

39. Ehrmann DA. Polycystic ovary syndrome. *N Engl J Med.* 2005;352:1223–1236.

40. Salmi DJ, Zisser HC, Jovanovic L. Screening for and treatment of polycystic ovary syndrome in teenagers: a mini review. *Exp Biol Med.* 2004;229:369–377.

41. Roett MA, Evans D. Ovarian cancer. *Am Fam Physician.* 2009;80(6):609–616.

42. Chobanian N, Dietrich CS. Ovarian cancer. *Surg Clin North Am.* 2008;88:285–299.

43. Vo C, Carney ME. Ovarian cancer hormonal and environmental risk effect. *Obstet Gynecol Clin North Am.* 2007;34:687–700.

44. Goff BA, Mandel LS, Drescher CW, et al. Development of an ovarian cancer symptom index: possibilities for earlier detection. *Cancer.* 2006;109:221–227.

45. Casablanca Y. Management of dysfunctional uterine bleeding. *Obstet Gynecol Clin North Am.* 2008;35:219–234.

46. Practice Committee of the American Society for Reproductive Medicine. Current evaluation of amenorrhea. *Fertil Steril.* 2006;86(suppl 4):S148–S155.

47. Morrow C, Naumburg E. Dysmenorrhea. *Prim Care Clin Office Pract.* 2009;36:10–32.

48. Minkin MJ, Moore AE. Identifying and managing premenstrual disorders: putting strategies into practice. *Clin Adv.* 2006;(suppl):4–15.

49. Dickerson VM. Premenstrual syndrome and premenstrual dysphoric disorder: individualizing therapy. *Fem Patient.* 2007;32(1):38–46.

50. Biggs WS, Demuth RH. Premenstrual syndrome and premenstrual dysphoric disorder. *Am Fam Physician.* 2011;84(8):918–924.

51. Braverman PK. Premenstrual syndrome and premenstrual dysphoric disorder. *J Pediatr Adolesc Gynecol.* 2007:203–212.

52. Rees M. Management of the menopause: integrated health-care pathway for the menopausal woman. *Menopause Int.* 2011;17(2):50–54.

53. Lyons J. Advice given to women undergoing gynaecological surgery in relation to menopause, symptoms and hormone replacement therapy: could and should we improve the service we provide? *Menopause Int.* 2011;17(2):59–62.

54. North American Menopause Society. The 2012 Hormone Therapy Position Statement of the North American Menopause Society. *Menopause.* 2012;19(3):257–271.

55. Rossouw JE, Manson JE, Kaunitz AM. Lessons learned from the Women's Health Initiative trials of menopausal hormone therapy. *Obstet Gynecol.* 2013;121(1):172–176.

56. Gadducci A; Guerrieri ME, Genazzani AR. Benign breast diseases, contraception and hormone replacement therapy. *Minerva Ginecol.* 2012;64(1):67–74.

57. Lester SC. The breast. In: Kumar V, Abbas AK, Fausto N, et al., eds. *Robbins and Cotran Pathologic Basis of Disease.* 8th ed. Philadelphia, PA: Saunders Elsevier; 2010:1065–1095.

58. Mulligan AM, O'Malley FP. The breast. In: Rubin R, Strayer DS, eds. *Rubin's Pathology: Clinicopathologic Foundations of Medicine.* 6th ed. Philadelphia, PA: Wolters Kluwer Health/ Lippincott Williams & Wilkins; 2012:923–945.

59. Barbieri, R. What is the gynecologist's role in the care of BRCA previvors? *OBG Manage.* 2013;25(9):10–14.

60. Hamilton R. Genetics: breast cancer as an exemplar. *Nurs Clin North Am.* 2009;44(3):327–338.

61. Maughan KL, Lutterbie MA, Ham PS. Treatment of breast cancer. *Am Fam Physician.* 2009;81(1):1339–1346.

62. American Cancer Society. Detailed guide: breast cancer. 2013. Available at: http://www.cancer.org/acs/groups/cid/documents. Accessed July 10, 2013.

63. Denkert, C, Huober J, Loibl S, et al. HER2 and ESR1 mRNA expression levels and response to neoadjuvant trastuzumab plus chemotherapy in patients with primary breast cancer. *Breast Cancer Res.* 2013;15(1):R11.

64. Lønning PE. The potency and clinical efficacy of aromatase inhibitors across the breast cancer continuum. *Ann Oncol.* 2011;22(3):503–514.

Porth Essentials Resources

Explore these additional resources to enhance learning for this chapter:

* NCLEX-Style Questions and Other Resources on thePoint, http://thePoint.lww.com/PorthEssentials4e
* Study Guide for Essentials of Pathophysiology
* Adaptive Learning | Powered by PrepU, http://thepoint.lww.com/prepu

C h a p t e r 41

Sexually Transmitted Infections

Sexually transmitted infections (STIs) encompass a broad range of infectious diseases that are spread by sexual contact.[1,2] Although the incidence of syphilis and gonorrhea as reported in the professional literature and public health statistics has decreased slightly, the incidence of other STIs is increasing. The actual figures are probably much higher than those reported because many STIs are not reportable or not reported. The agents of infection include bacteria, viruses, fungi, and other microorganisms (see Chapter 14). The initial site of an STI may be the urethra, genitalia, rectum, or oral pharynx. The organisms that cause these infections tend to be short lived outside the host, so they usually depend on person-to-person spread. The rates of many STIs are highest among adolescents; more common in persons who have more than one sexual partner; and it is not uncommon for a person to be concurrently infected with more than one type of STI.

Many factors contribute to the increased prevalence and the continued spread of STIs, including the fact that STIs are frequently asymptomatic, which promotes the spread of infection by persons who are unaware that they are carrying the infection. Furthermore, partners of infected persons are often difficult to notify and treat. Condoms could prevent the spread of many STIs, but they often are not used or are used improperly. In addition, there currently are no cures for viral STIs (e.g., human immunodeficiency virus [HIV], herpes simplex virus, and human papilloma virus [HPV]); although there are drugs available that may help to manage the infections, they do not entirely control the spread. Also, drug-resistant microorganisms are rapidly emerging, making treatment of many STIs more difficult.

This chapter discusses the manifestations of STIs in men and women in terms of infections of the external genitalia, vaginal infections, and infections that have genitourinary as well as systemic manifestations. HIV infection is presented in Chapter 16.

Infections of the External Genitalia

Sexually transmitted infections can selectively infect the mucocutaneous tissues of the external genitalia, rectum, and oral pharynx, or produce both genitourinary and systemic effects. These infections include condylomata acuminata, genital herpes, chancroid, and lymphogranuloma venereum.

Human Papillomavirus Infection and Genital Warts

Genital warts (condylomata acuminata) are caused by the human papillomavirus (HPV) that infects epithelial cells and can cause a number of benign and malignant growths.[2–8] Although recognized for centuries, HPV-induced genital warts have become one of the fastest-growing STIs of the past decade. The Centers for Disease Control and Prevention (CDC) estimates that 360,000 million Americans are currently infected with the HPV.[3]

Etiology and Pathogenesis

Transmission of HPV is usually through skin-to-skin contact, most often through penetration (oral–genital, manual–genital, and genital–genital contact). HPV can also be transmitted though nonsexual routes including mother to newborn (vertical transmission) and fomites (objects such as clothing, towels, or utensils that harbor the agent). Prevention of HPV transmission through condom use has not been adequately demonstrated. Most HPV infections are asymptomatic and transient, and resolve without treatment. In some cases, however, HPV infection results in genital warts, abnormal Papanicolaou (Pap) test abnormalities, or, rarely, cervical cancer.

Human papillomaviruses are nonenveloped double-stranded deoxyribonucleic acid (DNA) viruses that cause proliferative lesions of the squamous epithelium.[1,2] Human papillomavirus is species specific, meaning it only affects humans.[2] More than 100 distinct HPV subtypes have been identified, over 40 of which affect the anogenital area.[2–6] These subtypes are routinely classified into low-risk and high-risk categories. Low-risk types such as HPV 6 and 11 are typically associated with genital warts. Types 16, 18, 31, 33, and 45 are considered to be high risk because of their association with cervical dysplasia and cervical cancer. Of the high-risk types, HPV 16 and 18 account for approximately two thirds of cervical cancer.[2] Only a subset of women infected with HPV go on to develop cervical cancer, however, suggesting that even the most virulent HPV strains may vary in terms of their oncogenic potential. Cofactors that may increase the risk for cancer include smoking, immunosuppression, and exposure to hormonal alteration (e.g., pregnancy, oral contraceptives).[2]

Human papillomavirus infection begins with viral inoculation into squamous epithelial cells, where infection stimulates replication of the squamous epithelium, producing the various HPV-proliferative lesions.[5] The incubation period for HPV-induced genital warts ranges from 6 weeks to 8 months, with a mean of 2 to 3 months. Genital warts typically present as soft, raised, fleshy lesions on the external genitalia, including the penis (Fig. 41-1), vulva, scrotum, perineum, and perianal skin. External warts may appear as small bumps, or they may be flat, rough surfaced, or pedunculated. Less commonly, they can appear as smooth reddish or brown raised papules or as dome-shaped lesions on keratinized skin. Internal warts are cauliflower-shaped lesions that affect the mucous membranes of the vagina, urethra, anus, or mouth. They may cause discomfort, bleeding, or painful intercourse.[6]

Although warts can be a disturbing clinical feature of HPV infection, subclinical infection is common. Approximately 70% of women with HPV become HPV DNA negative within 1 year, and as many as 91% of them become negative within 2 years.[1] Many women with transient HPV infections develop atypical squamous cells of undetermined significance (ASC-US) or low-grade squamous intraepithelial lesions (LSILs) of the cervix as detected on a Pap test, colposcopy, or biopsy (see Chapter 40). In men, transient HPV infection may be associated with intraepithelial neoplasia of the penis and anus.[1] Although many individuals will clear the virus and become negative within 1 to 2 years, it is unclear if development of an effective immune response completely clears the infection. In some individuals the virus may remain dormant for years and reactivate at a later time. While some of these later lesions may be reactivations, others may be re-infections from an affected partner.

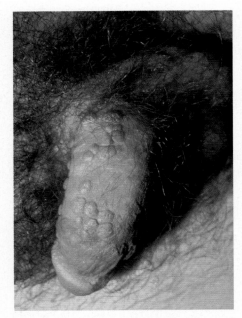

FIGURE 41-1. Condylomata of the penis. Raised circumscribed lesions are seen on the shaft of the penis. (From Damjanov I, McCue PA. The lower urinary tract and male reproductive system. In: Rubin R, Strayer DS, eds. *Rubin's Pathology: Clinicopathologic Foundations of Medicine.* 6th ed. Philadelphia, PA: Wolters Kluwer Health | Lippincott Williams & Wilkins; 2012:825.)

Diagnosis and Treatment

Diagnosis of genital warts is usually made by visualization or palpation of nontender papillomatous genital lesions. A diagnosis of genital warts may be confirmed by biopsy. There are no approved serologic tests for HPV or routine methods for culturing the virus.[7] As HPV infection is confined to the epithelium and cells are shed, the infection results in a minimal immune response and not all those infected produce antibodies to the virus that are detected using serology tests. HPV tests are available for women older than 30 years of age who are undergoing cervical cancer screening. These tests detect HPV nuclear DNA, ribonucleic acid (RNA), or capsid proteins. Four tests have been approved by the Food and Drug Administration (FDA), two of which indicate the presence of one or more high-risk HPV types, and two which provide individual detection of HPV 16 and 18.[7] None of these tests have been approved for use in men, for women older than 20 years of age, or as a general test for STIs.

The choice of treatment for genital warts is based on the number, size, site, and morphology of the lesions, as well the person's preference. If left untreated, the warts may resolve spontaneously, so expectant management is acceptable if the person is comfortable with this approach. Evaluation and treatment of sexual partners may be suggested, although this may be difficult considering that warts often do not become clinically apparent for several years after exposure.

Treatment regimens can be classified as patient-applied or provider-applied. Patient-applied products include cytoxic agents (podofilox [5%]), an immune enhancer (imiquimod), or a green tea extract (sinecatechin).[4–6] Podofilox is a topical antimitotic agent that results in visible necrosis of wart tissue. The safety of podofilox during pregnancy has not been established. Imiquimod stimulates the body's immune system (i.e., production of interferon-α and other cytokines). Imiquimod is a category B drug and therefore potentially safe for use in pregnancy. Sinecatechins are thought to destroy wart tissue by inducing cell cycle arrest and apoptosisis.[5] The safety of sinecatechins during pregnancy has not been established.[6]

Provider-administered treatments include podophyllin resin [10% or 25%], trichloroacetic acid (TCA), or bichloracetic acid (BCA). Podophyllin resin is a topical cytotoxic agent that has long been used for treatment of visible external growths. Multiple applications may be required for resolution of lesions. The amount of drug used and the surface area treated should be limited with each treatment session to avoid systemic absorption and toxicity. This treatment is contraindicated in pregnancy for the same reason. An alternative therapy involves the topical application of a solution of TCA or BCA. These weak destructive agents produce an initial burning in the affected area, followed in several days by a sloughing of the superficial tissue. Several applications at 1- to 2-week intervals may be necessary to eradicate the lesion. Sexual abstinence is suggested during any type of treatment to enhance healing.

Genital warts also may be removed using cryotherapy (i.e., freezing therapy) with liquid nitrogen or a cyroprobe, laser vaporization, electrocautery, or surgical excision.[4] Cryotherapy and BCA or TCA are the recommended treatments for cervical HPV lesions. Laser surgery can be used to remove large or widespread lesions of the cervix, vagina, or vulva, or lesions that have failed to respond to other first-line methods of treatment. Electrocautery treatment has become more widespread for these types of lesions because it does not require suturing and is beneficial for persons who have a large number of warts.[4]

Vaccination is currently regarded as one of the most effective strategies for controlling HPV-related diseases. Two vaccines are available to protect females against the type of HPV that causes cervical cancer—a quadrivalent vaccine (Gardasil) that protects against HPV types 6, 11, 16, and 18.[8] and a bivalent vaccine (Cevarix) that protects against HPV types 16 and 18.[7] The quadrivalent (Gardasil) vaccine can be given to males for protection from genital warts.[8] There is no treatment, however, to eradicate the virus once a person has become infected.

Genital Herpes

Genital herpes is a common cause of genital ulcers, affecting more than 50 million people in the United States.[1,2] Because herpesvirus infection is not reportable in all states, reliable data on its true incidence and prevalence are lacking.

Etiology and Pathogenesis

Genital herpes is caused by the herpes simplex virus (HSV), a large double-stranded DNA virus.[9–13] Herpes simplex infections are highly contagious. There are eight types of HSV; however, only two are considered sexually transmitted. These are HSV-1 (usually associated with fever blisters and cold sores) and HSV-2 (usually associated with genital herpes).[13] HSV-1 and HSV-2 are genetically similar; both cause a similar set of primary and recurrent infections; and both can cause oropharyngeal and genital lesions, but HSV-2 is most commonly found only in the genitals.[12]

HSV-1 and HSV-2 are *neurotropic* viruses, meaning that they grow in neurons and share the biologic property of latency.[9] Latency refers to the ability to maintain disease potential in the absence of clinical signs and symptoms. In genital herpes, the virus ascends through the peripheral nerves to the sacral dorsal root ganglia (Fig. 41-2). The virus can remain dormant in the dorsal root ganglia, or it can reactivate, in which case the viral particles are transported back down the nerve root to the skin, where they multiply and cause a lesion to develop. During the dormant or latent period, the virus replicates in a different manner so that the immune system or available treatments have no effect on it. It is not known what reactivates the virus. It may be that the body's defense mechanisms are altered. Numerous studies have shown that host responses to infection influence initial development of the disease, severity of

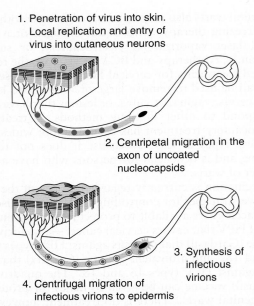

1. Penetration of virus into skin. Local replication and entry of virus into cutaneous neurons

2. Centripetal migration in the axon of uncoated nucleocapsids

3. Synthesis of infectious virions

4. Centrifugal migration of infectious virions to epidermis

FIGURE 41-2. Pathogenesis of primary mucocutaneous herpes simplex virus infection. (From Corey L, Spear PG. Infections with herpes simplex viruses: Part 1. *N Engl J Med.* 1986;314:686.)

infection, development and maintenance of latency, and frequency of HSV recurrences.

Herpes simplex virus is transmitted by contact with infectious lesions, but may also be transmitted when no symptoms or lesions are present. Although most HSV genital infections were once caused by HSV-2, it is now increasingly common for infections to be caused by both HSV-1 and HSV-2, particularly among adolescents and young women.[12] Persons infected with HSV-1 remain at risk for acquiring HSV-2. Most cases of HSV-2 infection are subclinical, manifesting as asymptomatic or symptomatic but unrecognized infections. These subclinical infections can occur in people who have never had a symptomatic outbreak or they can occur between recognized clinical recurrences. Up to 70% of genital herpes is spread through asymptomatic shedding by people who do not realize they have the infection.[11,12] This "unknown" transmission of the virus to sex partners explains why this infection has reached epidemic proportions throughout the world.[12]

The incubation period for HSV is 2 to 12 days.[11] Genital HSV infection may manifest as a first-episode or recurrent infection. The initial symptoms of primary genital herpes infections include tingling, itching, and pain in the genital area, followed by eruption of small pustules and vesicles. These lesions rupture on approximately the 5th day to form wet ulcers that are excruciatingly painful to touch and can be associated with dysuria, dyspareunia, and urine retention. This period is followed by a 10- to 12-day interval during which the lesions crust over and gradually heal. Involvement of the cervix, vagina, urethra, and inguinal lymph nodes is common in women with primary infections. In men, the infection can cause urethritis and lesions of the penis and scrotum. Rectal and perianal infections are possible with anal contact. Systemic symptoms associated with

primary infections include fever, headache, malaise, muscle ache, and lymphadenopathy. Primary infections may be debilitating enough to require hospitalization, particularly in women. First episodes of nonprimary infections (acquisition of HSV-2 in persons with preexisting antibodies to HSV-1 or, more rarely, acquisition of HSV-1 in persons with preexisting HSV-2 antibodies) are associated with fewer lesions, a shorter duration of disease, and a lower rate of complications than primary infections.

Recurrent HSV episodes are usually milder than the initial episode—there typically are fewer lesions, and viral shedding occurs at a lower concentration and for a shorter duration (about 3 days). However, the prodromal symptoms of itching, burning, and tingling at the lesion site are similar. Except for the greater tendency of HSV-2 to recur, the clinical manifestations of genital HSV-2 and HSV-1 infections are similar. The frequency and severity of recurrence vary from person to person. Numerous factors, including emotional stress, lack of sleep, overexertion, other infections, vigorous or prolonged coitus, and premenstrual or menstrual distress, have been identified as triggering mechanisms.

Diagnosis and Treatment

Diagnosis of genital herpes is based on symptoms, appearance of the lesions, and identification of the virus taken from the lesions. Viral culture can generally isolate the virus in 5 days, is relatively inexpensive, and is highly specific. However, it is not very sensitive, with false-negative results of 25% with primary infections and as high as 50% with recurrent infections. Polymerase chain reaction (PCR), which can detect single copies of viral DNA by amplifying the DNA many millions of times, has a higher sensitivity and has become the preferred method to confirm a diagnosis of genital HSV infection.[4,11] In addition to identifying the virus from a sample taken from the herpes lesion, detection of type-specific antibodies to HSV-1 and HSV-2 from a blood sample also can help to establish the diagnosis. These tests yield false-negative results when used in the early stages of infection, since it takes approximately 22 days for the body to produce antibodies to the virus.[2] Approximately 20% of patients may remain seronegative for 3 months, particularly if they have received antiviral medications.[2] This type of testing may prove useful in confirming infection in persons with recurrent genital symptoms and negative HSV testing, or in establishing a clinical diagnosis of genital herpes in a partner of a person with genital herpes.[4]

There is no known cure for genital herpes, and the methods of treatment are largely symptomatic. The oral antiviral drugs acyclovir, valacyclovir, and famciclovir have become the cornerstone for management of genital herpes.[2,11] By interfering with viral DNA replication, these drugs decrease the frequency of recurrences, shorten the duration of active lesions, reduce the number of new lesions formed, and decrease viral shedding. Valacyclovir, the active component of acyclovir, and famciclovir have greater bioavailability, which enables improved dosing schedules and increased compliance. Episodic intervention reduces the duration of viral shedding and the healing time for recurrent lesions. For individuals who wish to prevent transmission to a susceptible partner or wish to prevent outbreaks, continuous antiviral suppressive therapy may be advised. These drugs are well tolerated, with few adverse effects. This long-term suppressive therapy does not limit latency, and reactivation of the disease frequently occurs after the drug is discontinued. In 2002, the FDA approved long-term suppressive therapy with valacyclovir and condom use for the prevention of HSV-2 transmission to an uninfected sexual partner. Infection with HSV-2 may predispose an individual to HIV infection and antiviral therapy does not reduce this risk.[4]

Maternal/Neonatal Transmission

Herpes simplex virus may be transmitted from mother to child around the time of delivery causing potentially fatal disease in the newborn.[1,5,14,15] Women who experience their first genital HSV infection in pregnancy are at highest risk of transmitting the disease to their newborn. Disseminated neonatal infection carries high mortality and morbidity rates. Because of the risk involved, many authorities recommend that recently acquired HSV infections in pregnant women be treated with antiviral drugs (e.g., aciclovir or valaciclovir).

Active infection during labor may necessitate cesarean delivery, ideally before membranes rupture, but this is not a guarantee that the infant will not acquire infection. Pregnant women with a known history of HSV-2 infection should be treated with antiviral therapy from 36 weeks until delivery. If there are no active lesions at the time of labor, vaginal delivery is preferred. Neonatal HSV is treated with systemic antiviral therapy.

Chancroid

Chancroid is a disease of the external genitalia and lymph nodes caused by the gram-negative bacterium *Haemophilus ducreyi*.[2,4,11] The disease is most common in tropical and subtropical regions. It is one of the most common causes of genital ulcers in less developed countries, especially in Africa and parts of Asia, where it probably serves as an important cofactor in the transmission of HIV infection.[9] This STI has become uncommon in the United States. However, recent evidence suggests that chancroid may be underdiagnosed because many STI clinics do not have the facilities to test for *H. ducreyi*.

Chancroid is highly infectious and is usually transmitted by sexual intercourse or through skin and mucous membrane abrasions. Autoinoculation may lead to multiple chancres. Lesions begin as macules, progress to pustules, and then rupture. On physical examination, lesions and regional lymphadenopathy (i.e., buboes) may be found. Secondary infection may cause significant tissue destruction.

Diagnosis usually is made clinically, but may be confirmed through culture. Gram stain rarely is used today because it is insensitive and nonspecific. There are no FDA approved PCR tests for *H. ducreyi*.[4] The organism has shown resistance to treatment with sulfamethoxazole alone and to tetracycline.[4]

Lymphogranuloma Venereum

Lymphogranuloma venereum (LGV) is an acute and chronic venereal disease caused by *Chlamydia trachomatis* types L1, L2, and L3. The disease, although found worldwide, has a low incidence outside the tropics. Most cases reported in the United States are in men. There appears to be a new variant of L2 that is causing a resurgence of LGV in Europe and the United States, particularly in men who have sex with men.[4,11]

The lesions of LGV can incubate for a few days to several weeks and thereafter cause small, painless papules or vesicles that may go undetected. An important characteristic of the infection is the early (1 to 4 weeks later) development of large, tender, and sometimes fluctuant inguinal lymph nodes called *buboes*. There may be flulike symptoms with joint pain, rash, weight loss, pneumonitis, tachycardia, splenomegaly, and proctitis. In later stages of the disease, a small percentage of affected persons develop elephantiasis (hypertrophy, edema, and fibrosis of the skin and subcutaneous tissues) of the external genitalia, caused by lymphatic obstruction or fibrous strictures of the rectum or urethra from inflammation and scarring. Urethral involvement may cause pyuria and dysuria. Cervicitis is a common manifestation of primary LGV in women, and could extend to perimetritis or salpingitis, which are known to occur in other chlamydial infections.[4] Anorectal structures may be compromised to the point of incontinence. Complications of LGV may be minor or extensive, involving compromise of whole systems or progression to a cancerous state.

Diagnosis usually is accomplished by a complement fixation test for LGV-specific *Chlamydia* antibodies. High titers for this antibody differentiate this group from other chlamydial subgroups. PCR techniques, when more widely available, will provide a more practical, cost-effective tool for diagnosis.[4] Treatment involves 3 weeks of doxycycline, tetracycline, or erythromycin.[4] Because doxycycline is contraindicated in pregnancy, erythromycin should be used. Surgery may be required to correct sequelae such as strictures or fistulas or to drain fluctuant lymph nodes.

SUMMARY CONCEPTS

■ Sexually transmitted infections (STIs) are spread by sexual contact and involve both male and female partners. Portals of entry include the mouth, genitalia, urinary meatus, rectum, and skin. All STIs are more common in persons who have more than one sexual partner, and it is not uncommon for a person to be concurrently infected with more than one type of STI.

(continued)

Vaginal Infections

Candidiasis, trichomoniasis, and bacterial vaginosis are vaginal infections that can be associated with sexual activity. Trichomoniasis is the only form of vaginitis that is known to be sexually transmitted and requires partner treatment. A male partner usually is asymptomatic.

Candidiasis

Vulvovaginal candidiasis, also referred to as a *yeast infection*, *thrush*, or *moniliasis*, is one of the most frequent reasons that women visit a health care provider. *Candida albicans* is the most commonly identified organism in vaginal yeast infections, but other *Candida* species, such as *Candida glabrata* and *Candida tropicalis*, may also be present.[16–18] These organisms are present in 20% to 55% of healthy women without causing symptoms, and alteration of the host vaginal environment usually is necessary before the organism can cause pathologic effects.[18] Although vulvovaginal candidiasis usually is not transmitted sexually, it is included in the CDC STI treatment guidelines because it often is diagnosed in women being evaluated for STIs. The possibility of sexual transmission has been recognized for many years;

however, candidiasis requires a favorable environment for growth of the organism. Studies have documented the presence of *Candida* on the penis of male partners of women with vulvovaginal candidiasis, but few men develop balanoposthitis that requires treatment.[18] The gastrointestinal tract also serves as a reservoir for this organism, and candidiasis can develop through autoinoculation in women who are not sexually active.

Reported risk factors for the overgrowth of *C. albicans* include recent antibiotic therapy, which suppresses the normal protective bacterial flora; high hormone levels owing to pregnancy or the use of oral contraceptives, which cause an increase in vaginal glycogen stores; and uncontrolled diabetes mellitus, HIV infection, or other diseases, which compromise the immune system.[16–18] Women with vulvovaginal candidiasis commonly complain of vulvovaginal pruritus accompanied by irritation, erythema, swelling, dysuria, and dyspareunia. The characteristic discharge, when present, is usually thick, white, and odorless. In obese persons, *Candida* may grow in skin folds underneath the breast tissue, the abdominal flap, and the inguinal folds.

Accurate diagnosis is made by identification of budding yeast filaments (i.e., hyphae) or spores on a wet-mount slide using 10% potassium hydroxide (Fig. 41-3A). The pH of the discharge, which is checked with litmus paper, typically is less than 4.5. When the wet-mount technique is negative but the clinical manifestations are suggestive of candidiasis, a culture may be necessary.

For treatment purposes, vulvovaginitis is commonly classified as uncomplicated or complicated. Current choice of therapeutic agents is for the most part limited to the azole medications, fungistatic drugs that inhibit cell wall metabolism. Some of these antifungal medications (e.g., clotrimazole, miconazole) are available as topical preparations (creams or suppositories) that can be obtained without a prescription for treatment in women with uncomplicated cases of candidiasis. Topical terconazole and oral fluconazole are also available with prescription. Because of ease of use, oral fluconazole has become a preferred method for most women, but

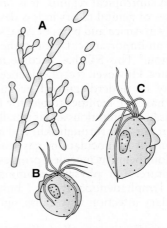

FIGURE 41-3. Organisms that cause vaginal infections. **(A)** *Candida albicans* (blastospores and pseudohyphae); **(B,C)** *Trichomonas vaginalis*.

usually requires a medical appointment to confirm the presence of vaginal candidiasis. Recurrent vulvovaginal candidiasis, defined as four or more mycologically confirmed episodes within 1 year, affects approximately 5% of women and is difficult to manage. Maintenance therapy with oral fluconazole often is required for long-term management of this problem.[16–18]

Trichomoniasis

Trichomoniasis affects an estimated 120 million people in the United States and is the most prevalent nonviral sexually transmitted infection worldwide.[4] *Trichomoniasis vaginalis* infections are commonly associated with other STIs and are therefore a marker for high-risk sexual behavior. Although the infection is commonly transmitted by sexual contact, it can occur via fomites and the organism has been shown to survive in swimming pools and hot tubs.[2]

The manifestations of infection with *T. vaginalis,* the causative agent of trichomoniasis, are primarily observed in women, and range from asymptomatic presentation to a copious, frothy, malodorous green or yellow discharge.[19–21] There often is erythema and edema of the affected mucosa, with occasional itching and irritation. Sometimes, small hemorrhagic punctations, called *strawberry spots*, appear on the cervix. Men can present with urethritis, prostatitis, and discharge, but most men are largely asymptomatic.[21]

Trichomoniasis vaginalis is an anaerobic protozoan that is shaped like a turnip and has three or four anterior flagella (see Fig. 41-3B, C). Trichomonads can reside in the paraurethral glands of both sexes. This extracellular parasite feeds on the vaginal mucosa and ingests bacteria and leukocytes. Trichomonads attach easily to mucous membranes. It may reduce the chorioamnionic membrane strength and predispose pregnant women to premature rupture of membranes and premature birth.[19] *Trichomoniasis vaginalis* infection has emerged as a cofactor for HIV transmission. Potential mechanisms for increased susceptibility include recruitment of HIV target cells, weakening of structural integrity of epithelial cells and their defense against HIV invasion, and creation of punctate microhemorrhages in mucosal genital tissue that serve as a portal of HIV entry.[19,20] Trichomonads may serve as vectors for the spread of other organisms, carrying pathogens attached to their surface into the fallopian tubes; infection has been associated with acute salpingitis and postpartum endometrial infection.[21] In men, it is a common cause of nongonococcal urethritis and is a risk factor for infertility, altering sperm motility and viability. It has also been associated with chronic prostatitis.

Diagnosis is made microscopically by identification of the motile protozoan on a wet-mount slide preparation. The pH of the discharge usually is greater than 6.0. Newer point-of-care tests include an antigen-based diagnostic test (OSOM *Trichomonas* Rapid Test), a DNA probe test (Affirm VP III), and a PCR-based test. The OSOM and DNA probes have greater sensitivity than a vaginal mount and results can be available in less than an hour.[4,19] Because the organism resides in other urogenital structures besides the vagina, systemic treatment is recommended. Metronidazole and tinidazole, which are the treatments of choice against anaerobic protozoans, can cure *T. vaginalis.*[19] Systemic treatment is preferred over topical application to achieve adequate drug concentrations in nonvaginal sites.[19] Because the organism responds to only one class of medication, mild drug resistance has been noted against metronidazole but not tinidazole.[24] Although metronidazole is considered safe for use during pregnancy, data on tinidazole use in pregnancy are limited. Sexual partners should be treated to avoid reinfection, and abstinence is recommended until the full course of therapy is completed.

Bacterial Vaginosis

Bacterial vaginosis is a polymicrobial infection characterized by lack of hydrogen peroxide–producing lactobacilli and an overgrowth of anaerobic organisms. It is the most prevalent vaginal disorder in women of reproductive age.[2] Bacterial vaginosis is associated with multiple male or female sex partners, a new sex partner, lack of condom use, and douching.[4,22–24] Sexual activity is believed to be a catalyst rather than a primary mode of transmission, and endogenous factors may play a role in the development of symptoms.

The predominant symptom of bacterial vaginosis is a thin, grayish-white discharge that has a foul, fishy odor. Burning, itching, and erythema usually are absent because the bacteria have only minimal inflammatory potential. Because of the lack of inflammation, the term *vaginosis* rather than *vaginitis* is used to describe the condition. The organisms associated with bacterial vaginosis may be carried asymptomatically by men and women.

The pathogenesis of bacterial vaginosis remains poorly understood. It is a complex disorder characterized by a shift in the vaginal flora from one dominated by hydrogen peroxide–producing lactobacilli to one with greatly reduced numbers of *Lactobacillus* species and an overgrowth of facultative anaerobic organisms, including *Gardnerella vaginalis, Mobiluncus* species, and *Mycoplasma hominis.*[2,22,24] The massive overgrowth of vaginal anaerobes is associated with the production of proteolytic enzymes that break down vaginal amines, which become volatile and malodorous in a high pH. The amines are associated with increased vaginal secretions and squamous epithelial cell exfoliation, creating the typical discharge. In conditions of elevated pH, the vaginal anaerobes more efficiently adhere to the exfoliating epithelial cells, creating what are called *clue cells* (Fig. 41-4).

In addition to causing bothersome symptoms, bacterial vaginosis is associated with an increased risk of pelvic inflammatory disease (PID), adverse pregnancy outcomes including premature rupture of membranes, preterm labor, preterm birth, and postpartum endometritis linked to the organisms associated with bacterial vaginosis. Postoperative infections, including postabortion

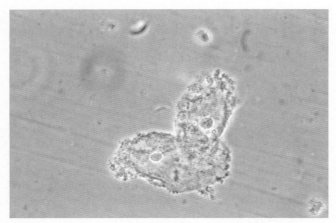

FIGURE 41-4. Clue cells. Clue cells are epithelial cells with clumps of bacteria clustered on their surface. Clue cells indicate the presence of bacterial vaginosis. (From the Centers for Disease Control and Prevention Public Health Image Library. No. 3720. Courtesy of M. Rein.)

- The manifestations of infection with *Trichomoniasis vaginalis,* the causative agent of trichomoniasis, are primarily observed in women, and range from asymptomatic presentation to a copious, frothy, malodorous green or yellow discharge. The disorder is associated with pelvic inflammatory disease, endometritis, infertility, and premature labor. It has also been shown to facilitate human immunodeficiency virus (HIV) infection.

- *Bacterial vaginosis* is a polymicrobial disorder characterized by a lack of hydrogen peroxide–producing lactobacilli and an overgrowth of anaerobic organisms, including *G. vaginalis, Mobiluncus* species, and *M. hominis.* It is the most prevalent vaginal disorder in women of reproductive age. The predominant symptom of bacterial vaginosis is a thin, grayish-white discharge that has a foul, fishy odor.

and postcesarean endometritis, have been shown to be associated with asymptomatic bacterial vaginosis. It has also been associated with increased risk of acquisition of HIV and HSV infection.

The diagnosis of bacterial vaginosis is made when at least three of the following signs or symptoms are present: abnormal gray discharge, vaginal pH above 4.5 (usually 5.0 to 6.0), positive fishy odor of vaginal discharge on addition of 10% potassium hydroxide, and appearance of characteristic "clue cells" on wet-mount microscopic studies.[4] Because *G. vaginalis* can be a part of the normal vaginal flora, cultures should not be done routinely.

Bacterial vaginosis may be treated with oral or topical metronidazole or clindamycin and oral tinidazole. Symptomatic pregnant women can also be treated with metronidazole or clindamycin.[2,4] Some studies have shown that screening for and treating bacterial vaginosis may reduce the incidence of adverse pregnancy outcomes. However, studies do not confirm a benefit from universal testing of low- and medium-risk pregnant women.

SUMMARY CONCEPTS

- Candidiasis, trichomoniasis, and bacterial vaginosis are common vaginal infections that become symptomatic because of changes in the vaginal ecosystem.

- *Candidiasis,* also called a *yeast infection,* is a frequent cause of vulvovaginitis. Candida can be present without producing symptoms; usually some host factor, such as altered immune status, contributes to the development of vulvovaginitis.

Vaginal-Urogenital-Systemic Infections

Some STIs infect male and female genital and extragenital structures. Among the infections of this type are chlamydial infections, gonorrhea, and syphilis. Many of these infections also pose a risk to infants born to infected mothers. Some infections, such as syphilis, may be spread to the unborn infant while in utero, whereas others, such as chlamydial and gonorrheal infections, can be spread to the infant during the birth process.

Chlamydial Infections

Chlamydial infection is the most frequently reported bacterial STI in the United States, with an incidence estimated to be more than twice that of gonorrhea. According the Centers for Disease Control and Prevention (CDC), an estimated 2.86 million infections occur annually.[25] A large number of cases go unreported because most people with chlamydia are asymptomatic and do not seek testing. If untreated, chlamydial infections can lead to serious complications including pelvic inflammatory disease, infertility, ectopic pregnancy, and chronic pelvic pain.[25]

Etiology and Pathogenesis

Chlamydia trachomatis is an obligate intracellular bacterial pathogen that is closely related to gram-negative bacteria.[9,10] It resembles a virus in that it requires tissue culture for isolation, but like bacteria, it has both DNA and RNA and is susceptible to some antimicrobial agents. Chlamydial infection exists in two morphologically distinct forms during its unique life—a small infectious elementary body and a large noninfectious reticulate body. Much like a spore, the *elementary body* is metabolically inactive and can survive outside the cell. It does not replicate. The *reticulate body* is metabolically active and cannot survive outside the cell. The 48-hour growth cycle starts with attachment of the elementary body to the susceptible host cell, after which it is ingested by a process that resembles phagocytosis (Fig. 41-5). Once inside the cell, the elementary body transforms into the larger *reticulate body*, which then commandeers the host cell's metabolic machinery to fuel its replication. The reticulate body divides repeatedly for up to 36 hours, forming new elementary bodies that are released when the infected cell bursts. Necrotic debris elicits inflammatory and immune processes that further damage infected tissue.

The signs and symptoms of chlamydial infection resemble those produced by gonorrhea. The most significant difference between chlamydial and gonococcal salpingitis is that chlamydial infections may be asymptomatic or clinically nonspecific. In women, chlamydial infections may cause urinary frequency, dysuria, and vaginal discharge.[25,26] The most common symptom is a mucopurulent cervical discharge. The cervix itself frequently hypertrophies and becomes erythematous, edematous, and extremely friable. This can lead to fallopian tube damage and increase the reservoir for further chlamydial infections. In men, chlamydial infections cause urethritis, including meatal erythema and tenderness, urethral discharge, dysuria, and urethral itching. Prostatitis and epididymitis with subsequent infertility may develop. The most serious complication of untreated chlamydial infection in men is the development of Reiter syndrome, a reactive arthritis that includes the triad of urethritis, conjunctivitis, and painless mucocutaneous lesions (see Chapter 44).

Diagnosis and Treatment

The CDC recommends annual screening of women who are sexually active and younger than 25 years; men who have sex with men and have receptive anal sex; and all HIV-infected individuals who participate in receptive anal sex.[25] Heterosexual individuals and men who have sex with men or have multiple and/or anonymous sex partners should be tested more frequently. A health care provider may choose to screen more frequently depending on a person's sexual risks. All pregnant women should be tested early in pregnancy; for women with increased risk factors, third-trimester screening is also recommended.[25]

Diagnosis of chlamydial infections takes several forms. The identification of polymorphonuclear leukocytes on Gram stain of penile discharge in the man or cervical discharge in the woman provides presumptive evidence. The direct fluorescent antibody test and the enzyme-linked immunosorbent assay, which use antibodies against an antigen in the *Chlamydia* cell wall, are rapid tests that are highly sensitive and specific. The positive predictive value of these tests is excellent among high-risk groups, but false-positive results occur more often in low-risk groups. The methodological challenges of culturing this organism have led to the development of non–culture-based tests that amplify and detect *C. trachomatis*–specific DNA and RNA sequences.[25] One of the newer sets of nonculture techniques, the nucleic acid amplification tests (NAATs), do not require viable organisms for detection, and can produce a positive signal from as little as a single copy of the target DNA or RNA.[25] These amplification methods are highly sensitive and, if properly monitored, very specific. Because NAATs can be performed on urine and self-collected swab specimens from the distal vagina as well as the traditional endocervical and urethral specimens, this easy, convenient means of accurate detection has become the diagnostic method of choice.[4] Detection rates (specificity) for chlamydiae in urine and vaginal samples are nearly identical to those for cervical and urethral samples.[24]

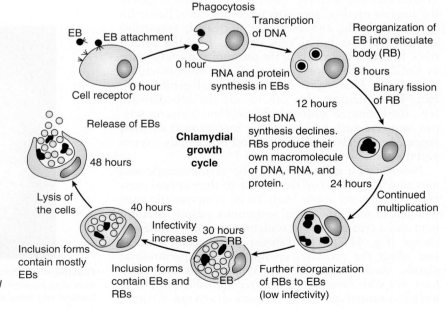

FIGURE 41-5. Chlamydial growth cycle. EB, elementary body; RB, reticulate body. (From Thompson SE, Washington AE. Epidemiology of sexually transmitted Chlamydia trachomatis infections. *Epidemiol Rev.* 1983;5:96–123.)

The CDC recommends the use of azithromycin or doxycycline in the treatment of chlamydial infection; penicillin is ineffective. Azithromycin or amoxicillin is the preferred choice in pregnancy.[4] Simultaneous antibiotic treatment of both sexual partners is recommended. Abstinence from sexual activity is encouraged to facilitate cure. With the exception of women who are pregnant, a test of cure 3 to 4 weeks after treatment is no longer recommended unless therapeutic compliance is in question.[4]

Gonorrhea

Gonorrhea is one of the oldest and still one of the most common STIs. Currently, it is the second most commonly reported communicable disease in the United States, with greater than 300,000 cases being reported in 2011.[4,27,28] The infection disproportionately affects vulnerable populations such as minorities, who are marginalized because of race, ethnicity, or sexual orientation.[4,27]

Etiology and Pathogenesis

The gonococcus is a pyogenic (i.e., pus-forming), gram-negative diplococcus that evokes inflammatory reactions characterized by purulent exudates.[9,10] Humans are the only natural host for *N. gonorrhoeae*. The organism grows best in warm, mucus-secreting epithelia. The portal of entry can be the genitourinary tract, eyes, oropharynx, anorectum, or skin. Transmission usually is by intercourse. Autoinoculation of the organism to the conjunctiva is possible. Neonates born to infected mothers can acquire the infection during passage through the birth canal and are in danger of developing gonorrheal conjunctivitis, with resultant blindness, unless treated promptly. Genital gonorrhea in young children should raise the possibility of sexual abuse.

Gonococcal infection commonly manifests 3 to 5 days after exposure, but asymptomatic infections are common in both men and women.[2] Gonorrhea typically begins in the anterior urethra, accessory urethral glands, Bartholin or Skene glands, and cervix. If untreated, gonorrhea spreads from its initial sites upward into the genital tract. In males, it spreads to the prostate and epididymis; in females, it commonly moves to the fallopian tubes (Fig. 41-6). Pharyngitis may follow oral–genital contact. The organism also can invade the bloodstream (i.e., disseminated gonococcal infection), causing serious sequelae such as bacteremic involvement of joint spaces, heart valves, meninges, and other body organs and tissues.

Persons with gonorrhea may be asymptomatic and may unwittingly spread the disease to their sexual partners.[29,30] Men are more likely to be symptomatic than women. In men, the initial symptoms include urethral pain and a creamy yellow, sometimes bloody, penile discharge (Fig. 41-7). The disorder may become chronic and affect the prostate, epididymis, and periurethral glands. Rectal infections are common in men who have sex with men. In women, recognizable symptoms include unusual genital or urinary discharge, dysuria,

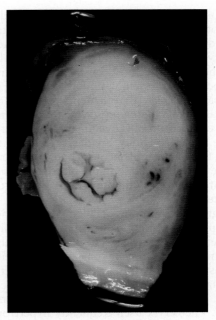

FIGURE 41-6. Gonorrhea of the fallopian tube. Cross-section of a "pus tube" shows thickening of the wall and lumen swollen with pus. (From Schwartz DA. Infectious and parasitic diseases. In: Rubin R, Strayer DS, eds. *Rubin's Pathology: Clinicopathologic Foundations of Medicine.* 6th ed. Philadelphia, PA: Wolters Kluwer Health | Lippincott Williams & Wilkins; 2012:356.)

dyspareunia, pelvic pain or tenderness, unusual vaginal bleeding (including bleeding after intercourse), fever, and proctitis. Symptoms may occur or increase during or immediately after menses because the bacterium is an intracellular diplococcus that thrives in menstrual blood but cannot survive long outside the human body. There may be infections of the uterus and development of acute or chronic infection of the fallopian tubes (i.e., salpingitis), with ultimate scarring and sterility.

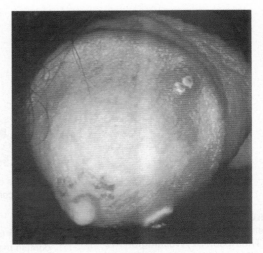

FIGURE 41-7. Purulent penile discharge due to gonorrhea with overlying pyodermal lesions. (From the Centers for Disease Control and Prevention Public Health Image Library. No. 4065.)

Diagnosis and Treatment

Diagnosis is based on the history of sexual exposure and symptoms. The presence of *N. gonorrhea* may be confirmed by identification of the organism on a gram stain or culture, but more rapid testing that can be done from a urine sample is becoming preferred. While culture remains the gold standard, detection by NAATs is possible using urine and urethral swab specimens.[29] The sensitivity of these tests is similar to that of culture, and they are cost effective in high-risk populations.

Updated recommendations from the U.S. Preventive Services Task Force (USPSTF) suggest that clinicians screen for gonorrhea in all sexually active men and women who are at increased risk for infection (i.e., younger than 25 years of age, new or multiple sexual partners, inconsistent condom use, sex work, men who have sex with men, or drug use).[31] Testing for other STIs, particularly syphilis and chlamydial infection, is suggested at the time of examination. Pregnant women are routinely screened at the time of their first prenatal visit; high-risk populations should have repeat cultures during the third trimester. Neonates are routinely treated with various antibacterial agents applied to the conjunctiva within 1 hour of birth to protect against undiagnosed gonorrhea and other diseases.

Strains of *N. gonorrhoeae* that are resistant to penicillin, tetracycline, and quinolone are prevalent worldwide, and strains with other kinds of antibiotic resistance continue to evolve and spread. The current treatment recommendation to combat penicillin- and tetracycline-resistant strains is ceftriaxone or cefixime in a single injection.[28,29] While a single injection of cefixime is still the standard treatment, some strains of *N. gonorrhoeae* have begun to show resistance to this dose. At this time the organism is responding to higher dosing (up to 1 gm) of cefixime. Because gonorrhea and chlamydia frequently occur together, treatment of cefixime should be followed with azithromycin or doxycycline for chlamydia. All sex partners within 60 days prior to discovery of the infection should be contacted, tested, and treated. Test of cure is not required with observed single-dose therapy. Patients are instructed to refrain from intercourse until therapy is completed and symptoms are no longer present.[4]

Syphilis

After declining every year from 1990 to 2000, the rates of primary and secondary syphilis have been increasing.[32,33] The CDC estimates that 55,400 people in the United States develop syphilis each year.[32] Increased rates were primarily in men, with men who have sex with men being particularly affected.[32] There has also been an increase in congenital syphilis.[32,33]

Etiology and Pathogenesis

Syphilis is caused by a spirochete, *Treponema pallidum*.[9,10] *T. pallidum* is spread by direct contact with an infectious moist lesion, usually through sexual intercourse. Bacterialaden secretions may transfer the organism during kissing

or intimate contact. Skin abrasions provide another possible portal of entry. There is rapid transplacental transmission of the organism from the mother to the fetus after 16 weeks' gestation, so that active infection in the mother during pregnancy can produce congenital syphilis in the fetus. Untreated syphilis can cause prematurity, stillbirth, and congenital defects and active infection in the infant (Fig. 41-8). Because the manifestations of maternal syphilis may be subtle, testing for syphilis is mandatory in all pregnancies. Once treated for syphilis, a pregnant woman usually is followed throughout pregnancy by repeat testing of serum titers.

The clinical disease is divided into three stages: primary, secondary, and tertiary. Primary syphilis is characterized by the appearance of a chancre at the site of exposure.[9,32–34] Chancres typically appear within 3 weeks of exposure but may incubate for 1 week to 3 months. The primary chancre begins as a single, indurated, buttonlike papule up to several centimeters in diameter that erodes to create a round or oval clean-based ulcerated lesion on an elevated base. These lesions usually are painless and located at the site of sexual contact. Primary syphilis is readily apparent in the male, where the lesion is on the scrotum or penis (Fig. 41-9). Although chancres can develop on the external genitalia in females, they are more common on the vagina or cervix, and primary syphilis therefore may go untreated. There usually is an accompanying regional lymphadenopathy. The infection is highly

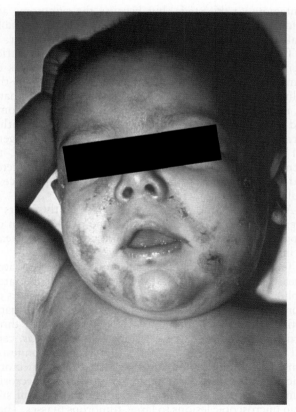

FIGURE 41-8. Infant who presented with congenital facial syphilitic lesions. (From the Centers for Disease Control and Prevention Public Health Image Library. No. 3503. Courtesy of Dr. Joseph Caldwell.)

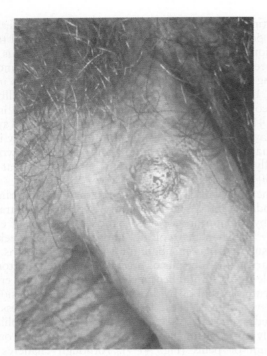

FIGURE 41-9. Syphilitic chancre of the penis shaft. (From the Centers for Disease Control and Prevention Public Health Image Library. No. 6758. Courtesy of Gavin Hart, N. J. Fiumara.)

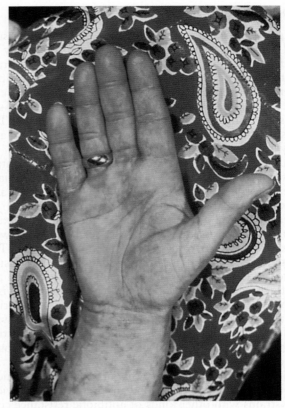

FIGURE 41-10. A maculopapular rash is present on the palm due to secondary syphilis. Note that some of the rash is sparsely distributed to areas of the forearm as well. (From the Centers for Disease Control and Prevention Public Health Image Library. No. 3478. Courtesy of Susan Lindsley.)

contagious at this stage, but because the symptoms are mild, it frequently goes unnoticed. The chancre usually heals within 3 to 12 weeks, with or without treatment.

The timing of the second stage of syphilis varies even more than that of the first, lasting from 1 week to 6 months. The symptoms of a rash (especially on the palms [Fig. 41-10] and soles), fever, sore throat, stomatitis, nausea, loss of appetite, and inflamed eyes may come and go for a year but usually last for 3 to 6 months. Secondary manifestations may include alopecia and genital lesions called *condylomata lata*. These elevated 2- to 3-cm red-brown lesions, which contain many spirocetes and are highly infectious, may ulcerate and produce a foul discharge.

After the second stage, syphilis frequently enters a latent phase that may last the lifetime of the person or progress to tertiary syphilis at some point. Persons can be infective during the first 1 to 2 years of latency.

Tertiary syphilis is a delayed response to the untreated disease. Approximately one third of people with untreated syphilis develop syphilis after a latent period of 5 years or more.[9] When syphilis does progress to the symptomatic tertiary stage, it commonly develops into one of three forms: localized destructive lesions called *gummas*, central nervous system lesions, or cardiovascular manifestations. The syphilitic gumma is a peculiar, rubbery, necrotic lesion that is caused by noninflammatory tissue necrosis. Gummas can occur singly or multiply and vary in size from microscopic lesions to large, tumorous masses. They most commonly are found in the liver, testes, and bone. Central nervous system lesions can produce dementia, blindness, or injury to the spinal cord, with ataxia and

sensory loss (i.e., tabes dorsalis). Cardiovascular manifestations usually result from scarring of the medial layer of the thoracic aorta with aneurysm formation. These aneurysms produce enlargement of the aortic valve ring with aortic valve insufficiency.

Diagnosis and Treatment

The diagnosis of syphilis can be made rapidly by darkfield microscopic examination of the exudate from skin lesions. However, the test is reliable only when a specimen with actively motile *T. pallidum* is examined immediately by a trained microscopist. *Treponema pallidum* does not survive transport to a laboratory and it cannot be cultured. It does, however, evoke a humoral immune response and production of antibodies that provide the basis for serologic tests.

Although PCR tests have been developed for syphilis, serology tests remain the mainstay for diagnosis. Two general types of serology tests are available: nonspecific (nontreponemal) tests and the specific treponemal tests.[4] The *nontreponemal tests* measure immunoglobin (Ig) G and IgM antibodies developed against molecules released from damaged cells during the early stages of the infection and present on the cell surface of treponemas. These antibodies are detected by tests such as the

Venereal Disease Research Laboratory (VDRL) or the rapid plasma reagin (RPR) tests. The tests, which are easy to perform, rapid, and inexpensive, are frequently used as screening tests for syphilis. Because these tests are nonspecific, positive results can occur for diseases other than syphilis. Results become positive 4 to 6 weeks after infection or 1 to 3 weeks after the appearance of the primary lesion. The disease's incubation period may delay test sensitivity; therefore, serologic tests usually are repeated after 6 weeks if the initial test results were negative.

The *specific treponemal* tests measure antibodies capable of reacting with *T. pallidum* antigens. These tests are used to determine whether a positive result on a nonspecific test such as the VDRL is attributable to syphilis. Some clinical laboratories and blood banks have begun to screen samples using automated treponemal tests, the enzyme-linked immunosorbent (EIA) or chemoiluminescence (CIA) assays, and then follow-up with a nontreponemal test (VDRL or RPR).[4] The CDC recommends that persons with a positive screening test should have a standard nontreponemal titer performed by the laboratory. If the test is negative, it is recommended that the laboratory perform a different test using a different antigen.[4]

The treatment of choice for syphilis is penicillin.[8] Because of the spirochetes' long generation time, effective tissue levels of penicillin must be maintained for several weeks. Long-acting injectable forms of penicillin are used. Tetracycline or doxycycline is used for treatment in persons who are sensitive to penicillin, but these medications cannot be used in pregnancy. Sexual partners should be evaluated and treated prophylactically even though they may show no sign of infection. All treated individuals should be reexamined clinically and serologically at 6 and 12 months after completing therapy; more frequent monitoring (3-month intervals) is suggested for individuals with HIV infection.[8]

SUMMARY CONCEPTS

- The vaginal-urogenital systemic STIs—chlamydial infections, gonorrhea, and syphilis—can severely affect the genital structures and manifest as systemic infections.

- Gonorrheal and chlamydial infections can cause a wide variety of genitourinary complications in men and women, and both can cause ocular disease and blindness in neonates born to infected mothers.

- Syphilis is caused by a spirochete, *T. pallidum*. It can produce widespread systemic effects and is transferred to the fetus of infected mothers through the placenta.

REVIEW EXERCISES

1. A 25-year-old woman has been told that her Pap test indicates infection with HPV type 16.

   A. What are the possible implications of infection with HPV 16?

   B. How might she have acquired this infection?

   C. What treatments are currently available for treatment of this infection?

2. A 35-year-old woman presents with vulvar pruritus, dysuria, dyspareunia, and an odorless, thick, cheesy vaginal discharge. She has diabetes mellitus and has recently recovered from a respiratory tract infection, which required antibiotic treatment.

   A. Given that these manifestations are consistent with a *Candida* infection, what tests might be used to confirm the diagnosis?

   B. What risk factors does this woman have that predispose her to this type of vaginitis?

   C. How might this infection be treated?

REFERENCES

1. Frenkl TL, Potts J. Sexually transmitted diseases. *Urol Clin North Am.* 2008;35:33–46.
2. Beckmann CRB, Ling FW, Barzansky BM, et al.; for American College of Obstetrics and Gynecology. *Obstet Gynecol.* 3rd ed. Philadelphia, PA: Wolters Kluwer Health/Lippincott Williams & Wilkins; 2010:241–258.
3. Centers for Disease Control and Prevention. Incidence, prevalence, and cost of sexually transmitted infections in the United States. 2013. Available at: http://www.cdc.gov/std/stats/STI-Estimates-Fact-Sheet-Feb-2013.pdf. Accessed July 24, 2013.
4. Centers for Disease Control and Prevention. Sexually transmitted diseases: treatment guidelines 2010. *MMWR Morb Mortal Wkly Rep.* 2010;59(RR12):1–116.
5. Stanley MA. Genital human papillomavirus infections: current and prospective therapies. *J Gen Virol.* 2012;93:681–695.
6. Hariri S, Dunna E, Saralya M, et al. Human papillomavirus. In: Centers for Disease Control and Prevention. *VPD Surveillance Manual.* 5th ed. Chapter 5. 2011. Available at: http://www.cdc.gov/vaccines/pubs/surv-manual/chpt05-hpv.pdf. Accessed July 29, 2013.
7. Center for Disease Control and Prevention. FDA licensure of bivalent human papillomavirus vaccine (HPV2, Cervarix) for use in females and updated HPV vaccination recommendations from the Advisory Committee on Immunization Practices (ACIP). *MMWR Morb Mortal Wkly Rep.* 2010;59(20):626–629.
8. Center for Disease Control and Prevention. FDA Licensure of qualivalent vaccine (HPV4, Gardasil) for use in males and guidance from the Advisory Committee on immunization practices (ACIP). *MMWR Morb Mortal Wkly Rep.* 2010;59(20):630–632.
9. McAdam AJ, Sharpe AH. Infectious diseases. In: Kumar V, Abbas AK, Fausto N, eds. *Robbins and Cotran Pathologic Basis of Disease.* 8th ed. Philadelphia, PA: Saunders Elsevier; 2010:351–352, 366, 374–377, 380.

10. Schwartz D. Infectious and parasitic diseases. In: Rubin E, Gorstein F, Rubin R, et al., eds. *Rubin's Pathology: Clinicopathologic Foundations of Medicine.* 6th ed. Philadelphia, PA: Wolters Kluwer Health/Lippincott Williams & Wilkins; 2012: 340–343.

11. Roett M, Mayor M, Uduhiri K. Diagnosis and management of genital ulcers. *Am Fam Physician.* 2012;8(3):254–262.

12. World Health Organization. An estimate of the global prevalence and incidence of herpes simplex virus type 2 infection. *Bull World Health Organ.* 2008;86(10):737–816.

13. Gilbert M, Petric M, Krajden M, et al. Using centralized laboratory data to monitor trends in herpes simplex virus-1 and 2 infection in British Columbia and the changing etiology of genital herpes. *Can J Public Health.* 2011:225–228.

14. American College of Obstetricians and Gynecologists. ACOG practice bulletin: management of herpes in pregnancy. *Obstet Gynecol.* 2007 (updated and reaffirmed in 2012):1489–1498.

15. Pinninti S, Kimberlin D. Maternal and neonatal herpes simplex virus infections. *Am J Perinatol.* 2013;30(2):113–119.

16. American College of Obstetricians and Gynecologists. ACOG practice bulletin: vaginitis. *Obstet Gynecol.* 2006 (revised/reaffirmed 2013);107:1195–1205.

17. Hainer BL, Gibson MA. Vaginitis: Diagnosis and treatment. *Am Fam Physician.* 2011;83(7):807–815.

18. Nyirjesy P, Sobel J. Genital mycotic infections in patients with diabetes. *Postgrad Med.* 2013;125(3):33–46.

19. Muzny C, Schwebke J. The clinical spectrum of Trichomonas vaginalis infection and challenges to management. *Sex Transm Infect.* 2013;89(6):423–425.

20. Secor WE. Trichomonas vaginalis: treatment questions and challenges. *Expert Rev Anti Infect Ther.* 2012;10(2):107–109.

21. Coleman JS, Gaydon CA, Witter F. Trichomonas vaginalis vaginitis in obstetrics and gynecology practice: new concepts and controversies. *Obstet Gynecol Surv.* 2013;68(1):43–50.

22. Verstraelen H, Swidsinski A. The biofilm in bacterial vaginosis: implications for epidemiology, diagnosis and treatment. *Curr Opin Infect Dis.* 2013;26(1):86–89.

23. Maraxxo JM. Interpreting the epidemiology and natural history of bacterial vaginosis: are we still confused? *Anaerobe.* 2011;17(4):186–190.

24. Turovskly Y, Noil KD, Chikindas ML. The etiology of bacterial vagiosis. *J Appl Microbiol.* 2011;110(5):1105–1128.

25. Centers for Disease Control and Prevention. Chlamydia—CDC fact sheet. 2013. Available at: http://www.cdc.gov/std/chlamydia/STDFact-Chlamydia-detailed.htm. Accessed July 25, 2013.

26. Mishori R, McClanskey EL, Windlerprins VJ. *Chlamydia trachomatis* infections: screening, diagnosis, and management. *Am Fam Physician.* 2012;86(12):1127–1132.

27. Centers for Disease Control and Prevention. CDC grand rounds: the growing threat of multi-drug resistant gonorrhea. *MMWR Morb Mortal Wkly Rep.* 2013;62(6):103–106.

28. Bolan GA, Sparling F, Wasserheit JN. The emerging threat of untreatable gonococcal infections. *N Engl J Med.* 2012;366(8):485–487.

29. Mayor M, Roett MA, Uduhiri KA. Diagnosis and management of gonococcal infections. *Am Fam Physician.* 2012;86(10):931–938.

30. Centers for Disease Control and Prevention. Gonorrhea—CDC Fact Sheet. 2013. Available at: http://www.cdc.gov/std/Gonorrhea/STDFact-gonorrhea.htm. Accessed July 23, 2013.

31. U.S. Preventive Services Task Force. Screening for gonorrhea: Recommendation statement. 2011. Available at: http://www.uspreventiveservicestaskforce.org/uspstf05/gonorrhea/gonrs.htm. Accessed July 23, 2013.

32. Centers for Disease Control and Prevention. Syphilis—CDC Fact Sheet. 2012. Available at: http://www.cdc.gov/std/syphilis/STDFact-Syphilis.htm. Accessed July 25, 2013.

33. Mattel PL, Beachkofsky TM, Gilson RT, et al. Syphilis: a reemerging infection. *Am Fam Physician.* 2012;86(5):433–440.

34. Ho EL, Lukehart SA. Syphilis: using modern approaches to understand an old disease. *J Clin Invest.* 2011;121(12):4584–4592.

Porth Essentials Resources

Explore these additional resources to enhance learning for this chapter:

- NCLEX-Style Questions and Other Resources on thePoint, http://thePoint.lww.com/PorthEssentials4e
- Study Guide for Essentials of Pathophysiology
- Adaptive Learning | Powered by PrepU, http://thepoint.lww.com/prepu

Chapter 42

Structure and Function of the Skeletal System

Without the skeletal system, movement in the external environment would not be possible. The bones of the skeletal system serve as a framework for skeletal muscle attachment and movement; protect and maintain vital structures in their proper position, provide stability for the body, and maintain the body's shape. The skeletal system also serves as a reservoir for ions such as calcium, phosphorous, and magnesium, and it houses the hematopoietic connective tissue in which blood cells are formed.

Structures of the Skeletal System

The skeletal system can be divided into two functional parts—the axial and appendicular skeletons (Fig. 42-1). The *axial skeleton*, which is composed of the bones of the skull, thorax, and vertebral column, forms the axis of the body. The *appendicular skeleton* consists of the bones of the upper and lower extremities, including those of the shoulder and hip girdles. In addition to bones, the skeletal system includes cartilage and ligaments that join bones together at joints, giving the body flexibility and allowing movement to occur.

Two types of connective tissue are found in the skeletal system: *cartilage* and *bone*. They both have living cells that secrete the extracellular matrix in which their cells are housed. The extracellular matrix in cartilage is firm but also somewhat pliable, providing the resilience needed for cushioning of bony structures. In contrast

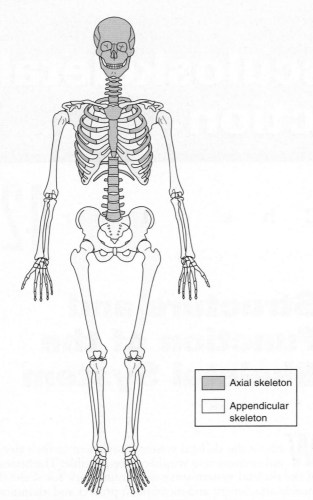

FIGURE 42-1. The axial (blue) and appendicular (uncolored) skeleton.

Axial skeleton

Appendicular skeleton

to cartilage, the extracellular matrix of bone is mineralized, producing a hard tissue capable of providing support for the body and protection for its vital structures.

Cartilage

Cartilage is an avascular tissue that consists of cells, called *chondrocytes*, and an extensive extracellular matrix composed of fibers and ground substance. The chondrocytes are sparse, but are essential to the production and maintenance of the matrix. A connective tissue sheath, called the *perichondrium*, overlies the free surfaces of most cartilage. The perichondrium is vascular and its blood vessels supply nutrients to the chrondrocytes. In areas where the cartilage has no perichondrium, such as the articular surfaces of moving joints, the chondrocytes receive their nourishment from the synovial fluid that bathes the joint surfaces.

Types of Cartilage

There are three types of cartilage, each exhibiting variations in matrix composition: elastic, fibrocartilage, and hyaline. *Elastic cartilage* has a dense network of elastic fibers scattered throughout its matrix. It is found in areas

where flexibility is important, such as in the auricle of the ear, the auditory canal, the epiglottis, and the larynx. *Fibrocartilage* is characterized by a matrix containing a combination of chrondrocytes and dense fibrous tissue. It is found in areas subjected to pulling forces such as attachments of ligaments to the cartilaginous surface of bones, the symphysis pubis, and intervertebral disks.

Hyaline cartilage is the most abundant and the best studied of the three types. It forms the articulating surfaces of the moveable joints in the body, costal cartilages that join the ribs to the sternum and vertebrae, and many of the cartilages of the respiratory tract. Hyaline cartilage is also essential for growth before and after birth. In the embryo, most of the axial and appendicular skeleton is formed first as a cartilage model and then is replaced by bone. In postnatal life, hyaline cartilage continues to play an essential role in the growth of long bones and persists as articular cartilage in the adult.

The matrix of hyaline cartilage is composed of collagen fibers embedded in a firm, hydrated gel of structural glycoproteins and proteoglycans, which have a high affinity for water. This high degree of hydration in the cartilage matrix contributes to the weight-bearing properties of cartilage and allows the cartilage matrix to respond to varying pressure loads. The multiadhesive glycoproteins influence interactions between the chondrocytes and matrix molecules and have clinical value as markers of cartilage turnover and degeneration.

Repair of Hyaline Cartilage

Hyaline cartilage can tolerate considerable amounts of intense and repetitive stress, but manifests a striking inability to heal from even the most minor injuries. This lack of response to injury is attributable to the avascular nature of cartilage, the immobility of chondrocytes, and the limited ability of chondrocytes to proliferate. Some repair can occur, but only if the defect involves the perichondrium, in which case chondrogenic cells from the perichondrium enter the defect and form new cartilage. If the defect is large, the cells form dense connective tissue to repair the injury. Hyaline cartilage is also subject to calcification, a process in which calcium phosphate crystals become embedded in the cartilage matrix. In most situations, given sufficient time, cartilage that calcifies will be replaced by bone. Chondrocytes normally derive all of their nutrients and dispose of waste materials through the extracellular matrix. When the matrix becomes heavily calcified, diffusion is impeded and the chondrocytes swell and die. The ultimate consequence of this event is removal of the calcified matrix and its replacement by bone.

Bones and Bone Structure

Bones are the major component of the skeletal system. Besides contributing to body shape and form, bones perform several other important functions. They provide the hard framework that supports the body and provides protection for its delicate soft tissues and organs. For example, the bones of lower limbs act as pillars to support the body trunk when we stand, and the fused bones of the skull provide protection for the brain. Skeletal muscles, which are attached to bones by tendons, use bones as levers to move the body and its parts. Bones also serve as reservoirs for storage of minerals such as calcium and phosphate; and the bulk of blood cells are formed within the marrow cavities of certain bones.

Classification of Bones

Bones can be classified according to type: compact (dense) or spongy (cancellous). They can also be classified according to their shape, and the effect that bone shape has on the location of compact and spongy bone.

Compact and Spongy Bone.
If a bone is cut, two distinct structural arrangements of bone tissue can be recognized—a dense layer of compact bone that forms the outside of the bone and a spongelike meshwork consisting of trabeculae (thin, anastomosing spicules of bone tissue) that forms the interior of bone (Fig. 42-2). Spongy bone is relatively light, but its structure is such that it has considerable tensile strength and weight-bearing properties. Although bones contain both compact and spongy elements, their proportions vary in different bones throughout the body and in different parts of the same bone, depending on the relative needs for strength and lightness.

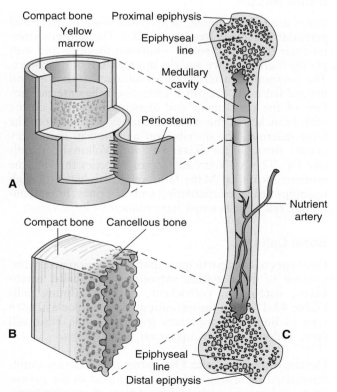

FIGURE 42-2. Diagram of bone structures. **(A)** Periosteum and bone marrow, **(B)** compact and spongy bone, and **(C)** a typical long bone showing the epiphysis, diaphysis, metaphysis, epiphyseal line, and sources of blood supply from the nutrient arteries.

Classification of Bones by Shape.
Bones are classified by shape as long, short, flat, and irregular. *Long bones* are found in the upper and lower extremities. *Short bones* are irregularly shaped bones located in the ankle and the wrist. Except for their surface, which is compact bone, these bones are spongy throughout. *Flat bones* are composed of a layer of spongy bone between two layers of compact bone. They are found in areas where extensive protection of underlying structures is needed such as the skull and rib cage, or where a broad surface for muscle attachment is needed, as in the scapula. *Irregular bones*, because of their shapes, cannot be classified in any of the previous groups. This group includes bones such as the vertebrae and the bones of the jaw.

Parts of a Long Bone

A typical long bone has a shaft, or *diaphysis*, and two ends, called *epiphyses* (Fig. 42-3). Long bones usually are narrow in the midportion and broad at the ends so that the weight they bear can be distributed over a wider surface. The shaft of a long bone is formed mainly of compact bone roughly hollowed out to form a marrow-filled medullary canal. The ends of long bones are covered with articular cartilage.

In growing bones, the part of the bone shaft that funnels out as it approaches the epiphysis is called the *metaphysis*. It is composed of bony trabeculae that have cores of cartilage. In the child, the *epiphysis* is separated from the metaphysis by the cartilaginous growth plate. After puberty, the metaphysis and epiphysis merge, and the growth plate is obliterated.

Bones are covered, except at their articular ends, by a membrane called the *periosteum* (see Fig. 42-2A). The periosteum consists of an outer layer of connective tissue

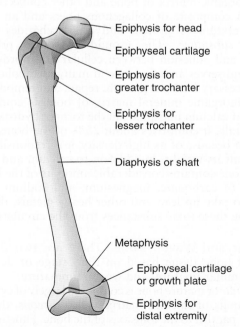

FIGURE 42-3. A femur, showing epiphyseal cartilages for the head, metaphysis, trochanters, and distal end of the bone.

and an inner, more cellular layer of osteoprogenitor cells which can differentiate into osteoblasts (bone-forming cells, to be discussed). The periosteum contains blood vessels and acts as an anchorage point for blood vessels as they enter and leave the bone. The *endosteum* is the membrane that lines the spaces of spongy bone, the marrow cavities, and the haversian canals of compact bone. It is considerably thinner than the periosteum and is composed of a single layer of flattened osteoprogenitor cells and small amounts of connective tissue. The principal functions of the periosteum and endosteum are the nutrition of bone tissue and continuous supply of new osteoblasts for repair and growth of bone.

Bone marrow occupies the medullary cavities of the long bones (see Fig. 42-2C) throughout the skeleton and the cavities of spongy bone in the vertebrae, ribs, sternum, and flat bones of the pelvis. The cellular composition of the bone marrow varies with age and skeletal location. Red bone marrow contains developing red blood cells and is the site of blood cell formation. Yellow bone marrow is composed largely of adipose cells. At birth, nearly all of the marrow is red and hematopoietically active. As the need for red blood cell production decreases during postnatal life, red marrow is gradually replaced with yellow bone marrow in most of the bones. In the adult, red marrow persists in the vertebrae, ribs, sternum, and ilia.

Bone Tissue

Bone, or *osseous*, tissue is perhaps one of the most distinctive tissues in the body. It is typical of other connective tissue in that it consists of cells, fibers, and an extracellular matrix. However, its extracellular components are hard and calcified, a feature that enables it to serve both supportive and protective functions. The extracellular bone matrix can be divided into two parts: the organic matrix and inorganic mineral matrix.

The organic matrix of bone and other connective tissues is a composite of collagenous fibers and an amorphous mixture of protein and polysaccharides called *ground substance*. The ground substance provides support and adhesion between cellular and fibrous elements and serves an active role in many metabolic functions necessary for bone growth, repair, and remodeling.

The inorganic mineral matrix of bone is composed largely of calcium phosphate in the form of hydroxyapatite crystals. It comprises about 25% of the bones' volume, but because of its high density, it is responsible for about half its weight. In addition to calcium and phosphate, bone contains considerable amounts of the body's content of carbonate, magnesium, and sodium. Bone may also take up lead and other heavy metals, thereby removing these toxic substances from the circulation.

Laminar and Woven Bone. There are two distinct types of bone tissue based on their stage of development: laminar (mature) and woven (immature).

Laminar or mature bone is composed largely of cylinder-shaped units of calcified matrix, called *osteons*, that are oriented parallel to the long axis of the bone. Functionally, osteons can be thought of as tiny weight-bearing pillars.

Running through the core of each osteon is a central canal, called a *haversian canal*, which contains the blood vessels and nerves that supply the osteon (Fig. 42-4A). Canals of a second type called *perforating*, or *Volkmann canals*, lie at right angles to the long axis of the bone, connecting the vascular and nerve supplies of the periosteum and medullary cavity. Spider-shaped osteocytes (mature bone cells) occupy small cavities, or *lacunae*, at the junctions of the lamellae (Fig. 42-4B). In compact bone (e.g., diaphysis of long bones), the lamellae exhibit a characteristic organization of outer circumferential lamellae, inner circumferential lamellae, and interstitial lamellae. *The outer circumferential lamellae* are located just beneath the periosteum and the *inner circumferential lamellae* are arranged concentrically around a central haversian canal. Between the two circumferential lamellae are the irregularly shaped *interstitial lamellae*. These are the remnants of haversian systems that have been destroyed during bone growth or remodeling. *Trabecular lamellar bone* forms the coarse spongy bone of the medullary cavity. It exhibits plates of lamellar bone perforated by marrow spaces.

In contrast to compact bone, *immature or woven bone*, consisting of trabeculae, looks like poorly organized bone. It is deposited more rapidly than lamellar bone, has low tensile strength, and serves as temporary scaffolding for support. It is found in the developing fetus, in areas surrounding tumors and infections, and as part of a healing fracture.

Blood Supply

Bones are richly supplied with blood from nutrient and perforating arteries (see Fig. 42-2C). The nutrient arteries enter the bone through a nutrient foramen and supply the marrow space and the internal half of the cortex. The perforating arteries are small arteries that extend inward from the periosteal arteries on the external surface of the periosteum and anastomose in the cortex with branches of the nutrient arteries coming from the bone marrow. The distribution of blood in the cortex occurs through the haversian and Volkmann canals (see Fig. 42-4A). Veins accompany arteries through the nutrient formania. Many large veins also leave through openings near the articulating ends of bones. Bones containing red bone marrow have numerous large veins.

Bone Cells

Five types of cells participate in the formation and maintenance of bone tissue: osteoprogenitor cells, osteoblasts, osteocytes, osteoclasts, and bone-lining cells (Table 42-1). With the exception of the osteoclast, each type of bone cell originates from the same basic cell type, undergoing transformation as it matures.

Osteoprogenitor Cells. Osteoprogenitor cells are undifferentiated or resting cells that are found in the periosteum, endosteum, and epiphyseal plate of growing bone. Derived from stem cells in the bone marrow, they have the potential to differentiate into many different cell types, including adipocytes, fibroblasts, and osteoblasts.

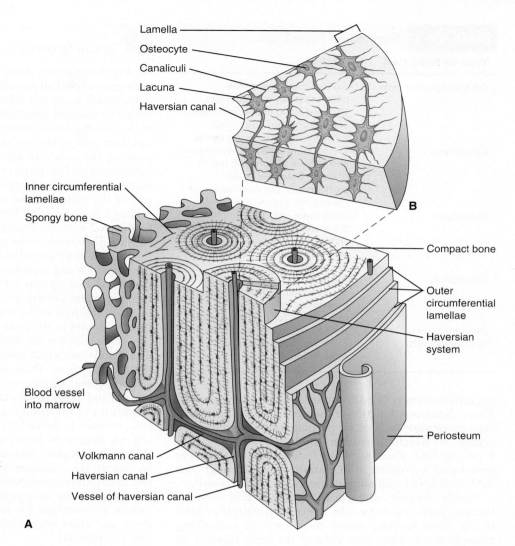

Lamella
Osteocyte
Canaliculi
Lacuna
Haversian canal

B

Inner circumferential lamellae
Spongy bone

Compact bone

Outer circumferential lamellae

Haversian system

Blood vessel into marrow

Periosteum

Volkmann canal
Haversian canal
Vessel of haversian canal

FIGURE 42-4. (A) Haversian systems as seen in a wedge of compact bone tissue. The periosteum has been peeled back to show a blood vessel entering a Volkmann canal. **(B)** Osteocytes lying within lacunae; canaliculi permit interstitial fluid to reach each lacuna.

A

When appropriately stimulated by bone morphogenic proteins (BMPs) and transforming growth factors, they undergo cell division and differentiate into osteoblasts.

Osteoblasts. Osteoblasts are cells that secrete bone matrix. Bone formation occurs in two stages: ossification and calcification. Ossification involves the formation of the initial unmineralized bone, or osteoid (also called prebone). Osteoblasts secrete both type I collagen (which constitutes 90% of the protein of bone) and bone matrix proteins, forming the osteoid. They also are responsible for calcification of the bone matrix. The calcification process appears to be initiated by the osteoblast through the secretion of the enzyme *alkaline phosphatase*, which is thought to act locally in bone tissue to raise calcium and phosphate levels to the point at which precipitation occurs. The activity of the osteoblasts undoubtedly contributes to the increase in serum levels of alkaline phosphatase that follows bone injury and fractures.

Osteocytes. Osteocytes are mature bone cells, derived from osteoblasts, which are housed in *lacunae* within the calcified bony matrix (see Fig. 42-4B). Extracellular

fluid-filled passageways permeate the calcified matrix and connect with the lacunae of adjacent osteocytes. These passageways are called *canaliculi*. Because diffusion does not occur through the calcified matrix of bone, the canaliculi serve as communicating channels for the exchange of nutrients and metabolites between the osteocytes and the blood vessels on the surface of the bone layer.

Osteocytes are the cells responsible for maintaining the bone matrix. They can synthesize new matrix, as well as participate in matrix degradation. Death of osteocytes through trauma, cell senescence, or apoptosis, results in resorption of the bone matrix by osteoclasts, followed by repair or remodeling of the bone tissue by osteoblasts.

Osteoclasts. Osteoclasts are large multinucleated "bone-chewing" cells that function in the resorption of bone, removing its mineral content and organic matrix. They are derived from the same mononuclear hematopoietic progenitor cells that give rise to blood monocytes and tissue macrophages. Osteoclast formation occurs in close association with the stromal cells of the bone marrow. These cells secrete essential cytokines that promote

TABLE 42-1	Function of Bone Cells
Type of Bone Cell	**Function**
Osteoprogenitor cells	Undifferentiated cells that differentiate into osteoblasts. They are found in the periosteum, endosteum, and epiphyseal growth plate of growing bones.
Osteoblasts	Bone-building cells that synthesize and secrete the organic matrix of bone. Osteoblasts also participate in the calcification of the organic matrix.
Osteocytes	Mature bone cells that function in the maintenance of bone matrix. Osteocytes also play an active role in releasing calcium into the blood.
Osteoclasts	Bone cells originating from mononuclear hematopoietic progenitor cells that are responsible for bone resorption.
Bone-lining cells (periosteal cells)	Cells derived from osteoblasts and cover bone that is not remodeling.

the differentiation of both osteoclasts and macrophages. These cytokines function either by stimulating osteoclast progenitor cells or by participating in a paracrine system in which osteoblasts and marrow cells play a central role. Recent studies indicate that substances promoting osteoclast differentiation act through the RANK–RANKL signaling pathway (to be discussed).

Newly formed osteoclasts undergo activation to become bone-resorbing cells. Once activated, they bind to the bone surface, where they form an underlying resorption pit. They then remove the bone mineral by generating an acidic environment and digest the organic bone matrix by releasing proteolytic enzymes.

Bone-Lining Cells. Bone-lining cells cover bone at sites where remodeling is not occurring. They are flat cells with an enlarged cytoplasm and a limited number of organelles. Bone-lining cells on external bone surfaces are called *periosteal cells*, and those lining the internal bone surfaces, *endosteal cells*. They represent a population of cells that are derived from osteoblasts and are thought to function in the maintenance and nutritional support of the osteocytes embedded in the underlying bone matrix and in the regulation of calcium and phosphate movement into and out of bone.

Bone Formation, Growth, and Remodeling

The development of skeletal structures begins in utero and continues to change throughout life. During childhood, skeletal structures grow in length and diameter, resulting in a bone having adult form and shape. Once skeletal growth has ceased, the process of bone *remodeling* is responsible for skeletal maintenance.

 ## Bone Growth in Childhood

During the first two decades of life, the skeleton undergoes general overall growth. The long bones of the skeleton, which grow at a relatively rapid rate, are provided with a specialized structure called the *epiphyseal growth plate*. As long bones grow in length, the deeper layers of cartilage cells in the growth plate multiply and enlarge, pushing the articular cartilage farther away from the metaphysis and diaphysis of the bone. As this occurs, the mature and enlarged cartilage cells at the metaphyseal end of the plate become metabolically inactive and are replaced by bone cells. This process allows bone growth to proceed without changing the shape of the bone or causing disruption of the articular cartilage. The cells in the growth plate stop dividing at puberty, at which time the epiphysis and metaphysis fuse.

Several factors can influence the growth of cells in the epiphyseal growth plate. Epiphyseal separation can occur in children as the result of trauma. The separation usually occurs in the zone of the mature enlarged cartilage cells, which is the weakest part of the growth plate. The blood vessels that nourish the epiphysis pass through the growth plate. These vessels are ruptured when the growth plate separates. This can cause cessation of growth and a shortened extremity. The growth plate also is sensitive to nutritional and metabolic changes. Scurvy (i.e., vitamin C deficiency) impairs the formation of the organic matrix of bone, causing slowing of growth at the epiphyseal plate and cessation of diaphyseal growth. In rickets (i.e., vitamin D deficiency), calcification of the newly developed bone on the metaphyseal side of the growth plate is impaired. Thyroid and growth hormones are required for normal growth. Alterations in these and other hormones can also affect bone growth (see Chapter 31).

Growth in the diameter of bones occurs as new bone is added to the outer surface of existing bone along with an accompanying resorption of bone on the endosteal or inner surface. Such oppositional growth allows for widening of the marrow cavity while preventing the cortex from becoming too thick and heavy. In this way, the shape of the bone is maintained. As a bone grows in diameter, concentric rings are added to the bone surface, much as rings are added to a tree trunk. These rings form the lamellar structure of mature bone. Osteocytes, which develop from osteoblasts, become buried in the rings.

Bone Remodeling

Peak bone mass is achieved during early adulthood. It is determined by a number of factors, including the type of vitamin D receptor inherited, nutrition, level of physical activity, age, and hormonal status. Once skeletal growth has attained its adult size, the breakdown and renewal of bone that is responsible for skeletal maintenance is initiated at sites that require replacement or repair. This process is called *bone remodeling*.

In bone remodeling, the processes of bone formation and resorption are tightly coupled, and their balance determines skeletal mass at any given time. The sequence of bone resorption and bone formation begins with osteoclastic resorption of existing bone, during which the organic (protein matrix) and the inorganic (mineral) components are removed. The sequence proceeds to the formation of new bone by osteoblasts. In the adult, the length of one sequence (i.e., bone resorption and formation) is approximately 4 months. Ideally, the replaced bone should equal the absorbed bone. If it does not, there is a net loss of bone. In the elderly, for example, bone resorption and formation no longer are perfectly coupled, and bone mass is lost.

Recently, significant progress has been made in understanding the phenomenon of bone remodeling as it relates to the coupling of bone resorption with bone formation. The pivotal paracrine pathway linking these two processes consists of three factors: RANKL (for *r*eceptor *a*ctivator of *n*uclear factor-κB *l*egend); its receptor, RANK; and a soluble inhibitor receptor for RANKL called *osteoprotegerin* (OPG). RANKL is expressed by osteoblasts and their immature precursors and is necessary for osteoclast differentiation and function. RANKL activates its receptor, RANK, which is expressed on osteoclasts and their precursors, thus promoting osteoclast differentiation and activation and prolonging osteoclast survival by suppressing apoptosis. The fact that RANKL is expressed on osteoblasts indicates that bone resorption and bone formation are linked through RANKL. The effects of RANKL are blocked by OPG, a soluble receptor protein, which acts as a decoy receptor that binds RANKL and prevents it from binding with RANK on osteoclasts.

It is now believed that dysregulation of the RANKL/RANK/OPG pathway plays a prominent role in the pathogenesis of bone diseases such as osteoporosis (low bone density). For example, it has been shown that postmenopausal women express higher levels of RANKL on their marrow stromal cells and lymphocytes than premenopausal women or postmenopausal women taking estrogen. It has also been shown that estrogens and the selective estrogen receptor modulator, raloxifene, stimulate OPG production in osteoblasts. Glucocorticoid exposure, which can contribute to steroid osteoporosis, enhances RANKL expression and suppresses OPG levels, thus elevating the RANKL-to-OPG ratio. There is also evidence linking the pathogenesis of inflammatory conditions such as rheumatoid arthritis to dysregulation of the RANKL/OPG system.

Hormonal Control of Bone Formation and Metabolism

The process of bone formation and mineral metabolism is complex. It involves the interplay among the actions of parathyroid hormone (PTH), calcitonin, and vitamin D (Table 42-2). Other hormones, such as corticosteroid hormone, growth hormone, thyroid hormone, and the sex hormones, also influence bone formation directly or indirectly.

Parathyroid Hormone. Parathyroid hormone, which is produced by the parathyroid glands embedded in the thyroid gland, is one of the important regulators of calcium and phosphate levels in the blood. Parathyroid hormone prevents serum calcium levels from falling below and serum phosphate levels from rising above normal physiologic concentrations (see Chapter 8). The secretion of PTH is regulated through negative feedback related to serum levels of ionized calcium, with decreased levels stimulating PTH release and increased levels inhibiting its release.

Parathyroid hormone maintains serum calcium levels by promoting bone resorption, conserving calcium by the kidney, enhancing intestinal absorption of calcium through activation of vitamin D, and reducing serum phosphate levels (Fig. 42-5). Parathyroid hormone also increases the movement of calcium and phosphate from bone into the extracellular fluid. In the kidney, PTH stimulates tubular reabsorption of calcium while reducing the reabsorption of phosphate. The latter effect ensures that the increased release of phosphate from bone during mobilization of calcium does not produce an elevation in serum phosphate levels. This is important because an increase in calcium and phosphate levels could lead to crystallization in soft tissues. Parathyroid hormone also stimulates the activation of vitamin D by the kidney, thereby increasing the absorption of calcium from the intestine.

(*text continues on page 1072*)

TABLE 42-2   Actions of Parathyroid Hormone, Calcitonin, and Vitamin D

Actions	Parathyroid Hormone	Calcitonin	Vitamin D
Intestinal absorption of calcium	Increases indirectly through increased activation of vitamin D	Probably has no effect	Increases
Intestinal absorption of phosphate	Increases	Probably has no effect	Increases
Renal excretion of calcium	Decreases	Minor effect	Probably increases, but less effect than PTH
Renal excretion of phosphate	Increases	Minor effect	Increases
Bone resorption	Increases	Decreases	$1,25\text{-}(OH)_2D_3$ increases
Bone formation	Decreases	Uncertain	$24,25\text{-}(OH)_2D_3$ increases
Serum calcium levels	Produces a prompt increase	Decreases with pharmacologic doses	No effect
Serum phosphate levels	Prevents an increase	Decreases with pharmacologic doses	No effect

UNDERSTANDING ➡ Bone Remodeling

Bone remodeling constitutes a process of skeletal maintenance once skeletal growth is complete. It takes place in the (1) osteons of mature bone and consists of a cycle of (2) bone resorption by osteoclasts, (3) followed by bone formation by osteoblasts. Bone remodeling is (4) controlled by cytokines and growth factors that interact with a paracrine system consisting of the RANK ligand (RANKL), the RANK receptor, and osteoprotegerin.

1 **Bone Remodeling Cycle.** Mature bone is made up of osteons or units of concentric lamellae (bone layers) and the haversian canal they surround. Bone remodeling consists of a sequence of bone resorption within an osteon by osteoclasts, followed by new bone formation by osteoblasts. In the adult, the length of one sequence (i.e., bone resorption and formation) is approximately 4 months. Ideally, the replaced bone should equal the resorbed bone. If it does not, there is net loss of bone. In the elderly, for example, bone resorption and formation no longer are perfectly coupled, and bone mass is lost.

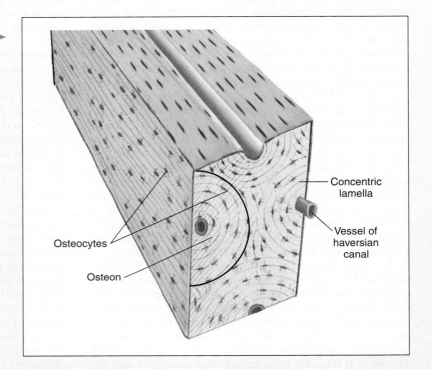

Concentric lamella

Vessel of haversian canal

Osteocytes

Osteon

2 **Bone Resorption.** The osteoclasts, which are bone-resorbing cells derived from monocyte/macrophage precursors, are the cells involved in the initiation of bone remodeling. The sequence of bone resorption and bone formation is activated by many stimuli, including the action of parathyroid hormone and calcitonin. It begins with osteoclastic resorption of existing bone, during which the organic (protein matrix) and inorganic (mineral) components are removed, creating a tunnel-like space in the osteon. Soluble factors released during resorption aid in the recruitment of osteoblasts to the site, thereby linking bone resorption to bone formation.

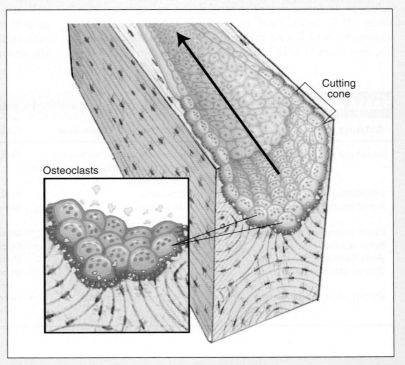

Cutting cone

Osteoclasts

3

Bone Formation. After osteoclastic activity has ceased, osteoblasts begin to deposit the organic matrix (osteoid) on the wall of the osteon canal. As successive lamellae of bone are deposited, the canal ultimately attains the relative proportions of the original osteon. In the formation and maintenance of bone, osteoblasts provide much of the local control because not only do they produce new bone matrix, they play an essential role in mediating osteoclast activity. Many of the primary stimulators of bone resorption, such as parathyroid hormone, have minimal or no direct effects on osteoclasts. Once the osteoblast, which has receptors for these substances, receives the appropriate signal, it releases a soluble mediator called *RANKL* that induces osteoclast activity.

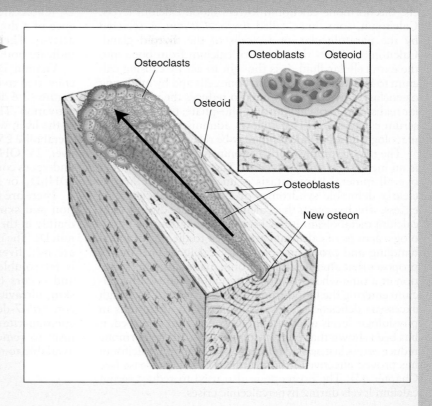

4

Control of Bone Metabolism and Remodeling. The pivotal pathway linking osteoclast-mediated bone resorption with osteoblast-mediated bone formation consists of a paracrine system that includes RANKL, its receptor RANK, and a soluble protein called *osteoprotegerin* (OPG). RANKL, which is produced by osteoblasts and their precursors, binds to RANK, promoting osteoclast differentiation and proliferation. The soluble OPG molecule, which is produced by a number of tissues, acts as a decoy receptor to block the action of RANKL. This system ensures the tight coupling of bone formation and resorption, and provides a means whereby a wide variety of biologic mediators (e.g., hormones, cytokines, growth factors) influence the homeostasis of bone.

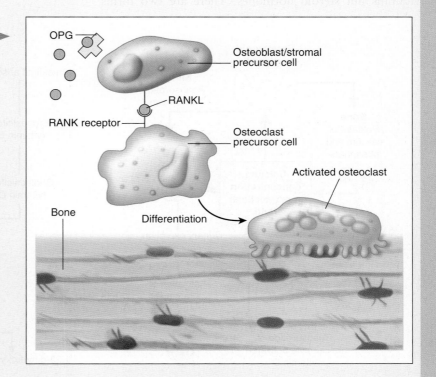

(text continued from page 1069)

Calcitonin. Whereas PTH increases blood calcium levels, the hormone calcitonin lowers blood calcium levels. Calcitonin, sometimes called *thyrocalcitonin*, is secreted by the parafollicular, or C, cells of the thyroid gland. Calcitonin inhibits the release of calcium from bone into the extracellular fluid. It is thought to act by causing calcium to become sequestered in bone cells and by inhibiting osteoclast activity. Calcitonin also reduces the renal tubular reabsorption of calcium and phosphate; the decrease in serum calcium level that follows administration of pharmacologic doses of calcitonin may be related to this action.

The major stimulus for calcitonin synthesis and release is an increase in serum calcium. The role of calcitonin in overall mineral homeostasis is uncertain. There are no clearly definable syndromes of calcitonin deficiency or excess, which suggests that calcitonin does not directly alter calcium metabolism. It has been suggested that the physiologic actions of calcitonin are related to the postprandial handling and processing of dietary calcium. This theory proposes that after meals, calcitonin maintains PTH secretion at a time when it normally would be reduced by calcium entering the blood from the digestive tract. Although excess or deficiency states associated with alterations in physiologic levels of calcitonin have not been observed, it has been shown that pharmacologic doses of the hormone reduce osteoclast activity. Because of this action, calcitonin has proved effective in the treatment of Paget disease (see Chapter 45). The hormone is also used to reduce serum calcium levels during hypercalcemic crises.

Vitamin D. Vitamin D and its metabolites are not true vitamins but steroid hormones. There are two forms of vitamin D: vitamin D_2 (ergocalciferol) and vitamin D_3 (cholecalciferol). The two forms differ by the presence of a double bond, but they have identical biologic activity. Therefore, the term *vitamin D* is often used to indicate both forms.

Vitamin D has little or no activity until it has been converted to its physiologically active form by the kidney. Figure 42-6 depicts sources of vitamin D and pathways for activation. The first step of the activation process occurs in the liver, where vitamin D is hydroxylated to form the metabolite 25-hydroxyvitamin D_3 [25-$(OH)D_3$]. From the liver, 25-$(OH)D_3$ is transported to the kidneys, where it undergoes conversion to 1,25-dihydroxyvitamin D_3 [1,25-$(OH)_2D_3$] or 24,25 hydroxyvitamin D_3 [24,25-$(OH)D_3$].

There are two sources of vitamin D: intestinal absorption and skin production. Intestinal absorption occurs mainly in the jejunum and includes vitamin D_2 and vitamin D_3. The most important dietary sources of vitamin D are fish, liver, and irradiated milk. Because vitamin D is fat soluble, its absorption is mediated by bile salts and occurs by means of the lymphatic vessels. In the skin, ultraviolet radiation from sunlight spontaneously converts 7-dehydrocholesterol D_3 to vitamin D_3. A circulating vitamin D–binding protein provides a mechanism to remove vitamin D from the skin and make it available to the rest of the body.

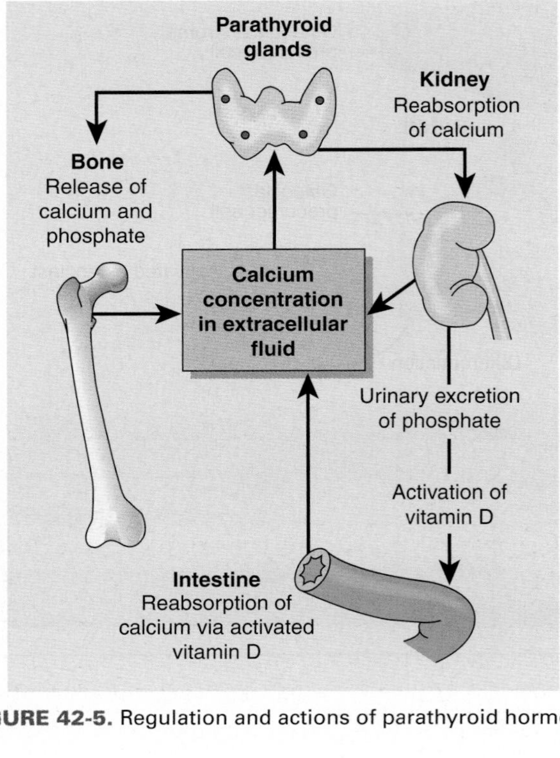

FIGURE 42-5. Regulation and actions of parathyroid hormone.

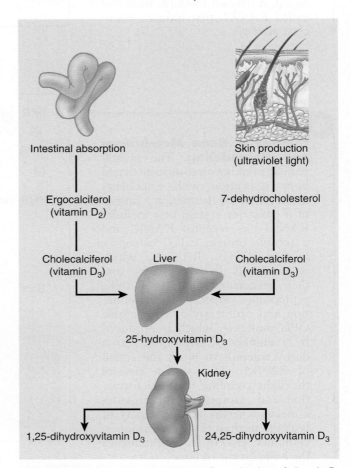

FIGURE 42-6. Sources and pathways for activation of vitamin D.

With adequate exposure to sunlight, the amount of vitamin D that can be produced by the skin is usually sufficient to meet physiologic requirements. Modern conditions of dress, lifestyle, and recommendations regarding sun screens and avoidance of sun exposure to reduce skin cancer risk may prevent a large proportion of the population from producing adequate amounts of vitamin D. Elderly persons who are housebound or institutionalized frequently have low vitamin D levels. The deficiency often goes undetected until there are problems such as pseudofractures or electrolyte imbalances. Seasonal variations in vitamin D levels probably reflect changes in sunlight exposure.

The most potent of the vitamin D metabolites is $1,25\text{-}(OH)_2D_3$. This metabolite increases intestinal absorption of calcium and promotes the actions of PTH on resorption of calcium and phosphate from bone. Bone resorption by the osteoclasts is increased and bone formation by the osteoblasts is decreased; there is also an increase in acid phosphatase and a decrease in alkaline phosphatase. Intestinal absorption and bone resorption increase the amount of calcium and phosphorus available to the mineralizing surface of the bone. The role of $24,25\text{-}(OH)_2D_3$ is less clear. There is evidence that $24,25\text{-}(OH)_2D_3$ in conjunction with $1,25\text{-}(OH)_2D_3$ may be involved in normal bone mineralization.

The regulation of vitamin D activity is influenced by several hormones. PTH and prolactin stimulate $1,25\text{-}(OH)_2D_3$ production by the kidney. States of hyperparathyroidism are associated with increased levels of $1,25\text{-}(OH)_2D_3$, and hypoparathyroidism leads to lowered levels of this metabolite. Prolactin may have an ancillary role in regulating vitamin D metabolism during pregnancy and lactation. Calcitonin inhibits $1,25\text{-}(OH)_2D_3$ production by the kidney. In addition to hormonal influences, changes in the concentration of ions such as calcium, phosphate, hydrogen, and potassium exert an effect on $1,25\text{-}(OH)_2D_3$ and $24,25\text{-}(OH)_2D_3$ production. Under conditions of phosphate and calcium deprivation, $1,25\text{-}(OH)_2D_3$ levels are increased, whereas hyperphosphatemia and hypercalcemia decrease the levels of metabolite.

SUMMARY CONCEPTS

- The skeletal system consists of the bones of the skull, thorax, and vertebral column, which form the axial skeleton, and the bones of the upper and lower extremities, which form the appendicular skeleton.

- Two types of connective tissue are found in the skeletal system: (1) cartilage, a semirigid and slightly flexible tissue that plays an essential role in prenatal and childhood development of the skeleton and serves as a surface for the articulating ends of skeletal joints; and (2) bone, which provides the firm structure of the skeleton and serves as a reservoir for calcium and phosphate storage.

- Bone tissue is classified as either spongy or compact according to the relative amount of solid matter and number and size of the spaces they contain. *Spongy* bone, which forms the interior of bones, is composed of spicules or trabeculae that form a latticelike pattern. *Compact bone*, which forms the outer shell of a bone, has a densely calcified intercellular matrix that makes it more rigid than spongy bone.

- Bone matrix is maintained by five types of cells: osteoprogenitor cells, which are resting cells that differentiate into osteoblasts; osteoblasts, which function as bone-building cells during bone remodeling; osteocytes, or mature bone cells; osteoclasts, which function as bone resorption cells during bone remodeling; and bone-lining cells, which cover the outer and inner surfaces of bone where remodeling is not occurring.

- The process of bone formation and mineral metabolism involves the interplay among the actions of parathyroid hormone (PTH), calcitonin, and vitamin D. PTH acts to maintain serum levels of ionized calcium by increasing the release of calcium and phosphate from bone, conserving calcium and increasing phosphate elimination by the kidney, and enhancing intestinal reabsorption of calcium through vitamin D. Calcitonin inhibits the release of calcium from bone and increases renal elimination of calcium and phosphate, thereby serving to lower serum calcium levels. Vitamin D, which functions as a hormone in regulating body calcium, increases absorption of calcium from the intestine and promotes the actions of PTH on bone.

Joints

Joints, or articulations, are places where adjacent bones or cartilages meet. Joints vary in the type and extent of movements they allow. Some joints have no movement; others allow only slight movement; and some such as the shoulder joint are freely moveable. There are three classes of joints based on their structure and function: fibrous (synarthroses), cartilaginous (amphiarthoses), and synovial (diarthroses).

Fibrous Joints (Synarthroses)

Fibrous joints, or synarthroses, are joints in which the bones are joined by dense fibrous tissue. They have little or no movement, depending on the length of the fibers connecting the articulating bone. The sutures of the skull are examples of fibrous joints. In children and young adults the bones of the skull are joined by dense connective tissue; and in older persons, by bone. Another type of fibrous joint that is partially moveable unites bones with a sheet of fibrous tissue, either a ligament or fibrous membrane. The interosseous membrane that joins the radius and the ulna of the forearm is an example of this type of joint. A unique type of fibrous joint is the one between the root of a tooth and the alveolar processes of the jaw. The fibrous tissue between the tooth and alveolar bone of the tooth socket is called the periodental ligament.

Cartilaginous Joints (Amphiarthoses)

Cartilaginous joints, or amphiarthroses, are connected by hyaline cartilage or fibrocartilage and have limited motion. In primary cartilaginous joints, the bones are joined by hyaline cartilage, which permits slight bending during early childhood. Primary cartilaginous joints are usually temporary articulations, such as those present during early development, where the epiphysis and the shaft are joined by cartilage or growth plate. Secondary cartilaginous joints are strong, slightly moveable joints united by fibrocartilage. The fibrocartilaginous intervertebral disks between the vertebrae consist of connective tissue that holds the vertebrae together. These joints provide strength and shock absorption as well as considerable flexibility.

Synovial Joints (Diarthroses)

Synovial joints, or *diarthroses*, are freely moveable joints in which the articulating bone ends are separated by a joint cavity containing synovial fluid. Most joints in the body are of this type. Although as a group they are classified as freely moveable, synovial joints include planar joints, which allow almost no movement (e.g., vertebrocostal joint), and hinge joints, which allow angular movement in one plane (e.g., interphalangeal, knee, and ankle joints). Only the *ball-and-socket joints* permit movement in all directions (e.g., shoulder and hip joint).

All synovial joints are covered with articular cartilage, a feature that allows the surfaces of these joints to slide freely past each other during movement. The articular cartilage, which is typically hyaline cartilage, is unique in that its free surface is not covered with perichondrium. It has only a peripheral rim of perichondrium, and calcification of the portion of cartilage abutting the bone may limit or preclude diffusion from blood vessels supplying the subchondral bone. Regeneration of most cartilage is slow; it is accomplished primarily by growth that requires the activity of perichondrium cells.

In synovial joints, the articulating ends of the bones are not connected directly but are indirectly linked by a strong fibrous capsule (i.e., joint capsule) that surrounds the joint and is continuous with the periosteum

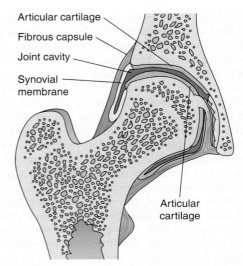

FIGURE 42-7. Synovial (diarthrodial) joint, showing the articular cartilage, fibrous joint capsule, joint cavity, and synovial membrane.

(Fig. 42-7). The joint capsule consists of two layers: an outer fibrous layer and an inner synovial membrane. The outer fibrous layer of the capsule supports the joint and helps to hold the bones in place. Additional support is provided by ligaments that extend between the bones and by tendons that attach to muscles supplying the joint. The synovium secretes a slippery fluid with the consistency of egg white called *synovial fluid*. In addition to supplying nutrients and oxygen to the chondrocytes in the articular cartilage, this fluid serves as a lubricant for the joint. Moreover, macrophages in the synovial fluid act to phagocytize debris in the joint space.

The collagen fibers in the articular surface cartilage are arranged to evenly distribute the forces generated by pressure to this tissue. The proteoglycan molecules of the cartilage, found isolated or aggregated in a network, contain large amounts of water. These matrix components, rich in hydrophylic glycosaminoglycans, function as a mechanical spring. When pressure is applied, water is forced out of the cartilage matrix into the synovial fluid. When the pressure is released, water is attracted back into the collagen matrix. These water movements, which are brought about by the use of a joint, are essential for the delivery of nutrients and the exchange of carbon dioxide, oxygen, and other molecules between the synovial fluid and articular cartilage.

Ligaments and Tendons

Ligaments and tendons are dense connective tissue structures that connect muscles and bone and support synovial joint structures. The dense connective tissue found in tendons and ligaments has a limited blood supply and is composed largely of intercellular bundles of collagen fibers arranged in the same direction and plane. Collagen is an inelastic and insoluble fibrous protein. Because of its molecular configuration, collagen has great tensile strength; the breaking point of collagenous fibers found in human tendons is reached with a force of several hundred kilograms per square centimeter.

Ligaments are fibrous thickenings of the articular capsule that join one bone to its articulating mate. They vary in size and shape depending on their specific role. Although most ligaments are considered inelastic, they are pliable enough to permit movement at the joints. However, ligaments tear rather than stretch when exposed to excess stress. Torn ligaments are extremely painful and accompanied by local swelling.

Tendons, which attach skeletal muscles to bone, are relatively inextensible because of their richness in collagen fibers. The intercellular bands of collagen fibers aggregate into bundles that are enveloped by loose connective tissue, blood vessels, and nerves. Tendons that may rub against bone or other friction-generating surfaces are enclosed in double-layered sheaths. An outer connective tissue tube is attached to the structures surrounding the tendon, and an inner sheath encloses the tendon and is attached to it. The space between the inner and outer sheath is filled with a fluid similar to synovial fluid. Overuse can result in *tendonitis* or inflammation of the tendon.

Joint Vasculature and Innervation

All the tissues of synovial joints, except the surfaces of the articulating cartilage, receive nourishment either directly or indirectly from blood vessels. The articulating areas are nourished indirectly by the synovial fluid that is distributed over the surface of the articular cartilage.

The blood supply to a joint arises from blood vessels that enter the subchondral bone at or near the attachment of the joint capsule and form an arterial circle around the joint. The synovial membrane has a rich blood supply, and constituents of plasma diffuse rapidly between these vessels and the joint cavity. Because many of the capillaries are near the surface of the synovium, blood may escape into the synovial fluid after relatively minor injuries. Healing and repair of the synovial membrane usually are rapid and complete. This is important because synovial tissue is injured in many surgical procedures that involve the joint.

The nerve supply to joints is provided by the same nerve trunks that supply the muscles that move the joints. These nerve trunks also supply the skin over the joints. As a rule, all the joints of an extremity are innervated by the same peripheral nerves as they travel down an extremity. This helps to explain the referral of pain from one joint to another. For example, hip pain may be perceived as pain in the knee.

The synovial membrane is innervated only by autonomic nerve fibers that control blood flow. It is relatively free of pain fibers, as evidenced by the fact that surgical procedures on the joint are often done under local anesthesia. The joint capsule and the ligaments have pain receptors; these receptors are more easily stimulated by stretching and twisting than are other joint structures. Pain arising from the capsule tends to be diffuse and poorly localized.

The tendons and ligaments of the joint capsule are sensitive to position and movement, particularly stretching and twisting. These structures are supplied by the large sensory nerve fibers that form proprioceptor endings for the deep tendon reflex (see Chapter 36). The proprioceptors function reflexively to adjust the tension of the muscles that support the joint and are particularly important in maintaining muscular support for the joint. For example, when a weight is lifted, there is a proprioceptor-mediated reflex contraction and relaxation of appropriate muscle groups to support the joint and protect the joint capsule and other joint structures. Loss of proprioception and reflex control of muscular support leads to destructive changes in the joint.

Bursae and Tendon Sheaths

In some synovial joints, the synovial membrane forms a closed sac that is not part of the joint. These sacs, called *bursae*, contain synovial fluid. Their purpose is to prevent friction on a tendon. Bursae occur in areas such as the knee where pressure is exerted because of close approximation of joint structures (Fig. 42-8).

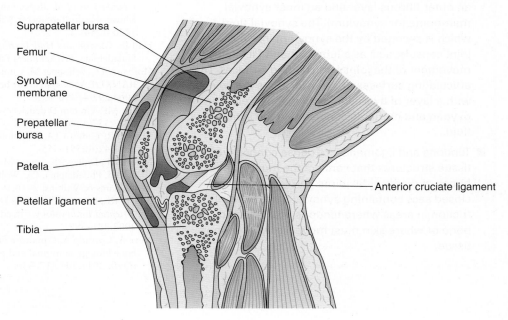

Suprapatellar bursa
Femur
Synovial membrane
Prepatellar bursa
Patella
Patellar ligament
Tibia
Anterior cruciate ligament

FIGURE 42-8. Sagittal section of knee joint, showing prepatellar and suprapatellar bursa.

Such conditions occur when tendons are deflected over bone or where skin must move freely over bony tissue. Bursae may become injured or inflamed, causing discomfort, swelling, and limitation in movement of the involved area.

In addition to bursae, structures called *tendon sheaths* also reduce friction at joints. Tendon sheaths are tubelike bursae that wrap around tendons where there is considerable friction. This occurs where tendons pass through synovial cavities, such as the tendon of the biceps brachi muscle at the shoulder joint. Similar areas of friction are found at the wrist and ankle, where many tendons come together in a confined space and may be torn as the result of an injury (see Chapter 44).

SUMMARY CONCEPTS

■ Joints (or articulations) are areas where two or more bones are joined together by fibrous tissue, cartilage, or bone. In fibrous joints, or synarthroses, such as those of the skull, the bones are joined by fibrous tissue. In cartilaginous joints, or amphiarthoses, bones are jointed by hyaline cartilage (as in the epiphyseal plate during childhood and early adolescence). In fibrocartilaginous joints (as in those that join the vertebrae and intervertebral disks) the articular surface is covered with hyaline cartilage, which in turn is fused to an intervening pad of fibrocartilage.

■ Synovial joints or diarthroses are freely moveable joints in which the surfaces of the articulating ends of bones are enclosed in a fibrous joint capsule. The joint capsule consists of two layers: an outer fibrous layer and an inner synovial membrane (or synovium). The synovial fluid, which is secreted by the synovium into the joint capsule, acts as a lubricant and facilitates movement of the joint's articulating surfaces. The articulating surfaces of synovial joints are covered with a layer of avascular cartilage that relies on oxygen and nutrients contained in the synovial fluid.

■ Tendons and ligaments are dense connective tissue structures that connect the muscles and bones of diarthroidal joints. Bursae, which are closed sacs containing synovial fluid, prevent friction in areas where tendons are deflected over bone or where skin must move freely over bony tissue.

REVIEW EXERCISES

1. Hyaline cartilage degenerates when the chondrocytes become metabolically inactive and die, causing the matrix to calcify and be replaced by bone.

   A. Explain how this process can contribute to normal skeletal growth during childhood and adolescence, but cause joint pain and immobility when it occurs during adulthood.

2. Persons with end-stage kidney disease have a deficiency of activated vitamin D.

   A. Explain why this occurs, and what effect it would have on the persons' bones.
   B. How might this deficiency be treated?

3. Recent studies have revealed that estrogen deficiency as well as normal aging may produce a decrease in osteoblast activity.

   A. Explain how this would contribute to a disruption in bone remodeling and the development of osteoporosis.

4. Often pain from injury to the knee is experienced as pain in the hip.

   A. Explain why this might occur.

BIBLIOGRAPHY

Cohen S. Role of RANK ligand in normal and pathologic bone remodeling and therapeutic potential of novel inhibitory molecules in musculoskeletal disease. *Arthritis Rheum.* 2006;55(1):15–18.

Garcia RA, Klein MJ, Schiller AL. Bones and joints. In: Rubin R, Strayer DS, eds. *Rubin's Pathology: Clinicopathologic Foundations of Medicine.* 6th ed. Philadelphia, PA: Wolters Kluwer Health/Lippincott Williams & Wilkins; 2012:1199–1218, 1250–1254.

Hall JE. *Guyton and Hall Textbook of Medical Physiology.* 12th ed. Philadelphia, PA: Saunders Elsevier; 2011:955–966.

Hofbauer LC, Schoppet M. Clinical implications of osteoprotegrin/RANKL/RANK system for bone and vascular disease. *JAMA.* 2004;292(4):490–495.

Holick MF. Vitamin D deficiency. *N Engl J Med.* 2007;357(3):266–281.

Marsall R, Einhorn TA. The biology of fracture healing. *Injury.* 2011;42(6):551–555.

Moore KL, Dalley AF, Agur AM. *Clinically Oriented Anatomy.* 6th ed. Philadelphia, PA: Wolters Kluwer Health/Lippincott Williams & Wilkins; 2010:19–29.

Moore KL, Persaud TVN. *The Developing Human: Clinically Oriented Embryology.* 7th ed. Philadelphia, PA: Saunders; 2003:381–399.

Neve A, Corrado A, Cantatore FP. Osteocytes: central conductors of bone biology in normal and pathological conditions. *Acta Physiol (Oxf).* 2011;204:317–330.

Rogers A, Eastell R. Review: circulating osteoprotegerin and receptor activator for nuclear factor κB ligand: clinical utility in metabolic bone disease assessment. *J Clin Endocrinol Metab.* 2005;90:6323–6331.

Rosenberg A. Bones, joints, and soft tissue tumors. In: Kumar V, Abbas AK, Fausto N, et al., eds. *Robbins and Cotran Pathologic Basis of Disease.* 8th ed. Philadelphia, PA: Elsevier Saunders; 2010:1205–1210.

Ross MH, Pawlina W. *Histology.* 6th ed. Philadelphia, PA: Wolters Kluwer Health/Lippincott Williams & Wilkins; 2011:218–232.

Seeman E, Delmas PD. Bone quality—The material and structural basis of bone strength and fragility. *N Engl J Med.* 2006;344(21):2250–2261.

Vega D, Maalouf NM, Sakhaee K. The role of receptor activator of nuclear factor-κB (Rank)/Rank ligand/osteoprotegerin: clinical implications. *J Clin Endocrinol Metab.* 2007;92(12):4514–4521.

Xiong J, O'Brien CA. Osteocyte RANKL: new insights into the control of bone remodeling. *J Bone Miner Res.* 2012;29(3):499–505.

Porth Essentials Resources

Explore these additional resources to enhance learning for this chapter:

- NCLEX-Style Questions and Other Resources on **thePoint**, http://thePoint.lww.com/PorthEssentials4e
- Study Guide for Essentials of Pathophysiology
- Adaptive Learning | Powered by PrepU, http://thepoint.lww.com/prepu

C h a p t e r 43

Disorders of the Skeletal System: Trauma, Infections, Neoplasms, and Childhood Disorders

The musculoskeletal system includes the bones, joints, and muscles of the body together with associated structures such as ligaments and tendons. This system, which constitutes more than 70% of the body, is subject to a large number of disorders causing pain and disability in people of all ages. The main discussion in this chapter focuses on injuries, infections, necrosis, and neoplasms of the musculoskeletal system. At the end of the chapter, disorders of skeletal growth and development in children are discussed.

Injury and Trauma of Musculoskeletal Structures

A broad spectrum of musculoskeletal injuries results from numerous physical forces, including blunt tissue trauma, disruption of tendons and ligaments, and fractures of bony structures. Many of the forces that cause these injuries are typical for a particular age group, activity, or environmental setting.[1] The most common causes of childhood injuries are falls, bicycle-related injuries, and sports injuries. Trauma resulting from motor vehicle accidents is ranked as the number one killer of adults younger than 45 years of age. Falls are the most common cause of injury in people 65 years of age and older, with fractures of the hip and proximal humerus particularly common in this age group.

Sports-Related Injuries

Sports and athletic activities are particularly common causes of acute and overuse injuries of the musculoskeletal system. Acute injuries are caused by sudden trauma and include injuries to soft tissues (contusion, strains, and sprains) and to bone (fractures).

Overuse injuries have been described as chronic injuries, including tendinopathies, stress fractures, compartment syndrome, and shin splints, that result from constant high levels of physiologic stress without sufficient recovery time.[2-4] They commonly occur in the elbow ("little league elbow" or "tennis elbow") and in tissue where tendons attach to the bone, such as the heel, knee, hip, and shoulder.

Factors that increase the likelihood of sports injuries include intrinsic and extrinsic risk factors.[4] Intrinsic risk factors are those that are unique to the individual that increase the likelihood of sustaining an injury, such as maturation status. Contact sports pose a greater threat for injury to the neck, spine, and growth plates in children and adolescents, who have not yet reached maturity. Extrinsic risk factors are those that, when applied to the athlete, may increase the risk of injury. They may include training methods, or equipment, and environment that may have an effect on the magnitude, stress, or force applied to the body. They include factors such as athletic activity that is repeated so often that areas of the body do not have enough time to heal between efforts. Injuries can often be prevented by proper training, use of safety equipment, and limiting the level of competition according to skill and size rather than chronologic age. Adequate warm-up time, hydration, and proper nutrition are also key factors in injury prevention.

Soft Tissue Injuries

Most skeletal injuries are accompanied by soft tissue (muscle, tendon, or ligament) injuries. These injuries include contusions and hematomas.

A contusion is an injury, or *bruise,* that results from direct trauma and is usually caused by striking a body part against a hard object.[5] Although the resulting disability is usually minor, some contusions can be quite painful. Muscle bruises are common in all athletic events, even the so-called noncontact sports. The thigh and the arm are the most commonly involved. In contusions, the skin overlying the injury remains intact while the injured tissue undergoes a well-defined sequence of events including microscopic rupture of blood vessels and damage to muscle cells, swelling, and inflammation. The area often becomes ecchymotic (i.e., black and blue) because of local hemorrhage; later, the discoloration gradually changes to brown and then to yellow as the blood is reabsorbed.

A large area of local hemorrhage is called a *hematoma.* Hematomas cause pain as blood accumulates and exerts pressure on nerve endings. The pain increases with movement or when pressure is applied to the area. The pain and swelling of a hematoma take longer to subside than those accompanying a contusion.

The treatment for a contusion and a hematoma consists of elevating the affected part and applying cold for the first 24 hours to reduce the bleeding into the area. A compression wrapping is sometimes helpful in the early stages. Reinjury is avoided by appropriately protecting the area and allowing for complete healing to occur before returning to activities.

Joint (Musculotendinous) Injuries

Joints, or articulations, are sites where two or more bones meet. Joints (i.e., diarthrodial) are supported by tough bundles of collagenous fibers called *ligaments* that attach to the joint capsule and hold the articular ends of bones together and by *tendons* that join muscles to the periosteum of the articulating bones (see Chapter 42). Joint injuries usually involve mechanical overloading or forcible twisting or stretching.

Strains and Sprains

Strains and sprains are both musculoskeletal injuries, but they differ in terms of the tissue that is affected.[5] Strains involve muscles, or more precisely the muscle–tendon unit. Sprains involve the supporting ligaments of a joint.

A *strain* is a stretching or partial tear in a muscle or a muscle–tendon unit. Strains commonly result from sudden stretch of a muscle that is actively contracting. Although there usually is no external evidence of a specific injury, an inflammatory response develops at the injured site, followed by fibrous tissue replacement of the damaged muscle fibers. Muscle strains are usually characterized by pain, stiffness, swelling, and local tenderness. Pain is increased with stretching of the muscle group. Strains can occur at any age but are more common in middle-aged and older adults. With aging, the collagen fibers in the muscle–tendon unit change; as a result, muscles have decreased elasticity and are more susceptible to injury. Common sites of muscle strains are the lower back and the cervical region of the spine. The elbow and the shoulder are also supported by muscle–tendon units that are subject to strains. Strains of muscle units around the hip, hamstring, and quadriceps are commonly associated with athletic activities. Proper warm-up exercises increase the flexibility of muscle–tendon units and help prevent these types of injuries.

A *sprain,* which involves the joint ligaments or capsule surrounding the joint, resembles a strain, but the pain and swelling subside more slowly. It usually is caused by abnormal or excessive movement of a joint. With a sprain, the ligaments may be incompletely torn or, in a severe sprain, completely torn or ruptured (Fig. 43-1). The signs of sprain are pain, rapid swelling, discoloration, and limitation of function. Any joint may be sprained, but the ankle joint is most commonly involved, especially in high-risk sports such as basketball. Most ankle sprains occur in the lateral ankle when the foot is turned inward under a person, forcing the ankle into inversion beyond its structural limits. Other common sites of sprain are the knee (the collateral

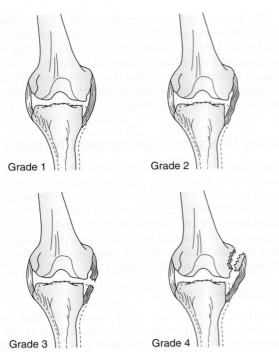

FIGURE 43-1. Degrees of sprain on the medial side of the right knee: grade 1, mild sprain of the medial collateral ligament; grade 2, moderate sprain with hematoma formation; grade 3, severe sprain with total disruption of the ligament; and grade 4, severe sprain with avulsion of the medial femoral condyle at the insertion of the medial collateral ligament.

ligament and anterior cruciate ligament) and elbow (the ulnar side). As with a strain, the soft tissue injury that occurs with a sprain is not evident on the radiograph. An MRI is the most sensitive test for evaluation of a soft tissue injury.

The treatment of muscle strains and ligamentous sprains involves rest, ice, compression, and elevation (RICE).[5] For an injured extremity such as the ankle, elevation of the injured body part followed by local application of cold may be sufficient. Compression, accomplished through the use of adhesive wraps, helps to reduce swelling and provide support. For a muscle strain, the affected joint is immobilized until the pain and swelling have subsided. In a sprain, the affected joint is immobilized for several weeks. Immobilization may be followed by graded active exercises. Early diagnosis, treatment, and rehabilitation are essential in preventing chronic ligamentous instability.

Healing of the dense connective tissues in tendons and ligaments is similar to that of other soft tissues. If properly treated, injuries usually heal with the restoration of the original tensile strength. Repair is accomplished by fibroblasts from the inner tendon sheath or, if the tendon has no sheath, from the loose connective tissue that surrounds the tendon.[6,7] Capillaries infiltrate the injured area during the initial healing process and supply the fibroblasts with the materials they need to produce large amounts of collagen. Formation of the long collagen bundles occurs within the first 2 weeks, and although tensile strength increases steadily thereafter, it

is not sufficient to permit strong tendon pulls for 6 to 8 weeks.[6] During the healing process, there is a danger that muscle contraction will pull the injured ends apart, causing the tendon to heal in the lengthened position. There is also a danger that adhesions will develop in areas where tendons pass through fibrous channels, such as in the distal palm of the hands, rendering the tendon useless.

Dislocations

A *dislocation* is the abnormal displacement of the articulating surfaces of a joint such that surfaces are not in contact. It usually follows a severe trauma that disrupts the holding ligaments. Dislocations are seen most often in the shoulder and acromioclavicular joints. A *subluxation* is a partial dislocation in which the bone ends in the joint are still in partial contact with each other.

Dislocations can be congenital, traumatic, or pathologic. Congenital dislocations occur in the hip or knee. Traumatic dislocations occur after falls, blows, or rotational injuries. For example, auto accidents often cause dislocations of the hip and accompanying acetabular fractures because of the direction of impact. In the shoulder and patella, dislocations may become recurrent, especially in athletes. They recur with the same motion but require less and less force each time. Less common sites of dislocation, seen mainly in young adults, are the wrist and midtarsal region. They usually are the result of direct force, such as a fall on an outstretched hand. Pathologic dislocation in the hip is a late complication of infection, rheumatoid arthritis, paralysis, and neuromuscular diseases.

Diagnosis of a dislocation is based on history, physical examination, and radiologic findings. The symptoms are pain, deformity, and limited movement. The treatment depends on the site, mechanism of injury, and associated injuries such as fractures. Dislocations that do not reduce spontaneously usually require manipulation or surgical repair. Immobilization is necessary for several weeks after reduction of a dislocation to allow healing of the joint structures. In dislocations affecting the knee, alternatives to surgery are isometric quadriceps-strengthening exercises and a temporary brace.

Shoulder and Rotator Cuff Injuries

The shoulder is a complex series of joints that produces extraordinary range of motion but lacks stability. This instability, combined with its relatively exposed position, makes the shoulder extremely vulnerable to injuries including fractures, dislocations, and degenerative processes such as rotator cuff disorders.[5,8,9]

The shoulder is composed of three bones: the scapula, the clavicle, and the humerus[10] (Fig. 43-2). The scapula is a thin bone that articulates widely and closely with the chest wall. It also articulates with the humerus by way of its small, shallow glenoid cavity and with the clavicle at the acromion process. The clavicle, which is held firmly in place by ligaments at the sternum and acromion, forms the only bony connection between the axial skeleton and the upper extremity. Clavicle fractures

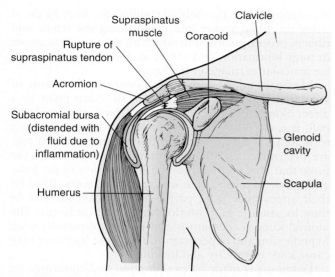

FIGURE 43-2. Structures of the glenohumeral shoulder joint, showing the location of common rotator cuff injuries. The supraspinatus muscle is the most commonly injured part of the rotator cuff. (Adapted from Moore KL, Dalley AF. *Clinically Oriented Anatomy*. 5th ed. Philadelphia, PA: Lippincott Williams & Wilkins; 2006:763.)

are among the most common fractures of childhood.[10] The typical mechanism of fracture is a fall on the lateral shoulder, or less commonly by a direct blow or by falling on an outstretched arm. Most clavicle fractures are treated nonoperatively, with either a simple arm sling or figure-of-eight clavicle strap.[5,8]

Three articulations form the shoulder joint—the acromioclavicular joint, which joins the clavicle to the acromion of the scapula; the glenohumeral joint, which connects the head of the humerus to the relatively shallow glenoid cavity in the scapula; and the sternoclavicular joint, which joins the sternum to the clavicle.[10] The stability of these joints is provided by a series of muscles and tendons. The acromioclavicular joint is a common site of sprains in athletes and physically active persons. The classic cause of an acromioclavicular joint injury is a direct blow to the acromion with the humerus in an adducted position. This force drives the acromion medially and inferiorly. Acromioclavicular joint injuries also may be caused by indirect trauma, such as falling on an outstretched arm or elbow. The glenohumeral joint is one of the most commonly dislocated joints. It is also the joint most likely to develop problems with instability. Most acute dislocations involve anterior displacement of the humeral head with respect to the glenoid cavity, the result of the shoulder being abducted and forcefully extended and rotated. Other mechanisms include a fall on an outstretched arm or a blow to the posterior shoulder.

Movement of the shoulder results from the coordinated efforts of the muscles of the rotator cuff: the supraspinous, teres minor, infraspinatus, and subscapularis.[5,8] These muscles and their musculotendinous attachments form a cover around the head of the humerus and function to rotate the arm and stabilize the humoral

head against the glenoid. The rotator cuff muscles are separated from the overlying "coracoacromial arch" by the subdeltoid and subcoracoid bursae.

Disorders of the rotator cuff, such as tendinitis, subacromial bursitis, and partial and complete tears, account for a substantial majority of shoulder problems (see Fig. 43-2). Rotator cuff injuries can result from excessive use, a direct blow, or stretch injury, usually involving throwing or swinging, as with baseball pitchers or tennis players.[5,8] While rotator cuff injuries sometimes occur with acute injury, most result from a combination of factors, including altered blood supply to the tendons, repeated mechanical insult as the tendon passes under the coracoacromial arch, and age-related degeneration. Repetitive overhead throwing, which produces significant stress on the glenohumeral complex of the rotator cuff, is a common cause of rotator cuff tendinitis. Full-thickness tears are more common in persons older than 40 years of age, although they can occur in athletes.[5,9,11] Tears generally originate in the supraspinous tendon and may progress posteriorly and anteriorly.

The major clinical features of rotator cuff disorders are pain (especially at night), tenderness, and occasionally muscle atrophy. Pain and impingement may be noted when motions of the arm squeeze and pinch cuff tendons between the humerus and the overlying arch. With rotator cuff tears, there may be difficulty abducting and rotating the arm.

Several physical examination maneuvers, including assessment of active and passive range of motion, are used to define shoulder pathology. The history and mechanism of injury are important. In addition to standard radiographs, an arthrogram or magnetic resonance imaging (MRI) scan may be obtained. Arthroscopic examination under anesthesia may be done for diagnostic purposes. Conservative treatment with anti-inflammatory agents, corticosteroid injections, and physical therapy often is used. A period of rest is followed by a customized exercise and rehabilitation program to improve strength, flexibility, and endurance. Surgical repair may be considered for persons with an acute traumatic rotator cuff tear or those with significant symptoms and failed rehabilitation.

Knee Injuries

The knee is a common site of injury, particularly sports-related injuries in which the knee is subjected to abnormal twisting and compression forces.[8,12,13] These forces can result in injury to the ligaments and menisci, patellar subluxation and dislocation, and the patellofemoral pain syndrome. Many knee injuries can predispose to osteoarthritis in later life.

The knee joint consists of lateral and medial femoral condyles, the lateral and medial femotibial condyles, and the patella[10] (Fig. 43-3). It is essentially a round bone (femoral condyles) sitting on a flat bone (tibial condyles) with no intrinsic bony stability and depends on its ligaments and menisci for support.[8] The most important ligaments are the medial and lateral collateral ligaments along with their associated posterior capsular structures

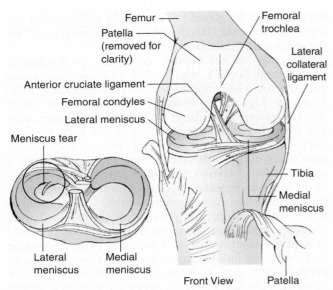

FIGURE 43-3. The knee, showing the lateral and medial condyles and menisci. The lateral and medial femotibial condyles are located between the lateral and medial femoral condyles and the tibial condyles (not shown). Inset (*lower left*) shows meniscus tear.

and the anterior cruciate ligament (ACL) and posterior cruciate ligament (PCL).

Ligamentous Injuries. Ligamentous injuries of the knee are among the most serious of all knee injuries. The mechanism is usually one of forceful stress against the knee when the extremity is bearing weight. A "pop" or tearing sensation along with sudden pain is often described, especially with ACL ruptures. After injury, the ability to bear weight on the extremity is often lost, and the knee becomes swollen because of hemorrhaging into the joint.

Initial treatment includes rest, ice, and use of crutches until the person is able to ambulate without a limp. A knee immobilizer or range-of-motion brace may be used for comfort until the acute pain subsides. Range-of-motion exercises are important. Definitive treatment depends on the ligaments that are involved, the person's age and activity level, and any associated injuries. Most isolated lateral ligament injuries and isolated ACL and PCL ruptures are treated nonsurgically, at least initially. Surgical reconstruction may be required in young, active persons. Older and less active individuals may be treated with physical therapy aimed at controlling the instability. A well-constructed brace may provide an option in some persons.

Meniscus Injuries. The menisci are C-shaped plates of fibrocartilage that are superimposed between the condyles of the femur and tibia. There are two menisci in each knee, a lateral and medial meniscus[5,8,12,13] (see Fig. 43-3). The menisci are thicker at their external margins and taper to thin, unattached edges at their interior margin. They are firmly attached at their ends to the intercondylar area of the tibia and are supported by the coronary and transverse ligaments of the knee. The menisci play a major role in load bearing and shock

absorption. They also help to stabilize the knee by deepening the tibial socket and maintaining the femur and tibia in proper position. In addition, the meniscus assists in joint lubrication and serves as a source of nutrition for articular cartilage in the knee.

Meniscus injury commonly occurs as the result of a rotational injury from a sudden or sharp pivot or a direct blow to the knee, as in hockey, basketball, or football. It is often associated with other injuries, such as a torn ACL. The type and location of the meniscal tear are determined by the magnitude and direction of the force that acts on the knee and the position of the knee at the time of injury. Meniscus tears can be described by their appearance (e.g., parrot-beak, bucket handle) or their location (e.g., posterior horn, anterior horn). The injured knee is edematous and painful, especially with hyperflexion and hyperextension. A loose fragment may cause knee instability and locking.

Diagnosis is made by examination and confirmed by MRI. A regular radiograph may be needed to rule out osteoarthritis. Initial treatment of meniscal injuries may be conservative. The knee may be placed in a removable knee immobilizer. Isometric quadriceps exercises may be prescribed. Activity usually is restricted until complete motion is recovered. Arthroscopic meniscectomy may be performed when there is recurrent or persistent locking, recurrent effusion, or disabling pain.

There is evidence that loss of meniscal function is associated with progressive deterioration of knee function and osteoarthritic changes.[13] Damaged articular cartilage has a limited capacity to heal because of its avascular nature and inadequate mobilization of regenerative cells. Meniscal reconstruction procedures have been developed to preserve these functions before significant degenerative changes develop, thus preventing the need for a total joint replacement later in life.[14]

Patellar Subluxation and Dislocations. Recurrent subluxation and dislocation of the patella are common in young adults.[5,8] Sports such as skiing or tennis involve external rotation of the foot and leg with knee flexion, a position that exerts rotational stresses on the knee. Congenital knee variations are also a predisposing factor. There is often a sensation of the patella "popping out" when the dislocation occurs. Other complaints include the knee giving out, swelling, crepitus, stiffness, and loss of range of motion. Treatment measures include immobilization with the knee extended, bracing, administration of anti-inflammatory agents, and isometric quadriceps-strengthening exercises. Surgical intervention often is necessary.

Patellofemoral Pain Syndrome. Patellofemoral pain syndrome is the most common cause of anterior knee pain.[5,10,15] It is caused by imbalances in the forces controlling movement of the patella during knee flexion and extension, particularly with overloading of the joint. The patellofemoral joint is composed of the patella and the central groove in the proximal femur, which is referred to as the patellar groove or femoral trochlea (see Fig. 43-3). Stability of the joint involves dynamic and static stabilizers, which control patellar tracking; that is, the movement of the patella within the femoral trochlea.[15] The disorder, also called "runner's knee," occurs most frequently in young adults and is often associated with jogging, volleyball, and basketball. Persons with this disorder typically complain of pain, particularly when climbing stairs or sitting with the knees bent. The pain is usually difficult to localize, and swelling of the knee is not characteristic of the disorder. Occasionally, the person experiences weakness of the knee.

Diagnosis is usually based on history and physical examination. Radiography may be used as an adjunct to the history and physical. Treatment consists of relative rest and physical therapy.[15] Reduction of loading of the patellofemoral joint and surrounding tissues is the first step to reduce pain. Inappropriate or excessively worn footwear may contribute to the problem and need to be replaced. Although a variety of braces, sleeves, and straps have been used in treatment of the disorder, studies have found no significant benefit from their use.

Hip Injuries

The hip is a ball-and-socket joint in which the femoral head articulates deeply in the acetabulum.[10] The proximal part of the femur consists of a head, neck, and greater trochanter. The vascular anatomy of the femoral head, which receives its main blood supply from the lateral and medial circumflex femoral arteries and the obturator artery, is of critical importance in any disorder of the hip (Fig. 43-4). Disease or injuries that compromise blood flow may damage the viability of the femoral head and lead to avascular necrosis or osteonecrosis.

Dislocations of the Hip. Dislocations of the hip in which the femoral head is displaced from the acetabulum are commonly the result of severe trauma and are usually posterior in direction. They typically result from the knee being struck while the hip and knee are in a flexed position.[8] This force drives the femoral head out of the acetabulum posteriorly. Anterior dislocations are less common and usually result from a force on the knee with the thigh abducted.

Hip dislocation is an emergency.[5,8] The disorder is typically accompanied by severe pain and inability to move the lower extremity. In the dislocated position, great tension is placed on the blood supply to the femoral head and avascular necrosis may result. To prevent this complication, early reduction is indicated. Weight bearing is usually limited after reduction to prevent the dislocation from reoccurring and allow healing to occur.

Fractures of the Hip. Hip fracture is a major public health problem in the Western world, particularly among the elderly.[16–18] It results in hospitalization, disability, and loss of independence. Risk factors for hip fracture include physical inactivity, excessive consumption of alcohol, use of certain psychotropic drugs, residence in an institution, visual impairment, and dementia.[16] Osteoporosis is an important contributing factor.

Most hip fractures result from falls. Occasionally, the person may actually fracture the hip before falling, the fracture representing the completion of an incomplete break. The characteristics of the fall (the direction, site of impact, and protective response) and environmental factors are recognized as important influences for the risk of hip fracture from a fall.

A hip fracture usually involves the proximal femur. Such fractures are commonly categorized according to the anatomic site in which they occur.[9,16–18] Femoral neck fractures are located in the area distal to the femoral head but proximal to the greater and lesser trochanters and are considered intracapsular because they are located

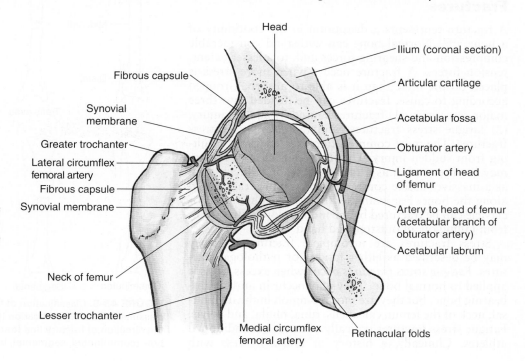

FIGURE 43-4. Blood supply of the head and neck of the femur (anterior view). A section of the bone has been removed from the femoral neck. (Modified from Moore KL, Agur AM, Dalley AF. *Essential Clinical Anatomy.* 4th ed. Philadelphia, PA: Wolters Kluwer Health | Lippincott Williams & Wilkins; 2010:380.)

Head

Ilium (coronal section)

Fibrous capsule

Articular cartilage

Synovial membrane

Acetabular fossa

Greater trochanter

Obturator artery

Lateral circumflex femoral artery

Ligament of head of femur

Fibrous capsule

Synovial membrane

Artery to head of femur (acetabular branch of obturator artery)

Acetabular labrum

Neck of femur

Lesser trochanter

Medial circumflex femoral artery

Retinacular folds

within the capsule of the hip joint. Intertrochanteric fractures occur in the metaphyseal region between the greater and lesser trochanter. Subtrochanteric fractures are those that occur just below the greater trochanter.

The location of a hip fracture is important in terms of blood flow to the femoral head, which receives its blood supply from vessels that course proximally up the femoral neck[10] (see Fig. 43-4). Subtrochanteric and intertrochanteric fractures that occur distal to these vessels do not usually disturb the blood supply to the femoral head, whereas femoral neck fractures, particularly those involving marked displacement, often disrupt the blood supply to the femoral head and are therefore associated with an increased incidence of complications (nonunion and avascular necrosis).

Most hip fractures are diagnosed based on clinical findings and standard radiographs. A bone scan or MRI may be done when the radiograph is negative, but the clinical findings support the diagnosis of hip fracture.

The primary goal of treatment for a hip fracture is a return to the preinjury level of function as soon as possible.[8] Undisplaced or impacted fractures have a better prognosis in terms of healing and are often treated nonoperatively or by simple internal fixation to provide stability. Displaced intracapsular fractures in the elderly are usually best treated by surgical hip replacement and early mobilization.[5] Young, healthy people are treated by reduction of the fracture (if needed) and internal fixation. This method allows for preservation of the femoral head, which in this age group is desirable because the long-term results are better than with prosthetic replacement. Intertrochanteric fractures are usually treated with open reduction and internal fixation. This allows for early ambulation by eliminating pain at the fracture site.

Fractures

A fracture represents a disruption in the continuity of a bone.[8,18,19] Normal bone can withstand considerable compression and shearing forces and, to a lesser extent, tension forces. A fracture occurs when more stress is placed on the bone than it is able to absorb. Grouped according to cause, fractures can be divided into three major categories: (1) fractures caused by sudden injury, (2) fatigue stress fractures, and (3) pathologic stress fractures. The most common fractures are those resulting from sudden injury. The force causing the fracture may be direct, such as a fall or blow, or indirect, such as a massive muscle contraction or trauma transmitted along the bone. For example, the head of the radius or clavicle can be fractured by the indirect forces that result from falling on an outstretched hand.

Stress fractures are incomplete fractures.[8,20] They may be described as either fatigue or pathologic fractures. *Fatigue stress fractures* occur when excess stress is applied to normal bone. They may occur in any weight-bearing bone, but they are most common in the metatarsal, neck of the femur, calcaneus, tibia, fibula, and pelvis. Fatigue stress fractures typically occur in unconditioned athletes. Clinically, a history of unusual stress with

subsequent pain over a bone is common in fatigue fractures. Stress fractures in the tibia may be confused with "shin splints," a nonspecific term for pain in the lower leg from overuse in walking and running, because they frequently are not apparent on x-ray films until 2 weeks after the onset of symptoms.[4,5]

Pathologic stress fractures occur when normal stress is applied to bones that have been weakened by disease or tumors.[8] Fractures of this type may occur spontaneously with little or no stress. The underlying disease state can be local, as with infections, cysts, or tumors, or it can be generalized, as in osteoporosis, Paget disease, or disseminated tumors.

Classification

Fractures usually are classified according to location, type, and direction or pattern of the fracture line[5,8] (Fig. 43-5). A fracture of the long bone is described in relation to its position in the bone—proximal, midshaft, and distal. Other descriptions are used when the fracture affects the head or neck of a bone, involves a joint, or is near a prominence such as a condyle or malleolus.

The type of fracture is determined by its communication with the external environment, the degree of break in continuity of the bone, and the character of the fracture pieces. A fracture can be classified as open or closed. When the bone fragments have broken through the skin, the fracture is called an *open* or *compound fracture*. In a closed fracture, there is no communication with the outside environment.

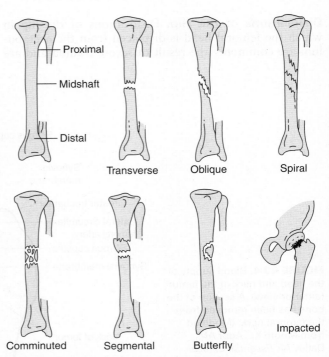

FIGURE 43-5. Classification of fractures. Fractures are classified according to location (proximal, midshaft, or distal), the direction of fracture line (transverse, oblique, spiral), and type (comminuted, segmental, butterfly, or impacted).

The degree of a fracture is described in terms of a complete or incomplete break in the continuity of bone.[5,8] A *greenstick fracture,* which is seen in children, is an example of a partial break in bone continuity and resembles that seen when a young sapling is broken. This kind of break occurs because children's bones, especially until approximately 10 years of age, are more resilient than the bones of adults.

The character of the fracture pieces may also be used to describe a fracture. A *comminuted fracture* has more than two pieces. A *compression fracture,* as occurs in the vertebral body, involves two bones that are crushed or squeezed together. A fracture is called *impacted* when the fracture fragments are wedged together. This type usually occurs in the humerus, often is less serious, and usually is treated without surgery.

The direction of the trauma or mechanism of injury produces a certain configuration or pattern of fracture. *Reduction* is the restoration of a fractured bone to its normal anatomic position. The pattern of a fracture indicates the nature of the trauma and provides information about the easiest method for reduction. *Transverse fractures* are caused by simple angulatory forces. A *spiral fracture* results from a twisting motion, or torque. A transverse fracture is not likely to become displaced or lose its position after it is reduced. On the other hand, spiral, oblique, and comminuted fractures often are unstable and may change position after reduction.

Manifestations

The signs and symptoms of a fracture include pain, tenderness at the site of bone disruption, swelling, loss of function, deformity of the affected part, and abnormal mobility.[5] The deformity varies according to the type of force applied, the area of the bone involved, the type of fracture produced, and the strength and balance of the surrounding muscles.

In long bones, three types of deformities—angulation, shortening, and rotation—are seen. Severely angulated fracture fragments may be felt at the fracture site and often push up against the soft tissue to cause a tenting effect on the skin. Bending forces and unequal muscle pulls cause angulation. Shortening of the extremity occurs as the bone fragments slide and override each other because of the pull of the muscles on the long axis of the extremity (Fig. 43-6). Rotational deformity occurs when the fracture fragments rotate out of their normal longitudinal axis; this can result from rotational strain produced by the fracture or unequal pull by the muscles that are attached to the fracture fragments. A crepitus, or grating

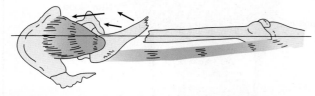

FIGURE 43-6. Displacement and overriding of fracture fragments of a long bone (femur) caused by severe muscle spasm.

sound, may be heard as the bone fragments rub against each other. In the case of an open fracture, there is bleeding from the wound where the bone protrudes. Blood loss from a pelvic fracture or multiple long bone fractures can cause hypovolemic shock in a trauma victim.

Shortly after the fracture has occurred, nerve function at the fracture site may be temporarily lost. The area may become numb, and the surrounding muscles may become flaccid. This condition has been called *local shock.* During this period, which may last for a few minutes to half an hour, fractured bones may be reduced with little or no pain. After this brief period, the pain sensation returns, and with it muscle spasms and contractions of the surrounding muscles.

Diagnosis and Treatment

Diagnosis is the first step in the care of fractures and is based on history and physical manifestations.[5,8] X-ray examination is used to confirm the diagnosis and direct the treatment. The ease of diagnosis varies with the location and severity of the fracture. In the trauma patient, the presence of other, more serious injuries may make diagnosis more difficult.

Treatment depends on the general condition of the person, the presence of associated injuries, the location of the fracture and its displacement, and whether the fracture is open or closed. A *splint* is a device for immobilizing the movable fragments of a fracture. When a fracture is suspected, the injured part always should be splinted before it is moved. This is essential for preventing further injury.[8]

There are three objectives for treatment of fractures: (1) reduction of the fracture, (2) immobilization, and (3) preservation and restoration of the function of the injured part.[8] Reduction of a fracture is directed toward manipulating the bone fragments to as near-normal an anatomic position as possible. This can be accomplished by closed or surgical (open) reduction. Closed reduction uses methods such as manual pressure and traction. Fractures are then held in place by external or internal fixation devices. Surgical reduction involves the use of various types of hardware to accomplish internal fixation of the fracture fragments.

Immobilization prevents movement of the injured parts and is the single most important element in obtaining union of the fracture fragments. Immobilization can be accomplished through the use of external devices, such as splints, casts, external fixation devices, or traction, or by means of internal fixation devices inserted during surgical reduction of the fracture. Preservation and restoration of the function of muscles and joints is an ongoing process in the unaffected and affected extremities during the period of immobilization required for fracture healing. Exercises designed to preserve function, maintain muscle strength, and reduce joint stiffness should be started early.

Bone Healing

Bone healing occurs in a manner similar to soft tissue healing. However, it is a more complex process and takes longer.[18–21] There are essentially four stages

(*text continues on page 1088*)

UNDERSTANDING ➡ Fracture Healing

A fracture, which is any break in a bone, undergoes a healing process to reestablish bone continuity and strength. The repair of simple fractures is commonly divided into four phases: (1) hematoma formation, (2) fibrocartilaginous callus formation, (3) bony callus formation, and (4) remodeling.

1 **Hematoma Formation.** When a bone breaks, blood vessels in the bone and surrounding tissues are torn and bleed into and around the fragments of the fractured bone, forming a blood clot, or hematoma. The hematoma facilitates the formation of the fibrin meshwork that seals off the fracture site and serves as a framework for the influx of inflammatory cells, the ingrowth of fibroblasts, and the development of new capillary buds (vessels). It is also the source of signaling molecules that initiate the cellular events that are critical to the healing process.

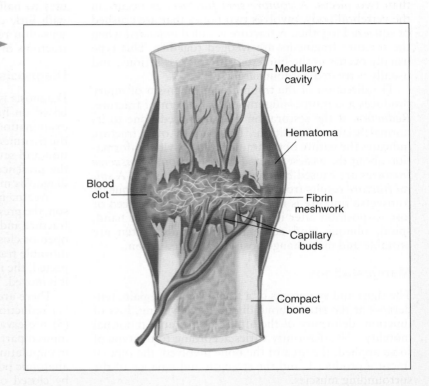

2 **Fibrocartilaginous Callus Formation.** As new capillaries infiltrate the hematoma at the fracture site, it becomes organized into a form of granulation tissue, called *procallus*. Fibroblasts from the periosteum, endosteum, and red bone marrow proliferate and invade the procallus. The fibroblasts produce a fibrocartilaginous soft callus bridge that connects the bone fragments. Although this repair tissue usually reaches its maximum girth at the end of the 2nd or 3rd week, it is not strong enough for weight bearing.

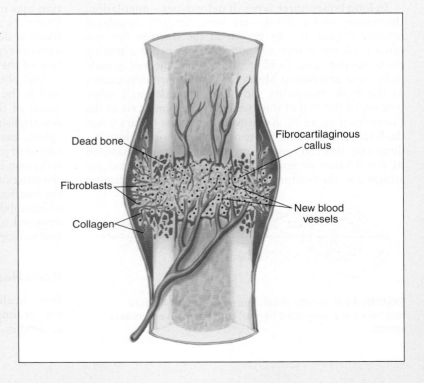

3

Bony Callus Formation. Ossification represents the conversion of the fibrocartilaginous cartilage to bony callus. In areas close to well-vascularized bone tissue, osteogenic cells develop into osteoblasts, or bone-building cells, which produce spongy bone trabeculae. The newly formed osteoblasts first deposit bone on the outer surface of the bone some distance from the fracture site. The formation of bone progresses toward the fracture site until a new bony sheath covers the fibrocartilaginous callus. In time, the fibrocartilage is converted to spongy bone, and the callus is then referred to as bony callus. Gradually, the bony callus calcifies and is replaced by mature bone. Bony callus formation begins 3 to 4 weeks after injury and continues until a firm bony union is formed months later.

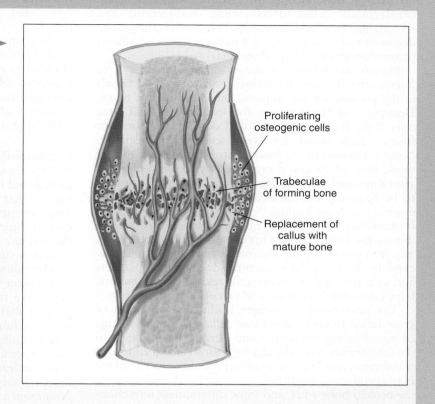

Proliferating osteogenic cells

Trabeculae of forming bone

Replacement of callus with mature bone

4

Remodeling. During remodeling of the bony callus, dead portions of the bone are gradually removed by osteoclasts. Compact bone replaces spongy bone around the periphery of the fracture, and there is reorganization of mineralized bone along the lines of mechanical stress. During this period, the excess material on the outside of the bone shaft and within the medullary cavity is removed and compact bone is laid down to reconstruct the shaft. The final structure of the remodeled area resembles that of the original unbroken bone; however, a thickened area on the surface of the bone may remain as evidence of a healed fracture.

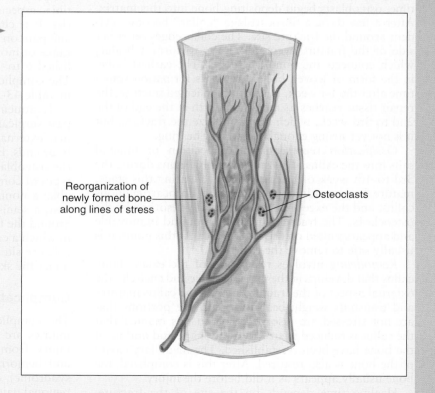

Reorganization of newly formed bone along lines of stress

Osteoclasts

(text continued from page 1085)

involved in bone healing: hematoma formation, fibrocartilaginous callus development, ossification, and remodeling (see Understanding Fracture Healing). The degree of response during each of these stages is in direct proportion to the extent of trauma.

Hematoma formation occurs during the first 1 to 2 days after fracture. It develops from torn blood vessels in the periosteum and adjacent muscles and soft tissue. Disruption of blood vessels also leads to death of bone cells at the fracture site. In 2 to 5 days, the hemorrhage forms a large blood clot. Neovascularization begins to occur peripheral to the blood clot. By the end of the 1st week, most of the clot is organized by invasion of blood vessels and early fibrosis. Hematoma formation is thought to be necessary for the initiation of the cellular events essential to bone healing.[18] As the result of hematoma formation, clotting factors remain in the injured area to initiate the formation of a fibrin meshwork, which serves as a framework for the ingrowth of fibroblasts and new capillary buds. At the same time, degranulated platelets and migrating inflammatory cells release growth factors, which stimulate osteoclast and osteoblast proliferation.[18]

The next event in fracture healing is formation of granulation tissue or *soft tissue callus*. During this stage of bone healing, fibroblasts and osteoblasts migrate into the fracture site from the nearby periosteal and endosteal membranes and begin reconstruction of bone. The fibroblasts produce collagen that spans the break and connects the broken bone ends, and some differentiate into chondrocytes that secrete collagen matrix. At about the same time, osteoblasts begin depositing bone into this matrix. After a few days, a fibrocartilage "collar" becomes evident around the fracture site. The collar edges on either side of the fracture eventually unite to form a bridge, which connects the bone fragments. The earliest bone, in the form of woven bone, begins its formation sometime after the 1st week. In an uncomplicated fracture, the repair tissue reaches its maximum girth at the end of the 2nd to 3rd week, which helps stabilize the fracture, but it is not yet strong enough for weight bearing.

Ossification represents the deposition of mineral salts into the callus. This stage usually begins during the 3rd to 4th week of fracture healing. During this stage, mature bone gradually replaces the fibrocartilaginous callus, and the excess callus is gradually resorbed by the osteoclasts. The fracture site feels firm and immovable and appears united on the radiograph. At this point, it is usually safe to remove the cast.

Remodeling involves resorption of the excess bony callus that develops in the marrow space and encircles the external aspect of the fracture site. As the callus matures and transmits weight-bearing forces, the portions that are not stressed are resorbed. It is in this manner that the callus is reduced in size until the shape and outline of the bone have been reestablished. The medullary cavity of the bone is also restored. After this is completed, the bone usually appears as it did before the injury.

Healing time depends on the site of the fracture, the condition of the fracture fragments, hematoma formation, and other local and host factors. In children,

fractures usually heal within 4 to 6 weeks; in adolescents, they heal within 6 to 8 weeks; and in adults, they heal within 10 to 18 weeks. The increased rate of healing among children compared with adults may be related to the increased cellularity and vascularity of the child's periosteum.[18] In general, fractures of long bones, displaced fractures, and fractures with less surface area heal more slowly. Function usually returns within 6 months after union is complete. However, return to complete function may take longer.

Impaired Bone Healing. Factors that influence bone healing are specific to the person, the type of injury sustained, and local factors that disrupt healing. Individual factors that may delay bone healing are the patient's age; current medications; debilitating diseases, such as diabetes and rheumatoid arthritis; local stress around the fracture site; circulatory problems and coagulation disorders; and poor nutrition.

Malunion is healing with deformity, angulation, or rotation that is visible on x-ray films.[5,22] Early and aggressive treatment, especially of the hand, can help prevent malunion and result in earlier alignment and return of function. *Delayed union* is the failure of a fracture to unite within the normal period (e.g., 20 weeks for a fracture of the tibia or femur in an adult). Intra-articular fractures (i.e., those through a joint) may heal more slowly and may eventually produce arthritis. *Nonunion* is failure to produce union and cessation of the processes of bone repair. It is seen most often in the tibia, especially with open fractures or crushing injuries. It is characterized by mobility of the fracture site and pain on weight bearing. Muscle atrophy and loss of range of motion may occur. Nonunion usually is established 6 to 12 months after the time of the fracture.[22] The complications of fracture healing are summarized in Table 43-1.

Treatment methods for impaired bone healing encompass surgical interventions, including bone grafts, bracing, external fixation, or electrical stimulation of the bone ends. Electrical stimulation is thought to stimulate the osteoblasts to lay down a network of bone. Three types of commercial bone growth stimulators are available: a noninvasive model, which is placed outside the cast; a semi-invasive model, in which pins are inserted around the fracture site; and a totally implantable type, in which a cathode coil is wound around the bone at the fracture site and operated by a battery pack implanted under the skin.[8]

Complications of Fractures and Other Injuries

The complications of fractures and other orthopedic injuries are associated with loss of skeletal continuity, injury from bone fragments, pressure from swelling and hemorrhage (e.g., fracture blisters, compartment syndrome), or development of fat emboli. The complex regional pain syndrome or reflex sympathetic dystrophy, caused by involvement of nerve fibers, is discussed in Chapter 35.

TABLE 43-1	**Complications of Fracture Healing**	
Complication	**Manifestations**	**Contributing Factors**
Delayed union	Failure of fracture to heal within predicted time as determined by x-ray	Large displaced fracture Inadequate immobilization Large hematoma Infection at fracture site Excessive loss of bone Inadequate circulation
Malunion	Deformity at fracture site Deformity or angulation on x-ray	Inadequate reduction Malalignment of fracture at time of immobilization
Nonunion	Failure of bone to heal before the process of bone repair stops Evidence on x-ray Motion at fracture site Pain on weight bearing	Inadequate reduction Mobility at fracture site Severe trauma Bone fragment separation Soft tissue between bone fragments Infection Extensive loss of bone Inadequate circulation Malignancy Bone necrosis Noncompliance with restrictions

Fracture Blisters. Fracture blisters are skin bullae and blisters representing areas of epidermal necrosis with separation of the epidermis from the underlying dermis by edema fluid. They are seen with more severe, twisting types of injuries (e.g., motor vehicle accidents and falls from heights) but can also occur after excessive joint manipulation, dependent positioning, and heat application, or from peripheral vascular disease. They can be solitary, multiple, or massive, depending on the extent of injury. Most fracture blisters occur in the ankle, elbow, foot, knee, or areas where there is little soft tissue between the bone and the skin. The development of fracture blisters reportedly is reduced by early surgical intervention in persons requiring operative repair.[23,24] This probably reflects the early operative release of the fracture hematoma, reapproximation of the disrupted soft tissues, ligation of bleeding vessels, and fixation of bleeding fracture surfaces. Prevention of fracture blisters is important because they pose an additional risk of infection.

Compartment Syndrome. The compartment syndrome has been described as a condition of increased pressure within a limited space (e.g., abdominal and limb compartments) that compromises the circulation and function of the tissues within the space.[25,26] The abdominal compartment syndrome alters cardiovascular hemodynamics, respiratory mechanics, and renal function. The discussion in this chapter is limited to the limb compartment syndromes.

The muscles and nerves of an extremity are enclosed in a tough, inelastic fascial envelope called a *muscle compartment* (Fig. 43-7). If the pressure in the compartment is sufficiently high, tissue circulation is compromised, causing death of nerve and muscle cells. Permanent loss of function may occur. Intracompartmental pressures greater than 30 mm Hg (normal is approximately 6 mm Hg) are considered

sufficient to impair capillary blood flow; however, the amount of pressure required to produce a compartment syndrome depends on many factors.[5]

Compartment syndrome can result from a decrease in compartment size, an increase in the volume of its contents, or a combination of the two factors. Among the causes of decreased compartment size are constrictive dressings and casts, closure of fascial defects, and burns. In persons with circumferential third-degree burns, the inelastic and constricting eschar (thick coagulated crust or slough) decreases the size of the underlying compartments.

An increase in compartment volume can be caused by trauma, including contusions and soft tissue injury,

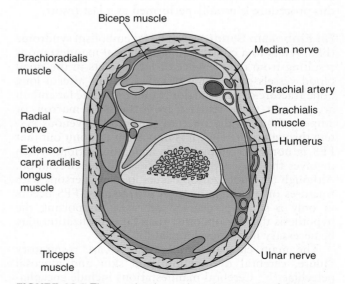

FIGURE 43-7. The proximal muscle compartment of the arm, showing the location of fascia, muscles, nerves, and blood vessels.

as well as a fracture, crushing injury, or bone surgery, when excessive swelling around the site of injury results in increased pressure in a closed compartment. Vascular injury and bleeding, and venous obstruction can also increase compartment volume. Exertional compartment syndrome is associated with walking or running.[5,26] Symptoms usually develop gradually with exercise, but resolve within 30 minutes of cessation of activity.[5]

The hallmark symptom of an acute compartment syndrome is severe pain that is out of proportion to the original injury or physical findings. Nerve compression may cause changes in sensation (e.g., paresthesias such as burning or tingling or loss of sensation), diminished reflexes, and eventually the loss of motor function. Symptoms usually begin within a few hours but can be delayed.

Because muscle necrosis can occur in as little as 4 to 8 hours, it is important that persons at risk for compartment syndrome be identified and proper treatment instituted.[5] Assessment should include pain, sensory function (i.e., light touch and two-point discrimination), motor function (i.e., movement and muscle strength), passive stretch, and palpation of the muscle compartments. Direct measurements of tissue pressure can be obtained using a needle or wick catheter inserted into the muscle compartment.

Treatment consists of reducing compartmental pressures. This entails cast splitting or removal of restrictive dressings. These procedures often are sufficient to relieve most of the underlying pressure and symptoms. Elevating the extremity on pillows can help to reduce edema. However, excessive elevation should be avoided because the effects of gravity can lower arterial pressure in the limb, thereby decreasing compartment perfusion.[5] When compartment syndrome cannot be relieved by conservative measures, a fasciotomy may become necessary. During this procedure, the fascia is incised longitudinally and separated so that the compartment volume can expand and blood flow can be reestablished. Because of potential problems with wound infection and closure, this procedure is usually performed as a last resort.

Fat Embolism Syndrome. The fat embolism syndrome (FES) refers to a constellation of clinical manifestations resulting from the presence of fat droplets in the small blood vessels of the lung or other organs after a long bone fracture or other major trauma.[27-29] The fat emboli are thought to be released from the bone marrow or adipose tissue at the fracture site into the venous system through torn veins. It is important to point out that FES is not synonymous with fat embolization, which involves the presence of fat particles in the circulation. Although fat embolization occurs in many persons with fractures or operative fixation of fractures, FES occurs in only a small percentage of cases, supporting the hypothesis that factors other than fat embolization may be necessary in the development of FES.

The main clinical features of FES are respiratory failure, cerebral dysfunction, and skin and mucosal petechiae.[24,32] Cerebral manifestations include encephalopathy, seizures, and focal neurologic deficits unrelated to head injury. Initial symptoms begin within a few hours to 3 to 4 days after injury and include a subtle change in behavior and signs of disorientation resulting from emboli in the cerebral circulation combined with respiratory depression. There may be complaints of substernal chest pain and dyspnea accompanied by tachycardia and a low-grade fever. Diaphoresis, pallor, and cyanosis become evident as respiratory function deteriorates. A petechial rash that does not blanch with pressure often occurs 2 to 3 days after the onset of symptoms. It is thought to be related to embolization of the skin capillaries or thrombocytopenia.

Three degrees of severity are seen: subclinical, overt clinical, and fulminating. Although the subclinical and overt clinical forms of FES respond well to treatment, the fulminating form often is fatal. Early diagnosis is critical. Arterial blood gases should be assayed immediately after recognition of clinical manifestations. Treatment is directed toward correcting hypoxemia and maintaining adequate fluid balance. Mechanical ventilation may be required. Corticosteroid drugs are administered to decrease the inflammatory response of lung tissues, decrease edema, stabilize the lipid membranes to reduce lipolysis, and combat bronchospasm. Corticosteroids are also given prophylactically to high-risk persons. The only preventive approach to FES is early stabilization of the fracture.

SUMMARY CONCEPTS

■ Many external physical agents can cause trauma to the musculoskeletal system. Some soft tissue injuries such as contusions, hematomas, and lacerations are relatively minor and easily treated. Muscle strains and ligamentous sprains are caused by mechanical overload on the connective tissue. They heal more slowly than the minor soft tissue injuries and require some degree of immobilization.

■ The shoulder and knee are common sites for injuries in athletes. Shoulder dislocations and rotator cuff injuries are common. Knee injuries include torn ligaments and menisci, patellar subluxation and dislocation, and patellofemoral pain syndrome. Hip dislocation is also common.

■ Fractures occur when more stress is placed on a bone than the bone can absorb. Healing of fractures is a complex process that takes place in four stages: hematoma formation, fibrocartilaginous callus formation, ossification, and remodeling. For satisfactory healing to take place, the affected bone has to be reduced and immobilized. This is accomplished with external fixation devices (e.g., splints, casts, or traction) or surgically implanted internal fixation devices.

■ The complications of fractures include a loss of skeletal continuity (malunion or nonunion), pressure from swelling and hemorrhage (fracture blisters and compartment syndrome), and fat embolism syndrome (FES). Compartment syndrome is a condition of increased pressure in a muscle compartment that compromises blood flow and potentially leads to death of nerve and muscle tissue. Fat embolism syndrome is a constellation of signs and symptoms including a petechial skin rash, respiratory failure, and cerebral dysfunction due to the presence of fat droplets in small blood vessels after a fracture.

Bone Infections and Osteonecrosis

Bone like other body tissues is susceptible to infection due to invasion by microorganisms. It also is susceptible to osteonecrosis (bone death) when it loses its blood supply.

Infections—Osteomyelitis

Osteomyelitis represents an acute or chronic infection of the bone and marrow.[18,19] Despite the common use of antibiotics, bone infections remain difficult to treat and eradicate. All types of organisms, including parasites, viruses, bacteria, and fungi, can cause osteomyelitis, but certain pyogenic bacteria and mycobacteria are the most common.

Pyogenic Osteomyelitis

Pyogenic osteomyelitis is almost always caused by bacteria. Organisms may reach the bone by seeding through the bloodstream (hematogenous spread), direct penetration or contamination of an open fracture or wound (exogenous origin), or extension from a contiguous site.

The specific agents isolated in pyogenic bacterial osteomyelitis are often associated with the age of the person or the inciting condition (e.g., trauma or surgery). *Staphylococcus aureus* is the most common cause, but organisms such as *Escherichia coli*, *Neisseria gonorrhoeae*, *Haemophilus influenzae*, and *Salmonella* species are also seen.[19,20] *Staphylococcus aureus* has two characteristics that favor its ability to produce osteomyelitis: (1) it has the ability to produce a collagen-binding adhesion molecule that allows it to adhere to the connective tissue elements of bone, and (2) it has the ability to evade host defenses, attack host cells, and colonize bone persistently.[31] Also, infection caused by methicillin-resistant *S. aureus* is becoming an increasingly common problem.[31]

Hematogenous Osteomyelitis. Hematogenous osteomyelitis originates with infectious organisms that reach the bone through the bloodstream.[8,19,20,30–32] Acute hematogenous osteomyelitis occurs predominantly in children. In adults, it is seen most commonly in debilitated persons and in those with a history of chronic skin infections, chronic urinary tract infections, and intravenous drug use and in those who are immunologically suppressed. Intravenous drug users are especially at risk for infections with *Streptococcus* and *Pseudomonas*.

The pathogenesis of hematogenous osteomyelitis differs in children and adults.[30] In children, the infection usually affects the long bones of the appendicular skeleton. It starts in the metaphyseal region close to the growth plate, where termination of nutrient blood vessels and sluggish blood flow favor the attachment of blood-borne bacteria (Fig. 43-8). With advancement of the infection, purulent exudate collects in the rigidly enclosed bony tissue. Because of the bone's rigid structure, there is little room for swelling and the purulent exudate finds its way beneath the periosteum, shearing off the perforating arteries that supply the cortex with blood, thereby leading to necrosis of cortical bone. The necrotic bone that is formed may separate from the viable surrounding bone

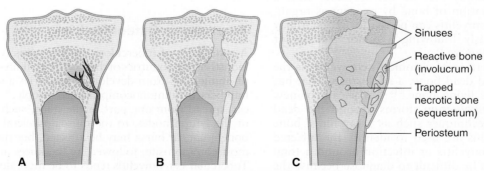

FIGURE 43-8. Hematogenous osteomyelitis. **(A)** Infectious organisms reach the metaphysis through a nutrient blood vessel. **(B)** Bacterial growth results in bone destruction and abscess formation. From the abscess cavity, the infection spreads between the trabeculae into the medullary cavity of compact bone and then through the cortex to the outside. **(C)** The purulent exudate finds its way beneath the periosteum, shearing off the perforating arteries that supply the cortex with blood, thereby leading to necrosis of cortical bone and formation of devascularized fragments, called *sequestra*.

Labels in figure: Sinuses; Reactive bone (involucrum); Trapped necrotic bone (sequestrum); Periosteum to form devascularized fragments, called *sequestra*.[18,19] Eventually, the purulent drainage may penetrate the periosteum and skin to form a draining sinus. In children 1 year of age and younger, the adjacent joint is often involved because the periosteum is not firmly attached to the cortex.[18,19] From 1 year of age to puberty, subperiosteal abscesses are more common. As the process continues, periosteal new bone formation and reactive bone formation in the marrow tend to wall off the infection.

In adults, the long bone microvasculature no longer favors seeding, and hematogenous infection rarely affects the appendicular skeleton. Instead, vertebrae, sternoclavicular and sacroiliac joints, and the symphysis pubis are involved. Infection typically first involves subchondral bone, then spreads to the joint space. With vertebral osteomyelitis, this causes sequential destruction of the endplate, adjoining disk, and contiguous vertebral body. Infection less commonly begins in the joint and spreads to the adjacent bone.

The signs and symptoms of acute hematogenous osteomyelitis are those of bacteremia accompanied by symptoms referable to the site of the bone lesion. Bacteremia is characterized by chills, fever, and malaise. There often is pain on movement of the affected extremity, loss of movement, and local tenderness followed by redness and swelling. X-ray studies may appear normal initially, but they show evidence of periosteal elevation and increased osteoclast activity after an abscess has formed. Radiographic bone scans and MRI can usually detect subtle changes at an earlier stage.

The treatment of hematogenous osteomyelitis begins with identification of the causative organism through blood and bone aspiration cultures. Antimicrobial agents are given first parenterally and then orally. The length of time the affected limb needs to be rested and the pain control measures used are based on the person's symptoms. Débridement and surgical drainage also may be necessary.

Chronic Osteomyelitis. Chronic osteomyelitis usually occurs in adults and is secondary to an open wound, most often to the bone or surrounding tissue. It may be the result of delayed or inadequate treatment of acute hematogenous osteomyelitis or osteomyelitis caused by direct contamination of bone by exogenous organisms. Chronic osteomyelitis can persist for years; it may appear spontaneously following a minor trauma, or when resistance is lowered.

The hallmark feature of chronic osteomyelitis is the presence of infected dead bone, a *sequestrum,* that has separated from the living bone.[8,18,19] A sheath of new bone, called the *involucrum,* forms around the dead bone. Radiologic techniques such as x-ray films, bone scans, and sinograms are used to identify the infected site. Chronic osteomyelitis or infection around a total joint prosthesis can be difficult to diagnose because the classic signs of infection are not apparent and the blood leukocyte count may not be elevated. A subclinical infection may exist for years. Bone scans are used with bone biopsy for a definitive diagnosis.

The treatment of chronic bone infections begins with wound cultures to identify the microorganism and its sensitivity to antibiotic therapy.[31-33] Initial antibiotic therapy is often followed by surgery to remove foreign bodies (e.g., metal plates, screws) or sequestra and by long-term antibiotic therapy. Immobilization of the affected part usually is necessary, with restriction of weight bearing on a lower extremity. External fixation devices are sometimes used.

Direct Penetration and Contiguous Spread Osteomyelitis. Direct penetration or extension of bacteria from an outside (exogenous) source is now the most common cause of osteomyelitis in the United States.[19] Bacteria may be introduced directly into the bone by a penetrating wound, an open fracture, or surgery. In persons with vascular insufficiency or poorly controlled diabetes, osteomyelitis may develop from a skin lesion.

Iatrogenic bone infections are those inadvertently brought about by surgery or other treatments. These complications include pin tract infection in skeletal traction, septic (infected) joints in joint replacement surgery, and wound infections after surgery. Risk factors for the development of a surgical site infection include both host factors and those related to the procedure.[34] Delays in wound healing, infection and failure of surgical implants cause greater morbidity and possibly the need for subsequent revision surgery.

Osteomyelitis after trauma or bone surgery usually is associated with persistent or recurrent fever, increased pain at the operative or trauma site, and poor incisional healing, which often is accompanied by continued wound drainage and wound separation. Prosthetic joint infections often present with joint pain, fever, and cutaneous drainage.

Treatment includes the use of antibiotics and selective use of surgical interventions. The choice of agents and method of administration depend on the microorganisms causing the infection. In acute osteomyelitis that does not respond to antibiotic therapy, surgical decompression is used to release intramedullary pressure and remove drainage from the periosteal area. Prosthesis removal may be necessary in cases of an infected prosthetic joint. The joint is left out while a 2- to 6-week course of therapy is given, after which another joint is implanted.[32]

Tuberculosis Osteomyelitis

A resurgence of tuberculosis osteomyelitis is occurring in industrialized countries of the world, attributed to the influx of immigrants from developing countries and the greater numbers of immunocompromised people.[19] Tuberculosis can spread from one part of the body, such as the lungs or the lymph nodes, to the musculoskeletal system. Any bone, joint, or bursa may be affected, but the spine is the most common site, followed by the knees and hips.[18,19,35] Tubercular osteomyelitis tends to be more destructive and difficult to control than pyogenic osteomyelitis. The infection spreads through large areas of the medullary cavity and causes extensive necrosis. In tuberculosis of the spine, also known as *Pott disease,* the infection spreads through the intervertebral disks to involve multiple vertebrae and extends into the soft tissue, forming abscesses.

Local symptoms include pain, immobility, and muscle atrophy; joint swelling, mild fever, and leukocytosis also may occur. The most feared complication of spinal tuberculosis is neurologic compromise due to spinal deformity and epidural abscess formation. Because there are no specific radiographic findings in tubercular osteomyelitis, the diagnosis is usually made by tissue biopsy or culture findings. In spinal tuberculosis, a computed tomography (CT)-guided biopsy is often used. The mainstay of treatment for tubercular osteomyelitis remains the appropriate three- or four-drug antimicrobial therapy based on current guidelines.[35] Conservative treatment is usually as effective as surgery, especially for earlier and milder cases.

Osteonecrosis

Osteonecrosis, also known as avascular necrosis, is an aseptic destruction of a segment of bone that is due to an interruption in blood flow rather than an infection.[18,19,36,37] It is relatively common and can occur in the medullary cavity of the metaphysis and the subchondral region of the epiphysis, especially in the hips, knees, shoulders, and ankles. Destruction of bone frequently is severe enough to require joint replacement surgery.

Bone has a rich blood supply that varies from site to site. The flow in the medullary portion of bone originates in nutrient vessels from an interconnecting plexus that supplies the marrow, trabecular bone, and endosteal half of the cortex. The outer cortex receives its blood supply from periosteal, muscular, metaphyseal, and epiphyseal vessels that surround the bone. Some bony sites, such as the head of the femur, have only limited collateral circulation so that interruption of the flow, such as with a hip fracture, can cause necrosis and irreversible damage to a substantial portion of medullary and cortical bone.

Although bone necrosis results from ischemia, the mechanisms producing the ischemia are varied and include mechanical interruption such as occurs with a fracture; thrombosis and embolism (e.g., sickle cell disease, nitrogen bubbles caused by inadequate decompression during deep sea diving); vessel injury (e.g., vasculitis, radiation therapy); and increased intraosseous pressure with vascular compression. Chart 43-1 lists some of the causes of osteonecrosis. Other than vessel injury and obstruction, the most common known cause is prior corticosteroid therapy.[38,39] Despite numerous studies, the mechanism of steroid-induced osteonecrosis remains unclear. The condition may develop after the administration of very high, short-term doses; during long-term treatment; or even from intra-articular injection. Although the risk increases with the dose and duration of treatment, it is difficult to predict who will be affected. Of recent concern is the development of osteonecrosis of the jaw with long-term use of bisphosphonates, drugs that are widely used for the treatment of postmenopausal osteoporosis, Paget disease of the bone, and cancer-related conditions.[40] The pathogenesis of bisphosphonate-associated osteonecrosis of the jaw remains largely unknown. The complication has mainly been reported in patients receiving the drugs intravenously for treatment of malignancies.

CHART 43-1	Causes of Osteonecrosis

Mechanical disruption of blood vessels
  Fractures
  Legg-Calvé-Perthes disease
  Blount disease
Thrombosis and embolism
  Sickle cell disease
  Nitrogen bubbles in decompression sickness
Vessel injury
  Vasculitis
  Connective tissue disease
    Systemic lupus erythematosus
    Rheumatoid arthritis
  Radiation therapy
  Gaucher disease
Corticosteroid therapy
Biphosphonate therapy (jaw osteonecrosis)

The pathologic features of bone necrosis are the same, regardless of cause. The site of the lesion is related to the vessels involved. There is necrosis of cancellous bone and marrow. The cortex usually is not involved because of collateral blood flow. In persons with subchondral infarcts (i.e., ischemia below the cartilage), a triangular or wedge-shaped segment of tissue that has the subchondral bone plate as its base and the center of the epiphysis as its apex undergoes necrosis (Fig. 43-9). In cases where medullary infarcts occur in fatty marrow, death of bone results in the release of calcium and necrosis of fat cells results in the release of free fatty acids.

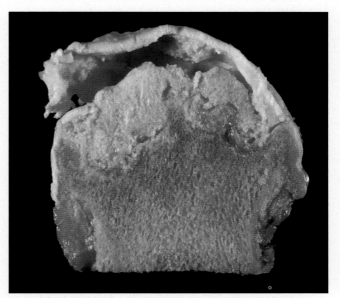

FIGURE 43-9. Osteonecrosis of the head of the femur. A coronal section shows a circumscribed area of subchondral infarction with partial detachment of the overlying articular cartilage and subarticular bone. (From Garcia RA, Klein MJ, Schiller AL. Bones and joints. In: Rubin R, Strayer DS, eds. *Rubin's Pathology: Clinicopathologic Foundations of Medicine.* 6th ed. Philadelphia, PA: Wolters Kluwer Health | Lippincott Williams & Wilkins; 2012:1217.)

The calcium and free fatty acids form lesions composed of an insoluble "soap." Because bone lacks mechanisms for resolving the infarct, the lesions remain for life.

The symptoms associated with osteonecrosis are varied and depend on the site and extent of infarction. Typically, subchondral infarcts cause chronic pain that is initially associated with activity but that gradually becomes more progressive until it is experienced at rest. Subchondral infarcts often collapse and predispose the patient to severe secondary osteoarthritis.

Diagnosis of osteonecrosis is based on history, physical findings, radiographic findings, and the results of special imaging studies, including CT scans and technetium-99 m bone scans. Treatment depends on the underlying pathologic process. In some cases, only short-term immobilization, nonsteroidal anti-inflammatory drugs, exercises, and limitation in weight bearing are used. Osteonecrosis of the hip is particularly difficult to treat. In persons with early disease, limitation of weight bearing through the use of a walker may allow the condition to stabilize. Although several surgical approaches have been used, the most definitive treatment of advanced osteonecrosis of the knee or hip is total joint replacement.

 SUMMARY CONCEPTS

■ Osteomyelitis, or infection of the bone and marrow, may be caused by a wide variety of microorganisms introduced during injury, operative procedures, or from the bloodstream. *Acute osteomyelitis* is seen most often as a result of direct contamination of bone by a foreign object. *Chronic osteomyelitis* represents an infection that continues beyond 6 to 8 weeks and may persist for years. *Tuberculosis osteomyelitis*, which is characterized by bone destruction and abscess formation, is caused by spread of infection from the lungs or lymph nodes.

■ Bone infections are difficult to treat and eradicate. Measures to prevent infection include careful cleaning and debridement of skeletal injuries and strict operating room procedures.

■ Osteonecrosis, or death of a segment of bone, is due to an interruption in blood flow rather than an infection. The mechanisms are varied and include mechanical interruption such as occurs with a fracture, vessel injury, increased intraosseous pressure with vascular compression, and corticosteroid therapy. Sites with poor collateral circulation, such as the femoral head, are most commonly affected. Symptoms include pain that varies in severity, depending on the extent of infarction. Total joint replacement is the most frequently used treatment for advanced osteonecrosis.

Neoplasms

Neoplasms of the skeletal system, often referred to as *bone tumors*, may be benign or malignant, and in the case of malignant neoplasms, may represent a primary tumor or secondary metastatic lesion.[5,8,18,19,41] Benign tumors greatly outnumber their malignant counterparts and occur with the greatest frequency in the first three decades of life, whereas in the elderly a bone tumor is more likely to be malignant.

Both benign and malignant tumors can develop from the cartilage (chondrogenic), bone (osteogenic), and supporting (fibrogenic) elements of bone, and bone tumors are generally classified according to their tissue counterpart. As a group, these tumors affect all age groups and arise in virtually every bone. Most develop during the first several decades of life and have a propensity to originate in the long bones of the extremities; however, certain types of tumors target specific age groups and anatomic sites. Thus, the location of the tumor provides important diagnostic information.

There are three major manifestations of bone tumors: pain, presence of a mass, and impairment of function.[5,8] Although benign tumors are frequently asymptomatic and are detected as an incidental finding, malignant tumors are associated with constant, deep aching pain that does not go away with rest and is present at night. However, certain benign tumors also cause night pain. A mass or hard lump may be the first sign of a bone tumor. A malignant tumor is suspected when a painful mass exists that is enlarging or eroding the cortex of the bone. The ease of discovery of a mass depends on the location of the tumor; a small lump arising on the surface of the tibia is easy to detect, whereas a tumor that is deep in the medial portion of the femur may grow to a considerable size before it is noticed. Benign and malignant tumors may cause the bone to erode to the point where it cannot withstand the strain of ordinary use. A sudden increase in pain followed by trivial trauma that is preceded by a history of mild, dull aching pain is suggestive of a pathologic fracture. A tumor also may produce pressure on a peripheral nerve, causing a decreased sensation, numbness, a limp, or limitation in movement.

The diagnosis of bone tumors relies on the history and physical examination, as well radiography, computed tomography, and MRI. Radiographs give the most general diagnostic information, such as malignant versus benign and primary versus metastatic status. The radiograph demonstrates the region of bone involvement, extent of destruction, and amount of reactive bone formed. CT scans further aid diagnosis and anatomic localization and can identify small pulmonary metastases not seen by conventional radiographs. Magnetic resonance imaging is the most accurate method of evaluating the intramedullary extent of bone tumor and can demarcate the soft structures in relation to neurovascular structures without the use of contrast media. It is best used in conjunction with a CT scan. Radionuclide bone scans are used to assess for metastasis. A biopsy may be done to determine the histologic characteristics of the tumor.

Benign Bone Tumors

Benign bone tumors usually are limited to the confines of the bone, have well-demarcated edges, and are surrounded by a thin rim of sclerotic bone. The most common benign tumors are of either fibrous or cartilaginous tissue origin. Benign fibrous tumors of the bone are common in growing bones. They are usually asymptomatic, resolve in 2 to 3 years, and do not require treatment.[8] Common cartilaginous tumors include chondromas and osteochondromas. Giant cell tumors, which contain mononuclear and osteoclast-type giant cells, are often classified as "intermediate" in nature between malignant and benign.

Chondromas are benign tumors of hyaline cartilage that usually occur in bones of endochondral origin.[18,19] They can arise within the medullary cavity, where they are known as *endochondromas*, or on the surface of bone, where they are called *subperiosteal* or *juxtacortical chondromas*. They are usually solitary lesions of and are most commonly found in short tubular bones of hands and feet. Most endochondromas are asymptomatic and detected incidentally. Occasionally they are painful and cause fractures. Treatment is usually simple observation, with surgical intervention reserved for cases in which pain or danger of fracture is present.

An *osteochondroma*, also known as an *exostosis*, is a benign cartilage-capped tumor that is attached to the underlying bone by a bony stalk. It is the most common benign bone tumor, about 85% of which occur as solitary tumors.[19] The remaining tumors are seen as part of a multiple hereditary exostosis syndrome, which is inherited as an autosomal dominant disorder. Solitary exostoses are usually first diagnosed in late adolescence or early adulthood, but multiple exostoses become apparent in childhood. Exostoses develop only in bones of endochondral origin, arising from the metaphysis near the growth plate of tubular bones, especially about the knee. Clinically, osteochondromas present as slow-growing masses, which can be painful if they impinge on a nerve or if the stalk is fractured. In many cases they are discovered incidentally. In multiple hereditary exostosis, the underlying bone may be bowed and shortened, reflecting an associated disturbance in epiphyseal growth. Osteochondromas usually stop growing at the time of growth plate closure. Malignant changes are rare, and excision of the tumor is done only when necessary.

A *giant cell tumor*, or *osteoclastoma*, is an aggressive tumor that often behaves like a malignant tumor, metastasizing through the bloodstream and recurring locally after excision.[19,42,43] The tumor is a mixture of mononuclear and multinucleated osteoclast-type giant cells. The mononuclear cells in the tumor express RANKL, and the giant osteoclast-like cells are believed to form via the RANK/RANKL signaling pathway (see Chapter 42).

Giant cell tumors usually arise in people in their thirties or forties.[19] The majority of tumors arise around the knee (distal femur and proximal tibia), but virtually any bone can be involved. The tumor begins in the metaphyseal region, grows into the epiphysis, and may extend into the joint surface. Pathologic fractures are common because the tumor destroys the bone substance.

Clinically, pain may occur at the tumor site, with gradually increasing swelling. X-ray films show destruction of the bone with expansion of the cortex. The biologic unpredictability of these tumors complicates their management. Conservative surgery such as curettage is associated with a 40% to 60% recurrence rate; up to 4% metastasize to the lungs.[19]

Malignant Bone Tumors

In contrast to benign tumors, primary malignant tumors tend to be ill defined, lack sharp borders, and extend beyond the confines of the bone. Primary malignant bone tumors occur in all age groups and may arise in any part of the skeleton. However, certain types of tumors tend to target certain age groups and anatomic sites (Fig. 43-10). For example, most osteosarcomas occur in adolescents and are particularly common around the knee joint. Also, people with certain conditions such as Paget disease are at increased risk for development of bone cancer.

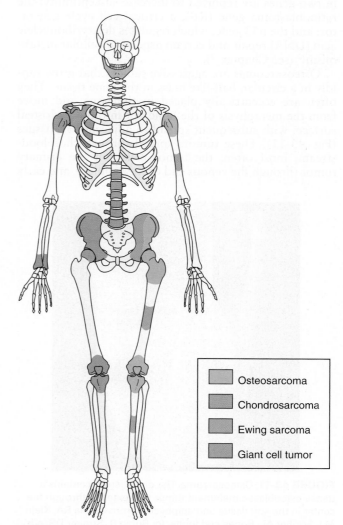

Osteosarcoma

Chondrosarcoma

Ewing sarcoma

Giant cell tumor

FIGURE 43-10. Common sites of primary malignant bone tumors (chondrosarcoma, osteosarcoma, and Ewing sarcoma) and giant cell tumor, a locally aggressive benign tumor.

Osteosarcoma

Osteosarcoma is an aggressive and highly malignant bone tumor.[18,19,44-46] It is the most common malignant bone tumor, representing one fifth of all primary bone tumors.[19] The tumor has a bimodal distribution, with 75% occurring in persons younger than 20 years of age.[19] A second peak occurs in the elderly with predisposing factors such as Paget disease, bone infarcts, or prior irradiation. Overall, men are more commonly affected than women.

The cause of osteosarcoma is unknown. The correlation of age and location of most of the tumors with the period of maximum growth suggests some relation to increased osteoblastic activity. In younger persons, the primary tumor most often is located at the anatomic sites associated with maximum growth velocity—the distal femur, proximal tibia, and proximal humerus. Bone tumors in the elderly are more common in the humerus, pelvis, and proximal femur. There are known genetic factors associated with osteosarcoma. Mutations in two genes are reported to increase susceptibility: the retinoblastoma gene (*RB*), a critical cell cycle generator; and the p53 gene, which regulates deoxyribonucleic acid (DNA) repair and certain aspects of cellular metabolism[19] (see Chapter 7).

Osteosarcomas are aggressive tumors that grow rapidly in a circular, ball-like mass in the bone tissue. They often are eccentrically placed in the bone and move from the metaphysis of the bone out into the periosteal surface, with subsequent spread to adjacent soft tissues (Fig. 43-11). These tumors spread through the bloodstream; most often, the tumor cells exit the primary tumor through the venous end of the capillary, and early metastasis to the lung is common. Lung metastases, even if massive, usually are relatively asymptomatic. The prognosis for a person with osteosarcoma depends on the aggressiveness of the disease, presence or absence of pathologic fractures, size of the tumor, and rapidity of tumor growth.

The primary clinical feature of osteosarcoma is deep, localized pain with nighttime awakening and swelling in the affected bone. Because the pain is often of sudden onset, patients and their families often associate the symptoms with recent trauma. The skin overlying the tumor may be warm, shiny, and stretched, with prominent superficial veins. The range of motion of the adjacent joint may be restricted.

The treatment of osteosarcoma is surgery in combination with multiagent chemotherapy, both before and after surgery.[45,46] In the past, treatment usually entailed amputation above the level of the tumor. Limb salvage surgical procedures, using a metal prosthesis or cadaver allograft, are now a standard alternative. In younger children who undergo arthroplasty, an expandable internal prosthesis is used to allow for bone growth. Amputation is another surgical option. It involves either the removal of expendable bones such as the fibula, toes, or ulna, or the complete removal of the tumor and the affected limb.

Chondrosarcoma

Chondrosarcoma consists of malignant tumors of cartilaginous lineage and is commonly subclassified according to site of origin as central (intramedullary) or peripheral (juxtacortical and surface).[18,19] Chondrosarcomas can arise as a primary tumor from preexisting benign cartilage tumors such as osteochondroma or chondroblastoma.[47] They commonly arise in the central portions of the skeleton, including the pelvis, shoulder, and ribs (see Fig. 43-10).

Chondrosarcomas develop about half as frequently as osteosarcomas. They occur primarily in middle or later life; however, there are chondromas that occur in younger persons. Chondrosarcomas are slow growing and metastasize late, and often are painless. They can remain hidden in an area such as the pelvis for a long period of time. This type of tumor, like many primary malignancies, tends to destroy bone and extend into the soft tissues beyond the confines of the bone of origin.

Early diagnosis is important because chondrosarcomas respond well to early radical surgical excision. It usually is resistant to radiation therapy and available chemotherapeutic agents. Not infrequently, these tumors transform into a highly malignant tumor, mesenchymal chondrosarcoma, which requires a more aggressive treatment, including combination chemotherapy.

Ewing Sarcoma

Ewing sarcoma is a member of a family of tumors that includes primitive neuroectodermal tumor (PNET). Both tumors are characterized by densely packed, regularly shaped, small cells with round or oval nuclei; and both share a specific reciprocal translocation of chromosomes 11 and 31, or variants thereof.[19,42,48,49]

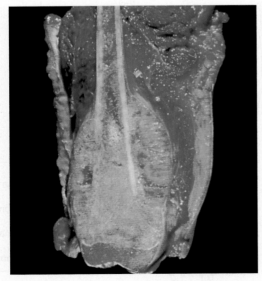

FIGURE 43-11. Osteosarcoma. The distal femur contains a dense osteoblastic malignant tumor that extends through the center in the soft tissue and epiphysis. (From Garcia RA, Klein MJ, Schiller AL. Bones and joints. In: Rubin R, Strayer DS, eds. *Rubin's Pathology: Clinicopathologic Foundations of Medicine.* 6th ed. Philadelphia, PA: Wolters Kluwer Health | Lippincott Williams & Wilkins; 2012:1244.)

Ewing sarcoma is primarily a disease of children and young adults and is rarely seen in older adults.[34,48,49] Males are affected slightly more frequently than females, and white children have an approximately ninefold higher incidence rate than black children. The most frequent site of Ewing sarcoma is the femur, usually in the diaphysis (see Fig. 43-10). The pelvis represents the second most common site; other sites include the pubis, sacrum, humerus, vertebrae, ribs, skull, and other flat bones. Manifestations of Ewing tumor include bone pain, limitation of movement, and tenderness over the involved bone or soft tissue. It often is accompanied by systemic manifestations such as fever or weight loss, which may serve to confuse the diagnosis. There may be a delay in diagnosis when the pain and swelling associated with the tumor are attributed to a sports injury, or when the tumor is located in the pelvis and the pain is not localized and the mass is not apparent. Pathologic fractures are common because of bone destruction. The most common sites of metastasis are the lungs, bone marrow, and other bones. Because Ewing sarcoma is a difficult diagnosis to establish, the diagnostic biopsy is very important.

Treatment methods incorporate a combination of multiagent chemotherapy, surgery, and radiation therapy.[34,48,49] Multiagent chemotherapy can shrink the tumor rapidly, and is generally given before local control measures are initiated. Ewing sarcoma is considered to be a radiosensitive tumor, and local control may be achieved through radiation or surgery. Patients with small, nonmetastatic, distally located tumors generally have the best prognosis.

Metastatic Bone Disease

Skeletal metastases are the most common malignancy of osseous tissue.[50,51] Approximately half of all people with cancer have bone metastasis at some point in their disease. Metastatic lesions are seen most often in the spine, femur, pelvis, ribs, sternum, proximal humerus, and skull, and are less common in anatomic sites more distant from the trunk of the body. Tumors that frequently spread to the skeletal system are those of the breast, lung, prostate, kidney, and thyroid, although any cancer can ultimately involve the skeleton.

The major symptom of bone metastasis is pain with evidence of an impending pathologic fracture. It usually develops gradually, over weeks, and is more severe at night. Pain is caused by stretching of the periosteum of the involved bone or by nerve entrapment, as when the nerve roots of the spinal cord are compressed by the vertebral body. Symptoms of hypercalcemia may occur in cases of bony destruction.

Radiographic examinations are used along with CT or bone scans to detect, diagnose, and localize metastatic bone lesions. A bone biopsy usually is done when there is a question regarding the diagnosis or treatment. Serum levels of alkaline phosphatase and calcium often are elevated in persons with metastatic bone disease.

The primary goals in treatment of metastatic bone disease are to prevent pathologic fractures and promote survival with maximum functioning, allowing the person to maintain as much mobility and pain control as possible. Standard treatment methods include chemotherapy, irradiation, and surgical stabilization. Radiation therapy is primarily used as a palliative treatment to alleviate pain and prevent pathologic fractures. After a pathologic fracture has occurred, bracing, intramedullary nailing of the femur, or spine stabilization may be done. Because adequate fixation often is difficult, bone cement often is used with internal fixation devices to stabilize the bone.

Recent research has focused on the role of osteoclastic and osteoblastic activity in the pathogenesis of metastatic bone disease and on the use of the bisphosphonates (e.g., pamidronate disodium, zoledronic acid) for its treatment.[52] The bisphosphonates, which are now well-established agents for the prevention and treatment of osteoporosis, have recently been shown to decrease symptoms associated with bone metastasis secondary to breast and prostate cancer. These agents bind preferentially to bone at sites of active bone metabolism, are released from the bone matrix during bone resorption, and potentially inhibit osteoclast activity and survival, thereby reducing osteoclast-mediated bone resorption. Recent studies suggest that besides their strong anti-osteoclastic activity, these agents may also have some direct antitumor effects.[41]

SUMMARY CONCEPTS

■ Both benign and malignant tumors can develop from the cartilage (chondrogenic), bone (osteogenic), and supporting (fibrogenic) elements of bone, and bone tumors are generally classified according to their tissue counterpart.

■ Benign bone tumors grow slowly and usually do not destroy the surrounding tissues. Malignant tumors can be primary or metastatic. Primary bone tumors are rare, grow rapidly, metastasize to the lungs and other parts of the body through the bloodstream. They include osteosarcoma, which begins in osteogenic cells of the bone and is the most common type of bone cancer; chondrosarcoma, which has its origin in the cartilaginous elements of bone; and Ewing sarcoma, which is characterized by small round cell tumors of bone and soft tissue origin.

■ Metastatic bone tumors usually are multiple in occurence, originating primarily from cancers of the breast, lung, and prostate. A primary goal in metastatic bone disease is the prevention of pathologic fractures.

Skeletal Disorders in Children

During childhood, skeletal structures grow in length and diameter and sustain a large increase in bone mass. Alterations in musculoskeletal structure and function may develop as a result of normal growth and developmental processes or as a result of impairment of skeletal development caused by hereditary or congenital influences.

Variations of Normal Growth and Development

Infants and children undergo changes in muscle tone and joint motion during growth and development. Intoeing, outtoeing, bowlegs, and knock-knees occur frequently in infancy and childhood. They usually cause few problems and are corrected during normal growth processes. The normal folded position of the fetus in utero causes physiologic flexion contractures of the hips and a froglike appearance of the lower extremities (Fig. 43-12). The hips are externally rotated and the patellae point outward, whereas the feet appear to point forward because of the internal pulling force of the tibiae. During the 1st year of life, the lower extremities begin to straighten out in preparation for walking. Internal and external rotations become equal, and the hips extend.

Musculoskeletal assessment of the newborn is important to identify abnormalities that require early intervention, facilitate treatment, establish baselines for future reference, and educate and counsel parents.[53–56] There are many clinical deviations that are easily correctable in a newborn. Many others correct spontaneously as the child grows.

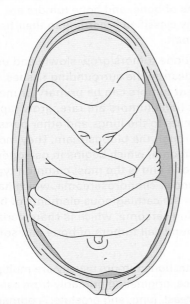

FIGURE 43-12. Position of fetus in utero, with tibial bowing and legs folded. (From Dunne KB, Clarren SK. The origin of prenatal and postnatal deformities. *Pediatr Clin North Am.* 1986;33(6):1277–1297; with permission from Elsevier Science.)

Angular and Torsional Deformities

All infants and toddlers have lax ligaments that become tighter with age and assumption of the weight-bearing posture. The hypermobility that accompanies joint laxity coupled with the torsional, or twisting, forces exerted on the limbs during growth are responsible for a number of variants seen in young children. Torsional forces caused by intrauterine positions or sleeping and sitting patterns twist the growing bones and can produce deformities as a child grows and develops.

In infants, the femur normally is rotated to an anteverted or forward position with the femoral head and neck rotated anteriorly with respect to the femoral condyles. Normally this angle is approximately 40 degrees at birth and declines to 15 to 29 degrees by 8 to 10 years of age.[55] A second source of rotation is found in the tibia. Infants can have 30 degrees of medial rotation of the tibia, and by maturity the rotation is between 5 degrees of medial rotation and 15 degrees of lateral rotation.[55] Abnormalities of rotation may include excessive adduction (turning in or toward the body) or abduction (turning out or away from the body).

Intoeing and Outtoeing. The foot progression angle describes the angle between the axis of the foot and the line of progression.[55] It is determined by watching the child walking and running, although it is usually less noticeable when the child is running or barefoot. Figure 43-13 illustrates the position of the foot in intoeing and outtoeing. Inward rotation of the foot is assigned a negative value and outward rotation is assigned a positive value. The normal value in children and adolescents is 10 degrees (range –3 to 20 degrees).

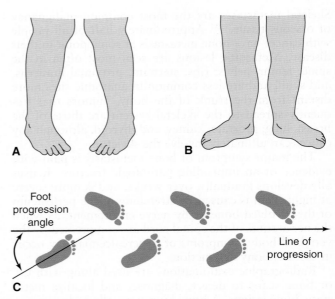

FIGURE 43-13. (A) Intoeing, **(B)** outtoeing, **(C)** intoeing and outtoeing can be determined by watching a child walk and comparing the long axis of the foot with the direction in which the child is walking. If the foot is directed inward, the angle is negative and indicative of intoeing; if it is positive, it is indicative of outtoeing.

The foot progression value serves only to define whether there is an intoeing or outtoeing gait.

Intoeing may be secondary to foot deformities or may be due to inward rotation of the femur or tibia, or a combination of the two.[54] Increased internal torsion of the femur (femoral anteversion) is the most common finding. In many cases intoeing is a variation of normal development. Outtoeing is a common problem in children and is caused by external femoral torsion. Because the femoral torsion persists when a child habitually sleeps in the prone position, an external tibial torsion also may develop. External tibial torsion rarely causes outtoeing; it only intensifies the condition. Outtoeing usually corrects itself as the child becomes proficient in walking.

Intoeing due to a condition called *metatarsus adductus* is a common congenital deformity characterized by forefoot adduction with a normal hindfoot, giving the foot a kidney-shaped appearance[55–57] (Fig. 43-14). It may occur in one foot or both feet. Diagnostic methods include examination of the plantar aspect of the foot, noting the overall shape of the foot and the presence or absence of an arch. The severity of the deformity can be determined by assessing the flexibility of the foot and using a heel bisection line. Normally, a line bisecting the heel crosses the forefoot between the second and third toes. In mild metatarsus adductus, the foot is flexible and can be passively manipulated and the line crosses the third toe; in a moderate deformity, the foot is less flexible and the line falls between the third and fourth toes; and in a severe deformity, the foot is more rigid and the line crosses between the fourth and fifth toes. Most infants do not require treatment, although parents are advised to avoid positioning the infant in the prone position with the feet turned in, a position that accentuates metatarsus adductus. Because the condition often corrects itself spontaneously, treatment is usually not instituted until the infant is 6 months of age.[56] When needed, treatment consists of serial long leg casting or a brace that pushes the metatarsals (not the hindfoot) into abduction.

Femoral Torsion. *Femoral torsion* refers to abnormal variations in hip rotation.[54] Hip rotation is measured at the pelvic level with the child in the prone position and the knees flexed at a 90-degree angle (Fig. 43-15A).

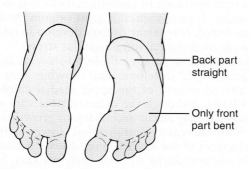

FIGURE 43-14. Shape of foot. The left foot is normal, whereas the right foot has metatarsus adductus.

- Back part straight
- Only front part bent

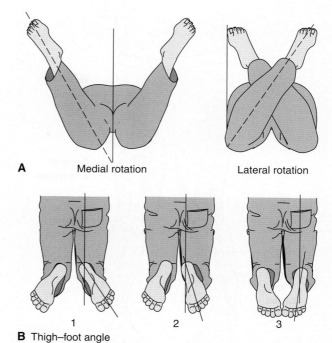

B Thigh–foot angle

FIGURE 43-15. (A) Hip rotation is measured with the child prone and knees flexed at a 90-degree angle. On outward rotation the leg produces internal (medial) hip and femoral rotation; on inward rotation the leg produces external hip and femoral rotation. **(B)** Assessment for tibial torsion using thigh–foot angle. When the child is in the prone position with the knee flexed, with normal alignment there is slight external rotation (2); internal tibial torsion produces inward rotation (3); external tibial torsion produces outward rotation (1). (Adapted from Staheli LT. Torsional deformity. *Pediatr Clin North Am.* 1986;33(6):1373–1383; and Kliegman RM, Neider MI, Super DM, eds. Practical strategies in pediatric diagnosis and therapy. Philadelphia, PA: W.B. Saunders; 1996.)

In this position, the hip is in a neutral position. Rotating the lower leg outward produces internal or medial femoral rotation; rotating it inward produces external or lateral rotation. During measurement of hip rotation, the legs are allowed to fall to full internal rotation by gravity alone; lateral rotation is measured by allowing the legs to fall inward and cross. Hip rotation in flexion and extension also can be measured with CT.

Excessive *internal femoral anteversion* is a normal variant commonly seen during the first 6 years of life, especially in 3- and 4-year-old girls.[55] Characteristically, there is 80 to 90 degrees of internal rotation of the hip in the prone position.[54,56] The condition is thought to be related to increased laxity of the anterior capsule of the hip such that it does not provide the stable pressure needed to correct the anteversion that is present at birth. Children are most comfortable sitting in the "W" position, with their hips between their knees. It is believed that this position allows the lower leg to act as a lever, producing torsional changes in the femur. When the child stands, the knees turn in and the feet appear to point straight ahead, and when the child walks, the

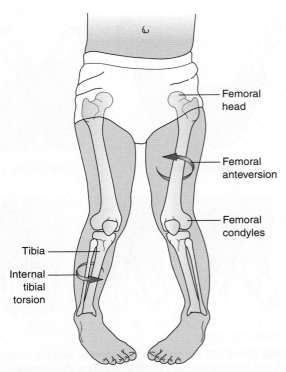

FIGURE 43-16. Femoral anteversion and internal tibial rotation. Femoral anteversion normally decreases from about 40 degrees at birth to 15 degrees at maturity, and internal tibial rotation from 5 degrees at birth to 15 degrees at maturity.

knees and toes point in (Fig. 43-16). Children with this problem are encouraged to sit cross-legged or in the so-called *tailor position* (with the knees touching and the legs folded under). If left untreated, the tibiae compensate by becoming externally rotated so that by 8 to 12 years of age, the knees may turn in but the feet no longer do so. A derotational osteotomy may be done in severe cases or if there is functional disability.

External femoral torsion is an uncommon disorder characterized by excessive external rotation of the hip. Bilateral external torsion is usually a benign condition, and treatment is observational. When the disorder is unilateral, slipped capital femoral epiphysis should be excluded (to be discussed).[54]

Tibial Torsion. Tibial rotation is determined by measuring the thigh–foot angle, which is done with the ankle and knee positioned at 90 degrees (see Fig. 43-15B). The angle is formed between the longitudinal axis of the femur and the longitudinal axis of the foot. Inward rotation, which is assigned a negative value, indicates internal tibial torsion, and outward rotation, which is given a positive value, represents external tibial rotation. Infants normally have a mean angle of –5 degrees as a consequence of normal in utero position.[54] In mid-childhood through adult life, the mean angle increases to about 10 degrees.

Internal or *medial tibial torsion* (i.e., bowing of the tibia) is a rotation of the tibia that makes the feet appear to turn inward. It is the most common cause of intoeing in children younger than 2 years of age.[55] It is present at birth and may fail to correct itself if children sleep on their knees with the feet turned in, or sit on in-turned feet. It is thought to be caused by genetic factors and intrauterine compression, such as an unstretched uterus during a first pregnancy or intrauterine crowding with twins or multiple fetuses. Tibial torsion improves naturally with growth, but this may take several years.[54]

External or *lateral tibial torsion* is a much less common disorder. It is usually seen between 4 and 7 years of age, and is often unilateral.[54] The natural growth rotates the tibia externally, and hence external tibial rotation can become worse with time.[54,55] Clinically, the patella faces outward when the foot is straight. There may be associated patellofemoral instability with knee pain. Although some correction may occur with growth, extremely symptomatic children may require surgical correction, which is usually done after 10 years of age.

Genu Varum and Genu Valgum

Genu varum and genu valgum are common pediatric deformities of the knee. As children grow, lower limb alignment usually follows a predicable pattern (Fig. 43-17). Genu varum, or bowlegs, is an outward bowing of the knees greater than 1 inch when the medial malleoli of the ankles are touching. Most infants and toddlers have some bowing of their legs up to 18 months of age. If there is a large separation between the knees (>15 degrees) after 2 years of age, the child may require bracing. Genu varum can cause gait awkwardness and increased risk for sprains and fractures. The child also should be evaluated for diseases such as rickets or tibia vara (i.e., Blount disease, to be discussed).

Genu valgum, or *knock-knees,* is a deformity in which there is decreased space between the knees.[58,59] The medial malleoli in the ankles cannot be brought in contact with each other when the knees are touching. Valgum normally develops after age 24 months and is most apparent between 3 and 4 years of age (see Fig. 43-17). By 7 years of age, the lower limb is in slight valgum and changes very little thereafter. Genu valgum can be ignored up to 7 years of age, unless it is more than 15 degrees, unilateral, or associated with short stature. It usually resolves spontaneously and rarely requires treatment. Uncorrected genu valgum may cause subluxation and recurrent dislocation of the patella, with a predisposition to chondromalacia and joint pain and fatigue. If genu varum or genu valgum persists and is uncorrected, osteoarthritis may develop in adulthood as a result of abnormal intra-articular stress.

Idiopathic tibia vara, or *Blount disease,* is an abnormal pathologic, developmental bowing that results from altered growth of the upper medial epiphysis[58,59] (Fig. 43-18). Although the cause of tibia vara remains unknown, it may occur secondary to growth suppression from increased compression forces across the medial aspect of the knee. Blount disease is more common in obese children who are early walkers. It is also more common in black children. It may be unilateral, in contrast to physiologic bowing, which is almost always

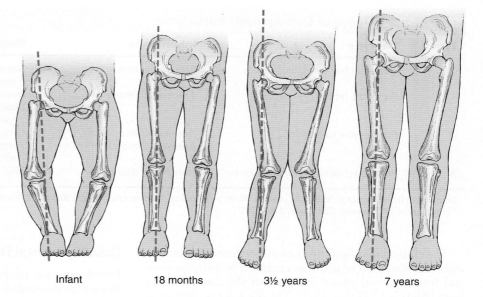

FIGURE 43-17. Lower limb alignment follows a predictable pattern. Infants typically have a gentle varum bow throughout the femur and tibia. By 18 to 24 months, the lower leg is nearly straight, with a neutral mechanical axis. Valgum gradually develops and is most apparent between 3 and 4 years of age. By 7 years of age, the lower limb is in slight valgus and changes very little thereafter. Varus should not recur, nor should valgus increase. (Adapted from Schoeneker PL, Rich MM. The lower extremity. In: Morrissy RT, Weinstein SL, eds. *Lovell & Winter's Pediatric Orthopaedics.* 6th ed. Philadelphia, PA: Lippincott Williams & Wilkins; 2006:1169.)

Infant   18 months   3½ years   7 years

bilateral. It has been classified into three types: infantile (1 to 3 years of age), juvenile (4 to 10 years of age), and adolescent (11 years or older). The juvenile and adolescent forms are commonly combined as late-onset tibia vara.

The infantile form of tibia vara, which is commonly bilateral, is the most common. Untreated infantile tibia vara is almost always progressive, with evidence of outward angulation, flexion, internal rotation, and abnormal lateral knee laxity. There is radiographic evidence of progressive depression of the medial metaphysis, the growth plate, and the epiphysis. Fusion of the metaphysis to the epiphysis may occur in severe cases. Night-brace treatment is used for mild early-onset disease. Valgum rotational osteotomy of the tibia is usually indicated if angulation persists beyond 3 years of age.

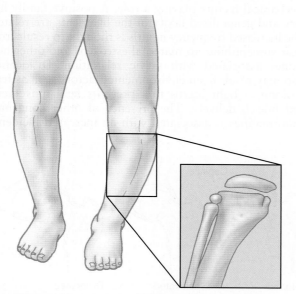

FIGURE 43-18. Rotational deformity of the proximal tibia, especially when unilateral, suggests tibia vara (Blount disease).

Persistent tibia vara leads to early degenerative changes of the knee.

Late-onset Blount disease is more common in obese boys who are of normal or greater-than-normal height. The condition may be bilateral or unilateral and characterized by pain rather than deformity as the primary initial complaint.[59] Radiography shows medial femoral and tibial bowing. Bracing is not practical in obese adolescents. Treatment includes osteotomy to realign the limb or lateral growth plate closure to allow growth to "catch up" medially.

Congenital Disorders

Congenital skeletal deformities can be caused by many factors, including hereditary influences, external agents that injure the fetus (e.g., radiation, alcohol, drugs, viruses), and intrauterine environmental factors. They range in severity from mild limb deformities, which are relatively common, to major limb malformations, which are relatively rare. The most common anomaly of the toes or fingers is *polydactyly,* or the presence of an extra digit on the hand or foot. There may also be a simple webbing of the fingers or toes (syndactyly) or the absence of a bone such as the phalanx, rib, or clavicle. Joint contractures and dislocations produce more severe deformity, as does the absence of entire bones, joints, or limbs.

Osteogenesis Imperfecta

Osteogenesis imperfecta, or brittle bone disease, is a hereditary disorder caused by deficiencies in the synthesis of type I collagen.[18,19,60,61] Although it is usually transmitted as an autosomal trait, a distinctive form of the disorder with multiple lethal defects is thought to be transmitted as an autosomal recessive trait.[19,61] In some cases, the disorder is caused by a spontaneous mutation.

TABLE 43-2 Types of Osteogenesis Imperfecta

Type	Subtype	Inheritance	Major Features
I	Postnatal fractures, blue sclera	Autosomal dominant	Normal stature, skeletal fragility, hearing impairment, joint laxity, blue sclera
II	Perinatal, lethal	Autosomal recessive	Death in utero, or during infancy Skeletal deformity with excessive fragility, multiple fractures, blue sclera
III	Progressive deformity	Autosomal dominant (75%) Autosomal recessive (25%)	Growth retardation, multiple fractures, progressive kyphoscoliosis, hearing impairment, blue sclera at birth
IV	Postnatal fractures, normal sclera	Autosomal dominant	Moderate skeletal fragility, short stature

Developed from Kumar V, Abbas AK, Fausto N, et al. *Robbins & Cotran Pathologic Basis of Disease*. 8th ed. Philadelphia, PA: Elsevier Saunders; 2010:1212.

The clinical manifestations of osteogenesis imperfecta include a spectrum of disorders marked by extreme skeletal fragility. Four major subtypes of the disorder have been identified[18] (Table 43-2). The disorder is characterized by thin and poorly developed bones that are prone to multiple fractures. These children have short limbs and a soft, thin cranium with bifrontal prominences that give a triangular appearance to the face. Other problems associated with defective connective tissue synthesis include thin skin, blue or gray sclera, abnormal tooth development, hypotonic muscles, loose-jointedness, scoliosis, and a tendency toward hernia formation. Hearing loss due to otosclerosis of the tiny bones in the middle ear is common in affected adults.

The most serious defects occur when the disorder is inherited as a recessive trait (type II). Severely affected fetuses have multiple intrauterine fractures and bowing and shortening of the extremities. Many of these infants are stillborn or die during infancy. Less severe forms occur when the disorder is inherited as a dominant trait. The skeletal system is not as weakened, and fractures often do not appear until the child becomes active and starts to walk, or even later in childhood. These fractures heal rapidly, although with a poor-quality callus. In some cases, parents may be suspected of child abuse when the child is admitted to the health care facility with multiple fractures. There also is an increased incidence of complications such as hernias and congenital heart abnormalities.

There is no definitive treatment for correction of the defective collagen synthesis that is characteristic of osteogenesis imperfecta. However, a short course of treatment with bisphosphonates has been shown to produce an increase in cortical bone width and cancellous bone volume, as well as increased bone strength and mineral content. In children treated with intravenous pamidronate, this has led to a decrease in fractures, improvements in mobility, and less pain.[62] Prevention and treatment of fractures is important. Precise alignment is necessary to prevent deformities. Nonunion is common, especially with repeated fractures. Surgical intervention often is needed to stabilize fractures and correct deformities (e.g., internal fixation of long bones may be done with an intramedullary rod that "grows" with the child).

Developmental Dysplasia of the Hip

Developmental dysplasia of the hip (DDH), formerly known as *congenital dislocation of the hip,* is an abnormality in hip development that leads to a wide spectrum of hip problems in infants and children, including hips that are unstable, malformed, subluxated, or dislocated.[63–65] In less-severe cases, the hip joint may be unstable, with excessive laxity of the joint capsule, or subluxated, so that the joint surfaces are separated and there is a partial dislocation (Fig. 43-19). With dislocated hips, the head of the femur is located outside of the acetabulum.

The results of newborn screening programs have shown that 1 of 250 infants have some evidence of hip instability, whereas actual dislocation of the hip is less common, being found in 1 to 1.5 of every 1000 live births.[55] The left hip is involved more frequently than the right hip because of the left occipital intrauterine positioning of most infants. The disorder occurs most frequently in first-born children and is six times more common in female than in male infants. The cause of DDH is multifactorial, with heredity, environmental, and mechanical factors playing a role. A positive family history and generalized laxity of the ligaments are related. The increased frequency in girls is thought to result from their susceptibility to maternal estrogens and other hormones associated with pelvic relaxation. Dislocation also may result from environmental factors such as fetal position, a tight uterus that prevents fetal movement, and breech delivery. The presence of other congenital abnormalities is associated with an increased incidence

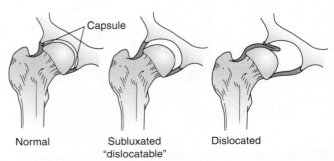

FIGURE 43-19. Normal *(left)* and abnormal relationships of hip joint structure in subluxation *(middle)* and dislocation (right).

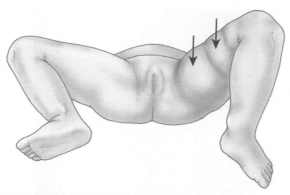

FIGURE 43-20. Congenital dysplasia of the left hip with shortening of the femur, as indicated by legs in abduction and asymmetric gluteal and thigh folds (*arrows*).

of DDH. Thus, the hips of children presenting with congenital abnormalities should be examined carefully.

Early diagnosis of DDH is important because treatment is easiest and most effective if begun during the first 6 months of life. Also, repeated dislocations cause damage to the femoral head and the acetabulum. In infants, signs of DDH include asymmetry of the hip or gluteal folds, shortening of the thigh so that one knee (on the affected side) is higher than the other knee, and limited abduction of the affected hip[63–67] (Fig. 43-20). The asymmetry of gluteal folds is not definitive but indicates the need for further evaluation. Physical examination remains the key to the diagnosis of DDH. However, the U.S. Preventive Services Task Force (USPSTF) recently concluded that evidence was insufficient to recommend routine screening of asymptomatic infants as a means of preventing adverse outcomes.[66] This recommendation applies only to infants who do not have obvious hip dislocation or other abnormalities evident without screening.

Several examination techniques can be used to screen for a dislocatable hip. Two provocative dynamic tests for assessing hip stability in the newborn are the Ortolani maneuver (for reducible dislocation) and the Barlow maneuver (for the dislocatable hip)[8,63–65] (Fig. 43-21). The Galeazzi test is a measurement of the length of the femurs that is done by comparing the height at the knees while they are flexed at 90 degrees. An inequality in the height of the knees is a positive Galeazzi sign and is usually caused by hip dislocation or congenital femoral shortening. This test is not useful in detecting bilateral DDH because both leg lengths will be equal. In an older child, instability of the hip may produce a delay in standing or walking and eventually cause a characteristic waddling gait. When the thumbs are placed over the anterior iliac crest and the hands are placed over the lateral pelvis in examination, the levels of the thumbs are not even; the child is unable to elevate the opposite side of the pelvis (positive Trendelenburg test).

Diagnosis of DDH is confirmed by ultrasonography or radiography. Ultrasonography is used in infants with high-risk factors (e.g., female infants born in the breech position) or an abnormal result on examination.[63–67] Radiographs of newborns with suspected DDH are of limited value because the femoral heads do not ossify until 4 to 6 months of age. After 6 months of age, the

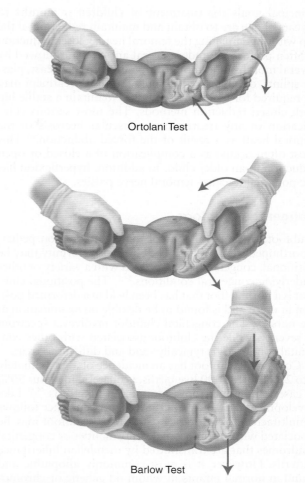

FIGURE 43-21. Examination for developmental dysplasia of the hip. In the newborn both hips should be able to be equally flexed, abducted, and rotated without producing a "click." A diagnosis of developmental dysplasia of the hip may be confirmed by the Ortolani "click" test (top), in which the involved hip cannot be abducted as far as the opposite one, and there is a "click" as the femoral head moves back into place. A positive Barlow test (bottom) is not diagnostic of developmental dyplasia of the hip, but indicates laxity and a dislocatable progressively, and a need for the baby to be re-examined in the future. A feeling of the head of the femur slipping out into the anterior lip of the acetabulum, constitutes a positive Barlow sign. This can be confirmed by abducting the hip by pressing with your index and middle fingers back inward and feeling for movement of the femoral head as it returns to the hip socket.

increasing ossification of the femur renders ultrasonography less reliable, and radiographs are preferred.

Treatment of DDH should be individualized and depends on whether the hip is subluxated or dislocated. Subluxation of the hip at birth often resolves without treatment and should be observed for 2 weeks. When subluxation persists beyond this time, treatment may be indicated and referral is recommended. The best results are obtained if the treatment is begun before changes in the hip structure (e.g., 2 to 3 months) prevent it from being reduced by gentle manipulation or abduction devices. The Pavlik harness is used on newborns (up to 6 months) to maintain the femoral head in the acetabulum.[63] The principal goals for treatment of children 6 months to 2 years of age are to obtain and maintain reduction of the hip without damaging the femoral head. Closed reduction is often performed under general anesthesia, followed by several months of immobilization in a hip spica cast, plaster splints, or an abduction splint. Surgical treatment may be required for children who fail to maintain a stable hip with closed reduction methods. The most serious complication of any treatment is avascular necrosis of the femoral head as a result of the forced abduction.[63] This most often occurs as a complication of a closed or open reduction in an older child. In addition, hyperflexion has the potential to cause femoral nerve palsies.

Congenital Clubfoot

Clubfoot, or talipes, is one of the most common pediatric orthopedic conditions. The clubfoot deformity may be positional, congenital, or associated with a variety of other underlying congenital conditions.[56,57] The positional clubfoot is a normal foot that has been held in a deformed position in utero and is found to be flexible on examination in the nursery. The congenital clubfoot involves a spectrum of severity, while the clubfoot associated with other congenital conditions is typically rigid and difficult to treat.

Congenital clubfoot has an incidence of approximately 1 to 2 cases per 1000 live births, is bilateral in about 50% of cases, and affects boys more often than girls.[56,57] Like developmental dysplasia of the hip, its occurrence follows a multifactorial inheritance pattern.[68,69] Clubfoot may be associated with chromosomal abnormalities or congenital syndromes that are transmitted by mendelian inheritance patterns. However, it is most commonly idiopathic and found in normal infants in whom no genetic or chromosomal abnormality or other extrinsic cause can be found.

In forefoot adduction, which accounts for approximately 95% of idiopathic cases, the foot is plantar flexed and inverted or twisted toward the midline of the leg.[56] This is the so-called *equinovarus type* of clubfoot (Fig. 43-22). The other 5% of cases are of the equinovalgus type, or reverse clubfoot, in which the foot is dorsiflexed and everted. Reverse clubfoot can occur as an isolated condition or in association with multiple congenital defects. At birth, the feet of many infants assume one of these two positions, but they can be passively overcorrected or brought back into the opposite position. If the foot cannot be overcorrected, some type of correction may be necessary.

Treatment of clubfoot is begun as soon as the diagnosis is made. When treatment is initiated during the first few weeks of life, a nonoperative procedure may be effective. Serial manipulations and casting are used gently to correct each component of the deformity. One method, called the *Ponseti method,* involves weekly gentle stretching and manipulation of the misaligned bones followed by application of a well-molded long leg plaster cast with the knee held at a right angle.[56,57,69–71] The cast maintains the correction and allows for further relaxation of tight structures in anticipation of the next week's casting. Correction of the deformity is usually obtained within 6 to 8 weeks. Frequently, a percutaneous Achilles tendon lengthening is performed using a topical

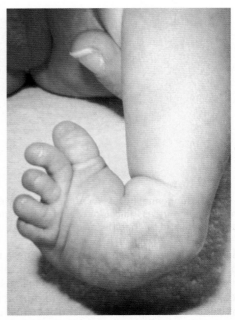

FIGURE 43-22. Newborn with clubbing of the left foot. (From the Centers for Disease Control and Prevention Public Health Images Library. No. 2632. Courtesy of James W. Hanson.)

anesthetic cream before application of the final cast to allow for complete correction of the equinus deformity. The correction is maintained by wearing a brace full time for 3 months and part-time wear during napping and at night for approximately 2 to 3 years.[56] Surgery may be required for severe deformities or when nonoperative treatment methods are unsuccessful. It is performed most commonly between 6 and 12 months of age.[56]

Juvenile Osteochondroses

Juvenile osteochondroses are a group of children's diseases in which one or more growth ossification centers undergo a period of degeneration, necrosis, or inactivity that is followed by regeneration and usually deformity. The osteochondroses are separated into two groups according to their causes. The first group consists of the true osteonecrotic osteochondroses, so called because the diseases are caused by localized osteonecrosis of an apophyseal or epiphyseal center (e.g., Legg-Calvé-Perthes disease, Freiberg infraction, Panner disease, Kienböck disease). The second group of juvenile osteochondroses is caused by abnormalities in ossification of cartilaginous tissue resulting from a genetically determined normal variation or from trauma (e.g., Osgood-Schlatter disease, Blount disease, Sever disease, Scheuermann disease). The discussion in this section focuses on Legg-Calvé-Perthes disease from the first group and Osgood-Schlatter disease from the second group. Slipped capital femoral epiphysis is a disorder of the growth plate.

Legg-Calvé-Perthes Disease

Legg-Calvé-Perthes disease is an idiopathic osteonecrotic disease of the proximal (capital) femoral epiphysis with later reabsorption.[72–74] The disorder usually (but not exclusively) affects children between the ages of 4 and 8 years. Boys are affected four to five times as often as girls and 10% to 15% of all cases are bilateral. Although no definite genetic pattern has been established, it occasionally affects more than one family member.

The cause of Legg-Calvé-Perthes disease is unknown. The disorder usually is insidious in onset and occurs in otherwise healthy children. It may, however, be associated with acute trauma. Affected children usually have a shorter stature. Recent evidence suggests that some cases may be caused by a subclinical hypercoagulable state such as deficiency in antithrombotic factors S or C or a decrease in fibrinolysis. When girls are affected, they usually have a poorer prognosis than boys because they are skeletally more mature and have a shorter period for growth and remodeling than boys of the same age.

The primary pathologic feature of Legg-Calvé-Perthes disease is an avascular necrosis of the bone and marrow involving the epiphyseal growth center in the femoral head. The disorder may be confined to part of the epiphysis, or it may involve the entire epiphysis. In severe cases, there is a disturbance in the growth pattern that leads to a broad, short femoral neck. The necrosis is followed by slow absorption of the dead bone over 2 to 3 years. Although the necrotic trabeculae eventually are replaced by healthy new bone, the epiphysis rarely regains its normal shape.

The main symptoms of Legg-Calvé-Perthes disease are pain in the groin, thigh, or knee and difficulty in walking. The child may have a painless limp with limited abduction and internal rotation and a flexion contracture of the affected hip. The age of onset is important because young children have a greater capability for remodeling of the femoral head and acetabulum, and thus less flattening of the femoral head occurs. Early diagnosis is important and is based on correlating physical symptoms with radiographic findings that are related to the stage of the disease.

The goal of treatment is to reduce deformity and preserve the integrity of the femoral head. Conservative and surgical interventions are used in the treatment of Legg-Calvé-Perthes disease. Children younger than 4 years of age with little or no involvement of the femoral head may require only periodic observation. In all other children, some intervention is needed to relieve the force of weight bearing, muscular tension, and subluxation of the femoral head. It is important to maintain the femur in a well-seated position in the concave acetabulum to prevent deformity. This is done by keeping the hip in abduction and mild internal rotation. Treatment involves periods of rest, use of assistive devices for walking, non–weight-bearing, and abduction braces to keep the legs separated in abduction with mild internal rotation. The Atlanta Scottish Rite brace, which does not extend below the knee, is the most widely used orthosis because it provides containment while allowing free knee motion and ambulation without crutches or external support[63] (Fig. 43-23). Surgery may be done to contain the femoral head in the acetabulum. This treatment usually is reserved for children older than 6 years of age who at the time of diagnosis have more serious involvement of the femoral head. The best surgical results are obtained when surgery is done early, before the epiphysis becomes necrotic.

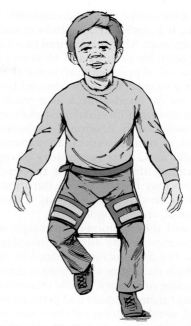

FIGURE 43-23. Scottish Rite brace for Legg-Calvé-Perthes disease produces containment for abduction and allows free knee motion. (From Crocetti M, Barone MA. *Oski's Essential Pediatrics*. 2nd ed. Philadelphia, PA: Lippincott Williams & Wilkins; 2004:679.)

Osgood-Schlatter Disease

Osgood-Schlatter disease involves microfractures in the area where the patellar tendon inserts into the tibial tubercle.[66] This area, which is an extension of the proximal tibial epiphysis, is particularly vulnerable to injury caused by sudden or continued strain from the patellar tendon during periods of growth. It occurs most frequently in boys between the ages of 10 and 15 years and in girls about 2 years before that in boys.[59]

The disorder is characterized by pain in the front of the knee that is associated with inflammation and thickening of the patellar tendon. The pain usually is associated with specific activities such as kneeling, running, bicycle riding, or stair climbing. There is swelling, tenderness, and increased prominence of the tibial tubercle. The symptoms usually are self-limiting. They may recur during growth periods, but usually resolve after closure of the tibial growth plate.

Treatment consists of rest, restriction of activities, and occasionally a knee immobilizer. Complete resolution of symptoms through healing (physical closure) of the tibial tubercle usually requires 12 to 24 months.[59] Occasionally, minor symptoms or an increased prominence of the tibial tubercle may continue into adulthood.

Slipped Capital Femoral Epiphysis

Slipped capital femoral epiphysis, or coxa vara, is a disorder of the growth plate that occurs near the age of skeletal maturity.[69] It involves a three-dimensional displacement of the epiphysis (posteriorly, medially, inferiorly), meaning that the femur is rotated externally from under the epiphysis. It is considered the most common hip disorder of adolescence with an increased prevalence among males, most often between 11 and 16 years of age.[72]

The cause of slipped capital femoral epiphysis is obscure, but it may be related to the child's susceptibility to stress on the femoral neck as a result of genetics or structural abnormalities. Affected children often are overweight with poorly developed secondary sex characteristics, or, in some instances, are extremely tall and thin. In many cases, there is a history of rapid skeletal growth preceding displacement of the epiphysis. The condition also may be affected by nutritional deficiencies or endocrine disorders such as hypothyroidism, hypopituitarism, and hypogonadism.

Children with the condition often complain of referred knee pain accompanied by difficulty in walking, fatigue, and stiffness. The diagnosis is confirmed by radiographic studies in which the degree of slipping is determined and graded according to severity.[72] Early treatment is imperative to prevent further slippage and permanent deformity. Avoidance of weight bearing on the femur and bed rest are essential parts of the treatment. Traction or gentle manipulation under anesthesia is used to reduce the slip. Surgical insertion of pins to keep the femoral neck and head of the femur aligned is a common method of treatment for children with moderate or severe slips. Crutches are used for several months after surgical correction to prevent full weight bearing until the growth plate closes.

Children with the disorder must be followed closely until the epiphyseal plate closes. Long-term prognosis depends on the amount of displacement that occurs. Complications include avascular necrosis, leg shortening, malunion, and problems with internal fixation. Degenerative arthritis may develop, requiring joint replacement later in life.

Scoliosis

Scoliosis is a lateral curvature of the spine in the upright position. Scoliosis is classified as postural or structural. With postural scoliosis, there is a small curve that corrects with bending. It can be corrected with passive and active exercises. Structural scoliosis does not correct with bending. It is a fixed deformity classified according to the cause: congenital, neuromuscular, or idiopathic.[75-79]

Types of Scoliosis

Congenital scoliosis is caused by disturbances in vertebral development during the sixth to eighth weeks of embryologic development.[75-79] It may involve failures of formation or failures of segmentation. Failures of formation indicate the absence of a portion of the vertebra, such as hemivertebra (absence of a whole side of the vertebra) and wedge vertebra (missing only a portion of the vertebra). Failure of segmentation is the absence of the normal separation between the vertebrae. The child may have other anomalies and neurologic complications if the spine is involved. Early diagnosis and treatment of progressive curves are essential for children

with congenital scoliosis. Surgical intervention is the treatment of choice for progressive congenital scoliosis.

In neuromuscular scoliosis, there is often a long, C-shaped curve from the cervical to the sacral region. It is seen in children with cerebral palsy, in whom severe deformity may make treatment difficult. It also develops in children with Duchenne muscular dystrophy and usually is not severe.

Idiopathic scoliosis is a structural spinal curvature for which no cause has been established. It occurs in healthy, neurologically normal children. Although the incidence is only slightly greater in girls than boys, it is more likely to progress and require treatment in girls.[8,77-79] It seems likely that heredity is involved because mother–daughter pairings are common, but identical twins are not uniformly affected, and the magnitude of the curvature in an affected individual is not related to magnitude of curvature in relatives. A recent study of the melatonin receptor 1B (MTNR1B) gene in persons with adolescent idiopathic scoliosis suggests that the MTNR1B gene may serve as a susceptibility gene.[81]

Idiopathic scoliosis usually appears clinically between the age of 10 and skeletal maturity, but may be seen at any age. By definition, the curve must be greater than 10 degrees—this has historically been used because 10 degrees is the limit that can be detected by physical examination.[8] Although the curve may be present in any area of the spine, the most common curve is a right thoracic curve.

Manifestations

Scoliosis usually is first noticed because of the deformity it causes. A high shoulder, prominent hip, or projecting scapula may be noticed by a parent or in a school-based screening program (Fig. 43-24). Idiopathic scoliosis

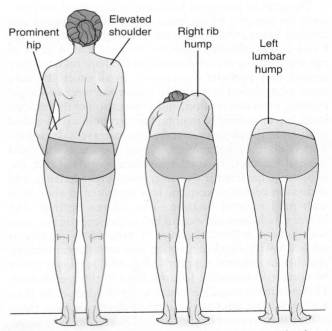

FIGURE 43-24. Scoliosis: Abnormalities to be determined at initial screening examination.

usually is a painless process, although pain may be present in severe cases, usually in the lumbar region. The pain may be caused by pressure on the ribs or on the crest of the ilium. There may be shortness of breath as a result of diminished chest expansion and gastrointestinal disturbances from crowding of the abdominal organs. Adults with less-severe deformity may experience mild backache. If scoliosis is left untreated, the curve may progress to an extent that compromises cardiopulmonary function and creates a risk for neurologic complications.

Diagnosis and Treatment

Early diagnosis of scoliosis can be important in the prevention of severe spinal deformity. The cardinal signs of scoliosis are uneven shoulders or iliac crest, prominent scapula on the convex side of the curve, misalignment of spinous processes, asymmetry of the flanks, asymmetry of the thoracic cage, and rib hump or paraspinal muscle prominence when bending forward[79–80] (see Fig. 43-24). A complete physical examination is necessary for children with scoliosis because the defect may be indicative of other, underlying pathologic processes.

Diagnosis of scoliosis is made by physical examination and confirmed by radiography. A scoliometer is used at the apex of the curvature to quantify a prominence; a scoliometer reading of greater than 10 degrees requires referral to a physician. The curve is measured by determining the amount of lateral deviation present on radiographs and is labeled "right" or "left" for the convex portion of the curve. Other radiographic procedures may be done, including CT scanning, MRI, and myelography.

Although school screening continues to be mandated in a number of states, the USPSTF recommends against the routine screening of asymptomatic adolescents for idiopathic scoliosis, indicating that the potential harms from screening include unnecessary follow-up visits and evaluations due to false-positive results, and adverse psychological effects, especially related to brace wear.[80] It is recommended, however, that health care professionals be prepared to evaluate idiopathic scoliosis when it is discovered incidentally or when an adolescent or parent expresses concern about scoliosis.

The treatment of scoliosis depends on the severity of the deformity and the likelihood of curve progression. The three determinants of progression are gender, the curve magnitude at the time of diagnosis, and skeletal growth potential.[82–83] In all cases, girls have a risk progression 10 times greater than that of boys. Larger curves are more likely to progress. Age of presentation also is important. Curves that are detected before menarche are more likely to progress than those detected after menarche. For persons with lesser degrees of curvature (10 to 20 degrees), the trend has been away from aggressive treatment and toward a "wait and see" approach, taking advantage of the more sophisticated diagnostic methods that now are available. Treatment is considered for physically immature patients with curves between 20 and 30 degrees. Curves between 30 and 40 degrees usually are considered for bracing, and those greater than 40 to 45 degrees are considered for surgery.

A brace may be used to control the progression of the curvature during growth and can provide some correction. In an effort to improve compliance, a number of new bracing techniques have been developed. These orthoses consist of easily more concealed, prefabricated forms that are modified to suit the patient.

The goals of surgery are to arrest progression of the deformity, improve appearance, and achieve a balanced spine, while limiting the number of vertebral segments that are stabilized. Instrumentation helps correct the curve and balance, and spinal fusion maintains the spine in the corrected position.[75–79] Several methods of instrumentation (i.e., rods that attach to the vertebral column and posterior fusion) are used. Combined anterior and posterior surgery is used for more severe curvatures. The newer systems provide better sagittal control and more stable fixation, which allow earlier mobility. Despite great advances in spinal surgery, no one method seems to be the best for all cases. There is recent interest in growth modulation approaches using minimally invasive techniques, which will result in curve correction while preserving spinal motion and intervertebral disk viability.[82]

SUMMARY CONCEPTS

■ Skeletal disorders can result from congenital or hereditary influences or from factors that occur during normal periods of skeletal growth and development. Newborn infants undergo normal changes in muscle tone and joint motion, causing torsional conditions of the femur or tibia. Many of these conditions are corrected as skeletal growth and development take place.

■ Osteogenesis imperfecta is a rare autosomal hereditary disorder characterized by defective synthesis of connective tissue, including bone matrix. It results in poorly developed bones that fracture easily.

■ Disorders such as developmental dysplasia of the hip and congenital clubfoot are present at birth. Both of these disorders are best treated during infancy. Regular examinations during the first year of life are recommended as a means of achieving early diagnosis.

■ Other childhood skeletal disorders, such as the juvenile osteochondroses and slipped capital femoral epiphysis, are not corrected by the growth process. These disorders are progressive, can cause permanent disability, and require treatment.

(continued)

SUMMARY CONCEPTS *(continued)*

■ Scoliosis is a lateral curvature of the spine. It is classified as congenital, which results from defects in vertebral development; neuromuscular, which is caused by diseases such as cerebral palsy; and idiopathic, which is the most common form. Idiopathic scoliosis affects girls more often than boys and usually becomes evident between age 10 years and skeletal maturity. The treatment of scoliosis depends on the severity of the deformity and the likelihood of curve progression. Curves between 30 and 40 degrees usually are considered for bracing, and those greater than 40 to 45 degrees are considered for surgery.

REVIEW EXERCISES

1. A 34-year-old football player dislocates his hip during a game.

A. Explain the need for immediate reduction of the dislocation based on the vascular anatomy of the hip.

2. A 39-year-old man is in intensive care after a motorcycle accident in which he skidded across the pavement on his right side. He has fractures of his right femur, pelvis, and several ribs on the right side. His right leg was crushed beneath the motorcycle, and he is beginning to lose movement in that leg.

A. What are the priorities in treating his orthopedic injuries? What are the available options for stabilizing his leg?
B. What risk factors for complications of fractures are present?
C. What are the symptoms of compartment syndrome, and how is it treated?

3. A 73-year-old woman with a history of breast cancer sustained a comminuted fracture in the mid-diaphysis of her left humerus when her husband lifted her up in bed. She has multiple lucent lesions scattered throughout her proximal humerus, radius, and ulna. She was recently hospitalized for confusion and found to have diffuse bone metastases.

A. What would you consider to be the most likely cause of her fracture?
B. What are the most common sites for bone metastasis?
C. Explain the treatment goals for persons with pathologic fractures.

4. A 14-year-old boy complains of recent pain and swelling of the knee, with some restriction in movement. Although he thinks he may have injured his knee playing football, his mother insists that he be seen by an orthopedic specialist and raises the possibility that the boy may have an osteosarcoma.

A. Use the information that osteosarcoma originates in sites of maximal growth velocity to explain the site of this boy's possible tumor.
B. What diagnostic tests could be used to establish a diagnosis of osteosarcoma?
C. The boy and his family are concerned that the boy will require radical surgery with amputation of the leg. How would you go about explaining possible treatment options to him?

5. A newborn girl was found to have developmental dysplasia of the hip during a routine screening examination.

A. Describe the anatomic abnormalities that are present in the disorder.
B. Explain the need for early treatment of developmental dysplasia of the hip.

REFERENCES

1. National Centers for Disease Control and Prevention, Centers for Disease Control and Prevention. *CDC Injury Fact Book.* Atlanta, GA: Centers for Disease Control and Prevention; 2006.
2. American Academy of Orthopaedic Surgeons. *Overuse injuries in children.* 2012. Available at: http://orthoinfo.aaos.org/topic.cfm?topic=A00613. Accessed August 21, 2013.
3. Paterno MV, Taylor-Haas JA, Myer GD, et al. Prevention of overuse sports injuries in young athletes. *Orthop Clin North Am.* 2013;44(4):553–564.
4. Landry GL. Sports medicine. In: Kliegman LM, Stanton BF, St. Genelli JW, et al., eds. *Nelson Textbook of Pediatrics.* 18th ed. Philadelphia, PA: Saunders Elsevier; 2011:2401–2418.
5. Sarwark JF, ed. *Essentials of Musculoskeletal Care.* 4th ed. Rosemont, IL: American Academy of Orthopedic Surgeons and American Academy of Pediatrics; 2010:58–66, 108–127, 230–240, 243–279, 303–327, 669–674, 684–691, 700–707.
6. Weintraub W. *Tendon and Ligament Healing: A New Approach to Sports and Overuse Injury.* Brookline, MA: Paradigm Publications; 2003:11–47.
7. Presti M, Kon E, Marcacci M. Nonoperative biologic treatment approached for partial Achilles tendon lesion. *Orthopedics.* 2010;33(2):120–124.
8. Mercier LR. *Practical Orthopedics.* 6th ed. Philadelphia, PA: Mosby Elsevier; 2008:7–28, 55–87, 158–161, 193–213, 215–241.
9. Quillen DM, Wuchner M, Hatch RL. Acute shoulder injuries. *Am Fam Physician.* 2004;70:1949–1954.
10. Moore KL, Dalley AR, Agur AMR. *Clinically Oriented Anatomy.* 6th ed. Philadelphia, PA: Wolters Kluwer Health/Lippincott Williams & Wilkins; 2010:508–510, 626–642, 663–685, 673–685.
11. Pujalte GG, Zaslow TL. A practical guide to shoulder injuries in throwing athletes. *J Fam Pract.* 2013;62(4):175–180.
12. Pimentel L. Orthopedic trauma: management of major joint injury. *Med Clin North Am.* 2006;90:355–382.

13. Englund M, Guermanzi A, Lohmander SL. The role of the meniscus in knee osteoarthritis: a cause or consequence. *Radiol Clin North Am.* 2009;47:703–712.

14. Scordino LE, DeBerardino TM. Biologic enhancement of meniscus repair. *Clin Sports Med.* 2012;31:91–100.

15. Dixit S, Burton M, Mines B. Management of patellofemoral pain syndrome. *Am Fam Physician.* 2007;75:194–204.

16. Brunner L, Eshilian-Oats L. Hip fractures in adults. *Am Fam Physician.* 2003;67:537–542.

17. Rocca GJD, Crist BD. Hip fracture protocols: what have we changed? *Orthop Clin North Am.* 2013;44:163–182.

18. Garcia RA, Klein MJ, Schiller AL. Bones and joints. In: Rubin R, Strayer DS, eds. *Rubin's Pathology: Clinicopathologic Foundations of Medicine.* 6th ed. Philadelphia, PA: Wolters Kluwer Health/Lippincott Williams & Wilkins; 2012:1199–1272.

19. Rosenberg AE. Bones, joints, and soft tissue tumors. In: Kumar V, Abbas AK, Fausto N, et al., eds. *Robbins and Cotran Pathologic Basis of Medicine.* 7th ed. Philadelphia, PA: Saunders Elsevier; 2010:1205–1256.

20. Patel DS, Roth M, Kaph N. Stress fractures. *Am Fam Physician.* 2011;83(1):39–46.

21. Marsell R, Einhorn TA. The biology of fracture healing. *Injury.* 2011;42(6):551–555.

22. Claes L, Recknagel S, Ignatius A. Fracture healing under healthy and inflammatory conditions. *Nat Rev Rheumatol.* 2012;8(3):133–143.

23. Hoover TJ, Siefert JA. Soft tissue complications of orthopedic emergencies. *Emerg Med Clin North Am.* 2000;18:115–139.

24. Tull F, Borrelli J, Jr. Soft-tissue injury associated with closed fractures: evaluation and management. *J Am Acad Orthop Surg.* 2003;11:431–438.

25. Köstler W, Strom PC, Sudkamp NP. Acute compartment syndrome of the limb. *Injury.* 2004;35:1221–1227.

26. King TW, Lerman OZ, Carter JJ, et al. Exertional compartmental syndrome of the thigh: a rare diagnosis and literature review. *J Emerg Med.* 2010;39(2):e93–e99.

27. Newton EJ. Acute complications of extremity trauma. *Emerg Med Clin North Am.* 2007;25:751–761.

28. Akhtar S. Fat embolism. *Anesthesiol Clin.* 2009;27:533–550.

29. Arai F, Kia T, Nakai T, et al. Histopathologic features of fat embolism in fulminant fat embolism syndrome. *Anesthesiology.* 2007;107:509–511.

30. Pääkkonen M, Peltola H. Bone and joint infections. *Pediatr Clin North Am.* 2013;60:425–436.

31. Hatzenbuehler J, Pulling TJ. Diagnosis and management of osteomyelitis. *Am Fam Physician.* 2011;84(9):1027–1033.

32. Chihara S, Segretti J. Osteomyelitis. *Dis Mon.* 2010;56:6–31.

33. Lew DP, Waldvogel FA. Osteomyelitis. *Lancet.* 2004;364:369–379.

34. Smith MA, Dahlen NR. Clinical practice guideline surgical site infection prevention. *Orthop Nurs.* 2013;32:242–250.

35. Ludwig B, Lazarus AA. Musculoskeletal tuberculosis. *Dis Mon.* 2007;53:39–45.

36. Childs SG. Osteonecrosis: death of bone cells. *Orthop Nurs.* 2005;24:295–301.

37. Banerjee S, Issa K, Pivec R, et al. Osteonecrosis of the hip: treatment options and outcomes. *Orthop Clin North Am.* 2013;44(4):463–476.

38. Weinstein RS. Glucocorticoid-induced bone disease. *N Engl J Med.* 2013;365(3):62–70.

39. Weinstein RS. Glucocorticoid-induced osteoporosis and osteonecrosis. *Endocrinol Metab Clin North Am.* 2012;41(3):595–611.

40. Goytia RN, Salama A, Khanuja HS. Bisphosphonates and osteonecrosis: potential treatment or serious complication? *Orthop Clin North Am.* 2009;40:223–234.

41. American Cancer Society. *What Is Bone Cancer?* 2013. Available at: http://www.cancer.org. Accessed October 4, 2013.

42. Arndt CAS. Neoplasms of bone. In: Kliegman LM, Stanton BF, St. Genelli JW, et al., eds. *Nelson Textbook of Pediatrics.* 18th ed. Philadelphia, PA: Saunders Elsevier; 2011:1763–1768.

43. Turcotte RE. Giant cell tumor of bone. *Orthop Clin North Am.* 2006;37:35–51.

44. American Cancer Society. *Osteosarcoma.* 2013. Available at: http://www.cancer.org/cancer/osteosarcoma/detailedguide/osteosarcoma-treating-general-info. Accessed October 1, 2013.

45. Hayden JB, Hoang BH. Osteosarcoma: basic science and clinical implications. *Orthop Clin North Am.* 2006;37:1–7.

46. Ritter J, Bielack SS. Osteosarcoma. *Ann Oncol.* 2010;27(suppl 7):vii320–v11325.

47. Terek RM. Recent advances in the basic science of chondrosarcomas. *Orthop Clin North Am.* 2006;37:9–14.

48. Balamuth NJ, Warner RB. Ewing sarcoma. *Lancet.* 2010;12:184–192.

49. Potratz J, Dirksen U, Jurgens H, et al. Ewing sarcoma: clinical state-of-the-art. *Pediatr Hematol Oncol.* 2011;29:1–11.

50. Roodman GD. Mechanisms of bone metastasis. *N Engl J Med.* 2004;350:1655–1664.

51. Juan J, Pollock CB, Kelly K. Mechanisms of cancer metastasis to the bone. *Cell Res.* 2005;15:57–62.

52. Hershey MS. Toward new horizons: the future of bisphosphonate therapy. *Oncologist.* 2004;9(suppl 4):38–47.

53. Schoeneker PL, Rich MM. The lower extremity. In: Morissy RT, Weinstein SL, eds. *Lovell & Winter's Pediatric Orthopaedics.* 6th ed. Philadelphia, PA: Lippincott Williams & Wilkins; 2006:1158–1213.

54. Wells L, Schgal K. Torsional and angular deformities. In: Kliegman RM, Stanton BF, St. Genelli JW, et al., eds. *Nelson Textbook of Pediatrics.* 18th ed. Philadelphia, PA: Saunders Elsevier; 2011:2344–2351.

55. Sass P, Hassan G. Lower extremity abnormalities in children. *Am Fam Physician.* 2003;68:461–468.

56. Hosalter HS, Spiegel D, Davidson RS. The foot and toes. In: Kliegman RM, Stanton BF, St. Genelli JW, et al., eds. *Nelson Textbook of Pediatrics.* 18th ed. Philadelphia, PA: Saunders Elsevier; 2011:2335–2344.

57. Gore AI, Spencer J. The newborn foot. *Am Fam Physician.* 2004;69:865–872.

58. Kim HW, Park HW. The pediatric leg and knee. In: Weinstein SL, Buckwalter JA, eds. *Turek's Orthopaedics: Principles and Their Application.* 6th ed. Philadelphia, PA: Lippincott Williams & Wilkins; 2005:575–588.

59. Wells L, Schgal K. The knee. In: Kliegman RM, Stanton BF, St. Genelli JW, et al., eds. *Nelson Textbook of Pediatrics.* 18th ed. Philadelphia, PA: Saunders Elsevier; 2011:2351–2555.

60. Marini JC. Osteogenesis imperfecta. In: Kliegman RM, Stanton BF, St. Genelli JW, et al., eds. *Nelson Textbook of Pediatrics.* 18th ed. Philadelphia, PA: Saunders Elsevier; 2011:2437–2440.

61. Amor MB, Rauch F, Monti E, et al. Osteogenesis imperfecta. *Pediatr Endocrinol Rev.* 2013;10:397–405.

62. Reid IR. Bisphosphonates: new indications and methods of administration. *Curr Opin Rheumatol.* 2003;15:458–463.

63. Holsalter HS, Horn D, Wells L, et al. The hip. In: Kliegman RM, Stanton BF, St. Genelli JW, et al., eds. *Nelson Textbook of Pediatrics.* 18th ed. Philadelphia, PA: Saunders Elsevier; 2011:2355–2365.

64. Bracen J, Tran T, Ditchfield M. Developmental dysplasia of the hip: controversies and current concepts. *J Paediatr Child Health.* 2012;46(11):963–972.

65. Storer S, Skaggs DL. Developmental dysplasia of the hip. *Am Fam Physician.* 2006;74:1310–1316.

66. U.S. Preventive Services Task Force. Screening for developmental dysplasia of the hip: Recommendation statement. *Pediatrics* 2006;117:898–902.

67. Sewell MD, Eastwood DM. Screening and treatment in developmental dysplasia of the hip—Where do we go from here? *Int Orthop.* 2011;35:1359–1367.

68. Dobbs MB, Gurnett CA. Genetics of clubfoot. *J Pediatr Orthop.* 2012;21(1):1–4.

69. Dobbs MB, Gurnett CA. Update on clubfoot: etiology and treatment. *Clin Orthop Relat Res.* 2009;467:1146–1153.

70. Horn BD, Davidson RS. Current treatment of clubfoot in infancy and childhood. *Foot Ankle Clin North Am.* 2010;15:235–243.

71. Faulks S. Changing paradigm for treatment of club feet. *Orthop Nurs.* 2005;26(1):25–30.

72. Kocher MS, Tucker R. Pediatric athlete hip disorders. *Clin Sports Med.* 2006;25:241–253.

73. Herring JA. Legg-Calvé-Perthes disease. In: Herring AJ, ed. *Tachdjian's Pediatric Orthopaedics.* 3rd ed. Vol 1. Philadelphia, PA: W.B. Saunders; 2002:655–709.

74. Shah H. Perthes disease: evaluation and management. *Orthoped Clin North Am.* 2013:1–13.

75. Reamy BV, Slakey JB. Adolescent scoliosis: review and current comments. *Am Fam Physician.* 2001;64:111–116.

76. Hresko MT. Idiopathic scoliosis in adolescents. *N Engl J Med.* 2013;368(9):834–841.

77. de Séze M, Cugy E. Pathogenesis of idiopathic scoliosis: a review. *Ann Phys Rehabil Med.* 2012;55:126–138.

78. Weinstein S. The thoracolumbar spine. In: Weinstein SL, Buckwalter JA, eds. *Turek's Orthopaedics: Principles and Their Application.* 6th ed. Philadelphia, PA: Lippincott Williams & Wilkins; 2005:477–518.

79. Spiegel DA, Dormans JP. The spine. In: Kliegman RM, Stanton BF, St. Genelli JW, et al., eds. *Nelson Textbook of Pediatrics.* 18th ed. Philadelphia, PA: Saunders Elsevier; 2011:2365–2377.

80. U.S. Preventive Services Task Force. Screening for idiopathic scoliosis in adolescents: Recommendation statement. *Am Fam Physician.* 2006;71:1975–1976.

81. Qiu XS, Tang NL, Yeung HY, et al. Melatonin receptor 1B (MTNR1B) gene polymorphism is associated with occurrence of adolescent idiopathic scoliosis. *Spine.* 2007;32:1748–1753.

82. Shaughnessy WJ. Advances in scoliosis brace treatment for adolescent idiopathic scoliosis. *Orthop Clin North Am.* 2007;38:469–475.

83. Lonner BS. Emerging minimally invasive technologies for management of scoliosis. *Orthop Clin North Am.* 2007;38:431–440.

Porth Essentials Resources

Explore these additional resources to enhance learning for this chapter:

- NCLEX-Style Questions and Other Resources on the Point, http://thePoint.lww.com/PorthEssentials4e
- Study Guide for Essentials of Pathophysiology Guide
- Concepts in Action Animations
- Adaptive Learning | Powered by PrepU, http://thepoint.lww.com/prepu

Chapter 44

Disorders of the Skeletal System: Metabolic and Rheumatic Disorders

The skeletal system plays an essential role in mineral homeostasis and mobility. The bones of the skeletal system provide the basic framework that supports the body, protects its organs, and provides for movement. Joints hold the bones of the skeleton together, making movement possible. Bone is also one of the few tissues that normally undergo mineralization. It is a storehouse for 99% of the body's calcium and 85% of its phosphorus. This chapter focuses on two types of skeletal disorders: metabolic bone diseases, which produce a decrease in bone mass and mineralization, and joint disorders, which disrupt mobility.

Metabolic Bone Disease

Metabolic bone disease represents disorders of bone metabolism that result in structural effects on the skeleton, including decreased bone density and diminished bone strength. The strength of bone is determined by its composition and structure.[1] It must be rigid enough to support the body, yet flexible enough to absorb energy by deforming, to shorten and widen when compressed, and to lengthen and narrow under tension without cracking.

There are two types of bone: cortical and trabecular. Cortical or compact bone is composed of densely packed layers of mineralized collagen; it provides rigidity and is the major component of tubular bones (see Chapter 42, Fig. 42-1). Trabecular or cancellous bone is spongy on cross-section; it provides strength and elasticity, and constitutes the major part of axial skeletal structures such as the vertebrae. Disorders in which cortical bone is defective or reduced in mass lead to fractures of the long bones, whereas those of cancellous bone lead preferentially to vertebral fractures.

Osteopenia

Osteopenia is a condition that is common to all metabolic bone diseases. It is characterized by a reduction in bone mineral density greater than expected for age, race, or gender, and occurs because of a decrease in bone formation, inadequate bone mineralization, or excessive bone deossification.[1] *Osteopenia* is not a diagnosis but a term used to describe an apparent loss of bone density seen on x-ray studies.[2] Approximately 60% of bone is mineral content, approximately 30% is organic matrix, and the remainder is living bone cells. Osteopenia can involve a decrease in bone matrix due to an imbalance between bone formation and destruction, or a decrease in mineralization. The major causes of osteopenia are osteoporosis, osteomalacia, malignancies such as multiple myeloma, and endocrine disorders such as hyperparathyroidism and hyperthyroidism.

Osteoporosis

Osteoporosis is a metabolic bone disease characterized by decreased bone density (i.e., increased porosity) and strength in which both the bone matrix and mineralization are decreased.[3–6] The World Health Organization has defined osteoporosis as a bone mineral density (BMD) value greater than 2.5 standard deviations (SD) below the mean for a young adult reference population.[7] The most useful methods of estimating fracture risk are BMD testing and consideration of clinical risk factors for fracture.[8] Fracture risk assessment tests, such as the International Osteoporosis Foundation one-minute osteoporosis risk test, are available online to estimate the fracture probability.[9]

Osteoporosis can occur as the result of a number of disorders, but is most often associated with the aging process. In the United States alone, osteoporosis affects approximately 10 million persons aged 50 years or older, and an additional 34 million have low bone mass (osteopenia) and are potentially at risk for development of osteoporosis and its complications.[10]

Etiology and Pathogenesis

The cause of osteoporosis remains largely unknown, but most data suggest an imbalance between bone resorption and formation such that bone resorption exceeds bone formation. Although both of these factors play a role in most cases of osteoporosis, their relative contribution to bone loss may vary depending on age, gender, genetic predisposition, activity level, and nutritional status.

Under normal conditions, bone mass increases steadily during childhood, reaching a peak in the young adult years. The peak bone mass, or BMD, is an important determinant of the subsequent risk for osteoporosis. It is determined in part by genetic factors, hormone (estrogen) levels, exercise, calcium intake and absorption, and environmental factors (Chart 44-1). Genetic factors are linked, in largest part, to the maximal amount of bone in a given person, referred to as *peak*

| CHART 44-1 | Risk Factors Associated with Osteoporosis* |

Personal Characteristics
Advanced age
Female
Gender
Ethnicity (white or Asian)
Small bone structure/low body weight
Postmenopausal
Family history

Lifestyle
Sedentary
Calcium/Vitamin D deficiency
High-protein diet
Excessive alcohol intake
Excessive caffeine intake
Smoking

Drug and Disease Related
Aluminum-containing antacids
Anticonvulsants
Heparin
Corticosteroids or Cushing disease
Gastrectomy
Celiac disease
Diabetes mellitus
Anorexia nervosa/female athlete triad
Hyperthyroidism
Hyperparathyroidism
Rheumatoid arthritis

*Not exclusive

bone mass. Race is a key determinant of BMD and the risk of fractures. Incidence rates obtained from studies among racial and ethnic groups demonstrate that although women have higher fracture rates compared with men overall, these differences vary by race and age. White and Asian women had higher rates for all age groups older than 50 years.[10] The highest BMD values and lowest fracture rates have been reported for black women.[10] Body size is another factor affecting the risk of osteoporosis and risk of fractures. Women with smaller body builds are at increased risk of hip fracture because of lower hip BMD.

Hormonal factors play a significant role in the development of osteoporosis, particularly in postmenopausal women.[11] Postmenopausal osteoporosis, which is caused by an estrogen deficiency, is manifested by a loss of cancellous bone and a predisposition to fractures of the vertebrae and distal radius. The loss of bone mass is greatest during early menopause, when estrogen levels are withdrawing. Several factors appear to influence the increased loss of bone mass associated with an estrogen deficiency, including an increased secretion of cytokines by monocytes and bone marrow cells. These cytokines stimulate osteoclast recruitment and activity by increasing the levels of RANK ligand (RANKL) while diminishing the expression of osteoprotegerin (OPG) (see Chapter 42, Understanding Bone Remodeling). Compensatory osteoblastic activity and new bone formation occurs, but does not keep pace with the bone that is lost.

Male sex hormone deficiency may contribute to age-related bone loss in men, although the effect is not of the same magnitude as that caused by estrogen deficiency. Unlike women, men do not have a midlife loss of sex hormone production.[12,13] Another factor that provides relative protection for men is the fact that they achieve 8% to 10% more peak bone mass than women.[13] Although androgens have long been assumed to be critical for growth and maintenance of the male skeleton, it has recently been suggested that estrogens obtained from peripheral conversion of testicular and adrenal hormone precursors may be even more important than androgens in the maintenance of bone mass in men.

Age-related changes in bone density occur in all individuals and contribute to the development of osteoporosis in both sexes. Age-related changes in bone cells and matrix have a strong impact on bone metabolism. Osteoblasts from elderly persons have reduced replicative and biosynthetic potential compared with those of younger persons. Growth factors that stimulate osteoblastic activity also lose their potential over time. The end result is a skeleton that has decreased ability to make bone. Reduced physical activity increases the rate of bone loss because mechanical forces are important stimuli for normal bone remodeling. Thus, the decreased physical activity that often accompanies aging may also contribute to the loss of bone mass in the elderly.

Secondary osteoporosis is associated with many conditions, including endocrine disorders, malabsorption disorders, malignancies, alcoholism, and certain medications.[14] Persons with endocrine disorders such as hyperthyroidism, hyperparathyroidism, Cushing syndrome, or diabetes mellitus are at high risk for development of osteoporosis.[15] Hyperthyroidism causes an acceleration of bone turnover. Some malignancies (e.g., multiple myeloma) secrete osteoclast-activating factor, causing significant bone loss. Alcohol is a direct inhibitor of osteoblasts and may also inhibit calcium absorption. Corticosteroid use is the most common cause of drug-related osteoporosis, and long-term corticosteroid use in the treatment of disorders such as rheumatoid arthritis and chronic obstructive lung disease is associated with a high rate of fractures.[16] The prolonged use of aluminum-containing antacids, which increase calcium excretion, and anticonvulsants, which impair vitamin D production, may also contribute to bone loss. Persons with human immunodeficiency virus (HIV) infection or acquired immunodeficiency syndrome (AIDS) who are being treated with antiretroviral therapy may develop a decrease in bone density and signs of osteopenia and osteoporosis.[17]

Several groups of children and adolescents are at particular risk for decreased bone mass, including premature infants and those with low birth weight who have lower-than-expected bone mass in the early weeks of life, and children who require treatment with corticosteroid drugs (e.g., those with childhood inflammatory diseases and transplant recipients).[18] Children with cystic fibrosis often have impaired gastrointestinal function that reduces the absorption of calcium and other nutrients, and many also require the frequent use of corticosteroid drugs.

Premature osteoporosis is increasingly being seen in female athletes due to an increased prevalence of eating disorders and amenorrhea.[19] It most frequently affects women engaged in endurance sports, such as running and swimming; in activities where appearance is important, such as figure skating, diving, and gymnastics; or in sports with weight restrictions, such as horse racing, martial arts, and rowing. The *female athlete triad* refers to a pattern of disordered eating that leads to amenorrhea and eventually osteoporosis. Poor nutrition, combined with intense training, can decrease the critical body fat–to–muscle ratio needed for normal menses and estrogen production by the ovary. The decreased levels of estrogen combined with the lack of calcium and vitamin D from dietary deficiencies result in a loss of bone density and increased risk for fractures. There is a concern that athletes with low BMD will be at increased risk for fractures during their competitive years. It is unclear whether osteoporosis induced by amenorrhea is reversible. Data are emerging that even having only one or two elements of the triad greatly increases the risk of these women for long-term morbidity.[19]

Clinical Features

Osteoporotic changes occur in the diaphysis and metaphysis of bone.[3,4] There is loss of trabeculae from cancellous bone and thinning of the cortex to such an extent that minimal stress causes fractures. The changes that occur with osteoporosis have been explained by two distinct disease processes: postmenopausal, or age-related, osteoporosis. In postmenopausal women, the increase in osteoclastic activity affects mainly bones or portions of bone that have increased surface area, such as the cancellous compartment of the vertebral bodies. The osteoporotic trabeculae become thinned and lose their interconnections, leading to microfractures and eventual vertebral collapse. In senile osteoporosis, the osteoporotic cortex is thinned by subperiosteal and endosteal resorption and the haversian systems are widened. In severe cases, the haversian systems are so enlarged that the cortex resembles cancellous bone[4] (Fig. 44-1). Hip fractures, which are seen later in life, are more commonly associated with senile osteoporosis.

Clinical Manifestations. Osteoporosis is usually a silent disorder. Often, the first manifestations of the disorder are those that accompany a skeletal fracture—a vertebral compression fracture or fracture of the hip, pelvis, humerus, or other bones (Fig. 44-2). Fractures are typically sudden in onset and may be caused by a fall, sudden movement, lifting, jumping, or even coughing. Hip fractures occur mainly in persons over age 65. Wedging and collapse of vertebrae cause a loss of height in the vertebral column and kyphosis, a condition

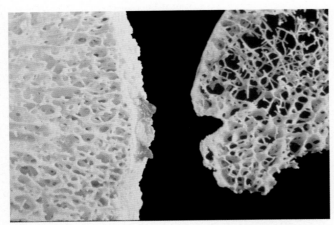

FIGURE 44-1. Osteoporosis. Femoral head of an 82-year-old woman with osteoporosis and femoral neck fracture *(right)*, compared with a normal control bone cut to the same thickness *(left)*. (From Garcia RA, Klein MJ, Schiller AL. Bones and joints. In: Rubin R, Strayer DS, eds. *Rubin's Pathology: Clinicopathologic Foundations of Medicine*. 6th ed. Philadelphia, PA: Wolters Kluwer Health | Lippincott Williams & Wilkins; 2012:1226.)

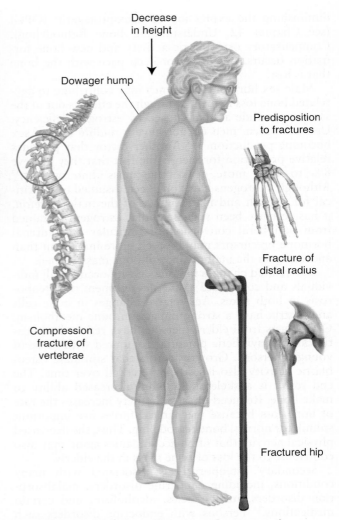

FIGURE 44-2. Clinical manifestations of osteoporosis.

commonly referred to as *dowager hump*. Usually, there is no generalized bone tenderness. When pain occurs, it usually is related to fractures. Systemic symptoms such as weakness and weight loss suggest that the osteoporosis may be caused by underlying disease.

Diagnosis and Treatment. An important advance in diagnostic methods used for the identification of osteoporosis has been the use of BMD assessment.[20–22] The clinical method of choice for BMD studies is dual-energy x-ray absorptiometry (DEXA) of the spine and hip. Measurement of serial heights in older adults is another simple way to screen for osteoporosis. A further advance in the diagnosis of osteoporosis is the refinement of risk factors, permitting better analysis of risk pertaining to particular persons. The U.S. Preventive Services Task Force (USPSTF) recommends a screening DEXA of all women 65 years of age and older, as well as women 60 to 64 years of age who have an increased fracture risk.[23] Although there are no USPSTF guidelines for BMD testing in men, the National Osteoporosis Foundation (NOF) recommends screening for all men 70 years of age and older and men 50 to 69 years of age with risk factors.[22]

Prevention and early detection of osteoporosis are essential to the prevention of associated deformities and fractures. It is important to identify persons in high-risk groups so that preventive measures can begin early (see Chart 44-1). Regular exercise and adequate calcium and vitamin D intake are important factors in preventing osteoporosis. Weight-bearing exercises such as walking, jogging, rowing, and weight lifting are important in the maintenance of bone mass. Studies have indicated that premenopausal women need more than 1000 mg/day of calcium, and postmenopausal women need at least 1200 mg of calcium daily.[20,22] Because most older American

women do not consume a sufficient quantity of dairy products to meet their calcium needs, calcium supplementation is recommended. A daily intake of 800 to 1000 IU of vitamin D is recommended for adults age 50 years and older. Many elderly persons are at high risk for vitamin D deficiency, especially those with chronic illness, malabsorption disorders (e.g., celiac disease), and limited exposure to sunlight. It is recommended that serum vitamin D levels be obtained for persons at risk of a deficiency and that supplemental vitamin D be prescribed for persons with low serum levels.[22]

There are five main types of drugs used in the treatment of osteoporosis: bisphosphonates, selective estrogen receptor modulators (SERMs), calcitonin, recombinant parathyroid hormone, and the RANKL inhibitor denosumab.[24] *Bisphosphonates* are effective inhibitors of bone resorption and the most effective agents for prevention and treatment of osteoporosis. The bisphosphonates (e.g., alendronate, risedronate, ibandronate, zoledronate) are analogs of endogenous inorganic pyrophosphate that the body cannot break down. In bone, they bind to hydroxyapatite and prevent bone resorption by inhibiting osteoclast activity. The most dramatic impact has been in the reduction of multiple spine fractures, showing that treatment can decrease progression of the disease. These drugs are effective in men as well women and for various causes of osteoporosis.[24]

Raloxifene, a selective estrogen receptor modulator (SERM) that acts only on specific estrogen receptors, has been approved for prevention and treatment of osteoporosis in postmenopausal women. Although hormone therapy (i.e., estrogen with or without progesterone) has been shown to slightly reduce the risk of hip and vertebral fractures in postmenopausal women, the use of hormone therapy has come under scrutiny after the release of data from the Women's Health Initiative, which linked hormone replacement therapy to an increased risk of stroke, venous thromboembolism, coronary heart disease, and breast cancer.[25] Raloxifene does not prevent hot flashes associated with menopause and it imposes the same risk of venous thrombosis as estrogen.[24]

Calcitonin is an endogenous peptide that partially inhibits osteoclastic activity. Nasal calcitonin has been approved for the treatment of postmenopausal osteoporosis. It has been shown to decrease the occurrence of vertebral fractures, but not nonvertebral or hip fractures. Because more effective drugs are available, it is not usually considered first-line treatment for osteoporosis.

Teriparatide, a recombinant human parathyroid hormone, stimulates bone remodeling by increasing osteoblast-mediated bone formation. Unlike the fluoride, this bone appears structurally normal and is associated with substantial reduction in the incidence of fractures. Teriparatide is given by injection and is approved for only 2 years of use.[24]

Denosumab, the RANKL inhibitor, has recently been approved for treatment of postmenopausal osteoporosis.[24] It is given subcutaneously every 6 months. Like the biphosphonates it suppresses bone resorption and secondary bone formation. Denosumab reduces the risk of both vertebral and nonvertebral fractures with comparable effectiveness to the potent biphosphonates.[24]

To reduce their fracture risk, persons with osteoporosis should correct conditions in their homes that predispose them to falls. They should follow their health care provider's prescribed diet and program of physical activity. In treating fractures, it is important to minimize immobility. Surgical interventions are used to provide stable fixation of lower extremity fractures and allow for early weight bearing and restoration of mobility and function. Vertebral fractures are treated symptomatically. Conservative treatment with bracing is most often seen, especially in fractures of the thoracic vertebra.

Osteomalacia and Rickets

In contrast to osteoporosis, which causes a loss of total bone mass and results in brittle bones, osteomalacia and rickets produce a softening of the bones resulting from an inadequate mineralization of newly formed bone matrix.[4] The term *rickets* refers to the disorder in children in which changes in bone growth produce characteristic skeletal abnormalities, and *osteomalacia* is used in adults because the bone that forms during the remodeling process is undermineralized.[4]

Osteomalacia

Osteomalacia is a generalized bone condition in which there is inadequate mineralization of bone.[3,4,15] There are two main causes of osteomalacia: (1) insufficient calcium absorption from the intestine because of a lack of dietary calcium or a deficiency of or resistance to the action of vitamin D and (2) phosphate deficiency caused by increased renal losses or decreased intestinal absorption. Vitamin D is ingested in the diet and synthesized in the skin from 7-dehydrocholesterol under the influence of ultraviolet B (UVB) sunlight. The vitamin is first hydroxylated in the liver to form its major metabolite, 25-hydroxyvitamin D. It is then hydroxylated in the kidney to produce the active hormone $1,25(OH)_2D$ (see Chapter 42). There are many causes of vitamin D deficiency including reduced skin synthesis, inadequate dietary intake, diminished intestinal absorption, and heritable and acquired disorders of vitamin D metabolism and responsiveness.[26,27]

The incidence of osteomalacia is high among the elderly because of diets deficient in calcium and vitamin D, a problem often compounded by the intestinal malabsorption that accompanies aging. Melanin is extremely efficient in absorbing UVB radiation; thus, decreased skin pigmentation markedly reduces vitamin D synthesis, as does the use of sunscreens. Osteomalacia also may occur in persons on long-term treatment with medications such as anticonvulsants (e.g., phenytoin, carbamazepine, valproate) that decrease the activation of vitamin D in the liver. There also is a greater incidence of osteomalacia in the colder regions of the world, particularly during the winter months when UVB radiation is inadequate to allow skin synthesis of vitamin D.

A form of osteomalacia called *renal rickets* occurs in persons with chronic renal failure. It is caused by the inability of the kidney to activate vitamin D and excrete phosphate and is accompanied by hyperparathyroidism, increased bone turnover, and increased bone resorption (see Chapter 26). Another form of osteomalacia results from renal tubular defects that cause excessive phosphate losses. This form of osteomalacia is commonly referred to as *vitamin D–resistant rickets*, and often is a familial disorder.[4] It is inherited as an X-linked dominant gene passed by mothers to one half of their children and by fathers to their daughters only. This form of osteomalacia affects boys more severely than girls. Long-standing primary hyperparathyroidism causes increased calcium resorption from bone and hypophosphatemia, which can lead to rickets in children and osteomalacia in adults.

The clinical manifestations of osteomalacia are bone pain, tenderness, and fractures as the disease progresses. In severe cases, muscle weakness often is an early sign. Osteomalacia predisposes a person to pathologic fractures in the weakened bones, especially those in the distal radius and the proximal femur. In contrast to osteoporosis, it is not a significant cause of hip fractures. There may be delayed healing and poor retention of internal fixation devices. Osteomalacia usually is accompanied by a compensatory or secondary hyperparathyroidism stimulated by low serum calcium levels. Parathyroid hormone reduces renal absorption of phosphate and removes calcium from the bone. Serum calcium levels are only slightly reduced in osteomalacia.

Diagnostic measures are directed toward identifying osteomalacia and establishing its cause. Diagnostic methods include x-ray studies, laboratory tests, bone scan, and bone biopsy. X-ray findings typical of osteomalacia are the development of transverse lines or pseudofractures called *Looser zones*. These apparently are caused by stress fractures that are inadequately healed or by the mechanical inadequacy of penetrating nutrient vessels.[4] A bone biopsy may be done to confirm the diagnosis of osteomalacia in a person with nonspecific osteopenia who shows no improvement after treatment with exercise, vitamin D, and calcium.

The treatment of osteomalacia is directed at the underlying cause. If the problem is nutritional, restoring adequate amounts of calcium and vitamin D to the diet may be sufficient. The elderly and persons with an inadequate dietary intake or sunlight exposure may require supplemental vitamin D. Supplemental vitamin D is specific for vitamin D–resistant rickets, but large doses usually are needed to overcome the resistance to calcium absorption action and to prevent renal loss of phosphate. The biologically active forms of vitamin D, 25-OH vitamin D (calciferol) or 1,25-(OH)$_2$ vitamin D (calcitriol), are available for use in the treatment of osteomalacia resistant to vitamin D (i.e., osteomalacia resulting from chronic liver disease and kidney failure). If osteomalacia is caused by malabsorption, the treatment is directed toward correcting the primary disease. For example, adequate replacement of pancreatic enzymes is of paramount importance in pancreatic insufficiency. In renal tubular disorders, the treatment is directed at the altered renal physiology.

Rickets

Rickets is a metabolic bone disorder characterized by a failure or delay in calcification of the cartilaginous growth plate in children whose epiphyses have not yet fused.[28–30] It is also manifested by widening and deformation of the metaphyseal regions of long bones and a delay in the mineralization of trabecular, endosteal, and periosteal bone surfaces. Rickets is not a reportable disease; however, case reports and hospital records suggest that, in the United States, its incidence has been rising during the past three decades.[31]

There are several forms of rickets, including nutritional rickets, vitamin D–dependent rickets, and vitamin D–resistant rickets. As with osteomalacia in the adult, rickets can result from kidney failure; malabsorptive syndromes such as celiac disease and cystic fibrosis; and medications such as anticonvulsants, which impair the activation of vitamin D in the liver; and aluminum-containing antacids, which bind phosphorus and prevent its absorption.

Etiology and Pathogenesis. Nutritional rickets results from inadequate sunlight exposure or inadequate intake of vitamin D, calcium, or phosphate. Although uncommon in developed countries of the world, rickets still can occur, particularly when an infant is solely breast fed, is dark skinned, or has limited exposure to sunlight. Modern conditions of dress, lifestyle, and recommendations regarding sun avoidance to reduce skin cancer risk may prevent a large proportion of the population from producing adequate amounts of vitamin D. In 2003, the American Academy of Pediatrics recommended a vitamin D supplement for breast-fed infants who do not consume at least 500 mL/day of vitamin D–fortified formula/beverages and non–breast-fed infants who do not consume greater than 500 mL of vitamin D–fortified beverages.[31] The supplementation should start during the first 2 months of life and continue throughout childhood and adolescence.

Vitamin D–dependent rickets can result from abnormalities in the gene coding for the enzyme that converts inactive vitamin D to the active form of vitamin D, or from an autosomal disorder caused by mutations in the vitamin D receptor.[29] Vitamin D–resistant rickets involves hypophosphatemia or a decrease in serum phosphate levels, the most common form being caused by mutations of the phosphate-regulating gene on the X chromosome.[29] The gene mutation causes renal wasting of phosphate at the proximal tubular level of the kidney.

Clinical Features. Rickets is characterized by changes in the growing bones of children with overgrowth of the epiphyseal cartilage due to inadequate provisional calcification and failure of the cartilage cells to disintegrate. Bones become deformed; ossification at the epiphyseal plates is delayed and disordered, resulting in widening of the epiphyseal cartilage plate. Any new bone that does grow is unmineralized. The conformation of the gross skeletal changes depends on the severity and duration of the rachitic process, and in particular on the stresses to which the individual bones are subjected. During the nonmobile stage of infancy, the head and chest undergo the greatest stresses. The skull is enlarged and soft, closure of the fontanels is delayed, and the teeth are slow to develop. When an ambulating child develops rickets, deformities are likely to affect the spine, pelvis, and long bones (i.e., tibia), causing, most notably, lumbar lordosis and bowing of the legs (Fig. 44-3). The ends of long bones and ribs are enlarged. The thorax may be abnormally shaped, with prominent rib cartilage (i.e., rachitic rosary). The child usually has stunted growth, with a height sometimes far below the normal range. Weight often is not affected so that the children, many of whom present with a protruding abdomen (i.e., rachitic potbelly), have been described as presenting a Buddha-like appearance when sitting.

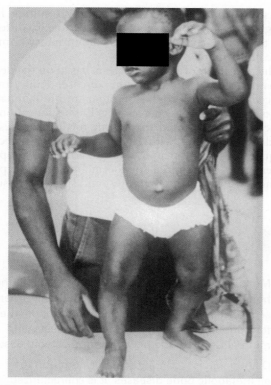

FIGURE 44-3. A child suffering from nutritional rickets. Note the bowed legs, protruding abdomen, and enlarged left wrist. (From the Centers for Disease Control and Prevention Public Health Images Library. No. 2435.)

Nutritional rickets is treated with a balanced diet sufficient in calcium, phosphorus, and vitamin D. Exposure to sunlight also is important, especially for premature infants and those on artificial milk feedings. Supplemental vitamin D in excess of normal requirements is given for several months. Children with vitamin D–dependent rickets caused by lack of the enzyme needed to convert vitamin D to its active form are treated with calcitriol, the active form of vitamin D.[29] Vitamin D–resistant forms of rickets are treated with oral phosphorus or oral phosphorus and calcitriol. Maintenance of good posture, positioning, and bracing in older children are used to prevent deformities. After the disease is controlled, deformities may have to be surgically corrected as the child grows.

Paget Disease

Paget disease (i.e., osteitis deformans) is the second most common bone disease after osteoporosis.[3,4,32,33] The disease, which has been described as a "collage of matrix madness," is characterized by focal areas of excessive osteoclast-mediated bone reabsorption preceding disorganized osteoblast-mediated bone repair. Paget disease usually begins during mid-adulthood and becomes progressively more common with increasing age, affecting about 5% of women and 8% of men by the eighth decade of life.[32] It is more common in people of Northern European heritage and is rare in Africans, people of the Indian subcontinent, and Asians.[32]

Etiology and Pathogenesis

Although the pathogenesis of Paget disease remains unclear, there is evidence of both genetic and environmental influences. It has been reported that 15% of persons with the disease have a positive family history[32] and numerous studies have described extended family members with the disease.[31] There is increasing evidence that Paget disease and some related diseases are caused by mutations in genes encoding proteins in the RANK signaling pathways.[3,4] Other evidence presents a probable association with a virus, possibly a paramyxovirus, suggesting that a viral infection may serve as a trigger for development of Paget disease in genetically predisposed individuals.[4,32] The incidence and severity of Paget disease of bone have decreased in recent years, possibly as a result of improved nutrition, reduced exposure to infections, and a more sedentary lifestyle, which has had the effect of reducing mechanical loading of the skeleton.[32]

Paget disease is a focal process with considerable variation in its stage of development in separate skeletal sites.[33] At the onset, the disease is marked by regions of furious osteoclastic bone resorption, followed by a period of hectic bone formation with increased numbers of osteoblasts rapidly depositing bone in a chaotic fashion such that the newly formed bone is of poor quality and is disorganized rather than lamellar. The poor quality of bone accounts for the bowing and fractures that occur in bones affected by the disease. The bone marrow adjacent to the bone-forming surface is replaced by loose connective tissue that contains osteoprogenitor cells and numerous blood vessels, which transport blood to and from these metabolically active sites. The lesions of Paget disease may be solitary or may occur in multiple sites. They tend to localize to the bones of the axial skeleton, including the skull, spine, and pelvis. The proximal femur and tibia may be involved in more widespread forms of the disease. Histologically, Paget lesions show increased vascularity and bone marrow fibrosis with intense cellular activity. Numerous osteoclasts, large active osteoblasts, and peritrabular fibrosis are encountered. The rapid remodeling leads to disruption of bone architecture. The bone has a somewhat mosaic-like pattern resembling pieces of jigsaw puzzle, separated by prominent areas of density, called *cement lines*[4] (Fig. 44-4).

Clinical Features

The clinical manifestations of Paget disease are extremely variable and depend on the extent and site of the disease (see Fig. 44-4). The disease is usually asymptomatic and discovered as an incidental radiograph finding.[32] Skeletal expansion and distortion may be obvious if the disease affects the skull, jaw, clavicle, or long bones of the leg. Involvement of the skull causes headaches, intermittent tinnitus, vertigo, and eventual hearing loss. The vertebrae of the spine may enlarge, weaken, and collapse, causing kyphosis of the thoracic spine and

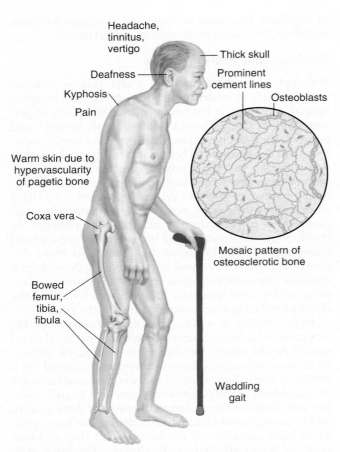

Headache, tinnitus, vertigo

Deafness

Kyphosis

Pain

Thick skull

Prominent cement lines

Osteoblasts

Warm skin due to hypervascularity of pagetic bone

Coxa vera

Bowed femur, tibia, fibula

Mosaic pattern of osteosclerotic bone

Waddling gait

FIGURE 44-4. Clinical manifestations of Paget disease.

nerve compression. Weight bearing may cause anterior bowings of the femur and tibia. Softening of the femoral neck can cause coxa vara (i.e., reduced angle of the femoral neck), which in combination with involvement of the pelvis can cause a waddling gait and secondary osteoarthritis. Mild to moderate deep, aching pain characteristically begins late in the course of the disease, persists throughout the day and at rest, and becomes worse at night. In some persons, the early hypervascularity of the pagetic bone produces warmth of the overlying skin and subcutaneous tissue. In persons with extensive disease, blood flow to the bones and subcutaneous tissue can increase remarkably, leading to high-output heart failure or exacerbation of underlying cardiac disease.[3]

A variety of tumor and tumorlike conditions develop in pagetic bone, the most dreaded of which is sarcoma. Osteogenic sarcomas occur in 5% to 10% of persons with extensive disease.[3] The bones most often affected, in order of frequency, are the femur, pelvis, and humerus.[4]

Diagnosis and Treatment. Diagnosis of Paget disease is based on characteristic bone deformities and x-ray changes. Elevated levels of serum alkaline phosphatase and urinary hydroxyproline support the diagnosis, and continued surveillance of these levels may be used to monitor the effectiveness of treatment. Bone scans are used to detect the rapid bone turnover indicative of active disease and to monitor the response to treatment.

The scan cannot identify bone activity resulting from malignant lesions. Bone biopsy may be done to differentiate the lesion from osteomyelitis or a primary or metastatic bone tumor.

The treatment of Paget disease is based on the degree of pain and the extent of the disease. Pain can be reduced with nonsteroidal or other anti-inflammatory agents. Suppressive agents such as the bisphosphonates and calcitonin are used to prevent further progress of the disease. Persons with Paget disease should receive adequate doses of calcium and vitamin D. Orthopedic surgery may be required for the management of pseudofractures, pathologic fractures, and spinal stenosis.[32]

SUMMARY CONCEPTS

■ Metabolic bone disorders have their origin in the bone remodeling process that involves an orderly sequence of osteoclastic bone reabsorption, the formation of new bone by the osteoblasts, and mineralization of the newly formed osteoid tissue.

■ Osteopenia is a condition that is common to all metabolic bone diseases. It is characterized by a reduction in bone mineral density greater than expected for age, race, or gender, and it occurs because of a decrease in bone formation, inadequate bone mineralization, or excessive bone deossification.

■ Osteoporosis represents an increased loss of total bone mass due to an imbalance between bone absorption and bone formation that results in a decrease in bone density and diminished bone strength and is associated with an increase in bone fragility and susceptibility to fractures. Although the disease can occur as the result of a number of disorders, the most common causes are age-related changes in bone metabolism and a relative absence of estrogen in postmenopausal women.

■ Osteomalacia and rickets represent a softening of bone due to inadequate mineralization of the bone matrix caused by a deficiency of calcium or phosphate. Osteomalacia is a disorder of adults and is caused by insufficient calcium absorption from the intestine because of lack of dietary vitamin D, resistance to the action of the vitamin, or a phosphate deficiency.

■ Rickets, which affects children, is characterized by failure or delay in calcification of the cartilaginous growth plate, widening and deformation of the metaphyseal regions in long bones, and a delay in mineralization of trabecular, endosteal, and periosteal bone surfaces.

■ Paget disease is a disorder involving excessive osteoclastic activity, and bone destruction and repair, resulting in structural deformities of the long bones, spine, pelvis, and cranium. Symptomatic disease may be manifest as skeletal changes and symptoms related to expansion of the skull, jaw, clavicle, spine, and long bones of the leg.

Rheumatic Disorders

Arthritis is a descriptive term applied to more than 100 rheumatic disorders, ranging from localized, self-limiting conditions to those that are systemic immune-mediated processes. The term, which is used to describe any disorder that affects the joints, oversimplifies the nature of the varied disease processes, the difficulty in differentiating one form of arthritis from another, and the complexity of treatment of these usually chronic conditions. These diverse rheumatic conditions share inflammation of the joint as a prominent or accompanying symptom. In the systemic rheumatic diseases, such as rheumatoid arthritis, the inflammation is primary, resulting from an immune response, probably autoimmune in origin. In rheumatic conditions limited to a single or few diarthrodial joints, such as osteoarthritis, the inflammation is secondary, resulting from the degenerative process and joint irregularities.

Systemic Autoimmune Rheumatic Diseases

Systemic autoimmune rheumatic diseases are a group of chronic disorders characterized by diffuse inflammatory vascular lesions and degenerative changes in connective tissue that share clinical features and may affect many of the same tissues and organs. They include rheumatoid arthritis, systemic lupus erythematosus, and systemic sclerosis, all of which share an immune-mediated pathogenesis.

Rheumatoid Arthritis

Rheumatoid arthritis (RA) is a chronic autoimmune systemic disease that affects all ethnic groups throughout the world, with women being affected more frequently than men. The onset of the disease can occur at any age, but its peak incidence is between 50 and 75 years of age.[34]

Etiology. Although the cause of RA remains uncertain, evidence points to a genetic predisposition and the development of joint inflammation that is immunologically mediated.[3,4,35] It has been suggested that the disease is initiated in a genetically predisposed individual by the activation of a T-cell–mediated

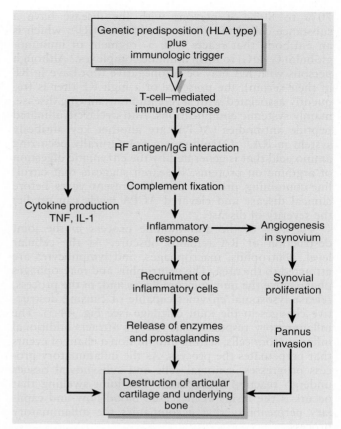

FIGURE 44-5. Disease process in rheumatoid arthritis. IL, interleukin; TNF, tumor necrosis factor.

response to an immunologic trigger, such as a microbial agent (Fig. 44-5). The importance of genetic factors in the pathogenesis of RA is supported by the increased frequency of the disease among first-degree relatives and monozygotic twins.[4] In addition, specific major histocompatibility complex (MHC) alleles or human leukocyte antigen (HLA) types have been associated with RA (see Chapter 15). An increased prevalence of RA has been associated with specific HLA DR alleles that share a sequence of amino acids located in the antigen-binding site of the DR molecule. This location is presumably the specific binding site of the immunologic trigger.[3] Cigarette smoking is a strong risk factor for the development of RA and may also influence the severity of the disease, especially in those with the shared epitope (HLA-DR4 marker) and a positive anti-citrullinated peptide antibody (ACPA) test, to be discussed.[35,36]

Pathogenesis. The pathogenesis of RA can be viewed as an aberrant immune response that leads to synovial inflammation and destruction of the joint architecture. It has been suggested that the disease is initiated by the activation of CD4⁺ helper T cells, the local release of inflammatory mediators and cytokines (e.g., tumor necrosis factor [TNF], interleukin [IL]-1) that destroy the joint, and formation of antibodies directed against joint-specific and systemic autoantigens. Approximately

70% to 80% of persons with the disease have a substance called the *rheumatoid factor* (RF), which is an antibody that reacts with a fragment of immunoglobulin G (IgG) to form immune complexes.[3] Although persons with RA may be seronegative (not have Ig RF in their serum), the presence of a high RF titer is frequently associated with severe and unremitting disease, mainly systemic complications. Anti-cyclic citrullinated peptide antibodies (ACPA) are another key antibody system in RA.[37] Citrulline is a nonnaturally occurring amino acid that is generated by the enzymatic digestion of arginine on proteins. Research suggests that citrulline-containing proteins may be present years before clinical disease and elevated ACPA levels can predict the severity of disease.

The role of the autoimmune process in the joint destruction of RA remains obscure. At the cellular level, neutrophils, macrophages, and lymphocytes are attracted to the area. The neutrophils and macrophages phagocytize the immune complexes and, in the process, release lysosomal enzymes capable of causing destructive changes in the joint cartilage (see Fig. 44-5). The inflammatory response that follows attracts additional inflammatory cells, setting into motion a chain of events that perpetuates the process. As the inflammatory process progresses, synovial cells and subsynovial tissues undergo reactive hyperplasia. The joint swelling that occurs is the result of increased blood flow and capillary permeability that accompanies the inflammatory process.

Characteristic of RA is the development of an extensive network of new blood vessels in the synovial membrane that contributes to the advancement of the rheumatoid synovitis. This destructive vascular granulation tissue, which is called *pannus,* extends from the synovium to involve the "bare area," a region of unprotected bone at the junction between cartilage and subchondral bone (Fig. 44-6B). Pannus is a feature of RA that differentiates it from other forms of inflammatory arthritis.[3,4] The inflammatory cells found in the pannus have a destructive effect on the adjacent cartilage and bone. Eventually, pannus develops between the joint margins, leading to reduced joint motion and the possibility of eventual ankylosis (joint fusion). With progression of the disease, joint inflammation and the resulting structural changes lead to joint instability, muscle atrophy from disuse, stretching of the ligaments, and involvement of the tendons and muscles. The effect of the pathologic changes on joint structure and function is related to the degree of disease activity, which can change at any time. Unfortunately, the destructive changes are irreversible.

Rheumatoid arthritis often is associated with articular as well as extra-articular (i.e., systemic) manifestations (see Fig. 44-6). It usually has an insidious onset marked by systemic manifestations such as fatigue, weakness, and generalized aching and stiffness.[37,38] The disease, which is characterized by exacerbations and remissions, may involve only a few joints for brief durations, or it may become relentlessly progressive and debilitating.

Articular Manifestations. Joint involvement usually is symmetric and polyarticular. Any diarthrodial joint can be involved. The person may complain of joint pain and stiffness that lasts for 30 minutes and frequently for several hours. The limitation of joint motion that occurs early in the disease usually is because of pain; later, it is because of fibrosis. In early disease, the wrists, metacarpophalangeal (MCP) joints, proximal interphalangeal (PIP) joints of the fingers, interphalangeal joints of the thumb, and metatarsophalangeal (MTP) joints are most commonly affected. Pain in the ball of the foot upon arising from bed and widening of the forefoot necessitating an increase in shoe size are frequently reported due to inflammation of the metatarsophalangeal joints.[34] Pain with turning door knobs, opening jars, and buttoning shirts is commonly reported due to swelling of the wrists and small joints of the hand. As the disease progresses, larger joints such as the ankles, knees, elbows, and shoulders become affected. Spinal involvement usually is limited to the cervical region.

Progressive joint destruction may lead to subluxation (i.e., a partial dislocation of the joint resulting in misalignment of the bone ends) with instability and limitation of movement. Swelling and thickening of the synovium can result in stretching of the joint capsule and ligaments. When this occurs, muscle and tendon imbalances develop, and mechanical forces applied to the joints through daily activities produce joint deformities. In the MCP joints, the extensor tendons can slip to the ulnar side of the metacarpal head, causing ulnar deviation of the fingers (see Fig. 44-6A). Hyperextension of the PIP joint and partial flexion of the distal interphalangeal (DIP) joint is called a *swan neck deformity.* After this condition becomes fixed, severe loss of function occurs because the person can no longer make a fist.

The knee is one of the most commonly affected joints and is responsible for much of the disability associated with the disease. Active synovitis may be apparent as visible swelling that obliterates the normal contour over the medial and lateral aspects of the patella. Joint contractures, instability, and genu valgus (knock-knee) deformity are other possible manifestations. Severe atrophy of the quadriceps muscles can contribute to the disability. A *Baker cyst* may develop in the popliteal area behind the knee. This is caused by enlargement of the bursa but does not usually cause symptoms unless the cyst ruptures, in which case symptoms mimicking thrombophlebitis appear. Ankle involvement can limit flexion and extension, which can create difficulty in walking. Involvement of the metatarsophalangeal joints can cause subluxation, hallux valgus, and hammertoe deformities. Neck pain and stiffness occur later in the disease.

Extra-Articular Manifestations. In addition to articular manifestations, persons with early RA frequently have constitutional symptoms such as fatigue, weakness, anorexia, and weight loss that are due to systemic inflammation.[37,38] The erythrocyte sedimentation rate (ESR) and C-reactive protein (CRP), which commonly are elevated during inflammatory processes, have been

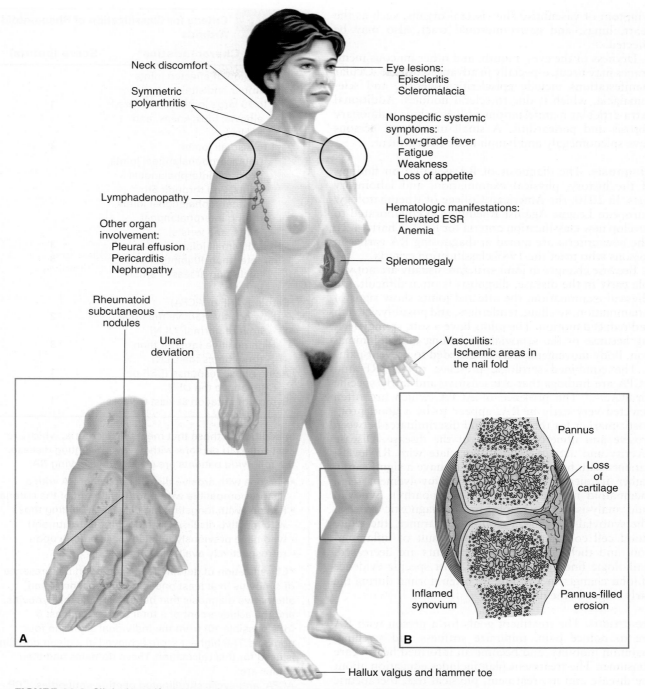

Neck discomfort

Symmetric polyarthritis

Lymphadenopathy

Other organ involvement:
    Pleural effusion
    Pericarditis
    Nephropathy

Rheumatoid subcutaneous nodules

Ulnar deviation

Eye lesions:
    Episcleritis
    Scleromalacia

Nonspecific systemic symptoms:
    Low-grade fever
    Fatigue
    Weakness
    Loss of appetite

Hematologic manifestations:
    Elevated ESR
    Anemia

Splenomegaly

Vasculitis:
    Ischemic areas in the nail fold

Pannus

Loss of cartilage

Inflamed synovium

Pannus-filled erosion

A

B

Hallux valgus and hammer toe

FIGURE 44-6. Clinical manifestations of rheumatoid arthritis featuring **(A)** hand and finger manifestations and **(B)** destructive joint changes. ESR, erythrocyte sedimentation rate.

found to correlate with the amount of disease activity. A moderate hypochromic anemia is common.

Extra-articular involvement occurring in long-standing disease include the development of rheumatic nodules (Fig. 44-6A). These granulomatous lesions have a central core of fibrinoid necrosis that is made up of a mixture of fibrin and other proteins such as degraded collagen.[4] The nodules may be tender or nontender, movable or immovable, and small or large. Typically,

they are found over pressure points such as the extensor surfaces of the ulna. The nodules may resolve spontaneously or be surgically removed.

Vasculitis, or inflammation of small and medium-sized arteries, is an uncommon manifestation that produces ischemic areas in the nail fold and digital pulp that appear as brown spots. Ulcerations may occur in the lower extremities, particularly around the malleolar areas. In some cases, neuropathy may be the only symptom of vasculitis. The visceral organs, such as the heart, lungs, and gastrointestinal tract, also may be affected.

Dryness of the eyes, mouth, and other mucous membranes may occur, especially in advanced disease. Ocular manifestations include episcleritis, scleritis, and scleromalacia, which is due to scleral nodules. Additional extra-articular manifestations of RA include pulmonary fibrosis and pericarditis. A small number of persons have splenomegaly and lymph node enlargement.

Diagnosis. The diagnosis of RA is based on findings of the history, physical examination, and laboratory tests. In 2010, the American College of Rheumatology/European League Against Rheumatism collaborated to develop new classification criteria for RA[39] (Chart 44-2). The new criteria are aimed at diagnosing RA earlier in persons who meet the 1987 classification criteria.

Because changes in joint structure usually are not visible early in the disease, diagnosis is often difficult. On physical examination, the affected joints show signs of inflammation, swelling, tenderness, and possibly warmth and reduced motion. The joints have a soft, spongy feeling because of the synovial thickening and inflammation. Body movements may be guarded to prevent pain.

The combined serologic presence of the RF and ACPA are findings that are sensitive and fairly specific for RA.[3,4,37] The presence of ACPA, which are often detected very early in RA, appear to be a good prognostic marker for the disease and discriminates between erosive and nonerosive forms of the disease. Disease severity and activity tend to correlate with RF levels; patients with high RF levels tend to have a significantly higher frequency of extra-articular involvement (e.g., rheumatoid nodules, vasculitis, neuropathy). Synovial fluid analysis can be helpful in the diagnostic process. The synovial fluid has a cloudy appearance, the white blood cell count is elevated as a result of inflammation, and the complement components are decreased. Radiologic findings provide the most specific evidence of joint changes in RA, but are often normal during the early stages of the disorder.

Treatment. The treatment goals for a person with RA are to reduce pain, minimize stiffness and swelling, maintain mobility, and become an informed health care consumer. The treatment plan includes education about the disease and its treatment, physical rest, therapeutic exercises, and medications. Because of the chronicity of the disease and the need for continuous, long-term adherence to the prescribed treatment modalities, it is important that the treatment be integrated with the person's lifestyle.

Both physical rest and therapeutic exercises are important aspects of care.[36] Physical rest reduces joint stress. Rest of specific joints is recommended to relieve pain. For example, sitting reduces the weight on an inflamed knee, and the use of lightweight splints reduces undue movement of the hand or wrist. Although rest is essential, therapeutic exercises also are important in maintaining joint motion and muscle strength.[37,38]

CHART 44-2 Criteria for Classification of Rheumatoid Arthritis

Patient Characteristics*	Score (points)
Distribution of affected joints (number and site)	
2 to 10 large joints (shoulders, elbows, hips, knees, and ankles)	1
1 to 3 small joints (metacarpophalangeal joints, proximal interphalangeal joints, 2nd through 5th metatarsophalangeal joints, thumb interphalangeal joints, and wrists)	2
4 to 10 small joints	3
Greater than 10 joints (including at least 1 small joint)	5
Serology (RF or ACPA)	
Low positive (above the upper limit of normal, ULN)	2
High positive (greater than three times the ULN)	3
Acute phase response (ESR or CRP) above the ULN	1
Symptom duration at least 6 weeks	1

In addition to those that meet these criteria, which are best suited to persons with newly presenting disease, the following patients are classified as having RA:

- Persons with erosive disease typical of RA with a history compatible with prior fulfillment of the criteria
- Persons with longstanding disease, including those with inactive disease (with or without treatment) who have previously fulfilled these criteria upon retrospectively available data

*Classification of definite RA based upon the presence of synovitis in at least one joint, the absence of an alternative diagnosis that better explains the synovitis, and the achievement of a total score of at least 6 (of a possible 10) from the individual scores in four domains. The highest score achieved in a given domain is used for this calculation. These domains and their values are:
ACPA, anti-cyclic citrullinated peptide antibodies; CRP, C-reactive protein; ESR, erythrocyte sedimentation rate; RF, rheumatoid factor.

Adapted from: Aletaha D, Neogi T, Silman AJ, et al. Rheumatoid arthritis classification criteria: an American College of Rheumatology/European League Against Rheumatism collaborative initiative. *Arth Rheum.* 2010;62(9):2569.

Proper posture, positioning, body mechanics, and the use of supportive shoes can provide further comfort. There often is a need for information about the principles of joint protection and work simplification. Some persons need assistive devices to reduce pain and improve their ability to perform activities of daily living. Instruction in the safe use of heat and cold modalities to relieve discomfort and in the use of relaxation techniques are also important.

The classes of drugs used in the treatment of RA include nonsteroidal anti-inflammatory drugs (NSAIDs) and selective cyclooxygenase (COX)-2 inhibitors; disease-modifying antirheumatic drugs (DMARDs); corticosteroids; and biologic agents.[38,40] The NSAIDs inhibit COX-mediated synthesis of prostaglandins, which have a damaging effect on joint structures (see Chapter 3, Fig. 3-4).

Corticosteroid drugs interrupt the inflammatory and immune cascade at several levels, such as interfering with inflammatory cell adhesion and migration, impairing prostaglandin synthesis, and inhibiting neutrophil superoxide production. To avoid long-term side effects, they are used only in specific situations for short-term therapy at a low dose level. The corticosteroids do not modify the disease and are unable to prevent joint destruction. Intra-articular corticosteroid injections can provide rapid relief of acute or subacute inflammatory synovitis (after infection is excluded) in a few joints. They should not be repeated more than a few times each year.

The DMARDs are a diverse group of therapeutic drugs that reduce the signs and symptoms of RA as well as retard progression of the disease. The DMARDs include hydroxychloroquine, sulfasalazine, methotrexate, and leflunomide. Methotrexate has become the drug of choice because of its potency, and it is relatively fast acting (i.e., improvement is seen in 1 month) compared with the slower-acting DMARDs, which can take 3 to 4 months to work. Methotrexate is thought to interfere with purine metabolism, leading to the release of adenosine, a potent anti-inflammatory compound. Leflunomide is a pyrimidine synthesis inhibitor that blocks the proliferation of T cells. All of the DMARDs can be toxic and require close monitoring for adverse effects, especially those related to bone marrow suppression.

The biologic agents are structurally engineered versions of natural molecules (e.g., monoclonal antibodies) designed to target specific pathogenic mediators of joint inflammation and damage. Etanercept, infliximab, adalimumab, certolizumab, and golimumab are biologic response–modifying agents that block tumor necrosis factor (TNF)-α, one of the key proinflammatory cytokines in RA. Abatacept is a recombinant protein that prevents the co-stimulatory signal that results in full T-cell activation. Rituximab is a chimeric antibody that causes B-cell depletion. Tocilizumab prevents IL-6 from interacting with its receptor and activating cells. The newest drug used in the treatment of RA is tofacitinib, a janus kinase 3 inhibitor which interrupts the signal from the cytokine receptors to the nucleus where inflammatory molecules are made.[41]

Surgery also may be a part of the treatment of RA. Synovectomy may be indicated to reduce pain and joint damage when synovitis does not respond to medical treatment. The most common soft tissue surgery is tenosynovectomy (i.e., repair of damaged tendons) of the hand to release nerve entrapments. Total joint replacements (i.e., arthroplasty) may be indicated to reduce pain and increase motion. Arthrodesis (i.e., joint fusion) is indicated only in extreme cases when there is so much soft tissue damage and scarring or infection that a replacement is impossible.

Systemic Lupus Erythematosus

Systemic lupus erythematosus (SLE) is a chronic inflammatory disease that can affect virtually any organ system, including the musculoskeletal system. It is a major rheumatic disease, with a prevalence of approximately 1 case per 2000 persons. Systemic lupus erythematosus is primarily a disease of young women, with a peak incidence between the ages of 15 and 40 years.[42] It is more common in African Americans, Hispanics, and Asians than whites, and the incidence in some families is higher than in others.

Etiology and Pathogenesis. The cause of SLE is largely unknown. It is characterized by the formation of autoantibodies and immune complexes (type III hypersensitivity; see Chapter 16).[44] Persons with SLE appear to have defective elimination of self-reactive B cells with a resultant increase in production of antibodies that can cause tissue damage. Autoantibodies have been identified against an array of self-molecules found in the plasma, cytoplasm, or on the surface of cells, but those directed against components of the cell nucleus (antinuclear antibodies [ANAs]) are the most characteristic. Antibodies to double-stranded DNA and a nuclear antigen called Sm is found in almost all persons with SLE and are part of the serologic classification of the disease.

The development of autoantibodies can result from a combination of genetic, hormonal, and environmental factors.[42] Genetic predisposition is evidenced by the occurrence of familial cases of SLE, especially among identical twins, and the increased incidence among African Americans compared with whites. As many as four genes may be involved in the expression of SLE.[42] Studies also suggest that an imbalance in sex hormone levels may play a role in the development of the disease, especially because the disease is so prevalent among women. Possible environmental triggers include ultraviolet (UV) light, certain foods, infectious agents, and toxic chemicals, including some drugs.[43,44] Photosensitivity frequently occurs in SLE.[43] Photosensitive persons may report a worsening of systemic disease symptoms such as fatigue and joint pain following sun exposure. Certain drugs may also provoke a lupus-like disorder in susceptible persons, particularly in the elderly. The most common of these drugs are hydralazine and procainamide.

Clinical Manifestations. Systemic lupus erythematosus can manifest in a variety of ways. The disease has been called the *great imitator* because it has the capacity to affect many different body systems, including the musculoskeletal system, skin, cardiovascular system, lungs, kidneys, central nervous system (CNS), and red

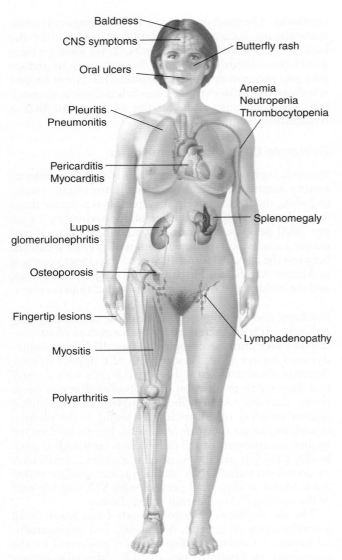

Baldness

CNS symptoms

Oral ulcers

Butterfly rash

Pleuritis
Pneumonitis

Anemia
Neutropenia
Thrombocytopenia

Pericarditis
Myocarditis

Lupus
glomerulonephritis

Splenomegaly

Osteoporosis

Fingertip lesions

Lymphadenopathy

Myositis

Polyarthritis

FIGURE 44-7. Clinical manifestations of systemic lupus erythematosus. CNS, central nervous system.

blood cells and platelets[43,45] (Fig. 44-7). The onset may be acute or insidious, and the course of the disease is characterized by exacerbations and remissions.

Arthralgias and arthritis, the most common manifestations of SLE, are present in up to 90% of persons at some point during the course of their disease.[46] Although the arthritis can affect any joint, it is most often symmetric with involvement of the small joints of the hands, wrists, and knees. Ligaments, tendons, and the joint capsule may be involved, causing varied deformities. Other musculoskeletal manifestations of SLE include tenosynovitis, rupture of the intrapatellar and Achilles tendons, and avascular necrosis, frequently of the femoral head.

Skin manifestations can vary greatly and may be classified as acute, subacute, or chronic. The acute skin lesions include the classic malar or "butterfly" rash on the nose and cheeks[43,45] (see Fig. 44-7). Other skin lesions that may occur include hives or livedo reticularis

(i.e., reticular cyanotic discoloration of the skin, often precipitated by cold), and fingertip lesions. Hair loss is common. Mucous membrane lesions tend to occur during periods of exacerbation. Sun sensitivity may occur in SLE even after mild exposure.

Renal involvement is common in SLE and a significant cause of morbidity and mortality.[45] Several forms of renal involvement may occur, including glomerulonephritis, tubulointerstitial nephritis, and vascular disease (see Chapter 25). The clinical manifestations of renal involvement range from asymptomatic hematuria and/or protinuria to frank nephrotic syndrome with progressive loss of renal function. Nephrotic syndrome causes proteinuria with resultant edema in the legs and abdomen, and around the eyes. Kidney biopsy is the best determinant of renal damage and the type of treatment needed.

Pulmonary involvement is manifested primarily by pleural effusions and/or pleuritis.[45] Pleural effusions are typically small, bilateral, and exudative. Up to 50% of persons with SLE develop pleuritis, which is manifested by pleuritic chest pain. The presence of pleuritis usually corresponds to active SLE in other organ systems.

Cardiovascular disease is a frequent complication of SLE. It can involve the pericardium, myocardium, or coronary arteries. Pericarditis, with or without effusion, is the most common cardiac manifestation in SLE, occurring in 50% of persons with SLE at some point during the course of their disease.[45] Coronary heart disease is also increased in persons with SLE. Hypertension may be associated with lupus nephritis and long-term corticosteroid use. Hematologic disorders may manifest as hemolytic anemia, leukopenia, lymphopenia, or thrombocytopenia.

The nervous system is involved in persons with SLE.[45] Involvement of both the central (CNS) and peripheral (PNS) nervous systems occurs. Central nervous system disorders range from diffuse processes such as headache, psychosis, and mood disorders to more focal processes such as seizures. Headaches are reported in more than 50% of persons with SLE, with both migrainous and tension-type headaches being described.[45] Psychotic manifestations include depression and unnatural euphoria, as well as decreased cognitive functioning, and confusion.

Chronic discoid cutaneous lupus is a disease characterized by plaquelike lesions on the head, scalp, and neck. These lesions first appear as red, swollen patches of skin, and later there can be scarring, depigmentation, and plugging of hair follicles. The disease is usually confined to the skin, but after many years 5% to 10% of persons with the disorder may develop multisystem manifestations.

Subacute cutaneous lupus erythematosus is a less-severe form of lupus that presents with skin lesions resembling psoriasis on sun-exposed areas such as the face, chest, upper back, and arms. Most persons have mild systemic manifestations of SLE, which usually are limited to joint and muscle pains. There is also a low incidence of lupus nephritis.

Diagnosis and Treatment. The diagnosis of SLE is based on a complete history, physical examination, and analysis of bloodwork. The most common laboratory test performed is the immunofluorescence test for ANA. The ANA test is not specific for SLE, and positive ANA results may be found in healthy persons or may be associated with other disorders. Other serum tests may reveal moderate to severe anemia, thrombocytopenia, and leukocytosis or leukopenia.

Treatment of SLE focuses on managing the acute and chronic symptoms of the disease.[46] Persons with photosensitivity should be cautioned against sun exposure and should apply a protective lotion when outdoors. Skin lesions often respond to local application of corticosteroids and minor joint symptoms are usually relieved by rest and NSAIDs.

An antimalarial drug (e.g., hydroxychloroquine) may be helpful in treating mucocutaneous manifestations, pleuritis, arthritis, and fatigue. Corticosteroids are used to treat more significant symptoms of SLE, such as renal and CNS disorders. High-dose corticosteroid treatment is used for acute symptoms, and the drug is tapered to the lowest therapeutic dose as soon as possible to minimize the adverse effects. Immunosuppressive drugs, such as azathioprine and cyclophosphamide, may be used in cases resistant to corticosteroids. Biologics, such as rituximab and belimumab, target B cells and are used for refractory symptoms.

Systemic Sclerosis/Scleroderma

Systemic sclerosis, commonly called *scleroderma,* is an autoimmune disease of connective tissues that causes extensive fibrosis throughout the body.[47–49] The disease affects women four times as frequently as men, with a peak incidence in the 35- to 50-year-old age group.[47]

The cause of systemic sclerosis is poorly understood, although there is evidence of both humoral and cellular immune system abnormalities.[47] Fibroblast activation with excessive fibrosis is a hallmark of the disease. Skin involvement is the usual presenting symptom, but it is the involvement of organs such as the gastrointestinal tract, heart, lungs, and kidneys that produces the major morbidity and mortality. Microvascular disease is also present early in the disease, with repeated cycles of endothelial damage followed by platelet activation and release of platelet factors that lead to fibrosis and narrowing of the microvasculature and tissue ischemia.

Clinical Manifestations. Scleroderma presents as two major clinical subsets: limited and diffuse scleroderma. The most common subset, which accounts for about half of the cases, is limited cutaneous scleroderma in which the skin changes are limited to the fingers, forearms, and face. Some persons with limited involvement also develop a condition called the *CREST* syndrome, characterized by a combination of *c*alcinosis (i.e., calcium deposits in the subcutaneous tissue that erupt through the skin), *R*aynaud phenomenon (a vascular disorder characterized by reversible vasospasm of the arteries supplying the fingers [see Chapter 18]), *e*sophageal dysmotility, *s*clerodactyly (localized scleroderma of the fingers), and *t*elangiectasia (dilated skin capillaries).[48]

Diffuse scleroderma, which accounts for approximately 35% of persons with scleroderma, is characterized by severe, widespread, and progressive skin involvement and early onset of organ involvement.[49] The typical person has a "stone facies" due to tightening of the facial skin with restricted motion of the mouth. Other cutaneous manifestations include hair loss on the involved skin and telangiectasis on the face, buccal mucosa, chest, and hands. Almost all persons with diffuse scleroderma develop Raynaud phenomenon. Musculoskeletal involvement is common. Puffy hands with arthralgia and myalgia may lead to difficulty forming a fist. There are palpable or audible friction rubs over the extensor and flexor tendons of the hands, knees, and ankles. Involvement of the esophagus that leads to difficulty swallowing is common, and malabsorption may develop if the disease affects the intestine. Pulmonary involvement leads to dyspnea and eventually respiratory failure. Vascular involvement of the kidneys is responsible for malignant hypertension and progressive renal insufficiency. Cardiac problems include pericarditis, heart block, and myocardial fibrosis.

Treatment. Treatment of systemic sclerosis is largely symptomatic and supportive.[48,49] Advances in treatment, primarily the use of angiotensin-converting enzyme (ACE) inhibitors in renal involvement, have led to a substantial decrease in the mortality from hypertensive renal disease.[50] Cardiopulmonary manifestations of scleroderma, specifically pulmonary hypertension, can be treated with prostanoids (or endothelial receptor antagonists [bosentan]). Disease modifying agents such as methotrexate, cyclophosphamide, azathioprine, and mycophenalate mofetil have been reported effective in limited case series or randomized controlled trials. These agents can be used in early diffuse disease.

Seronegative Spondyloarthropathies

The *spondyloarthropathies* are an interrelated group of multisystem inflammatory disorders that primarily affect the axial skeleton, particularly the spine.[3,4,51] Sacroiliitis is a pathologic hallmark of the disorders. Typically, the inflammation begins at sites, called *entheses,* where tendons and ligaments insert into bone rather than the synovium. There may also be inflammation and involvement of the peripheral joints, in which case the signs and symptoms overlap with other inflammatory types of arthritis.

The spondyloarthropathies are grouped into two subtypes: the axial spondyloarthropies, which include ankylosing spondylitis; and the peripheral spondyloarthropathies, which include psoriatic arthritis, reactive arthritis, inflammatory bowel disease–associated arthritis, and undifferentiated peripheral spondyloarthritis. Although they differ in terms of factors such as age and type of onset and extent of joint involvement, there is clinical evidence of overlap between the various disorders.

Ankylosing Spondylitis

Ankylosing spondylitis is a chronic, systemic inflammatory disease of the joints of the axial skeleton manifested by pain and progressive stiffening of the spine.[3,4,51] The disease usually begins in late adolescence or early adulthood. The incidence is greater in men than in women, and symptoms are generally more prominent in men.

Pathogenesis. Although the pathogenesis of ankylosing spondylitis has not been established, the presence of mononuclear cells in the acutely involved tissue suggests an immune response. Epidemiologic findings indicate that genetic and environmental factors play a role in the pathogenesis of the disease. The HLA-B27 allele remains one of the best-known examples of an association between a disease and a hereditary marker. Approximately 90% of those with ankylosing spondylitis possess the HLA-B27 allele, which also is present in approximately 5% to 15% of the normal population.[4] Several theories have been advanced to account for the association between HLA-B27 and ankylosing spondylitis. One possibility is that it predisposes to ankylosing spondylitis by influencing the body's endogenous flora.[52]

Clinical Manifestations. The typical musculoskeletal lesion associated with ankylosing spondylitis is inflammation, or *enthesitis*, at sites where tendons and ligaments attach to bones. Typically, the disease process begins with bilateral involvement of the sacroiliac joints and then moves to the smaller joints of the posterior elements of the spine (Fig. 44-8). The result is ultimate destruction of these joints with ankylosis or posterior fusion of the spine. The vertebrae take on a squared appearance and bone bridges fuse one vertebral body to the next across the intervertebral disks.[51] Progressive spinal changes usually begin with the sacroiliac area and then move up the spine to involve the costovertebral joints and cervical spine. Occasionally, large synovial joints (i.e., hips, knees, and shoulders) may be involved. The disease spectrum ranges from an asymptomatic sacroiliitis to a progressive disease that can affect many body systems.

The usual presenting symptom is back pain that may be persistent or intermittent.[3,4,51] The pain, which becomes worse when resting, particularly when lying in bed, may also involve the buttocks and hip areas, and can radiate to the thigh in a manner similar to that of sciatic pain. Mild physical activity or a hot shower helps reduce pain and stiffness. Sleep patterns frequently are interrupted because of these manifestations. Walking or exercise may be needed to provide the comfort needed to return to sleep. The most common extraskeletal involvement is acute anterior uveitis (iritis), which occurs in approximately 30% of persons sometime in the course of their disease. Systemic features of weight loss, fever, and fatigue may be apparent.

Osteoporosis may occur, especially in the spine, which contributes to the risk of spinal fracture. Loss of motion in the spinal column is characteristic of the disease (see Fig. 44-8). Loss of lumbar lordosis occurs as the disease progresses, and this is followed by kyphosis of the thoracic spine and extension of the neck. A spine fused

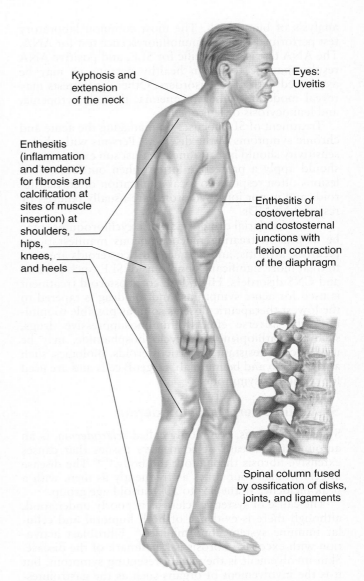

FIGURE 44-8. Clinical manifestations of ankylosing spondylitis.

in the flexed position is the end result of severe ankylosing spondylitis. A kyphotic spine makes it difficult for the patient to look ahead and to maintain balance while walking. The image is one of a person bent over looking at the floor and unable to straighten up. X-ray films show a rigid, bamboolike spine. The heart and lungs are constricted in the chest cavity. Abnormal weight bearing can lead to degeneration and destruction of the hip joint, necessitating joint replacement procedures. Peripheral arthritis is more common in the hips and shoulders.

Diagnosis and Treatment. The diagnosis of ankylosing spondylitis is based on history, physical examination, and x-ray examination.[51,53] The history and physical examination should include measures of physical function, pain, spinal mobility, duration of morning stiffness, involvement of peripheral joints and entheses, and fatigue. Laboratory findings frequently include an elevated ESR. The person also may have a mild normo-cytic normochromic anemia. HLA typing is not diagnostic of the disease and should not be used as a routine screening procedure. Radiologic evaluations help differentiate ankylosing spondylitis from sacroiliitis due to other diseases. However, x-ray images may be normal in early disease. One important advance in diagnosis of ankylosing spondylitis is the use of magnetic resonance imaging (MRI) to assess sacroiliac changes.[51] Whereas plain radiographic images can detect structural changes such as joint erosion and subchrondral bone sclerosis seen in the late stage of the disease, MRI allows for the visualization of synovial fluid, synovitis within the sacroiliac joint, and subchondral bone edema seen in earlier stages of the disease.[51]

Treatment of ankylosing spondylitis is directed at controlling pain and maintaining mobility by suppressing inflammation.[54] Proper posture and positioning are important. This includes sleeping in a supine position on a firm mattress and using one small pillow or no pillow. A bed board may be used to supply additional firmness. Therapeutic exercises are important to assist in maintaining motion in peripheral joints and in the spine. Muscle-strengthening exercises for extensor muscle groups also are prescribed. Swimming is an excellent general conditioning exercise that avoids joint stress and enhances muscle tone. Immobilizing joints is not recommended. Maintaining ideal weight reduces the stress on weight-bearing joints. Deep breathing exercises and avoidance or discontinuation of smoking should be emphasized.

Pharmacologic treatment includes the use of NSAIDs to reduce inflammation, relieve pain, and reduce muscle spasm. Disease-modifying antirheumatic drugs are potential second-line therapies, but their efficacy in ankylosing spondylitis is unproven. Sulfasalazine and methotrexate have not shown benefit for spondylitis-associated back pain, but have shown efficacy for peripheral joint involvement. Anti–TNF-α therapies, including etanercept, infliximab, adalimumab, and golimumab, have demonstrated rapid effectiveness in reducing both the axial and peripheral symptoms of ankylosing spondylitis, as well as improving quality of life.[54]

The disease process in ankylosing spondylitis varies considerably among individuals. Exacerbations and remissions are common; almost all persons have persistent symptoms over decades. Fortunately, most of those affected are able to lead productive lives. Progression during the first decade of the disease tends to predict the prognosis.

Reactive Arthritis

Reactive arthritis is an inflammatory joint disorder that arises after certain inciting gastrointestinal or genitourinary tract infections and manifests as a sterile oligoarthritis, typically of the lower extremities.[55] Most cases of reactive arthritis develop after either a gastrointestinal infection (*Salmonella, Shigella, Campylobacter,* or *Yersinia*) or sexually transmitted infection (*Chlamydia trachomatis*). The infecting agents cannot be cultured and are not viable after reaching the joints. A clinically indistinguishable syndrome can occur without antecedent infection, suggesting that subclinical infection or some other unrecognized agent can precipitate reactive arthritis. *Reiter syndrome* is a form of reactive arthritis defined by a triad of arthritis, nongonococcal urethritis or cervicitis, and conjunctivitis.[3] *Enteropathic arthritis* is a reactive arthritis that is associated with inflammatory bowel disease (i.e., Crohn disease and ulcerative colitis) or triggered by enterogenic bacteria.

Clinical Manifestations. Reactive arthritis is most commonly asymmetric and frequently involves the lower extremities. Symptoms typically start within 1 to 4 weeks of the initial infection. Hip disease is uncommon and involvement of the upper extremities is rare. The joints are typically warm, swollen, and tender. Systemic manifestations including fever and weight loss are common at the onset. Enthesitis is a common feature of reactive arthritis. The Achilles tendon and plantar fascia are the most common sites of involvement, but pain in the iliac crests, ischial tuberosities, and back may occur. This aspect of the disease can be disabling, with marked restriction in weight bearing and ambulation. Extra-articular lesions are common and include circinate balanitis (shallow ulcers on the glans or shaft of the penis), stomatitis (e.g., painless oral ulcers on the hard palate or tongue), and keratoderma blennorrhagicum (a papulosquamous rash most commonly affecting the palms of the hands and soles of the feet [Fig. 44-9]). While most of the signs and symptoms disappear within days or weeks, the arthritis may persist for several months, and in a small number of cases, it may follow a continuous and unremitting course.

Treatment. The treatment is largely symptomatic. NSAIDs are used in treating the arthritic symptoms.[55] Vigorous treatment of possible triggering infections is thought to prevent relapses of reactive arthritis, but in many cases the triggering infection passes unnoticed or

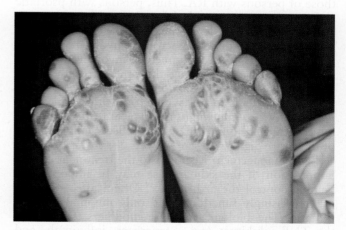

FIGURE 44-9. Keratoderma blennorrhagica of soles due to reactive arthritis (Reiter syndrome). (From the Centers for Disease Control and Prevention Public Health Images Library. No. 6950. Courtesy of M. F. Rein.)

is mild, and the person seeks medical care only with the onset of definite arthritis. Short antibiotic courses at this time are not effective.

Psoriatic Arthritis

Psoriatic arthritis is a seronegative inflammatory arthropathy that occurs with variable frequency in people with psoriasis.[56–58] It is a disease with various and similar features of the spondyloarthropathies in some persons, in whom an asymmetric sacroiliitis and spinal involvement predominate. In others, the disease is polyarticular and resembles RA, and in some, features of both disorders coexist. Although the arthritis can antedate a detectable skin rash, the definitive diagnosis of psoriatic arthritis cannot be made without evidence of skin or nail changes typical of psoriasis (see Chapter 46).

The etiology of psoriasis and psoriatic arthritis is unknown. Genetic, environmental, and immunologic factors appear to affect susceptibility and play a role in expression of the psoriatic skin disease and the arthritis. Environmental factors that may play a role in the pathogenesis of the disorder include infectious agents and physical trauma. T-cell–mediated immune responses seem to play an important role in the skin and joint manifestations of the disease, as indicated by the observation that there is improvement in disease status after treatment with immunosuppressant agents such as cyclosporine.

Psoriatic arthritis falls into five subgroups: (1) an oligoarticular form affecting four or fewer joints; (2) a spondylitis form in which sacroiliitis and spinal involvement predominate; (3) a polyarticular, or symmetric, form that resembles RA; (4) a form in which the distal interphalangeal joints are primarily affected; and (5) arthritis mutilans, a very destructive form of arthritis.[56,57] The joint involvement of peripheral psoriatic arthritis is inflammatory in nature, presenting with swelling and stiffness of the affected joints. Early in the disease, the arthritis tends to be oligoarticular, but may become polyarticular over time. The affected joints of persons with psoriatic arthritis are often less tender than those of persons with RA. Thus, persons with psoriatic arthritis may present with deformity and joint damage, not having perceived any pain during the inflammatory phase of the disease. Sacroiliac involvement, when it occurs, tends to be asymmetric, involving only one sacroiliac joint and sparing the other or with different degrees of radiologic involvement. Likewise, spinal involvement tends to be asymmetric, with skip lesions. *Dactylitis*, or *sausage digit*, is a typical feature of distal interphalangeal joint disease and reflects inflammation of the entire digit.[56,57]

Basic management is similar to the treatment of RA. Suppression of the skin disease may be important in helping control the arthritis.[56–58] Often, affected joints are surprisingly functional and only minimally symptomatic. The biologic response modifiers, specifically the TNF inhibitors (e.g., etanercept, infliximab, and adalimumab), have been found to be beneficial in controlling the arthritis as well as the psoriasis in patients with psoriatic arthritis.[56]

Osteoarthritis

Osteoarthritis (OA), also called *degenerative joint disease*, is the most prevalent type of joint disease and is one of the 10 most disabling conditions in developing nations.[3,4] The disorder, which is characterized by degenerative changes of the articular cartilage, can affect any one of 200 or so synovial joints in the body, and can occur as a primary idiopathic disorder or as a secondary disorder. In most instances, OA appears insidiously, without an apparent initiating cause, as an aging phenomenon (idiopathic or primary OA).[3,4] In these cases the disorder is usually oligoarticular, but may be generalized. Secondary OA has a known underlying cause such as congenital or acquired defects of joint structures, trauma, metabolic disorders, or inflammatory diseases.

Joint changes associated with OA include a gradual loss of articular cartilage, combined with thickening of the subchondral bone, bony outgrowths (osteophytes) at joint margins, and mild synovial inflammation. These changes are accompanied by joint pain, stiffness, and limitation of motion, and in some cases by joint instability and deformity.

Etiology and Pathogenesis

Osteoarthritis is a multifactorial disease that has genetic and environmental risk factors. Studies of families and twins suggest that the risk of OA is related to the net impact of multiple genes, each with a small effect.[3,4] Age, gender, and race interact to influence the time of onset and the pattern of joint involvement in OA. Age is one of the strongest risk factors for OA of all joints. The increase in incidence and prevalence with age probably is the consequence of cumulative exposure to the various risk factors and biologic changes that occur in a life time. Women are more likely to have OA than men, and they tend to have more severe OA as well. The prevalence of OA and pattern of joint involvement vary among racial and ethnic groups. Hand OA is more likely to affect white women, whereas knee OA is more common in black women. The incidence of hip OA is lower among the Chinese than Europeans, perhaps representing the influence of other factors such as occupation, obesity, or heredity. Bone mass may also influence the risk of developing OA. In theory, thinner subchondral bone mass may provide a greater shock-absorbing function than denser bone, allowing less direct trauma to the cartilage. Obesity is a particular risk factor for OA of the knee in women and a contributory biomechanical factor in the pathogenesis of the disease. Weight loss reduces the risk of developing symptomatic arthritis of the knee.

The pathogenesis of OA resides in the homeostatic mechanisms that maintain the articular cartilage.[3,4,59] Articular cartilage plays two essential mechanical roles in joint physiology. First, it serves as a remarkably smooth weight-bearing surface. In combination with synovial fluid, the articular cartilage provides extremely low friction during movement of the joint. Second, the cartilage transmits the load down to the bone, dissipating

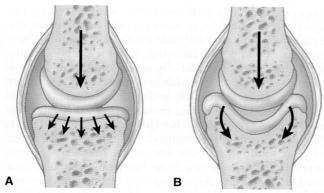

FIGURE 44-10. (A) A joint normally undergoes deformation of the articular cartilage and the subchondral bone when carrying a load. This maximizes the contact area and spreads the force of the load. **(B)** If the joint does not deform with a load, the stresses are concentrated and the joint breaks down.

the mechanical stress.[3] Thus, the subchondral bone protects the overlying articular cartilage, providing it with a pliable bed and absorbing the energy of the force (Fig. 44-10). Articular cartilage has two major components: an extracellular matrix, which is rich in proteoglycan and collagen fibers, and a limited number of chondrocytes, which produce the matrix.

Popularly known as *wear-and-tear* arthritis, OA is characterized by significant changes in both the composition and mechanical properties of cartilage.[3,4] The articular cartilage injury is thought to result from chondrocyte injury and release of cytokines such as

interleukin (IL)-1 and TNF (Fig. 44-11). These chemical messengers stimulate the production and release of proteases (enzymes) that are destructive to joint structures. The resulting damage predisposes the chondrocytes to additional injury and impairs their ability to maintain cartilage synthesis and repair the damage. The combined effects of inadequate repair mechanisms and imbalances between the proteases and their inhibitors contribute further to disease progression.

The earliest structural changes in OA include enlargement and reorganization of the chondrocytes in the superficial part of the articular cartilage.[3,4] This is accompanied by edematous changes in the cartilaginous matrix, principally the intermediate layer. The cartilage loses its smooth aspect and surface cracks or microfractures occur, allowing synovial fluid to enter and widen the crack. As the crack deepens, vertical clefts form and eventually extend through the full thickness of the articular surface and into the subchondral bone. Portions of the articular cartilage eventually become completely eroded and the exposed surface of the subchondral bone becomes thickened and polished to an ivory-like consistency (eburnation). Fragments of cartilage and bone often become dislodged, creating free-floating osteocartilaginous bodies ("joint mice") that enter the joint cavity. Synovial fluid may leak though the defects in the residual cartilage to form cysts within the bone (Fig. 44-12). As the disease progresses, the underlying subchondral bone becomes sclerotic and thickened in response to increased pressure on the surface of the joint, rendering it less effective as a shock absorber. Sclerosis, or formation of new bone and cysts, usually occurs at the joint margins, forming abnormal bony outgrowths called *osteophytes,* or *spurs* (see Fig. 44-12). As the joint begins to lose its integrity, there is trauma to the synovial membrane, which results in nonspecific inflammation. Compared with RA, however, the inflammatory

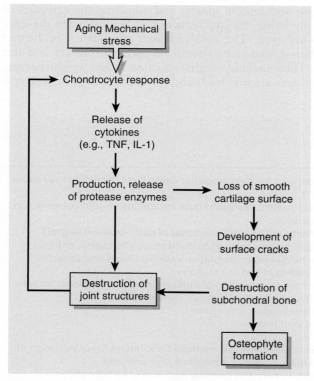

FIGURE 44-11. Disease process in osteoarthritis.

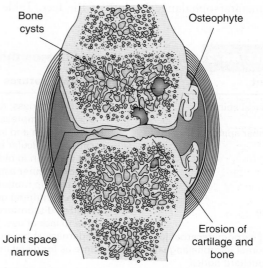

FIGURE 44-12. Joint changes in osteoarthritis. The left side denotes early changes and joint space narrowing with cartilage breakdown. The right side shows more severe disease progression with lost cartilage and osteophyte formation.

changes in the synovium that occur in OA are not as pronounced, nor do they occur as early.

In secondary forms of OA, repetitive impact loading contributes to joint failure, accounting for the high prevalence of OA specific to vocational or avocational sites, such as the shoulders and elbows of baseball pitchers, ankles of ballet dancers, and knees of basketball players. Immobilization also can produce degenerative changes in articular cartilage. Cartilage degeneration due to immobility may result from loss of the pumping action of lubrication that occurs with joint movement. These changes are more marked and appear earlier in areas of contact, but also occur in areas not subject to mechanical compression. Although cartilage atrophy is rapidly reversible with activity after a period of immobilization, impact exercise during the period of remobilization can prevent reversal of the atrophy. Therefore, slow and gradual remobilization may be important in preventing cartilage injury. Clinically, this has implications for instructions concerning the recommended level of physical activity after removal of a cast.

Clinical Features

Typically, OA presents with joint pain.[60,61] Initially, pain may be described as aching and may be somewhat difficult to localize. It usually worsens with use or activity and is relieved by rest. A common phenomenon, often referred to as "gelling," involves difficulty initiating joint movement after inactivity, epitomized by the problems older people with OA have in "getting started" after sitting down for a while. In later stages of disease activity, night pain may be experienced during rest. Cracking of joints (audible crepitus) and joint locking may occur when the joint is moved. As the disease advances, even minimal activity may cause pain.

The most frequently affected joints are the hips, knees, lumbar and cervical spine, proximal and distal joints of the hands, the first carpometacarpal joint, and the first metatarsophalangeal joints of the feet. Table 44-1

identifies the joints that commonly are affected by OA and the common clinical features correlated with the disease activity of each particular joint. A single joint or several may be affected. Although a single weight-bearing joint may be involved initially, other joints often become affected because of the additional stress placed on them while trying to protect the initial joint. It is not unusual for a person having a knee replacement to discover soon after the surgery is done that the second knee also needs to be replaced. Other clinical features are limitations of joint motion and joint instability. Joint enlargement usually results from new bone formation; the joint feels hard, in contrast to the soft, spongy feeling characteristic of the joint in RA. Sometimes, mild synovitis or increased synovial fluid can cause joint enlargement.

Diagnosis and Treatment. The diagnosis of OA usually is determined by history and physical examination, x-ray studies, and laboratory findings that exclude other diseases.[60–62] Although OA often is contrasted with RA for diagnostic purposes, the differences are not always readily apparent. Other rheumatic diseases may be superimposed on OA. Psychological factors, severity of joint disease, and educational level affect the expression of symptoms.

Because there is no cure, the treatment of OA is symptomatic and includes physical rehabilitative, pharmacologic, and surgical measures. Physical measures are aimed at improving the supporting structures of the joint and strengthening opposing muscle groups involved in cushioning weight-bearing forces. This includes a balance of rest and exercise, use of splints to protect and rest the joint, use of heat and cold to relieve pain and muscle spasm, and adjusting the activities of daily living. Weight reduction is helpful when the knee is involved. The involved joint should not be further abused, and steps should be taken to protect and rest it. These include weight reduction (when weight-bearing surfaces are involved) and the use of a cane or walker if

TABLE 44-1	Clinical Features of Osteoarthritis
Joint	**Clinical Features**
Cervical spine	Localized stiffness; radicular or nonradicular pain; posterior osteophyte formation may cause vascular compression
Lumbar spine	Low back pain and stiffness; muscle spasm; decreased back motion; nerve root compression causing radicular pain; spinal stenosis
Hip	Most common in older men; characterized by insidious onset of pain, localized to groin region or inner aspect of the thigh; may be referred to buttocks, sciatic region, or knee; reduced hip motion; leg may be held in external rotation with hip flexed and adducted; limp or shuffling gait; difficulty getting in and out of chairs
Knee	Localized discomfort with pain on motion; limitation of motion; crepitus; quadriceps atrophy due to lack of use; joint instability; genu varus or valgus; joint effusion
First carpometacarpal joint	Tenderness at base of thumb; squared appearance to joint
Proximal interphalangeal joint— Bouchard nodes	Same as for distal interphalangeal joint disease
Distal interphalangeal joint (DIP)—Heberden nodes	Occurs more frequently in women; usually involves multiple DIPs, lateral flexor deviation of joint, spur formation at joint margins, pain and discomfort after joint use
First metatarsophalangeal joint	Insidious onset; irregular joint contour; pain and swelling aggravated by tight shoes

the hips and knees are involved. Muscle-strengthening exercises may help protect the joint and decrease pain.

Several dietary supplements are available and advertised as beneficial for OA, but few have undergone rigorous testing. The most widely used supplements for OA are glucosamine and chondroitin sulfate. A recent multicenter trial funded by the National Institutes of Health found that glucosamine and chondroitin (alone or in combination) were no better than placebo in reducing pain in the total group of persons with knee pain, but that the combination may be effective in those with moderate to severe pain.[63] Topical capsaicin may have some pain-relieving effect in osteoarthritic knees and hands.

Oral medications are aimed at reducing inflammation or providing analgesia. The mainstay of treatment for mild osteoarthritis is acetaminophen. When acetaminophen fails to control symptoms , or if the symptoms are moderate to severe, NSAID therapy is recommended. Intra-articular corticosteroid injections may be used when other treatment measures have been unsuccessful in adequately relieving symptoms.[60,61] They are especially helpful in persons who have an effusion of the joint. Injections usually are limited to no more than three times a year in the same joint because their use is thought to accelerate joint destruction. Viscosupplementation is based on the hypothesis that joint lubrication is abnormal in OA.[64] Hyaluronate is injected into the joint weekly for 3 to 5 weeks.

Surgery is considered when the person is having severe pain and joint function is severely reduced.[60] Procedures include arthroscopic lavage and débridement, bunion resections, osteotomies to change alignment of the knee and hip joints, and decompression of the spinal roots in osteoarthritic vertebral stenosis. Total hip replacements have provided effective relief of symptoms and improved range of motion for many persons, as have total knee replacements, although the latter procedure has produced less-consistent results. Joint replacement is available for the first carpometacarpal joint. Arthrodesis (surgical stiffening of a joint) is used in advanced disease to reduce pain; however, this results in loss of motion.

Crystal-Induced Arthropathies

Crystal deposition in joints produces arthritis. In gout, monosodium urate or uric acid crystals are found in the joint cavity. Another condition in which calcium pyrophosphate dihydrate crystals are found in the joints sometimes is referred to as *pseudogout* or *chondrocalcinosis*. A brief discussion of pseudogout is found in the section on rheumatic diseases in the elderly.

Gout

Gout is actually a group of diseases known as the *gout syndrome*.[66–68] It includes acute gouty arthritis with recurrent attacks of severe articular and periarticular inflammation; tophi or the accumulation of crystalline deposits in articular surfaces, bones, soft tissue, and cartilage; gouty nephropathy or renal impairment; and uric acid kidney stones.

The term *primary gout* is used to designate cases in which the cause of the disorder is unknown or an inborn error in metabolism and is characterized primarily by hyperuricemia and gout. Primary gout is predominantly a disease of men, with a peak incidence in the fourth to sixth decade. In secondary gout, the cause of the hyperuricemia is known but the gout is not the main disorder. Asymptomatic hyperuricemia is a laboratory finding and not a disease. Most persons with hyperuricemia do not develop gout.

Pathogenesis. The pathogenesis of gout resides in an elevation of serum uric acid levels. Uric acid is the end product of purine (adenine and guanine from DNA and RNA) metabolism.[3,4] The elevation of uric acid and the subsequent development of gout can result from overproduction of purines, decreased salvage of free purine bases, augmented breakdown of nucleic acids as a result of increased cell turnover, or decreased urinary excretion of uric acid. Primary gout, which constitutes 90% of cases,[3] may be a consequence of enzyme defects that result in an overproduction of uric acid, inadequate elimination of uric acid by the kidney, or a combination of the two. In most cases, the reason is unknown. In secondary gout, hyperuricemia may be caused by increased breakdown of nucleic acids, as occurs with rapid tumor cell lysis during treatment for lymphoma or leukemia. Other cases of secondary gout result from chronic kidney disease. Some of the diuretics, including the thiazides, can interfere with the excretion of uric acid.

An attack of gout occurs when monosodium urate crystals precipitate in the joint and initiate an inflammatory response. Synovial fluid is a poorer solvent for uric acid than plasma. Moreover, uric acid crystals are even less soluble at temperatures below 37°C, and typically are deposited in peripheral areas of the body, such as the great toe, where the temperatures are cooler than other parts of the body.[3] With prolonged hyperuricemia, crystals and *microtophi* (i.e., small, hard nodules with irregular surfaces that contain crystalline deposits of monosodium urate) accumulate in the synovial lining cells and in the joint cartilage. The released crystals are chemotactic to leukocytes and also activate complement. Phagocytosis of urate crystals by polymorphonuclear leukocytes occurs and leads to polymorphonuclear cell death with the release of lysosomal enzymes. As this process continues, the inflammation causes destruction of the cartilage and subchondral bone.

Repeated attacks of acute arthritis eventually lead to chronic arthritis and the formation of the large, hard nodules called *tophi*[3,4] (Fig. 44-13). They are found most commonly in the synovium, olecranon bursa, Achilles tendon, subchondral bone, and extensor surface of the forearm and may be mistaken for rheumatoid nodules. Tophi usually do not appear until 10 years or more after the first gout attack. This stage of gout, called *chronic tophaceous gout,* is characterized by more frequent and prolonged attacks, which often are polyarticular.[67]

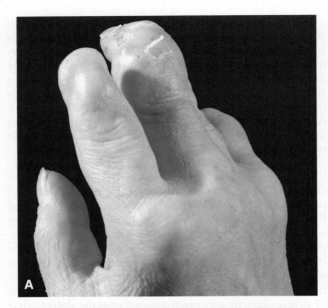

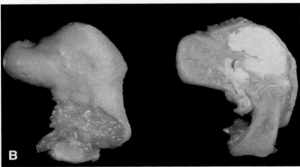

FIGURE 44-13. (A) Gouty tophi of the hands appear as multiple rubbery nodules, one of which is ulcerated. **(B)** A cross-section of a digit demonstrates the trophaceous collection of toothpaste-like urate crystals. (From: Garcia RA, Klein MJ, Schiller AL. Bones and joints. In: Rubin R, Strayer DS, eds. *Rubin's Pathology: Clinicopathologic Foundations of Medicine.* 6th ed. Philadelphia, PA: Wolters Kluwer Health | Lippincott Williams & Wilkins; 2012:1282.)

Clinical Manifestations. The typical acute attack of gout is monoarticular and usually affects the first metatarsophalangeal joint.[65,66] The tarsal joints, insteps, ankles, heels, knees, wrists, fingers, and elbows also may be initial sites of involvement. Acute gout often begins at night and may be precipitated by excessive exercise, certain medications or foods, alcohol, or dieting. The onset of pain typically is abrupt, and redness and swelling are observed. The attack may last for days or weeks. Pain may be severe enough to be aggravated even by the weight of a bed sheet covering the affected area.

In the early stages of gout after the initial attack has subsided, the person is asymptomatic, and joint abnormalities are not evident. This is referred to as *intercritical gout.* After the first attack, it may be months or years before another attack. As attacks recur with increased frequency, joint changes occur and become permanent.

Diagnosis and Treatment. Although hyperuricemia is the biochemical hallmark of gout, the presence of hyperuricemia cannot be equated with gout because many persons with this condition never develop gout. A definitive diagnosis of gout can be made only when monosodium urate crystals are present in the synovial fluid or in tissue sections of tophaceous deposits. Synovial fluid analysis is useful in excluding other conditions, such as septic arthritis, pseudogout, and RA.[65–68] Diagnostic methods also include measures to determine if the disorder is related to overproduction or to underexcretion of uric acid. This is done through measurement of serum uric acid levels and collection of a 24-hour urine sample for determination of urate excretion in the urine.

The objectives for treatment of gout include the termination and prevention of the acute attacks of gouty arthritis and the correction of hyperuricemia, with consequent inhibition of further precipitation of sodium urate and absorption of urate crystal deposits already in the tissues.

Pharmacologic management of acute gout is directed toward reducing joint inflammation.[65–68] Hyperuricemia and related problems of tophi, joint destruction, and renal problems are treated after the acute inflammatory process has subsided. Nonsteroidal anti-inflammatory drugs, particularly indomethacin and ibuprofen, are used for treating acute gouty arthritis.[68] Alternative therapies include colchicine and intra-articular deposition of corticosteroids. Colchicine produces its anti-inflammatory effects by inhibition of leukocyte migration and phagocytosis. Although the drug usually is given orally, a more rapid response is obtained when colchicine is given intravenously. The acute symptoms of gout usually subside within 48 hours after treatment with oral colchicine has been instituted and within 12 hours after intravenous administration of the drug. The corticosteroid drugs have not been systemically studied, but can be useful in the treatment of acute gout limited to a single joint or bursa.

Between acute attacks nonpharmacologic and pharmacologic measures are used to normalize uric acid levels as a means of reducing or preventing the frequency and severity of recurrence.[65–68] Nonpharmacologic methods include maintenance of ideal weight, moderation in alcohol consumption, and avoidance of purine-rich foods (e.g., liver, kidney, sardines, anchovies, and sweetbreads). Avoidance of medications that inhibit renal excretion of uric acid (e.g., loop and thiazide diuretics, low-dose aspirin, and niacin) is also needed.

Three classes of drugs may be used to lower the serum uric acid–xanthine oxidase inhibitors, uricosuric agents, and uricase agents. Xanthine oxidase inhibitors block the synthesis of uric acid. In this classification, the most commonly prescribed drug to lower urate levels is allopurinol. Another xanthine oxidase inhibitor, febuxostat, is used for treatment in persons with a hypersensitivity to allopurinol. The uricosuric agents (e.g., probenecid, sulfinpyrozone, and benzobromarone) prevent the tubular reabsorption of urate and increase its excretion in the urine. The serum urate concentrations are monitored to determine efficacy and dosage. Uricase agents convert insoluble uric acid to a soluble product that can be excreted easily. Pegloticase is an infusible uricase agent that works rapidly to reduce serum uric acid and tophaceous deposits of urate. Prophylactic colchicine may be used between gout attacks.

SUMMARY CONCEPTS

- Systemic autoimmune rheumatic disorders are a group of chronic disorders with overlapping symptoms that are characterized by diffuse inflammatory lesions and progressive changes in connective tissue.

- Rheumatoid arthritis (RA) is a chronic systemic inflammatory disorder affecting multiple joints. Joint involvement, which is symmetric, begins with inflammatory changes of the synovium and formation of a destructive granulation tissue called *pannus* that leads to joint instability and eventual deformity.

- Systemic lupus erythematosus is a chronic autoimmune disorder that affects multiple body systems, including the musculoskeletal system, skin, kidneys, cardiovascular system, hematologic system, and central nervous system. There is an exaggerated production of autoantibodies, which interact with antigens to produce an immune complex. These immune complexes produce an inflammatory response in affected tissues.

- Systemic sclerosis is an autoimmune disorder of connective tissues. It causes extensive fibrosis of many body organs and systems including the sheaths or fascia covering tendons and muscles.

- The seronegative spondyloarthropathies, which include ankylosing spondylitis, reactive arthropathies, and psoriatic arthritis, affect the axial skeleton, particularly the spine. The inflammatory process associated with the disorders commonly affects areas where ligaments and tendons attach to bone. Ankylosing spondylitis, which is characterized by bilateral sacroiliitis and loss of motion in the spinal column, is considered a prototype of this classification category. Although the cause of the disorders is unknown, there is a striking association between the HLA-B27 antigen and development of the spondyloarthropathies.

- Osteoarthritis (OA), often referred to as "wear-and-tear" arthritis, is a slowly destructive disorder of the articular cartilage. It can occur as a primary idiopathic disorder or as a secondary disorder due to congenital or acquired defects in joint structures. Risk factors for OA progression include older age, multiple joint involvement, neuropathy, and, for knees, obesity. The joint changes associated with OA, which include progressive loss of articular cartilage and subchondral bone, result from inflammatory changes that occur when cartilage tries to repair itself.

- Gout is a crystal-induced arthropathy caused by the presence of monosodium urate crystals in the joint cavity. It includes acute gouty arthritis with recurrent attacks of articular and periarticular inflammation, and the accumulation of crystalline deposits, called tophi, in articular surfaces, bones, and soft tissue surrounding joints. The disorder is accompanied by hyperuricemia, which results from overproduction of uric acid or from the reduced ability of the kidney to rid the body of excess uric acid.

Rheumatic Diseases in Children and the Elderly

Rheumatic diseases differ among children, adults, and the elderly in terms of diagnosis, impact of activities, and availability of treatment modalities. These conditions, which affect not only the child but also the family, can seriously impact a child's growth and development, limit their participation in childhood activities, and require an extensive plan of drug treatment and rehabilitation.

Weakness and gait disturbance that often accompany the rheumatic diseases in the elderly can contribute to the likelihood of falls and fracture, causing suffering, increased health care costs, further loss of independence, and the potential for a decreased life span.

Rheumatic Diseases in Children

Children can be affected by many of the same types of rheumatic diseases that occur in adults. About 1 child in every 1000 develops some type of juvenile arthritis.[69] It can affect a single joint or multiple joints, and cause systemic manifestations such as fevers, rash, and eye disorders. Rheumatic disorders of children include juvenile idiopathic arthritis, juvenile spondyloarthropathies, and juvenile dermatomyositis.

Juvenile Idiopathic Arthritis

Juvenile idiopathic arthritis (JIA), formerly known as *juvenile rheumatoid arthritis*, is the most common form of childhood arthritis, and one of the most common forms of chronic disease in children.[70–74] The disorder can be regarded not as a single disease but as a category of disorders, all involving chronic (long-term) joint inflammation, that begins before a child reaches the age of 16 and lasts for 6 weeks to 3 months. It may be present as an oligoarticular disorder (involving less than 5 joints) or as a polyarticular disorder (involving 5 or more joints), and may include other systemic manifestations such as fever, rash, and/or eye inflammation.

The initial symptoms of JIA may be subtle or acute, and often include morning stiffness and gelling; easy fatigability, particularly after school; and joint swelling. The involved joints are often warm, resist full range of motion, and are painful on motion, but not erythematous.[71] *Oligoarthritis*, which is the most common type of JIA, predominantly affects joints of the lower extremities, usually the knees or ankles. Involvement of upper extremity large joints and the hip is rarely a presenting sign. Often a single joint is affected at onset. The severity of joint symptoms is usually mild, and it is not uncommon for children to present with normal or near-normal overall function. Children with this form of JIA are usually younger (1 to 5 years at onset), more likely to be girls (girls outnumber boys by 4 to 1), often rheumatoid factor (RF) positive (discussed under rheumatoid arthritis), and at greater risk for developing chronic eye inflammation.[70] The inflammation primarily involves the anterior chamber of the eye and is associated with minimal, if any, symptoms in about 80% of cases. Because severe eye changes can occur, these children should be screened at regular intervals and treated by an experienced eye specialist.

The *polyarticular* form of the disorder is generally characterized by involvement of both large and small joints. This form of JIA may develop at any age up to 16 years of age, with girls outnumbering boys by 3 to 1.[70] This form of arthritis more closely resembles the adult form of the disease than the other two subgroups. The RF sometimes is present and may indicate a more active disease process. Clinical manifestations are highly variable and include fatigue, low-grade fever, weight loss, malaise, anemia, stunted growth, slight organomegaly (e.g., hepatosplenomegaly), and lymphadenopathy.

Systemic-onset disease, which affects approximately 2% to 17% of children with JIA, is characterized by arthritis and prominent visceral involvement that include hepatosplenomegaly, lymphadenopathy, and inflammation of serous membranes, such as in pericardial effusion.[70] The symptoms of systemic JIA include a daily intermittent high fever, which usually is accompanied by a characteristic faint, erythematous, macular rash. The salmon-colored lesions of the rash may be linear or circular, from 2 to 5 mm in size, and appear in groups with a linear distribution on the trunk and proximal extremities. The rash is not pruritic (it does not cause itching). The most prominent diagnostic feature is its transient nature, with a group of lesions lasting less than an hour. Systemic symptoms usually subside in 6 to 12 months.

The prognosis for most children with JIA is good. NSAIDs are the first-line drugs used in treating JIA. Most children with polyarticular or systemic JIA, however, need additional anti-inflammatory therapy.[74]

Corticosteroids are recommended only for overwhelming inflammation of systemic disease. Disease-modifying antirheumatic drugs (DMARDs), such as methotrexate, may also be used. Careful attention to growth and development and nutritional issues are additional aspects of treatment of children with JIA. Children are encouraged to lead as normal a life as possible.

Juvenile Spondyloarthropathies

Ankylosing spondylitis, reactive arthritis, psoriatic arthritis, and spondyloarthropathies associated with ulcerative colitis and regional enteritis can affect children as well as adults.[75–78] The arthropathies of inflammatory bowel disease and reactive arthritis are much less common in childhood.[75]

In children, spondyloarthropathy manifests in peripheral joints first, mimicking pauciarticular JIA, with no evidence of sacroiliac or spine involvement for months to years after onset. The spondyloarthropathies are more common in boys and commonly occur in children who have a positive family history. HLA-B27 typing is helpful in diagnosing children because of the unusual presentation of the disease. Juvenile ankylosing spondyloarthritis frequently begins with oligoarthritis and enthesitis or inflammation at the site where muscles insert into bone. The arthritis occurs predominantly in the lower extremities and frequently involves the hips.[75] Enthesitis is particularly common, manifesting as local and often severe tenderness over involved tendons and ligaments, especially those around the plantar surface of the foot, ankle, and knee. The disease course is variable and can include periods of low and high disease activity.

Juvenile psoriatic arthritis is composed of two subgroups, differentiated by age of onset. Older children have features of spondyloarthritis, including a relative male preponderance, increased risk of axial involvement, and enthesitis.[76] The mechanisms appear to involve autoinflammatory dysregulation centered at the synovial-entheseal complex. In contrast, children with early-onset disease bear similarities to children with early onset oligoarticular and polyarticular JIA disorders, including a female preponderance and positive RF factor, suggesting a possible role for autoimmune mechanisms. Inflammation of the fingers is seen in both groups, however.

Management of the disease involves physical therapy, education, and attention to growth and developmental issues.[77,78] Medication includes the use of salicylates or other NSAIDs. In children who are not responsive to these medications, sulfasalazine or methotrexate may be considered. Exercises to maintain range of motion of the back, thorax, and affected joints should be instituted early in the disease. Custom-fitted shoes are particularly useful in managing painful entheses of the feet.[75]

Juvenile Dermatomyositis

Juvenile dermatomyositis (JDM) is a rare, presumably autoimmune disorder that causes proximal muscle weakness and a characteristic rash.[79–81] The disorder can affect children of all ages, with an average age at onset of 7 years.[80,81] There is an increased incidence among girls. The cause is unknown, but there is a history of infection in the 3 months before disease onset in most affected children. Symmetric proximal muscle weakness, elevated muscle enzymes, evidence of vasculitis, and electromyographic changes confirming an inflammatory myopathy are diagnostic for JDM. The rash may precede or follow the onset of proximal muscle weakness. Periorbital edema with swelling and purple red discoloration of the upper eyelid is common. An erythematous (red) papulosquamous (containing both papules and scales) rash may also be present on the dorsal surfaces of the finger joints and on the extensor surfaces of the elbows and knees. Ulcerative skin disease is a serious and potentially life-threatening manifestation of JDM.

Calcifications can occur in 30% to 50% of children with JDM and are by far the most debilitating symptom. The calcifications appear at pressure points or sites of previous trauma. Juvenile dermatomyositis is treated primarily with corticosteroids to reduce inflammation. DMARDs, such as methotrexate, may be used as a steroid-sparing agent in cases of refractory disease. All children with JDM should avoid exposure to the sun, use a sunscreen with a sun protection factor (SPF) greater than 36, eat a calcium-sufficient diet, and take vitamin D therapy.[81]

Rheumatic Diseases in the Elderly

Rheumatic disorders are common causes for complaint among elderly persons.[82,83] Pain and severe limitations in function often threaten independence and quality of life. The weakness and gait disturbance that often accompany the rheumatic diseases can increase the risk of falls and fracture, causing suffering, increased health care costs, and further loss of independence.

Arthritic complaints in the elderly are most frequently associated with degenerative forms of arthritis, such as osteoarthritis, but forms of inflammatory arthritis such as rheumatoid and gouty arthritis are also seen. One form of rheumatic disease that has a predilection for the elderly is polymyalgia rheumatica.

Osteoarthritis

Osteoarthritis is by far the most common form of arthritis among the elderly.[82] It may affect any joint but is most common in the spine and small joints of the hand, particularly the distal interphalangeal joints, and knees, hip, ankle, and shoulder. When the upper extremity joints are affected, activities of daily living, such has holding on to an object, putting on a coat, buttoning a shirt, or turning a key may be a problem. When the lower extremities are involved, climbing and descending stairs and getting out of a chair are difficult.

Management of OA in older persons includes both conservative management and surgical correction or joint replacement.[82] Conservative management focuses on rehabilitative and pharmacologic measures. Rehabilitative measures are directed at reducing the load on the affected joint and maintaining joint mobility. Weight reduction significantly reduces the load in persons in whom weight-bearing joints are involved. Although resting painful arthritis joints is helpful in the short term, prolonged inactivity will lead to the more serious problem of immobility. Exercise programs are important to maintain joint motion and strength. Both passive and active exercises should be encouraged. The use of a cane will significantly reduce the loading force in all lower extremities and should be recommended to allow for continuation of a walking program. Attention to environmental hazards to prevent falls is essential. For persons with knee involvement, bracing and orthotics provide a shift in the medial knee compartment and, in so doing, may provide considerable relief of pain and improvement in function. The use of appropriate footwear may also reduce joint forces for persons with arthritic involvement of the lower extremities.

Pharmacologic treatment is accomplished mainly through the use of NSAIDS and analgesics.[82] As the disease progresses, these medications become less effective and other methods such intra-articular hydrocortisone injection may be used. Injection of hyaluronic acid preparations into the knee may be used as an alternative to steroids. Surgical treatment, including joint replacement, may be indicated for severely arthritic joints that are unresponsive to conservative treatment.

Rheumatoid Arthritis

The prevalence of RA increases with advancing age.[83,84] There are two distinct clinical presentations of RA in older persons: RA diagnosed before age 60, and elderly onset RA (EORA), in which the disease is first diagnosed after age 60. There is a slightly less female predominance and acute onset with marked elevations in inflammatory markers than in persons diagnosed at an earlier age. There is also significant morning stiffness, with prominent involvement of the upper extremities, particularly the shoulders. This is in contrast to older persons who have had disease activity for several decades and demonstrate advanced sequelae of the disease and its treatment.

Whether either form of RA has a better prognosis than the other is uncertain. Both forms require special considerations in terms of pharmacologic therapy, and both can have a negative impact on the functional status of the elderly.

Crystal-Induced Arthropathies

The two best-recognized forms of crystal-induced joint disease are caused by the deposition of monosodium urate (gout) and calcium pyrophosphate (pseudogout).[85] Gout typically has its onset in middle-aged adults, whereas pseudogout has an increasing prevalence in older adults and is often associated with unique and atypical features.

Gout. The incidence of clinical gout increases with advancing age, in part because of the increased involvement of joints after years of continued hyperuricemia.

High serum urate levels rarely occur in women before menopause; initial attacks of clinical gout occur around the age of 70 years, or 20 years after menopause. The treatment of gout is often more difficult in the elderly. Although colchicine may be effective in controlling the symptoms of chronic gout, it may cause diarrhea in some patients, limiting its effectiveness in maintenance therapy.

Pseudogout. As part of the tissue aging process, OA develops with associated cartilage degeneration and the shedding of calcium pyrophosphate crystals into the joint cavity. These crystals may produce a low-grade chronic inflammation—the chronic pseudogout syndrome. The accumulation of calcium pyrophosphate and related crystalline deposits in articular cartilage is common in the elderly. There are no medications that can remove the crystals from the joints. Although it may be asymptomatic, presence of the crystals may contribute to more rapid cartilage deterioration. This condition may coexist with severe OA. Calcium pyrophosphate deposition disease may also present with proximal muscle pain mimicking polymyalgia rheumatica.

Polymyalgia Rheumatica

Polymyalgia rheumatica is an inflammatory condition of unknown origin characterized by aching and morning stiffness in the cervical regions and shoulder and pelvic girdle areas.[86–88] Of the forms of arthritis affecting the elderly, it is one of the more difficult to diagnose and one of the most important to identify. Elderly women are especially at risk. Polymyalgia rheumatica is a common syndrome of older persons, rarely occurring before 50 years of age (and usually after age 60). The onset can be abrupt, with the patient going to bed feeling well and awakening with pain and stiffness in the neck, shoulders, and hips.

Diagnosis and Treatment. Diagnosis is based on the pain and stiffness persisting for at least 1 month and an elevated ESR. The diagnosis is confirmed when the symptoms respond dramatically to a small dose of prednisone, a corticosteroid. Biopsies have shown that the muscles are normal, despite the name, but that a nonspecific inflammation affecting the synovial tissue is present. It is possible that a number of patients are erroneously diagnosed as having RA or OA. For patients with an elevated ESR, the diagnosis usually is based on a 3-day trial of prednisone treatment.[87] Patients with polymyalgia rheumatica typically exhibit striking clinical improvement on the second day. Patients with RA also show improvement, although usually days later.

Treatment with NSAIDs provides relief for some patients, but most require continuing therapy with prednisone, with gradual reduction of the dose over the course of 1.5 to 2 years, using the person's symptoms as the primary guide. Patients need close monitoring during the maintenance phase with prednisone therapy. Because their symptoms are relieved, they often quit taking the prednisone and their symptoms recur, or doses are missed and the decreased dosage leads to an increase in symptoms. Unless careful assessment reveals the frequency of missed doses, the physician may be misled into increasing the dosage when it is not needed. Because of the side effects of the corticosteroids, the goal is to use the lowest dose of the drug necessary to control the symptoms. Weaning patients off low-dose prednisone therapy after this length of time can be a difficult and extended process.

Complications. A certain percentage of patients with polymyalgia rheumatica also develop *giant cell arteritis* (i.e., temporal arteritis) with involvement of the ophthalmic arteries.[89] The two conditions are considered to represent different manifestations of the same disease. Giant cell arteritis, a form of systemic vasculitis, is a systemic inflammatory disease of large and medium-sized arteries. The inflammatory response seems to be a T-cell response to an antigen.

Clinical manifestations of giant cell arteritis usually begin insidiously and may exist for some time before being recognized.[89] It is potentially dangerous if missed or mistreated, especially if the temporal artery or other vessels supplying the eye are involved, in which case blindness can ensue quickly without treatment. The condition is responsive to appropriate therapy. For those patients at risk, adherence to the medication program is critical, with preservation of sight being the goal. Because this complication can occur so quickly and is relatively asymptomatic, it is vital that the patient understand the importance of taking the correct dose regularly as prescribed. Initial treatment consists of large doses of prednisone. This dosage is continued for 4 to 6 weeks and then decreased gradually.

Management of Rheumatic Diseases in the Elderly

In addition to diagnosis-specific treatment, the elderly require special considerations.[82] Management techniques that rely on modalities other than drugs are particularly important. These include splints, walking aids, muscle-building exercise, and local heat. Muscle-strengthening and stretching exercises are particularly effective in the elderly person with age-related losses in muscle function and should be instituted early. Rest, the cornerstone of conservative therapy, is hazardous in the elderly, who can rapidly lose muscle strength.

In terms of medications, the NSAIDs may be less well tolerated by the elderly, and their side effects are more likely to be serious. In addition to bleeding from the gastrointestinal tract and renal insufficiency, there may be cognitive dysfunction manifested by forgetfulness, inability to concentrate, sleeplessness, paranoid ideation, and depression.

Joint arthroplasty can also be used for pain relief and increased function. Chronologic age is not a contraindication to surgical treatment of arthritis. In appropriately selected elderly candidates, survival and functional outcome after surgery are equivalent to those in younger age groups. The more sedentary activity level of the elderly makes them even better candidates for joint replacement because they put less stress and demand on the new joint.

SUMMARY CONCEPTS

■ Rheumatic diseases that affect children include juvenile idiopathic arthritis, juvenile dermatomyositis, and juvenile-onset spondyloarthropathies. Although the childhood form of the arthritis may be similar to that seen in the adult, there are manifestations and treatment issues that are unique to the younger population.

■ Arthritis is the most common complaint of the elderly population. There is a difference in the manifestations, diagnosis, and treatment of some of the rheumatic diseases in the elderly compared with those in the younger population. Osteoarthritis is the most common form of arthritis among the elderly. The prevalence of rheumatoid arthritis and gout increases with advancing age. One form of rheumatic disease that has a predilection for the elderly is polymyalgia rheumatica. A certain percentage of persons with polymyalgia rheumatica also develop giant cell arteritis (i.e., temporal arteritis) with involvement of the ophthalmic arteries, a condition that can cause blindness if not recognized and treated.

REVIEW EXERCISES

1. A 60-year-old postmenopausal woman presents with a compression fracture of the vertebrae. She has also noticed increased backache and loss of height over the last few years.

   A. Explain how aging and the lack of estrogen contribute to the development of osteoporosis.
   B. What other factors should be considered when assessing the risk for developing osteoporosis?
   C. What is the best way to measure bone density?
   D. Name the two most important factors in preventing osteoporosis.
   E. What medications might be used to treat this woman's condition?

2. A 30-year-old woman recently diagnosed with rheumatoid arthritis (RA) complains of general fatigue and weight loss along with symmetric joint swelling, stiffness, and pain. The stiffness is more prominent in the morning and subsides during the day. Laboratory measures reveal an elevated rheumatoid factor (RF).

   A. Describe the immunopathogenesis of the joint changes that occur with RA.
   B. How do these changes relate to this woman's symptoms?
   C. What is the significance of her RF test results?
   D. How do her complaints of general fatigue and weight loss relate to the RA disease process?

3. A 65-year-old obese woman with a diagnosis of osteoarthritis (OA) has been having increased pain in her right knee that is made worse with movement and weight bearing and is relieved by rest. Physical examination reveals an enlarged joint with a varus deformity; coarse crepitus is felt over the joint on passive movement.

   A. Compare the pathogenesis and articular structures involved in OA with those of RA.
   B. What is the origin of the enlargement of the affected joint, the varus deformity, and the crepitus that is felt on movement of the affected knee?
   C. Explain the predilection for involvement of the knee in persons such as this woman.
   D. What types of treatment are available for this woman?

4. A 75-year-old woman is seen by a health care provider because of complaints of fever, malaise, and weight loss. She is having trouble combing her hair, putting on a coat, and getting out of a chair because of the stiffness and pain in her shoulders, hip, and lower back. Because of her age and symptoms, the health care provider suspects the woman has polymyalgia rheumatica.

   A. What laboratory test can be used to substantiate the diagnosis?
   B. What other diagnostic strategies are used to confirm the diagnosis?
   C. How is the disease treated?

REFERENCES

1. Seeman E, Delmas PD. Bone quality—the material and structural basis of bone strength and fragility. *N Engl J Med.* 2006;354(21):2250–2261.
2. Khosia S, Melton LJ. Osteopenia. *N Engl J Med.* 2007;356(22):2293–2300.
3. Rosenberg AE. Bones, joints, and soft tissue tumors. In: Kumar V, Abbas AK, Fausto N, et al., eds. *Robbins and Cotran Pathologic Basis of Medicine.* 8th ed. Philadelphia, PA: Elsevier Saunders; 2010:1205–1219, 1235–1246.
4. Garcia RA, Klein MJ, Schiller AL. Bones and Joints. In: Rubin R, Strayer DS, eds. *Rubin's Pathology: Clinicopathologic Foundations of Medicine.* 6th ed. Philadelphia, PA: Wolters Kluwer Health/Lippincott Williams & Wilkins; 2012:1199–1272.
5. Simon LS. Osteoporosis. *Rheum Dis Clin North Am.* 2007;33:140–176.
6. Lewiecki CM. Managing osteoporosis: challenges and strategies. *Cleve Clin J Med.* 2009;26(8):457–466.
7. Kanis JA, for the World Health Organization Scientific Group. *Assessment of osteoporosis at the primary-care level. Technical report.* University of Sheffield, UK: World Health Organization Collaborating Centre for Metabolic Bone Diseases; 2008.
8. Lewiecki EM. Bone density measurement and assessment of fracture risk. *Clin Obstet Gynecol.* 2013;56(4):667–676.
9. International Osteoporosis Foundation. IOF one-minute osteoporosis risk test. Available at: https://www.iofbonehealth.org/sites/default/files/PDFs/2012-IOF_risk_test-english%5BWEB%5D_0.pdf. Accessed September 29, 2013.

10. Lane NE. Epidemiology, etiology, and diagnosis of osteoporosis. *Am J Obstet Gynecol*. 2006;194:S3–S11.

11. Rosen CJ. Postmenopausal osteoporosis. *N Engl J Med*. 2005;353:595–603.

12. Lambert JK, Zaidi M, Mechanick JI. Male osteoporosis: epidemiology and the pathogenesis of aging bones. *Curr Osteoporos Rep*. 2011;11(9):229–236.

13. Gennari L, Bilezikian JP. Osteoporosis in men. *Endocrinol Metab Clin North Am*. 2007;36:399–419.

14. Hudec SM, Camacho PM. Secondary osteoporosis. *Endocr Pract*. 2013;19(1):120–128.

15. Russell LA. Osteoporosis and osteomalacia. *Rheum Dis Clin North Am*. 2010;36:665–680.

16. Maricic M. Update on glucocorticoid-induced osteoporosis. *Rheum Dis Clin North Am*. 2011;37:415–431.

17. Rothman MS, Bessesen TB. HIV infection and osteoporosis: pathophysiology, diagnosis, and treatment options. *Curr Osteoporos Rep*. 2012;10(4):270–277.

18. Shaw NJ. Management of osteoporosis in children. *Eur J Endocrinol*. 2008;159:S33–S39.

19. Beals KA, Meyer NL. Female athlete triad update. *Clin Sports Med*. 2007;26:69–80.

20. Sweet MG, Sweet JM, Jeremiah MP, et al. Diagnosis and treatment of osteoporosis. *Am Fam Physician*. 2009;79(3):193–202.

21. Warriner AH, Saag KG. Osteoporosis diagnosis and medical treatment. *Orthop Clin North Am*. 2013;44(2): 125–135.

22. National Osteoporosis Foundation. *Clinician's Guide to Prevention and Treatment of Osteoporosis*. Washington, DC: National Osteoporosis Foundation; 2008.

23. U.S. Preventive Services Task Force. Screening for osteoporosis. Available at: http://www.uspreventiveservicestaskforce.org/uspstf10/osteoporosis/osteors.htm. Accessed September 29, 2013.

24. Katzung BG, Masters SB, Trevor AJ. *Basic & Clinical Pharmacology*. 12th ed. New York, NY: McGraw-Hill Lange; 2013:782–783.

25. Cauley JA, Robbins J, Chen Z, et al., for the Women's Health Initiative. Effects of estrogen plus progestin on risk of fracture and bone mineral density. *JAMA*. 2003;290:1729–1738.

26. Holick MF. Vitamin D deficiency. *N Engl J Med*. 2007;357(3):266–281.

27. Holick MF, Chen TC. Vitamin D deficiency: a worldwide problem with health consequences. *Am J Clin Nutr*. 2008;87(suppl):1080D–1086D.

28. Berg EE. Rickets. *Orthop Nurs*. 2004;23(1):53–55.

29. Nield LS, Mahajan P, Joshi A, et al. Rickets: not a disease of the past. *Am Fam Physician*. 2006;74:619–630.

30. Mughal MP. Rickets. *Curr Osteoporos Rep*. 2011;9:291–299.

31. Misra M, Pacaud D, Petryk A, et al. Vitamin D deficiency in children and its management: review of current knowledge and recommendations. *Pediatrics*. 2008;122:398–417.

32. Ralston SH. Paget's disease of bone. *N Engl J Med*. 2013;368(7):644–650.

33. Roodman GD, Windle JJ. Paget disease of bone. *J Clin Invest*. 2005;115:200–208.

34. Crowson CS, Matteson EL, Myasoedova E, et al. The lifetime risk of adult-onset rheumatoid arthritis and other inflammatory autoimmune rheumatic diseases. *Arthritis Rheum*. 2011;63(3):633–639.

35. McInnes IB, Schett G. The pathogenesis of rheumatoid arthritis. *N Engl J Med*. 2011;365(23):2205–2219.

36. Pedersen M, Jacobsen S, Garred P, et al. Strong combined gene-environment effects in anti-cyclic citrullinated peptide-positive rheumatoid arthritis: a nationwide case-control study in Denmark. *Arthritis Rheum*. 2007;56(5):1446–1453.

37. Sweeny SE, Harris ED, Firestein GS. Clinical features of rheumatoid arthritis. In: Firestein GS, Budd RC, Gabriel SE, et al., eds. *Kelley's Textbook of Rheumatology*. 9th ed. Philadelphia, PA: Elsevier Saunders; 2012:1108–1136.

38. Wasserman AM. Diagnosis and management of rheumatoid arthritis. *Am Fam Physician*. 2011;84(11):1245–1282.

39. Aletaha D, Neogi T, Silman AJ, et al. 2010 Rheumatoid arthritis classification criteria: an American College of Rheumatology/European League Against Rheumatism collaborative initiative. *Arthritis Rheum*. 2010;62(9):2569.

40. Oliver AM, St. Clair EW. Rheumatoid arthritis: treatment and assessment. In: Klippel JH, Stone JH, Crofford LJ, et al., eds. *Primer on the Rheumatic Diseases*. 13th ed. New York, NY: Springer; 2008:133–141.

41. Singh, JA, Furst DE, Bharat A, et al. 2012 update of the 2008 American College of Rheumatology recommendations for the use of disease-modifying anti-rheumatic drugs and biologic agents in the treatment of rheumatoid arthritis. *Arthritis Care Res*. 2012;64(5):625–639.

42. Pietsky DS. Systemic lupus erythematosus: epidemiology, pathology, and pathogenesis. In: Klippel JR, Stone JH, Crofford LJ, et al., eds. *Primer on the Rheumatic Diseases*. 13th ed. New York, NY: Springer; 2008:303–313.

43. Kumar V, Abbas AK, Fausto N, et al. *Robbins and Cotran Pathologic Basis of Disease*. 8th ed. Philadelphia, PA: Saunders Elsevier; 2010:213–226.

44. Schur P, Hahn B. Epidemiology and pathogenesis of systemic lupus erythematosus. January 2014. Available at: http://www.uptodate.com/contents/epidemiology-and-pathogenesis-of-systemic-lupus-erythematosus#H443498. Accessed February 21, 2014.

45. Dall'era M, Wofsy D. Clinical features of systemic lupus erythematosus. In: Firestein GS, Budd RC, Gabriel SE, et al., eds. *Kelley's Textbook of Rheumatology*. 9th ed. Philadelphia, PA: Elsevier Saunders; 2012:1283–1301.

46. Manzi S, Kao AH. Systemic lupus erythematosus: treatment and assessment. In: Klippel JR, Stone JH, Crofford LJ, et al., eds. *Primer on the Rheumatic Diseases*. 13th ed. New York, NY: Springer; 2008:303–313.

47. Gabrielli A, Avvedimento EV, Krieg T. Scleroderma. *N Engl J Med*. 2009; 360:1989–2008.

48. Boin F, Wigley FM. Clinical features and treatment of scleroderma. In: Firestein GS, Budd RC, Gabriel SE, et al., eds. *Kelley's Textbook of Rheumatology*. 9th ed. Philadelphia, PA: Elsevier Saunders; 2012:1366–1395.

49. Hinchcliff M, Varga J. Systemic sclerosis/scleroderma: a treatable multisystem disease. *Am Fam Physician*. 2008;78(8):961–969.

50. Buch MH, Seibold JR. Systemic sclerosis: treatment and assessment. In: Klippel JR, Stone JH, Crofford LJ, et al., eds. *Primer on the Rheumatic Diseases*. 13th ed. New York, NY: Springer; 2008:359–362.

51. Dougodos M, Baeten D. Spondyloarthritis. *Lancet*. 2011;377:2127–2137.

52. Rosenbaum, JT, Davey, MP. Time for a gut check: evidence for the hypotheses that HLA-B27 predisposes to ankylosing spondylitis by altering the microbiome. *Arthritis Rheum*. 2011;63(11):3195–3198.

53. Elyan M, Khan MA. Diagnosing ankylosing spondylitis. *J Rheumatol Suppl*. 2006;33(78):12–23.

54. Clegg DO. Treatment of ankylosing spondylitis. *J Rheumatol Suppl*. 2006;33(78):24–31.

55. Carter JD, Hudson AP. Reactive arthritis: clinical aspects and medical management. *Rheum Dis Clin North Am*. 2009;35:21–44.

56. Fitzgerald O. Psoriatic arthritis. In: Firestein GS, Budd RC, Gabriel SE, et al., eds. *Kelley's Textbook of Rheumatology*. 9th ed. Philadelphia, PA: Elsevier Saunders; 2012:1232–1249.

57. Gladman DD. Psoriatic arthritis. In: Klippel JR, Stone JH, Crofford LJ, et al., eds. *Primer on the Rheumatic Diseases*. 13th ed. New York, NY: Springer; 2008:170–177.

58. Mease PJ. Current treatment of psoriatic arthritis. *Rheum Dis Clin North Am*. 2003;29:495–511.

59. Loeser RF, Goldring SR, Scanzello CR, et al. Osteoarthritis: a disease of the joint as an organ. *Arthritis Rheum*. 2012;42(6):1697–1707.

60. Sinusas K. Osteoarthritis: diagnosis and treatment. *Am Fam Physician*. 2012;85(1):49–56.

61. Bijlsma JWJ, Berenbaum F, Lafeber FP. Osteoarthritis: an update with relevance for clinical practice. *Lancet*. 2011;377:2115–2126.

62. Hunter DJ, Lo GH. The management of osteoarthritis: an overview and call to appropriate conservative treatment. *Rheum Dis Clin North Am*. 2008;33:689–712.

63. Clegg DO, Reda DJ, Harris CL, et al. Glucosamine, chondroitin sulfate, and the two in combination for painful knee osteoarthritis. *N Engl J Med*. 2006;354:795–808.

64. Lo GH, LaValley M, McAllindon T, et al. Intra-articular hyaluronic acid in treatment of knee osteoarthritis: a meta-analysis. *JAMA*. 2003;290:3115–3121.

65. Burns CM, Wortman RL. Clinical features and treatment of gout. In: Firestein GS, Budd RC, Gabriel SE, et al., eds. *Kelley's Textbook of Rheumatology*. 9th ed. Philadelphia, PA: Elsevier Saunders; 2012:1554–1574.

66. Eggebeen AT. Gout: an update. *Am Fam Physician*. 2007;76:801–812.

67. Neogi T. Gout. *N Engl J Med*. 2011;364(5):443–452.

68. Khanna D, Fitzgerald JD, Khanna PP, et al. 2012 American College of Rheumatology guidelines for management of gout. Part 1: systematic nonpharmacologic and pharmacologic therapeutic approaches to hyperuricemia. *Arthritis Care Res (Hoboken)*. 2012;64(10):1431–1446.

69. Abramson L. Arthritis in children. American College of Rheumatology website. May 2013. Available at: http://www.rheumatology.org/Practice/Clinical/Patients/Diseases_And_Conditions/Arthritis_in_Children/. Accessed September 29, 2013.

70. Wu EY, Van Mater HA, Rabinovich CE. Juvenile idiopathic arthritis. In: Kliegman RM, Stanton BF, Schor NF, et al., eds. *Nelson Textbook of Pediatrics*. 19th ed. Philadelphia, PA: Elsevier Saunders; 2011:829.e1–839.e1.

71. Marzan KAB, Shaham B. Early juvenile idiopathic arthritis. *Rheum Dis Clin North Am*. 2012;38:355–373.

72. Growdie PJ, Tse SML. Juvenile idiopathic arthritis. *Pediatr Clin North Am*. 2012;59:301–327.

73. Kahn P. Juvenile idiopathic arthritis: an update for the clinician. *Bull NYU Hosp Jt Dis*. 2012;70(3):152–166.

74. Harris JG, Kessler EA, Verbsky JW. Update on the treatment of juvenile idiopathic arthritis. *Curr Allergy Asthma Rep*. 2013;13:337–346.

75. Birmingham J, Colbert RA. Ankylosing spondylitis and other spondyloarthritides. In: Kliegman RM, Stanton BF, Schor NF, et al., eds. *Nelson Textbook of Pediatrics*, 19th ed. Philadelphia, PA: Elsevier Saunders; 2011:837.e3–839.e3.

76. Colbert RA. Classification of juvenile spondyloarthritis: enthesitis-related arthritis. *Nat Rev Rheumatol*. 2010;6(8):477–485.

77. Tee SM, Laxer RM. New advances in juvenile spondyloarthritis. *Nat Rev Rheumatol*. 2012;8(5):269–279.

78. Gensler L, Davis JC Jr. Recognition and treatment of juvenile-set spondyloarthritis. *Curr Opin Rheumatol*. 2006;18(5):507–511.

79. Stoll ML, Punaro M. Psoriatic juvenile idiopathic arthritis: a tale of two subgroups. *Curr Opin Rheumatol*. 2011;23(5):437–443.

80. Huber AM. Juvenile dermatomyositis: advances in pathogenesis, evaluation, and treatment. *Paediatr Drugs*. 2009;11(6):361–374.

81. Batthish M, Feldman BM. Juvenile dermatomyositis. *Curr Rheumatol Rep*. 2011;13(3):216–224.

82. Cornell CN, Sculco TP. Orthopedic disorders. In: Duthie DH, Katz PR, Malone MI. *Duthie: Practice of Geriatrics*. 4th ed. Philadelphia, PA: Saunders Elsevier; 2007:521–527.

83. Tutuncu Z, Kavanaugh A. Rheumatic disease in the elderly: rheumatoid arthritis. *Rheum Dis Clin North Am*. 2007;33:57–70.

84. Majithia V, Peel C, Geraci SA. Rheumatoid arthritis in elderly patients. *Geriatrics*. 2009;64(9):22–28.

85. Wise CM. Crystal-induced arthritis in the elderly. *Rheum Dis Clin North Am*. 2007;33:33–55.

86. Kennedy S. Polymalgia rheumatica and giant cell arteritis: an in-depth look at diagnosis and treatment. *J Am Acad Nurse Pract*. 2012;24(6):277–285.

87. Kermani TA, Warrington KJ. Polymyalgia rheumatica. *Lancet*. 2013;383:63–72.

88. Van Hecke O. Polymyalgia rheumatica. *Aust Fam Physician*. 2011;40(5):303–306.

89. Falardeau J. Giant cell arteritis. *Neurol Clin*. 2010;28:581–591.

Porth Essentials Resources

Explore these additional resources to enhance learning for this chapter:

- NCLEX-Style Questions and Other Resources on thePoint, http://thePoint.lww.com/PorthEssentials4e
- Study Guide for Essentials of Pathophysiology
- Adaptive Learning | Powered by PrepU, http://thepoint.lww.com/prepu

C h a p t e r *45*

Structure and Function of the Integumentum

The integumentary system, including the skin and its appendages (sweat and sebaceous glands, hair follicles, and nails), constitutes a complex organ with many cell types. The diversity of these cells and their ability to work together provide many functions needed to cope with the constantly changing external environment.

Structure and Function of the Skin

The skin is one of the largest and most versatile organs in the body. It has a surface area of 1.5 to 2 square meters, weighs approximately 4 kg (9 pounds), and forms the major interface between the internal organs and the external environment. Besides providing a covering for the entire body surface, the skin performs many other functions, including protection against physical injury, sunlight, and microorganisms; prevention of loss of fluids from the internal environment; regulation of body temperature; continual reception of sensations from the environment, such as touch, temperature, and pain; and synthesis of vitamin D through the action of sunlight on the skin.

The properties of the skin, such as the thickness of skin layers, their cell types, the distribution of sweat and sebaceous glands, and the number and size of hair follicles, vary in different parts of the body. Nevertheless, certain properties are common to the skin on all areas of the body. Structurally, the skin consists of two main

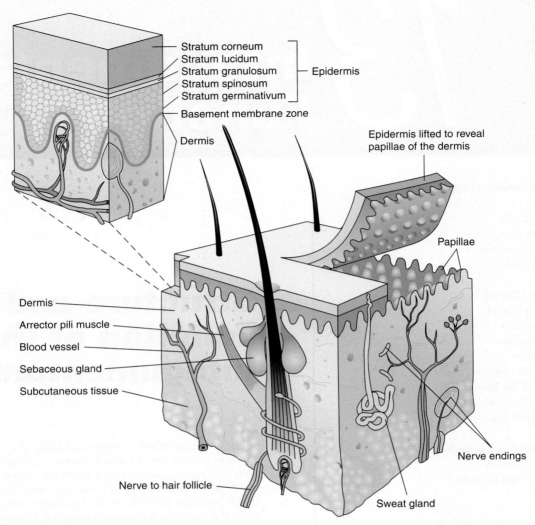

Stratum corneum
Stratum lucidum
Stratum granulosum
Stratum spinosum
Stratum germinativum — Epidermis

Basement membrane zone

Dermis

Epidermis lifted to reveal
papillae of the dermis

Papillae

Dermis

Arrector pili muscle

Blood vessel

Sebaceous gland

Subcutaneous tissue

Nerve endings

Nerve to hair follicle

Sweat gland

FIGURE 45-1. Three-dimensional view of the skin.

layers: a superficial and thinner epithelial tissue layer, called the *epidermis*, and a deeper and thicker connective tissue layer, called the *dermis* (Fig. 45-1). The basement membrane zone is an interface between the dermis and epidermis. A layer of subcutaneous tissue, sometimes called the *hypodermis*, serves as a storage site for fat and contains large blood vessels that supply the skin.

Epidermis

The functions of the skin depend largely on the properties of its epidermis, which is composed of stratified keratinized epithelium containing four types of cells: keratinocytes, melanocytes, Langerhans cells, and Merkel cells.

Keratinocytes

The keratinocytes are the predominant cell type of the epidermis. They produce a fibrous protein called *keratin,* which is essential to the protective function of skin and may be involved in the immune system and wound healing. As they divide and mature, the keratinocytes form five

distinct layers, or *strata*: the stratum germinativum, the stratum spinosum, the stratum granulosum, the stratum lucidum, and the stratum corneum.

The deepest layer, the *stratum germinativum* or *stratum basale,* consists of a single layer of basal cells that are attached to the basal lamina in the basement membrane zone (to be discussed). The basal cells are the only epidermal cells that are mitotically active. All cells of the epidermis arise from this layer. As new cells form in the basal layer, the older cells change shape and are pushed upward toward the skin surface (Fig. 45-2). As these cells approach the skin surface, their cytoplasm becomes converted to keratin and they form flattened plates of dead cells on the skin surface. It normally takes 3 to 4 weeks for the epidermis to replicate itself. The rate of cell division in the stratum germinativum is greatly accelerated when the outer layers of the epidermis are stripped away as occurs in abrasions and burns.

The remaining layers of epidermis are formed as cells from the basal cell layer move upward toward the skin surface. The second layer, the *stratum spinosum,* is two to four layers thick. The cells of this layer are commonly

Keratinized cells

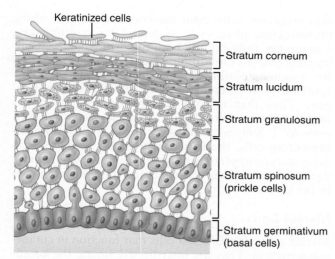

— Stratum corneum

— Stratum lucidum

— Stratum granulosum

— Stratum spinosum (prickle cells)

— Stratum germinativum (basal cells)

FIGURE 45-2. Epidermal cells. The basal cells undergo mitosis, producing keratinocytes that change their size and shape as they move upward, replacing cells that are lost during normal cell shedding.

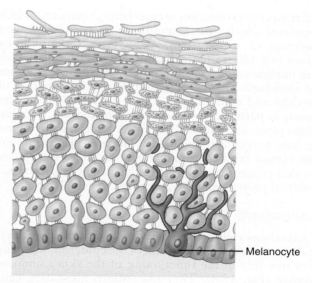

— Melanocyte

FIGURE 45-3. The melanocytes, which are located in the basal layer of the skin, produce melanin pigment granules that give skin its color. The melanocytes have threadlike, cytoplasm-filled extensions that are used in passing the pigment granules to the keratinocytes.

referred to as *prickle cells* because they develop a spiny appearance as their cell borders interact.

The third layer, the *stratum granulosum,* consists of three to five layers of flattened keratinocytes. The nuclei and organelles of these cells begin to degenerate and keratin filaments become more apparent. A distinctive feature of cells in this layer is the appearance of dark staining granules of a protein called *keratohyalin,* which serve as a support for the keratin filaments. The *stratum lucidum,* the fourth layer, which lies just superficial to the stratum granulosum, is a thin, transparent layer mostly confined to the palms of the hands and soles of the feet. It consists of transitional cells that retain some of the functions of living skin cells from the layers below but otherwise resemble the cells of the stratum corneum.

The top or surface layer of the epidermis is the *stratum corneum.* The cells in the stratum corneum are made up of numerous layers of dead keratinized cells. The interiors of the cells contain mostly keratin and keratohyalin. These cells are continuously shed and replaced by cells from the deeper strata. The stratum corneum is the layer that varies most in cell layers and thickness. It ranges from 15 layers of cells in areas such as the face to 25 or more layers on the arm. Specialized areas, such as the palms of the hand and soles of the feet, have 100 layers or more.

Melanocytes

Melanocytes are dendritic cells found scattered among the basal cells in the stratum germinativum. They function to produce pigment granules called *melanin,* the substance that is responsible for skin color, tanning, and protection against ultraviolet radiation.

During embryonic life, melanocyte precursor cells migrate from the neural crest and enter the developing epidermis. A specific functional association is then established in which one melanocyte maintains an association with a given number of keratinocytes. This association is called the *dermal melanin unit.* The ratio of

melanocytes to keratinocytes varies in different parts of the body and is constant in all races.

As dendritic cells, melanocytes are round to columnar cells with long undulating processes that extend between the keratinocytes of the stratum spinosum (Fig. 45-3). Melanocytes synthesize melanin from the amino acid tyrosine in the presence of an enzyme called *tyrosinase* that is activated by ultraviolet light. Synthesis of melanin occurs in membrane-bound structures called *premelanosomes,* which are derived from the Golgi complex. As melanin accumulates in the premelanosomes, they are transformed into mature melanin granules, called *melanosomes.* Premelanosomes are concentrated near the golgi apparatus, and nearly mature and mature melanocytes among the basal cells of stratum germinativum. Melanosomes and their melanin content are transferred to neighboring keratinocytes by pigment donation. This process involves the phagocytosis of the tips of the melanocyte process by keratinocytes. After pigment donation, the melanocyte process elongates and receives more melanosomes, and the process is repeated. Thus, a single melanocyte is able to provide melanin to all of the associated keratinocytes in its epidermal melanin unit.

Skin color is determined by the type, number, and size of the melanosomes transferred into the surrounding keratinocytes. Dark-skinned and light-skinned people have approximately the same number of melanocytes, but the production and packaging of pigment are different. In dark-skinned people, larger melanin-containing melanosomes are produced and transferred individually to the keratinocyte, whereas in light-skinned people, smaller melanosomes are produced and then packaged together in a membrane before being transferred to the keratinocyte.

There are two major forms of melanin: *eumelanin* and *pheomelanin.* Exposure to the sun's ultraviolet rays increases the production of eumelanin, a brownish-black pigment, which causes tanning to occur. The primary function of such melanin is to protect the skin by absorbing and scattering harmful ultraviolet rays, which are implicated in skin cancers. Localized concentrations of eumelanin are also responsible for the formation of freckles and moles. Pheomelanin, a reddish-yellow pigment, is particularly concentrated in the lips, nipples, glans penis, and vagina. Both types of melanin are found in hair, particularly red hair. It has been suggested that the reason fair-haired individuals are more susceptible to skin cancers may be due to the enhanced photoreactivity of pheomelanin, as compared to eumelanin.

Langerhans Cells

Langerhans cells are dendritic cells that reside principally in the stratum spinosum of the epidermis and play a major role in the functioning of the skin's immune system (Fig. 45-4). They are antigen-presenting cells

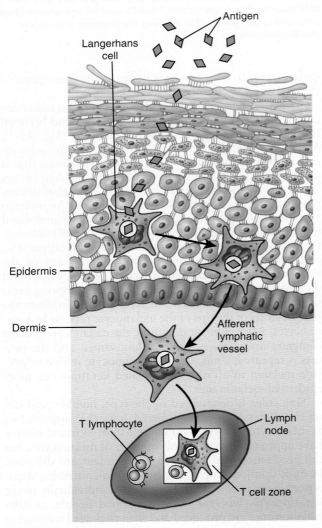

FIGURE 45-4. Langerhans cells, showing a multistep-process that includes capture and processing of the antigen, movement into a lymph node, and presentation of the antigen to a T lymphocyte.

that originate in the bone marrow and are part of the mononuclear phagocytic system. Like macrophages, Langerhans cells express both major histocompatibility class (MHC) I and II molecules as well as receptors for immunoglobulins (see Chapter 15). Their major function is to phagocytose and process foreign antigens. They then migrate into regional lymph nodes in the dermis, where they present the processed antigens to T lymphocytes (see Fig. 45-4). As antigen-presenting cells, the Langerhans cells are involved in delayed-type hypersensitivity reactions such as contact dermatitis and other cell-mediated immune responses in the skin.

Merkel Cells

Merkel cells are epidermal cells that function in cutaneous sensation. They are interspersed among the keratinocytes of the stratum germinativum of the epidermis, usually as single cells, and are particularly abundant in areas of the skin where sensory perception is acute, such as the fingertips. Myelinated sensory neurons traverse the basement membrane to approach the Merkel cell, forming a Merkel cell–neuron complex. These complexes may function as tactile mechanoreceptors. Merkel cells display distinctive, dense granules in their organelles and cytoplasm, suggesting that they possess neurosecretory function. These functions may include metabolic support of their associated neurons, neuron development, and regeneration after injury. These cells are also involved in a form of skin cancer called Merkel cell carcinoma.

Dermis

The dermis is the connective tissue layer that separates the epidermis from the subcutaneous fat layer (see Fig. 45-1). It supports the epidermis and serves as its primary source of nutrition. The main component of the dermis is collagen, a group of fibrous proteins. Collagen represents 70% of dry skin weight and serves as the major stress-resistant material of the skin. The hair follicles and glandular structures are embedded in the dermis and continue through the epidermis.

Based on its tissue structure, the dermis can be divided into a superficial papillary dermis and a deeper reticular dermis. Both layers contain fibroblasts that synthesize the tissue's ground substance and collagen, as well as immune cells, blood vessels, and nerves.

Papillary Dermis

The papillary layer of the dermis is a thin superficial layer that interdigitates directly with the epidermis, but is separated from it by the basement membrane zone. It consists of loosely arranged collagen fibers and ground substance. This layer is densely covered with conical projections called *dermal papillae* (see Fig. 45-1). The basal cells of the epidermis project into the papillary dermis, forming *rete ridges*. It is believed that the dense structure of the dermal papillae serves to maximize the adhesion of the dermis and the epidermis. This layer of the dermis is richly vascularized. It contains capillaries, end arterioles, and venules that nourish the epidermal layers of the skin. Lymph vessels and nerve tissue also are found in this layer.

Reticular Dermis

The reticular layer of the dermis is the thicker area of the dermis and forms the bulk of the dermal layer. This is the tough layer in animal hides from which leather is made. The reticular dermis is characterized by a complex meshwork of dense collagen bundles interconnected with large elastic fibers and ground substance, a viscid gel that is rich in mucopolysaccharides. The collagen fibers are oriented parallel to the body's surface in any given area. Collagen bundles may be organized lengthwise, as on the abdomen, or in round clusters, as on the heel. The direction of surgical incisions is often determined by this organizational pattern.

Immune Cells

Once thought to be composed primarily of fibroblasts, it is now believed that the dermis is mainly composed of dendritic cells called dermal dendrocytes. Believed to be one of the main cell types of the dermis, dermal dendrocytes are spindle-shaped cells that have both phagocytic and antigen-presenting functions and play an important part in the immunobiology of the dermis. In addition, it is possible that dermal dendrocytes may be able to initiate or respond to immunologic events in the epidermis. Dermal dendrocytes also are thought to be involved in processes such as wound healing, blood clotting, and inflammation.

The dermis also contains macrophages, T cells and mast cells. Dermal macrophages and venular epithelial cells may present antigen to T cells in the dermis, most of which are previously activated or memory T cells. T-cell responses to macrophage- or endothelium-associated antigens in the dermis are probably more important in generating an immune response to antigen challenge in previously exposed persons than in initiating a response to a new antigen. The major type of T-cell–mediated immune response in the skin is delayed-type hypersensitivity (see Chapter 16).

Mast cells, which have a prominent role in immunoglobulin E–mediated immediate hypersensitivity, also are present in the dermis. These cells are strategically located at body interfaces such as the skin and mucous membranes and are thought to interact with antigens that come in contact with the skin.

Blood Vessels

The arteries that nourish the skin form two plexuses (i.e., collections of blood vessels), one located between the dermis and the subcutaneous tissue and the other between the papillary and reticular layers of the dermis. The pink color of light skin results primarily from blood in the vessels of this latter plexus. Capillary flow that arises from vessels in this plexus also extends up and nourishes the overlying epidermis by diffusion. Blood leaves the skin through small veins that accompany the subcutaneous arteries. The lymphatic system of the skin, which aids in combating certain skin infections, also is limited to the dermis.

The skin is richly supplied with arteriovenous anastomoses in which blood flows directly between an artery and a vein, bypassing the capillary circulation. These anastomoses are important for temperature regulation. They can open up, letting blood flow through the skin vessels when there is a need to dissipate body heat, and close off, conserving body heat if the environmental temperature is cold.

Innervation

The innervation of the skin is complex. The dermis is well supplied with sensory receptors for temperature, pain, and touch (see Chapter 35), as well as nerves that supply the blood vessels, sweat glands, and arrector pili muscles.

The papillary layer of the dermis is supplied with free nerve endings that serve as nociceptors (i.e., pain receptors) and thermoreceptors. The dermis also contains encapsulated pressure-sensitive receptors that detect pressure and touch. The largest of these are the *pacinian corpuscles,* which are widely distributed in the dermis and subcutaneous tissue in the digits of the hands and breasts. These mechanoreceptors are specialized to perceive pressure, touch, and vibration. *Meissner corpuscles* are encapsulated mechanoreceptors specialized for tactile discrimination. They are concentrated on the fingertips and palms of the hands, where they account for about half of the tactile receptors. They are also located on the eyelids, lips, tongue, nipples, and skin of the foot and forearm. The deep dermis is supplied with small, oval mechanoreceptors called *Ruffini corpuscles.* They are slowly adapting receptors, responding to heavy pressure and joint movement. They are also believed to detect cold. The skin is also supplied by *Krause end bulbs,* nerve endings contained in a cylindrical or oval capsule. They are found most frequently in the oral cavity, conjunctiva, and genitalia. Although their function is uncertain, they are thought to act as mechanoreceptors and heat detectors.

Most of the skin's blood vessels are innervated by the sympathetic nervous system. The sweat glands are innervated by cholinergic fibers but controlled by the sympathetic nervous system. Likewise, the sympathetic nervous system controls the arrector pili (pilomotor) muscles that cause elevation of hairs on the skin (*pilo-* means hair). Contraction of these muscles tends to cause the skin to dimple, producing "goose bumps."

Basement Membrane Zone

The basement membrane zone is a layer of intercellular and extracellular matrices that serves as an interface between the dermis and the epidermis. It separates the epithelium from the underlying connective tissue, anchors the epithelium to the loose connective tissue underneath, and serves as a selective filter for molecules

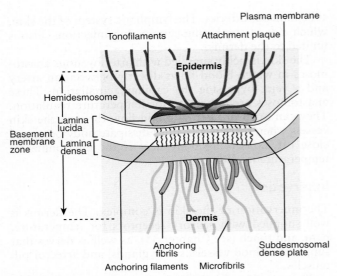

FIGURE 45-5. The dermal–epidermal interface and layers of the basement membrane zone. (Adapted from Storm CA, Elder DE. The skin. In: Rubin R, Strayer DS, eds. *Rubin's Pathology: Clinicopathologic Foundations of Medicine*. 6th ed. Philadelphia, PA: Wolters Kluwer Health | Lippincott Williams & Wilkins; 2012:1116.)

moving between the two layers. It is also a major site of immunoglobulin and complement deposition in skin disease.

Most of the structures of the basal membrane zone are produced by cells of the epidermis. The basal lamina is the zone's primary organizational structure. Its layers include the lamina lucida, lamina densa, and hemidesmosome (Fig. 45-5). The *lamina lucida* consists of fine anchoring filaments and a cell adhesion glycoprotein, called *laminin*, which plays a role in the organization of the macromolecules in the basement membrane zone and promotes attachment of cells to the extracellular matrix. The *lamina densa* contains an adhesive called *type IV collagen* as well as laminin. It is important in dermal–epidermal attachment. The hemidesmosome is similar in structure to half a desmosome, and serves as an attachment site for the dermis and epidermis. Bundles of tonofibrils, epidermal fibers similar to keratin filaments, converge and terminate in the hemidesmosomes. Because they form a continuous link between the intracellular tonofibrils of the epidermis and the extracellular basement membrane, the hemidesmosomes are also thought to be involved in relaying signals between the epidermis and dermis.

The basement membrane zone is often involved in skin disorders that cause bullae or blister formation. One of these disorders, bullous pemphigoid, is a blistering disease caused by antibodies against basement membrane proteins. The blisters of bullous pemphigoid are large and tense and may appear on skin that otherwise looks normal. The thighs and flexor tendons are most commonly affected. The disease is self-limited but chronic, and the person's general health is unaffected.

SUMMARY CONCEPTS

■ The skin is a complex organ that forms the major barrier between the internal and external environments. It consists of two primary layers, the epidermis and the dermis; is richly innervated with pain, temperature, and touch receptors; and plays an essential role in fluid and electrolyte balance.

■ The outer epidermis, which is avascular, is composed of four to five layers of stratified squamous epithelial cells, predominantly keratinocytes. The keratinocytes are formed in the deepest layer of the epidermis and migrate to the skin surface to replace cells that are lost during normal skin shedding.

■ The dermis is a connective tissue layer that separates the epidermis from the underlying subcutaneous fat layer. It contains the blood vessels and nerve fibers that supply the epidermis, as well as sensory receptors for pain, temperature, and touch.

■ The basement membrane zone is a layer of intercellular and extracellular matrices that serves as an interface between the dermis and the epidermis. It not only cements the epidermis to the dermis, but also serves as a selective filter for molecules moving between the two layers.

Appendages of the Skin

Skin appendages are derived from outgrowths of epidermal epithelium during development. They include the eccrine and apocrine sweat glands, sebaceous glands, hair follicles, and nails.

Sweat and Sebaceous Glands

Two types of exocrine glands originate in the dermis and release their products onto the skin surface. These are sweat (or sudoriferous) glands and sebaceous glands (commonly referred to as oil glands).

There are two types of sweat glands: eccrine and apocrine. Eccrine sweat glands are simple tubular structures that originate in the dermis and open directly to the skin surface. They are numerous (several million), vary in density, and are located over the entire body surface. Their purpose is to transport sweat to the outer skin surface to regulate body temperature. Apocrine sweat glands are less numerous than eccrine sweat glands. They are larger and located deep in the dermal layer. They open through a hair follicle, even though a hair may not be present, and are found primarily in the axillae and groin. The major difference between the two types of sweat glands is that the secretion of apocrine glands is oily. In many animals, apocrine secretions give rise to distinctive odors that enable animals to mark their territory and attract a mate. In humans, apocrine secretions are sterile and odorless until mixed with the bacteria on the skin surface; they then produce what is commonly known as "body odor."

The sebaceous glands are located over the entire skin surface except for the palms, soles, and sides of the feet. They are part of what is called the *pilosebaceous unit*, with their ducts opening into the upper third of the hair follicle. They secrete *sebum*, a waxlike mixture of triglycerides, cholesterol, and cellular debris. Sebum lubricates the hair and skin, prevents undue evaporation of moisture from the stratum corneum during cold weather, and helps to conserve body heat.

Sebum production is an example of holocrine secretion. The cytoplasm of the glandular epithelial cell produces and becomes filled with the fatty product. Eventually, the cell's plasma membrane ruptures, and the cell dies. Both the secretory product and the cell fragments, which together constitute sebum, are then discharged from the gland into the hair follicle. New cells are produced by mitosis of the basal cells in the gland.

Sebum production is under the control of genetic and hormonal influences. Sebaceous glands are relatively small and inactive until individuals approach adolescence. The glands then enlarge, stimulated by the rise in sex hormones. Gland size directly influences the amount of sebum produced, and the level of androgens influences gland size. The sebaceous glands are the structures that become inflamed in acne (see Chapter 46).

Hair and Hair Follicles

Hair is a filamentous, keratinized structure that consists of the hair follicle, sebaceous gland, hair muscle (arrector pili), and, in some instances, an apocrine gland (Fig. 45-6). Most hair follicles are associated with sebaceous glands,

and these structures combine to form the pilosebaceous unit. The arrector pili muscle, located under the sebaceous gland, provides a thermoregulatory function by contracting to cause goose bumps, thereby reducing the skin surface area that is available for the dissipation of body heat.

Hair color is attributable to the melanin pigments that the hair contains. Variations mainly reflect the quantity and ratio of the black to dark brown pigment eumelanin and the reddish-brown pigment pheomelanin.

The hair follicle is divided into three parts: the infundibulum, which extends from the surface opening to the level of the opening for the sebaceous gland; the isthmus, which extends from the infundibulum to the level of the arrector pili muscle; and the expanded inferior hair bulb, which is indented to conform to the shape of the dermal papilla occupying it. The dermal papilla contains a rich supply of nutrients and oxygen for the cells in the hair follicle.

Growth of the hair is centered in the bulb (i.e., base) of the hair follicle, and the hair undergoes changes as it is pushed outward. Hair growth goes through three cyclic phases: the anagen (growth), catagen (atrophy), and telogen (resting) phases. Anagen hair has long inner roots and outer root sheaths, is deeply rooted in the dermis, is difficult to detach, and does not come out with regular brushing. *Anagen* follicles are actively replicating and therefore especially susceptible to nutritional deficiencies and metabolic insults. The *catagen* phase represents degeneration of the root structure and migration of dermal papillae and the follicular unit toward the more superficial layers of the dermis. Catagen hair usually represents approximately 1% of all scalp hairs. *Telogen* hair has short, white, club-shaped roots. With formation of new anagen hair below the root, the developing follicle will eventually replace the telogen hair, leading to the shedding of approximately 50 to 100 hairs a day.

Nails

Nails are hardened keratinized plates that protect the fingers and toes and enhance dexterity. The nails grow out from a curved transverse groove called the *nail groove*. The floor of this groove, called the *nail matrix*, is the germinal region of the nail plate (Fig. 45-7). The underlying epidermis, attached to the nail plate, is called the *nail bed*.

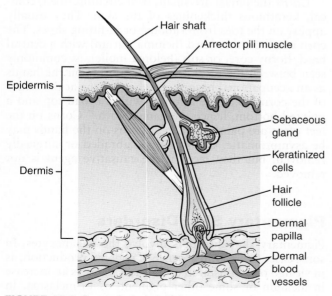

FIGURE 45-6. Parts of a hair follicle.

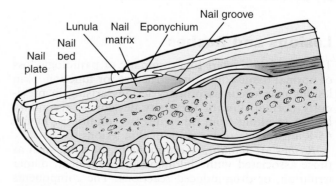

FIGURE 45-7. Parts of a fingernail.

Like hair, nails are the end product of dead cells that are pushed outward from the nail matrix. Unlike hair, nails grow continuously rather than cyclically, unless permanently damaged or diseased. The epithelium of the fold of skin that surrounds the nail consists of the usual layers of skin. The stratum corneum forms the *eponychium* or cuticle. The nearly transparent nail plate provides a useful window for viewing the amount of oxygen in the blood, and providing a view of the color of the blood in the dermal vessels. Changes or abnormalities of the nail can also serve to help diagnose skin or systemic diseases.

SUMMARY CONCEPTS

- Skin appendages, including the sweat glands, sebaceous glands, hair follicles, and nails, are derived from outgrowths of the epidermal epithelium during development.

- The skin glands are exocrine glands. Eccrine sweat glands secrete sweat directly onto the skin surface, whereas the apocrine sweat glands and sebaceous glands release an oily secretion into hair follicles.

- A hair is a keratin filament arising from a hair follicle, whereas a nail is a hardened keratinized plate emerging from a germinal region called the nail matrix.

Manifestations of Skin Disorders

No two skin disorders look exactly alike. Their appearance varies according to the causative agent, location, skin color, and many other factors, and may be further influenced by excessive scratching, secondary infection, or the effects of self-treatment. Nevertheless, most skin disorders have some common characteristics that can be used to describe them. This section of the chapter covers lesions and rashes, pigmentary skin disorders, pruritus, dry skin, and variations in dark skin.

Lesions and Rashes

The term *lesion* refers to a traumatic or pathologic loss of normal tissue continuity, structure, or function. Skin lesions may occur as primary lesions arising in previously normal skin, or they may develop as secondary lesions resulting from other disease conditions. Figure 45-8 illustrates various types of skin lesions.

Rashes are temporary eruptions of the skin, such as those associated with childhood diseases, heat, diaper irritation, or drug-induced reactions. The components of a rash often are referred to as lesions.

Lesions and rashes may range in size from a fraction of a millimeter (e.g., the pinpoint spots of petechiae) to many centimeters (e.g., pressure ulcer). They may be blanched (white), erythematous (reddened), hemorrhagic or purpuric (containing blood), or pigmented (colored). A *macule* is a small (≤ 1.0 cm in diameter) flat spot, such as a freckle; a *papule* is an elevated (≥ 1.0 cm) superficial lesion. *Plaques* are elevated lesions (≥ 1 cm), often formed by the coalescence of papules. *Nodules* are solid marblelike lesions (>0.5 cm) that are deeper and firmer than a papule. A *wheal* is a somewhat irregular, relatively transient area of localized skin edema, such as a mosquito bite. *Lichenification* is a thickened and leathery roughening of the skin with increased visibility of the normal skin furrows and excoriations caused by scratching.

Blisters are circumscribed elevations of the skin caused by fluid under or within the epidermis. *Pustules* are circumscribed pus-filled elevations of the skin. *Vesicles* are small (<1.0 cm in diameter) and *bullae* are large (1.0 cm or larger in diameter) fluid-filled blisters (see Fig. 45-8). Friction blisters most commonly occur on the palmar and plantar surfaces of the hands and feet where the skin is constantly exposed to mechanical trauma, such as from shoes and household tools and appliances.

An *erosion* is a loss of the superficial epidermis, the surface of which is moist but does not bleed. An *ulcer* is a skin defect in which there has been loss of the epidermis and papillary layer of dermis. It may extend into the subcutaneous tissue, and often occurs in pathologically damaged tissue.

A *callus* is a hyperkeratotic plaque of skin that develops because of chronic pressure or friction. It represents hyperplasia of the dead keratinocytes that make up the stratum corneum. Increased cohesion between cells results in hyperkeratosis and decreased skin shedding. A callus may be filed down but is likely to recur if pressure continues in the localized area.

Corns (helomas) are small, well-circumscribed, conical, keratinous thickenings of the skin. They usually appear on the toes from rubbing or ill-fitting shoes. The corn may be either hard (heloma durum) with a central hard, horny core, or soft (heloma molle), as commonly seen between the toes. They may appear on the hands as an occupational hazard. The hard tissue at the center of the corn looks like a funnel with a broad top and a pointed bottom, hence the name "corn." Corns on the feet often are painful, whereas corns on the hands may be asymptomatic. Corns may be abraded or surgically removed, but they recur if the causative agent is not removed.

Pigmentary Skin Disorders

Pigmentary skin disorders involve the melanocytes. In some cases, there is an absence of melanin production, as in vitiligo or albinism. In other cases, there is an increase in melanin or some other pigment, as in melasma. In either case, the emotional impact can be devastating.

Circumscribed, flat, nonpalpable changes in skin color	**Palpable elevated solid masses**	**Circumscribed superficial elevations of the skin formed by a fluid-filled cavity within the skin layers**
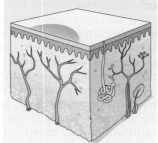	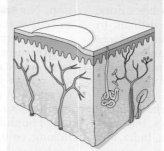	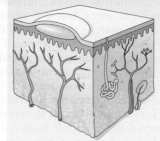
Macule—Small, flat spot, up to 1.0 cm Examples: freckle, petechia **Patch**—Larger than 1.0 cm Example: vitiligo	**Papule**—Up to 1.0 cm Example: an elevated nevis **Plaque**—Elevated superficial lesion 1.0 cm or larger, often formed by coalescence of papules **Nodule**—Marble-like lesion larger than 0.5 cm, often deeper and firmer than papule **Wheal**—A somewhat irregular, relatively transient, superficial area of skin edema Examples: mosquito bite, hive	**Vesicle**—Up to 1.0 cm; filled with serous fluid Example: herpes simplex **Bulla**—1.0 cm or larger; filled with serous fluid Example: 2nd degree burns **Pustule**—Filled with pus Examples: acne, impetigo

FIGURE 45-8. Primary lesions may arise in previously normal skin. Authorities vary somewhat on their definition of skin lesions by size. (Adapted from Bickley LS, Szilagyi PC. *Bates' Guide to Physical Assessment and History Taking.* 8th ed. Philadelphia, PA: Lippincott Williams & Wilkins; 2003:103.)

Albinism, a genetic disorder in which there is complete or partial congenital absence of pigment in the skin, hair, and eyes, is found in all races. Although there are over 10 different types of albinism, the most common type is recessively inherited oculocutaneous albinism, in which there is a normal number of melanocytes but they lack tyrosinase, the enzyme needed for synthesis of melanin. It affects the skin, hair, and eyes. Individuals have pale or pink skin, white or yellow hair, and light-colored or sometimes pink eyes. Persons with albinism have ocular problems, such as extreme sensitivity to light and refractive problems. Treatment efforts for people with albinism are aimed at reducing their risk for skin cancer through protection from solar radiation and screening for malignant changes. Efforts to manage the vision impairment, such as glasses, preferential seating in classrooms, and large-print books, are important.

Vitiligo is a pigmentary problem of concern to darkly pigmented persons of all races. It may be an autoimmune disease, a genetic defect, an excessive reactive oxygen species, a calcium imbalance, or any combination of these; all are being studied. Vitiligo also affects fair-skinned persons, but not as often, and the effects usually are not as socially problematic. The classic sign of vitiligo is the sudden appearance of white patches on the skin. The lesion is a depigmented macule with definite smooth borders on the face, axillae, neck, or extremities (Fig. 45-9). The patches vary in size from small macules to ones involving large skin surfaces. The large macular type is more common. Depigmented areas appear white, pale colored, or sometimes grayish-blue. Histologically, the depigmented areas may contain no melanocytes, greatly altered or decreased numbers of

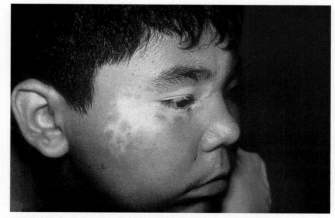

FIGURE 45-9. Vitiligo with various shades of hypopigmentation, depigmentation, and islands of spontaneous repigmentation. (From Goodheart HP. *Goodheart's Photoguide to Common Skin Disorders.* 3rd ed. Philadelphia, PA: Wolters Kluwer Health | Lippincott Williams & Wilkins; 2008:275.)

melanocytes, or, in some cases, melanocytes that no longer produce melanin. Although there are many treatment regimens for vitiligo, none is curative. Self-tanning lotions, skin stains, and cosmetics are used for camouflage. Micropigmentation (tattooing) has been done on smaller, recalcitrant areas, but it is often difficult to attain a correct color match. If extensive skin surfaces are involved, the treatment may be reversed and the pigmented areas bleached to match the remainder of the skin color. A melanocytotoxic agent is used to remove remaining melanocytes from skin areas.

Melasma is a disorder characterized by darkened macules on the face. It is common in all skin types, but most prominent in brown-skinned people from Asia, India, and South America. It occurs in men but is more common in women, particularly during pregnancy or while using oral contraceptives. It may or may not resolve after giving birth or discontinuing hormonal birth control. Melasma is exacerbated by sun exposure. Treatment measures are palliative, mostly consisting of limiting exposure to the sun and using sunscreens. Bleaching agents containing 2% to 4% hydroquinone are standard treatments.

Pruritus

Pruritus is an unpleasant sensation of itch leading to the desire to scratch. Symptoms of pruritus range from mild to so severe that it interrupts sleep and the general quality of life. While pruritus most commonly occurs in skin disorders, it may also occur with systemic disorders, such as chronic kidney disease, diabetes, and biliary disease. Pruritus is multidimensional and has been classified into four types: (a) pruritoceptive (generated in the skin: bug bites), (b) neurogenic (generated in the central nervous system: cholestasis), (c) neuropathic (due to lesions in the central nervous system blocking normal responses), and (d) psychogenic (emotional or stress related).

Pruritus originates within the skin's free nerve endings, is carried by small myelinated type C nerve fibers to the dorsal horn of the spinal cord, and is then transmitted to the somatosensory cortex through the spinothalamic tract (see Chapter 35). Many chemicals have been found to produce the itch sensation, including histamine, serotonin, and cytokines. Substances such as bradykinin and bile salts act locally to stimulate the itch sensation. Prostaglandins are modulators of the itch response, lowering the threshold for other mediators. Opioids produce pruritus in a number of patients who receive them while narcotic antagonists have been used successfully to relieve pruritus. Regardless of cause, pruritus is often exacerbated by skin inflammation, dry or hot ambient temperatures, skin vasodilation, and psychological stressors.

Scratching, the well-known response to itch, is a spinal reflex response that to varying degrees can be controlled by the individual. While providing momentary relief, scratching increases inflammation and stimulates nerve endings, leading to more itching and scratching. Repeated scratching also causes undesirable changes in the skin such as lichenification. Successful treatment of pruritus requires interruption of this cycle.

The focus of treatment measures for pruritus can be grouped into two categories: specific and nonspecific. Specific treatment involves finding and correcting the underlying disorder, thereby eliminating the itch sensation. Nonspecific measures involve the use of measures to relieve the itch sensation and prevent complications that arise from intense and persistent scratching.

Measures such as using the entire hand to rub over large areas and keeping the fingernails trimmed often can relieve itch and prevent skin damage. Self-limited or seasonal cases of pruritus may respond to treatment measures such as moisturizing lotions, bath oils, and the use of humidifiers. Because vasodilation tends to increase itching, cold applications may provide relief. Cool showers before bed, light sleepwear, and cool home temperatures also may be helpful. Also helpful can be cooling over-the-counter anti-itch agents containing menthol, camphor, or phenol. These substances stimulate nerve fibers that transmit the sensation of cold, thereby masking the itch sensation. Mild cutaneous disorders, such as bug bites, are mediated by histamine; therefore, topical antihistamines tend to be the treatment of choice. Topical corticosteroids are effective as antipruritics, particularly when used for urticaria (hives) or insect bites.

However, because most cases of pruritus are not histamine related, their management should be directed at the underlying cause. For example, systemic antihistamines and corticosteroids may be indicated for persons with severe pruritus or atopic dermatitis. Topical capsaicin cream and topical aspirin have been used for localized chronic pruritic disorders. Other modalities that have been used for pruritus with varying degrees of success are phototherapy, acupuncture, antidepressant medications, behavior modification, and alternative therapies (herbal, nutritional, and reflex therapies). In persons with pruritus due to a systemic cause, itching gradually recedes as the primary condition improves.

Dry Skin

Dry skin, also called *xerosis,* may be a natural occurrence, as in the drying of skin associated with aging, or it may be symptomatic of an underlying systemic disease or skin disorder such as contact dermatitis. Most cases of dry skin are caused by dehydration of the stratum corneum. The effects of aging on skin dryness include a change in the composition of sebaceous gland secretions and a decrease in the secretion of moisture from the sweat glands. Aging is also accompanied by a decrease in skin capillaries as well as a flattening of the dermal rete ridges, resulting in less surface area for exchange of fluids between the dermis, epidermis, and skin surface.

Dry skin appears rough and scaly; there may be increased wrinkles or lines. Persons with dry skin often experience severe pruritus, most commonly of the extremities, back, abdomen, or waist. They may resort to scratching, resulting in cracking, fissuring, and a number of other skin maladies.

Moisturizing agents are the cornerstone of treatment for dry skin. These agents exert their effects by repairing the skin barrier, increasing the water content of the skin, reducing transepidermal water loss, and restoring the lipid barrier's ability to attract, hold, and redistribute water. Moisturizing agents can be classified as emollients, humectants, and occlusives. *Emollients* are fatty acid–containing lotions that replenish the oils on the skin surface, but usually do not leave a residue on the skin. They have a short duration of action and need to be applied frequently. *Humectants* are the additives in lotions, such as α-hydroxy acids and urea, that draw out water from the deeper skin layers and hold it on the skin surface. However, the water that is drawn to the skin is transepidermal water, not atmospheric water; thus, continued evaporation from the skin can actually exacerbate dryness. α-Hydroxy acids are derived from fruits, hence the abundance of fruit additives in over-the-counter shampoos and lotions. Urea is a nitrogenous substance that has been quite effective in reducing xerosis when combined with lotions. It is a humectant at lower concentrations (10%), but in higher concentrations (20% to 30%) it is mildly keratolytic. Clinical trials of urea have indicated its utility compared with ammonium lactate (lactic acid) lotion and glycerin. *Occlusives* are thick creams that contain petroleum or some other moisture-proof material. They prevent water loss from the skin. They are the most effective agents for relieving skin dryness, but because of their greasiness and lack of cosmetic appeal, some people do not wish to use them.

Lotion or cream additives include corticosteroids or mild anesthetics, such as camphor, menthol, lidocaine, or benzocaine. These agents work by suppressing itching while moisturizing the skin. Using room humidifiers and keeping room temperatures as low as possible to prevent water loss from the skin also may be helpful. Soaps with moisturizers may be helpful. Glycerine soaps, although popular and visually appealing, are drying and can exacerbate the symptoms.

Variations in Dark-Skinned People

Some skin disorders common to people of African, Hispanic, or East Indian descent are not commonly found in those of European descent. Other skin disorders, such as skin cancers, affect light-skinned persons more commonly than dark-skinned persons. Because of these differences, serious skin disorders may be overlooked, and normal variations in darker skin may be mistaken for anomalies.

As noted earlier, skin color is determined by the melanin produced by the melanocytes. Although the number of melanosomes in dark and white skin is the same, black skin produces more melanin, and more quickly, than white skin. Because of their skin color, dark-skinned persons are better protected against skin cancer, premature wrinkling, and aging of the skin that occurs with sun exposure.

A condition common in people with dark skin is too much or too little color. Areas of the skin may darken after injury, such as a cut or scrape, or after disease conditions such as acne. These darkened areas may take many months or years to fade. Dry or "ashy" skin is also a common problem for people with dark skin. It often

TABLE 45-1	Common Normal Variations in Dark Skin
Variation	**Appearance**
Futcher (Voigt) line	Demarcation between darkly pigmented and lightly pigmented skin in upper arm; follows spinal nerve distribution; common in black and Japanese populations
Midline hypo-pigmentation	Line or band of hypopigmentation over the sternum, dark or faint, lessens with age; common in Latin American and black populations
Nail pigmentation	Linear dark bands down nails or diffuse nail pigmentation; brown, blue, or blue-black
Oral pigmentation	Blue to blue-gray pigmentation of oral mucosa; gingivae also affected
Palmar changes	Hyperpigmented creases, small hyperkeratotic papules, and tiny pits in creases
Plantar changes	Hyperpigmented macules; can be multiple with patchy distribution, irregular borders, and variance in color

Developed from information in Rosen T, Martin S. *Atlas of Black Dermatology.* Boston, MA: Little, Brown; 1981.

is uncomfortable, and it also is easily noticed because it gives the skin an ashen or grayish appearance. Although using a moisturizer may help relieve the discomfort, it may cause a worsening of acne in predisposed persons.

Normal variations in skin structure and skin tones often make evaluation of dark skin difficult. The darker pigmentation can make skin pallor, cyanosis, and erythema more difficult to observe. Therefore, verbal histories must be relied on to assess skin changes. The verbal history should include the client's description of her or his normal skin tones. Changes in skin color, in particular hypopigmentation and hyperpigmentation, often accompany disorders of dark skin and are very important signs to observe when diagnosing skin conditions. Common variations in dark skin and nails are described in Table 45-1.

SUMMARY CONCEPTS

■ Skin lesions are a loss of skin integrity and rashes are temporary skin eruptions. They are the most common manifestations of both skin and many systemic diseases. They vary in size and color; they can be flat (macule or patch), palpable (papule, plaque, or nodule), or fluid-filled elevations (vesicle or bullae).

■ Erosions involve a loss of the superficial epidermis, and an ulcer a loss of the epidermis and papillary layer of dermis.

(continued)

SUMMARY CONCEPTS *(continued)*

- Pigmentary skin disorders involve the melanocytes. In some cases, there is an absence of melanin production, as in vitiligo or albinism. In other cases, there is an increase in melanin or some other pigment, as in melasma.

- Pruritus, an unpleasant sensation of itch leading to the desire to scratch, may occur with both skin and systemic disorders.

- Dry skin, also called *xerosis,* may be a natural occurrence, as in the drying of skin associated with aging, or occur as a result of a skin or systemic disorder.

- Normal variations in skin structure and skin tones often make evaluation of dark skin difficult.

REVIEW EXERCISES

1. Bullous pemphigoid is an autoimmune blistering disease caused by autoantibodies to constituents of the dermal–epidermal junction.

   A. Explain how antibodies, which attack glycoproteins in the lamina lucida and their attachment to the hemidesmosomes, can cause blisters to form (hint: see Fig. 45-5).

2. "Allergy tests" involve the application of an antigen to the skin, either through a small scratch or intradermal injection.

   A. Explain how the body's immune system is able to detect and react to these antigens.

BIBLIOGRAPHY

Ali SM, Yosipovitch G. Skin pH: from basic science to basic skin care. *Acta Derm Venereol.* 2013;93:261–267.

Boissy RE, Spritz RA. Frontiers and controversies I. The pathobiology of vitiligo: separating the wheat from the chaff. *Exp Dermatol.* 2009;18:583–585.

Boulais N, Misery L. The epidermis: a sensory tissue. *Eur J Dermatol.* 2008;18(2):119–127.

Buddenkotte J, Steinhoff M. Pathophysiology and therapy of pruritus in allergic and atopic diseases. *Allergy.* 2010;65:805–821.

Colella G, Vicidomini A, Soro V, et al. Molecular insights into the effects of sodium hyaluronate preparations in keratinocytes. *Clin Exp Dermatol.* 2011;37:516–520.

Curtis BJ, Radek KA. Cholinergic regulation of keratinocyte innate immunity and permeability barrier integrity: new perspectives in epidermal immunity and disease. *J Invest Dermatol.* 2012;132:28–42.

Greaves MW. Pathogenesis and treatment of pruritus. *Curr Allergy Asthma Rep.* 2010;10:236–242.

Ilkovitch D. Role of immune-regulatory cells in skin pathology. *J Leukoc Biol.* 2011;89:41–49.

Kazmi P, Draelos ZD, Volz ED. Method of detection of ashen skin. *European Patent No. EP 2371349.* Munich, Germany: European Patent Office; 2012.

Kirkup MEM. Xerosis and stasis dermatitis. In: Norman R, ed. *Preventive Dermatology.* London, UK: Springer; 2010:71–79.

Lo KK. How to tackle my dry skin problem? *Hong Kong J Dermatol Venereol.* 2011;19:183–185.

Misery L, Stander S, eds. *Pruritus.* London, UK: Springer; 2010.

Nazarko L. Understanding and treating a common dermal problem: pruritus. *Br J Community Nurs.* 2008;13:302–308.

Schwanke J. Basic training: encourage proper skin care regimens before exploring alternatives. *Dermatol Times.* 2011:42–45.

Spritz RA. The genetics of vitiligo. *J Invest Dermatol.* 2011;17:E18–E20.

Storm CA, Elder DE. The skin. In: Rubin R, Strayer DS, eds. *Rubin's Pathology: Clinicopathologic Foundations of Medicine.* 5th ed. Philadelphia, PA: Lippincott Williams & Wilkins; 2008:999–1006.

Taïeb A, Picardo M. Vitiligo. *N Engl J Med.* 2009;360(2):160–169.

Vlahova L, Doerflinger Y, Houben R, et al. *Br J Dermatol.* 2012;166:1043–1052.

Zachariae R, Lei U, Haedersdal M, et al. Itch severity and quality of life in patients with pruritus: preliminary validity of a Danish adaptation of the itch severity scale. *Acta Derm Venereol.* 2012;29:508–514.

Porth Essentials Resources

Explore these additional resources to enhance learning for this chapter:

- NCLEX-Style Questions and Other Resources on thePoint, http://thePoint.lww.com/PorthEssentials4e
- Study Guide for Essentials of Pathophysiology
- Adaptive Learning | Powered by PrepU, http://thepoint.lww.com/prepu

Disorders of Skin Integrity and Function

The skin serves as the interface between the body's internal organs and the external environment. Therefore, skin disorders reflect a combination of environmental and internal factors. Sunlight, infectious organisms, chemicals, and physical agents all play a role in the pathogenesis of skin diseases. Although most of the disorders in this chapter are intrinsic to the skin and its integuments, the hair and nails, these structures also provide observable signs of many systemic disorders.

Primary Disorders of the Skin

A dermatosis is any skin condition involving acute or chronic lesions or eruptions. Primary dermatoses are those originating in the skin. They include infectious processes, acne, rosacea, papulosquamous dermatoses, allergic disorders, and drug reactions. Although most of these disorders are not life-threatening, they can affect the quality of life.

Infectious Processes

Normally, the skin flora, sebum, immune responses, and other protective mechanisms defend against serious systemic infections. However, the skin frequently succumbs to attack by microorganisms, including fungi, bacteria, and viruses.

Superficial Fungal Infections

Fungi are free-living, saprophytic, plantlike organisms, certain strains of which are considered part of the normal skin flora (see Chapter 14). There are two types of fungi: yeasts and molds. Yeasts, such as *Candida albicans*, grow as single cells and reproduce asexually. Molds grow in long filaments called hyphae. Fungal infections of the skin or mycoses are commonly classified as deep or superficial.[1-3] Deep fungal infections of the skin primarily involve the dermis and subcutaneous tissue, and may extend into deeper tissues. In contrast, superficial fungal infections, commonly known as tinea or ringworm, are confined to the epidermis and its integuments, the hair and nails.

Most of the superficial mycoses are *dermatophytoses*—dermatoses caused by the dermatophytes, a group of closely related fungi classified into three genera: *Microsporum, Epidermophyton,* and *Trichophyton.*[2,4] Some dermatophytes are anthropophilic; that is, they are parasitic in humans and are spread by other infected humans. These tend to cause chronic infections that are difficult to treat. *Zoophilic* species cause parasitic infections in animals, some of which can be spread to humans. *Geophilic* species originate in the soil, but may infect animals, which in turn serves as a source of infection for humans. These species tend to cause inflammatory lesions that respond well to therapy or may even resolve spontaneously.[2,4]

The fungi that cause superficial mycoses emit an enzyme that enables them to digest keratin, which results in superficial skin scaling, nail disintegration, or hair breakage, depending on the location of the infection. Deeper reactions involving vesicles, erythema, and infiltration are caused by the inflammation that results from exotoxins liberated by the fungus.

Diagnosis of superficial fungal infections is primarily done by microscopic examination of skin scrapings for fungal spores, the reproducing bodies of fungi.[2] Potassium hydroxide (KOH) preparations are used to prepare slides of skin scrapings. Potassium hydroxide disintegrates human tissue and leaves behind the thread-like filaments, or hyphae, that grow from the fungal spores. Cultures also may be done using a dermatophyte test medium or a microculture slide that allows for direct microscopic identification. The Wood light is an ultraviolet (UV) light that can assist with the diagnosis of tinea, as some types of fungi fluoresce yellow-green when the light is directed onto the affected area.

Topical agents are commonly used in the treatment of tinea infections; however, success often is limited because of the lengthy duration of treatment, poor compliance, and high rates of relapse at specific body sites. The principal agents are the azoles (ketoconazole, miconazole, clotrimazole, etc.) and the allylamines (naftifine and terbinafine). Both act by inhibiting the synthesis of ergosterol, which is an essential part of fungal cell membranes.[2,3] Topical corticosteroids may be used in conjunction with topical antifungal agents to relieve itching and erythema secondary to inflammation.

The systemic (i.e., oral) antifungal agents include griseofulvin, the azoles, and the allylamines.[2,3] Griseofulvin is an antifungal agent derived from a species of penicillium, whose only use is in the systemic treatment of dermatophytosis. It acts by binding to the keratin of newly formed skin, protecting the skin from new infection. It must be administered for 2 to 6 weeks to allow for skin and hair replacement, and nail infections often require months of treatment. Systemic azoles and allylamines are also used. In contrast to griseofulvin, the synthetic agents are fungicidal (i.e., kill the fungus) and therefore are more effective over shorter treatment periods. Some of the oral agents can produce serious side effects, such as hepatic toxicity, or interact adversely with other medications.

Tinea of the Body or Face.
Tinea corporis (ringworm of the body) can be caused by any of the dermatophyte species. Although it affects all ages, children seem most prone to infection. Transmission is most commonly from kittens, puppies, and other children who have infections. The most common types of lesions are oval or circular patches on exposed skin surfaces and the trunk, back, or buttocks (Fig. 46-1). Less common are foot and groin infections. The lesion begins as a red papule and enlarges, often with a central clearing. Patches have raised red borders consisting of vesicles, papules, or pustules. The borders are sharply defined, but lesions may coalesce. Pruritus, a mild burning sensation, and erythema frequently accompany the skin lesion.

Tinea faciale, or ringworm of the face, is typically caused by one of the *Trichophyton* species. Tinea faciale may mimic the annular, erythematous, scaling, pruritic lesions characteristic of tinea corporis. It also may appear as flat erythematous patches.

Topical antifungal agents usually are effective in treating tinea corporis and tinea faciale. Oral antifungal agents may be used in resistant cases.

Tinea of the Scalp.
Tinea capitis, the most common type of fungal infection in children, is an infection of the scalp and hairshaft. Children between the ages of 3 and 14 years are primarily affected. The primary lesions vary from grayish, round, hairless patches to balding spots. The lesions vary in size and are most commonly seen on the back of the head (Fig. 46-2). Mild erythema, crust, or scale may be present. The individual usually is asymptomatic, although pruritus may exist. Treatment is with oral griseofulvin or synthetic antifungal agents that penetrate the hair shafts.[5-7] Topical ointments or shampoos are sometimes indicated.

The inflammatory type of tinea capitis is caused by virulent strains of *T. mentagrophytes, T. verrucosum,* and *M. gypseum.* The onset is rapid, and inflamed lesions usually are localized to one area of the head. The inflammation is believed to be a delayed hypersensitivity reaction to the invading fungus. The initial lesion consists

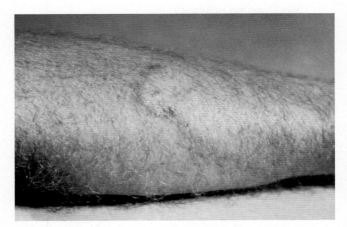

FIGURE 46-1. Tinea of the arm due to the dermatophytic fungus trichophyton rubrum. (From the Centers for Disease Control and Prevention Public Health Image Library. No. 4811.)

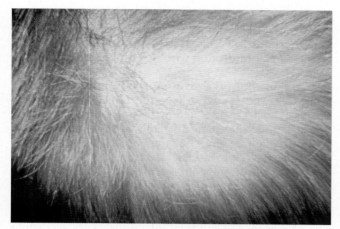

FIGURE 46-2. Ringworm or tinea of the scalp (tinea capitis) caused by the *Microsporum* species. (From the Centers for Disease Control and Prevention Public Health Image Library. No. 2940. Courtesy of Dr. Lucille K. Georg.)

of a pustular, scaly, round patch with broken hairs. A secondary bacterial infection is common and may lead to a painful, circumscribed, boggy, and indurated lesion called a *kerion*. The highest incidence is among children and farmers who work with infected animals.

Both the noninflammatory and inflammatory forms of tinea capitis are treated with oral griseofulvin or synthetic antifungal agents that penetrate the hair shafts.[5–7] Topical ointments or shampoos are sometimes indicated in addition to oral medications, both to decrease the spore population and to protect household members. Because of the lower fatty acid content in the sebum of young children, several of the topical antifungal agents are prepared with fatty acid bases. Wet packs, medicated shampoos, steroids, and antibiotics may be prescribed for secondary infections that occur.

Tinea of the Foot and Hand. Tinea pedis (athlete's foot) is the most common fungal dermatosis, primarily affecting the spaces between the toes, the soles, or the sides of the feet (Fig. 46-3). The lesions vary from a mildly scaling lesion to a painful, exudative, erosive, inflamed lesion with fissuring. Lesions often are accompanied by pruritus, pain, and foul odor. Mild forms are more common during dry environmental conditions. Exacerbations occur as a result of hot weather, sweating, and exercise or when the feet are exposed to moisture, occlusive shoes, and communal swimming.

Tinea of the hand (*Tinea manus*) is usually a secondary infection with tinea pedis as the primary infection. In contrast to other skin disorders, it usually occurs only on one hand. The characteristic lesion is a blister on the palm or finger surrounded by erythema. Chronic lesions are scaly and dry. Cracking and fissuring may occur. The lesions may spread to the plantar surfaces of the hand. If chronic, tinea manus may lead to tinea of the fingernails.

Simple forms of tinea pedis and tinea manus are treated with topical applications of antifungals. Complex cases are treated with oral antifungals. Other treatment and preventive measures include careful cleaning and drying of affected areas.

Tinea of the Nails. *Tinea unguium* is a dermatophyte infection of the nails. It is a subset of a condition called *onychomycosis*, which includes dermatophyte, nondermatophyte, and candidal infections of the nails.

The infection often begins at the tip of the nail, where the fungus digests the nail keratin (Fig. 46-4). In some cases, it may be caused by a crushing injury to a toenail or the spread of tinea pedis. Initially, the nail appears opaque, white, or silver. The nail then turns yellow or brown. The condition often remains unchanged for years. During this time it may involve only one or two nails and may produce little or no discomfort. As the infection spreads, the nail thickens and cracks and the nail plate separates from the nail bed.

The standard for the diagnosis of fungal nail disease is a positive result on microscopic examination and culture of nail clippings with subungual debris. Persons with minimal toenail involvement and no associated symptoms may not require treatment.

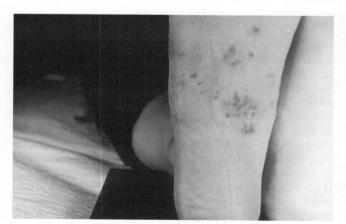

FIGURE 46-3. Chronic tinea of the sole caused by *Trichophyton rubrum*. (From the Centers for Disease Control and Prevention Public Health Image Library. No. 15441.)

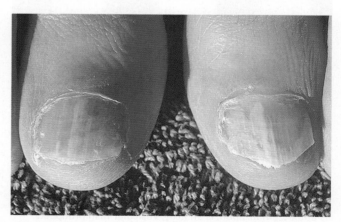

FIGURE 46-4. Onychomycosis due to *Trichophyton rubrum*, right and left great toes. (From the Centers for Disease Control and Prevention Public Health Image Library. No. 579. Courtesy of Edwin P. Ewing, Jr.)

Treatment of more severe cases usually requires oral antifungal therapy, such as terbenafine, administered for several months.[8] All of the oral agents require careful monitoring for side effects. A nail lacquer containing the antifungal agent ciclopirox is available for use in the topical management of mild to moderate infections of the fingernails and toenails caused by *T. rubrum*. A new nail may require 3 to 12 months to grow. Thus, people being treated with antifungal agents need to be reminded that the resolution of the infection requires 4 to 6 months for fingernails and longer for toenails.

Dermatophytid Reaction. A secondary skin eruption may occur in persons allergic to the fungus responsible for the dermatophytosis. This dermatophytid or allergic reaction may occur during an acute episode of a fungal infection. The most common reaction occurs on the hands in response to tinea pedis. The lesions are vesicles with erythema extending over the palms and fingers, sometimes extending to other areas (Fig. 46-5). Less commonly, papules or vesicles erupt on the trunk or extremities. These eruptions may resemble tinea corporis. Lesions may become excoriated and infected with bacteria. Treatment is directed at the primary site of infection. The intradermal reaction resolves in most cases without intervention if the primary site is cleared.

Candidal Infections. Candidiasis (moniliasis) is a fungal infection caused by *C. albicans*. This yeastlike fungus is a normal inhabitant of the gastrointestinal tract, mouth, and vagina (see Chapter 41). The skin problems result from the release of irritating toxins on the skin surface. *C. albicans* is almost always found only on the surface of the skin; it rarely penetrates deeper. Some persons are predisposed to candidal infections by

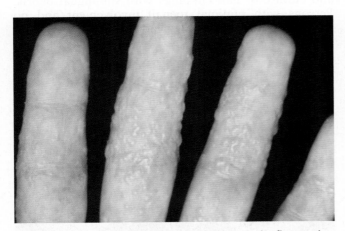

FIGURE 46-5. Dermatophytid or id reaction on the fingers due to a tinea infection. An id immunologic reaction, also known as *autoeczematization*, is an itchy, vesicular rash produced in response to an intense inflammatory process that can be located in another region of the body. (From the Centers for Disease Control and Prevention Public Health Image Library. No. 4805.)

conditions such as diabetes mellitus, antibiotic therapy, pregnancy, oral contraceptive use, poor nutrition, and immunosuppressive diseases.[9] Oral candidiasis may be the first sign of infection with human immunodeficiency virus (HIV).

Candida albicans thrives on warm, moist, intertriginous areas (i.e., between folds or adjacent surfaces) of the body. The rash is red with well-defined borders. Patches erode the epidermis, and there is scaling. Mild to severe itching and burning often accompany the infection. Severe forms of infection may involve pustules or vesiculopustules as well as maculopapular satellite lesions found outside the clearly demarcated borders of the candidal infection. Satellite lesions often are diagnostic of diaper rash complicated by *Candida*. The appearance of candidal infections varies according to the site (see Chapter 41 for a discussion of vaginal candidiasis).

Diagnosis usually is based on microscopic examination of skin or mucous membrane scrapings placed in a KOH solution. Treatment measures vary according to the location. Preventive measures such as wearing rubber gloves are encouraged for persons with infections of the hands. Intertriginous areas often are separated with clean cotton cloth and allowed to air dry as a means of decreasing the macerating effects of heat and moisture. Topical and oral antifungal agents, such as clotrimazole, econazole, ketoconazole, and miconazole, are used in treatment depending on the site and extent of involvement.

Bacterial Infections

Bacteria are considered normal flora of the skin. Most bacteria are not pathogenic, but when pathogenic bacteria invade the skin, superficial or systemic infections may develop. Bacterial skin infections are commonly classified as primary or secondary. Primary infections are superficial skin infections such as impetigo. Secondary infections consist of deeper cutaneous infections, such as infected ulcers. Diagnosis usually is based on cultures taken from the infected site. Treatment methods include antibiotic therapy and measures to promote comfort and prevent the spread of infection.

Impetigo. Impetigo is a common, superficial bacterial infection caused by staphylococci, group A β-hemolytic streptococci, or both.[10] It is common among infants and young children, although older children and adults occasionally contract the disease. Impetigo initially appears as a small vesicle or pustule or as a large bulla on the face or elsewhere on the body. As the primary lesion ruptures, it leaves a denuded area that discharges a honey-colored serous liquid that dries as a honey-colored crust with a "stuck-on" appearance (Fig. 46-6). New vesicles erupt within hours. Pruritus often accompanies the lesions, and skin excoriations that result from scratching multiply the infection sites. Although a very low risk, a possible complication of untreated streptococcal impetigo is poststreptococcal glomerulonephritis (see Chapter 25). Topical mupirocin

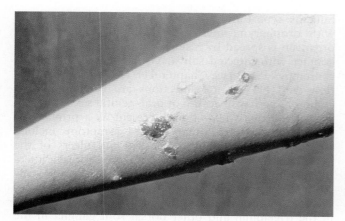

FIGURE 46-6. The lesions on this patient's forearm proved to be a dermatological condition caused by *Staphylococcus aureus* bacteria. Note the blister-like rash and the crusted lesion that resulted from the golden brown discharge as it dried. (From the Centers for Disease Control and Prevention Public Health Image Library. No. 14927. Courtesy of Dr. Herman Miranda, Univ. of Trujello, Peru; A. Chambers.)

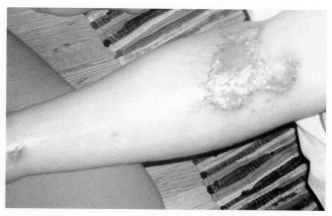

FIGURE 46-7. Cellulitis on leg infected with *Staphylococcus aureus* and *Pseudomonas*.

(Bactroban), which has few side effects, may be effective for limited infections. If the area is large or if there is concern about complications, systemic antibiotics are used.

Another form of impetigo exists, *bullous impetigo*, which is usually caused by *Staphylococcus aureus*.[10] Bullous impetigo is more common among children and occurs intermittently, with some cases transmitted among family members, but most often found among the institutionalized. Thin bullae erupt that appear clear to cloudy and coalesce. The bullae open, leaving the original bullous rim with central thin, flat, honey-colored crusts, or in some cases denuded areas. The face is often affected, but bullous impetigo may occur anywhere on the body. The treatment measures are the same as for nonbullous impetigo.

Cellulitis. Cellulitis is a deeper infection affecting the dermis and subcutaneous tissues.[11] It is usually caused by group A β-hemolytic streptococci or *S. aureus,* but can be caused by bacteria specific to certain activities, such as fish handling, swimming in fresh or salt water, or from animal bites or scratches. Preexisting wounds (e.g., ulcers, erosions) and tinea pedis are often portals of entry. Legs are the most common sites, followed by the hands and pinnae of the ears, but cellulitis may occur on many body sites. The lesion consists of an expanding red, swollen, tender plaque with an indefinite border, covering a variety of widths (Fig. 46-7). Cellulitis is frequently accompanied by fever, erythema, heat, edema, and pain. Cellulitis often involves the lymph system and, once compromised, repeat infections may impair lymphatic drainage, leading to chronically swollen legs, and eventually dermal fibrosis and lymphedema. Incorrectly treated, it may result in septicemia, nephritis, or death. Treatment measures (oral and intravenous antibiotics) are aimed at the invasive organisms and the extent of the infection.

Viral Infections

Viruses are intracellular pathogens that rely on live cells of the host for reproduction. They have no organized cell structure but consist of a deoxyribonucleic acid (DNA) or ribonucleic acid (RNA) core surrounded by a protein coat. The viruses seen in dermatoses tend to contain DNA. They invade the keratinocyte, begin to reproduce, and cause cellular proliferation or cellular death. The incidence of viral dermatoses is increasing. This has been attributed to the use of corticosteroid drugs, which have immunosuppressive properties, and the use of antibiotics, which alter the bacterial flora of the skin. As the number of bacterial infections has decreased, there has been a proportional rise in viral skin diseases.

Verrucae. Verrucae, or warts, are common benign papillomas caused by the DNA-containing human papillomavirus (HPV).[12] As benign papillomas, warts represent an exaggeration of the normal skin structures. There is an irregular thickening of the stratum spinosum and greatly increased thickening of the stratum corneum. The classification of warts is based largely on morphology and location.

Although warts vary in appearance depending on their location, it is now recognized that the clinically distinct types of warts result not simply because of the anatomic sites in which they arise, but also because of the distinct type of HPV. There are more than 80 types of HPV found on the skin and mucous membranes of humans that cause several different kinds of warts, including skin warts and genital warts. Many of the HPV types that cause genital warts are sexually transmitted, some of which (types 6, 11, 16, and 18) may increase the risk of cervical cancer (discussed in Chapter 41).

Nongenital warts often occur on the hands and feet. They are commonly caused by HPV types 1, 2, 3, 4, 27, and 57, and are not considered precancerous lesions. They are classified as common warts, flat warts, and plantar or palmar warts. Common warts, or verrucae vulgaris, are the most common type. The lesions can occur anywhere, but most frequently occur on dorsal surfaces of the hands, especially the periungual area,

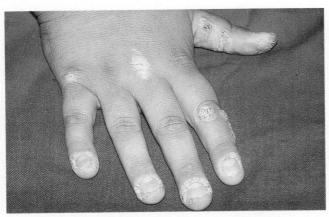

FIGURE 46-8. Common warts (verruca vulgaris). This young boy has multiple common warts. (From Goodheart HP. *Goodheart's Photoguide to Common Skin Disorders*. Philadelphia, PA: Wolters Kluwer Health | Lippincott Williams & Wilkins; 2009:141.)

where they appear as small, grayish-white to tan, flat to convex papules with a rough, pebblelike surface (Fig. 46-8). Verrucae plana, or flat warts, are common on the face or dorsal surfaces of the hands. These warts are slightly elevated, flat, smooth, tan papules that are slightly larger than verrucae vulgaris. Verrucae plantaris and verrucae palmaris (i.e., plantar and palmar warts, respectively) occur on the soles of the feet and palms of the hands, respectively. They appear as rough, scaly lesions that may reach 1 to 2 cm in diameter, coalesce, and be confused with ordinary calluses.

Transmission of HPV infection is largely by direct contact between individuals or by autoinoculation, usually through breaks in skin integrity. For example, plantar warts, which occur on the soles of the feet, frequently are transmitted to the abraded, softened heels of children in swimming areas. Common hand warts can be transmitted by biting the cuticles surrounding the nail.

Treatment is usually directed at inducing a "wart-free" period without producing scarring. Warts resolve spontaneously when immunity to the virus develops.[12] The immune response, however, may be delayed for years. Because of their appearance or discomfort, people usually desire their removal, rather than waiting for immunity to develop. Removal is usually done by applying a keratolytic agent, such as salicylic acid, which works by dissolving intercellular cement and producing desquamation of the horny layer of skin without affecting normal epidermal cells. Duct tape or "Ducto-Therapy" has been found effective for treatment of common warts. Intralesional bleomycin injections have been effective for recalcitrant warts.[12] Various types of laser surgery, electrosurgery, cryotherapy, immunotherapy (e.g., oral zinc sulfate), and antiviral therapy (e.g., cidofovir) also have been successful in wart eradication.

Herpes Simplex. Herpes simplex virus (HSV) infections of the skin and mucous membrane (i.e., cold sores or fever blisters) are common.[13] Two types of HSV infect humans: type 1 and type 2. HSV-1 is usually associated with oropharynx infections (labial herpes), and the organism is spread by respiratory droplets or by direct contact with infected saliva. Genital herpes usually is caused by HSV-2 (see Chapter 41). HSV-1 genital infections and HSV-2 oral infections are becoming more common, perhaps because of oral–genital sex.

Infection with HSV-1 may present as a primary or recurrent infection. Primary HSV-1 symptoms include fever, sore throat, painful vesicles, and ulcers of the lips, tongue, palate, and buccal mucosa. Primary infection results in the production of antibodies to the virus so that recurrent infections are more localized and less severe. After an initial infection, the herpesvirus persists in the trigeminal and other dorsal root ganglia in the latent state, periodically reactivating as recurrent infections. The symptoms of a primary HSV-1 infection most often occur in young children (1 to 5 years of age).

The recurrent lesions of HSV-1 are often found in the vicinity of the primary infection and usually begin with a burning or tingling sensation. Umbilicated vesicles and erythema follow and progress to pustules, ulcers, and crusts before healing (Fig. 46-9). Lesions are most common on the lips, face, mouth, nasal septum, and nose. When a lesion is active, HSV-1 is shed and there is risk of transmitting the virus to others. Pain is common, and healing takes place within 10 to 14 days. Precipitating factors include stress, menses, or injury. In particular, ultraviolet B exposure seems to be a trigger for recurrence. Individuals who are immunocompromised may have severe attacks.

There is no cure for oropharyngeal herpes; most treatment measures are palliative.[13] Over-the-counter topical preparations containing antihistamines, antipruritics, and anesthetic agents along with aspirin or acetaminophen may be used to relieve pain. Topical medications are best applied gently with a cotton-tipped applicator to prevent increased viral shedding and viral inoculation to another anatomic site. Oral acyclovir, valacyclovir,

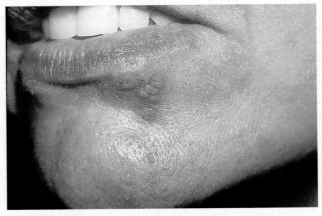

FIGURE 46-9. Recurrent herpes simplex virus infection (herpes labialis). Lesions are evident on the vermilion border of the lip and beyond. (From Goodheart HP. *Goodheart's Photoguide to Common Skin Disorders*. Philadelphia, PA: Wolters Kluwer Health | Lippincott Williams & Wilkins; 2009:157.)

and famciclovir may be used for prophylaxis. Sunscreen applied to the lips can prevent sun-induced herpes simplex. Efforts to develop vaccines to prevent HSV infections are in process.[13]

Herpes Zoster. Herpes zoster (shingles) is an acute, localized vesicular eruption distributed over a dermatomal segment of the skin.[14] It is caused by the same herpesvirus, varicella-zoster, that causes chickenpox. It is believed to be the result of reactivation of a latent varicella-zoster virus infection that was dormant in the sensory dorsal root ganglia since a primary childhood infection. During an episode of herpes zoster, the reactivated virus travels from the ganglia to the skin of the corresponding dermatome (Fig. 46-10A). Although herpes zoster is not as contagious as chickenpox, the reactivated virus can be transmitted to nonimmune contacts.

The incidence of herpes zoster increases with age; it occurs most frequently in persons older than 60 years of age. The normal age-related decrease in cell-mediated immunity is thought to account for the increased viral activation in this age group. Other persons at increased risk because of impaired cell-mediated immunity are persons with conditions such as HIV infection and certain malignancies, and those receiving long-term corticosteroid treatment, cancer chemotherapy, and radiation therapy.

The lesions of herpes zoster typically are preceded by a prodrome consisting of a burning pain, a tingling sensation, extreme sensitivity of the skin to touch, and pruritus along the affected dermatome (see Chapter 35). Among the dermatomes, the most frequently involved are the thoracic, the cervical, the trigeminal, and the lumbosacral.[14] Prodromal symptoms may be present for 1 to 3 days or longer before the appearance of the rash. During this time, the pain may be mistaken for a number of other conditions, such as heart disease, pleurisy, musculoskeletal disorders, or gastrointestinal disorders.

The lesions appear as an eruption of vesicles with erythematous bases that are restricted to skin areas supplied by sensory neurons of a single or associated group of dorsal root ganglia (Fig. 46-10B). In immunosuppressed persons, the lesions may extend beyond the dermatome. Eruptions usually are unilateral in the thoracic region, trunk, or face. New crops of vesicles erupt for 3 to 5 days along the nerve pathway. The vesicles dry, form crusts, and eventually fall off. The lesions usually clear in 2 to 3 weeks, although they can persist up to 6 weeks in some elderly persons.

Serious complications can accompany eruptions. Eye involvement can result in permanent blindness and occurs in a large percentage of cases involving the ophthalmic division of the trigeminal nerve (see Chapter 38). *Postherpetic neuralgia,* which is sharp, burning pain that persists longer than 1 to 3 months after the resolution of the rash, is seen most commonly in persons older than 60 years of age (see Chapter 35).

The treatment of choice for herpes zoster is the administration of an antiviral agent (e.g., acyclovir, valacyclovir, famciclovir).[14] Treatment is most effective when

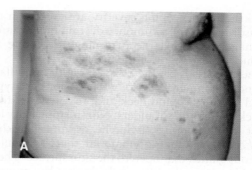

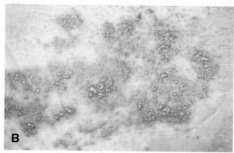

FIGURE 46-10. Acute herpes zoster. Panel **(A)** shows a cutaneous eruption in the right T7 dermatome. Panel **(B)** shows a close-up of fresh vesicular lesions. (From Gnann JW, Whitley RJ. Herpes zoster. *N Engl J Med.* 2002;347:341. Copyright © 2002. Massachusetts Medical Society.)

started within 72 hours of rash development. When given in the acute vesicular stage, the antiviral drugs have been shown to decrease the amount of lesion development and pain. Narcotic analgesics, tricyclic antidepressants, gabapentin, anticonvulsant drugs, and nerve blocks have been used for management of postherpetic neuralgia. Local application of capsaicin cream or lidocaine patches may be used in selected cases. Palliative treatments, such as heat and gentle pressure, may also be helpful.

A live herpes zoster vaccine is available to prevent both herpes zoster and postherpetic neuralgia. The vaccine is recommended for use in people 60 years of age and older, although the efficacy of the vaccine continues to be studied.[15,16]

Pustular Disorders

Although acne vulgaris, acne conglobata, and rosacea may present with a variety of skin lesions, they are characterized by the presence of pustules, which are circumscribed skin lesions filled with pus.

Acne Vulgaris

Acne vulgaris is a disorder of the pilosebaceous unit (see Chapter 45, Fig. 45-7) that results in formation of discrete papular or pustular lesions and may lead to scarring.[17-20] Acne can be cosmetically disfiguring and often psychologically disabling. It typically begins around puberty, as a result of increased androgen production. It may begin earlier and persist longer in females; however, overall the incidence and severity are greater in males. The disorder is very common, affecting more than 85% of teenagers, and a large percentage of young adults continue to show signs of the disorder.[20]

Acne vulgaris is characterized by both noninflammatory and inflammatory lesions. The lesions are typically located on the face and neck and, to a lesser extent, on the back, chest, and shoulders. Noninflammatory lesions consist of *comedones* (whiteheads and blackheads). *Blackheads* are plugs of material that accumulate in sebaceous glands that open to the skin surface. The color of blackheads results from melanin that has moved into the sebaceous glands from adjoining epidermal cells. *Whiteheads* are pale, slightly elevated papules with no visible orifice. Inflammatory lesions consist of papules, pustules, nodules, and, in severe cases, cysts. *Papules* are raised areas less than 5 mm in diameter. *Pustules* have a central core of purulent material. *Nodules* are larger than 5 mm in diameter and may become suppurative or hemorrhagic. Suppurative nodules often are referred to as *cysts* because of their resemblance to inflamed epidermal cysts. The inflammatory lesions are believed to develop from the escape of sebum into the dermis and the irritating effects of the fatty acids contained in the sebum.

The cause of acne vulgaris is largely unknown. There is a hereditary factor, multiple generations of family members being affected. Several factors are believed to contribute to acne, including (1) the influence of androgens on sebaceous gland activity; (2) increased proliferation of the keratinizing epidermal cells that form the sebaceous cells; (3) increased sebum production in relation to the severity of the disease; and (4) the presence of *Propionibacterium acnes*, the microorganism responsible for the inflammatory stage of the disorder. These factors are probably interrelated. Increased androgen production results in increased sebaceous cell activity, with resultant plugging of the pilosebaceous ducts. The excessive sebum provides a medium for *P. acnes* growth, and the organism contains lipases that break down the free fatty acids that produce the acne inflammation. *P. acnes* is also thought to form a biofilm (an extracellular polysaccharide lining in which the bacteria are encased) that acts as a protective barrier to antibiotic treatment (see Chapter 14), explaining why prolonged antibiotic treatments are necessary.[21] The sebaceous glands also may serve as sites for immune reactions.[22] Acne may be triggered or worsened by external factors such as obstructions (e.g., head bands, collars), manipulation of the lesions, cosmetics, and occupational exposures.

The diagnosis of acne is based on history and physical examination. The severity of the acne is generally assessed by the number, type, and distribution of lesions.[17] Mild acne is usually characterized by the presence of a small number (generally <10) of open and closed comedones, with a few inflammatory papules; moderate acne by the presence of a moderate number (10 to 40) of erythematous papules and pustules (Fig. 46-11), usually limited to the face; and moderately severe acne by the presence of numerous papules and pustules (40 to 100) and occasionally larger, deeper, nodular inflamed lesions

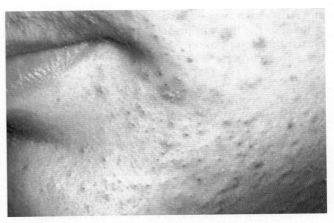

FIGURE 46-11. Moderate acne. Erythematous papules and pustules are the predominant lesions, and lesions are limited to the face. (From James WD. Acne. *N Engl J Med.* 2005;352:1464. Copyright © 2005. Massachusetts Medical Society.)

involving the face, chest, and back. Treatment of acne focuses on clearing up existing lesions, preventing new lesions, and limiting scar formation.[17–20]

Treatment measures include the use of topical antimicrobials, oral antibiotics, topical retinoids, and isotretinoin. Soaps are usually not effective in treating acne, and unless the skin is exceptionally oily, a mild soap should be used to avoid additional irritation that will limit the effectiveness of other topical treatments. Mild acne is usually treated with a topical preparation containing a combination of erythromycin or clindamycin and benzoyl peroxide. Topical antibiotics do not affect existing lesions but decrease the *P. acnes* on the skin, thereby reducing subsequent inflammation resulting from free fatty acid release and breakdown. Benzoyl peroxide, which is a bactericide, does not induce resistance, and when used with topical and oral antibiotics it protects against the development of lesions. Azelaic acid, products containing sodium sulfacetamide and sulfur, and salicylic acid preparations are also available. These agents are usually not considered as first-line therapies, but may be used in persons who cannot tolerate other topical agents.

Moderate to severe cases of acne may be managed with systemic antibiotics (e.g., tetracycline), topical vitamin A derivatives (retinoids), or oral retinoids (isotretinoin). Systemic antibiotics decrease *P. acnes* colonization and have intrinsic anti-inflammatory effects. The action of topical vitamin A (e.g., tretinoin) has been attributed to decreased cohesiveness of epidermal cells and increased epidermal cell turnover. This is thought to result in increased extrusion of open comedones and transformation of closed comedones into open ones. Isotretinoin is approved for treatment of recalcitrant cases of acne and cystic acnes. Although the exact mode of action is unknown, isotretinoin decreases sebaceous gland activity, prevents new comedones from forming, reduces the *P. acnes* count through sebum reduction, and has an anti-inflammatory effect. Because of its many side effects, it is used only in persons with severe acne. The oral retinoids are known teratogens and must not be used in women who are pregnant or may become pregnant.

A frequently seen adverse effect of acne in darker skinned persons is postinflammatory hyperpigmentation. Hence, treatment measures for persons of color may vary.[23]

Acne Conglobata

Acne conglobata occurs later in life as a severe, chronic form of acne. Comedones, papules, pustules, nodules, abscesses, cysts, and scars occur on the back, buttocks, and chest. Lesions occur to a lesser extent on the abdomen, shoulders, neck, face, upper arms, and thighs. The comedones or cysts have multiple openings, large abscesses, and interconnecting sinuses. Inflammatory nodules are not uncommon. Their discharge is odoriferous, serous or mucoid, and purulent. Healing often leaves deep keloidal lesions. Affected persons have anemia with elevated white blood cell counts, erythrocyte sedimentation rates, and neutrophil counts. The treatment is difficult and stringent. It often includes debridement, systemic corticosteroid therapy, oral retinoids, and systemic antibiotics.

Rosacea

Rosacea is a chronic skin disorder of middle-aged and older persons. The disease has a variety of clinical manifestations (blushing, presence of telangiectatic vessels, eruption of inflammatory papules and pustules) that primarily affect the central areas of the face. In the early stage of rosacea development, there are repeated episodes of blushing.[24,25] The blush eventually becomes a permanent, dark-red erythema on the nose and cheeks that sometimes extends to the forehead and chin (Fig. 46-12). This stage often occurs before 20 years of age. Ocular problems occur in at least 50% of persons with rosacea. Prominent symptoms include eyes that are itchy, burning,

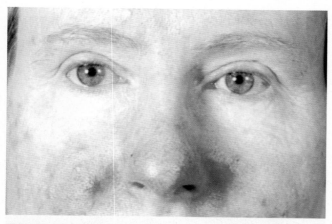

FIGURE 46-12. Papulopustular and ocular rosacea of moderate severity. The pustules are seen over the central portion of the face with sparing of the periocular area. Erythema and edema of the upper eyelids are also present. (From Powell FC. Rosacea. *N Engl J Med.* 2005;352:793–803. Copyright © 2005. Massachusetts Medical Society.)

or dry; a gritty or foreign body sensation; and erythema and swelling of the eyelid. As the person ages, the erythema persists, and telangiectasia with or without acne components (e.g., comedones, papules, pustules, nodules, erythema, and edema) develops. After years of affliction, rosacea may develop into an irregular bullous hyperplasia (thickening of the skin) of the nose, known as *rhinophyma*. Although rosacea is more common in women, rhinophyma is more common in men.

The cause of rosacea is unknown; however, it is believed to be a chronic inflammatory process involving the area surrounding the pilosebaceous units, accompanied by vascular instability with leakage of fluid and inflammatory mediators into the dermis. The lesions are accompanied by nonspecific perifollicular infiltrate of lymphocytes surrounded by dermal edema and dilated capillaries and terminal arterioles (telangiectases).[24,25] In the pustular phase, neutrophils may colonize the follicles, and follicular rupture may produce a granulomatous response. Rhinophyma is associated with hypertrophy of the sebaceous glands.

Rosacea is distinguished from acne vulgaris by the presence of the neurovascular component and absence of comedones. Treatment measures are similar to those used for acne vulgaris. Persons with rosacea are heat sensitive. They are instructed to avoid vascular stimulating agents such as heat, sunlight, hot liquids, foods, and alcohol. Topical metronidazole and azelaic acid creams have proved effective as treatment. Topical antibiotics (e.g., clindamycin, erythromycin), as well as systemic antibiotics (e.g., tetracycline and its derivatives) are also used in treatment of the disorder.[26] Pulsed dye laser therapy may be used for ablation of vessels in persons with prominent telangiectases. Rhinophyma can be treated by a number of surgical methods, including electrosurgery, laser ablation, dermabrasion, cryosurgery, and excision.

Allergic and Hypersensitivity Dermatoses

Allergic and hypersensitivity dermatoses involve the inflammatory response to multiple exogenous and endogenous agents. The disorders, which are usually characterized by epidermal edema with separation of epidermal cells, include atopic dermatitis, urticaria, drug-induced skin eruptions, and allergic contact dermatitis (discussed in Chapter 16).

Atopic Dermatitis

Atopic dermatitis (atopic eczema) is a highly pruritic chronic inflammatory skin disease. It usually begins early in life and often occurs in children with a personal or family history of other atopic disorders, such as allergic rhinitis and asthma.[27,28] The condition often remits during childhood, although it may reappear in adolescence and persist throughout adulthood.[28] The hallmarks of atopic dermatitis are a chronic, relapsing form of skin inflammation; a disturbance in the epidermal barrier function that leads to increased transepidermal water loss and dry skin; and immunoglobulin E (IgE)-mediated sensitization to food and environmental antigens.[27,28] Whether the primary defect is dermatologic or immunologic is uncertain. It has been suggested that the epidermal barrier disturbance allows increased antigen absorption and contributes to the hyperreactivity characteristic of atopic dermatitis.[27,28]

The lesions of atopic dermatitis are usually characterized by erythematous papules and vesicles, erosions, and serous exidates. Scratching causes crusted erosions. The clinical manifestations of the disorder often vary with age. In infancy the eczematous lesion usually appear on the cheeks and scalp (Fig. 46-13). The skin of the cheeks may be paler, with extra creases under the eyes, called *Dennie-Morgan folds*. During childhood, lesions involve flexures in the nape of the neck, and the dorsal aspects of the limbs.

Adolescents and adults usually have dry, red patches affecting the face, neck, and upper trunk. The bends of the elbows and knees are usually involved. In chronic cases, the skin is dry, leathery, and lichenified. Persons with dark skin may have a papular eruption and poorly demarcated hypopigmentation patches on the cheeks and extremities. In persons with black skin, pigmentation may be lost from lichenified skin. Acute flares may present with red patches that are weepy, shiny, or lichenified, and with plaques and papules. Itching may be severe and prolonged with both childhood and adult forms of atopic dermatitis. Secondary infections are common.

Treatment is designed to target the underlying abnormalities: dryness, pruritus, infection, and inflammation.[29] Basic therapy begins with optimal skin care, addressing the skin barrier defect with continuous use of emollients and skin hydration, along with avoiding exposure to irritants such as wool clothing, soaps, and hot water.

Topical corticosteroids remain an important treatment for acute flare-ups but can cause local and systemic side effects. Potency of topical corticosteroids is classified by the potential for vasoconstriction. In general, only preparations that have weak or moderate potency are used on the face and genital areas, whereas those that have moderate or high potency are used on other areas of the body. Lower-potency corticosteroids may be sufficient on all areas of the body in younger children. One of the main concerns of topical corticosteroid use is skin thinning. Another concern is secondary adrenal suppression and the suppression of growth in children resulting from systemic absorption. Wet-wrap therapy, in which a wet dressing is applied over emollients in combination with topical antiseptics or topical corticosteroids, has been shown to be beneficial in some cases of severe atopic dermatitis. Elimination of allergens in the living environment is a hallmark of therapy.

Systemic or adjuvant therapy is usually reserved for severe acute exacerbations. Short-term corticosteroids are also used during acute flare-ups in adults. Antihistamines may be used to relieve itching. Secondary infection with *S. aureus* is common and may be treated with systemic antimicrobial therapy. Phototherapy can be an important adjunct for severely affected adults and adolescents older than 12 years of age.

Urticaria

Urticaria, or hives, is a common skin disorder characterized by the development of edematous wheals accompanied by intense itching.[30,31] The lesions typically appear as raised pink or red areas surrounded by a paler halo (Fig. 46-14). They blanch with pressure and vary in size from a few millimeters to centimeters. Angioedema, which can occur alone or with urticaria, is characterized by nonpitting, nonpruritic, well-defined edematous swelling that involves subcutaneous tissues of the face, hands, feet, or genitals. It is more likely than urticaria to produce life-threatening swelling of the tongue and upper airways.

Urticaria can be acute or chronic and due to known or unknown causes. Numerous factors, both immunologic

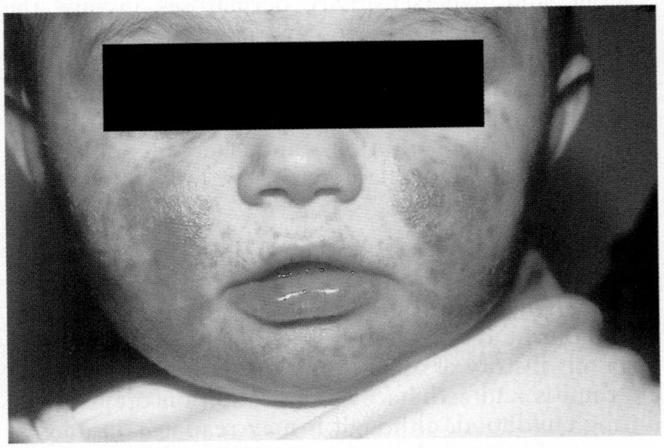

FIGURE 46-13. Atopic dermatitis. The cheeks are a typical location in an infant. (From Goodheart HP. *Goodheart's Photoguide to Common Skin Disorders.* Philadelphia, PA: Wolters Kluwer Health | Lippincott Williams & Wilkins; 2009:52.)

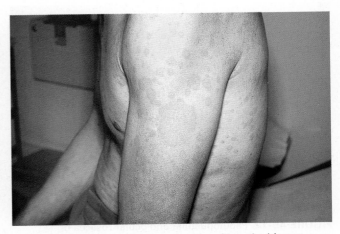

FIGURE 46-14. Urticarial drug eruption. Note the bizarre shapes of the urticarial plaques. (From Goodheart HP. *Goodheart's Photoguide to Common Skin Disorders.* Philadelphia, PA: Wolters Kluwer Health | Lippincott Williams & Wilkins; 2009:298.)

and nonimmunologic, can be involved in its pathogenesis. The urticarial wheal results from liberation of histamine from mast cells and basophils. Histamine causes hyperpermeability of the microvessels of the skin and surrounding tissue, allowing fluid to leak into the tissues, causing edema and wheal formation.

Acute immunologic urticaria is commonly the result of an IgE-mediated immune reaction that usually occurs within 1 hour of exposure to an antigen. The most common causes of acute urticaria are foods or drinks, medications (most notably penicillin and cephalosporin), insect stings, and exposure to pollens or chemicals. Although nonsteroidal anti-inflammatory drugs, including aspirin, do not normally cause urticaria, they may exacerbate the preexisting disease. In rare cases, urticaria is a manifestation of underlying disease, such as certain cancers, collagen diseases, and hepatitis. A hereditary deficiency of a C1 (complement 1) inhibitor also can cause a condition called *hereditary angioneurotic edema*.

The physical urticarias are a specific form of chronic urticaria, in which specific physical stimuli reproducibly elicit wheals.[30,31] Physical urticarias are intermittent, usually last less than 2 hours, are produced by appropriate stimuli, have distinctive appearances and locations, and are seen most frequently in young adults. Dermographism, or skin writing, is one form of physical urticaria in which wheals appear in response to simple rubbing of the skin. The wheals follow the pattern of the scratch or rubbing, appearing within 10 minutes and dissolving completely within 20 minutes. Other types of physical urticaria are induced by exercise, sunlight, water, vibration, cold, and heat. Appropriate challenge tests (e.g., application of an ice cube to the skin to initiate development of cold urticaria) are used to differentiate physical urticaria from chronic urticaria due to other causes.

Most types of urticaria are treated with nonsedating antihistamines that alleviate pruritus and decrease the incidence of hives without producing drowsiness. Leukotriene antagonists (zafirlukast and montelukast) may also be used. Oral corticosteroids may be used in the treatment of refractory urticaria. Tricyclic antidepressant drugs, particularly those with antihistamine actions, may also be used. Persons who have experienced angioedema of the larynx and pharynx should be counseled to carry a prescription of epinephrine in an autoinjectable syringe.

Drug-Induced Skin Eruptions

Most drugs can cause a localized or generalized skin eruption. Topical drugs are usually responsible for localized contact dermatitis types of rashes, whereas systemic drugs cause generalized skin lesions. Although many drug-induced skin eruptions are exanthematous or morbilliform (i.e., measleslike), they may mimic most of the skin disorders described in this chapter. Because the lesions vary greatly, the diagnosis depends almost entirely on an accurate patient report, including a full drug history. Early recognition and discontinuation of

the drug are essential. Management of mild cases is aimed at eliminating the offending drug while treating the symptoms. Severe cases require prompt medical attention.

Some drug reactions result in epidermal cell detachment and bullae (fluid-filled blisters) formation. The skin detachment seen with bullous skin lesions is different from the desquamation (i.e., peeling) that occurs with other skin disorders. In the bullous disorders, there is full-thickness detachment of the entire epidermis from the dermis. This leaves the person vulnerable to multiple problems, including loss of body fluids and electrolytes, impaired body temperature control, and a greatly increased risk of infection. Three types of drug reactions that result in bullous skin lesions are erythema multiforme minor, which is usually self-limiting, with a small amount of skin detachment at the lesion sites; Stevens-Johnson syndrome, which involves less than 10% of the body surface area; and toxic epidermal necrolysis, which involves detachment of more than 30% of the epidermis.[35] Detachment of 10% to 30% of the epidermis is considered an overlap of Stevens-Johnson syndrome and toxic epidermal necrolysis.

Etiology and Pathogenesis. Although the cause of erythema multiforme minor may be drug induced or unknown, it frequently occurs after infections, especially HSV infection. Stevens-Johnson syndrome and toxic epidermal necrolysis are caused by a hypersensitivity reaction to drugs, the most common being sulfonamides, anticonvulsants, nonsteroidal anti-inflammatory drugs, antimalarial agents, and allopurinol. The incidences of Stevens-Johnson syndrome and toxic epidermal necrolysis are rare, but mortality rates are high.[36] Recovery is based on the severity and quick, aggressive treatment.

Manifestations. The lesions of erythema multiforme minor and Stevens-Johnson syndrome are similar. The primary lesion of both is a round, erythematous papule resembling an insect bite. Within hours to days, these lesions change into several different patterns. The individual lesions may enlarge and coalesce, producing small plaques, or they may change to concentric zones of color appearing as "target" or "iris" lesions (Fig. 46-15). The outermost rings of the target lesions usually are erythematous; the central portion usually is opaque white, yellow, or gray (dusky). In the center, small blisters may form on the dusky purpuric macules, giving them their characteristic targetlike appearance. Although there is wide distribution of lesions over the body surface area, there is a propensity for them to occur on the face and trunk.

Toxic epidermal necrolysis is the most serious type of drug reaction, with mortality rates of 40%.[35] The person experiences a prodromal period of malaise, low-grade fever, and sore throat. Within a few days, widespread erythema and large, flaccid bullae appear, followed by the loss of the epidermis, leaving a denuded and painful dermis. The skin surrounding the large denuded areas may have the typical target-like lesions seen with

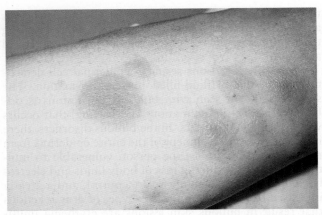

FIGURE 46-15. Erythema multiforme. Characteristic targetlike lesions are noted here. (From Goodheart HP. *Goodheart's Photoguide to Common Skin Disorders*. Philadelphia, PA: Wolters Kluwer Health | Lippincott Williams & Wilkins; 2009:311.)

Stevens-Johnson syndrome. Lateral pressure causes the surrounding skin to separate easily from the dermis (*Nikolsky sign*). The tracheobronchial mucosa and conjunctiva may be involved in severe cases with resultant scarring. Ophthalmologic consultation is required when ocular involvement in present.

Treatment. Treatment of erythema multiforme minor and less-severe cases of Stevens-Johnson syndrome includes relief of symptoms using compresses, antipruritic drugs, and topical anesthetics. Corticosteroid therapy may be indicated in moderate cases, although its use is controversial. For severe cases of Stevens-Johnson syndrome and toxic epidermal necrolysis, hospitalization is required for fluid replacement, respiratory care, administration of antibiotics and analgesics, and application of moist dressings. When large areas of skin are detached, the care is similar to that of a thermal burn. Intravenous immunoglobulin may hasten the healing response of the skin. Generally, healing is a slow process, taking 6 weeks or more to regenerate skin. The mucous membranes heal slowly and follow-up treatment is often needed for ophthalmologic and mucous membrane sequelae. Discontinuation of the responsible drug and chemically related compounds is imperative, as are measures to prevent future exposures to the drug.

Papulosquamous Dermatoses

Papulosquamous dermatoses are a group of skin disorders characterized by scaling papules and plaques. Among the major papulosquamous diseases are psoriasis, pityriasis rosea, and lichen planus.

Psoriasis

Psoriasis is a common, chronic, inflammatory skin disease characterized by raised erythematous plaques with silvery scales.[37–40] It affects approximately 2% of the population and occurs worldwide, although the incidence is lower in warmer, sunnier climates. The average age of onset is in the third decade; its prevalence increases with age. Approximately one third of persons have a genetic history, indicating a hereditary factor. Childhood onset of the disease is more strongly associated with a family history than psoriasis occurring in adults older than 30 years of age. In rare cases, psoriasis is associated with arthritis (see Chapter 44).

Etiology and Pathogenesis. Although the primary cause of psoriasis is uncertain, it is thought to be an immunological disorder in persons with a genetic predisposition. It is not known if the inciting antigen is of self or environment origin. A genetic component is supported by population studies indicating a greater incidence of psoriasis among relatives of persons with the disease than among the general population. There is a strong association between psoriasis and the human leukocyte antigen-C (HLA-C), particularly the HLA-Cw6 allele.[40] Immunologically, T lymphocytes may be the key to the pathogenesis of psoriasis.[40] Eruption of psoriatic lesions coincides with T-cell infiltration into the epidermis, and resolution of the lesions follows disappearance or reduction in epidermal T cells, suggesting a T-cell–mediated release of cytokines and growth factors that stimulate abnormal growth of keratinocytes and dermal blood vessels. Accompanying inflammatory changes are caused by infiltration of neutrophils and monocytes. Environmental stimuli may trigger the release of cytokines and growth factors from keratinocytes and other cells, with ensuing immune and inflammatory responses that lead to the full development of psoriatic lesions. For example, psoriatic lesions can be induced in susceptible individuals by trauma, a process known as the *Köbner phenomenon*.

Clinical Features. Histologically, psoriasis is characterized by increased epidermal cell turnover with marked epidermal thickening, a process called *hyperkeratosis*. The granular layer (stratum granulosum) of the epidermis is thinned or absent, and neutrophils are found in the stratum corneum. There also is an accompanying thinning of the epidermal cell layer that overlies the tips of the dermal papillae, and the blood vessels in the dermal papillae become tortuous and dilated. These capillary beds show permanent damage even when the disease is in remission or resolved. The close proximity of the vessels in the dermal papillae to the hyperkeratotic scale accounts for multiple, minute bleeding points that are seen when the scale is lifted.

Psoriasis most frequently affects the elbows, knees, scalp, lumbosacral area, and intragluteal cleft. The primary lesions are sharply demarcated, thick, red plaques covered by a silvery scale that varies in size and shape (Fig. 46-16). In darker-skinned persons, the plaques may appear purple. There may be excoriation, thickening, or oozing from the lesions. A differential diagnostic finding is that the plaques bleed from minute points when removed, which is known as the *Auspitz sign*.

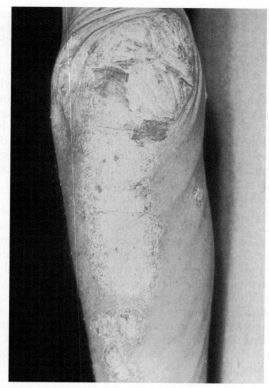

FIGURE 46-16. Psoriasis of the elbow. Note the irregular red patches covered by a dry scaly hyperkeratotic stratum corneum. (From the Centers for Disease Control and Prevention Public Health Image Library. No. 4055. Courtesy of Susan Lindsley.)

Treatment. The goals for psoriasis treatment focus on suppressing the hyperkeratosis, epidermal inflammation, and abnormal keratinocyte differentiation that are characteristic of the disease. Usually, topical agents are used first in any treatment regimen and when less than 20% of the body surface is involved. They include emollients, keratolytic agents, coal tar products, corticosteroids, and calcipotriene.[39] Emollients hydrate and soften the psoriatic plaques. Keratolytic agents are peeling agents that soften and remove plaques. Salicylic acid is the most widely used. Coal tar, the by-product of the processing of coke and gas from coal, is one of the oldest yet most effective forms of treatment. The exact mechanism of action of tar products is unknown, but side effects of the treatment are few. Newer preparations of coal tar lotions and shampoos are more aesthetically pleasing, but the odor remains a problem. *Calcipotriene* (a vitamin D derivative) *ointment* has been shown to inhibit epidermal cell proliferation and enhance cell differentiation. *Tazarotene,* a synthetic retinoid, also has been effective, but it is teratogenic and should be avoided in women of childbearing age.

Topical corticosteroids are widely used and relatively effective. They are generally more acceptable because they do not stain and are easy to use. Low-potency preparations usually are used on the face and on areas of the body, such as the groin and axilla, where the skin tends to be thinner. High-potency preparations are reserved for treatment of thick chronic plaques that do not respond to less-potent preparations. Although the corticosteroids are rapidly effective in the treatment of psoriasis, they are associated with flare-ups after discontinuation and they have many potential side effects. Their effectiveness is increased when used under occlusive dressings, but there is an increase in side effects.

Systemic treatments include phototherapy, photochemotherapy, methotrexate, corticosteroids, and cyclosporine. The positive effects of sunlight have long been established. Phototherapy with UVB radiation is a widely used treatment. Newly developed narrow-band UVB radiation is reportedly more effective than broad-band UVB.[39] Photochemotherapy involves using a light-activated form of the drug methoxsalen. Methoxsalen, a psoralen or phototoxic drug, exerts its actions when exposed to UVA radiation in 320- to 400-nm wavelengths. The combination treatment regimen of psoralen and UVA is known by the acronym *PUVA.* Methoxsalen is given orally before UVA exposure. Activated by the UVA energy, methoxsalen inhibits DNA synthesis, thereby preventing cell mitosis and decreasing the hyperkeratosis that occurs with psoriasis. Although viewed as one of the safest therapies since its introduction in the 1970s, PUVA increases the risk for squamous cell carcinoma, and it may increase the risk for development of melanoma.

Methotrexate, which is used for cancer treatment, is an antimetabolite that inhibits DNA synthesis and prevents cell mitosis. Oral methotrexate has been effective in treating psoriasis when other approaches have failed. The drug has many side effects, including nausea, malaise, leukopenia, thrombocytopenia, and liver function abnormalities. Cyclosporine is a potent immunosuppressive drug used to prevent rejection of organ transplants. It suppresses inflammation and the proliferation of T cells in persons with psoriasis. Its use is limited to severe psoriasis because of serious side effects, including nephrotoxicity, hypertension, and increased risk of cancers. Intralesional cyclosporine also has been effective. Biologic agents (drugs that are taken from or made of living tissues or cells instead of chemicals) that target the activity of T lymphocytes and cytokines responsible for the inflammatory nature of psoriasis have proven effective.[41]

Pityriasis Rosea

Pityriasis rosea is a rash that primarily affects children and young adults. The origin of the rash is unknown, but is thought to be caused by an infective agent, possibly a herpesvirus.[42] Its incidence is highest in winter. Cases occur in clusters and among persons who are in close contact; however, there are no data to support communicability, suggesting it may be an immune response to any number of agents.

The characteristic lesion is an oval macule or papule with surrounding erythema (Fig. 46-17). The lesion spreads with central clearing, much like tinea corporis. This initial lesion is called the *herald patch* and is usually on the trunk or neck. As the lesion enlarges and begins to fade (2 to 10 days), successive crops of lesions appear on the trunk and neck. The lesions on the back have a characteristic

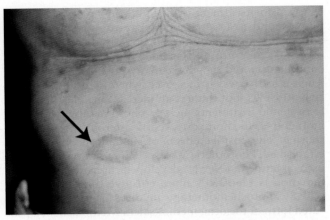

FIGURE 46-17. Pityriasis rosea. Note oval herald patch (*arrow*) on the abdomen as well as a more generalized rash. (From the Centers for Disease Control and Prevention Public Health Image Library. No. 4812.)

"Christmas tree" pattern. The extremities, face, and scalp may be involved. Mild to severe pruritus may occur. The disease is self-limited and usually disappears within 6 to 8 weeks. Treatment measures are palliative and include topical steroids, antihistamines, and colloid baths. Systemic corticosteroids may be indicated in severe cases.

Lichen Planus

The term *lichen* (Greek, "tree moss") refers to skin disorders characterized by small (2 to 10 mm), flat-topped papules with irregular, angulated borders. *Lichen planus* is a relatively common chronic pruritic disease.[43] It involves inflammation and papular eruption of the skin and mucous membranes. There are variations in the pattern of lesions (e.g., annular, linear) and differences in the sites (e.g., mucous membranes, genitalia, nails, scalp). The characteristic lesion is a purple, polygonal papule covered with a shiny, white, lacelike pattern (Fig. 46-18). The lesions appear on the wrist, ankles, and trunk of the body. Most persons who have skin lesions also have oral lesions, appearing as milky white lacework on the buccal mucosa or tongue. Other mucosal surfaces, such as

the genital, nasal, laryngeal, otic, gastric, and anal areas, may also be affected. As with psoriasis, lichen planus lesions can develop on scratches or skin injuries (Köbner phenomenon).

The etiology of lichen planus is unknown, but it is believed to be an abnormal immune response in which epithelial cells are recognized as foreign. The disorder involves the epidermal–dermal junction with damage to the basal cell layer. Some cases of lichen planus have been linked to hepatitis C virus infections or medication use. The most common medications include gold, antimalarial agents, thiazide diuretics, beta blockers, nonsteroidal anti-inflammatory agents, quinidine, and angiotensin-converting enzyme inhibitors.

Diagnosis is based on the clinical appearance of the lesions and the histopathologic findings from a punch biopsy. For most persons, lichen planus is a self-limited disease. Treatment measures include discontinuation of all medications, followed by treatment with topical corticosteroids and occlusive dressings. Antipruritic agents are helpful in reducing itch. Systemic corticosteroids may be indicated in severe cases. Photochemotherapy (i.e., PUVA) may also be used. Acitretin, an orally administered retinoid agent, also may be effective. Because retinoids are teratogenic, they should be avoided in women of childbearing age.

Lichen Simplex

Lichen simplex chronicus is a localized lichenoid pruritic dermatitis resulting from repeated rubbing and scratching.[44] It is characterized by the occurrence of itchy, reddened, thickened, and scaly patches of dry skin. Persons with the condition may have a single lesion or, less frequently, multiple lesions. The lesions are seen most commonly at the nape of the neck, wrists, ankles, or anal area. The condition usually begins as a small pruritic patch, which after a repetitive cycle of itching and scratching develops into a chronic dermatitis. Because of the chronic itching and scratching, excoriations and lichenification with thickening of the skin develops, often giving the appearance of tree bark.

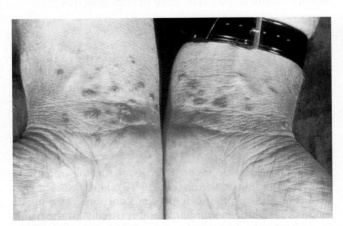

FIGURE 46-18. Lichen planus affecting both wrists. (From the Centers for Disease Control and Prevention Public Health Image Library. No. 6545. Courtesy of Susan Lindsley.)

SUMMARY CONCEPTS

- Primary dermatoses are conditions that have their origin in the skin.

- Infectious skin disorders are caused by fungi, bacteria, and viruses that invade the skin, incite inflammatory responses, and otherwise cause rashes and lesions that disrupt the skin surface.

- Superficial fungal infections or *dermatophytoses* are commonly known as *tinea* or *ringworm*. Tinea can affect the whole body (tinea corporis), scalp (tinea capitis), feet or hands (tinea pedis or manus), or nails (tinea unguium).

- Candidal skin infections due to *C. albicans* occur most often in persons with diabetes mellitus, those who are immunosuppressed, or those who have been treated with broad-spectrum antibiotics.

- Impetigo, which is caused by staphylococci or β-hemolytic streptococci, is the most common superficial bacterial infection.

- Viruses are responsible for verrucae (warts), herpes simplex type 1 lesions (cold sores or fever blisters), and herpes zoster (shingles).

- Disorders of the pilosebaceous unit include acne vulgaris, which is a common skin disorder of adolescents and young adults that involves increased sebum production and the presence of *P. acnes*; and rosacea, which is a chronic acneform disorder of middle-aged and older persons.

- Allergic skin responses involve the body's immune system and are caused by hypersensitivity reactions to allergens such as environmental agents, drugs, and other substances. They include atopic dermatitis, urticaria, and drug-induced skin eruptions (erythema multiforme, Stevens-Johnson syndrome, and toxic epidermal necrolysis).

- Papulosquamous dermatoses are characterized by scaling papules and plaques that result from uncontrolled keratinocyte proliferation. Psoriasis is a chronic proliferative skin disease characterized by epidermal hyperplasia. Lichen planus is a hypersensitivity reaction with lymphocytic infiltration at the dermal–epithelial junction.

Skin Disorders Due to Ultraviolet Radiation, Heat, and Pressure Injury

The skin is highly vulnerable to injury from excessive ultraviolet (UV) radiation, heat, and unrelieved pressure.

Ultraviolet Radiation

Sunlight is composed of a continuous spectrum of electromagnetic radiation that is divided into three main parts or wavelengths: ultraviolet (UV), visible, and infrared. The UV light region occurs between 100 and 400 nm (nm: one billionth of a meter).[45] Long-wave UVA radiation is 320 to 400 nm; medium-wave UVB is 280 to 320 nm; and short-wave UVC is 100 to 280 nm. The ozone layer effectively absorbs UV radiation up to 310 nm, absorbing all of UVC and much of UVB

radiation. However, damage to the protective ozone layer is allowing an increased amount of UVB to reach the earth. The ozone layer does not absorb UVA.

Ultraviolet Radiation Skin Damage

UVA makes up more than 95% of the solar radiation that reaches us. Compared to UVB, this long-wave radiation penetrates deep into the dermis of the skin and is more effective in producing an immediate tan. UVB radiation is a minor but more active constituent of sunlight. It is more genotoxic and about 1000 times more capable of causing sunburn than UVA light.[45] UVB acts mainly on the cells in the basal layer of the epidermis. It produces direct damage to the DNA and other nuclear proteins. It also provokes free radical production and induces a significant reduction in skin antioxidants, impairing the ability of the skin to protect itself against damage by the free radicals that are generated.

Etiology and Pathogenesis. Exposure to UVA and UVB produces acute effects that are short lived and reversible. They include erythema, pigmentation, and injury to Langerhans cells and keratinocytes in the epidermis. These reactions differ depending on whether the inciting agent is UVA or UVB. For example, UVA-induced erythema occurs immediately, fades within hours, and is believed to be due to the "heat load." UVB-induced erythema has a delayed response, peaking within 6 to 24 hours after exposure to sunlight and fading over 1 or 2 days. Pigmentation or tanning induced by UVA and UVB is due to increased synthesis of melanin by melanocytes, along with increased transfer of the melanin to keratinocytes (see Chapter 45). Small doses of UVA produce transient, immediate darkening of the skin that fades within 2 hours, whereas higher doses of UVA can produce pigmentary changes lasting for several hours to days.[45] Tanning induced by UVB is protective against subsequent exposures, whereas tanning induced by UVA provides limited protection.

Skin damage induced by UVB is believed to be caused by the generation of reactive oxygen species and by damage to melanocytes.[45] Cellular proteins and DNA are primarily damaged because of their abundance and ability to absorb UVB radiation. Both UVA and UVB also deplete Langerhans cells and immune cells. It is believed that these effects prevent immune cells from detecting and removing sun-damaged cells with malignant potential. Both UVA and UVB are now considered causes of skin cancer. UVA may actually be more carcinogenic than UVB. Although it causes less sunburn, UVA is present during all daylight hours, year-round. Artificial sources of UVA, such as tanning beds and therapeutic solar interventions (PUVA) for certain skin conditions, also produce the same effects as solar UVA in terms of skin cancer. This is of particular concern because of the increased use of indoor tanning, particularly among adolescents and young adults who are at greatest risk of melanoma.[45,46] Educating the population about avoiding tanning booths has not increased compliance; the number of people who use tanning booths continues to rise, while adherence of tanning booths to national guidelines is often violated.[46]

Clinical Features. Sunburn is caused by excessive exposure of the epidermal and dermal layers of the skin to UV radiation, resulting in an erythematous inflammatory reaction.[47] Sunburn ranges from mild to severe. Mild sunburn consists of various degrees of skin redness. The burn continues to develop for 24 to 72 hours, occasionally followed by peeling skin in 3 to 8 days. Some peeling and itching may continue for several weeks. Inflammation, blistering, weakness, chills, fever, malaise, and pain often accompany severe forms of sunburn. Scaling and peeling follow any overexposure to sunlight. Dark skin also burns and may appear grayish or gray-black. Severe sunburns are those that cover large portions of the body with blisters or are accompanied by a high fever or intense pain.

The UV rays of sunlight or other sources can be completely or partially blocked from the skin surface by sunscreens. There are two primary types of sunscreens available on the market—chemical (soluble) agents and physical (insoluble) agents.[45] Chemical agents (e.g., para-aminobenzoic acid [PABA] derivatives) protect the skin from absorbing sunlight, and physical agents (e.g., micronized titanium dioxide and microfine zinc) work by reflecting sunlight. The *sun protection factor* (SPF) rating of the various sunscreen products is based on their ability to obstruct UV radiation (UVR) absorption. The ratings usually are on a scale of 1 to 30+, with the higher ratings indicating greater blocking of UVR.[45] Products with a higher SPF screen out more UVB rays, which are primarily responsible for acute sun damage. Shielding the skin with protective clothing and hats or head coverings helps decrease UVR exposure.

Mild to moderate sunburns are treated with anti-inflammatory medications, such as aspirin or ibuprofen, until redness and pain subside. Cold compresses, cool baths, and applying a moisturizing cream, such as aloe, to affected skin help treat the symptoms. Steroid and nonsteroidal agents are used depending on the severity of the burn. Blisters should not be broken to preserve the protective layer of the skin, hasten the healing process, and decrease the risk of infection. Extensive second- and third-degree sunburns may require hospitalization and specialized burn care techniques, as described in the section on thermal injury.

Drug-Induced Photosensitivity

Some drugs are classified as photosensitive drugs because they produce an exaggerated response to UVR when the drug is taken in combination with sun exposure. Examples include some of the anti-infective agents (sulfonamides, tetracyclines, nalidixic acid), antihistamines (cyproheptadine, diphenhydramine), antipsychotic agents (phenothiazines, haloperidol), diuretics (thiazides, acetazolamide, amiloride), hypoglycemic agents (sulfonylureas), and nonsteroidal anti-inflammatory drugs (phenylbutazone, ketoprofen, naproxen).

Thermal Injury

About 450,000 people in the United States require medical care for burns each year, with 40,000 requiring hospitalization.[48] Flame burns occur because of exposure to direct fire. Scald burns result from hot liquids spilled or poured on the skin surface.

The effects and complications of burns fully illustrate the essential function that the skin performs in protecting the body from the many damaging elements in the environment while serving to maintain the constancy of the body's internal environment. The massive loss of skin tissue not only predisposes to attack by microorganisms that are present in the environment, but also allows for the massive loss of body fluids, interferes with temperature regulation, challenges the immune system, and imposes excessive demands on the metabolic and reparative processes that are needed to restore the body's interface with the environment.

Classification of Burns

Burns are typically classified according to the depth of involvement as first-degree, second-degree, and third-degree burns.[49,50] The depth of a burn is largely influenced by the duration of exposure to the heat source and the temperature of the heating agent. *First-degree burns* (superficial partial-thickness burns) involve only the outer layers of the epidermis. They are red or pink, dry, and painful. There usually is no blister formation, as with a mild sunburn. The skin maintains its ability to function as a water vapor and bacterial barrier and heals in 3 to 10 days. First-degree burns usually require only palliative treatment, such as pain-relief measures and adequate fluid intake. Extensive first-degree burns on infants, the elderly, and persons who receive radiation therapy for cancer may require more care.

Second-degree burns involve both the epidermis and dermis. *Second-degree partial-thickness burns* involve the epidermis and various degrees of the dermis. They are painful, moist, red, and blistered. Underneath the blisters is weeping, bright pink or red skin that is sensitive to temperature changes, air exposure, and touch. The blisters prevent the loss of body water and superficial dermal cells. Excluding excision of large burn areas, it is important to maintain intact blisters after injury because they serve as a good bandage and may promote wound healing. These burns heal in approximately 1 to 2 weeks.

Second-degree full-thickness burns involve the entire epidermis and dermis. Structures that originate in the subcutaneous layer, such as hair follicles and sweat glands, remain intact. These burns can be very painful because the pain sensors remain intact. Tactile sensation may be absent or greatly diminished in the areas of deepest destruction. These burns appear as mottled pink, red, or waxy white areas with blisters and edema. The blisters resemble flat, dry tissue paper, rather than the bullous blisters seen with superficial partial-thickness injury. After healing in approximately 1 month, these burns maintain their softness and elasticity, but there may be the loss of some sensation. Scar formation is common.

These burns heal with supportive medical care aimed at preventing further tissue damage, providing adequate hydration, and ensuring that the granular bed is adequate to support re-epithelialization.

Third-degree full-thickness burns extend into the subcutaneous tissue and may involve muscle and bone. Thrombosed vessels can be seen under the burned skin, indicating that the underlying vasculature is involved. Third-degree burns vary in color from waxy white or yellow to tan, brown, deep red, or black. These burns are hard, dry, and leathery. Edema is extensive in the burn area and surrounding tissues. There is no pain because the nerve sensors have been destroyed. However, there is no such thing as a "pure" third-degree burn. Third-degree burns are almost always surrounded by second-degree burns, which are surrounded by an area of first-degree burns. The injury sometimes has an almost targetlike appearance because of the various degrees of burn. Full-thickness burns wider than 1.5 inches usually require skin grafts because all the regenerative (i.e., dermal) elements have been destroyed. Smaller injuries usually heal from the margins inward toward the center, the dermal elements regenerating from the healthier margins. However, regeneration may take many weeks and leave a permanent scar, even in smaller burns.

In addition to the depth of the wound, the extent of the burn also is important. Extent is measured by estimating the amount of total body surface area (TBSA) involved.[49,50] Several tools exist for estimating the TBSA. For example, the *rule of nines* counts anatomic body parts as multiples of 9% (the head and neck is 9%, each arm 9%, each leg 18%, anterior trunk 18%, posterior trunk 18%), with the perineum 1%. The Lund and Browder chart includes a body diagram table that estimates the TBSA by age and anatomic part. Children are more accurately assessed using this method because it takes into account the difference in relative size of body parts. The estimates of TBSA are then converted to the American Burn Association Classification of Extent of Injury (Table 46-1).

Other factors, such as age, location, other injuries, and preexisting conditions, are taken into consideration for a full assessment of burn injury.[49,50] These factors can increase the assessed severity of the burn and the length of treatment. For example, a first-degree burn is reclassified as a more severe burn if other factors are present, such as burns to the hands, face, and feet; inhalation injury; other trauma; or existence of psychosocial problems. Genital burns almost always require hospitalization because edema may cause difficulty urinating and the location complicates maintenance of a bacteria-free environment.

Systemic Complications

Burn victims often are confronted with hemodynamic instability, impaired respiratory function, a hypermetabolic response, and sepsis.[49,50] The magnitude of the response is proportional to the extent of injury, usually reaching a plateau when approximately 60% of the body is burned. In addition to loss of skin, burn victims often have associated injuries or illnesses. The treatment challenge is to provide immediate resuscitation efforts and long-term maintenance of physiologic function. Pain and emotional problems are additional challenges faced by persons with burns.

Hemodynamic Instability. Hemodynamic instability begins almost immediately with injury to capillaries in the burned area and surrounding tissue. Fluid is lost from the vascular, interstitial, and cellular compartments. Because of a loss of vascular volume, major burn victims often present in the emergency department in a form of hypovolemic shock (Chapter 20) known as *burn shock*. Because proteins from the blood are lost into the interstitial compartment, generalized edema, including pulmonary edema, can be severe.

TABLE 46-1	American Burn Association Grading System for Burn Severity and Disposition		
	Type of Burn		
	Minor	**Moderate**	**Major**
Criteria	<10% TBSA in adult	10%–20% TBSA in adult	>20% TBSA in adult
	<5% TBSA in young (<10 years) or old (>50 years)	5%–10% TBSA in young or old	>10% TBSA in young or old
	<2% Full-thickness burn	2%–5% Full-thickness burn	>5% Full-thickness burn
		High-voltage injury	High-voltage burn
		Suspected inhalation injury	Known inhalation injury
		Circumferential burn	Any significant burn to face, eyes, ears, genitalia, hands, feet, or major joints
		Concomitant medical problem predisposing to infection (e.g., diabetes, sickle cell disease)	Significant associated injuries (e.g., major trauma)
Disposition	Outpatient management	Hospital admission	Referral to burn center

TBSA, total body surface area.

From American Burn Association. Hospital and prehospital resources for optimal care of patients with burn injury: guidelines for development and operation of burn centers. *J Burn Care Rehabil.* 1990;11:98–104.

Respiratory System Dysfunction. Another injury commonly associated with burns is postburn lung injury from smoke inhalation. Victims often are trapped in a burning structure and inhale significant amounts of smoke, carbon monoxide, and other toxic fumes. Water-soluble gases found in smoke from burning plastics and rubber, such as ammonia, sulfur dioxide, and chlorine, react with mucous membranes to form strong acids and alkalis that induce ulceration of the mucous membrane, bronchospasm, and edema. Lipid-soluble gases, such as nitrous oxide and hydrogen chloride, are transported to the lower airways, where they damage lung tissue. There also may be thermal injury to the respiratory passages. Manifestations of inhalation injury include hoarseness, drooling and inability to handle secretions, hacking cough, and labored, shallow breathing. Serial blood gases show a fall in the partial pressure of arterial oxygen (PO_2). Signs of mucosal injury and airway obstruction often are delayed for 24 to 48 hours after a burn. Other pulmonary conditions, such as pneumonia, pulmonary embolism, or pneumothorax, may occur secondarily to the burn.

Hypermetabolic Response. The stress of burn injury increases metabolic and nutritional requirements. Secretion of stress-related hormones such as catecholamines and cortisol is increased in an effort to maintain homeostasis. Heat production is increased in an effort to balance heat losses from the burned area. Hypermetabolism, characterized by increased oxygen consumption, increased glucose use, and protein and fat wasting, is a characteristic response to burn trauma and infection. The hypermetabolic state peaks at approximately 7 to 17 days after the burn, and tissue breakdown diminishes as the wounds heal. Nutritional support is essential to recovery from burn injury. Enteral and parenteral hyperalimentation may be used during this time to deliver sufficient nutrients to prevent tissue breakdown and postburn weight loss.

Sepsis. Immunologically, the skin is the body's first line of defense. When the skin is no longer intact, the body is open to bacterial infection. Destruction of the skin also prevents the delivery of cellular components of the immune system to the site of injury. There also is loss of normal protective skin flora and a shift to colonization by more pathogenic flora. Thus, a significant complication of the acute phase of burn injury is sepsis. It may arise from the burn wound, pneumonia, urinary tract infection, infection elsewhere in the body, or the use of invasive procedures or monitoring devices. The burn site is an ideal growth area for microorganisms; the serum and debris provide nutrients, and the burn injury compromises blood flow.

Emergency and Long-Term Treatment

Regardless of the type of burn, the first step in any burn situation is to stop the burning process, cool the burn, provide pain relief, and cover the burn. Active cooling removes the heat and prevents progression of the burn. Immersion or irrigation with lukewarm water for at least 20 minutes can be extremely helpful. Immediate submersion is more important than removal of clothing, which may delay cooling the involved areas. The application of ice or cold water is not recommended because it can further limit blood flow to an area, turning a partial-thickness into a full-thickness burn.

Depending on the depth and extent of the burn, medical treatment may be necessary. Emergency care consists of resuscitation and stabilization with intravenous fluids while maintaining cardiac and respiratory function. Once hospitalized, the immediate treatment regimen focuses on continued maintenance of cardiorespiratory function, pain alleviation, wound care, and emotional support. After hemodynamic and pulmonary stability have been established, treatment is directed toward initial care of the wound. Treatment of the burn wound focuses on protection from desiccation and further injury of those burn areas that re-epithelialize in 7 to 10 days (superficial second-degree burns). "Nature's own blister" is the best protection for these burns. Topical antimicrobial preparations (e.g., silver sulfadiazine) and dressings are used to cover the wound when the blister has been broken. Wounds that will not heal spontaneously in 7 to 10 days (deep second-degree and third-degree burns) are usually treated by excision and skin grafts. The sloughed tissue, or *eschar*, produced by the burn is excised as soon as possible. This decreases the chance of infection and allows the skin to regenerate faster.

Burns that encircle the entire surface of the body or a body part (e.g., arms, legs, torso) can act as a tourniquet, causing major tissue damage to the muscles, tendons, and vascular under the area of the leathery burn eschar. These burns are called *circumferential burns*. The eschar is incised longitudinally (escharotomy), and sometimes a fasciotomy (surgical incision through the fascia of the muscle) is performed.

Systemic infection remains a leading cause of morbidity among persons with extensive burns. Continuous microbiologic surveillance is necessary; protective isolation measures are often instituted. There is an increasing trend toward use of prophylactic antibiotic treatment in persons with major burns.

Skin grafts are surgically implanted as soon as possible, often at the same time the burn tissue is excised, to promote new skin growth, limit fluid loss, and act as a dressing.[51] Skin grafts can be permanent or temporary, and split thickness or full thickness. Permanent skin grafts are used over newly excised tissue. Temporary skin grafts are used to cover a burned area until the tissue underneath it has healed. Various sources of skin grafts exist: *autograft* (skin obtained from the person's own body), *homograft* (skin obtained from another human being, alive or recently dead), and *heterograft* (skin obtained from another species, such as pigs). The best choice is autografting when there is enough uninterrupted skin on the person's body. The thickness of these grafts depends on the donor site and the needs of the burn patient. A *split-thickness skin graft* is one that includes the epidermis and part of the dermis.

A split-thickness skin graft can be sent through a skin mesher that cuts tiny slits into the skin, allowing it to expand up to nine times its original size. These grafts are used frequently because they can cover large surface areas and there is less autorejection. *Full-thickness skin grafts* include the entire thickness of the dermal layer. They are used primarily for reconstructive surgery or for small deep areas. The donor site of a full-thickness skin graft requires a split-thickness skin graft to help it heal.

Two-layered synthetic skin grafts, such as *Apligraf* or *Integra*, are composed of a layer of silicone, mimicking the properties of the epidermis, and a layer or matrix of fibers.[52] Skin cells attach to the fibers, enabling dermal skin growth. Once the dermal skin has regenerated, the silicone layer is removed and a thin epidermal skin graft is applied, thus requiring less skin grafting overall.

Other treatment measures include positioning, splinting, and physical therapy to prevent contractures and maintain muscle tone. Because the normal body response to disuse is flexion, the contractures that occur with a burn are disfiguring and cause loss of limb or appendage use. Once the wounds have healed sufficiently, elastic pressure garments, sometimes for the full body, often are used to prevent hypertrophic scarring.

Pressure Ulcers

Pressure ulcers are ischemic lesions of the skin and underlying structures caused by unrelieved pressure that impairs the flow of blood and lymph. Pressure ulcers often are referred to as decubitus ulcers or bedsores. The word decubitus comes from the Latin term meaning "lying down." However, a pressure ulcer may result from pressure exerted when seated or lying down. Pressure ulcers are most likely to develop over a bony prominence, but they may occur on any part of the body that is subjected to external pressure, friction, or shearing forces.

Approximately 2.2 million people in the United States develop pressure ulcers annually.[53] Several subpopulations are at particular risk, including persons with quadriplegia, elderly persons with restricted activity and hip fractures, and persons in the critical care setting.

Mechanisms of Development

Many factors contribute to the development of pressure ulcers, such as length of stay in the hospital, vasopressure infusion, spinal cord injury, age, and body mass index.[54] Pressure, shearing forces, friction, and moisture contribute to the incidence of pressure ulcers. External pressures that exceed capillary pressure interrupt blood flow in the capillary beds. When the pressure between a bony prominence and a support surface exceeds the normal capillary filling pressure, capillary flow essentially is obstructed. If this pressure is applied constantly for 2 hours, oxygen deprivation coupled with an accumulation of metabolic end products leads to irreversible tissue damage. While pressure magnitude and duration are important in the creation of a pressure ulcer, no specific amount of pressure necessary to compress capillaries and interrupt blood flow has been determined.[55] Tolerance to pressure loads differs according to tissue, location, and metabolism.[55] Persons with impaired circulation require less pressure to interrupt circulation. The same amount of pressure causes more damage when it is distributed over a small area than over a larger area.

Whether a person is sitting or lying down, the weight of the body is borne by tissues covering the bony prominences. Most pressure ulcers are located on the lower part of the body, such as the sacrum, the coccygeal area, the ischial tuberosities, and the greater trochanters. Pressure over a bony area is transmitted from the surface to the underlying dense bone, compressing all of the intervening tissue. As a result, the greatest pressure occurs at the surface of the bone and dissipates outward in a cone-like manner toward the surface of the skin (Fig. 46-19). Thus, extensive underlying tissue damage can be present when a small superficial skin lesion is first noticed.

Altering the distribution of pressure from one skin area to another prevents tissue injury. Pressure ulcers most commonly occur in persons with conditions such as spinal cord injury in which normal sensation and the ability to move to redistribute body weight are impaired. Normally, persons unconsciously shift their weight to redistribute pressure on the skin and underlying tissues. For example, during the night, people turn in their sleep, preventing ischemic injury of tissues that overlie the bony prominences that support the weight of the body; the same is true for sitting for any length of time.

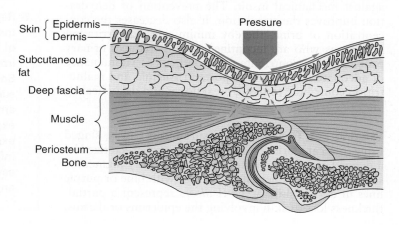

FIGURE 46-19. Pressure over a bony prominence compresses all intervening soft tissue, with a resulting wide, three-dimensional pressure gradient that causes various degrees of tissue damage. (From Shea JD. Pressure sores: classification and management. *Clin Orthop Relat Res.* 1975;112:90.)

The movements needed to shift the body weight are made unconsciously, and only when movement is restricted do people become aware of discomfort.

Shearing forces are caused by the sliding of one tissue layer over another with stretching and angulation of blood vessels, causing injury and thrombosis. Shear occurs when the skeleton moves, but the skin remains fixed to an external surface, such as occurs with transfer from a stretcher to a bed or pulling a person up in bed. The same thing happens when the head of the bed is elevated, causing the torso to move toward the foot of the bed while friction and moisture cause the skin to remain fixed to the bed linens. *Friction* contributes to pressure ulceration by damaging the skin at the epidermal–dermal interface. It occurs as persons who are bedridden use their elbows and heels to aid in movement. *Moisture* contributes to pressure ulcer formation by weakening the cell wall of individual skin cells and by changing the protective pH of the skin. This makes the skin more susceptible to pressure, shear, and friction injury.

Prevention and Treatment

The prevention of pressure ulcers is preferable to their treatment.[53] Preventive measures include identifying at-risk persons and the specific factors placing them at risk, maintaining and improving tissue tolerance to prevent injury, and protecting the skin and underlying tissue against the adverse effects of external mechanical forces (i.e., pressure, friction, shear). Risk factors contributing to the development of pressure ulcers are those related to sensory perception and the ability to respond meaningfully to pressure-related discomfort, level of skin moisture, urine and fecal continence, nutrition and hydration status, mobility, and circulatory status.

Prevention Methods. Methods for preventing pressure ulcers include frequent position changes, meticulous skin care, and frequent and careful observation to detect early signs of skin breakdown. Moisture macerates and injures skin. Sources of moisture include sweat, wound drainage, urine, and feces. Both urinary and fecal incontinence increase the risk of pressure ulcers. Food crumbs, intravenous tubing, and other debris in the bed can greatly increase local skin pressure points. Adequate hydration of the stratum corneum appears to protect the skin against mechanical insult. The prevention of dehydration improves the circulation. It also decreases the concentration of urine, thereby minimizing skin irritation in persons who are incontinent, and it reduces urinary problems that contribute to incontinence. Maintenance of adequate nutrition is important. Anemia and malnutrition contribute to tissue breakdown and delay healing after tissue injury has occurred.[56]

Staging and Treatment. Pressure ulcers can be staged using four categories.[57] *Stage I ulcers* are characterized by a defined area of persistent redness in lightly pigmented skin or an area of persistent redness with blue or purple hues in darker skin. *Stage II ulcers* represent a partial-thickness loss of skin involving the epidermis or dermis, or both. The ulcer is superficial and presents clinically as an abrasion, a blister, or a shallow crater. *Stage III ulcers* represent a full-thickness skin loss involving damage and necrosis of subcutaneous tissue that may extend down to but not through underlying fascia. The ulcer manifests as a deep crater with or without undermining of adjacent tissue. *Stage IV ulcers* involve full-thickness skin loss and necrosis with extensive destruction or damage to the underlying subcutaneous tissues that may extend to involve muscle, bone, and supporting structures (e.g., tendon or joint capsule).

After skin breakdown has occurred, special treatment measures are needed to prevent further ischemic damage, reduce bacterial contamination and infection, and promote healing. Treatment methods are selected based on the stage of the ulcer. Stage I ulcers usually are treated with frequent turning and measures to remove pressure. Stage II or III ulcers with little exudate are treated with semipermeable or occlusive dressings. Occlusive dressings are credited with preventing the loss of wound fluid and maintaining a moist environment that is necessary for epithelial cell migration. Wound fluid is thought to contain a variety of growth factors that enhance wound healing. Occlusive dressings may also relieve wound pain and prevent bacterial contamination. Several types of occlusive dressings are available, and each has advantages and disadvantages. Finally, vasopressure infusions may be important in the healing of pressure ulcers.[54]

Necrotic debris increases the possibility of bacterial infection and delays wound healing. Stage III ulcers with exudate and necrotic debris and stage IV ulcers usually require débridement (i.e., removal of necrotic tissue and eschar). This can be done surgically, with wet-to-dry dressings, or through the use of proteolytic enzymes. Stage IV wounds often require packing to obliterate dead space and are covered with nonadherent dressings. Stage IV ulcers may require surgical interventions, such as skin grafts or myocutaneous flaps.

SUMMARY CONCEPTS

- Because the skin covers the body, it is exposed to a number of potentially damaging agents in the external environment.

- Repeated exposure to the ultraviolet (UV) rays of the sun predisposes to sunburn, premature aging of the skin (wrinkling, degenerative changes, and irregularities in pigmentation), and skin cancer. Solar and artificial sources of UV radiation, such as from a tanning bed, contribute to the amount of radiation to which human beings are exposed. Sunburn, which is caused by excessive exposure to UV radiation, is an erythematous inflammatory reaction, ranging from mild to severe. Photosensitive drugs can also produce an exaggerated response to UV radiation when they are taken in combination with sun exposure. Sunscreens are protective agents that work by either reflecting sunlight or preventing its absorption.

■ Thermal injury can damage the skin and subcutaneous tissues, destroying the barrier function of the skin. The extent of injury is determined by the thickness of the burn and the total body surface area involved. Treatment methods vary with the severity of injury and include immediate resuscitation and maintenance of physiologic function, wound cleaning and débridement, application of antimicrobial agents and dressings, and skin grafting.

■ Pressure ulcers are ischemic lesions of the skin and underlying structures caused by unrelieved pressure that impairs the flow of blood and lymph. Pressure ulcers are divided into four stages, according to the depth of tissue involvement. The prevention of pressure ulcers is preferable to their treatment. The goals of prevention should include identifying at-risk persons along with the specific factors placing them at risk, maintaining and improving tissue tolerance to pressure to prevent injury, and protecting against the adverse effects of external mechanical forces (i.e., pressure, friction, and shear).

Nevi and Skin Cancers

Nevi, or moles, are common congenital or acquired tumors of the skin that are benign. However, some nevi can become malignant.

Nevi

Almost all adults have nevi, some in greater numbers than others. Nevi can be pigmented or nonpigmented, flat or elevated, and hairy or nonhairy.

Melanocytic nevi are pigmented skin lesions resulting from proliferation of melanocytes in the epidermis or dermis.[58] Melanocytic nevi are tan to deep brown, uniformly pigmented, small papules with well-defined, rounded borders (Fig. 46-20A). They are formed initially by melanocytes with their long dendritic extensions that are normally interspersed among the basal keratinocytes (see Chapter 45, Fig. 45-3). The melanocytes are transformed into round or oval melanin-containing cells that grow in nests or clusters along the dermal–epidermal junction. Because of their location, these lesions are called *junctional nevi* (see Fig. 46-20B). Most junctional nevi eventually grow into the surrounding dermis as nests or cords of cells. *Compound nevi* contain epidermal and dermal components. In older lesions, the epidermal nests may disappear entirely, leaving *dermal nevi*. Compound and dermal nevi usually are more elevated than junctional nevi.

Another form of nevus, the *dysplastic nevus*, is important because of its capacity to transform into malignant melanoma.[59,60] Dysplastic nevi are usually larger than other nevi (often >5 mm in diameter). Their appearance is a flat, slightly raised plaque with a pebbly surface, or a targetlike lesion with a darker, raised center and irregular border (Fig. 46-21). They vary in shade from brown and red to flesh tones. A person may have hundreds of these lesions. Although dysplastic nevi can give rise to melanoma, the vast majority are stable and never progress, suggesting that they are best viewed as markers for melanoma risk. Dysplastic nevi have been documented in multiple members of families prone to development of malignant melanoma.

Because of the possibility of malignant transformation, any mole that undergoes a change warrants immediate medical attention. Observe and report changes in size, thickness, or color; itching; and bleeding.

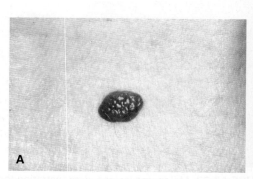
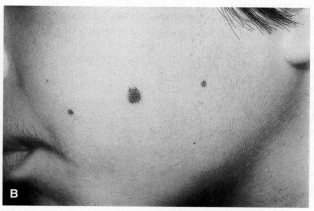

FIGURE 46-20. (A) Normal mole, with no different shades of brown, black, or tan. (From National Cancer Institute Visuals. No. AV-8809-4032. Courtesy of Skin Cancer Foundation.) **(B)** Junctional melanocytic nevi. These small, flat lesions are uniform in color. (From Goodheart HP. *Goodheart's Photoguide to Common Skin Disorders*. Philadelphia, PA: Wolters Kluwer Health | Lippincott Williams & Wilkins; 2009:364.)

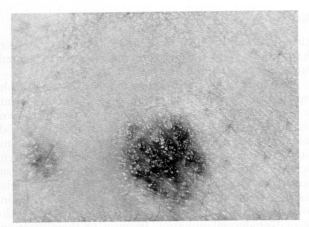

FIGURE 46-21. Dysplastic nevi. Lesion has a dark brown "pebbly" elevated surface against a lighter tan, macular background. The irregular, indistinct margin helps to distinguish it from the small congenital pattern nevus, which some dysplastic nevi closely resemble. Its distinct morphology, rather than its size (6 × 6 mm), identifies it as a dysplastic nevus (From National Cancer Institute Visuals. No. AV-8500-3696.)

Skin Cancer

Skin cancer represents the most common malignancy in white-skinned people in the Western world.[61] The majority of skin cancers are nonmelanomas, either basal cell or squamous cell carcinoma, which are not associated with a high risk of morbidity or mortality. Although malignant melanoma represents a small subset of skin cancers, it is the most deadly. In 2009 61,646 people in the United States were diagnosed with malignant melanoma—35,436 men and 26,210 women.[61] In the United States, 9199 people also died from melanomas of the skin (5992 men and 3207 women).[61] The rising incidence of melanoma and other skin cancers has been attributed to increased sun exposure associated with social and lifestyle changes.[62]

The factors linking sun exposure to skin cancer are not completely understood, but both total cumulative exposure and altered patterns of exposure are strongly implicated. Basal cell and squamous cell carcinomas are often associated with total cumulative exposure to UV radiation. Thus, basal cell and squamous cell carcinomas occur more commonly on maximally sun-exposed parts of the body, such as the face and back of the hands and forearms. Melanomas occur most commonly on areas of the body that are exposed to the sun intermittently, such as the back in men and the lower legs in women.[62] They are more common in persons with indoor occupations whose exposure to sun is limited to weekends and vacations. Excessive childhood sun exposure is an important risk factor for melanoma, particularly blistering sunburns.[63]

Malignant Melanoma

Malignant melanoma is a cancerous tumor of the melanocytes.[64,65] It is a rapidly progressing, metastatic form of cancer. The dramatic increase in the incidence of

malignant melanoma over the past several decades has been credited to increased UV light exposure, including tanning salons. Other risk factors include a family history of malignant melanoma, fair hair and skin, tendency to freckle, and a history of blistering sunburns as a child. Still other significant risk factors for melanoma are atypical moles/dysplastic nevus syndrome, immunosuppression, and prior PUVA therapy.

Roughly 90% of malignant melanomas in whites occur on sun-exposed skin. However, in darker-skinned people melanomas often occur on non–sun-exposed areas, such as the mucous membranes and subungual, palmar, and plantar surfaces. Malignant melanomas differ in size and shape. Usually, they are slightly raised and black or brown. Borders are irregular and surfaces are uneven. Most appear to arise from preexisting nevi or new molelike growths (Fig. 46-22). There may be surrounding erythema, inflammation, and tenderness. Periodically, melanomas ulcerate and bleed. Dark melanomas are often mottled with shades of red, blue, and white. These three colors represent three concurrent processes: melanoma growth (blue), inflammation and the body's attempt to localize and destroy the tumor (red), and scar tissue formation (white).

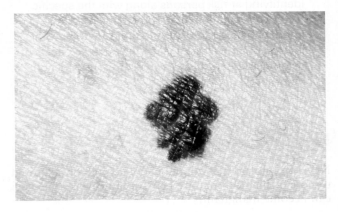

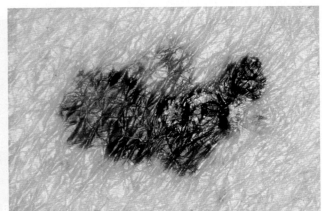

FIGURE 46-22. Melanoma lesions, demonstrating the ABCD rule: A (asymmetry), B (irregular borders), C (different colors), and D (diameter change in size). (From National Cancer Institute Visuals. Nos. AV-8809-4036, AV-8809-4037. Courtesy of Skin Cancer Foundation.)

Pathogenesis. Four types of melanomas have been identified based on their radial and vertical growth progression: lentigo maligna, superficial spreading, acral lentiginous, and nodular. Radial growth describes the horizontal spread of the melanoma within the epidermis and superficial dermis. During this initial stage, the tumor seems to lack the ability to metastasize. Lentigo maligna melanomas, superficial spreading melanomas, and acral lentiginous melanomas are tumors that are in the radial growth phase. *Lentigo maligna melanomas* are flat, slow-growing nevi that may remain in the radial growth phase for several decades. They are seen primarily on sun-exposed skin of elderly persons. *Superficial spreading melanoma,* the most common type of melanoma, is seen most commonly in persons who sunburn easily and have intermittent sun exposure. It is characterized by a raised-edged nevus with lateral growth and a disorderly appearance in color and outline. It typically ulcerates and bleeds with growth. *Acral lentiginous melanoma* has an appearance similar to that of lentigo maligna, and is seen primarily on the palms, soles, nail beds, and mucous membranes. Its occurrence is unrelated to sun exposure.

After a variable and unpredictable period of time, melanomas shift from a radial to vertical growth phase, during which the tumor cells invade downward into the deeper dermis layers.[11] This growth phase is heralded by the nodular phase and correlates with the emergence of a clone of cells with metastatic potential. *Nodular melanomas* are raised, dome-shaped lesions that can occur anywhere on the body. They are commonly a uniform blue-black color and tend to look like blood blisters. Nodular melanomas tend to rapidly invade the dermis from the start, with no apparent horizontal growth phase.

Diagnosis and Treatment. Early detection is critical with malignant melanoma. Regular self-examination of the total skin surface in front of a well-lighted mirror provides a method for early detection. It requires that a person undress completely and examine all areas of the body using a full mirror, handheld mirror, and handheld hair dryer (to examine the scalp). An *ABCD* rule has been developed to aid in early diagnosis and timely treatment of malignant melanoma.[64] The ABCD acronym stands for *a*symmetry, *b*order irregularity, *c*olor variegation, and *d*iameter greater than 6 mm (1/4 inch or pencil eraser size). People should be taught to watch for these changes in existing nevi or the development of new nevi, as well as other alterations such as bleeding or itching. Because of the existence of small-diameter melanomas (i.e., <6 mm in diameter), it has been suggested that people routinely screen their skin for all possible manifestations of skin cancer. Since their description over 20 years ago, evidence has accumulated to add an E for "evolving" to the ABCD rule.[68] The E for evolving is intended to encourage the recognition of melanomas at an earlier stage by emphasizing the dynamic nature of their growth.

Diagnosis of melanoma is based on biopsy findings from a lesion.[64–66] Because most melanomas initially metastasize to regional lymph nodes, additional information may be obtained through lymph node biopsy. Consistent with other cancerous tumors, melanoma is commonly staged using the TNM (tumor, lymph node, and metastasis) staging system (see Chapter 7) or the American Joint Committee on Cancer Staging System for Cutaneous Melanoma, in which the tumor is rated 0 to 4 depending on numerous factors, including extent of tumor invasion, ulceration, and metastasis.[64] Ulceration and invasion of the tumor into the deeper skin tissue result in a poorer prognosis. The degree and number of lymph nodes involved correlate well with overall survival.

Treatment of melanoma is usually surgical excision, the extent of which is determined by the thickness of the lesion, invasion into the deeper skin layers, and spread to the regional lymph nodes.[64–66] Deep, wide excisions with elective removal of lymph tissue and the use of skin grafts were once the hallmarks of treatment. When diagnosed in a premetastatic phase, melanoma is now treated in ambulatory settings, lessening the cost and inconvenience of care. Current capability allows for mapping lymph flow to a regional lymph node that receives lymphatic drainage from tumor sites on the skin. This lymph node, which is called the *sentinel lymph node,* is then sampled for biopsy. If tumor cells have spread from the primary tumor to the regional lymph nodes, the sentinel node will be the first node in which tumor cells appear. Therefore, sentinel node biopsy can be used to test for the presence of melanoma cells and determine if radical lymph node dissection is necessary. When nodes are positive, consideration is also given to systemic adjuvant therapy. Although no effective chemotherapy is available for melanoma, interferon alfa-2b is a biologic therapy available for adjuvant treatment of melanoma. At this time, however, the use of interferon is controversial. Clinical trials with other therapies, including combination chemotherapies, vaccines, and hyperthermic isolation limb perfusion, are ongoing.[64–66]

Basal Cell Carcinoma

Basal cell carcinoma is a neoplasm of the nonkeratinizing cells of the basal layer of the epidermis.[67] It is the most common invasive cancer in humans; approximately 75% of all skin cancers are basal cell carcinomas.[67] Basal cell carcinomas have a tendency to occur in fair-skinned persons with a history of significant long-term sun exposure. They are most frequently seen on the head and neck, most often occurring on skin that has hair.

Basal cell carcinomas are slow-growing tumors that extend wide and deep if left untreated, but rarely metastasize. Advanced lesions are often invasive and ulcerative. Risk factors for extensive spread include a tumor diameter greater than 2 cm, location on the central part of the face or ears, long-standing duration, incomplete excision, and perineural or perivascular involvement.

Histologically, the tumor cells resemble those in the normal basal layer from the epidermis or follicular epithelium and do not occur on mucosal surfaces.[67]

There are two types of basal cell carcinoma, determined by their pattern of growth: superficial basal cell carcinomas originating from the epidermis and extending upward, and nodular basal cell carcinomas in which the tumor grows downward into the dermis. *Nodular basal cell carcinoma,* the classic type, presents as a small, flesh-colored or pink, smooth, translucent nodule that enlarges over time (Fig. 46-23). Telangiectatic vessels frequently are seen beneath the surface. Over the years, there is a central depression that forms and develops into an ulcer surrounded by the original shiny, waxy border. *Superficial basal cell carcinoma* presents as a scaly erythematous patch or plaque. Both nodular and superficial forms may contain melanin, imparting a brown, blue, or black color to the lesions.

Since basal cell carcinoma is highly curable if detected and treated early, all suspected lesions should undergo biopsy for diagnosis. The treatment depends on the site and extent of the lesion. The most important treatment goal is complete elimination of the lesion. Also important is the maintenance of function and optimal cosmetic effect. Curettage with electrodesiccation, surgical excision, irradiation, laser, cryosurgery, and chemosurgery are effective in removing all cancerous cells. Immune therapy, gene therapy, and photodynamic therapy are emerging treatments. Persons should be checked at regular intervals for recurrences.

Squamous Cell Carcinoma

Squamous cell carcinomas are the second most common malignant tumors arising on sun-exposed sites in older people, exceeded only by basal cell carcinoma. In addition to sun exposure, occupational exposure to arsenic (i.e., Bowen disease), industrial tars, coal, and paraffin increase the risk for squamous cell carcinoma. Men are twice as likely as women to have squamous cell carcinoma. Black persons are rarely affected.

Squamous cell cancers are composed of tumor cells that resemble the epidermal cells of the stratum spinosum to varying degrees and extend into the adjacent dermis.[68] There are two types of squamous cell carcinomas: intraepidermal (termed in situ carcinoma) and invasive carcinoma. *Intraepidermal squamous cell carcinoma* remains confined to the epidermis for a long time. However, at some unpredictable time, it penetrates the basement membrane to the dermis and metastasizes to the regional lymph nodes. It then converts to *invasive squamous cell carcinoma.* The invasive type of squamous cell carcinoma can develop from intraepidermal carcinoma or from a premalignant lesion (e.g., actinic keratoses). It may be slow growing or fast growing with metastasis.

Squamous cell carcinoma is a red, scaling, keratotic, slightly elevated lesion with an irregular border, usually with a shallow chronic ulcer (Fig. 46-24). The lesions usually lack the pearly rolled border and superficial

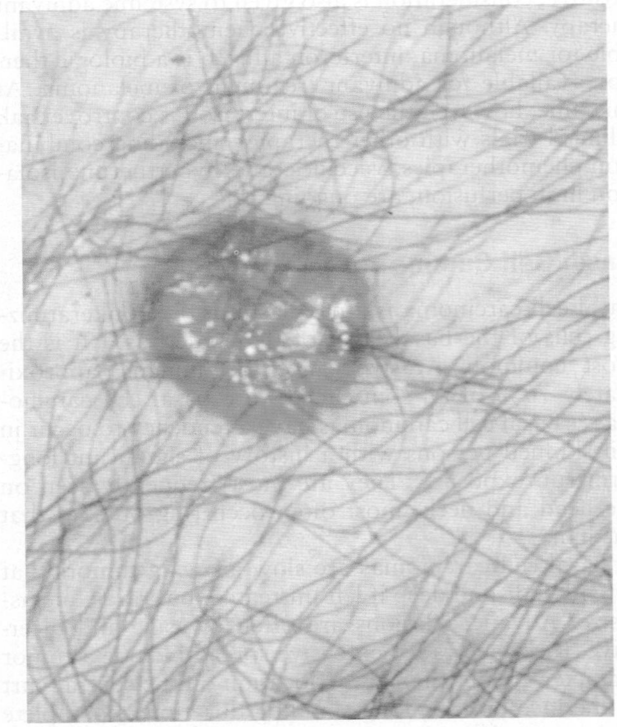

FIGURE 46-23. Nodular basal cell carcinoma, which presents as a reddish-brown papule, often with telangiectatic blood vessels, and a central depression with rolled borders. (From National Cancer Institute Visuals. No. AV-8500-3608.)

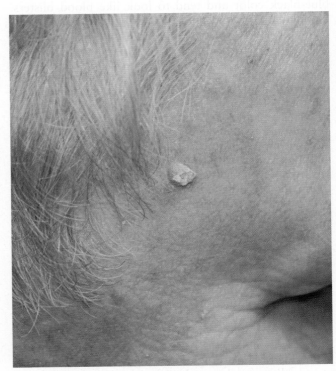

FIGURE 46-24. Squamous cell carcinoma as manifested by a raised lesion of the skin of the face. (From National Cancer Institute Visuals. No. AV-CDR728323. Courtesy of Kelly Nelson, photographer.)

telangiectases found on basal cell carcinomas. Later, lesions grow outward, show large ulcerations, and have persistent crusts and raised erythematous borders. The lesions occur on sun-exposed areas of the skin, particularly the nose, forehead, helix of the ear, lower lip, and back of the hand. Invasive squamous cell carcinoma has the potential to recur and metastasize. Chief among the risk factors for tumor recurrence and metastasis are the size and location of the tumor.[70] Large lesions (>2 cm in diameter), tumors of the lip and ear, tumors arising in injured or chronically diseased skin, and rapidly growing lesions are at particular risk.

Treatment measures are aimed at the removal of all cancerous tissue using methods such as electrosurgery, excision surgery, chemosurgery, or radiation therapy. After treatment, the person is observed for the remainder of his or her life for signs of recurrence.

SUMMARY CONCEPTS

■ Nevi or moles usually are benign neoplasms of the skin. Because they may undergo cancerous transformation, any mole that changes warrants immediate medical attention.

■ Repeated exposure to the UV rays of the sun has been implicated as the principal cause of skin cancer.

■ The melanocytes, which protect against sunburn through increased production of melanin, are particularly vulnerable to the adverse effects of unprotected exposure to ultraviolet light. Malignant melanoma, which is a cancerous tumor of melanocytes, is a rapidly progressive and metastatic form of skin cancer. The most important clinical sign is the change in size, shape, and color of pigmented skin lesions, such as moles. As the result of increased public awareness, melanomas are now more likely to be diagnosed at an earlier stage, when they can be cured surgically.

■ Basal cell carcinoma, which is a neoplasm of the nonkeratinizing cells of the basal layer of the epidermis, is the most common skin cancer in light-skinned people. It is slow-growing and rarely metastasizes.

■ Squamous cell tumors resemble the epidermal cells of the stratum spinosum to varying degrees and extend into the adjacent dermis. Squamous cell carcinoma may remain confined to the epidermis for a period of time, but at some unpredictable time, it becomes invasive and metastasizes to the regional lymph nodes. Chief among the risk factors for tumor invasion and metastasis are the size and location of the tumor.

Age-Related Skin Conditions

Some skin problems occur in specific age groups. These include not only birthmarks, but also disorders characteristic of childhood, as well as skin changes common in the elderly.

Skin Manifestations of Infancy and Childhood

Infancy connotes the image of perfect, unblemished skin. For the most part, this is true. However, several acquired skin conditions, including diaper dermatitis, prickly heat, and cradle cap, are relatively common in infants. Moreover, congenital skin lesions, such as Mongolian spots, hemangiomas, and nevi, are associated with the neonatal period, and many childhood infections are commonly accompanied by skin changes.

Skin Disorders of Infancy

Throughout infancy, the skin is especially sensitive to irritation from harsh chemicals, humidity, and heat.

Diaper Dermatitis. Irritant diaper dermatitis, or *diaper rash*, is a form of contact dermatitis caused by the interaction of several factors, including prolonged contact of the skin with a mixture of urine and feces. The appearance of diaper rash ranges from simple (i.e., widely distributed macules on the buttocks and anogenital areas) to severe (i.e., beefy, red, excoriated skin surfaces in the diaper area). Secondary infections with bacteria and yeasts are common; discomfort may be marked because of intense inflammation. Such conditions as contact dermatitis, seborrheic dermatitis, candidiasis, and atopic dermatitis should be considered when the eruption is persistent and recalcitrant to simple therapeutic measures.

Diaper dermatitis often responds to simple measures, including frequent diaper changes with careful cleansing of the irritated area to remove all waste products. Feces in particular should be removed from the skin as soon as possible after the diaper has been soiled. Because soap and lipid solvents remove protective lipids from the stratum corneum, using water or an alcohol-free baby wipe is recommended. Exposing the irritated area to air is helpful. It has been shown that application of a barrier ointment after each diaper change is a valuable component of therapy. Topical corticosteroid therapy is usually effective, but should be used cautiously because infants absorb proportionately greater quantities through their skin than adults. Antifungal therapy should not be used routinely, but can be helpful when *Candida* infection is established or suspected. Antibacterial agents should not be used because bacterial infections are rarely involved in diaper dermatitis, and the normal microflora should be preserved.

Intractable and severe cases of diaper dermatitis should be seen by a health care provider for treatment of any secondary infections. Secondary candidal or other skin manifestations discussed in this chapter may occur in the diaper area. It is important to differentiate between normal diaper dermatitis and more serious skin problems.

Prickly Heat. Prickly heat (heat rash) results from constant maceration of the skin because of prolonged exposure to a warm, humid environment. Maceration leads to midepidermal obstruction and rupture of the sweat glands. Although commonly seen during infancy, prickly heat may occur at any age. The treatment includes removing excessive clothing, cooling the skin with warm water baths, drying the skin with powders, and avoiding hot, humid environments.

Cradle Cap. Cradle cap is a greasy crust or scale formation on the scalp. It usually is attributed to infrequent and inadequate washing of the scalp. Cradle cap is treated using mild shampoo and gentle combing to remove the scales. Sometimes oil can be left on the head for minutes to several hours, softening the scales before scrubbing. Other emulsifying ointments or creams may be helpful in difficult cases. The scalp may need to be rubbed firmly to remove the buildup of keratinized cells. Recalcitrant cases need to be seen by a health care provider; serious or chronic forms of seborrheic dermatitis may exist.

Pigmented and Vascular Birthmarks

Pigmented birthmarks represent abnormal migration or proliferation of melanocytes. For example, *Mongolian spots* are caused by selective pigmentation. They usually occur on the buttocks or sacral area and are seen commonly in Asian and black persons. *Nevi* or moles are small, tan to brown, uniformly pigmented solid macules. *Melanocytic nevi* are formed initially from aggregates of melanocytes and keratinocytes along the dermal–epidermal border. *Congenital melanocytic nevi* are collections of melanocytes that are present at birth or develop within the first year of life. They present as macular, papular, or plaquelike pigmented lesions of various shades of brown, with a black or blue focus. The texture of the lesions varies and they may be with or without hair. They usually are found on the hands, shoulders, buttocks, entire arm, or trunk of the body. Some involve large areas of the body in garmentlike fashion. They usually grow proportionately with the child. Congenital melanocytic nevi are clinically significant because of their association with malignant melanoma.

Vascular birthmarks are cutaneous anomalies of angiogenesis and vascular development.[69] Two types of vascular birthmarks commonly are seen in infants and small children: bright red, raised hemangiomas of infancy and flat, reddish-purple port-wine stains.

Hemangiomas of infancy (formerly called *strawberry hemangiomas*) are small, red lesions that are noticed shortly after birth.[69] Hemangiomas of infancy are generally benign vascular tumors produced by prolifera-

tion of endothelial cells. They are seen in approximately 10% of children in the 1st year of life, with about 60% being located on the head and neck.[69] Although they can occur anywhere on the body, they can be life-threatening when they occur in the airway. Approximately 30% of these lesions are present at birth while the remainder develop within a few weeks after birth.[69] Hemangiomas of infancy typically undergo an early period of proliferation during which they enlarge, followed by a period of slow involution during which the growth is reversed until complete resolution occurs. Most hemangiomas of infancy disappear before 5 to 9 years of age without leaving an appreciable scar. A small percentage of hemangiomas develop complications. Ulceration, the most frequent complication, can be painful and carries the risk of infection, hemorrhage, and scarring. Some hemangiomas are located in anatomic regions associated with other anomalies requiring careful monitoring and early intervention.

Port-wine stains are pink or red patches that can occur anywhere on the body and are very noticeable (Fig. 46-25). They represent slow-growing capillary malformations that grow proportionately with the child and persist throughout life.[69] There is progressive dilation of the dermal capillaries, which initially is confined to the immediate epidermis, with gradual involvement of deeper dermal blood vessels, although the greater number is always in the upper dermis. Distribution of lesions on the face roughly corresponds to the sensory branches of the trigeminal nerve. Port-wine stains usually are confined to the skin, but may be associated with vascular malformations of the eye, resulting primarily in glaucoma, or leptomeningeal involvement, leading to cognitive disorders, seizures, and other neurologic deficits (Sturge-Weber syndrome). Cover-up cosmetics are useful in concealing the stains. Laser surgery has revolutionized the treatment of port-wine stains.

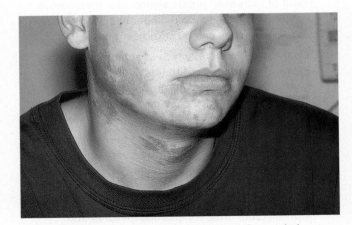

FIGURE 46-25. Port-wine stain on the face. Congenital malformation of blood vessels. Usually appears at birth. (From Goodheart HP. *Goodheart's Photoguide to Common Skin Disorders.* Philadelphia, PA: Wolters Kluwer Health | Lippincott Williams & Wilkins; 2009:521.)

Skin Manifestations of Common Infectious Diseases

Infectious childhood diseases that produce rashes include roseola infantum, rubella, rubeola, and varicella. Because these diseases are seen less frequently than in the past because of successful immunization programs and the use of antibiotics, they may be misdiagnosed or their diagnosis may be delayed.

Roseola Infantum. Roseola infantum (exanthem subitum or sixth disease) is a contagious disease caused by human herpes virus type 6 (HHV-6).[70] Because HHV-6 is the etiologic agent, the condition is often referred to as *sixth disease*. Primary HHV-6 infection occurs early in life. More than 95% of roseola cases occur in children younger than 3 years of age, with a peak at 6 to 15 months of age.[70] Transplacental antibodies likely protect most infants until 6 months of age. Roseola produces a characteristic maculopapular rash covering the trunk and spreading to the appendages. The rash is preceded by an abrupt onset of high fever ($\leq$105°F), inflamed tympanic membranes, and coldlike symptoms usually lasting 3 to 4 days. These symptoms improve at approximately the same time the rash appears. Because infants with roseola exhibit a unique constellation of symptoms over a short time, the infection may be confused with other childhood illnesses. Blood antibody titers may be taken to determine the actual diagnosis. In most cases, there are no long-term effects from this disease. Infants who spike high temperatures should be seen by their health care providers.

Rubella. Rubella (i.e., 3-day measles or German measles) is a childhood disease caused by the rubella virus. It is characterized by a diffuse, punctate, macular rash that begins on the trunk and spreads to the arms and legs (Fig. 46-26). Mild febrile states occur (usually <100°F). Postauricular, suboccipital, and cervical lymph node adenopathy is common. Coldlike symptoms usually accompany the disease in the form of cough, congestion, and coryza (i.e., nasal discharge).

Rubella usually has no long-lasting sequelae; however, the transmission of the disease to pregnant women early in their gestation periods may result in congenital rubella syndrome. Among the clinical signs of congenital rubella syndrome are cataracts, microcephaly, mental retardation, deafness, patent ductus arteriosus, glaucoma, purpura, and bone defects. Most states have laws requiring immunization to prevent transmission of rubella. Immunization is accomplished by live-virus injection. Rubella vaccination has close to a 100% immunity response in treated children. Many states require a second preschool or later dose of rubella vaccine to increase immunity. Cases and outbreaks of rubella occur in the United States, especially among foreign-born unvaccinated adults.

Rubeola. Rubeola (measles, 7-day measles) is an acute, highly communicable viral disease caused by a morbillivirus.[71] The characteristic rash is macular and blotchy;

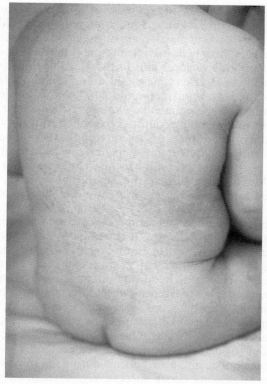

FIGURE 46-26. Rash of rubella on a child's back. Distribution is similar to measles (rubeola), but not as intense. (From the Centers for Disease Control and Prevention Public Health Image Library. No. 712.)

sometimes the macules become confluent (Fig. 46-27). The rubeola rash usually begins on the face and spreads to the appendages. There are several accompanying symptoms: a fever of 100°F or greater, *Koplik spots* (i.e., small, irregular red spots with a bluish-white speck

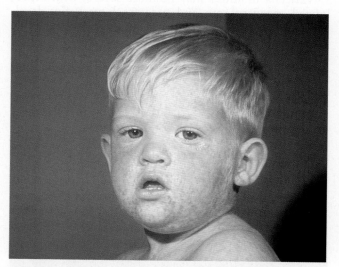

FIGURE 46-27. Child with measles (rubeola) showing the characteristic conjunctivitis, coryza, and red, blotchy rash that appear around day 3 of illness, first on the face and then becoming more generalized. (From the Centers for Disease Control and Prevention Public Health Image Library. No. 1150.)

in the center) on the buccal mucosa, and mild to severe photosensitivity. The person commonly has coldlike symptoms, general malaise, and myalgia. In severe cases, the macules may hemorrhage into the skin tissue or onto the outer body surface. This form is called *hemorrhagic measles*. The course of measles is more severe in infants, adults, and malnourished children. The World Health Organization recommends vitamin A treatment for measles in developing countries to reduce morbidity and mortality. There may be severe complications, including otitis media, pneumonia, and encephalitis. Antibody titers are determined for a conclusive diagnosis of rubeola. Measles is a disease preventable by vaccine, and immunization is required by law in the United States.

Varicella. Varicella (chickenpox) is a common communicable childhood disease. It is caused by the varicellazoster virus, which also is the agent in herpes zoster (shingles). The characteristic skin lesion occurs in three stages: macule, vesicle, and granular scab. The macular stage is characterized by development within hours of macules over the trunk, spreading to the limbs, buccal mucosa, scalp, axillae, upper respiratory tract, and conjunctiva (Fig. 46-28). During the second stage, the macules form vesicles with depressed centers. The vesicles break open and a scab forms during the third stage. Crops of lesions occur successively, so that all three forms of the lesion usually are visible by the 3rd day of the illness.

Mild to extreme pruritus accompanies the lesions, which can lead to scratching and subsequent development of secondary bacterial infections. Chickenpox also is accompanied by coldlike symptoms, including cough, coryza, and sometimes photosensitivity. Mild febrile states usually occur, typically beginning 24 hours before lesion outbreak. Side effects, such as pneumonia, septic complications, and encephalitis, are rare.

Varicella in adults may be more severe, with a prolonged recovery rate and greater chances for development of varicella pneumonitis or encephalitis.

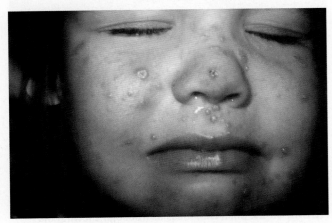

FIGURE 46-28. Blisterlike lesions of varicella (i.e., chickenpox) on the face of a young child. (From the Centers for Disease Control and Prevention Public Health Image Library. No. 10486. Courtesy of John Noble, Jr.)

Immunocompromised persons may experience a chronic, painful form of the infection.

Despite breakthrough cases and lower efficacy rates overall than in other vaccines, live attenuated varicella vaccine has been demonstrated to have dramatically decreased varicella morbidity and mortality since 1995, when the vaccine was introduced in the United States.[72] The vaccine is most effective in children under 10 years of age.[72] One dose of the vaccine is required by law in the United States; however, a second dose is now recommended to address what is called *primary vaccine failure*. It is believed that a single dose of varicella vaccine may only prime the host response, without inducing protective immunity. Outbreaks of mild cases of varicella, called *breakthrough varicella*, have occurred in vaccinated populations. The breakthrough infection is difficult to diagnose because the maculopapular rash does not have the classic sign of vesicles.

Skin Manifestations and Disorders in the Elderly

Elderly persons experience a variety of age-related skin disorders and exacerbations of earlier skin problems. Aging skin is believed to involve a complex process of actinic (solar) damage, normal aging, and hormonal influences. Actinic changes primarily involve increased occurrence of lesions on sun-exposed surfaces of the body.

Normal Age-Related Changes

Normal skin changes associated with aging are seen on areas of the body that have not been exposed to the sun. They include thinning of the dermis and the epidermis, diminution in subcutaneous tissue, a decrease and thickening of blood vessels, and a decrease in the number of melanocytes, Langerhans cells, and Merkel cells. The keratinocytes shrink, but the number of dead keratinized cells at the surface increases. This results in less padding and thinner skin, with color and elasticity changes. The skin also loses its resistance to environmental and mechanical trauma. Tissue repair takes longer.

With aging, there is also less hair and nail growth, and there is permanent hair pigment loss. Hormonally, there is less sebaceous gland activity, although the glands in the facial skin may increase in size. Hair growth reduction also may be hormonally influenced. Although the reason is poorly understood, the skin in most elderly persons older than 70 years of age becomes dry, rough, scaly, and itchy. When there is no underlying pathologic process, it is called *senile pruritus*. Itching and dryness become worse during the winter, when the need for home heating lowers the humidity.

The aging of skin, however, is not just a manifestation of age itself. Most skin changes associated with the elderly are the result of cumulative actinic or environmental damage. For example, the wrinkled, leathery look of aged skin, as well as odd scars and ecchymotic spots, are due to solar elastotic degenerative change.

Skin Lesions Common Among the Elderly

Among the most common benign skin lesions in the elderly are skin tags, seborrheic keratoses, solar lentigines, and vascular lesions. Most are actinic manifestations; they occur as a result of exposure to sun and weather over the years.

Skin Tags. *Skin tags* are soft, brown, or flesh-colored papules. They occur on any skin surface, but most frequently the neck, axilla, and intertriginous areas. They range in size from a pinhead to the size of a pea. Skin tags have the normal texture of the skin. They are benign and can be removed with scissors or electrodesiccation for cosmetic purposes.

Seborrheic Keratosis. A keratosis is a circumscribed overgrowth of the horny layer of keratinocytes. *Seborrheic keratoses* are common benign tumors that arise spontaneously and are particularly numerous on the trunk, although they can also occur on the extremities, head, and neck. In people of color, multiple small lesions on the face are termed dermatoses papulosa nigra. The lesions characteristically appear as round, flat, coin-shaped waxy plaques that vary in diameter from a few millimeters to several centimeters in diameter.[73] Seborrheic keratoses are benign, but they must be watched for changes in color, texture, or size, which may indicate malignant transformation.

Actinic Keratoses. *Actinic keratoses* are the most common premalignant skin lesions that develop on sun-exposed areas. The lesions usually are less than 1 cm in diameter and appear as dry, brown, scaly areas, often with a reddish tinge (Fig. 46-29). Actinic keratoses often are multiple and more easily felt than seen. They often are indistinguishable from squamous cell carcinoma without biopsy. Actinic keratoses may accumulate dense scale on the surface of the skin and become hyperkeratotic (i.e., developing cutaneous growths of fingernail-type tissue that grow into hornlike appendages). This form is more prominent and palpable. Often, there is a weathered appearance to the surrounding skin. Slight changes, such as enlargement or ulceration, may indicate malignant transformation. Roughly 20% of actinic keratoses convert to squamous cell carcinomas. There is controversy regarding the classification of actinic keratoses. Most experts agree that they are capable of converting to cancerous growths; however, some believe that actinic keratoses do not convert or progress to cancerous cells, but that they are actual early malignancies.[73]

Actinic keratoses are removed with cryosurgery, electrodesiccation, or lasers. When surgery is not indicated, they are treated with topical chemotherapy agents, such as 5-fluorouracil or imiquimod creams, which erode the lesions.

Solar Lentigines. Also referred to as *liver spots*, solar lentigines are small (5- to 10-mm), benign, oval or round, tan-brown macules or patches resulting from localized hyperplasia of melanocytes. *Solar lentigines* gradually appear on sun-exposed areas, particularly the dorsum of the hand. They do not fade with cessation of sun exposure. Like all pigmented lesions, they should be evaluated. If the pigmentation is homogenous and they are symmetric and flat, they are most likely benign. Solar lentigines can be treated with a topical bleaching agent such as hydroquinone (e.g., Eldoquin, Solaquin), laser therapy, or cryotherapy.

Lentigo maligna (i.e., Hutchinson freckle) is a slowly progressive preneoplastic disorder of melanocytes, also referred to as lentigo maligna melanoma in situ. It occurs on sun-exposed areas, particularly the face. The lesion is a pigmented macule with an irregular border and grows to 5 cm or sometimes larger. As it grows over the years, it may become slightly raised and wartlike. If untreated, a true malignant melanoma often develops. Surgery, curettage, and cryotherapy have been effective at removing the lentigines. Careful monitoring for conversion to melanoma is important.

Vascular Lesions. Vascular lesions include angiomas, telangiectases, and venous lakes. *Cherry angiomas* are smooth, cherry-red or purple, dome-shaped papules that occur in nearly all people older than 30 years of age. They usually are found on the trunk and are generally benign unless there is a sudden appearance of many cherry angiomas. *Telangiectases* are single, dilated blood vessels, capillaries, or terminal arteries that appear on areas exposed to sun or harsh weather, such as the cheeks and the nose. They occur individually or in clusters, measure 1 cm or less, are nonpalpable, and easily blanch. They can become large and disfiguring. Pulsed dye lasers have been effective in removing them. *Venous lakes* are small, dark blue, slightly raised papules. They occur on exposed body parts, particularly the backs of the hands, ears, and lips. They are smooth and compressible. Venous lakes can be removed by electrosurgery, laser therapy, or surgical excision if desired.

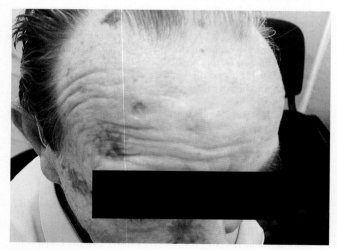

FIGURE 46-29. Nonhyperkeratotic actinic keratosis of scalp, forehead, and cheek in a 74-year-old man. (From Sanmartin O, Guillen C. Fluorescence diagnosis of subclinical actinic keratosis. *N Eng J Med.* 2008;358(19):e21. Copyright © 2008. Massachusetts Medical Society.)

SUMMARY CONCEPTS

■ Some skin problems occur in specific age groups. Common in infants are diaper rash, prickly heat, and cradle cap. Nevi, hemangiomas, and port-wine stains may be present at birth. Infectious childhood diseases that are characterized by rashes include roseola infantum, rubella, rubeola, and varicella. Vaccines are available to protect against rubella, rubeola, and varicella.

■ With aging, there is thinning of the dermis and the epidermis, diminution in subcutaneous tissue, loss and thickening of blood vessels, and slowing of hair and nail growth. Dry skin is common among the elderly, becoming worse during the winter months. Among the skin lesions seen in the elderly are skin tags, keratoses, lentigines, and vascular lesions.

REVIEW EXERCISES

1. The mother of a 7-year-old boy notices that he is scratching his head frequently. On close examination she notices a grayish, round, and roughened area where the hair has broken off. Examination by the child's pediatrician produces a diagnosis of tinea capitis.

   A. Explain the cause of the infection and propose possible mechanisms for spread of this infection in school-age children, particularly during winter months.
   B. Referring to Chapter 14, explain the preference of the superficial mycoses (dermatophytoses) for the skin-covered areas of the body.
   C. What methods are commonly used in the diagnosis of superficial fungal infections?

2. A 75-year-old woman presents with severe burning pain and a vesicular rash covering a strip over the rib cage on one side of the chest. She is diagnosed with herpes zoster or shingles.

   A. What is the source of this woman's rash and pain?
   B. Explain the dermatomal distribution of the lesions.

3. Psoriasis is a chronically recurring papulosquamous skin disorder, characterized by circumscribed red, thickened plaques with an overlying silvery-white scale.

   A. Explain the development of the plaques in terms of epidermal cell turnover.
   B. Persons with psoriasis are instructed to refrain from rubbing or scratching the lesions. Explain the rationale for these instructions.
   C. Among the methods used in the treatment of psoriasis are the use of topical keratolytic agents and corticosteroid skin preparations. Explain how these two different types of agents exert their effect on the plaque lesions.

4. During the past several decades there has been an alarming increase in the incidence of skin cancers, including malignant melanoma, that has been attributed to increased sun exposure.

   A. Explain the possible mechanisms whereby ultraviolet radiation promotes the development of malignant skin lesions.
   B. Cite two important clinical signs that aid in distinguishing a dysplastic nevus from a malignant melanoma.

REFERENCES

1. Likeness LO. Common dermatologic infections in athletes and return-to-play guidelines. *J Am Osteopath Assoc.* 2011;111(6):373–379.
2. Wolff K, Johnson RA, Saavedra AP, eds. *Fitzpatrick's Color Atlas and Synopsis of Clinical Dermatology.* 7th ed. Chicago, IL: McGraw-Hill; 2013:607–610.
3. Goodheart HP. *Goodheart's Photoguide to Common Skin Disorders.* Philadelphia, PA: Wolters Kluwer Health | Lippincott Williams & Wilkins; 2009:167–187.
4. DermNet NZ. *Mycology of Dermatophyte Infections.* 2013. Available at: http://www.dermnetnz.org/fungal/mycology.html. Accessed September 25, 2013.
5. Patel GA, Schwartz RA. Tinea capatitis: still an unsolved problem? *Mycoses.* 2011;51:183–188.
6. Grover C, Arora P, Manchada V. Comparative evaluation of griseofulvin, terbenafine, and fluconazole in the treatment of tinea capitis. *Int J Dermatol.* 2012;51:455–458.
7. Gonzalez U, Seaton T, Bergus G, et al. Systemic antifungal therapy for tinea capitis in children: a summarized Cochrane review. *Clin Exp Dermatol.* 2010;36:826–827.
8. Graham LVD, Elewski BE. Recent updates in oral terbenafine: its use in onychomycosis and tinea capitis in the US. *Mycoses.* 2011;54:e679–e685.
9. Wolff K, Johnson RA, Saavedra AP, eds. *Fitzpatrick's Color Atlas and Synopsis of Clinical Dermatology.* 7th ed. Chicago, IL: McGraw-Hill; 2013:591.
10. Wolff K, Johnson RA, Saavedra AP, eds. *Fitzpatrick's Color Atlas and Synopsis of Clinical Dermatology.* 7th ed. Chicago, IL: McGraw-Hill; 2013:524.
11. Wolff K, Johnson RA, Saavedra AP, eds. *Fitzpatrick's Color Atlas and Synopsis of Clinical Dermatology.* 7th ed. Chicago, IL: McGraw-Hill; 2013:534.
12. Goodheart HP. *Goodheart's Photoguide to Common Skin Disorders.* Philadelphia, PA: Wolters Kluwer Health | Lippincott Williams & Wilkins; 2009:140–150.
13. Goodheart HP. *Goodheart's Photoguide to Common Skin Disorders.* Philadelphia, PA: Wolters Kluwer Health | Lippincott Williams & Wilkins; 2009:155–161.

14. Forbes HJ, Thomas SL, Langan SM. The epidemiology and prevention of herpes zoster. *Curr Dermatol Rep.* 2012;1:39–47.

15. Tseng HF, Smith N, Harpaz R, et al. Herpes zoster vaccine in older adults and the risk of subsequent herpes zoster disease. *JAMA.* 2011;305(2):160–166.

16. Goldman GS, King PG. Review of the United States universal varicella vaccination program: herpes zoster incidence rates, cost effectiveness, and vaccine efficacy based primarily on the Antelope Valley Varicella Active Surveillance Project Data. *Vaccine.* 2013;31(13):1680–1694.

17. Ramli R, Malik AS, Hani AFH, et al. Acne analysis, grading and computational assessment methods: an overview. *Skin Res Technol.* 2012;18:1–14.

18. Archer CB, Cohen SN, Baron SE. Guidance on the diagnosis and clinical management of acne. *Clin Exp Dermatol.* 2012;37:1–6.

19. Steventon K. Expert opinion and review article: the timing of comedone extraction in the treatment of premenstrual acne—a proposed therapeutic approach. *Int J Cosmet Sci.* 2010;33:99–104.

20. Perkins AC, Maglione J, Hillebrand GG, et al. Acne vulgaris in women: prevalence across the lifespan. *J Womens Health.* 2010;21(2):223–230.

21. Jahns AC, Lundskog B, Ganceviciene R, et al. An increased incidence of *Propionibacterium acnes* biofilms in acne vulgaris: a case-control study. *Br J Dermatol.* 2012;167:150–158.

22. Kurokawa I, Danby W, Ju Q, et al. New developments in our understanding of acne pathogenesis and treatment. *Exp Dermatol.* 2009;18:821–832.

23. Shah SK, Alexis AF. Acne in skin color: practical approaches to treatment. *J Dermatolog Treat.* 2010;21:206–211.

24. Chauhan N, Ellis DA. Rosacea: pathophysiology and management principles. *Facial Plast Surg Clin North Am.* 2013;21(1):127–136.

25. Torpy JM, Schwartz LA, Golub RM. Rosacea. *JAMA.* 2012;307(21):3942.

26. van Zuuren EJ, Kramer SF, Carter BR, et al. Effective and evidence-based management strategies for rosacea: summary of a Cochrane systematic review. *Br J Dermatol.* 2011;165:760–781.

27. Rustemeyer T, van Hoogstraten MW, von Blomberg BME, et al. Mechanisms of irritant and allergic contact dermatitis. In: Johansen JD, Frosh PJ, Lepoittevin JP, eds. *Contact Dermatitis.* 5th ed. Dortmund, Germany: Springer; 2011:43–90.

28. Goodheart HP. *Goodheart's Photoguide to Common Skin Disorders.* Philadelphia, PA: Wolters Kluwer Health | Lippincott Williams & Wilkins; 2009:51–59.

29. Cheong WK. Gentle cleansing and moisturizing for patients with atopic dermatitis and sensitive skin. *Am J Clin Dermatol.* 2009;10:13–17.

30. Zitelli KB, Cordoro KM. Evidence-based evaluation and management of chronic urticaria in children. *Pediatr Dermatol.* 2011;28(6):629–639.

31. Axelrod S, Davis-Lorton M. Urticaria and angioedema. *Mt Sinai J Med.* 2011;78:784–802.

32. Sokumbi O, Wetter DA. Clinical features, diagnosis, and treatment of erythema multiforme: a review for the practicing dermatologist. *Int J Dermatol.* 2012;51:889–902.

33. Diaz L, Ciurea AM. Cutaneous and systemic adverse reactions to antibiotics. *Dermatol Ther.* 2012;25:12–22.

34. Wolff K, Johnson RA, Saavedra AP, eds. *Fitzpatrick's Color Atlas and Synopsis of Clinical Dermatology.* 7th ed. Chicago, IL: McGraw-Hill; 2013:488–507.

35. Khalili R, Bahria SL. Pathogenesis and recent therapeutic trends in Stevens-Johnson syndrome and toxic epidermal necrolysis. Ann Allergy Asthma Immunol. 2006;97:272–281.

36. Ziemer M, Kardaun SH, Liss Y, et al. Stevens-Johnson syndrome and toxic epidermal necrolysis in patients with lupus erythematosus: a descriptive study of 17 cases from a national registry and review of the literature. *Br J Dermatol.* 2012;166:575–600.

37. Nestle FO, Kaplan DH, Barker J. Psoriasis. *N Engl J Med.* 2009;361(15):496–509.

38. Raho G, Koleva DM, Garattini L, et al. The burden of moderate to severe psoriasis: an overview. *Pharmacoeconomics.* 2012;30(11):1005–1013.

39. Cohen SN, Baron SE, Archer CB. Guidance on the diagnosis and clinical management of psoriasis. *Clin Exp Dermatol.* 2012;37:13–18.

40. Herrier RN. Advances in the treatment of moderate-to-severe plaque psoriasis. *Am J Health Syst Pharm.* 2011;68:795–806.

41. Kim IH, West CE, Kwatra SG, et al. Comparative efficacy of biologics in psoriasis: a review. *Am J Clin Dermatol.* 2012;3(6):365–374.

42. Goodheart HP. *Goodheart's Photoguide to Common Skin Disorders.* Philadelphia, PA: Wolters Kluwer Health | Lippincott Williams & Wilkins; 2009:114–118.

43. Lehman JS, Tollefson MM, Gibson LE. Lichen planus. *Int J Dermatol.* 2009;48:682–694.

44. Martin-Brufau R, Corbalan-Berna J, Ramirez-Andreo A, et al. Personality differences between patients with lichen simplex chronicus and normal population: a study of pruritus. *Eur J Dermatol.* 2010;20(3):359–363.

45. Galadari HI, Gilchrest BA. Skin cancer prevention and sunscreens. In: Nouri K, ed. *Skin Cancer.* Chicago, IL: McGraw-Hill; 2008:643–647.

46. Bouzari N, Nouri K. Indoor tanning. In: Nouri K, ed. *Skin Cancer.* Chicago, IL: McGraw-Hill; 2008:672–678.

47. Land V, Small L. The evidence on how to best treat sunburn in children: a common treatment dilemma. *Pediatr Nurs.* 2008;34(4):343–348.

48. American Burn Association. Burn incidence and treatment in the United States: 2012 Fact Sheet. 2012. Available at: http://ameriburn.org/resources_factsheet.php. Accessed October 5, 2013.

49. Price LA, Milner SM. The totality of burn care. *Trauma.* 2012;15(1):16–28.

50. Evers LH, Bhavsar D, Mailander P. The biology of burn injury. *Exp Dermatol.* 2010;19:777–783.

51. Orgill DP. Excision and skin grafting of thermal burns. *N Engl J Med.* 2009;360(9):891–901.

52. van der Veen VC, Boekema BKHL, Ulrich MMW, et al. New dermal substitutes. *Wound Repair Regen.* 2011;19:S59–S65.

53. Agency for Healthcare Research and Quality. Preventing pressure ulcers in hospital: a toolkit for improving quality of care. 2013. Available at: http://www.ahqr.gov/reserach/ltc/pressureulcertoolkit. Accessed October 13, 2013.

54. Alderden J, Whitney JD, Taylor SM, et al. Risk profile characteristics associated with outcomes of hospital-acquired pressure ulcers: a retrospective review. *Crit Care Nurse.* 2011;31(4):30–43.

55. Sprigle S, Sonenblum S. Assessing evidence supporting redistribution of pressure for pressure ulcer prevention: a review. *J Rehabil Res Dev.* 2011;48(3):203–214.

56. Reddy M. Pressure ulcers. *Clin Evid* (Online) 2011:1901.

57. National Pressure Ulcer Advisory Panel. NPUAP pressure ulcer stages/categories. 2013. Available at: http://www.npuap.org/resources/educational-and-clinical-resources/npuap-pressure-ulcer-stagescategories/. Accessed October 5, 2013.

58. Goodheart HP. *Goodheart's Photoguide to Common Skin Disorders.* Philadelphia, PA: Wolters Kluwer Health | Lippincott Williams & Wilkins; 2009:364–369.

59. Goodheart HP. *Goodheart's Photoguide to Common Skin Disorders.* Philadelphia, PA: Wolters Kluwer Health | Lippincott Williams & Wilkins; 2009:370–374.

60. Clarke LE. Dyplastic nevi. *Clin Lab Med.* 2011;31(2):255–265.

61. Centers for Disease Control and Prevention. Skin cancer statistics. 2013. Available at: http://www.cdc.gov/cancer/skin/statistics/index.htm. Accessed October 5, 2013.

62. Gonzalez M, Erdel E, Berwick M. Epidemiology of skin cancer. In: Nouri K, ed. *Skin Cancer*. Chicago, IL: McGraw-Hill; 2008:32–38.

63. Nouri K, Patel SS, Singh A. Etiology of skin cancer. In: Nouri K, ed. *Skin Cancer*. Chicago, IL: McGraw-Hill; 2008:29–45.

64. Barnhill RL, Mihm MC, Elgart G. Malignant melanoma. In: Nouri K, ed. *Skin Cancer*. Chicago, IL: McGraw-Hill; 2008:140–167.

65. Lazar AJF, Murphy GF. The skin. In: Kumar V, Abbas AK, Fausto N, et al., eds. *Robbins and Cotran Pathologic Basis of Disease*, 8th ed. Philadelphia, PA: Saunders Elsevier; 2010:1185–1204.

66. Argenziano G, Albertini G, Castagnetti F, et al. Early diagnosis of melanoma: what is the impact of dermoscopy? *Dermatol Ther.* 2012;25:403–409.

67. Nouri K, Ballard CJ, Patel A, et al. Basal cell carcinoma. In: Nouri K, ed. *Skin Cancer*. Chicago, IL: McGraw-Hill; 2008:61–85.

68. Anadolu-Brasie R, Patel AR, Patel SS, et al. Squamous cell carcinoma of the skin. In: Nouri K, ed. *Skin Cancer*. Chicago, IL: McGraw-Hill; 2008:86–114.

69. Wolff K, Johnson RA, Saavedra AP, eds. *Fitzpatrick's Color Atlas and Synopsis of Clinical Dermatology*. 7th ed. Chicago, IL: McGraw-Hill; 2013:155–157, 162–163.

70. Wolz MM, Sciallis GF, Pittelkow MR. Human herpesviruses 6, 7, and 8 from a dermatologic perspective. *Mayo Clin Proc.* 2012;87(10):1004–1014.

71. Sabella C. Measles: not just a childhood rash. *Cleve Clin J Med.* 2010;77(3):207–213.

72. Schmid DS, Jumaan AO. Impact of varicella vaccine on varicella-zoster virus dynamics. *Clin Microbiol Rev.* 2010;23(1):202–217.

73. Goodheart HP. *Goodheart's Photoguide to Common Skin Disorders*. Philadelphia, PA: Wolters Kluwer Health | Lippincott Williams & Wilkins; 2009:372–374, 392–398.

Porth Essentials Resources

Explore these additional resources to enhance learning for this chapter:

- NCLEX-Style Questions and Other Resources on thePoint, http://thePoint.lww.com/PorthEssentials4e
- Study Guide for Essentials of Pathophysiology
- Adaptive Learning | Powered by PrepU, http://thepoint.lww.com/prepu

Glossary

Abduction The act of abducting (moving or spreading away from a position near the midline of the body or the axial line of a limb) or the state of being abducted.

Abrasion The wearing or scraping away of a substance or structure, such as the skin, through an unusual or abnormal mechanical process.

Abscess A collection of pus that is restricted to a specific area in tissues, organs, or confined spaces.

Accommodation The adjustment of the lens (eye) to variations in distance.

Acromion The lateral extension of the spine of the scapula, forming the highest point of the shoulder. (Adjective: acromial)

Acuity The clearness or sharpness of perception, especially of vision.

Adaptation The adjustment of an organism to its physical or psychological environment, through changes and responses to stress of any kind.

Adduction The act of adducting (moving or drawing toward a position near the midline of the body or the axial line of a limb) or the state of being adducted.

Adhesin The molecular components of the bacterial cell wall that are involved in the adhesion processes.

Adrenergic Activated by or characteristic of the sympathetic nervous system or its neurotransmitters (i.e., epinephrine and norepinephrine).

Aerobic Growing, living, or occurring only in the presence of air or oxygen.

Afferent Bearing or conducting inward or toward a center, as an afferent neuron.

Agglutination The clumping together of particles, microorganisms, or blood cells in response to an antigen–antibody reaction.

Agonist A muscle whose action is opposed by another muscle (antagonist) with which it is paired or a drug or other chemical substance that has affinity for or stimulates a predictable physiologic function.

Akinesia An abnormal state in which there is an absence or poverty of movement.

Allele One of two or more different forms of a gene that can occupy a particular locus on a chromosome.

Alveolus A small saclike structure, as in the alveolus of the lung.

Ambient The surrounding, encompassing, or prevailing area or environment; especially of or pertaining to the area immediately around the body.

Amblyopia A condition of vision impairment without a detectable organic lesion of the eye.

Amine An organic compound containing nitrogen.

Amorphous Without a definite form; shapeless.

Amphoteric Capable of reacting chemically as an acid or a base.

Ampulla A saclike dilatation of a duct, canal, or any other tubular structure.

Anabolism A constructive metabolic process characterized by the conversion of simple substances into larger, complex molecules.

Anaerobic Growing, living, or occurring only in the absence of air or oxygen.

Analog A part, organ, or chemical having the same function or appearance but differing in respect to a certain component, such as origin or development.

Anaplasia A change in the structure of cells and in their orientation to each other that is characterized by a loss of cell differentiation, as in cancerous cell growth.

Anastomosis The connection or joining between two vessels; or an opening created by surgical, traumatic, or pathologic means.

Androgen Any substance, such as a male sex hormone, that increases male characteristics.

Anergy A state of absent or diminished reaction to an antigen or group of antigens.

Aneuploidy A variation in the number of chromosomes within a cell involving one or more missing chromosomes rather than entire sets.

Aneurysm An outpouching or dilation in the wall of a blood vessel or the heart.

Ankylosis Stiffness or fixation of separate bones of a joint, resulting from disease, injury, or surgical procedure. (Verb: ankylose)

Anorexia Lack or loss of appetite for food. (Adjective: anorexic)

Anoxia An abnormal condition characterized by the total lack of oxygen.

Antagonist A muscle whose action directly opposes that of another muscle (agonist) with which it is paired, or a drug or other chemical substance that can diminish or nullify the action of a neuromediator or body function.

Anterior Pertaining to a surface or part that is situated near or toward the front.

Antigen A substance that generates an immune response by causing the formation of an antibody or reacting with antibodies or T-cell receptors.

Apex The uppermost point, the narrowed or pointed end, or the highest point of a structure, such as an organ.

Aphagia A condition characterized by the refusal or the loss of ability to swallow.

Aplasia The absence of an organ or tissue due to a developmental failure.

Apnea The absence of spontaneous respiration.

Apoptosis A mechanism of programmed cell death, marked by shrinkage of the cell, condensation of chromatin, formation of cytoplasmic blebs, and fragmentation of the cell into membrane-bound bodies eliminated by phagocytosis.

Apraxia Loss of the ability to carry out familiar, purposeful acts or to manipulate objects in the absence of paralysis or other motor or sensory impairment.

Articulation The place of connection or junction between two or more bones of a skeletal joint.

Ascites An abnormal accumulation of serous fluid in the peritoneal cavity.

Asepsis The condition of being free or freed from pathogenic microorganisms.

Astereognosis A neurologic disorder characterized by an inability to identify objects by touch.

Asterixis A motor disturbance characterized by a hand-flapping tremor, which results when the prolonged contraction of groups of muscles lapses intermittently.

Ataxia An abnormal condition characterized by an inability to coordinate voluntary muscular movement.

Athetosis A neuromuscular condition characterized by the continuous occurrence of slow, sinuous, writhing movements that are performed involuntarily. (Adjective: athetoid)

Atopy Genetic predisposition toward the development of hypersensitivity or an allergic reaction to common environmental allergens.

Atresia The absence or closure of a normal body orifice or tubular organ, such as the esophagus.

Atrophy A wasting or diminution of size, often accompanied by a decrease in function, of a cell, tissue, or organ.

Aura A distinct subjective feeling, sensation, or motor phenomenon that precedes and marks the onset of an episode of a neurological condition, such as a migraine or epileptic seizure.

Autocrine A mode of hormone action in which a chemical messenger acts on the same cell that secretes it.

Autophagy Segregation of part of the cell's own damaged cytoplasmic material within a vacuole and its disposal.

Autosome Any chromosome other than a sex chromosome.

Axillary Of or pertaining to the axilla, or armpit.

Bacteremia The presence of bacteria in the blood.

Bactericide An agent that destroys bacteria. (Adjective: bactericidal)

Bacteriostat An agent that inhibits bacterial growth. (Adjective: bacteriostatic)

Ballismus An abnormal condition characterized by violent flailing motions of the arms and, occasionally, the head, resulting from injury to or destruction of the subthalamic nucleus or its fiber connections.

Baroreceptor A type of sensory nerve ending, such as those found in the aorta and the carotid sinus, that is stimulated by changes in pressure.

Basal Pertaining to, situated at, or forming the base; or the fundamental or basic.

Benign Not malignant; or of the character that does not threaten health or life.

Bipolar neuron A nerve cell that has an afferent process at one end and an efferent process at the other end.

Bolus A rounded mass of food ready to swallow or such a mass passing through the gastrointestinal tract; or a concentrated mass of medicinal material or other pharmaceutical preparation injected all at once intravenously for diagnostic purposes.

Borborygmus The rumbling, gurgling, or tinkling noise produced by the propulsion of gas through the intestine.

Bruit A sound or murmur heard while auscultating an organ or blood vessel, especially an abnormal one.

Buccal Pertaining to or directed toward the inside of the cheek.

Buffer A substance or group of substances that prevents change in the concentration of another chemical substance.

Bulla A thin-walled blister of the skin or mucous membranes greater than 5 mm in diameter containing serous or seropurulent fluid.

Bursa A fluid-filled sac or saclike cavity situated in places in the tissues at which friction would otherwise develop, such as between certain tendons and the bones beneath them.

Cachexia A condition of general ill health and malnutrition, marked by weakness and emaciation.

Calculus A stony mass formed within body tissues, usually composed of mineral salts.

Capsid The protein shell that envelops and protects the nucleic acid of a virus.

Carcinogen Any substance or agent that causes the development or increases the incidence of cancer.

Carpal Of or pertaining to the carpus, or wrist.

Caseation A form of tissue necrosis in which the tissue is changed into a dry, amorphous mass resembling crumbly cheese.

Catabolism A metabolic process through which living organisms break down complex substances to simple compounds, liberating energy for use in work, energy storage, or heat production.

Catalyst A substance that increases the velocity of a chemical reaction without being consumed by the process.

Catecholamines Any one of a group of biogenic amines having a sympathomimetic action and composed of a catechol molecule and the aliphatic portion of an amine.

Caudal Signifying an inferior position, toward the distal end of the spine.

Cellulitis An acute, diffuse, spreading, edematous inflammation of the deep subcutaneous tissues and sometimes muscle, characterized most commonly by an area of heat, redness, pain, and swelling, and occasionally by fever, malaise, chills, and headache.

Cephalic Of or pertaining to the head, or to the head end of the body.

Cerumen The waxlike secretion produced by vestigial apocrine sweat glands in the external ear canal.

Cheilosis A noninflammatory disorder of the lips and mouth characterized by chapping and fissuring.

Chelate A chemical compound composed of a central metal ion and an organic molecule with multiple bonds, arranged in ring formation, used especially in treatment of metal poisoning.

Chemoreceptor A sensory nerve cell activated by chemical stimuli; for example, a chemoreceptor in the carotid artery is sensitive to changes in the oxygen content in the blood and reflexly increases or decreases respiration and blood pressure.

Chemosis Excessive edema of the mucous membrane of the eyeball and eyelid lining (conjunctiva).

Chemotaxis A response involving cell orientation or cell movement that is either toward (positive chemotaxis) or away from (negative chemotaxis) a chemical stimulus.

Chimeric Relating to, derived from, or being an individual possessing one's own immunologic characteristics and that of another individual; a phenomenon that can occur as the result of procedures such as a bone marrow graft.

Chondrocyte Any one of the mature polymorphic cells that form the cartilage of the body.

Chromatid One of the paired threadlike chromosome filaments, joined at the centromere, that make up a metaphase chromosome.

Chromosome Any one of the structures in the nucleus of a cell containing a linear thread of DNA, which functions in the transmission of genetic information.

Chyme The creamy, viscous, semifluid material produced during digestion of a meal that is expelled by the stomach into the duodenum.

Cilia A minute, hairlike process projecting from a cell, composed of nine microtubules arrayed around a single pair. Cilia beat rhythmically to move the cell around in its environment, or they move mucus or fluids over the surface.

Circadian Being, having, pertaining to, or occurring in a period or cycle of approximately 24 hours.

Circumduction The active or passive circular movement of a limb or of the eye.

Cisterna An enclosed space, such as a cavity, that serves as a reservoir for lymph or other body fluids.

Clathrin The major structural coat protein of the coated vesicles involved in the intracellular transport between membranous organelles.

Clone One or a group of genetically identical cells or organisms derived from a single parent.

Coagulation The process of transforming a liquid into a semisolid mass, especially of blood clot formation.

Coarctation A condition of stricture or contraction of the walls of a vessel.

Cofactor A substance that must unite with another substance in order to function.

Colic Sharp, intermittent abdominal pain localized in a hollow or tubular organ, resulting from torsion, obstruction, or smooth muscle spasm. (Adjective: colicky)

Collagen The protein substance of the white, glistening, inelastic fibers of the skin, tendons, bone, cartilage, and all other connective tissue.

Collateral Secondary or accessory rather than direct or immediate; or a small branch, as of a blood vessel or nerve.

Complement Any one of the complex, enzymatic serum proteins that are involved in physiologic reactions, including antigen–antibody reaction and anaphylaxis.

Confluent Flowing or coming together; not discrete.

Congenital Present at, and usually before, birth.

Conjugate To pair and fuse in conjugation; or a form of sexual reproduction seen in unicellular organisms in which genetic material is exchanged during the temporary fusion of two cells.

Contiguous In contact (or nearly so) in an unbroken sequence along a boundary or at a point.

Contralateral Affecting, pertaining to, or originating in the opposite side of a point or reference.

Contusion An injury of a part without a break in the skin, characterized by swelling, discoloration, and pain.

Convolution An elevation or tortuous winding, such as one of the irregular ridges on the surface of the brain, formed by a structure being folded in upon itself.

Corpuscle Any small mass, cell, or body, such as a red or white blood cell.

Costal Pertaining to a rib or ribs.

Crepitus A sound or sensation that resembles a crackling or grating noise.

Cutaneous Pertaining to the skin.

Cyanosis A bluish discoloration, especially of the skin and mucous membranes, caused by an excess of deoxygenated hemoglobin in the blood.

Cytokine Any of a class of polypeptide immunoregulatory substances that are secreted by cells, usually of the immune system, that affect other cells.

Cytology The study of cells, including their origin, structure, function, and pathology.

Cytosol Cytoplasm exclusive of membranous components (e.g., mitochondria, endoplasmic reticulum) and nonmembranous insoluble components.

Decibel A unit for expressing the relative power sound intensity that is equal to one tenth of a bel.

Defecation The evacuation of feces from the digestive tract through the rectum.

Deformation The process of adapting in form or shape; also, the product of such alteration.

Degeneration The deterioration of a normal cell, tissue, or organ to a less functionally active form. (Adjective: degenerative)

Deglutition The act or process of swallowing.

Degradation The reduction of a chemical compound to a compound-less complex, usually by splitting off one or more groups.

Dehydration The condition that results from excessive loss of water from the body tissues.

Delirium An acute, reversible organic mental syndrome characterized by confusion, disorientation, restlessness, incoherence, fear, and often illusions.

Dendrite One of the branching processes that extends and transmits impulses toward a cell body of a neuron. (Adjective: dendritic)

De novo Anew; often applied to the biochemical pathway where a complex biomolecule is synthesized in a new or different form from simple molecules.

Depolarization The reduction of a cell membrane potential to a less-negative value than that of the potential outside the cell.

Dermatome The area of the skin supplied with afferent nerve fibers of a single dorsal root of a spinal nerve.

Desmosome A small, circular, dense area within the intercellular bridge that forms the site of adhesion between intermediate filaments and cell membranes.

Desquamation A normal process in which the cornified layer of the epidermis is shed in fine scales or sheets.

Dialysis The process of separating colloids and crystalline substances in solution, which involves the two distinct physical processes of diffusion and ultrafiltration; or a medical procedure for the removal of urea and other elements from the blood or lymph.

Diapedesis The outward passage of red or white blood corpuscles through the intact walls of the vessels.

Diaphoresis Perspiration, especially the profuse perspiration associated with elevated body temperature, physical exertion, exposure to heat, and mental or emotional stress.

Diarthrosis A specialized articulation that permits, to some extent, free joint movement. (Adjective: diarthrodial)

Diastole The dilatation of the heart; or the period of dilatation, which is the interval between the second and the first heart sound and is the time during which blood enters the relaxed chambers of the heart from the systemic circulation and the lungs.

Differentiation The act or process in development in which unspecialized cells or tissues acquire more specialized characteristics, including those of physical form, physiologic function, and chemical properties.

Diffusion The process of becoming widely spread, as in the spontaneous movement of molecules or other particles in solution from an area of higher concentration to an area of lower concentration, resulting in an even distribution of the particles in the fluid.

Dimer A compound or unit formed by the combination of two identical molecules or radicals of a simpler compound. (Adjective: dimeric)

Diopter A unit of measurement of the refractive power of lenses equal to the reciprocal of the focal length in meters.

Diploid Pertaining to an individual, organism, strain, or cell that has two full sets of homologous chromosomes.

Disseminate To scatter or distribute over a considerable area.

Distal Away from or being the farthest from a point of reference.

Diurnal Of, relating to, or occurring in the daytime.

Diverticulum A pouch or sac of variable size occurring naturally or through herniation of the muscular wall of a tubular organ.

Dorsum The back or posterior. (Adjective: dorsal)

Dysgenesis Defective or abnormal development of an organ or part, typically occurring during embryonic development. (Also called dysgenesia.)

Dyslexia A disturbance in the ability to read, spell, and write words.

Dyspepsia The impairment of the power or function of digestion, especially epigastric discomfort following eating.

Dysphagia A difficulty in swallowing.

Dysphonia Any impairment of the voice that is experienced as difficulty in speaking.

Dysplasia The alteration in size, shape, and organization of adult cell types.

Eburnation The conversion of bone or cartilage, through thinning or loss, into a hard and dense mass with a worn, polished, ivorylike surface.

Ecchymosis A small hemorrhagic spot, larger than a petechia, in the skin or mucous membrane caused by the extravasation of blood into the subcutaneous tissues.

Ectoderm The outermost of the three primary germ layers of the embryo, and from which the epidermis and epidermal tissues, such as nails, hair, and glands of the skin, develop.

Ectopic Relating to or characterized by an object or organ being situated in an unusual place, away from its normal location.

Edema The presence of an abnormal accumulation of fluid in interstitial spaces of tissues. (Adjective: edematous)

Efferent Conveyed or directed away from a center.

Effusion The escape of fluid from blood vessels into a part or tissue, as an exudation or a transudation.

Embolus A mass of clotted blood or other formed elements, such as bubbles of air, calcium fragments, or a bit of tissue or tumor, that circulates in the bloodstream until it becomes lodged in a vessel, obstructing the circulation. (Plural: emboli)

Empyema An accumulation of pus in a cavity of the body, especially the pleural space.

Emulsify To disperse one liquid throughout the body of another liquid, making a colloidal suspension, or emulsion.

Endocytosis The uptake or incorporation of substances into a cell by invagination of its plasma membrane, as in the processes of phagocytosis and pinocytosis.

Endoderm The innermost of the three primary germ layers of the embryo, and from which epithelium arises.

Endogenous Growing within the body; or developing or originating from within the body or produced from internal causes.

Endoscopy The visualization of any cavity of the body with an endoscope.

Enteral Within or pertaining to the intestine.

Enteropathic Relating to any disease of the intestinal tract.

Enzyme A protein molecule produced by living cells that catalyzes chemical reactions of other organic substances without itself being destroyed or altered.

Epiphysis The expanded articular end of a long bone (head) that is separated from the shaft of the bone by the epiphyseal plate until the bone stops growing, the plate is obliterated, and the shaft and the head become united.

Epithelium The covering of the internal and external surfaces of the body, including the lining of vessels and other small cavities.

Epitope The simplest form of an antigenic determinant that combines with an antibody or a T-cell receptor to cause a specific reaction by an immunoglobulin.

Epizootic A diffuse, rapidly spreading outbreak of a disease affecting many animals in any region at the same time, often with the implication that it may extend to humans, such as bird flu.

Erectile Capable of being erected or raised to an erect position.

Erythema The redness or inflammation of the skin or mucous membranes produced by the congestion of superficial capillaries. (Adjective: erythematous)

Etiology The study or theory of all factors that may be involved in the development of a disease, including susceptibility of an individual, the nature of the disease agent, and the way in which an individual's body is invaded by the agent; or the cause of a disease.

Eukaryotic Pertaining to an organism with cells having a true nucleus; that is, a highly complex, organized nucleus surrounded by a nuclear membrane containing organelles and exhibiting mitosis.

Euploid Pertaining to an individual, organism, strain, or cell with a balanced set or sets of chromosomes, in any number, that is an exact multiple of the normal, basic haploid number characteristic of the species; or such an individual, organism, strain, or cell.

Evisceration The removal of the viscera from the abdominal cavity, or disembowelment; or the extrusion of an internal organ through a wound or surgical incision.

Exacerbation An increase in the severity of a disease as marked by greater intensity in any of its signs and symptoms.

Exfoliation Peeling and sloughing off of tissue cells in scales or layers. (Adjective: exfoliative)

Exocytosis The discharge of cell particles, which are packaged in membrane-bound vesicles, by fusion of the vesicular membrane with the plasma membrane and subsequent release of the particles to the exterior of the cell.

Exogenous Developed or originating outside the body, as a disease caused by a bacterial or viral agent foreign to the body.

Exophthalmos A marked or abnormal protrusion of the eyeball.

Extension A movement that allows the two elements of any jointed part to be drawn apart, increasing the angle between them, as extending the leg increases the angle between the femur and the tibia.

Extrapyramidal Pertaining to motor systems supplied by fibers outside the corticospinal or pyramidal tracts.

Extravasation A discharge or escape, usually of blood, serum, or lymph, from a vessel into the tissues.

Extubation The process of withdrawing a previously inserted tube from an orifice or cavity of the body.

Exudate Fluid, cells, or other substances that have been slowly exuded or have escaped from blood vessels and have been deposited in tissues or on tissue surfaces. (Adjective: exudation)

Fascia A sheet or band of fibrous connective tissue that may be separated from other specifically organized structures, such as the tendons, aponeuroses, and ligaments.

Febrile Pertaining to or characterized by an elevated body temperature, or fever.

Fibrillation A small, local, involuntary contraction of muscle resulting from spontaneous activation of a single muscle fiber or of an isolated bundle of nerve fibers.

Fibrin A stringy, insoluble protein formed by the action of thrombin on fibrinogen during the clotting process.

Fibrosis The formation of fibrous connective tissue, as in the repair or replacement of parenchymatous elements.

Filtration The process of passing a liquid through or as if through a filter, which is accomplished by gravity, pressure, or vacuum.

Fimbria Any structure that forms a fringe, border, or edge or the processes that resemble such a structure.

Fissure A cleft or a groove, normal or otherwise, on the surface of an organ or a bony structure.

Fistula An abnormal passage or communication from an internal organ to the body surface or between two internal organs.

Flaccid Weak, soft, and lax; lacking normal muscle tone.

Flatus Air or gas in the intestinal tract that is expelled through the anus. (Adjective: flatulent)

Flexion A movement that allows the two elements of any jointed part to be brought together, decreasing the angle between them, as bending the elbow.

Flora The microorganisms, such as bacteria and fungi, both normally occurring and pathologic, inhabiting the external or internal surfaces of the body.

Focal Relating to, having, or occupying a focus.

Follicle A sac or pouchlike depression or cavity.

Fontanel A membrane-covered opening in or between bones, such as the soft spot covered by tough membranes between the bones of an infant's incompletely ossified skull.

Foramen A natural opening or aperture in a membranous structure or bone.

Fossa A hollow or depressed area, especially on the surface of the end of a bone.

Fovea A small pit or depression in the surface of a structure or organ.

Fundus The base or bottom of an organ or the portion farthest from the mouth of an organ.

Ganglion One of the nerve cell bodies, chiefly collected in groups outside the central nervous system. (Plural: ganglia)

Genotype The entire genetic constitution of an individual, as determined by the particular combination and location of the genes on the chromosomes; or the alleles present at one or more sites on homologous chromosomes.

Glia The neuroglia, or supporting structure of nervous tissue.

Globulin One of a broad group of proteins classified by solubility, electrophoretic mobility, and size.

Gluconeogenesis The formation of glucose from any of the substances of glycolysis other than carbohydrates.

Glycolysis A series of enzymatically catalyzed reactions, occurring within cells, by which glucose is converted to adenosine triphosphate (ATP) and pyruvic acid during aerobic metabolism.

Gonad A gamete-producing gland, as an ovary or a testis.

Gradient The rate of increase or decrease of a measurable phenomenon expressed as a function of a second; or the visual representation of such a change.

Granuloma A small mass of nodular granulation tissue resulting from chronic inflammation, injury, or infection. (Adjective: granulomatous)

Hapten A small, nonproteinaceous substance that is not antigenic by itself but that can act as an antigen when combined with a larger molecule.

Haustrum A structure resembling a recess or sacculation. (Plural: haustra)

Hematoma A localized collection of extravasated blood trapped in an organ, space, or tissue, resulting from a break in the wall of a blood vessel.

Hematopoiesis The normal formation and development of blood cells.

Hemianopia Defective vision or blindness in half of the visual field of one or both eyes.

Heterogeneous Consisting of or composed of dissimilar elements or parts; or not having a uniform quality throughout. (Noun: heterogeneity)

Heterophagy The taking into the cell of an exogenous substance by phagocytosis or pinocytosis and the subsequent digestion of the newly formed vacuole by a lysosome.

Heterozygous Having two different alleles at corresponding loci on homologous chromosomes.

Histology The branch of anatomy that deals with the minute (microscopic) structure, composition, and function of cells and tissue. (Adjective: histologic)

Homolog Any organ or part corresponding in function, position, origin, and structure to another organ or part, as the flippers of a seal correspond to human hands. (Adjective: homologous)

Homozygous Having two identical alleles at corresponding loci on homologous chromosomes.

Humoral Relating to elements dissolved in the blood or body fluids.

Hybridoma A tumor of hybrid cells produced by fusion of normal lymphocytes and tumor cells.

Hydrolysis The chemical alteration or decomposition of a compound into fragments by the addition of water.

Hypercapnia Excess amounts of carbon dioxide in the blood.

Hyperemia An excess or engorgement of blood in a part of the body.

Hyperesthesia An unusual or pathologic increase in sensitivity of a part, especially the skin, or of a particular sense.

Hyperplasia An abnormal multiplication or increase in the number of normal cells of a body part.

Hypertonic A solution having a greater concentration of solute than another solution with which it is compared, hence exerting more osmotic pressure than that solution.

Hypertrophy The enlargement or overgrowth of an organ that is due to an increase in the size of its cells rather than the number of its cells.

Hypesthesia An abnormal decrease of sensation in response to stimulation of the sensory nerves. (Also called hypoesthesia.)

Hypocapnia A deficiency of carbon dioxide in the blood.

Hypotonic A solution having a lesser concentration of solute than another solution with which it is compared, hence exerting less osmotic pressure than that solution.

Hypoxia An inadequate supply of oxygen to tissue that is below physiologic levels despite adequate perfusion of the tissue by blood.

Iatrogenic Induced inadvertently through the activity of a physician or by medical treatment or diagnostic procedures.

Idiopathic Arising spontaneously or from an unknown cause.

Idiosyncrasy A physical or behavioral characteristic or manner that is unique to an individual or group. (Adjective: idiosyncratic)

Immunogenicity The property that provides a substance with the capacity to produce an immune response. (Adjective: immunogenic)

Incidence The rate at which a certain event occurs (e.g., the number of new cases of a specific disease during a particular period of time in a population at risk).

Inclusion The act of enclosing or the condition of being enclosed; or anything that is enclosed.

Indigenous Native, or natural, to a particular country or region.

Infarction Necrosis or death of tissues due to local ischemia resulting from obstruction of blood flow.

Inotropic Influencing the force or energy of muscular contractions.

In situ In the natural or normal place; or something, such as cancer, that is confined to its place of origin and has not invaded neighboring tissues.

Interferon Any one of a group of small glycoproteins (cytokines) produced in response to viral infection and which inhibit viral replication.

Interleukin Any of several multifunctional cytokines produced by a variety of lymphoid and nonlymphoid cells, including immune cells, that stimulate or otherwise affect the function of lymphopoietic and other cells and systems in the body.

Interstitial Relating to or situated between parts or in the interspaces of a tissue.

Intramural Situated or occurring within the wall of an organ.

Intrinsic Pertaining exclusively to a part or situated entirely within an organ or tissue.

In vitro A biologic reaction occurring in an artificial environment, such as a test tube.

In vivo A biologic reaction occurring within the living body.

Involution The act or instance of enfolding, entangling, or turning inward.

Ionize To separate or change into ions.

Ipsilateral Situated on, pertaining to, or affecting the same side of the body.

Ischemia Decreased blood supply to a body organ or part, usually due to functional constriction or actual obstruction of a blood vessel.

Juxta-articular Situated near a joint or in the region of a joint.

Juxtaglomerular Near to or adjoining a glomerulus of the kidney.

Karyotype The total chromosomal characteristics of a cell; or the micrograph of chromosomes arranged in pairs in descending order of size.

Keratin A fibrous, sulfur-containing protein that is the primary component of the epidermis, hair, and horny tissues. (Adjective: keratinous)

Keratosis Any skin condition in which there is overgrowth and thickening of the cornified epithelium.

Ketosis A condition characterized by the abnormal accumulation of ketones (organic compounds with a carboxyl group attached to two carbon atoms) in the body tissues and fluid.

Kinesthesia The sense of movement, weight, tension, and position of body parts mediated by input from joint and muscle receptors and hair cells. (Adjective: kinesthetic)

Kyphosis An abnormal condition of the vertebral column, characterized by increased convexity in the curvature of the thoracic spine as viewed from the side.

Lacuna A small pit or cavity within a structure, especially bony tissue; or a defect or gap, as in the field of vision.

Lateral A position farther from the median plane or midline of the body or a structure; or situated on, coming from, or directed toward the side.

Lesion Any wound, injury, or pathologic change in body tissue.

Lethargy The lowered level of consciousness characterized by listlessness, drowsiness, and apathy; or a state of indifference.

Ligament One of many predominantly white, shiny, flexible bands of fibrous tissue that binds joints together and connects bones or cartilages.

Ligand A group, ion, or molecule that binds to the central atom or molecule in a chemical complex.

Lipid Any of the group of fats and fatlike substances characterized by being insoluble in water and soluble in nonpolar organic solvents, such as chloroform and ether.

Lipoprotein Any one of the conjugated proteins that is a complex of protein and lipid.

Lobule A small lobe.

Lordosis The anterior concavity in the curvature of the lumbar and cervical spine as observed from the side.

Lumen A cavity or the channel within a tube or tubular organ of the body.

Luteal Of, pertaining to, or having the properties of the corpus luteum.

Lysis Destruction or dissolution of a cell or molecule through the action of a specific agent.

Maceration Softening of tissue by soaking, especially in acidic solutions.

Macroscopic Large enough to be visible with the unaided eye without a microscope.

Macula A small, flat blemish, thickening, or discoloration that is flush with the skin surface; or a structure having the form of a spot differentiated from surrounding tissues (e.g., macula lutea). (Adjective: macular)

Malaise A vague feeling of bodily fatigue and discomfort.

Manometry The measurement of tension or pressure of a liquid or gas using a device called a manometer.

Marasmus A condition of extreme protein-calorie malnutrition that is characterized by growth retardation and progressive wasting of subcutaneous tissue and muscle and occurs chiefly during the first year of life.

Matrix The intracellular substance of a tissue or the basic substance from which a specific organ or kind of tissue develops.

Meatus An opening or passage through any body part.

Medial Pertaining to the middle; or situated or oriented toward the midline of the body.

Mediastinum The mass of tissues and organs in the middle of the thorax, separating the pleural sacs containing the two lungs.

Meiosis The division of a sex cell as it matures, so that each daughter nucleus receives one half of the number of chromosomes characteristic of the somatic cells of the species.

Mesoderm The middle layer of the three primary germ layers of the developing embryo, lying between the ectoderm and the endoderm.

Metabolism The sum of all the physical and chemical processes by which living organisms are produced and maintained, and also the transformation by which energy is provided for vital processes and activities.

Metaplasia Change in type of adult cells in a tissue to a form that is not normal for that tissue.

Metastasis The transfer of disease (e.g., cancer) from one organ or part to another not directly connected with it. (Adjective: metastatic)

Miosis Contraction of the pupil of the eye.

Mitosis A type of indirect cell division that occurs in somatic cells and results in the formation of two daughter nuclei containing the identical complements of the number of chromosomes characteristic of the somatic cells of the species.

Molecule The smallest mass of matter that exhibits the properties of an element or compound.

Morbidity A diseased condition or state; the relative incidence of a disease or of all diseases in a population.

Morphology The study of the physical form and structure of an organism; or the form and structure of a particular organism. (Adjective: morphologic)

Mosaicism In genetics, the presence in an individual or in an organism of cell cultures having two or more cell lines that differ in genetic constitution but are derived from a single zygote.

Mutagen Any chemical or physical agent that induces a genetic mutation (an unusual change in form, quality, or some other characteristic) or increases the mutation rate by causing changes in DNA.

Mydriasis Physiologic dilatation of the pupil of the eye.

Myoclonus A spasm of a portion of a muscle, an entire muscle, or a group of muscles.

Myoglobin The oxygen-transporting pigment of muscle consisting of one heme molecule containing one iron molecule attached to a single globin chain.

Myopathy Any disease or abnormal condition of skeletal muscle, usually characterized by muscle weakness, wasting, and histologic changes within muscle tissue.

Myotome The muscle plate or portion of an embryonic somite that develops into a voluntary muscle; or a group of muscles innervated by a single spinal segment.

Necrosis Localized tissue death that occurs in groups of cells or part of a structure or an organ in response to disease or injury.

Neutropenia An abnormal decrease in the number of neutrophilic leukocytes in the blood.

Nidus The point where a morbid process originates, develops, or is located.

Nociception The reception of painful stimuli from the physical or mechanical injury to body tissues by nociceptors (receptors usually found in either the skin or the walls of the viscera).

Nosocomial Pertaining to or originating in a hospital, such as a nosocomial infection; an infection acquired during hospitalization.

Nystagmus Involuntary, rapid, rhythmic movements of the eyeball.

Oncogene A gene that is capable of causing the initial and continuing conversion of normal cells into cancer cells.

Oncotic Relating to, caused by, or marked by edema or any swelling.

Oocyte A primordial or incompletely developed ovum.

Oogenesis The process of the growth and maturation of the female gametes, or ova.

Opacification An act or process of becoming or rendering impenetrable to light rays, x-rays, or other electromagnetic radiations.

Opsonization The process of making cells, such as bacteria, more susceptible to the action of phagocytes.

Organelle Any one of the various membrane-bound particles of distinctive morphology and function present within most cells, such as the mitochondria, Golgi complex, and lysosomes.

Orthopnea An abnormal condition in which a person must be in an upright position in order to breathe deeply or comfortably.

Orthosis An external orthopedic appliance or apparatus, as a brace or splint, used to support, align, prevent, or correct deformities, or to improve the function of movable parts of the body.

Osmolality The concentration of osmotically active particles in solution expressed in osmols or milliosmols per kilogram of solvent.

Osmolarity The concentration of osmotically active particles in solution expressed in osmols or milliosmols per liter of solution.

Osmosis The movement or passage of a pure solvent, such as water, through a semipermeable membrane from a solution that has a lower solute concentration to one that has a higher solute concentration.

Osteophyte A bony project or outgrowth.

Palpable Perceptible by touch.

Pandemic A sudden outbreak, or epidemic, of a disease occurring over a widespread geographic area and affecting a high proportion of the population.

Papilla A small, nipple-shaped projection, elevation, or structure, such as the conoid papillae of the tongue.

Papule A small, circumscribed, solid elevation of the skin less than one centimeter in diameter. (Adjective: papular)

Paracrine A mode of hormone action in which a chemical messenger that is synthesized and released from a cell acts on nearby cells of a different type and affects their function.

Paralysis An abnormal condition characterized by the impairment or loss of motor function due to a lesion of the neural or muscular mechanism.

Paraneoplastic Relating to alterations produced in tissue remote from a tumor or its metastases.

Parenchyma The basic tissue or elements of an organ as distinguished from supporting or connective tissue or elements. (Adjective: parenchymal)

Paresis Slight or partial paralysis.

Paresthesia Any abnormal touch sensation, which can be experienced as numbness, tingling, or a "pins and needles" feeling, often in the absence of external stimuli.

Parietal Pertaining to the outer wall of a cavity or organ; or pertaining to the parietal bone of the skull or the parietal lobe of the brain.

Parous Having borne one or more viable offspring.

Pathogen Any microorganism capable of producing disease.

Pedigree A systematic presentation, such as in a table, chart, or list, of an individual's ancestors that is used in human genetics in the analysis of inheritance.

Peptide Any of a class of molecular chain compounds composed of two or more amino acids joined by peptide bonds.

Perfusion The process or act of pouring over or through, especially the passage of a fluid through a specific organ or an area of the body.

Peripheral Pertaining to the outside, surface, or surrounding area of an organ or other structure; or located away from a center or central structure.

Permeable A condition of being pervious, or permitting passage, so that fluids and certain other substances can pass through, as in a permeable membrane.

Pervasive Pertaining to something that becomes diffused throughout every part.

Petechia A tiny, perfectly round, purplish-red spot that appears on the skin as a result of minute intradermal or submucous hemorrhage. (Plural: petechiae)

Phagocytosis The process by which certain cells engulf and consume foreign material and cell debris.

Phalanx Any one of the bones composing the fingers of each hand and the toes of each foot.

Phenotype The complete physical, biochemical, and physiologic makeup of an individual, as determined by the interaction of both genetic makeup and environmental factors.

Pheresis A procedure in which blood is withdrawn from a donor, a portion (plasma, leukocytes, etc.) is separated and retained, and the remainder is reperfused into the donor. It includes plasmapheresis and leukophoresis.

Pili Hair; or in microbiology, the minute filamentous appendages of certain bacteria. (Singular: pilus)

Plethora A body condition characterized by an excess of any of the body fluids, especially blood, marked by distention and a beefy red coloration. (Adjective: plethoric)

Plexus A network of intersecting nerves, blood vessels, or lymphatic vessels.

Polygene Any of a group of nonallelic genes that interact to influence the same character in the same way so that the effect is cumulative, usually of a quantitative nature, as size, weight, or skin pigmentation. (Adjective: polygenic)

Polymorph One of several, or many, forms of an organism or cell. (Adjective: polymorphic)

Polyp A small, tumor-like growth that protrudes from a mucous membrane surface.

Polypeptide A molecular chain of more than two amino acids joined by peptide bonds.

Presbyopia A visual condition (farsightedness) that commonly develops with advancing years or old age in which the lens loses elasticity, causing defective accommodation and inability to focus sharply for near vision.

Prevalence The number of new and old cases of a disease that are present in a population at a given time, or occurrences of an event during a particular period of time.

Prodrome An early symptom indicating the onset of a condition or disease. (Adjective: prodromal)

Prokaryotic Pertaining to an organism, such as bacterium, with cells lacking a true nucleus and nuclear membrane that reproduces through simple fission.

Prolapse The falling down, sinking, or sliding of an organ from its normal position or location in the body.

Proliferation The reproduction or multiplication of similar forms, especially cells.

Pronation Assumption of a position in which the ventral, or front, surface of the body or part of the body faces downward. (Adjective: prone)

Propagation The act or action of reproduction.

Proprioception The reception of stimuli originating from within the body regarding body position and muscular activity by proprioceptors (sensory nerve endings found in muscles, tendons, joints).

Prosthesis An artificial replacement for a missing body part; or a device designed and applied to improve function, such as a hearing aid.

Proteoglycans Any one of a group of polysaccharide-protein conjugates occurring primarily in the matrix of connective tissue and cartilage.

Proto-oncogene A normal cellular gene that with alteration, such as by mutation, becomes an active oncogene.

Proximal Closer to a point of reference, usually the trunk of the body, than other parts of the body.

Pruritus The symptom of itching, an uncomfortable sensation leading to the urge to rub or scratch the skin to obtain relief. (Adjective: pruritic)

Purpura A small hemorrhage, up to about 1 cm in diameter, in the skin, mucous membrane, or serosal surface; or any of several bleeding disorders characterized by the presence of purpuric lesions.

Purulent Producing or containing pus.

Quiescent Quiet, causing no disturbance, activity, or symptoms.

Reflux An abnormal backward or return flow of a fluid, such as stomach contents, blood, or urine.

Regurgitation A flow of material that is in the opposite direction from normal, as in the return of swallowed food into the mouth or the backward flow of blood through a defective heart valve.

Remission The partial or complete disappearance of the symptoms of a chronic or malignant disease; or the period of time during which the abatement of symptoms occurs.

Resorption The loss of substance or bone by physiologic or pathologic means; for example, the loss of dentin and cementum of a tooth.

Retrograde Moving backward or against the usual direction of flow; reverting to an earlier state or worse condition (degenerating); catabolic.

Retroversion A condition in which an entire organ is tipped backward or in a posterior direction, usually without flexion or other distortion.

Rhabdomyolysis Destruction or degeneration of muscle, associated with myoglobinuria (excretion of myoglobin in the urine).

Rostral Situated near a beak (oral or nasal region).

Sacroiliitis Inflammation in the sacroiliac joint.

Saprophyte An organism that obtains nourishment from the products of organic breakdown and decay. (Adjective: saprophytic)

Sclerosis A condition characterized by induration or hardening of tissue resulting from any of several causes, including inflammation, diseases of the interstitial substance, and increased formation of connective tissues.

Scotopic vision Describes vision, especially night vision, when the eye is dark adapted.

Semipermeable Partially but not wholly permeable, especially a membrane that permits the passage of some (usually small) molecules but not the passage of other (usually larger) particles.

Senescence The process or condition of aging or growing old.

Sepsis The presence in the blood or other tissues of pathogenic microorganisms or their toxins; or the condition resulting from the spread of microorganisms or their products. (Adjective: septic)

Serous Relating to or resembling serum; or containing or producing serum, such as a serous gland.

Shunt To divert or bypass bodily fluid from one channel, path, or part to another; a passage or anastomosis between two natural channels, especially between blood vessels, established by surgery or occurring as an abnormality.

Soma The body of an organism as distinguished from the mind; all of an organism, excluding germ cells; the body of a cell.

Spasticity The condition characterized by spasms or other uncontrolled contractions of the skeletal muscles. (Adjective: spastic)

Spatial Relating to, having the character of, or occupying space.

Sphincter A ringlike band of muscle fibers that constricts a passage or closes a natural orifice of the body.

Stenosis An abnormal condition characterized by the narrowing or stricture of a duct or canal.

Stochastic Involving a random process.

Stria A streak or a linear scarlike lesion that often results from rapidly developing tension in the skin; or a narrow bandlike structure, especially the longitudinal collections of nerve fibers in the brain.

Stricture An abnormal temporary or permanent narrowing of the lumen of a duct, canal, or other passage, as the esophagus, because of inflammation, external pressure, or scarring.

Stroma The supporting tissue or the matrix of an organ as distinguished from its functional element, or parenchyma.

Stupor A lowered level of consciousness characterized by lethargy and unresponsiveness in which a person seems unaware of his or her surroundings.

Subchondral Beneath a cartilage.

Subcutaneous Beneath the skin.

Subluxation An incomplete or partial dislocation in which the relationship between joint surfaces is altered, but contact remains.

Sulcus A shallow groove, depression, or furrow on the surface of an organ, such as a sulcus on the surface of the brain, separating the gyri.

Supination Assuming the position of lying horizontally on the back, or with the face upward. (Adjective: supine)

Suppuration The formation of pus, or purulent matter.

Symbiosis Mode of living characterized by close association between organisms of different species, usually in a mutually beneficial relationship.

Sympathomimetic An agent or substance that produces stimulating effects on organs and structures similar to those produced by the sympathetic nervous system.

Syncope A brief lapse of consciousness due to generalized cerebral ischemia.

Syncytium A multinucleate mass of protoplasm produced by the merging of a group of cells.

Syndrome A complex of signs and symptoms that occur together to present a clinical picture of a disease or inherited abnormality.

Synergist An organ, agent, or substance that aids or cooperates with another organ, agent, or substance.

Synthesis An integration or combination of various parts or elements to create a unified whole.

Systemic Pertaining to the whole body rather than to a localized area or region of the body.

Systole The contraction, or period of contraction, of the heart that drives the blood onward into the aorta and pulmonary arteries.

Tamponade Stoppage of the flow of blood to an organ or a part of the body by pathologic compression, such as the compression of the heart by an accumulation of pericardial fluid.

Teratogen Any agent or factor that induces or increases the incidence of developmental abnormalities in the fetus.

Thermistor A device that is used to measure extremely small changes in temperature.

Thrombus A stationary mass of clotted blood or other formed elements that remains attached to its place of origin along the wall of a blood vessel, frequently obstructing the circulation. (Plural: thrombi)

Tinnitus A tinkling, buzzing, or ringing noise heard in one or both ears.

Tophus A chalky deposit containing sodium urate that most often develops in periarticular fibrous tissue, typically in individuals with gout. (Plural: tophi)

Torsion The act or process of twisting in either a positive (clockwise) or negative (counterclockwise) direction.

Trabecula A supporting or anchoring stand of connective tissue, such as the delicate fibrous threads connecting the inner surface of the arachnoid to the pia mater.

Transmural Situated or occurring through the wall of an organ.

Transudate A fluid substance passed through a membrane or extruded from the blood.

Tremor Involuntary quivering or trembling movements caused by the alternating contraction and relaxation of opposing groups of skeletal muscles.

Trigone A triangular-shaped area.

Ubiquitous The condition or state of existing or being everywhere at the same time.

Ulcer A circumscribed excavation of the surface of an organ or tissue, which results from necrosis that accompanies some inflammatory, infectious, or malignant processes. (Adjective: ulcerative)

Urticaria A pruritic skin eruption of the upper dermis, usually transient, characterized by wheals (hives) of various shapes and sizes.

Uveitis An inflammation of all or part of the uveal tract of the eye.

Vector An invertebrate animal (e.g., tick, mite, mosquito) that serves as a carrier, transferring an infective agent from one vertebrate host to another.

Ventral Pertaining to a position toward the belly of the body; or situated or oriented toward the front or anterior of the body.

Vertigo An illusory sensation that the environment or one's own body is revolving.

Vesicle A small bladder or sac, as a small, thin-walled, raised skin lesion, containing liquid.

Visceral Pertaining to the viscera, or internal organs of the body.

Viscosity Pertaining to the physical property of fluids, caused by the adhesion of adjacent molecules, that determines the internal resistance to shear forces.

Zoonosis A disease of animals that may be transmitted to humans from its primary animal host under natural conditions. (Adjective: zoonotic)

A p p e n d i x A

Lab Values

TABLE A-1 Prefixes Denoting Decimal Factors

Prefix	Symbol	Factor
mega	M	10^6
kilo	k	10^3
hecto	h	10^2
deci	d	10^{-1}
centi	c	10^{-2}
milli	m	10^{-3}
micro	μ	10^{-6}
nano	n	10^{-9}
pico	p	10^{-12}
femto	f	10^{-15}

TABLE A-2 Hematology

Test	Conventional Units	Conversion Factor	SI Units
Erythrocyte count (RBC count)	M. 4.2–5.4 × 10^6/μL F. 3.6–5.0 × 10^6/μL	1.0	M. 4.2–5.4 × 10^{12}/L F. 3.6–5.0 × 10^{12}/L
Hematocrit (Hct)	M. 40–50% F. 37–47%	0.01	M. 0.40–0.50 F. 0.37–0.47
Hemoglobin (Hb)	M. 14.0–16.5 g/dL F. 12.0–15.0 g/dL	10.0	M. 140–165 g/L F. 120–150 g/L
Mean corpuscular hemoglobin (MHC)	27–34 pg/cell		0.40–0.53 fmol/cell
Mean corpuscular hemoglobin concentration (MCHC)	31–35 g/dL	10.0	310–350 g/L
Mean corpuscular volume (MCV)	85–100 fL/cell		
Reticulocyte count	1.0–1.5% total RBC	1.0	
Platelet count	150–400 × 10^3/μL	1.0	150–400 × 10^9/L
Leukocyte count (WBC count)	4.8–10.8 × 10^3/μL	1.0	4.8–10.8 × 10^9/L
Basophils	0.3–0.5%		
Eosinophils	1–3%		
Lymphocytes	25–33%		
Monocytes	3–7%		
Neutrophils (segmented [Segs])	60–65%		
Neutrophils (bands)	0–4%		

M = Male; F = Female.

TABLE A-3   Blood Chemistry*

Test	Conventional Units	Conversion Factor	SI Units
Alanine aminotransferase (ALT, SGPT, GPT)	0–35 units/L[†]	0.02	0-0.7 µkat/L[†]
Alkaline phosphatase	41–133 units/L[†,‡]	0.02	0.7–2.2 µkat/L[†,‡]
Ammonia	18–60 µg/dL	0.590	11–35 µmol/L
Amylase	20–110 units/L[†]	0.02	0.33–1.83 µkat/L[†]
Aspartase aminotransferase (AST, SGOT, GOT)	0–35 units/L[†]	0.02	0–0.58 µkat/L[†]
Bicarbonate	24–31 mEq/L	1.0	24–31 mmol/L
Bilirubin (total)	0.1–1.2 mg/dL	17.100	2–21 µmol/L
Direct	0.1–0.5 mg/dL		<8 µmol/L
Indirect	0.1–0.7 mg/dL		<12 µmol/L
Blood urea nitrogen (BUN)	8–20 mg/dL	0.360	2.9–7.1 mmol/L
Calcium (Ca^{2+})	8.5–10.5 mg/dL	0.250	2.1–2.6 mmol/L
Chloride	98–106 mEq/L	1.000	98–106 mmol/L
Creatine kinase (CK, CPK)	32–267 units/L[†]	0.017	0.53–4.45 µkat/L[†]
Creatinine (serum)	0.6–1.2 mg/dL[‡]	83.300	50–100 µmol/L[‡]
Gamma-glutamyl-transpeptidase (GGT)	9–85 units/L[†]	0.02	0.15–1.42 µkat/L[†]
Glucose (plasma, fasting)	<100 mg/dL	0.055	<5.6 mmol/L
Glycosylated hemoglobin (HbA$_{1c}$)	3.9–6.9%		
Lactate dehydrogenase (LDH)	88–230 units/L[†]	0.02	1.46–3.82 µkat/L[†]
Lipids			
Cholesterol	<200 mg/dL (optimal)	0.26	<5.2 mmol/L (optimal)
	200–239 mg/dL (borderline)		5.2–6.1 mmol/L (borderline)
	≥240 (high)		>6.2 mmol/L (high)
LDL cholesterol	<130 mg/dL	0.026	<3.37 mmol/L
HDL cholesterol	<40 low	0.026	1.04 mmol/L
	>60 high		1.56 mmol/L
Triglycerides	<165 mg/dL	0.01	<1.8 mmol/L (fasting)
Lipase	0–160 units/L[†]	0.02	0-2.66 µkat/L[†]
Magnesium	1.3–2.1 mg/dL	0.50	0.65–1.05 mmol/L
Osmolality	275–295 mOsm/kg H_2O		275–295 mmol/kg H_2O
pH (arterial)	7.35–7.45		
Phosphorus (inorganic)	2.5–4.5 mg/dL	0.32	0.80–1.45 mmol/L
Potassium	3.5–5.0 mEq/L	1.0	3.5–5.0 mmol/L
Prostate specific antigen (PSA)	0–4 ng/mL	1.0	0–4 µg/L
Protein total	6.0–8.0 g/dL	10.0	60–80 g/L
Albumin	3.4–4.7 g/dL	10.0	34–47 g/L
Globulin	2.3–3.5 g/dL	10.0	23–35 g/L
A/G ratio	1.0–2.2	10.0	10–22
Thyroid tests			
Thyroxine (T$_4$) total	5.0–11.0 µg/dL	12.80	64–142 nmol/L
Thyroxine, free (FT$_4$)	0.7–1.86 ng/dL	12.87	9–24 pmol/L[†]
Triiodothyronine (T$_3$) total	95–190 ng/dL	0.015	1.5–2.9 nmol/L
Thyroid-stimulating hormone (TSH)	0.4–4.2 µU/mL	1.0	0.4–4.2 mU/L
Thyroglobin	3–42 ng/mL	1.0	3–42 µg/L
Sodium	135–145 mEq/L	1.0	135–145 mmol/L
Uric acid	Male: 2.4–7.4 mg/dL	59.48	Male: 140–440 µmol/L
	Female: 1.4–5.8 mg/dL		Female: 88–345 µmol/L

*Values may vary with laboratory. The values supplied by the laboratory performing the test should always be used since the ranges may be method specific.

[†]Laboratory and/or method specific.

[‡]Varies with age and muscle mass.

Values obtained from Papadakis MA, McPhee SJ. *Current Medical Diagnosis and Treatment.* 52nd ed. New York: McGraw Medical; 2013:1722–1736; Fischbach F, Dunning MB. *A Manual of Laboratory and Diagnostic Tests.* 8th ed. Philadelphia, PA: Wolters Kluwer Health/Lippincott Williams & Wilkins; 2009; and other sources.

Index

Note: Page numbers followed by the letter *f* refer to figures; those followed by the letter *t* refer to tables; those followed by the letter *b* refer to boxes, and those followed by the letter *c* refer to charts.